AMERICA'S
TOP DOCTORS

A Castle Connolly Guide

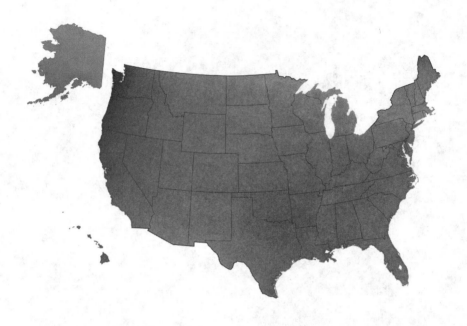

Printed in the United States of America

TABLE OF CONTENTS

HIPPOCRATIC OATH

I swear by Apollo the physician, and Asklepios, and health, and All-Heal and all the gods and goddesses, that, according to my ability and judgement, I will keep this Oath and this stipulation — to reckon him who taught me this Art equally dear to me as my parents, to share my substance with him, and relieve his necessities if required; to look upon his offspring in the same footing as my own brothers, and to teach them this Art, if they should wish to learn it, without fee or stipulation; and that by precept, lecture and every other mode of instruction, I will impart a knowledge of the Art to my own sons, and those of my teachers, and to disciples bound by a stipulation and oath according to the law of medicine, but to none others.

I will follow that system of regimen which, according to my ability and judgement, I consider for the benefit of my patients, and abstain from whatever is deleterious and mischievous. I will give no deadly medicine to anyone if asked nor suggest any such counsel; and in like manner I will not give to a woman a pessary to produce abortion. With purity and wholeness I will pass my life and practice my Art.

I will not cut persons labouring under the stone, but will leave this to be done by men who are practitioners of this work. Into whatever houses I enter, I will go into them for the benefit of the sick, and will abstain from every voluntary act of mischief and corruption; and, further, from the seduction of females or males, of freemen and slaves. Whatever, in connection with my professional practice, or not in connection with it, I see or hear, in the life of men, which ought not to be spoken of abroad, I will not divulge, as reckoning that all such should be kept secret. While I continue to keep this Oath unviolated, may it be granted to me to enjoy life and the practice of the art, respected by all men, in all times! But should I trespass and violate this Oath, may the reverse be my lot!

from Dorland's Illustrated Medical Dictionary. 27th ed. (Philadelphia) W.B. Saunders Co., 1988. Hippocratic Oath. [Hippocrates. Greek physician, 460-377 B.C.]

ABOUT THE PUBLISHERS

John K. Castle, the Chairman of Castle Connolly Medical Ltd., has spent much of the last two decades involved with healthcare institutions and issues. Mr. Castle served as Chairman of the Board of New York Medical College for eleven years, an institution at which he has continued on the Board for more than twenty years.

Mr. Castle has been extensively involved in other healthcare and voluntary activities as well. He served for five years as a public commissioner on the Joint Commission on Accreditation of Healthcare Organizations (JCAHO), the body which accredits most public and private hospitals throughout the United States. Mr. Castle has also served as a trustee of five different hospitals in the metropolitan New York region and is a director emeritus of the United Hospital Fund as well as a trustee of the Whitehead Institute.

In addition to his healthcare activities, Mr. Castle has served on many voluntary boards including the Corporation of the Massachusetts Institute of Technology, as well as numerous corporate boards of directors, including the Equitable Life Assurance Society of the United States. He is chairman of a leading merchant bank and has been chief executive of a major investment bank.

Mr. Castle holds a Bachelor of Science degree from MIT, an MBA with High Distinction from the Harvard Business School, where he was a Baker Scholar, and an honorary doctorate from New York Medical College.

ABOUT THE PUBLISHERS

John J. Connolly, Ed.D., served as President of New York Medical College, the state's largest private medical college, for more than ten years. He is a Fellow of the New York Academy of Medicine, a Fellow of the New York Academy of Sciences, a Director of the New York Business Group on Health, a member of the President's Council of the United Hospital Fund, and a member of the Executive Committee of Funding First. Dr. Connolly has served as a trustee of two hospitals and as Chairman of the Board of one. He is extensively involved in healthcare and community activities, and serves on a number of voluntary and corporate boards including the Board of the American Lyme Disease Foundation, of which he is a founder and past chairman, and the Board of Advisors of the Whitehead Institute. He holds a Bachelor of Science degree from Worcester State College, a Master's degree from the University of Connecticut, and a Doctor of Education degree in College and University Administration from Teacher's College, Columbia University.

MEDICAL ADVISORY BOARD

We are pleased to have associated with Castle Connolly Medical Ltd. a distinguished group of medical leaders who offer invaluable advice and wisdom in our efforts to assist consumers in making the best healthcare choices. We thank each member of the Medical Advisory Board for their valuable contributions.

Charles Bechert, M.D.
Director
The Sight Foundation
Fort Lauderdale, FL

Roger Bulger, M.D.
President
Association of Academic Health Centers
Washington, DC

Harry J. Buncke, M.D.
Davies Medical Center
San Francisco, CA

Paul T. Calabresi, M.D.
Professor of Medicine and Medical Science
Chairman Emeritus
Department of Medicine
  Brown University
Rhode Island Hospital
Providence, RI

Joseph Cimino, M.D.
Professor and Chairman
Community and Preventive Medicine
  New York Medical College
Valhalla, NY

Jane Clark, M.D.
Ear, Nose, Throat,
  and Hearing Center of Framingham
61 Lincoln St.
Framingham, MA

John C. Duffy, M.D.
Medical Director for Youth Services
Charter Pines Behavioral Health System
Charlotte, NC

J. Richard Gaintner, M.D.
Chief Executive Officer
Shands Health Care
  University of Florida
Gainesville, FL

Menard M. Gertler, M.D., D.Sc.
Clinical Professor of Medicine
Cornell University Medical School
New York, NY

Leo Hennikoff, M.D.
President and CEO
Rush Presbyterian-St.Luke's Medical Center
Chicago, IL

Yutaka KikaOwa, M.D.
Professor and Chairman
Department of Pathology
University of California,
  Irvine College of Medicine
Irvine, CA

Nicholas F. LaRusso, M.D.
Chairman
Division of Gastroenterology
Mayo Medical School Clinic and Foundation
Rochester, MN

MEDICAL ADVISORY BOARD

FOREWORD

The challenge of finding the best healthcare is a formidable one for most Americans and for others who seek medical care in the United States. While this country offers the best medical care in the world, many people are overwhelmed by its complexity and bureaucracy.

While most of us are fortunate and never need venture beyond our local communities to find medical specialists able to meet our healthcare needs, the needs of many patients' cannot be met in their local areas. For them, the search for the top specialists can be as important as life itself!

This great nation is fortunate in possessing some of the world's leading medical centers and specialty hospitals where cutting edge research is conducted and innovative new therapies are practiced daily. These health centers employ and train many of the world's most skilled physicians. My organization, the Association of Academic Health Centers, serves as a forum of exchange for these centers of medical excellence and, therefore, I know them well. However, I also know well the difficulty and challenges that patients and their families face in identifying and locating the tremendous wealth of medical talent and dedication that lies within the walls of these outstanding facilities.

Castle Connolly Medical Ltd. has dedicated extensive time and resources to identifying the best healthcare this nation has to offer. They have done this not to serve physicians or hospitals, but to serve healthcare consumers. Their efforts will be vital and important resources to Americans and others who seek the best medical care available in this country—wherever it is being practiced.

Roger Bulger, M.D.
President, Association of Academic Health Centers
Washington DC

INTRODUCTION

There are times in life when the nature of a disease or medical condition that afflicts you or a loved one warrants identifying the top doctor—the very best specialist anywhere in the nation—to diagnose or treat that particular medical problem. It's at times like these that you need *America's Top Doctors*, the national guide designed to assist you under just these circumstances.

While the overall quality of medical care throughout the United States is generally of very high quality, and in many places is superb, there are still those rare, complex or extremely difficult problems that demand resources beyond the ordinary or that require talents that are exceptional.

This guide identifies those top medical specialists throughout the country who possess the skill and experience to address these problems. Top specialists who provide excellent care tend to be located predominantly, although not exclusively, at major medical centers, specialty hospitals and leading teaching hospitals. These exceptional physicians are acknowledged as such by their peers and are recognized for their expertise by the medical profession.

The top specialists we have identified are not the only excellent physicians who are caring for patients in this nation. Since there are more than 650,000 doctors in the United States, we cannot identify every top specialist. Therefore, we have included narrative to assist those using this guide who may not find the specialist they need within its listings. Clearly, there are many primary care physicians and other well-trained specialists in communities and hospitals throughout the United States. Most of these physicians not only are board certified in a specialty, but also are board certified in a subspecialty or in multiple subspecialties. Board or subspecialty certification alone, however, does not distinguish them from excellent specialists at hospitals in your community, many of whom also are board certified in both a specialty and a subspecialty.

INTRODUCTION

Physicians who are included in this guide have trained at the top medical centers under medical pioneers who possess state-of-the-art knowledge in a specific disease or problem and have often devised new techniques and therapeutic approaches, many of which are life-saving procedures or cures. These doctors most often practice their science and art at leading hospitals and, more specifically, in programs at hospitals that are recognized for their excellence in a given field. Many others have been trained at leading centers in other nations since the U.S. is not alone in pioneering new medical knowledge, although its position as the leader in "high-tech" medicine is generally acknowledged.

A major characteristic distinguishing the physicians in this guide from those at local hospitals is their continued focus and training. Rather than practicing at a community hospital (or even at a leading regional hospital) and developing a general, broad-based practice, these physicians continued their training in a particular disease, syndrome or problem to such degree that they developed extensive knowledge and unique skills in treating that particular problem.

Often that focused, advanced training is accompanied by active involvement in clinical research. This is an additional reason why the physicians listed in this guide are located at only a few hundred of the more than six thousand hospitals in the United States. It is difficult, although not impossible, to conduct important clinical research in isolation or without an environment supportive of research. It takes time, money, residents, research associates, technicians, equipment and more to produce significant clinical research. Certainly there have been individuals who have made important and lasting contributions to research with little or none of this support, but those instances are rare. Today, for the most part, major advances in medicine occur in the labs and on the floors of major medical centers and specialty hospitals, in medical schools and in clinical labs created and financed for that purpose by commercial enterprises.

How Physicians Were Selected For Inclusion In This Guide

The basis of the Castle Connolly selection process is peer nomination. In some ways, the process may be viewed as an enhanced referral process similar to that of a patient who asks a personal physician to provide a referral to another physician for a particular problem. However, we have enhanced and strengthened that process: if the recommendation of one doctor is good, the recommendation of many doctors is even better. And we asked many doctors for their recommendations; in fact, over 250,000 doctors!

How did we accomplish this enormous task? First, the Castle Connolly research team surveyed over 200,000 doctors by mail asking them to nominate the top people in their specialties and in related specialties, especially those to whom they would refer their own patients. Thousands of telephone interviews were also conducted, primarily with leaders in medical specialties and leading physicians at major medical centers. In addition to physicians throughout the country surveyed by the Castle Connolly physician-led research team, online surveys were conducted with members of Physicians' OnLine (POL), the nation's largest community of physicians connected through the Internet.

To augment these large samplings contacted by mail, telephone and online, additional surveys were conducted among the following carefully selected groups: directors of graduate medical programs; directors of clinical services at member hospitals of the Council of Teaching Hospitals (COTH); board members of various medical specialty academies, associations and societies; and deans and chairs of departments at medical schools.

Moreover, thousands of phone interviews were subsequently conducted with those leaders in medical specialties who were identified by their peers through the survey process.

INTRODUCTION

Focus then shifted to the 3,969 physicians selected from over 17,924 physicians nominated. Extensive biographical forms were sent to those physicians for completion. After careful review of their professional backgrounds, the Castle Connolly research staff conducted further research to check disciplinary and license histories.

The result is a carefully researched and highly selective list of the top specialists in the nation. This select group of physicians, identified through our extensive research process, constitutes a list of physicians recognized by their peers for their excellence in providing care for specific diseases and problems.

Undoubtedly, there will be comments that we have missed some terrific doctors who should be included. That is inevitable, since this guide is designed to identify only those doctors noted for excellence in diagnosing or treating a specific problem or disease.

What we intentionally have not done is include physicians simply because they have an important title. While a position as a chief of service or a department head at a teaching hospital is an important post, such positions are achieved through a combination of many talents including administrative skills, seniority and factors that are not as important for inclusion in this guide as is skill in clinical care. The same is true of leaders of county medical societies, professional associations or even specialty groups. While these are significant positions and acknowledge leadership among peers, they are not essentially recognition of clinical skills.

The same perspective applies to research expertise. Many physicians listed in the Guide are engaged in clinical research and make significant contributions to their fields, with some devoting a substantial portion of their time to research. However, we avoided including those physicians who solely conduct research and who do not provide patient care.

The result of this extensive research effort is a list of outstanding, highly skilled physicians who are recognized as among the best in their specialties and in the nation; a list which consumers/patients can use to find the very best specialists to meet their particular needs.

Lastly, this book differs from the regional Castle Connolly Guides, Top Doctors: New York, Chicago and Florida, in two important ways. First, **America's Top Doctors** is national, not regional, in scope. Second, the regional Guides are based on the generally accurate premise that healthcare is local and most people find their healthcare where they live and work. However, **America's Top Doctors** is designed to meet the needs of those people who cannot find the right specialists locally but who can and will travel anywhere in the country to be cared for by a top specialist at an outstanding hospital. This guide will assist readers in that important search.

INTRODUCTION

USING THIS GUIDE TO FIND TOP SPECIALISTS

This guide is organized and planned to be as user-friendly as possible. Still, as with anything as complex as medical specialties, subspecialties and the myriad diseases and problems that specialists treat, there needs to be a system to organize the physicians' names, the diseases and problems they manage and their special expertise.

To organize the specialists in this guide, we have followed the American Board of Medical Specialties (ABMS) format. The ABMS is the authoritative body for the recognition of medical specialties. Without the ABMS as the official controlling body there would be hundreds of unregulated medical specialties.

The ABMS recognizes twenty-five specialties and over ninety subspecialties. The listing of ABMS specialties and subspecialties can be found in Appendix B. In addition to ABMS recognized specialties, there are at least one hundred other groups calling themselves "medical specialists" that are not recognized by the ABMS. Some of these groups are working toward recognition and have exams and other standards for membership. Others are organizations of physicians interested in a particular problem or area of medicine that exist to exchange information but have no intention of seeking ABMS recognition. Some groups calling themselves "boards" really have little authority or meaningful standards. Thus, while a physician may state he/she is, for example, a specialist in cosmetic surgery, there is no ABMS recognized specialty by that name. Therefore, you have no idea whether this physician has any special training and expertise or is simply trying to recruit paying patients to a lucrative aspect of surgical practice.

You can get information on a doctor's credentials from the doctor, from the doctor's hospital (medical affairs office) or from your health plan if a doctor is in the network. You can also get this information from numerous Web sites, including www.castleconnolly.com. You can check on a physician's board certification by calling the ABMS at 847-481-9091 or by logging on to its Web site at www.abms.org.

If you seek a particular kind of specialist or subspecialist, turn to the section of this guide covering that medical specialty or subspecialty. There you will be able to further restrict your search to a specific geographic region or, if you prefer, search throughout the nation.

To make your search easier, we have organized the specialties and subspecialties into the following regions: New England, Mid-Atlantic, Midwest, Southeast, Southwest, Great Plains and Mountains and West Coast and Pacific. To find an outstanding cardiologist in St. Louis, for example, look under cardiology and then under the Midwest region.

A second way to use this guide is to look at the Special Expertise Index, which lists the areas of special expertise of included physicians. This list of special expertises indicates over 2,000 medical topics including diseases, therapeutic approaches and techniques. You can look up the particular disease, problem or technique you are interested in and locate a physician in that manner. We assume that many people using this guide will know what their particular problem is and will begin their exploration with this index. However, we encourage you to read the entire text since it will help you to better understand how to find the right physician for yourself or a family member, especially if one is not found in this guide.

CHOOSING AN APPROPRIATE SPECIALIST

It may seem that choosing the correct specialist to treat a particular medical problem is simply a matter of finding a top doctor in a specific medical specialty. For treatment of a problem with your vision, you would choose an ophthalmologist. A skin or hair problem would require treatment by a dermatologist and a broken bone would need the care of an orthopaedist.

INTRODUCTION

Sometimes, however, the type of specialist needed may not be obvious. For example, back surgery may be performed by either an orthopaedist or a neurosurgeon. Different aspects of sports medicine, as another example, are practiced by orthopaedists who treat sports-related injuries in both adults and children, pediatricians who treat only children or internists and family practitioners whose focus is on prevention of injuries.

In some cases, several specialists with expertise in different areas of medical practice all become involved in treating the same patient's health problem. For example, a person with diabetes might need care from an endocrinologist, a cardiologist and an ophthalmologist. In other situations, doctors trained in different specialties may use varied approaches or differing therapies to manage a disease or condition. Such is the case, for example, with prostate cancer: a patient could be treated by a urologist, a medical oncologist, or a radiotherapist. The urologist might provide the patient with a surgical treatment option, while the medical oncologist would treat the patient with chemotherapy and the radiotherapist would use radiation therapy and/or radioactive seed implantation. All approaches could be successful, or one might be preferable to another, depending on the patient and his condition. Therefore, a wise patient will thoroughly explore all options before making a choice.

Finding the right specialist is also important in terms of the quality of your care. For example, many orthopaedic surgeons will operate on hands, but it is clearly much better to have someone trained and certified specifically in hand surgery (a subspecialty of both orthopaedics and plastic surgery) to perform that delicate surgery. Similarly, a dermatologist may indicate that his/her practice includes cosmetic surgery, however, there is no approved ABMS dermatology subspecialty or fellowship training in cosmetic surgery. While many dermatologists do pursue additional training in cosmetic surgery, it should be understood that dermatologic practice is limited to cutaneous procedures ranging from the removal of skin tumors to laser resurfacing. On the other hand, some board certified otolaryngologists have additional training that enables them to perform plastic and cosmetic surgery procedures on the head and neck.

Using the right type of specialist is as important as selecting the right doctor. For example, the diagnosis of melanoma, a very serious, potentially life threatening form of skin cancer, is missed in many cases. Therefore, if you have a skin lesion that might possibly be melanoma, you should be certain that the pathologist reading your slides is board certified in the subspecialty of dermatopathology.

These examples illustrate this important principle: always seek the best healthcare. Look for the best-trained doctors, not those who simply can do the job. That doesn't mean that you need to consult a doctor listed in this guide every time you have a health problem. It does mean you should be certain that the physicians who care for you, whether in your community or at a world-class medical center, are trained appropriately and are qualified to provide the care you require. Remember, when it comes to healthcare no one wants second best!

Given this complexity, how do you find the right specialist to provide your care? The first and most important person to look to for guidance is your primary care physician. He/she will assess your medical condition, determine the appropriate type of specialist to recommend and perhaps refer you to a specific doctor or doctors. You should always ask your primary care physician why a particular specialist is being recommended, since that specialist may be a colleague in your doctor's medical group or may be the only (or the most conveniently located) specialist of the type in your health plan. Ask how well your primary care physician knows the specialist, whether they have a long-standing professional relationship and if other patients referred to the specialist had successful outcomes. Be sure to ask for several recommendations, if possible, to provide you with some choice among specialists.

INTRODUCTION

If you do not have a primary care doctor, try to learn as much as you can about your medical problem and the type of specialist best suited to treat it. However, keep in mind that many diseases or conditions present with symptoms that often are indistinguishable from those of other diseases or conditions (Lupus and Lyme disease, for example) making them difficult to diagnose precisely even for physicians armed with the results of diagnostic tests.

JUDGING THE QUALIFICATIONS OF A PHYSICIAN

The specialists listed in *America's Top Doctors* are clearly among the best in the nation and have been identified through a rigorous research process and thorough screening by the Castle Connolly research team. Through our extensive surveys and research we have done much of the work in finding a top referral specialist for you. But how do you judge the qualifications of a physician who may not be listed in this Guide? If you are trying to find a specialist on your own, how should you go about it? How can you tell when a physician has the appropriate training in a specialty and how do you distinguish what is meaningful and what is not from among all those plaques and certificates on a doctor's wall?

The following pages will outline that process for you. In fact, what is written here reflects much of the logic that underlies the selection of physicians for this book.

The following material will help you not only in finding a top specialist in this Guide, but it also should be helpful to you in choosing among the many specialists, primary care doctors and other physicians that you will need to consult throughout your life.

The reality is that few of us see only one doctor in our lifetime. Each of us may be cared for by a primary care physician, an ophthalmologist, an orthopaedist, a dermatologist, a surgeon or a number of other specialists. The choices can be many and they can be among the most important choices that we make in our lives.

Education

Your review of your prospective doctor's education and training should begin with medical school. While you may feel that the institution at which someone earned a bachelor's degree could be an indication of the quality of the doctor, most people in the medical field do not believe it plays a major role. A degree from a highly selective undergraduate college or university will help an aspiring doctor gain admission to a medical school, but once there, all students are peers. However, the information on undergraduate colleges, if important to you, is available in the American Board of Medical Specialties (ABMS) Compendium of Certified Medical Specialists and other medical directories.

American medical schools are highly standardized, at least in terms of minimal quality. A group known as the Liaison Committee for Medical Education (LCME) accredits all U.S. medical schools that grant medical degrees (MDs) and osteopathic degrees (DOs). Most also are accredited by the appropriate state agency, if one exists, and by regional accrediting agencies that accredit colleges and universities of all kinds.

Furthermore, U.S. medical schools have universally high standards for admission, including success on the undergraduate level and on the Medical College Admissions Tests (MCATs). Although frequently criticized for being slow to change and for training too many specialists, the system of medical education in the United States has insured high quality in medical practice. One recent positive change is a strong effort in most medical schools to diversify the composition of the student body. While these schools have been less successful in enrolling racial minorities, the number of women in U.S. medical schools has increased to the point that women now make up about 40 percent of most classes. In certain specialties preferred by women medical graduates (pediatrics, for example) it is possible that in coming years the majority of specialists will be female.

INTRODUCTION

Most doctors practicing in the United States are graduates of U.S. medical schools, but there are two other groups of doctors who make up a relatively small portion of the total physician population. They are (1) foreign nationals who graduated from foreign schools and (2) U.S. nationals who graduated from foreign schools. (Canadian medical schools are not considered foreign.)

Foreign Medical Graduates

Foreign medical schools vary greatly in quality. Even some of the oldest and finest European schools have become virtually "open door," with huge numbers of unscreened students making teaching and learning difficult. Others are excellent and provided the model for our system of medical education.

The fact that someone graduated from a foreign school does not mean that he/she is a poor doctor. Foreign schools, like U.S. schools, produce good doctors and poor doctors. Foreign medical graduates must pass the same exam taken by U.S. graduates for licensure, but the failure rate for foreign graduates is significantly higher. In the first year of using the new United States Medical Licensing Exam (USMLE), 93 percent of U.S. medical school graduates passed Step II, the clinical exam, as compared with 39 percent of the foreign graduates. It is clear that the quality of foreign schools, if not individual doctors, is not the same as U.S. medical schools, at least as measured by our standards. Nonetheless, many communities and patients have been well served by foreign medical graduates practicing in this country—often in areas where it has been difficult to attract graduates of American schools.

In addition, many foreign medical schools and their teaching hospitals are world renowned for their leadership in medical care, research and teaching and many of the technologies and techniques we utilize in the U.S. today have been developed and perfected in foreign countries.

Residency

Most doctors practicing today have at least three years of postgraduate training (following the MD or DO) in an approved residency program. This not only is an important step in the process of becoming a competent doctor, but it is also a requirement for board (specialty) certification. Most people assume that a prospective doctor needs to complete a three-year residency program to obtain a medical license. That is not an accurate assumption! New York State, for example, requires only one postgraduate year. However, since all approved residencies last at least three years and some, such as those in neurosurgery, general surgery, orthopaedic surgery and urology, may extend for five or more years, it is important to know the details of a doctor's training. Licensure alone is not enough of a basis on which to make a decision.

Without undertaking extensive and detailed research on every residency program, the best assessment you can make of a doctor's residency program is to see if it took place in a large medical center whose name you recognize. The more prestigious institutions tend to attract the best medical students, sometimes regardless of the quality of the individual residency program. If in doubt about a doctor's training, ask the doctor if the residency he/she completed was in the specialty of the practice; if not, ask why not.

It is also important to be certain that a doctor completed a residency that has been approved by the appropriate governing board of the specialty, such as the American Board of Surgery, the American Board of Radiology, or the American Osteopathic Board of Pediatrics. These board groups are listed in Appendices B and C. If you are really concerned about a doctor's training, you should call the hospital that offered the residency and ask if the residency program was approved by the appropriate specialty group. If still in doubt, consult the publication Directory of Graduate Medical Education Programs, often called the "green book," found in medical school or hospital libraries, which lists all approved residencies.

Board Certification

With an MD or DO degree and a license, an individual may practice in any medical specialty with or without additional training. For example, doctors with a license but no special training may call themselves cardiologists, pediatricians or gynecologists. This is why board certification is such an important factor. The American Board of Medical Specialties (ABMS) recognizes 25 specialties and over 90 subspecialties. Eighteen boards certify in 106 specialties under the aegis of the American Osteopathic Association (AOA). Doctors who have qualified for such specialization are called board certified; they have completed an approved residency and passed the board's exam. (See Appendix B for an approved ABMS list; see Appendix C for the AOA list. While many doctors who are not board certified do call themselves "specialists," board certification is the best standard by which to measure competence and training. Throughout this Guide a description of each specialty and subspecialty is provided as an introduction to the listing of physicians in that specialty.

You can be confident that doctors who are board certified have, at a minimum, the proper training in their specialty and have demonstrated their proficiency through supervision and testing. While there are many non-board certified doctors who are highly competent, it is more difficult to assess the level of their training. While board certification alone does not guarantee competence, it is a standard that reflects successful completion of an appropriate training program. If it is impossible to find a doctor in your area who is board certified in a particular subspecialty, for example, geriatric medicine or sports medicine, at least be certain the physician is board certified in a related specialty such as internal medicine or orthopaedics.

Board certified doctors are referred to as Diplomates of the Board. Some of the colleges of medical specialties (e.g., the American College of Radiology, the American College of Surgeons) have multiple levels of recognition. The first is basic membership and the second, more prestigious and difficult to obtain, is status as a Fellow. Fellowship status in the colleges is meaningful and is based on experience, professional achievement and recognition by one's peers, including extensive experience in patient care. It should be viewed as a significant professional qualification.

Board Eligibility

Many doctors who have been more recently trained are waiting to take the boards. They are sometimes described as "board eligible," a common term that the ABMS advocates abandoning because of its ambiguity. Board eligible means that the doctor has completed an approved residency and is qualified to sit for the related board's exam.

Each member board of the ABMS has its own policy regarding the use and recognition of the board eligible term. Therefore, the description "board eligible" should not be viewed as a genuine qualification, especially if a doctor has been out of medical school long enough to have taken the certification exam. To the boards, a doctor is either board certified or not. Furthermore, most of the specialty boards permit unlimited attempts to pass the exam and, in some cases, doctors who have failed the exam twice or even ten times continue to call themselves board eligible. In osteopathic medicine, the board eligible status is recognized only for the first six years after completion of a residency.

In addition to the approved lists of specialties and subspecialties of the ABMS and AOA, there are a wide variety of other doctors and groups of doctors who call themselves specialists. At present there are at least 100 such groups called "self-

INTRODUCTION

designated medical specialties." They range from doctors who are working to create a recognized body of knowledge and subspecialty training to less formal groups interested in a particular approach to the practice of medicine. These groups may or may not have standards for membership. There is no way to determine the true extent of their members' training and the ABMS or the AOA does not recognize them. While you should be cautious of doctors who claim they are specialists in these areas, many do have advanced training and the groups at least offer a listing of people interested in a particular approach to medical care. Rely on board certification to assure yourself of basic competence, and use membership in one of these groups to indicate strong interest and possible additional training in a particular aspect of medicine. A list of these self-designated medical specialties may be found in Appendix D.

Recertification

A relatively new focus of the specialty boards is the area of recertification. Until recently, board certification lasted for an unlimited time. Now, almost all the boards have put time limits on the certification period. For example, in Internal Medicine and Anesthesiology, the time limit is ten years; in Family Practice, six, and under some circumstances, seven years. These more stringent standards reflect an increasing emphasis, by both the medical boards and state agencies responsible for licensing doctors, on recertification.

Since the policies of the boards vary widely, it is a good procedure to ask a doctor if certification was awarded and when. If the date was seven to ten years ago, ask if he/she has been recertified. Unfortunately, many boards permit "grandfathering," whereby already certified doctors do not have to be recertified, and recertification requirements apply only to newly certified doctors. Appendix B contains a list of the names and addresses of the boards and the certification period for each board specialty. Even if recertification is not required, it is good professional practice for doctors to undertake the process. It assures you, the patient, that they are attempting to stay current.

Many states have a continuing medical education requirement for doctors. These states typically require a minimum number of continuing medical education (CME) credits for a doctor to maintain a medical license. Twenty-eight states require 150 CME credits over a three-year period. Osteopathic doctors are required to take 150 hours of CME credits within three years to maintain certification.

Fellowships

The purpose of a fellowship is to provide advanced training in the clinical techniques and research of a particular specialty. Fellowships usually, but not always, are designed to lead to board certification in a subspecialty, such as cardiology, which is a subspecialty of internal medicine. Many physicians listed in this Guide have had fellowship training. In the U.S. there are a variety of fellowship programs available to doctors, which fall into two broad categories: approved and unapproved. Approved fellowships are those that are approved by the appropriate medical specialty board (e.g., the American Board of Radiology) and lead to subspecialty certificates. Fellowship programs that are unapproved are often in the same areas of training as those that are approved, but they do not lead to subspecialty certificates. Unfortunately, all too often, an unapproved fellowship exists only to provide relatively inexpensive labor for the research and/or patient care activities of a clinical department in a medical school or hospital. In such cases, the learning that takes place is secondary and may be a good deal less than in an approved fellowship. On the other hand, any fellowship is better than none at all and some unapproved fellowships have that status for a valid reason that should not reflect negatively on the program. For example, the fellowship may have been recently created, with approval being sought. To check that a fellowship is an

INTRODUCTION

approved one, call the hospital where the training took place or call the medical board for that specialty.

Some physicians may have completed more than one fellowship and may be boarded in two or more subspecialties. Also, some physicians may pursue fellowship training and subspecialty certification, but then choose to practice in their primary field of certification. For example, a doctor who is board certified in internal medicine also may have obtained board certification in cardiology, but may choose to practice primarily internal medicine rather than cardiology. For the most part, the physicians in this Guide practice in their subspecialties.

Professional Reputation

There are doctors who meet every professional standard on paper, but who are simply not good doctors. In all probability the medical community has ascertained that and, while the individual may still practice medicine, his/her reputation will reflect that collective assessment. There are also doctors who are outstanding leaders in their fields because of research or professional activities but who are not particularly strong, or perhaps even active, in patient care. It is important to distinguish that kind of professional reputation from a reputation as a competent, caring doctor in delivering patient care, or in the case of this Guide, as an outstanding practitioner in a given specialty.

Hospital Appointment

Most doctors are on the medical staff of one or more hospitals and are known as "attendings;" some are not. If a doctor does not have admitting privileges or is not on the attending staff of a hospital, you may wish to consider choosing a different doctor. It can be very difficult to ascertain whether or not the lack of hospital appointment is for a good reason. For example, it is understandable that some doctors who are raising families or heading toward retirement choose not to meet

18

the demands (meetings, committees, etc.) of being an attending. However, if you need care in a hospital, the lack of such an appointment means that another doctor will have to oversee that care. In some specialties, such as dermatology and psychiatry, doctors may conduct their entire practice in the office and a hospital appointment is not as essential, or as good a criterion for assessment, as in other specialties.

While mistakes are made, most hospitals are quite careful about admissions to their medical staffs. The best hospitals are highly selective, so a degree of screening (or "credentialing") has been done for you. In other words, the best doctors practice at the best hospitals. Since caring for a patient in a hospital is often a team effort involving a number of specialists, the reputation of the hospital to which the doctor admits patients carries special weight. Hospital medical staffs review their colleagues and authorize those who can perform specific procedures. In addition, they typically review and reappoint their medical staff every two or three years. In effect, this is an additional screening to protect patients. It is especially true of hospitals that have what are known as closed staffs, where it is impossible to obtain admitting privileges unless there is a vacancy that the administration and medical staff deem necessary to fill. If you are having a surgical procedure and are concerned about the doctor's skill or experience, it may be worthwhile to call the medical affairs office at the doctor's hospital to see if he/she is authorized to perform that procedure in that hospital.

The reasons for a hospital's selectivity are easy to understand: no hospital wishes to expose itself to liability and every hospital wants to have the best reputation possible in order to attract patients. Obviously, the quality of the medical staff is immensely important in creating that reputation. Unfortunately, some hospitals are less diligent when a major group practice of doctors, all of whom have previously been affiliated with the institution, adds new members. In such cases, the

INTRODUCTION

hospital may almost automatically grant privileges without conducting the same intensive review given to individual doctors who are not members of a group practice. Also, some hospitals are less selective in granting privileges when beds are empty than when beds are full.

A last and very important reason why a hospital appointment is an essential requirement in your choice of doctor is that some states permit doctors to practice without malpractice insurance. If you are injured as a result of a doctor's poor care, you could be without recourse. However, few hospitals permit doctors to practice in them unless they carry malpractice insurance. This not only protects the hospital, but the patient as well.

Medical School Faculty Appointment

Many doctors have appointments on the faculties of medical schools. There is a range of categories from "straight" appointments, meaning full-time appointment as professor, associate professor, assistant professor or instructor, to clinical ranks that may reflect lesser degrees of involvement in teaching or research. If someone carries what is known as a straight academic rank (i.e. professor of surgery, without clinical in the title), this usually means that the individual is engaged full-time in medical school research, teaching activities and patient care. The title "clinical professor of surgery" usually identifies a part-time or adjunct appointment and less direct involvement in medical school activities such as teaching and research.

Doctors who are full-time academicians may be in the forefront of new techniques and research, but they are not necessarily better doctors. Nonetheless, you would be assured that they have the support of other faculty, residents and medical students.

When you are seeking a subspecialist, a doctor's relationship to a medical school becomes more meaningful since medical school faculties tend to be made up of subspecialists. You are less likely to find large numbers of general or primary care practitioners engaged full-time on a medical school faculty. The newest approaches and techniques in medicine, for the most part, are explored and developed by medical school faculties in their laboratories and clinical practice settings. This is where they practice their subspecialties, as well as teach and perform research. Such leading specialists are not necessarily better doctors than community doctors; rather, they are trained to provide a different kind of medical care. Obviously the type of medical care users of this guide are seeking is that different kind of care available primarily from top subspecialists at leading hospitals and medical centers.

Medical Society Membership

Most medical society memberships sound very prestigious and some are; however, there are many societies that are not selective and which virtually any doctor can join. In addition, membership in many of the more prestigious societies is based on research and publication or on leadership in the field and may have little to do with direct patient care. While it is clearly an honor to be invited to join these groups, membership may be less than helpful in discerning whether a doctor can meet your needs.

Experience

Experience is difficult to assess. Obviously, in most cases, an older doctor has more experience; on the other hand, a younger doctor has been more recently immersed in the challenge of medical school, residency, or even a fellowship, and may be the most up-to-date. If a doctor is board certified, you may assume that assures at least a minimal amount of experience, but since it could be as little as

INTRODUCTION

a year, check the date of graduation from medical school or completion of residency to know precisely how long a doctor has been in practice.

There is a good deal of evidence that there is a positive relationship between quantity of experience and quality of care. That is, the more a doctor performs a procedure, the better he/she becomes at it. That is why it is important to ask a doctor about his or her experience with the procedure that you need. Does the doctor see and treat similar cases every day, every week or only rarely? Of course, with some rare diseases, rarely is the only possible answer, but it is relative frequency that is critical. Major metropolitan areas, especially New York and San Francisco, became leaders in the treatment of AIDS because of the number of patients seen in those metropolitan areas. Doctors in the suburbs of New York City (especially in New York's Westchester, Nassau and Suffolk counties) and in Fairfield County, Connecticut became leaders in the research and treatment of Lyme disease because that region is the epicenter of the disease.

In some states, data is available on volume or numbers of certain procedures performed at hospitals. For this information in New York you can call the Center for Medical Consumers, a non-profit advocacy organization, or visit its Web site at www.medicalconsumers.org. For volume and outcome information in other states, visit the Web site of Health Care Choices at www.healthcarechoices.org. There is a good deal of controversy, however, on the validity and usefulness of such data. Opponents cite the fact that some of the data is produced from Medicare patient records only and, thus, is based solely on an elderly population that does not represent the total activity of a hospital or doctor. Proponents of the use of such volume data agree that it is not perfect, but suggest it can be one useful criterion in selecting the best places to receive care for these specific problems. Recognizing the limitations of such data, the healthcare consumer may, nonetheless, find it of interest and use.

The one type of experience you should specifically want to know about is that dealing with any special procedure, particularly a surgical one, that has recently been developed and introduced into practice. For example, in the 1980's many doctors using laparoscopic cholecystectomy, a then new surgical technique for removing gallbladders, experienced a high percentage of problems because they were not properly trained. This prompted the American Board of Surgery to promulgate new standards for the training of surgeons using this technique. Do not hesitate to ask about your doctor's training in a procedure and how frequently and with what degree of success he/she has performed it. Practice may not lead to perfection, but it does improve skills and enhance the probability of success.

In some cases, relatively young doctors have recently completed residency or fellowship training under recognized leaders who have developed new approaches or techniques for dealing with a particular problem. They may have learned the new techniques from their mentors and may be far ahead of the field (and ahead of more senior and distinguished colleagues) in using those approaches. So age and experience must be considered and weighed along with other factors when choosing a physician.

OTHER CONSIDERATIONS

Second Opinions

Second opinions are a valuable medical tool, too infrequently used in many instances and overused in others. Clearly, you do not want to seek another doctor's opinion on every ailment or problem that you face, but a second opinion should be pursued in the following situations:

• before major surgery

• if the diagnosis is serious or life threatening

• if a rare disease is diagnosed

INTRODUCTION

- if a diagnosis is uncertain
- if the number of tests or procedures recommended might be excessive
- if a test result has serious implications (e.g., a positive Pap smear)
- if the treatment suggested is risky or expensive
- if you are uncomfortable with the prescribed diagnosis and treatment
- if a course of treatment is not successful
- if you question your doctor's competence
- if your insurance company requires it

Most doctors will be supportive if you request a second opinion and many will recommend it. In many cases, insurance companies will pay for second opinions, but check ahead of time to make sure your insurance plan does cover them. In an HMO you may have to be more assertive because one way HMOs control costs is by limiting second opinions. Often, the opinion of a second doctor will confirm the opinion of the first, but the reassurance may be worth the time and extra cost. On the other hand, if the second opinion differs from the first, you have two alternatives: seek the opinion of a third doctor, or educate yourself as much as possible by talking to both doctors, reading up on the problem, and trusting your instincts about which diagnosis is correct.

Office and Practice Arrangements

Although clearly not as important as training or reputation, a specialist's office and practice arrangements often are of significance to patients. Practice arrangements include office hours, office location, billing procedures and accessibility among the many factors that result in how well the office is run.

Some specialists only will see new patients who are referred to them by another doctor. Therefore, you may need to have your treating physician contact the specialist's office to arrange for your initial visit. Your health plan may also require that your primary care doctor provide a referral.

If English is not your first language, it may be advisable to determine whether someone in the specialist's office speaks your primary language or if a translator can be present during appointments. This will ease communication and assure that all questions, responses and instructions are understood.

Accessibility of the specialist's office may be a concern if you are wheelchair-bound, are elderly or cannot climb stairs or negotiate narrow corridors. Convenient parking may also be important to you.

Other arrangements that may need to be made in advance of your first visit or discussed with the specialist's office staff concern payment. You may wish to ask the following:

- Does the specialist accept your health insurance coverage?
- Is the specialist within your plan's network and will you need to pay a co-payment? Or, is the specialist out-of-network and will you have to pay for your care out-of-pocket, meet a deductible or submit a form for reimbursement?
- Are credit cards an acceptable mode of payment?
- Does the specialist accept Medicare, Medicaid or no-fault insurance? Does the specialist treat worker's compensation cases?
- If you are a non-resident of the United States, will you need to arrange for the transfer or exchange of currency to pay the specialist's fee?

When you are choosing a top specialist, these issues may be of lesser or greater importance, depending on the problem and type of care warranted. If you are traveling a great distance to have a specific procedure performed by a top specialist at a major medical center, continuing long-term monitoring or follow-up care by that physician may not be required or may not be feasible and such things as office practice arrangements are of less importance. On the other hand, if you have a chronic problem that needs to be monitored with follow-up care provided by the same top specialist, then such issues as accessibility of the doctor's office, appointment hours, waiting times and courtesy and professionalism of the staff become more significant.

INTRODUCTION

Personal Chemistry

One element of the doctor-patient relationship that we stress in our guides is chemistry between doctor and patient, a part of which is often referred to as a doctor's "bedside manner." While this factor is of major import in a long-term relationship such as one you would have with your primary care physician, it is of less importance when you see a specialist only once or twice. However, since many people using this book may have chronic conditions that require ongoing care, it is important to give the matter some consideration.

It is vital that there is a sense of mutual trust and respect between patient and doctor; a judgment that individuals must make for themselves. Among the many talented doctors listed in this guide, there are very likely some to whom you would relate well and others with whom you may not feel as comfortable.

Patients prefer doctors who listen, demonstrate concern, are responsive to patient needs and spend sufficient time with them. The qualities of physicians in this regard, even the excellent ones in this guide, vary immensely.

You, the patient, are the only one who can assess these qualities because individuals react differently to various personalities. It is important for you to carefully judge your feelings towards a physician, especially if you are embarking on a long-term relationship. You should feel you can be open, trusting and responsive to your physician and that your relationship will be a positive one. Otherwise, find another doctor, since not doing so could adversely affect your care.

Once you have used this guide to identify the top specialist(s) best suited to treat your condition, there is much you can do to maximize the value of your first visit.

MAXIMIZING YOUR FIRST APPOINTMENT WITH A TOP DOCTOR

After your research is done and you've secured an appointment for an initial consultation with a top doctor known for his/her expertise in the diagnosis or treatment of your particular medical condition, what should you do?

Whether your visit to the specialist's office is a car ride or a plane trip away, there undoubtedly will be arrangements to make before your appointment. You may have to take time off from work, arrange for childcare while you are away and make travel plans and hotel reservations, but there are a number of other important steps to take to assure that you and the specialist make the best use of the time you spend together.

Have you done everything you can to prepare yourself and the specialist for the consultation? The following checklist will help you maximize the value of your visit to the specialist and will go a long way toward focusing you on the task at hand—getting the best advice or treatment for your health problem from one of the top doctors in the medical specialty related to your condition.

Gathering the facts

- Does the specialist have all the information needed to make a diagnosis of or treatment plan for your condition?

- Have your medical records, test results and X-rays been sent ahead of time to allow for their review by the specialist in advance of your first appointment?

- Have you written out your medical history emphasizing the particular problem for which you are visiting this specialist?

- Are you prepared with a written list of questions?

- Do you understand the answers?

A specialist becoming newly involved in your care needs to learn as much as possible about the state of your health in a very limited time. Since top doctors are extremely busy people with many demands on their time, you should make certain that all relevant records and case summaries are obtained and sent to the specialist well in advance of your appointment.

Obtaining Your Records

All healthcare providers including hospitals, doctors and their staffs are under legal obligation to maintain the privacy of your medical records. In order to obtain release of those records, you must make a request in writing. If you need to obtain records from a number of providers, you should write one clear and concise letter authorizing release of your records and including your name, address, telephone number, date of birth, social security number and any other identifying information such as a hospital chart number. You then can make photocopies of this letter, but be sure to sign and date each copy as if it were an original. You also may want to specifically name those test results (e.g., pathology slides) or X-ray films (not just written reports or summaries) that must be included in addition to making a general request for your records. It's also a good idea to indicate the date of your appointment so the office staff can respond in a timely manner.

Although state laws require the timely release of medical records, hospital medical records departments and doctors' offices often take several weeks to pull and review patient charts and get them in the mail either to you or to another doctor. In addition to written authorization, you may be asked to pay the costs involved in copying your records, test results and X-ray films because many doctors' offices will not release the originals. Consider placing a call in advance to determine the procedure for releasing your records, how long you can expect it to take and the costs involved so that you can save time by including payment with your release authorization letter. Be sure to allow sufficient time in advance of your consultation appointment for your request to be processed. Since you often must wait several weeks for an appointment with a specialist, allow at least that amount of time to obtain your records.

Even after making your written requests, you should follow up each letter with a telephone call to be sure that your records actually are sent. You should not assume that your request for records will be promptly fulfilled by an often over-burdened, although well-intentioned, office staff.

Remember, the more information the specialist has about your condition, the fewer repeat or additional tests or procedures you will need to undergo, the lower the costs of your consultation and, most important, the more expeditiously the specialist will be able to render an opinion.

THE FACTS AND ONLY THE FACTS

Be thorough and organized in documenting your personal and familial medical histories, the medications you take and in relaying information about your condition. Even seemingly minor bits of information may provide subtle clues to the nature of your medical problem and the optimal way in which to treat it. It's also advisable to bring a list with you of names, addresses and telephone numbers of all physicians who have cared for you, especially those you have seen regarding your current medical problem.

Even though thoroughness is essential to presenting a clear picture of your medical condition, bear in mind that the specialist needs to get to your core health concerns as quickly as possible. Therefore, if you have a complex medical history, you may want to ask your current doctors to provide treatment summaries in addition to copies of your medical records. Hospital records should include your admission history and physical exam, dictated consultation and operation notes and discharge summaries for all hospitalizations. You may also be able to get a cumulative lab and X-ray summary for your hospital stays.

Unlike X-rays, which can be copied at reasonable cost, original pathology slides must be transported by mail or hand-carried. Your specialist may wish to have the pathologist with whom he/she works speak directly with the pathologist who initially interpreted your slides as part of the process of evaluating your case.

BEING PREPARED

You are likely to be a bit nervous when you meet with the specialist you have chosen. Anxiety about your health and concern about your future care may cause you to forget information you should provide or miss hearing or understanding important information that the specialist communicates. Therefore, you may want to write down all relevant information so that you do not leave out anything of importance when you meet with the specialist or complete forms in the office. You also may want to write out your questions in advance so you don't forget anything.

To avoid leaving out important details of your condition or past treatment, prepare a concise, chronological summary before your consultation takes place. You may wish to type it and provide a copy to the specialist for inclusion in your chart. Highlight major medical results or significant events in the course of an illness or treatment if these will enlighten the doctor about your condition. Your personal perspective on the state of your health is vital to a full understanding of your medical problem.

It is possible that the specialist will use language that you do not understand or may speak quickly assuming certain knowledge on your part about your condition or its treatment. Don't hesitate to ask for clarification as often or repeatedly as you may need to in order to fully comprehend what you are being told. If you are concerned that you may forget what the doctor tells you, ask the doctor's permission to take notes or ask if you might bring along a tape recorder so you can later replay what was said, especially any instructions you are given. You may prefer to bring along a relative or close friend to serve as a "second set of ears," but, again, seek the doctor's permission to do so in advance of your appointment.

Following this process will assure that you and the specialist you are consulting get the most from your appointment. After all, you both have the same goal: restoring you to optimal health and well being.

INTRODUCTION

UTILIZING SPECIAL RESOURCES

The following information on special resources has been included to meet the needs of healthcare consumers who have extraordinarily difficult or unique health problems, and have been unable to identify the resources to address their problems. These patients and their doctors may need to search for very new, cutting-edge, perhaps even experimental and not yet approved therapies. In such cases the search may lead to clinical trials; tests of new drugs and new medical devices or innovative therapeutic approaches. Fortunately, these situations are rare, but when they do occur, they are critical.

In addition to the outstanding private and public hospitals recognized in this guide, the U.S. government maintains its own unique, expert source of patient care and clinical research at the National Institutes of Health (NIH). In fact, the NIH operates its own hospital at which the care provided is usually related to clinical studies its researchers are undertaking.

In addition to those at the NIH, clinical trials also are conducted at leading medical centers and other organizations throughout the country. These facilities may be testing a new drug therapy, a new use for an existing medication or a medical device to deal with a problem that is not being resolved through the use of more traditional approaches.

This section will guide you in utilizing these special resources.

ABOUT CLINICAL TRIALS

The Clinical Trial as a Treatment Option

For some patients the best medical treatment may only be available through clinical trials (also called treatment studies), which are designed to develop improved ways to use current medical treatments or to find new medical treatments by studying their effects on humans. Treatments are studied to determine if they are safe, effective and better treatments than conventional or standard therapies. Only if they meet all three of these criteria are they made available to the general public.

Many people are frightened by the term "clinical trial" because it conveys the notion of being a "guinea pig" in an experiment. Contrary to popular belief, however, most new treatments are extensively studied by scientists in the laboratory before they are ever tested by physicians in clinical settings. Among the factors that keep patients from participating in clinical trials are: lack of awareness about clinical trials as a treatment option; fear of side effects or adverse reactions to treatment; refusal of insurance companies to pay for experimental treatments; failure of a physician to inform the patient about clinical trials; difficulty finding suitable clinical trials; unavailability of clinical trials for certain medical problems; distance of the patient from major medical centers conducting clinical trials; disruption of personal and family life; and the decision to stop medical treatment altogether.

Despite these and other obstacles, many people do seek out clinical trials. One of the most pressing reasons to participate is the opportunity to obtain treatment that might not be available otherwise. New medical treatments can offer participants hope for a cure, an extended lifespan, or an improvement in how they feel. Some participants also take comfort in knowing that others may benefit from their contribution to medical knowledge.

Deciding if a clinical trial is the right treatment option for you is no simple matter. Certainly, you will want to talk about it with your doctor(s) and other professionals involved in your care, as well as with family members and friends. But in order to fully benefit from what others have to say — based on either their professional knowledge or personal experience — you need to understand exactly what a clinical trial is and what your role as a volunteer will be.

INTRODUCTION

Understanding Clinical Trials

Clinical trials are conducted for just about every medical condition, including life-threatening diseases such as AIDS or cancer; chronic illnesses such as diabetes and asthma; psychiatric disorders such as depression or anxiety; behavioral problems such as smoking and substance abuse; and even common ailments such as hair loss and acne. Chances are, there is at least one trial (and probably more) that may be appropriate for you.

With more than 100 different types of cancer, it is understandable that a large number of clinical trials are cancer-related. Extensive information about clinical trials for cancer can be found on the Web site of the National Cancer Institute (NCI) which is part of the NIH. CenterWatch, an online clinical trials listing service, identifies 5,200 clinical trials that are actively recruiting patients. Veritas Medicine, another useful online organization, allows individuals to perform personalized searches of its clinical trials database. See "Resources" in Appendix G for more information on clinical trials.

Most clinical trials study new medical treatments, combinations of treatments, or improvements in conventional treatments using drugs, surgery and other medical procedures, medical devices, radiation or other therapies. Newer types of clinical trials, called screening or prevention trials, study how to prevent the incidence or recurrence of disease through the use of medicines, vitamins, minerals or other supplements; and how to screen for disease, especially in its early stages. Another type of trial studies how to improve the quality of life for patients, including both their physical and emotional well-being.

Clinical trials are sponsored both by the federal government (through the National Institutes of Health, the National Cancer Institute and many others) and by private industry through pharmaceutical and biotechnology companies,

34

and through healthcare institutions (hospitals or health maintenance organizations) and community-based physician-investigators. The National Cancer Institute sponsors clinical trials at more than 1000 sites in the United States. Trials are carried out in major medical research centers such as teaching hospitals as well as in community hospitals, specialized medical clinics (for example, those for the treatment of AIDS or Alzheimer's disease) and in doctors' offices.

Though clinical trials often involve hospitalized patients, a fair number of trials are conducted on an outpatient basis. Many trials are part of a cooperative network which may include as few as one or two sites or hundreds of locations, although one center generally assumes responsibility for overall coordination of the research. More than 45 research-oriented institutions, recognized for their scientific excellence, have been designated by the NCI as comprehensive or clinical cancer centers. See "Resources" in Appendix G to find out how to locate these centers.

Clinical research is based on a protocol (established rules or procedures) describing who will be studied, how and when medications, procedures and/or treatments will be administered and how long the study will last. Trials that are conducted simultaneously at different sites use the same protocol to ensure that all patients are treated identically and all data are collected uniformly so that study findings can be compared.

Clinical trials generally are conducted in three phases, as outlined in the study protocol. The first phase begins testing of the treatment on a small group of human subjects after rigorous and successful animal testing has been concluded. The interim phase varies, but usually involves a broader test group and is designed to further evaluate the treatment's safety and more accurately determine appropriate dosage, application methods and side effects. In some trials there may be a fourth phase, conducted after the treatment is in widespread use, to monitor the results of long-term use and the occurrence of any serious side effects.

Some clinical trials test one treatment on one group of subjects, while others compare two or more groups of subjects. In such comparison studies participants are divided into two groups: the control group that receives the standard treatment and the experimental or treatment group which receives the new treatment. For example, the control group may undergo a surgical procedure while the experimental or treatment group undergoes a surgical procedure plus radiation to determine which treatment modality is more effective. To ensure that patient characteristics do not unduly influence the study findings, patients may be randomly assigned to either the control or the experimental group, meaning that each patient's assignment is based purely on chance. In cases in which a standard treatment does not exist for a particular disease, the experimental group of patients receives the new treatment and the control group receives no treatment at all, or receives a placebo, an inactive medicine or procedure that has no treatment value and is sometimes called a "dummy" pill or a "sugar" pill. It is important to keep in mind that patients are never put into a control group without any treatment if there is a known treatment that could help them. Also, whether a patient is receiving an investigational drug or a placebo, he/she receives the same level and quality of medical care as those receiving the investigational treatment.

Questions to ask your doctor and the trial's research team if you are considering participating in a clinical trial:

- Who is sponsoring the trial?
- How many patients will be involved?
- Will the trial be testing a single treatment or a combination of treatments?
- Will there be one treatment group or more than one treatment group?

• If more than one treatment group, how are patients assigned to each group?

• Has this treatment been studied in previous clinical trials? What were the findings?

Protecting the Rights of Participants

The safety of those who participate in clinical trials is a serious matter and is the number one priority of medical investigators. All clinical research, regardless of type of sponsorship, is guided by the same ethical and legal codes that govern the medical profession and the practice of medicine. Most clinical research is federally funded or federally regulated (at least in part) with built-in safeguards for patients. According to federal government regulations (and some state laws), every clinical trial in the United States must be approved and monitored by an Institutional Review Board (IRB), which is an independent committee of physicians, statisticians, community advocates and others (representing at least five distinct disciplines) to ensure that the protocol is being followed.

Government regulations require researchers to fully inform participants about all aspects of a clinical trial before they agree to participate through a process called informed consent. To be sure that you understand your role in a clinical trial, you should jot down any questions beforehand so as not to forget them. You should also consider bringing along a friend or family member for support and additional input, and perhaps even tape recording the conversation (after asking permission to do so) to make sure you do not forget or misunderstand anything. Each participant in a clinical trial must be given a written consent form, which should be available in English and other languages. The consent form explains the following:

• Why the research is being done.

• What the researchers hope to accomplish.

• What types of treatment interventions (and other tests or procedures) will be performed.

INTRODUCTION

- How long the study will continue.
- What the expected benefits and the possible risks are.
- What other treatments are available.
- What costs will be covered by the study, by the patient or by third-party payers such as Medicare, Medicaid or private insurance.

Patients also are informed that they may leave the trial, or exclude themselves from any part of it, at any time. Informed consent means exactly what the term implies: you agree to join a clinical trial only after you completely understand exactly what your participation will involve for the duration of the study. By law, each patient must be provided with a copy of the signed consent form, which also must include the name and telephone number of a contact person for questions or additional information. Informed consent is a continuous process, so do not hesitate to ask questions before, during or after the trial.

The investigators must protect the privacy of each participant in a clinical trial by ensuring that all medical records are kept confidential except for inspection by the sponsoring agency, the Food and Drug Administration and other agencies involved in regulating the drug or treatment, and all data are collected anonymously by assigning a numeric code or initials to each individual.

During the course of the trial, participants are regularly seen by members of the research team to monitor their health and well-being. Participants also should be responsible for their own health by following the treatment plan (such as taking the proper dosage of medications on time), keeping all scheduled visits and informing members of the healthcare team about any symptoms that occur. If during the course of the trial, the treatment proves to be ineffective or harmful, the patient is free to leave the study and still obtain conventional care. Conversely, as soon as there is evidence that one treatment modality is better than another, all patients in the trial are given the benefit of the new information.

Questions to ask the sponsors about your rights as a participant in a clinical trial:

- Who is responsible for approving and monitoring this research? Is there an IRB?

- Who informs me about the trial process? Do I sign a consent form? Will I receive a copy?

- May I leave the trial at any time? Have previous patients dropped out? Why?

- Whom do I contact if I am experiencing any difficulty with this trial?

Enrolling in Clinical Trials

Each clinical trial has its own guidelines, called eligibility criteria, for determining who can participate. Treatment studies recruit participants who have a disease or other medical condition, while screening and prevention studies generally recruit healthy volunteers. Inclusion criteria (those that allow you to participate in a study) and exclusion criteria (those that keep you from participating in a study) ensure that the study will answer the research questions posed in the research protocol while maintaining the safety of participants. The disease being studied is a primary factor in selecting suitable patients, but other factors such as the patient's gender, age, treatment history and other diagnosed medical conditions may also be important. Unfortunately, eligibility also may depend upon ability to pay. Many health plans do not cover all of the costs associated with clinical trials because they define these trials as experimental procedures. However, trials some-times pay volunteers for their time and/or reimburse them for travel, childcare, meals and lodging.

To prevent people who qualify from being excluded from clinical trials for finan-cial reasons, agencies such as the National Cancer Institute are working with health plans to find solutions and a growing number of states require insurance companies to pay for all routine patient care costs in cancer trials. To encourage more senior citizens to participate in cancer trials, Medicare plans to revise its payment policy to cover those trials.

INTRODUCTION

When choosing a clinical trial you should determine the factors that are most important to you. For instance, patients generally prefer to participate in trials near their homes so that they can maintain their usual day-to-day activities, be surrounded by family and friends and avoid travel and lodging costs. If travel or temporary relocation becomes necessary, try to find a trial site that is near to some family member or friend or one that is in a locale similar to your own city or town. Many organizations, such as the National Cancer Institute, will work with patients and their families to identify support networks for them wherever they participate.

Questions to ask the trial's sponsor about eligibility criteria:

- What are the inclusion and exclusion criteria for the clinical trial(s) I am considering?
- How can I improve my chances of being accepted? Can I change my health plan to one that will cover the trial's costs? Can I relocate to another city or state?
- If I am not eligible for one trial, what other trials are being conducted for my condition?
- Will I be paid for my time or reimbursed for my out-of-pocket expenses?

Participating in a Clinical Trial

Clinical trials are conducted by a research team led by a principal investigator (usually a physician) and are comprised of physicians, nurses and other health professionals such as social workers, psychologists and nutritionists. As a participant you may be required to commit a fair amount of time to a clinical trial, often more than with standard treatment. Initially, you will probably be given a physical examination and asked for your medical history. During the trial, you will have regular or periodic visits to the trial site which may include diagnostic and laboratory tests. You also may be asked to follow fixed schedules for medications and other interventions and to keep detailed records of your symptoms and

40

health condition. Generally, clinical trials last from six to twenty-six weeks, though some (called maintenance trials) can last up to a year to determine if a treatment will prevent the relapse of a medical condition.

Participants in clinical trials should remain under the care of their regular physician(s) since clinical trials tend to provide short-term treatment for a specific medical condition and do not generally provide comprehensive primary care. In fact, some trials require that a patient's regular physician sign a consent form before the patient is enrolled. In addition, your regular physician can collaborate with the research team to make sure there are no adverse reactions between your other medications or treatments and the investigational treatment.

Questions to ask the research team or your physician about your role in a clinical trial:

- Who are the members of the health team? Who will be in charge of my care?
- How long will the trial last?
- How does treatment in the trial compare with or differ from the standard treatment?
- Will I be hospitalized? How often? For how long a period of time?
- What will occur during each visit? What treatments or procedures will I be given?
- Will I still be able to see my regular physician(s)? Will my doctor and the research team collaborate?
- Can I be put in touch with other patients who have participated in this trial?

Weighing the Benefits and Risks of a Clinical Trial

If you are considering participation in a clinical trial, you need to consider the medical, emotional and financial ramifications of participation. Of course, the obvious benefit of a clinical trial is the chance that a new treatment may improve your health and prognosis. You will have access to drugs and other medical interventions before they are widely available to the public and you will obtain expert and specialized medical care at leading healthcare facilities. Many patients receive an added psychological benefit by taking an active role in their treatment .

It is important to bear in mind that some medical interventions used in clinical trials may carry potential risks depending upon the type of treatment and the patient's condition. While many side effects or adverse reactions are temporary (such as hair loss and nausea caused by some anticancer drugs), other more serious reactions can be permanent and even life-threatening (for example, heart, liver or kidney damage).

Deciding whether or not to participate in a clinical trial is often a matter of determining if the trial's potential benefits outweigh its possible risks. This is a highly personal decision that may be difficult to make in situations involving experimental treatment in which limited medical information may be available.

Questions to ask the research team about the benefits and risks of a clinical trial:

- What other treatment option(s) do I have at this time? Is there any chance that a more promising treatment may be available soon?
- What are the short and long-term benefits and risks as compared with standard treatment?
- Will I experience any known side effects or adverse reactions? Will these be temporary, long-term or permanent? Relatively minor or perhaps life-threatening?
- If I am harmed in any way by the new treatment, what other treatments will I be entitled to? Who will pay for subsequent treatment?

Getting Information on Clinical Trials

The more information you have about a clinical trial, the easier it will be to make a decision about whether or not it is right for you, and the more confident you will be that you made an appropriate decision. In addition to the "Resources" appendix in this guide, the staff at your local public library, community hospital, or major medical center can assist you in locating the information you need from books, consumer organizations and on the Internet.

LEARNING ABOUT THE NATIONAL INSTITUTES OF HEALTH (NIH)

The National Institutes of Health (NIH) comprise one the world's leading medical research centers and the Federal government's principal agency for biomedical research. An agency of the United States Department of Health, United States Public Health Service, NIH encompasses 25 separate institutions and centers with its main campus located in Bethesda, Maryland. Research is also conducted at several field units across the country and abroad.

PATIENT CARE AT THE NIH

The Warren Grant Magnuson Clinical Center, NIH's principal medical research center and hospital located in Bethesda, Maryland, provides medical care only to patients participating in clinical research programs. Two categories of patients participate in the Clinical Center studies: children and adults who wish to improve their own health, such as those with newly diagnosed medical problems, ongoing medical problems or family history of disease; and healthy volunteers wishing to advance knowledge about the causes, progress and treatment of disease. The patient's case must fit into an ongoing NIH research project for which the patient has the precise kind or stage of illness under investigation. General diagnostic and treatment services common to community hospitals are not available.

The Magnuson Clinical Center is the world's largest biomedical research hospital and ambulatory care facility, housing 1,600 laboratories conducting basic and clinical research. There are 1,200 physicians, dentists and researchers on staff along with 660 nurses and 570 allied healthcare professionals (dieticians, imaging technologists, medical technologists, medical records and clerical staff, pharmacists and therapists).

The Center's hospital is specially designed for medical research and accommodates 540 carefully selected patients who are participating in clinical research programs. Its 350-bed facility has 24 inpatient care units to which 7,000 patients are admitted annually. The Center also has an Ambulatory Care Research Facility (ACRF) that serves 68,000 outpatient visits each year. A new facility, called the Mark O. Hatfield Clinical Research Center, is currently under construction and, when completed in 2002, will include 250 beds for inpatient care and 100 day-hospital stations for outpatient care.

The Clinical Center also maintains a Children's Inn for pediatric outpatients and their families. This family-centered residence operates 24 hours a day, 7 days a week, 365 days a year. Adult outpatients without adequate childcare may make use of a childcare program for their children ages three to seven during the hours of 8:00 AM and 5:00 PM.

In an effort to bring clinical research to the community, NIH supports approximately 77 General Clinical Research Centers (GCRCs) around the country, located within hospitals of major academic medical centers.

It is important to note that, as part of the federal government, the Warren Grant Magnuson Clinical Center provides treatment in clinical trials at no cost to its patients. In some cases, patients receive a stipend to help cover the costs of traveling to Bethesda for treatment and follow-up care. Travel costs for the initial screening visit, however, are not covered.

INTRODUCTION

AREAS OF CLINICAL STUDY AT THE NIH

At the Magnuson Clinical Center alone, NIH physician-scientists conduct about 1,000 studies each year. Among the areas of study are:

- AIDS
- Aging
- Alcohol abuse and alcoholism
- Allergy
- Arthritis, musculoskeletal and-skin diseases
- Cancer
- Child
- Chronic pain
- Deafness and other communication disorders

- Dental and orafacial disorders
- Diabetes
- Digestive and kidney diseases
- Eye disorders
- Heart, lung and blood diseases
- Infectious diseases
- Medical genetics
- Mental health
- Neurological disorders
- Stroke

Not all of these clinical areas are under investigation at any given time, however. The Patient Recruitment and Public Liaison Office (PRPL) at the NIH Clinical Center assists patients, their families and their physicians in obtaining information about participation in NIH clinical trials. Trained nurses are available to answer questions about the research programs and admission procedures.

CANCER CARE AT THE WARREN GRANT MAGNUSON CLINICAL CENTER

The National Cancer Institute (NCI) is the largest of the biomedical research institutes and centers at NIH. There, clinical studies are designed to evaluate new and promising ways to prevent, detect, diagnose and treat cancer. The Warren Grant Magnuson Clinical Center provides a separate outpatient division for cancer patients and also has several designated inpatient units.

46

If you are interested in entering a cancer study at the Magnuson Clinical Center (or at the General Clinical Research Centers), you should first discuss treatment options with a physician. As a general rule, patients interested in participating in clinical studies must be referred by a physician. However, in some instances, self-referral may be permitted.

If your physician concurs that a clinical study might be appropriate for you, the NIH recommends that the following steps be taken:

- Contact NCI's Clinical Studies Support Center (CSSC), which is staffed by trained oncology (cancer) nurses who can identify appropriate clinical studies for you. Summaries of these trials and other pertinent information about the type of treatment being offered and the type of patients eligible for inclusion can be mailed or faxed to you and/or your physician.

- Review the clinical trials summaries and other information with your physician to decide which study or studies you should consider. Your physician also can contact the CSSC to communicate directly with the investigator in charge of the study.

- In cases in which you meet the initial eligibility requirements, it may be necessary for you to schedule a screening visit at the Clinical Center to learn more about the trial and possibly undergo some medical tests.

- If accepted for a clinical trial, make sure that you understand the details about the treatment and any possible risks and benefits.

Patients with medical problems other than cancer or healthy volunteers who wish to participate in a clinical study should contact the particular NIH institute responsible for the clinical area involved.

Cancer care at the NCI Clinical Centers and Comprehensive Cancer Centers

You may also obtain clinical oncology services (education, screening, diagnosis or treatment) or participate in clinical trials at one of the 13 Clinical Cancer Centers or 37 Comprehensive Cancer Centers designated by the NCI for their scientific

INTRODUCTION

excellence and extensive resources devoted to cancer and cancer-related problems. Centers are located in 29 states, with the majority of sites in California, New York and Pennsylvania. You can find out about clinical trials at the NCI-designated centers by contacting NCI's Clinical Studies Support Center (CSSC) or by calling each center directly. Information about other cancer-related services at these centers also may be obtained from the center itself.

WHAT TO DO IF YOU CAN'T GET AN APPOINTMENT

At times it may be difficult, perhaps even impossible, to secure an appointment with the specific specialist you have identified. There are a number of reasons why this may occur. For example, the specialist may not be taking any new patients or may have such a busy schedule that it takes several weeks or months to get an appointment. He/she may only see patients during very limited hours because of teaching, research or other responsibilities or currently may have other limitations related to the acceptance of new patients.

However, bear in mind that the doctors in this guide are the leaders in their specialties and therefore they work with and train the very best and brightest in their specialties. So, if you are unable to consult with a particular doctor, consider making an appointment with one of his/her outstanding colleagues. You can do this by asking a member of the doctor's office staff to refer you to an associate who is a member of the practice group or to another excellent physician who is specially trained to address your particular medical issue.

You can be comfortable knowing that you will receive high quality care from another specialist who practices in the same top setting.

GEOGRAPHIC REGIONS AND STATES

To assist you in using **America's Top Doctors** in the most efficient and effective manner, the Guide is divided into seven geographic regions. This will help you to locate a specialist in your local or neighboring region. For example, if you live in Mississippi in the Southeast region and you are willing and able to travel to Louisiana in the Southwest region to consult with a specialist in neurology, you can review just those two regions, under the section headed **"NEUROLOGY."** However, if you prefer to review the information on neurologists *throughout* the country, you can search the entire neurology section. Or, you can consult the **"SPECIAL EXPERTISE INDEX"** in the back of this Guide and choose a neurologist who has specific expertise to meet your particular needs.

The geographic sections are as follows:

> *New England*
> *Mid Atlantic*
> *Southeast*
> *Midwest*
> *Great Plains and Mountains*
> *Southwest*
> *West Coast and Pacific*

The states that are included in each region are listed on the following page and a map of the regions is also provided. Please note that not all regions are represented in all specialties. For example, in Adolescent Medicine there are no listings in the Southwest region.

GEOGRAPHIC REGIONS AND STATES

New England:
Connecticut
Maine
Massachusetts
New Hampshire
Rhode Island
Vermont

Mid Atlantic:
Delaware
Maryland
New Jersey
New York
Pennsylvania
Washington, DC
West Virginia

Southeast:
Alabama
Florida
Georgia
Kentucky
Mississippi
North Carolina
South Carolina
Tennessee
Virginia

Midwest:
Illinois
Indiana
Iowa
Michigan
Minnesota
Missouri
Ohio
Wisconsin

Great Plains and Mountains:
Colorado
Idaho
Kansas
Montana
Nebraska
North Dakota
South Dakota
Utah
Wyoming

Southwest:
Arizona
Arkansas
Louisiana
New Mexico
Oklahoma
Texas

West Coast and Pacific:
Alaska
California
Hawaii
Nevada
Oregon
Washington

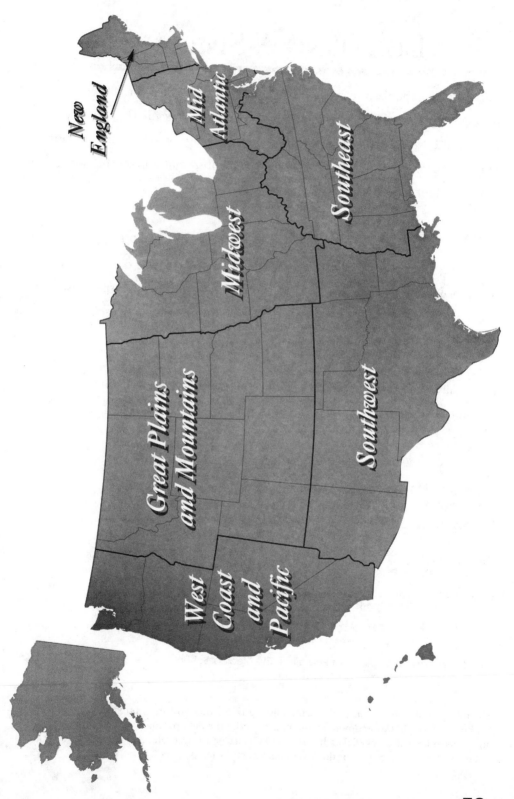

New England

Mid Atlantic

Southeast

Midwest

Great Plains and Mountains

Southwest

West Coast and Pacific

53

LOCATING A SPECIALIST

This guide is organized to make finding the right specialists for you or your loved ones as simple as possible. Physicians' biographies are presented by specialty and are organized by geographic region within each specialty or subspecialty. Thus, you may search for a particular type of specialist or subspecialist in one or more regions or throughout the nation.

A second way to locate the right specialist is to use the **Special Expertise Index** beginning on page 951. This index is organized according to diseases, conditions and procedures or techniques. For example, you can locate a top specialist for diabetes or for Mohs' surgery by looking for those terms in the **Special Expertise Index**.

If you already know a specialist's name, you can find his/her listing by using the **Alphabetical Listing of Doctors** beginning on page 1057.

SAMPLE PHYSICIAN LISTING

Smith, John MD (Adolescent Medicine) - *Special Expertise: Asthma Allergy;*
Physician's Name   Physician's Specialty   Physician's Special Expertise

Admitting Hospital: Children's Hospital; **Office Address:** 300 Ridge Road Boston, MA 12345;
    Physician's Admitting Hospital   Physician's Office Address

Office Phone: (617) 555-2343; **Board Certifications:** Pediatrics 1975, Adolescent Medicine 1994;
    Physician's Office Phone   Physician's Board Certification(s)

Medical School: Harvard Med Sch 1970; **Residency:** Children's Hospital, Boston, MA 1971-1973;
    Physician's Medical School   Physician's Residency(ies)

Fellowship: Adolescent Medicine, Children's Hospital, Boston, MA 1973-1974;
                Physician's Fellowship(s)

Faculty Appointment: Assoc Prof Pediatrics, The Medical School
                Physician's Faculty Appointment

The information reported in each doctor's listing is, for the most part, provided by the doctor or his/her office staff. Castle Connolly attempts to verify the data through other sources but cannot guarantee that in all cases all data have been so verified or are accurate. All such information is subject to change from time to time due to changes in physician practices.

HOSPITAL INFORMATION PROGRAM

Among the more than 6,000 acute care and specialty hospitals in the United States, many have extraordinary capabilities for superior patient care. These hospitals, renowned for their use of state-of-the-art equipment and up-to-the-minute technology, also attract outstanding physicians and other healthcare professionals. Many of their physicians are among those in the listings in this Guide.

To further assist you in your search for top specialists and to supplement the information contained in the physician listings that follow, we invited a select group of these fine institutions to profile their services, special programs and centers of excellence in *The Hospital Information Program*. This special section contains pages sponsored by the included hospitals. Participation in this section is totally separate from the physician selection process, which is based upon a completely independent review.

The Hospital Information Program provides an overview of the programs and services offered by the included hospitals with information related to their accreditation and sponsorship. Most also provide their physician referral numbers, should you wish to ask the hospitals for recommendations of doctors not listed in *America's Top Doctors*.

In addition to *The Hospital Information Program*, profiled hospitals were also invited to highlight their special programs or services that focus on a particular disease or medical condition. These can be found in the *Centers of Excellence* sections that are interspersed throughout this book following the medical specialties and/or subspecialties to which they relate. Sponsored pages in the centers of excellence sections reflect the depth of commitment of these hospitals, which provide the staff, resources and financial support necessary to develop these special programs.

We believe you will find this information helpful in your search for the best healthcare—from both physicians and hospitals—throughout the United States!

HOSPITAL LISTINGS:

BETH ISRAEL DEACONESS MEDICAL CENTER
A member of CAREGROUP
Where the patient comes first.

330 Brookline Ave.
Boston, MA 02215
Tel. 617.667.7000
www.bidmc.caregroup.org

Beds: 549 licensed beds
Accreditation: Joint Commission on Accreditation of Healthcare Organization

ABOUT BETH ISRAEL DEACONESS MEDICAL CENTER

A major teaching affiliate of Harvard Medical School and a member of CareGroup Healthcare System, Beth Israel Deaconess Medical Center is renowned for excellence in patient care, biomedical research, teaching, and community service. Located in the heart of Boston's medical community, it cares for more than half a million patients annually in Boston and communities north, west and south of the city. It serves as the principal tertiary/academic resource for the CareGroup Healthcare System, an organized system of health care that comprises six hospitals and more than 1,800 physicians.

MEDICAL EXCELLENCE

The Beth Israel Deaconess Medical Center is known for clinical expertise in the following areas: solid organ transplantation, cancer (with emphasis on breast cancer), diabetes/vascular surgery, obstetrics, cardiology, cardiac surgery, women's health, and AIDS. Its long list of medical milestones includes developing the first implantable cardiac pacemaker in 1960 (Beth Israel Hospital), performing New England's first minimally invasive coronary bypass surgery in 1995 (Deaconess Hospital) and performing the first living donor liver transplant in New England in 1998.

PATIENT CARE

Beth Israel Deaconess Medical Center is a nonprofit health care institution that provides care for patients of any race, creed, color, or nationality. It features a full range of emergency services, including a Level 1 Trauma Center and roof-top heliport; Boston's first hospital-based Palliative Care Unit, providing care, support and comfort for terminally ill patients and their families; The state's largest hospital-based Transitional Care Unit, allowing inpatients to regain their mobility, function, and independence before returning home; and The Beth Israel Deaconess Learning Center, offering patients and families up-to-date health information and access to current research on a wide range of medical conditions.

BIOMEDICAL RESEARCH

Cutting-edge clinical and biomedical research is supported by grants from private foundations and government agencies. Among independent teaching hospitals, Beth Israel Deaconess Medical Center is the third-largest recipient of biomedical research funding from the National Institutes of Health. The Harvard-Thorndike Laboratory, the nation's oldest clinical research laboratory, has been located on this site since 1973. Beth Israel Deaconess Medical Center shares important clinical and research programs with other world-renowned institutions such as the Dana-Farber Cancer Institute, the Joslin Diabetes Center and Boston's Children's Hospital.

TEACHING

Beth Israel Deaconess Medical Center has 1,178 physicians on the active medical staff. Most physicians hold faculty appointments at Harvard Medical School. The Carl J. Shapiro Institute For Education and Research provides medical students with innovative clinical education programs, including interdepartmental courses focusing on the whole patient and a state-of-the-art computer lab that lets students diagnose and manage simulated patients. Located on site, it is the first program of its kind in the country.

For help choosing a doctor, call the CareConnection at 800-667-5356.

CONTINUUM HEALTH PARTNERS, INC.

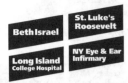

555 West 57th Street
New York, NY 10019
Phone: 800-420-4004
www.WeHealNewYork.org

Sponsorship: Voluntary Not-for-Profit
Beds: 3,048 certified beds
Accreditation: Joint Commission on Accreditation of Healthcare Organizations (JCAHO), Accreditation Council for Graduate Medical Education, Medical Society of New York, in cooperation with the Accreditation Council for Continuing Medical Education

A STRONG PARTNERSHIP WITH A PROUD HERITAGE

Continuum Health Partners, Inc. is a partnership of four venerable health care providers, Beth Israel Medical Center, St. Luke's-Roosevelt Hospital Center, Long Island College Hospital, and the New York Eye and Ear Infirmary. Each of the four partner institutions was established more than a century ago by individuals committed to improving health and health care in their communities. Today, the system represents more than 4,700 physicians and dentists and is superbly equipped to respond to the health care needs of the populations we serve. Continuum providers also see patients in group and private practice settings and in ambulatory centers in New York City and Westchester County.

LOCATIONS

Continuum Health Partners has campuses throughout Manhattan and Brooklyn. Beth Israel Medical Center has three divisions: the Milton and Caroll Petrie Division on the Lower East Side, the Herbert and Nell Singer Division on the Upper East Side, and the Kings Highway Division in Brooklyn. The Phillips Ambulatory Care Center, a state-of-the-art outpatient center, is located at Union Square. St. Luke's-Roosevelt Hospital Center has two campuses on Manhattan's West Side: the St. Luke's Division in Morningside Heights and the Roosevelt Division in Midtown. Long Island College Hospital is located in the Brooklyn Heights/Cobble Hill section of Brooklyn. The New York Eye and Ear Infirmary is located on the Lower East Side.

ACADEMIC AFFILIATIONS

Beth Israel Medical Center is University Hospital and Manhattan Campus for the Albert Einstein College of Medicine. St. Luke's-Roosevelt Hospital Center is University Hospital for Columbia University College of Physicians and Surgeons. Long Island College Hospital is the primary teaching affiliate of the SUNY–Health Science Center at Brooklyn. The New York Eye and Ear Infirmary is the primary teaching center of the New York Medical College and affiliated teaching hospitals in the areas of ophthalmology and otolaryngology.

PHYSICIAN REFERRAL SERVICE: For a referral to a doctor in your neighborhood, call (800) 420-4004. Continuum's Referral Service can help you find a primary care physician or specialist affiliated with Beth Israel, St. Luke's-Roosevelt, Long Island College Hospital, or the New York Eye and Ear Infirmary. Visit our web site at www.WeHealNewYork.org.

DETROIT MEDICAL CENTER

3663 Woodward Ave., Suite 200   Detroit, Michigan 48201
Tel. 1-888-DMC-2500
www.dmc.org

DMC
Detroit Medical Center
Wayne State University

The Detroit Medical Center is the largest health care provider in Southeast Michigan.

GENERAL OVERVIEW

The Detroit Medical Center operates seven hospitals, two nursing homes and more than 100 outpatient facilities throughout southeast Michigan. Established as a non-profit corporation in 1985, the Detroit Medical Center has become a leading regional health care system with a mission of excellence in clinical care, research and medical education.

ACADEMIC & CLINICAL AFFILIATIONS

With over 2,000 licensed beds, the Detroit Medical Center serves as the teaching and clinical research site for Wayne State University School of Medicine and Nursing and Allied Health Services. Wayne State University is the largest single-campus medical school in the country.

MEDICAL STAFF

The Detroit Medical Center's world-class medical staff consists of 3,000 affiliated physicians, many of whom teach and conduct research at Wayne State University, providing their patients with the most up-to-date and cutting-edge clinical care. The *"1999 Best Doctors in America: Midwest Region"* includes more than 150 Detroit Medical Center's physicians chosen by their peers as the "best and brightest in their fields."

PIONEERING, COMPREHENSIVE MEDICAL CARE

The relationship between the Detroit Medical Center and Wayne State University has already pioneered many treatments for cancer, birth defects, heart disease, and neurological disorders— and innovative diagnostic methods and treatments are being developed every day. On the cutting edge of developments in artificial vision research is the Kresge Eye Institute's Ligon Research Center of Vision, a partnership between Wayne State University, the Detroit Medical Center and the Institute. The research center plans to test a retinal implant within two years.

INTERNATIONAL SERVICES

International patients and physicians readily utilize the Detroit Medical Center's International Center for services ranging from health care to education. The International Center also provides housing for patients and their families, medical staff and health care specialists from other countries who visit the Detroit Medical Center to observe internationally renowned physicians, participate in research, and explore new technologies.

ACCREDITATION, COMMENDATIONS & NATIONAL RECOGNITION

In 1999, the Michigan Minority Business Development Council honored the Detroit Medical Center with its Corporation of the Year — Health Care Sector award in recognition of its excellent minority supplier-purchasing program. The Detroit Medical Center's Hutzel Hospital is an active participant in the national **Women's Health Initiative** research study along with Sinai-Grace Hospital and Huron Valley-Sinai Hospital. The program focuses on the health care issues of women.

Children's Hospital of Michigan • Detroit Receiving Hospital and University Health Center • DMC Physician Services • Harper Hospital • Huron Valley-Sinai Hospital • Hutzel Hospital • Karmanos Cancer Institute • Kresge Eye Institute • Rehabilitation Institute of Michigan • Sinai-Grace Hospital

DUKE UNIVERSITY HEALTH SYSTEM

Durham, NC 27710   *Tel. 1.800.ASK.DUKE*   *www.mc.duke.edu*

Beds: Duke University Hospital: 1,124; Durham Regional Hospital: 446 acute care beds; Raleigh Community Hospital: 218 acute care beds
Accreditation: Accredited with commendation by JCAHO

The Duke University Health System is a world-class health care network dedicated to providing outstanding patient care, educating tomorrow's health care leaders, and discovering new and better ways to treat disease through biomedical research. Duke offers every level of health service--from wellness and preventive care to the most advanced specialty services—in an atmosphere of caring and compassion.

The hub of the Health System—Duke University Medical Center, in Durham, North Carolina—is consistently rated one of the top five hospitals in the country by U.S. News & World Report. The youngest of the nation's leading medical centers, Duke University Medical Center earned its reputation as a world-class health care institution through ground-breaking clinical care and research. Duke operates one of the country's largest clinical and biomedical research enterprises, and quickly translates advances in technology and medical knowledge into improved patient care. It is the leading medical center in the Southeast, with a medical school ranked among the top three in the nation.

The Health System also provides high-quality clinical services in convenient locations throughout the surrounding region. Included in the Health System are three hospitals, ambulatory surgery centers, primary and specialty care clinics, home care, hospice, skilled nursing care, wellness centers, and community-based clinical partnerships.

Duke provides a range of respected clinical programs to meet every patient's needs. Among them are the Duke Comprehensive Cancer Center, known for its multidisciplinary approach to treating large tumors and its innovative therapies using bone marrow transplantation and hyperthermia; the Duke Heart Center, which has conducted many of the leading studies on the effectiveness of new treatments for heart disease; an experienced organ transplant team which performs hundreds of transplants each year; Duke Women's Services, offering comprehensive care for normal and high-risk pregnancies, reproductive and endocrinology services including the most advanced fertilization techniques, genetic testing, and fetal assessment; a Children's Hospital & Health Center offering the full range of primary care and specialty services, including leading programs in bone marrow transplant, pediatric AIDS, and severe combined immunodeficiency syndrome (SCIDS); and an orthopaedic program providing expert care in such areas as major joint reconstruction, sports medicine, and reconstructive microsurgery.

In addition, Duke is a leader in the field of human genetics. Researchers have helped identify genes associated with obesity and with people's susceptibility to such diseases as breast cancer, colon cancer, Lou Gehrig's disease, and Alzheimer's disease, opening new avenues toward curing and treating these devastating diseases.

To make an appointment with a Duke physician, call 1-888-ASK-DUKE.

FOUR WINDS HOSPITAL

800 Cross River Road   *Katonah, New York 10536*
Tel. 914-763-8151   *Fax. 914-763-9598*
www.fourwindshospital.com

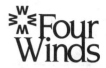

Beds: 175, Westchester, 92 Saratoga, 107 Syracuse

GENERAL OVERVIEW

Four Winds is a psychiatric health system specializing in inpatient and outpatient mental health treatment services for children (5-12), adolescents (13-17) and adults (18 and older). Four Winds Hospital is the leading provider of child and adolescent mental health services in the Northeast. In addition to a broad range of inpatient treatment services, including dual diagnosis treatment for adolescents and adults, Four Winds provides child, adolescent and adult outpatient Partial Hospitalization Programs. CHOICES, an alcohol/substance abuse outpatient treatment center provides ambulatory detoxification along with a full range of comprehensive clinic services. Four Winds operates two other sites in Saratoga Springs, NY (518-584-3600) and Syracuse, NY (315-476-2161).

ACADEMIC & CLINICAL AFFILIATIONS

An affiliate of the Albert Einstein College of Medicine, Four Winds Hospital provides internship trainings and psychiatric rotations for medical students, clinical social workers, clinical art therapists and a year-long pre-doctoral clinical internship training program in child and adolescent psychology.

ADMISSION AND REFERRAL INFORMATION

Four Winds admits patients 24 hours a day, 7 days a week, with 24 hour triage services. Upon admission, each patient is triaged to the appropriate level of care. Four Winds accepts third party insurance, empire blue cross/blue shield, medicaid (NYS), and medicare. Admission can be voluntary or involuntary, and our referring community includes clinicians, managed care organizations, schools, employers, employee assistance personnel, clergy, family members, community agencies and self-referrals. Four Winds maintains regular contact with the referring professional during the admission process, and throughout the treatment experience.

OUTCOME STUDIES

For over 10 years, Four Winds Hospital has evaluated the effectiveness of the treatment that we provide. There are many uses for the outcome data collected at Four Winds, the most important of which is to establish a continuous process of evaluation of the care that is provided at the hospital. Four Winds Hospital has made over 75 presentations at scientific meetings with these data, including the American Psychiatric Association, The Institute on Psychiatric Services, The Society for Biological Psychiatry, The American Psychological Association, The Society for Research in Psychopathology, The Association of Private Psychiatric Hospitals, Eastern Psychological Association, and the New York Neuropsychological Group.

ACCREDITATIONS AND LICENSURES

Treatment services at Four Winds are accredited by the Joint Commission on the Accreditation of Healthcare Organizations (JCAHO) and licensed by the New York State Office of Mental Health. CHOICES is JCAHO accredited and licensed by the NYS Office of Alcoholism and Substance Abuse Services (OASAS).

HENRY FORD HOSPITAL

2799 W. GRAND BOULEVARD
DETROIT, MICH. 48202

85 Years of Healing

Henry Ford Hospital is a 903-bed tertiary care hospital, a multi-organ transplantation center and a Level 1 trauma center, teaching and research institution. It is the flagship of Henry Ford Health System, which consists of a dozen owned or affiliated hospitals, more than 25 medical centers, the state's largest health maintenance organization and a wide range of other health services.

The Henry Ford Medical Group, one of the nation's largest group practices with 900 physicians and research staff in more than 40 medical specialties, staffs Henry Ford Hospital and 25 Henry Ford Medical Centers.The health system is also affiliated with 1,800 private practice physicians.

Henry Ford Guest Services representatives assist out-of-town patients and visitors from throughout Michigan, the U.S. and abroad with a variety of arrangements. The service provides assistance in coordinating hospital admissions, family lodging, travel and transportation. Language translation services are also available.

Teaching Institution

Henry Ford has academic affiliations with Case Western Reserve University School of Medicine in Cleveland; Michigan State University School of Osteopathic Medicine; the University of Michigan School of Medicine; Oakland University School of Nursing; and Oakland University's Biomedical Physics Program.

Research

More than 150 medical specialists and research scientists, including 55 full-time researchers, are involved in more than 1,500 individual research projects. Areas include stroke, hypertension, heart disease, cancer, osteoporosis, arthritis, sleep disorders, diabetes and lung diseases. Henry Ford ranks in the top 6 percent of all institutions granted funding by the National Institutes of Health and U.S. Public Heart Service.

www.HenryFord.com
1-888-291-8304

CENTERS OF EXCELLENCE

*The **Heart and Vascular Institute** offers one of the nation's most successful heart failure treatment, transplant and rehab programs.*

***Neurosciences Institute** includes a stroke care and research center, epilepsy program, headache center, spine program and Hermelin Brain Tumor Center.*

***Bone and Joint Center** provides the latest advances in joint replacement and treatment of bone and joint-related disorders.*

*The **Multi-Organ Transplantation Center** has nationally recognized programs for heart, lung, kidney, kidney-pancreas, liver and cornea tranplants.*

*The **Josephine Ford Cancer Center** offers a continuum of care, from prevention and bone marrow transplantation to hospice.*

*The **Department of Medical Genetics** provides genetic counseling and prenatal diagnoses.*

***Maplegrove center** is a nationally recognized treatment program for adults and adolescents.*

HOSPITAL FOR SPECIAL SURGERY

HOSPITAL
FOR
SPECIAL
SURGERY

535 East 70th Street
Tel.: 212.606.1779

New York, NY 10021
Website: www.hss.edu

Sponsorship: Private, Non-Profit
Beds: 160
Accreditation: Awarded Accreditation With Commendation from the Joint Commission on Accreditation of Healthcare Organizations (JCAHO).

PROFILE

Hospital for Special Surgery is one of the world's leading orthopedic, rheumatologic and rehabilitation specialty hospitals. US News and World Report has selected the Hospital as the top ranked hospital in the Northeast for its specialties.

Founded in 1863, the Hospital is dedicated to the prevention and treatment of diseases of the musculoskeletal system. HSS is a voluntary, not for profit teaching hospital, affiliated with the New York Presbyterian Health System and the Weill Medical College of Cornell University.

MEDICAL STAFF

There are more than 200 board certified attending medical staff at the Hospital. All physicians have appointments at Weill Medical College of Cornell University, and a large number of the staff are actively engaged in groundbreaking research.

RESEARCH

The mission of research at Hospital for Special Surgery is to attain the highest level of scientific excellence in orthopedics, rheumatology and related scientific disciplines. Expert scientists and clinicians work in close proximity in three integrated levels of research—basic, applied and clinical—with the goal of preventing musculoskeletal conditions and enhancing the quality of life for those afffected by them.

TEACHING PROGRAMS

The Hospital for Special Surgery has had a continuous postgraduate training program ("Residency") for more than 100 years. The four-year Orthopedic Surgery Residency has 8 Residents in each class. In addition, HSS postgraduate programs include Fellowships in Orthopedic Surgery subspecialties, Rheumatic Disease Medicine, Musculoskeletal Radiology and MRI, Neurology, and Anesthesiology. About 100 third year and fourth year medical students rotate through HSS each year, receiving instruction from Residents, Fellows, and Attending Staff.

SPECIALTIES

The Hospital addresses all problems of the elbow, foot, hand, hip, knee, shoulder, and spine. Specialties include: Arthroscopy, Back Pain, Bone Tumors, Carpal Tunnel Syndrome, Cerebral Palsy, Club Foot, Congenital Dislocation of the Hip, Fibromyalgia, Joint Replacement Surgery, Juvenile Rheumatoid Arthritis, Ligament Injuries, Lyme Disease, Muscular Dystrophy, Occupational Therapy, Orthopedic Trauma, Osteoporosis, Paget's Disease, Pain Management, Pediatric Orthopedics, Pediatric Rheumatology, Physical Therapy, Physiatry, Podiatry, Rheumatoid Arthritis, Scoliosis, Spina Bifida, Sports Medicine, Systemic Lupus Erythematosus, Rehabilitation, Women's Sports Medicine.

Physician Referral: Call 1.800.854.0071 for a referral to one of our specialists,
Monday - Friday 9:00 am - 5:00 pm.

ILLINOIS MASONIC MEDICAL CENTER

836 West Wellington Avenue   *Chicago, Illinois 60657*
phone (773) 975-1600   *Web Site:*   *http://www.immc.org* ·

Sponsorship: Voluntary Not-for-Profit
Beds: 801 (Licensed)
Accreditation: Joint Commission on Accreditation of Healthcare Organizations   All 14 graduate medical education programs fully accredited

GENERAL DESCRIPTION

Illinois Masonic Medical Center (IMMC) is located on the north side of Chicago. The Medical Center consists of a 507-bed teaching hospital; a 294-bed skilled care facility serving older adults in need of medical attention, long-term care or rehabilitative services; and a health network of services featuring numerous primary care centers located on the north and northwest sides of Chicago. The mission of IMMC is to improve the health of its patients and the community it serves.

EDUCATION PROGRAMS

Almost 200 residency and fellowship positions are offered annually to new doctors in the fields of pathology, internal medicine, dentistry, primary care, family medicine, anesthesiology, obstetrics/gynecology, radiology.

CANCER CARE

The Angelo P. Creticos, M.D. Cancer Center offers an interdisciplinary approach to the diagnosis and treatment of cancer, allowing patients to take advantage of the latest techniques in surgery, chemotherapy and radiation therapy.

CARDIAC CARE

Cardiac specialists provide a full range of services for diagnosing and treating patients with cardiovascular disease, including diagnostic tests, traditional treatments and innovative investigational therapies, as well as patient and family support programs.

EMERGENCY CARE

One of four Level I Trauma Centers in Chicago, IMMC provides immediate assessment and care for severely injured patients. The Emergency Department features 17 exam rooms, and a state-of-the-art trauma suite to provide medical care more quickly and with greater privacy. The newest digital x-ray equipment and a complete laboratory reduce waiting time by as much as one hour.

HIV/AIDS CARE

IMMC had the first designated AIDS unit in Chicago, and today remains the only designated inpatient unit on the north side. A cadre of more than 80 healthcare professionals in both inpatient and outpatient settings help people with HIV/AIDS live healthier, more fulfilling lives. Among these professionals is an internal medicine health practice specializing in this area. Services include research, infusion, transfusion, dietary, podiatry, pharmacy and wellness activities.

WOMEN'S CARE

In 1982, IMMC responded to the growing need for alternative and specialized care for women by opening Women's Health Resources, the first such program in the country. This program provides comprehensive care for women, by women. This includes providing complete physical examinations, obstetric/gynecological care, family planning, nutritional assessments, mid-life women's services and counseling. In addition, IMMC offers a full range of reproductive health services, including the Alternative Birthing Center, the first such center in the Midwest (1978); a Level III Perinatal Facility, which treats low birth weight and high risk babies; an Antenatal Resource Center, providing comprehensive antepartum care for both mother and fetus.

Physician Referral: Call (773) 296-7091 if you are looking for a primary care or specialist physician at IMMC.

JOHNS HOPKINS
M E D I C I N E

600 N. Wolfe St.   Baltimore, MD 21287
1.800.507.9952 ext 76   www.hopkinsmedicine.org

Beds: 875
Sponsorship: Private, Non-Profit
Accreditation: Joint Commission on Accreditation of Healthcare Organizations (JCAHO)

JOHNS HOPKINS MEDICINE

As leaders and pioneers in their fields, Hopkins physicians have been responsible for many of this century's key discoveries and innovations in patient care. Patients at Johns Hopkins are the first to benefit from these new technologies and treatments developed by physicians here. Recent advances include new sight-saving procedures for disorders of the eye, nerve-sparing surgery for prostate and colo-rectal cancer, the first successful treatment for sickle-cell anemia, and new diagnosis, treatment and prevention techniques for colon and other cancers.

After more than a century of extraordinary progress in medicine and health, the quest for new knowledge leading to better health care remains the defining mission of Johns Hopkins Medicine. Johns Hopkins Centers of Excellence include:
- Blaustein Pain Center
- Brady Urologic Institute
- Cardiovascular Institute
- Children's Center
- Comprehensive Cancer Center
- Kelly Gynecologic Service
- Kelly Ripken Center for Thyroid Disease
- Meyer Neurosciences Center
- Meyerhoff Digestive Disease Center
- Nathans and McKusick Institute for Genetics
- Phipps Psychiatric Institute
- Wilmer Eye Institute

Patients are seen at either The Johns Hopkins Hospital, Johns Hopkins Bayview Medical Center or at our outpatient facilities. The Marburg Pavilion, a special group of patient rooms offering five star hotel-like accommodations and amenities, is available to many patients at The Johns Hopkins Hospital.

ARRANGING MEDICAL CARE AT JOHNS HOPKINS IS EASY.

Johns Hopkins USA offers a single point of contact for the hospital repeatedly ranked #1 in the nation by *U.S. News & World Report*. Our experienced staff members can help you locate the right specialist at Hopkins, schedule an appointment and coordinate every other aspect of your visit to Johns Hopkins.

To find a specialist or receive a copy of the U.S. News 2000 "America's Best Hospitals" guide, Call 1-800-507-9952, ext. 76. Appointments also can be requested on-line, www.hopkinsmedicine.org

THE UNIVERSITY OF TEXAS
MD ANDERSON
CANCER CENTER
Making Cancer History™

1515 Holcombe Boulevard
Houston, Texas 77030
Tel.: 713.792.6161
Toll Free: 800.392.1611
www.mdanderson.org

Beds: 450

GENERAL OVERVIEW

Located in Houston, Texas, on the sprawling campus of the Texas Medical Center, The University of Texas M. D. Anderson Cancer Center is one of the world's most respected centers devoted exclusively to cancer patient care, research, education and prevention.

M. D. Anderson was created by the Texas Legislature in 1941 as a component of The University of Texas System, and the faculty exceeds 900 - both M.D.s and Ph.D.s. M. D. Anderson is one of the nation's original three Comprehensive Cancer Centers designated by the National Cancer Act of 1971 and is one of only 37 such centers today.

M. D. Anderson was ranked the top hospital for cancer care in the annual "Best Hospitals" survey published by *U.S. News & World Report* magazine in July 2000. M. D. Anderson has ranked among the top two cancer hospitals since the survey began 11 years ago.

The institution has increased about 50 percent in size in the last five years. The physical plant includes a 249-bed hospital pavilion, for a total of 450 beds, and a clinical research building which opened in 1998. A 13-story faculty office tower has opened recently, and a 126-room expansion to M. D. Anderson's 198-room patient/family hotel is nearing completion. Another research building and an ambulatory clinical building are in the planning stages.

PATIENT CARE

Since 1944, more than 400,000 patients have turned to M. D. Anderson for cancer care in the form of surgery, chemotherapy, radiation therapy, immunotherapy or combinations of these and other treatments. This multidisciplinary approach to treating cancer was pioneered at M. D. Anderson. And because they focus only on cancer, experts here are renowned for their ability to treat uncommon or rare cancers as well as they treat common cancers.

This year, about 65,000 persons with cancer will receive care at M. D. Anderson, and about 18,000 of them will be new patients. More than half of these patients come from outside Texas seeking the research-based care that has made M. D. Anderson so widely respected. Approximately 15 percent of all patients will participate in clinical trials of new therapies at some time during their illnesses.

M. D. Anderson holds Accreditation with Commendation from the Joint Commission on Accreditation of Healthcare Organizations (JCAHO), the highest level of accreditation given by the nation's oldest body charged with improving the quality of healthcare given to the public.

RESEARCH

M. D. Anderson contributes more research to patient care than any other academic center. Important scientific knowledge gained in the laboratory is rapidly translated into clinical care through research trials. The institution currently spends more than $150 million per year in research. M. D. Anderson now ranks first in the number of grants awarded nationwide by both the National Cancer Institute and the American Cancer Society. The research program is considered one of the most productive efforts in the world aimed solely at cancer.

PREVENTION

Recognizing that, ultimately, prevention is the best way to eliminate the threat of cancer, M. D. Anderson has initiated a multifaceted effort. Expanded research efforts in epidemiology and behavioral sciences complement achievements made in the clinical cancer arena. Laboratory activities support developmental and practical applications of cancer prevention. Cancer prevention services are offered in individual and corporate programs, from personalized risk assessments to screening and genetic counseling.

MAIMONIDES MEDICAL CENTER

4802 Tenth Avenue   *Brooklyn, NY 11219*
Phone: (718) 283-8200   *Fax: (718) 283-8848*
Physician Referral: (888) MMC-DOCS
www.maimonidesmed.org

Maimonides
MEDICAL CENTER

Sponsorship: Voluntary Not-for-Profit
Beds: 705 acute, 70 psychiatric
Accreditation: Joint Commission on Accreditation of Healthcare Organizations (JCAHO),
American College of Surgeons, American Council of Graduate Medical Education (ACGME)

GENERAL DESCRIPTION

Maimonides Medical Center is the nation's third largest independent teaching hospital. A nonsectarian institution under Jewish auspices, it serves patients from the New York metropolitan area and beyond. Maimonides is a major teaching affiliate of the SUNY-Health Science Center at Brooklyn.

MEDICAL STAFF AND TEACHING PROGRAMS

Maimonides Medical Center has 851 active physicians, including internationally renowned specialists. The hospital offers 24 residency programs in various areas, including anesthesiology, cardiology, dentistry, internal medicine, obstetrics and gynecology, orthopaedic surgery, pediatrics, psychiatry, radiology, surgery, urology, and various subspecialties of medicine and surgery. The hospital's resident staff is composed of 380 physicians.

CENTERS OF EXCELLENCE

Ambulatory Health Services: 30 primary care and specialty sites, including cardiac rehab program and women's healthcare at Brooklyn Women's Services

Brooklyn IVF: Comprehensive diagnostic testing and intervention, including hormone replacement therapy, laparoscopy, microsurgery, ovulation induction, in-vitro fertilization and other assisted reproductive techniques

The Cardiac Institute: World-renowned excellence in cardiac surgery (1,000+ procedures annually); pioneers many new angiographic techniques (e.g., atherectomy and percutaneous transmyocardial revascularization)

Infants and Children's Hospital: Pediatric subspecialty services, including adolescent medicine, allergy, behavioral psychology, cardiology, endocrinology, gastroenterology, genetics, hematology/oncology, infectious disease, neonatology, otolaryngology and surgery

Community Mental Health Center: Specialized programs targeted to specific groups, including FACES, an innovative teen theater network, and programs for ethnic communities

The Orthopaedic Institute: Complex procedures, e.g., limb-lengthening techniques, correction of congenital deformities, endoscopic spinal surgery, repair of traumatic sports injuries

Stella and Joseph Payson Birthing Center: Warm environment with life-saving technologies, 40 physicians and 10 midwives

Rehabilitation Medicine: Comprehensive services at three Brooklyn sites, including a new state-of-the-art center equipped with a full lap pool and advanced exercise equipment

The Vascular Institute: Comprehensive diagnostic and surgical services for treatment of vascular diseases

Weinberg Emergency Center: More than 80,000 cases annually; separate pediatric area provides emergency services for children from infants to teens

Massachusetts Eye and Ear Infirmary

A Teaching Affiliate of Harvard Medical School

243 Charles Street
Tel. 617.523.7900
617.573.4545 (TDD)
toll free 877.222.MEEI (6334)
www.meei.harvard.edu

Boston, MA 02114
Fax. 617.573.3091

Sponsorship: Voluntary, not-for-profit academic teaching hospital
Accreditation: Consistently receives perfect or high commendation scores from the Joint Commission on Accreditation of Healthcare Organizations (JCAHO). Fewer than 2% of all hospitals achieve these scores.
Affiliations: Primary teaching hospital of the Harvard Medical School in our specialties of eye, ear, nose, throat, head and neck care.

A LEADING ACADEMIC MEDICAL CENTER

Founded in 1824, the Massachusetts Eye and Ear Infirmary is home to the world's most accomplished researchers and clinicians, and attracts bright young physicians and scientists from across the globe to participate in its very effective partnership between basic science, clinical research, and patient care. Infirmary staff also provides services at many community centers and other hospitals in the region such as the Brigham and Women's Hospital and the Massachusetts General Hospital. Every full-time physician is a faculty member of the Harvard Medical School. The Chairmen of the Harvard Departments of Ophthalmology and Otology and Laryngology for all of the Harvard teaching hospitals are based at the Infirmary. The Infirmary's teaching programs are highly sought after by the best and brightest aspiring physicians.

GENERAL DESCRIPTION

Each year, the Infirmary treats hundreds of thousands of patients, from as near as downtown Boston to as far as Tokyo, Japan. From our specialty walk-in clinics and emergency room services, to our state-of-the-art operating rooms, patients receive the highest quality care. As a specialty hospital, the Infirmary provides the most highly trained nurses, radiologists and anesthesiologists. Our International Department services the needs of thousand of patients from other countries seeking medical assistance.

RESEARCH

The Infirmary has generated some of the most important advances in medical history, including the first successful treatment of Pannus (the patient, Annie Sullivan, went on to work with Helen Keller), the first applications of proton beam irradiation for malignant eye tumors, the first treatment for herpes simplex to prevent blindness, numerous prostheses and procedures for voice, sleep, and hearing disorders, and the first successful application of photodynamic therapy for age-related macular degeneration patients. Researchers at the Infirmary are beginning to unlock the mysteries of some of the most devastating diseases of the eye and ear: the blinding diseases, retinitis pigmentosa; and the bone disease, otosclerosis, a common cause of hearing loss.

MEDICAL STAFF

The Massachusetts Eye and Ear Infirmary has a medical staff of nearly 1,000 physicians, including experts recognized nationally and internationally for their excellence by their peers as well as by publications such as U.S. News and World Report, Boston Magazine, Town and Country, and "America's Best Doctors."

SERVICES AND CENTERS

Audiology, Cataract Consultation and General Eye, Cornea, Cranial Base, Electroretinography, Eye Emergency, Eye Oncology, Eye Plastics/Orbital Surgery, Facial and Cosmetic Surgery, Glaucoma, General Otolaryngology, Head and Neck Surgical Oncology, Hyperbaric Oxygen Therapy (HBO), Immunology/Uveitis, Laryngology and Voice Disorders, Laser Vision Correction/Refractive Surgery, Neuro-Ophthalmology, Optical Shop/Contact Lens, Otolaryngology (Ear, Nose, Throat) Walk-In Center, Otology, Pediatric Eye, Pediatric Otolaryngology, Retina, Rhinology/Sinus, Thyroid, Vision Rehabilitation, Voice and Speech.

Physician Referral: For eye-related referrals, contact 1-617-573-4199. For ear, nose, throat, head and neck related referrals, contact 1-617-573-3954. Referral numbers can also be requested by calling the Infirmary's toll free number, 1-877-222-MEEI (6334). For more information on our physicians, research, and services, please visit our website: www.meei.harvard.edu.

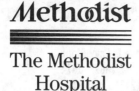

Methodist

The Methodist Hospital

6565 Fannin St.
Houston, TX 77030
Tel. 713.790.3333
www.methodisthealth.com

Beds: 1,269
Sponsorship/Network Affiliation: Private, Non-profit; Methodist Health Care System
Accreditation: Joint Commission on Accreditation of Healthcare Organizations (JCAHO)

GENERAL OVERVIEW

The Methodist Hospital is recognized as one of the country's leading hospitals, serving as the primary adult teaching facility for the distinguished Baylor College of Medicine. The Houston hospital has been recognized as a top center for cardiology, urology, orthopedics, geriatrics, gynecology, ophthalmology, otolaryngology, neurology/neurosurgery and rheumatology.

ACADEMIC & CLINICAL AFFILIATIONS

The Methodist Hospital is the flagship of Methodist Health Care System, which offers comprehensive services through community hospitals, a health plan and a home health care agency. Methodist has been affiliated with Baylor - a leading center for research and education - since 1950.

MEDICAL STAFF

The Methodist Hospital has more than 1,700 physicians on its medical staff, with many nationally recognized in their fields. For 50 years, The Methodist Hospital has been the home of heart pioneer Michael E. DeBakey, M.D.

CENTERS OF EXCELLENCE

The Methodist Hospital offers comprehensive heart care through the **Methodist DeBakey Heart Center**, from surgery to cardiac catherterization. Annually, our world-class physicians perform more than 2,500 angioplasties, 6,000 cardiac catheterizations, and 1,300 open-heart surgeries.

Neurosurgeons at Methodist were among the country's first to offer surgical treatments for Parkinson's disease and continue to be recognized for their expertise. Methodist neurology services have been ranked among the country's best by *U.S. News & World Report*. In 2000, neurology was ranked 15th.

The hospital's Urology Institute offers comprehensive treatment of urologic disorders with more than 30 board-certified physicians, leaders in their fields. Urology was ranked 13th in *U.S. News & World Report* this year.

INNOVATION

Methodist and Baylor's partnership has produced the Center for Cell and Gene Therapy and the Breast Care Center. These programs will revolutionize approaches to the treatment of many diseases.

Methodist also has a strong commitment to serving patients through information technology by being one of the first in the nation to offer online registration.

To reach physician referral, call 713-790-3333
or visit our website at www.methodisthealth.com

THE MOUNT SINAI HOSPITAL

MOUNT SINAI NYU
HEALTH

One Gustave L. Levy Place
New York, NY 10029-6574
Phone: (212) 241-6500
Physician Referral: (800) MD-SINAI (800-637-4624)
www.msnyuhealth.org

Sponsorship: Voluntary Not-for-Profit
Beds: 1,171
Accreditation: Joint Commission on Accreditation of Healthcare Organizations (JCAHO), Commission for Accreditation of Rehabilitation Facilites (CARF)

The Mount Sinai Hospital of is one of the country's oldest and largest hospitals. Since its founding in 1852, Mount Sinai has been the source of some of the most important advances in medical history. Today, that tradition of innovation continues as the hospital embraces its mission to provide superb patient care, conduct groundbreaking research, provide outstanding medical education, and service the neighboring community.

The Mount Sinai Hospital is one of the five world-class hospital centers that make up Mount Sinai NYU Health. The other member institutions include NYU Hospitals Center (Tisch Hospital and Rusk Institute of Rehabilitation Medicine), Hospital for Joint Diseases, NYU Downtown Hospital and The Mount Sinai Hospital of Queens.

Among the departments and services most frequently singled out for excellence are:

• The **Zena and Michael A. Wiener Cardiovascular Institute,** which offers the latest technologies and procedures for those at risk for heart disease and those with acute cardiac illnesses.

• The **Henry L. Schwartz Department of Geriatrics and Adult Development** which offers a full range of preventive care, inpatient, and outpatient services for older adults.

• The **Recanati/Miller Transplantation Institute of Mount Sinai** is renowned for transplantation surgery including combined organ transplantation. The Institute is recognized nationally as a leader in organ transplantation, with an emphasis on liver and combined organ transplantation.

• At the **Derald H. Ruttenberg Cancer Center,** pioneering scientists work assiduously to translate basic science findings into clinical applications.

• The **Samuel Bronfman Department of Medicine's Division of Grastroenterology** is heir to a great tradition in the field, dating back to the beginning of the 20th Century. Today, its physicians are equipped with latest knowledge to treat patients with inflammatory bowel disease, peptic ulcer disease, gastrointestinal cancer, and other diseases of the gastrointestinal tract.

Some of Mount Sinai's other special services include its Women's Health Program, a full range of inpatient and outpatient rehabilitation services, home care, and a growing number of minimally invasive surgical procedures. The Mount Sinai Hospital also offers special services for individuals with Alzheimer's disease, for women with high-risk pregnancies, and for children. Its affiliated hospitals and long-term-care facilities offer services throughout the New York/New Jersey metropolitan area.

Physician Referral (800) MD-SINAI - (800-637-4624) - The Mount Sinai Hospital provides a free Physician Referral and Health Resource Service from 8:30 a.m. to 6 p.m. weekdays. The service is offered to the public and gives access to over 10,000 physicians.

THE NEW YORK EYE & EAR INFIRMARY

310 East Fourteenth St.   *New York, New York 10003*
Tel.: 212.979.4000   *Fax.: 212.228.0664*
Web: www.nyee.edu

NY Eye & Ear Infirmary

Continuum Health Partners, Inc.

Sponsorship: Voluntary Not-for-Profit
Beds: 103
Accreditation: Joint Commission on Accreditation of Healthcare Organizations, College of American Pathologists

ABOUT THE NEW YORK EYE AND EAR INFIRMARY

The New York Eye and Ear Infirmary is one of the world's leading facilities for the diagnosis and treatment of diseases of the eyes, ears, nose, throat and related conditions. A voluntary, not-for-profit institution, the Infirmary is an affiliated teaching hospital of New York Medical College and a member of Continuum Health Partners.

THE MEDICAL STAFF

The Medical Staff includes more than 500 attending physicians and surgeons throughout the metropolitan area. Many are renowned for their breakthrough research introducing widely practiced techniques.

RESEARCH AND EDUCATION

The New York Eye and Ear Infirmary is a national and international leader in research in its specialties, achieving many "firsts" in successful procedures and medical treatments. Laboratories include Cell Culture, Temporal Bone and the Aborn Center for Eye Research.

SPECIALTIES

Ophthalmology: Within this area are subspecialties of cataract, glaucoma, retina, cornea and refractive surgery, ocular plastic surgery, pediatric ophthalmology and strabismus, neuro-ophthalmology and ocular tumor. Laser, photography, fluorescein angiography and electro-physiological testing are among the most advanced services available anywhere.

Otolaryngology: The department is in the forefront of treatment modalities using highly sophisticated endoscopic and laser equipment, Subspecialties include allergy, voice, rhinology, head & neck surgery, otology, neurotology, pediatric otolaryngology, audiology, speech therapy and hearing aid dispensing.

Plastic & Reconstructive Surgery: Microsurgical capabilities and premium patient accommodations provide an optimum environment for facial plasty, liposuction and repair of defects from disease or trauma.

RELATED SERVICES

New York Eye Trauma Center: An advanced program for emergency treatment of eye injuries, it handles a significant percentage of all cases reported to the National Eye Trauma Center.

Vision Correction Center: State-of-the-art facility dedicated to all forms of laser refractive surgery performed in an academic medical center in the forefront of teaching and research in vision correction.

Ambulatory Surgery: A comprehensive Ambulatory Surgery Center is designed to expedite admission testing, pre-op preparation and post-op recovery in an efficient and comfortable setting.

Pediatric Specialty Care: The city's only such center coordinating the services of eye and ear, nose and throat specialists with other staff especially sensitive to the youngest patients.

Physician Referral: Call 1-800-449-HOPE (4673)

NewYork-Presbyterian

THE UNIVERSITY HOSPITALS OF COLUMBIA AND CORNELL

NewYork Weill Cornell Medical Center   *Columbia Presbyterian Medical Center*
525 East 68th Street   *622 West 168th Street*
New York, NY 10021   *New York, NY 10032*

Sponsorship: Voluntary Not-for-Profit
Beds: 2,369
Accreditation: Joint Commission on Accreditation of Healthcare Organizations (JCAHO), Commission on Accreditation of Rehabilitation Facilities (CARF) and College of American Pathologists (CAP)

The U.S. News & World Report has ranked NewYork-Presbyterian higher in more specialties than any other hospital in the New York area.

OVERVIEW:

NewYork-Presbyterian Hospital — created from the merger of The New York Hospital and The Presbyterian Hospital — is the largest hospital in New York and one of the most comprehensive health-care institutions in the world with 5,500 physicians, approximately 92,000 discharges, over 856,4000 outpatient visits annually, and with its affiliated medical schools, more than $293 million in research support. The Hospital's world-class medical staff provides state-of-the-art diagnosis and treatment in all areas of medicine—including preventive and primary care—and in all specialties and subspecialties. The Hospital also offers inpatient and outpatient services at the Allen Pavilion in northern Manhattan and inpatient and outpatient psychiatric services at the Westchester Division, one of the nation's top ranked and the region's largest psychiatric facility.

AMONG ITS RENOWNED CENTERS OF EXCELLENCE ARE:

Columbia Weill Cornell Cancer Centers — offering coordinated, multidisciplinary care and the latest therapeutic options and clinical trials available for all types of cancer.

Columbia Weill Cornell Heart Institute — providing expert diagnostic capabilities and medical and surgical innovations for simple to complex heart conditions.

Columbia Weill Cornell Neuroscience Centers — the latest research, diagnosis and treatment capabilities in Alzheimer's disease, multiple sclerosis, Parkinson's disease, aneurysms, brain tumors, strokes and other neurological disorders.

Columbia Weill Cornell Transplant Institute — pioneering life-saving surgical techniques for adult and pediatric heart, heart/lung, liver, and kidney transplantation and researching new medications to enhance quality of life following a transplant or following transplantation.

Pediatric Cardiovascular Center — outstanding cardiology, interventional cardiology and cardiac surgery care for children with heart disease.

Randolph Hearst Burn Center — the largest and busiest burn center in the nation which also conducts research to improve survival and enhance quality of life for burn victims.

Children's Hospital of New York — one of the largest, most comprehensive children's hospitals in the world providing highly sophisticated pediatric medical, surgical and intensive care in a compassionate environment.

Trauma Center — Level 1 designations as an Adult Trauma Unit and a Pediatric Trauma Unit ensure the Hospital upholds the highest standards of 24-hour preparedness and treatment.

In addition, the Hospital offers extraordinary expertise, comprehensive programs and specialized resources in the fields of: *AIDS, Complementary Medicine, Gene Therapy, Psychiatry and Behavioral Health, Reproductive Medicine and Infertility, Women's Health Care.*

ACADEMIC AFFILIATIONS:

As a leading academic medical center, NewYork-Presbyterian Hospital is the only hospital in the world affiliated with two Ivy League medical schools: the Joan and Sanford I. Weill Medical College of Cornell University and the Columbia University College of Physicians & Surgeons. Physicians with the Hospital serve as faculty for their affiliated medical school, sharing a commitment to quality patient care, biomedical research, medical education and community service.

Physician Referral: To find a NewYork-Presbyterian Hospital affiliated physician to meet your needs, call toll free 1-877-NYP-WELL (1-877-697-9355) or visit our Web site at www.nyp.org.

NYU HOSPITALS CENTER
Tisch Hospital & Rusk Institute of Rehabilitation Medicine

550 First Avenue (at 31st Street)
New York, NY 10016
Physician Referral: (888) 7-NYU-MED (888-769-8633)
www.msnyuhealth.org

MOUNT SINAI NYU
HEALTH

Sponsorship: Private, Not-for-Profit
Beds: 878 beds
Accreditation: Joint Commission on Accreditation of Healthcare Organizations (JCAHO)
Commission for Accreditation of Rehabilitation Facilities (CARF)

NYU Hospitals Center is one of the nation's leading biomedical resources, combining excellence in patient care, research and medical education. NYU Hospitals Center includes **Tisch Hospital,** a voluntary 704-bed tertiary care facility serving more than 28,000 inpatients and 172,000 outpatients annually, and **Rusk Institute of Rehabilitation Medicine,** which has 174 beds and serves nearly 3,000 inpatients and more than 50,000 outpatients annually.

SPECIAL PROGRAMS AT TISCH HOSPITAL

Cancer — One of the country's elite NCI-designated comprehensive cancer centers

Cardiac Surgery — A leader in minimally invasive techniques and robotic procedures

Cardiology — A full range of diagnostic, prognostic and treatment sevices for patients of all ages

Epilepsy — The largest facility of its kind on the East Coast

Gamma Knife — Non-surgical presicion treatment for many neurological disorders

Pain Management — Specialties: acute cancer and chronic pain management services

Plastic Surgery — The largest facility of its kind in the world

Pregnancy (High-Risk) — Unparalleled diagnostic techniques and surgical innovations for those with trouble conceiving or with special risks

Skin Diseases — Renowned for treating serious and rare skin disorders

Surgery — Leading the nation in advancement of minimally invasive procedures and surgical techniques.

Transplant — Some of the nation's best patient and graft survival statistics

Urology — Leaders in treating prostate disorders and other urological problems

RUSK INSTITUTE OF REHABILITATION MEDICINE
The world's first and still one of the largest university centers for adult and pediatric rehabilitation.

Physician Referral (888) 7-NYU-MED - (888-769-8633) - **NYU Hospitals Center provides a free telephone referral service from 9 a.m. to 5 p.m. weekdays. The service is offered to the public and gives access to nearly 4,000 NYU physicians.**

RUSH-PRESBYTERIAN-ST. LUKE'S MEDICAL CENTER

1653 W. CONGRESS PARKWAY   CHICAGO, IL 60612
Tel. 312.942.5000   *www.rush.edu*

Beds: 963
Sponsorship/Network Affiliation: Rush-Presbyterian St.-Luke's Medical Center, the heart of the Rush System for Health, is a private, not-for-profit organization.

GENERAL OVERVIEW

For more than 160 years, Rush-Presbyterian-St. Luke's Medical Center has been recognized as a leader in patient care, teaching and research. Located minutes from downtown Chicago on the city's near West Side, Rush is the largest private hospital in Illinois and home of one of the first medical centers in the Midwest. This medical academic center includes the 809-bed Presbyterian-St. Luke's Hospital (including Rush Children's Hospital) and the 154-bed Johnston R. Bowman Health Center for the Elderly as well as Rush University. Its seven Rush institutes draw together patient care and research to address major health problems and offer primary health care services as well as latest treatments for arthritis and orthopedic problems, cancer, heart disease, mental illness, diseases associated with aging and neurological problems.

ACADEMIC & CLINICAL AFFILIATIONS

Integral to the Medical Center is Rush University, which includes Rush Medical College, the College of Nursing, the College of Health Sciences, the Graduate College and a cooperative educational network of 14 liberal arts colleges and universities in six states from Tennessee to Colorado. Rush-Presbyterian-St. Luke's Medical Center is the hub of one of the largest health care networks in the Chicago area, which encompasses five affiliated hospitals in Illinois and a wide range of health services, including alternative health care, hospice services, behavioral health and home health care. These hospitals include, Oak Park Hospital, Riverside HealthCare in Kankakee, Rush-Copley Medical Center in Aurora and Rush North Shore Medical Center in Skokie.

MEDICAL STAFF

Rush-Presbyterian-St. Luke's has 1,241 physicians who represent virtually all medical specialties and sub-specialties. Many of Rush's physicians are also leaders in research, pioneering innovative treatments and improving patient care. The Medical Center's multidisciplinary approach has allowed the development of integrated therapies for patients with diseases such as multiple sclerosis, rheumatoid arthritis and Alzheimer's disease.

COMPREHENSIVE CARE

Rush-Presbyterian-St. Luke's, a major referral center, provides care from the most basic to the most advanced for patients from metropolitan Chicago and across the country. The Medical Center includes seven institutes—comprehensive, multidisciplinary centers that offer primary health care services along with leading-edge diagnostic techniques and treatments for a variety of problems, including arthritis and orthopedic problems, heart disease, mental illness, diseases associated with aging and neurological disorders.

PIONEERING RESEARCH

As one of the largest centers for basic and clinical research in the Midwest, Rush is involved in more than 2,000 investigations of promising technologies and therapies aimed at achieving a better understanding of disease, and in fiscal year 2000 Rush researchers received $63.5 million in outside funding. By rapidly transferring knowledge from the laboratory to the bedside, Rush is continually helping patients at Rush and across the country.

ACCREDITATION, COMMENDATIONS & NATIONAL RECOGNITION

Rush-Presbyterian-St. Luke's Medical Center is accredited by the Joint Commission on Accreditation of Healthcare Organizations, the Commission for Accreditation of Rehabilitation Facilities, the Liaison Committee on Medical Education and numerous other organizations. In 2000, *U.S. News & World Report* ranked Rush in the top 50 in 11 medical specialties and tops in heart care in Chicago.

Rush-Presbyterian-St. Luke's Medical Center—Where world-class medicine revolves around you. www.rush.edu

ST. FRANCIS HOSPITAL
THE HEART CENTER®

100 PORT WASHINGTON BLVD. ROSLYN, NEW YORK 11576
Tel. 516. 562.6000 Fax. 516.562.6909
www.stfrancisheartcenter.com

Beds: 279
Sponsorship/Network Affiliation: A voluntary not-for-profit organization, St. Francis Hospital is a Member of Catholic Health Services of Long Island.

OVERVIEW

St. Francis Hospital, The Heart Center is New York State's only specialty designated cardiac center and has the highest cardiac caseload in the Northeast. Founded in 1922 by the Sisters of the Franciscan Missionaries of Mary, St. Francis Hospital is recognized as an innovator in delivering specialized cardiac services in a cost-efficient and caring environment. More than 95% of patients report that the Hospital met or exceeded their expectations; over 99% would recommend it to a friend.

EXPERIENCED IN CARDIAC CARE AND SURGERY

Open Heart Surgery: Performed 2,589 open heart surgeries in 1999; only New York hospital with a risk-adjusted mortality rate significantly below the statewide average for coronary bypass surgery, for all three-year periods analyzed by the NY State Department of Health. (1989-1997).

Cardiac Catheterization: Site of 9,342 diagnostic catheterizations and 2,990 coronary angioplasties in 1999 (mortality rate for angioplasty is less than half the statewide average.)

Arrhythmia & Pacemakers: Largest pacemaker and arrhythmia program in the United States; Expertise in radiofrequency ablation.

Minimally Invasive Surgery: Leading center experienced in the Port-Access™ device for coronary bypass and valve surgery. Alternative methods include off-pump bypass surgery and catheter-based treatments for congenital heart defects.

RESEARCH & TECHNOLOGY

Cardiac Research Institute offers leading edge technology and medications, including electron beam computed tomography, 3-D echocardiography, MRI and nuclear studies.

INTERNATIONAL PATIENTS

Located 17 miles from JFK International Airport, on Long Island, works with organizations such as the Knights of Malta and Rotary International's Gift of Life program to offer cardiac treatment to individuals from around the world.

ACCREDITATION AND AFFILIATION

Awarded *Accreditation With Commendation* from the Joint Commission on Accreditation of Healthcare Organizations for the third consecutive, three-year period. Received Consumer Choice Award for Heart Care Service (National Research Corporation, 1999). A teaching affiliate of the Columbia University College of Physicians and Surgeons and New York-Presbyterian Hospital.

St. Francis Hospital, The Heart Center
The Experience Matters

ST. LUKE'S EPISCOPAL HOSPITAL

ST. LUKE'S®
EPISCOPAL
HEALTH
SYSTEM

6720 Bertner Ave. Houston, TX 77030
Tel. 713.791.4343 www.stlukestexas.com

Beds: 949
St. Luke's Episcopal Hospital is a faith-based, non-profit hospital located in the heart of the Texas Medical Center.

ST. LUKE'S MISSION

Guided by the faith and support of the Episcopal Diocese of Texas and the Houston community, St. Luke's opened in 1954 with a promise to provide the type of care that would enhance the quality of its patients' lives. With this promise came a vision to advance the medical profession through education. The hospital's collaborative research and education efforts with the Texas Heart Institute®, established in 1962, have led to innovations in patient care and international recognition for advances in cardiovascular medicine and technology. For ten years in a row, *U.S.News & World Report* has ranked the Texas Heart Institute at St. Luke's as one of the nation's top ten centers for cardiology and heart surgery - and #1 in the Southwest.

PROVIDING SPECIALTY CARE

One of the nation's premiere teaching and research hospitals, St. Luke's cares for more than 32,000 adult inpatients, 188,000 outpatients, 2,500 newborns, and 2,000 home health patients each year. St. Luke's also has a network of 1,800 community-based physicians and world-renowned specialists. But numbers alone do not tell the full story of St. Luke's unique commitment to patient care. As a faith-based, non-profit hospital, St. Luke's believes that true healing involves the body, mind and spirit.

PIONEERING, COMPREHENSIVE MEDICAL CARE

Pioneering research programs at the Texas Heart Institute have consistently proven there is high-tech hope for the limitations and defects of the human body. Invaluable heart-assist devices and artificial grafts and valves have been developed and tested at the Texas Heart Institute. New drug treatments and diagnostic and surgical techniques are being refined daily as well. Following in the spirit of its invaluable relationship with the Texas Heart Institute, St. Luke's recently founded the St. Luke's Texas Liver Institute℠ and the St. Luke's Texas Cancer Institute®. St. Luke's also boasts experienced, world-class specialists in orthopaedics, urology, high-risk obstetrics, radiology, ophthalmology, internal medicine, neuroscience, otolaryngology, pathology and general surgery.

DOING WELL BY DOING GOOD

St. Luke's Episcopal Health System founded St. Luke's Episcopal Health Charities in 1997 by creating a foundation endowed with $150 million. St. Luke's Episcopal Health Charities is the seventh largest charity in Houston in annual distribution of funds and the largest focused on health care.

CONTACTING ST. LUKE'S EPISCOPAL HOSPITAL

To obtain information about our physicians, wellness programs, executive physicals or other health services, call St. Luke's Health Resource Line at (713) 791-4343 or (800) 872-9355 or visit our Web site at www.stlukestexas.com.

SHANDS AT THE UNIVERSITY OF FLORIDA

1600 SW Archer Road *Gainesville, FL 32610*
Tel. 352.265.0111 *Physician-to-physician referral: 800.633.2122*
Patient referral to access our services: 800.749.7424 *shands.org*

Sponsorship: Not-for-profit teaching hospital affiliated with the University of Florida
Accreditation: Joint Commission on Accreditation of HealthCare Organizations

HISTORY

Shands at the University of Florida (UF) was established in 1958 and named in honor of State Sen. William A. Shands, who was instrumental in promoting the legislation to complete funding for Florida's first teaching hospital, affiliated with the state's first medical college at UF.

Despite being one of the youngest academic health systems in the country, its youth has not kept Shands at UF from becoming one of the most prominent and well-respected institutions of learning and healing in the nation.

A COMPREHENSIVE HEALTHCARE RESOURCE FOR THE SOUTHEAST

Shands at UF is the nationally recognized medical center within the Shands HealthCare system of hospitals and affiliated physician practices located throughout north Florida. The 570-bed private, not-for-profit facility is one of the most comprehensive hospitals in the Southeast, offering highly specialized complex medical care. At the heart of Shands at UF are four centers of excellence -- in cardiovascular services, neurological services, cancer care and transplantation -- as well as Shands Children's Hospital, nationally recognized for its innovative and family-friendly environmental design. It also offers the Shands Arts In Medicine program, one of the most comprehensive hospital-based arts programs in the nation.

As the academic health center's leading teaching hospital, Shands at UF provides exclusive support to the six colleges of the UF Health Science Center: dentistry, health professions, medicine, nursing, pharmacy and veterinary medicine.

WORLD-CLASS MEDICAL STAFF

More than 500 University of Florida faculty physicians representing 110 medical specialties work with teams of highly skilled nurses and health professionals to provide quality care for our patients. These multidisciplinary teams have pioneered numerous "firsts" for Shands at UF. Accomplishments include:
- Florida's first adult liver transplant (1986)
- Florida's first radiosurgery procedure (1988)
- Florida's first neonatal/infant heart transplant (1993)
- Florida's first adult (1994) and pediatric lung transplant (1996)
- North Florida's first pancreas transplant (1995)
- World's fifth, nation's third and Southeast's first placenta-umbilical cord blood bank (1995)
- Florida's first pediatric (1995) and adult (1996) umbilical cord blood transplants for treatment of rare blood diseases including cancer
- United States' second and Southeast's first gene therapy for cystic fibrosis (1996)
- United States' first embryonic tissue transplant for spinal-cord repair (1997)
- The Southeast's first live-donor hand-assisted laparoscopic donor nephrectomy - minimally invasive kidney removal for transplantation (1998)
- United States' first minimally invasive hemodynamic monitoring procedure (1999)
- Southeast's first ethanol non-surgical septal reduction for hypertrophic obstructive cardiomyopathy (2000)

PHYSICIAN REFERRAL: The Shands Consultation Center is your link to more than 500 UF physicians and the programs and services offered by Shands HealthCare.
For more information or to schedule an appointment, please call our toll-free number 800.749.7424 or visit us on the Web at shands.org

THE UNIVERSITY OF CHICAGO HOSPITALS

5841 S. Maryland Avenue • For general information: 1-888-UCH-0200
Chicago, IL 60637-1470 • Web address: www.uchospitals.edu

Beds: 890
Sponsorship: Private. Not-for profit
Accreditation: Joint Commission on Accreditaiton of Healthcare Organizations

AT THE FOREFRONT OF MEDICINE ™

We have been at the forefront of medicine for decades -- delivering extraordinary care to patients who come from the Chicago area, as well as from all parts of the world. According to *U.S. News & World Report*'s ranking of America's best hospitals, the University of Chicago Hospitals rank 14th in the nation and first in Illinois. We were named among the best in the country and best in Illinois in eight specialty areas: cancer, endocrinology, gastroenterology, geriatrics, nephrology, neurology/neurosurgery, otolaryngology, and pulmonary medicine.

Our mission is to provide superior health care in a compassionate manner, ever mindful of each patient's dignity and individuality. To accomplish our mission, we call upon the skills and expertise of all our medical professionals, who work together to advance biomedical innovation, serve the health needs of the community, and further the knowledge of medical students, physicians, and others dedicated to caring.

WORLD-RENOWNED UNIVERSITY OF CHICAGO PHYSICIANS

All patients are encouraged to establish an ongoing relationship with a personal University of Chicago physician. Should the need arise, this physician will collaborate with or refer to any one of over 400 U of C board-certified specialists, many of whom are world leaders in their areas of expertise. Our faculty physicians see patients at the main Hospitals' campus, as well as at several other locations in the Chicago area. At the main campus, adult inpatient care is provided at Bernard Mitchell Hospital and Chicago Lying-in Hospital.

THE CENTER FOR ADVANCED MEDICINE

The Duchossois Center for Advanced Medicine is home to nearly all specialty clinics of the University of Chicago physicians, along with an unparalleled range of outpatient diagnostic and treatment services. The Center for Advanced Medicine is designed with the patient's best interests in mind. Physician offices are conveniently located next to related diagnostic and treatment suites, enabling patients to receive care for all related medical conditions within the same area of the building.

At the Center, patients have access to significant advances in medical treatment. Our physicians bring to its outpatient setting all of the knowledge and resources of the University of Chicago: virtually every clinical trial available and more research funded by the National Institutes of Health than any other place in the state.

THE UNIVERSITY OF CHICAGO CHILDREN'S HOSPITAL

Staffed by more than 100 faculty physicians, the University of Chicago Children's Hospital is dedicated to helping children with medical problems ranging from the routine to the complex. Our pediatricians provide advanced therapies in virtually all clinical areas. Critically ill or injured children are cared for in the state-of-the-art Frankel Pediatric Intensive Care Unit. In addition, a 53-bassinet neonatal intensive medical care and life support systems. The pediatric liver transplantation program is one of the largest in the country and was the first living-donor program in the world. The University of Chicago Children's Hospital offers every available form of therapy, both conventional and investigational, for a child afflicted with cancer.

WEISS MEMORIAL HOSPITAL AND OTHER OFF-CAMPUS LOCATIONS

Off-campus, care is provided at Louis A. Weiss Memorial Hospital, a 225-bed hospital on Chicago's North Side, and through a network of more than 25 physician offices located throughout Chicago, Chicago's suburbs, and northwest Indiana.

**Call 1-888-UCH-0200 for help in choosing a physician suitable to your needs.
Visit our website: www.uchospitals.edu.**

Washington Hospital Center

MedStar Health

WASHINGTON HOSPITAL CENTER

110 Irving St. NW Washington, D.C. 20010
Phone: 202-877-7000 (main)
Physician Referral: 202-877-DOCS (3627)
Website: www.WHCenter.org

Sponsorship: Private, not for profit • **Beds**: 907 • **Accreditation**: Joint Commission on Accreditation of Healthcare Organizations, member American Hospital Association, Council of Teaching Hospitals, a division of the Association of American Medical Colleges.

EXPERIENCE IS THE DIFFERENCE

Washington Hospital Center is a 907-bed, acute care teaching and research hospital based in Northwest Washington, D.C. It is the largest private non-profit hospital in the nation's capital and has the thirteenth highest patient volume in the United States. The Hospital Center is home to the nation's third largest cardiac program. It also has a comprehensive Cancer Institute; a full range of women's services; an extensive organ transplantation program; one of the nation's top shock/trauma centers; and the most advanced burn facility in the region. Washington Hospital Center is one of the nation's top 100 hospitals according to HCIA and is listed by *US News & World Report* as one of the best hospitals for heart services, hormonal disorders, neurology and neurorsurgery and kidney disorders.

WORLD CLASS CARDIOVASCULAR SERVICES

Our internationally recognized cardiovascular program, Washington Heart, is ranked as third-largest in the United States by *US News & World Report*. Our world-class facilities are equipped with some of the most advanced technology housed in dedicated diagnostic, EP, cardiac cath, peripheral vascular and cardiac OR facilities. Our internationally respected team works collaboratively across a number of specialties to care for some of the most complex cases to provide patients with the best outcomes. Nearly 15,700 cardiac catheterization procedures and 2,800 open heart procedures were performed last year, including more "off pump" open heart procedures than any other facility. All this experience means a quicker recovery for our patients and faster return to normal living. Call **202-877-3627** to obtain a free video brochure about our cardiovascular program.

THE PAVILION

Modeled after the world's best luxury hotels, this private wing is available to meet the needs of the most discriminating patient. Each private room includes a kitchenette; guest accommodations, 24-hour private chef services, heated towel racks and high tea served every afternoon. Call 202-877-7174 for more information or reservations.

INTERNATIONAL SERVICES

Our international services department serves a variety of needs including translation, scheduling and escorting guests to physician appointments and working with private security or international groups or delegations. Call 202-877-2100 or e-mail worldmed@mhg.edu for a private tour or more information.

TO MAKE AN APPOINTMENT WITH A TOP DOCTOR

Washington Hospital Center's physician referral service, DOCtorsLine, offers a convenient and fast way to make an appointment with over 1,500 physicians throughout the area. This free service can help find a top specialist based on education, office location or insurance coverage. And, most appointments are made within 48 hours of your call.
Call **202-877-DOCS (3627)**.

THE TRAINING OF A SPECIALIST

Excerpted from "**Which Medical Specialist For You?**"
American Board of Medical Specialties, Evanston, IL, Revised 2000

Everyone knows that a "medical doctor" is a physician who has had years of training to understand the diagnosis, treatment and prevention of disease. The basic training for a physician specialist includes four years of premedical education in a college or university, four years of medical school, and after receiving the M.D. degree, at least three years of specialty training under supervision (called a "residency"). Training in subspecialties can take an additional one to three years.

Some specialists are primary care doctors such as family physicians, general internists and general pediatricians. Other specialists concentrate on certain body systems, specific age groups, or complex scientific techniques developed to diagnose or treat certain types of disorders. Specialties in medicine developed because of the rapidly expanding body of knowledge about health and illness and the constantly evolving new treatment techniques for disease.

A subspecialist is a physician who has completed training in a general medical specialty and then takes additional training in a more specific area of that specialty called a subspecialty. This training increases the depth of knowledge and expertise of the specialist in that particular field. For example, cardiology is a subspecialty of internal medicine and pediatrics, pediatric surgery is a subspecialty of surgery and child and adolescent psychiatry is a subspecialty of psychiatry. The training of a subspecialist within a specialty requires an additional one or more years of full-time education.

The training, or residency, of a specialist begins after the doctor has received the M.D. degree from a medical school. Resident physicians dedicate themselves for three to seven years to full-time experience in hospital and/or ambulatory care settings, caring for patients under the supervision of experienced specialists. Educational conferences and research experience are often part of that training. In years past, the first year of post-medical school training was called an internship, but is now called residency.

Licensure

The legal privilege to practice medicine is governed by state law and is not designed to recognize the knowledge and skills of a trained specialist. A physician is licensed to practice general medicine and surgery by a state board of medical examiners after passing a state or national licensure examination. Each state or territory has its own procedures to license physicians and sets the general standards for all physicians in that state or territory.

Who credentials a specialist and/or subspecialist?

Specialty boards certify physicians as having met certain published standards. There are 24 specialty boards that are recognized by the American Board of Medical Specialties (ABMS) and the American Medical Association (AMA). All of the specialties and subspecialties recognized by the ABMS and the AMA are listed in the brief descriptions that follow. Remember, *a subspecialist first must be trained and certified as a specialist.*

In order to be certified as a medical specialist by one of these recognized boards a physician must complete certain requirements. Generally, these include:
(1) Completion of a course of study leading to the M.D. or D.O. (Doctor of Osteopathy) degree from a recognized school of medicine.

(2) Completion of three to seven years of full-time training in an accredited residency program designed to train specialists in the field.

(3) Many specialty boards require assessments and documentation of individual performance from the residency training director, or from the chief of service in the hospital where the specialist has practiced.

(4) All of the ABMS Member Boards require that a person seeking certification have an unrestricted license to practice medicine in order to take the certification examination.

(5) Finally, each candidate for certification must pass a written examination given by the specialty board. Fifteen of the 24 specialty boards also require an oral examination conducted by senior specialists in that field. Candidates who have passed the exams and other requirements are then given the status of "Diplomate" and are certified as specialists. A similar process is followed for specialists who want to become subspecialists.

All of the ABMS Member Boards now, or will soon, issue only time-limited certificates which are valid for six to ten years. In order to retain certification, diplomates must become "recertified," and must periodically go through an additional process involving continuing education in the specialty, review of credentials and further examination. Boards that may not yet require recertification have provided voluntary recertification with similar requirements.

How to determine if a physician is a certified specialist

Certified specialists are listed in *The Official ABMS Directory of Board Certified Medical Specialists* published by Marquis Who's Who. The *ABMS Directory* can be found in most public libraries, hospital libraries, university libraries and medical libraries, and is also available on CD-ROM. Alternatively, you could ask for that information from your county medical society, the American Board of Medical Specialties, or one of the specialty boards.

The ABMS operates an 800 phone line (1-800-776-2378) to verify the certification status of individual physicians. Additionally, information about the ABMS organization and links to an electronic directory of certified specialists can be accessed through the ABMS Web site at www.abms.org.

Almost all board certified specialists also are members of their medical specialty societies. These societies are dedicated to furthering standards, practice and professional and public education within individual medical specialties. Some, such as the American College of Surgeons and the American College of Obstetricians and Gynecologists, require board certification for full membership. A physician who has attained full membership is called a "Fellow" of the society and is entitled to use this designation in all formal communications such as certificates, publications, business cards, stationery and signage. Thus, "John Doe, M.D., F.A.C.S. (Fellow of the American College of Surgeons) is a board certified surgeon. Similarly, F.A.A.D. (Fellow of the American Academy of Dermatology) following the M.D. or D.O. in a physician's title would likely indicate board certification in that specialty.

PREFACE TO MEDICAL SPECIALTIES

In the pages that follow, each list of doctors in a medical specialty or subspecialty is preceded by a brief description of that specialty (or subspecialty) and the training required for board certification.

A few specialties have not been included since they are specialties for which patients generally do not search beyond their local communities (e.g., Family Practice Medicine) or are specialties for which patients must depend on the expertise of their treating doctors for selection (e.g. Anesthesiology). In addition, Critical Care Medicine (and its subspecialties) has been excluded because in emergency situations there is neither time nor opportunity for choice.

Descriptions of those medical specialties and subspecialties that are not included in the main sections of the Guide may be found in Appendix A.

The following descriptions of medical specialties and subspecialties were provided by the American Board of Medical Specialties (ABMS), an organization comprised of the 24 medical specialty boards that provide certification in 25 medical specialties. A complete listing of all specialists certified by the ABMS can be found in *The Official ABMS Directory of Board Certified Medical Specialists*, published by Marquis Who's Who. It is available (either in a multi-volume directory or on CD-ROM) in most public libraries, hospital libraries, university libraries and medical libraries. The ABMS also operates a toll-free phone line at 1-800-776-2378 to verify the certification status of individual doctors.

The following important policy statement, approved by the ABMS Assembly on March 19, 1987, remains valid.

The Purpose of Certification:
The intent of the certification process, as defined by the member boards of the American Board of Medical Specialties, is to provide assurance to the public that a certified medical specialist has successfully completed an approved educational program and an evaluation, including an examination process designed to assess the knowledge, experience and skills requisite to the provision of high quality patient care in that specialty.

ADOLESCENT MEDICINE

(a subspecialty of either INTERNAL MEDICINE or PEDIATRICS)

An internist or pediatrician who specializes in adolescent medicine is a multi-disciplinary healthcare specialist trained in the unique physical, psychological and social characteristics of adolescents, their healthcare problems and needs.

INTERNAL MEDICINE

A personal physician who provides long-term, comprehensive care in the office and the hospital, managing both common and complex illness of adolescents, adults and the elderly. Internists are trained in the diagnosis and treatment of cancer, infections and diseases affecting the heart, blood, kidneys, joints and digestive, respiratory and vascular systems. They are also trained in the essentials of primary care internal medicine which incorporates an understanding of disease prevention, wellness, substance abuse, mental health and effective treatment of common problems of the eyes, ears, skin, nervous system and reproductive organs.

PEDIATRICS

A physician concerned with the physical, emotional and social health of children from birth to young adulthood. Care encompasses a broad spectrum of health services ranging from preventive healthcare to the diagnosis and treatment of acute and chronic diseases. A pediatrician deals with biological, social and environmental influences on the developing child, and with the impact of disease and dysfunction on development.

Training required: Three years in internal medicine *OR* three years in pediatrics *plus* additional training and examination for certification in adolescent medicine

PHYSICIAN LISTINGS

Adolescent Medicine

New England

Emans, Sarah Jean Herriot MD (Adolescent Medicine) - *Special Expertise:* Pediatric & Adolscent Gynecology; **Admitting Hospital:** Children's Hospital; **Office Address:** 300 Longwood Avenue Boston, MA 02115; **Office Phone:** (617) 355-5482; **Board Certifications:** Pediatrics 1975, Adolescent Medicine 1994; **Medical School:** Harvard Med Sch 1970; **Residency:** Children's Hospital, Boston, MA 1971-1973; **Fellowship:** Adolescent Medicine, Children's Hospital, Boston, MA 1973-1974; **Faculty Appointment:** Assoc Prof Pediatrics, Harvard Med Sch

Mid Atlantic

Diaz, Angela MD (Adolescent Medicine) - *Special Expertise:* Adolescent Medicine - General; **Admitting Hospital:** Mount Sinai Hospital (Page 70); **Office Address:** 312 E 94th St New York, NY 10128-5604; **Office Phone:** (212) 423-2900; **Board Certifications:** Pediatrics 1987, Adolescent Medicine 1994; **Medical School:** Columbia P&S 1981; **Residency:** Pediatrics, Mt Sinai Med Ctr, New York, NY 1981-1984; **Fellowship:** Adolescent Medicine, Mt Sinai Med Ctr, New York, NY 1984-1985; **Faculty Appointment:** Assoc Prof Pediatrics, Mount Sinai Sch Med

Schwarz, Donald F. MD (Adolescent Medicine) - *Special Expertise:* Adolescent Mothers; Adolescent Chronic Illness; **Admitting Hospital:** The Children's Hospital of Philadelphia; **Office Address:** Children's Hosp-Philadelphia, Main Bldg 34th St & Civic Ctr Blvd, Fl 9 Philadelphia, PA 19104-4399; **Office Phone:** (215) 590-1462; **Board Certifications:** Pediatrics 1987, Adolescent Medicine 1994; **Medical School:** Johns Hopkins Univ 1982; **Residency:** Pediatrics, Yale-New Haven Hospital, New Haven, CT 1983-1985; **Fellowship:** Adolescent Medicine, Chldn's Hosp, Philadelphia, PA 1985-1987; **Faculty Appointment:** Prof Pediatrics, Univ Penn

Southeast

Ford, Carol Ann MD (Adolescent Medicine) - *Special Expertise:* Adolescent Medicine - General; **Admitting Hospital:** University of North Carolina Hospitals; **Office Address:** UNC at Chapel Hill, Dept Ped Adol Med CB#7225, Wing C, Med School Chapel Hill, NC 27599-7225; **Office Phone:** (919) 966-2504; **Board Certifications:** Pediatrics 1989, Adolescent Medicine 1994; **Medical School:** Univ Fla Coll Med 1983; **Residencies:** Internal Medicine, Univ North Carolina Hosp, Chapel Hill, NC 1983-1987; Pediatrics, Univ North Carolina Hosp, Chapel Hill, NC 1983-1987; **Fellowship:** Adolescent Medicine, UC San Francisco Med Ctr, San Francisco, CA 1992-1995; **Faculty Appointment:** Asst Prof Pediatrics, Univ NC Sch Med

Midwest

Blum, Robert W MD/PhD (Adolescent Medicine) - *Special Expertise:* Adolescent Medicine - General; **Admitting Hospital:** Fairview Southdale Hospital; **Office Address:** Univ Minn, Adolescent Hlth Prgm 200 Oak St SE, Ste 260 Minneapolis, MN 55455; **Office Phone:** (612) 626-2820; **Board Certifications:** Pediatrics 1993, Adolescent Medicine 1994; **Medical School:** Howard Univ 1973; **Residency:** Pediatrics, Univ Minn, Minneapolis, MN 1974-1976; **Fellowship:** Adolescent Medicine, Univ Minn, Minneapolis, MN 1976-1978; **Faculty Appointment:** Assoc Prof Pediatrics, Univ Minn

Slap, Gail MD (Adolescent Medicine) - *Special Expertise:* Chronic Disease; **Admitting Hospital:** Children's Hospital Medical Center; **Office Address:** Children's Hosp Med Ctr, Div of Adolescent Med 3333 Burnet Ave, Bldg PAV Cincinnati, OH 45229-3039; **Office Phone:** (513) 636-8602; **Board Certifications:** Internal Medicine 1980, Adolescent Medicine 1994; **Medical School:** Univ Penn 1977; **Residency:** Internal Medicine, Univ Penn, Philadelphia, PA 1977-1980; **Fellowship:** Adolescent Medicine, Children's Hosp, Philadelphia, PA 1980-1982; **Faculty Appointment:** Prof Pediatrics, Univ Cincinnati

Great Plains and Mountains

Kaplan, David William MD (Adolescent Medicine) - *Special Expertise:* Eating Disorders; **Admitting Hospital:** The Children's Hospital - Denver; **Office Address:** Children's Hospital 1056 E 19th Ave, Ste B025 Denver, CO 80218-1007; **Office Phone:** (303) 861-6131; **Board Certifications:** Pediatrics 1975, Adolescent Medicine 1994; **Medical School:** Case West Res Univ 1970; **Residencies:** Pediatrics, Univ Colorado Med Ctr, Denver, CO 1970-1972; Pediatrics, Chldns Hosp Med Ctr, Boston, MA 1974-1975; **Fellowship:** Public Health & General Preventive Medicine, Harvard Sch Pub Hlth, Boston, MA 1975-1976; **Faculty Appointment:** Prof Pediatrics, Univ Colo

West Coast and Pacific

Anderson, Martin Mathew MD (Adolescent Medicine) - *Special Expertise:* Adolescent Medicine - General; **Admitting Hospital:** UCLA Medical Center; **Office Address:** UCLA Med Ctr, Dept Pediatrics 10833 Le Conte Ave Los Angeles, CA 90095; **Office Phone:** (310) 825-5803; **Board Certifications:** Pediatrics 1986, Adolescent Medicine 1994; **Medical School:** UC Davis 1980; **Residency:** Pediatrics, Mott Chldns Hosp, Ann Arbor, MI 1981-1983; **Fellowships:** Adolescent Medicine, UCSF, San Francisco, CA 1984-1986; Substance Abuse Training Program, UCLA Med Ctr, Los Angeles, CA 1993; **Faculty Appointment:** Assoc Prof Pediatrics, UCLA

Fuster, Carlos Daniel MD (Adolescent Medicine) - *Special Expertise:* Adolescent Medicine - General; **Admitting Hospital:** KPH Panorama City Medical Center; **Office Address:** Kaiser Permanente Panorama City Med Ctr, Dept Peds 13652 Cantara St Panorama City, CA 91402; **Office Phone:** (818) 375-2652; **Board Certifications:** Pediatrics 1986, Adolescent Medicine 1997; **Medical School:** Mount Sinai Sch Med 1980; **Residency:** Pediatrics, Children's Hosp, Los Angeles, CA 1981-1983; **Fellowship:** Adolescent Medicine, Children's Hosp, Los Angeles, CA 1983-1985

Irwin Jr, Charles Edwin MD (Adolescent Medicine) - *Special Expertise:* Adolescent Medicine - General; **Admitting Hospital:** University of California - San Francisco Medical Center; **Office Address:** 3333 California St, Ste 245 San Francisco, CA 94118; **Office Phone:** (415) 476-2184; **Board Certifications:** Pediatrics 1993, Adolescent Medicine 1994; **Medical School:** UCSF 1971; **Residency:** Pediatrics, UCSF, San Francisco, CA 1972-1974; **Fellowship:** Adolescent Medicine, UCSF, San Francisco, CA 1974-1977; **Faculty Appointment:** Prof Pediatrics, UCSF

Litt, Iris F MD (Adolescent Medicine) - *Special Expertise:* Adolescent Medicine - General; **Admitting Hospital:** Stanford Medical Center; **Office Address:** Stanford Univ, Div Adolescent Medicine 750 Welch Rd, Ste 325 Palo Alto, CA 94304; **Office Phone:** (415) 725-8293; **Board Certifications:** Pediatrics 1993, Adolescent Medicine 1994; **Medical School:** SUNY Downstate 1965; **Residency:** Pediatrics, NY Hosp, New York, NY 1966-1968; **Faculty Appointment:** Prof Pediatrics, Stanford Univ

MacKenzie, Richard G MD (Adolescent Medicine) - *Special Expertise:* Eating Disorders; **Admitting Hospital:** Children's Hospital - Los Angeles; **Office Address:** 5000 Sunset Blvd, Fl 4 Los Angeles, CA 90027; **Office Phone:** (323) 669-2112; **Medical School:** McGill Univ 1966; **Residency:** Internal Medicine, Royal Victoria Hosp, Montreal Canada 1966-1967; **Fellowship:** Adolescent Medicine, Childrens Hosp, Los Angeles, CA 1969-1970; **Faculty Appointment:** Assoc Prof Pediatrics, USC Sch Med

Morris, Robert Edward MD (Adolescent Medicine) - *Special Expertise:* Adolescent *Medicine - General;* **Admitting Hospital:** UCLA Medical Center; **Office Address:** Pediatric & Adolescent Medicine 200 UCLA Medical Plaza, Ste 265 Los Angeles, CA 90095; **Office Phone:** (310) 825-1844; **Board Certifications:** Pediatrics 1986, Adolescent Medicine 1997; **Medical School:** Temple Univ 1971; **Residencies:** Pediatrics, Univ Wash, Seattle, WA 1972-1974; Pediatric Gastroenterology, UCLA, Los Angeles, CA 1981-1982; **Faculty Appointment:** Prof Pediatrics, UCLA

ALLERGY & IMMUNOLOGY

An allergist-immunologist is trained in evaluation, physical and laboratory diagnosis and management of disorders involving the immune system. Selected examples of such conditions include asthma, anaphylaxis, rhinitis, eczema and adverse reactions to drugs, foods and insect stings as well as immune deficiency diseases (both acquired and congenital), defects in host defense and problems related to autoimmune disease, organ transplantation or malignancies of the immune system. As our understanding of the immune system develops, the scope of this specialty is widening.

Training programs are available at some medical centers to provide individuals with expertise in both allergy/immunology and adult rheumatology, or in both allergy/immunology and pediatric pulmonology. Such individuals are candidates for dual certification.

Training required: Two years in allergy/immunology OR prior certification in internal medicine or pediatrics *plus* additional training and examination.

PHYSICIAN LISTINGS

Allergy & Immunology

New England

MacLean, James Andrew MD (Allergy & Immunology) - *Special Expertise:* Asthma; Allergy; **Admitting Hospital:** Massachusetts General Hospital; **Office Address:** Mass Genl Hosp 55 Fruit St, Bldg Wang - rm 622 Boston, MA 02114; **Office Phone:** (617) 726-3850; **Board Certifications:** Internal Medicine 1988, Allergy & Immunology 1991; **Medical School:** McGill Univ 1985; **Residency:** Internal Medicine, Royal Victoria Hosp, Montreal, CN 1986-1989; **Fellowship:** Allergy & Immunology, Mass Genl Hosp, Boston, MA 1989-1991; **Faculty Appointment:** Clin Inst Allergy & Immunology, Harvard Med Sch

Wong, Johnson T MD (Allergy & Immunology) - *Special Expertise:* Asthma; Rhinitis; Sinus Disorders; **Admitting Hospital:** Massachusetts General Hospital; **Office Address:** Allergy & Asthma Assoc 5 Long Fellow Pl, Ste 201 Boston, MA 02114; **Office Phone:** (617) 726-3850; **Board Certifications:** Internal Medicine 1983, Allergy & Immunology 1985; **Medical School:** UCSF 1980; **Residency:** Internal Medicine, UCLA-Wadsworth VA Hosp, Los Angeles, CA 1981-1983; **Fellowship:** Allergy & Immunology, Mass Genl Hosp, Boston, MA 1983-1986; **Faculty Appointment:** Asst Prof Medicine, Harvard Med Sch

Mid Atlantic

Adkinson, Franklin MD (Allergy & Immunology) - *Special Expertise:* Drug Sensitivity; Asthma; **Admitting Hospital:** Johns Hopkins Hospital - Baltimore (Page 65); **Office Address:** 5501 Hopkins Bayview Circle Baltimore, MD 21224; **Office Phone:** (410) 550-2051; **Medical School:** Johns Hopkins Univ 1969; **Faculty Appointment:** Prof Medicine, Johns Hopkins Univ

Atkins, Paul Charles MD (Allergy & Immunology) - *Special Expertise:* Asthma; Sinus Disorders; **Admitting Hospital:** Hospital of the University of Pennsylvania; **Office Address:** Hosp Of Univ Penn, Dept A&I 3400 Spruce St, Fl 3 - Ste G Philadelphia, PA 19143; **Office Phone:** (215) 662-2425; **Board Certifications:** Internal Medicine 1974, Allergy & Immunology 1975; **Medical School:** NY Med Coll 1967; **Residency:** Internal Medicine, NY Med-Metro Hosp Ctr, New York, NY 1968-1970; **Fellowship:** Allergy & Immunology, Hosp Univ Penn, Philadelphia, PA 1970-1972; **Faculty Appointment:** Prof Univ Penn

Baraniuk, James N MD (Allergy & Immunology) - *Special Expertise:* Asthma and Sinusitis; Immune Deficiency; Neural Regulation of Mucosal Secretion; **Admitting Hospital:** Georgetown University Hospital; **Office Address:** GUMC-Lower Level, Gorman Building 3800 Reservoir Rd NW Washington, DC 20007; **Office Phone:** (202) 687-8233; **Board Certifications:** Internal Medicine 1984, Allergy & Immunology 1987; **Residencies:** Internal Medicine, St Thomas Hosp, Akron, OH 1982-1984; Internal Medicine, Duke Univ, Durham, NC 1984-1985; **Fellowships:** Allergy & Immunology, Duke Univ, Durham, NC 1987-1989; Allergy & Immunology, Natnl Heart Lung Instt, London England 1989-1991; **Faculty Appointment:** Asst Clin Prof Georgetown Univ

Buchbinder, Ellen MD (Allergy & Immunology) - *Special Expertise:* Asthma; **Admitting Hospital:** Mount Sinai Hospital (Page 70); **Office Address:** 111 E 88th St, Ste B New York, NY 10128; **Office Phone:** (212) 410-3246; **Board Certifications:** Internal Medicine 1981, Allergy & Immunology 1983; **Medical School:** Tulane Univ 1978; **Residency:** Internal Medicine, New England Deaconess Hosp, Boston, MA 1978-1981; **Fellowship:** Allergy & Immunology, Mass Genl Hosp, Boston, MA 1981-1983; **Faculty Appointment:** Asst Clin Prof Medicine, Mount Sinai Sch Med

Chandler, Michael MD (Allergy & Immunology) - *Special Expertise: Asthma;* **Admitting Hospital:** Mount Sinai Hospital (Page 70); **Office Address:** 115 E 61st St, Bldg Fl 12 New York, NY 10021-8101; **Office Phone:** (212) 486-6715; **Board Certifications:** Internal Medicine 1984, Allergy & Immunology 1987; **Medical School:** Wayne State Univ 1981; **Residency:** Internal Medicine, Northwestern, Chicago, IL 1981-1984; **Fellowship:** Allergy & Immunology, Northwestern, Chicago, IL 1984-1986; **Faculty Appointment:** Clin Inst Medicine, Mount Sinai Sch Med

Cunningham-Rundles, Charlotte MD/PhD (Allergy & Immunology) - *Special Expertise: Immune Deficiency;* **Admitting Hospital:** Mount Sinai Hospital (Page 70); **Office Address:** 5 E 98th St New York, NY 10029; **Office Phone:** (212) 659-9268; **Board Certification:** Internal Medicine 1972; **Medical School:** Columbia P&S 1969; **Residency:** Internal Medicine, Bellevue Hosp, New York, NY 1970-1972; **Fellowship:** Allergy & Immunology, NYU, New York, NY 1972-1974; **Faculty Appointment:** Prof Medicine, Mount Sinai Sch Med

Dattwyler, Raymond MD (Allergy & Immunology) - *Special Expertise: Lyme Disease;* **Admitting Hospital:** University Hospital & Medical Center at Stony Brook; **Office Address:** Hlth Sci Ctr Div A&I, Bldg Tower 16 - rm 040 Stony Brook, NY 11794-8161; **Office Phone:** (631) 444-3808; **Board Certifications:** Internal Medicine 1977, Allergy & Immunology 1979; **Medical School:** SUNY Buffalo 1973; **Residency:** Internal Medicine, Tufts-New England Med, Boston, MA 1976-1977; **Fellowships:** Immunology, Mayo Clinic, Rochester, MN 1974-1976; Clinical Immunology, Mass Genl Hosp-Harvard, Boston, MA 1977-1978; **Faculty Appointment:** Prof Medicine, SUNY Stony Brook

Levinson, Arnold MD (Allergy & Immunology) - *Special Expertise: Autoimmune Disease; Immune Deficiency; Allergy;* **Admitting Hospital:** Hospital of the University of Pennsylvania; **Office Address:** Hosp of Univ Penn, Div A&I 3400 Spruce St- 3 Silverstein, Ste B Philadelphia, PA 19104-4219; **Office Phone:** (215) 662-2425; **Board Certifications:** Internal Medicine 1972, Allergy & Immunology 1975; **Medical School:** Univ MD Sch Med 1969; **Residency:** Internal Medicine, Baltimore City Hosp, Baltimore, MD 1970-1971; **Fellowships:** Clinical Immunology, UCSF, San Francisco, PA 1972-1973; Clinical Immunology, Univ Penn, Philadelphia, PA 1973-1975; **Faculty Appointment:** Prof Medicine, Univ Penn

Macris, Nicholas T MD (Allergy & Immunology) - *Special Expertise: Asthma;* **Admitting Hospital:** Lenox Hill Hospital; **Office Address:** 1430 2nd Ave, Ste 102 New York, NY 10021; **Office Phone:** (212) 249-2940; **Board Certification:** Allergy & Immunology 1974; **Medical School:** SUNY Hlth Sci Ctr 1958; **Residency:** Internal Medicine, Lenox Hill Hosp, New York, NY 1961-1963; **Fellowship:** Allergy & Immunology, Rockefeller Univ, New York, NY 1963-1965; **Faculty Appointment:** Clin Prof Medicine, Cornell Univ-Weil Med Coll

Mazza, David S MD (Allergy & Immunology) - *Special Expertise: Asthma - Adult & Pediatric; Sinus Disorders;* **Admitting Hospital:** St Luke's - Roosevelt Hospital Center - Roosevelt Division (Page 58); **Office Address:** 7 Lexington Ave, Ste 3 New York, NY 10010-5517; **Office Phone:** (212) 677-7170; **Board Certifications:** Pediatrics 1983, Allergy & Immunology 1989; **Medical School:** Univ VT Coll Med 1977; **Residency:** Pediatrics, New York Univ, New York, NY 1977-1980; **Fellowships:** Pediatrics, Bellevue Hosp, New York, NY 1980-1982; Allergy & Immunology, St Luke's, New York, NY 1987-1989; **Faculty Appointment:** Assoc Prof Columbia P&S

Metcalfe, Dean D MD (Allergy & Immunology) - *Special Expertise: Mast Cell Diseases; Food Allergy;* **Admitting Hospital:** National Institutes of Health - Clinical Center; **Office Address:** Natl Inst Allergy and Inf Disease, Lab Allergic Dis 9000 Rockville Poke, Bldg 10 - rm 11C205 Bethesda, MD 20892-1881; **Office Phone:** (301) 496-2165; **Board Certifications:** Internal Medicine 1975, Allergy & Immunology 1977; **Medical School:** Univ Tenn Coll Med, Memphis 1972; **Residencies:** Internal Medicine, Mich Hosp, Ann Arbor, MI 1973-1974; Allergy & Immunology, Natl Inst Allergy & Infectious Dis-NIH, Bethesda, MD 1974-1977; **Fellowship:** Rheumatology, PB Brigham Hosp, Boston, MA 1977-1979

Reisman, Robert E MD (Allergy & Immunology) - *Special Expertise: Insect Sting Allergy;* **Admitting Hospital:** Buffalo General Hospital; **Office Address:** Buffalo Med Grp 295 Essjay Williamsville, NY 14221-8216; **Office Phone:** (716) 630-1130; **Board Certifications:** Internal Medicine 1969, Allergy & Immunology 1972; **Medical School:** SUNY Buffalo 1956; **Residency:** Internal Medicine, Buffalo Genl Hosp, Buffalo, NY 1957-1959; **Fellowship:** Allergy & Immunology, Buffalo Genl Hosp, Buffalo, NY 1959-1961; **Faculty Appointment:** Clin Prof Medicine, SUNY Buffalo

Shepherd, Gillian M MD (Allergy & Immunology) - *Special Expertise: Allergy & Immunology - General;* **Admitting Hospital:** New York Weill Cornell Medical Center - NY Presbyterian Hospital (Page 72); **Office Address:** 235 E 67th St, Ste 203 New York, NY 10021; **Office Phone:** (212) 288-9300; **Board Certifications:** Internal Medicine 1979, Allergy & Immunology 1981; **Medical School:** NY Med Coll 1976; **Residency:** Internal Medicine, Lenox Hill Hosp, New York, NY 1976-1979; **Fellowship:** Allergy & Immunology, NY Hosp-Cornell, New York, NY 1979-1981; **Faculty Appointment:** Medicine, Cornell Univ-Weil Med Coll

Slankard, Marjorie MD (Allergy & Immunology) - *Special Expertise: Rhinitis; Asthma;* **Admitting Hospital:** Columbia Presbyterian Medical Center (Page 72); **Office Address:** 16 E 60th St New York, NY 10022; **Office Phone:** (212) 326-8410; **Board Certifications:** Internal Medicine 1974, Allergy & Immunology 1977; **Medical School:** Univ MO-Columbia Sch Med 1971; **Residencies:** Internal Medicine, NY Hosp-Cornell Med Ctr, New York, NY 1972-1974; Internal Medicine, Rockefeller Univ Hosp, New York, NY 1973-1974; **Fellowships:** Allergy & Immunology, NY Hosp-Cornell Med Ctr, New York, NY 1974-1976; Immunology, Mount Sinai Med Ctr, New York, NY 1976-1980; **Faculty Appointment:** Assoc Clin Prof Medicine, Columbia P&S

Strober, Warren MD (Allergy & Immunology) - *Special Expertise: Immune Deficiency; Inflammatory Bowel Disease;* **Admitting Hospital:** National Institutes of Health - Clinical Center; **Office Address:** NIH - Laboratory of Clinical Investigation Bldg 10 - rm 11N238 Bethesda, MD 20892; **Office Phone:** (301) 496-6810; **Board Certifications:** Internal Medicine 1974, Allergy & Immunology 1977; **Medical School:** Univ Rochester 1962; **Residencies:** Internal Medicine, Strong Meml Hosp, Rochester, NY 1963-1964; Allergy & Immunology, Natl Inst Hlth, Bethesda, MD 1964-1972

Togias, Alkis George MD (Allergy & Immunology) - *Special Expertise: Asthma; Occupational Asthma; Rhinitis;* **Admitting Hospital:** Johns Hopkins Medical Center - Bayview; **Office Address:** Johns Hopkins Asthma & Allergy Ctr 5501 Hopkins Bayview Circle Baltimore, MD 21224; **Office Phone:** (410) 550-2191; **Board Certifications:** Internal Medicine 1990, Allergy & Immunology 1995; **Medical School:** Greece 1983; **Residencies:** Internal Medicine, Johns Hopkins Hosp, Baltimore, MD 1983-1985; Internal Medicine, Johns Hopkins Hosp, Baltimore, MD 1985-1986; **Fellowship:** Clinical Immunology, Johns Hopkins Hosp, Baltimore, MD 1986-1988; **Faculty Appointment:** Assoc Prof Medicine, Johns Hopkins Univ

97

Southeast

Benenati, Susan MD (Allergy & Immunology) - *Special Expertise: Asthma; Latex Allergy; Sinus Disorders;* **Admitting Hospital:** Baptist Hospital - Miami; **Office Address:** 7000 SW 62nd Ave, Ste 510 South Miami, FL 33143-4721; **Office Phone:** (305) 665-1623; **Board Certifications:** Internal Medicine 1988, Allergy & Immunology 1991; **Medical School:** Univ S Fla Coll Med 1984; **Residencies:** Internal Medicine, Indiana Univ Med Ctr, Indianapolis, IN 1984-1987; Medical Oncology, Indiana Univ Med Ctr, Indianapolis, IN 1987-1988; **Fellowship:** Allergy & Immunology, Johns Hopkins Hosp, Baltimore, MD 1988-1990; **Faculty Appointment:** Asst Prof Medicine, Univ Miami Sch Med

de Shazo, Richard Denson MD (Allergy & Immunology) - *Special Expertise: Insect Allergy; Geriatric Medicine; Rheumatology;* **Admitting Hospital:** University Hospital & Clinics- Mississippi; **Office Address:** Univ Miss Med Ctr 2500 N State St Jackson, MS 39216-4505; **Office Phone:** (601) 984-5600; **Board Certifications:** Allergy & Immunology 1977, Geriatric Medicine 1994; **Medical School:** Univ Ala 1971; **Residencies:** Internal Medicine, Walter Reed Genl Hosp., Washington, DC 1972-1974; Rheumatology, Walter Reed Genl Hosp, Washington, DC 1975-1977; **Fellowship:** Clinical Immunology, Walter Reed Genl Hosp., Washington, DC 1974-1975; **Faculty Appointment:** Prof Medicine, Univ Miss

Fox, Roger W MD (Allergy & Immunology) - *Special Expertise: Allergy & Immunology - General;* **Admitting Hospital:** University Community Hospital; **Office Address:** 13801 Bruce B Downs Blvd, Ste 502 Tampa, FL 33613; **Office Phone:** (813) 971-9743; **Board Certifications:** Internal Medicine 1978, Allergy & Immunology 1981; **Medical School:** St Louis Univ 1975; **Residency:** Internal Medicine, Univ South Florida, Tampa, FL 1976-1978; **Fellowship:** Allergy & Immunology, Univ South Florida, Tampa, FL 1978-1980; **Faculty Appointment:** Assoc Prof Medicine, Univ S Fla Coll Med

Friedman, Stuart MD (Allergy & Immunology) - *Special Expertise: Asthma; Sinus Disorders;* **Admitting Hospital:** Boca Raton Community Hosp; **Office Address:** Stuart A. Friedman, MD 5162 Linton Blvd #201 Delray Beach, FL 33484-6567; **Office Phone:** (561) 495-2580; **Board Certifications:** Internal Medicine 1980, Allergy & Immunology 1983; **Medical School:** Spain 1976; **Residency:** Internal Medicine, Winthrop Univ Hosp, Mineola, NY 1977-1980; **Fellowship:** Allergy & Immunology, Univ Cincinnati Med Ctr, Cincinnati, OH 1980-1982

Gluck, Joan MD (Allergy & Immunology) - *Special Expertise: Asthma in Pregnancy; Asthma/Allergies-Pediatric;* **Admitting Hospital:** Baptist Hospital - Miami; **Office Address:** Allergy & Asthma Assoc 8970 SW 87th Ct, Ste 100 Miami, FL 33176-2205; **Office Phone:** (305) 279-3366; **Board Certification:** Allergy & Immunology; **Medical School:** NYU Sch Med 1972; **Residency:** Pediatrics, U Of Miami Jackson Meml, Miami, FL 1972-1974; **Fellowship:** Allergy & Immunology, U Of Miami Jackson Meml, Miami, FL 1974-1976

Good, Robert MD/PhD (Allergy & Immunology) - *Special Expertise: Immune Deficiency; Bone Marrow Transplant; Nutrition in Aging - Associated Diseases;* **Admitting Hospital:** All Children's Hospital; **Office Address:** 801 Sixth St S, Box 9350 St Petersburg, FL 33701; **Office Phone:** (727) 892-4470; **Medical School:** Univ Minn 1947; **Residencies:** Pediatrics, Univ Minn Hosps, Minneapolis, MN 1947-1949; Pediatrics, Univ Minn Hosps, Minneapolis, MN 1950-1951; **Fellowship:** Research, Rockefeller Inst, New York, NY 1949-1950; **Faculty Appointment:** Prof Pediatrics, Univ S Fla Coll Med

Kaplan, Allen MD (Allergy & Immunology) - *Special Expertise:* Urticaria; **Admitting Hospital:** MUSC Medical Center; **Office Address:** MUSC, Div of Allergy 172 Ashley Ave Charleston, SC 29425-2220; **Office Phone:** (843) 792-3712; **Board Certifications:** Allergy & Immunology 1974, Clinical & Laboratory Dematologic Immunology 1986; **Medical School:** SUNY Downstate 1965; **Residency:** Internal Medicine, Strong Meml Hosp, Rochester 1966-1967; **Faculty Appointment:** Prof Medicine, Univ SC Sch Med

Ledford, Dennis MD (Allergy & Immunology) - *Special Expertise:* Asthma; **Admitting Hospital:** University Community Hospital of Carrollwood; **Office Address:** 13801 Bruce B Downs Blvd, Ste 502 Tampa, FL 33613-3923; **Office Phone:** (813) 971-9743; **Board Certifications:** Rheumatology 1984, Allergy & Immunology 1985; **Medical School:** Univ Tenn Coll Med, Memphis 1976; **Residency:** Internal Medicine, City of Memphis Hosp, Memphis, TN 1978-1980; **Fellowships:** Rheumatology, NYU Hosp-Bellevue, New York, NY 1980-1982; Allergy & Immunology, Univ South Florida, Tampa, FL 1983-1985; **Faculty Appointment:** Assoc Prof Allergy & Immunology, Univ S Fla Coll Med

Lockey, Richard MD (Allergy & Immunology) - *Special Expertise:* Immune Deficiency; **Admitting Hospital:** University Community Hospital; **Office Address:** 13801 Bruce B Downs Blvd, Ste 502 Tampa, FL 33613-3946; **Office Phone:** (813) 971-9743; **Board Certifications:** Internal Medicine 1970, Allergy & Immunology 1974; **Medical School:** Temple Univ 1965; **Residency:** Internal Medicine, Univ Mich Hosp, Ann Arbor, MI 1966-1968; **Fellowship:** Allergy & Immunology, Univ Mich Hosp, Ann Arbor, MI 1969-1970; **Faculty Appointment:** Prof Medicine, Univ S Fla Coll Med

Pacin, Michael MD (Allergy & Immunology) - *Special Expertise:* Insect Allergies; **Admitting Hospital:** Baptist Hospital - Miami; **Office Address:** 8970 SW 87th Court, Ste 100 Miami, FL 33175; **Office Phone:** (305) 932-3252; **Board Certifications:** Internal Medicine 1974, Allergy & Immunology 1979; **Medical School:** Washington Univ, St Louis 1969; **Residencies:** Internal Medicine, Jewish Hosp, St Louis, MO 1970-1971; Internal Medicine, Jackson Meml Hosp, Miami, FL 1971-1972; **Fellowship:** Allergy & Immunology, Long Beach VA Hosp 1972-1974

Stein, Mark R MD (Allergy & Immunology) - *Special Expertise:* Allergy & Immunology - General; **Admitting Hospital:** St Mary's Medical Center - West Palm Beach; **Office Address:** Allergy Associates 840 US Hwy 1, Ste 235 North Palm Beach, FL 33408-3835; **Office Phone:** (561) 626-2006; **Board Certifications:** Internal Medicine 1975, Allergy & Immunology 1977; **Medical School:** Jefferson Med Coll 1968; **Residency:** Internal Medicine, Letterman Army Med Ctr, San Francisco, CA 1972-1975; **Fellowship:** Allergy & Immunology, Fitzsimmons Army Med Ctr, Denver, CO 1975-1977; **Faculty Appointment:** Asst Clin Prof Allergy & Immunology, Univ S Fla Coll Med

Midwest

Aaronson, Donald W MD (Allergy & Immunology) - *Special Expertise:* Asthma; Sinus Disorders; **Admitting Hospital:** Advocate Lutheran General Hospital; **Office Address:** 9301 W Golf Rd, Ste 301 Des Plaines, IL 60016; **Office Phone:** (847) 635-7300; **Board Certification:** Allergy & Immunology 1975; **Medical School:** Univ IL Coll Med 1961; **Residency:** Internal Medicine, Hines VA Hosp, Chicago, IL 1962-1965; **Fellowship:** Allergy & Immunology, Northwestern Univ, Chicago, IL 1965-1966; **Faculty Appointment:** Clin Prof Medicine, Univ Hlth Sci/Chicago Med Sch

ALLERGY & IMMUNOLOGY

Baker Jr., James Russell MD (Allergy & Immunology) - *Special Expertise:* Immune Deficiency - Thyroid; **Admitting Hospital:** University of Michigan Health Center; **Office Address:** Taubman Health Care Ctr 1500 E Medical Center Drive, Fl 3 - Ste 3918, Box 0380 Ann Arbor, MI 48109-0380; **Office Phone:** (734) 647-2777; **Board Certifications:** Internal Medicine 1981, Allergy & Immunology 1983; **Medical School:** Loyola Univ-Stritch Sch Med 1978; **Residency:** Internal Medicine, Walter Reed Army Med Ctr, Washington, DC 1979-1981; **Fellowship:** Allergy & Immunology, Walter Reed Army Med Ctr/NIAID, Bethesda, MD 1981-1984; **Faculty Appointment:** Prof Allergy & Immunology, Univ Mich Med Sch

Bush, Robert MD (Allergy & Immunology) - *Special Expertise:* Allergy & Immunology - General; **Admitting Hospital:** University of Wisconsin Hospital & Clinics; **Office Address:** 2500 Overlook Terrace Madison, WI 53705-2254; **Office Phone:** (608) 263-6180; **Board Certifications:** Internal Medicine 1975, Allergy & Immunology 1977; **Medical School:** W VA Univ 1970; **Residencies:** Internal Medicine, Univ Wisc, Madison, WI 1973-1975; Allergy & Immunology, Univ Wisc, Madison, WI 1975-1977; **Faculty Appointment:** Prof Medicine, Univ Wisc

Busse, William MD (Allergy & Immunology) - *Special Expertise:* Asthma; Autoimmune Disease; **Admitting Hospital:** University of Wisconsin Hospital & Clinics; **Office Address:** Univ Wisc Hosp, Dept Allergy 600 Highland Ave B6/242 Madison, WI 53792-0001; **Office Phone:** (608) 263-6180; **Board Certifications:** Internal Medicine 1972, Allergy & Immumnology 1974; **Medical School:** Univ Wisc 1966; **Residencies:** Internal Medicine, Cincinnati Genl Hosp, Cincinnati, OH 1967-1968; Internal Medicine, Cincinnati Genl Hosp, Cincinnati, OH 1970-1971; **Fellowship:** Allergy & Immunology, Univ Wisc, Madison, WI 1971-1973; **Faculty Appointment:** Prof Medicine, Univ Wisc

Frigas, Evangelo MD (Allergy & Immunology) - *Special Expertise:* Urticaria; Angioedema; **Admitting Hospital:** St Mary's Hospital; **Office Address:** Mayo Clinic 200 First St SW Rochester, MN 55905; **Office Phone:** (507) 284-2511; **Board Certification:** Allergy & Immunology 1981; **Medical School:** Italy 1970; **Residency:** Internal Medicine, Morristown Mem Hosp, Rutger 1976-1978; **Fellowship:** Allergy & Immunology, Mayo Clinic, Rochester 1978-1980; **Faculty Appointment:** Assoc Prof Medicine, Mayo Med Sch

Grammer, Leslie C MD (Allergy & Immunology) - *Special Expertise:* Asthma; Occupational Allergy; **Admitting Hospital:** Northwestern Memorial Hospital; **Office Address:** Northwestern Med Faculty Fdtn - Ambulatory Care Ctr 675 N St Clare, Fl 18 - Ste 18250 Chicago, IL 60611-3008; **Office Phone:** (312) 695-8624; **Board Certifications:** Allergy & Immunology 1981, Occupational Medicine 1989; **Medical School:** Northwestern Univ 1976; **Residency:** Internal Medicine, Northwestern Univ, Chicago, IL 1977-1979; **Fellowship:** Allergy & Immunology, Northwestern Univ, Chicago, IL 1979-1981; **Faculty Appointment:** Prof Medicine, Northwestern Univ

Grant, Evalyn N MD (Allergy & Immunology) - *Special Expertise:* Asthma; **Admitting Hospital:** Rush/Presbyterian - St Luke's Medical Center - Chicago (Page 74); **Office Address:** Univ Consultants A & I 1725 W Harrison, Ste 207 Chicago, IL 60612; **Office Phone:** (312) 942-6296; **Board Certifications:** Pediatrics 1989, Allergy & Immunology 1995; **Medical School:** Rush Med Coll 1986; **Residency:** Pediatrics, Univ of Chicago, Chicago, IL 1986-1989; **Fellowship:** Allergy & Immunology, Rush Pres/St Luke's, Chicago, IL 1993-1996; **Faculty Appointment:** Asst Prof Rush Med Coll

Greenberger, Paul A MD (Allergy & Immunology) - *Special Expertise:* Asthma; Anaphylaxis; **Admitting Hospital:** Northwestern Memorial Hospital; **Office Address:** Northwestern Med Faculty Fdtn - Ambulatory Care Ctr 675 N St Clare, Fl 18 - Ste 18250 Chicago, IL 60611; **Office Phone:** (312) 695-8624; **Board Certifications:** Internal Medicine 1976, Allergy & Immunology 1979; **Medical School:** Indiana Univ 1973; **Residency:** Internal Medicine, Jewish Hosp, St Louis, MO 1974-1976; **Fellowship:** Allergy & Immunology, Northwestern Meml Hosp, Chicago, IL 1976-1978; **Faculty Appointment:** Prof Medicine, Northwestern Univ

Kaiser, Harold MD (Allergy & Immunology) - *Special Expertise:* Allergy & Immunology - General; **Admitting Hospital:** Fairview-University Medical Center - University Campus; **Office Address:** 825 Nicollett Mall, Ste 1149 Minneapolis, MN 55402; **Office Phone:** (612) 338-3333; **Board Certifications:** Internal Medicine 1963, Allergy & Immunology 1972; **Medical School:** Univ Minn 1956; **Residencies:** Internal Medicine, Wadsworth VA Hosp, Los Angeles, CA 1957-1958; Allergy & Immunology, VA Hosp-Univ Minn Hosp, Minneapolis, MN 1960-1962; **Fellowship:** Allergy & Immunology, UCLA Med Ctr, Los Angeles, CA 1964-1965; **Faculty Appointment:** Clin Prof Medicine, Univ Minn

Korenblat, Phillip Erwin MD (Allergy & Immunology) - *Special Expertise:* Allergy; Asthma; **Admitting Hospital:** Barnes - Jewish Hospital; **Office Address:** 1040 N Mason Rd, Ste 115 St. Louis, MO 63141; **Office Phone:** (314) 542-0606; **Board Certifications:** Internal Medicine 1971, Allergy & Immunology 1974; **Medical School:** Univ Ark 1960; **Residency:** Internal Medicine, Jewish Hosp, St Louis, MO 1961-1965; **Fellowship:** Allergy & Immunology, Scripps Clin Rsch Fdn, La Jolla, CA 1965-1966

Sanders, Georgiana MD (Allergy & Immunology) - *Special Expertise:* Asthma; Allergy; Lung Disease -Pediatric; **Admitting Hospital:** University of Michigan Health Center; **Office Address:** 1500 E Med Ctr Dr A. Alfred Taubman Health Care Center, rm 3918, Box 0380 Ann Arbor, MI 48109-0380; **Office Phone:** (734) 936-5634; **Board Certifications:** Pediatrics 1983, Allergy & Immunology 1985; **Medical School:** Univ Cincinnati 1975; **Residencies:** Pediatrics, Children's Hosp of Mich, Detroit, MI 1975-1978; Pediatrics, Boston City Hospi, Boston, MA 1978-1979; **Fellowship:** Allergy & Immunology, Univ of Michigan Hosp, Ann Arbor, MI 1981-1984; **Faculty Appointment:** Asst Clin Prof Pediatrics, Univ Mich Med Sch

Slavin, Raymond MD (Allergy & Immunology) - *Special Expertise:* Asthma; Sinus Disorders; Immune Deficiency-Lung; **Admitting Hospital:** St Louis University Hospital; **Office Address:** St Louis Univ Hlth Scis Ctr, Div Allergy & Immunology 3635 Vista Ave @Grand Blvd St.Louis, MO 63110; **Office Phone:** (314) 577-6070; **Board Certifications:** Internal Medicine 1964, Allergy & Immunology 1987; **Medical School:** St Louis Univ 1967; **Residency:** Internal Medicine, St Louis Univ Hosp, St Louis, MO 1959-1961; **Fellowship:** Allergy & Immunology, Northwestern Univ, Chicago, IL 1961-1964; **Faculty Appointment:** Prof Medicine, St Louis Univ

Ten, Rosa Maria MD/PhD (Allergy & Immunology) - *Special Expertise:* Immune Deficiency; Asthma; **Admitting Hospital:** Mayo Medical Center & Clinic - Rochester; **Office Address:** Mayo Clinic 200 1st St SW Rochester, MN 55905; **Office Phone:** (507) 284-9077; **Board Certifications:** Internal Medicine 1995, Allergy & Immunology 1997; **Medical School:** Spain 1982; **Residency:** Internal Medicine, Mayo Clinic, Rochester, MN 1992-1994; **Fellowships:** Immunology, Inst Pasteur, Paris France 1989-1991; Allergy & Immunology, Mayo Clinic, Rochester, MN 1995-1996; **Faculty Appointment:** Assoc Prof Allergy & Immunology, Mayo Med Sch

Wood, John MD (Allergy & Immunology) - *Special Expertise:* Allergy; Asthma; **Admitting Hospital:** Barnes - Jewish Hospital; **Office Address:** 224 S Woodsmill Rd, Ste 500 Chesterfield, MO 63017; **Office Phone:** (314) 878-6260; **Board Certifications:** Pulmonary Disease 1978, Allergy & Immunology 1979; **Medical School:** Univ Okla Coll Med 1968; **Residencies:** Internal Medicine, Univ Hosp, Oklahoma City, OK 1969-1970; Internal Medicine, Barnes Hosp-Wash Univ Sch Med, St Louis, MO 1970-1971; **Fellowships:** Pulmonary Disease, Wash Univ Sch Med, St Louis, MO 1975-1977; Allergy & Immunology, Wash Univ Sch Med, St Louis, MO 1976-1977; **Faculty Appointment:** Asst Prof Medicine, Washington Univ, St Louis

Great Plains and Mountains

Jones, James F MD (Allergy & Immunology) - *Special Expertise: Chronic Fatigue Syndrome;* **Admitting Hospital:** National Jewish Medical & Research Center; **Office Address:** National Jewish Medical & Research Center 1400 Jackson St Denver, CO 80206; **Office Phone:** (303) 398-1195; **Board Certifications:** Pediatrics 1974, Allergy & Immunology 1977; **Medical School:** Univ Tex Med Br, Galveston 1968; **Residencies:** Surgery, Univ Arizona Hosp, Tucson, AZ 1970; Plastic Surgery, Univ Arizona Hosp, Tucson, AZ 1971; **Fellowships:** Immunology, Univ Tex Med, TX 1969-1970; Immunology, Univ Arizona Hosp, Tucson, AZ 1971-1975; **Faculty Appointment:** Assoc Prof Univ Colo

Nelson, Harold MD (Allergy & Immunology) - *Special Expertise: Asthma; Allergies-Pediatric;* **Admitting Hospital:** National Jewish Medical & Research Center; **Office Address:** National Jewish Med & Rsch Ctr 1400 Jackson St Denver, CO 80206; **Office Phone:** (303) 398-1562; **Board Certifications:** Internal Medicine 1963, Allergy & Immunology 1983; **Medical School:** Emory Univ 1955; **Residency:** Internal Medicine, Letterman Genl Hosp, San Francisco, CA 1959-1962; **Fellowship:** Allergy & Immunology, Univ Mich Med Ctr, Ann Arbor, MI 1967-1969; **Faculty Appointment:** Prof Medicine, Univ Colo

Neustrom, Mark Ray DO (Allergy & Immunology) - *Special Expertise: Asthma; Rhinitis;* **Admitting Hospital:** Overland Park Regional Medical Center; **Office Address:** Kansas City A & I 4500 College Blvd, Ste 200 Overland Park, KS 66211; **Office Phone:** (913) 491-5501; **Board Certifications:** Internal Medicine 1991, Allergy & Immunology 1995; **Medical School:** Univ Osteo Med & Hlth Sci 1987; **Residency:** Internal Medicine, Univ South Dakota-VA Hosp, Sioux Falls, SD 1987-1990; **Fellowship:** Allergy & Immunology, Med Coll Wisc, Milwaukee, WI 1992-1994

Rosenwasser, Lanny Jeffrey MD (Allergy & Immunology) - *Special Expertise: Asthma;* **Admitting Hospital:** National Jewish Medical & Research Center; **Office Address:** 1400 Jackson St Denver, CO 80206; **Office Phone:** (800) 222-5864; **Board Certifications:** Internal Medicine 1975, Allergy & Immunology 1977; **Medical School:** NYU Sch Med 1972; **Residency:** Univ Calif Affil Hosps, San Francisco, CA 1973-1974

Wald, Jeffrey A MD (Allergy & Immunology) - *Special Expertise: Asthma; Rhinitis;* **Admitting Hospital:** Overland Park Regional Medical Center; **Office Address:** Kansas City Allergy & Asthma 4500 College Blvd, Ste 200 Overland Park, KS 66211; **Office Phone:** (913) 491-5501; **Board Certifications:** Internal Medicine 1983, Allergy & Immunology 1987; **Medical School:** Univ MO-Columbia Sch Med 1980; **Residencies:** Internal Medicine, Jewish Hosp, St. Louis, MO 1980-1983; Allergy & Immunology, Natl Jewish Hosp, Denver, CO 1981-1983; **Fellowship:** Allergy & Immunology, Natl Jewish Hosp, Denver, CO 1984-1986

Southwest

Freeman, Theodore MD (Allergy & Immunology) - *Special Expertise: Insect Allergies;* **Admitting Hospital:** Wilford Hall Medical Center; **Office Address:** Wilford Hall Med Ctr, 59th Medical Wing 220 Bergquist Dr, Ste 1 Lackland AFB, TX 78236; **Office Phone:** (210) 292-5378; **Board Certifications:** Internal Medicine 1983, Allergy & Immunology 1987; **Medical School:** Univ S Fla Coll Med 1980; **Residencies:** Internal Medicine, Keesler Med Ctr, Biloxi, MS 1981-1983; Allergy & Immunology, Wilford Hall Med Ctr, San Antonio, TX 1984-1986; **Fellowship:** Diagnostic Lab Immunology, Mass Genl Hosp, Boston, MA 1986-1987; **Faculty Appointment:** Assoc Prof Medicine

West Coast and Pacific

Beall, Gildon N MD (Allergy & Immunology) - *Special Expertise: AIDS/HIV; Immune Deficiency;* **Admitting Hospital:** LAC - Harbor - UCLA Medical Center; **Office Address:** 1000 W Carson St Torrance, CA 90509-2910; **Office Phone:** (310) 222-5101; **Board Certifications:** Internal Medicine 1974, Allergy & Immunology 1983; **Medical School:** Univ Wash 1953; **Residencies:** Internal Medicine, Seattle VA Hosp, Seattle, WA 1957; Internal Medicine, Univ Wash Affl Hosp, Seattle, WA 1959-1960; **Fellowship:** Allergy & Immunology, Univ Wash, Seattle, WA 1957-1959; **Faculty Appointment:** Prof Medicine, UCLA

Tamaroff, Marc A MD (Allergy & Immunology) - *Special Expertise: Allergy & Immunology - General;* **Admitting Hospital:** Long Beach Memorial Medical Center; **Office Address:** 3816 Woodruff Ave, Ste 209 Long Beach, CA 90808; **Office Phone:** (310) 496-4749; **Board Certifications:** Allergy & Immunology 1983, Internal Medicine 1979; **Medical School:** Univ Ariz Coll Med 1974; **Residency:** Internal Medicine, St Mary Med Ctr, Long Beach, CA 1974-1977; **Fellowship:** Allergy & Immunology, UCLA Med Ctr, Los Angeles, CA 1977-1979; **Faculty Appointment:** Assoc Clin Prof Medicine, UCLA

Wasserman, Stephen MD (Allergy & Immunology) - *Special Expertise: Anaphylaxis; Sinus Disorders;* **Admitting Hospital:** University of California - San Diego Healthcare; **Office Address:** UCSD Med Ctr, Dept Med 9500 Gilman St, rm 244 Lajolla, CA 92093; **Office Phone:** (858) 822-4261; **Board Certifications:** Internal Medicine 1973, Allergy & Immunology 1975; **Medical School:** UCLA 1968; **Residency:** Internal Medicine, Peter Bent Brigham Hosp, Boston, MA 1968-1970; **Fellowship:** Allergy & Immunology, R Breck-PB Brigham Hosp, Boston, MA 1972-1974; **Faculty Appointment:** Prof Medicine, UCSD

CARDIOLOGY

(a subspecialty of INTERNAL MEDICINE)

Cardiology: A cardiologist specializes in diseases of the heart, lungs and blood vessels and manages complex cardiac conditions such as heart attacks and life-threatening, abnormal heartbeat rhythms.

Cardiac Electrophysiology: A field of special interest within the subspecialty of cardiovascular disease which involves intricate technical procedures to evaluate heart rhythms and determine appropriate treatment for them.

Interventional Cardiology: An area of medicine within the subspecialty of cardiology which uses specialized imaging and other diagnostic techniques to evaluate blood flow and pressure in the coronary arteries and chambers of the heart, and uses technical procedures and medications to treat abnormalities that impair the function of the heart.

INTERNAL MEDICINE

A personal physician who provides long-term, comprehensive care in the office and the hospital, managing both common and complex illness of adolescents, adults and the elderly. Internists are trained in the diagnosis and treatment of cancer, infections and diseases affecting the heart, blood, kidneys, joints and digestive, respiratory and vascular systems. They are also trained in the essentials of primary care internal medicine which incorporates an understanding of disease prevention, wellness, substance abuse, mental health and effective treatment of common problems of the eyes, ears, skin, nervous system and reproductive organs.

Training required: Three years in internal medicine *plus* additional training and examination for certification in cardiovascular disease, clinical electrophysiology or interventional cardiology.

CONTINUUM HEALTH PARTNERS, INC.

CONTINUUM HEART INSTITUTE

Administrative Offices: First Ave. at 16th St.
New York, NY 10003
Phone (212) 420-HEART

The Continuum Heart Institute combines the strengths of the cardiac programs at Beth Israel Medical Center, St. Luke's-Roosevelt Hospital Center and Long Island College Hospital for clinical, technological and innovative excellence. The skill and caliber of its cardiologists, cardiovascular surgeons, primary care physicians and other physician specialists is matched only by its state-of-the-art facilities—including the most technologically advanced cardiac care units, catheterization and electrophysiology labs, cardiac surgery suites, open heart recovery units, and cardiopulmonary stepdown telemetry units.

The Continuum Heart Institute offers every heart care service needed to prevent, diagnose, and treat heart disease, including leading-edge cardiac surgery, catheter-based diagnosis and treatment, hypertension diagnosis and treatment, heart failure diagnosis and treatment, and a hypertropic cardiomyopathy program. Strong believers in prevention and early detection, the professionals throughout the Continuum Heart Institute also provide complete medical evaluations, echocardiography, nuclear cardiology services, coronary artery disease prevention, treatment centers for obesity and diabetes, smoking cessation programs, and complementary techniques for relaxation and stress reduction, such as massage therapy and therapeutic touch.

Some of the unique features available at the hospitals of the Continuum Heart Institute include New York City's first robotic surgical suite for closed-chest coronary artery bypass surgery; the Ross procedure—a pulmonary autograft replacement of the aortic valve; and a nationally recognized arrhythmia service.

The program is recognized by the New York State Department of Health as having one of the lowest mortality rates of any New York City hospital, and is consistently ranked among the top five programs in New York State.

CONTINUUM HEART INSTITUTE

In an effort to bridge its many cardiac care programs and provide patients with more streamlined access to its full range of services, the Continuum Heart Institute was established. This interdisciplinary cardiology, cardiac surgery and cardiac rehabilitation team consists of clinicians, surgeons, nurses and nurse practitioners, physician assistants, social workers, complementary care experts and rehabilitation specialists—all working together to give patients a full range of individualized treatment choices and services.

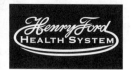

HENRY FORD HOSPITAL
HEART & VASCULAR INSTITUTE

The Henry Ford Heart and Vascular Institute is a recognized leader and innovator in cardiovascular care. Recently ranked 14th among top cardiac centers in the nation by *U.S. News & World* Report, it is a comprehensive program with nearly 40 physicians practicing at seven locations throughout southeast Michigan.

Each year the Institute treats more than 20,000 patients. It offers a full spectrum of cardiovascular care including cardiology, cardiac surgery, cardiac wellness, vascular surgery, as well one of only two programs in Michigan for advanced heart failure treatment and heart transplantation. The heart transplant survival rates are the best in the state and significantly above the national average.

A history of excellence
- First in Michigan to perform open-heart surgery using a heart-lung machine.
- First to perform a heart transplant in Detroit.
- First in the state to introduce an advanced echocardiography system that combines ultrasound with digital imaging to help diagnose heart conditions.
- One of the first centers in the world to perform aortic aneurysm repair.

Research
The Heart and Vascular Institute is a premier site for heart failure and hypertension research. As a clinical trials coordinating center, the Institute oversees major pharmaceutical research for national multi-center trials.

Its world-recognized heart failure research lab is exploring treatments that may induce new cell growth in heart tissue deadened by heart attack. And through a major National Institutes of Health grant, the hypertension lab is investigating the role of hormones in lowering blood pressure.

LEADING-EDGE PATIENT CARE

The Henry Ford Heart and Vascular Institutte houses a recently renovated Electrophysiology Laboratory for the diagnosis and treatment of electrical heart defects.

There, patients are offered the latest in advanced technology - from pacemakers the size of a microchip that regulate electrical impulses, to implanted defibrilators that control abnormal heart beat and help prevent a heart attack.

The lab is the only one in Michigan that uses two state-of-the-art mapping systems. The computer programs take signals received from electrodes on the chest and a catheter placed inside the heart to create a high-resolution, 3-D color map of the patient's heart. The variations in color allow the cardiologists to see how electrical pulses of the heart travel through the heart muscle.

www.HenryFord.com
1 • 888 • 291 - 8304

THE CARDIAC INSTITUTE
MAIMONIDES MEDICAL CENTER

4802 Tenth Avenue   Brooklyn, NY 11219
Tel. 718.283.8902   Fax. 718.283.8069   www.maimonidesmed.org

CARDIOLOGY

The cardiologists of Maimonides Medical Center are expertly trained to provide cardiac care, from diagnosis to medical treatment. They have at their fingertips the most sophisticated testing and monitoring technology. They know and understand the most progressive treatments available. They have immediate access to some of the best cardiac resources in the country. And they also offer the largest hospital-based cardiac rehabilitation program in the nation.

INTERVENTIONAL CARDIOLOGY

When a patient with heart disease needs a more involved diagnostic workup or therapeutic procedure, Maimonides Medical Center's interventional cardiology program is considered second to none. New York State statistics have repeatedly confirmed that its catheterization lab yields the best possible outcomes for patients. And its collaboration with the Department of Emergency Medicine ensures that chest pain patients are evaluated immediately—with intervention to stop a heart attack in progress when necessary.

CARDIOTHORACIC SURGERY

With approximately 1,200 surgical procedures a year, the Division of Cardiothoracic Surgery has one of the busiest programs in the New York metropolitan area. As a regional training center for cardiac surgeons, it conducts one of the largest residency programs in the country. And as a major research facility, it continually investigates unsolved problems in cardiac surgery. Maimonides' cardiothoracic surgeons not only have the best in mind for their patients—they are guiding the future of cardiac care.

THE CARDIAC INSTITUTE

Heart disease...it can strike suddenly. Its symptoms can be mild or debilitating, intermittent or persistent. It can be diagnosed as a mild, easily treatable condition or it can be found to be life-threatening, requiring major, complex surgery. That is why the best cardiac programs are those that are prepared for any contingency...from a medical evaluation of chest pain, to intervention to open a blocked artery or surgery to save a life.

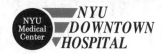

Cardiac Care

Cardiology and Interventional Cardiology

AT MOUNT SINAI HOSPITAL:
- NIH-designated Specialized Center of Research in both Thrombosis and Cardiovascular Disease
- International leadership in MRI diagnosis

· AT NYU HOSPITALS CENTER:
- First biventricular heart pacer in New York
- Pioneered interventional therapy for heart attacks, enhanced safety of stenting procedures, using stents with biologic and pharmacologic coatings
- Specialized therapies for diabetics and the elderly

AT NYU DOWNTOWN HOSPITAL:
- First dedicated chest pain emergency center in New York City
- Intervention and treatment administered 53 minutes faster than the national average; third fastest in the US

Cardiovascular Surgery

AT NYU HOSPITALS CENTER:
- The nation's first robotically-assisted mitral valve surgery
- More experience in minimally invasive valve repair than any other group of surgeons in the world—the world's first minimally invasive mitral valve repair surgery in 1996 and the world's first minimally invasive triple bypass surgery, also in 1996

AT MOUNT SINAI HOSPITAL:
- One of a handful of centers performing heart and lung transplant and implanting artificial heart assist devicesin the tri-state area
- Internationally recognized expertise in aortic anecurysm surgery, more experience than any other center in the region

Pediatric Cardiology

AT MOUNT SINAI HOSPITAL:
- One of the few hospitals in the tri-state area to perform open-heart surgery on newborns and infants, including heart transplantation
- Leaders in fetal echocardiography

AT NYU HOSPITALS CENTER:
- Pioneering use of MRI to precisely define anatomy in complex congenital heart defects
- Internationally-recognized center for pediatric cardiac surgery

The Mount Sinai Hospital's Zena and Michael A. Wiener Cardiovascular Institute and NYU Hospitals Center are world leaders in mending broken hearts. In 1936, the worlds first cardiac stress test was developed at Mount Sinai, and recently NYU Hospitals Center was the first to introduce 2-D echocardiography and color Doppler in New York City.

Both provide superior adult and pediatric cardiology services along with the latest in cardiovascular surgical techniques. And both offer superb inpatient and outpatient cardiac rehabilitation services that include exercise, education, counseling and ongoing support. Together, the hospitals of Mount Sinai NYU Health provide the rare wealth of resources and depth of expertise that you deserve.

800-MD-YOURS
(800-639-6877)
www.msnyuhealth.org

MOUNT SINAI NYU
HEALTH

RUSH HEART INSTITUTE
RUSH-PRESBYTERIAN-ST. LUKE'S MEDICAL CENTER

1725 W. Harrison Street, Suite 1159   Chicago, IL 60612
Tel. 312.563.2230   Fax. 312.733.1221

A LEADER IN THE MIDWEST

Staffed by world-renowned physicians, scientists and other health care professionals, the Rush Heart Institute is ranked among the country's top medical centers for the diagnosis and treatment of heart disease.

Serving both adults and children, the Rush Heart Institute provides the most advanced and comprehensive medical and surgical cardiovascular care in the Midwest. The Rush Heart Institute has several programs that are available at only a handful of medical centers in the United States. These include the Rush Heart Failure and Cardiac Transplant Program, which provides innovative medical and surgical treatment for advanced heart failure patients; the Pulmonary Heart Disease Program, which provides advanced treatment for one of the most deadly and unusual heart diseases; the Rush Interventional Cardiology Program, which offers some of the country's most innovative nonsurgical treatments for blocked coronary arteries; the Rush Preventive Cardiology Program, which offers advanced cholesterol management and risk modification services; and the Rush Electrophysiology Program, which provides advanced treatment for complex cardiac arrhythmias.

COMPREHENSIVE CARDIAC CARE

Cardiovascular surgeons at the Rush Heart Institute are experts in performing all types of heart surgery—from the more routine (bypass surgeries and new minimally invasive procedures) to the more complex (valve repair and replacement procedures and heart transplantation). Recently, the Rush Heart Institute opened the Thoracic Aortic Center, which will be dedicated to treating the complex and challenging problems related to the thoracic aorta. For patients with chest pain who have not been helped by other treatments, the Rush Heart Institute offers a revolutionary new procedure known as transmyocardial laser revascularization that restores blood flow to damaged areas of the heart. Only a few medical centers in the nation provide this technology.

When time is of the essence, the Rush Emergent Transfer System is available—24 hours a day, 7 days a week—to transport cardiovascular patients in immediate need of advanced therapies and expert care to the Rush Heart Institute by land or air.

RESEARCH & CLINICAL TRIALS

Physicians and scientists at the Institute have received numerous research grants from the National Institutes of Health for pioneering work regarding the causes and treatment of heart disease. More than 60 clinical trials are under way at the Institute to evaluate drugs, devices and technical advances in cardiac care.

CUTTING-EDGE TECHNOLOGY AND TREATMENT

To ensure the accurate diagnosis of cardiac problems, the Rush Heart Institute offers cutting-edge technologies such as the Rush Heart Scan, which uses electron beam computed tomography to detect heart disease long before the onset of problems; three-dimensional and contrast echocardiography, which provides pinpoint accuracy in diagnosing cardiac problems; and positron emission tomography, or PET scanning, which enables physicians to identify damaged, nonfunctioning heart muscle that can be saved with surgical repair.

As a research facility, the Rush Heart Institute has pioneered many innovative treatments. These include procedures performed in the cardiac catheterization laboratory, such as percutaneous (nonsurgical) myocardial channeling for persistent chest pain and low-dose beta radiation to prevent reclosing of coronary vessels after angioplasty. In addition, Rush researchers have investigated the use of DNA to stimulate the growth of healthy new blood vessels in damaged areas of the heart.

To speak to a Rush Heart Institute representative, please call (312) 563-2230.

TEXAS HEART® INSTITUTE

at St. Luke's Episcopal Hospital

6720 Bertner Ave. Houston, TX 77030 Tel. (713) 791-4011 <u>www.texasheartinstitute.org</u>

LEADING WITH THE HEART®

Founded in 1962 by world-renowned cardiovascular surgeon Denton A. Cooley, M.D., the Texas Heart Institute at St. Luke's Episcopal Hospital is a non-profit organization dedicated to the study and treatment of diseases of the heart and blood vessels.

CLINICAL EXCELLENCE

The Texas Heart Institute and its clinical partner, St. Luke's, have become the largest cardio-vascular center in the world and have been ranked among the nation's top ten heart centers in an annual survey published by *U.S.News & World Report* for the past ten years - and #1 in the Southwest.

PIONEERING RESEARCH

Cutting edge research programs produce or refine new devices, drug therapies and diagnos-tic testing methods that are directly applied to patient care. Two of the most notable surgical achievements by Texas Heart Institute and St. Luke's physicians are the first successful heart transplant in the United States and the first implantation in the world of a total artificial heart in a human. Innovations in interventional cardiology treatments include the evaluation of the first generation of stents, mesh-like tubes used to support the walls of arteries, as well as the recently approved fabric-covered stents, called stent-grafts, for the repair of abdominal aortic aneurysms.

CURRENT BREAKTHROUGHS

Current research includes the implantations of the Jarvik 2000®, a small, axial-flow, assist pump that sustains patients as they wait for heart transplants; the development of specialized catheters which may be used to detect, and possibly treat, unstable, or "vulnerable" plaque in arteries-the rupturing of such plaque is the major cause of heart attacks; the use of radiation to prevent the repeated buildup of arterial plaque; and the development of a new total artifi-cial heart. The Texas Heart Institute and St. Luke's also hosted the first open-heart surgery simulcast live on the Internet and cable television.

COMMUNITY EDUCATION

Another facet of the Texas Heart Institute at St. Luke's mission is education. The public can learn more about heart disease and its prevention through the free Heart Information Service which can be accessed through a toll-free telephone number (1-800-292-2221) or the Internet (www.texasheartinstitute.org).

APPOINTMENTS AND INFORMATION

For more information about the Texas Heart Institute, dial (713) 791-4011. To make an appoint-ment with a cardiologist, call St. Luke's Health Resource Line at (713) 791-4343, or visit the St. Luke's Web site at www.stlukestexas.com.

The University of Chicago Hospitals
Heart Program

5841 S. Maryland Avenue
Chicago, IL 60637-1470
For help finding a physician: 1-888-UCH-0200

AT THE FOREFRONT OF CARDIAC CARE

The University of Chicago Hospitals' cardiac center is among the finest in the nation. Our team of cardiologists and cardiac surgeons at the University of Chicago Hospitals has two goals: to provide state-of-the-art, high quality care to all patients, and to develop new therapies that improve health and prolong lives.

Our team of clinicians, scientists, and medical staff work in the most modern facilities to provide patients with up-to-date treatments often before they are generally available in the community. The new 525,000-square-foot Center for Advanced Medicine houses our outpatient cardiovascular center and offers patients numerous efficiencies, including easier scheduling. And, with all cardiology and related clinics on one floor, multiple tests and procedures can often be performed on the same day.

NEW AND EFFECTIVE TREATMENTS

Our physicians are at the forefront of exciting advances in clinical cardiology:

- New three-dimensional, non-invasive imaging techniques, which enable physicians to better diagnose, evaluate, and treat cardiac conditions.

- Enhanced electrophysiology capabilities for the treatment of abnormal heart rhythms, including the non-surgical implantation of smart defibrillators.

- The use of newly developed interventional techniques to revascularize patients with severe three vessel coronary artery disease without open-heart surgery.

- Innovative medical and surgical therapies for patients with severe ventricular dysfunction and congestive heart failure.

As part of the oldest and most successful National Institutes of Health-funded cardiovascular research program in the country, our physician-scientists benefit from millions of dollars in annual research support to study and cure heart disease. Spanning molecular biology, physiology, pharmacology, and biochemistry of the cardiovascular system, this research helps to develop novel therapies for hyperlipidemias, atherosclerosis, cardiac arrythmias, and heart failure.

**To Find a University of Chicago Heart Specialist,
Call 1-888-UCH-0200**

FINDING NEW THERAPIES FOR HEART DISEASES

University of Chicago experts are unraveling the genetic basis of heart diseases such as hyperlipidemias, atherosclerosis, and congestive heart failure and are devising new genetic and pharmacological therapies for these disorders.

Physician Listings

New England

McGovern, Brian Anthony MD (Cardiac Electrophysiology) - *Special Expertise:* Cardiac Electrophysiology - General; **Admitting Hospital:** Massachusetts General Hospital; **Office Address:** Mass Genl Hosp Grey Bldg, Fl 1 - rm 109 Boston, MA 02114; **Office Phone:** (617) 726-5557; **Board Certifications:** Cardiology (Cardiovascular Disease) 1989; Cardiac Electrophysiology 1992; **Medical School:** Ireland 1979; **Residency:** Internal Medicine, Mass Genl Hosp, Boston, MA 1986-1987; **Fellowship:** Cardiology (Cardiovascular Disease), Mass Genl Hosp, Boston, MA 1981-1984; **Faculty Appointment:** Asst Prof Medicine, Harvard Med Sch

Stevenson, William G. MD (Cardiac Electrophysiology) - *Special Expertise:* Arrhythmias; **Admitting Hospital:** Brigham & Women's Hospital; **Office Address:** Brigham-Womens Hosp, Dept Cardio Vasc 75 Francis St Boston, MA 02115; **Office Phone:** (617) 732-7517; **Board Certifications:** Cardiology (Cardiovascular Disease) 1985, Cardiac Electrophysiology 1992; **Medical School:** Tulane Univ 1979; **Residency:** Internal Medicine, UCLA Ctr Health Sci, Los Angeles, CA 1980-1982; **Fellowship:** Cardiology (Cardiovascular Disease), UCLA Ctr Health Sci, Los Angeles, CA 1982-1984; **Faculty Appointment:** Assoc Prof Medicine

Mid Atlantic

Cohen, Martin MD (Cardiac Electrophysiology) - *Special Expertise:* Interventional Cardiology; **Admitting Hospital:** Westchester Medical Center; **Office Address:** Cardiology Consultants of Westchester 19 Bradhurst Ave Hawthorne, NY 10532; **Office Phone:** (914) 593-7800; **Board Certifications:** Cardiac Electrophysiology 1996, Cardiology (Cardiovascular Disease) 1985; **Medical School:** SUNY Hlth Sci Ctr 1980; **Residency:** Internal Medicine, Univ Hosp, Brooklyn, NY 1980-1983; **Fellowships:** Cardiology (Cardiovascular Disease), Univ Hosp, Brooklyn, NY 1983-1985; Westchester, Valhalla, NY 1985-1986; **Faculty Appointment:** Assoc Clin Prof Medicine, NY Med Coll

Gomes, J Anthony MD (Cardiac Electrophysiology) - *Special Expertise:* Arrhythmias; Heart Attack/ Sudden Death; **Admitting Hospital:** Mount Sinai Hospital (Page 70); **Office Address:** Mt Sinai Med Ctr One Gustave Levy Pl, Box 1054 New York, NY 10029; **Office Phone:** (212) 241-7272; **Board Certifications:** Cardiology (Cardiovascular Disease) 1975, Cardiac Electrophysiology 1994; **Medical School:** India 1970; **Residency:** Internal Medicine, Mt Sinai Med Ctr, New York, NY 1970-1973; **Fellowship:** Cardiology (Cardiovascular Disease), Mt Sinai Med Ctr, New York, NY 1973-1975; **Faculty Appointment:** Prof Medicine, Mount Sinai Sch Med

Lerman, Bruce MD (Cardiac Electrophysiology) - *Special Expertise:* Cardiac Electrophysiology - General; **Admitting Hospital:** New York Weill Cornell Medical Center - NY Presbyterian Hospital (Page 72); **Office Address:** 520 E 70th St New York, NY 10021; **Office Phone:** (212) 746-2169; **Board Certifications:** Cardiology (Cardiovascular Disease) 1985, Cardiac Electrophysiology 1992; **Medical School:** Loyola Univ-Stritch Sch Med 1977; **Residencies:** Internal Medicine, NorthWestern Univ, Chicago, IL 1977-1980; Internal Medicine, Univ Michigan, Ann Harbor, MI 1980-1981; **Fellowships:** Cardiology (Cardiovascular Disease), Univ Penn, Philadelphia, PA 1981-1982; Cardiology (Cardiovascular Disease), Johns Hopkins Hosp, Baltimore, MD 1982-1983; **Faculty Appointment:** Prof Medicine, Cornell Univ-Weil Med Coll

Levine, Joseph H MD (Cardiac Electrophysiology) - *Special Expertise:* Arrhythmias; Pacemakers; **Admitting Hospital:** St Francis Hospital (Page 75); **Office Address:** St Francis Hosp 100 Port Washington Blvd Roslyn, NY 11576; **Office Phone:** (516) 562-6672; **Board Certifications:** Cardiology (Cardiovascular Disease) 1987; Cardiac Electrophysiology 1992; **Medical School:** Univ Rochester 1980; **Residencies:** Internal Medicine, Yale-New Haven Hosp, New Haven, CT 1980-1983; Cardiology (Cardiovascular Disease), Johns Hopkins Hosp, Baltimore, MD 1983-1986

Marchlinski, Francis Edward MD (Cardiac Electrophysiology) - *Special Expertise:* Pacemakers; Arrhythmias; **Admitting Hospital:** Hospital of the University of Pennsylvania; **Office Address:** Univ Penns Healthcare System 3400 Spruce St Philadelphia, PA 19104; **Office Phone:** (215) 662-6005; **Board Certifications:** Cardiology (Cardiovascular Disease) 1981, Cardiac Electrophysiology 1992; **Medical School:** Univ Penn 1976; **Residency:** Internal Medicine, Hosp Univ Penn, Philadelphia, PA 1977-1979; **Fellowship:** Cardiology (Cardiovascular Disease), Hosp Univ Penn, Philadelphia, PA 1979-1982; **Faculty Appointment:** Clin Prof Medicine, Univ Penn

Rothman, Steven Alan MD (Cardiac Electrophysiology) - *Special Expertise:* Arrhythmias; **Admitting Hospital:** Temple University Hospital; **Office Address:** Temple Univ Hosp 3401 N Broad St, Bldg Parkinson - Ste 9 Philadelphia, PA 19140; **Office Phone:** (215) 707-4724; **Board Certifications:** Cardiology (Cardiovascular Disease) 1995; Cardiac Electrophysiology 1996; **Medical School:** Temple Univ 1988; **Residencies:** Internal Medicine, Univ Maryland Med System, Baltimore, MD 1988-1991; Cardiology (Cardiovascular Disease), Temple Univ Hosp, Philadelphia, PA 1991-1995

Southeast

Anderson, Mark MD (Cardiac Electrophysiology) - *Special Expertise:* Cardiac Electrophysiology - General; **Admitting Hospital:** Vanderbilt University Medical Center; **Office Address:** Vanderbilt Univ Med Ctr 315 Med Rsch Bldg II Nashville, TN 37232-6300; **Office Phone:** (615) 322-2318; **Board Certifications:** Internal Medicine 1992, Cardiac Electrophysiology 1996; **Medical School:** Univ Mich Med Sch 1989; **Residency:** Internal Medicine, Stanford Univ Sch Med, Stanford, CA 1990-1991; **Fellowships:** Cardiology (Cardiovascular Disease), Stanford Univ Sch Med, Stanford, CA 1991-1994; Cardiac Electrophysiology, Stanford Univ Sch Med, Stanford, CA 1994-1996

Curtis, Anne B MD (Cardiac Electrophysiology) - *Special Expertise:* Pacemakers; **Admitting Hospital:** Shands Healthcare at University Florida (Page 77); **Office Address:** Department of Medicine 1600 SW Archer Rd, Box 100277 Gainesville, FL 32610; **Office Phone:** (352) 392-2469; **Board Certifications:** Cardiology (Cardiovascular Disease) 1985, Cardiac Electrophysiology 1992; **Medical School:** Columbia P&S 1979; **Residency:** Internal Medicine, NY Presby Hosp, New York, NY 1979-1982; **Fellowship:** Cardiology (Cardiovascular Disease), Duke Univ Med Ctr, Durham, NC 1982-1986; **Faculty Appointment:** Prof Medicine, Univ Fla Coll Med

DiMarco, John Philip MD/PhD (Cardiac Electrophysiology) - *Special Expertise:* Arrhythmias; Pacemakers; Defibrillators; **Admitting Hospital:** University of Virginia Health Systems; **Office Address:** Univ Virginia Hlth Scis Ctr PO Box 800158 Charlottesville, VA 22908-0158; **Office Phone:** (804) 924-2031; **Board Certifications:** Cardiology (Cardiovascular Disease) 1981, Cardiac Electrophysiology 1998; **Medical School:** Case West Res Univ 1975; **Residencies:** Internal Medicine, Mass Genl Hosp, Boston, MA 1975-1977; Critical Care Medicine, Case West Res Univ, Cleveland, OH 1977-1978; **Fellowship:** Cardiology (Cardiovascular Disease), Mass Genl Hosp, Boston, MA 1978-1981; **Faculty Appointment:** Prof Medicine, Univ VA Sch Med

Ellenbogen, Kenneth A. MD (Cardiac Electrophysiology) - *Special Expertise:* Arrhythmias; **Admitting Hospital:** Medical College of Virginia Hospitals; **Office Address:** Med College of Virginia/ Electrophysiology P.O.Box 980053, Box 980053 Richmond, VA 23219; **Office Phone:** (804) 828-7565; **Board Certifications:** Cardiology (Cardiovascular Disease) 1985, Cardiac Electrophysiology 1992; **Medical School:** Johns Hopkins Univ 1980; **Residency:** Internal Medicine, Johns Hopkins Hosp, Baltimore, MD 1981-1983; **Fellowship:** Cardiology (Cardiovascular Disease), Duke Univ Med Ctr, Durham, NC 1983-1986; **Faculty Appointment:** Asst Prof Cardiology (Cardiovascular Disease), Med Coll VA

Epstein, Andrew Ernest MD (Cardiac Electrophysiology) - *Special Expertise:* Arrhythmias; Implantable ICD; **Admitting Hospital:** University of Alabama Hospital at Birmingham; **Office Address:** Kirklin Clinic/Univ Ala @ Birmingham 2000 6th Ave S Birmingham, AL 35233; **Office Phone:** (205) 934-7114; **Board Certifications:** Cardiac Electrophysiology 1996, Cardiology (Cardiovascular Disease) 1983; **Medical School:** Univ Rochester 1977; **Residency:** Internal Medicine, Barnes Hosp, St Louis, MO 1978-1980; **Fellowship:** Cardiology (Cardiovascular Disease), Univ Ala Hosp, Birmingham, AL 1980-1982; **Faculty Appointment:** Prof Medicine, Univ Ala

Interian Jr, Alberto MD (Cardiac Electrophysiology) - *Special Expertise:* Cardiac Electrophysiology - General; **Admitting Hospital:** University of Miami - Jackson Memorial Hospital; **Office Address:** 1611 NW 12th Ave Bldg Central - rm 401 Miami, FL 33136; **Office Phone:** (305) 585-5532; **Board Certifications:** Internal Medicine 1985, Cardiology (Cardiovascular Disease) 1987; **Medical School:** Univ Miami Sch Med 1982; **Residency:** Internal Medicine, Univ Miami, Miami, FL; **Fellowship:** Cardiology (Cardiovascular Disease), Univ Miami, Miami, FL 1986-1988; **Faculty Appointment:** Prof Medicine, Univ Miami Sch Med

Sorrentino, Robert A. MD (Cardiac Electrophysiology) - *Special Expertise:* Pacemakers; **Admitting Hospital:** Duke University Medical Center (Page 60); **Office Address:** Duke Univ Med Ctr 7623 Erwin Rd, Box 3330 Durham, NC 27710; **Office Phone:** (919) 681-4358; **Board Certifications:** Cardiology (Cardiovascular Disease) 1991, Cardiac Electrophysiology 1996; **Medical School:** Albany Med Coll 1985; **Residency:** Internal Medicine, Duke Univ Med Ctr, Durham, NC 1985-1988; **Fellowships:** Cardiology (Cardiovascular Disease), Duke Univ Med Ctr, Durham, NC 1988-1991; Cardiac Electrophysiology, Duke Univ Med Ctr, Durham, NC 1988-1991; **Faculty Appointment:** Asst Prof Medicine, Duke Univ

Midwest

Cain, Michael Edwin MD (Cardiac Electrophysiology) - *Special Expertise:* Arrhythmias; **Admitting Hospital:** Barnes - Jewish Hospital; **Office Address:** Washington Univ 660 S Euclid Ave, Box 8086 St Louis, MO 63110-1010; **Office Phone:** (314) 747-3032; **Board Certifications:** Cardiology (Cardiovascular Disease) 1983, Cardiac Electrophysiology 1992; **Medical School:** Geo Wash Univ 1975; **Residency:** Internal Medicine, Barnes Hosp, St Louis, MO 1976-1977; **Fellowship:** Cardiology (Cardiovascular Disease), Barnes Hosp, St Louis, MO 1977-1979; **Faculty Appointment:** Prof Washington Univ, St Louis

Hammill, Stephen Charles MD (Cardiac Electrophysiology) - *Special Expertise:* Pacemakers; **Admitting Hospital:** Mayo Medical Center & Clinic - Rochester; **Office Address:** Mayo Clinic, Div Card Dis 200 1st St SW Rochester, MN 55905; **Office Phone:** (507) 284-4888; **Board Certifications:** Cardiology (Cardiovascular Disease) 1981, Cardiac Electrophysiology 1992; **Medical School:** Univ Colo **Residency:** Internal Medicine, Univ Col Sch Med, Denver, CO 1974-1977; **Fellowship:** Cardiology (Cardiovascular Disease), Duke Univ, Durham, NC 1978-1981; **Faculty Appointment:** Prof Medicine, Mayo Med Sch

Morady, Fred MD (Cardiac Electrophysiology) - *Special Expertise:* Arrhythmias - Atrial; WPW Syndrome; Arrhythmias; **Admitting Hospital:** University of Michigan Health Center; **Office Address:** University Michigan Hospital 1500 E Medical Center Dr, rm B1-F245, Box 0022 Ann Arbor, MI 48109-0022; **Office Phone:** (734) 647-7321; **Board Certifications:** Cardiology (Cardiovascular Disease) 1981, Cardiac Electrophysiology 1994; **Medical School:** UCSF 1975; **Residency:** Internal Medicine, UC-San Francisco, San Francisco, CA 1976-1978; **Fellowship:** Cardiology (Cardiovascular Disease), UC-San Francisco, San Francisco, CA 1978-1980; **Faculty Appointment:** Prof Cardiology (Cardiovascular Disease), Univ Mich Med Sch

CARDIAC ELECTROPHYSIOLOGY

Prystowsky, Eric Neal MD (Cardiac Electrophysiology) - *Special Expertise:* Arrhythmias; **Admitting Hospital:** St Vincent's Hospital and Health Center - Indianapolis; **Office Address:** The Care Group 8333 Naab Rd., Ste 200 Indianapolis, IN 46260; **Office Phone:** (317) 338-6024; **Board Certifications:** Cardiology (Cardiovascular Disease) 1979, Cardiac Electrophysiology 1992; **Medical School:** Mount Sinai Sch Med 1973; **Residency:** Internal Medicine, Mt. Sinai Hosp., New York, NY 1974-1976; **Fellowship:** Cardiology (Cardiovascular Disease), Duke U. Med Ctr., Durham, NC 1976-1979; **Faculty Appointment:** Prof Medicine, Duke Univ

Schuger, Claudio David MD (Cardiac Electrophysiology) - *Special Expertise:* Cardiac Electrophysiology - General; **Admitting Hospital:** Henry Ford Health System (Page 62); **Office Address:** 2799 W Grand Blvd, rm B1451 Detroit, MI 48202-2608; **Office Phone:** (313) 916-2417; **Board Certifications:** Cardiology (Cardiovascular Disease) 1997, Cardiac Electrophysiology 1998; **Medical School:** Argentina 1977; **Residency:** Internal Medicine, Hacarmel Hosp, Haifa, Israel 1980-1982; **Fellowships:** Cardiology (Cardiovascular Disease), Bikur Cholim Hosp, Jerusalem, Israel 1983-1985; Cardiac Electrophysiology, Harper Hosp-Wayne State Univ, Detroit, MI 1987-1990; **Faculty Appointment:** Asst Prof Medicine, Wayne State Univ

Waldo, Albert MD (Cardiac Electrophysiology) - *Special Expertise:* Cardiac Electrophysiology - General; **Admitting Hospital:** University Hospital - Cleveland; **Office Address:** Univ Hosp Cleveland- Dept Cardio 11100 Euclid Ave Cleveland, OH 44106; **Office Phone:** (216) 844-7690; **Board Certifications:** Cardiac Electrophysiology 1992, Cardiology (Cardiovascular Disease) 1975; **Medical School:** NYU Sch Med 1962; **Residencies:** Internal Medicine, Baltimore City Hosp, Baltimore, MD 1963-1965; Internal Medicine, Kings Co Hosp, Brooklyn, MD 1965-1966; **Fellowships:** Cardiac Electrophysiology, Columbia Presby Med Ctr, New York, NY 1966-1968; Cardiology (Cardiovascular Disease), Columbia Presby Med Ctr, New York, NY 1968-1969; **Faculty Appointment:** Prof Emeritus Medicine, Case West Res Univ

Wilber, David James MD (Cardiac Electrophysiology) - *Special Expertise:* Ventricular Tachycardia; Defibrillators - Implantable; Cardiac Catheter Ablation; **Admitting Hospital:** University of Chicago Hospitals (Page 78); **Office Address:** Center for Advanced Medicine 5758 S Maryland Ave Chicago, IL 60637; **Office Phone:** (773) 702-9372; **Board Certifications:** Cardiology (Cardiovascular Disease) 1985, Cardiac Electrophysiology 1992; **Medical School:** Northwestern Univ 1977; **Residency:** Internal Medicine, Northwestern Meml Hosp, Chicago, IL 1978-1980; **Fellowships:** Cardiology (Cardiovascular Disease), Univ Mich Med Sch, Ann Arbor, MI 1982-1984; Cardiology (Cardiovascular Disease), Mass Genl Hosp, Boston, MA 1984-1986; **Faculty Appointment:** Prof Medicine, Univ Chicago-Pritzker Sch Med

Southwest

Jackman, Warren MD (Cardiac Electrophysiology) - *Special Expertise:* Cardiac Electrophysiology - General; **Admitting Hospital:** University of Oklahoma Health Science Center; **Office Address:** 1200 Everette Rd Oklahoma City, OK 73190-3048; **Office Phone:** (405) 271-8764; **Board Certifications:** Cardiology (Cardiovascular Disease) 1981, Cardiac Electrophysiology 1992; **Medical School:** Univ Fla Coll Med 1976; **Residency:** Internal Medicine, Wake Fores U Hosp, Winston-Salem, NC 1977-1979; **Fellowship:** Cardiology (Cardiovascular Disease), Ind U Hosp, Indianapolis, IN 1979; **Faculty Appointment:** Prof Medicine, Univ Okla Coll Med

West Coast and Pacific

Cannom, David S MD (Cardiac Electrophysiology) - *Special Expertise:* Cardiac Electrophysiology - General; **Admitting Hospital:** Good Samaritan Hospital - Los Angeles; **Office Address:** 1245 Wilshire Blvd, Ste 703 Los Angeles, CA 90017-4806; **Office Phone:** (213) 977-0419; **Board Certifications:** Cardiology (Cardiovascular Disease) 1975, Internal Medicine 1980; **Medical School:** Univ Minn 1967; **Residency:** Internal Medicine, Yale- New Haven Hosp, New Haven, CT 1968-1969; **Fellowship:** Cardiology (Cardiovascular Disease), Stanford Unv, Palo Alto, CA 1971-1973; **Faculty Appointment:** Clin Prof Medicine, UCLA

Gang, Eli Shimshon MD (Cardiac Electrophysiology) - *Special Expertise:* Cardiac Electrophysiology - General; **Admitting Hospital:** Cedars-Sinai Medical Center; **Office Address:** 414 N Camden drive, Ste 1100 Beverly Hills, CA 90210-4532; **Office Phone:** (310) 278-3400; **Board Certifications:** Cardiology (Cardiovascular Disease) 1981, Cardiac Electrophysiology 1996; **Medical School:** Columbia P&S 1975; **Residency:** Internal Medicine, Roosevelt Hosp, New York, NY 1976-1978; **Fellowship:** Cardiology (Cardiovascular Disease), Columbia Presby Hosp, New York, NY 1978

Swerdlow, Charles Dennis MD (Cardiac Electrophysiology) - *Special Expertise:* Defibrillators; Arrhythmias; **Admitting Hospital:** Cedars-Sinai Medical Center; **Office Address:** 8635 W 3rd St, Ste 1190W Los Angeles, CA 90048-6101; **Office Phone:** (310) 652-4600; **Board Certifications:** Cardiac Electrophysiology 1994, Cardiology (Cardiovascular Disease) 1981; **Medical School:** Harvard Med Sch 1976; **Residency:** Internal Medicine, LA Co- Harbor Genl Hosp, Los Angeles, CA 1977-1979; **Fellowship:** Cardiac Electrophysiology, Stanford Med Ctr, Stanford, CA 1979-1981; **Faculty Appointment:** Clin Prof Medicine, UCLA

CARDIOLOGY (CARDIOVASCULAR DISEASE)

New England

Balady, Gary MD (Cardiology (Cardiovascular Disease)) - *Special Expertise:* Preventive Cardiology; **Admitting Hospital:** Boston University Medical Center-East Newton Street Campus; **Office Address:** Boston Medical Ctr, Dept Cardiology 88 East Newton St, Bldg C8 Boston, MA 02118; **Office Phone:** (617) 638-7490; **Board Certifications:** Internal Medicine 1982, Cardiology (Cardiovascular Disease) 1985; **Medical School:** Rutgers Univ 1979; **Residency:** Internal Medicine, Univ Hosp-Boston Univ, Boston, MA 1980-1982; **Fellowship:** Cardiology (Cardiovascular Disease), Boston Univ Med Ctr, Boston, MA 1982-1985; **Faculty Appointment:** Prof Medicine, Boston Univ

Batsford, William P MD (Cardiology (Cardiovascular Disease)) - *Special Expertise:* Cardiac Electrophysiology; **Admitting Hospital:** Yale - New Haven Hospital; **Office Address:** Yale Univ Sch Med 333 Cedar St, 3 FMP New Haven, CT 06520; **Office Phone:** (203) 785-4126; **Board Certifications:** Internal Medicine 1972, Cardiology (Cardiovascular Disease) 1977; **Medical School:** Albany Med Coll 1969; **Residency:** Internal Medicine, Hosp Univ Penn, Pennsylvalnia, PA 1969-1972; **Faculty Appointment:** Prof Medicine, Yale Univ

Braunwald, Eugene MD (Cardiology (Cardiovascular Disease)) - *Special Expertise:* Cardiology Research; **Admitting Hospital:** Brigham & Women's Hospital; **Office Address:** Brigham & Womens Hosp, Dept Med 75 Francis St Boston, MA 02115-6110; **Office Phone:** (617) 278-1086; **Board Certifications:** Internal Medicine 1960, Cardiology (Cardiovascular Disease) 1965; **Medical School:** NYU Sch Med 1952; **Residency:** Internal Medicine, John Hopkins Hosp, Baltimore, MD 1957-1958; **Fellowships:** Cardiology (Cardiovascular Disease), Bellvue Hosp, New York, NY 1954-1955; Cardiology (Cardiovascular Disease), Natl Inst Health, Bethesda, MD 1957; **Faculty Appointment:** Prof Medicine, Harvard Med Sch

Cohen, Lawrence Sorel MD (Cardiology (Cardiovascular Disease)) - *Special Expertise:* Cardiology (Cardiovascular Disease) - General; **Admitting Hospital:** Yale - New Haven Hospital; **Office Address:** Yale Univ Sch Med, Dept Med 333 Cedar St New Haven, CT 06520-8017; **Office Phone:** (203) 785-4128; **Board Certifications:** Internal Medicine 1966, Cardiology (Cardiovascular Disease) 1967; **Medical School:** NYU Sch Med 1958; **Residencies:** Internal Medicine, Yale Univ Sch Med, New Haven, CT 1959-1960; Internal Medicine, Yale Univ Sch Med, New Haven, CT 1964-1965; **Fellowship:** Research, Peter Bent Brigham Hosp, Cambridge, MA 1962-1964; **Faculty Appointment:** Prof Medicine, Yale Univ

De Sanctis, Roman MD (Cardiology (Cardiovascular Disease)) - *Special Expertise:* Cardiology (Cardiovascular Disease) - General; **Admitting Hospital:** Massachusetts General Hospital; **Office Address:** Mass Genl Hosp 15 Parkman St, Bldg WACC - rm 467 Boston, MA 02114; **Office Phone:** (617) 726-2889; **Board Certifications:** Internal Medicine 1962, Cardiology (Cardiovascular Disease) 1971; **Medical School:** Harvard Med Sch 1955; **Residency:** Internal Medicine, Mass Genl Hosp, Boston, MA 1958-1960; **Fellowship:** Cardiology (Cardiovascular Disease), Mass Genl Hosp, Boston, MA 1960-1962; **Faculty Appointment:** Prof Medicine, Harvard Med Sch

Dzau, Victor J MD (Cardiology (Cardiovascular Disease)) - *Special Expertise: Vascular Medicine;* **Admitting Hospital:** Brigham & Women's Hospital; **Office Address:** Brigham & Women's Hosp, Dept of Medicine 75 Francis St Boston, MA 02115; **Office Phone:** (617) 732-6340; **Board Certifications:** Internal Medicine 1976, Cardiology (Cardiovascular Disease) 1981; **Medical School:** McGill Univ 1972; **Residencies:** Internal Medicine, PB Brigham Hosp, Boston, MA 1974-1976; PB Brigham Hospital, Boston, MA 1978-1979; **Fellowships:** Research, Mass Genl Hosp, Boston, MA 1976-1978; Cardiology (Cardiovascular Disease), Mass Genl Hosp, Boston, MA 1979-1980; **Faculty Appointment:** Prof Medicine, Harvard Med Sch

Hutter Jr, Adolph M MD (Cardiology (Cardiovascular Disease)) - *Special Expertise: Cardiology (Cardiovascular Disease) - General;* **Admitting Hospital:** Massachusetts General Hospital; **Office Address:** Mass Genl Hosp 55 Fruit St, Bldg ACC - Ste 467 Boston, MA 02114-3139; **Office Phone:** (617) 726-2884; **Board Certifications:** Internal Medicine 1969, Cardiology (Cardiovascular Disease) 1971; **Medical School:** Univ Wisc 1963; **Residency:** Internal Medicine, Strong Meml Hosp, Rochester, MN 1966-1968; **Fellowship:** Cardiology (Cardiovascular Disease), Mass Genl Hosp, Boston, MA 1968-1970; **Faculty Appointment:** Assoc Prof Medicine, Harvard Med Sch

Isner, Jeffrey Michael MD (Cardiology (Cardiovascular Disease)) - *Special Expertise: Cardiac Catheterization; Angioplasty;* **Admitting Hospital:** St Elizabeth's Medical Center; **Office Address:** 736 Cambridge St Boston, MA 02135; **Office Phone:** (617) 789-2392; **Board Certifications:** Internal Medicine 1976, Cardiology (Cardiovascular Disease) 1977; **Medical School:** Tufts Univ 1973; **Residency:** Internal Medicine, Georgetown Hosp 1974-1975; **Fellowship:** Cardiology (Cardiovascular Disease), Georgetown Hosp 1975-1977

Josephson, Mark Eric MD (Cardiology (Cardiovascular Disease)) - *Special Expertise: Cardiac Electrophysiology; Arrhythmias;* **Admitting Hospital:** Beth Israel Deaconess Medical Center - Boston (Page 57); **Office Address:** Beth Israel Deaconess Med Ctr 330 Brookline Ave Boston, MA 02215; **Office Phone:** (617) 667-4387; **Board Certifications:** Cardiology (Cardiovascular Disease) 1975, Cardiac Electrophysiology 1992; **Medical School:** Columbia P&S 1969; **Residency:** Internal Medicine, Mt Sinai Med Ctr, New York, NY 1970-1971; **Fellowship:** Cardiology (Cardiovascular Disease), Hosp Univ Penn, Philadelphia, PA 1973-1975; **Faculty Appointment:** Prof Medicine, Harvard Med Sch

Kirshenbaum, James M MD (Cardiology (Cardiovascular Disease)) - *Special Expertise: Cardiac Catheterization/Angioplasty;* **Admitting Hospital:** Brigham & Women's Hospital; **Office Address:** Brigham & Womens Hosp, Div Card 75 Francis St Boston, MA 02115; **Office Phone:** (617) 732-7173; **Board Certifications:** Internal Medicine 1982, Cardiology (Cardiovascular Disease) 1985; **Medical School:** Harvard Med Sch 1979; **Residency:** Internal Medicine, Peter Bent Brigham & Womens, Boston, MA 1980-1982; **Fellowship:** Cardiology (Cardiovascular Disease), Brigham & Womens, Boston, MA 1982-1985; **Faculty Appointment:** Assoc Prof Medicine, Harvard Med Sch

Konstam, Marvin Amnon MD (Cardiology (Cardiovascular Disease)) - *Special Expertise: Transplant Medicine-Heart; Congestive Heart Failure; Coronary Angioplasty;* **Admitting Hospital:** New England Medical Center; **Office Address:** New England Med Ctr, Div Card 750 Washington St Boston, MA 02111; **Office Phone:** (617) 636-6293; **Board Certifications:** Internal Medicine 1979, Cardiology (Cardiovascular Disease) 1981; **Medical School:** Columbia P&S 1975; **Residencies:** Diagnostic Radiology, Mass Genl Hosp, Boston, MA 1976-1978; Internal Medicine, Mass Genl Hosp, Boston, MA 1978-1979; **Fellowship:** Cardiology (Cardiovascular Disease), Brigham & Women's Hosp, Boston, MA 1979-1981; **Faculty Appointment:** Prof Medicine, Tufts Univ

Libby, Peter MD (Cardiology (Cardiovascular Disease)) - *Special Expertise:* *Atherosclerosis;* **Admitting Hospital:** Brigham & Women's Hospital; **Office Address:** Brigham & Women's Hosp 75 Francis St Boston, MA 02115-5822; **Office Phone:** (617) 732-8086; **Board Certifications:** Internal Medicine 1976, Cardiology (Cardiovascular Disease) 1981; **Medical School:** UCSD 1973; **Residency:** Internal Medicine, Peter Bent Brigham Hosp, Boston, MA 1974-1976; **Fellowships:** Physiology, Harvard Med Sch, Boston, MA 1976-1979; Cardiology (Cardiovascular Disease), Brigham & Woman's Hosp, Boston, MA 1979-1980; **Faculty Appointment:** Prof Medicine, Harvard Med Sch

Loscalzo, Joseph MD (Cardiology (Cardiovascular Disease)) - *Special Expertise:* *Cardiology (Cardiovascular Disease) - General;* **Admitting Hospital:** Boston University Medical Center-East Newton Street Campus; **Office Address:** Boston Univ Med Ctr Hosp-Cardiol Sect Dept Med 88 E Newton St Boston, MA 02118-2394; **Office Phone:** (617) 638-7254; **Board Certifications:** Cardiology (Cardiovascular Disease) 1983, Internal Medicine 1981; **Medical School:** Univ Penn 1978; **Residency:** Internal Medicine, Peter Bent Brigham Hosp., Boston, MA 1979-1981; **Fellowship:** Cardiology (Cardiovascular Disease), Brigham & Women's Hosp, Boston, MA 1981-1983; **Faculty Appointment:** Prof Medicine, Boston Univ

Manning, Warren MD (Cardiology (Cardiovascular Disease)) - *Special Expertise:* *Arrhythmias-Atrial; Echocardiography;* **Admitting Hospital:** Beth Israel Deaconess Medical Center - Boston (Page 57); **Office Address:** Beth Israel Deaconess Med Ctr, Dept Cardiology 330 Brookline Ave Boston, MA 02215-5400; **Office Phone:** (617) 667-2192; **Board Certifications:** Cardiology (Cardiovascular Disease) 1989, Internal Medicine 1986; **Medical School:** Harvard Med Sch 1983; **Residency:** Internal Medicine, Beth Israel Hosp., Boston, MA 1984-1986; **Fellowship:** Cardiology (Cardiovascular Disease), Beth Israel Hosp., Boston, MA 1986-1989; **Faculty Appointment:** Assoc Prof Medicine, Harvard Med Sch

O'Gara, Patrick Thomas MD (Cardiology (Cardiovascular Disease)) - *Special Expertise:* *Heart Valve Disease; Coronary Artery Disease;* **Admitting Hospital:** Brigham & Women's Hospital; **Office Address:** Brigham & Womens Hosp, Cardiovascular Div 75 Francis St Boston, MA 02115; **Office Phone:** (617) 732-8380; **Board Certifications:** Internal Medicine 1981, Cardiology (Cardiovascular Disease) 1983; **Medical School:** Northwestern Univ 1978; **Residency:** Internal Medicine, Mass Genl Hosp, Boston, MA 1984-1986; **Fellowship:** Cardiology (Cardiovascular Disease), Mass Genl Hosp, Boston, MA 1981-1983; **Faculty Appointment:** Assoc Prof Medicine, Harvard Med Sch

Palacios, Igor F MD (Cardiology (Cardiovascular Disease)) - *Special Expertise:* *Interventional Cardiology;* **Admitting Hospital:** Massachusetts General Hospital; **Office Address:** Mass Gen Hosp 55 Fruit St Boston, MA 02114; **Office Phone:** (617) 726-8424; **Board Certifications:** Internal Medicine 1979, Cardiology (Cardiovascular Disease) 1981; **Medical School:** Venezuela 1969; **Residency:** Cardiology (Cardiovascular Disease), Hosp. U de Caracas, Venezuela 1972-1973; **Faculty Appointment:** Assoc Prof Medicine, Harvard Med Sch

Stevenson, Lynne W MD (Cardiology (Cardiovascular Disease)) - *Special Expertise:* *Congestive Heart Failure;* **Admitting Hospital:** Brigham & Women's Hospital; **Office Address:** Brigham & Women's Hosp, Tower 3 75 Francis St Boston, MA 02115; **Office Phone:** (617) 732-7406; **Board Certifications:** Internal Medicine 1982, Cardiology (Cardiovascular Disease) 1985; **Medical School:** Stanford Univ 1979; **Residency:** Internal Medicine, UCLA Med Ctr, Los Angeles, CA 1980-1982; **Fellowship:** Cardiology (Cardiovascular Disease), UCLA Med Ctr, Los Angeles, CA 1982-1984; **Faculty Appointment:** Assoc Prof Medicine, Harvard Med Sch

Weyman, Arthur Edward MD (Cardiology (Cardiovascular Disease)) - *Special Expertise:* *Echocardiography;* **Admitting Hospital:** Massachusetts General Hospital; **Office Address:** Mass Genl Hosp, Cardiac Ultrasound Lab 55 Fruit St Boston, MA 02114; **Office Phone:** (617) 724-7738; **Board Certifications:** Internal Medicine 1973, Cardiology (Cardiovascular Disease) 1975; **Medical School:** UMDNJ-NJ Med Sch, Newark 1966; **Residency:** Internal Medicine, St Vincent's Hosp, New York, NY 1971-1973; **Fellowships:** Cardiology (Cardiovascular Disease), Indiana Univ Med Ctr, Bloomington, IN 1973-1974; Cardiology (Cardiovascular Disease), Indiana Univ Med Ctr, Bloomington, IN 1974-1975; **Faculty Appointment:** Prof Medicine, Harvard Med Sch

Williams, David MD (Cardiology (Cardiovascular Disease)) - *Special Expertise:* *Interventional Cardiology;* **Admitting Hospital:** Rhode Island Hospital; **Office Address:** 2 Dudley St, Ste 360 Providence, RI 02905; **Office Phone:** (401) 444-4581; **Board Certifications:** Internal Medicine 1972, Cardiology (Cardiovascular Disease) 1975; **Medical School:** Hahnemann Univ 1969; **Residency:** Internal Medicine, Hahnemann Univ Hosp, Philadelphia, PA 1970-1972; **Fellowship:** Cardiology (Cardiovascular Disease), UC Davis Med Ctr, Sacramento, CA 1972-1974; **Faculty Appointment:** Prof Medicine, Brown Univ

Zaret, Barry L. MD (Cardiology (Cardiovascular Disease)) - *Special Expertise:* *Nuclear Cardiology; Heart Failure; Coronary Artery Disease;* **Admitting Hospital:** Yale - New Haven Hospital; **Office Address:** 333 Cedar St New Haven, CT 06520; **Office Phone:** (203) 785-4127; **Board Certifications:** Cardiology (Cardiovascular Disease) 1973, Internal Medicine 1973; **Medical School:** NYU Sch Med 1966; **Residency:** Internal Medicine, Bellevue Hosp Ctr, New York, NY 1967-1969; **Fellowship:** Cardiology (Cardiovascular Disease), Johns Hopkins Hosp, Baltimore, MD 1969-1971; **Faculty Appointment:** Prof Medicine, Yale Univ

Mid Atlantic

Abittan, Meyer H MD (Cardiology (Cardiovascular Disease)) - *Special Expertise:* *Angiography - Coronary;* **Admitting Hospital:** St Francis Hospital (Page 75); **Office Address:** 100 Port Washington Blvd Roslyn, NY 11576; **Office Phone:** (516) 365-6444; **Board Certifications:** Cardiology (Cardiovascular Disease) 1991, Interventional Cardiology 1999; **Medical School:** Mount Sinai Sch Med 1984; **Residencies:** Internal Medicine, Brookdale Univ Hosp Med Ctr, Brooklyn, NY 1986-1989; Cardiology (Cardiovascular Disease), Mt Sinai Med Ctr, New York, NY 1989-1990; **Fellowship:** Cardiology (Cardiovascular Disease), Mt Sinai Med Ctr, New York, NY 1989-1990

Achuff, Stephen Charles MD (Cardiology (Cardiovascular Disease)) - *Special Expertise:* *Angina; Heart Valve Disease;* **Admitting Hospital:** Johns Hopkins Hospital - Baltimore (Page 65); **Office Address:** Johns Hopkins Hosp 600 N Wolfe St, Carnegie Bldg, rm 568 Baltimore, MD 21287; **Office Phone:** (410) 955-7670; **Board Certifications:** Internal Medicine 1974, Cardiology (Cardiovascular Disease) 1977; **Medical School:** Univ MO-Columbia Sch Med 1969; **Residencies:** Internal Medicine, Johns Hopkins Hosp, Baltimore, MD 1969-1971; Internal Medicine, Johns Hopkins Hosp, Baltimore, MD 1973-1974; **Fellowships:** Cardiology (Cardiovascular Disease), MD 1971-1973; Cardiology (Cardiovascular Disease), Royal Infirmary, Scotland 1974-1975; **Faculty Appointment:** Prof Medicine, Johns Hopkins Univ

Ambrose, John MD (Cardiology (Cardiovascular Disease)) - *Special Expertise:* *Cardiac Catheterization;* **Admitting Hospital:** St Vincents Catholic Medical Center of New York; **Office Address:** 170 W 12th St New York, NY 10011; **Office Phone:** (212) 604-2818; **Board Certifications:** Internal Medicine 1975, Cardiology (Cardiovascular Disease) 1977; **Medical School:** NY Med Coll 1972; **Residency:** Internal Medicine, Mount Sinai, New York, NY 1972-1975; **Fellowship:** Cardiology (Cardiovascular Disease), Mount Sinai, New York, NY 1975-1977; **Faculty Appointment:** Prof Medicine, NY Med Coll

CARDIOLOGY

Baughman, Kenneth MD (Cardiology (Cardiovascular Disease)) - *Special Expertise:* *Congestive Heart Failure; Cardiomyopathy;* **Admitting Hospital:** Johns Hopkins Hospital - Baltimore (Page 65); **Office Address:** Johns Hopkins Hosp, Dept Cardiology 600 N Wolfe St Baltimore, MD 21287; **Office Phone:** (410) 955-3097; **Board Certifications:** Internal Medicine 1975, Cardiology (Cardiovascular Disease) 1979; **Medical School:** Univ MO-Columbia Sch Med 1972; **Residencies:** Internal Medicine, John Hopkins Hosp, Baltimore, MD 1973-1975; Internal Medicine, John Hopkins Hosp, Baltimore, MD 1975-1977; **Fellowship:** Cardiology (Cardiovascular Disease), Mass Genl Hosp, Boston, MA 1977-1979; **Faculty Appointment:** Prof Medicine, Johns Hopkins Univ

Blumenthal, David S MD (Cardiology (Cardiovascular Disease)) - *Special Expertise:* *Heart Valve Disease;* **Admitting Hospital:** New York Weill Cornell Medical Center - NY Presbyterian Hospital (Page 72); **Office Address:** 407 E 70th St, Fl 1 New York, NY 10021; **Office Phone:** (212) 861-3222; **Board Certifications:** Internal Medicine 1978, Cardiology (Cardiovascular Disease) 1981; **Medical School:** Cornell Univ-Weil Med Coll 1975; **Residencies:** Internal Medicine, NY Hosp-Cornell Univ, New York, NY 1975-1978; Internal Medicine, NY Hosp-Cornell Univ, New York, NY 1980-1981; **Fellowship:** Cardiology (Cardiovascular Disease), Johns Hopkins Hosp, Baltimore, MD 1978-1980; **Faculty Appointment:** Assoc Clin Prof Medicine, Cornell Univ-Weil Med Coll

Borer, Jeffrey MD (Cardiology (Cardiovascular Disease)) - *Special Expertise:* *Heart Valve Disease;* **Admitting Hospital:** New York Weill Cornell Medical Center - NY Presbyterian Hospital (Page 72); **Office Address:** 525 E 68th St New York, NY 10021; **Office Phone:** (212) 746-4646; **Board Certifications:** Internal Medicine 1973, Cardiology (Cardiovascular Disease) 1975; **Medical School:** Cornell Univ-Weil Med Coll 1969; **Residencies:** Internal Medicine, Mass Gen Hosp, Boston, MA 1969-1970; Internal Medicine, Mass Gen Hosp, Boston, MA 1970-1971; **Fellowships:** Cardiology (Cardiovascular Disease), Nat Heart, Lung & Blood Inst, Bethesda, MD 1971-1974; Cardiology (Cardiovascular Disease), Guy's Hosp, London, England 1974-1975; **Faculty Appointment:** Prof Cardiology (Cardiovascular Disease), Cornell Univ-Weil Med Coll

Brozena, Susan Celia MD (Cardiology (Cardiovascular Disease)) - *Special Expertise:* *Transplant Medicine-Heart; Congestive Heart Failure;* **Admitting Hospital:** Hospital of the University of Pennsylvania; **Office Address:** Univ Penn Med Ctr, Div Cardiovascular 3400 Spruce St, 6 Penn Tower Philadelphia, PA 19104; **Office Phone:** (800) 789-7366; **Board Certifications:** Internal Medicine 1984, Cardiology (Cardiovascular Disease) 1987; **Medical School:** Temple Univ 1981; **Residency:** Internal Medicine, Temple Univ Hosp, Philadelphia, PA 1981-1984; **Fellowship:** Cardiology (Cardiovascular Disease), Temple Univ Hosp, Philadelphia, PA 1984-1986; **Faculty Appointment:** Asst Prof Medicine, Hahnemann Univ

Cerqueira, Manuel MD (Cardiology (Cardiovascular Disease)) - *Special Expertise:* *Cardiac Imaging;* **Admitting Hospital:** Georgetown University Hospital; **Office Address:** Georgetown Univ Hosp, Dept Cardiology 3800 Reservoir Rd NW, Fl 5-PHC Washington, DC 20007-2197; **Office Phone:** (202) 687-7190; **Board Certifications:** Nuclear Medicine 1984, Cardiology (Cardiovascular Disease) 1989; **Medical School:** NYU Sch Med 1976; **Residencies:** Cardiology (Cardiovascular Disease), Yale-New Haven Hosp, CT 1980-1982; Internal Medicine, Bellvue Hosp Ctr, New York, NY 1979-1980; **Fellowship:** Nuclear Medicine, Yale-New Haven Hosp, CT 1982-1983; **Faculty Appointment:** Prof Medicine, Georgetown Univ

Cohen, Howard Arthur MD (Cardiology (Cardiovascular Disease)) - *Special Expertise:* *Interventional Cardiology;* **Admitting Hospital:** UPMC - Presbyterian University Hospital; **Office Address:** UPP-Cardiovascular Institute 200 Lothrop St, Bldg S566 - Scaife Hall Pittsburgh, PA 15213; **Office Phone:** (412) 647-6000; **Board Certifications:** Internal Medicine 1974, Cardiology (Cardiovascular Disease) 1977; **Medical School:** NYU Sch Med 1970; **Residency:** Internal Medicine, Bellevue Hosp Ctr, New York, NY 1971-1974; **Fellowship:** Cardiology (Cardiovascular Disease), Johns Hopkins Hosp, Baltimore, MD 1974-1976

Coppola, John MD (Cardiology (Cardiovascular Disease)) - *Special Expertise: Cardiac Catheterization;* **Admitting Hospital:** St Vincents Catholic Medical Center of New York; **Office Address:** 32 W 18th St, FL 4 New York, NY 10011; **Office Phone:** (212) 647-6420; **Board Certifications:** Cardiology (Cardiovascular Disease) 1983, Interventional Cardiology 1999; **Medical School:** NY Med Coll 1978; **Residency:** Internal Medicine, St Vincent's Hosp, New York, NY 1979-1981; **Fellowship:** Cardiology (Cardiovascular Disease), St Vincent's Hosp, New York, NY 1982-1983

Eisen, Howard J MD (Cardiology (Cardiovascular Disease)) - *Special Expertise: Transplant Medicine-Heart; Congestive Heart Failure;* **Admitting Hospital:** Temple University Hospital; **Office Address:** Temple Univ Cardi Transpl Prgm 3401 N Broad St, Ste 320 Philadelphia, PA 19140; **Office Phone:** (215) 707-5900; **Board Certifications:** Internal Medicine 1984, Cardiology (Cardiovascular Disease) 1987; **Medical School:** Univ Penn 1981; **Residency:** Internal Medicine, Hosp Univ Penn, Philadelphia, PA 1982-1984; **Fellowship:** Cardiology (Cardiovascular Disease), Barnes Hosp-Wash Univ, St Louis, MO 1984-1987; **Faculty Appointment:** Prof Medicine, Temple Univ

Follansbee, William MD (Cardiology (Cardiovascular Disease)) - *Special Expertise: Cardiology (Cardiovascular Disease) - General;* **Admitting Hospital:** UPMC - Presbyterian University Hospital; **Office Address:** 200 Lothrop St, Scaife Hall, Ste A382 Pittsburgh, PA 15213; **Office Phone:** (412) 647-3437; **Board Certifications:** Internal Medicine 1977, Cardiology (Cardiovascular Disease) 1981; **Medical School:** Univ Penn 1974; **Residency:** Internal Medicine, Hosp Univ Penn, Philadelphia, PA 1975-1979; **Fellowship:** Cardiology (Cardiovascular Disease), Hosp Univ Penn, Philadelphia, PA 1977-1978

Fuster, Valentin MD (Cardiology (Cardiovascular Disease)) - *Special Expertise: Heart Disease - Congenital; Atherosclerosis;* **Admitting Hospital:** Mount Sinai Hospital (Page 70); **Office Address:** 1 Gustave L Levy Pl, Box 1030 New York, NY 10029; **Office Phone:** (212) 241-7911; **Board Certifications:** Internal Medicine 1976, Cardiology (Cardiovascular Disease) 1977; **Medical School:** Spain 1967; **Residencies:** Internal Medicine, Mayo Clinic, Rochester, MN 1971-1972; Cardiology (Cardiovascular Disease), Mayo Clinic, Rochester, MN 1972-1974; **Fellowship:** Cardiology (Cardiovascular Disease), Univ Edinburgh, Scotland 1968-1971; **Faculty Appointment:** Prof Medicine, Mount Sinai Sch Med

Gliklich, Jerry MD (Cardiology (Cardiovascular Disease)) - *Special Expertise: Heart Valve Disease;* **Admitting Hospital:** Columbia Presbyterian Medical Center (Page 72); **Office Address:** 161 Fort Washington Ave, Ste 645 New York, NY 10032; **Office Phone:** (212) 305-5588; **Board Certifications:** Internal Medicine 1978, Cardiology (Cardiovascular Disease) 1981; **Medical School:** Columbia P&S 1975; **Residency:** Internal Medicine, NY Hosp-Cornell, New York, NY 1975-1978; **Fellowship:** Columbia-Presby, New York, NY 1978-1981; **Faculty Appointment:** Clin Prof Medicine, Columbia P&S

Gottdiener, John MD (Cardiology (Cardiovascular Disease)) - *Special Expertise: Cardiology (Cardiovascular Disease) - General;* **Admitting Hospital:** St Francis Hospital (Page 75); **Office Address:** St Francis Hosp, Dematteis Ctr for Research 100 Port Washington Blvd, Admin Bldg Roslyn, NY 11576; **Office Phone:** (516) 622-4555; **Board Certifications:** Internal Medicine 1975, Cardiology (Cardiovascular Disease) 1979; **Medical School:** Georgetown Univ 1970; **Residency:** Internal Medicine, UNC Hosp, Chapel Hill, NC 1971-1972; **Fellowship:** Cardiology (Cardiovascular Disease), Georgetown Univ Hosp, Washington, DC 1974-1976

Gulotta, Stephen J MD (Cardiology (Cardiovascular Disease)) - *Special Expertise:*
Cardiology (Cardiovascular Disease) - General; **Admitting Hospital:** St Francis Hospital (Page 75); **Office Address:** 100 Port Washington Blvd Roslyn, NY 11576; **Office Phone:** (516) 365-5599; **Board Certifications:** Cardiology (Cardiovascular Disease) 1968, Internal Medicine 1965; **Medical School:** SUNY Hlth Sci Ctr 1958; **Residency:** Montefiore Hosp Med Ctr, Bronx, NY 1959-1961; **Fellowship:** Cardiology (Cardiovascular Disease), NY Hosp, New York, NY 1961-1962

Halperin, Jonathan MD (Cardiology (Cardiovascular Disease)) - *Special Expertise:*
Peripheral Vascular Disease; **Admitting Hospital:** Mount Sinai Hospital (Page 70); **Office Address:** 5 E 98th St, Fl 3 New York, NY 10029; **Office Phone:** (212) 427-1540; **Board Certifications:** Internal Medicine 1980, Cardiology (Cardiovascular Disease) 1981; **Medical School:** Boston Univ 1975; **Residency:** Boston Univ, Boston, MA 1975-1977; **Faculty Appointment:** Prof Medicine

Herling, Irving M MD (Cardiology (Cardiovascular Disease)) - *Special Expertise:*
Cholesterol/Lipid Disorders; Cardiology - Geriatric; **Admitting Hospital:** Hospital of the University of Pennsylvania; **Office Address:** Hosp Univ Penn, Dept Card Med 3400 Spruce St, Penn Tower, Ste 800 Philadelphia, PA 19104-4219; **Office Phone:** (215) 662-6020; **Board Certifications:** Internal Medicine 1977, Cardiology (Cardiovascular Disease) 1979; **Medical School:** Univ Penn 1974; **Residency:** Internal Medicine, Hosp Univ Penn, Philadelphia, PA 1975-1977; **Fellowship:** Cardiology (Cardiovascular Disease), Hosp Univ Penn, Philadelphia, PA 1977; **Faculty Appointment:** Asst Prof Medicine, Univ Penn

Killip, Thomas MD (Cardiology (Cardiovascular Disease)) - *Special Expertise: Cardiology (Cardiovascular Disease) - General;* **Admitting Hospital:** Beth Israel Medical Center - New York; **Office Address:** 1st Ave and 16th St New York, NY 10003; **Office Phone:** (212) 420-4010; **Board Certifications:** Internal Medicine 1977, Cardiology (Cardiovascular Disease) 1968; **Medical School:** Cornell Univ-Weil Med Coll 1952; **Residencies:** Internal Medicine, NY Hospital, New York, NY 1957-1958; Cardiology (Cardiovascular Disease), NY Hospital, New York, NY 1954-1955; **Fellowship:** Cardiac Respiratory Physiology, NY Hospital, New York, NY 1955-1957; **Faculty Appointment:** Prof Medicine, Albert Einstein Coll Med

Klapholz, Marc MD (Cardiology (Cardiovascular Disease)) - *Special Expertise:*
Congestive Heart Failure; Angioplasty; **Admitting Hospital:** St Vincents Hospital & Med Center of N.Y.- Westchester Branch; **Office Address:** St Vincents Catholic Med Ctr, Spellman Bldg 153 W 11th St, Fl 790 New York, NY 10011; **Office Phone:** (212) 604-7380; **Board Certifications:** Internal Medicine 1989, Cardiology (Cardiovascular Disease) 1991; **Medical School:** Albert Einstein Coll Med 1986; **Residency:** Internal Medicine, Bronx Municipal Hosp, Bronx, NY 1986-1989; **Fellowship:** Cardiology (Cardiovascular Disease), Bronx Municipal Hosp, Bronx, NY 1989-1992

Kostis, John B MD (Cardiology (Cardiovascular Disease)) - *Special Expertise:*
Hypertension; **Admitting Hospital:** Robert Wood Johnson University Hospital @ New Brunswick; **Office Address:** 125 Paterson St, Fl 5 New Brunswick, NJ 08903-0019; **Office Phone:** (732) 235-7208; **Board Certifications:** Cardiology (Cardiovascular Disease) 1973, Internal Medicine 1973; **Medical School:** Greece 1960; **Residencies:** Internal Medicine, Evangelism, Athens, Greece 1963-1964; Internal Medicine, Cumberland Med Ctr, Brooklyn, NY 1965-1967; **Fellowship:** Cardiology (Cardiovascular Disease), Philadelphia Genl Hosp, Philadelphia, PA 1967-1969; **Faculty Appointment:** Prof Medicine, UMDNJ-RW Johnson Med Sch

Lindsay Jr, Joseph MD (Cardiology (Cardiovascular Disease)) - *Special Expertise:* *Cardiology (Cardiovascular Disease) - General;* **Admitting Hospital:** Washington Hospital Center - DC (Page 79); **Office Address:** Washington Hosp Ctr, Div Cardiology 110 Irving St NW Washington, DC 20010; **Office Phone:** (202) 877-7597; **Board Certifications:** Internal Medicine 1966, Cardiology (Cardiovascular Disease) 1968; **Medical School:** Emory Univ 1958; **Residencies:** Internal Medicine, Grady Meml Hosp, Atlanta, GA 1959-1960; Cardiology (Cardiovascular Disease), Grady Meml Hosp, Atlanta, GA 1963-1966; **Faculty Appointment:** Prof Medicine, Geo Wash Univ

Moses, Jeffrey W MD (Cardiology (Cardiovascular Disease)) - *Special Expertise:* *Angiography - Coronary; Vascular Medicine;* **Admitting Hospital:** Lenox Hill Hospital; **Office Address:** Advanced Heart Physicians & Surgeons Network 130 E 77th St New York, NY 10021; **Office Phone:** (212) 434-2606; **Board Certifications:** Internal Medicine 1977, Cardiology (Cardiovascular Disease) 1981; **Medical School:** Univ Penn 1974; **Residency:** Internal Medicine, Presby Univ Med Ctr, Philadelphia, PA 1975-1977; **Fellowship:** Cardiology (Cardiovascular Disease), Presby Univ Penn Med Ctr, Philadelphia, PA 1978-1980; **Faculty Appointment:** Clin Prof Medicine, Cornell Univ-Weil Med Coll

Naccarelli, Gerald V MD (Cardiology (Cardiovascular Disease)) - *Special Expertise:* *Cardiac Electrophysiology; Pacemakers;* **Admitting Hospital:** Penn State University Hospital - Milton S.Hershey Medical Center; **Office Address:** Penn State Univ Coll Med 500 University Drive, Box 850 Hershey, PA 17033; **Office Phone:** (717) 531-3907; **Board Certifications:** Internal Medicine 1979, Cardiac Electrophysiology 1992; **Medical School:** Penn State Univ-Hershey Med Ctr 1976; **Residencies:** Internal Medicine, NC Bapt Hosp, Winston-Salem, NC 1977-1978; Internal Medicine, Hershey Med Ctr, Hershey, PA 1979; **Fellowship:** Cardiology (Cardiovascular Disease), Indiana Univ Med Ctr, Indianapolis, IN 1980-1982

Packer, Milton MD (Cardiology (Cardiovascular Disease)) - *Special Expertise:* *Congestive Heart Failure;* **Admitting Hospital:** Columbia Presbyterian Medical Center (Page 72); **Office Address:** Columbia-Prebyterian Med Ctr 177 Ft Washington Ave, Bldg Milstein - Fl 5 New York, NY 10032-3713; **Office Phone:** (212) 305-9260; **Board Certifications:** Internal Medicine 1976, Cardiology (Cardiovascular Disease) 1979; **Medical School:** Jefferson Med Coll 1973; **Residency:** Internal Medicine, Bronx Muni Hosp Ctr, Bronx, NY 1973-1976; **Fellowship:** Cardiology (Cardiovascular Disease), Mount Sinai Hosp, New York, NY 1976-1978

Plehn, Jonathan MD (Cardiology (Cardiovascular Disease)) - *Special Expertise:* *Echocardiography; Congestive Heart Failure;* **Admitting Hospital:** St Francis Hospital (Page 75); **Office Address:** St Francis Hosp, Div Research and Education 100 Port Washington Blvd Roslyn, NY 11576; **Office Phone:** (516) 622-4550; **Board Certifications:** Internal Medicine 1981, Cardiology (Cardiovascular Disease) 1983; **Medical School:** NYU Sch Med 1977; **Residencies:** Internal Medicine, Montefiore Hosp, Pittsburgh, PA 1978-1980; Cardiology (Cardiovascular Disease), Montefiore Hosp, Pittsburgh, PA 1980-1981; **Fellowship:** Cardiology (Cardiovascular Disease), St Lukes Hosp, Chicago, IL 1981-1983; **Faculty Appointment:** Assoc Prof Medicine, SUNY Stony Brook

Sacchi, Terrence J MD (Cardiology (Cardiovascular Disease)) - *Special Expertise:* *Arrhythmias; Cardiac Catheterization; Angiography - Coronary;* **Admitting Hospital:** Long Island College Hospital (Page 58); **Office Address:** 339 Hicks St Brooklyn, NY 11201; **Office Phone:** (718) 780-4626; **Board Certifications:** Internal Medicine 1979, Cardiology (Cardiovascular Disease) 1981; **Medical School:** Albany Med Coll 1976; **Residency:** Internal Medicine, St Vincent's Hosp & Med Ctr, New York, NY 1976-1979; **Fellowships:** Cardiology (Cardiovascular Disease), Georgetown Univ Hosp, Washington, DC 1979-1981; Interventional Cardiology, Mercy Hospital, Des Moines, IA 1986; **Faculty Appointment:** Asst Prof Medicine, SUNY Downstate

CARDIOLOGY

Schulman, Steven Paul MD (Cardiology (Cardiovascular Disease)) - *Special Expertise:* *Cardiology (Cardiovascular Disease) - General;* **Admitting Hospital:** Johns Hopkins Hospital - Baltimore (Page 65); **Office Address:** Johns Hopkins Hosp 600 N Wolfe St, Bldg Carnegie - rm 568 Baltimore, MD 21287-6568; **Office Phone:** (410) 955-7378; **Board Certifications:** Internal Medicine 1986, Cardiology (Cardiovascular Disease) 1989; **Medical School:** Johns Hopkins Univ 1981; **Residency:** Internal Medicine, Johns Hopkins Hosp, Baltimore, MD 1982-1984; **Fellowships:** Cardiology (Cardiovascular Disease), Johns Hopkins Hosp, Baltimore, MD 1984-1985; Cardiology (Cardiovascular Disease), Johns Hopkins Hops, Baltimore, MD 1986-1988; **Faculty Appointment:** Assoc Prof Medicine, Johns Hopkins Univ

Schwartz, Allan MD (Cardiology (Cardiovascular Disease)) - *Special Expertise:* *Interventional Cardiology; Cardiac Catheterization;* **Admitting Hospital:** Columbia Presbyterian Medical Center (Page 72); **Office Address:** 161 Ft Washington Ave, Ste 551 New York, NY 10032-3713; **Office Phone:** (212) 305-5367; **Board Certifications:** Internal Medicine 1977, Cardiology (Cardiovascular Disease) 1979; **Medical School:** Columbia P&S 1974; **Residency:** Internal Medicine, Columbia-Presby Med Ctr, New York, NY 1975-1976; **Fellowship:** Cardiology (Cardiovascular Disease), Mass Genl Hosp, Boston, MA 1976-1978

Segal, Bernard L MD (Cardiology (Cardiovascular Disease)) - *Special Expertise: Stroke; Heart Disease; Non-Invasive Cardiology;* **Admitting Hospital:** Thomas Jefferson University Hospital; **Office Address:** 111 S 11th St, Fl 6215 Philadelphia, PA 19104; **Office Phone:** (215) 955-5050; **Board Certifications:** Internal Medicine 1962, Cardiology (Cardiovascular Disease) 1964; **Medical School:** McGill Univ 1955; **Residencies:** Internal Medicine, Johns Hopkins Hosp, Baltimore, MD 1956-1957; Internal Medicine, Beth Israel Hosp, Boston, MA 1957-1958; **Fellowships:** Cardiology (Cardiovascular Disease), Georgetown Univ Hosp, Washington, DC 1958-1959; Cardiology (Cardiovascular Disease), St George's Hosp, London, England 1959-1960; **Faculty Appointment:** Prof Medicine, Jefferson Med Coll

Shani, Jacob MD (Cardiology (Cardiovascular Disease)) - *Special Expertise: Cardiac Catheterization; Angioplasty; Interventional Cardiology;* **Admitting Hospital:** Maimonides Medical Center (Page 67); **Office Address:** Maimonides Med Ctr, Dept Cardiac Cath Lab 4802 10th Ave Brooklyn, NY 11219-2916; **Office Phone:** (718) 283-7480; **Board Certifications:** Internal Medicine 1981, Cardiology (Cardiovascular Disease) 1983; **Medical School:** Israel 1977; **Residency:** Internal Medicine, Maimonides Med Ctr, Brooklyn, NY 1977-1981; **Fellowship:** Cardiology (Cardiovascular Disease), Beth Israel-Harvard, Boston, MA 1981-1983; **Faculty Appointment:** Clin Prof Medicine, SUNY Downstate

Shlofmitz, Richard A MD (Cardiology (Cardiovascular Disease)) - *Special Expertise:* *Heart Disease; Hypertension;* **Admitting Hospital:** St Francis Hospital (Page 75); **Office Address:** Long Island Interventional Cardiology 100 Port Washington Blvd, Ste 105 Roslyn, NY 11576; **Office Phone:** (516) 365-2900; **Board Certifications:** Internal Medicine 1984, Cardiology (Cardiovascular Disease) 1987; **Medical School:** NYU Sch Med 1980; **Residencies:** Internal Medicine, North Shore Univ Hosp, Manhasset, NY 1980-1984; Cardiology (Cardiovascular Disease), Columbia-Presby Med Ctr, New York, NY 1984-1987

Sonnenblick, Edmund MD (Cardiology (Cardiovascular Disease)) - *Special Expertise:* *Cardiology (Cardiovascular Disease) - General;* **Admitting Hospital:** Montefiore Medical Center - Weiler/Einstein Division; **Office Address:** 1825 Eastchester Rd Bronx, NY 10461-1926; **Office Phone:** (718) 904-2932; **Board Certification:** Internal Medicine 1968; **Medical School:** Harvard Med Sch 1958; **Residency:** Internal Medicine, Columbia-Presby Med Ctr, New York, NY 1959-1963; **Fellowship:** Cardiology (Cardiovascular Disease), Natl Heart Inst, Bethesda, MD 1963-1967; **Faculty Appointment:** Prof Medicine, Albert Einstein Coll Med

Tenenbaum, Joseph MD (Cardiology (Cardiovascular Disease)) - *Special Expertise:* *Cardiology (Cardiovascular Disease) - General;* **Admitting Hospital:** Columbia Presbyterian Medical Center (Page 72); **Office Address:** 161 Ft Washington Ave New York, NY 10032; **Office Phone:** (212) 305-5288; **Board Certifications:** Internal Medicine 1977, Cardiology (Cardiovascular Disease) 1979; **Medical School:** Harvard Med Sch 1974; **Residencies:** Internal Medicine, Columbia-Presby Med Ctr, New York, NY 1974-1977; Mt Sinai Hosp, New York, NY 1977-1979; **Fellowship:** Cardiology (Cardiovascular Disease), Mt Sinai Hosp, New York, NY 1977-1979; **Faculty Appointment:** Prof Medicine, Columbia P&S

Thames, Marc MD (Cardiology (Cardiovascular Disease)) - *Special Expertise: Coronary Artery Disease; Congestive Heart Failure;* **Admitting Hospital:** Temple University Hospital; **Office Address:** Temple Univ Health System, Dept Cardio 3401 N Broad St, Fl 9 Philadelphia, PA 19140; **Office Phone:** (215) 707-3346; **Board Certifications:** Internal Medicine 1974, Cardiology (Cardiovascular Disease) 1979; **Medical School:** Med Coll VA 1970; **Residency:** Internal Medicine, Peter Bent Brigham Hosp, Boston, MA 1971-1974; **Fellowships:** Cardiology Research, Peter Bent Brigham Hosp, Boston, MA 1974-1975; Cardiology (Cardiovascular Disease), Mayo Clinic, Rochester, MN 1975-1977; **Faculty Appointment:** Prof Medicine, Temple Univ

Southeast

Bashore, Thomas MD (Cardiology (Cardiovascular Disease)) - *Special Expertise: Heart Valve Disease;* **Admitting Hospital:** Duke University Medical Center (Page 60); **Office Address:** Duke Univ Med Ctr PO Box 3012 Durham, NC 27710; **Office Phone:** (919) 681-2407; **Board Certifications:** Internal Medicine 1975, Cardiology (Cardiovascular Disease) 1977; **Medical School:** Ohio State Univ 1972; **Residency:** NC Meml Hosp, Chapel Hill, NC 1973-1975; **Fellowship:** Cardiology (Cardiovascular Disease), Duke Univ Med Ctr, Durham, NC 1975-1977; **Faculty Appointment:** Prof Medicine, Duke Univ

Bass, Theodore Adam MD (Cardiology (Cardiovascular Disease)) - *Special Expertise:* *Cardiology (Cardiovascular Disease) - General;* **Admitting Hospital:** Shands Jacksonville Medical Center; **Office Address:** 655 W 8th St, Bldg ACC - Fl 5 Jacksonville, FL 32209-6511; **Office Phone:** (904) 244-2655; **Board Certifications:** Internal Medicine 1979, Cardiology (Cardiovascular Disease) 1981; **Medical School:** Brown Univ 1976; **Residency:** Internal Medicine, Mayo Clinic, Rochester, NY 1977-1979; **Fellowship:** Cardiology (Cardiovascular Disease), Univ Hosp, Boston, MA 1979-1981; **Faculty Appointment:** Prof Medicine, Univ Fla Coll Med

Behar, Victor Samuel MD (Cardiology (Cardiovascular Disease)) - *Special Expertise:* *Cardiac Catheterization; Angioplasty;* **Admitting Hospital:** Duke University Medical Center (Page 60); **Office Address:** Duke Univ Med Ctr Box 3126 Durham, NC 27710-3126; **Office Phone:** (919) 684-4295; **Board Certifications:** Internal Medicine 1968, Cardiology (Cardiovascular Disease) 1973; **Medical School:** Duke Univ 1961; **Residencies:** Internal Medicine, Duke Univ Med Ctr, Durham, NC 1962-1963; Internal Medicine, Duke Univ Med Ctr, Durham, NC 1967-1968; **Fellowship:** Cardiology (Cardiovascular Disease), Duke Univ Med Ctr, Durham, NC 1965-1967; **Faculty Appointment:** Prof Medicine, Duke Univ

Beller, George Allan MD (Cardiology (Cardiovascular Disease)) - *Special Expertise:* *Coronary Artery Disease; Nuclear Cardiology;* **Admitting Hospital:** University of Virginia Health Systems; **Office Address:** Univ VA Health Systems Box 800158 Charlottesville, VA 22908; **Office Phone:** (804) 924-2134; **Board Certifications:** Internal Medicine 1971, Cardiology (Cardiovascular Disease) 1977; **Medical School:** Univ VA Sch Med 1966; **Residencies:** Internal Medicine, Wisc Hosps, Madison, WI 1967-1968; Cardiology (Cardiovascular Disease), Boston City Hosp, Boston, MA 1968-1970; **Fellowship:** Cardiology (Cardiovascular Disease), Mass Genl Hosp, Boston, MA 1973-1974

Bourge, Robert Charles MD (Cardiology (Cardiovascular Disease)) - *Special Expertise:* *Transplant Medicine-Heart;* **Admitting Hospital:** University of Alabama Hospital at Birmingham; **Office Address:** 1900 University Blvd, Bldg 311 Birmingham, AL 35294; **Office Phone:** (205) 934-4011; **Board Certifications:** Internal Medicine 1982, Cardiology (Cardiovascular Disease) 1985; **Medical School:** Louisiana State Univ 1979; **Residency:** Internal Medicine, Univ Alabama Hosp, Birmingham, AL 1979-1982; **Fellowship:** Cardiology (Cardiovascular Disease), Univ Alabama Hosp, Birmingham, AL 1982-1984; **Faculty Appointment:** Prof Medicine, Univ Ala

Byrd III, Benjamin F MD (Cardiology (Cardiovascular Disease)) - *Special Expertise:* *Heart Disease-Congenital; Echocardiography;* **Admitting Hospital:** Vanderbilt University Medical Center; **Office Address:** 2311 Pierce Ave Nashville, TN 37232-8802; **Office Phone:** (615) 322-2318; **Board Certifications:** Internal Medicine 1981, Cardiology (Cardiovascular Disease) 1983; **Medical School:** Vanderbilt Univ 1977; **Residencies:** Psychiatry, Harvard Univ, Boston, MA 1978-1979; Internal Medicine, Vanderbilt Univ Hosp, Nashville, TN 1979-1981; **Fellowships:** Cardiology (Cardiovascular Disease), Vanderbilt Univ Hosp, Nashville, TN 1981-1983; Cardiology (Cardiovascular Disease), UCSF, San Francisco, CA 1983-1984; **Faculty Appointment:** Assoc Prof Cardiology (Cardiovascular Disease), Vanderbilt Univ

Califf, Robert M MD (Cardiology (Cardiovascular Disease)) - *Special Expertise:* *Interventional Cardiology; Heart Failure;* **Admitting Hospital:** Duke University Medical Center (Page 60); **Office Address:** 2400 Pratt St, rm 0311 Terrace Level Durham, NC 27705; **Office Phone:** (919) 681-5816; **Board Certifications:** Internal Medicine 1984, Cardiology (Cardiovascular Disease) 1985; **Medical School:** Duke Univ 1978; **Residency:** Internal Medicine, UCSF, San Francisco, CA 1979-1980; **Fellowships:** Cardiology (Cardiovascular Disease), Duke Univ Med Ctr, Durham, NC 1978; Cardiology (Cardiovascular Disease), Duke Univ Med Ctr, Durham, NC 1980-1983; **Faculty Appointment:** Prof Medicine, Duke Univ

Clements, Stephen MD (Cardiology (Cardiovascular Disease)) - *Special Expertise:* *Cardiacatheterization; Echocardiography;* **Admitting Hospital:** Emory University Hospital; **Office Address:** Emory Clinic 1365 Clifton Rd NE Atlanta, GA 30322; **Office Phone:** (404) 778-4368; **Board Certifications:** Internal Medicine 1971, Cardiology (Cardiovascular Disease) 1975; **Medical School:** Med Coll GA 1966; **Residency:** Internal Medicine, Grady Meml Hosp, Atlanta, GA 1967-1970; **Fellowship:** Cardiology (Cardiovascular Disease), Emory Univ Sch Med, Atlanta, GA 1969-1971; **Faculty Appointment:** Prof Cardiology (Cardiovascular Disease), Emory Univ

Conti, Charles Richard MD (Cardiology (Cardiovascular Disease)) - *Special Expertise:* *Angioplasty; Myocardial Infarction;* **Admitting Hospital:** Shands Healthcare at University Florida (Page 77); **Office Address:** Shands Healthcare Univ FL, Dept Cardio 1600 SW Archer Rd, rm M438 Gainesville, FL 32610; **Office Phone:** (352) 392-4383; **Board Certifications:** Internal Medicine 1967, Cardiology (Cardiovascular Disease) 1971; **Medical School:** Johns Hopkins Univ 1960; **Residencies:** Internal Medicine, Johns Hopkins, Baltimore, MD 1961-1965; Internal Medicine, Johns Hopkins, Baltimore, MD 1967-1968; **Fellowship:** Cardiology (Cardiovascular Disease), Johns Hopkins, Baltimore, MD 1965-1967

Del Negro, Albert Anthony MD (Cardiology (Cardiovascular Disease)) - *Special Expertise:* *Irregular Heartbeat;* **Admitting Hospital:** Fairfax Hospital; **Office Address:** Arrhythmia Assoc, Prosperity Plz 3020 Hamaker Ct, Ste 401 Fairfax, VA 22031-2220; **Office Phone:** (703) 849-0770; **Board Certifications:** Cardiology (Cardiovascular Disease) 1981, Cardiac Electrophysiology 1994; **Medical School:** Georgetown Univ 1969; **Residency:** Internal Medicine, DC Genl Hosp, Washington, DC 1970-1972; **Fellowships:** Cardiology (Cardiovascular Disease), Georgetown Univ Med Ctr, Washington, DC 1972-1973; Cardiology (Cardiovascular Disease), VA Med Ctr, Washington, DC 1973-1974; **Faculty Appointment:** Asst Clin Prof Medicine, Georgetown Univ

Douglas Jr, John Simonton MD (Cardiology (Cardiovascular Disease)) - *Special Expertise:* Congestive Heart Failure; Angiography - Coronary; **Admitting Hospital:** Emory University Hospital; **Office Address:** Emory University Hospital 1364 Clifton Rd, rm c430 Atlanta, GA 30322; **Office Phone:** (404) 727-7040; **Board Certifications:** Cardiology (Cardiovascular Disease) 1975, Interventional Cardiology 1999; **Medical School:** Washington Univ, St Louis 1967; **Residencies:** Internal Medicine, Grady Mem Hosp, Atlanta, GA 1971-1972; Internal Medicine, NC Mem Hosp, Chapel Hill, NC 1968-1969; **Fellowship:** Cardiology (Cardiovascular Disease), Emory Affil Hosps, Atlanta, GA 1972-1974; **Faculty Appointment:** Prof Medicine, Emory Univ

Harrison, John Kevin MD (Cardiology (Cardiovascular Disease)) - *Special Expertise:* Interventional Cardiology; Heart Valve Disease; **Admitting Hospital:** Duke University Medical Center (Page 60); **Office Address:** Duke Univ Med Ctr PO Box 3331 Durham, NC 27710; **Office Phone:** (919) 681-3763; **Board Certifications:** Internal Medicine 1988, Cardiology (Cardiovascular Disease) 1991; **Medical School:** NYU Sch Med 1984; **Residency:** Internal Medicine, Johns Hopkins Hosp, Baltimore, MD 1984-1987; **Fellowship:** Cardiology (Cardiovascular Disease), Duke Univ Med Ctr, Durham, NC 1988-1990; **Faculty Appointment:** Assoc Prof Cardiology (Cardiovascular Disease), Duke Univ

Margolis, James MD (Cardiology (Cardiovascular Disease)) - *Special Expertise:* Cardiac Catherization; Invasive Cardiology; **Admitting Hospital:** Miami Heart Institute - North Campus; **Office Address:** Miami Intl Cardiac Consultants 4701 N Meridian Ave, Bldg Adams - Ste 440 Miami Beach, FL 33140-2910; **Office Phone:** (305) 674-3117; **Board Certifications:** Cardiology (Cardiovascular Disease) 1975, Interventional Cardiology 1999; **Medical School:** Univ IL Coll Med 1968; **Residency:** Internal Medicine, Barnes Hosp, St Louis, MO 1971-1972; **Fellowship:** Cardiology (Cardiovascular Disease), Duke Med Ctr, Durham, NC 1972-1974; **Faculty Appointment:** Clin Prof Medicine, Univ Miami Sch Med

Myerburg, Robert MD (Cardiology (Cardiovascular Disease)) - *Special Expertise:* Cardiac Electrophysiology; Arrhythmias - Defibrillators/Pacemakers; Sudden Cardiac Death; **Admitting Hospital:** University of Miami - Jackson Memorial Hospital; **Office Address:** Univ Miami Sch Med, Div Cardio, D-39, Box 16960 Miami, FL 33101-6960; **Office Phone:** (305) 585-5523; **Board Certifications:** Cardiology (Cardiovascular Disease) 1970; Cardiac Electrophysiology 1998; **Medical School:** Univ MD Sch Med 1961; **Residency:** Internal Medicine, Charity Hosp, New Orleans, LA 1964-1966; **Fellowships:** Cardiology (Cardiovascular Disease), Grady Meml Hosp, Atlanta, GA 1966-1968; Cardiac Electrophysiology, Columbia Univ Coll P & S, New York, NY 1968-1970; **Faculty Appointment:** Prof Medicine, Univ Miami Sch Med

Nocero, Michael MD (Cardiology (Cardiovascular Disease)) - *Special Expertise:* Nuclear Cardiology; **Admitting Hospital:** Florida Hospital; **Office Address:** Central Fla Cardi Group 500 E Colonial Drive Orlando, FL 32803-4504; **Office Phone:** (407) 841-7151; **Board Certifications:** Internal Medicine 1972, Cardiology (Cardiovascular Disease) 1976; **Medical School:** NYU Sch Med 1966; **Residencies:** Internal Medicine, Bellevue Hosp Ctr NYU, New York, NY 1967-1968; Internal Medicine, Bellevue Hosp Ctr NYU, New York, NY 1970-1971; **Fellowship:** Cardiology (Cardiovascular Disease), Bellevue Hosp Ctr NYU, New York, NY 1971-1973

Pepine, Carl J MD (Cardiology (Cardiovascular Disease)) - *Special Expertise:* Heart Disease - Ischemic; **Admitting Hospital:** Shands Healthcare at University Florida (Page 77); **Office Address:** Univ Florida Coll Med, Div Cardio 1600 Archer Rd, Box 100277 Gainesville, FL 32610-0277; **Office Phone:** (352) 846-0620; **Board Certifications:** Internal Medicine 1971, Cardiology (Cardiovascular Disease) 1973; **Medical School:** UMDNJ-NJ Med Sch, Newark 1966; **Residencies:** Internal Medicine, Jefferson Univ Hosp, Philadelphia, PA 1967-1968; Internal Medicine, Naval Hosp-Thomas Jefferson Univ, Philadelphia, PA 1968-1969; **Fellowship:** Cardiology (Cardiovascular Disease), Naval Hosp-Thomas Jeff Univ, Philadelphia, PA 1969-1971; **Faculty Appointment:** Prof Medicine, Univ Fla Coll Med

CARDIOLOGY Southeast

Phillips III, Harry Rissler MD (Cardiology (Cardiovascular Disease)) - *Special Expertise:* Angioplasty; Cardiac Catheterization; **Admitting Hospital:** Duke University Medical Center (Page 60); **Office Address:** Duke Univ Med Ctr, Cardio Assocs 7412 Hospital N, Box 3126 Durham, NC 27710; **Office Phone:** (919) 681-4804; **Board Certifications:** Internal Medicine 1978, Cardiology (Cardiovascular Disease) 1979; **Medical School:** Duke Univ 1975; **Residency:** Internal Medicine, Mass Genl Hosp, Boston, MA 1976-1977; **Fellowship:** Cardiology (Cardiovascular Disease), Mass Genl Hosp, Boston, MA 1977-1979

Powers, Eric Randall MD (Cardiology (Cardiovascular Disease)) - *Special Expertise:* Heart Valve Disease; Interventional Cardiology; **Admitting Hospital:** University of Virginia Health Systems; **Office Address:** Univ VA Hlth Scis Ctr Box 80062 Charlottesville, VA 22908-0001; **Office Phone:** (804) 924-5204; **Board Certifications:** Internal Medicine 1977, Cardiology (Cardiovascular Disease) 1979; **Medical School:** Harvard Med Sch 1974; **Residency:** Internal Medicine, Mass Genl Hosp, Boston, MA 1974-1976; **Fellowship:** Cardiology (Cardiovascular Disease), Mass Genl Hosp, Boston, MA 1976-1979; **Faculty Appointment:** Prof Medicine, Univ VA Sch Med

Robertson, Rose Marie MD (Cardiology (Cardiovascular Disease)) - *Special Expertise:* Autonomic Disorders; Syncope; **Admitting Hospital:** Vanderbilt University Medical Center; **Office Address:** Vanderbilt Univ Med Ctr, Div of Cardiology 2200 Pierce Ave, Bldg MRB II - rm 315 Nashville, TN 37232-6300; **Office Phone:** (615) 322-2318; **Board Certifications:** Internal Medicine 1974, Cardiology (Cardiovascular Disease) 1975; **Medical School:** Harvard Med Sch 1970; **Residency:** Internal Medicine, Mass Gen'l Hosp, Boston, MA 1971-1972; **Fellowship:** Cardiology (Cardiovascular Disease), Johns Hopkins Hosp, Baltimore, MD 1973-1975; **Faculty Appointment:** Prof Medicine, Vanderbilt Univ

Russell Jr, Richard MD (Cardiology (Cardiovascular Disease)) - *Special Expertise:* Mitral Valve Disease; **Admitting Hospital:** Montclair - Baptist Medical Center; **Office Address:** Cardiovasc Associates PC 880 Montclair Rd, Fl 1 Birmingham, AL 35213; **Office Phone:** (205) 599-3500; **Board Certifications:** Internal Medicine 1965, Cardiology (Cardiovascular Disease) 1967; **Medical School:** Vanderbilt Univ 1956; **Residencies:** Internal Medicine, Peter Bent Brigham Hosp, Boston, MA 1959-1960; Internal Medicine, Peter Bent Brigham Hosp, Boston, MA 1963-1964; **Fellowship:** Cardiology (Cardiovascular Disease), Med Coll Alabama Hosp, Birmingham, AL 1960-1962; **Faculty Appointment:** Clin Prof Medicine, Univ Ala

Smith Jr, Sidney C MD (Cardiology (Cardiovascular Disease)) - *Special Expertise:* Cardiology (Cardiovascular Disease) - General; **Admitting Hospital:** University of North Carolina Hospitals; **Office Address:** Univ NC-Chapel Hill, Div Cardiology 324 Barnett-Womack Bldg, Campus Box 7075 Chapel Hill, NC 27599-7075; **Office Phone:** (919) 966-0732; **Board Certifications:** Internal Medicine 1972, Cardiology (Cardiovascular Disease) 1973; **Medical School:** Yale Univ 1967; **Residency:** Internal Medicine, Peter Bent Brigham Hosp, Boston, MA 1968-1969; **Fellowships:** Cardiology (Cardiovascular Disease), Peter Bent Brigham Hosp, Boston, MA 1969-1971; Research, Harvard Med Sch, Boston, MA 1969-1971; **Faculty Appointment:** Prof Medicine, Univ NC Sch Med

Vetrovec, George MD (Cardiology (Cardiovascular Disease)) - *Special Expertise:* Interventional Cardiology; **Admitting Hospital:** Medical College of Virginia Hospitals; **Office Address:** 1200 E Broad St, Fl 6th, Box 980036 Richmond, VA 23298; **Office Phone:** (804) 828-8885; **Board Certifications:** Cardiology (Cardiovascular Disease) 1977, Interventional Cardiology 1999; **Medical School:** Univ VA Sch Med 1970; **Residency:** Internal Medicine, Med Coll Virginia Hosp, Richmond, VA 1971-1974; **Fellowship:** Cardiology (Cardiovascular Disease), Med Coll Virginia Hosp, Richmond, VA 1974-1976; **Faculty Appointment:** Prof Medicine, Med Coll VA

Vignola, Paul MD (Cardiology (Cardiovascular Disease)) - *Special Expertise:*
Interventional Cardiology; **Admitting Hospital:** Mount Sinai Medical Center; **Office Address:**
MSMC Invasive Cardiology Group 4300 Alton Rd Miami Beach, FL 33140-2800; **Office Phone:**
(305) 674-2533; **Board Certifications:** Cardiology (Cardiovascular Disease) 1977, Interventional
Cardiology 1999; **Medical School:** Yale Univ 1971; **Residency:** Infectious Disease, Yale-New
Haven Hosp, New Haven, CT 1972-1974; **Fellowship:** Cardiology (Cardiovascular Disease), Mass
Genl Hospital-Harvard, Boston, MA 1974-1976

Wenger, Nanette Kass MD (Cardiology (Cardiovascular Disease)) - *Special Expertise:*
Heart Disease in Women; Heart Disease in the Elderly; **Admitting Hospital:** Grady Health System;
Office Address: Univ Sch of Med 69 Butler St SE Atlanta, GA 30303; **Office Phone:** (404) 616-4420;
Medical School: Harvard Med Sch 1954; **Residency:** Internal Medicine, Mt Sinai Med Ctr, New
York, NY 1954-1957; **Fellowship:** Cardiology (Cardiovascular Disease), Emory Univ Sch Med,
Atlanta, GA 1958-1959; **Faculty Appointment:** Prof Medicine, Emory Univ

Midwest

Armstrong, William F MD (Cardiology (Cardiovascular Disease)) - *Special Expertise:*
Non-Invasive Cardiology; **Admitting Hospital:** University of Michigan Health Center; **Office
Address:** Briarwood Specialty Center 325 Briarwood Circle-Bldg 5 Ann Arbor, MI 48108; **Office
Phone:** (734) 647-9000; **Board Certifications:** Internal Medicine 1979, Cardiology (Cardiovascular
Disease) 1981; **Medical School:** Va Commonwealth Univ 1976; **Residency:** Internal Medicine,
Med Coll of Virginia Hosp, VA 1977-1979; **Fellowship:** Cardiology (Cardiovascular Disease),
Indiana University Hosp 1979-1982; **Faculty Appointment:** Prof Medicine, Univ Mich Med Sch

Bonow, Robert O MD (Cardiology (Cardiovascular Disease)) - *Special Expertise:*
Cardiology (Cardiovascular Disease) - General; **Admitting Hospital:** Northwestern Memorial
Hospital; **Office Address:** 675 N St Clair St, Bldg Galter - Fl 19 Chicago, IL 60611; **Office Phone:**
(312) 908-1052; **Board Certifications:** Internal Medicine 1976, Cardiology (Cardiovascular
Disease) 1981; **Medical School:** Univ Penn 1973; **Residency:** Internal Medicine, Hosp Univ Penn,
Philadelphia, PA 1974-1976; **Fellowship:** Cardiology (Cardiovascular Disease), Nat Heart Inst,
Bethesda, MD 1976-1979; **Faculty Appointment:** Prof Medicine, Northwestern Univ

Borzak, Steven MD (Cardiology (Cardiovascular Disease)) - *Special Expertise:*
Myocardial Infarction; Angina-Unstable; **Admitting Hospital:** Henry Ford Health System (Page
62); **Office Address:** Henry Ford Hospital 2799 W Grand Blvd Detroit, MI 48202; **Office Phone:**
(313) 916-9406; **Board Certifications:** Internal Medicine 1987, Cardiology (Cardiovascular
Disease) 1991; **Medical School:** Univ IL Coll Med 1984; **Residency:** Internal Medicine, Michael
Reese Hosp, Chicago, IL 1985-1988; **Fellowship:** Cardiology (Cardiovascular Disease), Brigham &
Women's Hosp, Boston, MA 1988-1991; **Faculty Appointment:** Asst Prof Medicine, Case West Res
Univ

Braverman, Alan Charles MD (Cardiology (Cardiovascular Disease)) - *Special
Expertise:* *Marfan's syndrome; Aortic Diseases & Dissection;* **Admitting Hospital:** Barnes - Jewish
Hospital; **Office Address:** Barnes-Jewish Hosp 1 Barnes Hospital Plaza, Ste 16419 St Louis, MO
63110; **Office Phone:** (314) 362-1291; **Board Certifications:** Internal Medicine 1988, Cardiology
(Cardiovascular Disease) 1991; **Medical School:** Univ MO-Kansas City 1985; **Residencies:** Internal
Medicine, Brigham-Women's Hosp, Boston, MA 1985-1988; Internal Medicine, Brigham-Women's
Hosp, Boston, MA 1990-1991; **Fellowship:** Cardiology (Cardiovascular Disease), Brigham-
Women's Hosp/Harvard, Boston, MA 1988-1990; **Faculty Appointment:** Assoc Prof Medicine,
Washington Univ, St Louis

CARDIOLOGY

Burket, Mark W. MD (Cardiology (Cardiovascular Disease)) - *Special Expertise:*
Peripheral Vascular Intervention; **Admitting Hospital:** Medical College of Ohio Hospitals; **Office Address:** 3000 Arlington Ave Dept Med Toledo, OH 43614-5809; **Office Phone:** (419) 383-3697; **Board Certifications:** Internal Medicine 1982, Cardiology (Cardiovascular Disease) 1985; **Medical School:** Ohio State Univ 1979; **Residency:** Internal Medicine, Ohio State Univ, Columbus, OH 1980-1982; **Fellowship:** Cardiology (Cardiovascular Disease), Med Coll Ohio, Toledo, OH 1982-1985

Chaitman, Bernard R. MD (Cardiology (Cardiovascular Disease)) - *Special Expertise:*
Nuclear Cardiology; **Admitting Hospital:** St Louis University Hospital; **Office Address:** St Louis Univ Sch Med 3635 Vista Ave at Grand Blvd St.Louis, MO 63110; **Office Phone:** (314) 577-6190; **Board Certifications:** Internal Medicine 1973, Cardiology (Cardiovascular Disease) 1975; **Medical School:** McGill Univ 1969; **Residency:** Internal Medicine, Royal Victoria Hosp, Montreal Canada 1970-1972; **Fellowship:** Cardiology (Cardiovascular Disease), Univ Oregon Hosp, Portland, OR 1972-1974; **Faculty Appointment:** Prof Medicine, St Louis Univ

Cody Jr., Robert James MD (Cardiology (Cardiovascular Disease)) - *Special Expertise:*
Congestive Heart Failure; Transplant Medicine-Heart; **Admitting Hospital:** University of Michigan Health Center; **Office Address:** 1500 E Medical Ctr Dr , Bldg Women's - rm L3623 Ann Arbor, MI 48109-0271; **Office Phone:** (734) 936-5255; **Board Certifications:** Internal Medicine 1977, Cardiology (Cardiovascular Disease) 1981; **Medical School:** Penn State Univ-Hershey Med Ctr 1974; **Residency:** Internal Medicine, Cleveland Clinic Hospital, Cleveland, OH 1974-1978; **Fellowship:** Cardiology (Cardiovascular Disease), Mass Genl Hosp, Boston, MA 1978-1980; **Faculty Appointment:** Prof Cardiology (Cardiovascular Disease), Univ Mich Med Sch

Cooper, Christopher MD (Cardiology (Cardiovascular Disease)) - *Special Expertise:*
Radial Artery Catherization; **Admitting Hospital:** Medical College of Ohio Hospitals; **Office Address:** 3000 Arlington Ave Toledo, OH 43614; **Office Phone:** (419) 383-3925; **Board Certifications:** Internal Medicine 1991, Cardiology (Cardiovascular Disease) 1995; **Medical School:** Univ Cincinnati 1988; **Residency:** Internal Medicine, Brigham & Womens Hosp, Boston, MA 1989-1991; **Fellowship:** Cardiology (Cardiovascular Disease), Brigham & Women's Hosp-Harvard Med Sch, Boston, MA 1991-1994

Costanzo, Maria Rosa MD (Cardiology (Cardiovascular Disease)) - *Special Expertise:*
Transplant Medicine-Heart; Congestive Heart Failure; **Admitting Hospital:** Rush/Presbyterian - St Luke's Medical Center - Chicago (Page 74); **Office Address:** Rush Presby St Luke's Med Ctr, Cardiac Transplant Program 1725 West Harrison St, rm 439 Chicago, IL 60612; **Office Phone:** (312) 563-2121; **Board Certifications:** Internal Medicine 1982, Cardiology (Cardiovascular Disease) 1985; **Medical School:** Italy 1978; **Residency:** Internal Medicine, Lutheran Genl Hosp, Park Ridge, IL 1980-1982; **Fellowship:** Cardiology (Cardiovascular Disease), Loyola Univ Med Ctr, Chicago, IL 1982-1984; **Faculty Appointment:** Prof Medicine, Rush Med Coll

De Franco, Anthony MD (Cardiology (Cardiovascular Disease)) - *Special Expertise:*
Electron Beam Tomography; **Admitting Hospital:** McLaren Regional Medical Center; **Office Address:** McLaren Regional Med Ctr 401 S Ballenger Hwy Flint, MI 48532; **Office Phone:** (810) 342-3029; **Board Certifications:** Internal Medicine 1989, Cardiology (Cardiovascular Disease) 1993; **Medical School:** Tufts Univ 1985; **Residency:** Internal Medicine, Univ Chicago Med Ctr, Chicago, IL 1986-1988; **Fellowship:** Cardiology (Cardiovascular Disease), Cleveland Clinic, Cleveland, OH 1990-1993

Eagle, Kim A MD (Cardiology (Cardiovascular Disease)) - *Special Expertise:* Cardiology *(Cardiovascular Disease) - General;* **Admitting Hospital:** University of Michigan Health Center; **Office Address:** Univ Mich Med Ctr, Dept Int Med-Cardio 1500 E Medical Center Drive, Bldg TC - Ste 3910 Ann Arbor, MI 48109-0366; **Office Phone:** (734) 936-5275; **Board Certifications:** Internal Medicine 1982, Cardiology (Cardiovascular Disease) 1987; **Medical School:** Tufts Univ 1979; **Residency:** Internal Medicine, Yale New Haven Hosp-Yale Univ, New Haven, CT 1980-1983; **Fellowship:** Cardiology (Cardiovascular Disease), Mass Genl Hosp-Harvard, Boston, MA 1983-1986; **Faculty Appointment:** Asst Prof Medicine, Univ Mich Med Sch

Faxon, David P MD (Cardiology (Cardiovascular Disease)) - *Special Expertise:* Interventional Cardiology; **Admitting Hospital:** University of Chicago Hospitals (Page 78); **Office Address:** Univ Chicago Hosps 5841 S Maryland Ave, MC-6080 Chicago, IL 60637; **Office Phone:** (773) 702-1919; **Board Certifications:** Internal Medicine 1974, Cardiology (Cardiovascular Disease) 1977; **Medical School:** Boston Univ 1971; **Residency:** Internal Medicine, Mary Hitchcock Meml Hosp 1972-1974; **Fellowship:** Cardiology (Cardiovascular Disease), Mary Hitchcock Meml Hosp 1974-1976; **Faculty Appointment:** Assoc Prof Medicine

Gardin, Julius Markus MD (Cardiology (Cardiovascular Disease)) - *Special Expertise:* Cardiology *(Cardiovascular Disease) - General;* **Admitting Hospital:** St John Hospital and Medical Center; **Office Address:** St John's Medical Center 22151 Moross Rd, PB1, Ste 105 Detroit, MI 48236; **Office Phone:** (313) 343-6390; **Board Certifications:** Internal Medicine 1975, Cardiology (Cardiovascular Disease) 1977; **Medical School:** Univ Mich Med Sch 1972; **Residency:** Internal Medicine, Univ Mich Hosp, Ann Arbor, MI 1973-1975; **Fellowship:** Cardiology (Cardiovascular Disease), Georgetown Univ Hosp, Washington, DC 1975-1977; **Faculty Appointment:** Prof Medicine, Univ Mich Med Sch

Gibbons, Raymond John MD (Cardiology (Cardiovascular Disease)) - *Special Expertise:* Nuclear Cardiology; **Admitting Hospital:** Mayo Medical Center & Clinic - Rochester; **Office Address:** Mayo Clinic 200 1st St SW Rochester, MN 55905; **Office Phone:** (507) 284-2541; **Board Certifications:** Internal Medicine 1979, Cardiology (Cardiovascular Disease) 1981; **Medical School:** Harvard Med Sch 1976; **Residency:** Internal Medicine, Mass Genl Hosp, Boston, MA 1977-1978; **Fellowship:** Cardiology (Cardiovascular Disease), Duke Univ Med Ctr, Durham, NC 1978-1981; **Faculty Appointment:** Prof Medicine, Mayo Med Sch

Grubb, Blair Paul MD (Cardiology (Cardiovascular Disease)) - *Special Expertise:* Autonomic Disorders; Cardiac Electrophysiology; **Admitting Hospital:** Medical College of Ohio Hospitals; **Office Address:** Medical College of Ohio - Cardiac Clinic 3000 Arlington Ave, Fl 3 Toledo, OH 43614; **Office Phone:** (419) 383-3925; **Board Certifications:** Internal Medicine 1985, Cardiac Electrophysiology 1987; **Medical School:** Dominican Republic 1980; **Residency:** Grtr Baltimore Med Ctr, Baltimore, MD 1982-1985; **Fellowship:** Cardiology (Cardiovascular Disease), MS Hershey Med Ctr/Penn State, PA 1985-1988; **Faculty Appointment:** Asst Prof Medicine, Univ SD Sch Med

Jaffe, Allan S. MD (Cardiology (Cardiovascular Disease)) - *Special Expertise:* Cardiology *(Cardiovascular Disease) - General;* **Admitting Hospital:** Mayo Medical Center & Clinic - Rochester; **Office Address:** Mayo Clinic-Cardiovascular Disease 200 First St SW Rochester, MN 55905; **Office Phone:** (507) 284-9325; **Board Certifications:** Internal Medicine 1976, Cardiology (Cardiovascular Disease) 1979; **Medical School:** Univ MD Sch Med 1973; **Residencies:** Internal Medicine, Barnes Hosp Wash U, St Louis, MO 1974-1975; Internal Medicine, Washington Univ, St Louis, MO 1976; **Fellowship:** Cardiology (Cardiovascular Disease), Barnes Hosp Wash U, St Louis, MO 1976-1978; **Faculty Appointment:** Prof Medicine, Washington Univ, St Louis

Johnson, Maryl R MD (Cardiology (Cardiovascular Disease)) - *Special Expertise:* *Congestive Heart Failure; Transplant-Heart;* **Admitting Hospital:** Northwestern Memorial Hospital; **Office Address:** 675 N St Claire Fl 19 Chicago, IL 60611; **Office Phone:** (312) 695-4965; **Board Certifications:** Cardiology (Cardiovascular Disease) 1983, Internal Medicine 1981; **Medical School:** Univ Iowa Coll Med 1977; **Residency:** Internal Medicine, U IA Hosp, Iowa City, IA 1978-1981; **Fellowship:** Cardiology (Cardiovascular Disease), U IA Hosp, Iowa City, IA 1979-1982; **Faculty Appointment:** Medicine, Northwestern Univ

Kereiakes, Dean J MD (Cardiology (Cardiovascular Disease)) - *Special Expertise:* *Interventional Cardiology;* **Admitting Hospital:** Christ Hospital; **Office Address:** 2123 Auburn Ave, Ste 139 Cincinnati, OH 45219-2966; **Office Phone:** (513) 721-8881; **Board Certifications:** Cardiology (Cardiovascular Disease) 1985, Internal Medicine 1981; **Medical School:** Univ Cincinnati 1978; **Residencies:** Internal Medicine, Mass Genl Hospital, Boston, MA 1980-1981; Internal Medicine, UC San Francisco, San Francisco, CA 1981-1982; **Fellowship:** Cardiology (Cardiovascular Disease), UC San Francisco, San Francisco, CA 1982-1984; **Faculty Appointment:** Clin Prof Medicine, Univ Cincinnati

Mehlman, David J MD (Cardiology (Cardiovascular Disease)) - *Special Expertise:* *Echocardiography;* **Admitting Hospital:** Northwestern Memorial Hospital; **Office Address:** Northwestern Univ Med Ctr 250 E Superior St, Wesley Bldg, Ste 586 Chicago, IL 60611-2914; **Office Phone:** (312) 695-4965; **Board Certifications:** Internal Medicine 1976, Cardiology (Cardiovascular Disease) 1979; **Medical School:** Johns Hopkins Univ 1973; **Residency:** Internal Medicine, Johns Hopkins Hosp, Baltimore, MD 1974-1976; **Fellowship:** Cardiology (Cardiovascular Disease), Univ Chicago Hosps, Chicago, IL 1976-1978; **Faculty Appointment:** Assoc Prof Medicine, Northwestern Univ

Moran, John MD (Cardiology (Cardiovascular Disease)) - *Special Expertise:* *Coronary Artery Disease;* **Admitting Hospital:** Loyola University Health System; **Office Address:** Loyola University Medical Center 2160 S 1st Avenue Maywood, IL 60153; **Office Phone:** (708) 327-3600; **Board Certifications:** Internal Medicine 1971, Cardiology (Cardiovascular Disease) 1973; **Medical School:** Loyola Univ-Stritch Sch Med 1964; **Residency:** Internal Medicine, Univ Ill Rsch Ed Hosp, Chicago, IL 1965-1967; **Fellowship:** Cardiology (Cardiovascular Disease), Univ Ill Rsch Ed Hosp, Chicago, IL 1967-1969; **Faculty Appointment:** Prof Medicine, Loyola Univ-Stritch Sch Med

Nemickas, Rimgaudas MD (Cardiology (Cardiovascular Disease)) - *Special Expertise:* *Cardiology (Cardiovascular Disease) - General;* **Admitting Hospital:** Illinois Masonic Medical Center (Page 64); **Office Address:** 3000 N Halsted St, Ste 703 Cardiac Diagnosis Ltd Chicago, IL 60657-5194; **Office Phone:** (773) 296-3600; **Board Certifications:** Internal Medicine 1969, Cardiology (Cardiovascular Disease) 1973; **Medical School:** Loyola Univ-Stritch Sch Med 1961; **Residency:** Internal Medicine, Univ Ill Med Clinic, Chicago, IL 1966-1967; **Fellowships:** Cardiology (Cardiovascular Disease), Cook County Hosp, Chicago, IL 1962-1963; Cardiology (Cardiovascular Disease), Univ Chicago Hosp, Chicago, IL 1967-1969; **Faculty Appointment:** Clin Prof Medicine, Loyola Univ-Stritch Sch Med

O'Neill, William MD (Cardiology (Cardiovascular Disease)) - *Special Expertise:* *Interventional Cardiology;* **Admitting Hospital:** William Beaumont Hospital; **Office Address:** 3601 W 13 Mile Rd, Fl 3 Heart Center Royal Oak, MI 48073; **Office Phone:** (248) 551-4163; **Board Certifications:** Internal Medicine 1980, Cardiology (Cardiovascular Disease) 1983; **Medical School:** Wayne State Univ 1977; **Residency:** Internal Medicine, Wayne State U Affil Hosps, MI 1978-1980

Rahko, Peter MD (Cardiology (Cardiovascular Disease)) - *Special Expertise:* Congestive *Heart Failure; Heart Valve Disease; Echocardiography;* **Admitting Hospital:** University of Wisconsin Hospital & Clinics; **Office Address:** Univ Wisc Hosp & Clin 600 Highland Ave, Ste 86 Madison, WI 53792; **Office Phone:** (608) 263-1530; **Board Certifications:** Internal Medicine 1982; Cardiology (Cardiovascular Disease) 1985; **Medical School:** Univ Minn 1979; **Residency:** Internal Medicine, Indiana Univ Med Ctr, Indianapolis, IN 1979-1982; **Fellowship:** Cardiology (Cardiovascular Disease), Univ Pittsburgh, Pittsburgh, PA 1982-1985; **Faculty Appointment:** Assoc Prof Medicine, Univ Wisc

Reiss, Craig MD (Cardiology (Cardiovascular Disease)) - *Special Expertise:* Heart Disease *- Ischemic; Coronary Artery Disease;* **Admitting Hospital:** Barnes - Jewish Hospital; **Office Address:** 1 Barnes Hosp Plz, Ste 16419 St Louis, MO 63110-1036; **Office Phone:** (314) 362-1291; **Board Certifications:** Internal Medicine 1986, Cardiology (Cardiovascular Disease) 1989; **Medical School:** Univ MO-Kansas City 1983; **Residencies:** Internal Medicine, Brigham & Women's Hosp, Boston, MA 1984-1986; Internal Medicine, Brigham & Women's Hosp, Boston, MA 1988-1989; **Fellowship:** Cardiology (Cardiovascular Disease), Brigham& Women's Hosp, Boston, MA 1986-1988; **Faculty Appointment:** Assoc Prof Medicine, Washington Univ, St Louis

Rich, Stuart MD (Cardiology (Cardiovascular Disease)) - *Special Expertise:* Pulmonary *Hypertension; Congestive Heart Failure;* **Admitting Hospital:** Rush/Presbyterian - St Luke's Medical Center - Chicago (Page 74); **Office Address:** Rush Heart Inst Ctr Pulm Heart Disease 1725 W Harrison St, Ste 020 Chicago, IL 60612; **Office Phone:** (312) 563-2169; **Board Certifications:** Internal Medicine 1978, Cardiology (Cardiovascular Disease) 1981; **Medical School:** Loyola Univ-Stritch Sch Med 1974; **Residency:** Internal Medicine, Jewish Hosp, St Louis, MO 1975-1978; **Fellowship:** Cardiology (Cardiovascular Disease), Univ Chicago, Chicago, IL 1978-1980; **Faculty Appointment:** Prof Medicine, Rush Med Coll

Rogers, Joseph MD (Cardiology (Cardiovascular Disease)) - *Special Expertise:* Congestive *Heart Failure; Transplant Medicine-Heart;* **Admitting Hospital:** Barnes - Jewish Hospital; **Office Address:** Barnes Jewish Heart Failure Transplant Svcs Ste 4455, MC-903161 St Louis, MO 63110; **Office Phone:** (314) 454-7687; **Board Certifications:** Internal Medicine 1991, Cardiology (Cardiovascular Disease) 1995; **Medical School:** Univ Nebr Coll Med 1988; **Residency:** Internal Medicine, Univ Nebraska Med Ctr, Omaha, NE 1988-1991; **Fellowship:** Cardiology (Cardiovascular Disease), Wash Univ Med Ctr, St Louis, MO 1991-1995; **Faculty Appointment:** Cardiology (Cardiovascular Disease), Washington Univ, St Louis

Safian, Robert D MD (Cardiology (Cardiovascular Disease)) - *Special Expertise:* Interventional *Cardiology;* **Admitting Hospital:** William Beaumont Hospital; **Office Address:** William Beaumont Hosp, Div Cardio 3601 W 13 Mile Rd, Heart Ctr Bldg, 3rd FL Royal oak, MI 48073; **Office Phone:** (248) 551-5482; **Board Certifications:** Internal Medicine 1983, Cardiology (Cardiovascular Disease) 1987; **Medical School:** Univ Fla Coll Med 1979; **Residencies:** Pathology, Univ Miami Med Ctr, Miami, FL 1980-1981; Internal Medicine, UC San Diego Med Ctr, San Diego, CA 1981-1983; **Fellowship:** Cardiology (Cardiovascular Disease), Beth Israel Hosp-Harvard, Boston, MA 1984-1987

Seward, James Bernard MD (Cardiology (Cardiovascular Disease)) - *Special Expertise:* Cardiology - Pediatric; Echocardiography; **Admitting Hospital:** Mayo Medical Center & Clinic - Rochester; **Office Address:** Mayo Clinic 200 First St SW Rochester, MN 55905; **Office Phone:** (507) 284-3581; **Board Certifications:** Internal Medicine 1974, Cardiology (Cardiovascular Disease) 1975; **Medical School:** Univ Mich Med Sch 1968; **Residencies:** Internal Medicine, Boston City Hosp, Boston, MA 1968-1971; Internal Medicine, Mayo Clinic, Rochester, MN 1972; **Fellowship:** Cardiology (Cardiovascular Disease), Mayo Clinic, Rochester, MN 1973-1975; **Faculty Appointment:** Prof Pediatrics, Mayo Med Sch

Stewart, William MD (Cardiology (Cardiovascular Disease)) - *Special Expertise:* Heart *Valve Disease; Heart Valve Surgery - Aortic & Mitral;* **Admitting Hospital:** Cleveland Clinic Foundation; **Office Address:** 9500 Euclid Ave, Ste F15 Cleveland, OH 44195; **Office Phone:** (216) 444-5923; **Board Certifications:** Internal Medicine 1980, Cardiology (Cardiovascular Disease) 1983; **Medical School:** Univ Cincinnati 1977; **Residency:** Internal Medicine, Univ Mich Hosp, Ann Arbor, MI 1977-1980; **Fellowships:** Cardiology (Cardiovascular Disease), Boston Med Ctr, Boston, MA 1980-1982; Cardiology (Cardiovascular Disease), Mass Genl Hosp, Boston, MA 1982-1984; **Faculty Appointment:** Assoc Prof Medicine, Ohio State Univ

Topol, Eric Jeffrey MD (Cardiology (Cardiovascular Disease)) - *Special Expertise:* *Coronary Artery Disease; Interventional Cardiology;* **Admitting Hospital:** Cleveland Clinic Foundation; **Office Address:** Cleveland Clinic Heart Ctr 9500 Euclid Ave Cleveland, OH 44195; **Office Phone:** (216) 445-9490; **Board Certifications:** Internal Medicine 1982, Cardiology (Cardiovascular Disease) 1985; **Medical School:** Univ Rochester 1979; **Residency:** Internal Medicine, Univ California Sch Med, San Francisco, CA 1979-1982; **Fellowship:** Cardiology (Cardiovascular Disease), Johns Hopkins Hospital, Baltimore, MD 1982-1985

Vander Ark, Condon R MD (Cardiology (Cardiovascular Disease)) - *Special Expertise:* *Congestive Heart Failure;* **Admitting Hospital:** University of Wisconsin Hospital & Clinics; **Office Address:** Univ WI Hosp and Clinics 600 Highland Ave, Ste H6 - rm 356, Box CSC Madison, WI 53792; **Office Phone:** (608) 263-1530; **Board Certification:** Internal Medicine 1971; **Medical School:** Univ Mich Med Sch 1961; **Residencies:** Internal Medicine, Butterworth Hosp, Grand Rapids, MI 1962-1963; Internal Medicine, Mich Med Ctr, Ann Arbor, MI 1965-1966; **Fellowship:** Cardiology (Cardiovascular Disease), Mich Med Ctr, Ann Arbor, MI 1966-1968; **Faculty Appointment:** Assoc Prof Medicine, Univ Wisc

Vander Laan, Ronald Lee MD (Cardiology (Cardiovascular Disease)) - *Special Expertise:* Cardiac Rehabilitation;* **Admitting Hospital:** Spectrum Health East; **Office Address:** West Michigan Heart 1900 Wealthy St SE, Ste 200 Grand Rapids, MI 49506; **Office Phone:** (616) 454-5551; **Board Certifications:** Internal Medicine 1985, Cardiology (Cardiovascular Disease) 1987; **Medical School:** Univ Mich Med Sch 1982; **Residency:** Internal Medicine, Blodgett Meml Hosp, Grand Rapids, MI 1982-1985; **Fellowship:** Cardiology (Cardiovascular Disease), Cleveland Clinic Fdn, Cleveland, OH 1985-1987

Williams, Kim A MD (Cardiology (Cardiovascular Disease)) - *Special Expertise:* Nuclear *Cardiology; Heart Disease - Ischemic;* **Admitting Hospital:** University of Chicago Hospitals (Page 78); **Office Address:** 5758 S Maryland Ave, Ste 5C, MC-9025 Chicago, IL 60637; **Office Phone:** (773) 702-9461; **Board Certifications:** Internal Medicine 1982, Cardiology (Cardiovascular Disease) 1985; **Medical School:** Univ Chicago-Pritzker Sch Med 1975; **Residency:** Internal Medicine, Emory Univ, Atlanta, GA 1980-1982; **Fellowships:** Cardiology (Cardiovascular Disease), Univ Chicago, Chicago, IL 1982-1984; Nuclear Medicine, Univ Chicago, Chicago, IL 1984-1986; **Faculty Appointment:** Assoc Prof Cardiology (Cardiovascular Disease), Univ Chicago-Pritzker Sch Med

Young, James B MD (Cardiology (Cardiovascular Disease)) - *Special Expertise:* *Congestive Heart Failure;* **Admitting Hospital:** Cleveland Clinic Foundation; **Office Address:** Cleveland Clin Fdn 9500 Euclid Ave, Ste F-25 Cleveland, OH 44195; **Office Phone:** (216) 444-2270; **Board Certifications:** Internal Medicine 1977, Cardiology (Cardiovascular Disease) 1979; **Medical School:** Baylor Coll Med 1974; **Residencies:** Internal Medicine, Baylor Affl Hosp, Houston, TX 1975-1977; Internal Medicine, Methodist Hosp, Houston, TX 1980; **Fellowship:** Cardiology (Cardiovascular Disease), Baylor Affl Hosp, Houston, TX 1977-1979

Zipes, Douglas P MD (Cardiology (Cardiovascular Disease)) - *Special Expertise:* Cardiology (Cardiovascular Disease) - *General;* **Admitting Hospital:** Methodist Hospital - Indianapolis; **Office Address:** Ind U Sch Med-Krannert Inst Cardio 1111 W 10th St Indianapolis, IN 46202-4800; **Office Phone:** (317) 630-6640; **Board Certifications:** Cardiac Electrophysiology 1988, Cardiology (Cardiovascular Disease) 1972; **Medical School:** Harvard Med Sch 1964; **Residency:** Cardiology (Cardiovascular Disease), Duke Univ Med Ctr 1966-1968; **Faculty Appointment:** Prof Medicine, Indiana Univ

Great Plains and Mountains

Lindenfeld, JoAnn MD (Cardiology (Cardiovascular Disease)) - *Special Expertise:* Congestive Heart Failure; Transplant Medicine-Heart; **Admitting Hospital:** University of Colorado Health & Science Center; **Office Address:** 4200 E Ninth Ave #B130 Denver, CO 80262; **Office Phone:** (303) 315-4410; **Board Certifications:** Cardiology (Cardiovascular Disease) 1979, Internal Medicine 1976; **Medical School:** Univ Mich Med Sch 1973; **Residencies:** Internal Medicine, University California, San Diego, CA 1973-1977; Cardiology (Cardiovascular Disease), University Texas, San Antonio, TX 1977-1979; **Faculty Appointment:** Prof Medicine, Univ Colo

Southwest

Freeman, Gregory Lane MD (Cardiology (Cardiovascular Disease)) - *Special Expertise:* Interventional Cardiology; **Admitting Hospital:** University of Texas Health & Science Center; **Office Address:** Univ Texas Hlth Sci Ctr, Dept Cardiology 7703 Floyd Curl Dr San Antonio, TX 78284; **Office Phone:** (210) 567-4600; **Board Certifications:** Internal Medicine 1979, Cardiology (Cardiovascular Disease) 1983; **Medical School:** Loyola Univ-Stritch Sch Med 1976; **Residency:** Internal Medicine, Cook County Hosp, Chicago, IL 1977-1979; **Fellowships:** Cardiology (Cardiovascular Disease), Loyola Univ Med Ctr, Maywood, IL 1979-1981; Research, UCSD Sch Med, CA 1981-1983; **Faculty Appointment:** Prof Medicine, Univ Tex, San Antonio

Garcia-Gonzalez, Efrain MD (Cardiology (Cardiovascular Disease)) - *Special Expertise:* Cardiac Catheterization; **Admitting Hospital:** St Luke's Episcopal Hospital - Houston (Page 76); **Office Address:** 6624 Fannin St, Ste 2480 Houston, TX 77030-2309; **Office Phone:** (713) 529-5530; **Board Certifications:** Internal Medicine 1963, Cardiology (Cardiovascular Disease) 1964; **Medical School:** Univ Puerto Rico 1955; **Residency:** Internal Medicine, Brooke Genl Hosp 1957-1959; **Fellowship:** Cardiology (Cardiovascular Disease), Brooke Genl Hosp, Ft. Sam Houston, TX 1960-1961; **Faculty Appointment:** Clin Prof Medicine

Gould, K Lance MD (Cardiology (Cardiovascular Disease)) - *Special Expertise:* Preventive Cardiology; PET Imaging; **Admitting Hospital:** Memorial Hermann Healthcare System; **Office Address:** Univ Texas Med Sch - PET Imaging Ctr 6431 Fannin, Rm 4256 MSB Houston, TX 77030; **Office Phone:** (713) 500-6611; **Board Certifications:** Cardiology (Cardiovascular Disease), Internal Medicine; **Medical School:** Case West Res Univ 1964; **Residencies:** Internal Medicine, U Washington Med Ctr, Seattle, WA 1965-1967; Cardiology (Cardiovascular Disease), U Washington Med Ctr, Seattle, WA 1964-1964; **Fellowship:** Cardiology (Cardiovascular Disease), U Washington Med Ctr, Seattle, WA 1969-1971; **Faculty Appointment:** Prof Medicine, Univ Tex, Houston

Massin, Edward Krauss MD (Cardiology (Cardiovascular Disease)) - *Special Expertise:* *Congestive Heart Failure; Transplant Medicine-Heart;* **Admitting Hospital:** St Luke's Episcopal Hospital - Houston (Page 76); **Office Address:** Cardiology Consultants of Houston 6624 Fannin St, Fl 2310 Houston, TX 77030-2335; **Office Phone:** (713) 796-2668; **Board Certifications:** Internal Medicine 1973, Cardiology (Cardiovascular Disease) 1973; **Medical School:** Washington Univ, St Louis 1965; **Residency:** Internal Medicine, Barnes Hosp, St Louis, MO 1966-1967; **Fellowship:** Cardiology (Cardiovascular Disease), Univ Colo Med Ctr, Denver, CO 1969-1971; **Faculty Appointment:** Clin Prof Medicine, Baylor Coll Med

Ramee, Stephen Robert MD (Cardiology (Cardiovascular Disease)) - *Special Expertise:* *Angiography - Coronary;* **Admitting Hospital:** Ochsner Foundation Hospital; **Office Address:** Ochsner Clinic 1514 Jefferson Hwy New Orleans, LA 70121; **Office Phone:** (504) 842-4135; **Board Certifications:** Cardiology (Cardiovascular Disease) 1985, Interventional Cardiology 1999; **Medical School:** Geo Wash Univ 1980; **Residency:** Internal Medicine, Letterman Army Med Ctr, San Francisco, CA 1981-1983; **Fellowship:** Cardiology (Cardiovascular Disease), Letterman Army Med Ctr, San Francisco, CA 1983-1985

Wilansky, Susan MD (Cardiology (Cardiovascular Disease)) - *Special Expertise: Women's Health - Heart Disease; Heart Disease in Pregnancy;* **Admitting Hospital:** St Luke's Episcopal Hospital - Houston (Page 76); **Office Address:** 6624 Fannin St, Ste 2480 Houston, TX 77030-2309; **Office Phone:** (713) 529-5530; **Board Certification:** Cardiology (Cardiovascular Disease) 1989; **Medical School:** McMaster Univ 1979; **Residencies:** Internal Medicine, Toronto Hosp-Univ Toronto, Toronto Canada 1980-1983; Cardiology (Cardiovascular Disease), Toronto Hosp-Univ Toronto, Toronto Canada 1983-1985; **Fellowship:** Electrocardiograph, Toronto Hosp-Univ Toronto, Toronto Canada 1985-1986; **Faculty Appointment:** Assoc Clin Prof Medicine, Baylor Coll Med

Willerson, James Thorton MD (Cardiology (Cardiovascular Disease)) - *Special Expertise:* *Cardiology (Cardiovascular Disease) - General;* **Admitting Hospital:** St Luke's Episcopal Hospital - Houston (Page 76); **Office Address:** 6431 Fannin St, Ste 1.150 MSB Houston, TX 77030-1501; **Office Phone:** (713) 500-6500; **Board Certifications:** Internal Medicine 1972, Cardiology (Cardiovascular Disease) 1974; **Medical School:** Baylor Coll Med 1965; **Residency:** Internal Medicine, Mass Genl Hosp, Boston, MA 1966-1967; **Fellowship:** Cardiology (Cardiovascular Disease), Mass Genl Hosp, Boston, MA 1966-1967; **Faculty Appointment:** Prof Medicine, Univ Tex, Houston

West Coast and Pacific

Barr, Mark Lee MD (Cardiology (Cardiovascular Disease)) - *Special Expertise: Thoracic Surgery - General;* **Admitting Hospital:** USC University Hospital - Richard K. Eamer Medical Plaza; **Office Address:** USC Cardiothoracic Surg 1510 San Pablo St #415 Los Angeles, Ca 90033-4612; **Office Phone:** (323) 442-5849; **Board Certification:** Critical Care Medicine 1987; Cardiology (Cardiovascular Disease) 1989; **Medical School:** Mount Sinai Sch Med 1981; **Residencies:** Surgery, Bellevue Hosp Ctr, New York, NY 1983-1984; Cardiothoracic Surgery, Colum-Presby Med, New York, NY 1985-1987; Cardiology (Cardiovascular Disease), Colum-Presby Med, New York, NY 1987-1990; **Faculty Appointment:** Assoc Prof Thoracic Surgery, USC Sch Med

Bleifer, Selvyn Burton MD (Cardiology (Cardiovascular Disease)) - *Special Expertise:* *Non-Invasive Cardiology;* **Admitting Hospital:** Cedars-Sinai Medical Center; **Office Address:** 414 N Camden #1100 Beverly Hills, CA 90210-4532; **Office Phone:** (310) 278-3400; **Board Certifications:** Internal Medicine 1962, Cardiology (Cardiovascular Disease) 1975; **Medical School:** UCSF 1955; **Residencies:** Internal Medicine, VA Hosp, Boston, MA 1956-1958; Cardiology (Cardiovascular Disease), Mt Sinai Hosp, New York, NY 1958; **Faculty Appointment:** Assoc Clin Prof Medicine, UCLA

Brindis, Ralph Gerard MD (Cardiology (Cardiovascular Disease)) - *Special Expertise:* Cardiology (Cardiovascular Disease) - *General;* **Admitting Hospital:** Kaiser Permanente Medical Center; **Office Address:** 2350 Geary Blvd, rm 218 San Francisco, CA 94115; **Office Phone:** (415) 202-2616; **Board Certifications:** Internal Medicine 1980, Cardiology (Cardiovascular Disease) 1999; **Medical School:** Emory Univ 1977; **Residencies:** Internal Medicine, Fort Miley VA Hosp, San Francisco, CA 1980-1981; Internal Medicine, Herbert C Moffitt Hosp, San Francisco, CA 1978-1980; **Fellowship:** Cardiology (Cardiovascular Disease), Herbert C Moffitt Hosp, San Francisco, CA 1981-1983; **Faculty Appointment:** Prof Medicine, UCSF

Chatterjee, Kanu MD (Cardiology (Cardiovascular Disease)) - *Special Expertise:* Coronary Artery Disease; Congestive Heart Failure; **Admitting Hospital:** University of California - San Francisco Medical Center; **Office Address:** 1182 Moffitt Hospital 505 Parnassus Ave, Box 0124 San Francisco, CA 94143-0327; **Office Phone:** (415) 476-1326; **Board Certifications:** Internal Medicine 1973, Cardiology (Cardiovascular Disease) 1975; **Medical School:** India 1956; **Fellowship:** Cardiology (Cardiovascular Disease), Brompton Hosp, London, England 1969-1971; **Faculty Appointment:** Prof Cardiology (Cardiovascular Disease), UCSF

Choe, Soo-Sang MD (Cardiology (Cardiovascular Disease)) - *Special Expertise:* Cardiology (Cardiovascular Disease) - *General;* **Admitting Hospital:** Loma Linda University Medical Center; **Office Address:** 903 E Devovshire Ave, Ste A Hemet, CA 92543; **Office Phone:** (909) 925-0571; **Board Certifications:** Internal Medicine 1984, Cardiology (Cardiovascular Disease) 1995; **Medical School:** South Korea 1967; **Residencies:** Internal Medicine, Hahnemann Med Coll Hosp Hosp, Philadelphia, PA 1972-1974; Cardiology (Cardiovascular Disease), Sloan-Kettering Meml Hosp, New YorK, NY 1974-1975; **Fellowship:** Cardiology (Cardiovascular Disease), Bronx VA Hosp, New York, NY 1975-1977

Criley, John Michael MD (Cardiology (Cardiovascular Disease)) - *Special Expertise:* Cardiac Catheterization; **Admitting Hospital:** LAC - Harbor - UCLA Medical Center; **Office Address:** St John's Cardiovascular Rsch Ctr 1000 W Carson St Torrance, CA 90502; **Office Phone:** (310) 222-5101; **Medical School:** Stanford Univ 1956; **Residency:** Internal Medicine, Johns Hospkins Hosp, Baltimore, MD 1956-1960; **Faculty Appointment:** Prof Medicine, UCLA

Elkayam, Uri MD (Cardiology (Cardiovascular Disease)) - *Special Expertise:* Congestive Heart Failure; **Admitting Hospital:** LAC + USC Medical Center; **Office Address:** LAC-USC Med Ctr, Div Cardiology 2025 Zonal Ave, rm 7440 Los Angeles, CA 90033; **Office Phone:** (323) 226-7541; **Board Certifications:** Internal Medicine 1989, Cardiology (Cardiovascular Disease) 1991; **Medical School:** Israel 1973; **Residency:** Internal Medicine, Ichilov Hosp, Tel-Aviv, Israel 1976; **Fellowships:** Cardiology (Cardiovascular Disease), Albert Einstein Hosp, New York, NY 1978; Cardiology (Cardiovascular Disease), Cedars Sinai Med Ctr, Los Angeles, CA 1978-1979; **Faculty Appointment:** Prof Medicine, Univ SC Sch Med

Fishbein, Daniel P MD (Cardiology (Cardiovascular Disease)) - *Special Expertise:* Congestive Heart Failure; Transplant Medicine-Heart; **Admitting Hospital:** University of Washington Medical Center; **Office Address:** Univ Wash Med Ctr, Div Cardiology 1959 NE Pacific St, Box 356422 Seattle, WA 98195-6043; **Office Phone:** (206) 598-4300; **Board Certifications:** Internal Medicine 1983, Cardiology (Cardiovascular Disease) 1987; **Medical School:** Albert Einstein Coll Med 1980; **Residencies:** Internal Medicine, Lankenau Hosp, Wynnewood, PA 1980-1981; Internal Medicine, Univ Wash Med Ctr, Seattle, WA 1981-1983; **Fellowship:** Cardiology (Cardiovascular Disease), Univ Wash Med Ctr, Seattle, WA 1984-1987

CARDIOLOGY West Coast and Pacific

Gershengorn, Kent N MD (Cardiology (Cardiovascular Disease)) - *Special Expertise:*
Cardiology (Cardiovascular Disease) - General; **Admitting Hospital:** University of California - San Francisco Medical Center; **Office Address:** 350 Parnassus Ave, Ste 410 San Francisco, CA 94117; **Office Phone:** (415) 476-6388; **Board Certifications:** Internal Medicine 1973, Cardiology (Cardiovascular Disease) 1973; **Medical School:** SUNY Buffalo 1965; **Residencies:** Internal Medicine, Mt Sinai Hosp, New York, NY 1968-1970; Cardiology (Cardiovascular Disease), Mt Sinai Hosp, New York, NY 1970-1971; **Fellowship:** Cardiology (Cardiovascular Disease), Herbert C Moffitt Hosp-UCSF, San Francisco, CA 1971-1972; **Faculty Appointment:** Clin Prof Medicine, UCSF

Heger, Joel William MD (Cardiology (Cardiovascular Disease)) - *Special Expertise:*
Cardiology (Cardiovascular Disease) - General; **Admitting Hospital:** LAC + USC Medical Center; **Office Address:** 10 Congress St, Ste 507 Passadena, CA 91105-3023; **Office Phone:** (626) 792-5300; **Board Certifications:** Cardiology (Cardiovascular Disease) 1979, Interventional Cardiology 1999; **Medical School:** USC Sch Med 1972; **Residency:** Internal Medicine, USC Med Ctr, Los Angeles, CA 1973-1975; **Fellowships:** Cardiology (Cardiovascular Disease), USC Med Ctr, Los Angeles, CA 1975-1976; Cardiology (Cardiovascular Disease), UCLA Med Ctr, Torrance, CA 1976-1978; **Faculty Appointment:** Clin Prof Medicine, USC Sch Med

Hunt, Sharon Ann MD (Cardiology (Cardiovascular Disease)) - *Special Expertise:*
Transplant Medicine-Heart; **Admitting Hospital:** Stanford Medical Center; **Office Address:** Stanford Med Ctr, Dept Cardiovascular Rsch 300 Pasteur Drive, Bldg FALK - rm CV213 Stanford, CA 94305; **Office Phone:** (650) 723-5771; **Board Certifications:** Internal Medicine 1977, Cardiology (Cardiovascular Disease) 1979; **Medical School:** Stanford Univ 1972; **Residency:** Internal Medicine, Stanford Univ Hosp, Stanford, CA 1972-1974; **Fellowship:** Cardiology (Cardiovascular Disease), Stanford Univ Hosp, Stanford, CA 1974-1976; **Faculty Appointment:** Prof Medicine, Stanford Univ

Kobashigawa, Jon Akira MD (Cardiology (Cardiovascular Disease)) - *Special Expertise:*
Transplant Medicine-Heart; **Admitting Hospital:** UCLA Medical Center; **Office Address:** 100 UCLA Med Plaza, Ste 630 Los Angeles, CA 90095; **Office Phone:** (310) 794-1200; **Board Certifications:** Internal Medicine 1983, Cardiology (Cardiovascular Disease) 1987; **Medical School:** Mount Sinai Sch Med 1980; **Residency:** Internal Medicine, UCLA Med Ctr, Los Angeles, CA 1981-1983; **Fellowship:** Cardiology (Cardiovascular Disease), UCLA Med Ctr, Los Angeles, CA 1984-1986; **Faculty Appointment:** Assoc Clin Prof Cardiology (Cardiovascular Disease), UCLA

Parmley, William Watts MD (Cardiology (Cardiovascular Disease)) - *Special Expertise:*
Coronary Artery Disease; Heart Failure; **Admitting Hospital:** University of California - San Francisco Medical Center; **Office Address:** 505 Parnassus Ave, rm 1180 San Francisco, CA 94143-0124; **Office Phone:** (415) 476-1326; **Board Certifications:** Internal Medicine 1970, Cardiology (Cardiovascular Disease) 1972; **Medical School:** Johns Hopkins Univ 1963; **Residency:** Internal Medicine, Johns Hopkins Hosp, Baltimore, MD 1963-1965; **Fellowships:** Cardiology (Cardiovascular Disease), Natl Heart Institute, Bethesda, MD 1965-1967; Cardiology (Cardiovascular Disease), Peter Bent Brigham, Boston, MA 1967-1969; **Faculty Appointment:** Prof Medicine, UCSF

Perloff, Joseph Kayle MD (Cardiology (Cardiovascular Disease)) - *Special Expertise:*
Heart Disease - Congenital; **Admitting Hospital:** UCLA Medical Center; **Office Address:** UCLA Med Ctr 650 Charles E. Young Drive S, rm 47-123 CHS, Box 951679 Los Angeles, CA 90095-1679; **Office Phone:** (310) 825-2019; **Board Certifications:** Internal Medicine 1960, Cardiology (Cardiovascular Disease) 1967; **Medical School:** Louisiana State Univ 1951; **Residencies:** Internal Medicine, Mt Sinai Hosp, New York, NY 1951-1954; Internal Medicine, Georgetown Univ Hosp, Washington, DC 1955-1956; **Fellowship:** Cardiology (Cardiovascular Disease), Natl Heart Hosp, London, England 1954-1955; **Faculty Appointment:** Prof Pediatric Cardiology, UCLA

Ritchie, James L. MD (Cardiology (Cardiovascular Disease)) - *Special Expertise:* Cardiology (Cardiovascular Disease) - General; **Admitting Hospital:** University of Washington Medical Center; **Office Address:** Univ of Wash Sch Med 1959 NE Pacific St, Box 356422 Seattle, WA 98195; **Office Phone:** (206) 543-8584; **Board Certifications:** Internal Medicine 1972, Cardiology (Cardiovascular Disease) 1975; **Medical School:** Case West Res Univ 1967; **Residency:** Internal Medicine, Univ Washington Med Ctr, Seattle, WA 1970-1972; **Fellowship:** Cardiology (Cardiovascular Disease), Univ Washington Med Ctr, Seattle, WA 1972-1974; **Faculty Appointment:** Prof Medicine, Univ Wash

Scheinman, Melvin M MD (Cardiology (Cardiovascular Disease)) - *Special Expertise:* Stroke; **Admitting Hospital:** University of California - San Francisco Medical Center; **Office Address:** UCSF Cardiology Faculty Practice 400 Parnassus Ave San Francisco, CA 94143-0327; **Office Phone:** (415) 476-5706; **Board Certifications:** Cardiology (Cardiovascular Disease) 1971, Cardiac Electrophysiology 1992; **Medical School:** Albert Einstein Coll Med 1960; **Residency:** Internal Medicine, NC Meml Hosp, Chapel Hill, NC 1963-1965; **Fellowship:** Cardiology (Cardiovascular Disease), UCSF, San Francisco, CA 1965-1967

Schnittger, Ingela MD (Cardiology (Cardiovascular Disease)) - *Special Expertise:* Cardiovascular Imaging - Non-Invasive; **Admitting Hospital:** Stanford Medical Center; **Office Address:** Stanford Univ Sch Med 300 Pasteur Rd, rm H2157, MC-5233 Stanford, CA 94305-5233; **Office Phone:** (650) 723-5196; **Board Certifications:** Internal Medicine 1980, Cardiology (Cardiovascular Disease) 1983; **Medical School:** Sweden 1975; **Residency:** Internal Medicine, Stanford Univ Hosp, Stanford, CA 1979-1980; **Fellowship:** Cardiology (Cardiovascular Disease), Stanford Univ Hosp, Stanford, CA 1980-1983; **Faculty Appointment:** Assoc Prof Medicine, Stanford Univ

Schroeder, John S MD (Cardiology (Cardiovascular Disease)) - *Special Expertise:* Congestive Heart Failure; Coronary Artery Disease; **Admitting Hospital:** Stanford Medical Center; **Office Address:** Stanford U Sch Med, Div CVRB #293 300 Pasteur Rd Palo Alto, CA 94304-5406; **Office Phone:** (650) 723-5561; **Board Certifications:** Internal Medicine 1969, Cardiology (Cardiovascular Disease) 1973; **Medical School:** Univ Mich Med Sch 1962; **Residency:** Internal Medicine, Stanford U Med Ctr 1965-1967; **Fellowship:** Cardiology (Cardiovascular Disease), Stanford U Med Ctr 1967-1969; **Faculty Appointment:** Prof Cardiology (Cardiovascular Disease), Stanford Univ

Shah, Prediman K MD (Cardiology (Cardiovascular Disease)) - *Special Expertise:* Cardiology (Cardiovascular Disease) - General; **Admitting Hospital:** Cedars-Sinai Medical Center; **Office Address:** Cedars-Sinai Med Ctr 8700 Beverly Blvd, rm 5347 Los Angeles, CA 90048-1865; **Office Phone:** (310) 423-3884; **Board Certifications:** Internal Medicine 1975, Cardiology (Cardiovascular Disease) 1977; **Medical School:** India 1969; **Residencies:** All India Inst Med Scis, New Delhi, India 1970-1971; Internal Medicine, Montefiore Hosp, New York, NY 1973-1974; **Fellowship:** Cardiology (Cardiovascular Disease), Montefiore Hosp, New York, NY 1974-1976; **Faculty Appointment:** Prof Medicine, UCLA

INTERVENTIONAL CARDIOLOGY

New England

Diver, Daniel Joseph MD (Interventional Cardiology) - *Special Expertise:* *Angioplasty;* *Coronary Artery Disease;* **Admitting Hospital:** St Francis Hospital & Medical Center; **Office Address:** Division of Cardiology 114 Woodland St Hartford, CT 06105; **Office Phone:** (860) 714-5900; **Board Certifications:** Cardiology (Cardiovascular Disease) 1989, Interventional Cardiology 1999; **Medical School:** Johns Hopkins Univ 1981; **Residency:** Internal Medicine, Johns Hopkins Hosp, Baltimore, MD 1982-1984; **Fellowship:** Cardiology (Cardiovascular Disease), Beth Israel Hosp/Harvard, Boston, MA 1984-1987; **Faculty Appointment:** Prof Medicine, Univ Conn

Jacobs, Alice K MD (Interventional Cardiology) - *Special Expertise:* *Cardiac Catheterization;* **Admitting Hospital:** Boston University Medical Center-East Newton Street Campus; **Office Address:** Boston Univ Medical Center-Cardiology 88 E Newton St Boston, MA 02118; **Office Phone:** (617) 638-7490; **Board Certifications:** Internal Medicine 1978, Cardiology (Cardiovascular Disease) 1985; **Medical School:** St Louis Univ 1975; **Residency:** Internal Medicine, St Louis Univ Hosp, St Louis, MO 1976-1978; **Fellowships:** Endocrinology, UCSD Med Ctr, San Diego, Ca 1978-1980; Cardiology (Cardiovascular Disease), Boston Univ Med Ctr, Boston, MA 1980-1982; **Faculty Appointment:** Prof Medicine, Boston Univ

Weiner, Bonnie H MD (Interventional Cardiology) - *Special Expertise:* *Interventional Cardiology - General;* **Admitting Hospital:** UMASS Memorial Health Care - Worcester; **Office Address:** UMASS Memorial Hosp 55 Lake Ave N Worcester, MA 01655-0002; **Office Phone:** (508) 856-3691; **Board Certifications:** Internal Medicine 1977, Interventional Cardiology 1999; **Residency:** Internal Medicine, Norwalk Hosp, Norwalk, CT 1975-1977; **Fellowship:** Cardiology (Cardiovascular Disease), Univ Mass, Worcester, MA

Mid Atlantic

Leon, Martin MD (Interventional Cardiology) - *Special Expertise:* *Interventional Cardiology - General;* **Admitting Hospital:** Lenox Hill Hospital; **Office Address:** Lenox Hill Hospital 130 E 77th St, Fl 9th New York, NY 10021; **Office Phone:** (212) 434-6300; **Board Certifications:** Internal Medicine 1979, Cardiology (Cardiovascular Disease) 1983; **Medical School:** Yale Univ 1975; **Residency:** Internal Medicine, Yale-New Haven Hosp, New Haven, CT 1976-1978; **Fellowship:** Cardiology (Cardiovascular Disease), Yale-New Haven Hosp, New Haven, CT

Pichard, Augusto MD (Interventional Cardiology) - *Special Expertise:* *Angioplasty;* **Admitting Hospital:** Washington Hospital Center - DC (Page 79); **Office Address:** Washington Cardiology Ctr 110 Irving St NW, Ste 4B1 Washington, DC 20010; **Office Phone:** (202) 877-5975; **Board Certification:** Cardiology (Cardiovascular Disease) 1977; **Medical School:** Chile 1969; **Residencies:** Internal Medicine, Catholic U 1970-1971; Internal Medicine, U Chile 1969-1970

Southeast

Applegate, Robert Joseph MD (Interventional Cardiology) - *Special Expertise:* *Cardiac Catheterization; Angioplasty;* **Admitting Hospital:** Wake Forest University Baptist Medical Center; **Office Address:** Wake Forest Univ Baptist Med Ctr Medical Center Blvd Winston-Salem, NC 27157; **Office Phone:** (336) 716-6674; **Board Certifications:** Cardiology (Cardiovascular Disease) 1987, Interventional Cardiology 1999; **Medical School:** Univ VA Sch Med 1980; **Residency:** Internal Medicine, Oregon Hlth Sci Univ Hosp, Portland, OR 1981-1983; **Fellowships:** Pharmacology, Univ Texas Hlth Sci Ctr, San Antonio, TX 1983-1984; Cardiology (Cardiovascular Disease), Univ Texas Hlth Sci Ctr, San Antonio, TX 1984-1986; **Faculty Appointment:** Prof Medicine, Wake Forest Univ Sch Med

Braden, Gregory Alan MD (Interventional Cardiology) - *Special Expertise:* Cardiac Catheterization; **Admitting Hospital:** Wake Forest University Baptist Medical Center; **Office Address:** Wake Forest Univ Baptist Med Ctr Medical Center Blvd Winston Salem, NC 27157; **Office Phone:** (336) 716-6674; **Board Certifications:** Cardiology (Cardiovascular Disease) 1989, Interventional Cardiology 1999; **Medical School:** Wake Forest Univ Sch Med 1982; **Residency:** Internal Medicine, Univ Texas Med Br Hosp, Galveston, TX 1982-1985; **Fellowship:** Cardiology (Cardiovascular Disease), Vanderbilt Univ Med, Nashville, TN 1986-1989

King III, Spencer MD (Interventional Cardiology) - *Special Expertise:* Interventional Cardiology - General; **Admitting Hospital:** Piedmont Hospital; **Office Address:** 95 Collier Rd NW, Ste 2075 Atlanta, GA 30309; **Office Phone:** (404) 351-4353; **Board Certifications:** Internal Medicine 1970, Cardiology (Cardiovascular Disease) 1971; **Medical School:** Med Coll GA 1963; **Residency:** Internal Medicine, Emory Univ Hosp, GA 1966-1968; **Fellowship:** Cardiology (Cardiovascular Disease), Emory U Sch Med, GA 1968-1970

Matar, Fadi MD (Interventional Cardiology) - *Special Expertise:* Angioplasty; **Admitting Hospital:** Tampa General Hospital; **Office Address:** 508 South Habana, Ste 340 Tampa, FL 33609-3568; **Office Phone:** (813) 353-1515; **Board Certifications:** Cardiology (Cardiovascular Disease) 1993, Interventional Cardiology 1999; **Medical School:** Lebanon 1987; **Residency:** Internal Medicine, Maryland Genl Hosp, Baltimore, MD 1987-1990; **Fellowship:** Cardiology (Cardiovascular Disease), Wash Hosp Ctr, Washington DC, WA 1990-1994; **Faculty Appointment:** Asst Prof Medicine, Univ S Fla Coll Med

Morris, Douglas MD (Interventional Cardiology) - *Special Expertise:* Interventional Cardiology; **Admitting Hospital:** Emory University Hospital; **Office Address:** The Emory Clinic 1365-A Clifton Rd NE Atlanta, GA 30322; **Board Certifications:** Internal Medicine 1973, Cardiology (Cardiovascular Disease) 1975; **Medical School:** Baylor Coll Med 1968; **Residency:** Internal Medicine, Vanderbilt University, Nashville, TN 1969-1970; **Fellowship:** Cardiology (Cardiovascular Disease), Emory University, Atlanta, GA 1973-1975; **Faculty Appointment:** Prof Cardiology (Cardiovascular Disease), Emory Univ

Midwest

Clark, Vivian MD (Interventional Cardiology) - *Special Expertise:* Cardiac Catheterization; **Admitting Hospital:** Henry Ford Health System (Page 62); **Office Address:** Cardiovascular Henry Ford Hospital 2799 W Grand Blvd Detroit, MI 48202; **Office Phone:** (313) 876-2737; **Board Certifications:** Internal Medicine 1982, Cardiology (Cardiovascular Disease) 1985; **Medical School:** Ohio State Univ 1979; **Residency:** Internal Medicine, Akron City Hospital 1980-1982; **Fellowship:** Cardiology (Cardiovascular Disease), Henry Ford Hospital, Detroit, MI 1982-1984

Ellis, Stephen Geoffrey MD (Interventional Cardiology) - *Special Expertise:* Interventional Cardiology - General; **Admitting Hospital:** Cleveland Clinic Foundation; **Office Address:** Cleveland Clinic 9500 Euclid Ave, Ste F25 Cleveland, OH 44195; **Office Phone:** (216) 445-6712; **Board Certifications:** Internal Medicine 1981, Cardiology (Cardiovascular Disease) 1985; **Medical School:** UCLA 1978; **Residency:** Infectious Disease, Cedars-Sinai, Los Angeles, CA 1978-1981; **Fellowships:** Cardiology (Cardiovascular Disease), Stanford University, Stanford, CA 1982-1985; Interventional Cardiology, Emory University, Atlanta, GA 1985-1986; **Faculty Appointment:** Prof Medicine, Ohio State Univ

Feldman, Ted MD (Interventional Cardiology) - *Special Expertise:* *Interventional Cardiology - General;* **Admitting Hospital:** University of Chicago Hospitals (Page 78); **Office Address:** Univ Chicago Hosp 5841 S Maryland Ave, MC-567 Chicago, IL 60637-1463; **Office Phone:** (773) 702-9461; **Board Certifications:** Internal Medicine 1981, Cardiology (Cardiovascular Disease) 1985; **Medical School:** Indiana Univ 1978; **Residency:** Internal Medicine, Rush-Presby-St Luke's Hosp, Chicago, IL 1978-1982; **Fellowship:** Cardiology (Cardiovascular Disease), Univ Chicago, Chicago, IL 1982-1985; **Faculty Appointment:** Prof Medicine, Univ Chicago-Pritzker Sch Med

Holmes Jr., David Richard MD (Interventional Cardiology) - *Special Expertise:* *Interventional Cardiology; Myocardial Infarction;* **Admitting Hospital:** Mayo Medical Center & Clinic - Rochester; **Office Address:** 200 First St SW Mayo Medical Center & Clinic Rochester, MN 55905; **Office Phone:** (507) 255-2504; **Board Certification:** Cardiology (Cardiovascular Disease) 1977; **Medical School:** Med Coll Wisc 1971; **Residency:** Mayo Clinic, Rochester, MN 1972; **Faculty Appointment:** Prof Medicine, Mayo Med Sch

Klein, Lloyd MD (Interventional Cardiology) - *Special Expertise:* *Coronary Disease - Complex;* **Admitting Hospital:** Rush/Presbyterian - St Luke's Medical Center - Chicago (Page 74); **Office Address:** Rush Presby-St Luke's Med Ctr 1653 W Congress Pkwy, Ste 1035 Chicago, IL 60612-3835; **Office Phone:** (312) 942-5020; **Board Certifications:** Internal Medicine 1980, Cardiology (Cardiovascular Disease) 1983; **Medical School:** Univ Cincinnati 1977; **Residency:** Internal Medicine, Einstein-Bronx Muni Hosp, Bronx, NY 1977-1980; **Fellowship:** Cardiology (Cardiovascular Disease), Mt Sinai Med Ctr, New York, NY 1980-1982; **Faculty Appointment:** Prof Medicine, Rush Med Coll

Pitt, Bertram MD (Interventional Cardiology) - *Special Expertise:* *Interventional Cardiology - General;* **Admitting Hospital:** University of Michigan Health Center; **Office Address:** Univ Mich Med Ctr, Div Cardiology 1500 E Med Ctr Dr Ann Arbor, MI 48109-0366; **Office Phone:** (734) 936-5260; **Board Certifications:** Internal Medicine 1973, Cardiology (Cardiovascular Disease) 1975; **Medical School:** Switzerland 1959; **Residency:** Internal Medicine, Beth Israel Hosp, Boston, MA 1960-1963; **Fellowship:** Cardiology (Cardiovascular Disease), Johns Hopkins Hosp, Baltimore, MD 1966-1968; **Faculty Appointment:** Prof Medicine, Univ Mich Med Sch

Weaver, Wayne Douglas MD (Interventional Cardiology) - *Special Expertise:* *Interventional Cardiology - General;* **Admitting Hospital:** Henry Ford Health System (Page 62); **Office Address:** Henry Ford Hosp, K-14 2799 W Grand Blvd Detriot, MI 48202; **Office Phone:** (313) 876-4420; **Board Certifications:** Internal Medicine 1974, Cardiology (Cardiovascular Disease) 1977; **Medical School:** Tufts Univ 1971; **Residency:** Internal Medicine, Univ Wash Hosps, Seattle, WA 1972-1974; **Fellowship:** Cardiology (Cardiovascular Disease), Univ Wash Hosp, Seattle, WA 1974-1976

White, Carl W MD (Interventional Cardiology) - *Special Expertise:* *Interventional Cardiology - General;* **Admitting Hospital:** Fairview-University Medical Center - University Campus; **Office Address:** 420 Delaware St Minneapolis, MN 55455; **Office Phone:** (612) 625-9100; **Board Certifications:** Cardiology (Cardiovascular Disease) 1973, Interventional Cardiology 1999; **Medical School:** Univ Nebr Coll Med 1964; **Residency:** Internal Medicine, Univ Iowa Hosp, Des Moines, IA 1967-1970; **Fellowship:** Cardiology (Cardiovascular Disease), Univ Iowa Hosp, Des Moines, IA 1970-1972; **Faculty Appointment:** Prof Medicine, Univ Minn

Southwest

Bailey, Steven Roderick MD (Interventional Cardiology) - *Special Expertise:* *Interventional Cardiology - General;* **Admitting Hospital:** University of Texas Health & Science Center; **Office Address:** 7703 Floyd Curl, MC-7872 San Antonio, TX 78229-3900; **Office Phone:** (710) 567-4601; **Board Certifications:** Cardiology (Cardiovascular Disease) 1983, Interventional Cardiology 1999; **Medical School:** Oregon Hlth Scis Univ 1978; **Residency:** Internal Medicine, Fitzsimmons AMC, Denver, CO 1979-1981; **Fellowship:** Cardiology (Cardiovascular Disease), Fitzsimmons AMC, Denver, CO 1981-1983; **Faculty Appointment:** Prof Medicine, Univ Tex, San Antonio

Kleiman, Neal Stephen MD (Interventional Cardiology) - *Special Expertise:* *Angioplasty;* **Admitting Hospital:** Methodist Hospital - Houston (Page 69); **Office Address:** 6565 Fannin, MS F-1090 Houston, TX 77030; **Office Phone:** (713) 790-4952; **Board Certifications:** Interventional Cardiology 1999, Cardiology (Cardiovascular Disease) 1987; **Medical School:** Columbia P&S 1981; **Residency:** Internal Medicine, Baylor Coll Med, Houston, TX 1981-1984; **Fellowship:** Interventional Cardiology, Baylor Coll Med, Houston, TX 1984-1987; **Faculty Appointment:** Assoc Prof Medicine, Baylor Coll Med

Smalling, Richard Warren MD/PhD (Interventional Cardiology) - *Special Expertise:* *Stroke;* **Admitting Hospital:** Memorial Hermann Healthcare System; **Office Address:** 6431 Fannin St, MS 1246 Houston, TX 77030-1501; **Office Phone:** (713) 500-6559; **Board Certifications:** Cardiology (Cardiovascular Disease) 1981, Internal Medicine 1978; **Medical School:** Univ Tex, Houston **Residency:** Internal Medicine, UCSD, San Diego, CA 1975-1978; **Fellowship:** UCSD, San Diego, CA 1978-1981; **Faculty Appointment:** Prof Medicine, Univ Tex, Houston

West Coast and Pacific

Teirstein, Paul Shepherd MD (Interventional Cardiology) - *Special Expertise:* *Interventional Cardiology - General;* **Admitting Hospital:** Scripps Hospital - La Jolla; **Office Address:** Scripps Clinic - Torrey Pines 10666 N Torrey Pines Rd La Jolla, CA 92037; **Office Phone:** (858) 455-9100; **Board Certifications:** Cardiology (Cardiovascular Disease) 1987, Interventional Cardiology 1999; **Medical School:** Mount Sinai Sch Med 1980; **Residency:** Internal Medicine, Brigham & Women's Hosp, Boston, MA 1981-1983; **Fellowships:** Cardiology (Cardiovascular Disease), Stanford Univ, Stanford, CA 1983-1986; Cardiology (Cardiovascular Disease), Mid-Amer Heart Inst, Kansas City, MO 1986-1987

CHILD NEUROLOGY

(a subspecialty of NEUROLOGY)

A neurologist specializes in the diagnosis and treatment of all types of disease or impaired function of the brain, spinal cord, peripheral nerves, muscles and autonomic nervous system, as well as the blood vessels that relate to these structures. A child neurologist has special skills in the diagnosis and management of neurologic disorders of the neonatal period, infancy, early childhood and adolescence.

Training required: Four years

Physician Listings

Child Neurology

New England

Darras, Basil Theodore MD (Child Neurology) - *Special Expertise:* Neuromuscular Disorders; **Admitting Hospital:** Children's Hospital; **Office Address:** Children's Hospital, Dept Neur 300 Longwood Ave Boston, MA 02115; **Office Phone:** (617) 355-8235; **Board Certifications:** Pediatrics 1988, Neurology 1992; **Medical School:** Other Foreign Country 1977; **Residencies:** Pediatrics, Nassau County Med Ctr, East Meadow, NY 1980-1982; Child Neurology, Tufts-New England Med Ctr, Boston, MA 1982-1985; **Fellowship:** Clinical Genetics, Yale Univ Sch Med, New Haven, CT 1985-1988; **Faculty Appointment:** Assoc Prof Neurology, Harvard Med Sch

Holmes, Gregory Lawrence MD (Child Neurology) - *Special Expertise:* Epilepsy/Seizure Disorders; Neurologic Disorders; **Admitting Hospital:** Children's Hospital; **Office Address:** Children's Hospital, Neurophysiology Lab 300 Longwood Ave Boston, MA 02115; **Office Phone:** (617) 355-8461; **Board Certifications:** Pediatrics 1979, Neurology 1980; **Medical School:** Univ VA Sch Med 1974; **Residency:** Pediatrics, Yale-New Haven Hosp, New Haven, CT 1975-1976; **Fellowship:** Neurology, Univ Va, Charlottesville, VA 1976-1979; **Faculty Appointment:** Prof Harvard Med Sch

Shaywitz, Bennett MD (Child Neurology) - *Special Expertise:* Learning Disorders; Dyslexia; **Admitting Hospital:** Yale - New Haven Hospital; **Office Address:** Yale U School of Med-Pediatric Dept 333 Cedar St, rm LMP3089 New Haven, CT 06520; **Office Phone:** (203) 785-4641; **Board Certifications:** Pediatrics 1968, Child & Adolescent Psychiatry 1973; **Medical School:** Washington Univ, St Louis 1963; **Residencies:** Pediatrics, Bronx Municipal Hosp Ctr, Bronx, NY 1963-1966; Pediatrics, Bronx Municipal Hosp, Bronx, NY 1966-1967; **Fellowship:** Child Neurology, Albert Einstein Coll Med 1967-1970; **Faculty Appointment:** Prof Child Neurology, Yale Univ

Volpe, Joseph J. MD (Child Neurology) - *Special Expertise:* Neonatal Neurology; Cerebral Palsy; **Admitting Hospital:** Children's Hospital; **Office Address:** Children's Hospital 300 Longwood Ave, Segan Bldg, Fl 11 Boston, MA 02115-5724; **Office Phone:** (617) 355-6386; **Board Certifications:** Pediatrics 1970, Neurology 1974; **Medical School:** Harvard Med Sch 1964; **Residencies:** Pediatrics, Mass Genl Hosp, Boston, MA 1965-1966; Neurology, Mass Genl Hosp, Boston, MA 1968-1971; **Fellowship:** Natl Inst Child Hlth Human Dev, Bethesda, MD 1966-1968; **Faculty Appointment:** Prof Neurology, Harvard Med Sch

Mid Atlantic

Aron, Alan MD (Child Neurology) - *Special Expertise:* Neurofibromatosis; Seizure Disorders; **Admitting Hospital:** Mount Sinai Hospital (Page 70); **Office Address:** 5 E 98th St New York, NY 10029; **Office Phone:** (212) 831-4393; **Board Certifications:** Pediatrics 1963, Neurology 1967; **Medical School:** Columbia P&S 1958; **Residency:** Pediatrics, Babies Hosp-Columbia Presby, New York, NY 1959-1961; **Fellowship:** Child Neurology, Babies Hosp-Columbia Presby, New York, NY 1961-1964; **Faculty Appointment:** Prof Pediatric Endocrinology, Mount Sinai Sch Med

Chutorian, Abraham MD (Child Neurology) - *Special Expertise:* Child Neurology - General; **Admitting Hospital:** New York Weill Cornell Medical Center - NY Presbyterian Hospital (Page 72); **Office Address:** 525 E 68th St, Box 91 New York, NY 10021; **Office Phone:** (212) 746-3278; **Board Certifications:** Pediatrics 1962, Neurology 1965; **Medical School:** Univ Manitoba 1957; **Residency:** Pediatrics, Children's Hosp, Los Angeles, CA 1958-1960; **Fellowship:** Neurology, Columbia-Presby Med Ctr, New York, NY 1960-1963; **Faculty Appointment:** Prof Neurology, Cornell Univ-Weil Med Coll

Crawford, Thomas Owen MD (Child Neurology) - *Special Expertise: Neuromuscular Disorders; Muscular Dystrophy;* **Admitting Hospital:** Johns Hopkins Hospital - Baltimore (Page 65); **Office Address:** Johns Hopkins Hosp 600 N Wolfe St, Harvey Bldg, rm 811 Baltimore, MD 21287-8811; **Office Phone:** (410) 955-4259; **Board Certifications:** Pediatrics 1986, Neurology 1990; **Medical School:** USC Sch Med 1980; **Residencies:** Neurology, Children's Hosp, Los Angeles, CA 1984-1987; Pediatrics, LAC-USC Med Ctr, Los Angeles, CA 1981-1984; **Fellowship:** Neurology, Johns Hopkins Hosp, Baltimore, MD 1987-1988; **Faculty Appointment:** Asst Prof Neurology, Johns Hopkins Univ

De Vivo, Darryl C MD (Child Neurology) - *Special Expertise: Child Neurology - General;* **Admitting Hospital:** Columbia Presbyterian Medical Center (Page 72); **Office Address:** 710 W 168TH St New York, NY 10032; **Office Phone:** (212) 305-5244; **Board Certification:** Child Neurology 1972; **Medical School:** Univ VA Sch Med 1964; **Residencies:** Pediatrics, Mass Genl Hosp, Boston, MA 1965-1966; Neurology, Mass Genl Hosp, Boston, MA 1966-1967; **Fellowships:** Neurology, NIH, Bethesda, MD 1967-1969; Child Neurology, Children's Hosp-Wash Univ, St Louis, MO 1969-1970; **Faculty Appointment:** Prof Neurology, Columbia P&S

Eviatar, Lydia MD (Child Neurology) - *Special Expertise: Tourette's Syndrome; Epilepsy/Seizure Disorders;* **Admitting Hospital:** Long Island Jewish Medical Center; **Office Address:** 269-01 76th Ave, rm 267 New Hyde Park, NY 11040-1433; **Office Phone:** (718) 470-3450; **Board Certifications:** Pediatrics 1968, Child Neurology 1977; **Medical School:** Israel 1961; **Residency:** Pediatrics, Israel 1961-1966; **Fellowships:** Child Neurology, UCLA Med Ctr, Los Angeles, CA 1966-1967; Neurology, UCLA Med Ctr, Los Angeles, CA 1967-1969; **Faculty Appointment:** Prof Neurology, Albert Einstein Coll Med

Freeman, John M MD (Child Neurology) - *Special Expertise: Epilepsy/Seizure Disorders;* **Admitting Hospital:** Johns Hopkins Hospital - Baltimore (Page 65); **Office Address:** Johns Hopkins Hospital 600 N Wolfe St, Meyer Bldg 2-147 Baltimore, MD 21287; **Office Phone:** (410) 955-9100; **Board Certifications:** Pediatrics 1963, Child Neurology 1969; **Medical School:** Johns Hopkins Univ 1958; **Residency:** Pediatrics, Johns Hopkins Hosp, Baltimore, MD 1959-1961; **Fellowship:** Child Neurology, Columbia-Presby Med Ctr, New York, NY 1961-1964; **Faculty Appointment:** Prof Pediatrics, Johns Hopkins Univ

Lell, Mary-Elizabeth MD (Child Neurology) - *Special Expertise: Neonatal Neurology; Learning Disorders;* **Admitting Hospital:** St Vincents Catholic Medical Center of New York; **Office Address:** St Vincent's Hosp, Dept Neuro 153 W 11th St, rm 457 New York, NY 10011; **Office Phone:** (212) 604-7494; **Board Certifications:** Child Neurology 1976, Pediatrics 1980; **Medical School:** Univ Penn 1968; **Residencies:** Neurology, Univ Vermont, Burlington, VT 1969-1971; Pediatrics, St Louis Univ-Chldns Hosp, St Louis, MO 1971-1972; **Fellowship:** Child Neurology, Columbia Presby Hosp, New York, NY 1972-1974; **Faculty Appointment:** Assoc Clin Prof Neurology, NY Med Coll

Maytal, Joseph MD (Child Neurology) - *Special Expertise: Epilepsy/Seizure Disorders; Migraine;* **Admitting Hospital:** Schneider Children's Hospital; **Office Address:** Schneider Children's Hospital 269-01 76th Ave, Fl 2ND - rm 267 New Hyde Park, NY 11040; **Office Phone:** (718) 470-3450; **Board Certifications:** Pediatrics 1986, Child Neurology 1988; **Medical School:** Israel 1978; **Residencies:** Pediatrics, Brookdale Hosp, Brooklyn, NY 1982-1983; Child Neurology, Albert Einstein Coll Med Coll, Bronx, NY 1983-1986; **Fellowship:** Neurological Physiology, Albert Einstein Med Coll, Bronx, NY 1986-1987; **Faculty Appointment:** Clin Prof Neurology, Albert Einstein Coll Med

Packer, Roger MD (Child Neurology) - *Special Expertise:* Brain Tumors; **Admitting Hospital:** Children's National Medical Center - DC; **Office Address:** Children's Natl Med Ctr, Div Neur 111 Michigan Ave NW Washington, DC 20010-2970; **Office Phone:** (202) 884-2120; **Board Certifications:** Child Neurology 1982, Pediatrics 1982; **Medical School:** Northwestern Univ 1976; **Residencies:** Pediatrics, Chldns Med Ctr, Cincinnati, OH 1976-1978; Neurology, U Penn Chldns, Philadelphia, PA 1978-1981; **Faculty Appointment:** Prof Neurology, Geo Wash Univ

Southeast

Fenichel, Gerald M MD (Child Neurology) - *Special Expertise:* Amyotrophic Lateral Sclerosis(ALS); Neuromuscular Disorders; **Admitting Hospital:** Vanderbilt University Medical Center; **Office Address:** Univ Vanderbuilt Sch Med, Dept Neurology 2100 Pierce Ave, rm 362 Nashville, TN 37212; **Office Phone:** (615) 936-2024; **Board Certifications:** Neurology 1966, Child Neurology 1968; **Medical School:** Yale Univ 1959; **Residencies:** Neurology, Natnl Inst Neuro Disorders-NIHspital, Bethesda, MD 1961-1963; Neurology, Yale-New Haven Hosp, New Haven, CT 1963-1964; **Faculty Appointment:** Prof Neurology, Vanderbilt Univ

Greenwood, Robert Samuel MD (Child Neurology) - *Special Expertise:* Child Neurology - General; **Admitting Hospital:** University of North Carolina Hospitals; **Office Address:** U NC Sch Med Dept. Neurology 751 Burnett Womack, MC-CB 7025 Chapel Hill, NC 27599; **Office Phone:** (919) 966-2528; **Board Certifications:** Neurology 1979, Pediatrics 1974; **Medical School:** Univ Tex Med Br, Galveston 1968; **Residencies:** Child Neurology, Chldns Hosp., St. Louis, MO 1973-1975; Pediatrics, Chldns Hosp, St. Louis, MO 1970-1971; **Fellowship:** Child Neurology, Childrens Hosp, St Louis, MO 1976-1977; **Faculty Appointment:** Prof Neurology, Univ NC Sch Med

Turk, William MD (Child Neurology) - *Special Expertise:* Epilepsy/Seizure Disorders; Headache; **Admitting Hospital:** Wolfson Children's Hospital @ Baptist Medical Center; **Office Address:** 807 Nira St Jacksonville, FL 32207-8426; **Office Phone:** (904) 390-3780; **Board Certifications:** Pediatrics 1981, Pediatrics 1984; **Medical School:** Case West Res Univ 1976; **Residencies:** Pediatrics, NC Meml Hosp, Chapel Hill, NC 1977-1979; Neurology, Barnes Hospital, St Louis, MO 1979-1980; **Fellowship:** Child Neurology, St Louis Chldns Hosp, St Louis, MO 1980-1983; **Faculty Appointment:** Asst Prof Neurology, Mayo Med Sch

Midwest

Epstein, Leon G MD (Child Neurology) - *Special Expertise:* AIDS/HIV; **Admitting Hospital:** Children's Memorial Hospital; **Office Address:** Chldns Mem Hosp 2300 Children's Plaza Chicago, IL 60614; **Office Phone:** (773) 880-4352; **Board Certification:** Child Neurology 1979; **Medical School:** Wayne State Univ 1973; **Residencies:** Neurology, St Joseph's Mercy-Univ Michigan, Ann Arbor, MI 1973-1974; Neurology, Univ Arizona, Tucson, AZ 1974-1976; **Fellowship:** Neurology, Columbia Presby Med Ctr, New York, NY 1976-1978; **Faculty Appointment:** Prof Pediatrics, Northwestern Univ

Nigro, Michael A DO (Child Neurology) - *Special Expertise:* Neurologic Disorders; Neuromuscular Disorders; **Admitting Hospital:** Children's Hospital of Michigan; **Office Address:** Michigan Institute For Neurological Disorders 28595 Orchard Lake Rd, Ste 200 Farmington Hill, MI 48334; **Office Phone:** (248) 553-0010; **Board Certifications:** Neurology 1975, Clinical Neurophysiology 1996; **Medical School:** Philadelphia Coll Osteo Med 1966; **Residencies:** Neurology, Detroit Osteo Hosp, Highland Park, MI 1967-1970; Child Neurology, Univ Penn Chldns Hosp, Philadelphia, PA 1970-1972; **Faculty Appointment:** Prof Child Neurology, Wayne State Univ

CHILD NEUROLOGY

Noetzel, Michael MD (Child Neurology) - *Special Expertise:* Cerebral Palsy; Epilepsy/Seizure Disorders; Movement Disorders; **Admitting Hospital:** St Louis Children's Hospital; **Office Address:** Washington University, Dept of Neurology One Chldns Place St Louis, MO 63310-1014; **Office Phone:** (314) 454-6120; **Board Certifications:** Child Neurology 1984, Pediatrics 1984; **Medical School:** Univ VA Sch Med 1977; **Residencies:** Pediatrics, St Louis Chldns Hosp, St Louis, MO 1978-1979; Neurology, Barnes Hosp, St Louis, MO 1979-1980; **Fellowship:** Child Neurology, St Louis Chldns Hosp, St Louis, MO 1980-1982; **Faculty Appointment:** Assoc Prof Child Neurology, Washington Univ, St Louis

Patterson, Marc MD (Child Neurology) - *Special Expertise:* Hereditary Metabolic Diseases; Niemann-Pick Disease Type C; **Admitting Hospital:** Mayo Medical Center & Clinic - Rochester; **Office Address:** Mayo Clin, Dept Child Neur 200 First St SW Rochester, MN 55905; **Office Phone:** (507) 284-2091; **Board Certification:** Neurology 1994; **Medical School:** Australia 1981; **Residencies:** Neurology, Univ Queenland, Brisbane, Australia 1986-1988; Child Neurology, Mayo Clinic, Rochester, MN 1988-1990; **Fellowships:** Metabolic Neurology, Natl Inst Health, Bethesda, MD 1990-1992; Pediatrics, Mayo Cilnic, Rochester, MN 1992-1993; **Faculty Appointment:** Assoc Prof Child Neurology, Mayo Med Sch

Prensky, Arthur MD (Child Neurology) - *Special Expertise:* Headache; **Admitting Hospital:** St Louis Children's Hospital; **Office Address:** St Louis Chldns Hosp 1 Children's Pl, rm 12E25 St Louis, MO 63110; **Office Phone:** (314) 454-6120; **Board Certifications:** Neurology 1966, Child Neurology 1969; **Medical School:** NYU Sch Med 1955; **Residency:** Neurology, Mass Genl Hosp, Boston, Ma 1960-1963; **Fellowship:** Neurology, Mass Genl Hosp, Boston, Ma 1963-1966; **Faculty Appointment:** Prof Neurology, Washington Univ, St Louis

Stumpf, David A MD (Child Neurology) - *Special Expertise:* Ataxia; Epilepsy/Seizure Disorders; **Admitting Hospital:** Northwestern Memorial Hospital; **Office Address:** 675 N Saint Clair St, Fl 20 - Ste 100 Chicago, IL 60611-5935; **Office Phone:** (312) 695-7950; **Board Certifications:** Pediatrics 1978, Child Neurology 1979; **Medical School:** Univ Colo 1972; **Residencies:** Pediatrics, Strong Meml Hosp, Rochester, NY 1973-1974; Neurology, Childrens Hosp, Boston, MA 1974-1977

Wyllie, Elaine MD (Child Neurology) - *Special Expertise:* Epilepsy/Seizure Disorders; **Admitting Hospital:** Cleveland Clinic Foundation; **Office Address:** 9500 Euclid Ave, MC-Desk S51 Cleveland, OH 44195; **Office Phone:** (216) 444-2095; **Board Certifications:** Pediatrics 1982, Child Neurology 1986; **Medical School:** Indiana Univ 1978; **Residencies:** Pediatrics, Indiana Univ Sch Med, Indianapolis, IN 1978-1980; Pediatrics, Case West Res Med Sch, Cleveland, OH 1980-1981; **Fellowships:** Child Neurology, Cleveland Clinic Fdn, Cleveland, OH 1981-1984; Clinical Neurophysiology, Cleveland Clinic Fdn, Cleveland, OH 1984-1985

Great Plains and Mountains

Bale Jr, James MD (Child Neurology) - *Special Expertise:* Epilepsy/Seizure Disorders; **Admitting Hospital:** Primary Children's Medical Center; **Office Address:** Primary Chldns Med Ctr 100 N Medical Dr Salt Lake City, UT 84113; **Office Phone:** (801) 588-3385; **Board Certifications:** Child Neurology 1982, Pediatrics 1993; **Medical School:** Univ Mich Med Sch 1975; **Residencies:** Pediatrics, Univ Utah, Salt Lake City, UT 1975-1977; Neurology, Univ Utah, Salt Lake City, UT 1977-1980; **Fellowships:** Infectious Disease, Univ Utah, Salt Lake City, UT 1980-1981; Neurological Virus, UC San Fran-VAMC, San Francisco, CA 1981-1982; **Faculty Appointment:** Prof Univ Utah

Southwest

Edgar, Terence MD (Child Neurology) - *Special Expertise:* Neuromuscular Disorders; Cerebral Palsy; **Admitting Hospital:** Arkansas Children's Hospital; **Office Address:** Arkansas Children's Hosp, Dept Neuro 800 Marshall St, Box 512 Little Rock, AR 72202; **Office Phone:** (501) 320-1850; **Board Certifications:** Pediatrics 1995, Child Neurology 1997; **Medical School:** South Africa 1984; **Residencies:** Pediatrics, Univ of Pretoria, Pretoria, South Africa 1989-1992; Pediatrics, Univ Wisconsin Hosp & Clin, Madison, WI 1992-1993; **Fellowship:** Child Neurology, Univ Wisconsin Hosp & Clin, Madison, WI 1993-1996; **Faculty Appointment:** Asst Prof Pediatrics, Univ Ark

Fishman, Marvin Allen MD (Child Neurology) - *Special Expertise:* Child Neurology - General; **Admitting Hospital:** Texas Children's Hospital - Houston; **Office Address:** Texas Childns Hosp 6621 Fannin MC3-3311 Houston, TX 77030; **Office Phone:** (832) 824-3960; **Board Certifications:** Pediatrics 1966, Child Neurology 1972; **Medical School:** Univ IL Coll Med 1961; **Residencies:** Pediatrics, Michael Reese Hosp, Chicago, IL 1962-1964; Child Neurology, Mass Genl Hosp, Boston, MA 1966-1967; **Fellowship:** Child Neurology, Chldns Hosp, St Louis, MO 1967-1969; **Faculty Appointment:** Prof Child Neurology, Baylor Coll Med

Iannaccone, Susan MD (Child Neurology) - *Special Expertise:* Neuromuscular Disorders; **Admitting Hospital:** Texas Scottish Rite Hospital for Children - Dallas; **Office Address:** 2222 Welborn St Dallas, TX 75219-3924; **Office Phone:** (214) 559-7830; **Board Certifications:** Pediatrics 1975, Child Neurology 1976; **Medical School:** SUNY Hlth Sci Ctr 1969; **Residencies:** Pediatrics, St Louis Childrens Hosp-Washington 1971-1972; Neurology, Strong Meml Hosp, Rochester, NY 1972-1975; **Fellowship:** Neurology, Strong Meml Hosp, Rochester, NY 1972-1975; **Faculty Appointment:** Assoc Prof Neurology, Univ Cincinnati

West Coast and Pacific

Ashwal, Stephen MD (Child Neurology) - *Special Expertise:* Child Neurology - General; **Admitting Hospital:** Loma Linda University Medical Center; **Office Address:** Loma Linda Pediatric Medical Group 11262 Campus, Bldg West Hall Loma Linda, CA 92354; **Office Phone:** (909) 796-4848; **Board Certifications:** Pediatrics 1975, Child Neurology 1978; **Medical School:** NYU Sch Med 1970; **Residency:** Pediatrics, Bellevue Hosp, New York, NY 1971-1973; **Fellowship:** Child Neurology, Univ Minn, Minneapolis, MN 1973-1976; **Faculty Appointment:** Prof Pediatrics, Loma Linda Univ

Ferriero, Donna Marie MD (Child Neurology) - *Special Expertise:* Neuro-Endocrinology; **Admitting Hospital:** St Francis Memorial Hospital; **Office Address:** San Francisco Genl Hosp, Neuro Svc 4M65 1001 Potrero San Francisco, CA 94110; **Office Phone:** (415) 353-7789; **Board Certifications:** Pediatrics 1986, Child Neurology 1987; **Medical School:** UCSF 1979; **Residencies:** Pediatrics, Mass Genl Hosp, Boston, MA 1981-1982; Child Neurology, UCSF, San Francisco, CA 1982-1985; **Fellowship:** UCSF, San Francisco, CA 1985-1987

Haas, Richard H MD (Child Neurology) - *Special Expertise:* Mitochondrial Disorders; **Admitting Hospital:** University of California - San Diego Healthcare; **Office Address:** UCSD Med Ctr, Div Ped Neuro 9500 Gilman La Jolla, CA 92093-0935; **Office Phone:** (858) 587-4004; **Board Certifications:** Child Neurology 1983, Pediatrics 1985; **Medical School:** England 1972; **Residencies:** Pediatrics, Univ London, London, UK 1976-1979; Child Neurology, Univ Colorado, Denver, CO 1979-1981; **Fellowship:** Biochemical Mental Retardation, Univ Colorado, Denver, CO 1979-1981; **Faculty Appointment:** Assoc Prof Child Neurology, UCSD

Lott, Ira T MD (Child Neurology) - *Special Expertise:* Down Syndrome; **Admitting Hospital:** University of California - Irvine Medical Center; **Office Address:** UC Irvine Med Ctr, Dept Ped/Neurology 101 City Dr S Orange, CA 92868-3201; **Office Phone:** (714) 456-7002; **Board Certifications:** Pediatrics 1975, Child Neurology 1977; **Medical School:** Ohio State Univ 1967; **Residency:** Pediatrics, Mass Genl Hosp, Boston, MA 1967-1969; **Fellowships:** Research, Natl Inst Hlth, Bethesda, MD 1969-1971; Neurology, Harvard-Mass Genl Hosp, Boston, MA 1971-1974; **Faculty Appointment:** Prof Child Neurology, UC Irvine

Menkes, John H MD (Child Neurology) - *Special Expertise:* Genetic Disorders; Movement Disorders; **Admitting Hospital:** Cedars-Sinai Medical Center; **Office Address:** 9320 Wilshire Blvd, Ste 202 Beverly Hills, CA 90212-3216; **Office Phone:** (310) 246-6582; **Board Certifications:** Pediatrics 1958, Neurology 1962; **Medical School:** Johns Hopkins Univ 1952; **Residencies:** Pediatrics, Boston Children's Hosp, Boston, MA 1952-1954; Pediatrics, Bellevue Hosp Ctr, New York, NY 1956-1957; **Fellowship:** Child Neurology, Neurological Inst, New York, NY 1957-1960; **Faculty Appointment:** Prof Emeritus Child Neurology, UCLA

Mitchell, Wendy Gayle MD (Child Neurology) - *Special Expertise:* Epilepsy/Seizure Disorders; Developmental Disabilities, Autism; Cysticercosis; **Admitting Hospital:** Children's Hospital - Los Angeles; **Office Address:** Children's Hosp Los Angeles, Dept Neuro 4650 Sunset Blvd, Box 82 Los Angeles, CA 90027; **Office Phone:** (323) 669-2471; **Board Certifications:** Pediatrics 1978, Child Neurology 1983; **Medical School:** UCSF 1973; **Residencies:** Pediatrics, Moffit Hosp-UCSF, San Francisco, CA 1973-1975; Child Neurology, Univ NC, Chapel Hill, NC 1978-1981; **Fellowship:** Child Psychiatry, Mt Zion Hosp, San Francisco, CA 1975-1976; **Faculty Appointment:** Prof Neurology, USC Sch Med

Mobley, William Charles MD (Child Neurology) - *Special Expertise:* Child Neurology - General; **Admitting Hospital:** Stanford Medical Center; **Office Address:** 300 Pasteur Dr SHS H3160, MC 5235 Stanford, CA 94305-5235; **Office Phone:** (650) 723-6424; **Board Certifications:** Pediatrics 1983, Child Neurology 1987; **Medical School:** Stanford Univ 1976; **Residencies:** Pediatrics, Stanford Univ Schl Med, Stanford, CA 1977-1979; Neurology, John Hopkins Hosp, Baltimore, MD 1979-1982; **Faculty Appointment:** Prof Neurology, UCSF

Shields, William Donald MD (Child Neurology) - *Special Expertise:* Epilepsy/Seizure Disorders; **Admitting Hospital:** UCLA Medical Center; **Office Address:** UCLA Med Ctr, Dept Ped/Neurology 10833 Le Conte Ave Los Angeles, CA 90095; **Office Phone:** (310) 825-6196; **Board Certifications:** Child Neurology 1977, Pediatrics 1978; **Medical School:** Univ Utah 1971; **Residencies:** Pediatrics, USC Med Ctr, Los Angeles, CA 1972-1973; Neurology, Univ Utah Med Ctr, Salt Lake City, UT 1973-1976; **Faculty Appointment:** Prof Pediatrics, UCLA

Trauner, Doris Ann MD (Child Neurology) - *Special Expertise:* Autism; Speech Disorders; **Admitting Hospital:** University of California - San Diego Healthcare; **Office Address:** UCSD Med Ctr, Div Ped Neuro 9500 Gilman Dr, MC-0935 La Jolla, CA 92093-0935; **Office Phone:** (858) 587-4004; **Board Certifications:** Pediatrics 1978, Child Neurology 1979; **Medical School:** Med Coll VA 1972; **Residencies:** Neurology, UCSD Med Ctr, San Diego, CA 1974-1975; Pediatrics, UCSD Med Ctr, San Diego, CA 1973-1974; **Fellowship:** Child Neurology, Univ Chicago, Chicago, IL 1975-1977; **Faculty Appointment:** Prof Pediatrics, UCSD

CLINICAL GENETICS

A specialist trained in diagnostic and therapeutic procedures for patients with genetically-linked diseases. This specialist uses modern cytogenetic, radiologic and biochemical testing to assist in specialized genetic counseling, implements needed therapeutic interventions and provides prevention through prenatal diagnosis.

A clinical geneticist demonstrates competence in providing comprehensive diagnostic, management and counseling services for genetic disorders.

A medical geneticist plans and coordinates large scale screening programs for inborn errors of metabolism, hemoglobinopathies, chromosome abnormalities and neural tube defects.

Training required: Two or four years

PHYSICIAN LISTINGS

Clinical Genetics

New England

Holmes, Lewis B MD (Clinical Genetics) - *Special Expertise:* Birth Defects; Inherited Diseases; **Admitting Hospital:** Massachusetts General Hospital; **Office Address:** Mass Gen Hosp 55 Fruit St, Bldg Warren 801 Boston, MA 02114-2696; **Office Phone:** (617) 726-1742; **Board Certifications:** Pediatrics 1968, Clinical Genetics 1982; **Medical School:** Duke Univ 1963; **Residency:** Pediatrics, Mass Genl Hosp, Boston, MA; **Faculty Appointment:** Prof Pediatrics, Harvard Med Sch

Korf, Bruce MD/PhD (Clinical Genetics) - *Special Expertise:* Inherited Diseases; Neuro-Genetics; **Admitting Hospital:** Brigham & Women's Hospital; **Office Address:** Partners Center for Human Genetics 77 Avenue Louis Pasteur, Bldg HIM - Fl 6 - Ste 642 Boston, MA 02115; **Office Phone:** (617) 525-5750; **Board Certifications:** Clinical Genetics 1984, Child Neurology 1986; **Medical School:** Cornell Univ-Weil Med Coll 1980; **Residencies:** Pediatrics, Chldns Hosp, Boston, MA 1981-1982; Neurology, Chldns Hosp, Boston, MA 1982-1985; **Fellowship:** Clinical Genetics, Chldns Hosp, Boston, MA 1982-1985; **Faculty Appointment:** Assoc Prof Neurology, Harvard Med Sch

Nussbaum, Robert MD (Clinical Genetics) - *Special Expertise:* Genetic Disorders; **Admitting Hospital:** National Institutes of Health - Clinical Center; **Office Address:** Natl Human Gen Res Inst 49 Convent Dr MSC 4472 Bethesda, MA 20892; **Office Phone:** (301) 402-2039; **Board Certifications:** Internal Medicine 1978, Clinical Genetics 1982; **Medical School:** Harvard Med Sch 1975; **Residency:** Internal Medicine, Barnes Hospital, St Louis, MO 1976-1978; **Fellowship:** Clinical Genetics, Baylor, Houston, TX 1978-1983; **Faculty Appointment:** Prof Clinical Genetics, Univ Penn

Seashore, Margretta MD (Clinical Genetics) - *Special Expertise:* Inherited Metabolic Disorders; **Admitting Hospital:** Yale - New Haven Hospital; **Office Address:** Yale Univ Sch Med, Dept Genetics 333 Cedar St, rm 305 New Haven, CT 06520-8005; **Office Phone:** (203) 785-2660; **Board Certifications:** Pediatrics 1970, Clinical Genetics 1982; **Medical School:** Yale Univ 1965; **Residency:** Pediatrics, Yale-New Haven Hosp, New Haven, CT 1966-1968; **Fellowship:** Clinical Genetics, Yale-New Haven Hosp, New Haven, CT 1968-1970; **Faculty Appointment:** Prof Clinical Genetics, Yale Univ

Mid Atlantic

Anyane-Yeboa, Kwame MD (Clinical Genetics) - *Special Expertise:* Syndromology; Prenatal Genetic Diagnosis; **Admitting Hospital:** Columbia Presbyterian Medical Center (Page 72); **Office Address:** Columbia Presby Med Ctr 622 W 168th St New York, NY 10032-3702; **Office Phone:** (212) 305-6731; **Board Certifications:** Clinical Genetics 1982, Pediatrics 1979; **Medical School:** Ghana 1972; **Residency:** Pediatrics, Harlem Hosp, New York, NY 1974-1977; **Fellowship:** Clinical Genetics, Babies Hosp-Columbia, New York, NY 1977-1980; **Faculty Appointment:** Assoc Prof Pediatrics, Coll Physicians & Surgeons

Biesecker, Leslie Glenn MD (Clinical Genetics) - *Special Expertise:* Clinical Genetics - General; **Admitting Hospital:** National Institutes of Health - Clinical Center; **Office Address:** NIH Nat Hum Gen Res Int 9000 Rockville Pike, Bldg 49 - rm 4A80 Bethesda, MD 20892; **Office Phone:** (301) 402-2041; **Board Certifications:** Pediatrics 1987, Clinical Genetics 1990; **Medical School:** Univ IL Coll Med 1983; **Residency:** Pediatrics, Univ Wisc Hosp, Madison, WI 1984-1986; **Fellowship:** Clinical Genetics, Univ Mich Med Ctr, Ann Arbor, MI 1988-1990

Davis, Jessica S MD (Clinical Genetics) - *Special Expertise:* Marfan's Syndrome; Mental Retardation; **Admitting Hospital:** New York Weill Cornell Medical Center - NY Presbyterian Hospital (Page 72); **Office Address:** 525 E 68th St, Bldg HT150 New York, NY 10021; **Office Phone:** (212) 746-1496; **Board Certification:** Clinical Genetics 1984; **Medical School:** Columbia P&S 1959; **Residency:** Pediatrics, St Luke's Hosp, New York, NY 1961-1962; **Fellowships:** Clinical Genetics, Albert Einstein Coll Med, Bronx, NY 1961-1965; Cytogenetics, Albert Einstein Col Med, Bronx, NY 1965-1966; **Faculty Appointment:** Assoc Clin Prof Pediatrics, Cornell Univ-Weil Med Coll

Desnick, Robert J MD/PhD (Clinical Genetics) - *Special Expertise:* Porphyria; Fabry's Disease; Inherited Metabolic Diseases; **Admitting Hospital:** Mount Sinai Hospital (Page 70); **Office Address:** Mt Sinai Sch Med, Box 1498 Fifth Ave @ 100th Street New York, NY 10029; **Office Phone:** (212) 659-6700; **Board Certifications:** Clinical Genetics 1982, Clinical Molecular Genetics 1999; **Medical School:** Univ Minn 1971; **Residency:** Pediatrics, Univ Minn Hosps, Minneapolis, MN 1972-1973; **Faculty Appointment:** Prof Clinical Genetics, Mount Sinai Sch Med

Desposito, Franklin MD (Clinical Genetics) - *Special Expertise:* Birth Defects; Genetic Disorders; **Admitting Hospital:** UMDNJ-University Hospital-Newark; **Office Address:** UMDNJ Univ Hosp 185 S Orange Ave Newark, NJ 07103; **Office Phone:** (973) 972-3300; **Board Certifications:** Clinical Genetics 1982, Pediatrics 1986; **Medical School:** Univ Hlth Sci/Chicago Med Sch 1957; **Residency:** Pediatrics, Long Island Jewish Hosp, New Hyde Park, NY 1958-1961; **Fellowship:** Hematology, Univ Wisc Sch Med, Milwaukee, WI 1961-1963; **Faculty Appointment:** Prof Pediatrics, UMDNJ-NJ Med Sch, Newark

Rosenbaum, Kenneth MD (Clinical Genetics) - *Special Expertise:* Clinical Genetics - General; **Admitting Hospital:** Children's National Medical Center - DC; **Office Address:** 111 Michigan Avenue NW Washington, DC 20010; **Office Phone:** (202) 884-2187; **Board Certifications:** Pediatrics 1976, Clinical Genetics 1982; **Medical School:** Univ Louisville Sch Med 1971

Shapiro, Lawrence R MD (Clinical Genetics) - *Special Expertise:* Clinical Genetics - General; **Admitting Hospital:** Westchester Medical Center; **Office Address:** Regional Med Genetics Ctr 19 Bradhurst Ave Hawthorne, NY 10532; **Office Phone:** (914) 347-3010; **Board Certifications:** Pediatrics 1967, Clinical Genetics 1982; **Medical School:** NYU Sch Med 1962; **Residencies:** Pediatrics, Los Angeles Chldns Hosp, Los Angeles, CA 1962-1964; Pediatrics, Bellevue Hosp, New York, NY 1964-1965; **Fellowships:** Clinical Genetics, NYU, New York, NY 1965; Clinical Genetics, Mount Sinai Med Ctr, New York, NY 1967-1968; **Faculty Appointment:** Prof Pediatrics, NY Med Coll

Willner, Judith P MD (Clinical Genetics) - *Special Expertise:* Dysmorphology; Birth Defects; Metabolic Genetic Disorders; **Admitting Hospital:** Mount Sinai Hospital (Page 70); **Office Address:** One Gustave Levy Pl New York, NY 10029; **Office Phone:** (212) 241-6947; **Board Certifications:** Pediatrics 1977, Clinical Genetics 1982; **Medical School:** NYU Sch Med 1971; **Residency:** Pediatrics, Children's Hosp Natl Med Ctr, Washington, DC 1972-1973; **Fellowship:** Clinical Genetics, Mount Sinai Hosp, New York, NY 1974-1977; **Faculty Appointment:** Prof Clinical Genetics, Mount Sinai Sch Med

Zackai, Elaine MD (Clinical Genetics) - *Special Expertise:* Craniosynostosis; Cytogenetics; **Admitting Hospital:** The Children's Hospital of Philadelphia; **Office Address:** 34th & Civic Center Blvd Philadelphia, PA 19104; **Office Phone:** (215) 590-2920; **Board Certifications:** Pediatrics 1977, Clinical Genetics 1982; **Medical School:** NYU Sch Med 1968; **Residencies:** Pediatrics, Albert Einstein Med Sch, Bronx, NY 1968-1969; Pediatrics, Chldns Hosp, St Louis, MO 1969-1970; **Fellowships:** Clinical Genetics, Chldns Hosp, St Louis, MO 1970-1971; Clinical Genetics, Yale Univ Med Sch, New Haven, CT 1971-1972; **Faculty Appointment:** Prof Pediatrics, Univ Penn

Southeast

Driscoll, Daniel J MD (Clinical Genetics) - *Special Expertise: Angelman Syndrome; Prader-Willi Syndrome; Obesity;* **Admitting Hospital:** Shands Healthcare at University Florida (Page 77); **Office Address:** Univ Florida-Pediatric Genetics 1600 SW ARcher Rd, Bldg RG232, Box 100296 Gainesville, FL 32610-0296; **Office Phone:** (352) 392-4104; **Board Certifications:** Pediatrics 1987, Clinical Genetics 1990; **Medical School:** Albany Med Coll 1983; **Residency:** Pediatrics, John Hopkins Hospital, Baltimore, MD 1983-1986; **Fellowship:** Clinical Genetics, John Hopkins Hospital, Baltimore, MD 1986-1989; **Faculty Appointment:** Assoc Prof Pediatrics, Univ Fla Coll Med

Elsas II, Louis Jacob MD (Clinical Genetics) - *Special Expertise: Maple Syrup Urine Disease;* **Admitting Hospital:** Emory University Hospital; **Office Address:** Emory Univ, Div Med Genetics 2040 Ridgewood Dr Atlanta, GA 30322; **Office Phone:** (404) 727-5863; **Board Certifications:** Internal Medicine 1972, Clinical Genetics 1982; **Medical School:** Univ VA Sch Med 1962; **Residency:** Internal Medicine, Yale-New Haven Hosp, New Haven, CT 1963-1965; **Fellowship:** Clinical Genetics, New HAven Hosp-Yale, New Haven, CT 1965-1968; **Faculty Appointment:** Prof Pediatrics, Emory Univ

Hall, Bryan Davis MD (Clinical Genetics) - *Special Expertise: Birth Defects; Dysmorphology;* **Admitting Hospital:** University of Kentucky Medical Center; **Office Address:** Univ Kentucky Chldns Hosp, Dept Ped/Div Genetics 800 Rose St Lexington, KY 40536-0284; **Office Phone:** (859) 257-5559; **Board Certification:** Pediatrics 1970; **Medical School:** Univ Louisville Sch Med 1965; **Residencies:** Pediatrics, St Hosp Sick Chldn, London, England 1966-1967; Pediatrics, Chldns Hosp, Louisville, KY 1967-1968; **Fellowship:** Clinical Genetics, Univ Wash, Seattle, WA 1970-1972; **Faculty Appointment:** Prof Pediatrics, Univ KY Coll Med

Saul, Robert MD (Clinical Genetics) - *Special Expertise: Birth Defects;* **Admitting Hospital:** Self Memorial Hospital; **Office Address:** Greenwood Genetic Ctr One Gregor Mendel Cir Greenwood, SC 29646-2307; **Office Phone:** (888) 442-4363; **Board Certifications:** Pediatrics 1981, Clinical Genetics 1982; **Medical School:** Univ Colo 1976; **Residency:** Pediatrics, Duke Med Ctr, Durham, NC 1976-1979; **Fellowship:** Clinical Genetics, Greenwood Genetics Ctr, Greenwood, SC 1979-1981

Seaver, Laurie Heron MD (Clinical Genetics) - *Special Expertise: Fetal Pathology; Fetal Alcohol Syndrome;* **Admitting Hospital:** Self Memorial Hospital; **Office Address:** Greenwood Genetic Ctr One Gregor Mendel Cir Greenwood, SC 29646; **Office Phone:** (894) 941-8100; **Board Certifications:** Pediatrics 1998, Clinical Genetics 1993; **Medical School:** Univ Ariz Coll Med 1987; **Residency:** Pediatrics, Univ Ariz, Tucson, AZ 1988-1990; **Fellowship:** Clinical Genetics, U Ariz Coll Med, Tucson, AZ 1990-1993

Stevenson, Roger E MD (Clinical Genetics) - *Special Expertise: Birth Defects; Mental Retardation;* **Admitting Hospital:** Self Memorial Hospital; **Office Address:** Greenwood Genetic Ctr One Gregor Mendel Cir Greenwood, SC 29646-2307; **Office Phone:** (864) 941-8100; **Board Certifications:** Pediatrics 1971, Clinical Genetics 1982; **Medical School:** Wake Forest Univ Sch Med 1966; **Residency:** Pediatrics, Johns Hopkins Hosp, Baltimore, MD 1967-1969; **Fellowship:** Clinical Genetics, Johns Hopkins Hosp, Baltimore, MD 1971-1972

Midwest

Cassidy, Suzanne MD (Clinical Genetics) - *Special Expertise:* Prader-Willi Syndrome; Connective Tissue Disorders; Neurocutaneous Disorders; **Admitting Hospital:** Rainbow Babies & Children's Hospital; **Office Address:** Center for Human Genetics, Lakeside 1500 11100 Euclid Ave Cleveland, OH 44106; **Office Phone:** (216) 844-7236; **Board Certifications:** Pediatrics 1983, Clinical Genetics 1982; **Medical School:** Vanderbilt Univ 1976; **Residency:** Pediatrics, Univ Wash Affil Prgms, Seattle, WA 1978-1979; **Fellowship:** Clinical Genetics, Univ Wash, Seattle, WA 1979-1981; **Faculty Appointment:** Prof Clinical Genetics, Case West Res Univ

Charrow, Joel MD (Clinical Genetics) - *Special Expertise:* Biochemical Genetics; **Admitting Hospital:** Children's Memorial Hospital; **Office Address:** Childrens Meml Hosp. - Div Genetics 2300 Childrens Plaza Chicago, IL 60614-3318; **Office Phone:** (773) 880-4462; **Board Certifications:** Clinical Genetics 1987, Clinical Genetics 1982; **Medical School:** Mount Sinai Sch Med 1976; **Residency:** Pediatrics, Chldns Meml Hosp-Northwestern, Chicago, IL 1977-1979; **Fellowship:** Clinical Genetics, Chldns Meml Hosp-Northwestern, Chicago, IL 1979-1981; **Faculty Appointment:** Assoc Prof Pediatrics, Northwestern Univ

Gray, Diana Lee MD (Clinical Genetics) - *Special Expertise:* Prenatal Diagnosis; **Admitting Hospital:** Barnes - Jewish Hospital; **Office Address:** Barnes-Jewish Hosp, Dept ObGyn 216 S Kingshighway Blvd, Ste 5300, MS 90-31-644 St Louis, MO 63110; **Office Phone:** (314) 454-8135; **Board Certifications:** Obstetrics & Gynecology 1996, Clinical Genetics 1993; **Medical School:** Univ IL Coll Med 1981; **Residencies:** Obstetrics & Gynecology, Wash Univ, St Louis, MO 1982-1985; Obstetrics & Gynecology, Wash Univ, St Louis, MO 1985-1987; **Fellowships:** Obstetrics & Gynecology, Wash Univ, St Louis, MO 1985-1987; Clinical Genetics, Wash Univ, St Louis, MO 1988-1990; **Faculty Appointment:** Assoc Prof Clinical Genetics, Washington Univ, St Louis

Martin, Rick A MD (Clinical Genetics) - *Special Expertise:* Dysmorphology; **Admitting Hospital:** St Louis Children's Hospital; **Office Address:** St Louis Chldrn's Hosp 1 Children's Place St Louis, MO 63110; **Office Phone:** (314) 454-6093; **Board Certifications:** Pediatrics 1998, Clinical Genetics 1993; **Medical School:** Univ Utah 1987; **Residency:** Pediatrics, UCSD, San Diego, CA 1988-1990; **Fellowship:** Clinical Genetics, UCSD, San Diego, CA 1990-1992; **Faculty Appointment:** Assoc Prof Clinical Genetics, Washington Univ, St Louis

Saal, Howard MD (Clinical Genetics) - *Special Expertise:* Craniofacial Disorders; Cleft Palate/Lip; Neurofibromatosis; **Admitting Hospital:** Children's Hospital Medical Center; **Office Address:** Chldns Hosp Med Ctr, Div Human Genetics 3333 Burnet Ave Cinncinnati, OH 45229-2899; **Office Phone:** (513) 636-4760; **Board Certifications:** Clinical Genetics 1984, Pediatrics 1985; **Medical School:** Wayne State Univ 1979; **Residency:** Pediatrics, Univ Conn Hlth Ctr, Farmington, CT 1979-1982; **Fellowship:** Clinical Genetics, Univ Wash, Seattle, WA 1982-1984; **Faculty Appointment:** Prof Pediatrics, Univ Cincinnati

Weaver, David Dawson MD (Clinical Genetics) - *Special Expertise:* Inherited Bone Disorders; Genetic Disorders; Prenatal Diagnosis; **Admitting Hospital:** Indiana University Hospital & Medical Center - Indianapolis; **Office Address:** Ind Univ Sch Med, Dept Med Genetics 975 W Walnut St, Bldg IB - rm 130 Indianapolis, IN 46202-5251; **Office Phone:** (317) 274-2241; **Board Certifications:** Pediatrics 1978, Clinical Genetics 1982; **Medical School:** Oregon Hlth Scis Univ 1966; **Residency:** Pediatrics, Oregon Hlth Scis Univ Sch Med, Portland, OR 1970-1972; **Fellowships:** Metabolic Diseases, Oregon Hlth Scis Univ Sch Med, Portland, OR 1974-1976; Clinical Genetics, Univ WA Sch Med, Seattle, WA; **Faculty Appointment:** Prof Clinical Genetics, Indiana Univ

Whelan, Alison MD (Clinical Genetics) - *Special Expertise:* Clinical Genetics - General; **Admitting Hospital:** Barnes - Jewish Hospital; **Office Address:** Wash U Sch Med 660 S Euclid, Box 8073 St Louis, MO 63110; **Office Phone:** (314) 454-6093; **Board Certification:** Clinical Genetics 1996; **Medical School:** Washington Univ, St Louis 1986; **Residencies:** Internal Medicine, Barnes Hosp, St Louis, MO 1987-1989; Pediatrics, Wash U Sch Med, St Louis, MO 1992-1994; **Fellowships:** Research, Wash U Sch Med, St Louis, MO 1989-1991; Clinical Genetics, Wash U Sch Med, St Louis, MO 1993-1994; **Faculty Appointment:** Asst Prof Medicine, Washington Univ, St Louis

Great Plains and Mountains

Carey, John MD (Clinical Genetics) - *Special Expertise:* Neurofibromatosis; Birth Defects; **Admitting Hospital:** University of Utah Hospital and Clinics; **Office Address:** Univ Utah Med Ctr-Div of Med Gen 50 N Med Dr, 2C412SOM Salt Lake City, UT 84132; **Office Phone:** (801) 581-8943; **Board Certifications:** Pediatrics 1979, Clinical Genetics 1982; **Medical School:** Georgetown Univ 1972; **Residency:** Pediatrics, UCSF Med Ctr, CA 1973-1975; **Fellowship:** Clinical Genetics, UCSF Med Ctr, CA 1976-1979; **Faculty Appointment:** Prof Medicine, Univ Utah

Southwest

Craigen, William MD (Clinical Genetics) - *Special Expertise:* Biochemical Genetics; **Admitting Hospital:** Texas Children's Hospital - Houston; **Office Address:** Dept Molecular Human Genetics 1 Baylor Plaza Houston, TX 77030; **Office Phone:** (713) 798-8305; **Board Certifications:** Pediatrics 1992, Clinical Genetics 1993; **Medical School:** Baylor Coll Med 1988; **Residencies:** Pediatrics, Baylor Coll Med, Houston, TX 1988-1990; Pediatrics, Baylor Coll Med, Houston, TX 1990-1992; **Fellowship:** Clinical Genetics, Baylor Coll Med, Houston, TX 1988-1990; **Faculty Appointment:** Assoc Prof Clinical Genetics, Baylor Coll Med

Cunniff, Christopher MD (Clinical Genetics) - *Special Expertise:* Birth Defects; **Admitting Hospital:** University Medical Center; **Office Address:** U Ariz Coll Med-Dept Ped, Sect Med Genetics 1501 N Campbell Ave Tucson, AZ 85724; **Office Phone:** (520) 626-5175; **Board Certifications:** Pediatrics 1996, Clinical Genetics 1990; **Medical School:** Univ Ala 1984; **Residency:** Pediatrics, MC Hosp Of Vt, Burlington, VT 1985-1987; **Fellowship:** Clinical Genetics, UCSD Med Ctr, San Diego, CA 1987-1989; **Faculty Appointment:** Assoc Prof Pediatrics, Univ Ariz Coll Med

Northrup, Hope MD (Clinical Genetics) - *Special Expertise:* Biochemical Genetics; Neuro-Genetics; **Admitting Hospital:** Memorial Hermann Healthcare System; **Office Address:** Univ TX Med Sch-Houston-Dept Peds-Div Med Genetics 6431 Fannin St Houston, TX 77030; **Office Phone:** (713) 500-5760; **Board Certifications:** Pediatrics 1988, Clinical Genetics 1990; **Medical School:** Med Univ SC 1983; **Residency:** Pediatrics, Children's MC-Southwestern Med Sch, Dallas, TX 1983-1986; **Fellowship:** Clinical Genetics, Baylor Coll of Medicine, Houston, TX 1986-1989; **Faculty Appointment:** Prof Pediatrics

West Coast and Pacific

Boles, Richard Gregory MD (Clinical Genetics) - *Special Expertise:* Mitochondrial Disorders; Mitochondrial Dis/Maternal Inheritance; **Admitting Hospital:** Children's Hospital - Los Angeles; **Office Address:** Childrens Hosp-Div Med Genetics 4650 Sunset Blvd, MS 90 Los Angeles, CA 90027; **Office Phone:** (323) 669-2290; **Board Certifications:** Pediatrics 1994, Clinical Genetics 1993; **Medical School:** UCLA 1987; **Residency:** Pediatrics, Harbor-UCLA Med Ctr, Torrance, CA 1988-1990; **Fellowship:** Clinical Genetics, Yale Univ Sch Med, New Haven, CT 1991-1993; **Faculty Appointment:** Asst Prof Pediatrics, USC Sch Med

CLINICAL GENETICS

Cederbaum, Stephen D MD (Clinical Genetics) - *Special Expertise: Inborn Errors of Metabolism;* **Admitting Hospital:** UCLA Medical Center; **Office Address:** UCLA Ctr Hlth Sci 760 Westwood Los Angeles, CA 90024-1759; **Office Phone:** (310) 206-6581; **Board Certifications:** Clinical Genetics 1982, Clinical Biochemical Genetics 1982; **Medical School:** NYU Sch Med 1964; **Residency:** Internal Medicine, Barnes Hosp, St. Louis, MO 1965-1966; **Fellowship:** Clinical Genetics, Univ Wash, Seattle, WA 1968-1970; **Faculty Appointment:** Prof Pediatrics, UCLA

Curry, Cynthia J MD (Clinical Genetics) - *Special Expertise: Clinical Genetics - General;* **Admitting Hospital:** Valley Children's Hospital; **Office Address:** Valley Chldns Hosp-Genetic Med 9300 Valley Childrens Pl Madera, CA 93638; **Office Phone:** (559) 353-6626; **Board Certifications:** Pediatrics 1973, Clinical Genetics 1982; **Medical School:** Yale Univ 1967; **Residencies:** Pediatrics, Univ Minn Hosp, Seattle, WA 1968-1969; Pediatrics, Univ Wash Orth Chldns Hosp, Minneapolis, MN 1969-1970; **Fellowship:** Clinical Genetics, UCSF Med Ctr, San Francisco, CA 1975-1976; **Faculty Appointment:** Prof Clinical Genetics, UCSF

Falk, Rena Ellen MD (Clinical Genetics) - *Special Expertise: Clinical Genetics - General;* **Admitting Hospital:** Cedars-Sinai Medical Center; **Office Address:** Genetics-Birth Defects Ctr 444 S San Vicente Blvd, Ste 1001 Los Angeles, CA 90048; **Office Phone:** (310) 423-9942; **Board Certifications:** Clinical Genetics 1982, Pediatrics 1976; **Medical School:** UCLA 1971; **Residency:** Pediatrics, Cedars-Sinai Med Ctr, Los Angeles, CA 1971-1973; **Fellowships:** Clinical Genetics, UCLA Med School, Los Angeles, CA 1973-1975; UCLA, Los Angeles, CA 1975-1977; **Faculty Appointment:** Prof Pediatrics, UCLA

Graham Jr, John M MD (Clinical Genetics) - *Special Expertise: Dysmorphology; Craniofacial Disorders;* **Admitting Hospital:** Cedars-Sinai Medical Center; **Office Address:** 444 S San Vicente Blvd, Ste 1001 Los Angeles, CA 90048-4175; **Office Phone:** (310) 423-9914; **Board Certifications:** Pediatrics 1982, Clinical Genetics 1982; **Medical School:** Med Univ SC 1975; **Residency:** Pediatrics, Boston Chldns Hosp-Harvard Med Sch, Boston, MA 1976-1977; **Fellowships:** Developmental Pediatrics, Boston Chldns Hosp, Boston, MA 1977-1978; Dysmorphology, Univ Wash, Seattle, WA 1978-1980; **Faculty Appointment:** Prof Pediatrics, UCLA

Grody, Wayne W MD (Clinical Genetics) - *Special Expertise: Genetic Disorders; Familial Cancer;* **Admitting Hospital:** UCLA Medical Center; **Office Address:** UCLA Med Ctr 10833 Le Conte Ave Los Angeles, CA 90095-1732; **Office Phone:** (310) 825-5648; **Board Certifications:** Clinical Genetics 1990, Pathology 1987; **Medical School:** Baylor Coll Med 1977; **Residency:** Pathology, UCLA Med Ctr, Los Angeles, CA 1982-1986; **Fellowship:** Clinical Genetics, UCLA Med Ctr, Los Angeles, CA 1985-1987; **Faculty Appointment:** Prof Clinical Genetics, UCLA

Hoyme, Harold Eugene MD (Clinical Genetics) - *Special Expertise: Fetal Alcohol Syndrome; Cytogenetic Disorders; Dysmorphology;* **Admitting Hospital:** Stanford Medical Center; **Office Address:** Stanford Univ-Div Med Genetics, Dept Ped 300 Pasteur Dr, Rm H315 Palo Alto, CA 94305-5208; **Office Phone:** (650) 723-6858; **Board Certifications:** Pediatrics 1980, Clinical Genetics 1984; **Medical School:** Univ Chicago-Pritzker Sch Med 1976; **Residency:** Pediatrics, UCSD Med Ctr, San Diego, CA 1977-1979; **Faculty Appointment:** Prof Clinical Genetics, Stanford Univ

Hudgins, Louanne MD (Clinical Genetics) - *Special Expertise: Congenital Abnormalities-Limb;* **Admitting Hospital:** Stanford Medical Center; **Office Address:** 300 Pasteur Dr, rm h315 Palo Alto, CA 94305-5208; **Office Phone:** (650) 723-6858; **Board Certifications:** Pediatrics 1997, Clinical Genetics 1993; **Medical School:** Univ Kans 1984; **Residency:** Pediatrics, Univ Conn Hlth Ctr, Farmington, CT 1984-1987; **Fellowship:** Clinical Genetics, Univ Conn Hlth Ctr, Farmington, CT 1987-1990; **Faculty Appointment:** Assoc Prof Pediatrics, Stanford Univ

Jonas, Adam Jonathan MD (Clinical Genetics) - *Special Expertise: Biochemical Genetics; Inherited Diseases;* **Admitting Hospital:** LAC - Harbor - UCLA Medical Center; **Office Address:** Harbor-UCLA Med Ctr, Dept Med Genetics 1000 W Carson St, Box 17 Torrance, CA 90502-2006; **Office Phone:** (310) 222-2301; **Board Certifications:** Pediatrics 1982, Clinical Genetics 1990; **Medical School:** UCSD 1976; **Residencies:** Pediatrics, Chldns Ortho Hosp, Seattle, WA 1976-1978; Pediatrics, Univ Hosp, San Diego, CA 1978-1979; **Fellowship:** Genetics and Metabolism, UCSD Sch Med, San Diego, CA 1979-1982; **Faculty Appointment:** Prof Pediatrics, UCLA

Jones, Kenneth L. MD (Clinical Genetics) - *Special Expertise: Dysmorphology;* **Admitting Hospital:** University of California - San Diego Healthcare; **Office Address:** Univ Cal San Diego 200 W Arbor Dr San Diego, CA 92103; **Office Phone:** (619) 543-2040; **Board Certification:** Pediatrics 1971; **Medical School:** Hahnemann Univ 1966; **Residencies:** Pediatrics, Chldns Ortho Hosp, Seattle, WA 1967-1969; Pediatrics, Chldns Ortho Hosp, Seattle, WA 1971-1972; **Faculty Appointment:** Prof Pediatrics, UCSD

Jones, Marilyn MD (Clinical Genetics) - *Special Expertise: Dysmorphology; Craniofacial Disorders;* **Admitting Hospital:** Children's Hospital and Health Center; **Office Address:** Chldns Assoc Med Grp - Div Dysmorphology & Genetics 3020 Childrens Way, MC 5031 San Diego, CA 92123-2746; **Office Phone:** (858) 576-5840; **Board Certifications:** Pediatrics 1979, Clinical Genetics 1982; **Medical School:** Columbia P&S 1974; **Residencies:** Internal Medicine, UCSD Med Ctr, San Diego, CA 1975-1977; Pediatrics, UCSD Med Ctr, San Diego, CA 1977; **Fellowship:** Dysmorphology, UCSD Med Ctr, San Diego, CA 1977-1979; **Faculty Appointment:** Adjct Prof Pediatrics, UCSD

Morris, Colleen A. MD (Clinical Genetics) - *Special Expertise: Williams Syndrome; Inherited Diseases;* **Admitting Hospital:** University Medical Center; **Office Address:** Univ of Nevada Sch of Medicine, Dept Pediatrics 2040 W Charleston, Ste 401 Las Vegas, NV 89102; **Office Phone:** (702) 671-2200; **Board Certifications:** Clinical Genetics 1987, Pediatrics 1986; **Medical School:** Loyola Univ-Stritch Sch Med 1981; **Residency:** Pediatrics, Phoenix Hosp Affil Ped Prgm, Phoenix, AZ 1981-1984; **Fellowship:** Clinical Genetics, Univ Utah Sch Med, Salt Lake City, UT 1984-1986; **Faculty Appointment:** Prof Pediatrics, Univ Nevada

Pagon, Roberta Anderson MD (Clinical Genetics) - *Special Expertise: Eye Diseases - Hereditary;* **Admitting Hospital:** Children's Hospital and Regional Medical Center - Seattle; **Office Address:** Chldns Hosp Med Ctr.-Div Med Genetics CH-25 4800 Sand Point Way NE Seattle, WA 98105-0371; **Office Phone:** (206) 526-2056; **Board Certifications:** Clinical Genetics 1982, Pediatrics 1978; **Medical School:** Harvard Med Sch 1972; **Residency:** Pediatrics, U Wash Affil Hosp, Seattle, WA 1973-1975; **Fellowship:** Clinical Genetics, U Wash, Seattle, WA 1976-1979; **Faculty Appointment:** Prof Pediatrics, Univ Wash

Rimoin, David L MD/PhD (Clinical Genetics) - *Special Expertise: Skeletal Dysplasias; Marfan's Syndrome; Birth Defects;* **Admitting Hospital:** Cedars-Sinai Medical Center; **Office Address:** Cedars-Sinai Med Ctr 444 S San Vicente, Ste 1001 Los Angeles, CA 90048; **Office Phone:** (310) 423-4461; **Board Certifications:** Internal Medicine 1968, Clinical Genetics 1984; **Medical School:** McGill Univ 1961; **Residencies:** Internal Medicine, Royal Victoria Hosp, Montreal, Canada 1962-1963; Internal Medicine, Johns Hopkins Hosp, Baltimore, MD 1963-1964; **Fellowship:** Clinical Genetics, Johns Hopkins Hosp, Baltimore, MD 1964-1967; **Faculty Appointment:** Prof Pediatrics, UCLA

Wilcox, William MD (Clinical Genetics) - *Special Expertise:* *Inborn Errors of Metabolism;* *Skeletal Dysplasias;* **Admitting Hospital:** Cedars-Sinai Medical Center; **Office Address:** Cedars Sinai Med Ctr, Dept Med Genetics 444 S San Vincente Blvd, Ste 101 Los Angeles, CA 90048; **Office Phone:** (310) 423-9914; **Board Certifications:** Pediatrics 1999, Clinical Genetics 1993; **Medical School:** UCLA 1988; **Residency:** Pediatrics, UCLA Med Ctr, Los Angeles, CA 1989-1991; **Fellowship:** Clinical Genetics, Cedars-Sinai Med Ctr, Los Angeles, CA 1991; **Faculty Appointment:** Asst Prof Pediatrics, UCLA

COLON & RECTAL SURGERY

A colon and rectal surgeon is trained to diagnose and treat various diseases of the intestinal tract, colon, rectum, anal canal and perianal area by medical and surgical means. This specialist also deals with other organs and tissues (such as the liver, urinary and female reproductive system) involved with primary intestinal disease.

Colon and rectal surgeons have the expertise to diagnose and often manage anorectal conditions such as hemorrhoids, fissures (painful tears in the anal lining), abscesses and fistulae (infections located around the anus and rectum) in the office setting. They also treat problems of the intestine and colon and perform endoscopic procedures to evaluate and treat problems such as cancer, polyps (precancerous growths) and inflammatory conditions.

Training required: Six years (including general surgery)

PHYSICIAN LISTINGS

Colon & Rectal Surgery

New England

Becker, James MD (Colon & Rectal Surgery) - *Special Expertise:* Inflammatory Bowel Disease; Colon Cancer; **Admitting Hospital:** Boston Medical Center; **Office Address:** Boston Med Ctr-Dept Surgery 88 E Newton St, rm C500 Boston, MA 02118-2393; **Office Phone:** (617) 638-8600; **Board Certification:** Surgery 1999; **Medical School:** Case West Res Univ 1975; **Residency:** Surgery, U Utah Med Ctr, Salt Lake City, UT 1975-1980; **Fellowship:** Research, Mayo Clinic, Rochester, MN 1980-1982; **Faculty Appointment:** Prof Surgery, Boston Univ

Bleday, Ronald MD (Colon & Rectal Surgery) - *Special Expertise:* Colon Cancer; **Admitting Hospital:** Beth Israel Deaconess Medical Center - Boston (Page 57); **Office Address:** Brigham & Women's Hosp 45 Francis St, Bldg ASB2 Boston, MA 02115; **Office Phone:** (617) 732-8460; **Board Certifications:** Colon & Rectal Surgery 1992, Surgery 1999; **Medical School:** McGill Univ 1982; **Residencies:** Surgery, Brown Univ-RI Hosp, Providence, RI 1982-1989; Surgical Oncology, Brigham & Women's Hosp, Boston, MA 1984-1986; **Fellowships:** Endoscopy, Mass Genl Hosp, Boston, MA 1990; Colon & Rectal Surgery, Univ Minn, Minneapolis, MN 1990-1991; **Faculty Appointment:** Asst Prof Surgery, Harvard Med Sch

Coller, John MD (Colon & Rectal Surgery) - *Special Expertise:* Colon Cancer; **Admitting Hospital:** Lahey Clinic; **Office Address:** Lahey Clinic, Dept Colon & Rectal 41 Mall Rd Burlington, MA 01805; **Office Phone:** (781) 744-8581; **Board Certifications:** Surgery 1973, Colon & Rectal Surgery 1973; **Medical School:** Univ Penn 1965; **Residency:** Surgery, Hosp Univ Penn, Philadelphia, PA 1966-1972; **Fellowship:** Colon & Rectal Surgery, Lahey Clinic Fdtn, Boston, MA 1972-1973; **Faculty Appointment:** Clin Inst Surgery, Harvard Med Sch

Littlejohn, Charles MD (Colon & Rectal Surgery) - *Special Expertise:* Colon & Rectal Surgery - General; **Admitting Hospital:** Stamford Hospital (Page 72); **Office Address:** 70 Mill River St Stamford, CT 06902-3725; **Office Phone:** (203) 323-8989; **Board Certifications:** Surgery 1994, Colon & Rectal Surgery 1985; **Medical School:** Dartmouth Med Sch 1978; **Residencies:** Surgery, Univ Rochester Affil Hosps, Rochester, NY 1979-1980; Surgery, UMDNJ-Rutgers Affil Hosp, Newark, NJ 1980-1983; **Fellowship:** Colon & Rectal Surgery, UMDNJ-Rutgers Affil Hosp, Newark, NJ 1983-1984; **Faculty Appointment:** Asst Clin Prof Surgery, NY Med Coll

Roberts, Patricia L MD (Colon & Rectal Surgery) - *Special Expertise:* Diverticulitis; Colon Cancer; **Admitting Hospital:** Lahey Clinic; **Office Address:** Lahey Clin, Dept Colon & Rectal 41 Mall Rd Burlington, MA 01805; **Office Phone:** (781) 744-8243; **Board Certifications:** Colon & Rectal Surgery 1988, Surgery 1996; **Medical School:** Boston Univ 1981; **Residency:** Surgery, Boston Univ-Boston City Hosp, Boston, MA 1981-1986; **Fellowship:** Colon & Rectal Surgery, Lahey Clinic, Burlington, MA 1986-1988; **Faculty Appointment:** Asst Clin Prof Colon & Rectal Surgery, Tufts Univ

Schoetz, David MD (Colon & Rectal Surgery) - *Special Expertise:* Inflammatory Bowel Disease; Colorectal Cancer; **Admitting Hospital:** Lahey Clinic; **Office Address:** Lahey Clinic Medical Center, Dept of Colon Rectal Surgery 41 Mall Rd Burlington, MA 01805; **Office Phone:** (781) 744-8889; **Board Certifications:** Colon & Rectal Surgery 1983, Surgery 1991; **Medical School:** Med Coll Wisc 1974; **Residency:** Surgery, Boston Univ Med Ctr., Boston, MA 1975-1981; **Fellowship:** Colon & Rectal Surgery, Lahey Clin Med Ctr., Burlington, MA 1981-1982; **Faculty Appointment:** Prof Surgery, Tufts Univ

Shellito, Paul C MD (Colon & Rectal Surgery) - *Special Expertise:* Colorectal Cancer; *Ulcerative Colitis; Anorectal Disorders;* **Admitting Hospital:** Massachusetts General Hospital; **Office Address:** 15 Parkman St, Ste 336 Boston, MA 02114; **Office Phone:** (617) 724-0365; **Board Certifications:** Colon & Rectal Surgery 1994, Surgery 1992; **Medical School:** Harvard Med Sch 1977; **Residencies:** Surgery, Mass Genl Hosp., Boston, MA 1982-1983; Surgery, Auckland U Med Sch. 1981; **Fellowship:** Colon & Rectal Surgery, U Minn., Minneapolis, MN 1984-1985; **Faculty Appointment:** Asst Prof Surgery, Harvard Med Sch

Mid Atlantic

Forde, Kenneth MD (Colon & Rectal Surgery) - *Special Expertise:* Colonoscopy/Polypectomy; Laparoscopic Surgery; **Admitting Hospital:** Columbia Presbyterian Medical Center (Page 72); **Office Address:** 161 Fort Washington Ave, rm 812 New York, NY 10032-3713; **Office Phone:** (212) 305-5394; **Board Certification:** Surgery 1967; **Medical School:** Columbia P&S 1959; **Residencies:** Surgery, Bellevue Hosp Ctr, New York, NY 1960-1964; Surgery, Columbia Presby Hosp, New York, NY 1961-1963; **Faculty Appointment:** Clin Prof Surgery, Columbia P&S

Fry, Robert Dean MD (Colon & Rectal Surgery) - *Special Expertise:* Rectal Cancer; *Inflammatory Bowel Disease;* **Admitting Hospital:** Thomas Jefferson University Hospital; **Office Address:** Thomas Jefferson Univ Hosp 1100 Walnut St, Ste 702 Philadelphia, PA 19107; **Office Phone:** (215) 955-5869; **Board Certifications:** Surgery 1996, Colon & Rectal Surgery 1998; **Medical School:** Washington Univ, St Louis 1972; **Residency:** Surgery, Jewish Hosp, St Louis, MO 1973-1977; **Fellowship:** Colon & Rectal Surgery, Cleveland Clin Fdn, Cleveland, OH 1977-1978; **Faculty Appointment:** Prof Surgery

Gingold, Bruce MD (Colon & Rectal Surgery) - *Special Expertise:* Colostomy Avoidance; *Inflammatory Bowel Disease;* **Admitting Hospital:** St Vincents Catholic Medical Center of New York; **Office Address:** 36 7th Ave, Ste 507 New York, NY 10011; **Office Phone:** (212) 675-2997; **Board Certifications:** Colon & Rectal Surgery 1976, Surgery 1977; **Medical School:** Jefferson Med Coll 1970; **Residency:** Surgery, St Vincent's Hosp & Med Ctr, New York, NY 1970-1975; **Fellowship:** Colon & Rectal Surgery, Cleveland Clinic, Cleveland, OH 1975-1976; **Faculty Appointment:** Assoc Clin Prof Surgery, NY Med Coll

Golub, Richard MD (Colon & Rectal Surgery) - *Special Expertise:* Colorectal Cancer; *Endoscopy;* **Admitting Hospital:** University Hospital - Brooklyn; **Office Address:** Downstate Surgical Associates 450 Clarkson Ave, Box 40 Brooklyn, NY 11203-2012; **Office Phone:** (718) 270-3349; **Board Certifications:** Surgery 1991, Colon & Rectal Surgery 1992; **Medical School:** Albert Einstein Coll Med 1984; **Residency:** Surgery, Univ Hosp Stony Brook, Stony Brook, NY 1984-1990; **Fellowship:** Colon & Rectal Surgery, Grant Medical Center, Columbus, OH 1990-1991; **Faculty Appointment:** Assoc Prof Surgery, SUNY Downstate

Gorfine, Stephen MD (Colon & Rectal Surgery) - *Special Expertise:* Anal Fissure; **Admitting Hospital:** Mount Sinai Hospital (Page 70); **Office Address:** 25 E 69th St New York, NY 10021; **Office Phone:** (212) 517-8600; **Board Certifications:** Surgery 1987, Colon & Rectal Surgery 1988; **Medical School:** Univ Mass Sch Med 1978; **Residencies:** Internal Medicine, Mount Sinai Hosp, New York, NY 1978-1981; Surgery, Mount Sinai Hosp, New York, NY 1981-1985; **Fellowship:** Colon & Rectal Surgery, Ferguson Hosp, Grand Rapids, MI 1986-1987; **Faculty Appointment:** Assoc Clin Prof Surgery, Mount Sinai Sch Med

Medich, David MD (Colon & Rectal Surgery) - *Special Expertise:* Rectal Cancer; Ulcerative Colitis; Inflammatory Bowel Disease - Crohn's; **Admitting Hospital:** Allegheny General Hospital; **Office Address:** 320 E North Ave, Ste 312 Pittsburgh, PA 15212; **Office Phone:** (412) 359-3901; **Board Certifications:** Surgery 1994, Colon & Rectal Surgery 1995; **Medical School:** Ohio State Univ 1987; **Residency:** Surgery, Univ of Pittsburgh, Pittsburgh, PA 1987-1990; **Fellowships:** Research, Univ of Pittsburgh, Pittsburgh, PA 1990-1993; Colon & Rectal Surgery, Cleveland Clin Fdn, Cleveland, OH 1993-1994; **Faculty Appointment:** Assoc Prof Surgery

Milsom, Jeffrey MD (Colon & Rectal Surgery) - *Special Expertise:* Colon & Rectal Surgery; **Admitting Hospital:** Mount Sinai Hospital (Page 70); **Office Address:** 5 E 98th St, rm 15, Box 1259 New York, NY 10029; **Office Phone:** (212) 241-9289; **Board Certifications:** Colon & Rectal Surgery 1986, Surgery 1992; **Medical School:** Univ Pittsburgh 1979; **Residencies:** Surgery, Roosevelt Hosp, New York, NY 1980-1981; Surgery, Univ Virginia Med Ctr, Charlottesville, VA 1981-1984; **Fellowship:** Colon & Rectal Surgery, Ferguson Hosp, Grand Rapids, MI 1984-1985; **Faculty Appointment:** Prof Surgery, Mount Sinai Sch Med

Salvati, Eugene MD (Colon & Rectal Surgery) - *Special Expertise:* Colon & Rectal Surgery - General; **Admitting Hospital:** Muhlenberg Regional Medical Center; **Office Address:** Toranco Bldg 3900 Park Ave, Ste 101 Edison, NJ 08820; **Office Phone:** (732) 494-6640; **Board Certifications:** Colon & Rectal Surgery 1956, Surgery 1962; **Medical School:** Univ MD Sch Med 1947; **Residencies:** Surgery, St Vincent Hosp, Indianapolis, IN 1950-1951; Surgery, Veterans Hosp, Indianapolis, IN 1951-1952; **Fellowship:** Colon & Rectal Surgery, Allentown Genl Hosp, Allentown, PA 1954-1956; **Faculty Appointment:** Clin Prof Surgery, UMDNJ-RW Johnson Med Sch

Smith, Lee MD (Colon & Rectal Surgery) - *Special Expertise:* Colon Cancer; **Admitting Hospital:** Washington Hospital Center - DC (Page 79); **Office Address:** 110 Irving St NW, Ste 3B-31 Washington, DC 20010-2975; **Office Phone:** (202) 877-8484; **Board Certifications:** Surgery 1971, Colon & Rectal Surgery 1973; **Medical School:** UCSF 1962; **Residencies:** Surgery, Univ Minn, Minneapolis, MN 1966-1970; Colon & Rectal Surgery, Naval Hosp, San Diego, CA 1972-1973; **Faculty Appointment:** Prof Surgery, Geo Wash Univ

Steinhagen, Randolph MD (Colon & Rectal Surgery) - *Special Expertise:* Diverticulitis; Colon & Rectal Cancer; Ulcerative Colitis/Crohn's Disease; **Admitting Hospital:** Mount Sinai Hospital (Page 70); **Office Address:** Surgical Associates 5 E 98th St, Fl 11, Box 1263 New York, NY 10029; **Office Phone:** (212) 241-3336; **Board Certifications:** Colon & Rectal Surgery 1985, Surgery 1992; **Medical School:** Wayne State Univ 1977; **Residency:** Surgery, Mount Sinai Hosp, New York, NY 1977-1982; **Fellowship:** Colon & Rectal Surgery, Cleveland Clinic, Cleveland, OH 1982-1983; **Faculty Appointment:** Assoc Prof Surgery, Mount Sinai Sch Med

Whelan, Richard MD (Colon & Rectal Surgery) - *Special Expertise:* Laparoscopic Surgery; Colon Cancer; **Admitting Hospital:** Columbia Presbyterian Medical Center (Page 72); **Office Address:** 161 Ft Washington Ave, Rm 817 New York, NY 10032; **Office Phone:** (212) 305-6136; **Board Certifications:** Surgery 1988, Colon & Rectal Surgery 1990; **Medical School:** Columbia P&S 1982; **Residency:** Surgery, Columbia Presby, New York, NY 1982-1987; **Fellowship:** Colon & Rectal Surgery, Univ Minn Med Ctr, Minneapolis, MN 1987-1988; **Faculty Appointment:** Assoc Clin Prof Surgery, Columbia P&S

Wong, Westley Douglas MD (Colon & Rectal Surgery) - *Special Expertise:* Incontinence-Fecal; Artificial Sphincter - Anal; Rectal Cancer; **Admitting Hospital:** Memorial Sloan Kettering Cancer Center; **Office Address:** Meml Sloan Kettering Cancer Ctr 1275 York Ave, rm C991 New York, NY 10021; **Office Phone:** (212) 639-5117; **Board Certifications:** Surgery 1997, Colon & Rectal Surgery 1985; **Medical School:** Canada 1972; **Residency:** Surgery, Univ Manitoba Hosp, Canada 1973-1977; **Fellowship:** Colon & Rectal Surgery, Univ Minn Med Ctr, Minneapolis, MN 1983-1984; **Faculty Appointment:** Assoc Clin Prof Surgery, Cornell Univ-Weil Med Coll

Southeast

Carbonell, Manuel MD (Colon & Rectal Surgery) - *Special Expertise: Colon & Rectal Surgery - General;* **Admitting Hospital:** Mercy Hospital - Miami; **Office Address:** 3661 S Miami Ave, Apt 1006 Carbonell & Alvarez Miami, FL 33133-4214; **Office Phone:** (305) 854-2432; **Board Certification:** Colon & Rectal Surgery 1971; **Medical School:** Med Coll Wisc 1958; **Residency:** Surgery, Jackson Meml Hosp, Miami, FL 1959-1963; **Fellowship:** Colon & Rectal Surgery, Mercy Hosp, Miami, FL 1963-1965

Christie, John MD (Colon & Rectal Surgery) - *Special Expertise: Colonoscopy;* **Admitting Hospital:** Baptist Hospital - Miami; **Office Address:** Gastroenterology Care Center 7500 SE 87th Ave, Ste 200 Miami, FL 33173-2131; **Office Phone:** (305) 913-0666; **Board Certification:** Surgery 1971; **Medical School:** Univ Cincinnati 1965; **Residency:** Surgery, Wadsworth VA Hosp-UCLA, Los Angeles, CA 1966-1970; **Fellowship:** Endoscopy, Beth Israel Med Ctr, New York, NY 1972; **Faculty Appointment:** Assoc Clin Prof Colon & Rectal Surgery, Univ Miami Sch Med

Cohen, Alfred M MD (Colon & Rectal Surgery) - *Special Expertise: Colorectal Cancer - Liver Metastasis;* **Admitting Hospital:** University of Kentucky Medical Center; **Office Address:** Markey Cancer Ctr 800 Rose St, Bldg MRISC - Ste 105 Lexington, KY 40536-0098; **Office Phone:** (859) 323-6556; **Board Certification:** Surgery 1976; **Medical School:** Johns Hopkins Univ 1967; **Residencies:** Surgical Oncology, Surg Branch Natl Cancer Inst, Bethesda, MD 1969-1971; Surgery, Mass Genl Hosp, Boston, MA 1972-1975; **Faculty Appointment:** Prof Surgery, Univ KY Coll Med

Foley, Eugene F MD (Colon & Rectal Surgery) - *Special Expertise: Colon & Rectal Surgery; Ulcerated Colitis;* **Admitting Hospital:** University of Virginia Health Systems; **Office Address:** Univ of VA Hlth Scis Ctr Charlottesville, VA 22901-0709; **Office Phone:** (804) 924-9304; **Board Certifications:** Surgery 1994, Colon & Rectal Surgery 1993; **Medical School:** Harvard Med Sch 1985; **Residency:** Surgery, New England Deaconess Hosp, Boston, MA; **Fellowship:** Colon & Rectal Surgery, Lahey Clinic, Burlington, MA; **Faculty Appointment:** Assoc Prof Surgery, Univ VA Sch Med

Galandiuk, Susan MD (Colon & Rectal Surgery) - *Special Expertise: Colon & Rectal Cancer; Inflammatory Bowel Disease;* **Admitting Hospital:** University of Louisville Hospital; **Office Address:** Univ Louisville Sch Med, Dept Surgery 550 S Jackson, Ambulatory Care Bldg Louisville, KY 40292; **Office Phone:** (502) 852-4568; **Board Certifications:** Colon & Rectal Surgery 1991, Surgery 1998; **Medical School:** Germany 1982; **Residency:** Surgery, Cleveland Clinic Fdtn, Cleveland, OH 1984-1988; **Fellowships:** Surgery, Univ Louisville Hosp, Louisville, KY 1988-1989; Colon & Rectal Surgery, Mayo Clinic, Rochester, MN 1989-1990; **Faculty Appointment:** Assoc Prof Surgery, Univ Louisville Sch Med

Hartmann, Rene MD (Colon & Rectal Surgery) - *Special Expertise: Colon & Rectal Surgery - General;* **Admitting Hospital:** Baptist Hospital - Miami; **Office Address:** 9195 Sunset Dr, ste 230 Miami, FL 33173-3488; **Office Phone:** (305) 271-0300; **Board Certifications:** Surgery 1978, Colon & Rectal Surgery 1994; **Medical School:** Venezuela 1971; **Residencies:** Surgery, Jackson Meml Hoso, Miami, FL 1973-1976; Surgery, Orange Meml Hosp, Orlando, FL 1976-1977; **Fellowship:** Colon & Rectal Surgery, Grant Hosp, Columbus, OH 1977-1978; **Faculty Appointment:** Assoc Clin Prof Surgery, Univ Miami Sch Med

Larach, Sergio MD (Colon & Rectal Surgery) - *Special Expertise:* Colon Cancer; inflammatory Bowel Disease; **Admitting Hospital:** Orlando Regional Medical Center; **Office Address:** 110 W Underwood St, Ste A Orlando, FL 32806-1132; **Office Phone:** (407) 422-3790; **Board Certification:** Colon & Rectal Surgery 1979; **Medical School:** Chile 1968; **Residencies:** Surgery, Hosp de Salvador, Santiago, Chile 1968-1973; Surgery, Orlando Reg Med Ctr, Orlando, FL 1973-1976; **Fellowship:** Colon & Rectal Surgery, Univ Texas Med Sch, Houston, TX 1976-1977; **Faculty Appointment:** Assoc Prof Surgery, Univ Fla Coll Med

Nogueras, Juan Jose MD (Colon & Rectal Surgery) - *Special Expertise:* Colon & Rectal Surgery - General; **Admitting Hospital:** Cleveland Clinic Florida; **Office Address:** Cleveland Clinic Florida 3000 W Cypress Creek Rd Fort Lauderdale, FL 33309-1710; **Office Phone:** (954) 978-5266; **Board Certifications:** Surgery 1988, Colon & Rectal Surgery 1993; **Medical School:** Jefferson Med Coll 1982; **Residency:** Surgery, Columbia Presby Med Ctr, New York, NY 1983-1987; **Fellowship:** Colon & Rectal Surgery, Univ Minn, Minneapolis, MN 1990-1991

Wexner, Steven MD (Colon & Rectal Surgery) - *Special Expertise:* Rectal Cancer; Inflammatory Bowel Disease; **Admitting Hospital:** Cleveland Clinic Florida; **Office Address:** Cleveland Clinic Florida 3000 W Cypress Creek Rd Fort Lauderdale, FL 33309-1743; **Office Phone:** (954) 978-5251; **Board Certifications:** Surgery 1996, Colon & Rectal Surgery 1989; **Medical School:** Cornell Univ-Weil Med Coll 1982; **Residency:** Surgery, Roosevelt Hosp, New York, NY 1982-1987; **Fellowship:** Colon & Rectal Surgery, Univ Minn, Minneapolis, MN 1987-1988; **Faculty Appointment:** Prof Surgery, Ohio State Univ

Midwest

Abcarian, Herand MD (Colon & Rectal Surgery) - *Special Expertise:* Rectal Cancer/Sphincter Saving Surgery; Inflammatory Bowel Disease; Anorectal Disorders; **Admitting Hospital:** University of Illinois at Chicago Medical Center; **Office Address:** 30 N Michigan Ave, Fl 1118 Chicago, IL 60602; **Office Phone:** (312) 782-4828; **Board Certifications:** Colon & Rectal Surgery 1972, Surgery 1972; **Medical School:** Iran 1965; **Residencies:** Surgery, Cook County Hosp, Chicago, IL 1967-1971; Colon & Rectal Surgery, Cook County Hosp, Chicago, IL 1971-1972; **Faculty Appointment:** Prof Surgery, Univ IL Coll Med

Dozois, Roger R MD (Colon & Rectal Surgery) - *Special Expertise:* Inflammatory Bowel Disease; Polyposis Syndromes; **Admitting Hospital:** Mayo Medical Center & Clinic - Rochester; **Office Address:** Mayo Clinic, Div Colon & Rectal Surg 200 1st St SW Rochester, MN 55905; **Office Phone:** (507) 284-2622; **Board Certifications:** Surgery 1974, Colon & Rectal Surgery 1984; **Medical School:** Laval Univ, Quebec 1965; **Residency:** Surgery, Mayo Grad Sch Med, Rochester, MN 1966-1971

Fazio, Victor MD (Colon & Rectal Surgery) - *Special Expertise:* Inflammatory Bowel Disease; Colorectal Cancer; **Admitting Hospital:** Cleveland Clinic Foundation; **Office Address:** Cleveland Clinic, Dept Colorectal Surg 9500 Euclid Ave, Box A111 Cleveland, OH 44195; **Office Phone:** (216) 444-6672; **Board Certification:** Colon & Rectal Surgery 1976; **Medical School:** Australia 1964; **Residencies:** Surgery, St Vincents Hosp, Sidney, Australia 1967-1971; Surgery, Lahey Clinic, Boston, MA 1972; **Fellowship:** Colon & Rectal Surgery, Cleveland Clinic, Cleveland, OH 1973

Fleshman, James MD (Colon & Rectal Surgery) - *Special Expertise:* Incontinence-Fecal; Colon & Rectal Surgery; **Admitting Hospital:** Barnes - Jewish Hospital; **Office Address:** Washington Univ Sch Med 660 S Euclid Ave, Box 8109 St Louis, MO 63110; **Office Phone:** (314) 454-7177; **Board Certifications:** Colon & Rectal Surgery 1988, Surgery 1996; **Medical School:** Washington Univ, St Louis 1980; **Residency:** Surgery, Jewish Hospital, St. Louis, MO 1980-1986; **Fellowship:** Colon & Rectal Surgery, Univ Toronto, Toronto, CN 1986-1987; **Faculty Appointment:** Assoc Prof Surgery, Washington Univ, St Louis

Goldberg, Stanley MD (Colon & Rectal Surgery) - *Special Expertise: Diverticulitis;* **Admitting Hospital:** Abbott - Northwestern Hospital; **Office Address:** 1731 Medical Arts Bldg-Div Colorectal Surgery 825 Nicollet Mall Minneapolis, MN 55402; **Office Phone:** (612) 339-4534; **Board Certifications:** Colon & Rectal Surgery 1963, Surgery 1964; **Medical School:** Univ Minn 1956; **Residencies:** Surgery, Minneapolis VA Hosp, Minneapolis, MN 1957-1960; Colon & Rectal Surgery, Univ Minnesota Hosps, Minneapolis, MN 1960-1963; **Faculty Appointment:** Clin Prof Surgery, Univ Minn

Kodner, Ira Joe MD (Colon & Rectal Surgery) - *Special Expertise: Colorectal Cancer; Inflammatory Bowel Disease;* **Admitting Hospital:** Barnes - Jewish Hospital; **Office Address:** 216 S Kingshighway St. Louis, MO 63110; **Office Phone:** (314) 454-7177; **Board Certifications:** Colon & Rectal Surgery 1975, Surgery 1975; **Medical School:** Washington Univ, St Louis 1967; **Residency:** Surgery, Jewish Hosp, St. Louis, MO 1971-1974; **Fellowship:** Colon & Rectal Surgery, Cleveland Clinic, Cleveland, OH 1974-1975; **Faculty Appointment:** Prof Surgery, Washington Univ, St Louis

Lowry, Ann MD (Colon & Rectal Surgery) - *Special Expertise: Anal Sphincter Repair; Rectovaginal Fistula;* **Admitting Hospital:** Fairview Southdale Hospital; **Office Address:** 6545 France Avenue S Edina, MN 55435; **Office Phone:** (612) 920-6111; **Board Certifications:** Colon & Rectal Surgery 1988, Surgery 1993; **Medical School:** Tufts Univ 1977; **Residency:** Surgery, New England Hosp, Boston, MA 1978-1982; **Fellowship:** Colon & Rectal Surgery, University Minn, Minneapolis, TN 1986-1987; **Faculty Appointment:** Assoc Clin Prof Surgery, Univ Minn

MacKeigan, John MD (Colon & Rectal Surgery) - *Special Expertise: Rectal Cancer;* **Admitting Hospital:** Spectrum Health East; **Office Address:** 75 Sheldon Blvd, Ste 201 Grand Rapids, MI 49503-4224; **Office Phone:** (616) 356-4100; **Board Certification:** Colon & Rectal Surgery 1974; **Medical School:** Dalhousie Univ 1969; **Residencies:** Surgery, Dalhousie Univ, Halifax, Nova Scotia 1969-1973; Colon & Rectal Surgery, Ferguson Hosp, Grand Rapids, MI 1973-1974; **Faculty Appointment:** Assoc Prof Surgery, Mich State Univ

Nelson, Heidi MD (Colon & Rectal Surgery) - *Special Expertise: Colorectal Cancer;* **Admitting Hospital:** Mayo Medical Center & Clinic - Rochester; **Office Address:** Mayo Clinic, Div Col & Rec Surg 200 First St SW, Fl E6A Rochester, MN 55905; **Office Phone:** (507) 284-3329; **Board Certifications:** Colon & Rectal Surgery 1989, Surgery 1995; **Medical School:** Univ Wash 1981; **Residencies:** Surgery, Oregan Health Science Univ, Portland, OR 1981-1987; Oregan Health Science Univ, Portland, OR 1984-1985; **Fellowship:** Colon & Rectal Surgery, Mayo Clinic, Rochester, MN 1987-1988; **Faculty Appointment:** Prof Surgery, Mayo Med Sch

Nivatvongs, Santhat MD (Colon & Rectal Surgery) - *Special Expertise: Colon & Rectal Cancer; Anorectal Disorders;* **Admitting Hospital:** Mayo Medical Center & Clinic - Rochester; **Office Address:** Mayo Clinic, CRS Sect 200 First St SW Rochester, MN 55905; **Office Phone:** (507) 284-4985; **Board Certifications:** Colon & Rectal Surgery 1971, Surgery 1971; **Medical School:** Thailand 1964; **Residency:** Surgery, United Hosp, St. Paul, MN 1965-1970; **Fellowship:** Colon & Rectal Surgery, Univ Minn, Minneapolis, MN 1970-1971; **Faculty Appointment:** Prof Surgery, Mayo Med Sch

Pemberton, John MD (Colon & Rectal Surgery) - *Special Expertise: Rectal Surgery; Inflammatory Bowel Disease;* **Admitting Hospital:** Mayo Medical Center & Clinic - Rochester; **Office Address:** Mayo Clinic-Dept Surgery 200 First St SW Rochester, MN 55905; **Office Phone:** (507) 284-2359; **Board Certifications:** Surgery 1984, Colon & Rectal Surgery 1985; **Medical School:** Tulane Univ 1976; **Residency:** Surgery, Mayo Clinic, Rochester, MN 1977-1983; **Fellowship:** Colon & Rectal Surgery, Mayo Clinic, Rochester, MN 1983-1984; **Faculty Appointment:** Prof Surgery, Mayo Med Sch

Rothenberger, David MD (Colon & Rectal Surgery) - *Special Expertise: Colorectal Cancer;* **Admitting Hospital:** Fairview-University Medical Center - University Campus; **Office Address:** 420 Delaware St SE, MC-450 Minneapolis, MN 55114-1084; **Office Phone:** (612) 625-3288; **Board Certifications:** Surgery 1979, Colon & Rectal Surgery 1979; **Medical School:** Tufts Univ 1973; **Residency:** Surgery, St Paul-Ramsey Med Ctr, St Paul, MN 1974-1978; **Fellowship:** Colon & Rectal Surgery, Univ Minn, Minneapolis, MN 1978-1979; **Faculty Appointment:** Clin Prof Surgery, Univ Minn

Saclarides, Theodore John MD (Colon & Rectal Surgery) - *Special Expertise: Rectal Cancer - Sphincter Preservation; Incontinence - Fecal;* **Admitting Hospital:** Rush/Presbyterian - St Luke's Medical Center - Chicago (Page 74); **Office Address:** University Surgeons 1725 W Harrison St, Ste 810 Chicago, IL 60612-3832; **Office Phone:** (312) 942-6543; **Board Certifications:** Colon & Rectal Surgery 1989, Surgery 1996; **Medical School:** Univ Miami Sch Med 1982; **Residency:** Surgery, Rush Presby-St Lukes Hosp, Chicago, IL 1982-1987; **Fellowship:** Colon & Rectal Surgery, Mayo Clinic, Rochester, MN 1987-1988; **Faculty Appointment:** Assoc Prof Rush Med Coll

Senagore, Anthony MD (Colon & Rectal Surgery) - *Special Expertise: Laparoscopic Surgery; Colorectal Cancer;* **Admitting Hospital:** Cleveland Clinic Foundation; **Office Address:** Cleveland Clinic 9500 Euclid Ave, rm A111 Cleveland, OH 44195; **Office Phone:** (216) 445-7882; **Board Certifications:** Surgery 1988, Colon & Rectal Surgery 1990; **Medical School:** Mich State Univ 1981; **Residencies:** Surgery, Butterworth Hospital-Michigan State University, Grand Rapids, MI 1982-1987; Colon & Rectal Surgery, Ferguson Hospital, Grand Rapids, MI 1987-1989

Stryker, Steven J MD (Colon & Rectal Surgery) - *Special Expertise: Colon Cancer; Crohn's Disease;* **Admitting Hospital:** Northwestern Memorial Hospital; **Office Address:** Northwestern Meml Hosp 676 N Saint Clair St, Ste 1525 Chicago, IL 60611; **Office Phone:** (312) 943-5427; **Board Certifications:** Colon & Rectal Surgery 1986, Surgery 1992; **Medical School:** Northwestern Univ 1978; **Residency:** Surgery, Northwestern Meml Hosp, Chicago, IL 1978-1983; **Fellowship:** Colon & Rectal Surgery, Mayo Clinic, Rochester, MN 1983-1985; **Faculty Appointment:** Assoc Clin Prof Surgery, Northwestern Univ

Wolff, Bruce MD (Colon & Rectal Surgery) - *Special Expertise: Inflammatory Bowel Disease; Colorectal Cancer;* **Admitting Hospital:** Mayo Medical Center & Clinic - Rochester; **Office Address:** Mayo Clinic, Div Colon & Rectal Surgery 200 First St SW Rochester, MN 55905; **Office Phone:** (507) 284-2472; **Board Certifications:** Colon & Rectal Surgery 1983, Surgery 1990; **Medical School:** Duke Univ 1973; **Residency:** Surgery, Cornell Med Ctr, New York, NY 1977-1981; **Fellowship:** Colon & Rectal Surgery, Mayo Med Sch, Rochester, NY 1981-1982; **Faculty Appointment:** Prof Surgery, Mayo Med Sch

Great Plains and Mountains

Thorson, Alan MD (Colon & Rectal Surgery) - *Special Expertise: Artificial Bowel Sphincter; Ulcerative Colitis; Incontinence - Fecal;* **Admitting Hospital:** Bergen Regional Medical Center; **Office Address:** Colon & Rectal Surg Inc 8712 W Dodge Rd, Ste 240 Omaha, NE 68114-3419; **Office Phone:** (402) 343-1122; **Board Certifications:** Surgery 1994, Colon & Rectal Surgery 1999; **Medical School:** Univ Nebr Coll Med 1979; **Residency:** Surgery, Univ of Nebraska, Omaha, NE 1979-1984; **Fellowship:** Colon & Rectal Surgery, Univ Minn, Minneapolis, MN 1984-1985; **Faculty Appointment:** Assoc Prof Surgery, Creighton Univ

Southwest

Bailey, Harold Randolph MD (Colon & Rectal Surgery) - *Special Expertise: Endometriosis - Intestine; Laparoscopic Surgery; Fistula;* **Admitting Hospital:** Methodist Hospital - Houston (Page 69); **Office Address:** Colon & Rectal Clinic, Smith Tower 6550 Fannin St, Ste 2307 Houston, TX 77030-2717; **Office Phone:** (713) 790-9250; **Board Certifications:** Surgery 1974, Colon & Rectal Surgery 1994; **Medical School:** Univ Tex SW, Dallas 1968; **Residency:** Surgery, Hermann Hosp-Univ Tex Med Sch, Houston, TX 1969-1973; **Fellowship:** Colon & Rectal Surgery, Ferguson-Droste Hosp, Grand Rapids, MI 1973-1974; **Faculty Appointment:** Assoc Clin Prof Surgery, Baylor Coll Med

Beck, David MD (Colon & Rectal Surgery) - *Special Expertise: Colon Cancer;* **Admitting Hospital:** Ochsner Foundation Hospital; **Office Address:** Ochsner Cancer Institute 1514 Jefferson Hwy New Orleans, LA 70121; **Office Phone:** (504) 842-4060; **Board Certifications:** Colon & Rectal Surgery 1987, Surgery 1996; **Medical School:** Univ Miami Sch Med 1979; **Residency:** Surgery, Wilford Hall USAF Med Ctr, Lackland AFB, TX 1980-1984; **Fellowship:** Colon & Rectal Surgery, Cleveland Clinic Fdn, Cleveland, OH 1985-1986; **Faculty Appointment:** Assoc Clin Prof Surgery, F Edward Herbert Sch Med

Huber, Philip MD (Colon & Rectal Surgery) - *Special Expertise: GI Surgery;* **Admitting Hospital:** St Paul Medical Center; **Office Address:** St Paul Hosp, Dept Surg Ste 530 5939 Harry Hines Blvd Dallas, TX 75221; **Office Phone:** (214) 879-3787; **Board Certifications:** Colon & Rectal Surgery 1993, Surgery 1997; **Medical School:** Columbia P&S 1972; **Residencies:** Surgery, Parkland Hosp, Dallas, TX 1973-1977; Colon & Rectal Surgery, Presby Hosp, Dallas, TX 1978; **Faculty Appointment:** Prof Surgery, Univ Tex SW, Dallas

Opelka, Frank MD (Colon & Rectal Surgery) - *Special Expertise: Colon & Rectal Surgery; Colon Cancer;* **Admitting Hospital:** Ochsner Foundation Hospital; **Office Address:** Ochsner Cancer Institute, Dept Colon & Rectal Surg 1514 Jefferson Hwy, Fl 4 New Orleans, LA 70121; **Office Phone:** (504) 842-4060; **Board Certification:** Colon & Rectal Surgery 1991; **Medical School:** Univ Hlth Sci/Chicago Med Sch **Residencies:** Surgery, Eisenhower AMC, Augusta, GA 1982-1986; Colon & Rectal Surgery, Ochsner Clinic, New Orleans, LA 1989-1990

West Coast and Pacific

Beart Jr, Robert W MD (Colon & Rectal Surgery) - *Special Expertise: Colon & Rectal Cancer; Inflammatory Bowel Disease;* **Admitting Hospital:** USC Norris Cancer Comprehensive Center; **Office Address:** USC, Dept Surg 1450 San Pablo St, Ste 5400 Los Angeles, CA 90033-4612; **Office Phone:** (323) 442-5751; **Board Certifications:** Surgery 1993, Colon & Rectal Surgery 1995; **Medical School:** Harvard Med Sch 1971; **Residencies:** Surgery, Univ Colorado Medical Center, Denver, CO 1972-1976; Colon & Rectal Surgery, Mayo Clinic, Rochester, MN 1977-1978; **Fellowship:** Transplant Surgery, Univ Colorado Medical Center, Denver, CO 1974-1975; **Faculty Appointment:** Prof Surgery, USC Sch Med

Coutsoftides, Theodore MD (Colon & Rectal Surgery) - *Special Expertise: Colon & Rectal Surgery - General;* **Admitting Hospital:** St Joseph's Hospital - Orange; **Office Address:** 1310 W Stewart, Ste 605 Orange, CA 92868-3857; **Office Phone:** (714) 532-2544; **Board Certifications:** Colon & Rectal Surgery 1977, Surgery 1987; **Medical School:** Israel 1970; **Residencies:** Surgery, Cleveland Clinic, Cleveland, OH 1971-1973; Surgery, Royal Victoria Hosp, Montreal, Canada 1973-1976; **Fellowship:** Colon & Rectal Surgery, Cleveland Clinic, Cleveland, OH 1976-1977; **Faculty Appointment:** Assoc Prof Surgery, UC Irvine

Schrock, Theodore R MD (Colon & Rectal Surgery) - *Special Expertise:* Colon & Rectal Surgery - *General;* **Admitting Hospital:** University of California - San Francisco Medical Center; **Office Address:** UCSF, Dept Surg 513 Parnassus Ave S-320 San Francisco, CA 94143; **Office Phone:** (415) 353-2760; **Board Certification:** Surgery 1972; **Medical School:** UCSF 1964; **Residencies:** Surgery, Moffit Hosp - Univ CA 1965-1967; Surgery, Moffit Hosp - Univ CA 1969-1971; **Fellowship:** Surgery, Mass Genl Hosp, Boston, MA 1967-1969

Stamos, Michael Jerry MD (Colon & Rectal Surgery) - *Special Expertise:* Colon & Rectal Surgery - *General;* **Admitting Hospital:** LAC - Harbor - UCLA Medical Center; **Office Address:** 3400 Lomita Blvd, Ste 500 Torrance, CA 90505; **Office Phone:** (310) 539-2630; **Board Certifications:** Surgery 1991, Colon & Rectal Surgery 1992; **Medical School:** Case West Res Univ 1985; **Residencies:** Surgery, Jackson Meml Hosp, Miami, Fl 1985-1990; Colon & Rectal Surgery, Ochsner Clinic, New Orleans, LA 1990-1991; **Faculty Appointment:** Assoc Prof Surgery, UCLA

Volpe, Peter Anthony MD (Colon & Rectal Surgery) - *Special Expertise:* Colon & Rectal Surgery - *General;* **Admitting Hospital:** California Pacific Medical Center; **Office Address:** 3838 California St, Ste 616 San Francisco, CA 94118; **Office Phone:** (415) 668-0411; **Board Certifications:** Surgery 1970, Colon & Rectal Surgery 1971; **Medical School:** Ohio State Univ 1961; **Residency:** Surgery, UCSF Hosp, San Francisco, CA 1964-1969; **Faculty Appointment:** Clin Prof Surgery, UCSF

DERMATOLOGY

A dermatologist is trained to diagnose and treat pediatric and adult patients with benign and malignant disorders of the skin, mouth, external genitalia, hair and nails, as well as a number of sexually transmitted diseases. The dermatologist has had additional training and experience in the diagnosis and treatment of skin cancers, melanomas, moles and other tumors of the skin, the management of contact dermatitis and other allergic and nonallergic skin disorders, and in the recognition of the skin manifestations of systemic (including internal malignancy) and infectious diseases. Dermatologists have special training in dermatopathology and in the surgical techniques used in dermatology. They also have expertise in the management of cosmetic disorders of the skin such as hair loss and scars, and the skin changes associated with aging.

Training required: Four years

PHYSICIAN LISTINGS

New England

Anderson, Richard Rox MD (Dermatology) - *Special Expertise:* Skin Laser Surgery; Skin Cancer; **Admitting Hospital:** Massachusetts General Hospital; **Office Address:** 275 Cambridge St, Ste 501 Boston, MA 02114; **Office Phone:** (617) 724-6960; **Board Certification:** Dermatology 1991; **Medical School:** Harvard Med Sch 1984; **Residency:** Dermatology, Mass Gen Hosp, Boston, MA 1988-1991; **Fellowship:** Dermatologic Research, Mass Gen Hosp, Boston, MA 1986-1988; **Faculty Appointment:** Assoc Prof Dermatology, Harvard Med Sch

Arndt, Kenneth MD (Dermatology) - *Special Expertise:* Skin Laser Surgery; Cosmetic Dermatology; Dermatologic Therapeutics; **Admitting Hospital:** Beth Israel Deaconess Medical Center - Boston (Page 57); **Office Address:** Skincare Phys of Chestnut Hill 1244 Boylston St, Route 9, Ste 302 Chestnut Hill, MA 02467; **Office Phone:** (617) 731-1600; **Board Certification:** Dermatology 1966; **Medical School:** Yale Univ 1961; **Residency:** Dermatology, Mass Genl Hosp-Harvard Med Sch, Boston, MA 1962-1965; **Fellowship:** Dermatology, Harvard Med Sch, Boston, MA 1964-1965; **Faculty Appointment:** Prof Dermatology, Harvard Med Sch

Braverman, Irwin MD (Dermatology) - *Special Expertise:* Psoriasis/Lupus; Skin Diseases; **Admitting Hospital:** Yale - New Haven Hospital; **Office Address:** Yale Faculty Practice - Yale Phys Bldg 800 Ave, Fl 4th New Haven, CT 06520-8059; **Office Phone:** (203) 785-4092; **Board Certifications:** Dermatology 1963, Dermatopathology 1982; **Medical School:** Yale Univ 1955; **Residencies:** Internal Medicine, Yale, New Haven, CT 1955-1956; Internal Medicine, Yale, New Haven, CT 1958-1959; **Fellowship:** Dermatology, Yale, New Haven, CT 1959-1962; **Faculty Appointment:** Prof Dermatology, Yale Univ

Dover, Jeffrey MD (Dermatology) - *Special Expertise:* Skin Resurfacing - Laser; Photomedicine; **Admitting Hospital:** Beth Israel Deaconess Medical Center - Boston (Page 57); **Office Address:** Skin Care Physicians of Chestnut Hill 1244 Boylston St, Ste 302 Chestnut Hill, MA 02467; **Office Phone:** (617) 731-1600; **Board Certification:** Dermatology 1985; **Medical School:** Univ Ottawa 1981; **Residencies:** Dermatology, Univ Toronto, Toronto, Canada 1982-1984; Dermatology, St Johns Hosp, London 1984-1985; **Fellowship:** Dermatology, Mass Genl Hosp-Harvard, Boston, MA 1985-1987; **Faculty Appointment:** Assoc Prof Dermatology, Harvard Med Sch

Edelson, Richard MD (Dermatology) - *Special Expertise:* Skin Cancer; Skin Diseases-Immunologic; **Admitting Hospital:** Yale - New Haven Hospital; **Office Address:** Yale Dermatology Assoc 800 Howard Ave New Haven, CT 06520; **Office Phone:** (203) 785-4632; **Board Certification:** Dermatology 1977; **Medical School:** Yale Univ 1970; **Residencies:** Dermatology, Mass Genl Hosp, Boston, MA 1971-1972; Dermatology, Natnl Inst Hlth, Bethesda, MD 1972-1975; **Faculty Appointment:** Prof Dermatology, Yale Univ

Gilchrest, Barbara (Dermatology) - *Special Expertise:* Photoaging; Melanoma; **Admitting Hospital:** Boston University Medical Center-East Newton Street Campus; **Office Address:** Boston Univ School of Medicine, Dept Dermatology 609 Albany St, rm 507 Boston, MA 02118-2394; **Office Phone:** (617) 638-5538; **Board Certifications:** Internal Medicine 1975, Dermatology 1978; **Medical School:** Harvard Med Sch 1971; **Residencies:** Internal Medicine, Boston City Hosp, Boston, MA 1972-1973; Dermatology, Harvard Med Sch, Boston, MA 1973-1976; **Fellowship:** Photo Biology, Harvard Med Sch, Boston, MA 1974-1975; **Faculty Appointment:** Prof Dermatology, Boston Univ

DERMATOLOGY

New England

Maloney, Mary MD (Dermatology) - *Special Expertise:* Mohs' Surgery; Skin Laser Surgery; **Admitting Hospital:** UMASS Memorial Health Care - Worcester; **Office Address:** Univ Mass Med Ctr 281 Lincoln St, Ste 4 Worcester, MA 01605; **Office Phone:** (508) 334-5962; **Board Certification:** Dermatology 1982; **Medical School:** Univ VT Coll Med 1977; **Residencies:** Internal Medicine, Hartford Hospital, Hartford, CT 1978-1979; Dermatology, Dartmouth Med Ctr, Lebanon, NH 1979-1982; **Fellowship:** Dermatologic Surgery, UCSF, San Francisco, CA 1983; **Faculty Appointment:** Prof Medicine, Univ Mass Sch Med

McDonald, Charles J MD (Dermatology) - *Special Expertise:* Skin Cancer; Skin Cancer; **Admitting Hospital:** Rhode Island Hospital; **Office Address:** RI Hosp Dept Derm 593 Eddy St APC 10 Providence, RI 02903; **Office Phone:** (401) 444-7816; **Board Certification:** Dermatology 1966; **Medical School:** Howard Univ 1960; **Residencies:** Internal Medicine, Hosp St Raphael, New Haven, CT 1961-1963; Dermatology, Yale New Haven Hosp, New Haven, CT 1963-1965; **Fellowship:** Clinical Oncology, Yale New Haven Hosp, New Haven, CT 1965-1966; **Faculty Appointment:** Prof Dermatology, Brown Univ

Mihm Jr., Martin C. MD (Dermatology) - *Special Expertise:* Melanoma; Vascular Birthmarks; **Admitting Hospital:** Massachusetts General Hospital; **Office Address:** Mass General Hospital 55 Fruit St, Bldg Warren 827 ACC 4 Boston, MA 02114; **Office Phone:** (617) 724-1350; **Board Certifications:** Anatomic Pathology 1974, Dermatopathology 1974; **Medical School:** Univ Pittsburgh 1961; **Residencies:** Internal Medicine, Mt Sinai Hosp, New York, NY 1962-1964; Dermatology, Mass General Hosp, Boston, MA 1964-1967; **Fellowship:** Anatomic Pathology, Mass General Hosp, Boston, MA 1969-1972; **Faculty Appointment:** Clin Prof Pathology, Harvard Med Sch

Mid Atlantic

Ackerman, A Bernard MD (Dermatology) - *Special Expertise:* Dermatopathology; Melanoma; Inflammatory Diseases of Skin; **Admitting Hospital:** St Luke's - Roosevelt Hospital Center - Roosevelt Division (Page 58); **Office Address:** Ackerman Academy of Dermatopathology 145 E 32nd St, Fl 10th New York, NY 10016; **Office Phone:** (212) 889-6225; **Board Certifications:** Dermatology 1970, Dermatopathology 1974; **Medical School:** Coll Physicians & Surgeons 1962; **Residencies:** Dermatology, Univ Penn, Philadelphia, PA 1966-1967; Dermatology, Mass Genl Hosp, Boston, MA 1967-1968; **Fellowship:** Dermatopathology, Mass Genl Hosp, Boston, MA 1968-1969

Alster, Tina MD (Dermatology) - *Special Expertise:* Skin Resurfacing - Laser; **Admitting Hospital:** Washington Hospital; **Office Address:** Washington Inst. Derm Laser Surg. 2311 M St NW, Ste 200 Washington, DC 20037-1445; **Office Phone:** (202) 785-8855; **Board Certification:** Dermatology 1990; **Medical School:** Duke Univ 1986; **Residency:** Dermatology, Yale Univ, New Haven, CT 1987-1989; **Fellowship:** Dermatologic Laser Surgery, Boston Univ Hosp, Boston, MA 1989-1990; **Faculty Appointment:** Asst Clin Prof Dermatology, Georgetown Univ

Anhalt, Grant James MD (Dermatology) - *Special Expertise:* Blistering Diseases; Pemphigus; **Admitting Hospital:** Johns Hopkins Hospital - Baltimore (Page 65); **Office Address:** Richard S. Ross Rsch Bldg 720 Rutlend Ave, rm 771 Baltimore, MD 21205-2196; **Office Phone:** (410) 955-2992; **Board Certification:** Dermatology 1980; **Medical School:** Canada 1975; **Residencies:** Internal Medicine, Hlth Scis Ctr, Winnipeg, Canada 1976-1977; Dermatology, Univ Mich Med Ctr, Ann Arbor, MI 1977-1980; **Fellowship:** Allergy & Immunology, Univ Mich Med Ctr, Ann Arbor, MI 1980-1981; **Faculty Appointment:** Prof Dermatology, Johns Hopkins Univ

182

Bernstein, Robert M MD (Dermatology) - *Special Expertise:* Hair Restoration/Transplant; **Admitting Hospital:** Columbia Presbyterian Medical Center (Page 72); **Office Address:** 125 E 63rd St New York, NY 10021; **Office Phone:** (212) 826-2400; **Board Certification:** Dermatology 1982; **Medical School:** UMDNJ-NJ Med Sch, Newark 1978; **Residency:** Dermatology, Albert Einstein Med Ctr, Bronx, NY 1979-1982; **Faculty Appointment:** Asst Clin Prof Dermatology, Columbia P&S

Bystryn, Jean-Claude MD (Dermatology) - *Special Expertise:* Vitiligo; Blistering Diseases; Pemphigus; **Admitting Hospital:** NYU Medical Center (Page 70); **Office Address:** 530 1st Ave, Ste 7F New York, NY 10016; **Office Phone:** (212) 889-3846; **Board Certifications:** Dermatology 1970, Clinical & Laboratory Dematologic Immunology 1984; **Medical School:** NYU Sch Med 1962; **Residencies:** Internal Medicine, Montefiore Hosp, Bronx, NY 1963-1964; Dermatology, New York Univ, New York, NY 1966-1969; **Fellowship:** Immunology, New York Univ, New York, NY 1969-1972; **Faculty Appointment:** Prof Dermatology, NYU Sch Med

DeLeo, Vincent A. MD (Dermatology) - *Special Expertise:* Photoaging; Contact Dermatitis; Exzema; **Admitting Hospital:** St Luke's - Roosevelt Hospital Center - Roosevelt Division (Page 58); **Office Address:** 425 West 59th Street, Ste 5C New York, NY 10019; **Office Phone:** (212) 523-6003; **Board Certification:** Dermatology 1977; **Medical School:** Louisiana State Univ 1969; **Residencies:** Obstetrics & Gynecology, USPHS Hosp, New Orleans, LA 1970-1972; Dermatology, USPHS Hosp, Staten Island, NY 1972-1974; **Fellowships:** Photo Biology, Cornell Univ, New York, NY 1975; Dermatologic Research, Cornell Univ, New York, NY 1982-1984; **Faculty Appointment:** Assoc Prof Dermatology, Columbia P&S

Dzubow, Leonard MD (Dermatology) - *Special Expertise:* Mohs' Surgery; Skin Laser Surgery; **Admitting Hospital:** Hospital of the University of Pennsylvania; **Office Address:** 3400 Spruce St Philadelphia, PA 19104-4211; **Office Phone:** (215) 662-6534; **Board Certifications:** Internal Medicine 1978, Dermatology 1980; **Medical School:** Univ Penn 1975; **Residencies:** Internal Medicine, Upstate Med Ctr, Syracuse, NY 1976-1977; Internal Medicine, Hosp Penn, Philadelphia, PA 1977-1978; **Fellowship:** Dermatology, NYU-Skin Cancer Unit, New York, NY 1978-1980; **Faculty Appointment:** Prof Dermatology, Univ Penn

Fisher, Michael MD (Dermatology) - *Special Expertise:* Dermatology - General; **Admitting Hospital:** Montefiore Medical Center - Weiler/Einstein Division; **Office Address:** 1575 Blondell Ave Bronx, NY 10461; **Office Phone:** (718) 405-8300; **Board Certification:** Dermatology 1970; **Medical School:** SUNY Hlth Sci Ctr 1963; **Residency:** Dermatology, Mass Genl Hosp-Harvard, Boston, MA 1966-1969; **Faculty Appointment:** Prof Dermatology, Albert Einstein Coll Med

Freedberg, Irwin M MD (Dermatology) - *Special Expertise:* Psoriasis; **Admitting Hospital:** NYU Medical Center (Page 70); **Office Address:** NYU Dermatologic Associates 530 1st Ave, Ste 7R New York, NY 10016; **Office Phone:** (212) 263-5889; **Board Certification:** Dermatology 1963; **Medical School:** Harvard Med Sch 1956; **Residencies:** Internal Medicine, Beth Israel, Boston, MA 1957-1958; Dermatology, Mass Genl. Hosp., Boston, MA 1959-1961; **Fellowship:** Internal Medicine, Beth Israel Hosp, Boston, MA 1958-1959; **Faculty Appointment:** Prof Dermatology, NYU Sch Med

Geronemus, Roy MD (Dermatology) - *Special Expertise:* Skin Laser Surgery; Mohs' Surgery; **Admitting Hospital:** NYU Medical Center (Page 70); **Office Address:** Laser & Skin Surg Ctr 317 E 34th St, Ste 11N New York, NY 10016; **Office Phone:** (212) 686-7306; **Board Certification:** Dermatology 1983; **Medical School:** Univ Miami Sch Med 1979; **Residency:** Dermatology, NYU-Skin Cancer Unit, New York, NY 1980-1983; **Fellowship:** Mohs Surgery, NYU-Skin Cancer Unit, New York, NY 1983-1984

Gordon, Marsha MD (Dermatology) - *Special Expertise:* Photoaging; Acne; **Admitting Hospital:** Mount Sinai Hospital (Page 70); **Office Address:** Mt Sinai Dermatology Assoc 5 E 98th St, Fl 12, Box 1048 New York, NY 10029; **Office Phone:** (212) 831-4119; **Board Certification:** Dermatology 1988; **Medical School:** Univ Penn 1984; **Residency:** Dermatology, Mount Sinai, New York, NY 1985-1988; **Faculty Appointment:** Assoc Clin Prof Dermatology, Mount Sinai Sch Med

Granstein, Richard MD (Dermatology) - *Special Expertise:* Acne; ImmunoDermatology; **Admitting Hospital:** New York Weill Cornell Medical Center - NY Presbyterian Hospital (Page 72); **Office Address:** Cornell Dermatology Consultants 520 E 70th St, Fl 3 New York, NY 10021; **Office Phone:** (212) 746-2007; **Board Certifications:** Dermatology 1983, Clinical & Laboratory Dematologic Immunology 1985; **Medical School:** UCLA 1978; **Residency:** Dermatology, Mass Genl Hosp, Boston, MA 1979-1981; **Fellowships:** Research, Natnl Cancer Inst-Frederick Cancer Resch Facilitys, Frederick, MD 1981-1982; Dermatology, Mass Genl Hosp, Boston, MA 1982-1983; **Faculty Appointment:** Prof Dermatology, Cornell Univ-Weil Med Coll

Grossman, Melanie MD (Dermatology) - *Special Expertise:* Skin Laser Surgery; Hair Removal; **Admitting Hospital:** NYU Downtown Hospital; **Office Address:** 161 Madison Ave, Fl 4 nw New York, NY 10016; **Office Phone:** (212) 725-8600; **Board Certification:** Dermatology 1999; **Medical School:** NYU Sch Med 1988; **Residencies:** Internal Medicine, Yale-New Haven Hosp, New Haven, CT 1988-1989; Dermatology, NY Hosp-Cornell Univ, New York, NY 1989-1992

Katz, Stephen (Dermatology) - *Special Expertise:* Immune Deficiency-Skin; **Admitting Hospital:** National Institutes of Health - Clinical Center; **Office Address:** NIH- Dermatology Branch Bldg 10 - rm r13c404 Bethesda, MD 20892-0001; **Office Phone:** (301) 496-2481; **Board Certifications:** Dermatology 1971, Clinical & Laboratory Dematologic Immunology 1985; **Medical School:** Tulane Univ 1966; **Residency:** Dermatology, Univ Miami, Miami, FL 1967-1970; **Fellowship:** Research, London, England 1972-1974

Kopf, Alfred MD (Dermatology) - *Special Expertise:* Skin Cancer - Melanoma; **Admitting Hospital:** NYU Medical Center (Page 70); **Office Address:** Dermatology Medical Assoc 350 5th Ave, Ste 7805 New York, NY 10118; **Office Phone:** (212) 689-5050; **Board Certification:** Dermatology 1957; **Medical School:** Cornell Univ-Weil Med Coll 1951; **Residency:** Dermatology, NYU Sch Med, New York, NY 1952-1955; **Faculty Appointment:** Clin Prof Dermatology, NYU Sch Med

Lebwohl, Mark MD (Dermatology) - *Special Expertise:* Psoriasis; Skin Cancer; **Admitting Hospital:** Mount Sinai Hospital (Page 70); **Office Address:** 5 E 98th St, Fl 12 New York, NY 10029; **Office Phone:** (212) 876-7199; **Board Certifications:** Internal Medicine 1981, Dermatology 1983; **Medical School:** Harvard Med Sch 1978; **Residency:** Internal Medicine, Mount Sinai Hosp, New York, NY 1979-1981; **Fellowship:** Dermatology, Mount Sinai Hosp, New York, NY 1981-1983; **Faculty Appointment:** Prof Dermatology, Mount Sinai Sch Med

Leyden, James MD (Dermatology) - *Special Expertise:* Infectious Disease; Acne; **Admitting Hospital:** Hospital of the University of Pennsylvania; **Office Address:** University of Pennsylvania Hospital 3600 Spruce St, Bldg Rhoads - Fl 2nd Philadelphia, PA 19104; **Office Phone:** (215) 662-6151; **Board Certification:** Dermatology 1973; **Medical School:** Univ Penn 1966; **Residencies:** Dermatology, Univ Penn, Philadelphia, PA 1967-1968; Dermatology, Univ Penn, Philadelphia, PA 1970-1971; **Faculty Appointment:** Prof Dermatology, Univ Penn

Miller, Stanley MD (Dermatology) - *Special Expertise: Dermatologic Surgery; Skin Cancer;* **Admitting Hospital:** Johns Hopkins Hospital - Baltimore (Page 65); **Office Address:** John Hopkins Outpat Ctr 601 N Caroline St Baltimore, MD 21287-0900; **Office Phone:** (410) 551-1588; **Board Certification:** Dermatology 1989; **Medical School:** Univ VT Coll Med 1984; **Residency:** Dermatology, UC San Diego, San Diego, CA 1986-1989; **Fellowship:** Surgery, U Penn, Philadelphia, PA 1989-1991; **Faculty Appointment:** Prof Dermatology, Johns Hopkins Univ

Nigra, Thomas P MD (Dermatology) - *Special Expertise: Hair Problems; Vitiligo; Psoriasis;* **Admitting Hospital:** Washington Hospital Center - DC (Page 79); **Office Address:** Washington Hosp Ctr 110 Irving St NW, Fl 2B-44 Washington, DC 20010-2976; **Office Phone:** (202) 877-6227; **Board Certification:** Dermatology 1973; **Medical School:** Univ Penn 1967; **Residencies:** Dermatology, Mass Genl Hosp, Boston, MA 1968-1969; Dermatology, Mass Genl Hosp, Boston, MA 1972-1973

Orlow, Seth MD (Dermatology) - *Special Expertise: Dermatology - Pediatric; Hemangioma;* **Admitting Hospital:** NYU Medical Center (Page 70); **Office Address:** 530 1st Ave, Ste 7R New York, NY 10016; **Office Phone:** (212) 263-5889; **Board Certification:** Dermatology 1990; **Medical School:** Albert Einstein Coll Med 1986; **Residencies:** Pediatrics, Mt Sinai, New York, NY 1986-1987; Dermatology, Yale Med Sch, New Haven, CT 1987-1989; **Fellowship:** Dermatology, Yale Med Sch, New Haven, CT 1989-1990; **Faculty Appointment:** Assoc Prof Dermatology, NYU Sch Med

Rigel, Darrell MD (Dermatology) - *Special Expertise: Dermatology - General;* **Admitting Hospital:** NYU Medical Center (Page 70); **Office Address:** 35 E 35th Street, Ste 208 New York, NY 10016; **Office Phone:** (212) 684-5964; **Board Certification:** Dermatology 1983; **Medical School:** Geo Wash Univ 1978; **Residency:** Dermatology, New York Univ, New york, NY 1979-1982; **Fellowship:** Dermatology, New York Univ, New York, NY 1982-1983; **Faculty Appointment:** Clin Prof Dermatology, NYU Sch Med

Robins, Perry MD (Dermatology) - *Special Expertise: Mohs' Surgery; Skin Cancer - Melanoma;* **Admitting Hospital:** NYU Medical Center (Page 70); **Office Address:** 530 First Ave, Ste 7H New York, NY 10016; **Office Phone:** (212) 263-7222; **Board Certification:** Dermatology 1991; **Medical School:** Germany 1960; **Residencies:** Dermatology, VA Med Ctr/nyu/bellevue, Bronx, NY 1961-1962; Dermatology, NYU Med Ctr, New York, NY 1963; **Faculty Appointment:** Prof Dermatology, NYU Sch Med

Safai, Bijan MD (Dermatology) - *Special Expertise: Dermatologic Surgery; Cosmetic Dematology; Cosmetic Dermatology;* **Admitting Hospital:** Westchester Medical Center; **Office Address:** NY Med Coll, rm 217 Vosburgh Pavillion Valhalla, NY 10595; **Office Phone:** (914) 594-4566; **Board Certification:** Dermatology 1974; **Medical School:** Iran 1965; **Residencies:** Internal Medicine, VA Med Ctr/NYU/Bellevue, New York, NY 1969-1970; Dermatology, NYU Med Ctr, New York, NY 1970-1973; **Fellowship:** Immunology, Mem Sloan-Kettering Cancer Ctr, New York, NY 1973-1974; **Faculty Appointment:** Prof Dermatology, NY Med Coll

Scher, Richard K MD (Dermatology) - *Special Expertise: Nail Diseases;* **Admitting Hospital:** Columbia Presbyterian Medical Center (Page 72); **Office Address:** 16 E 60th St New York, NY 10022; **Office Phone:** (212) 326-8465; **Board Certification:** Dermatology 1960; **Medical School:** Howard Univ 1955; **Residency:** Dermatology, New York Univ, New York, NY 1956-1959; **Faculty Appointment:** Prof Dermatology, Columbia P&S

DERMATOLOGY

Shalita, Alan MD (Dermatology) - *Special Expertise:* Acne; Rosacea; **Admitting Hospital:** University Hospital - SUNY Health Sciences Center - Syracuse; **Office Address:** Downstate Derm Assoc 450 Clarkson Ave Brooklyn, NY 11203-2012; **Office Phone:** (718) 270-1230; **Board Certification:** Dermatology 1971; **Medical School:** Wake Forest Univ Sch Med 1964; **Residency:** Dermatology, NYU Med Ctr, New York, NY 1967-1970; **Fellowship:** Dermatologic Research, NYU Med Ctr, New York, NY 1970-1973; **Faculty Appointment:** Prof Dermatology, SUNY Hlth Sci Ctr

Shupack, Jerome L MD (Dermatology) - *Special Expertise:* Skin Diseases; Melanoma; **Admitting Hospital:** Bellevue Hospital Center; **Office Address:** NYU Med Ctr 530 1st Ave New York, NY 10016-6402; **Office Phone:** (212) 263-7344; **Board Certification:** Dermatology 1970; **Medical School:** Columbia P&S 1963; **Residencies:** Internal Medicine, Mt Sinai Hosp, New York, NY 1964-1965; Dermatology, NYU, New York, NY 1967-1970; **Faculty Appointment:** Clin Prof Dermatology, NYU Sch Med

Spielvogel, Richard Lee MD (Dermatology) - *Special Expertise:* Melanoma; Skin Cancer; **Admitting Hospital:** Hahnemann University Hospital; **Office Address:** MCP Hahnemann Univ, Dept Derm 401 Broad & Vine, MC-401 Philadelphia, PA 19101; **Office Phone:** (215) 762-8252; **Board Certifications:** Dermatopathology 1981, Clinical & Laboratory Dematologic Immunology 1985; **Medical School:** Univ Rochester 1972; **Residency:** Dermatology, Univ Minn Hosp, Minneapolis, MN 1974-1977; **Fellowship:** Dermatopathology, NYU Med Ctr, New York, NY 1980-1981; **Faculty Appointment:** Prof Dermatology, Hahnemann Univ

Stanley, John R MD (Dermatology) - *Special Expertise:* Blistering Diseases; Pemphigus; **Admitting Hospital:** Hospital of the University of Pennsylvania; **Office Address:** Hosp Univ Penn, Dept Derm 3600 Spruce St, 2 Rhoads Pavilion Philadelphia, PA 19104; **Office Phone:** (215) 662-3626; **Board Certifications:** Dermatology 1978, Clinical & Laboratory Dematologic Immunology 1985; **Medical School:** Harvard Med Sch 1974; **Residency:** Dermatology, NYU Med Ctr, New York, NY 1975-1978; **Faculty Appointment:** Prof Dermatology, Univ Penn

Zitelli, John MD (Dermatology) - *Special Expertise:* Mohs' Surgery; Skin Cancer; **Admitting Hospital:** UPMC - Presbyterian University Hospital; **Office Address:** Shadyside Med Ctr 5200 Centre Ave, Ste 303 Pittsburgh, PA 15232; **Office Phone:** (412) 681-9400; **Board Certification:** Dermatology 1980; **Medical School:** Univ Pittsburgh 1976; **Residency:** Dermatology, Univ Hlth Ctr Hosp, Pittsburgh, PA 1977-1979; **Fellowship:** Mohs Surgery, Univ Wisconsin, Madison, WI 1980

Southeast

Amonette, Rex A MD (Dermatology) - *Special Expertise:* Skin Cancer; Mohs' Surgery; **Admitting Hospital:** University of Tennessee Bowld Hospital; **Office Address:** Memphis Derm Clinic 1455 Union Ave Memphis, TN 38104-6727; **Office Phone:** (901) 726-6655; **Board Certification:** Dermatology 1974; **Medical School:** Univ Ark 1966; **Residency:** Dermatology, Univ Tenn, Memphis, TN 1969-1971; **Fellowship:** Mohs Surgery, NYU, New York, NY 1971-1972

Burton III, Claude Shreve MD (Dermatology) - *Special Expertise:* Leg Ulcers; Wound Healing/Care; Hemangioma; **Admitting Hospital:** Duke University Medical Center (Page 60); **Office Address:** Duke Univ Med Ctr Box 3511 Durham, NC 27710; **Office Phone:** (919) 681-5421; **Board Certifications:** Internal Medicine 1982, Dermatology 1984; **Medical School:** Duke Univ 1979; **Residencies:** Internal Medicine, Duke Univ, Durham, NC 1980-1982; Dermatology, Duke Univ, Durham, NC 1982-1984; **Faculty Appointment:** Assoc Prof Medicine, Duke Univ

Callen, Jeffrey P MD (Dermatology) - *Special Expertise:* Lupus Dermatomysitis Vasculitis; **Admitting Hospital:** Jewish Hospital & Medical Center - Louisville; **Office Address:** 310 E Broadway Louisville, KY 40202; **Office Phone:** (502) 583-1749; **Board Certifications:** Internal Medicine 1975, Dermatology 1977; **Medical School:** Univ Mich Med Sch 1972; **Residencies:** Internal Medicine, Univ Michigan Med Ctr, Ann Arbor 1972-1975; Dermatology, Univ Michigan Med Ctr, Ann Arbor 1975-1977; **Faculty Appointment:** Prof Medicine, Univ Louisville Sch Med

Cohen, Bernard Hershel MD (Dermatology) - *Special Expertise:* Skin Cancer; Hair Loss & Restoration Surgery; Cosmetic Dermatology; **Admitting Hospital:** Baptist Hospital - Miami; **Office Address:** 9150 SW 87th Ave, Ste 208 Miami, FL 33176-2313; **Office Phone:** (305) 274-1040; **Board Certification:** Dermatology 1972; **Medical School:** Columbia P&S 1967; **Residency:** Dermatology, NYU, New York, NY 1968-1971; **Faculty Appointment:** Clin Prof Dermatology, Univ Miami Sch Med

Eaglstein, William MD (Dermatology) - *Special Expertise:* Wound Healing/Care; **Admitting Hospital:** University of Miami - Jackson Memorial Hospital; **Office Address:** 1444 NW Ninth Avenue Miami, FL 33136; **Office Phone:** (305) 243-6704; **Board Certification:** Dermatology 1971; **Medical School:** Univ MO-Kansas City 1965; **Residency:** Dermatology, Univ Miami/Jackson Meml, Miami, FL 1966-1969; **Faculty Appointment:** Prof Dermatology, Univ Miami Sch Med

Eichler, Craig MD (Dermatology) - *Special Expertise:* Skin Cancer; Dermatologic Surgery; Dermatologic Infectious Disease; **Admitting Hospital:** Cleveland Clinic Florida; **Office Address:** Cleveland Clinic-Naples 6101 Pine Ridge Road Naples, FL 34119; **Office Phone:** (877) 675-7223; **Board Certification:** Dermatology 1993; **Medical School:** Univ Fla Coll Med 1989; **Residency:** Dermatology, Univ Texas, Galveston, TX 1989-1993

Fenske, Neil MD (Dermatology) - *Special Expertise:* Skin Cancer; Aging Skin; Psoriasis; **Admitting Hospital:** Tampa General Hospital; **Office Address:** 12901 Bruce B Downs Blvd MDC-33 Tampa, FL 33612-4742; **Office Phone:** (813) 974-2920; **Board Certifications:** Dermatology 1977, Dermatopathology 1984; **Medical School:** St Louis Univ 1973; **Residency:** Dermatology, Wisc Hlth Sci Ctr, Madison, WI 1974-1977; **Faculty Appointment:** Prof Medicine, Univ S Fla Coll Med

Flowers, Franklin P MD (Dermatology) - *Special Expertise:* Mohs' Surgery; Dermatopathology; **Admitting Hospital:** Shands Healthcare at University Florida (Page 77); **Office Address:** 1600 SW Archer Rd Gainesville, FL 32610; **Office Phone:** (352) 395-8001; **Board Certifications:** Dermatology 1976, Dermatopathology 1981; **Medical School:** Univ Fla Coll Med 1971; **Residency:** Dermatology, Ohio State Univ, Columbus, OH 1972-1975; **Fellowship:** Mohs Surgery, Univ Alabama, Birmingham, AL 1992-1993; **Faculty Appointment:** Prof Medicine, Univ Fla Coll Med

Green, Howard MD (Dermatology) - *Special Expertise:* Mohs' Surgery; **Admitting Hospital:** St Mary's Medical Center - West Palm Beach; **Office Address:** Dermatology Assocs PA of Palm Beaches 120A Butler St West Palm Beach, FL 33407; **Office Phone:** (561) 622-6976; **Board Certification:** Dermatology 1992; **Medical School:** Boston Univ 1985; **Residencies:** Internal Medicine, Jefferson Univ Hosp, Philadelphia, PA 1986-1988; Dermatology, Harvard Med Sch, Boston, MA 1988-1992; **Fellowship:** Mohs Surgery, Boston Univ Med Ctr, Boston, MA 1992-1993

Johr, Robert MD (Dermatology) - *Special Expertise:* Skin Cancer; **Admitting Hospital:** Boca Raton Community Hosp; **Office Address:** 1050 NW 15th St, Apt 201A Boca Raton, FL 33486-1341; **Office Phone:** (561) 368-4545; **Board Certification:** Dermatology 1981; **Medical School:** Mexico 1975; **Residencies:** Dermatology, Roswell Pk Cancer, Cleveland, NY 1976-1977; Dermatology, Metro Med Ctr, Buffalo, NY 1977-1979

Jorizzo, Joseph L. MD (Dermatology) - *Special Expertise:* Dermatology; Rheumatologic & Immunologic Dermatology; **Admitting Hospital:** Wake Forest University Baptist Medical Center; **Office Address:** Wake Forest Univ Baptist Med Ctr Med Ctr Blvd Winston-Salem, NC 27157; **Office Phone:** (336) 716-2768; **Board Certification:** Dermatology 1979; **Medical School:** Boston Univ 1975; **Residency:** Dermatology, Univ NC, Chapel Hill, NC 1976-1979; **Fellowship:** Dermatology, Derm Inst, London, UK 1979-1980; **Faculty Appointment:** Prof Dermatology, Wake Forest Univ Sch Med

Leshin, Barry MD (Dermatology) - *Special Expertise:* Dermatologic Surgery; Mohs' Surgery; **Admitting Hospital:** Wake Forest University Baptist Medical Center; **Office Address:** Wake Forest Univ Sch Med, Dept Derm Med Ctr Blvd Winston-Salem, NC 27157-0001; **Office Phone:** (336) 716-3926; **Board Certification:** Dermatology 1985; **Medical School:** Univ Tex, Houston 1981; **Residency:** Dermatology, Univ IA Hosp, Iowa City, IA 1982-1985; **Fellowship:** Dermatologic Surgery, Univ IA Hosp, Iowa City, IA 1985-1986; **Faculty Appointment:** Assoc Prof Dermatology, Wake Forest Univ Sch Med

Pinnell, Sheldon MD (Dermatology) - *Special Expertise:* Skin & Collagen Disorders; Melanoma/Skin Cancer; **Admitting Hospital:** Duke University Medical Center (Page 60); **Office Address:** Duke Univ Med Ctr, Dept of Dermatology Trent Drive S, Box 3135 Durham, NC 27710; **Office Phone:** (919) 684-5337; **Board Certification:** Dermatology; **Medical School:** Yale Univ 1963; **Residency:** Internal Medicine, Minn Hosp, Minneapolis, MN 1964-1965; **Fellowship:** Dermatology, Mass Genl Hosp, Boston, MA 1968-1971; **Faculty Appointment:** Prof Dermatology, Duke Univ

Sherertz, Elizabeth F MD (Dermatology) - *Special Expertise:* Dermatitis; **Admitting Hospital:** Wake Forest University Baptist Medical Center; **Office Address:** Med Ctr Blvd Winston Salem, NC 27157-1071; **Office Phone:** (336) 716-3203; **Board Certification:** Dermatology 1982; **Medical School:** Univ VA Sch Med 1978; **Residencies:** Internal Medicine, Univ VA Hosp, Charlottesville, VA 1978-1979; Dermatology, Duke Univ, Durham, NC 1979-1982; **Faculty Appointment:** Prof Dermatology, Wake Forest Univ Sch Med

Sobel, Stuart MD (Dermatology) - *Special Expertise:* Skin Cancer; Blistering Diseases; **Admitting Hospital:** Memorial Regional Hospital- Hollywood; **Office Address:** 4340 Sheridan St, Ste 101 Hollywood, FL 33021-3511; **Office Phone:** (954) 983-5533; **Board Certification:** Dermatology 1977; **Medical School:** Tufts Univ 1972; **Residency:** Dermatology, Mt Sinai Hosp, New York, NY 1973-1976

Sokoloff, Daniel MD (Dermatology) - *Special Expertise:* Dermatology - General; **Admitting Hospital:** St Mary's Medical Center - West Palm Beach; **Office Address:** 1000 45th St, Ste 1 West Palm Beach, FL 33407-2416; **Office Phone:** (561) 863-1000; **Board Certification:** Dermatology 1982; **Medical School:** Geo Wash Univ 1977; **Residency:** Dermatology, Baylor Coll Med, Houston, TX 1979

Midwest

Bailin, Philip Lawrence MD (Dermatology) - *Special Expertise:* Mohs' Surgery; Skin Laser Surgery; **Admitting Hospital:** Cleveland Clinic Foundation; **Office Address:** Cleveland Clinic Foundation 9500 Euclid Ave, MC-A61 Cleveland, OH 44195; **Office Phone:** (216) 444-2115; **Board Certification:** Dermatology 1975; **Medical School:** Northwestern Univ 1968; **Residency:** Dermatology, Cleveland Clinic Fdn, Cleveland, OH 1971-1974; **Fellowship:** Dermatopathology, AFIP, Washignton, DC 1974-1975

Camisa, Charles MD (Dermatology) - *Special Expertise:* Dermatology - General; **Admitting Hospital:** Cleveland Clinic Foundation; **Office Address:** Cleveland Clinic Foundation Dept. Dermatology 9500 Euclid Ave Cleveland, OH 44195-0001; **Office Phone:** (216) 444-8377; **Board Certifications:** Dermatology 1981, Clinical & Laboratory Dematologic Immunology 1987; **Medical School:** Mount Sinai Sch Med 1981; **Residency:** Dermatology, NYU Hospital, New York, NY 1978-1981; **Faculty Appointment:** Assoc Prof Medicine, Ohio State Univ

Cornelius, Lynne A MD (Dermatology) - *Special Expertise:* Melanoma; **Admitting Hospital:** Barnes - Jewish Hospital; **Office Address:** 969 N Mason St, Ste 220 St Louis, MO 63141; **Office Phone:** (314) 362-8187; **Board Certification:** Dermatology 1989; **Medical School:** Univ MO-Columbia Sch Med 1984; **Residency:** Dermatology, Wash Univ, St Louis, MO 1986-1989; **Fellowship:** Dermatology, Emory, Atlanta, GA 1989-1992; **Faculty Appointment:** Asst Prof Dermatology, Washington Univ, St Louis

Fivenson, David MD (Dermatology) - *Special Expertise:* Blistering Diseases; Wound Healing/Care; Lupus/SLE; **Admitting Hospital:** Henry Ford Health System (Page 62); **Office Address:** Henry Ford Hospital-Dept Derm 2799 W Grand Blvd Detroit, MI 48202; **Office Phone:** (313) 876-2972; **Board Certification:** Dermatology 1989; **Medical School:** Univ Mich Med Sch 1984; **Residency:** Dermatology, Univ Cincinnati, OH 1986-1989; **Fellowship:** Dermatology, Univ Cal-San Diego, San Diego, CA 1985-1986

Garden, Jerome MD (Dermatology) - *Special Expertise:* Skin Laser Surgery; Skin Resurfacing; **Admitting Hospital:** Northwestern Memorial Hospital; **Office Address:** 150 E Huron St, Ste 910 Chicago, IL 60611-2946; **Office Phone:** (312) 280-0890; **Board Certification:** Dermatology 1984; **Medical School:** Northwestern Univ 1980; **Residencies:** Internal Medicine, Northwestern Univ, Chicago, IL 1980-1981; Dermatology, Northwestern Univ, Chicago, IL 1981-1984; **Faculty Appointment:** Assoc Clin Prof Dermatology, Northwestern Univ

Hanke, C William MD (Dermatology) - *Special Expertise:* Skin Cancer; Dermatologic Surgery; **Admitting Hospital:** St Vincent's Hospital - Carmel; **Office Address:** Carmel Medical Center 13450 N Meridian St, Ste 355 Carmel, IN 46032; **Office Phone:** (317) 582-8484; **Board Certifications:** Dermatology 1978, Dermatopathology 1982; **Medical School:** Univ Iowa Coll Med 1971; **Residencies:** Dermatology, Cleveland Clinic, Cleveland, OH 1975-1978; Dermatopathology, Indiana Univ, Indianapolis, IN 1981-1982; **Fellowship:** Cutaneous Oncology, Cleveland Clinic, Cleveland, OH 1978-1979

Hruza, George J MD (Dermatology) - *Special Expertise:* Skin Laser Surgery; Mohs' Surgery; **Admitting Hospital:** St Lukes Hospital; **Office Address:** Laser & Derm Surg Ctr 14377 Woodlake Dr., Ste 111 St. Louis, MO 63017; **Office Phone:** (314) 878-3839; **Board Certification:** Dermatology 1986; **Medical School:** NYU Sch Med 1982; **Residencies:** Internal Medicine, New York Hosp-Cornell Univ, New York City, NY 1982-1983; Dermatology, NYU Med Ctr-Skin Cancer Unit, New York City, NY 1983-1986; **Fellowships:** Surgery, Mass Genl Hosp-Harvard, Boston, MA 1986-1987; Surgery, Univ Wisc Med Sch, Madison, WI 1987-1988; **Faculty Appointment:** Prof Dermatology, St Louis Univ

Johnson, Timothy M MD (Dermatology) - *Special Expertise:* Melanoma; Cosmetic Surgery - Face; **Admitting Hospital:** University of Michigan Health Center; **Office Address:** 1147 Cancer Ctr Univ Hosp Ann Arbor, MI 48109-0314; **Office Phone:** (734) 936-4068; **Board Certification:** Dermatology 1988; **Medical School:** Univ Tex, Houston 1984; **Residencies:** Surgery, Univ Mich, Ann Arbor, MI 1988-1989; Dermatology, Univ Texas, Houston, TX 1985-1988; **Fellowship:** Surgery, Univ Oregon, Portland, OR 1989-1990; **Faculty Appointment:** Assoc Prof Dermatology, Univ Mich Med Sch

DERMATOLOGY

Neuberg, Marcy MD (Dermatology) - *Special Expertise:* Mohs' Surgery; Skin Cancer; Pigmented Lesions; **Admitting Hospital:** Froedtert Memorial Lutheran Hospital; **Office Address:** Froedtert & Medical College Clinics 9200 West Wisconsin Avenue Milwaukee, WI 53226; **Office Phone:** (414) 805-3666; **Board Certifications:** Internal Medicine 1985, Dermatology 1988; **Medical School:** Oregon Hlth Scis Univ 1982; **Residencies:** Internal Medicine, Georgetown Univ, Washington, DC 1982-1985; Dermatology, Boston Univ Sch of Med Ctr, Boston, MA 1985-1988; **Fellowship:** Mohs Surgery, Tufts New England Med Ctr, Boston, MA 1988-1990; **Faculty Appointment:** Assoc Prof Dermatology, Med Coll Wisc

Paller, Amy Susan MD (Dermatology) - *Special Expertise:* Acne; Rosacea; **Admitting Hospital:** Children's Memorial Hospital; **Office Address:** Children's Meml Hospital 2300 Chldns Plaza #107 Chicago, IL 60614-3394; **Office Phone:** (773) 880-4698; **Board Certifications:** Pediatrics 1982, Dermatology 1983; **Medical School:** Stanford Univ 1978; **Residencies:** Pediatrics, Chldns Meml Hosp, Chicago, IL 1979-1981; Dermatology, Northwestern, Chicago, IL 1981-1983; **Fellowship:** U NC Hosp, Chapel Hill, NC 1983-1984; **Faculty Appointment:** Prof Pediatrics, Northwestern Univ

Shwayder, Tor A MD (Dermatology) - *Special Expertise:* Dermatology - Pediatric; Skin Laser Surgery - Birthmarks; **Admitting Hospital:** Henry Ford Health System (Page 62); **Office Address:** Henry Ford Hosp, Dept Derm 2799 W Grand Blvd Detroit, MI 48202; **Office Phone:** (313) 876-2161; **Board Certifications:** Pediatrics 1986, Dermatology 1987; **Medical School:** Univ Mich Med Sch 1980; **Residencies:** Pediatrics, Univ of Michigan, Ann Arbor, MI 1980-1983; Dermatology, Strong Meml Hosp Univ of Rochester, Rochester, MI 1984-1987; **Faculty Appointment:** Asst Prof Dermatology, Wayne State Univ

Sontheimer, Richard MD (Dermatology) - *Special Expertise:* Dermatologic Immunology; Lupus/SLE; **Admitting Hospital:** University of Iowa Hospitals and Clinics; **Office Address:** Univ Ia Hosps & Clins, Dept Derm 200 Hawkins Dr Iowa City, IA 52242-1090; **Office Phone:** (319) 356-3609; **Board Certifications:** Dermatology 1979, Clinical & Laboratory Dematologic Immunology 1985; **Medical School:** Univ Tex SW, Dallas 1972; **Residencies:** Internal Medicine, Univ Utah Affil Hosps, Salt Lake City, UT 1974-1976; Dermatology, Parkland Meml Hosp, Dallas, TX 1978-1979; **Fellowship:** Research, Southwestern Med Sch, Dallas, TX 1976-1978; **Faculty Appointment:** Prof Dermatology, Univ Iowa Coll Med

Treadwell, Patricia MD (Dermatology) - *Special Expertise:* Dermatology - Pediatric; Birthmarks; **Admitting Hospital:** Riley Hospital for Children; **Office Address:** U H 3240 550 N Univ Blvd Indianapolis, IN 46202; **Office Phone:** (317) 274-7744; **Board Certifications:** Pediatrics 1982, Dermatology 1983; **Medical School:** Cornell Univ-Weil Med Coll 1977; **Residencies:** Pediatrics, James Whitcomb Riley Hosp, Indianapolis, IN 1978-1980; Dermatology, Indiana Univ Med Ctr, Indianapolis, IN 1980-1983

Voorhees, John MD (Dermatology) - *Special Expertise:* Aging Skin; Psoriasis; Photoaging; **Admitting Hospital:** University of Michigan Health Center; **Office Address:** Taubman Hlth Care Ctr 1500 E Med Ctr Dr, rm 1910, Box 0314 Ann Arbor, MI 48109-0314; **Office Phone:** (734) 936-4054; **Board Certification:** Dermatology 1970; **Medical School:** Univ Mich Med Sch 1963; **Residency:** Dermatology, Univ Mich Hosp, Ann Arbor, MI 1966-1969; **Faculty Appointment:** Prof Dermatology, Univ Mich Med Sch

Zelickson, Brian D MD (Dermatology) - *Special Expertise:* Skin Laser Surgery; **Admitting Hospital:** Abbott - Northwestern Hospital; **Office Address:** Med Arts Bldg 825 Nicollet Mall, Ste 1002 Minneapolis, MN 55402-2614; **Office Phone:** (612) 338-0711; **Board Certification:** Dermatology 1999; **Medical School:** Mayo Med Sch 1986; **Residency:** Dermatology, Mayo Clinic, Rochester, MN 1988-1990; **Faculty Appointment:** Asst Prof Dermatology, Univ Minn

Great Plains and Mountains

Krueger, Gerald MD (Dermatology) - *Special Expertise:* Psoriasis; **Admitting Hospital:** University of Utah Hospital and Clinics; **Office Address:** Univ Utah Hlth Sci Ctr, Dept Derm 50 N Medical Dr, Ste 4B454 Salt Lake City, UT 84132; **Office Phone:** (801) 581-6465; **Board Certification:** Dermatology 1973; **Medical School:** Loma Linda Univ 1966; **Residency:** Dermatology, Univ Colorado Med Ctr, Denver, Co 1969-1972; **Faculty Appointment:** Prof Dermatology, Univ Utah

Weston, William Lee MD (Dermatology) - *Special Expertise:* Lupus/SLE - Neonatal; **Admitting Hospital:** University of Colorado Health & Science Center; **Office Address:** 4200 E 9th Ave, Box E-153 Denver, CO 80262; **Office Phone:** (303) 372-1111; **Board Certifications:** Dermatology 1973, Pediatrics 1970; **Medical School:** Univ Colo 1965; **Residencies:** Dermatology, Colo Med Ctr, Denver, CO 1970-1972; Pediatrics, UCSF, San Francisco, CA 1967-1968; **Faculty Appointment:** Prof Dermatology, Univ Colo

Southwest

Butler, David F MD (Dermatology) - *Special Expertise:* Skin Cancer; **Admitting Hospital:** University Medical Center; **Office Address:** Dept Dermatology 3601 4th St Lubbock, TX 79430; **Office Phone:** (806) 743-1842; **Board Certification:** Dermatology 1985; **Medical School:** Univ Tex Med Br, Galveston 1980; **Residency:** Dermatology, Walter Reed Army Med Ctr, Washington, DC 1982-1985; **Faculty Appointment:** Asst Clin Prof Medicine, Texas Tech Univ

Cockerell, Clay J MD (Dermatology) - *Special Expertise:* Dermatopathology; **Admitting Hospital:** Zale Lipshy University Hospital; **Office Address:** Cockerell & Assocs DermPath 2330 Butler St, Ste 115 Dallas, TX 75235; **Office Phone:** (214) 638-2222; **Board Certifications:** Dermatology 1985, Dermatopathology 1986; **Medical School:** Baylor Coll Med 1981; **Residency:** Dermatology, NYU, New York, NY 1982-1985; **Fellowship:** Dermatopathology, NYU, New York, NY 1985-1986; **Faculty Appointment:** Prof Dermatopathology, Univ Tex SW, Dallas

Duvic, Madeleine MD (Dermatology) - *Special Expertise:* Cutaneous T-Cell Lymphoma; Skin Cancer; **Admitting Hospital:** University of Texas MD Anderson Cancer Center (Page 66); **Office Address:** UT MD Anderson Cancer Ctr, Dept Derm 1515 Holcombe Blvd, Box 28 Houston, TX 77030; **Office Phone:** (713) 745-1113; **Board Certifications:** Dermatology 1981, Internal Medicine 1982; **Medical School:** E Carolina Univ 1977; **Residencies:** Dermatology, Duke Univ, Durham, NC 1978-1980; Internal Medicine, Duke Univ, Durham, NC 1980-1982; **Fellowship:** Geriatric Medicine, Duke Univ, Durham, NC 1982-1984; **Faculty Appointment:** Prof Dermatology, Univ Tex, Houston

Hansen, Ronald MD (Dermatology) - *Special Expertise:* Dermatology - Pediatric; **Admitting Hospital:** University Medical Center; **Office Address:** Univ Arizona Hlth Sci Ctr, Dept Dermatology 1501 N Campbell St, Box 245038 Tucson, AZ 85724; **Office Phone:** (520) 626-7783; **Board Certifications:** Pediatrics 1974, Dermatology 1980; **Medical School:** Univ Iowa Coll Med 1968; **Residencies:** Pediatrics, Childrens Hosp, Los Angeles, CA 1969-1970; Pediatrics, Stanford Univ Med Ctr, CA 1970-1972

Horn, Thomas MD (Dermatology) - *Special Expertise:* Graft vs. Host Disease; Skin Cancer; **Admitting Hospital:** University of Arkansas for Medical Sciences; **Office Address:** Univ Hosp Arkansas Med Scis 4301 W Markham Dr # 576 Little Rock, AR 72205; **Office Phone:** (501) 686-5110; **Board Certifications:** Dermatology 1987, Dermatopathology 1988; **Medical School:** Univ VA Sch Med 1982; **Residency:** Dermatology, Univ Maryland, Baltimore, MD 1984-1987; **Fellowship:** Dermatopathology, John Hopkins Hosp, Baltimore, MD 1987-1989

DERMATOLOGY

Levy, Moise MD (Dermatology) - *Special Expertise:* Dermatology - Pediatrics; Vascular
Malformations; **Admitting Hospital:** Texas Children's Hospital - Houston; **Office Address:** Texas
Chldns Hosp 6621 Fannin St #MC3-3315 Houston, TX 77030-2303; **Office Phone:** (832) 824-3720;
Board Certifications: Pediatrics 1985, Dermatology 1986; **Medical School:** Univ Tex, Houston
1979; **Residencies:** Pediatrics, Univ Texas Affil Hosp, Houston, TX 1980-1983; Dermatology, Baylor
Coll Med, Houston, TX 1983-1986; **Faculty Appointment:** Prof Dermatology, Baylor Coll Med

Menter, M Alan MD (Dermatology) - *Special Expertise:* Psoriasis; **Admitting Hospital:** Baylor
University Medical Center; **Office Address:** 5310 Harvest Hill Rd, Ste 260 Dallas, TX 75230-5891;
Office Phone: (972) 386-7546; **Board Certification:** Dermatology 1978; **Medical School:** Africa
1978; **Residencies:** Dermatology, Pretoria General Hospital 1968-1971; Dermatology, Guys
Hospital, London, England 1972; **Fellowships:** Dermatology, St Johns Hospital, London, England
1973; Dermatology, Univ Texas-Southwestern, Dallas, TX 1977; **Faculty Appointment:** Clin Prof
Dermatology, Univ Tex SW, Dallas

Taylor, R Stan MD (Dermatology) - *Special Expertise:* Mohs' Surgery; Melanoma; Skin
Cancer; **Admitting Hospital:** Zale Lipshy University Hospital; **Office Address:** Univ Tex SW Med Ctr
5323 Harry Hines Blvd Dallas, TX 75390-9069; **Office Phone:** (214) 648-8085; **Board Certification:**
Dermatology 1989; **Medical School:** Univ Tex Med Br, Galveston 1985; **Residency:** Dermatology,
Univ Mich, Ann Arbor, MI 1986-1989; **Fellowships:** Immunological Dermatology, Univ Mich, Ann
Arbor, MI 1989-1990; Mohs Surgery, Oreg Hlth Sci Univ, Portland, OR 1990-1991; **Faculty
Appointment:** Assoc Prof Dermatology, Univ Tex SW, Dallas

Wheeland, Ronald MD (Dermatology) - *Special Expertise:* Skin Laser Surgery; Mohs' Surgery;
Cosmetic Dematology; **Admitting Hospital:** University of New Mexico Hospital; **Office Address:**
1651 Galisteo St, Fl 8 Santa Fe, NM 87505; **Office Phone:** (505) 992-3400; **Board Certifications:**
Dermatology 1977, Dermatopathology 1978; **Medical School:** Univ Ariz Coll Med 1973;
Residency: Dermatology, Univ OK Hlth Sci Ctr, Oklahoma City, OK 1974-1977; **Fellowships:**
Dermatopathology, Univ OK Hlth Sci Ctr, Oklahoma City, OK 1977-1978; Dermatologic Surgery,
Cleveland Clin Fnd, Cleveland, OH 1983-1984; **Faculty Appointment:** Prof Dermatology, Univ Ariz
Coll Med

West Coast and Pacific

Berg, Daniel MD (Geriatric Psychiatry) - *Special Expertise:* Dermatological & Laser Surgery;
Skin Cancer; **Admitting Hospital:** University of Washington Medical Center; **Office Address:** Univ
Washington Med Ctr Box 356166 Seattle, WA 98195; **Office Phone:** (206) 598-2112; **Board
Certification:** Dermatology 1991; **Medical School:** Univ Toronto 1985; **Residencies:** Internal
Medicine, Sunnybrook Med Ctr, Toronto, CN 1987-1988; Dermatology, Duke Univ Med Ctr,
Durham, NC 1988-1991; **Fellowships:** Dermatology, Univ Toronto, Toronto, CN 1992;
Dermatology, Univ British Columbia 1993-1994; **Faculy Appointment:** Prof Dermatology, Univ
Wash

Conant, Marcus A MD (Dermatology) - *Special Expertise:* AIDS/HIV-Kaposi's Sarcoma;
Admitting Hospital: University of California - San Francisco Medical Center; **Office Address:** 350
Parnassus Ave, Ste 808 San Francisco, CA 94117; **Office Phone:** (415) 661-2613; **Board
Certification:** Dermatology 1969; **Medical School:** Duke Univ 1961; **Residency:** Dermatology,
UCSF, San Francisco, CA 1964-1967; **Faculty Appointment:** Clin Prof Dermatology, UCSF

Fitzpatrick, Richard MD (Dermatology) - *Special Expertise:* Hair Transplantation & Laser
Surgery; Photoaging; **Admitting Hospital:** University of California - San Diego Healthcare; **Office
Address:** 477 N El Camino Real, Ste B303 Encinitas, CA 92024; **Office Phone:** (760) 753-1027;
Board Certification: Dermatology 1978; **Medical School:** Emory Univ 1970; **Residency:**
Dermatology, UCLA, Los Angeles, CA 1975-1978

Frieden, Ilona J MD (Dermatology) - *Special Expertise:* *Dermatology - General;* **Admitting Hospital:** UCSF - Mount Zion Medical Center; **Office Address:** 1701 Divisadero St, Box 0316 Department of Dermatology San Francisco, CA 94143-0316; **Office Phone:** (415) 353-7800; **Board Certifications:** Dermatology 1983, Pediatrics 1983; **Medical School:** UCSF 1977; **Residencies:** Pediatrics, UCSF Med Ctr, San Francisco, CA 1978-1980; Dermatology, UCSF Med Ctr, San Fransisco, CA 1980-1983; **Faculty Appointment:** Clin Prof Dermatology

Glogau, Richard Gordon MD (Dermatology) - *Special Expertise:* *Mohs' Surgery; Cosmetic Dermatology;* **Admitting Hospital:** University of California - San Francisco Medical Center; **Office Address:** Richard G Glogau, M.D. & Assocs 350 Parnassus Ave, Ste 400 San Francisco, CA 94117-3685; **Office Phone:** (415) 564-1261; **Board Certifications:** Dermatology 1978, Dermatopathology 1982; **Medical School:** Harvard Med Sch 1973; **Residency:** Dermatology, UCSF Med Ctr, San Francisco, CA 1974-1977; **Fellowship:** Chemosurgery, UCSF Med Ctr, San Francisco, CA 1977-1978; **Faculty Appointment:** Clin Prof Dermatology, UCSF

Grimes, Pearl E MD (Dermatology) - *Special Expertise:* *Pigment Disorders;* **Admitting Hospital:** UCLA Medical Center; **Office Address:** Vitiligo & Pigmentation Ctr - Southern Cali 321 N Larchment Blvd, Ste 609 Los Angeles, CA 90004-6405; **Office Phone:** (323) 467-4389; **Board Certification:** Dermatology 1979; **Medical School:** Washington Univ, St Louis 1974; **Residency:** Dermatology, Howard Univ, Washington, DC 1976-1979; **Faculty Appointment:** Assoc Prof Dermatology, UCLA

Gurevitch, Arnold William MD (Dermatology) - *Special Expertise:* *Infectious Disease; Atopic Dermatitis;* **Admitting Hospital:** USC University Hospital - Richard K. Eamer Medical Plaza; **Office Address:** USC Ambulatory Health Center 1355 San Pablo St Los Angeles, CA 90033-1026; **Office Phone:** (323) 442-5100; **Board Certification:** Dermatology 1967; **Medical School:** UCLA 1962; **Residency:** Dermatology, Harbor-UCLA Med Ctr, Torrance, CA 1963-1966; **Faculty Appointment:** Prof Dermatology, Univ SC Sch Med

Kane, Bryna MD (Dermatology) - *Special Expertise:* *Cosmetic Dematology; Dermatology - Pediatric;* **Admitting Hospital:** Long Beach Memorial Medical Center; **Office Address:** 701 E 28th St, Ste 418 Long Beach, CA 90806; **Office Phone:** (562) 989-5512; **Board Certification:** Dermatology; **Medical School:** UC Davis 1980; **Residency:** Pediatrics, UCLA, Los Angeles, CA 1981-1983; **Fellowship:** Dermatology, LAC-Harbor UCLA, Los Angeles, CA 1983-1986

Kilmer, Suzanne L MD (Dermatology) - *Special Expertise:* *Skin Laser Surgery;* **Admitting Hospital:** University of California - Davis Medical Center; **Office Address:** Laser & Skin Surg Ctr N Cal 3835 J St Sacramento, CA 95816; **Office Phone:** (916) 456-0400; **Board Certification:** Dermatology 1999; **Medical School:** UC Davis 1987; **Residency:** Dermatology, UC Davis Med Ctr, Sacramento, CA 1988-1991; **Fellowship:** Laser Surgery, Mass Genl Hosp, Boston, MA 1991-1992; **Faculty Appointment:** Asst Clin Prof Dermatology, UC Davis

Lask, Gary P MD (Dermatology) - *Special Expertise:* *Skin Laser Surgery - Resurfacing; Cosmetic Dermatology;* **Admitting Hospital:** UCLA Medical Center; **Office Address:** 16260 Ventura Blvd, Ste 530 Encino, CA 91436-4603; **Office Phone:** (818) 788-4022; **Board Certification:** Dermatology 1983; **Medical School:** Mexico 1977; **Residency:** Dermatology, Martin Luther King Jr Hosp, Los Angeles, CA 1980-1983; **Faculty Appointment:** Clin Prof Dermatology, UCLA

Lowe, Nicholas J MD (Dermatology) - *Special Expertise:* Psoriasis; **Admitting Hospital:** UCLA Medical Center; **Office Address:** S Calif Derm/Psoriasis Ctr Inc 2001 Santa Monica Blvd, Ste 490w Santa Monica, CA 90404-2104; **Office Phone:** (310) 264-2434; **Board Certification:** Dermatology 1978; **Medical School:** England 1968; **Residencies:** Dermatology, Univ Southhampton, England, UK 1972-1974; Dermatology, Liverpool Univ, England, UK 1974-1977; **Fellowship:** Dermatology, Scripps Clin, La Jolla, CA 1975-1976; **Faculty Appointment:** Clin Prof Dermatology, UCLA

Tabak, Brian MD (Dermatology) - *Special Expertise:* Skin Cancer; **Admitting Hospital:** Long Beach Memorial Medical Center; **Office Address:** 2865 Atlantic Ave #152 Long Beach, CA 90806; **Office Phone:** (562) 595-7581; **Board Certification:** Dermatology 1981; **Medical School:** McGill Univ 1977; **Residency:** Dermatology, USC Med Ctr, Los Angeles, CA 1978-1981; **Faculty Appointment:** Asst Clin Prof Medicine, USC Sch Med

ENDOCRINOLOGY, DIABETES & METABOLISM

(a subspecialty of INTERNAL MEDICINE)

An internist who concentrates on disorders of the internal (endocrine) glands such as the thyroid and adrenal glands. This specialist also deals with disorders such as diabetes, metabolic and nutritional disorders, pituitary diseases, menstrual and sexual problems.

INTERNAL MEDICINE

An internist is a personal physician who provides long-term, comprehensive care in the office and the hospital, managing both common and complex illness of adolescents, adults and the elderly. Internists are trained in the diagnosis and treatment of cancer, infections and diseases affecting the heart, blood, kidneys, joints and digestive, respiratory and vascular systems. They are also trained in the essentials of primary care internal medicine which incorporates an understanding of disease prevention, wellness, substance abuse, mental health and effective treatment of common problems of the eyes, ears, skin, nervous system and reproductive organs.

Training required: Three years in internal medicine *plus* additional training and examination for certification in endocrinology, diabetes and metabolism

PHYSICIAN LISTINGS

Endocrinology, Diabetes & Metabolism

New England

Axelrod, Lloyd MD (Endocrinology, Diabetes & Metabolism) - *Special Expertise:* *Diabetes; Geriatric Endocrinology;* **Admitting Hospital:** Massachusetts General Hospital; **Office Address:** Diabetes Ctr 50 Staniford St, Fl 3 - Ste 340 Boston, MA; **Office Phone:** (617) 726-8722; **Board Certifications:** Internal Medicine 1973, Endocrinology, Diabetes & Metabolism 1973; **Medical School:** Harvard Med Sch 1967; **Residencies:** Internal Medicine, Peter Bent Brigham Hosp, Boston, MA 1968-1969; Internal Medicine, Mass Genl Hosp, Boston, MA 1970-1971; **Fellowships:** Endocrinology, Diabetes & Metabolism, Peter Bent Brigham Hosp, Boston, MA 1969-1970; Endocrinology, Diabetes & Metabolism, Mass Genl Hosp, Boston, MA 1971-1972; **Faculty Appointment:** Assoc Prof Medicine, Harvard Med Sch

Biller, Beverly M K MD (Endocrinology, Diabetes & Metabolism) - *Special Expertise:* *Pituitary Disorders; Cushing's Syndrome; Acromegaly;* **Admitting Hospital:** Massachusetts General Hospital; **Office Address:** Mass Genl Hosp WAC 730S Boston, MA 02114; **Office Phone:** (617) 726-3870; **Board Certifications:** Internal Medicine 1986, Endocrinology, Diabetes & Metabolism 1989; **Medical School:** Univ Okla Coll Med 1983; **Residency:** Internal Medicine, Beth Israel Deaconness Hosp, Boston, MA 1983-1986; **Fellowship:** Endocrinology, Diabetes & Metabolism, Mass Genl Hosp, Boston, MA 1989

Daniels, Gilbert MD (Endocrinology, Diabetes & Metabolism) - *Special Expertise:* Thyroid *Disorders;* **Admitting Hospital:** Massachusetts General Hospital; **Office Address:** 15 Parkman St, Bldg WACC - Ste 730 Boston, MA 02114; **Office Phone:** (617) 726-8430; **Board Certifications:** Internal Medicine 1972, Endocrinology, Diabetes & Metabolism 1975; **Medical School:** Harvard Med Sch 1966; **Residency:** Internal Medicine, Mass Genl Hosp, Boston, MA 1972; **Fellowships:** Biochemistry, NIH, Bethesda, MD 1970; Endocrinology, Diabetes & Metabolism, UCSF Med Ctr, San Francisco 1971; **Faculty Appointment:** Assoc Prof Medicine, Harvard Med Sch

Godine, John Elliott MD/PhD (Endocrinology, Diabetes & Metabolism) - *Special Expertise:* *Diabetes;* **Admitting Hospital:** Massachusetts General Hospital; **Office Address:** Mass General Hospital, Diabetes Center 50 Staniford St, Ste 340 Boston, MA 02114; **Office Phone:** (617) 726-8722; **Board Certifications:** Internal Medicine 1979, Endocrinology, Diabetes & Metabolism 1981; **Medical School:** Harvard Med Sch 1976; **Residency:** Internal Medicine, Mass Genl Hosp, Boston, MA 1977-1978; **Fellowship:** Endocrinology, Diabetes & Metabolism, Mass Genl Hosp, Boston, MA 1978-1981; **Faculty Appointment:** Asst Prof Medicine, Harvard Med Sch

Hare, John W MD (Endocrinology, Diabetes & Metabolism) - *Special Expertise:* Diabetes; **Admitting Hospital:** Beth Israel Deaconess Medical Center - Boston (Page 57); **Office Address:** Joslin Diabetes Ctr One Joslin Pl Boston, MA 02215; **Office Phone:** (617) 732-2645; **Board Certifications:** Internal Medicine 1972, Endocrinology, Diabetes & Metabolism 1975; **Medical School:** Indiana Univ 1965; **Residencies:** Internal Medicine, VA Rsch Hosp, Chicago, IL 1969-1970; Internal Medicine, New England Deaconess Hosp, Boston, MA 1966-1967; **Fellowship:** Endocrinology, Diabetes & Metabolism, Northwestern Univ, Chicago, IL 1970-1973; **Faculty Appointment:** Assoc Clin Prof Medicine, Harvard Med Sch

Klibanski, Anne MD (Endocrinology, Diabetes & Metabolism) - *Special Expertise:* Pituitary *Disorders; Prolactin Disorders;* **Admitting Hospital:** Massachusetts General Hospital; **Office Address:** Mass Genl Hosp, Neuro-endocrine Ctr 15 Parkman St, WAC 730S Boston, MA 02114; **Office Phone:** (617) 726-3870; **Board Certifications:** Internal Medicine 1978, Endocrinology, Diabetes & Metabolism 1981; **Medical School:** NYU Sch Med 1975; **Residency:** Internal Medicine, Bellevue Hosp Ctr, New York, NY 1976-1978; **Fellowship:** Endocrinology, Mass Genl Hosp-Harvard, Boston, MA 1978-1981; **Faculty Appointment:** Assoc Prof Endocrinology, Diabetes & Metabolism, Harvard Med Sch

Lechan, Ronald MD/PhD (Endocrinology, Diabetes & Metabolism) - *Special Expertise:* *Pituitary Disorders; Hypoithalamic Dysfunction;* **Admitting Hospital:** New England Medical Center; **Office Address:** New England Med Ctr 750 Washington St, Box 268 Boston, MA 02111-1854; **Office Phone:** (617) 636-5689; **Board Certifications:** Internal Medicine 1979, Endocrinology, Diabetes & Metabolism 1981; **Medical School:** Univ VA Sch Med 1976; **Residency:** Internal Medicine, Beth Israel Hosp, Boston, MA 1977-1978; **Fellowship:** Endocrinology, Diabetes & Metabolism, Tufts-New England Med Ctr., Boston, MA 1978-1981; **Faculty Appointment:** Prof Medicine, Tufts Univ

Moses, Alan Charles MD (Endocrinology, Diabetes & Metabolism) - *Special Expertise:* *Diabetes; Metabolic Disorders;* **Admitting Hospital:** Beth Israel Deaconess Medical Center - Boston (Page 57); **Office Address:** Joslin Diabetes Center One Joslin Pl Boston, MA 02215; **Office Phone:** (617) 732-2501; **Board Certifications:** Internal Medicine 1976, Endocrinology, Diabetes & Metabolism 1981; **Medical School:** Washington Univ, St Louis 1973; **Residency:** Internal Medicine, Barnes Hosp, St Louis, MO 1974-1975; **Fellowships:** Endocrinology, Diabetes & Metabolism, National Cancer Inst 1975-1978; Endocrinology, Diabetes & Metabolism, Tufts-NEMC, Boston, MA 1978-1979; **Faculty Appointment:** Assoc Prof Medicine, Harvard Med Sch

Seely, Ellen Wells MD (Endocrinology, Diabetes & Metabolism) - *Special Expertise:* *Endocrinology, Diabetes & Metabolism - General;* **Admitting Hospital:** Brigham & Women's Hospital; **Office Address:** Brigham and Womens Hosp 221 Longwood Ave Boston, MA 02115-5804; **Office Phone:** (617) 732-5661; **Board Certifications:** Internal Medicine 1984, Endocrinology, Diabetes & Metabolism 1987; **Medical School:** Columbia P&S 1981; **Residency:** Internal Medicine, Brigham & Womens Hosp, Boston, MA 1982-1984; **Fellowship:** Endocrinology, Diabetes & Metabolism, Brigham & Womens Hosp, Boston, MA 1984-1987; **Faculty Appointment:** Assoc Prof Medicine, Harvard Med Sch

Sherwin, Robert MD (Endocrinology, Diabetes & Metabolism) - *Special Expertise:* *Diabetes;* **Admitting Hospital:** Yale - New Haven Hospital; **Office Address:** Yale University Box 208020 New Haven, CT 06520-8020; **Office Phone:** (203) 785-4183; **Board Certification:** Internal Medicine 1972; **Medical School:** Albert Einstein Coll Med 1967; **Residencies:** Internal Medicine, Mt Sinai Hosp, New York, NY 1968-1969; Internal Medicine, Mt Sinai Hosp, New York, NY 1971-1972; **Fellowship:** Metabolism, Yale-New Haven Hosp, New Haven, CT 1972-1973; **Faculty Appointment:** Prof Medicine, Yale Univ

Williams, Gordon H MD (Endocrinology, Diabetes & Metabolism) - *Special Expertise:* *Hypertension; Pituitary Disorders;* **Admitting Hospital:** Brigham & Women's Hospital; **Office Address:** Brigham&Womens Hosp, Div Endo Hypertension 221 Longwood Ave Boston, MA 02115-5817; **Office Phone:** (617) 732-5666; **Board Certifications:** Internal Medicine 1970, Endocrinology, Diabetes & Metabolism 1975; **Medical School:** Harvard Med Sch 1963; **Residency:** Internal Medicine, Peter Bent Brigham Hosp, Boston, MA 1966-1967; **Fellowship:** Endocrinology, Diabetes & Metabolism, Peter Bent Brigham Hosp, Boston, MA 1967-1970; **Faculty Appointment:** Prof Medicine, Harvard Med Sch

Mid Atlantic

Blum, Manfred MD (Endocrinology, Diabetes & Metabolism) - *Special Expertise:* Thyroid Disorders; Parathyroid Disease; **Admitting Hospital:** NYU Medical Center (Page 70); **Office Address:** 530 1st Ave, Ste 4E New York, NY 10016; **Office Phone:** (212) 263-7444; **Board Certifications:** Internal Medicine 1964, Endocrinology, Diabetes & Metabolism 1975; **Medical School:** NYU Sch Med 1957; **Residencies:** Internal Medicine, Montefiore Hosp, New York, NY 1958-1959; Internal Medicine, Bellevue Hosp, New York, NY 1959-1960; **Fellowship:** Endocrinology, Diabetes & Metabolism, Harvard-Beth Israel Hosp, Boston, MA 1960-1961; **Faculty Appointment:** Clin Prof NYU Sch Med

Bockman, Richard MD/PhD (Endocrinology, Diabetes & Metabolism) - *Special*
Expertise: Bone Disorders-Metabolic; Osteoporosis; **Admitting Hospital:** Hospital for Special Surgery (Page 63); **Office Address:** Hospital for Special Surgery 535 E 70th St New York, NY 10021; **Office Phone:** (212) 606-1458; **Board Certification:** Internal Medicine 1975; **Medical School:** Yale Univ 1968; **Residency:** Internal Medicine, NYU, New York, NY 1973-1975; **Fellowship:** Internal Medicine, Weill Med Coll-Cornell, New York, NY 1971-1973; **Faculty Appointment:** Prof Medicine, Cornell Univ-Weil Med Coll

Cooper, David Stephen MD (Endocrinology, Diabetes & Metabolism) - *Special*
Expertise: Thyroid Disorders; **Admitting Hospital:** Sinai Hospital - Baltimore; **Office Address:** Sinai Hospital, Div Endo 2401 W Belvedere Ave Baltimore, MD 21215-5216; **Office Phone:** (410) 601-5961; **Board Certifications:** Internal Medicine 1987, Endocrinology, Diabetes & Metabolism 1979; **Medical School:** Tufts Univ 1973; **Residency:** Internal Medicine, Barnes Hosp, St Louis, MO 1974-1976; **Fellowship:** Endocrinology, Diabetes & Metabolism, Mass Genl Hosp, Boston, MA 1976-1978; **Faculty Appointment:** Prof Medicine, Johns Hopkins Univ

Davies, Terry MD (Endocrinology, Diabetes & Metabolism) - *Special Expertise:* Thyroid Disorders; **Admitting Hospital:** Mount Sinai Hospital (Page 70); **Office Address:** 1 Gustave Levy Pl, Box 1055 New York, NY 10029-6504; **Office Phone:** (212) 241-6627; **Medical School:** England 1971; **Residency:** Internal Medicine, Univ of Newcastle Upon Tyne, UK 1971-1975; **Fellowships:** Endocrinology, Diabetes & Metabolism, Univ of Newcastle Upon Tyne, UK 1975-1977; Endocrinology, Diabetes & Metabolism, Natl Inst Hlth, Bethesda, MD 1977-1979; **Faculty Appointment:** Prof Medicine, Mount Sinai Sch Med

Dobs, Adrian Sandra MD (Endocrinology, Diabetes & Metabolism) - *Special Expertise:* Hormonal Disorders; **Admitting Hospital:** Johns Hopkins Hospital - Baltimore (Page 65); **Office Address:** Johns Hopkins Hosp 1830 E Monument St, Fl 3 - Ste 328 Baltimore, MD 21287-4904; **Office Phone:** (410) 955-2130; **Board Certifications:** Internal Medicine 1981, Endocrinology, Diabetes & Metabolism 1987; **Medical School:** Albany Med Coll 1978; **Residency:** Internal Medicine, Montefiore Hosp, Bronx, NY 1979-1982; **Fellowship:** Endocrinology, Diabetes & Metabolism, John Hopkins, Baltimore, MD 1982-1984; **Faculty Appointment:** Assoc Prof Medicine, Johns Hopkins Univ

Drexler, Andrew Jay MD (Endocrinology, Diabetes & Metabolism) - *Special Expertise:* Endocrinology, Diabetes & Metabolism - General; **Admitting Hospital:** Mount Sinai Hospital (Page 70); **Office Address:** 1200 5th Ave New York, NY 10029-6574; **Office Phone:** (212) 241-2000; **Board Certifications:** Internal Medicine 1977, Endocrinology, Diabetes & Metabolism 1981; **Medical School:** NYU Sch Med 1972; **Residency:** Internal Medicine, Barnes Hosp, St Louis, MO 1975-1976; **Fellowship:** Endocrinology, Diabetes & Metabolism, Wash Univ Med Ctr, St Louis, MO 1976-1978; **Faculty Appointment:** Assoc Clin Prof Medicine, Mount Sinai Sch Med

Felig, Philip MD (Endocrinology, Diabetes & Metabolism) - *Special Expertise:* Endocrinology, Diabetes & Metabolism - General; **Admitting Hospital:** Lenox Hill Hospital; **Office Address:** 1056 5th Ave New York, NY 10028-0112; **Office Phone:** (212) 534-5900; **Board Certification:** Internal Medicine 1968; **Medical School:** Yale Univ 1961; **Residency:** Internal Medicine, Yale-New Haven Hosp, New Haven, CT 1961-1967; **Fellowship:** Endocrinology, Diabetes & Metabolism, Peter Bent Brigham Hosp-Harvard, Boston, MA 1967-1969

Fleischer, Norman MD (Endocrinology, Diabetes & Metabolism) - *Special Expertise:* *Thyroid Disorders; Adrenal Disorders;* **Admitting Hospital:** Montefiore Medical Center - Weiler/Einstein Division; **Office Address:** Endocrinology 1575 Blondell Ave, Ste 200 Bronx, NY 10461-2601; **Office Phone:** (718) 405-8260; **Board Certifications:** Internal Medicine 1968, Endocrinology, Diabetes & Metabolism 1973; **Medical School:** Vanderbilt Univ 1961; **Residency:** Internal Medicine, Bronx Muni Hosp Ctr, Bronx, NY 1961-1964; **Fellowship:** Endocrinology, Diabetes & Metabolism, Vanderbilt Univ, Nashville, TN 1964-1966; **Faculty Appointment:** Prof Medicine, Albert Einstein Coll Med

Greene, Loren Wissner MD (Endocrinology, Diabetes & Metabolism) - *Special Expertise:* *Diabetes;* **Admitting Hospital:** NYU Medical Center (Page 70); **Office Address:** 530 1st Ave, Ste 4B New York, NY 10016; **Office Phone:** (212) 263-7449; **Board Certifications:** Internal Medicine 1978, Endocrinology, Diabetes & Metabolism 1981; **Medical School:** NYU Sch Med 1975; **Residency:** Internal Medicine, Bellevue Hosp Ctr-NYU, New York, NY 1976-1978; **Fellowship:** Endocrinology, Diabetes & Metabolism, Bellevue Hosp Ctr-NYU, New York, NY 1978-1980; **Faculty Appointment:** Assoc Clin Prof Medicine, NYU Sch Med

Hurley, James MD (Endocrinology, Diabetes & Metabolism) - *Special Expertise:* *Thyroid Disorders; Graves' Disease;* **Admitting Hospital:** New York Weill Cornell Medical Center - NY Presbyterian Hospital (Page 72); **Office Address:** 525 E 68th St, Box 136 New York, NY 10021-4873; **Office Phone:** (212) 746-6290; **Board Certifications:** Internal Medicine 1968, Nuclear Medicine 1972; **Medical School:** Cornell Univ-Weil Med Coll 1961; **Residency:** Internal Medicine, NY Hosp, New York, NY 1961-1964; **Fellowship:** Endocrinology, Diabetes & Metabolism, NY Hosp, New York, NY 1964-1965; **Faculty Appointment:** Assoc Prof Medicine, Cornell Univ-Weil Med Coll

Jacobs, Thomas MD (Endocrinology, Diabetes & Metabolism) - *Special Expertise:* *Adrenal Disorders; Pituitary Disorders; Bone-Calcium Problems;* **Admitting Hospital:** Columbia Presbyterian Medical Center (Page 72); **Office Address:** 161 Fort Washington Ave, rm 210 New York, NY 10032-3713; **Office Phone:** (212) 305-5578; **Board Certifications:** Internal Medicine 1973, Endocrinology, Diabetes & Metabolism 1975; **Medical School:** Johns Hopkins Univ 1968; **Residency:** Internal Medicine, Columbia Presby, New York, NY 1968-1973; **Fellowship:** Endocrinology, Diabetes & Metabolism, Univ WA Med Ctr, Seattle, WA 1973-1975; **Faculty Appointment:** Clin Prof Medicine, Columbia P&S

Korytkowski, Mary T MD (Endocrinology, Diabetes & Metabolism) - *Special Expertise:* *Diabetes; Polycystic Ovary Disease;* **Admitting Hospital:** UPMC - Presbyterian University Hospital; **Office Address:** Univ Pitts Phys, Div EDM 3601 Fifth Ave, Bldg Falk - rm 2B Pittsburgh, PA 15213; **Office Phone:** (412) 383-8700; **Board Certifications:** Endocrinology, Diabetes & Metabolism 1989, Internal Medicine 1985; **Medical School:** Univ NC Sch Med 1982; **Residency:** Internal Medicine, Francis Scott Key Med Ctr, Baltimore, MD 1982-1985; **Fellowships:** Endocrinology, Diabetes & Metabolism, Sinai Hosp, Baltimore, MD 1983-1985; Endocrinology, Johns Hopkins Hosp, Baltimore, MD 1986-1988; **Faculty Appointment:** Assoc Prof Medicine, Univ Pittsburgh

Ladenson, Paul William MD (Endocrinology, Diabetes & Metabolism) - *Special Expertise:* *Thyroid Disorders;* **Admitting Hospital:** Johns Hopkins Hospital - Baltimore (Page 65); **Office Address:** Johns Hopkins, Dept Endocrin & Metab 1830 E Monument St, rm 333 Baltimore, MD 21287-0003; **Office Phone:** (410) 955-3663; **Board Certifications:** Internal Medicine 1978, Endocrinology, Diabetes & Metabolism 1981; **Medical School:** Harvard Med Sch 1975; **Residency:** Internal Medicine, Mass Genl Hosp, Boston, MA 1975-1978; **Fellowship:** Endocrinology, Diabetes & Metabolism, Mass Genl Hosp, Boston, MA 1978-1980; **Faculty Appointment:** Prof Medicine, Johns Hopkins Univ

Mahler, Richard J MD (Endocrinology, Diabetes & Metabolism) - *Special Expertise:* *Thyroid Disorders;* **Admitting Hospital:** New York Weill Cornell Medical Center - NY Presbyterian Hospital (Page 72); **Office Address:** 220 E 69th St New York, NY 10021; **Office Phone:** (212) 879-4073; **Board Certification:** Internal Medicine 1987; **Medical School:** NY Med Coll 1959; **Residencies:** Internal Medicine, NY Med-Metro Med, New York, NY 1960-1962; Endocrinology, Diabetes & Metabolism, NY Med Coll, New York, NY 1962-1963; **Fellowship:** Endocrinology, Diabetes & Metabolism, Univ Durham, Durham, NC 1963-1964; **Faculty Appointment:** Assoc Clin Prof Medicine, Cornell Univ-Weil Med Coll

Mandel, Susan MD (Endocrinology, Diabetes & Metabolism) - *Special Expertise:* *Thyroid Disorders; Calcium Disorders;* **Admitting Hospital:** Hospital of the University of Pennsylvania; **Office Address:** Hospital of Univ of Pa-Dept Endocrinology 3400 Spruce St Philadelphia, PA 19104; **Office Phone:** (215) 662-2300; **Board Certifications:** Internal Medicine 1989, Endocrinology 1991; **Medical School:** Columbia P&S 1986; **Residency:** Internal Medicine, Columbia Presby Hosp, New York, NY 1987-1989; **Fellowship:** Endocrinology, Barigham & Womens Hosp, Boston, MA 1989-1992; **Faculty Appointment:** Asst Prof Medicine, Univ Penn

McConnell, Robert John MD (Endocrinology, Diabetes & Metabolism) - *Special Expertise:* *Thyroid Disorders;* **Admitting Hospital:** Columbia Presbyterian Medical Center (Page 72); **Office Address:** 161 Fort Washington Ave New York, NY 10032-3713; **Office Phone:** (212) 305-5579; **Board Certifications:** Endocrinology, Diabetes & Metabolism 1981, Internal Medicine 1978; **Medical School:** Columbia P&S 1973; **Residency:** Wash-Barnes Hosp., St. Louis, MO 1974-1975; **Fellowship:** Endocrinology, Diabetes & Metabolism, Colum-Presby Hosp., New York, NY 1975-1978; **Faculty Appointment:** Assoc Prof Medicine, Columbia P&S

Mersey, James Harris MD (Endocrinology, Diabetes & Metabolism) - *Special Expertise:* *Diabetes;* **Admitting Hospital:** Greater Baltimore Medical Center; **Office Address:** 6565 N Charles St, Ste 411 Baltimore, MD 21204-5803; **Office Phone:** (410) 828-7417; **Board Certifications:** Internal Medicine 1975, Endocrinology, Diabetes & Metabolism 1977; **Medical School:** Johns Hopkins Univ 1972; **Residencies:** Internal Medicine, Johns Hopkins Hosp, Baltimore, MD 1973-1974; Internal Medicine, Johns Hopkins Hosp, Baltimore, MD 1976-1977; **Fellowship:** Endocrinology, Diabetes & Metabolism, Peter Bent Brigham Hosp., Boston, MA 1974-1976; **Faculty Appointment:** Asst Prof Medicine, Johns Hopkins Univ

Ratner, Robert MD (Endocrinology, Diabetes & Metabolism) - *Special Expertise:* *Diabetes in Pregnancy; Thyroid/Lipid Disorders; Diabetes;* **Admitting Hospital:** Washington Hospital Center - DC (Page 79); **Office Address:** Medlantic Clin Rsch Ctr 650 Pennsylvania SE Ave, Fl 50 Washington, DC 20003; **Office Phone:** (202) 675-1042; **Board Certifications:** Internal Medicine 1980, Endocrinology, Diabetes & Metabolism 1983; **Medical School:** Baylor Coll Med 1977; **Residency:** Internal Medicine, Baylor Affil Hosps, Houston, TX 1978-1980; **Fellowship:** Endocrinology, Diabetes & Metabolism, Lahey Clin/Joslin Clin, Boston, MA 1980-1982; **Faculty Appointment:** Assoc Prof Endocrinology, Diabetes & Metabolism, Geo Wash Univ

Resnick, Lawrence MD (Endocrinology, Diabetes & Metabolism) - *Special Expertise:* *Endocrinology, Diabetes & Metabolism - General;* **Admitting Hospital:** New York Weill Cornell Medical Center - NY Presbyterian Hospital (Page 72); **Office Address:** NY Presbyterian Hypertension Ctr 520 E 70th St, Fl 4 New York, NY 10021; **Office Phone:** (212) 746-2210; **Board Certifications:** Internal Medicine 1973, Endocrinology, Diabetes & Metabolism 1975; **Medical School:** Northwestern Univ 1970; **Residency:** Internal Medicine, Univ Chicago Hosps, Chicago, IL 1971-1973; **Fellowships:** Endocrinology, Diabetes & Metabolism, Columbia-Presby Hosp, New York, NY 1973-1974; Cardiology (Cardiovascular Disease), Peter Bent Brigham Hosp, Boston, MA 1979-1980; **Faculty Appointment:** Prof Medicine, Cornell Univ-Weil Med Coll

Saudek, Christopher D MD (Endocrinology, Diabetes & Metabolism) - *Special Expertise:* Diabetes; **Admitting Hospital:** Johns Hopkins Hospital - Baltimore (Page 65); **Office Address:** 600 N Wolfe St, Olser Bldg, Ste 576 Baltimore, MD 2120872104; **Office Phone:** (410) 955-2132; **Board Certification:** Internal Medicine 1972; **Medical School:** Cornell Univ-Weil Med Coll 1967; **Residencies:** Internal Medicine, Rush-Presby-St Lukes Hosp, Chicago, IL 1968-1969; Internal Medicine, Boston City Hosp-Harvard, Boston, MA 1969-1970; **Fellowship:** Endocrinology, Diabetes & Metabolism, Thorndale Lab-Harvard Med Sch, MA 1970-1972; **Faculty Appointment:** Prof Medicine

Schwartz, Stanley MD (Endocrinology, Diabetes & Metabolism) - *Special Expertise:* Diabetes; **Admitting Hospital:** Hospital of the University of Pennsylvania; **Office Address:** Univ Penn Med Ctr, EDM Division, Suite 8 3400 Spruce St, 3 Ravdin Bldg Philadelphia, PA 19104; **Office Phone:** (215) 662-2517; **Board Certifications:** Internal Medicine 1976, Endocrinology, Diabetes & Metabolism 1979; **Medical School:** Univ Chicago-Pritzker Sch Med 1973; **Residency:** Internal Medicine, Univ Penn Hosp, Philadelphia, PA 1974-1976; **Fellowship:** Endocrinology, Diabetes & Metabolism, Univ Chicago, Chicago, IL 1976-1978

Shuldiner, Alan Rodney MD (Endocrinology, Diabetes & Metabolism) - *Special Expertise:* Diabetes; Eating Disorders - Obesity; **Admitting Hospital:** University of Maryland Medical System; **Office Address:** Univ Maryland Sch Med 725 W Lombard St, rm S-422 Baltimore, MD 21201; **Office Phone:** (410) 706-1623; **Board Certifications:** Internal Medicine 1988, Endocrinology, Diabetes & Metabolism 1989; **Medical School:** Harvard Med Sch 1984; **Residency:** Internal Medicine, Columbia-Presbyterian Hosp, New York, NY 1984-1986; **Fellowship:** Endocrinology, Diabetes & Metabolism, NIH, Bethesda, MD 1986-1990; **Faculty Appointment:** Prof Medicine, Univ MD Sch Med

Snyder, Peter Joseph MD (Endocrinology, Diabetes & Metabolism) - *Special Expertise:* Pituitary Adenomas; Reproductive Endocrinology - Male; **Admitting Hospital:** Hospital of the University of Pennsylvania; **Office Address:** Univ Penn Med Grp 3400 Spruce St Philadelphia, PA 19104; **Office Phone:** (215) 898-0208; **Board Certifications:** Internal Medicine 1972, Endocrinology, Diabetes & Metabolism 1972; **Medical School:** Harvard Med Sch 1965; **Residencies:** Internal Medicine, Beth Israel Hosp, Boston, MA 1966-1967; Internal Medicine, Beth Israel Hosp, Boston, MA 1969-1970; **Fellowship:** Endocrinology, Diabetes & Metabolism, Penn Hosp, Philadelphia, PA 1970-1971; **Faculty Appointment:** Prof Medicine, Univ Penn

Surks, Martin MD (Endocrinology, Diabetes & Metabolism) - *Special Expertise:* Thyroid Disorders; **Admitting Hospital:** Montefiore Medical Center; **Office Address:** Montefiore Med Ctr 111 E 210th St Bronx, NY 10467-2490; **Office Phone:** (718) 920-4331; **Board Certifications:** Internal Medicine 1967, Endocrinology, Diabetes & Metabolism 1977; **Medical School:** NYU Sch Med 1960; **Residencies:** Internal Medicine, Montefiore Hosp Med Ctr, Bronx, NY 1961-1962; Internal Medicine, VA Hosp, Bronx, NY 1963-1964; **Fellowship:** Research, NIMAS, Bethesda, MD 1963-1964; **Faculty Appointment:** Prof Medicine, Albert Einstein Coll Med

Wartofsky, Leonard MD (Endocrinology, Diabetes & Metabolism) - *Special Expertise:* Thyroid Cancer; **Admitting Hospital:** Washington Hospital Center - DC (Page 79); **Office Address:** Washington Hosp Ctr, Dept Med 110 Irving St NW Washington, DC 20010-2975; **Office Phone:** (202) 877-3109; **Board Certifications:** Internal Medicine 1971, Endocrinology, Diabetes & Metabolism 1972; **Medical School:** Geo Wash Univ 1964; **Residencies:** Internal Medicine, Barnes Hosp, New York, NY 1965-1966; Internal Medicine, Bronx Muni Hosp Ctr, New York, NY 1966-1967; **Fellowship:** Endocrinology, Diabetes & Metabolism, Boston City Hosp, Boston, MA 1967-1969; **Faculty Appointment:** Prof Medicine, Uniformed Srvs Univ, Bethesda

Young, Iven MD (Endocrinology, Diabetes & Metabolism) - *Special Expertise:* Thyroid Disorders; **Admitting Hospital:** St Vincents Catholic Medical Center of New York; **Office Address:** 130 W 12th St, Ste 7D New York, NY 10011-8270; **Office Phone:** (212) 675-9332; **Board Certifications:** Internal Medicine 1966, Endocrinology, Diabetes & Metabolism 1973; **Medical School:** NYU Sch Med 1959; **Residency:** Internal Medicine, VA Med Ctr/NYU/Bellevue, New York, NY 1960-1963; **Fellowship:** Endocrinology, Diabetes & Metabolism, NYU Med Ctr, New York, NY 1963-1966; **Faculty Appointment:** Asst Clin Prof Medicine, NY Med Coll

Southeast

Barrett, Eugene Joseph MD (Endocrinology, Diabetes & Metabolism) - *Special Expertise:* Diabetes; Cholesterol/Lipid Disorders; **Admitting Hospital:** University of Virginia Health Systems; **Office Address:** Univ VA Hlth Sys, Endocrine Clinic@ Bldg Private Clinic - Fl 5, Box 379 Charlottesville, VA 22908; **Office Phone:** (804) 924-1175; **Board Certifications:** Internal Medicine 1978, Endocrinology, Diabetes & Metabolism 1995; **Medical School:** Univ Rochester 1975; **Residency:** Internal Medicine, Strong Meml Hosp, Rochester, NY 1975-1977; **Fellowship:** Endocrinology, Diabetes & Metabolism, Yale Univ Hosp, New Haven, CT 1977; **Faculty Appointment:** Prof Medicine, Univ VA Sch Med

Bell, David S H MD (Endocrinology, Diabetes & Metabolism) - *Special Expertise:* Diabetes - Insulin-dependent; Diabetes - Insulin Pump Therapy; **Admitting Hospital:** University of Alabama Hospital at Birmingham; **Office Address:** Univ Alabama-Boshell Diabetes Rsch Bldg 1808 7th Avenue South Birmingham, AL 35294; **Office Phone:** (205) 975-2404; **Board Certifications:** Internal Medicine 1987, Endocrinology, Diabetes & Metabolism 1981; **Medical School:** Ireland 1970; **Residencies:** Internal Medicine, Royal Victoria Hosp, Ireland 1972-1973; Endocrinology, Diabetes & Metabolism, Univ Saskatchewan Hosp, Saskatchewan, Canada 1973-1975; **Fellowship:** Endocrinology, Diabetes & Metabolism, Greater Baltimore Med Ctr, Baltimore, MD 1975-1976; **Faculty Appointment:** Prof Medicine, Univ Ala

Dalkin, Alan Craig MD (Endocrinology, Diabetes & Metabolism) - *Special Expertise:* Bone Disorders-Metabolic; Osteoporosis; **Admitting Hospital:** University of Virginia Health Systems; **Office Address:** Univ Virginia Hlth Scis Ctr 5041 MR4 Bldg Charlottesville, VA 22908; **Office Phone:** (804) 924-5629; **Board Certifications:** Internal Medicine 1987, Endocrinology, Diabetes & Metabolism 1989; **Medical School:** Univ Mich Med Sch 1984; **Residency:** Internal Medicine, Univ Chicago, Chicago, IL 1985-1987; **Fellowship:** Endocrinology, Diabetes & Metabolism, Univ Michigan Med Ctr, Ann Harbor, MI 1987-1990; **Faculty Appointment:** Assoc Prof Endocrinology, Diabetes & Metabolism, Univ VA Sch Med

Earp III, Henry Shelton MD (Endocrinology, Diabetes & Metabolism) - *Special Expertise:* Cancer - Hormonal Influences; **Admitting Hospital:** University of North Carolina Hospitals; **Office Address:** University NC Highgate Specialty Clinic 5316 Highgate Dr, Ste 125 Durham, NC 27713; **Office Phone:** (919) 484-1015; **Board Certifications:** Internal Medicine 1976, Endocrinology, Diabetes & Metabolism 1977; **Medical School:** Univ NC Sch Med 1970; **Residency:** Internal Medicine, NC Meml Hosp, Chapel Hill, NC 1974-1975; **Fellowship:** Endocrinology, Diabetes & Metabolism, Univ North Carolina, Chapel Hill, NC 1975-1977; **Faculty Appointment:** Prof Medicine, Univ NC Sch Med

Ellis III, George John MD (Endocrinology, Diabetes & Metabolism) - *Special Expertise:* Endocrinology, Diabetes & Metabolism - General; **Admitting Hospital:** Duke University Medical Center (Page 60); **Office Address:** Duke Univ Med Ctr, Div Endo 278 Baker House, Box 2924 Durham, NC 27710; **Office Phone:** (919) 684-5568; **Board Certification:** Internal Medicine 1969; **Medical School:** Harvard Med Sch 1963; **Residency:** Internal Medicine, Duke Med Ctr, Durham, NC 1965-1968; **Fellowship:** Endocrinology, Diabetes & Metabolism, Duke Med Ctr, Durham, NC 1964-1967; **Faculty Appointment:** Assoc Prof Medicine, Duke Univ

Feinglos, Mark MD (Endocrinology, Diabetes & Metabolism) - *Special Expertise:* *Diabetes;* **Admitting Hospital:** Duke University Medical Center (Page 60); **Office Address:** Duke Univ Med Ctr Box 3921 Durham, NC 27710; **Office Phone:** (919) 684-3208; **Board Certifications:** Internal Medicine 1976, Endocrinology, Diabetes & Metabolism 1977; **Medical School:** McGill Univ 1973; **Residency:** Internal Medicine, Duke Univ, Durham, NC 1973-1975; **Fellowship:** Endocrinology, Diabetes & Metabolism, Duke Univ, Durham, NC 1975-1978; **Faculty Appointment:** Prof Medicine, Duke Univ

Graber, Alan MD (Endocrinology, Diabetes & Metabolism) - *Special Expertise:* *Diabetes;* *Thyroid Disorders;* **Admitting Hospital:** Vanderbilt University Medical Center; **Office Address:** Vanderbilt Univ Med Ctr 2501A The Vanderbilt Clinic Nashville, TN 37232-5356; **Office Phone:** (615) 322-4752; **Board Certifications:** Endocrinology, Diabetes & Metabolism 1972, Internal Medicine 1968; **Medical School:** Washington Univ, St Louis 1961; **Residencies:** Internal Medicine, Vanderbilt Univ Hosp, Nashville, TN 1962-1963; Internal Medicine, Univ Washington Hosp, Seattle, WA 1965-1966; **Fellowships:** Endocrinology, Diabetes & Metabolism, Vanderbilt Univ Hosp, Nashville, TN 1963-1964; Endocrinology, Diabetes & Metabolism, Univ Washington Hosp, Seattle, WA 1964-1965; **Faculty Appointment:** Prof Medicine, Vanderbilt Univ

Kreisberg, Robert Alan MD (Endocrinology, Diabetes & Metabolism) - *Special Expertise:* *Diabetes;* **Admitting Hospital:** University of Alabama Hospital at Birmingham; **Office Address:** Univ Southern Alabama 307 University Blvd, Bldg CSAB 170 Mobile, AL 36688; **Office Phone:** (334) 460-7187; **Board Certification:** Internal Medicine 1987; **Medical School:** Northwestern Univ 1958; **Residency:** Internal Medicine, Northwestern Univ, Chicago, IL 1959-1962; **Fellowship:** Endocrinology, Diabetes & Metabolism, Peter Bent Brigham Hosp, Boston, MA 1962-1964; **Faculty Appointment:** Prof Medicine, Univ Ala

Marshall, John Crook MD/PhD (Endocrinology, Diabetes & Metabolism) - *Special Expertise:* *Neuro-Endocrinology; Hypothalamic Dysfunction; Reproductive Endocrinology;* **Admitting Hospital:** University of Virginia Health Systems; **Office Address:** Univ VA Hlth Scis Ctr Hospital Dr, Box 800612 Charlottesville, VA 22908; **Office Phone:** (804) 924-2431; **Board Certifications:** Internal Medicine 1978, Endocrinology, Diabetes & Metabolism 1981; **Medical School:** England 1973; **Residencies:** Neurology, Natl Hosp Queen Square, London, England 1967-1968; Cardiology (Cardiovascular Disease), Natl Heart Hosp, London, England 1968-1969; **Fellowships:** Endocrinology, Diabetes & Metabolism, Hammersmith Hospital, London, England; Endocrinology, Diabetes & Metabolism, Harbor Genl Hosp-UCLA, Los Angeles, CA 1973-1974

Ontjes, David A MD (Endocrinology, Diabetes & Metabolism) - *Special Expertise:* *Osteoporosis; Thyroid & Pituitary Disorders; Adrenal Disorders;* **Admitting Hospital:** University of North Carolina Hospitals; **Office Address:** Univ of NC Chapel Hill Dept of Medicine - CB 7527 Chapell Hill, NC 27599-7527; **Office Phone:** (919) 966-3336; **Board Certifications:** Internal Medicine 1972, Endocrinology, Diabetes & Metabolism 1972; **Medical School:** Harvard Med Sch 1964; **Residency:** Internal Medicine, Boston Clty Hosp, Boston, MA 1965-1966; **Faculty Appointment:** Prof Medical Toxicology, Univ NC Sch Med

Ovalle, Fernando MD (Endocrinology, Diabetes & Metabolism) - *Special Expertise:* *Diabetes; Hypoglycemia;* **Admitting Hospital:** University of Alabama Hospital at Birmingham; **Office Address:** UAB Sch Med 2000 6th Ave, Ste S Birmingham, AL 35233; **Office Phone:** (205) 801-8490; **Board Certifications:** Internal Medicine 1995, Endocrinology, Diabetes & Metabolism 1997; **Medical School:** Mexico 1989; **Residency:** Internal Medicine, Henry Ford Hosp, Detroit, MI 1991-1995; **Fellowship:** Endocrinology, Diabetes & Metabolism, Barnes Hosp-Wash Univ Sch Med, St Louis, MO 1995-1997; **Faculty Appointment:** Asst Prof Medicine, Univ Ala

Powers, Alvin C MD (Endocrinology, Diabetes & Metabolism) - *Special Expertise:* Diabetes; **Admitting Hospital:** Vanderbilt University Medical Center; **Office Address:** Vanderbilt Univ Med Ctr, Endo Ctr 1211 22nd Ave S, rm 715 MRB II Nashville, TN 37232-6303; **Office Phone:** (615) 936-1653; **Board Certifications:** Internal Medicine 1982, Endocrinology, Diabetes & Metabolism 1985; **Medical School:** Univ Tenn Coll Med, Memphis 1979; **Residency:** Internal Medicine, Duke Univ Med Ctr, Durham, NC 1980-1982; **Fellowship:** Endocrinology, Diabetes & Metabolism, Mass Genl Hosp, Boston, MA 1983-1985; **Faculty Appointment:** Assoc Prof Medicine, Vanderbilt Univ

Quinn, Suzanne Lorraine MD (Endocrinology, Diabetes & Metabolism) - *Special Expertise:* Endocrinology, Diabetes & Metabolism - General; **Admitting Hospital:** Shands at Jacksonville; **Office Address:** 655 W 8th St Jacksonville, FL 32209-6533; **Office Phone:** (904) 244-4704; **Board Certifications:** Internal Medicine 1988, Endocrinology, Diabetes & Metabolism 1993; **Medical School:** Univ Fla Coll Med 1985; **Residency:** Internal Medicine, Univ Fla Coll Med, Gainesville, FL 1985-1988; **Fellowship:** Endocrinology, Diabetes & Metabolism, Univ Fla Coll Med, Gainesville, FL 1989-1992; **Faculty Appointment:** Assoc Prof Medicine, Univ Fla Coll Med

Skyler, Jay S MD (Endocrinology, Diabetes & Metabolism) - *Special Expertise:* Diabetes; **Admitting Hospital:** University of Miami - Jackson Memorial Hospital; **Office Address:** Univ Miami D-110 PO Box 16960 Miami, FL 33101-6960; **Office Phone:** (305) 243-6146; **Board Certifications:** Internal Medicine 1972, Endocrinology, Diabetes & Metabolism 1973; **Medical School:** Jefferson Med Coll 1969; **Residency:** Internal Medicine, Duke Med Ctr, Durham, NC 1969-1971; **Fellowship:** Endocrinology, Diabetes & Metabolism, Duke Med Ctr, Durham, NC 1971-1973; **Faculty Appointment:** Prof Medicine, Univ Miami Sch Med

Veldhuis, Johannes D MD (Endocrinology, Diabetes & Metabolism) - *Special Expertise:* Reproductive Endocrinology; Pituitary Disorders; Adrenal & Gonadal Disorders; **Admitting Hospital:** University of Virginia Health Systems; **Office Address:** Jordan Hall Annex Jefferson Park Ave, rm 1230, Box 800202 Charlottesville, VA 22908; **Office Phone:** (804) 924-9697; **Board Certifications:** Internal Medicine 1977, Endocrinology, Diabetes & Metabolism 1979; **Medical School:** Penn State Univ-Hershey Med Ctr 1974; **Residency:** Internal Medicine, Mayo Grad Sch Med, Rochester, MN 1975-1977; **Fellowship:** Endocrinology, Diabetes & Metabolism, Penn State Univ Hosp, Hershey, PA 1977-1978; **Faculty Appointment:** Prof Medicine, Univ VA Sch Med

Watts, Nelson B MD (Endocrinology, Diabetes & Metabolism) - *Special Expertise:* Bone Disorders-Metabolic; Osteoporosis; **Admitting Hospital:** Emory University Hospital; **Office Address:** Emory Clinic 1365 Clifton Rd NE, Bldg A - Fl 4 - rm 4424 Atlanta, GA 30322-1013; **Office Phone:** (404) 778-3269; **Board Certifications:** Internal Medicine 1972, Endocrinology, Diabetes & Metabolism 1985; **Medical School:** Univ NC Sch Med 1969; **Residency:** Internal Medicine, Charlotte Meml Hosp, Charlotte, NC 1971-1972; **Fellowship:** Endocrinology, Diabetes & Metabolism, NC Meml Hosp, Chapel Hill, NC 1970-1971; **Faculty Appointment:** Prof Endocrinology, Diabetes & Metabolism, Emory Univ

Weissman, Peter MD (Endocrinology, Diabetes & Metabolism) - *Special Expertise:* Diabetes; **Admitting Hospital:** Baptist Hospital - Miami; **Office Address:** Endocrinolgy Assoc 8940 SW 88th St, Ste 804E Miami, FL 33176-2148; **Office Phone:** (305) 595-0777; **Board Certifications:** Internal Medicine 1972, Endocrinology, Diabetes & Metabolism 1972; **Medical School:** NYU Sch Med 1966; **Residency:** Internal Medicine, Barnes Hosp/Wash Univ, St Louis, MO 1966-1968; **Fellowships:** Geriatric Medicine, Gerontology Rsch Ctr, Baltimore, MD 1968-1970; Endocrinology, Diabetes & Metabolism, Univ Mich Hosp, Ann Arbor, MI 1970-1972; **Faculty Appointment:** Assoc Clin Prof Endocrinology, Diabetes & Metabolism, Univ Miami Sch Med

Midwest

Bahn, Rebecca Sue MD (Endocrinology, Diabetes & Metabolism) - *Special Expertise:*
Thyroid Disorders; Graves' Disease; **Admitting Hospital:** Mayo Medical Center & Clinic -
Rochester; **Office Address:** Mayo Clinic, Div Endo 200 1st St SW Rochester, MN 55905; **Office
Phone:** (507) 284-0051; **Board Certifications:** Internal Medicine 1985, Endocrinology, Diabetes &
Metabolism 1987; **Medical School:** Mayo Med Sch 1981; **Residency:** Internal Medicine, Mayo
Grad Sch Med., Rochester, MN 1982-1984; **Fellowship:** Endocrinology, Diabetes & Metabolism,
Mayo Grad Sch Med., Rochester, MN 1984-1986; **Faculty Appointment:** Prof Medicine, Mayo
Med Sch

Brennan, Michael Desmond MD (Endocrinology, Diabetes & Metabolism) - *Special*
Expertise: Thyroid Disorders; Diabetes; **Admitting Hospital:** Mayo Medical Center & Clinic -
Rochester; **Office Address:** Mayo Clinic 200 1st St SW Rochester, MN 55905; **Office Phone:** (507)
284-7246; **Board Certifications:** Internal Medicine 1975, Endocrinology, Diabetes & Metabolism
1977; **Medical School:** Ireland 1969; **Residencies:** Internal Medicine, Mayo Grad Sch, Rochester,
MN 1972-1975; Internal Medicine, Henry Ford Hosp, Detroit, MI 1971-1972; **Fellowship:**
Endocrinology, Diabetes & Metabolism, Mayo Grad Sch, Rochester, MN 1975-1977; **Faculty
Appointment:** Assoc Prof Medicine, Mayo Med Sch

Burke, Susan F MD (Endocrinology, Diabetes & Metabolism) - *Special Expertise:*
Diabetes; Thyroid Disorders; **Admitting Hospital:** Northwestern Memorial Hospital; **Office Address:**
676 N Saint Clair St, Apt 2020 Chicago, IL 60611-2941; **Office Phone:** (312) 280-4700; **Board
Certifications:** Internal Medicine 1981, Endocrinology, Diabetes & Metabolism 1983; **Medical
School:** Northwestern Univ 1978; **Residency:** Internal Medicine, Northwestern Meml Hosp,
Chicago, IL 1979-1981; **Fellowship:** Endocrinology, Diabetes & Metabolism, Northwestern Univ
Med Sch, Chicago, IL 1981-1984

Collins, Francis M MD (Endocrinology, Diabetes & Metabolism) - *Special Expertise:*
Hormonal Disorders; Diabetes; **Admitting Hospital:** Good Samaritan Hosp - Cincinnati; **Office
Address:** Queen City Phys 463 Ohio Pike, Ste 300 Cincinnati, OH 45255; **Office Phone:** (513) 528-
5600; **Board Certifications:** Internal Medicine 1978, Endocrinology, Diabetes & Metabolism 1981;
Medical School: Univ Chicago-Pritzker Sch Med 1975; **Residency:** Internal Medicine, Univ
Pittsburgh, Pittsburgh, PA 1978-1978; **Fellowship:** Endocrinology, Diabetes & Metabolism, Ohio
State Univ, Columbus, OH 1978-1980; **Faculty Appointment:** Asst Clin Prof Endocrinology,
Diabetes & Metabolism, Univ Cincinnati

Cryer, Philip E MD (Endocrinology, Diabetes & Metabolism) - *Special Expertise: Diabetes;*
Admitting Hospital: Barnes - Jewish Hospital; **Office Address:** 45-70 Children's Pl St Louis, MO
63110-1010; **Office Phone:** (314) 362-7617; **Board Certifications:** Internal Medicine 1972,
Endocrinology, Diabetes & Metabolism 1972; **Medical School:** Northwestern Univ 1962;
Residency: Internal Medicine, Barnes Jewish Hosp, St Louis, MO 1966-1972; **Fellowship:**
Endocrinology, Diabetes & Metabolism, Wash Univ Sch Med, St Louis, MO 1967-1968; **Faculty
Appointment:** Prof Medicine, Washington Univ, St Louis

De Groot, Leslie MD (Endocrinology, Diabetes & Metabolism) - *Special Expertise: Thyroid*
Cancer; Graves' Disease; **Admitting Hospital:** University of Chicago Hospitals (Page 78); **Office
Address:** 5758 S Maryland Ave Chicago, IL 60637; **Office Phone:** (773) 702-6138; **Board
Certification:** Internal Medicine 1960; **Medical School:** Columbia P&S 1952; **Residencies:** Internal
Medicine, Columbia-Presby, New York, NY 1952-1954; Internal Medicine, Mass Genl Hosp,
Boston, MA 1957; **Fellowship:** Endocrinology, Diabetes & Metabolism, Mass Genl Hosp, Boston,
MA 1957-1959; **Faculty Appointment:** Prof Medicine, Univ Chicago-Pritzker Sch Med

Ehrmann, David Alan MD (Endocrinology, Diabetes & Metabolism) - *Special Expertise:*
Polycystic Ovary Disease; Diabetes; **Admitting Hospital:** University of Chicago Hospitals (Page
78); **Office Address:** Univ Chicago Hosps 5841 S Maryland Ave, Box MC1027 Chicago, IL 60637;
Office Phone: (773) 702-9653; **Board Certifications:** Internal Medicine 1985, Endocrinology,
Diabetes & Metabolism 1987; **Medical School:** Univ Mich Med Sch 1985; **Residency:** Internal
Medicine, Univ Mich Med Ctr, Ann Arbor, MI 1983-1985; **Fellowship:** Endocrinology, Diabetes &
Metabolism, Univ Chicago Hosps, Chicago, IL 1985-1988; **Faculty Appointment:** Assoc Prof
Endocrinology, Diabetes & Metabolism, Univ Chicago-Pritzker Sch Med

Emanuele, Mary Ann MD (Endocrinology, Diabetes & Metabolism) - *Special Expertise:*
Diabetes; **Admitting Hospital:** Loyola University Health System; **Office Address:** Loyola Univ Hlth
Sys 2160 S 1st Ave, Ste 117N Maywood, IL 60153-3304; **Office Phone:** (708) 216-0406; **Board
Certifications:** Internal Medicine 1978, Endocrinology, Diabetes & Metabolism 1983; **Medical
School:** Loyola Univ-Stritch Sch Med 1975; **Residencies:** Internal Medicine, Northwestern Univ,
Chicago, IL 1975-1976; Internal Medicine, Univ of Hawaii, Honolulu, HI 1976-1978; **Fellowship:**
Endocrinology, Edward Hines Jr VA Hosp, Hines, IL 1978-1980; **Faculty Appointment:** Prof
Medicine, Loyola Univ-Stritch Sch Med

Emanuele, Nicholas Victor MD (Endocrinology, Diabetes & Metabolism) - *Special
Expertise:* Endocrinology, Diabetes & Metabolism - General;* **Admitting Hospital:** Loyola
University Health System; **Office Address:** Loyola Univ Med Center 2160 S First Ave Maywood, IL
60153; **Office Phone:** (708) 216-6200; **Board Certifications:** Internal Medicine 1975,
Endocrinology, Diabetes & Metabolism 1979; **Medical School:** Northwestern Univ 1967;
Residency: Internal Medicine, Hines VA Hosp, Chicago, IL 1972-1974; **Fellowship:** Endocrinology,
Diabetes & Metabolism, Northwestern Univ, Chicago, IL 1974-1976

Gorman, Colum MD (Endocrinology, Diabetes & Metabolism) - *Special Expertise:* Thyroid
Disorders; **Admitting Hospital:** Mayo Medical Center & Clinic - Rochester; **Office Address:** Mayo
Clinic 200 1st St SW Rochester, MN 55905; **Office Phone:** (507) 284-4738; **Board Certifications:**
Internal Medicine 1980, Endocrinology, Diabetes & Metabolism 1972; **Medical School:** Ireland
1959; **Residency:** Internal Medicine, Mayo Clinic, Rochester, MN 1961-1964; **Fellowship:**
Endocrinology, Diabetes & Metabolism, Mayo Clinic, Rochester, MN 1964-1966; **Faculty
Appointment:** Prof Medicine, Mayo Med Sch

Herman, William H MD (Endocrinology, Diabetes & Metabolism) - *Special Expertise:*
Diabetes; **Admitting Hospital:** University of Michigan Health Center; **Office Address:** 1500 Med
Ctr Dr 3920 Taubman Center, Box 0354 Ann Arbor, MI 48109; **Office Phone:** (734) 647-5922; **Board
Certifications:** Internal Medicine 1982, Endocrinology, Diabetes & Metabolism 1989; **Medical
School:** Boston Univ 1979; **Residencies:** Internal Medicine, Univ Michigan, Ann Arbor, MI 1980-
1982; Preventive Medicine, Ctrs Dis Control, Atlanta, GA 1984-1985; **Fellowship:** Endocrinology,
Diabetes & Metabolism, Univ Michigan, Ann Arbor, MI 1985-1988; **Faculty Appointment:** Assoc
Prof Medicine, Univ Mich Med Sch

Jensen, Michael D. MD (Endocrinology, Diabetes & Metabolism) - *Special Expertise:*
Eating Disorders - Obesity; Eating Disorders; **Admitting Hospital:** Mayo Medical Center & Clinic -
Rochester; **Office Address:** Mayo Clinic 200 W 1st St, Fl 18 Rochester, MN 55905; **Office Phone:**
(507) 284-2462; **Board Certifications:** Internal Medicine 1982, Endocrinology, Diabetes &
Metabolism 1985; **Medical School:** Univ MO-Kansas City 1979; **Residency:** Internal Medicine,
Mayo Clinic, Rochester, MN 1980-1982; **Fellowship:** Endocrinology, Diabetes & Metabolism,
Mayo Clinic, Rochester, MN 1982-1985; **Faculty Appointment:** Prof Medicine, Mayo Med Sch

Khosla, Sundeep MD (Endocrinology, Diabetes & Metabolism) - *Special Expertise:* *Osteoporosis; Bone Disorders-Metabolic;* **Admitting Hospital:** Mayo Medical Center & Clinic - Rochester; **Office Address:** Mayo Clinic 200 1st St SW Rochester, MN 55905; **Office Phone:** (507) 284-3707; **Board Certifications:** Internal Medicine 1985, Endocrinology 1987; **Medical School:** Harvard Med Sch 1982; **Residency:** Internal Medicine, Mass Genl Hosp, Boston, MA 1983-1985; **Fellowship:** Endocrinology, Diabetes & Metabolism, Mass Genl Hosp, Boston, MA 1985-1988; **Faculty Appointment:** Asst Prof Medicine, Mayo Med Sch

Licata, Angelo A MD (Endocrinology, Diabetes & Metabolism) - *Special Expertise:* Bone *Disorders-Metabolic;* **Admitting Hospital:** Cleveland Clinic Foundation; **Office Address:** 9500 Euclid Ave, Ste A30 Cleveland, OH 44195; **Office Phone:** (216) 444-6248; **Board Certification:** Internal Medicine 1983; **Medical School:** Univ Rochester 1973; **Residency:** Internal Medicine, Georgetown Univ Hosps, Washigton, DC 1976; **Fellowship:** Endocrinology, Diabetes & Metabolism, Natl Inst Hlth, Washington, DC 1974; **Faculty Appointment:** Asst Clin Prof Case West Res Univ

Mazzone, Theodore MD (Endocrinology, Diabetes & Metabolism) - *Special Expertise:* *Metabolic Disorders;* **Admitting Hospital:** Rush/Presbyterian - St Luke's Medical Center - Chicago (Page 74); **Office Address:** Rush Presby, Dept Endocrin 1725 W Harrison St, Ste 250 Chicago, IL 60612; **Office Phone:** (312) 942-6163; **Board Certifications:** Internal Medicine 1980, Endocrinology, Diabetes & Metabolism 1983; **Medical School:** Northwestern Univ 1977; **Residency:** Internal Medicine, UCLA Med Ctr, Los Angeles, CA 1978-1980; **Fellowship:** Metabolism, Univ WA Med Ctr, Seattle, WA 1980-1983; **Faculty Appointment:** Prof Endocrinology, Diabetes & Metabolism, Rush Med Coll

McMahon, Marion MD (Endocrinology, Diabetes & Metabolism) - *Special Expertise:* *Nutrition;* **Admitting Hospital:** Mayo Medical Center & Clinic - Rochester; **Office Address:** Mayo Clinic 200 1st St SW Rochester, MN 55902; **Office Phone:** (507) 284-1600; **Board Certifications:** Internal Medicine 1985, Endocrinology, Diabetes & Metabolism 1987; **Medical School:** Univ Wisc 1981; **Residency:** Internal Medicine, Med Coll Wisconsin, Milwaukee, WI 1981-1984; **Fellowships:** Endocrinology, Diabetes & Metabolism, Mayo Clinic, Rochester, MN 1984-1987; Nutrition, New England Deaconess Hosp, Boston, MA 1987-1988

Polonsky, Kenneth S MD (Endocrinology, Diabetes & Metabolism) - *Special Expertise:* *Diabetes;* **Admitting Hospital:** Barnes - Jewish Hospital; **Office Address:** Washington Univ Med Ctr 660 S Euclid, Box 8066 St Louis, MO 60637-2602; **Office Phone:** (314) 362-8060; **Board Certification:** Internal Medicine 1978; **Medical School:** South Africa 1973; **Residencies:** Internal Medicine, Michael Reese Hosp & Med Ctr, Chicago, IL 1976; Internal Medicine, VA Hosp, Hines, IL 1976; **Fellowship:** Internal Medicine, Univ Chicago, Chicago, IL 1978; **Faculty Appointment:** Prof Endocrinology, Diabetes & Metabolism, Univ Chicago-Pritzker Sch Med

Rizza, Robert Alan MD (Endocrinology, Diabetes & Metabolism) - *Special Expertise:* *Diabetes mellitus - Lipid Disorders; Hypoglycemia;* **Admitting Hospital:** St Mary's Hospital; **Office Address:** Mayo Clinic 200 First St SW, Fl W18B Rochester, MN 55905; **Office Phone:** (507) 284-2784; **Board Certifications:** Internal Medicine 1976, Endocrinology, Diabetes & Metabolism 1979; **Medical School:** Univ Fla Coll Med 1971; **Residency:** Internal Medicine, Johns Hopkins Hosp, Baltimore, MD 1971-1973; **Fellowship:** Endocrinology, Diabetes & Metabolism, Mayo Clinic, Rochester, MN 1976-1979; **Faculty Appointment:** Prof Medicine, Mayo Med Sch

Robertson, Gary Lee MD (Endocrinology, Diabetes & Metabolism) - *Special Expertise:* *Diabetes Insipidus; Pituitary/Hypothalamic Disease;* **Admitting Hospital:** Northwestern Memorial Hospital; **Office Address:** Northwestern Med Fac Fdn 675 N Sinclair, Ste 250 Chicago, IL 60611; **Office Phone:** (312) 695-7970; **Medical School:** Harvard Med Sch 1961; **Residency:** Internal Medicine, Univ Louisville Hosp, Louisville, KY 1961-1964; **Fellowship:** Internal Medicine, Brigham & Women's Hosp, Boston, MA 1964-1967

Semenkovich, Clay F MD (Endocrinology, Diabetes & Metabolism) - *Special Expertise:* *Cholesterol/Lipid Disorders; Diabetes;* **Admitting Hospital:** Barnes - Jewish Hospital; **Office Address:** 4570 Children's Pl St Louis, MO 63110; **Office Phone:** (314) 362-3500; **Board Certifications:** Internal Medicine 1984, Endocrinology, Diabetes & Metabolism 1987; **Medical School:** Washington Univ, St Louis 1981; **Residency:** Internal Medicine, Barnes Hosp, St Louis, MO 1981-1984; **Fellowship:** Endocrinology, Diabetes & Metabolism, Wash Univ, St Louis, MO 1984-1986; **Faculty Appointment:** Assoc Prof Medicine, Washington Univ, St Louis

Sizemore, Glenn MD (Endocrinology, Diabetes & Metabolism) - *Special Expertise:* Bone *Disorders-Metabolic; Osteoporosis;* **Admitting Hospital:** Loyola University Health System; **Office Address:** 2160 S First Ave Maywood, IL 60153; **Office Phone:** (708) 216-0406; **Board Certifications:** Internal Medicine 1972, Endocrinology, Diabetes & Metabolism 1973; **Medical School:** Univ Rochester 1963; **Residency:** Internal Medicine, Univ Kentucky Hosp 1963-1970; **Fellowship:** Endocrinology, Diabetes & Metabolism, Mayo Clinic, Rochester, MN 1969-1972; **Faculty Appointment:** Prof Emeritus Medicine, Loyola Univ-Stritch Sch Med

Werner, Phillip Ladd MD (Endocrinology, Diabetes & Metabolism) - *Special Expertise:* *Diabetes;* **Admitting Hospital:** Advocate Lutheran General Hospital; **Office Address:** Advocate Medical Group 1775 Ballard Rd Park Ridge, IL 60068; **Office Phone:** (847) 318-2400; **Board Certifications:** Endocrinology, Diabetes & Metabolism 1977, Internal Medicine 1975; **Medical School:** Univ IL Coll Med 1972; **Residency:** Internal Medicine, Univ IL Affl Hosp, Chicago, IL 1973-1974; **Fellowship:** Endocrinology, Diabetes & Metabolism, Univ WA, Seattle, WA 1975-1977; **Faculty Appointment:** Prof Medicine, Chicago Coll Osteo Med

Great Plains and Mountains

Eckel, Robert MD (Endocrinology, Diabetes & Metabolism) - *Special Expertise:* Diabetes; *Eating Disorders - Obesity;* **Admitting Hospital:** University of Colorado Health & Science Center; **Office Address:** Univ Colorado Hlth Scis Ctr 4200 E 9th Ave, Fl 1W, Box B151 Denver, CO 80262; **Office Phone:** (303) 372-7240; **Board Certifications:** Internal Medicine 1976, Endocrinology, Diabetes & Metabolism 1979; **Medical School:** Univ Cincinnati 1973; **Residency:** Internal Medicine, University Wisc Hosp, Madison, WI 1974-1976; **Fellowship:** Endocrinology, Diabetes & Metabolism, Univ Washington, Seattle, WA 1976-1979; **Faculty Appointment:** Prof Medicine, Univ Colo

Southwest

Griffin, James Emmet MD (Endocrinology, Diabetes & Metabolism) - *Special Expertise:* *Hypogonadism - Male; Thyroid Disorders;* **Admitting Hospital:** Parkland Memorial Hospital; **Office Address:** Univ Texas SW Med Ctr, Dept Med 5323 Harry Hines Blvd Dallas, TX 75390-8857; **Office Phone:** (214) 648-3494; **Board Certifications:** Endocrinology, Diabetes & Metabolism 1977, Internal Medicine 1975; **Medical School:** Univ Kans 1970; **Residency:** Internal Medicine, Univ Kansas Med Ctr, Kansas City, KS 1971-1972; **Fellowship:** Endocrinology, Diabetes & Metabolism, Univ Texas Hlth Sci Med Ctr, Dallas, TX 1974-1976; **Faculty Appointment:** Prof Medicine, Univ Tex SW, Dallas

Lavis, Victor Ralph MD (Endocrinology, Diabetes & Metabolism) - *Special Expertise:* *Diabetes;* **Admitting Hospital:** Memorial Hermann Healthcare System; **Office Address:** Adult Diabetes and Endo Ctr 6410 Fannin, Bldg Hermann Prof - Fl 6 Houston, TX 77030; **Office Phone:** (713) 704-6661; **Board Certifications:** Endocrinology, Diabetes & Metabolism 1998, Internal Medicine 1969; **Medical School:** Stanford Univ 1962; **Residencies:** Internal Medicine, UCLA Med Ctr, Los Angeles, CA 1966-1967; Internal Medicine, Boston City Hosp, Boston, MA 1963-1964; **Fellowship:** Endocrinology, Diabetes & Metabolism, Univ Washington, Washington, DC 1967-1969; **Faculty Appointment:** Prof Endocrinology, Diabetes & Metabolism, Univ Tex, Houston

Levy, Philip MD (Endocrinology, Diabetes & Metabolism) - *Special Expertise:* *Diabetes;* *Thyroid Disorders;* **Admitting Hospital:** Good Samaritan Regional Medical Center - Phoenix; **Office Address:** Phoenix Endocrinology Clin 1300 N 12th St, Ste 600 Phoenix, AZ 85006-2850; **Office Phone:** (602) 252-3699; **Board Certifications:** Endocrinology, Diabetes & Metabolism 1972, Nuclear Medicine 1976; **Medical School:** Univ Pittsburgh 1956; **Residencies:** Internal Medicine, Michael Reese Hosp, Chicago, IL 1957-1960; Endocrinology, Diabetes & Metabolism, Guys Hosp Med Sch, London, England 1961-1962; **Fellowship:** Endocrinology, Diabetes & Metabolism, Michael Reese Hosp, Chicago, IL 1960-1961; **Faculty Appointment:** Clin Prof Medicine, Univ Ariz Coll Med

Mundy, Gregory Robert MD (Endocrinology, Diabetes & Metabolism) - *Special Expertise:* *Osteoporosis; Bone Disorders-Metabolic;* **Admitting Hospital:** University of Texas Health & Science Center; **Office Address:** Univ TX Hlth Sci Ctr, Dept Med 7703 Floyd Curl Dr San Antonio, TX 78229-3900; **Office Phone:** (210) 567-4900; **Board Certifications:** Endocrinology, Diabetes & Metabolism 1977, Internal Medicine 1975; **Medical School:** Australia 1973; **Residency:** Internal Medicine, Royal Hobart Hosp, Tasmania, Australia 1968-1970; **Faculty Appointment:** Prof Medicine, Univ Tex, San Antonio

Raskin, Philip MD (Endocrinology, Diabetes & Metabolism) - *Special Expertise:* *Diabetes;* **Admitting Hospital:** Zale Lipshy University Hospital; **Office Address:** Univ Tex SW Med Ctr at Dallas 5323 Harry Hines Blvd Dallas, TX 75390-8858; **Office Phone:** (214) 648-2017; **Board Certifications:** Internal Medicine 1972, Endocrinology, Diabetes & Metabolism 1973; **Medical School:** Univ Pittsburgh 1966; **Residency:** Internal Medicine, Hlth Ctr Hosps-Univ Pittsburgh, Pittburgh, PA 1967-1968; **Fellowship:** Endocrinology, Diabetes & Metabolism, Southwestern Med Sch, Dallas, TX 1970-1972; **Faculty Appointment:** Prof Medicine, Univ Tex SW, Dallas

Reasner, Charles A MD (Endocrinology, Diabetes & Metabolism) - *Special Expertise:* *Thyroid Disorders; Thyroid Tumors;* **Admitting Hospital:** University of Texas Health & Science Center; **Office Address:** Texas Diabetes Inst 701 Zarzamora St San Antonio, TX 78207; **Office Phone:** (210) 358-7402; **Board Certifications:** Endocrinology, Diabetes & Metabolism 1985, Internal Medicine 1983; **Medical School:** Loma Linda Univ 1979; **Residency:** Internal Medicine, USAF Med Ctr, Keesler AFB, MS 1981-1983; **Fellowship:** Endocrinology, Diabetes & Metabolism, Wilford Hall Med Ctr, Lackland AFB, TX 1983-1985; **Faculty Appointment:** Assoc Prof Medicine, Univ Tex, San Antonio

West Coast and Pacific

Berkson, Richard Alan MD (Endocrinology, Diabetes & Metabolism) - *Special Expertise:* *Diabetes; Thyroid Disorders;* **Admitting Hospital:** St Mary's Medical Center; **Office Address:** 1868 Pacific Ave Long Beach, CA 90806-6113; **Office Phone:** (562) 595-4718; **Board Certifications:** Internal Medicine 1975, Endocrinology, Diabetes & Metabolism 1977; **Medical School:** SUNY Buffalo 1972; **Residency:** Internal Medicine, Univ Program, Buffalo, NY 1972-1975; **Fellowships:** Endocrinology, Diabetes & Metabolism, Joslin Clinic, Boston, MA 1975-1976; Endocrinology, Diabetes & Metabolism, UCLA Ctr Hlth Scis, Los Angeles, CA 1976-1977; **Faculty Appointment:** Assoc Clin Prof Medicine, UCLA

Chopra, Inder Jit MD (Endocrinology, Diabetes & Metabolism) - *Special Expertise:* Endocrinology, Diabetes & Metabolism - General; **Admitting Hospital:** UCLA Medical Center; **Office Address:** 900 Dteran Ave Los Angeles, CA 90024-1301; **Office Phone:** (310) 825-2346; **Board Certifications:** Internal Medicine 1972, Endocrinology, Diabetes & Metabolism 1973; **Medical School:** India 1961; **Residencies:** Internal Medicine, Queens Medical Center, Honolulu, HI 1962; Internal Medicine, Inst Med Sci, New Delhi India 1967; **Fellowship:** Endocrinology, Diabetes & Metabolism, Harbor-UCLA, Torrance, CA 1968-1971; **Faculty Appointment:** Prof Medicine, UCLA

Fitzgerald, Paul Anthony MD (Endocrinology, Diabetes & Metabolism) - *Special Expertise:* Endocrinology, Diabetes & Metabolism - General; **Admitting Hospital:** University of California - San Francisco Medical Center; **Office Address:** 350 Parnassus Ave, Ste 710 San Francisco, CA 94117; **Office Phone:** (415) 665-1136; **Board Certifications:** Internal Medicine 1975, Endocrinology, Diabetes & Metabolism 1981; **Medical School:** Jefferson Med Coll 1972; **Residency:** Internal Medicine, Presby Med Ctr-Univ Colo, Denver, CO 1973-1975; **Fellowship:** Endocrinology, Diabetes & Metabolism, UC San Francisco Med Ctr, San Francisco, CA 1976-1978; **Faculty Appointment:** Clin Prof Medicine, UCSF

Gonzalez, Martha MD/PhD (Endocrinology, Diabetes & Metabolism) - *Special Expertise:* Osteoporosis/ Menopause; Thyroid Disorders & Diabetes; **Admitting Hospital:** Ventura County Medical Center; **Office Address:** 116 N Brent St Ventura, CA 93003; **Office Phone:** (805) 656-4311; **Board Certifications:** Internal Medicine 1995, Endocrinology, Diabetes & Metabolism 1997; **Medical School:** UCLA 1986; **Residency:** Internal Medicine, UCLA-Wadsworth VA Med Ctr, West Los Angeles, CA 1988-1990; **Fellowship:** Endocrinology, Diabetes & Metabolism, LA Co-USC Med Ctr, Los Angeles, CA 1990-1992

Greenspan, Francis S MD (Endocrinology, Diabetes & Metabolism) - *Special Expertise:* Endocrinology, Diabetes & Metabolism - General; **Admitting Hospital:** University of California - San Francisco Medical Center; **Office Address:** 350 Parnassus Ave, Ste 609 U Calif Med Ctr San Francisco, CA 94117; **Office Phone:** (415) 476-1121; **Board Certifications:** Internal Medicine 1977, Endocrinology, Diabetes & Metabolism 1972; **Medical School:** Cornell Univ-Weil Med Coll 1943; **Residencies:** Internal Medicine, New York Hosp, New York, NY 1944-1947; Internal Medicine, Stanford Univ Hosp, San Francisco, CA 1947-1948; **Fellowship:** Endocrinology, Diabetes & Metabolism, Univ CA, Berkeley, CA 1947-1948; **Faculty Appointment:** Clin Prof Medicine, UCSF

Hoffman, Andrew R MD (Endocrinology, Diabetes & Metabolism) - *Special Expertise:* Pituitary Disorders; **Admitting Hospital:** Stanford Medical Center; **Office Address:** VA-Palo Alto Healthcare System, MC-111 3801 Miranda Ave Palo Alto, CA 94304; **Office Phone:** (650) 858-3930; **Board Certifications:** Internal Medicine 1979, Endocrinology, Diabetes & Metabolism 1981; **Medical School:** Stanford Univ 1976; **Residency:** Internal Medicine, Mass Genl Hosp, Boston, MA 1977-1978; **Fellowships:** Pharmacology, Mass Genl Hosp, Boston, MA 1978-1980; Endocrinology, Diabetes & Metabolism, Mass Genl Hosp, Boston, MA 1980-1982; **Faculty Appointment:** Prof Medicine, Stanford Univ

Hsueh, Willa Ann MD (Endocrinology, Diabetes & Metabolism) - *Special Expertise:* Diabetes; Hypertension; **Admitting Hospital:** UCLA Medical Center; **Office Address:** UCLA Med Ctr, Div Endocrinology 10833 Le Conte Ave Los Angeles, CA 90095; **Office Phone:** (310) 825-8611; **Board Certifications:** Internal Medicine 1976, Endocrinology, Diabetes & Metabolism 1977; **Medical School:** Ohio State Univ 1973; **Residency:** Internal Medicine, Johns Hopkins Hosp, Baltimore, MD 1974-1975; **Fellowship:** Endocrinology, Diabetes & Metabolism, Johns Hopkins Hosp, Baltimore, MD 1975-1976; **Faculty Appointment:** Prof Medicine, UCLA

Ipp, Eli MD (Endocrinology, Diabetes & Metabolism) - *Special Expertise:* Diabetes; **Admitting Hospital:** LAC - Harbor - UCLA Medical Center; **Office Address:** Harbor-UCLA Professional Bldg 21840 S Normandy Ave, Ste 700 Torrance, CA 90502; **Office Phone:** (310) 222-5101; **Board Certifications:** Internal Medicine 1979, Endocrinology, Diabetes & Metabolism 1981; **Medical School:** South Africa 1968; **Residency:** Internal Medicine, Tel Hashomer Hosp, Tel Aviv, Israel 1970-1974; **Fellowship:** Endocrinology, Diabetes & Metabolism, Univ Tex SW, Dallas, TX 1976-1978; **Faculty Appointment:** Prof Medicine, UCLA

Kamdar, Vikram V MD (Endocrinology, Diabetes & Metabolism) - *Special Expertise:* Diabetes; Amputee Rehabilitation; **Admitting Hospital:** LAC - Rancho Los Amigos Medical Center; **Office Address:** Rancho Los Amigos Med Ctr 7601 E Imperial Hwy, rm 145-HB Downey, CA 90242; **Office Phone:** (562) 401-7225; **Board Certifications:** Internal Medicine 1978, Endocrinology, Diabetes & Metabolism 1979; **Medical School:** India 1971; **Residencies:** Internal Medicine, Lemuel Shattuck Hosp, Boston, MA 1972; Endocrinology, Diabetes & Metabolism, Cedars-Sinai Med Ctr, Los Angeles, CA 1975-1977; **Fellowship:** Endocrinology, Diabetes & Metabolism, LA Co-USC Med Ctr, Los Angeles, CA 1973-1975; **Faculty Appointment:** Assoc Clin Prof Medicine, USC Sch Med

Marcus, Robert A MD (Endocrinology, Diabetes & Metabolism) - *Special Expertise:* Osteoporosis; Thyroid Disorders; Eating Disorders; **Admitting Hospital:** VA Medical Center - Palo Alto; **Office Address:** Stanford Univ 900 Blake Wilbur, rm 3045 Palo Alto, CA 94304; **Office Phone:** (650) 498-6910; **Board Certifications:** Internal Medicine 1972, Endocrinology, Diabetes & Metabolism 1973; **Medical School:** Stanford Univ 1966; **Residencies:** Internal Medicine, Stanford Univ Hosp, Stanford, CA 1967-1968; Internal Medicine, Washington Hosp, Washington, DC 1971-1973; **Faculty Appointment:** Prof Medicine, Stanford Univ

Melmed, Shlomo MD (Endocrinology, Diabetes & Metabolism) - *Special Expertise:* Pituitary Tumors; Acromegaly; **Admitting Hospital:** Cedars-Sinai Medical Center; **Office Address:** Cedars Sinai Med Ctr, Pituitary Ctr 8700 Beverly Blvd Los Angeles, CA 90048; **Office Phone:** (310) 423-4691; **Board Certifications:** Internal Medicine 1979, Endocrinology, Diabetes & Metabolism 1983; **Medical School:** South Africa 1970; **Residency:** Internal Medicine, Sheba Med Ctr, Tel Hashomer 1972-1976; **Fellowship:** Endocrinology, Diabetes & Metabolism, Wadsworth VA Hosp, Los Angeles, CA 1978-1980; **Faculty Appointment:** Prof Medicine, UCLA

Rudnick, Paul Arthur MD (Endocrinology, Diabetes & Metabolism) - *Special Expertise:* Diabetes; **Admitting Hospital:** Cedars-Sinai Medical Center; **Office Address:** 8920 Wilshire Blvd, Ste 635 Beverly Hills, CA 90211-2007; **Office Phone:** (310) 652-3870; **Board Certifications:** Endocrinology, Diabetes & Metabolism 1973, Internal Medicine 1977; **Medical School:** Yale Univ 1958; **Residency:** Internal Medicine, Peter Bent Brigham Hosp, Boston, MA 1961-1962 **Fellowship:** Endocrinology, Diabetes & Metabolism, Mass Genl Hosp, Boston, MA 1962-1963

Singer, Peter Albert MD (Endocrinology, Diabetes & Metabolism) - *Special Expertise:* Thyroid Disorders; **Admitting Hospital:** LAC + USC Medical Center; **Office Address:** USC - Keck Sch Med, Dept Med Diabetes AHC 119 Bldg, MC-9233 Los Angeles, CA 90033; **Office Phone:** (323) 442-5575; **Board Certifications:** Internal Medicine 1972, Endocrinology, Diabetes & Metabolism 1973; **Medical School:** UCSF 1965; **Residency:** Internal Medicine, LA Co-USC Med Ctr, Los Angeles, CA 1968-1971; **Fellowship:** Endocrinology, Diabetes & Metabolism, LA Co-USC Med Ctr, Los Angeles, CA 1971-1973; **Faculty Appointment:** Clin Prof Medicine, USC Sch Med

Swerdloff, Ronald Sherwin MD (Endocrinology, Diabetes & Metabolism) - *Special Expertise:* Andrology; Pituitary Tumors; **Admitting Hospital:** LAC - Harbor - UCLA Medical Center; **Office Address:** Harbor-UCLA Med Ctr 1000 W Carson St, Box 446 Torrance, CA 90509; **Office Phone:** (310) 222-1867; **Board Certifications:** Internal Medicine 1968, Endocrinology, Diabetes & Metabolism 1972; **Medical School:** UCSF 1962; **Residencies:** Univ Washington, Seattle, WA 1963-1964; UCLA, Los Angeles, CA 1966-1967; **Fellowships:** Endocrinology, Diabetes & Metabolism, Natl Inst Health Ger Branch, Baltimore, MD 1964-1966; Endocrinology, Diabetes & Metabolism, Harbor-UCLA Med Ctr, Torrance, CA 1967-1969; **Faculty Appointment:** Prof Medicine, UCLA

Woeber, Kenneth Alois MD (Endocrinology, Diabetes & Metabolism) - *Special Expertise:* Thyroid Disorders; **Admitting Hospital:** University of California - San Francisco Medical Center; **Office Address:** UCSF Mt Zion San Francisco, CA 94143-1640; **Office Phone:** (415) 885-7574; **Board Certifications:** Internal Medicine 1980, Endocrinology, Diabetes & Metabolism 1973; **Medical School:** South Africa 1957; **Residency:** Internal Medicine, Jackson Miami Hosp, Miami, FL 1959-1962; **Fellowship:** Endocrinology, Diabetes & Metabolism, Harvard Med unit-Boston City Hosp, Boston, MA 1962-1964; **Faculty Appointment:** Prof Medicine, UCSF

GASTROENTEROLOGY

(a subspecialty of INTERNAL MEDICINE)

An internist who specializes in diagnosis and treatment of diseases of the digestive organs including the stomach, bowels, liver and gallbladder. This specialist treats conditions such as abdominal pain, ulcers, diarrhea, cancer and jaundice and performs complex diagnostic and therapeutic procedures using endoscopes to see internal organs.

INTERNAL MEDICINE

An internist is a personal physician who provides long-term, comprehensive care in the office and the hospital, managing both common and complex illness of adolescents, adults and the elderly. Internists are trained in the diagnosis and treatment of cancer, infections and diseases affecting the heart, blood, kidneys, joints and digestive, respiratory and vascular systems. They are also trained in the essentials of primary care internal medicine which incorporates an understanding of disease prevention, wellness, substance abuse, mental health and effective treatment of common problems of the eyes, ears, skin, nervous system and reproductive organs.

Training required: Three years in internal medicine *plus* additional training and examination for certification in gastroenterology

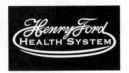

HENRY FORD HOSPITAL
DIVISION OF GASTROENTEROLOGY

The Division of Gastroenterology is consistently recognized for its excellence in treating gastrointestinal conditions by *U.S. News & World Report*. Areas of expertiseinclude esophageal reflux, colitis, hepatitis and colon cancer.

Patient Care

Physicians perform highly specialized, diagnostic and theraputic endoscopic procedures, including endoscopic ultrsound and laser therapy. With endoscopic ultrasound, patients can be diagnosed and staged for cancer treatment without going through the discomfort of surgery.

The Division is on the forefront of delivering patient education through an on-line forum, which is available through Med-Help International.

Hepatitis C

One of only two liver transplantation centers in Michigan, Henry Ford offers the most comprehensive support group in the Midwest for patients with hepatitis C.

Research

The Division is internationally known for its research in the areas of colon cancer, abdominal pain, hepatitis and bleeding from ulcers. Henry Ford's Viral Hepatitis Clinic also is examining the effectiveness of such therapies as interferon non-responders and relapsers and immune-regulatory cytokine.

Many patients participate in National Cancer Institute trials, in-house trials for new treatments and innovative applications of surgical, radiation and chemotherapeutic treatments for gastointestinal malignancies. They include combined modality therapy for esophageal cancer and photodynamic therapy in Barrett's esophagus.

LEADING-EDGE PATIENT CARE

Henry Ford is the only Michigan hospital offering a new treatment for people suffering from chronic heartburn or gastroesophageal acid reflux disease (GERD), in which stomach acid backs up into the esophagus.

Until now, GERD had been typically controlled with prescription medications or through open surgery.

An endoscopic suturing system has been developed to strenghten the area where the stomach connects to the esophagus.The non-invasive procedure is performed on an outpatient basis and usually without general anesthesia. Patients typically are able to return to normal activities the next day.

Henry Ford is one of several regional training sites in the United States where physicians can learn how to perform the procedure.

---

www.HenryFord.com
1-888-291-8304

ST. LUKE'S TEXAS LIVER INSTITUTE^{SM}

ST. LUKE'S EPISCOPAL HOSPITAL

6720 Bertner Ave., 23rd Floor   Houston, TX 77030
Tel. 1-877-LIVER-SL   www.texasliverinstitute.com

A TRADITION OF EXCELLENCE

For more than four decades, St. Luke's Episcopal Hospital has been a center of quality clinical care, research, and education. St. Luke's has recently taken the treatment of liver disease a step further by dedicating an institution exclusively to treating patients with all forms of liver disease - ranging from screening for abnormal liver function to liver transplantation. St. Luke's Texas Liver Institute offers unsurpassed medical expertise and state-of-the-art facilities matched with the latest medical technology that provides the most effective treatment options available.

WORLD-CLASS PHYSICIANS

Doctors at St. Luke's Texas Liver Institute are the most experienced group of liver specialists in the Texas Medical Center. The St. Luke's physicians providing services are all board certified in internal medicine and gastroenterology, or surgery. The physicians and surgeons at St. Luke's Texas Liver Institute have unmatched experience in treating patients with all forms of liver disease - and are experts in handling all facets of care, ranging from screening for abnormal liver function to liver transplantation.

CARING THROUGH CLINICAL SERVICE

In addition, a multidisciplinary team of specially trained nurses, dieticians, social workers, physician assistants, and other healthcare professionals provide unsurpassed care, in a caring environment, for patients with liver conditions. St. Luke's Texas Liver Institute's specialized staff and state-of-the-art facilities ensure than patients receive the most accurate diagnosis, the most up-to-date care, and the most effective treatments anywhere - all backed by St. Luke's Episcopal Hospital's reputation for world-class care, compassion, and confidentiality.

SERVICES PROVIDED

Services provided by the healthcare professionals at St. Luke's Texas Liver Institute include:

- diagnosis and management of viral hepatitis
- evaluation of abnormal liver tests
- treatment of alcoholic and metabolic liver disease
- management of patients with cirrhosis and portal hypertension
- large volume paracentesis
- liver transplantation
- treatment of liver tumors (malignant and benign)

APPOINTMENTS AND INFORMATION

To make an appointment, or for additional information about how to maintain good liver health, call St. Luke's Texas Liver Institute at its toll-free telephone number: (877) LIVER-SL (877-548-3775). Send e-mail to liver@sleh.com. Or visit the Texas Liver Institute's Web site at www.texasliverinstitute.com.

Accreditation: The St. Luke's Texas Liver Institute is accredited by the Joint Commission on Accreditation of Healthcare Organizations.

The University of Chicago Hospitals
Gastroenterology Program

5841 S. Maryland Avenue
Chicago, Illinois 60637-1470
For help finding a physician: 1-888-UCH-0200

AT THE FOREFRONT OF GASTROENTEROLOGY

The University of Chicago Hospitals' gastroenterology program ranks seventh in the nation and first in Illinois, according to *U.S. News & World Report*. With more than 25 GI specialists on staff, the program plays a leading role in the understanding of digestive diseases and in developing innovative and successful treatments.

Since forming the nation's first full-time department of gastroenterology in 1927, University of Chicago physicians have continually improved treatments for digestive tract and related disorders, including inflammatory bowel disease, hepatitis and other liver diseases, pancreatic disease, and nutrition disorders.

INFLAMMATORY BOWEL DISEASE

The University of Chicago Hospitals have an international reputation in the diagnosis and treatment of inflammatory bowel diseases: Crohn's disease and ulcerative colitis. Because physicians here study the causes of these diseases and continually evaluate new therapies, patients often have access to new medications before they are available elsewhere. Surgery, when necessary, is performed by specialists in complex gastro-intestinal surgery and who work closely with their colleagues on the GI team.

HEPATITIS, OTHER LIVER DISEASES, AND PANCREATIC DISEASE

Here, our primary focus is to develop new therapies for fulminant and chronic hepatitis B and C, as well as for cirrhosis and pancreatic disease. When appropriate, specialists call upon the University of Chicago's Liver Transplant Program, established in 1984 and the oldest in the Midwest. More than 1,000 liver transplants have been successfully performed in adult patients.

NUTRITION DISORDERS

The Clinical Nutrition Support Team has extensive experience in the treatment of complicated nutritional problems, including obesity disorders. It is one of just eight in the country supported by the National Institutes of Health.

**To Find a University of Chicago
Gastroenterology Specialist,
call 1-888-UCH-0200
Visit our web site: www.uchospitals.edu**

Physician Listings

New England

Banks, Peter Alan MD (Gastroenterology) - *Special Expertise: Inflammatory Bowel Disease;* **Admitting Hospital:** Brigham & Women's Hospital; **Office Address:** Div Gastro 45 Francis St, Bldg ASBII - Fl 2 Boston, MA 02115; **Office Phone:** (617) 732-6389; **Board Certifications:** Internal Medicine 1968, Gastroenterology 1970; **Medical School:** Columbia P&S 1961; **Residency:** Internal Medicine, Beth Israel Hosp, Boston, MA 1962-1963; **Fellowship:** Gastroenterology, Mt Sinai Hosp, New York, NY 1965-1967; **Faculty Appointment:** Assoc Prof Medicine, Harvard Med Sch

Bonkovsky, Herbert MD (Gastroenterology) - *Special Expertise: Porphyria; Liver Disease; Nutrition;* **Admitting Hospital:** UMASS Memorial Health Care - Worcester; **Office Address:** Univ Mass Meml Med Ctr 55 Lake Ave N Worcester, MA 01655-0002; **Office Phone:** (508) 856-3068; **Board Certifications:** Internal Medicine 1973, Gastroenterology 1977; **Medical School:** Case West Res Univ 1967; **Residencies:** Internal Medicine, MetroHealth Med Ctr, Cleveland, OH 1968-1969; Internal Medicine, Dartmouth-Hitchcock Med Ctr, Lebanon, NH 1971-1973; **Fellowships:** Gastroenterology, Dartmouth Med Sch, Lebanon, NH 1971-1973; Hepatology, Yale Univ Sch Med, New Haven, CT 1973-1974; **Faculty Appointment:** Prof Medicine, Emory Univ

Carr-Locke, David L MD (Gastroenterology) - *Special Expertise: ERCP-Biliary Endoscopy; Pancreatic & Biliary Disease;* **Admitting Hospital:** Brigham & Women's Hospital; **Office Address:** Brigham & Women's Hosp, Endoscopy Ctr 75 Francis St Boston, MA 02115; **Office Phone:** (617) 732-7414; **Board Certification:** Internal Medicine 1974; **Medical School:** England 1972; **Residencies:** Obstetrics & Gynecology, Orsett Hosp, Essex, UK 1974; Leicester Hosp, UK 1976-1978; **Fellowships:** New England Baptist Hosp, Boston, MA 1976; New England Baptist Hosp, Boston, MA 1979; **Faculty Appointment:** Assoc Prof Medicine

Chuttani, Ram MD (Gastroenterology) - *Special Expertise: Pancreatic/Biliary Disease; Endoscopy(ERC; Gastrointestinal Cancer;* **Admitting Hospital:** Brigham & Women's Hospital; **Office Address:** 330 Brookline Ave, Ste 116 Boston, MA 02215; **Office Phone:** (617) 667-0162; **Board Certifications:** Internal Medicine 1990, Gastroenterology 1991; **Medical School:** India 1983; **Residency:** Internal Medicine, Norwalk Hosp-Yale Univ, New Haven, CT 1984-1987; **Fellowship:** Gastroenterology, Brigham & Women's Hosp, W Roxbury, VA 1987-1990; **Faculty Appointment:** Asst Prof Medicine, Boston Univ

Dienstag, Jules Leonard MD (Gastroenterology) - *Special Expertise: Liver Disease; Hepatitis; Liver/Pancreas Diseases;* **Admitting Hospital:** Massachusetts General Hospital; **Office Address:** Mass Genl Hosp 55 Fruit St. GI Unit-GRJ 825 Boston, MA 02114; **Office Phone:** (617) 726-7450; **Board Certification:** Internal Medicine 1975; **Medical School:** Columbia P&S 1972; **Residencies:** Internal Medicine, University of Chicago Hospitals/Clinics, Chicago, IL 1972-1974; National Institutes of Health; **Fellowships:** Infectious Disease, National Institutes of Health, Bethesda, MD 1974-1976; Gastroenterology, Mass General Hospital, Boston, MA 1976-1978; **Faculty Appointment:** Assoc Prof Medicine, Harvard Med Sch

Friedman, Lawrence S. MD (Gastroenterology) - *Special Expertise: Liver Disease;* **Admitting Hospital:** Massachusetts General Hospital; **Office Address:** Mass Genl Hosp, Gastro Unit 55 Fruit St Blake 456D Boston, MA 02114; **Office Phone:** (617) 724-6005; **Board Certifications:** Internal Medicine 1981, Gastroenterology 1983; **Medical School:** Johns Hopkins Univ 1978; **Residency:** Internal Medicine, Johns Hopkins Hosp, Baltimore, MD 1979-1981; **Fellowship:** Gastroenterology, Mass Genl Hosp, Boston, MA 1981-1984; **Faculty Appointment:** Assoc Prof Medicine, Harvard Med Sch

Peppercorn, Mark MD (Gastroenterology) - *Special Expertise:* Inflammatory Bowel Disease; **Admitting Hospital:** Beth Israel Deaconess Medical Center - Boston (Page 57); **Office Address:** Beth Israel Deconess Med Ctr 330 Brookline Ave Boston, MA 02215; **Office Phone:** (617) 667-2153; **Board Certifications:** Internal Medicine 1974, Gastroenterology 1977; **Medical School:** Harvard Med Sch 1968; **Residencies:** Internal Medicine, Beth Isreal Hosp, Boston, MA 1969-1974; Metabolic Diseases, Natl Inst Hlth, Bethesda, MD 1970-1972; **Fellowship:** Gastroenterology, Beth Israe Hospl, Boston, MA 1972-1973; **Faculty Appointment:** Prof Medicine, Harvard Med Sch

Mid Atlantic

Aronchick, Craig Alan MD (Gastroenterology) - *Special Expertise:* Barrett's Esophagus; Pancreatic/Biliary Disease.Endoscopy(ERC; **Admitting Hospital:** Pennsylvania Hospital; **Office Address:** 800 Spruce St Philadelphia, PA 19107; **Office Phone:** (215) 829-3561; **Board Certifications:** Internal Medicine 1981, Gastroenterology 1983; **Medical School:** Temple Univ 1978; **Residency:** Internal Medicine, Temple Univ Hosp, Philadelphia, PA 1978-1981

Bayless, Theodore MD (Gastroenterology) - *Special Expertise:* Crohn's Disease; Ulcerative Colitis; **Admitting Hospital:** Johns Hopkins Hospital - Baltimore (Page 65); **Office Address:** Johns Hopkins Medical Center 600 N Wolfe St Blalock Bldg 461 Baltimore, MD 21287; **Office Phone:** (410) 955-4916; **Board Certification:** Internal Medicine 1966; **Medical School:** Univ Hlth Sci/Chicago Med Sch 1957; **Residency:** Internal Medicine, Memorial Sloan Kettering Hosp, New York, NY 1958-1960; **Fellowship:** Gastroenterology, Johns Hopkins Hospl, Baltimore, MD 1960-1962; **Faculty Appointment:** Prof Medicine, Johns Hopkins Univ

Benjamin, Stanley MD (Gastroenterology) - *Special Expertise:* Esophageal Disorders; Pancreatic/Biliary Disease.Endoscopy(ERC; Esophageal/Biliary Disease; **Admitting Hospital:** Georgetown University Hospital; **Office Address:** GUMC - Second Floor, Main Hospital 3800 Reservoir Rd NW Washington, DC 20007; **Office Phone:** (202) 687-8684; **Board Certifications:** Internal Medicine 1977, Gastroenterology 1979; **Medical School:** Univ Pittsburgh 1974; **Faculty Appointment:** Prof Medicine, Georgetown Univ

Brandt, Lawrence MD (Gastroenterology) - *Special Expertise:* AIDS/HIV; Ischemic Bowel Disease; **Admitting Hospital:** Montefiore Medical Center; **Office Address:** 111 E 210th St Montefiore Med Ctr, Div of Gastroenterology Bronx, NY 10467-2490; **Office Phone:** (718) 920-4476; **Board Certifications:** Internal Medicine 1972, Gastroenterology 1975; **Medical School:** SUNY Downstate 1968; **Residency:** Internal Medicine, Mount Sinai Hosp, New York, NY 1968-1972; **Fellowship:** Gastroenterology, Mount Sinai Hosp, New York, NY 1971-1972; **Faculty Appointment:** Prof Medicine, Albert Einstein Coll Med

Cohen, Jonathan MD (Gastroenterology) - *Special Expertise:* Gastroenterology - General; **Admitting Hospital:** New York Weill Cornell Medical Center - NY Presbyterian Hospital (Page 72); **Office Address:** Concorde Med Group 232 E 30th St New York, NY 10016; **Office Phone:** (212) 889-5544; **Board Certifications:** Internal Medicine 1993, Gastroenterology 1995; **Medical School:** Harvard Med Sch 1990; **Residency:** Internal Medicine, Beth Israel Hosp, Boston, MA 1991-1993; **Fellowships:** Gastroenterology, UCLA, Los Angeles, CA 1993-1995; Gastroenterology, Wellesley Hosp Univ Toronto, Toronto, Canada

Deren, Julius Jay MD (Gastroenterology) - *Special Expertise:* Inflammatory Bowel Disease - Crohn's; **Admitting Hospital:** University of Pennsylvania - Presbyterian Medical Center; **Office Address:** Wright Saunder Bldg, Ste W-218 39th & Market St Philadelphia, PA 19104; **Office Phone:** (215) 662-8900; **Board Certifications:** Internal Medicine 1968, Gastroenterology 1970; **Medical School:** SUNY Downstate 1958; **Residencies:** Gastroenterology, Boston City Hosp/Harvard, Boston, MA 1961-1962; Internal Medicine, Maimonides Hosp, Brooklyn, NY 1959-1961; **Fellowship:** Physiology, Harvard, Boston, MA 1962-1964; **Faculty Appointment:** Prof Medicine, Univ Penn

Dieterich, Douglas MD (Gastroenterology) - *Special Expertise:* Hepatitis; AIDS/HIV; **Admitting Hospital:** Cabrini Medical Center; **Office Address:** 232 E 20th St, Fl 2 New York, NY 10003; **Office Phone:** (212) 995-6904; **Board Certifications:** Internal Medicine 1981, Gastroenterology 1987; **Medical School:** NYU Sch Med 1978; **Residency:** Internal Medicine, Bellevue Hosp Ctr-NYU, New York, NY 1978-1981; **Fellowship:** Gastroenterology, Bellevue Hosp Ctr-NYU, New York, NY 1981-1983; **Faculty Appointment:** Assoc Prof Medicine, NYU Sch Med

Farmer, Richard G MD (Gastroenterology) - *Special Expertise:* Inflammatory Bowel Disease; **Admitting Hospital:** Georgetown University Hospital; **Office Address:** GUMC - Second Floor, Main Hospital 3800 Reservoir Rd NW, rm 2122 Washington, DC 20007; **Office Phone:** (202) 687-8035; **Board Certifications:** Gastroenterology 1968, Internal Medicine 1963; **Medical School:** Univ Minn 1960; **Residency:** Internal Medicine, Mayo Clinic, Rochester, MN 1957-1960; **Fellowship:** Gastroenterology, Mayo Clinic, Rochester, MN 1960; **Faculty Appointment:** Clin Prof Medicine, Georgetown Univ

Fleischer, David MD (Gastroenterology) - *Special Expertise:* Barrett's Esophagus; Esophageal Cancer; **Admitting Hospital:** Georgetown University Hospital; **Office Address:** GUMC-Main Hospital 3800 Reservoir Rd NW, Fl 2nd - Ste 2122 Washington, DC 20007-2197; **Office Phone:** (202) 687-8741; **Board Certifications:** Internal Medicine 1975, Gastroenterology 1977; **Medical School:** Vanderbilt Univ 1970; **Residencies:** Internal Medicine, Wellington Hosp 1973-1974; Internal Medicine, Metro General Hosp CWRU, Cleveland, OH 1974-1975; **Fellowship:** Gastroenterology, LA Co Harbor-UCLA Medical Center, Torrance, CA 1975-1977; **Faculty Appointment:** Prof Medicine, Georgetown Univ

Holt, Peter R MD (Gastroenterology) - *Special Expertise:* Diarrhea; Inflammatory Bowel Disease; **Admitting Hospital:** St Luke's - Roosevelt Hospital Center - Roosevelt Division (Page 58); **Office Address:** 1111 Amsterdam Ave, Ste 1216 St Lukes's Roosevelt Hospital Center New York, NY 10025; **Office Phone:** (212) 523-3680; **Board Certification:** Internal Medicine 1966; **Medical School:** England 1954; **Residencies:** London Hosp, London, England 1954-1955; Internal Medicine, St Luke's Hosp, New York, NY 1957-1959; **Fellowship:** Gastroenterology, Mass Genl Hosp, Boston, MA 1959-1961; **Faculty Appointment:** Prof Medicine, Columbia P&S

Jacobson, Ira MD (Gastroenterology) - *Special Expertise:* Pancreatic Disease; Liver Disease; **Admitting Hospital:** New York Weill Cornell Medical Center - NY Presbyterian Hospital (Page 72); **Office Address:** 50 E 69th St New York, NY 10021; **Office Phone:** (212) 746-2115; **Board Certifications:** Internal Medicine 1982, Gastroenterology 1985; **Medical School:** Columbia P&S 1979; **Residency:** Internal Medicine, Univ Cal San Francisco, San Francisco, CA 1979-1982; **Fellowship:** Gastroenterology, Mass Gen Hosp, Boston, MA 1982-1984; **Faculty Appointment:** Assoc Clin Prof Medicine, Cornell Univ-Weil Med Coll

Kalloo, Anthony Nicholas MD (Gastroenterology) - *Special Expertise:* Endoscopy; **Admitting Hospital:** Johns Hopkins Hospital - Baltimore (Page 65); **Office Address:** 1835 E Monument St, rm 419 Baltimore, MD; **Office Phone:** (410) 955-9697; **Board Certifications:** Internal Medicine 1985, Gastroenterology 1987; **Medical School:** Other Foreign Country 1979; **Residency:** Internal Medicine, Howard Univ Hosp, Washington, DC 1983-1985; **Fellowship:** Gastroenterology, VA Med Coll, Washington, DC 1985; **Faculty Appointment:** Assoc Prof Gastroenterology, Johns Hopkins Univ

Kodsi, Baroukh MD (Gastroenterology) - *Special Expertise:* Endoscopy; Peptic Ulcer Reflux Disease; **Admitting Hospital:** Maimonides Medical Center (Page 67); **Office Address:** 925 48th St Brooklyn, NY 11219; **Office Phone:** (718) 851-6767; **Board Certification:** Gastroenterology 1963; **Medical School:** Egypt 1945; **Residency:** Boston Med Ctr, Boston, MA 1959-1961; **Fellowship:** Gastroenterology, Boston Med Ctr, Boston, MA 1961-1963; **Faculty Appointment:** Assoc Clin Prof SUNY Downstate

Korelitz, Burton I MD (Gastroenterology) - *Special Expertise:* Inflammatory Bowel Disease; **Admitting Hospital:** Lenox Hill Hospital; **Office Address:** 45 E 85th St, Ste 1E New York, NY 10028-0957; **Office Phone:** (212) 988-3800; **Board Certifications:** Internal Medicine 1958, Gastroenterology 1961; **Medical School:** Boston Univ 1951; **Residencies:** Internal Medicine, VA Hosp, Boston, MA 1952-1953; Gastroenterology, Beth Isreal Hosp, Boston, MA 1953-1954; **Fellowship:** Gastroenterology, Mt Sinai Hosp, New York, NY 1956; **Faculty Appointment:** Clin Prof Medicine, NYU Sch Med

Kotler, Donald P MD (Gastroenterology) - *Special Expertise:* Esophageal Disease; AIDS/HIV-Nutrition; **Admitting Hospital:** St Luke's - Roosevelt Hospital Center - Roosevelt Division (Page 58); **Office Address:** G I Immunology 421 W 113th St Ste 1301 New York, NY 10025; **Office Phone:** (212) 523-3670; **Board Certifications:** Internal Medicine 1976, Gastroenterology 1979; **Medical School:** Albert Einstein Coll Med 1973; **Residency:** Internal Medicine, Jacobi Med Ctr, Bronx, NY 1973-1976; **Fellowship:** Gastroenterology, Hosp of Univ of Penn, Philadelphia, PA 1976-1978; **Faculty Appointment:** Assoc Prof Medicine, Columbia P&S

Lightdale, Charles MD (Gastroenterology) - *Special Expertise:* Barrett's Esophagus; Photodynamic Therapy; **Admitting Hospital:** Columbia Presbyterian Medical Center (Page 72); **Office Address:** Columbia-Presbyterian Medical Center 161 Fort Washington Ave, Bldg DAP - rm 812 New York, NY 10032; **Office Phone:** (212) 305-3423; **Board Certifications:** Internal Medicine 1972, Gastroenterology 1973; **Medical School:** Columbia P&S 1966; **Residencies:** Internal Medicine, Yale-New Haven, New Haven, CT 1966-1968; Internal Medicine, NY Hosp, New York, NY 1968-1969; **Fellowship:** Gastroenterology, NY Hosp-Cornell, New York, NY 1971-1973; **Faculty Appointment:** Clin Prof Medicine, Columbia P&S

Lipshutz, William H. MD (Gastroenterology) - *Special Expertise:* Colon Cancer; Esophageal Disorders; **Admitting Hospital:** Pennsylvania Hospital; **Office Address:** Penn Hosp 8th & Spruce Philadelphia, PA 19107; **Office Phone:** (215) 829-3561; **Board Certifications:** Gastroenterology 1973, Internal Medicine 1972; **Medical School:** Univ Penn 1967; **Residencies:** Internal Medicine, Penn Hospital, Philadelphia, PA 1971-1972; Internal Medicine, Penn Hospital, Philadelphia, PA 1968-1969; **Fellowship:** Gastroenterology, Univ Penn, Philadelphia, PA 1969-1971; **Faculty Appointment:** Clin Prof Medicine, Univ Penn

Markowitz, David MD (Gastroenterology) - *Special Expertise:* Gastroenterology - General; **Admitting Hospital:** Columbia Presbyterian Medical Center (Page 72); **Office Address:** 161 Ft Washington Ave New York, NY 10032; **Office Phone:** (212) 305-1024; **Board Certifications:** Internal Medicine 1988, Gastroenterology 1991; **Medical School:** Columbia P&S 1985; **Residency:** Internal Medicine, Columbia-Presby, New York, NY 1985-1988; **Fellowship:** Gastroenterology, Columbia-Presby, New York, NY 1988-1991

Mayer, Lloyd MD (Gastroenterology) - *Special Expertise:* Crohn's Disease; Ulcerative Colitis; **Admitting Hospital:** Mount Sinai Hospital (Page 70); **Office Address:** 5 E 98th St, Fl 10th, Box 1473 New York, NY 10029; **Office Phone:** (212) 659-9266; **Board Certifications:** Internal Medicine 1979, Gastroenterology 1981; **Medical School:** Mount Sinai Sch Med 1976; **Residency:** Internal Medicine, Bellevue Hosp, New York, NY 1976-1979; **Fellowship:** Gastroenterology, Mount Sinai Med Ctr, New York, NY 1979-1981; **Faculty Appointment:** Prof Medicine, Mount Sinai Sch Med

Metz, David C. MD (Gastroenterology) - *Special Expertise:* Peptic Ulceration; Neuroendocrine Tumors; **Admitting Hospital:** Hospital of the University of Pennsylvania; **Office Address:** Univ of Penn MC, Gastro Div 3400 Spruce St, 3 Dulles Philadelphia, PA 19104; **Office Phone:** (215) 662-3541; **Board Certifications:** Internal Medicine 1989, Gastroenterology 1991; **Medical School:** South Africa 1982; **Residency:** Internal Medicine, Albert Einstein Med Center, Philadelphia, PA 1986-1988; **Fellowship:** Gastroenterology, Natl Naval Med Ctr, Bethesda, MD 1989-1991; **Faculty Appointment:** Assoc Prof Medicine, Univ Penn

Miskovitz, Paul MD (Gastroenterology) - *Special Expertise:* *Gastroenterology - General;* **Admitting Hospital:** New York Weill Cornell Medical Center - NY Presbyterian Hospital (Page 72); **Office Address:** 50 E 70th St New York, NY 10021-4928; **Office Phone:** (212) 717-4966; **Board Certifications:** Internal Medicine 1978, Gastroenterology 1981; **Medical School:** Cornell Univ-Weil Med Coll 1975; **Residency:** Internal Medicine, NY Hosp, New York, NY 1975-1978; **Fellowship:** Gastroenterology, NY Hosp, New York, NY 1978-1980; **Faculty Appointment:** Clin Prof Medicine, Cornell Univ-Weil Med Coll

Present, Daniel MD (Gastroenterology) - *Special Expertise:* *Inflammatory Bowel Disease - Crohn's; Inflammatory Bowel Disease; Ulcerative Colitis;* **Admitting Hospital:** Mount Sinai Hospital (Page 70); **Office Address:** 12 E 86th St New York, NY 10028-0506; **Office Phone:** (212) 861-2000; **Board Certifications:** Internal Medicine 1966, Gastroenterology 1969; **Medical School:** SUNY Downstate 1959; **Residency:** Internal Medicine, Mount Sinai Med Ctr, New York, NY 1962-1964; **Fellowship:** Gastroenterology, Mount Sinai Med Ctr, New York, NY 1964-1966; **Faculty Appointment:** Clin Prof Medicine, Mount Sinai Sch Med

Ravich, William Jay MD (Gastroenterology) - *Special Expertise:* *Dysphagia; Achalasia;* **Admitting Hospital:** Johns Hopkins Hospital - Baltimore (Page 65); **Office Address:** Johns Hopkins Hospital- Div Gastroenterology 600 N Wolfe St, Ste 4 - rm 465 Baltimore, MD 21287-6417; **Office Phone:** (410) 955-4910; **Board Certifications:** Internal Medicine 1978, Gastroenterology 1981; **Medical School:** Univ Hlth Sci/Chicago Med Sch 1975; **Residencies:** Gastroenterology, Montefiore Hosp., Bronx, NY 1977-1978; Internal Medicine, Montefiore Hosp., Bronx, NY 1976-1978; **Fellowship:** Gastroenterology, Johns Hopkins Hosp., Baltimore, MD 1978-1981; **Faculty Appointment:** Assoc Prof Gastroenterology, Johns Hopkins Univ

Sachar, David MD (Gastroenterology) - *Special Expertise:* *Inflammatory Bowel Disease; Inflammatory Bowel Disease - Crohn's; Ulceractive Colitis;* **Admitting Hospital:** Mount Sinai Hospital (Page 70); **Office Address:** Gastroenterology Consultants 5 E 98th St, Ste 11 New York, NY 10029; **Office Phone:** (212) 241-4299; **Board Certifications:** Gastroenterology 1972, Internal Medicine 1969; **Medical School:** Harvard Med Sch 1963; **Residencies:** Internal Medicine, Beth Israel Hosp, Boston, MA 1964-1965; Internal Medicine, Beth Israel Hosp, Boston, MA 1967-1968; **Fellowship:** Gastroenterology, Mount Sinai Hosp, New York, NY 1968-1970; **Faculty Appointment:** Clin Prof Medicine, Mount Sinai Sch Med

Siegel, Jerome MD (Gastroenterology) - *Special Expertise:* *Pancreatic/Biliary Disease.Endoscopy(ERC;* **Admitting Hospital:** Beth Israel Medical Center - New York; **Office Address:** 60 E End Ave New York, NY 10028-7907; **Office Phone:** (212) 734-8874; **Board Certifications:** Internal Medicine 1978, Gastroenterology 1979; **Medical School:** Med Coll GA 1960; **Residencies:** Internal Medicine, NY VA Med Ctr, New York, NY 1963-1965; Gastroenterology, NY VA Med Ctr, New York, NY 1965-1966; **Fellowship:** Gastroenterology, Royal Free Hosp, London/England 1973-1975; **Faculty Appointment:** Assoc Clin Prof Medicine, Albert Einstein Coll Med

Wald, Arnold MD (Gastroenterology) - *Special Expertise:* *Constipation; Gastrointestinal Motility Disorders; Irritable Bowel Syndrome;* **Admitting Hospital:** UPMC - Presbyterian University Hospital; **Office Address:** Univ Pitt Med Ctr, Dept Gastro 200 Lothrop St Pittsburgh, PA 15213; **Office Phone:** (412) 648-9241; **Board Certifications:** Internal Medicine 1972, Gastroenterology 1975; **Medical School:** SUNY Downstate 1968; **Residency:** Internal Medicine, SUNY - Downstate Med Ctr, Brooklyn, NY 1968-1971; **Fellowship:** Gastroenterology, Johns Hopkins Hosp, Baltimore, MD 1973-1975; **Faculty Appointment:** Prof Medicine, Univ Pittsburgh

Waye, Jerome MD (Gastroenterology) - *Special Expertise:* Endoscopy; Colon Cancer; **Admitting Hospital:** Mount Sinai Hospital (Page 70); **Office Address:** 650 Park Ave First Fl New York, NY 10021-6115; **Office Phone:** (212) 439-7779; **Board Certifications:** Internal Medicine 1965, Gastroenterology 1970; **Medical School:** Boston Univ 1958; **Residency:** Internal Medicine, Mount Sinai Hosp, New York, NY 1959-1961; **Fellowship:** Gastroenterology, Mount Sinai Hosp, New York, NY 1961-1962

Winawer, Sidney J MD (Gastroenterology) - *Special Expertise:* Endoscopy; Colon Cancer; Colonoscopy/Polypectomy; **Admitting Hospital:** Memorial Sloan Kettering Cancer Center; **Office Address:** Meml Sloan Kettering Cancer Ctr 1275 York Ave, Box 90 New York, NY 10021; **Office Phone:** (212) 639-7678; **Board Certifications:** Internal Medicine 1965, Gastroenterology 1973; **Medical School:** SUNY Hlth Sci Ctr 1956; **Residencies:** Internal Medicine, VA Med Ctr/nyu/bellevue, New York, NY 1959-1961; Internal Medicine, Maimonides Hosp, Brooklyn, NY 1961-1962; **Fellowship:** Gastroenterology, Boston City Hosp, Boston, MA 1962-1964; **Faculty Appointment:** Prof Medicine, Cornell Univ-Weil Med Coll

Southeast

Barkin, Jamie MD (Gastroenterology) - *Special Expertise:* Pancreatic & Biliary Disease; Gastrointestinal Cancer; **Admitting Hospital:** Mount Sinai Medical Center; **Office Address:** Mount Sinai Medical Center 4300 Alton Rd, Ste G22 Miami Beach, FL 33140-2800; **Office Phone:** (305) 674-2240; **Board Certifications:** Internal Medicine 1973, Gastroenterology 1975; **Medical School:** Univ Miami Sch Med 1970; **Residency:** Internal Medicine, Univ Miami Hosp, Miami, FL 1971-1973; **Fellowship:** Gastroenterology, Univ Miami Hosp, Miami, FL 1973-1975; **Faculty Appointment:** Prof Medicine, Univ Miami Sch Med

Bloomer, Joseph MD (Gastroenterology) - *Special Expertise:* Porphyria; Liver Disease; **Admitting Hospital:** University of Alabama Hospital at Birmingham; **Office Address:** Univ of Ala @ Birmingham, 395 MCLM 1918 University Blvd Birmingham, AL 35294; **Office Phone:** (205) 975-9699; **Board Certifications:** Internal Medicine 1972, Gastroenterology 1985; **Medical School:** Case West Res Univ 1966; **Residency:** Internal Medicine, UC/San Francisco Med Ctr, San Francisco, CA 1966-1968; **Faculty Appointment:** Prof Medicine, Univ Ala

Boyce Jr, H Worth MD (Gastroenterology) - *Special Expertise:* Swallowing Disorders; Barrett's Esophagus; **Admitting Hospital:** H Lee Moffitt Cancer Center & Research Institute; **Office Address:** USF College of Medicine, Ctr for Swallowing Disorders 12901 Bruce B Downs Blvd, MC-72 Tampa, FL 33612; **Office Phone:** (813) 974-3374; **Board Certifications:** Gastroenterology 1965, Internal Medicine 1977; **Medical School:** Wake Forest Univ Sch Med 1955; **Residencies:** Internal Medicine, Brooke Army Hosp, Fort Sam Houston, TX 1956-1959; Gastroenterology, Brooke Army Hosp, Fort Sam Houston, TX 1959-1960; **Faculty Appointment:** Prof Medicine, Univ S Fla Coll Med

Brazer, Scott Robert MD (Gastroenterology) - *Special Expertise:* Barrett's Esophagus; Dysphagia; Esophageal Cancer; **Admitting Hospital:** Duke University Medical Center (Page 60); **Office Address:** Duke Univ Med Ctr P.O. Box 3662 Durham, NC 27710; **Office Phone:** (919) 684-6437; **Board Certifications:** Internal Medicine 1984, Gastroenterology 1987; **Medical School:** Case West Res Univ 1981; **Residencies:** Internal Medicine, Duke Univ, Durham, NC 1982-1984; Internal Medicine, Duke Univ, Durham, NC 1987-1988; **Fellowship:** Gastroenterology, Duke Univ, Durham, NC 1985-1987; **Faculty Appointment:** Assoc Prof Gastroenterology, Duke Univ

Brenner, David Allen MD (Gastroenterology) - *Special Expertise:* Gastroenterology - General; **Admitting Hospital:** University of North Carolina Hospitals; **Office Address:** UNC-Chapel Hill 156 Glaxo Bldg ,CB# 7038 Chapel Hill, NC 27599-7038; **Office Phone:** (919) 966-0650; **Board Certifications:** Internal Medicine 1982, Gastroenterology 1986; **Medical School:** Yale Univ 1979; **Residency:** Internal Medicine, Yale, New Haven, CT 1979-1982; **Fellowships:** Research, NIH, Bethesda, MD 1982-1985; Gastroenterology, Univ California, San Diego, CA 1985-1986; **Faculty Appointment:** Prof Emeritus Medicine, Univ NC Sch Med

Cominelli, Fabio MD/PhD (Gastroenterology) - *Special Expertise:* Inflammatory Bowel Disease; Crohn's Disease; Ulcerative Colitis; **Admitting Hospital:** University of Virginia Health Systems; **Office Address:** Dept of Medicine - Digestive Health Center UVA P. O. BOX 800708 Charlottesville, VA 22908; **Office Phone:** (804) 243-6400; **Board Certification:** Gastroenterology 1986; **Medical School:** Italy 1983; **Residency:** Gastroenterology, Careggi Hosp-Univ of Italy, Florence, Italy 1983-1986; **Fellowship:** Gastroenterology, Harbor-UCLA Med Ctr, Torrance, CA 1987-1989; **Faculty Appointment:** Prof Medicine, Univ VA Sch Med

Cotton, Peter MD (Gastroenterology) - *Special Expertise:* Pancreatc Disease; Biliary Disease; **Admitting Hospital:** MUSC Medical Center; **Office Address:** MUSC - Digestive Disease Center - 210 CSB 96 Jonathon Lucas St, Box 250327 Charleston, SC 29425; **Office Phone:** (843) 792-6865; **Medical School:** England 1963; **Residencies:** Internal Medicine, St Thomas' Hosp, London, UK 1966-1970; Gastroenterology, St Thomas' Hosp, London, UK 1970-1973; **Faculty Appointment:** Prof Medicine, Med Univ SC

Cunningham, John MD (Gastroenterology) - *Special Expertise:* Sphincter of Oddi Dysfunction; Pancreatitis; Bleeding - Gastrointestinal; **Admitting Hospital:** MUSC Medical Center; **Office Address:** Med Univ of South Carolina 96 Johnathan Lucas 210 CSB Box 250-327 Charleston, SC 29425-0001; **Office Phone:** (843) 792-7896; **Board Certifications:** Internal Medicine 1975, Gastroenterology 1977; **Medical School:** Med Coll VA 1970; **Residency:** Internal Medicine, Med Univ SC, Charleston, SC 1973-1975; **Fellowship:** Gastroenterology, Med Univ SC, Charleston, SC 1975-1977; **Faculty Appointment:** Prof Medicine, Univ SC Sch Med

Davis, Gary L MD (Gastroenterology) - *Special Expertise:* Liver Disease; Hepatitis; Transplant Medicine-Liver; **Admitting Hospital:** Shands Healthcare at University Florida (Page 77); **Office Address:** University of Florida 1600 SW Archer Road, P.O. Box 100214 Gainesville, FL 32610-0214; **Office Phone:** (352) 392-7353; **Board Certifications:** Internal Medicine 1979, Gastroenterology 1983; **Medical School:** Univ Minn 1976; **Residency:** Internal Medicine, Mayo Grad Sch Med, Minneapolis, MN 1977-1979; **Fellowships:** Gastroenterology, Mayo Grad Sch Med, Minneapolis, MN 1979-1981; Natl Inst of Hlth, Bethesda, MD 1982-1984; **Faculty Appointment:** Prof Medicine, Univ Fla Coll Med

Diamond, Jeffrey MD (Gastroenterology) - *Special Expertise:* Inflammatory Bowel Disease - Crohn's; Ulcerative Colitis; Gastroesophageal Reflex; **Admitting Hospital:** Memorial Regional Hospital- Hollywood; **Office Address:** Gastroenterology Consultants 4700 Sheridan St, Ste M Hollywood, FL 33021; **Office Phone:** (954) 431-7724; **Board Certifications:** Internal Medicine 1972, Gastroenterology 1993; **Medical School:** NYU Sch Med 1965; **Residencies:** Internal Medicine, Kings County Hosp, Brooklyn, NY 1966-1968; Gastroenterology, Univ of Miami Jackson Mem Hosp, Miami, FL 1968-1969; **Fellowship:** Gastroenterology, Jackson Mem Hosp, Miami, FL 1968-1969; **Faculty Appointment:** Clin Prof Medicine, Univ Miami Sch Med

Drossman, Douglas Arnold MD (Gastroenterology) - *Special Expertise: Digestion - Motility Disorders;* **Admitting Hospital:** University of North Carolina Hospitals; **Office Address:** Box 7080 726 Burnett Womack Building, Box cb7080 Chapell Hill, NC 27599-7080; **Office Phone:** (919) 966-0141; **Board Certifications:** Internal Medicine 1973, Gastroenterology 1979; **Medical School:** Albert Einstein Coll Med 1970; **Residencies:** Internal Medicine, NC Meml Hosp-UNC, Chapel Hill, NC 1971-1972; Internal Medicine, Bellevue Hosp Ctr-NYU, New York, NY 1972-1973; **Fellowships:** Psychiatry, Univ Rochester, Rochester, NY 1975-1976; Gastroenterology, NC Meml Hosp-UNC, Chapel, NY 1976-1978; **Faculty Appointment:** Prof Medicine, Univ NC Sch Med

Forsmark, Christopher MD (Gastroenterology) - *Special Expertise: AIDS/HIV-Gastrointestinal Complications; Gastrointestinal Cancer; Pancreatic Cancer;* **Admitting Hospital:** Shands Healthcare at University Florida (Page 77); **Office Address:** University of Florida 1600 SW Archer Rd, Box 100214 Gainesville, FL 32610-0214; **Office Phone:** (352) 392-2877; **Board Certifications:** Internal Medicine 1986, Gastroenterology 1989; **Medical School:** Johns Hopkins Univ 1983; **Residency:** Internal Medicine, Univ Calif-San Fran, San Francisco, CA 1984-1987; **Fellowship:** Gastroenterology, Univ Calif-San Fran, San Francisco, CA 1987-1990; **Faculty Appointment:** Assoc Prof Gastroenterology, Univ Fla Coll Med

Hoffman, Brenda MD (Gastroenterology) - *Special Expertise: Liver & Biliary Disease; Endoscopic Ultrasound;* **Admitting Hospital:** MUSC Medical Center; **Office Address:** Digestive Disease Center 96 Johnathan Lucas St 210 CSB, Box 250327 Charleston, SC 29425-0001; **Office Phone:** (843) 792-7896; **Board Certifications:** Internal Medicine 1986, Gastroenterology 1989; **Medical School:** Univ KY Coll Med 1993; **Residency:** Internal Medicine, MUSC Med Ctr, Charleston, SC 1984-1987; **Fellowship:** Gastroenterology, MUSC Med Ctr, Charleston, SC 1987-1989; **Faculty Appointment:** Asst Prof Medicine, Univ SC Sch Med

Hunter, Ellen B MD (Gastroenterology) - *Special Expertise: Hepatitis;* **Admitting Hospital:** Vanderbilt University Medical Center; **Office Address:** Liver Transplant 801 Oxford House 1312 21 Ave. S Nashville, TN 37232-4753; **Office Phone:** (615) 936-2573; **Board Certifications:** Internal Medicine 1986, Gastroenterology 1989; **Medical School:** Georgetown Univ 1983; **Residency:** Internal Medicine, Vanderbilt University Medical Center, Nashville, TN 1984-1986; **Fellowship:** Gastroenterology, Mayo Clinic, Rochester, MN 1986-1989; **Faculty Appointment:** Asst Prof Medicine, Vanderbilt Univ

Lambiase, Louis MD (Gastroenterology) - *Special Expertise: Pancreatitis;* **Admitting Hospital:** Shands Jacksonville Medical Center; **Office Address:** 653 W 8th St Jacksonville, FL; **Office Phone:** (904) 244-3273; **Board Certifications:** Gastroenterology 1993, Internal Medicine 1990; **Medical School:** Univ Miami Sch Med 1987; **Residency:** Internal Medicine, Univ Pittsburgh-Presby VA, Pittsburgh, PA 1987-1990; **Fellowship:** Gastroenterology, Univ Fla, Gainsville, Fl 1990; **Faculty Appointment:** Assoc Prof Medicine, Univ Fla Coll Med

Liddle, Rodger Alan MD (Gastroenterology) - *Special Expertise: Gastrointestinal Cancer;* **Admitting Hospital:** Duke University Medical Center (Page 60); **Office Address:** Duke Univ Med Ctr, Dept Gastroenterology Box 3913 Durhama, NC 27710; **Office Phone:** (919) 684-5066; **Board Certifications:** Gastroenterology 1983, Internal Medicine 1981; **Medical School:** Vanderbilt Univ 1978; **Residency:** Internal Medicine, UCSF, San Francisco, CA 1979-1981; **Fellowship:** Gastroenterology, UCSF, San Francisco, CA 1981-1984; **Faculty Appointment:** Prof Medicine, Duke Univ

Raiford, David S MD (Gastroenterology) - *Special Expertise:* Liver Disease; Drug Hepatotoxicity; Liver Tumors; **Admitting Hospital:** Vanderbilt University Medical Center; **Office Address:** The Vanderbilt Clinic- GI Div Box 1501 Nashville, TN 37232; **Office Phone:** (615) 322-0128; **Board Certifications:** Gastroenterology 1991, Internal Medicine 1989; **Medical School:** Johns Hopkins Univ 1985; **Residency:** Internal Medicine, Johns Hopkins Hosp, Baltimore, MD 1985-1988; **Faculty Appointment:** Prof Gastroenterology, Vanderbilt Univ

Roche, James Kenneth MD/PhD (Gastroenterology) - *Special Expertise:* Intestinal Chronic Inflammatory Disorder; Diarrhea; **Admitting Hospital:** University of Virginia Health Systems; **Office Address:** Univ VA Hlth Sci Ctr, IM-Div Gastro Bldg MR-4, Box 801317 Charlottesville, VA 22908; **Office Phone:** (804) 243-2655; **Board Certification:** Internal Medicine 1975; **Medical School:** Univ Penn 1969; **Residencies:** Internal Medicine, Univ Hlth Ctr Penn, Pittsburgh, PA 1970-1971; Internal Medicine, Duke Univ Med Ctr, Durham, NC 1973-1974; **Fellowship:** Gastroenterology, Duke Univ Med Ctr, Durham, NC 1974-1977; **Faculty Appointment:** Assoc Prof Gastroenterology, Univ VA Sch Med

Rogers, Arvey MD (Gastroenterology) - *Special Expertise:* Endoscopy; Crohn's Disease; **Admitting Hospital:** University of Miami - Jackson Memorial Hospital; **Office Address:** Univ Miami Hosp and Clinics 1425 NW 12th Ave, Ste D1007 Miami, FL 33136-1002; **Office Phone:** (305) 324-3162; **Board Certification:** Internal Medicine 1965; **Medical School:** Univ Tex Med Br, Galveston 1958; **Residencies:** Internal Medicine, Jackson Meml Hosp, Miami, FL 1959-1962; Gastroenterology, Coral Gables VA Med Ctr, Miami, FL 1962-1964; **Faculty Appointment:** Prof Medicine, Univ Miami Sch Med

Schiff, Eugene MD (Gastroenterology) - *Special Expertise:* Hepatitis; Liver Disease; **Admitting Hospital:** Cedars Medical Center - Miami; **Office Address:** Univ Miami Ctr for Liver Disease 1500 NW 12th Ave, Ste 1101 Miami, FL 33136-3877; **Office Phone:** (305) 243-5787; **Board Certifications:** Internal Medicine 1980, Gastroenterology 1972; **Medical School:** Columbia P&S 1962; **Residencies:** Internal Medicine, Cincinnati Genl Hosp, Cincinati, OH 1963-1964; Internal Medicine, Parkland Meml Hosp, Dallas, TX 1966-1967; **Fellowship:** Gastroenterology, Univ Tex Med Ctr, Dallas, TX 1967-1969; **Faculty Appointment:** Prof Gastroenterology, Univ Miami Sch Med

Scudera, Peter MD (Gastroenterology) - *Special Expertise:* Transplant Medicine-Liver; **Admitting Hospital:** Fairfax Hospital; **Office Address:** 3700 Joseph Siewick Dr, Ste 308 Fairfax, VA 22033-1739; **Office Phone:** (703) 716-8700; **Board Certifications:** Internal Medicine 1987, Gastroenterology 1989; **Medical School:** Cornell Univ-Weil Med Coll 1984; **Residency:** Internal Medicine, New York Hosp-Cornell, New York, NY 1985-1987; **Fellowship:** Gastroenterology, NewYork Hosp-Cornell, New York, NY 1987-1989

Shenk, Ian MD (Gastroenterology) - *Special Expertise:* Irritable Bowel Syndrome; **Admitting Hospital:** Fairfax Hospital; **Office Address:** Gastro Assoc of NVA 3027 Javier Rd Fairfax, VA 22031; **Office Phone:** (703) 435-8535; **Board Certifications:** Internal Medicine 1970, Gastroenterology 1973; **Medical School:** Johns Hopkins Univ 1965; **Residencies:** Internal Medicine, Johns Hopkins Hosp, Baltimore, MD 1965-1967; Surgery, Yale-New Haven Hosp, New Haven, CT 1967-1968

Sninsky, Charles MD (Gastroenterology) - *Special Expertise:* Diabetes- Gastrointestinal Complications; Irritable Bowel Syndrome; **Admitting Hospital:** Vanderbilt University Medical Center; **Office Address:** 1501 The Vanderbilt Clinic Nashville, TN 37232-5280; **Office Phone:** (615) 322-0128; **Board Certifications:** Internal Medicine 1979, Gastroenterology 1983; **Medical School:** Temple Univ 1976; **Residency:** Internal Medicine, Shands Tchg Hosps, Gainesville, FL 1976-1979; **Fellowship:** Gastroenterology, Shands Tchg Hosps, Gainesville, FL 1979; **Faculty Appointment:** Prof Medicine, Vanderbilt Univ

Toskes, Phillip MD (Gastroenterology) - *Special Expertise:* Nutrition; Malabsorption; Pancreatitis; **Admitting Hospital:** Shands Healthcare at University Florida (Page 77); **Office Address:** Univ of Fla 1600 SW Archer Rd Gainesville, FL 32610-0214; **Office Phone:** (352) 392-2877; **Board Certifications:** Internal Medicine 1970, Gastroenterology 1973; **Medical School:** Univ MD Sch Med 1965; **Residency:** Internal Medicine, Univ of Maryland Hosp, Baltimore, MD 1966-1968; **Fellowship:** Gastroenterology, Hosp Univ Penn, Philadelphia, PA 1968-1970; **Faculty Appointment:** Prof Medicine, Univ Fla Coll Med

Midwest

Achkar, Edgar MD (Gastroenterology) - *Special Expertise:* Esophageal Disorders; Motility Disorders; **Admitting Hospital:** Cleveland Clinic Foundation; **Office Address:** 9500 Euclid Ave, rm s40 Cleveland, OH 44195; **Office Phone:** (216) 444-6523; **Board Certifications:** Internal Medicine 1978, Gastroenterology 1979; **Medical School:** France 1964; **Residency:** Internal Medicine, Lahey Clin, Boston, MA 1965-1967; **Fellowships:** Gastroenterology, Lahey Clin, Boston, MA 1967-1968; Gastroenterology, Clevland Clin, Cleveland, OH 1968-1969; **Faculty Appointment:** Asst Prof Medicine, Ohio State Univ

Bacon, Bruce MD (Gastroenterology) - *Special Expertise:* Hepatitis; Hepatic Iron Metabolism; **Admitting Hospital:** St Louis University Hospital; **Office Address:** 3660 Vista Ave St Louis, MO 63110; **Office Phone:** (314) 577-6150; **Board Certifications:** Internal Medicine 1978, Gastroenterology 1983; **Medical School:** Case West Res Univ 1975; **Residency:** Internal Medicine, Metro Genl Hosp, Cleveland, OH 1976-1979; **Fellowship:** Gastroenterology, Metro Genl Hosp, Cleveland, OH 1979-1982; **Faculty Appointment:** Prof Medicine, St Louis Univ

Blei, Andres T MD (Gastroenterology) - *Special Expertise:* Hepatitis C; Liver Disease; **Admitting Hospital:** Northwestern Memorial Hospital; **Office Address:** NW Faculty Foundation 675 N Sinclair, rm 15-, Box 250 Chicago, IL 60611; **Office Phone:** (312) 695-5620; **Board Certifications:** Gastroenterology 1985, Internal Medicine 1981; **Medical School:** Argentina 1973; **Residencies:** Internal Medicine, Police Posadas, Buenos Aires, Argentina 1974-1976; Hepatology, Yale Univ Sch Med, New Haven, CT 1976-1978; **Fellowships:** Gastroenterology, Yale Univ Sch Med, New Haven, CT 1976-1978; Internal Medicine, Univ Chicago Hosp, Chicago, IL 1978-1980; **Faculty Appointment:** Prof Medicine, Northwestern Univ

Bresalier, Robert MD (Gastroenterology) - *Special Expertise:* Gastrointestinal Cancer; Peptic Acid Disorders; **Admitting Hospital:** Henry Ford Health System (Page 62); **Office Address:** Henry Ford Hosp, Dept of Gastro 2799 W Grand Blvd Detroit, MI 48202; **Office Phone:** (313) 876-2600; **Board Certifications:** Internal Medicine 1981, Gastroenterology 1983; **Medical School:** Univ Chicago-Pritzker Sch Med 1978; **Residency:** Internal Medicine, Barnes Hosp-Washington Univ, Saint Louis, MO 1978-1981; **Fellowship:** Gastroenterology, Univ Calif-San Fran, San Francisco, CA 1981-1983; **Faculty Appointment:** Assoc Prof Medicine, Univ Mich Med Sch

Brown, Kimberly A MD (Gastroenterology) - *Special Expertise:* Liver Disease; **Admitting Hospital:** Henry Ford Health System (Page 62); **Office Address:** 2799 W Grand Blvd Gastro k-7 Detroit, MI 48202; **Office Phone:** (313) 916-2393; **Board Certification:** Internal Medicine 1988; **Medical School:** Wayne State Univ 1985; **Residencies:** Internal Medicine, Univ Michigan, Ann Arbor, MI 1985-1988; Internal Medicine, Univ Michigan, Ann Arbor, MI 1988-1989; **Fellowship:** Gastroenterology, Univ Michigan, Ann Arbor, MI 1989-1992

Clouse, Ray Eugene MD (Gastroenterology) - *Special Expertise: Gastroesophageal Reflux; Esophageal Disorders;* **Admitting Hospital:** Barnes - Jewish Hospital; **Office Address:** 4570 Children's Pl St Louis, MO 63110; **Office Phone:** (314) 747-2066; **Board Certification:** Internal Medicine 1979; **Medical School:** Indiana Univ 1976; **Residency:** Internal Medicine, Barnes Hosp/Washington Univ Sch Med, Saint Louis, MO 1976-1978; **Fellowship:** Gastroenterology, Barnes Hosp/Washington Univ Sch Med, Saint Louis, MO 1978-1979; **Faculty Appointment:** Prof Medicine, Washington Univ, St Louis

Craig, Robert M MD (Gastroenterology) - *Special Expertise: Inflammatory Bowel Disease - Crohn's; Gallbladder & Swallowing Disorders; Inflammatory Bowel Disease;* **Admitting Hospital:** Northwestern Memorial Hospital; **Office Address:** 233 E Erie St Ste 206 Chicago, IL 60611; **Office Phone:** (312) 908-9644; **Board Certifications:** Internal Medicine 1972, Gastroenterology 1975; **Medical School:** Northwestern Univ 1967; **Residencies:** Internal Medicine, VA Rsch Hosp, Chicago, IL 1968-1969; Internal Medicine, VA Rsch Hosp, Chicago, IL 1971-1972; **Fellowship:** Gastroenterology, Northwestern U, Chicago, IL 1972-1974; **Faculty Appointment:** Prof Medicine, Northwestern Univ

Di Magno, Eugene MD (Gastroenterology) - *Special Expertise: Pancreatic Disease;* **Admitting Hospital:** Mayo Medical Center & Clinic - Rochester; **Office Address:** Mayo Clinic 200 1st St SW Rochester, MN 55905; **Office Phone:** (507) 255-5713; **Board Certifications:** Gastroenterology 1972, Internal Medicine 1969; **Medical School:** Univ Penn 1962; **Residency:** Internal Medicine, Mayo Grad Sch Med, Rochester, MN 1966-1968; **Fellowship:** Gastroenterology, Mayo Grad Sch Med, Rochester, MN 1968-1970; **Faculty Appointment:** Prof Medicine, Mayo Med Sch

Edmundowicz, Steven MD (Gastroenterology) - *Special Expertise: Endoscopy; Biliary Disease;* **Admitting Hospital:** Barnes - Jewish Hospital; **Office Address:** WUSM 4570 Children's Pl St. Louis, MO 63110; **Office Phone:** (314) 747-2066; **Board Certifications:** Internal Medicine 1986, Gastroenterology 1989; **Medical School:** Jefferson Med Coll 1983; **Residency:** Internal Medicine, Barnes Hosp/Wash Univ, St Louis, MO 1984-1986; **Fellowship:** Gastroenterology, Barnes Hosp/Wash Univ, St Louis, MO 1986; **Faculty Appointment:** Asst Clin Prof Medicine, Jefferson Med Coll

Elliott, David MD (Gastroenterology) - *Special Expertise: Celiac Disease; Inflammatory Bowel Disease; Intestinal Parasites;* **Admitting Hospital:** University of Iowa Hospitals and Clinics; **Office Address:** University of Iowa Hospitals and Clinics 200 Hawkins Dr Iowa City, IA 52242; **Office Phone:** (319) 356-4060; **Board Certifications:** Internal Medicine 1991, Gastroenterology 1993; **Medical School:** Wayne State Univ 1988; **Residency:** Internal Medicine, Johns Hopkins Hosp, Baltimore, MD 1989-1991; **Fellowship:** Gastroenterology, Univ Iowa Hosps, Iowa City, IA 1991; **Faculty Appointment:** Asst Prof Medicine, Univ Iowa Coll Med

Elta, Grace Helen MD (Gastroenterology) - *Special Expertise: Biliary Disease; Inflammatory Bowel Disease;* **Admitting Hospital:** University of Michigan Health Center; **Office Address:** Taubman Hlth Care Ctr 1500 E Medical Ctr Dr, rm 3912 Ann Arbor, MI 48109-0362; **Office Phone:** (888) 229-7408; **Board Certifications:** Gastroenterology 1983, Internal Medicine 1980; **Medical School:** Univ Mich Med Sch 1977; **Residency:** Internal Medicine, Tufts-New England Med Ctr., Boston, MA 1978-1980; **Fellowship:** Gastroenterology, Tufts-New England Med Ctr., Boston, MA 1980-1982; **Faculty Appointment:** Prof Medicine, Univ Mich Med Sch

Gostout, Christopher John MD (Gastroenterology) - *Special Expertise: Gastroscopy;* **Admitting Hospital:** Mayo Medical Center & Clinic - Rochester; **Office Address:** Mayo Clinic 200 First St SW Rochester, MN 55905; **Office Phone:** (507) 284-2141; **Board Certifications:** Internal Medicine 1979, Gastroenterology 1981; **Medical School:** SUNY Downstate 1976; **Residency:** Mayo Grad Sch Med Hosp, Rochester, MN 1977-1979; **Fellowship:** Gastroenterology, Mayo Grad Sch Med Hosp, Rochester, MN 1979-1981

Hanauer, Stephen MD (Gastroenterology) - *Special Expertise: Inflammatory Bowel Disease; Inflammatory Bowel Disease - Crohn's;* **Admitting Hospital:** University of Chicago Hospitals (Page 78); **Office Address:** Univ Chicago Hosps 5758 S Maryland Ave, MC-9028 Chicago, IL 60637; **Office Phone:** (773) 702-1466; **Board Certifications:** Gastroenterology 1983, Internal Medicine 1980; **Medical School:** Univ IL Coll Med 1977; **Residency:** Internal Medicine, Univ Chicago Hosps, Chicago, IL 1978-1980; **Fellowship:** Gastroenterology, Univ Chicago Hosps, Chicago, IL 1980-1982; **Faculty Appointment:** Prof Medicine, Univ Chicago-Pritzker Sch Med

Kahrilas, Peter MD (Gastroenterology) - *Special Expertise: Esophageal Disorders; Swallowing Disorders;* **Admitting Hospital:** Northwestern Memorial Hospital; **Office Address:** 675 N St Claire 17th Floor Ste 250 Chicago, IL 60611; **Office Phone:** (312) 695-0606; **Board Certifications:** Internal Medicine 1982, Gastroenterology 1987; **Medical School:** Univ Rochester 1979; **Residency:** Internal Medicine, Univ Hosp, Cleveland, OH 1979-1982; **Fellowships:** Gastroenterology, Northwestern Univ, Chicago, IL 1982-1984; Research, Med Coll Wisc, Milwaukee, WI 1984-1986; **Faculty Appointment:** Prof Medicine, Northwestern Univ

Klamut, Michael MD (Gastroenterology) - *Special Expertise: Gastroenterology - General;* **Admitting Hospital:** Loyola University Health System; **Office Address:** Loyola Univ 2160 S 1st Avenue, Bldg 117 - Ste 20A Maywood, IL 60153-5500; **Office Phone:** (708) 216-8563; **Board Certification:** Internal Medicine 1976; **Medical School:** Loyola Univ-Stritch Sch Med 1973; **Residency:** Internal Medicine, Loyola Univ Med, Maywood, IL 1974-1976; **Fellowship:** Gastroenterology, Loyola Univ Med, Maywood, IL 1976-1978; **Faculty Appointment:** Assoc Prof Medicine, Loyola Univ-Stritch Sch Med

Konicek, Frank MD (Gastroenterology) - *Special Expertise: Gastroenterology - General;* **Admitting Hospital:** Illinois Masonic Medical Center (Page 64); **Office Address:** Ill Masonic Med Ctr 836 W Wellington, Ste 1423 Chicago, IL 60657-5192; **Office Phone:** (773) 296-7071; **Board Certifications:** Gastroenterology 1975, Internal Medicine 1977; **Medical School:** Loyola Univ-Stritch Sch Med 1963; **Residencies:** Internal Medicine, St Francis, Evanston, IL 1964-1965; Internal Medicine, Hines VA Hosp, Chicago, IL 1967-1969; **Fellowship:** Gastroenterology, Hines VA Hosp, Chicago, IL 1969-1971; **Faculty Appointment:** Medicine, Loyola Univ-Stritch Sch Med

La Russo, Nicholas Francis MD (Gastroenterology) - *Special Expertise: Transplant Medicine-Liver; Liver & Biliary Disease;* **Admitting Hospital:** Mayo Medical Center & Clinic - Rochester; **Office Address:** Mayo Medical Center 200 1st St SW Rochester, MN 55905-0001; **Office Phone:** (507) 284-8700; **Board Certifications:** Gastroenterology 1979, Internal Medicine 1972; **Medical School:** NY Med Coll 1969; **Residency:** Mayo Med Grad Sch., Rochester, MN 1970-1972; **Fellowship:** Gastroenterology, Mayo Med Grad Sch., Rochester, MN 1972-1975; **Faculty Appointment:** Prof Medicine, Mayo Med Sch

Levitan, Ruven MD (Gastroenterology) - *Special Expertise:* Gastroenterology - General; **Admitting Hospital:** Advocate Lutheran General Hospital; **Office Address:** North Shore Gastroenterology 4709 Golf Rd, Ste 1000 Skokie, IL 60076-1260; **Office Phone:** (847) 677-1170; **Board Certifications:** Gastroenterology 1968, Internal Medicine 1980; **Medical School:** Israel 1953; **Residencies:** Internal Medicine, Mount Sinai Med Ctr, New York, NY 1956-1957; Gastroenterology, Beth Israel Med Ctr, Boston, MA 1958-1959; **Fellowship:** Internal Medicine, Mem Sloan Kettering Cancer Ctr, New York, NY 1957-1958; **Faculty Appointment:** Clin Prof Univ Chicago-Pritzker Sch Med

Lindor, Keith Douglas MD (Gastroenterology) - *Special Expertise:* Liver Disease/Biliary Cirrhosis; Sclerosing Cholangitis; **Admitting Hospital:** Mayo Medical Center & Clinic - Rochester; **Office Address:** Mayo Clinic-Div of Gastro and Hepatology 200 1st St SW Rochester, MN 55905; **Office Phone:** (507) 284-2511; **Board Certifications:** Gastroenterology 1987, Internal Medicine 1983; **Medical School:** Mayo Med Sch 1979; **Residency:** Internal Medicine, NC Bapt Hosp, Winston-Salem, NC 1979-1982; **Fellowship:** Gastroenterology, Mayo Clin, Rochester, MN 1983-1986; **Faculty Appointment:** Prof Medicine, Mayo Med Sch

Owyang, Chung MD (Gastroenterology) - *Special Expertise:* Motility Disorders; Digestion; **Admitting Hospital:** University of Michigan Health Center; **Office Address:** 1500 E Medical Ctr. Dr., rm 3912, Box 0362 Taubman Health Care Center Ann Arbor, MI 48109-0362; **Office Phone:** (888) 229-7408; **Board Certifications:** Internal Medicine 1976, Gastroenterology 1981; **Medical School:** McGill Univ 1972; **Residency:** Internal Medicine, Montreal Genl-Hosp, Montreal, CN 1973-1975; **Fellowship:** Gastroenterology, Mayo Grad Sch., Rochester, MN 1975-1978; **Faculty Appointment:** Prof Medicine, Univ Mich Med Sch

Rao, Satish S C MD (Gastroenterology) - *Special Expertise:* Constipation; Incontinence, fecal; Non-Cardiac Chest Pain; **Admitting Hospital:** University of Iowa Hospitals and Clinics; **Office Address:** Univ Iowa Coll Med, Div Gastroenterology 4612 JCP, 200 Hawkins Drive Iowa City, IA 52242; **Office Phone:** (319) 353-6602; **Board Certifications:** Internal Medicine 1996, Gastroenterology 1998; **Medical School:** India 1978; **Residencies:** Internal Medicine, Sunderland Hosps, Sunderland, England 1980-1982; Internal Medicine, York Dist Hosp, York, England 1982-1984; **Fellowships:** Royal Hallamshire Hosp, Sheffield, England 1984-1986; Gastroenterology, Royal Liverpool Hosp, Liverpool, England 1987-1988; **Faculty Appointment:** Assoc Prof Medicine, Univ Iowa Coll Med

Reichelderfer, Mark MD (Gastroenterology) - *Special Expertise:* Endoscopy; **Admitting Hospital:** University of Wisconsin Hospital & Clinics; **Office Address:** Univ Wisc Hosp & Clin 600 Highland Ave, Ste H6 - rm 516 Madison, WI 53792; **Office Phone:** (608) 263-8094; **Board Certifications:** Internal Medicine 1977, Gastroenterology 1979; **Medical School:** Coll Physicians & Surgeons 1974; **Residency:** Internal Medicine, Mary Imogene Bassett Hosp, Cooperstown, NY 1975-1977; **Fellowship:** Gastroenterology, Univ Wisc Hosps & Clin, Madison, WI 1977-1979; **Faculty Appointment:** Prof Medicine, Univ Wisc

Rex, Douglas Kevin MD (Gastroenterology) - *Special Expertise:* Endoscopy; **Admitting Hospital:** Indiana University Hospital & Medical Center - Indianapolis; **Office Address:** University Hosp 550 N University Blvd, Ste 2300 Indianapolis, IN 46202; **Office Phone:** (317) 274-0912; **Board Certifications:** Internal Medicine 1985, Gastroenterology 1987; **Medical School:** Indiana Univ 1980; **Residencies:** Internal Medicine, Indiana Univ Med Ctr, Indianapolis, IN 1981-1982; Internal Medicine, Indiana Univ Hosp, Indianapolis, IN 1984-1985; **Fellowship:** Gastroenterology, Indiana Univ Med Ctr, Indianapolis, IN 1982-1984; **Faculty Appointment:** Assoc Prof Medicine, Indiana Univ

Richter, Joel MD (Gastroenterology) - *Special Expertise:* Gastroesophageal Reflux; *Esophageal Disorders;* **Admitting Hospital:** Cleveland Clinic Foundation; **Office Address:** Cleveland Clinic 9500 Euclid Ave Ste 40 Cleveland, OH 44195; **Office Phone:** (216) 445-9102; **Board Certifications:** Internal Medicine 1978, Gastroenterology 1981; **Medical School:** Univ Tex SW, Dallas 1975; **Residency:** Internal Medicine, Natl Naval Med Ctr, Bethesda, MD 1976-1978; **Fellowship:** Gastroenterology, Natl Naval Med Ctr, Bethesda, MD 1978-1980; **Faculty Appointment:** Prof Medicine, Ohio State Univ

Sandborn, William Jeffery MD (Gastroenterology) - *Special Expertise:* Inflammatory Bowel *Disease; Ulcerative Colitis;* **Admitting Hospital:** Mayo Medical Center & Clinic - Rochester; **Office Address:** Mayo Clinic 200 First St SW Rochester, MN 55905; **Office Phone:** (507) 284-0959; **Board Certifications:** Infectious Disease 1990, Gastroenterology 1993; **Medical School:** Loma Linda Univ 1987; **Residency:** Internal Medicine, Loma Linda U., Loma Linda, CA 1987-1990; **Fellowship:** Gastroenterology, Mayo Clinic, Rochester, MN 1990-1993; **Faculty Appointment:** Assoc Prof Medicine, Mayo Med Sch

Schmidt, Warren Norman MD (Gastroenterology) - *Special Expertise:* Liver Disease; **Admitting Hospital:** University of Iowa Hospitals and Clinics; **Office Address:** U Iowa Hosp & Clin-Div Gastroenterology-Hepatology 200 Hawkins Drive, 4544 JCP Iowa City, IA 52242-1081; **Office Phone:** (319) 353-7048; **Board Certifications:** Internal Medicine 1993, Gastroenterology 1997; **Medical School:** Univ Tenn Coll Med, Memphis 1989; **Residency:** Internal Medicine, U Tenn Ctr Hlth Sci, Memphis, TN 1990-1992; **Fellowship:** Gastroenterology, U Iowa Hosp & Clin, Iowa City, IA 1992

Schulze, Konrad S MD (Gastroenterology) - *Special Expertise:* Reflux Esophagitis; Gastric *Diseases; Gastroparesis;* **Admitting Hospital:** University of Iowa Hospitals and Clinics; **Office Address:** 200 Hawkins Dr Iowa City, IA 52242; **Office Phone:** (319) 356-4060; **Board Certifications:** Internal Medicine 1987, Gastroenterology 1975; **Medical School:** Germany 1968; **Residencies:** Psychiatry, Boston City Hosp, Boston, MA 1970-1971; Internal Medicine, Montreal General Hosp, Montreal, Canada 1971-1974; **Fellowship:** Gastroenterology, Univ IA, Iowa City, IA 1975-1977

Silverman, William Bruce MD (Gastroenterology) - *Special Expertise:* Liver Disease; *Pancreatic/Biliary Disease; Endoscopy(ERCP);* **Admitting Hospital:** University of Iowa Hospitals and Clinics; **Office Address:** Univ Iowa Hospital and Clinics 200 Hawkins Dr Iowa City, IA 52242; **Office Phone:** (319) 384-9995; **Board Certifications:** Internal Medicine 1988, Gastroenterology 2007; **Medical School:** Belgium 1984; **Residency:** Internal Medicine, Lutheran Hosp-Univ Ill, Chicago, IL 1985-1987; **Fellowships:** Gastroenterology, Univ Hosp-Case West Res, Cleveland, OH 1988-1989; Gastroenterology, Univ Brussels, Brussels Belgium 1989-1990; **Faculty Appointment:** Assoc Prof Medicine, Univ Iowa Coll Med

Sivak, Michael MD (Gastroenterology) - *Special Expertise:* Endoscopy; Endoscopic *Ultrasound;* **Admitting Hospital:** University Hospital - Cleveland; **Office Address:** 11100 Euclid Ave Cleveland, OH 44106-5066; **Office Phone:** (216) 844-7344; **Board Certification:** Internal Medicine 1977; **Medical School:** Hahnemann Univ 1969; **Residency:** Internal Medicine, Cleveland Clinic, Cleveland, OH 1970-1972; **Fellowship:** Gastroenterology, Cleveland Clinic, Cleveland, OH 1972-1974; **Faculty Appointment:** Prof Medicine, Case West Res Univ

Tremaine, William John MD (Gastroenterology) - *Special Expertise:* Inflammatory Bowel *Disease - Crohn's; Ulcerative Colitis;* **Admitting Hospital:** Mayo Medical Center & Clinic - Rochester; **Office Address:** Mayo Clinic 200 1st St SW Rochester, MN 55905; **Office Phone:** (507) 284-2469; **Board Certifications:** Internal Medicine 1979, Gastroenterology 1981; **Medical School:** Univ Miss 1976; **Residency:** Internal Medicine, Mayo Clinic, Rochester, MN 1978-1980; **Fellowship:** Gastroenterology, Mayo Clinic, Rochester, MN 1980-1981; **Faculty Appointment:** Assoc Prof Medicine, Mayo Med Sch

Van Thiel, David MD (Gastroenterology) - *Special Expertise: Transplant Medicine-Liver; Hepatitis;* **Admitting Hospital:** Loyola University Health System; **Office Address:** Loyola Univ Med Ctr 2160 S First Ave, Bldg 114 - rm 54 Maywood, IL 60153; **Office Phone:** (708) 216-0364; **Board Certifications:** Internal Medicine 1972, Gastroenterology 1975; **Medical School:** UCLA 1967; **Residencies:** Internal Medicine, NY Hosp, New York, NY 1968-1969; Gastroenterology, Univ Hosp, Boston, MA 1971-1972; **Fellowship:** Gastroenterology, Univ Hosp, Boston, MA 1972-1974; **Faculty Appointment:** Prof Medicine, Loyola Univ-Stritch Sch Med

Winans, Charles MD (Gastroenterology) - *Special Expertise: Esophageal & Swallowing Disorders; Gastroesophageal Reflux;* **Admitting Hospital:** University of Chicago Hospitals (Page 78); **Office Address:** University Chicago Hospitals 5758 S Maryland Ave, MC-9028 Chicago, IL 60637; **Office Phone:** (773) 702-6137; **Board Certifications:** Internal Medicine 1968, Gastroenterology 1970; **Medical School:** Case West Res Univ 1961; **Residency:** Internal Medicine, Univ Hosp Cleveland, Cleveland, OH 1962-1964; **Fellowship:** Gastroenterology, Boston Univ Med Ctr, Boston, MA 1964-1966; **Faculty Appointment:** Prof Medicine, Univ Chicago-Pritzker Sch Med

Great Plains and Mountains

Fitz, John Gregory MD (Gastroenterology) - *Special Expertise: Gastroenterology - General;* **Admitting Hospital:** University of Colorado Health & Science Center; **Office Address:** 4200 E 9th Ave, Box B158 Denver, CO 80262; **Office Phone:** (303) 315-2537; **Board Certifications:** Internal Medicine 1982, Gastroenterology 1985; **Medical School:** Duke Univ 1979; **Residency:** Internal Medicine, Univ Calif, San Francisco, CA 1979-1982; **Fellowship:** Gastroenterology, Univ Calif, San Francisco, CA 1982-1985; **Faculty Appointment:** Prof Gastroenterology, Univ Colo

Sorrell, Michael MD (Gastroenterology) - *Special Expertise: Transplant Medicine-Liver; Hepatitis;* **Admitting Hospital:** University of Nebraska Medical Center; **Office Address:** Univ Nebr Med Ctr 600 S 42nd St Omaha, NE 68198-3285; **Office Phone:** (402) 559-7912; **Board Certification:** Internal Medicine 1972; **Medical School:** Univ Nebr Coll Med 1959; **Residencies:** Internal Medicine, Univ Nebr Hosp, Omaha, NE 1966-1968; Gastroenterology, Univ Nebr Hosp, Omaha, NE 1968-1969; **Faculty Appointment:** Prof Medicine, Univ Nebr Coll Med

Southwest

Anderson, Karl MD (Gastroenterology) - *Special Expertise: Porphyria;* **Admitting Hospital:** University of Texas Medical Branch Hospitals at Galveston; **Office Address:** Univ Tex Med Br-Ewing Hall 700 Harborside Dr Galveston, TX 77555-1109; **Office Phone:** (409) 772-4661; **Board Certifications:** Internal Medicine 1972, Gastroenterology 1972; **Medical School:** Johns Hopkins Univ 1965; **Residencies:** Internal Medicine, Vanderbilt U Hosp, Nashville, TN 1966-1967; Internal Medicine, NY Hosp-Cornell Med Ctr, New York, NY 1967-1968; **Fellowship:** Gastroenterology, NY Hosp-Cornell Med Ctr, New York, NY 1968-1970; **Faculty Appointment:** Prof Medicine, Univ Tex Med Br, Galveston

Brady III, Charles Elmer MD (Gastroenterology) - *Special Expertise: Esophageal Disorders;* **Admitting Hospital:** University of Texas Health & Science Center; **Office Address:** Univ Texas, Dept Med/GI (MC7878) 7703 Floyd Curl Dr San Antonio, TX 78229-3900; **Office Phone:** (210) 567-4876; **Board Certifications:** Gastroenterology 1977, Internal Medicine 1974; **Medical School:** Med Coll VA 1971; **Residency:** Internal Medicine, Wilford Hall Med Ctr, Lackland AFB, TX 1972-1974; **Fellowship:** Gastroenterology, Univ Tex, Dallas, TX 1974-1976; **Faculty Appointment:** Assoc Prof Medicine, Univ Tex, San Antonio

Feldman, Mark MD (Gastroenterology) - *Special Expertise:* Peptic Acid Disorders; **Admitting Hospital:** VA Medical Center - Dallas; **Office Address:** 4500 S Lancaster Rd #111 Dallas, TX 75216-7256; **Office Phone:** (214) 376-9500; **Board Certifications:** Internal Medicine 1976, Gastroenterology 1989; **Medical School:** Temple Univ 1972; **Residency:** Internal Medicine, Temple Univ, Philadelphia, PA 1972-1977; **Fellowship:** Gastroenterology, Univ SW Texas, Dallas, TX 1975-1976; **Faculty Appointment:** Prof Medicine, Univ Tex SW, Dallas

Fordtran, John MD (Gastroenterology) - *Special Expertise:* Malabsorption; Diarrhea; **Admitting Hospital:** Baylor University Medical Center; **Office Address:** Baylor Univ Med Ctr, Dept Med 3500 Gaston Ave Dallas, TX 75246; **Office Phone:** (214) 820-2672; **Medical School:** Tulane Univ 1956; **Residency:** Internal Medicine, Parkland Hosp, Dallas, TX 1956-1958; **Fellowship:** Gastroenterology, Mass Meml Hosp, Boston, MA 1960-1962

Galati, Joseph Steven MD (Gastroenterology) - *Special Expertise:* Liver Disease; Transplant Medicine-Liver; **Admitting Hospital:** St Luke's Episcopal Hospital - Houston (Page 76); **Office Address:** Gastroenterology & Liver Assocs 1200 Binz, Ste 480 Houston, TX 77004; **Office Phone:** (713) 521-0039; **Board Certifications:** Gastroenterology 1995, Internal Medicine 1990; **Medical School:** Grenada 1987; **Residencies:** Internal Medicine, SUNY Hlth Sci Ctr-Kings Co, Brooklyn, NY 1988-1990; Internal Medicine, SUNY Hlth Sci Ctr-Kings Co, Brooklyn, NY 1990-1991; **Fellowship:** Gastroenterology, Univ Nebraska, Omaha, NE 1991-1994

Glombicki, Alan Paul MD (Gastroenterology) - *Special Expertise:* Hepatitis - Antiviral Therapy; Transplant Medicine-Liver; **Admitting Hospital:** St Luke's Episcopal Hospital - Houston (Page 76); **Office Address:** 7737 SW Freeway, Ste 840 Hosuton, TX 77074; **Office Phone:** (713) 777-2555; **Board Certifications:** Internal Medicine 1986, Gastroenterology 1987; **Medical School:** Univ IL Coll Med 1981; **Residencies:** Internal Medicine, Baylor Coll Med, Houston, TX 1982-1984; Hepatology, Baylor Coll Med, Houston, TX 1986-1987; **Fellowship:** Gastroenterology, Baylor Coll Med, Houston, TX 1984-1986; **Faculty Appointment:** Asst Clin Prof Medicine, Univ Tex, Houston

Hodges, David S MD (Gastroenterology) - *Special Expertise:* Inflammatory Bowel Disease; **Admitting Hospital:** University Medical Center; **Office Address:** Med Office Plaza 3502 9th St Lubbock, TX 79415; **Office Phone:** (806) 743-3085; **Board Certifications:** Internal Medicine 1986, Gastroenterology 1989; **Medical School:** Texas Tech Univ 1983; **Residency:** Internal Medicine, Lubbock Genl Hosp, Lubbock, TX 1983-1986; **Fellowship:** Gastroenterology, Lubbock Genl Hosp, Lubbock, TX 1987-1989; **Faculty Appointment:** Assoc Prof Medicine, Texas Tech Univ

Levin, Bernard MD (Gastroenterology) - *Special Expertise:* Gastrointestinal Cancer; Colorectal Cancer; **Admitting Hospital:** University of Texas MD Anderson Cancer Center (Page 66); **Office Address:** UT MD Anderson Cancer Ctr 1515 Holcombe Blvd, Box 0203 Houston, TX 77030-4095; **Office Phone:** (713) 792-3900; **Board Certifications:** Internal Medicine 1972, Gastroenterology 1972; **Medical School:** South Africa 1964; **Residency:** Internal Medicine, Rush Presby-St Lukes Hosp, Chicago, IL 1966-1968; **Fellowships:** Pathology, Univ Chicago, Chicago, IL 1968-1970; Gastroenterology, Univ Chicago, Chicago, IL 1970-1972; **Faculty Appointment:** Prof Emeritus Medicine, Univ Tex, Houston

Maddrey, Willis Crocker MD (Gastroenterology) - *Special Expertise:* Hepatitis C & B; Liver Disease - Drug Induced; **Admitting Hospital:** Zale Lipshy University Hospital; **Office Address:** Univ Tex SW Med Ctr 5323 Harry Hines Blvd Dallas, TX 75235-8570; **Office Phone:** (214) 648-2024; **Board Certification:** Internal Medicine 1971; **Medical School:** Johns Hopkins Univ 1964; **Residencies:** Internal Medicine, Johns Hopkins Hosp, Baltimore, MD 1968-1970; Internal Medicine, Johns Hopkins Hosp, Baltimore, MD 1965-1966; **Fellowship:** Hepatology, Yale, New Haven, CT 1970-1971; **Faculty Appointment:** Prof Medicine, Univ Tex SW, Dallas

Speeg, Kermit Vincent MD/PhD (Gastroenterology) - *Special Expertise:* Transplant Medicine-Liver; **Admitting Hospital:** Southwest Texas Methodist Hospital; **Office Address:** SW Tex Meth Hosp, Dept Med 7703 Floyd Curl Dr, MC-7878 San Antonio, TX 78299-3900; **Office Phone:** (210) 567-4882; **Board Certification:** Internal Medicine 1976; **Medical School:** Univ Tex SW, Dallas 1972; **Residency:** Internal Medicine, Vanderbilt Univ Hosp, Nashville, TN 1973-1974; **Fellowship:** Gastroenterology, Vanderbilt Univ Hosp, Nashville, TN 1976-1977; **Faculty Appointment:** Prof Medicine, Univ Tex, San Antonio

West Coast and Pacific

Cello, John Patrick MD (Gastroenterology) - *Special Expertise:* Gastroenterology - General; **Admitting Hospital:** University of California - San Francisco Medical Center; **Office Address:** San Francisco Genl Hosp, Div GI 1001 Potrero Ave San Francisco, CA 94110; **Office Phone:** (415) 206-4767; **Board Certifications:** Internal Medicine 1972, Gastroenterology 1977; **Medical School:** UCSF 1969; **Residency:** Internal Medicine, Peter Bent Brigham Hosp, Boston, MA 1970-1972; **Fellowship:** Gastroenterology, UC San Francisco, San Francisco, CA 1975-1977; **Faculty Appointment:** Prof Surgery, UCSF

Ellis, Jonathan C MD (Gastroenterology) - *Special Expertise:* Gastroenterology - General; **Admitting Hospital:** Cedars-Sinai Medical Center; **Office Address:** Gastro Med Group 8631 W Third St, Ste 540E Los Angeles, CA 90048; **Office Phone:** (310) 659-9600; **Board Certifications:** Internal Medicine 1985, Gastroenterology 1989; **Medical School:** Stanford Univ 1982; **Residencies:** Internal Medicine, Cedars Sinai Med Ctr, Los Angeles, CA 1983-1985; Internal Medicine, Cedars Sinai Med Ctr, Los Angeles, CA 1985-1986; **Fellowship:** Gastroenterology, Harbor UCLA, Torrance, CA 1986-1988

Keeffe, Emmet B MD (Gastroenterology) - *Special Expertise:* Hepatitis - Antiviral Therapy; Liver Disease; **Admitting Hospital:** Stanford Medical Center; **Office Address:** 750 Welch Rd, Ste 210 Palo Alto, CA 94304; **Office Phone:** (650) 498-5691; **Board Certifications:** Gastroenterology 1975, Internal Medicine 1972; **Medical School:** Creighton Univ 1969; **Residencies:** Internal Medicine, Oreg Hlth Sci Univ, Portland, OR 1972-1973; Internal Medicine, Oreg Hlth Sci Univ, Portland, OR 1970-1972; **Fellowships:** Gastroenterology, Oreg Hlth Sci, Portland, OR 1973-1974; Gastroenterology, UnivU Calif San Francisco, San Francisco, CA 1977-1979; **Faculty Appointment:** Prof Medicine, Stanford Univ

Kimmey, Michael Bryant MD (Gastroenterology) - *Special Expertise:* ERCP-Biliary Endoscopy; Endoscopy; **Admitting Hospital:** University of Washington Medical Center; **Office Address:** Univ WA Div GE-Box 356424 Seattle, WA 98195; **Office Phone:** (206) 543-4404; **Board Certifications:** Internal Medicine 1982, Gastroenterology 1987; **Medical School:** Washington Univ, St Louis 1979; **Residency:** Internal Medicine, Univ Wash, Seattle, WA 1980-1982; **Fellowship:** Gastroenterology, Univ Wash, Seattle, WA 1984-1987; **Faculty Appointment:** Prof Medicine, Univ Wash

Kozarek, Richard MD (Gastroenterology) - *Special Expertise:* Endoscopy; **Admitting Hospital:** Virginia Mason Medical Center; **Office Address:** 1100 9th Ave Seattle, WA 98101-2756; **Office Phone:** (206) 223-6939; **Board Certifications:** Internal Medicine 1977, Gastroenterology 1979; **Medical School:** Univ Wisc 1973; **Residency:** Internal Medicine, Good Samaritan Hosp, Phoenix, AZ 1974-1976; **Fellowship:** Gastroenterology, Univ Arizona VA Hosp, Phoenix, AZ 1976-1978; **Faculty Appointment:** Clin Prof Medicine, Univ Wash

Martin, Paul MD (Gastroenterology) - *Special Expertise:* *Liver Disease;* **Admitting Hospital:** Cedars-Sinai Medical Center; **Office Address:** 8635 W Third Street Ste 590 West Los Angeles, CA 90048; **Office Phone:** (310) 423-2641; **Board Certifications:** Internal Medicine 1984, Gastroenterology 1987; **Medical School:** Ireland 1978; **Residencies:** Internal Medicine, St Vincent's Hosp, Dublin, Ireland 1979-1982; Internal Medicine, Univ of Alberta, Edmonton Alberta, Canada 1982-1984; **Fellowships:** Gastroenterology, Queen Univ, Ontario, Canada 1984-1986; Hepatology, NIH, Bethesda, MD 1987-1989; **Faculty Appointment:** Assoc Prof Medicine, UCLA

Ostroff, James Warren MD (Gastroenterology) - *Special Expertise:* *Pancreatic/Biliary Disease; Endoscopy(ERCP); Colonoscopy;* **Admitting Hospital:** University of California - San Francisco Medical Center; **Office Address:** 350 Parnassus Ave, Ste 410 San Francisco, CA 94117; **Office Phone:** (415) 502-2112; **Board Certifications:** Internal Medicine 1980, Gastroenterology 1983; **Medical School:** Cornell Univ-Weil Med Coll 1977; **Residency:** Internal Medicine, New York Hospital-Cornell Med, New York, NY 1978-1980; **Fellowship:** Gastroenterology, UCSF, Hospitals, San Francisco, CA 1980-1982; **Faculty Appointment:** Clin Prof Medicine, UCSF

Pimstone, Neville R MD (Gastroenterology) - *Special Expertise:* *Porphyria; Hepatitis C;* **Admitting Hospital:** University of California - Davis Medical Center; **Office Address:** UC Davis Med Ctr 4150 V St, Ste 3500 Sacramento, CA 95817; **Office Phone:** (916) 734-3751; **Medical School:** South Africa 1960; **Residency:** Gastroenterology, Moffit Hosp- Univ Ca, San Francisco, CA; **Faculty Appointment:** Prof Medicine, UC Davis

Surawicz, Christina MD (Gastroenterology) - *Special Expertise:* *Clostridium Difficile Disease;* **Admitting Hospital:** University of Washington Medical Center; **Office Address:** Harborview Medical Center 325 9th Ave, Box 359773 Seattle, WA 98104; **Office Phone:** (206) 731-5917; **Board Certifications:** Internal Medicine 1976, Gastroenterology 1979; **Medical School:** Univ KY Coll Med 1973; **Residency:** Internal Medicine, U Washington Med Ctr, Seattle, WA 1973-1976; **Fellowship:** Gastroenterology, U Washington Med Ctr, Seattle, WA 1976-1979; **Faculty Appointment:** Prof Medicine, Univ Wash

Targan, Stephan Raoul MD (Gastroenterology) - *Special Expertise:* *Inflammatory Bowel Disease; Crohn's Disease;* **Admitting Hospital:** Cedars-Sinai Medical Center; **Office Address:** Cedars-Sinai IBD Center 8631 W Third St, Ste 430E Los Angeles, CA 90048; **Office Phone:** (310) 423-4100; **Board Certifications:** Infectious Disease 1976, Gastroenterology 1979; **Medical School:** Johns Hopkins Univ 1971; **Residency:** Internal Medicine, Harbor-UCLA Med Ctr, Torrance, CA 1971-1976; **Fellowships:** Infectious Disease, Harbor-UCLA Med Ctr, Torrance, CA 1975-1976; Gastroenterology, UCLA Med Ctr, Los Angeles, CA 1976-1978; **Faculty Appointment:** Prof Gastroenterology, UCLA

Vierling, John Moore MD (Gastroenterology) - *Special Expertise:* *Liver Disease; Transplant Medicine-Liver;* **Admitting Hospital:** Cedars-Sinai Medical Center; **Office Address:** 8635 W 3rd St #590W Los Angeles, CA 90048; **Office Phone:** (310) 423-6140; **Board Certifications:** Internal Medicine 1975, Gastroenterology 1979; **Medical School:** Stanford Univ 1972; **Residencies:** Internal Medicine, Strong Meml Hosp, Rochester, NY 1973-1974; Hepatology, NIH-Liver Unit, Bethesda, MD 1974-1977; **Fellowship:** Gastroenterology, UCSF Med Ctr, San Francisco, CA 1977-1978

GERIATRIC MEDICINE

(a subspecialty of INTERNAL MEDICINE or FAMILY PRACTICE)

An internist with special knowledge of the aging process and special skills in the diagnostic, therapeutic, preventive and rehabilitative aspects of illness in the elderly. This specialist cares for geriatric patients in the patient's home, the office, long-term care settings such as nursing homes and the hospital.

INTERNAL MEDICINE

An internist is a personal physician who provides long-term, comprehensive care in the office and the hospital, managing both common and complex illness of adolescents, adults and the elderly. Internists are trained in the diagnosis and treatment of cancer, infections and diseases affecting the heart, blood, kidneys, joints and digestive, respiratory and vascular systems. They are also trained in the essentials of primary care internal medicine which incorporates an understanding of disease prevention, wellness, substance abuse, mental health and effective treatment of common problems of the eyes, ears, skin, nervous system and reproductive organs.

FAMILY PRACTICE

A family physician is concerned with the total healthcare of the individual and the family, and is trained to diagnose and treat a wide variety of ailments in patients of all ages. The family physician receives a broad range of training that includes internal medicine, pediatrics, obstetrics and gynecology, psychiatry and geriatrics. Special emphasis is placed on prevention and the primary care of entire families, utilizing consultations and community resources when appropriate.

Training required: Three years in internal medicine or family pratice *plus* additional training and examination for certification in geriatric medicine.

Geriatrics

Together, the geriatricians of Mount Sinai and of NYU Hospitals Center are working hard to improve life and longevity for New York's elderly. Both hospitals offer unparalleled inpatient and out-patient care and numerous treatment programs designed to meet the unique needs of older adults. And both hospitals are home to the world-class researchers dedicated to advancing our understanding of Alzheimer's disease. By fostering an environment of mutual respect and contant consultation between physicians and researchers, both The Mount Sinai Hospital and NYU Hospitals Center are able to give patients an unsurpassed understanding of the illnesses they face and with it the most advanced care available anywhere.

The Mount Sinai Hospital has long been a pioneer in geriatric medicine. A Mount Sinai physician coined the term "geriatrics" in 1909 and wrote the first textbook on medical care for older adults in 1914. Today, Mount Sinai offers comprehensive care, disease prevention and health promotion with a focus on healthy and productive aging. It offers the full spectrum of patient care, including a specialized care unit for the elderly (to minimize complications sometimes associated with an older person's hospital stay); the Orthopaedic-Geriatric Service, dedicated to the prevention and treatment of bone fractures; the Geriatrics Home Medical Program, which provides optimal care for homebound older adults; and a Palliative Care team dedicated to assuring quality end-of-life care. In addition, Mount Sinai's National-Institute-on-Aging-Sponsored researchers continue to break ground in the understanding, prevention and treatment of age-related disorders.

NYU Hospitals Center has a similar history of distinction. The William and Sylvia Silberstein Aging and Dementia Research Center is one of the oldest and largest aging and dementia centers in the nation. It is a National-Institute-on-Aging-designated Center of Excellence devoted to the diagnosis and treatment of Alzheimer's disease. Established in 1973, the center provides comprehensive diagnostic evaluations to determine if memory loss is "normal" or more serious; a memory enhancement program for age-related memory decline; pharmaceutical clinical trials for mild memory loss and for Alzheimer's treatment; state-of-the-art brain imaging techniques; methods to prevent excess disability in Alzheimer's disease patients; and comprehensive, on-going counseling and support groups for patients, caregivers and family members. Its longitudinal study of Alzheimer's patients is the most comprehensive, ongoing study of its kind.

In recognition of the care offered to older patients, Mount Sinai NYU Health specialists are cited time and time again as the finest in the nation. U.S. News & World Reports has consistently ranked The Mount Sinai Hospital as number one in New York for geriatric care. And the pioneering longitudinal Alzheimer's study currently underway at NYU Hospitals Center is the first and most comprehensive in the world.

800-MD-YOURS
(800-639-6877)
www.msnyuhealth.org

MOUNT SINAI NYU
HEALTH

PHYSICIAN LISTINGS

New England

Cooney, Leo MD (Geriatric Medicine) - *Special Expertise:* Geriatric Medicine - General; **Admitting Hospital:** Yale - New Haven Hospital; **Office Address:** 20 York St, Ste TMP17 New Haven, CT 06504; **Office Phone:** (203) 785-2204; **Board Certifications:** Rheumatology 1978, Geriatric Medicine 1988; **Medical School:** Yale Univ 1969; **Residencies:** Internal Medicine, Boston City Hosp, Boston, MA 1970-1971; Internal Medicine, Boston City Hosp, Boston, MA 1973-1974; **Fellowship:** Rheumatology, Boston Med Ctr, Boston, MA 1974-1975; **Faculty Appointment:** Prof Medicine

Lipsitz, Lewis Arnold MD (Geriatric Medicine) - *Special Expertise:* Falls; Fainting; **Admitting Hospital:** Hebrew Rehabilitation Center for the Aged; **Office Address:** 1200 Center St Roslindale, MA 02131; **Office Phone:** (617) 363-8293; **Board Certifications:** Internal Medicine 1980, Geriatric Medicine 2009; **Medical School:** Univ Penn 1977; **Residency:** Internal Medicine, Beth Israel Hosp, Boston, MA 1978-1980; **Fellowship:** Geriatric Medicine, Harvard, New Haven, CT 1980-1983; **Faculty Appointment:** Prof Medicine, Harvard Med Sch

Minaker, Kenneth MD (Geriatric Medicine) - *Special Expertise:* Aging; Neuroendocrine Disease; Cardiovascular Disease; **Admitting Hospital:** Massachusetts General Hospital; **Office Address:** Beacon Hill Senior Health 100 Charles River Plaza Boston, MA 02114; **Office Phone:** (617) 726-4600; **Board Certifications:** Internal Medicine 1979, Geriatric Medicine 1985; **Medical School:** Univ Toronto 1972; **Residency:** Internal Medicine, Univ Toronto, Canada 1979; **Fellowship:** Geriatric Medicine, Mass Gen Hosp-Harvard, Boston, MA 1982

Resnick, Neil M. MD (Geriatric Medicine) - *Special Expertise:* Voiding Dysfunction; **Admitting Hospital:** Brigham & Women's Hospital; **Office Address:** Brigham & Womens Hosp 75 Francis St Boston, MA 02115; **Office Phone:** (617) 732-6844; **Board Certifications:** Internal Medicine 1980, Geriatric Medicine 1988; **Medical School:** Stanford Univ 1977; **Residency:** Infectious Disease, Beth Israel Hosp, Boston, MA 1978-1980; **Fellowships:** Geriatric Medicine, Harvard, Boston, MA 1980-1982; Urology, Harvard, Boston, MA 1982-1984; **Faculty Appointment:** Assoc Prof Medicine, Harvard Med Sch

Tinetti, Mary MD (Geriatric Medicine) - *Special Expertise:* Fall Injuries; **Admitting Hospital:** Yale - New Haven Hospital; **Office Address:** Adler Geriatric Assessment Ctr 789 Howard Ave, Box 208025 New Haven, CT 06519; **Office Phone:** (203) 688-6361; **Board Certifications:** Geriatric Medicine 1988, Internal Medicine 1981; **Medical School:** Univ Mich Med Sch 1978; **Residency:** Internal Medicine, Univ Minnesota, Minneapolis, MN 1978-1981; **Fellowship:** Geriatric Medicine, Univ Rochester, Rochester, NY 1981-1984; **Faculty Appointment:** Prof Medicine, Yale Univ

Mid Atlantic

Bennett, Richard Gordan MD (Geriatric Medicine) - *Special Expertise:* Geriatric Medicine - General; **Admitting Hospital:** Johns Hopkins Hospital - Baltimore (Page 65); **Office Address:** 5505 Hopkins Bayview Rd Baltimore, MD 21224; **Office Phone:** (410) 550-0781; **Board Certifications:** Internal Medicine 1985, Geriatric Medicine 1998; **Medical School:** Johns Hopkins Univ 1982; **Residency:** Internal Medicine, Johns Hopkins Hosp, Baltimore, MD 1983-1985; **Fellowship:** Geriatric Medicine, Johns Hopkins Hosp, Baltimore, MD 1985-1987; **Faculty Appointment:** Assoc Prof Medicine, Johns Hopkins Univ

GERIATRIC MEDICINE

Blass, John MD/PhD (Geriatric Medicine) - *Special Expertise:* *Alzheimer's Disease;* *Dementia;* **Admitting Hospital:** Burke Rehabilitation Hospital; **Office Address:** Burke Rehabilitation Hospital & Research Inst 785 Mamaroneck Ave White Plains, NY 10605-2523; **Office Phone:** (914) 597-2359; **Medical School:** Colombia 1965; **Residencies:** Internal Medicine, Mass Gen Hosp, Boston, MA 1965-1967; Nat Heart Inst-NIH, Bethesda, MD 1967-1970; **Faculty Appointment:** Prof Neurology, Cornell Univ-Weil Med Coll

Bloom, Harrison MD (Geriatric Medicine) - *Special Expertise:* *Dementia;* **Admitting Hospital:** Mount Sinai Hospital (Page 70); **Office Address:** Mt Sinai Med Ctr, Dept of Geriatrics 1424 Madison Ave New York, NY 10029; **Office Phone:** (212) 824-7646; **Board Certifications:** Internal Medicine 1978, Geriatric Medicine 1988; **Medical School:** Univ Minn 1975; **Residency:** Internal Medicine, Montefiore Med Ctr, Bronx, NY 1976-1978; **Faculty Appointment:** Assoc Clin Prof Medicine, Albert Einstein Coll Med

Bloom, Patricia MD (Geriatric Medicine) - *Special Expertise:* *Dementia;* **Admitting Hospital:** St Luke's - Roosevelt Hospital Center - Roosevelt Division (Page 58); **Office Address:** University Medical Practice Associates 190 Amsterdam Blvd New York, NY 10025; **Office Phone:** (646) 375-0486; **Board Certifications:** Internal Medicine 1978, Geriatric Medicine 1988; **Medical School:** Univ Minn 1975; **Residency:** Internal Medicine, Montefiore Hosp, Bronx, NY 1975-1978; **Faculty Appointment:** Assoc Clin Prof Medicine, Columbia P&S

Burton, John Russell MD (Geriatric Medicine) - *Special Expertise:* *Geriatric Medicine - General;* **Admitting Hospital:** Johns Hopkins Hospital - Baltimore (Page 65); **Office Address:** Johns Hopkins Geriatric Ctr 5505 Hopkins Bayview Cir Baltimore, MD 21224-6821; **Office Phone:** (410) 550-0520; **Board Certifications:** Internal Medicine 1980, Geriatric Medicine 1990; **Medical School:** McGill Univ 1965; **Residencies:** Internal Medicine, Baltimore City Hosp, Baltimore, MD 1969-1970; Internal Medicine, Baltimore City Hosp, Baltimore, MD 1970-1971; **Fellowship:** Nephrology, Mass Genl Hosp, Boston, MA 1971-1972; **Faculty Appointment:** Prof Medicine, Johns Hopkins Univ

Cassel, Christine MD (Geriatric Medicine) - *Special Expertise:* *Geriatric Medicine - General;* **Admitting Hospital:** Mount Sinai Hospital (Page 70); **Office Address:** Mount Sinai Hospital, Dept of Geriatrics & Adult Development 1 Gustave Levy Pl New York, NY 10029; **Office Phone:** (212) 241-4840; **Board Certifications:** Internal Medicine 1979, Geriatric Medicine 1998; **Medical School:** Univ Mass Sch Med 1976; **Residencies:** Internal Medicine, Children's Hosp, San Francisco, CA 1977-1979; Internal Medicine, UC San Francisco Med Ctr, San Francisco, CA 1978-1979; **Fellowship:** Geriatric Medicine, Portland VA Hosp, Portland, OR 1979-1981; **Faculty Appointment:** Prof Geriatric Medicine, Mount Sinai Sch Med

Freedman, Michael L MD (Geriatric Medicine) - *Special Expertise:* *Alzheimer's Disease;* **Admitting Hospital:** NYU Medical Center (Page 70); **Office Address:** 530 First Ave, Ste 4J New York, NY 10016; **Office Phone:** (212) 263-7043; **Board Certifications:** Hematology 1972, Geriatric Medicine 1988; **Medical School:** Tufts Univ 1963; **Residencies:** Internal Medicine, Bellevue Hosp, New York, NY 1964-1965; Internal Medicine, Bellevue Hosp, New York, NY 1968-1969; **Fellowship:** Hematology, Natl Inst Hlth-NCI, Bethesda, MD 1965-1968; **Faculty Appointment:** Prof Medicine, NYU Sch Med

Gambert, Steven MD (Geriatric Medicine) - *Special Expertise:* *Endocrinology; Aging;* **Admitting Hospital:** Sinai Hospital - Baltimore; **Office Address:** Sinai Hosp Baltimore, Hoffberger Bldg 2401 W Belvedere Ave, Ste 56 Baltimore, MD 21215; **Office Phone:** (410) 601-6340; **Board Certifications:** Internal Medicine 1978, Geriatric Medicine 1988; **Medical School:** Columbia P&S 1975; **Residency:** Internal Medicine, Dartmouth Affl Hosp, Lebanon, NH 1975-1977; **Fellowship:** Geriatric Medicine, Harvard/Beth Israel Med Ctr, Boston, MA 1977-1979; **Faculty Appointment:** Prof Medicine, Johns Hopkins Univ

Libow, Leslie MD (Geriatric Medicine) - *Special Expertise:* Geriatric Medicine - General; **Admitting Hospital:** Mount Sinai Hospital (Page 70); **Office Address:** Mount Sinai Hospital 1 Gustave Levy Pl, Box 1070 New York, NY 10029; **Office Phone:** (212) 824-7646; **Board Certifications:** Internal Medicine 1977, Geriatric Medicine 1988; **Medical School:** Univ Hlth Sci/Chicago Med Sch 1958; **Residencies:** Internal Medicine, Bronx VA Hosp, Bronx, NY 1959-1960; Internal Medicine, Mt Sinai Hosp, New York, NY 1963-1964; **Faculty Appointment:** Prof Geriatric Medicine, Mount Sinai Sch Med

Meier, Diane MD (Geriatric Medicine) - *Special Expertise:* Geriatric Medicine - General; **Admitting Hospital:** Mount Sinai Hospital (Page 70); **Office Address:** 5 E 98th St, Bldg FL 5 New York, NY 10029; **Office Phone:** (212) 241-8258; **Board Certifications:** Internal Medicine 1981, Geriatric Medicine 1999; **Medical School:** Northwestern Univ 1977; **Residency:** Internal Medicine, Oregon Hlth Sci Univ, Portland, OR 1981; **Fellowship:** Geriatric Medicine, VA Med Ctr/nyu/bellevue, Portland, OR 1983; **Faculty Appointment:** Prof Geriatric Medicine, Mount Sinai Sch Med

Paris, Barbara MD (Geriatric Medicine) - *Special Expertise:* Geriatric Medicine - General; **Admitting Hospital:** Mount Sinai Hospital (Page 70); **Office Address:** Mount Sinai Hosp One Gustave Levy L Pl, Box 1070 New York, NY 10029-6574; **Office Phone:** (212) 241-1305; **Board Certifications:** Geriatric Medicine 1998, Internal Medicine 1982; **Medical School:** SUNY Downstate 1977; **Residency:** Internal Medicine, St Vincents Hosp, New York, NY 1978-1981; **Fellowship:** Geriatric Medicine, Mount Sinai Hosp, New York, NY 1983-1986; **Faculty Appointment:** Assoc Clin Prof Geriatric Medicine, Mount Sinai Sch Med

Southeast

Applegate, William MD (Geriatric Medicine) - *Special Expertise:* Hypertension; **Admitting Hospital:** Wake Forest University Baptist Medical Center; **Office Address:** Wake Forest Univ Baptist Med Ctr Medical Center Blvd Winston-Salem, NC 27157; **Office Phone:** (336) 716-2020; **Board Certifications:** Internal Medicine 1976, Geriatric Medicine 1988; **Medical School:** Univ Louisville Sch Med 1972; **Residencies:** Internal Medicine, Boston City, Boston, MA 1973-1975; Internal Medicine, NC Meml Hosp, Chapel Hill, NC 1975-1977; **Faculty Appointment:** Prof Medicine, Wake Forest Univ Sch Med

Ciocon, Jerry MD (Geriatric Medicine) - *Special Expertise:* Geriatric Medicine - General; **Admitting Hospital:** Cleveland Clinic Florida; **Office Address:** Cleveland Clinic Florida 2900 W Cypress Creek Rd Fort Lauderdale, FL 33309-1743; **Office Phone:** (954) 978-5153; **Board Certifications:** Internal Medicine 1985, Geriatric Medicine 1990; **Medical School:** Philippines 1980; **Residency:** Internal Medicine, Mercy Hosp, Buffalo, NY 1983-1985; **Fellowship:** Geriatric Medicine, LI Jewish Med Ctr, New Hyde Park, NY 1985-1987; **Faculty Appointment:** Asst Prof Medicine, Univ Nebr Coll Med

Cohen, Harvey MD (Geriatric Medicine) - *Special Expertise:* Oncology; **Admitting Hospital:** Duke University Medical Center (Page 60); **Office Address:** Ctr for Study of Aging & Human Development Box 3003 Durham, NC 27710; **Office Phone:** (919) 660-7502; **Board Certifications:** Internal Medicine 1972, Hematology 1972; **Medical School:** SUNY Downstate 1965; **Residency:** Internal Medicine, Duke Univ Med Ctr, Durham, NC 1966-1967; **Fellowships:** Hematology, Duke Univ Med Ctr, Durham, NC 1969-1971; Medical Oncology, Duke Univ Med Ctr, Durham, NC 1969-1971; **Faculty Appointment:** Prof Medicine, Duke Univ

Greganti, Mac Andrew MD (Geriatric Medicine) - *Special Expertise: Geriatric Medicine - General;* **Admitting Hospital:** University of North Carolina Hospitals; **Office Address:** Univ North Carolina Hosp 5039 Old Clinic Bldg, Box 7110 Chapel Hill, NC 27599; **Office Phone:** (919) 966-3063; **Board Certifications:** Internal Medicine 1987, Geriatric Medicine 1988; **Medical School:** Univ Miss 1972; **Residency:** Internal Medicine, Strong Meml Hosp, Rochester, NY 1973-1975; **Faculty Appointment:** Prof Medicine, Univ NC Sch Med

Groene, Linda A MD (Geriatric Medicine) - *Special Expertise: Vitamin B-12 Metabolism; Sleep Disorders;* **Admitting Hospital:** Cleveland Clinic Florida; **Office Address:** Cleveland Clinic Florida 3000 W Cypress Creek Rd Ft Lauderdale, FL 33309-1710; **Office Phone:** (954) 978-5154; **Board Certifications:** Internal Medicine 1986, Geriatric Medicine 1990; **Medical School:** Louisiana State Univ 1981; **Residencies:** Pathology, Jackson Meml Hosp- Univ Miami, Miami, FL 1982-1983; Internal Medicine, Mt Sinai Med Ctr, Miami Beach, FL 1984-1986

Hanson, Laura Catherine (Geriatric Medicine) - *Special Expertise: Frail Elderly; Palliative Care;* **Admitting Hospital:** University of North Carolina Hospitals; **Office Address:** Univ North Carolina 5039 Old Clinic Building, Box 7110 Chapel Hill, NC 27599; **Office Phone:** (919) 966-2276; **Board Certifications:** Internal Medicine 1989, Geriatric Medicine 1992; **Medical School:** Harvard Med Sch 1986; **Residencies:** Internal Medicine, Brigham & Women's Hosp, Boston, MA 1986-1988; Internal Medicine, UNC Hosp, Chapel Hill, NC 1988-1989; **Fellowship:** Geriatric Medicine, UNC Hosp, Chapel Hill, NC 1989-1991; **Faculty Appointment:** Assoc Prof Medicine, Univ NC Sch Med

Lyles, Kenneth W MD (Geriatric Medicine) - *Special Expertise: Bone Disorders-Metabolic; Tumoral Calcinosis; Parathyroid Disease;* **Admitting Hospital:** Duke University Medical Center (Page 60); **Office Address:** Duke Univ Med Ctr Box 3881 Durham, NC 27710; **Office Phone:** (919) 668-7630; **Board Certifications:** Endocrinology, Diabetes & Metabolism 1979, Internal Medicine 1977; **Medical School:** Med Coll VA 1974; **Residency:** Internal Medicine, Med Coll VA, Richmond, VA 1975-1977; **Fellowships:** Endocrinology, Diabetes & Metabolism, Duke Univ Med Ctr, Durham, NC 1977-1979; Geriatric Medicine, VA Med Ctr-Duke Univ, Durham, NC 1979-1981; **Faculty Appointment:** Prof Medicine, Duke Univ

Ouslander, Joseph MD (Geriatric Medicine) - *Special Expertise: Incontinence;* **Admitting Hospital:** Emory University Hospital; **Office Address:** Emory University Wessleywood 1841 Clifton Rd Atlanta, GA 30329; **Office Phone:** (404) 728-6363; **Board Certifications:** Internal Medicine 1980, Geriatric Medicine 1998; **Medical School:** Case West Res Univ 1977; **Residencies:** Internal Medicine, University Hosp Cleveland 1978-1979; Internal Medicine, Sepulveda Med Ctr 1979-1980; **Fellowship:** Geriatric Medicine, UCLA 1980-1982

Snustad, Diane Gail MD (Geriatric Medicine) - *Special Expertise: Osteoporosis; Dementia;* **Admitting Hospital:** University of Virginia Health Systems; **Office Address:** Colonnades Medical Associates 2610 Barracks Rd Charlottesville, VA 22901; **Office Phone:** (804) 924-1212; **Board Certifications:** Internal Medicine 1982, Geriatric Medicine 1988; **Medical School:** Univ Minn 1979; **Residency:** Internal Medicine, West VA Univ, Morgantown, WV 1980-1982; **Faculty Appointment:** Assoc Prof Geriatric Medicine, Univ VA Sch Med

Tenover, Joyce Sander MD/PhD (Geriatric Medicine) - *Special Expertise: Hormonal Disorders;* **Admitting Hospital:** Wesley Woods Geriatric Hospital; **Office Address:** Wesley Woods Health Center 1841 Clifton Rd NE Atlanta, GA 30329; **Office Phone:** (404) 728-6331; **Board Certifications:** Internal Medicine 1983, Geriatric Medicine 1997; **Medical School:** Geo Wash Univ 1980; **Residencies:** Internal Medicine, U Wash Alffil Hosp, Seattle, WA 1981-1983; Internal Medicine, VA Med Ctr, Seattle, WA 1983-1984; **Fellowship:** Geriatric Medicine, VA Med Ctr, Seattle, WA 1984-1987; **Faculty Appointment:** Assoc Prof Medicine, Emory Univ

Weinberg, Andrew David MD (Geriatric Medicine) - *Special Expertise:* Elderly Long Term Care; **Admitting Hospital:** Wesley Woods Geriatric Hospital; **Office Address:** Wesley Woods Ctr for Geriatrics 1841 Clifton Rd NE Atlanta, GA 30329; **Office Phone:** (404) 728-6901; **Board Certifications:** Internal Medicine 1981, Geriatric Medicine 1992; **Medical School:** SUNY Syracuse 1978; **Residency:** Internal Medicine, Mayo Clin, Rochester, MN 1979-1981; **Fellowship:** Endocrinology, Diabetes & Metabolism, Yale Sch Med, New Haven, CT 1981-1982; **Faculty Appointment:** Prof Medicine, Emory Univ

Midwest

Barnhart, William MD (Geriatric Medicine) - *Special Expertise:* Preventive Medicine; **Admitting Hospital:** University of Chicago Hospitals (Page 78); **Office Address:** Medical Education 4646 N Marine St, Fl 4th Chicago, IL 60640; **Office Phone:** (773) 564-5446; **Board Certifications:** Geriatric Medicine 1994, Internal Medicine 1974; **Medical School:** Northwestern Univ 1971; **Residencies:** Internal Medicine, Emory University, Atlanta, GA 1972-1974; Internal Medicine, Grady Meml Hosp, Atlanta, GA 1972-1974; **Faculty Appointment:** Assoc Clin Prof Geriatric Medicine, Univ Chicago-Pritzker Sch Med

Bentley, David Warren MD (Geriatric Medicine) - *Special Expertise:* Infectious Disease in Elderly; **Admitting Hospital:** St Louis University Hospital; **Office Address:** St Louis Univ Hlth Sci Ctr, Div Geriatric Med 1402 S Grand Blvd, rm M238 St Louis, MO 63104; **Office Phone:** (314) 894-6510; **Board Certifications:** Geriatric Medicine 1969, Geriatric Medicine 1998; **Medical School:** Univ Rochester 1963; **Residency:** Internal Medicine, Vanderbilt Univ Hosp, Nashville, TN 1964-1966; **Fellowship:** Infectious Disease, Univ IL, Chicago, IL 1966-1968; **Faculty Appointment:** Prof Medicine, St Louis Univ

Carr, David Brian MD (Geriatric Medicine) - *Special Expertise:* Geriatric Medicine - General; **Admitting Hospital:** Barnes - Jewish Hospital; **Office Address:** Wash Univ, Div Ger Med 4488 Forest Park Ave St Louis, MO 63108; **Office Phone:** (314) 286-2700; **Board Certifications:** Internal Medicine 1989, Geriatric Medicine 2002; **Medical School:** Univ MO-Columbia Sch Med 1985; **Residency:** Internal Medicine, Mich State Assoc Hosp, Lansing, MI 1986-1988; **Fellowship:** Geriatric Medicine, Duke Univ, Durham, NC 1988-1990; **Faculty Appointment:** Prof Geriatric Medicine, Washington Univ, St Louis

Couch, Nancy MD (Geriatric Medicine) - *Special Expertise:* Geriatric Medicine - General; **Admitting Hospital:** Henry Ford Health System (Page 62); **Office Address:** Henry Ford MC-Hamtramck 9100 Brombach Hamtramck, MI 48212; **Office Phone:** (313) 972-9000; **Board Certifications:** Internal Medicine 1986, Geriatric Medicine 1988; **Medical School:** Wayne State Univ 1982; **Residencies:** Internal Medicine, Wayne State Univ Affil Hosps, Detroit, MI 1982-1984; Internal Medicine, Henry Ford Hosp, Detroit, MI 1984-1985; **Fellowship:** Geriatric Medicine, Univ of Mich/VA Medical Ctr, Ann Arbor, MI 1985-1987

Dale, Lowell C MD (Geriatric Medicine) - *Special Expertise:* Tobacco Abuse; Nutrition; **Admitting Hospital:** Mayo Medical Center & Clinic - Rochester; **Office Address:** 200 1st St SW Rochester, MN 55902; **Office Phone:** (507) 266-5032; **Board Certifications:** Internal Medicine 1984, Geriatric Medicine 1992; **Medical School:** Univ Minn 1981; **Residency:** Internal Medicine, Mayo Clin, Rochester, MN 1981-1984; **Fellowship:** Internal Medicine, Mayo Clin, Rochester, MN 1984-1985

Gorbien, Martin MD (Geriatric Medicine) - *Special Expertise:* Geriatric Medicine - General; **Admitting Hospital:** Rush/Presbyterian - St Luke's Medical Center - Chicago (Page 74); **Office Address:** 1725 W Harrison St, Fl 319 1725 W Harrison St, Ste 319 Chicago, IL 60612; **Office Phone:** (312) 942-7030; **Board Certifications:** Geriatric Medicine 1998, Internal Medicine 1996; **Medical School:** Mexico 1983; **Residency:** Internal Medicine, Mercy Hosp & Med Ctr, Chicago, IL 1984-1987; **Fellowship:** Geriatric Medicine, UCLA, Los Angeles, CA 1987-1989; **Faculty Appointment:** Assoc Prof Medicine, Rush Med Coll

Halter, Jeffrey Brian MD (Geriatric Medicine) - *Special Expertise:* Endocrinology; **Admitting Hospital:** University of Michigan Health Center; **Office Address:** University of Michigan - CCGCB Room 1111 1500 E Medical Center Ann Arbor, MI 48109; **Office Phone:** (734) 763-4002; **Board Certifications:** Internal Medicine 1974, Endocrinology, Diabetes & Metabolism 1977; **Medical School:** Univ Minn 1969; **Residencies:** Internal Medicine, LA Co Harbor Gen Hosp, Torrance, CA 1970-1971; Internal Medicine, Univ Wash Affil Hosp, Seattle, WA 1973-1974; **Fellowship:** Seattle VA Hospital, Seattle, WA 1975-1977; **Faculty Appointment:** Prof Medicine, Univ Mich Med Sch

Miller, Douglas Kent MD (Geriatric Medicine) - *Special Expertise:* Geriatric Medicine - General; **Admitting Hospital:** St Louis University Hospital; **Office Address:** St Louis Univ Health Sciences Ctr - Div of Ger Med 1402 S Grand Blvd, rm M 238 St Louis, MO 63104; **Office Phone:** (314) 577-6055; **Board Certifications:** Internal Medicine 1978, Geriatric Medicine 1998; **Medical School:** Washington Univ, St Louis 1972; **Residencies:** Internal Medicine, Jewish Hosp, St Louis, MO 1972-1973; Internal Medicine, Hosp Univ Pa, Philadelphia, PA 1977-1978; **Fellowship:** Geriatric Medicine, UCLA, Los Angeles, CA 1987-1988; **Faculty Appointment:** Prof Medicine, St Louis Univ

Morley, John MD (Geriatric Medicine) - *Special Expertise:* Nutrition; Endocrinology; **Admitting Hospital:** St Louis University Hospital; **Office Address:** St Louis Univ Hlth Sci Ctr, Div Ger Med 1402 S Grand Blvd, rm M 238 St Louis, MO 63104; **Office Phone:** (314) 577-6055; **Board Certifications:** Internal Medicine 1978, Geriatric Medicine 1998; **Medical School:** South Africa 1972; **Residencies:** Internal Medicine, Johannesburg Genl Hosp, Johannesburg, South Africa 1974; Internal Medicine, Baragwanath Hosp, Johannesburg, South Africa 1975-1976; **Fellowship:** Endocrinology, Diabetes & Metabolism, Wadsworth VA Hosp UCLA, Los Angeles, CA 1977-1979; **Faculty Appointment:** Assoc Prof Geriatric Medicine, Univ Minn

Olson, Jack Conrad MD (Geriatric Medicine) - *Special Expertise:* Geriatric Medicine - General; **Admitting Hospital:** Rush/Presbyterian - St Luke's Medical Center - Chicago (Page 74); **Office Address:** 1725 W Harrison St, Ste 319 Chicago, IL 60612; **Office Phone:** (312) 942-7030; **Board Certifications:** Internal Medicine 1987, Geriatric Medicine 2000; **Medical School:** Univ Mich Med Sch 1984; **Residency:** Internal Medicine, Univ Wisc Med Sch, Madison, WI 1985-1987; **Fellowship:** Geriatric Medicine, Univ Wisc Med Sch, Madison, WI 1987-1989; **Faculty Appointment:** Assoc Prof Geriatric Medicine, Univ Chicago-Pritzker Sch Med

Palmer, Robert MD (Geriatric Medicine) - *Special Expertise:* Geriatric Medicine - General; **Admitting Hospital:** Cleveland Clinic Foundation; **Office Address:** Cleveland Clinic Foundation 9500 Euclid Ave, MC-A-91 Cleveland, OH 44195; **Office Phone:** (216) 444-8091; **Board Certifications:** Internal Medicine 1975, Geriatric Medicine 1998; **Medical School:** Univ Mich Med Sch 1971; **Residency:** Internal Medicine, LA Co Med Ctr, Los Angeles, CA 1972-1975; **Fellowship:** Geriatric Medicine, UCLA, Los Angeles, CA 1985-1986; **Faculty Appointment:** Assoc Prof Medicine, Ohio State Univ

Sachs, Greg MD (Geriatric Medicine) - *Special Expertise: Memory Disorders/Alzheimer's;* **Admitting Hospital:** University of Chicago Hospitals (Page 78); **Office Address:** Windermere Senior Health Center 5549 S Cornell Ave Chicago, IL 60637; **Office Phone:** (773) 702-8840; **Board Certifications:** Internal Medicine 1988, Geriatric Medicine 1990; **Medical School:** Yale Univ 1985; **Residency:** Internal Medicine, Univ Chicago Hosps, Chicago, IL 1985-1987; **Fellowship:** Geriatric Medicine, Univ Chicago Hosps, Chicago, IL 1987-1990; **Faculty Appointment:** Assoc Prof Medicine, Univ Chicago-Pritzker Sch Med

Sheehan, Myles MD (Geriatric Medicine) - *Special Expertise: Geriatric Medicine - General;* **Admitting Hospital:** Loyola University Health System; **Office Address:** Loyola Univ Med Ctr 2160 S 1st Ave Ste 7604 Maywood, IL, 60153; **Office Phone:** (708) 216-8887; **Board Certifications:** Internal Medicine 1984, Geriatric Medicine 1992; **Medical School:** Dartmouth Med Sch 1981; **Residencies:** Internal Medicine, Beth Israel Deaconcess Med Ctr, Boston, MA 1981-1985; Pathology, Beth Israel Deaconess Med Ctr, Boston, MA 1989-1991; **Fellowship:** Geriatric Medicine, Beth Israel Deaconess Med Ctr, Boston, MA 1989-1991; **Faculty Appointment:** Asst Prof Medicine, Loyola Univ-Stritch Sch Med

Supiano, Mark A. MD (Geriatric Medicine) - *Special Expertise: Hypertension; Congestive Heart Failure; Hypertension;* **Admitting Hospital:** University of Michigan Health Center; **Office Address:** Turner Geriatric Ctr 1500 E Med Ctr Dr Ann Arbor, MI 48109-0926; **Office Phone:** (734) 764-6831; **Board Certifications:** Internal Medicine 1985, Geriatric Medicine 1988; **Medical School:** Univ Wisc 1982; **Residency:** Internal Medicine, Univ Mich, Ann Arbor, MI 1983-1985; **Fellowship:** Geriatric Medicine, Univ Mich, Ann Arbor, MI 1985-1986; **Faculty Appointment:** Assoc Prof Medicine, Univ Mich Med Sch

Von Sternberg, Thomas MD (Geriatric Medicine) - *Special Expertise: Dementia;* **Admitting Hospital:** Fairview-University Medical Center - University Campus; **Office Address:** Adult Medicine 2220 Riverside Ave S, Fl 1st Minneapolis, MN 55454; **Office Phone:** (612) 371-1610; **Board Certifications:** Family Practice 1997, Geriatric Medicine 1998; **Medical School:** Ohio State Univ 1980; **Residency:** Family Practice, Fairview-Univ Minn, Minneapolis, MN 1980-1983; **Fellowship:** Geriatric Medicine, Westminster Med Sch, London 1983

Williamson, Wayne MD (Geriatric Medicine) - *Special Expertise: Hypertension; Asthma;* **Admitting Hospital:** Northwestern Memorial Hospital; **Office Address:** 150 East Huron, Ste 805 Chicago, IL 61611; **Office Phone:** (312) 649-6565; **Board Certifications:** Internal Medicine 1984, Geriatric Medicine 1992; **Medical School:** Univ Cincinnati 1978; **Residency:** Internal Medicine, Rush Presby St Lukes Med Ctr, Chicago, IL 1979-1981; **Faculty Appointment:** Asst Prof Geriatric Medicine, Rush Med Coll

Great Plains and Mountains

Schwartz, Robert S MD (Geriatric Medicine) - *Special Expertise: Diabetes; Eating Disorders - Obesity; Exercise Therapy;* **Admitting Hospital:** University of Colorado Health & Science Center; **Office Address:** Univ Colo Hlth Scis Ctr 4200 E Ninth Ave, Box B179 Denver, CO 80262; **Office Phone:** (303) 315-8668; **Board Certifications:** Endocrinology, Diabetes & Metabolism 1981, Geriatric Medicine 1990; **Medical School:** Ohio State Univ 1974; **Residency:** Internal Medicine, Univ Wash, Seattle, WA 1975-1977; **Fellowship:** Endocrinology, Diabetes & Metabolism, Univ Wash, Seattle, WA 1977-1980; **Faculty Appointment:** Prof Medicine, Univ Wash

Southwest

Carter, William Jerry MD (Geriatric Medicine) - *Special Expertise:* *Geriatric Endocrinology;* **Admitting Hospital:** University of Arkansas for Medical Sciences; **Office Address:** VA Hospital, Dept Geriatrics 2200 Fort Root Dr Little Rock, AR 72114; **Office Phone:** (501) 257-2061; **Board Certifications:** Geriatric Medicine 1994, Endocrinology, Diabetes & Metabolism 1975; **Medical School:** Univ Ark 1963; **Residency:** Internal Medicine, University Ark, Little Rock, AR 1964-1967; **Fellowship:** Endocrinology, Diabetes & Metabolism, University Ark, Little Rock, AR 1969-1971; **Faculty Appointment:** Prof Medicine, Univ Ark

Garb, Leslie Julian MD (Geriatric Medicine) - *Special Expertise:* *Sigmoidoscopy;* **Admitting Hospital:** Methodist Hospital - Houston (Page 69); **Office Address:** Baylor Methodist Primary Care Assocs 5420 Dashwood Dr, Ste 100 Houston, TX 77081; **Office Phone:** (713) 664-0719; **Board Certifications:** Family Practice 1997, Geriatric Medicine 1997; **Medical School:** South Africa 1963

Lichtenstein, Michael Joseph MD (Geriatric Medicine) - *Special Expertise:* *Alzheimer's Disease;* **Admitting Hospital:** University of Texas Health & Science Center; **Office Address:** Univ TX Hlth Sci Ctr, Dept Med 7703 Floyd Curl Dr San Antonio, TX 78229-3900; **Office Phone:** (210) 617-5237; **Board Certifications:** Geriatric Medicine 1988, Internal Medicine 1982; **Medical School:** Baylor Coll Med 1978; **Faculty Appointment:** Prof Medicine, Univ Tex, San Antonio

Liem, Pham MD (Geriatric Medicine) - *Special Expertise:* *Dementia; Alzheimer's Disease;* **Admitting Hospital:** University of Arkansas for Medical Sciences; **Office Address:** Univ Hosp Arkansas Med Sci 4301 W Markham #748 Little Rock, AR 77205; **Office Phone:** (501) 686-8948; **Board Certifications:** Family Practice 1980, Geriatric Medicine 1988; **Medical School:** Vietnam 1973; **Residency:** Family Practice, Univ Ark Med Sch, Little Rock, AR 1977-1980; **Fellowship:** Geriatric Medicine, Univ Ark Med Sch, Little Rock, AR 1980-1982; **Faculty Appointment:** Assoc Prof Geriatric Medicine, Univ Ark

Lipschitz, David Arnold MD/PhD (Geriatric Medicine) - *Special Expertise:* *Nutrition;* **Admitting Hospital:** University of Arkansas for Medical Sciences; **Office Address:** Univ Hosp of AR for Med Sci 4301 W Markham St, Ste 748 Little Rock, AR 72205-7101; **Office Phone:** (501) 296-1000; **Board Certifications:** Hematology 1976, Internal Medicine 1976; **Medical School:** Africa 1966; **Residency:** Internal Medicine, Johannesburg General Hosp, Johannesburg 1966-1972; **Fellowships:** Hematology, Univ of Washington, Seattle, WA 1972-1974; Internal Medicine, Montefiore Hosp, New York, NY 1974-1975; **Faculty Appointment:** Prof Geriatric Medicine, Univ Ark

Vicioso, Belinda Angelica MD (Geriatric Medicine) - *Special Expertise:* *Geriatric Medicine - General;* **Admitting Hospital:** Parkland Memorial Hospital; **Office Address:** 5323 Harry Hines Blvd Dallas, TX 75390-8889; **Office Phone:** (214) 648-9012; **Board Certifications:** Internal Medicine 1989, Geriatric Medicine 1990; **Medical School:** Dominican Republic 1979; **Residency:** Internal Medicine, St Francis Med Ctr, Trenton, NJ 1981-1983; **Fellowship:** Geriatric Medicine, Univ Penn Med Sch, Philadelphia, PA 1984-1986

West Coast and Pacific

Abrass, Itamar MD (Geriatric Medicine) - *Special Expertise:* *Endocrinology;* **Admitting Hospital:** University of Washington Medical Center; **Office Address:** Harborview Med Ctr 325 9th Ave, Box 359755 Seattle, WA 98104-2499; **Office Phone:** (206) 731-4191; **Board Certifications:** Geriatric Medicine 1988, Endocrinology, Diabetes & Metabolism 1975; **Medical School:** UCSF 1966; **Residency:** Internal Medicine, Columbia-Pesby Med Ctr, New York, NY 1967-1968; **Fellowship:** Endocrinology, Diabetes & Metabolism, UC SanDiego Med Ctr, SanDiego, CA 1970-1971; **Faculty Appointment:** Prof Medicine, Univ Wash

Davis Jr, James William MD (Geriatric Medicine) - *Special Expertise:* Geriatric Medicine - General; **Admitting Hospital:** UCLA Medical Center; **Office Address:** 200 UCLA Medical Plaza, Ste 420 Los Angeles, CA 90095; **Office Phone:** (310) 206-8272; **Board Certifications:** Internal Medicine 1979, Geriatric Medicine 2000; **Medical School:** Med Univ SC 1975; **Residencies:** Internal Medicine, Mount Zion MC Univ, San Fransisco, CA; Geriatric Medicine, Mount Zion MC Univ, San Francisco, CA

Landefeld, Charles Seth MD (Geriatric Medicine) - *Special Expertise:* Geriatric Medicine - General; **Admitting Hospital:** University of California - San Francisco Medical Center; **Office Address:** 3333 California St, Ste 380 San Francisco, CA 94118; **Office Phone:** (415) 750-6625; **Board Certifications:** Internal Medicine 1982, Geriatric Medicine 2000; **Medical School:** Yale Univ 1979; **Residency:** Internal Medicine, UCSF, San Francisco, CA 1980-1983; **Fellowship:** Geriatric Medicine, Brigham-Womens Hosp, Boston, MA 1983-1985; **Faculty Appointment:** Prof Medicine, UCSF

McCormick, Wayne MD (Geriatric Medicine) - *Special Expertise:* Dementia; AIDS/HIV; Elderly Long Term Care; **Admitting Hospital:** University of Washington Medical Center; **Office Address:** Harborview Med Ctr 325 9th Ave Seattle, WA 98104; **Office Phone:** (206) 731-4191; **Board Certifications:** Internal Medicine 1986, Geriatric Medicine 1992; **Medical School:** Washington Univ, St Louis 1983; **Residencies:** Internal Medicine, Michael Reese Hosp, Chicago, IL 1984-1986; Internal Medicine, Michael Reese Hosp, Chicago, IL 1986-1987; **Fellowship:** Geriatric Medicine, Univ Wash Med Ctr, Seattle, WA 1987-1990; **Faculty Appointment:** Asst Prof Medicine, Univ Wash

Reuben, David MD (Geriatric Medicine) - *Special Expertise:* Aging; **Admitting Hospital:** UCLA Medical Center; **Office Address:** UCLA Dept Med, Div Geriatrics 10945 Le Conte Ave, Ste 2339 Los Angeles, CA 90095; **Office Phone:** (310) 825-8253; **Board Certifications:** Geriatric Medicine 1988, Internal Medicine 1980; **Medical School:** Emory Univ 1977; **Residency:** Internal Medicine, Rhode Island Hosp, Providence, RI 1977-1980; **Fellowship:** Geriatric Medicine, John A. Hartford Foundation, Los Angeles, CA 1987; **Faculty Appointment:** Prof Medicine, UCLA

GYNECOLOGIC ONCOLOGY

(a subspecialty of OBSTETRICS AND GYNECOLOGY)

An obstetrician/gynecologist possesses special knowledge, skills and professional capability in the medical and surgical care of the female reproductive system and associated disorders. This physician serves as a consultant to other physicians and as a primary physician for women.

OBSTETRICS/GYNECOLOGY

An obstetrician/gynecologist who provides consultation and comprehensive management of patients with gynecologic cancer, including those diagnostic and therapeutic procedures necessary for the total care of the patient with gynecologic cancer and resulting complications.

Training required: Four years plus two years in clinical practice before certification in obstetrics and gynecology is complete *plus* additional training and examination in gynecologic oncology

Physician Listings

Gynecologic Oncology

New England

Fuller, Arlan F. MD (Gynecologic Oncology) - *Special Expertise:* Ovarian Cancer; Cervical Cancer; **Admitting Hospital:** Massachusetts General Hospital; **Office Address:** Gillette Ctr. For Womens Cancer 100 Blossom St, Bldg Cox - Fl 120 Boston, MA 02114; **Office Phone:** (617) 724-6880; **Board Certifications:** Obstetrics & Gynecology 1979, Gynecologic Oncology 1982; **Medical School:** Harvard Med Sch 1971; **Residencies:** Surgery, Mass Genl Hosp, Boston, MA 1971-1974; Obstetrics & Gynecology, Brigham and Womens Hosp, Boston, MA 1974-1977; **Fellowship:** Gynecologic Oncology, Memorial Sloan Kettering Cancer Ctr, New York, NY 1977-1979; **Faculty Appointment:** Assoc Prof Obstetrics & Gynecology, Harvard Med Sch

Goodman, Annekathryn MD (Gynecologic Oncology) - *Special Expertise:* Cervical Cancer; AIDS/HIV; **Admitting Hospital:** Massachusetts General Hospital; **Office Address:** Mass Genl Hosp 15 Parkman St Wang 231 Boston, MA 02114; **Office Phone:** (617) 726-2429; **Board Certifications:** Obstetrics & Gynecology 1991, Gynecologic Oncology 1994; **Medical School:** Tufts Univ 1983; **Residency:** Obstetrics & Gynecology, Tufts, Boston, MA 1983-1987; **Fellowship:** Gynecologic Oncology, Mass Genl Hosp., Boston, MA 1987-1990; **Faculty Appointment:** Asst Prof Obstetrics & Gynecology, Harvard Med Sch

Niloff, Jonathan Mitchell MD (Gynecologic Oncology) - *Special Expertise:* Gynecologic Oncology - General; **Admitting Hospital:** Beth Israel Deaconess Medical Center - Boston (Page 57); **Office Address:** Beth Israel Deaconess Med Ctr 330 Brookline Ave, rm KS-330 Boston, MA 02215; **Office Phone:** (617) 667-4040; **Board Certifications:** Obstetrics & Gynecology 1987, Gynecologic Oncology 1987; **Medical School:** McGill Univ 1978; **Residency:** Obstetrics & Gynecology, Brigham & Women's Hosp, Boston, MA 1979-1982; **Fellowship:** Gynecologic Oncology, Brigham & Women's Hosp, Boston, MA 1982-1984; **Faculty Appointment:** Assoc Prof Obstetrics & Gynecology, Harvard Med Sch

Schwartz, Peter MD (Gynecologic Oncology) - *Special Expertise:* Gynecologic Oncology - General; **Admitting Hospital:** Yale - New Haven Hospital; **Office Address:** Yale University School of Medicine 333 Cedar St, Ste FM13316 New Haven, CT 06520; **Office Phone:** (203) 785-4135; **Board Certifications:** Obstetrics & Gynecology 1973, Gynecologic Oncology 1979; **Medical School:** Albert Einstein Coll Med 1966; **Residency:** Obstetrics & Gynecology, Yale-New Haven Hosp, New Haven, CT 1967-1970; **Fellowship:** Gynecologic Oncology, MD Anderson Cancer Ctr, Houston, TX 1973-1975; **Faculty Appointment:** Prof Obstetrics & Gynecology, Yale Univ

Mid Atlantic

Barnes, Willard MD (Gynecologic Oncology) - *Special Expertise:* Pelvic Tumors; **Admitting Hospital:** Georgetown University Hospital; **Office Address:** GUMC - Lombardi Cancer Center 3800 Reservoir Rd NW Washington, DC 20007-2194; **Office Phone:** (202) 687-2114; **Board Certifications:** Obstetrics & Gynecology 1997, Gynecologic Oncology 1997; **Medical School:** Univ Miss 1979; **Residency:** Obstetrics & Gynecology, Univ Miss Med Ctr, Jackson, MS 1979-1983; **Fellowship:** Gynecologic Oncology, Georgetown Univ Med Ctr, Washington, DC 1983-1985; **Faculty Appointment:** Assoc Prof Obstetrics & Gynecology, Georgetown Univ

Barter, James MD (Gynecologic Oncology) - *Special Expertise:* Laparoscopic Surgery; **Admitting Hospital:** Georgetown University Hospital; **Office Address:** Georgetown Univ Hosp, Lombardi Cancer Ctr 3800 Reservoir Rd NW Washington, DC 20007; **Office Phone:** (202) 687-2114; **Board Certifications:** Obstetrics & Gynecology 1997, Gynecologic Oncology 1997; **Medical School:** Univ VA Sch Med 1977; **Residencies:** Internal Medicine, Univ of KY, Lexington, KY 1978-1979; Obstetrics & Gynecology, Duke Univ, Durham, NC 1980-1983; **Fellowship:** Gynecologic Oncology, Univ of Alabama, Birmingham, AL 1983-1986; **Faculty Appointment:** Assoc Prof Obstetrics & Gynecology, Georgetown Univ

Caputo, Thomas A MD (Gynecologic Oncology) - *Special Expertise: Cervical Cancer; Ovarian Cancer; Uterine Cancer;* **Admitting Hospital:** New York Weill Cornell Medical Center - NY Presbyterian Hospital (Page 72); **Office Address:** 525 E 68th St, Ste J130 New York, NY 10021; **Office Phone:** (212) 746-3179; **Board Certifications:** Obstetrics & Gynecology 1971, Gynecologic Oncology 1977; **Medical School:** UMDNJ-NJ Med Sch, Newark 1965; **Residency:** Obstetrics & Gynecology, Martland Hosp-NJ Coll, Newark, NJ 1966-1969; **Fellowship:** Gynecologic Oncology, Emory Univ Hosp, Atlanta, GA 1972-1974; **Faculty Appointment:** Clin Prof Obstetrics & Gynecology, Cornell Univ-Weil Med Coll

Carlson, John MD (Gynecologic Oncology) - *Special Expertise: Oncology;* **Admitting Hospital:** Thomas Jefferson University Hospital; **Office Address:** Thomas Jefferson Univ. Hosp. 111 S 11th St, Bldg Gibbons - rm 6200 Philadelphia, PA 19107; **Office Phone:** (215) 955-6200; **Board Certifications:** Gynecologic Oncology 1981, Obstetrics & Gynecology 1982; **Medical School:** Georgetown Univ 1974; **Residencies:** Obstetrics & Gynecology, Hartford Hosp, Hartford, CT 1974-1975; Obstetrics & Gynecology, Hosp Univ Penn, Philadelphia, PA 1975-1978; **Fellowship:** Gynecologic Oncology, MD Anderson Hosp, Houston, TX 1978-1980; **Faculty Appointment:** Prof Obstetrics & Gynecology, Jefferson Med Coll

Chalas, Eva MD (Gynecologic Oncology) - *Special Expertise: Gynecologic Cancer;* **Admitting Hospital:** University Hospital & Medical Center at Stony Brook; **Office Address:** Long Island Gynecologic Oncologists PC 994 Jericho Tpke Smithtown, NY 11787; **Office Phone:** (631) 864-5440; **Board Certifications:** Obstetrics & Gynecology 1998, Gynecologic Oncology 1998; **Medical School:** SUNY Stony Brook 1981; **Residency:** Obstetrics & Gynecology, Univ Hosp, Stony Brook, NY 1981-1985; **Fellowship:** Gynecologic Oncology, Mem Sloan, New York, NY 1985-1987

Cohen, Carmel MD (Gynecologic Oncology) - *Special Expertise: Ovarian Cancer; Cervical Cancer;* **Admitting Hospital:** Mount Sinai Hospital (Page 70); **Office Address:** Mt Sinai Hosp 5 E 98th St Fl 2nd New York, NY 10029; **Office Phone:** (212) 427-9898; **Board Certifications:** Obstetrics & Gynecology 1967, Gynecologic Oncology 1974; **Medical School:** Tulane Univ 1958; **Residency:** Obstetrics & Gynecology, Mount Sinai, New York, NY 1959-1964; **Fellowship:** Gynecologic Oncology, Mount Sinai Hosp, New York, NY 1964-1965; **Faculty Appointment:** Prof Obstetrics & Gynecology, Mount Sinai Sch Med

Curtin, John P MD (Gynecologic Oncology) - *Special Expertise: Uterine Cancer; Ovarian Cancer; Laparoscopic Surgery;* **Admitting Hospital:** NYU Medical Center (Page 70); **Office Address:** NYU Sch Med, Dept Gyn/Onc 530 First Ave, Ste 9R New York, NY 10016; **Office Phone:** (212) 263-2353; **Board Certifications:** Gynecologic Oncology 1990, Obstetrics & Gynecology 1996; **Medical School:** Creighton Univ 1979; **Residency:** Obstetrics & Gynecology, Univ Minn Med Ctr, Minneapolis, MN 1979-1984; **Fellowship:** Gynecologic Oncology, Meml Sloan-Kettering Cancer Ctr, New York, NY 1986-1988; **Faculty Appointment:** Prof Gynecologic Oncology, NYU Sch Med

Hoskins, William MD (Gynecologic Oncology) - *Special Expertise: Gynecologic Oncology - General;* **Admitting Hospital:** Memorial Sloan Kettering Cancer Center; **Office Address:** Memorial Sloan Kettering Cancer Center 1275 York Ave New York, NY 10021-0014; **Office Phone:** (212) 639-7766; **Board Certifications:** Obstetrics & Gynecology 1993, Gynecologic Oncology 1979; **Medical School:** Univ Tenn Coll Med, Memphis 1965; **Residency:** Obstetrics & Gynecology, Naval Med Ctr, New York, NY 1968-1971; **Fellowship:** Gynecologic Oncology, Univ Miami Hosp, Miami, FL 1974-1975; **Faculty Appointment:** Prof Obstetrics & Gynecology, Cornell Univ-Weil Med Coll

Kwon, Tae MD (Gynecologic Oncology) - *Special Expertise:* Uterine Cancer; Cervical Cancer; Ovarian Cancer; **Admitting Hospital:** Our Lady of Mercy Medical Center; **Office Address:** 305 North St White Plains, NY 10605; **Office Phone:** (914) 681-7171; **Board Certifications:** Obstetrics & Gynecology 1978, Gynecologic Oncology 1981; **Medical School:** South Korea 1965; **Residencies:** Obstetrics & Gynecology, Lenox Hill Hosp, New York, NY 1970-1974; Gynecologic Oncology, Lenox Hill Hosp, New York, NY 1974-1976; **Fellowship:** Gynecologic Oncology, Univ Mississippi Hosp, Jackson, MS 1976-1978; **Faculty Appointment:** Assoc Clin Prof Obstetrics & Gynecology, NY Med Coll

Montz, Fredrick John MD (Gynecologic Oncology) - *Special Expertise:* Gynecologic Oncology - General; **Admitting Hospital:** Johns Hopkins Hospital - Baltimore (Page 65); **Office Address:** Johns Hopkins Med Inst. 600 N Wolfe St, rm 248 Baltimore, MD 21287; **Office Phone:** (410) 955-8240; **Board Certifications:** Obstetrics & Gynecology 1999, Gynecologic Oncology 1997; **Medical School:** Baylor Coll Med 1980; **Residency:** Obstetrics & Gynecology, LA Co-USC Med Ctr., Los Angeles, CA 1980-1984; **Fellowship:** Gynecologic Oncology, LA Co-USC Med. Ctr., Los Angeles, CA 1985-1987; **Faculty Appointment:** Prof Obstetrics & Gynecology, Johns Hopkins Univ

Smith, Daniel MD (Gynecologic Oncology) - *Special Expertise:* Gynecologic Oncology - General; **Admitting Hospital:** Columbia Presbyterian Medical Center (Page 72); **Office Address:** Herbert Irving Pavillion 161 Fort Washington Ave, Ste 837 New York, NY 10032; **Office Phone:** (212) 305-3410; **Board Certifications:** Obstetrics & Gynecology 1994, Gynecologic Oncology 1983; **Medical School:** Harvard Med Sch 1972; **Residencies:** Surgery, Mass Gen Hosp, Boston, MA 1978-1979; Obstetrics & Gynecology, LA Co USC Med Ctr, Los Angeles, CA 1975-1978; **Fellowship:** Gynecologic Oncology, Mem Sloan Kettering Cancer Ctr, New York, NY 1979-1981; **Faculty Appointment:** Assoc Prof Obstetrics & Gynecology, Columbia P&S

Wallach, Robert C MD (Gynecologic Oncology) - *Special Expertise:* Gynecologic Oncology - General; **Admitting Hospital:** NYU Medical Center (Page 70); **Office Address:** 700 Park Ave New York, NY 10021-4930; **Office Phone:** (212) 666-5566; **Board Certifications:** Obstetrics & Gynecology 1967, Gynecologic Oncology 1974; **Medical School:** Yale Univ 1969; **Residency:** Obstetrics & Gynecology, Beth Israel Med Ctr, New York, NY 1961-1965; **Fellowship:** Gynecologic Oncology, SUNY Brooklyn Med Ctr, Brooklyn, NY 1965-1966; **Faculty Appointment:** Clin Prof Obstetrics & Gynecology, NYU Sch Med

Southeast

Alleyn, James MD (Gynecologic Oncology) - *Special Expertise:* Gynecologic Oncology - General; **Admitting Hospital:** Baptist Hospital - Miami; **Office Address:** 3661 S Miami Ave, Ste 308 Miami, FL 33133-4206; **Office Phone:** (305) 854-3603; **Board Certification:** Obstetrics & Gynecology 1978; **Medical School:** Indiana Univ 1972; **Residency:** Obstetrics & Gynecology, Miami-Jackson Meml Hosp, Miami, FL 1973-1976; **Fellowship:** Gynecologic Oncology, Miami-Jackson Meml Hosp, Miami, FL 1976-1978

Berchuck, Andrew (Gynecologic Oncology) - *Special Expertise:* Ovarian Cancer - Hereditary; Uterine Cancer; **Admitting Hospital:** Duke University Medical Center (Page 60); **Office Address:** Duke Univ Med Ctr Box 3079 Durham, NC 27710; **Office Phone:** (919) 684-3765; **Board Certifications:** Obstetrics & Gynecology 1998, Gynecologic Oncology 1998; **Medical School:** Case West Res Univ 1980; **Residency:** Obstetrics & Gynecology, Case Western Resrv, Cleveland, OH 1980-1984; **Fellowships:** Gynecology, UT Southwestern, Dallas, TX 1984-1985; Gynecology, Meml Sloan-Kettering, New York, NY 1985-1987; **Faculty Appointment:** Prof Obstetrics & Gynecology, Duke Univ

Clarke-Pearson, Daniel L MD (Gynecologic Oncology) - *Special Expertise:* Pelvic Reconstruction; Gynecologic Surgery - Complex; **Admitting Hospital:** Duke University Medical Center (Page 60); **Office Address:** Duke Univ Med Ctr, Box 3079 Durham, NC 27710; **Office Phone:** (919) 684-3765; **Board Certifications:** Obstetrics & Gynecology 1982, Gynecologic Oncology 1983; **Medical School:** Case West Res Univ 1975; **Residency:** Obstetrics & Gynecology, Duke Med Ctr, NC 1975-1979; **Fellowship:** Gynecologic Oncology, Duke Med Ctr 1979-1981; **Faculty Appointment:** Prof Obstetrics & Gynecology, Duke Univ

Fiorica, James Vincent MD (Gynecologic Oncology) - *Special Expertise:* Gynecologic Cancer; Breast Cancer; **Admitting Hospital:** H Lee Moffitt Cancer Center & Research Institute; **Office Address:** H Lee Moffitt Cancer Ctr 12902 Magnolia Drive Tampa, FL 33612; **Office Phone:** (813) 972-8450; **Board Certifications:** Obstetrics & Gynecology 1999, Gynecologic Oncology 1999; **Medical School:** Tufts Univ 1982; **Residency:** Obstetrics & Gynecology, Univ of S Fla Affil Hosp, Tampa, FL 1982-1986; **Fellowships:** Gynecologic Oncology, Univ of S Fla Affil Hosp, Tampa, FL 1986-1989; Breast Disease, Tufts Univ, Boston, MA 1990; **Faculty Appointment:** Prof Obstetrics & Gynecology, Univ S Fla Coll Med

Fowler Jr, Wesley C MD (Gynecologic Oncology) - *Special Expertise:* Vulva Disease/Neoplasia; DES-Exposed Females; **Admitting Hospital:** University of North Carolina Hospitals; **Office Address:** U NC Chapel Hill, Div of Ob/Gyn MacNider - CB 7570 Chapel Hill, NC 27599-7570; **Office Phone:** (919) 966-1196; **Board Certifications:** Obstetrics & Gynecology 1991, Gynecologic Oncology 1979; **Medical School:** Univ NC Sch Med 1966; **Residency:** Obstetrics & Gynecology, NC Meml Hosp, Chapel Hill, NC 1967-1971; **Faculty Appointment:** Prof Obstetrics & Gynecology, Univ NC Sch Med

Jones III, Howard Wilbur MD (Gynecologic Oncology) - *Special Expertise:* Gynecologic Oncology - General; **Admitting Hospital:** Vanderbilt University Medical Center; **Office Address:** Vanderbilt Univ Med Ctr Medical Center North, Box 1100 Nashville, TN 37232-2519; **Office Phone:** (615) 322-2114; **Board Certifications:** Obstetrics & Gynecology 1999, Gynecologic Oncology 1999; **Medical School:** Duke Univ 1968; **Residency:** Obstetrics & Gynecology, Univ Colo Med Ctr, Denver, CO 1969-1972; **Fellowship:** Gynecologic Oncology, Univ Tex-MD Anderson Hosp, Houston, TX 1972-1974; **Faculty Appointment:** Prof Emeritus Gynecologic Oncology, Vanderbilt Univ

Partridge, Edward E MD (Gynecologic Oncology) - *Special Expertise:* Ovarian Cancer; **Admitting Hospital:** University of Alabama Hospital at Birmingham; **Office Address:** UAB, Div Gyn Onc 619 19th St, Bldg Old Hillman - rm 538 Birmingham, AL 35249-7333; **Office Phone:** (205) 934-4986; **Board Certifications:** Obstetrics & Gynecology 1980, Gynecologic Oncology 1981; **Medical School:** Univ Ala 1973; **Residency:** Obstetrics & Gynecology, Univ Ala Sch Med, Birmingham, AL 1974-1977; **Fellowship:** Gynecologic Oncology, Univ Ala Sch Med, Brimingham, AL 1978-1979; **Faculty Appointment:** Prof Obstetrics & Gynecology, Univ Ala

Poliakoff, Steven MD (Gynecologic Oncology) - *Special Expertise:* Gynecologic Oncology - General; **Admitting Hospital:** Mount Sinai Medical Center; **Office Address:** 6280 Sunset Dr, Ste 502 South Miami, FL 33143-4843; **Office Phone:** (305) 596-0870; **Board Certification:** Obstetrics & Gynecology 1983; **Medical School:** Univ NC Sch Med 1975; **Residencies:** Obstetrics & Gynecology, Johns Hopkins Hosp, Baltimore, MD 1976-1979; Gynecologic Oncology, Jackson Meml Hosp, Miami, FL 1979-1981

Taylor Jr., Peyton T. MD (Gynecologic Oncology) - *Special Expertise:* Gynecologic Surgery-Complex; Gynecologic Cancer; **Admitting Hospital:** University of Virginia Health Systems; **Office Address:** Univ VA, Dept OB/GYN P.O. Box #800712 Charlottesville, VA 22908; **Office Phone:** (804) 924-9933; **Board Certifications:** Obstetrics & Gynecology 1994, Gynecologic Oncology 1981; **Medical School:** Univ Ala 1968; **Residencies:** Obstetrics & Gynecology, Univ VA Hosp, Charlottesville, VA 1969-1970; Obstetrics & Gynecology, Univ VA Hosp, Charlottesville, VA 1972-1975; **Fellowships:** Gynecologic Oncology, Univ Va Hosp, Charlottesville, VA 1975-1977; Surgical Oncology, Natl Cancer Inst, Bethesda, MD 1970-1972; **Faculty Appointment:** Prof Obstetrics & Gynecology, Univ VA Sch Med

Van Nagell Jr., John R. MD (Gynecologic Oncology) - *Special Expertise:* Ovarian Cancer; Cervical Cancer; **Admitting Hospital:** University of Kentucky Medical Center; **Office Address:** Univ Hosp, Dept Ob/Gyn 800 Rose St, rm MN308 Lexington, KY 40536; **Office Phone:** (859) 323-5553; **Board Certifications:** Obstetrics & Gynecology 1973, Gynecologic Oncology 1976; **Medical School:** Univ Penn 1967; **Residency:** Obstetrics & Gynecology, Kentucky Med Ctr, Lexington, KY 1968-1971; **Faculty Appointment:** Prof Obstetrics & Gynecology, Univ KY Coll Med

Midwest

Belinson, Jerome Leslie MD (Gynecologic Oncology) - *Special Expertise:* Ovarian Cancer; Cervical Cancer; **Admitting Hospital:** Cleveland Clinic Foundation; **Office Address:** Cleveland Clinic Foundation-OB/Gyn Euclid Ave, Bldg A - Ste 8 Cleveland, OH 44195; **Office Phone:** (216) 444-7933; **Board Certifications:** Obstetrics & Gynecology 1998, Gynecologic Oncology 1980; **Medical School:** Univ MO-Columbia Sch Med 1968; **Residency:** Obstetrics & Gynecology, Columbia Presby Med Ctr, New York, NY 1969-1973; **Fellowship:** Gynecologic Oncology, Univ Miami- Jackson Meml Hosp, Miami, Florida, FL 1975-1977; **Faculty Appointment:** Prof Obstetrics & Gynecology, Ohio State Univ

Copeland, Larry James MD (Gynecologic Oncology) - *Special Expertise:* Ovarian Cancer; Pelvic Surgery; **Admitting Hospital:** Arthur G. James Cancer Hospital & Research Institute; **Office Address:** Ohio St. Univ College of Medicine and Public Health 1654 Upham, Fl 505 Columbus, OH 43210-1250; **Office Phone:** (614) 293-8697; **Board Certifications:** Obstetrics & Gynecology 1991, Gynecologic Oncology 1981; **Medical School:** Canada 1973; **Residency:** Obstetrics & Gynecology, McMaster Univ Affiliated Hosp, Hamilton, CN 1973-1977; **Fellowship:** Gynecologic Oncology, Univ Texas M.D. Anderson Cancer Center, Houston, TX 1977-1979; **Faculty Appointment:** Prof Obstetrics & Gynecology, Ohio State Univ

De Geest, Koen MD (Gynecologic Oncology) - *Special Expertise:* Ovarian Cancer; Cervical Cancer; Clinical Trials; **Admitting Hospital:** Rush/Presbyterian - St Luke's Medical Center - Chicago (Page 74); **Office Address:** 1725 W Harrison St, Ste 863 Chicago, IL 60612; **Office Phone:** (312) 942-6723; **Board Certifications:** Gynecologic Oncology 1997, Obstetrics & Gynecology 1997; **Medical School:** Belgium 1977; **Residency:** Obstetrics & Gynecology, Univ Ghent, Ghent, Belgium 1977-1982; **Fellowship:** Gynecologic Oncology, Penn State/Hershey Med Ctr, Hershey, PA 1987-1990; **Faculty Appointment:** Assoc Prof Obstetrics & Gynecology, Rush Med Coll

Herbst, Arthur MD (Gynecologic Oncology) - *Special Expertise:* Ovarian Cancer; **Admitting Hospital:** University of Chicago Hospitals (Page 78); **Office Address:** OB/GYN Dept 5841 S Maryland Ave, MS 2050 Chicago, IL 60637; **Office Phone:** (773) 702-6127; **Board Certifications:** Obstetrics & Gynecology 1983, Gynecologic Oncology 1974; **Medical School:** Harvard Med Sch 1959; **Residencies:** Surgery, Mass Genl Hosp, Boston, MA 1960-1962; Obstetrics & Gynecology, Women'sHosp, Boston, MA 1962-1965; **Faculty Appointment:** Prof Obstetrics & Gynecology, Univ Chicago-Pritzker Sch Med

Johnston, Carolyn Marie MD (Gynecologic Oncology) - *Special Expertise:* Gynecologic Cancer; Gynecologic Surgery - Complex; **Admitting Hospital:** University of Michigan Health Center; **Office Address:** Womens Hosp 1500 E Medical Center Dr Ann Arbor, MI 48109-0276; **Office Phone:** (734) 647-8906; **Board Certifications:** Gynecologic Oncology 2005, Obstetrics & Gynecology 2001; **Medical School:** Yale Univ 1984; **Residency:** Obstetrics & Gynecology, Univ Chicago Hosp, Chicago, IL 1985-1988; **Fellowship:** Gynecologic Oncology, Mt Sinai Hosp, New York, NY 1988-1990; **Faculty Appointment:** Asst Clin Prof Gynecologic Oncology, Univ Mich Med Sch

Kim, Woo Shin MD (Gynecologic Oncology) - *Special Expertise:* Ovarian Cancer; Cervical Cancer; **Admitting Hospital:** Henry Ford Health System (Page 62); **Office Address:** 2799 W Grand Blvd, Fl 9 Detroit, MI 48202; **Office Phone:** (313) 876-2465; **Board Certifications:** Obstetrics & Gynecology 1977, Gynecologic Oncology 1979; **Medical School:** South Korea 1966; **Residency:** Obstetrics & Gynecology, Boston City Hosp, Boston, MA 1970-1973; **Fellowship:** Gynecologic Oncology, Meml Sloan-Kettering Cancer Ctr, New York, NY 1973-1976

Look, Katherine MD (Gynecologic Oncology) - *Special Expertise:* Ovarian Cancer; **Admitting Hospital:** Indiana University Hospital & Medical Center - Indianapolis; **Office Address:** 535 Barnhill Dr, rm 434 Indianapolis, IN 46202; **Office Phone:** (317) 274-8987; **Board Certifications:** Obstetrics & Gynecology 1996, Gynecologic Oncology 1996; **Medical School:** Univ Mich Med Sch 1979; **Residency:** Obstetrics & Gynecology, Univ Illinois, Chicago, IL 1979-1983; **Fellowship:** Gynecologic Oncology, Meml Sloan Kettering Cancer Ctr, New York, NY 1984-1986; **Faculty Appointment:** Prof Obstetrics & Gynecology, Indiana Univ

Lurain, John R MD (Gynecologic Oncology) - *Special Expertise:* Trophoblastic Disease; LEEP Procedure; **Admitting Hospital:** Northwestern Memorial Hospital; **Office Address:** Northwestern Meml Hosp 333 E Superior St Chicago, IL 60611-3056; **Office Phone:** (312) 926-7365; **Board Certifications:** Obstetrics & Gynecology 1977, Gynecologic Oncology 1981; **Medical School:** Univ NC Sch Med 1972; **Residency:** Obstetrics & Gynecology, Univ Pittsburgh, Pittsburgh, PA 1972-1975; **Fellowship:** Gynecologic Oncology, Roswell Cancer Ctr, Buffalo, NY 1977-1979; **Faculty Appointment:** Prof Obstetrics & Gynecology, Northwestern Univ

Massad, L Stewart MD (Gynecologic Oncology) - *Special Expertise:* Gynecologic Surgery; **Admitting Hospital:** Rush/Presbyterian - St Luke's Medical Center - Chicago (Page 74); **Office Address:** Cook Co Hosp, Dept Gyn Onc 1835 W Harrison St Chicago, IL 60612; **Office Phone:** (312) 942-2233; **Board Certifications:** Gynecologic Oncology 1995, Obstetrics & Gynecology 1993; **Medical School:** Duke Univ 1984; **Residency:** Obstetrics & Gynecology, Duke Univ, Durham, NC 1985-1989; **Fellowship:** Gynecologic Oncology, Washington Univ, St. Louis, MO 1989-1992; **Faculty Appointment:** Asst Prof Gynecologic Oncology, Rush Med Coll

Moore, David H MD (Gynecologic Oncology) - *Special Expertise:* Cervical Cancer; Ovarian Cancer; **Admitting Hospital:** Indiana University Hospital & Medical Center - Indianapolis; **Office Address:** Clarian Hlth Partners I-65 at 21st St Indianapolis, IN 46202; **Office Phone:** (317) 274-2422; **Board Certifications:** Obstetrics & Gynecology 1989, Gynecologic Oncology 1990; **Medical School:** Indiana Univ 1982; **Residency:** Obstetrics & Gynecology, Indiana Univ, Indianapolis, IN 1982-1986; **Fellowship:** Gynecologic Oncology, Univ North Carolina, Chapel Hill, NC 1986-1988; **Faculty Appointment:** Assoc Prof Gynecologic Oncology, Indiana Univ

Mutch, David MD (Gynecologic Oncology) - *Special Expertise:* Pelvic Reconstruction; **Admitting Hospital:** Barnes - Jewish Hospital; **Office Address:** 4911 Barnes Hospital Plaza St. Louis, MO 63110; **Office Phone:** (314) 362-3181; **Board Certifications:** Obstetrics & Gynecology 1999, Gynecologic Oncology 1996; **Medical School:** Washington Univ, St Louis 1980; **Residency:** Obstetrics & Gynecology, Barnes Hosp/Wash Univ of St Louis, St Louis, MO 1981-1984; **Fellowship:** Gynecologic Oncology, Duke Univ Med Ctr, Durham, NC 1984-1987; **Faculty Appointment:** Assoc Prof Obstetrics & Gynecology, Washington Univ, St Louis

Podratz, Karl C MD/PhD (Gynecologic Oncology) - *Special Expertise:* Pelvic Reconstruction; **Admitting Hospital:** Mayo Medical Center & Clinic - Rochester; **Office Address:** Mayo Clinic 200 1st St SW Rochester, MN 55905; **Office Phone:** (507) 266-7712; **Board Certifications:** Obstetrics & Gynecology 1993, Gynecologic Oncology 1982; **Medical School:** St Louis Univ 1974; **Residency:** Obstetrics & Gynecology, Univ Chicago Hosp, Chicago, IL 1974-1977; **Fellowship:** Gynecologic Oncology, Mayo Clinic, Rochester, MN 1977-1979; **Faculty Appointment:** Prof Obstetrics & Gynecology, Mayo Med Sch

Potkul, Ronald MD (Gynecologic Oncology) - *Special Expertise:* Ovarian Cancer; Cervical Cancer; **Admitting Hospital:** Loyola University Health System; **Office Address:** 2160 S First Ave, Bldg 112 - rm 267 Maywood, IL 60153; **Office Phone:** (708) 327-3314; **Board Certifications:** Obstetrics & Gynecology 1989, Gynecologic Oncology 1990; **Medical School:** Univ Chicago-Pritzker Sch Med 1981; **Residency:** Obstetrics & Gynecology, Univ of Chicago, Chicago, IL 1981-1985; **Fellowship:** Gynecologic Oncology, Georgetown Univ, Washington, DC 1985-1988; **Faculty Appointment:** Prof Obstetrics & Gynecology, Loyola Univ-Stritch Sch Med

Rader, Janet Sue MD (Gynecologic Oncology) - *Special Expertise:* Gynecologic Oncology - General; **Admitting Hospital:** Barnes - Jewish Hospital; **Office Address:** 4911 Barnes Hospital Plaza St. Louis, MO 63110; **Office Phone:** (314) 362-3181; **Board Certifications:** Obstetrics & Gynecology 1991, Gynecologic Oncology 1992; **Medical School:** Univ MO-Columbia Sch Med 1983; **Residency:** Obstetrics & Gynecology, Michael Reese Hosp, Chicago, IL 1983-1987; **Fellowship:** Gynecologic Oncology, Johns Hopkins Hosp, Baltimore, MD 1988-1990; **Faculty Appointment:** Asst Prof Obstetrics & Gynecology, Washington Univ, St Louis

Reynolds, R Kevin MD (Gynecologic Oncology) - *Special Expertise:* Gynecologic Oncology - General; **Admitting Hospital:** University of Michigan Health Center; **Office Address:** University of MI Medical Center / GYN Oncology 1500 E Medical Center Rd, Box 0276 Ann Arbor, MI 48109-0276; **Office Phone:** (734) 764-9106; **Board Certifications:** Gynecologic Oncology 1998, Obstetrics & Gynecology 1998; **Medical School:** Univ New Mexico 1982; **Residency:** Obstetrics & Gynecology, Univ Vt Hosp, Burlington, VT 1983-1986; **Fellowship:** Gynecologic Oncology, Univ Michigan Med Ctr, Ann Arbor, MI 1988-1991; **Faculty Appointment:** Asst Prof Obstetrics & Gynecology, Univ Mich Med Sch

Schink, Julian C MD (Gynecologic Oncology) - *Special Expertise:* Gynecologic Oncology - General; **Admitting Hospital:** University of Wisconsin Hospital & Clinics; **Office Address:** Univ Hosp 600 Highland Ave, Ste H4 - rm 636 Madison, WI 53792; **Office Phone:** (608) 263-1209; **Board Certifications:** Obstetrics & Gynecology 1989, Gynecologic Oncology 1990; **Medical School:** Univ Tex, San Antonio 1982; **Residency:** Obstetrics & Gynecology, Northwestern Univ Med Sch, Chicago, IL 1982-1986; **Fellowship:** Gynecologic Oncology, UCLA Med Ctr, Los Angeles, CA 1986-1988; **Faculty Appointment:** Prof Gynecologic Oncology, Univ Wisc

Smith, Donna Marie MD (Gynecologic Oncology) - *Special Expertise:* Cervical Cancer; Ovarian Cancer; **Admitting Hospital:** Foster G McGaw Hospital/Loyola Univ Med Ctr; **Office Address:** 2160 S First Ave, Bldg 112 - rm 340 Maywood, IL 60153; **Office Phone:** (708) 327-3314; **Board Certifications:** Obstetrics & Gynecology 1997, Gynecologic Oncology 1997; **Medical School:** Univ MO-Kansas City 1980; **Residency:** Obstetrics & Gynecology, Emory Univ Hosp, Atlanta, GA 1981-1984; **Fellowship:** Georgetown Univ Med Ctr, Washington, DC 1984-1987; **Faculty Appointment:** Assoc Prof Obstetrics & Gynecology, Loyola Univ-Stritch Sch Med

Waggoner, Steven MD (Gynecologic Oncology) - *Special Expertise:* Ovarian Cancer; Cervical Cancer; **Admitting Hospital:** University of Chicago Hospitals (Page 78); **Office Address:** Univ of Chicago Hosp, Dept of OB/GYN 5841 S Maryland Ave, MS 2050 Chicago, IL 60637; **Office Phone:** (773) 702-6722; **Board Certifications:** Obstetrics & Gynecology 1992, Gynecologic Oncology 1994; **Medical School:** Univ Wash 1984; **Residency:** Obstetrics & Gynecology, U Chicago, Chicago, IL 1984-1988; **Fellowship:** Gynecologic Oncology, Georgetown, Washington, DC 1988-1991; **Faculty Appointment:** Prof Gynecologic Oncology, Univ Chicago-Pritzker Sch Med

Webb, Maurice James MD (Gynecologic Oncology) - *Special Expertise:* Ovarian Cancer; Pelvic Reconstruction; **Admitting Hospital:** Mayo Medical Center & Clinic - Rochester; **Office Address:** Mayo Clinic 200 1st St SW Rochester, MN 55905; **Office Phone:** (507) 266-8683; **Board Certifications:** Obstetrics & Gynecology 1974, Gynecologic Oncology 1976; **Medical School:** Australia 1965; **Residencies:** Obstetrics & Gynecology, Univ Queensland-Royal Hosp, England, UK 1968-1969; Obstetrics & Gynecology, St Marys Hosp, Portsmouth, UK 1970-1971; **Fellowship:** Gynecologic Oncology, Mayo Clinic, Rochester, MN 1971-1972; **Faculty Appointment:** Prof Obstetrics & Gynecology, Mayo Med Sch

Yordan, Edgardo MD (Gynecologic Oncology) - *Special Expertise:* Gynecologic Cancer; **Admitting Hospital:** Advocate Lutheran General Hospital; **Office Address:** Luth Gen Hosp-Canc Care Ctr, Advocate Med Gp 1700 Luther Ln Park Ridge, IL 60068; **Office Phone:** (847) 723-8110; **Board Certifications:** Obstetrics & Gynecology 1980, Gynecologic Oncology 1983; **Medical School:** Univ MD Sch Med 1972; **Residencies:** Obstetrics & Gynecology, Columbia Presby, New York, NY 1973-1977; Gynecologic Oncology, Meml Sloan-Kettering, New York, NY 1976; **Fellowship:** Gynecologic Oncology, USC Med Ctr, Los Angeles, CA 1977-1979; **Faculty Appointment:** Prof Obstetrics & Gynecology, Rush Med Coll

Southwest

Finan, Michael A MD (Gynecologic Oncology) - *Special Expertise:* Pelvic Cancer; **Admitting Hospital:** Ochsner Foundation Hospital; **Office Address:** Ochsner Clinical Division - Gyneclogic Oncology 1514 Jefferson Hwy New Orleans, LA 70121-2429; **Office Phone:** (504) 842-4165; **Board Certifications:** Obstetrics & Gynecology 1993, Gynecologic Oncology 1997; **Medical School:** Louisiana State Univ 1986; **Residency:** Obstetrics & Gynecology, Univ South Fla Affiliated Hosps, Tampa, FL 1986-1990; **Fellowship:** Gynecologic Oncology, Univ Soutt Fla Affiliated Hosps, Tampa, FL 1990-1992

Freedman, Ralph MD (Gynecologic Oncology) - *Special Expertise:* Immune Deficiency; Ovarian Cancer; **Admitting Hospital:** University of Texas MD Anderson Cancer Center (Page 66); **Office Address:** Univ Texas MD Anderson Canc Ctr, Dept Gyn Onc 1515 Holcombe Blvd, Box 67 Houston, TX 77030; **Office Phone:** (713) 792-2764; **Board Certification:** Obstetrics & Gynecology 1980; **Medical School:** South Africa 1965; **Residency:** Obstetrics & Gynecology, Queen Victoria-Johannesburg-Baragwanath Hosps, Johannesburg, S Africa 1968-1971; **Fellowship:** Gynecologic Oncology, Univ Texas MD Anderson Canc Ctr, Houston, TX 1976; **Faculty Appointment:** Prof Gynecologic Oncology, Univ Tex, Houston

Fromm, Geri Lynn MD (Gynecologic Oncology) - *Special Expertise:* Gynecologic Oncology - General; **Admitting Hospital:** St Luke's Episcopal Hospital - Houston (Page 76); **Office Address:** 2223 Dorrington St Houston, TX 77030; **Office Phone:** (713) 665-0404; **Board Certifications:** Obstetrics & Gynecology 1998, Gynecologic Oncology 1991; **Medical School:** Northwestern Univ 1981; **Residency:** Obstetrics & Gynecology, Magee Womens-Univ Pittsburgh, Pittsburgh, PA 1981-1985; **Fellowship:** Gynecologic Oncology, MD Anderson-Univ Texas, Houston, TX 1985-1987

Gershenson, David Marc MD (Gynecologic Oncology) - *Special Expertise:* Ovarian Cancer; Uterine Cancer; **Admitting Hospital:** University of Texas MD Anderson Cancer Center (Page 66); **Office Address:** Univ Tex-MD Anderson Cancer Ctr 1515 Holcombe Blvd, Box 0067 Houston, TX 77030; **Office Phone:** (713) 745-2565; **Board Certifications:** Obstetrics & Gynecology 1991, Gynecologic Oncology 1981; **Medical School:** Vanderbilt Univ 1971; **Residency:** Obstetrics & Gynecology, Yale-New Haven Hosp, New Haven, CT 1972-1975; **Fellowship:** Gynecologic Oncology, MD Anderson Hosp, Houston, TX 1977-1979; **Faculty Appointment:** Clin Prof Obstetrics & Gynecology, Univ Tex, Houston

Parham, Groesbeck Preer MD (Gynecologic Oncology) - *Special Expertise:* Cervical Cancer; **Admitting Hospital:** University of Arkansas for Medical Sciences; **Office Address:** Univ Hosp of Arkansas for Med Sci 4301 W Markham St Little Rock, AR 72205; **Office Phone:** (501) 296-1099; **Board Certifications:** Obstetrics & Gynecology 1999, Gynecologic Oncology 1999; **Medical School:** Univ Ala 1981; **Residency:** Obstetrics & Gynecology, Univ Ala Hosp, Birmingham, AL 1981-1985; **Fellowship:** Gynecologic Oncology, UC Irvine Med Ctr, Orange, CA 1986-1988; **Faculty Appointment:** Prof Obstetrics & Gynecology, Univ Ark

Roman-Lopez, Juan J MD (Gynecologic Oncology) - *Special Expertise:* Gynecologic Oncology - General; **Admitting Hospital:** University of Arkansas for Medical Sciences; **Office Address:** Univ Hosp for Med Sciences 4301 W Markham St, Ste 518 Little Rock, AR 72205-7101; **Office Phone:** (501) 661-0596; **Board Certification:** Obstetrics & Gynecology 1971; **Medical School:** Univ Puerto Rico 1963; **Residencies:** Obstetrics & Gynecology, San Juan City Hosp, Puerto Rico 1966-1967; Obstetrics & Gynecology, Tulane-Charity Hosp, New Orleans, LA 1967-1969; **Fellowship:** Gynecologic Oncology, Tulane-LSU Med Ctr, New Orleans, LA 1969-1970; **Faculty Appointment:** Assoc Clin Prof Obstetrics & Gynecology, Univ Ark

West Coast and Pacific

Berek, Jonathan S MD (Gynecologic Oncology) - *Special Expertise:* Ovarian Cancer; **Admitting Hospital:** UCLA Medical Center; **Office Address:** UCLA ObGyn Consultations Suites 760 Westwood Plaza, Bldg 300 Los Angeles, CA 90090; **Office Phone:** (310) 794-7274; **Board Certifications:** Gynecologic Oncology 1983, Obstetrics & Gynecology 1991; **Medical School:** Johns Hopkins Univ 1975; **Residency:** Obstetrics & Gynecology, Harvard Med Sch-Brigham & Woman's Hosp, Boston, MA 1976-1979; **Fellowship:** Gynecologic Oncology, UCLA Sch Med, Los Angeles, CA 1979-1981; **Faculty Appointment:** Prof Obstetrics & Gynecology, UCLA

Greer, Benjamin MD (Gynecologic Oncology) - *Special Expertise:* Gynecologic Oncology - General; **Admitting Hospital:** University of Washington Medical Center; **Office Address:** Univ Washington Med Ctr, Dept OB/GYN Box 356460 Seattle, WA 98195-6460; **Office Phone:** (206) 685-2463; **Board Certifications:** Obstetrics & Gynecology 1989, Gynecologic Oncology 1983; **Medical School:** Univ Penn 1966; **Residency:** Obstetrics & Gynecology, Univ Colorado Med Ctr, Denver, CO 1967-1970; **Faculty Appointment:** Prof Obstetrics & Gynecology, Univ Wash

Lagasse, Leo D MD (Gynecologic Oncology) - *Special Expertise:* Ovarian Cancer; **Admitting Hospital:** Cedars-Sinai Medical Center; **Office Address:** Cedars-Sinai Med Ctr 8700 Beverly Blvd Ste 160W Los Angeles, CA 90048-1804; **Office Phone:** (310) 423-3373; **Board Certifications:** Obstetrics & Gynecology 1967, Gynecologic Oncology 1974; **Medical School:** Univ VA Sch Med 1959; **Residency:** Obstetrics & Gynecology, UCLA Med Ctr, Los Angeles, CA 1960-1964; **Faculty Appointment:** Prof Obstetrics & Gynecology, UCLA

Morrow, Charles Paul MD (Gynecologic Oncology) - *Special Expertise:* Gynecologic Oncology - General; **Admitting Hospital:** USC Norris Cancer Comprehensive Center; **Office Address:** USC K Norris, Jr Cancer Hosp 1441 Eastlake Ave, Ste 7419 Los Angeles, CA 90033; **Office Phone:** (323) 865-3922; **Board Certifications:** Obstetrics & Gynecology 1970, Gynecologic Oncology 1974; **Medical School:** Loyola Univ-Stritch Sch Med 1962; **Residencies:** Obstetrics & Gynecology, Little Co Mary Hosp, Evergreen, IL 1965-1966; Obstetrics & Gynecology, Chicago Mercy Hosp, Chicago, IL 1966-1968; **Fellowship:** Gynecologic Oncology, MD Anderson Hosp Houston, Houston, TX 1968-1970; **Faculty Appointment:** Prof Obstetrics & Gynecology, UCLA

Roberts, James A MD (Gynecologic Oncology) - *Special Expertise:* Gynecologic Cancer; **Admitting Hospital:** Stanford Medical Center; **Office Address:** Stanford Univ Med Ctr 300 Pasteur Drive, GYN Clinic, Fl 3 Stanford, CA 94305-5317; **Office Phone:** (650) 498-8080; **Board Certifications:** Obstetrics & Gynecology 1999, Gynecologic Oncology 1999; **Medical School:** Med Coll Wisc 1973; **Residency:** Obstetrics & Gynecology, UCLA, Los Angeles, CA 1973-1977; **Fellowship:** Gynecologic Oncology, UCLA-City of Hope Med Ctr, Los Angeles, CA 1977-1979; **Faculty Appointment:** Prof Obstetrics & Gynecology, Stanford Univ

Stern, Jeffrey L MD (Gynecologic Oncology) - *Special Expertise:* Gynecologic Oncology - General; **Admitting Hospital:** Alta Bates Summit Medical Center; **Office Address:** Womens Cancer Ctr Northern Calif 2100 Webster St, Fl 319 San Francisco, CA 94115; **Office Phone:** (415) 202-1570; **Board Certifications:** Obstetrics & Gynecology 1983, Gynecologic Oncology 1984; **Medical School:** SUNY Syracuse 1976; **Residency:** Obstetrics & Gynecology, Johns Hopkins Hosp, Baltimore, MD 1977-1980; **Fellowship:** Gynecologic Oncology, USC Med Ctr, Los Angeles, CA 1980-1982; **Faculty Appointment:** Assoc Prof Obstetrics & Gynecology, UCSF

Teng, Nelson NH MD/PhD (Gynecologic Oncology) - *Special Expertise:* Gynecologic Cancer; **Admitting Hospital:** Stanford Medical Center; **Office Address:** Stanford Univ Sch Med, Dept Gyn Onc 300 Pasteur Dr, Rm H302 Stanford, CA 94305-5317; **Office Phone:** (650) 498-8080; **Board Certifications:** Obstetrics & Gynecology 1985, Gynecologic Oncology 1987; **Medical School:** Univ Miami Sch Med 1977; **Residency:** Obstetrics & Gynecology, UCLA, Los Angeles, CA 1978-1981; **Fellowship:** Gynecologic Oncology, Stanford Univ Sch Med, Stanford, CA 1984; **Faculty Appointment:** Assoc Prof Gynecologic Oncology, Stanford Univ

HAND SURGERY

(a subspecialty of ORTHOPAEDICS, SURGERY or PLASTIC SURGERY)

A specialist trained in the investigation, preservation and restoration by medical, surgical and rehabilitative means of all structures of the upper extremity directly affecting the form and function of the hand and wrist.

ORTHOPAEDICS
An orthopaedic surgeon is involved with the care of patients whose musculoskeletal problems include congenital deformities, trauma, infections, tumors, metabolic disturbances of the musculoskeletal system, deformities, injuries and degenerative diseases of the spine, hands, feet, knee, hip, shoulder and elbow in children and adults. An orthopaedic surgeon is also concerned with primary and secondary muscular problems and the effects of central or peripheral nervous system lesions of the musculoskeletal system.

SURGERY
A surgeon manages a broad spectrum of surgical conditions affecting almost any area of the body. The surgeon establishes the diagnosis and provides the preoperative, operative and postoperative care to surgical patients and is usually responsible for the comprehensive management of the trauma victim and the critically ill surgical patient. The surgeon uses a variety of diagnostic techniques, including endoscopy, for observing internal structures, and may use specialized instruments during operative procedures. A general surgeon is expected to be familiar with the salient features of other surgical specialties in order to recognize problems in those areas and to know when to refer a patient to another specialist.

PLASTIC SURGERY
A plastic surgeon deals with the repair, reconstruction or replacement of physical defects of form or function involving the skin, musculoskeletal system, craniomaxillofacial structures, hand, extremities, breast and trunk and external genitalia. He/she uses aesthetic surgical principles not only to improve undesirable qualities of normal structures but in all reconstructive procedures as well.

Training required: Five years (including general surgery) in orthopaedics *plus* two years in clinical practice before final certification is achieved *plus* additional training and examination in hand surgery OR five to seven years in plastic surgery *plus* additional training and examination in hand surgery.

265

PHYSICIAN LISTINGS

New England

Belsky, Mark R MD (Hand Surgery) - *Special Expertise:* Hand Surgery - General; **Admitting Hospital:** Newton - Wellesley Hospital; **Office Address:** Surgery 2000 Washington St, Ste 553 Newton, MA 02462-1628; **Office Phone:** (617) 965-4263; **Board Certifications:** Orthopaedic Surgery 1982, Hand Surgery 1990; **Medical School:** Tufts Univ 1974; **Residencies:** Surgery, Peter Bent Brigham Hosp, Boston, MA 1975-1976; Orthopaedic Surgery, Tufts-New Eng Med Ctr, Boston, MA 1976-1979; **Fellowship:** Hand Surgery, Roosevelt Hosp, New York, NY 1980; **Faculty Appointment:** Assoc Clin Prof Orthopaedic Surgery, Tufts Univ

Upton, Joseph MD (Hand Surgery) - *Special Expertise:* Hand-Congenital Anomaly; Hand Microsurgical Reconstruction; **Admitting Hospital:** Children's Hospital; **Office Address:** 830 Boylston St, Ste 212 Chestnut Hill, MA 02467; **Office Phone:** (617) 739-1972; **Board Certifications:** Plastic Surgery 1981, Hand Surgery 1992; **Medical School:** Baylor Coll Med 1970; **Residencies:** Orthopaedic Surgery, Eisenhower Med Ctr, Augusta, GA 1972-1974; Surgery, St Joseph Hosp, Houston, TX 1974-1976; **Fellowship:** Hand Surgery, Roosevelt Hosp, New York, NY 1976-1977; **Faculty Appointment:** Assoc Prof Surgery, Harvard Med Sch

Waters, Peter Michael MD (Hand Surgery) - *Special Expertise:* Brachial Plexus; Hand-Congenital Anomaly; **Admitting Hospital:** Children's Hospital; **Office Address:** Chldrns Hosp, Dept Ortho Surg 300 Longwood Ave Boston, MA 02115; **Office Phone:** (617) 355-6021; **Board Certifications:** Orthopaedic Surgery 1991, Hand Surgery 1992; **Medical School:** Tufts Univ 1981; **Residencies:** Pediatrics, Mass Genl Hosp, Boston, MA 1981-1983; Orthopaedic Surgery, Harvard Combined Prog, Boston, MA 1984-1988; **Fellowship:** Hand Surgery, Brigham/Childrens Hosp, Boston, MA 1988-1989; **Faculty Appointment:** Assoc Prof Orthopaedic Surgery, Harvard Med Sch

Weiss, Arnold Peter MD (Hand Surgery) - *Special Expertise:* Carpal Tunnel Syndrome; **Admitting Hospital:** Rhode Island Hospital; **Office Address:** Univ Orth Inc 2 Dudley St, Ste 200 Providence, RI 02905; **Office Phone:** (401) 457-1520; **Board Certifications:** Orthopaedic Surgery 1993, Hand Surgery 1994; **Medical School:** Johns Hopkins Univ 1985; **Residency:** Orthopaedic Surgery, Johns Hopkins Hosp, Baltimore, MD 1986-1990; **Fellowship:** Hand Surgery, Ind Hand Ctr, Indianapolis, IN 1990-1991; **Faculty Appointment:** Prof Orthopaedic Surgery, Brown Univ

Mid Atlantic

Beasley, Robert MD (Hand Surgery) - *Special Expertise:* Plastic Surgery of Hand; Paralytic Disorders; Arthritis Hand Surgery; **Admitting Hospital:** NYU Medical Center (Page 70); **Office Address:** 345 E 37th St, Ste 306 New York, NY 10016; **Office Phone:** (212) 986-9494; **Board Certification:** Plastic Surgery 1968; **Medical School:** Univ Tenn Coll Med, Memphis 1955; **Residencies:** Surgery, St Luke's Roosevelt Hosp, New York, NY 1957-1959; Hand Surgery, Presbyterian Hosp, New York, NY 1960-1961; **Fellowship:** Plastic Surgery, Columbia-Presby Med Ctr, New York, NY 1962-1963; **Faculty Appointment:** Prof Surgery, NYU Sch Med

Chiu, David MD (Hand Surgery) - *Special Expertise:* Hand & Microvascular Surgery; Cosmetic Surgery; **Admitting Hospital:** Columbia Presbyterian Medical Center (Page 72); **Office Address:** 900 Park Ave at 79th St New York, NY 10021; **Office Phone:** (212) 879-8880; **Board Certifications:** Plastic Surgery 1982, Hand Surgery 1990; **Medical School:** Columbia P&S 1973; **Residencies:** Surgery, Columbia-Presby Med Ctr, New York, NY 1973-1977; Plastic Surgery, Barnes Hosp-Washington Univ, St Louis, MO 1977-1979; **Fellowship:** Hand Surgery, NYU Med Ctr, New York, NY 1980; **Faculty Appointment:** Prof Surgery, Columbia P&S

HAND SURGERY

Mid Atlantic

Culp, Randall MD (Hand Surgery) - *Special Expertise:* Microsurgery; **Admitting Hospital:** Thomas Jefferson University Hospital; **Office Address:** The Philadelphia Hand Center PC 700 S Henderson Rd, Ste 200 King of Prussia, PA 19406; **Office Phone:** (610) 768-4474; **Board Certifications:** Orthopaedic Surgery 1990, Hand Surgery 1992; **Medical School:** Penn State Univ-Hershey Med Ctr 1982; **Residency:** Orthopaedic Surgery, Hosp Univ Penn, Philadelphia, PA 1983-1987; **Fellowship:** Hand Surgery, Hosp Univ Penn, Philadelphia, PA 1987-1988; **Faculty Appointment:** Assoc Prof Orthopaedic Surgery, Jefferson Med Coll

Glickel, Steven MD (Hand Surgery) - *Special Expertise:* Hand & Wrist Surgery; Elbow Disorders/Surgery; **Admitting Hospital:** St Luke's - Roosevelt Hospital Center - Roosevelt Division (Page 58); **Office Address:** 1000 10th Ave New York, NY 10019; **Office Phone:** (212) 523-7590; **Board Certifications:** Orthopaedic Surgery 1985, Hand Surgery 1998; **Medical School:** Harvard Med Sch 1976; **Residencies:** Surgery, Columbia Presby Hosp, New York, NY 1976-1978; Orthopaedic Surgery, Harvard Comb Ortho, Boston, MA 1978-1981; **Fellowship:** Hand Surgery, St Luke's-Roosevelt Hosp Ctr, New York, NY 1982-1983; **Faculty Appointment:** Assoc Clin Prof Orthopaedic Surgery, Columbia P&S

Lubahn, John D MD (Hand Surgery) - *Special Expertise:* Microsurgery; **Admitting Hospital:** Hamot Medical Center; **Office Address:** 300 State St, Ste 205 Erie, PA 16507-1429; **Office Phone:** (814) 456-6022; **Board Certifications:** Orthopaedic Surgery 1992, Hand Surgery 1998; **Medical School:** Case West Res Univ 1975; **Residencies:** Surgery, Univ Rochester Med Ctr, Rochester, MN 1976-1977; Orthopaedic Surgery, Univ Rochester Med Ctr, Rochester, MN 1977-1980; **Fellowship:** Hand Surgery, Univ Louisville Hosp, Louisville, KY 1980-1981

McCormack Jr, Richard R MD (Hand Surgery) - *Special Expertise:* Dupuytren's Contracture; Arthritis Hand Surgery; Hand & Wrist Fractures; **Admitting Hospital:** Hospital for Special Surgery (Page 63); **Office Address:** 523 E 72nd St, Fl 4 New York, NY 10021; **Office Phone:** (212) 606-1230; **Board Certifications:** Orthopaedic Surgery 1983, Hand Surgery 1992; **Medical School:** Cornell Univ-Weil Med Coll 1975; **Residencies:** Surgery, Roosevelt Hosp, New York, NY 1976-1977; Orthopaedic Surgery, Hosp For Special Surg, New York, NY 1977-1980; **Fellowship:** Hand Surgery, Roosevelt Hosp, New York, NY 1980-1981; **Faculty Appointment:** Assoc Clin Prof Orthopaedic Surgery, Cornell Univ-Weil Med Coll

Melone Jr, Charles P MD (Hand Surgery) - *Special Expertise:* Arthritis Hand Surgery; Wrist Surgery; **Admitting Hospital:** Beth Israel Medical Center - New York; **Office Address:** 321 E 34th St New York, NY 10016; **Office Phone:** (212) 340-0000; **Board Certifications:** Orthopaedic Surgery 1976, Hand Surgery 1993; **Medical School:** Georgetown Univ 1969; **Residencies:** Surgery, Nassau County Med Ctr, East Meadow, NY 1970-1971; Orthopaedic Surgery, Nassau County Med Ctr, East Meadow, NY 1971-1974; **Fellowship:** Hand Surgery, NYU Med Ctr, New York, NY 1974-1975; **Faculty Appointment:** Clin Prof Orthopaedic Surgery, Albert Einstein Coll Med

Patel, Mukund MD (Hand Surgery) - *Special Expertise:* Hand Surgery - General; **Admitting Hospital:** Staten Island University Hospital - South; **Office Address:** Orthopedic Surg Assocs 4901 Fort Hamilton Pkwy Brooklyn, NY 11219; **Office Phone:** (718) 435-4944; **Board Certifications:** Orthopaedic Surgery 1972, Hand Surgery 2000; **Medical School:** India 1966; **Residency:** Orthopaedic Surgery, Maimonides Med Ctr, Brooklyn, NY 1968-1970; **Fellowship:** Hand Surgery, Mass Gen Hosp, Boston, MA 1970-1971; **Faculty Appointment:** Asst Clin Prof Surgery, SUNY Hlth Sci Ctr

Peimer, Clayton Austin MD (Hand Surgery) - *Special Expertise:* Hand Surgery - General; **Admitting Hospital:** Millard Fillmore Hospitals; **Office Address:** Hand Center of Western New York 3 Gates Cir Buffalo, NY 14209-1120; **Office Phone:** (716) 887-4599; **Board Certifications:** Orthopaedic Surgery 1978, Hand Surgery 2000; **Medical School:** SUNY Syracuse 1971; **Residencies:** Surgery, Beth Israel Med Ctr, NY, NY 1972-1973; Orthopaedic Surgery, SUNY Upstate Med tr, Syracuse, NY 1973-1976; **Fellowship:** Hand Surgery, Mass Gen Hosp, Boston, MA 1976-1977; **Faculty Appointment:** Assoc Prof Orthopaedic Surgery, SUNY Buffalo

Strauch, Robert MD (Hand Surgery) - *Special Expertise:* Hand Surgery - General; **Admitting Hospital:** Columbia Presbyterian Medical Center (Page 72); **Office Address:** 161 Fort Washington Ave New York, NY 10032; **Office Phone:** (212) 305-4272; **Board Certifications:** Orthopaedic Surgery 1994, Hand Surgery 1995; **Medical School:** Columbia P&S 1986; **Residency:** Orthopaedic Surgery, Columbia-Presby Hosp, New York, NY 1988-1991; **Fellowship:** Hand Surgery, Indiana Hand Center, Indianapolis, IN 1991-1992; **Faculty Appointment:** Asst Prof Orthopaedic Surgery, Columbia P&S

Weiland, Andrew J MD (Hand Surgery) - *Special Expertise:* Wrist/Hand Injuries; **Admitting Hospital:** Hospital for Special Surgery (Page 63); **Office Address:** 535 E 70th St New York, NY 10021; **Office Phone:** (212) 606-1575; **Board Certifications:** Hand Surgery 1989, Orthopaedic Surgery 1992; **Medical School:** Wake Forest Univ Sch Med 1968; **Residencies:** Surgery, Univ Michigan Med Ctr, Ann Arbor, MI 1969-1970; Orthopaedic Surgery, Johns Hopkins Hosp, Baltimore, MD 1972-1975; **Fellowship:** Hand Surgery, Kleinert Hosp, Louisville, KY 1975; **Faculty Appointment:** Prof Orthopaedic Surgery, Cornell Univ-Weil Med Coll

Wolfe, Scott W MD (Hand Surgery) - *Special Expertise:* Hand Surgery - General; **Admitting Hospital:** Hospital for Special Surgery (Page 63); **Office Address:** 523 E 72nd St New York, NY 10021; **Office Phone:** (212) 606-1529; **Board Certifications:** Orthopaedic Surgery 1992, Hand Surgery 1993; **Medical School:** Cornell Univ-Weil Med Coll 1984; **Residency:** Orthopaedic Surgery, Hosp Special Surg, New York, NY 1986-1989; **Fellowship:** Hand Surgery, Columbia Presby Med Ctr, New York, NY 1989-1990; **Faculty Appointment:** Prof Orthopaedic Surgery, Cornell Univ-Weil Med Coll

Southeast

Carneiro, Ronaldo Dos Santos MD (Hand Surgery) - *Special Expertise:* Hand Surgery - General; **Admitting Hospital:** Cleveland Clinic Florida; **Office Address:** Cleveland Clinic-Florida 6101 Pine Ridge Rd Naples, FL 34119; **Office Phone:** (941) 348-4000; **Board Certifications:** Plastic Surgery 1990, Hand Surgery 1994; **Medical School:** Brazil 1970; **Residencies:** Surgery, Union Meml Hosp, Baltimore, MD 1971-1975; Plastic Surgery, Allentown & Sacred Heart Hosp Ctr, Allentown, PA 1975-1977; **Fellowships:** Hand Surgery, Jackson Meml Hosp-Univ Miami Hosp, Miami, FL 1977; Plastic Surgery, Univ Miami Sch Med, Miami, FL 1978

Freeland, Alan Edward MD (Hand Surgery) - *Special Expertise:* Hand Surgery - General; **Admitting Hospital:** University Hospital & Clinics- Mississippi; **Office Address:** Univ Mississippi Med Ctr, Orthopaedic Assocs 2500 N State St Jackson, MS 39216-4505; **Office Phone:** (601) 984-5144; **Board Certifications:** Orthopaedic Surgery 1977, Hand Surgery 2000; **Medical School:** Geo Wash Univ 1965; **Residencies:** Orthopaedic Surgery, Letterman AMC, San Francisco, CA 1973-1976; Orthopaedic Surgery, Johns Hopkins Hosp, Baltimore, MD 1967-1970; **Fellowship:** Hand Surgery, Jackson Meml Hosp-Univ Miami Med Ctr, Miami, FL 1973-1976; **Faculty Appointment:** Prof Surgery, Univ Miss

Freshwater, M Felix MD (Hand Surgery) - *Special Expertise:* Plastic Surgery of Hand; **Admitting Hospital:** Baptist Hospital - Miami; **Office Address:** Miami Inst of Hand & Microsurgery 9100 S Dadeland Blvd, Ste 502 Miami, FL 33156-7815; **Office Phone:** (305) 670-9988; **Board Certifications:** Plastic Surgery 1980, Hand Surgery 1997; **Medical School:** Yale Univ 1972; **Residencies:** Surgery, Yale-New Haven Hosp, New Haven, CT 1972-1974; Plastic Surgery, Jackson Meml Hosp, Miami, FL 1977-1978; **Fellowships:** John Hopkins University, Baltimore, MD 1974-1977; Hand Surgery, Univ Louisville, Louisville, KY 1979; **Faculty Appointment:** Asst Clin Prof Surgery, Univ Miami Sch Med

Greene, Thomas MD (Hand Surgery) - *Special Expertise:* Hand Surgery - General; **Admitting Hospital:** Tampa General Hospital; **Office Address:** Tampa Bay Surgery Specialists, PA 2727 W Dr Martin Luther King Jr Blvd, Ste 560 Tampa, FL 33607; **Office Phone:** (813) 873-0337; **Board Certifications:** Orthopaedic Surgery 1983, Hand Surgery 2000; **Medical School:** Ohio State Univ 1975; **Residencies:** Surgery, Univ Michigan, Ann Arbor, MI 1976-1977; Orthopaedic Surgery, Univ Michigan, Ann Arbor, MI 1977-1980; **Fellowship:** Hand Surgery, St Vincent's Hosp, Indianapolis, IN 1980-1981

Koman, L Andrew MD (Hand Surgery) - *Special Expertise:* Carpal Tunnel Syndrome; Wrist/Hand Injuries; **Admitting Hospital:** Wake Forest University Baptist Medical Center; **Office Address:** Wake Forest University Baptist Medical Center Medical Center Blvd Winston-Salem, NC 27157; **Office Phone:** (336) 716-2878; **Board Certifications:** Orthopaedic Surgery 1981, Hand Surgery 2000; **Medical School:** Duke Univ 1974; **Residencies:** Surgery, Duke Univ Med Ctr., Durham, NC 1974-1975; Orthopaedic Surgery, Duke Univ Med Ctr., Durham, NC 1975-1979; **Fellowship:** Hand Surgery, Duke Univ Med Ctr, Durham, NC 1979-1980; **Faculty Appointment:** Prof Orthopaedic Surgery, Wake Forest Univ Sch Med

McAuliffe, John A MD (Hand Surgery) - *Special Expertise:* Hand Surgery - General; **Admitting Hospital:** Cleveland Clinic Florida; **Office Address:** 3000 West Cypress Creek Rd Fort Lauderdale, FL 33109; **Office Phone:** (954) 978-7425; **Board Certifications:** Orthopaedic Surgery 1991, Hand Surgery 1992; **Medical School:** Univ Fla Coll Med 1982; **Residency:** Orthopaedic Surgery, Univ Fla Affil Hosp, Gainsville, FL 1983-1988; **Fellowship:** Hand Surgery, Univ Miami, Miami, FL 1988-1989; **Faculty Appointment:** Asst Prof Orthopaedic Surgery, Univ Miami Sch Med

Nunley, James MD (Hand Surgery) - *Special Expertise:* Arthritis Hand Surgery; Ankle Joint Replacement; **Admitting Hospital:** Duke University Medical Center (Page 60); **Office Address:** Orthopaedic Surgery, Duke Univ. Med. Ctr. Box 2923 Durham, NC 27710-0001; **Office Phone:** (919) 684-4033; **Board Certifications:** Orthopaedic Surgery 1981, Hand Surgery 1989; **Medical School:** Tulane Univ 1973; **Residency:** Orthopaedic Surgery, Duke Univ Med Ctr, Durham, NC 1975-1979; **Fellowship:** Hand Surgery, Duke Univ Med Ctr, Durham, NC 1979-1980; **Faculty Appointment:** Prof Orthopaedic Surgery, Duke Univ

Ouellette, Elizabeth Anne MD (Hand Surgery) - *Special Expertise:* Hand Surgery - General; **Admitting Hospital:** University of Miami - Jackson Memorial Hospital; **Office Address:** 900 NW 17th St, Ste 549 Miami, FL 33136; **Office Phone:** (305) 326-6590; **Board Certifications:** Orthopaedic Surgery 2000, Hand Surgery 2000; **Medical School:** Univ Tex, San Antonio 1978; **Residency:** Orthopaedic Surgery, Univ Wash Hosp, Seattle, WA 1978-1983; **Fellowship:** Hand Surgery, Jackson Meml Hosp, Miami, FL 1984-1985; **Faculty Appointment:** Assoc Prof Orthopaedic Surgery, Univ Miami Sch Med

Tsai, Tsu-Min MD (Hand Surgery) - *Special Expertise:* Microsurgery; **Admitting Hospital:** Jewish Hospital & Medical Center - Louisville; **Office Address:** One Med Ctr Plaza 225 Abraham Flexner Way, Ste 700 Louisville, KY 40202; **Office Phone:** (502) 561-4263; **Board Certifications:** Orthopaedic Surgery 1984, Hand Surgery 1990; **Medical School:** Taiwan 1961; **Residencies:** Surgery, Natl Taiwan Univ Hosp, Taipei, Taiwan 1964-1970; Orthopaedic Surgery, Univ Louisville Hosp, Louisville, KY 1976-1979; **Fellowship:** Hand Surgery, Univ Louisville Hosp, Louisville, KY 1976; **Faculty Appointment:** Clin Prof Orthopaedic Surgery, Univ Louisville Sch Med

Urbaniak, James R MD (Hand Surgery) - *Special Expertise:* Hand, Wrist, Elbow Microsurgery; Peripheral nerve repair; **Admitting Hospital:** Duke University Medical Center (Page 60); **Office Address:** Duke Univ Med Ctr Box 2912 Durham, NC 27712; **Office Phone:** (919) 684-5388; **Board Certification:** Orthopaedic Surgery 1992; **Medical School:** Duke Univ 1962; **Residency:** Orthopaedic Surgery, Duke Univ Affl Hosps, Durham, NC 1965-1969; **Faculty Appointment:** Prof Orthopaedic Surgery, Duke Univ

Midwest

Bishop, Allen Thorp MD (Hand Surgery) - *Special Expertise:* Hand Surgery - General; **Admitting Hospital:** Mayo Medical Center & Clinic - Rochester; **Office Address:** Mayo Clinic 200 1st St SW Rochester, MN 55905; **Office Phone:** (507) 284-4149; **Board Certifications:** Orthopaedic Surgery 2000, Hand Surgery 2000; **Medical School:** Mayo Med Sch 1981; **Residency:** Orthopaedic Surgery, Mayo Grad Sch Med, Rochester, MN 1981-1986; **Fellowship:** Hand Surgery, St Vincent Hosp, Indianapolis, IN 1986-1987; **Faculty Appointment:** Prof Orthopaedic Surgery, Mayo Med Sch

Carroll, Charles MD (Hand Surgery) - *Special Expertise:* Carpal Tunnel Syndrome; Hand Surgery; Elbow Disorders/Surgery; **Admitting Hospital:** Northwestern Memorial Hospital; **Office Address:** Northwestern Center for Orthopedics 676 N Saint Clair Rd, Ste 450 Chicago, IL 60611-2983; **Office Phone:** (312) 943-7850; **Board Certifications:** Orthopaedic Surgery 1990, Hand Surgery 1992; **Medical School:** Univ MD Sch Med 1982; **Residencies:** Surgery, Johns Hopkins Hosp, Baltimore, MD 1983-1984; Orthopaedic Surgery, Johns Hopkins Hosp, Baltimore, MD 1984-1987; **Fellowship:** Hand Surgery, Indiana Univ Med Ctr, Indianapolis, IN 1987-1988; **Faculty Appointment:** Assoc Clin Prof Orthopaedic Surgery, Northwestern Univ

Chung, Kevin MD (Hand Surgery) - *Special Expertise:* Hand-Congenital Anomaly; Hand & Microvascular Surgery; Upper Extremity Trauma; **Admitting Hospital:** University of Michigan Health Center; **Office Address:** U of M Plastic Surgery-Domino's Farms 24 Frank Lloyd Wright Dr, Fl D Ann Arbor, MI 48106; **Office Phone:** (734) 998-6022; **Board Certifications:** Plastic Surgery 1997, Hand Surgery 1997; **Medical School:** Emory Univ 1987; **Residencies:** Plastic Surgery, Univ Michigan Hosp & Hlth Ctr, Ann Arbor, MI 1992-1994; Hand Surgery, Union Meml Hosp, Baltimore, MD 1994-1995

Cooney, William MD (Hand Surgery) - *Special Expertise:* Wrist/Hand Injuries; **Admitting Hospital:** Mayo Medical Center & Clinic - Rochester; **Office Address:** Mayo Clinic 200 1st St SW Rochester, MN 55905; **Office Phone:** (507) 284-2994; **Board Certifications:** Orthopaedic Surgery 1978, Hand Surgery 1989; **Medical School:** St Louis Univ 1969; **Residencies:** Surgery, Mich Hosp 1969-1970; Orthopaedic Surgery, Mayo Fdn Hosp., Rochester, MN 1971-1975; **Fellowship:** Hand Surgery, Mayo Fdn Hosp., Rochester, MN 1975-1976; **Faculty Appointment:** Prof Orthopaedic Surgery, Mayo Med Sch

HAND SURGERY _Midwest_

Derman, Gordon Harris MD (Hand Surgery) - *Special Expertise:* Carpal Tunnel Syndrome; Tendon Repair/ Reattachment; Repetitive Motion Injuries; **Admitting Hospital:** Rush/Presbyterian - St Luke's Medical Center - Chicago (Page 74); **Office Address:** 800 S Wells St, Ste 105 Chicago, IL 60607; **Office Phone:** (312) 408-0800; **Board Certifications:** Plastic Surgery 1984, Hand Surgery 1999; **Medical School:** Rush Med Coll 1975; **Residencies:** Surgery, Loyola Univ Med Ctr, Maywood, IL 1977-1981; Plastic Surgery, Univ Mich Hosp, Ann Arbor, IL 1981-1983; **Fellowship:** Microsurgery, Rush/Presby St Luke's, Chicago, IL 1976; **Faculty Appointment:** Asst Prof Surgery, Rush Med Coll

Failla, Joseph M MD (Hand Surgery) - *Special Expertise:* Hand Surgery; Hand Reconstruction; **Admitting Hospital:** Henry Ford Health System (Page 62); **Office Address:** 2799 W Grand Blvd Detroit, MI 48202; **Office Phone:** (313) 876-2181; **Board Certifications:** Orthopaedic Surgery 1990, Hand Surgery 1992; **Medical School:** SUNY Buffalo 1982; **Residency:** Orthopaedic Surgery, SUNY-Buffalo, Buffalo, NY 1983-1987; **Fellowship:** Hand Surgery, Mayo Clinic, Rochester, NY 1987-1988

Fischer, Thomas James MD (Hand Surgery) - *Special Expertise:* Hand Surgery - General; **Admitting Hospital:** St Vincent's Hospital and Health Center - Indianapolis; **Office Address:** The Indiana Hand Center Box 80434 indianapolis, IN 46280-0434; **Office Phone:** (315) 875-9105; **Board Certifications:** Orthopaedic Surgery 2000, Hand Surgery 2000; **Medical School:** Indiana Univ 1979; **Residencies:** Orthopaedic Surgery, Univ Wash Affil Hosp, Seattle, WA 1980-1984; Hand Surgery, Duke Univ Med Ctr, Durham, NC 1986; **Fellowships:** Hand Surgery, Hand Surg Assoc, Indianapolis, IN 1984-1985; Hand Surgery, Duke Univ Med Ctr, Durham, NC 1986; **Faculty Appointment:** Asst Clin Prof Orthopaedic Surgery, Indiana Univ

Gelberman, Richard MD (Hand Surgery) - *Special Expertise:* Flexor Tendon Surgery; Peripheral Nerve Surgery; **Admitting Hospital:** Barnes - Jewish Hospital; **Office Address:** 1 Barnes Hospital Plaza, Ste 11300 St Louis, MO 63110; **Office Phone:** (314) 747-2531; **Board Certifications:** Orthopaedic Surgery 1997, Hand Surgery 1996; **Medical School:** Univ Tenn Coll Med, Memphis 1969; **Residency:** Surgery, Univ Wisc Med Ctr, Madison, WI 1971-1975; **Fellowships:** Hand Surgery, Duke Univ Med Ctr, Durham, NC 1976-1977; Pediatric Orthopedic Surgery, Harvard Univ/Children's Hosp, Boston, MA 1985-1986; **Faculty Appointment:** Prof Orthopaedic Surgery, Washington Univ, St Louis

Hastings II, Hill MD (Hand Surgery) - *Special Expertise:* Hand Surgery - General; **Admitting Hospital:** St Vincent's Hospital and Health Center - Indianapolis; **Office Address:** The Indiana Hand Center 8501 Harcourt Rd Indianapolis, IN 46280; **Office Phone:** (317) 471-4338; **Board Certifications:** Orthopaedic Surgery 1982, Hand Surgery 2000; **Medical School:** USC Sch Med 1974; **Residencies:** Surgery, Univ Colorado Med Ctr, Denver, CO 1975-1976; Orthopaedic Surgery, Mass Genl Hosp, Boston, MA 1977-1980; **Fellowship:** Hand Surgery, St Vincent Hosp, Indianapolis, IN 1980-1981; **Faculty Appointment:** Assoc Clin Prof Orthopaedic Surgery, Indiana Univ

Hunt III, Thomas MD (Hand Surgery) - *Special Expertise:* Hand Surgery; Wrist Surgery; **Admitting Hospital:** Cleveland Clinic Foundation; **Office Address:** The Cleveland Clinic Dept of Orthopaedic Surgery 9500 Euclid Ave, MC-A40 Cleveland, OH 44195; **Office Phone:** (216) 445-6426; **Board Certifications:** Orthopaedic Surgery 1995, Hand Surgery 1996; **Medical School:** Vanderbilt Univ 1986; **Residency:** Orthopaedic Surgery, Univ Kansas Med Ctr, Kansas City, KS 1987-1992; **Fellowship:** Hand Surgery, Hospital of the Univ. of Pennsylvania, Philadelphia, PA 1992-1993

Idler, Richard S. MD (Hand Surgery) - *Special Expertise:* Hand Surgery; **Admitting Hospital:** Indiana University Hospital & Medical Center - Indianapolis; **Office Address:** The Indiana Hand Ctr 8501 Harcourt Rd Indianapolis, IN 46260; **Office Phone:** (317) 471-4334; **Board Certifications:** Orthopaedic Surgery 1985, Hand Surgery 1989; **Medical School:** Dartmouth Med Sch 1975; **Residencies:** Surgery, UCLA Med Ctr, Los Angeles, CA 1976-1977; Plastic Surgery, UCLA Med Ctr, Los Angeles, CA 1977-1978; **Fellowship:** Hand Surgery, St Vincent Hosp, Indianapolis, IN 1981-1982; **Faculty Appointment:** Asst Clin Prof Orthopaedic Surgery, Indiana Univ

Light, Terry MD (Hand Surgery) - *Special Expertise:* Hand Surgery - General; **Admitting Hospital:** Loyola University Health System; **Office Address:** Loyola University Medical Center 2160 S First Ave Maywood, IL 60153-5590; **Office Phone:** (708) 216-4570; **Board Certifications:** Orthopaedic Surgery 1979, Hand Surgery 2000; **Medical School:** Univ Hlth Sci/Chicago Med Sch 1973; **Residency:** Orthopaedic Surgery, Yale-New Haven Hosp, New Haven, CT 1974-1977; **Fellowship:** Hand Surgery, Hartford Hosp, Hartford, CT 1977; **Faculty Appointment:** Prof Surgery, Loyola Univ-Stritch Sch Med

Louis, Dean MD (Hand Surgery) - *Special Expertise:* Hand-Congenital Anomaly; **Admitting Hospital:** University of Michigan Health Center; **Office Address:** A.Alfred Taubman Health Care Ctr.Rm2912 Box 0328 1500 E. Medical Center Drive Ann Arbor, MI 48109-0328; **Office Phone:** (734) 936-5200; **Board Certifications:** Orthopaedic Surgery 1998, Hand Surgery 1998; **Medical School:** Univ VT Coll Med 1962; **Residency:** Orthopaedic Surgery, Univ Michigan, Ann Arbor, MI 1967-1970; **Fellowship:** Hand Surgery, Columbia Presby, New York, NY 1970-1971; **Faculty Appointment:** Prof Surgery, Univ Mich Med Sch

Manske, Paul MD (Hand Surgery) - *Special Expertise:* Hand Surgery - General; **Admitting Hospital:** Barnes - Jewish Hospital; **Office Address:** One Barnes Hospital Plaza West Pavilion, Ste 11300 St. Louis, MO 63110; **Office Phone:** (314) 747-2500; **Board Certifications:** Orthopaedic Surgery 1974, Hand Surgery 2000; **Medical School:** Washington Univ, St Louis 1964; **Residencies:** Surgery, Univ Wash Med Ctr, Seattle, WA 1965-1966; Orthopaedic Surgery, Wash Univ/Barnes Hosp, St Louis, MO 1969-1972; **Fellowship:** Hand Surgery, Univ Louisville Hosp, Louisville, KY 1971; **Faculty Appointment:** Prof Orthopaedic Surgery, Washington Univ, St Louis

Mass, Daniel MD (Hand Surgery) - *Special Expertise:* Tendon/nerve injuries; Arthritis Hand Surgery; **Admitting Hospital:** University of Chicago Hospitals (Page 78); **Office Address:** 5841 S Maryland Ave, MS 3079 Chicago, IL 60637; **Office Phone:** (773) 702-6306; **Board Certifications:** Orthopaedic Surgery 1994, Hand Surgery 2000; **Medical School:** Univ Chicago-Pritzker Sch Med 1975; **Residency:** Orthopaedic Surgery, Univ Chicago Hosp, Chicago, IL 1976-1979; **Fellowship:** Hand Surgery, St Francis Hosp, San Francisco, CA 1980; **Faculty Appointment:** Clin Prof Surgery, Univ Chicago-Pritzker Sch Med

Mih, Alexander MD (Hand Surgery) - *Special Expertise:* Microsurgery; **Admitting Hospital:** Indiana University Hospital & Medical Center - Indianapolis; **Office Address:** The Indiana Hand Ctr 541 Clinical Dr Indianapolis, IN 46202-5111; **Office Phone:** (317) 274-5648; **Board Certifications:** Orthopaedic Surgery 1992, Hand Surgery 1993; **Medical School:** Johns Hopkins Univ 1984; **Residency:** Orthopaedic Surgery, Mayo Clinic, Rochester, MN 1984-1989; **Fellowship:** Hand Surgery, Indiana Ctr for Hand Surg, Indianapolis, IA 1989-1990; **Faculty Appointment:** Assoc Prof Orthopaedic Surgery, Indiana Univ

Putnam, Matthew Douglas MD (Hand Surgery) - *Special Expertise:* Hand Surgery - General; **Admitting Hospital:** Fairview-University Medical Center - University Campus; **Office Address:** 401 E River Rd Minneapolis, MN 55455; **Office Phone:** (612) 625-1192; **Board Certifications:** Hand Surgery 1990, Orthopaedic Surgery 1998; **Medical School:** Dartmouth Med Sch 1977; **Residencies:** Surgery, Roosevelt Hosp, New York, NY 1978-1979; Orthopaedic Surgery, Univ Pittsburgh, Pittsburgh, PA 1981-1984; **Fellowship:** Hand Surgery, NVOH, New York, NY 1984-1985; **Faculty Appointment:** Assoc Prof Orthopaedic Surgery, Univ Minn

Schenck, Robert Roy MD (Hand Surgery) - *Special Expertise:* Carpal Tunnel Syndrome; Trigger Finger; **Admitting Hospital:** Rush/Presbyterian - St Luke's Medical Center - Chicago (Page 74); **Office Address:** 1725 W Harrison St Rm 263 Chicago, IL 60612; **Office Phone:** (312) 738-3426; **Board Certifications:** Hand Surgery 1998, Plastic Surgery 1973; **Medical School:** Univ IL Coll Med 1955; **Residencies:** Surgery, Western Penn Hosp, Pittsburgh, PA 1967-1969; Plastic Surgery, Columbia-Presby, New York, NY 1969-1971; **Fellowships:** Hand Surgery, Rooselvelt Hosp, New York, NY 1971-1972; Roosevelt, Edison, NJ 1971-1972; **Faculty Appointment:** Assoc Prof Surgery, Rush Med Coll

Stern, Peter MD (Hand Surgery) - *Special Expertise:* Hand Injuries; Microsurgery; **Admitting Hospital:** University Hospital - Cincinnati; **Office Address:** 2800 Winslow Ave, Ste 401 Cincinnati, OH 45206-1174; **Office Phone:** (513) 961-4263; **Board Certifications:** Orthopaedic Surgery 1993, Hand Surgery 2000; **Medical School:** Washington Univ, St Louis 1970; **Residencies:** Surgery, Beth Israel Hosp, Boston, MA 1970-1972; Orthopaedic Surgery, Harvard Combined Pgrm., Boston, MA 1975-1977; **Fellowship:** Hand Surgery, Univ Louisville Hosp, Loisville, KY 1978; **Faculty Appointment:** Prof Orthopaedic Surgery, Univ Cincinnati

Great Plains and Mountains

Ferlic, Donald C. MD (Hand Surgery) - *Special Expertise:* Hand Surgery - General; **Admitting Hospital:** Presbyterian - St Luke's Medical Center; **Office Address:** Denver Orthopedic Specialists 1601 E 19th Avenue #5000 Denver, CO 80218; **Office Phone:** (303) 839-5383; **Board Certifications:** Orthopaedic Surgery 1992, Hand Surgery 1989; **Medical School:** Johns Hopkins Univ 1961; **Residencies:** Orthopaedic Surgery, Duke Univ Med Ctr, Durham, NC 1962-1968; Pediatric Orthopedic Surgery, NC Ortho Hosp, NC 1966-1967; **Faculty Appointment:** Assoc Clin Prof Orthopaedic Surgery, Univ Colo

Southwest

Ezaki, Marybeth MD (Hand Surgery) - *Special Expertise:* Hand-Congenital Anomaly; Hand Reconstruction-Pediatric; **Admitting Hospital:** Texas Scottish Rite Hospital for Children - Dallas; **Office Address:** Scottish Rite Hosp for Children/ Dir of Upper Extremities 2222 Welborn St Dallas, TX 75219; **Office Phone:** (214) 559-7842; **Board Certifications:** Orthopaedic Surgery 1993, Hand Surgery 2000; **Medical School:** Yale Univ 1977; **Residency:** Orthopaedic Surgery, U Tex SW AFfil Hosp, Dallas, TX 1978-1982; **Fellowship:** Hand Surgery, Weyham Pk Hosp, Slough, England 1982; **Faculty Appointment:** Assoc Prof Orthopaedic Surgery, Univ Tex SW, Dallas

Moneim, Moheb S.A. MD (Hand Surgery) - *Special Expertise:* Hand/Forearm Surgery; **Admitting Hospital:** University of New Mexico Hospital; **Office Address:** Univ. New Mexico Health Sciences Center Dept Orthopaedics Albuquerque, NM 87131-5296; **Office Phone:** (505) 272-4107; **Board Certifications:** Orthopaedic Surgery 1998, Hand Surgery 1998; **Medical School:** Egypt 1963; **Residency:** Orthopaedic Surgery, Duke Univ, Durham, NC 1972-1975; **Fellowship:** Hand Surgery, Cornell-Hosp Spec Surg, New York, NY 1975-1976; **Faculty Appointment:** Prof Orthopaedic Surgery, Univ New Mexico

Rayan, Ghazi M. MD (Hand Surgery) - *Special Expertise:* Microsurgery; **Admitting Hospital:** Intergris Baptist Medical Center - Oklahoma; **Office Address:** Physicians Building D 3366 NW Expressway #700 Oklahoma City, OK 73112; **Office Phone:** (405) 945-4888; **Board Certification:** Orthopaedic Surgery 1983; **Medical School:** Egypt 1973; **Residencies:** Surgery, S Baltimore Genl Hosp-U Md Sch Med, Baltimore, MD 1976-1977; Orthopaedic Surgery, Johns Hopkins Hosp, Baltimore, MD 1977-1980; **Fellowship:** Hand Surgery, Union Mem'l Hosp, Baltimore, MD 1980; **Faculty Appointment:** Clin Prof Orthopaedic Surgery, Univ Okla Coll Med

West Coast and Pacific

Diao, Edward MD (Hand Surgery) - *Special Expertise:* Hand Surgery - General; **Admitting Hospital:** VA Medical Center - San Francisco; **Office Address:** UC San Francisco 500 Parnassus-Orth Surg Ave, Bldg West - Fl 3rd - rm 323 San Francisco, CA 94143; **Office Phone:** (415) 761-1167; **Board Certifications:** Orthopaedic Surgery 1992, Hand Surgery 1993; **Medical School:** Columbia P&S 1981; **Residencies:** Surgery, Beth Isreal Hospital, Boston, MA 1981-1983; Orthopaedic Surgery, Howard Combined/MA General, Boston, MA 1983-1987; **Fellowship:** Hand Surgery, Roosevelt Hospital, New York, NY 1988-1988; **Faculty Appointment:** Assoc Prof Hand Surgery, UCSF

Godzik, Cathleen MD (Hand Surgery) - *Special Expertise:* Hand Surgery - General; **Admitting Hospital:** Orthopaedic Hospital; **Office Address:** Inst Hand & Upper Ext Surg 2300 S Hope St, Bldg 300 Los Angeles, CA 90007-2613; **Office Phone:** (213) 742-9708; **Board Certifications:** Orthopaedic Surgery 1990, Hand Surgery 1992; **Medical School:** NY Med Coll 1981; **Residencies:** Surgery, Brown Univ Sch Med, Providence, RI 1982-1983; Orthopaedic Surgery, Univ Conn Sch Med, Farmington, CT 1983-1984; **Fellowship:** Hand Surgery, USC, Los Angeles, CA 1986-1987

Hanel, Douglas MD (Hand Surgery) - *Special Expertise:* Microvascular Surgery; **Admitting Hospital:** University of Washington Medical Center; **Office Address:** Harborview Medical Center-Orthopaedic Clinic 325 9th Ave Seattle, WA 98104; **Office Phone:** (206) 731-3462; **Board Certifications:** Orthopaedic Surgery 1997, Hand Surgery 1997; **Medical School:** St Louis Univ 1977; **Residencies:** Orthopaedic Surgery, St Louis Univ Hosp, St Louis, MO; Hand Surgery, Univ Louisville Hosp, Louisville, KY 1982-1983; **Fellowship:** Microsurgery, Univ Louisville Hosp, Louisville, KY 1983; **Faculty Appointment:** Assoc Prof Orthopaedic Surgery, Univ Wash

Hentz, Vincent R MD (Hand Surgery) - *Special Expertise:* Hand Surgery - General; **Admitting Hospital:** Stanford Medical Center; **Office Address:** Stanford Med Ctr-Hand & Upper Extremity Surg Clin 900 Blake Wilbur Dr Stanford, CA 94305; **Office Phone:** (650) 723-5256; **Board Certification:** Plastic Surgery 1977; **Medical School:** Univ Fla Coll Med 1968; **Residency:** Plastic Surgery, Stanford Univ Hosp, Stanford, CA 1969-1974; **Fellowship:** Hand Surgery, Roosevelt Hosp, New York, NY 1974-1975; **Faculty Appointment:** Prof Surgery, Stanford Univ

Jones, Neil MD (Hand Surgery) - *Special Expertise:* Hand Surgery - General; **Admitting Hospital:** UCLA Medical Center; **Office Address:** 200 UCLA Med Plz , Ste 140 Los Angeles, CA 90095; **Office Phone:** (310) 794-7784; **Board Certifications:** Plastic Surgery 1985, Hand Surgery 1990; **Medical School:** England 1974; **Residencies:** Surgery, Nat Inst Health, Bethesda, MD 1976-1979; Plastic Surgery, Univ Mich Med Ctr, Ann Arbor, MI 1979-1981; **Fellowships:** Plastic Surgery, St Bartholomew's, London, England 1982; Hand Surgery, Mass Gen Hosp/Harvard, Boston, MA 1983; **Faculty Appointment:** Prof Plastic Surgery, UCLA

Meals, Roy Allen MD (Hand Surgery) - *Special Expertise:* Hand Surgery - General; **Admitting Hospital:** UCLA Medical Center; **Office Address:** 100 UCLA Medical Plaza Ste 305 Los Angeles, CA 90024; **Office Phone:** (310) 206-6337; **Board Certifications:** Orthopaedic Surgery 1980, Hand Surgery 2000; **Medical School:** Vanderbilt Univ 1971; **Residencies:** Surgery, John Hopkins Hosp, Baltimore, MD 1972-1973; Orthopaedic Surgery, John Hopkins Hosp, Baltimore, MD 1974-1978; **Fellowship:** Hand Surgery, Mass General Hosp, Boston, MA 1978-1979; **Faculty Appointment:** Assoc Prof Surgery, UCLA

Szabo, Robert MD (Hand Surgery) - *Special Expertise:* Peripheral Nerve Surgery; Hand *Injuries;* **Admitting Hospital:** University of California - Davis Medical Center; **Office Address:** UC Davis, Dept Ortho 4860 Y St, Ste 1700 Sacramento, CA 95817; **Office Phone:** (916) 734-3678; **Board Certifications:** Orthopaedic Surgery 1998, Hand Surgery 1998; **Medical School:** SUNY Buffalo 1977; **Residencies:** Surgery, Mt Sinai Med Ctr, New York, NY 1978-1979; Orthopaedic Surgery, Mt Sinai Med Ctr, New York, NY 1978-1982; **Fellowship:** Vascular Surgery (General), UCSD, San Diego, CA 1982-1983; **Faculty Appointment:** Prof Orthopaedic Surgery, UC Davis

Taleisnik, Julio MD (Hand Surgery) - *Special Expertise:* Wrist/Hand Injuries; Arthritis Hand *Surgery;* **Admitting Hospital:** St Joseph's Hospital - Orange; **Office Address:** The Hand Care Center 1140 W La Veta Ave, Ste 860 Orange, CA 92868; **Office Phone:** (714) 835-6500; **Board Certification:** Orthopaedic Surgery 1968; **Medical School:** Argentina 1957; **Residency:** Orthopaedic Surgery, Mayo Clinic, Rochester, MN 1961-1966; **Faculty Appointment:** Clin Prof Orthopaedic Surgery, UC Davis

Trumble, Thomas MD (Hand Surgery) - *Special Expertise:* Nerve Regeneration; Upper *Extremity Trauma; Biomechanics - Arms;* **Admitting Hospital:** University of Washington Medical Center; **Office Address:** Bone and Joint Center 4245 Roosevelt Way NE Seattle, WA 98105-4740; **Office Phone:** (206) 598-4288; **Board Certifications:** Orthopaedic Surgery 1999, Hand Surgery 1999; **Medical School:** Yale Univ 1979; **Residency:** Orthopaedic Surgery, Yale-New Haven Hosp, New Haven, CT 1980-1984; **Fellowships:** Microvascular Surgery, Duke Univ Med Ctr, Durham, NC 1984; Hand Surgery, Mass Genl Hosp, Boston, MA 1985; **Faculty Appointment:** Assoc Prof Surgery, Univ Wash

HEMATOLOGY & MEDICALONCOLOGY

(a subspecialty of INTERNAL MEDICINE)

Hematology: An internist with additional training who specializes in diseases of the blood, spleen and lymph glands. This specialist treats conditions such as anemia, clotting disorders, sickle cell disease, hemophilia, leukemia and lymphoma.

Medical Oncology: An internist who specializes in the diagnosis and treatment of all types of cancer and other benign and malignant tumors. This specialist decides on and administers chemotherapy for malignancy, as well as consulting with surgeons and radiotherapists on other treatments for cancer.

INTERNAL MEDICINE

An internist is a personal physician who provides long-term, comprehensive care in the office and the hospital, managing both common and complex illness of adolescents, adults and the elderly. Internists are trained in the diagnosis and treatment of cancer, infections and diseases affecting the heart, blood, kidneys, joints and digestive, respiratory and vascular systems. They are also trained in the essentials of primary care internal medicine which incorporates an understanding of disease prevention, wellness, substance abuse, mental health and effective treatment of common problems of the eyes, ears, skin, nervous system and reproductive organs.

Training required: Three years in internal medicine *plus* additional training and examination for certification in hematology or medical oncology.

CONTINUUM HEALTH PARTNERS, INC.

THE CONTINUUM CANCER CENTERS OF NEW YORK

Phone (800) 420-4004

The hospitals of Continuum — Beth Israel Medical Center, St. Luke's-Roosevelt Hospital Center, Long Island College Hospital and the New York Eye and Ear Infirmary — are leading providers of cancer care through the Continuum Cancer Centers of New York. Our integrated system allows us to build on the clinical strengths found at our four partner hospitals.

The goal — and result — is delivery of care in ways that are more efficient, more attractive and more convenient for patients. Specifically, it means that cancer patients at any Continuum hospital can benefit from system-wide cancer expertise, facilities and resources. The Cancer Centers feature world-renowned cancer specialists, including top-rated surgeons, medical oncologists, physicians, radiation oncologists, radiologists, and oncology nurses.

Comprehensive diagnostic and treatment services are available for breast cancer, prostate cancers, head and neck cancers, skin cancer, lung cancer, colorectal and other gastrointestinal cancers, Lymphoma/Hodgkin's Disease, gynecological cancers, and cancers of the brain and central nervous system. Delivered efficiently in a friendly and supportive environment, services include prevention programs—such as community education, screenings and early detection—expert diagnosis, outpatient treatment, inpatient services, home care and, when necessary, hospice care. In addition, the Cancer Centers Research Program offers patients access to investigational protocols through a wide number of clinical trials.

Support services play an important role at The Cancer Centers. Nurses, social workers, psychiatrists, chaplains, pharmacists, rehabilitation therapists and nutritionists—each with specialized knowledge and expertise in the field of oncology—work together to ensure that patients' medical, emotional and family needs are addressed appropriately and in a timely manner.

COMPREHENSIVE BREAST CENTER

The Comprehensive Breast Center at St. Luke's-Roosevelt combines state-of-the-art diagnosis and treatment of breast cancer with a supportive approach to health care that addresses emotional as well as physical needs. With radiology, pathology and consultation services available on site, a suspected malignancy can be confirmed or ruled out quickly and treatment options—including plastic surgery—can be outlined in a single visit. Services also include genetic testing, gynecologic cancer screening, referral to complementary therapies, psychiatric care and support groups.

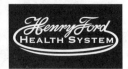

HENRY FORD HOSPITAL
JOSEPHINE FORD CANCER CENTER

The Josephine Ford Cancer Center (JFCC) is the focus of all cancer-related activities within the Henry Ford Health System. It is one of the largest cancer centers in Michigan, where more than 15,000 patients are seen annually. The JFCC, which is ranked among the top 50 cancer centers in the United States by *U.S. News & World Report*, provides a full continuum of care to patients, from cancer prevention to specialized care for the terminally ill. More than 15 percent of people in southeast Michigan diagnosed with cancer are treated by the JFCC, and more than 3,000 newly-diagnosed patients are treated here annually.

Research
The JFCC is involved in more than 200 cancer research trials, including the use of the promising suicide gene therapy for colon, prostate and brain cancer, and promotes patient recruiting for clinical trials and research.

Specialty Services
The JFCC provides majority of services at seven treatment facilities located throughout southeastern Michigan, making quality care available for patients close to home. Services include radiation therapy, chemotherapy, a variety of surgical oncology and support groups.

The center offers the largest and most clinically advanced breast cancer treatment in Michigan, which is why more patients receive a mammography with the JFCC than any other health care institution.

The pediatric cancer program is recognized as a Blue Quality Center for Pediatric Cancer. Pediatric oncologists treat children with many types of cancer, including acute leukemia, brain tumors, and solid tumors like Hodgkin's disease, lymphoma, neuroblastoma and Wilms' tumor.

The Bone Marrow Transplant Program is one of only four in Michigan to offer both autologous and allogeneic bone marrow transplantation.

LEADING EDGE PATIENT CARE

The sentinel lymph node biopsy, a new, innovative way to diagnose the spread of breast cancer, is among the latest breast cancer care treatments available at the JFCC.

The procedure enhances physicians' ability to diagnose where breast cancer might spread. This is done by injecting a blue dye near the breast tumor and tracking its path through the lymph nodes. The dye accumulates in the sentinel lymph node, which is then removed and analyzed.

Sentinel lymph node biopsy is less invasive than the standard treatment, which usually involved removing a tumor by either lumpectomy or mastectomy, and removing most of the lymph nodes in the armpit. Removing most of the lymph nodes can cause swelling in the arm, a persistent burning sensation, infection and restricted use of the shoulder.

THE UNIVERSITY OF TEXAS
MD ANDERSON
CANCER CENTER
Making Cancer History™

1515 Holcombe Boulevard
Houston, Texas 77030
Tel. 713-792-6161
Toll Free 800-392-1611
www.mdanderson.org

GENERAL OVERVIEW

Located in Houston, Texas, on the sprawling campus of the Texas Medical Center, The University of Texas M. D. Anderson Cancer Center is one of the world's most respected centers devoted exclusively to cancer patient care, research, education and prevention.

M. D. Anderson was created by the Texas Legislature in 1941 as a component of The University of Texas System, and the faculty exceeds 900 - both M.D.s and Ph.D.s. M. D. Anderson is one of the nation's original three Comprehensive Cancer Centers designated by the National Cancer Act of 1971 and is one of only 37 such centers today.

M. D. Anderson was ranked the top hospital for cancer care in the annual "Best Hospitals" survey published by *U.S. News & World Report* magazine in July 2000. M. D. Anderson has ranked among the top two cancer hospitals since the survey began 11 years ago.

The institution has increased about 50 percent in size in the last five years. The physical plant includes a 249-bed hospital pavilion, for a total of 450 beds, and a clinical research building which opened in 1998. A 13-story faculty office tower has opened recently, and a 126-room expansion to M. D. Anderson's 198-room patient/family hotel is nearing completion. Another research building and an ambulatory clinical building are in the planning stages.

PATIENT CARE

Since 1944, more than 400,000 patients have turned to M. D. Anderson for cancer care in the form of surgery, chemotherapy, radiation therapy, immunotherapy or combinations of these and other treatments. This multidisciplinary approach to treating cancer was pioneered at M. D. Anderson. And because they focus only on cancer, experts here are renowned for their ability to treat uncommon or rare cancers as well as they treat common cancers.

This year, about 65,000 persons with cancer will receive care at M. D. Anderson, and about 18,000 of them will be new patients. More than half of these patients come from outside Texas seeking the research-based care that has made M. D. Anderson so widely respected. Approximately 15 percent of all patients will participate in clinical trials of new therapies at some time during their illnesses.

M. D. Anderson holds Accreditation with Commendation from the Joint Commission on Accreditation of Healthcare Organizations (JCAHO), the highest level of accreditation given by the nation's oldest body charged with improving the quality of healthcare given to the public.

RESEARCH

M. D. Anderson contributes more research to patient care than any other academic center. Important scientific knowledge gained in the laboratory is rapidly translated into clinical care through research trials. The institution currently spends more than $150 million per year in research. M. D. Anderson now ranks first in the number of grants awarded nationwide by both the National Cancer Institute and the American Cancer Society. The research program is considered one of the most productive efforts in the world aimed solely at cancer.

PREVENTION

Recognizing that, ultimately, prevention is the best way to eliminate the threat of cancer, M. D. Anderson has initiated a multifaceted effort. Expanded research efforts in epidemiology and behavioral sciences complement achievements made in the clinical cancer arena. Laboratory activities support developmental and practical applications of cancer prevention. Cancer prevention services are offered in individual and corporate programs, from personalized risk assessments to screening and genetic counseling.

TEXAS CANCER INSTITUTE®

ST. LUKE'S® ST. LUKE'S EPISCOPAL HOSPITAL
TEXAS CANCER INSTITUTE®

6624 Fannin, 2nd Floor Mezzanine Houston, TX 77030
Tel. (713) 791-3490 www.texascancerinstitute.com

MISSION OF ST. LUKE'S TEXAS CANCER INSTITUTE

The mission of St. Luke's Texas Cancer Institute is to provide high quality, personalized cancer care to each patient through a full range of integrated services. St. Luke's Texas Cancer Institute is located in state-of-the-art facilities and supported by private practice oncology specialists, a multidisciplinary team of skilled nursing professionals, and a corps of supportive Partners in Healing volunteers. Through a full continuum of care, St. Luke's Texas Cancer Institute emphasizes the special needs of cancer patients and ministers to the whole patient: body, mind and spirit.

PERSONALIZED PATIENT CARE

We offer optimal, personalized cancer care in a private hospital setting. Private-practice cancer specialists employ a full range of leading-edge diagnostic technologies and treatment modalities as they provide treatment excellence to patients. Members of St. Luke's academically oriented medical staff and nursing staff remain abreast of current, effective therapies and research and are skilled in minimizing the discomfort patients may experience.

CARING THROUGH CLINICAL SERVICE

St. Luke's Texas Cancer Institute's new outpatient clinic features chemotherapy and multidisciplinary programs in breast, melanoma, lung, prostate, GI and other cancer sites. Our patients benefit from a full range of diagnostic technologies and treatment modalities, which are continuously enhanced and customized to meet the needs of patients, physicians and researchers:

- Sentinel lymph node mapping for melanoma and for breast surgery
- PET scanning
- X-knife radiosurgery
- Stereotactic biopsy and fine-needle biopsy
- Three magnetic resonance imaging machines and digitized radiologic film imaging
- Breast-conservation surgery
- Mastectomy with immediate reconstructive surgery using TRAM flap procedure
- Chemotherapy, biochemotherapy, hormone therapy, chemoprevention therapy
- Mobile mammography coach with bone densitometry
- Dedicated 34-bed oncology inpatient unit with oncology nurses, pharmacist, social worker, care coordinator, and case manager
- Frontline cancer research: original and co-ops for melanoma, prostate, lung, and other sites
- STAR breast cancer prevention trial – NSABP
- Palliative care services

Call (713) 791-4343 to make an appointment with a St. Luke's Texas Cancer Institute physician.

Accreditation: The St. Luke's Texas Cancer Institute is accredited by the Commission on Cancer of the American College of Surgeons and the Joint Commission on Accreditation of Healthcare Organizations and a member of ACCC.

The University of Chicago Hospitals
Cancer Program

5841 S. Maryland Avenue
Chicago, Illinois 60637-1470
For help finding a physician: 1-888-UCH-0200

AT THE FOREFRONT OF CANCER CARE

The University of Chicago Hospitals' cancer program ranks sixth in the nation and first in Illinois, according to *U.S. News & World Report*. More than 500 scientists, physicians, and other professionals from 20 different academic and clinical departments fight cancer here. Their work encompasses all aspects of the disease: prevention, detection, diagnosis, and treatment.

Designated by the National Cancer Institute (NCI) as a Comprehensive Cancer Center, the University of Chicago Hospitals are currently working with more than $30 million in cancer research grants -- more funding than any other hospital in Illinois. We are one of only a few centers in the United States selected by the NCI for Phase I and II clinical trials on new cancer-fighting drugs. Our cancer experts -- among the most renowned in the world -- can quickly translate new knowledge from the scientific lab to the patient's bedside, providing innovative treatments long before they are available at most other hospitals.

NEW, EFFECTIVE TREATMENTS AND CLINICAL TRIALS

- Sophisticated diagnostics, including a computerized system that combines an MRI, PET scan and CT scan to produce a three-dimensional image of the brain. This detailed image allows doctors to pinpoint tumor location before radiation therapy or surgery.

- Advanced techniques that preserve organ function and healthy tissue whenever possible, so patients with colon, rectal, head and neck, and other cancers can maintain normal body functioning and appearance.

- Bone marrow transplants for treatment of Hodgkin's and non-Hodgkin's lymphomas, and all types of leukemia in children and adults. Bone marrow transplants are also used to treat solid tumors in the breasts, testicles, and other areas. Stem-cell transplants are provided as well.

**To Find a University of Chicago
Cancer Specialist,
Call 1-888-UCH-0200**

Physician Listings

New England

Benz, Edward MD (Hematology) - *Special Expertise:* Anemias & Red Cell Disorders; Bone Marrow Transplant; **Admitting Hospital:** Dana Farber Cancer Institute; **Office Address:** 44 Binney St, Ste 1628 Boston, MA 02115; **Office Phone:** (617) 632-2159; **Board Certifications:** Internal Medicine 1979, Hematology 1982; **Medical School:** Harvard Med Sch 1973; **Residencies:** Internal Medicine, Peter Bent Brigham Hosp, Boston, MA 1973-1975; Hematology, Yale New Haven Hosp, New Haven, CT 1978-1980; **Fellowship:** Hematology, Natl Inst of Hlth, Bethesda, MD 1975-1978; **Faculty Appointment:** Prof Medicine, Harvard Med Sch

Duffy, Thomas MD (Hematology) - *Special Expertise:* Hematology - General; **Admitting Hospital:** Yale - New Haven Hospital; **Office Address:** Yale Physicians Building 800 Howard Avenue New Haven, CT 06520-8021; **Office Phone:** (203) 785-4744; **Board Certifications:** Internal Medicine 1972, Hematology 1974; **Medical School:** Johns Hopkins Univ 1962; **Residency:** Internal Medicine, Johns Hopkins Hosp, Baltimore, MD 1963-1965; **Fellowship:** Hematology, Johns Hopkins Hosp, Baltimore, MD 1968-1970; **Faculty Appointment:** Prof Medicine, Yale Univ

Miller, Kenneth B. MD (Hematology) - *Special Expertise:* Bone Marrow Transplant; Leukemia; **Admitting Hospital:** New England Medical Center; **Office Address:** New England Medical Center 860 Washington St, Box 542 Boston, MA 02111; **Office Phone:** (617) 636-5144; **Board Certifications:** Internal Medicine 1976, Hematology 1980; **Medical School:** NY Med Coll 1972; **Residencies:** Internal Medicine, NYU Med Ctr/VA Hosp, New York, NY 1973-1976; Internal Medicine, NYU Med Ctr, New York, NY 1975-1976; **Fellowship:** Hematology, New England Med Ctr., Boston, MA 1976-1979; **Faculty Appointment:** Assoc Prof Medicine, Tufts Univ

Stone, Richard Maury MD (Hematology) - *Special Expertise:* Leukemia - Adult; **Admitting Hospital:** Massachusetts General Hospital; **Office Address:** Dana Farber Cancer Inst 44 Binney St, rm D-840B Boston, MA 02115-6013; **Office Phone:** (617) 632-2214; **Board Certifications:** Medical Oncology 1987, Hematology 1988; **Medical School:** Harvard Med Sch 1981; **Residency:** Internal Medicine, Brigham & Womens Hosp, Boston, MA 1982-1984; **Fellowship:** Medical Oncology, Dana Farber Cancer Inst, Boston, MA 1984-1987; **Faculty Appointment:** Assoc Prof Medicine, Harvard Med Sch

Mid Atlantic

Coller, Barry MD (Hematology) - *Special Expertise:* Bleeding/Coagulation Disorders; Thrombotic Disorders; Glanzmann's Thrombasthenia; **Admitting Hospital:** Mount Sinai Hospital (Page 70); **Office Address:** Mount Sinai Sch Med, Dept Medicine 1 Gustave Levy Pl, Box 118 New York, NY 10029; **Office Phone:** (212) 241-4200; **Board Certifications:** Internal Medicine 1973, Hematology 1975; **Medical School:** NYU Sch Med 1970; **Residency:** Internal Medicine, Bellevue Hosp, New York, NY 1970-1974; **Faculty Appointment:** Prof Medicine, Mount Sinai Sch Med

Diuguid, David Lincoln MD (Hematology) - *Special Expertise:* Bleeding/Coagulation Disorders; **Admitting Hospital:** Columbia Presbyterian Medical Center (Page 72); **Office Address:** 161 Ft Washington Ave, Rm 862 New York, NY 10032; **Office Phone:** (212) 305-0527; **Board Certifications:** Hematology 1986, Medical Oncology 1985; **Medical School:** Cornell Univ-Weil Med Coll 1979; **Residency:** Internal Medicine, Boston Univ Med Ctr, Boston, MA 1980-1983; **Fellowship:** Hematology, New England Med Ctr, Boston, MA 1983-1986; **Faculty Appointment:** Asst Prof Clinical Pathology, Columbia P&S

Kempin, Sanford Jay MD (Hematology) - *Special Expertise:* Leukemia; Lymphoma; **Admitting Hospital:** St Vincents Catholic Medical Center of New York; **Office Address:** St Vincents Cancer Ctr 325 W 15th St New York, NY 10011; **Office Phone:** (212) 604-6010; **Board Certifications:** Hematology 1978, Medical Oncology 1977; **Medical School:** Belgium 1971; **Residency:** Internal Medicine, Lemuel Shattuck Hosp, Boston, MA 1971-1972; **Fellowship:** Hematology, St Jude Chldns Hosp, Memphis, TN 1973-1975; **Faculty Appointment:** Assoc Clin Prof Medicine, NY Med Coll

Schuster, Michael MD (Hematology) - *Special Expertise:* Bone Marrow Transplant; **Admitting Hospital:** New York Weill Cornell Medical Center - NY Presbyterian Hospital (Page 72); **Office Address:** 525 E 68th St New York, NY 10044; **Office Phone:** (212) 746-2119; **Board Certifications:** Internal Medicine 1984, Hematology 1986; **Medical School:** Dartmouth Med Sch 1980; **Residency:** Internal Medicine, New England Deaconess Hosp, Boston, MA 1980-1983; **Fellowship:** Hematology and Oncology, Beth Israel Hosp-Harvard, Boston, MA 1983-1987; **Faculty Appointment:** Assoc Prof Medicine, Cornell Univ-Weil Med Coll

Silverstein, Roy MD (Hematology) - *Special Expertise:* Aplastic Anemia; Thrombotic Disorders; **Admitting Hospital:** New York Weill Cornell Medical Center - NY Presbyterian Hospital (Page 72); **Office Address:** Starr Pavillion 520 E 70th St, Ste 341 New York, NY 10021; **Office Phone:** (212) 746-2075; **Board Certifications:** Hematology 1984, Medical Oncology 1985; **Medical School:** Emory Univ 1979; **Residencies:** Internal Medicine, New York Hosp-Cornell Med Ctr, New York, NY 1979-1982; Hematology, New York Hosp-Cornell Med Ctr, New York, NY 1982-1984; **Faculty Appointment:** Prof Hematology, Cornell Univ-Weil Med Coll

Spivak, Jerry L. MD (Hematology) - *Special Expertise:* Myeloproliferative Disorders; Polycythemia Vera; **Admitting Hospital:** Johns Hopkins Hospital - Baltimore (Page 65); **Office Address:** Johns Hopkins Hospital 720 Rutland Ave, Traylor 924 Baltimore, MD 21205; **Office Phone:** (410) 955-5454; **Board Certifications:** Internal Medicine 1971, Hematology 1974; **Medical School:** Cornell Univ-Weil Med Coll 1964; **Residencies:** Internal Medicine, New York Hosp, New York, NY 1968-1969; Internal Medicine, Johns Hopkins Hosp., Baltimore, MD 1965-1966; **Fellowship:** Hematology, Johns Hopkins Hosp., Baltimore, MD 1969-1971; **Faculty Appointment:** Prof Hematology, Johns Hopkins Univ

Wisch, Nathaniel MD (Hematology) - *Special Expertise:* Lymphoma; **Admitting Hospital:** Lenox Hill Hospital; **Office Address:** 12 E 86th St New York, NY 10028-0506; **Office Phone:** (212) 861-6660; **Board Certifications:** Medical Oncology 1977, Hematology 1972; **Medical School:** Northwestern Univ 1958; **Residencies:** Internal Medicine, VA Hosp, Brooklyn, NY 1959-1960; Internal Medicine, Montefiore Hosp, Bronx, NY 1961-1962; **Fellowship:** Hematology, Mount Sinai Hosp, New York, NY 1960-1961; **Faculty Appointment:** Assoc Prof Medicine, Mount Sinai Sch Med

Zalusky, Ralph MD (Hematology) - *Special Expertise:* Anemia; **Admitting Hospital:** Beth Israel Medical Center - New York; **Office Address:** 1st Ave & 16th St New York, NY 10003; **Office Phone:** (212) 420-4185; **Board Certifications:** Internal Medicine 1964, Hematology 1972; **Medical School:** Boston Univ 1957; **Residencies:** Internal Medicine, Duke Univ Med, Durham, NC 1957-1959; Internal Medicine, Duke Univ Med, Durham, NC 1961-1962; **Fellowship:** Hematology, Boston Med Ctr, Boston, MA 1959-1961; **Faculty Appointment:** Prof Medicine, Albert Einstein Coll Med

Southeast

De Simone, Philip A MD (Hematology) - *Special Expertise:* Hematology - General; **Admitting Hospital:** University of Kentucky Medical Center; **Office Address:** Markey Cancer Ctr, U Of Kentucky CC454 800 Rose St Lexington, KY 40537; **Office Phone:** (859) 323-6562; **Board Certifications:** Internal Medicine 1972, Hematology 1974; **Medical School:** Univ VT Coll Med 1967; **Residency:** Internal Medicine, Univ Kentucky Hosp, Lexington, KY 1968-1974; **Faculty Appointment:** Prof Medicine, Univ KY Coll Med

Lutcher, Charles MD (Hematology) - *Special Expertise:* Hemophilia - Adult; **Admitting Hospital:** Medical College of Georgia Hospital; **Office Address:** Med Coll Georgia 1120 15th St Augusta, GA 30912-3125; **Office Phone:** (706) 721-2505; **Board Certifications:** Internal Medicine 1987, Hematology 1974; **Medical School:** Washington Univ, St Louis 1961; **Residencies:** Hematology, Univ Oregon Hosp, Eugene, OR 1963-1964; Internal Medicine, Univ Wash City Hosp, St Louis, MO 1962-1963; **Fellowship:** Hematology, Univ Oregon Hosp, Eugene, OR 1964-1966; **Faculty Appointment:** Prof Medicine, Med Coll GA

Solberg, Lawrence MD (Hematology) - *Special Expertise:* Bone Marrow Transplant; **Admitting Hospital:** Mayo/St Luke's Hospital; **Office Address:** Mayo Clinic - Jacksonville 4500 San Pablo Rd Jacksonville, FL 32224; **Office Phone:** (904) 953-7292; **Board Certifications:** Internal Medicine 1978, Hematology 1980; **Medical School:** St Louis Univ 1975; **Residency:** Internal Medicine, Mayo Grad Sch, Rochester, MN 1976-1978; **Fellowship:** Hematology, Mayo Grad Sch, Rochester, MN 1978-1980; **Faculty Appointment:** Assoc Prof Medicine, Mayo Med Sch

Telen, Marilyn J MD (Hematology) - *Special Expertise:* Transfusion Medicine; Hemolytic Onemia; **Admitting Hospital:** Duke University Medical Center (Page 60); **Office Address:** Duke Univ Med Ctr 3333 MSRB Durham, NC 27710; **Office Phone:** (919) 684-5426; **Board Certifications:** Internal Medicine 1980, Hematology 1984; **Medical School:** NYU Sch Med 1977; **Residency:** Internal Medicine, Erie Co Med Cr-SUNY-Buffalo, Buffalo, NY 1978-1980; **Fellowship:** Hematology, Duke Univ Med Ctr, Durham, NC 1980-1982; **Faculty Appointment:** Prof Medicine, Duke Univ

Zuckerman, Kenneth MD (Hematology) - *Special Expertise:* Leukemia; Myeloproliferative Disorders; **Admitting Hospital:** H Lee Moffitt Cancer Center & Research Institute; **Office Address:** 12902 Magnolia Dr Tampa, FL 33612-9416; **Office Phone:** (813) 972-8470; **Board Certifications:** Internal Medicine 1975, Hematology 1978; **Medical School:** Ohio State Univ 1972; **Residency:** Internal Medicine, Ohio State Univ Hosp, Columbus, OH 1973-1975; **Fellowship:** Hematology, Peter Bent Brigham Hosp, Boston, MA 1975-1978; **Faculty Appointment:** Prof Medical Oncology, Univ S Fla Coll Med

Midwest

Adler, Solomon Stanley MD (Hematology) - *Special Expertise:* Lymphoma; Leukemia; Myelodysplastic Syndromes; **Admitting Hospital:** Rush/Presbyterian - St Luke's Medical Center - Chicago (Page 74); **Office Address:** 1725 W Harrison St, Ste 862 Chicago, IL 60612; **Office Phone:** (312) 563-2320; **Board Certifications:** Hematology 1973, Medical Oncology 1975; **Medical School:** Albert Einstein Coll Med 1970; **Residencies:** Internal Medicine, Brookdale Hosp Med Ctr, Brooklyn, NY 1971-1972; Hematology, Brookdale Hosp Med Ctr, Brooklyn, NY 1972-1973; **Fellowship:** Hematology, Rush Presby/St Lukes Hosp, Chicago, IL 1973-1975; **Faculty Appointment:** Prof Medicine, Rush Med Coll

Baron, Joseph M MD (Hematology) - *Special Expertise:* *Bleeding/Coagulation Disorders;*
Lymphoma; Myeloproliferative Disorders; **Admitting Hospital:** University of Chicago Hospitals
(Page 78); **Office Address:** Ctr for Advanced Med 5758 S Maryland Ave Chicago, IL 60637;
Office Phone: (773) 702-6149; **Board Certifications:** Hematology 1972, Medical Oncology 1975;
Medical School: Univ Chicago-Pritzker Sch Med 1962; **Residency:** Internal Medicine, Univ
Chicago, Chicago, IL 1963-1968; **Fellowship:** Hematology, Univ Chicago, Chicago, IL 1967-1968;
Faculty Appointment: Assoc Prof Medicine, Univ Chicago-Pritzker Sch Med

Bitran, Jacob MD (Hematology) - *Special Expertise:* *Breast Cancer; Bone Marrow Transplant;*
Admitting Hospital: Advocate Lutheran General Hospital; **Office Address:** Advocate Medical
Group 1700 Luther Ln Park Ridge, IL 60068-1270; **Office Phone:** (847) 723-2500; **Board
Certifications:** Hematology 1985, Medical Oncology 1977; **Medical School:** Univ IL Coll Med
1971; **Residencies:** Pathology, Rush Presby St Luke's Hosp, Chicago, IL 1972-1973; Internal
Medicine, Michael Reese Hosp, Chicago, IL 1972-1973; **Fellowship:** Hematology and Oncology,
Univ Chicago Hosp, Chicago, IL 1975-1977

Blinder, Morey MD (Hematology) - *Special Expertise:* *Bleeding/Coagulation Disorders;*
Anemia; **Admitting Hospital:** Barnes - Jewish Hospital; **Office Address:** Dept of Internal Medicine
4960 Children's Pl, Fl 4, MC-8125 St. Louis, MO 63110; **Office Phone:** (314) 362-8808; **Board
Certifications:** Hematology 1987, Medical Oncology 1988; **Medical School:** St Louis Univ 1981;
Residency: Internal Medicine, Univ Illinois Hosp, Chicago, IL 1981-1984; **Faculty Appointment:**
Assoc Prof Medicine, Washington Univ, St Louis

Bockenstedt, Paula MD (Hematology) - *Special Expertise:* *Bleeding/Coagulation Disorders;*
Leukemia/Hematopoietic Malignancy; Von Willebrand's Disease; **Admitting Hospital:** University
of Michigan Health Center; **Office Address:** Medical Science Research Bldg III 1150 W Medical
Center Dr, Rm 5301,Box 0640 Ann Arbor, MI 48109-0640; **Office Phone:** (734) 647-8901; **Board
Certifications:** Internal Medicine 1981, Hematology 1984; **Medical School:** Harvard Med Sch
1978; **Residency:** Internal Medicine, Brigham-Womens Hosp, Boston, MA 1979-1981; **Fellowship:**
Hematology, Brigham-Womens Hosp, Boston, MA 1981-1984; **Faculty Appointment:** Asst Clin Prof
Hematology, Univ Mich Med Sch

Bricker, Leslie J MD (Hematology) - *Special Expertise:* *Hospice Care; Palliative Care;*
Admitting Hospital: Henry Ford Health System (Page 62); **Office Address:** 2799 W Grand Blvd
Detroit, MI 48202; **Office Phone:** (313) 876-1841; **Board Certifications:** Hematology 1982, Medical
Oncology 1983; **Medical School:** Wayne State Univ 1977; **Residency:** Internal Medicine, Sinai
Hosp, Detroit, MI 1978-1980; **Fellowship:** Hematology, Univ Mich Hosp, Ann Arbor, MI 1980

Bukowski, Ronald Mathew MD (Hematology) - *Special Expertise:* *Kidney Cancer - Renal
Cell;* **Admitting Hospital:** Cleveland Clinic Foundation; **Office Address:** Cleveland Clinic-Dept.
Hem/Onc. 9500 Euclid Ave Cleveland, OH 44195-0001; **Office Phone:** (216) 444-6825; **Board
Certifications:** Medical Oncology 1975, Hematology 1976; **Medical School:** Northwestern Univ
1967; **Residencies:** Internal Medicine, Cleveland Clinic, Cleveland, OH 1968-1969; Internal
Medicine, Cleveland Clinic, Cleveland, OH 1972-1973; **Fellowship:** Hematology, Cleveland
Clinic, Cleveland, OH 1973

Gaynor, Ellen MD (Hematology) - *Special Expertise:* *Lymphoma;* **Admitting Hospital:** Loyola
University Health System; **Office Address:** 2160 S First Ave Maywood, IL 60153; **Office Phone:**
(708) 327-3214; **Board Certifications:** Medical Oncology 1985, Hematology 1986; **Medical
School:** Univ Wisc 1978; **Residency:** Internal Medicine, Loyola Univ Med Ctr, Maywood, IL 1979-
1982; **Fellowships:** Medical Oncology, Loyola Univ Med Ctr, Maywood, IL 1980-1981;
Hematology and Oncology, Univ Chicago Hosp, Chicago, IL 1982-1984; **Faculty Appointment:**
Prof Medicine, Loyola Univ-Stritch Sch Med

Godwin, John MD (Hematology) - *Special Expertise:* Hematology - General; **Admitting Hospital:** Loyola University Health System; **Office Address:** Loyola Univ Med Ctr, Dept Hematology 2160 S First Ave, Bldg 112 Maywood, IL 60153; **Office Phone:** (708) 216-4655; **Board Certifications:** Hematology 1986, Internal Medicine 1981; **Medical School:** Univ Ala 1978; **Residencies:** Internal Medicine, Baylor Coll Med, Houston, TX 1979-1981; Hematology, Baylor Coll Med, Houston, TX 1981-1983; **Fellowship:** Hematology, NC Meml Hosp-UNC, Chapel Hill, NC 1983-1985; **Faculty Appointment:** Assoc Prof Medicine, Loyola Univ-Stritch Sch Med

Green, David MD (Hematology) - *Special Expertise:* Bleeding/Coagulation Disorders; Blood Disorders; **Admitting Hospital:** Northwestern Memorial Hospital; **Office Address:** Rehab Inst Chicago 345 E Superior St, rm 1407 Chicago, IL 60611; **Office Phone:** (312) 238-4701; **Board Certifications:** Hematology 1972, Internal Medicine 1987; **Medical School:** Jefferson Med Coll 1960; **Residency:** Internal Medicine, Jefferson Hosp, Philadelphia, PA 1961-1963; **Fellowship:** Hematology, Jefferson Hosp, Philadelphia, PA 1963-1964; **Faculty Appointment:** Prof Medicine, Northwestern Univ

Gregory, Stephanie MD/PhD (Hematology) - *Special Expertise:* Lymphoma; Leukemia; **Admitting Hospital:** Rush/Presbyterian - St Luke's Medical Center - Chicago (Page 74); **Office Address:** 1725 W Harrison St, Ste 809 Chicago, IL 60612; **Office Phone:** (312) 563-2320; **Board Certifications:** Hematology 1972, Internal Medicine 1972; **Medical School:** Med Coll PA Hahnemann 1965; **Residency:** Internal Medicine, Rush Presb, Chicago, IL 1966-1969; **Fellowship:** Hematology, Rush Presb, Chicago, IL 1969-1972; **Faculty Appointment:** Prof Medicine, Southern IL Univ

Greipp, Philip R MD (Hematology) - *Special Expertise:* Multiple Myeloma; **Admitting Hospital:** Mayo Medical Center & Clinic - Rochester; **Office Address:** Mayo Clinic-Div Hematology 200 1st St SW Rochester, MN 55905; **Office Phone:** (507) 284-3159; **Board Certifications:** Internal Medicine 1974, Hematology 1994; **Medical School:** Georgetown Univ 1968; **Residency:** Internal Medicine, Mayo Clinic, Rochester, MN 1971-1973; **Fellowship:** Hematology, Mayo Clinic, Rochester, MN 1973-1975; **Faculty Appointment:** Prof Medicine, Mayo Med Sch

Litzow, Mark Robert MD (Hematology) - *Special Expertise:* Bone Marrow Transplant; **Admitting Hospital:** Mayo Medical Center & Clinic - Rochester; **Office Address:** Mayo Clinic 200 1st St SW Rochester, MN 55905; **Office Phone:** (507) 284-5302; **Board Certifications:** Medical Oncology 1989, Hematology 1988; **Medical School:** Univ Chicago-Pritzker Sch Med 1980; **Residencies:** Internal Medicine, Mayo Clinic, Rochester, MN 1983-1984; Internal Medicine, Mayo Clinic, Rochester, MN 1980-1983; **Fellowship:** Medical Oncology, Mayo Clinic, Rochester, MN 1985-1990; **Faculty Appointment:** Asst Prof Medicine, Mayo Med Sch

Mosher, Deane F MD (Hematology) - *Special Expertise:* Hematology - General; **Admitting Hospital:** University of Wisconsin Hospital & Clinics; **Office Address:** Univ Wisc Hosp, Dept Hematology 600 Highland Avenue Madison, WI 53792; **Office Phone:** (608) 263-7022; **Board Certifications:** Internal Medicine 1973, Hematology 1980; **Medical School:** Harvard Med Sch 1968; **Residency:** Internal Medicine, Beth Israel Hosp, Boston, MA 1969-1970; **Fellowship:** Hematology, Harvard, Boston, MA 1970-1972; **Faculty Appointment:** Prof Medicine, Univ Wisc

Nand, Sucha MD (Hematology) - *Special Expertise:* Hematology - General; **Admitting Hospital:** Loyola University Health System; **Office Address:** Cardinal Bernardin Cancer Center 2160 S First Ave Maywood, IL 60153-3304; **Office Phone:** (708) 327-3217; **Board Certifications:** Hematology 1982, Medical Oncology 1981; **Medical School:** India 1971; **Residencies:** Internal Medicine, Northwestern Meml Hosp, Chicago, IL 1975-1976; Hematology, North Chicago VA Hospital, Chicago, IL 1977-1978; **Fellowship:** Medical Oncology, Northwestern Meml Hosp, Chicago, IL 1979-1981; **Faculty Appointment:** Prof Medicine, Loyola Univ-Stritch Sch Med

Preisler, Harvey D MD (Hematology) - *Special Expertise:* Lymphoma; **Admitting Hospital:** Rush/Presbyterian - St Luke's Medical Center - Chicago (Page 74); **Office Address:** 1725 W Harrison St, Ste 862 Chicago, IL 60612; **Office Phone:** (312) 563-2328; **Board Certifications:** Internal Medicine 1972, Medical Oncology 1975; **Medical School:** Univ Rochester 1965; **Residencies:** Internal Medicine, Buffalo Genl, Buffalo, NY 1966-1967; Internal Medicine, Roswell Cancer Ctr, Buffalo, NY 1966-1967; **Fellowship:** Hematology, Columbia-Presby Hosp, New York, NY 1969-1971; **Faculty Appointment:** Prof Medicine, Univ Chicago-Pritzker Sch Med

Stiff, Patrick J MD (Hematology) - *Special Expertise:* Bone Marrow Transplant; Non-Hodgkin's Lymphoma; **Admitting Hospital:** Loyola University Health System; **Office Address:** 2160 S First Ave Maywood, IL 60153; **Office Phone:** (708) 169-9000; **Board Certifications:** Medical Oncology 1981, Hematology 1982; **Medical School:** Loyola Univ-Stritch Sch Med 1975; **Residency:** Internal Medicine, Cleveland Clin, Cleveland, OH 1976-1978; **Fellowship:** Medical Oncology, Meml Sloan Kettering Med Ctr, New York, NY 1978-1981; **Faculty Appointment:** Prof Medicine, Loyola Univ-Stritch Sch Med

White, Peter MD (Hematology) - *Special Expertise:* Porphyria; **Admitting Hospital:** Medical College of Ohio Hospitals; **Office Address:** Rupert Health Ctr 3120 Glendale Ave Toledo, OH 43614; **Office Phone:** (419) 383-3747; **Board Certifications:** Internal Medicine 1974, Hematology 1974; **Medical School:** Univ Penn 1955; **Residency:** Internal Medicine, Hosp Univ Penn, Philadelphia, PA 1956-1960; **Fellowship:** Hematology, Hosp Univ Penn, Philadelphia, PA 1963-1965; **Faculty Appointment:** Prof Medicine, Med Coll OH

Winter, Jane N. MD (Hematology) - *Special Expertise:* Hodgkin's Disease; Bone Marrow Transplant; **Admitting Hospital:** Northwestern Memorial Hospital; **Office Address:** 223 East Eire, Ste 700 Chicago, IL 60611; **Office Phone:** (312) 695-8697; **Board Certifications:** Internal Medicine 1980, Hematology 1982; **Medical School:** Univ Penn 1977; **Residency:** Internal Medicine, Univ Chicago Hosp, Chcago, IL 1978-1980; **Fellowships:** Hematology and Oncology, Columbia Presby Hosp, New York, NY 1980-1981; Hematology, Northwestern Univ Hosp, Chicago, IL 1981-1983; **Faculty Appointment:** Prof Medicine, Northwestern Univ

Southwest

Barlogie, Bartholomew MD/PhD (Hematology) - *Special Expertise:* Bone Marrow Transplant; Plasma Cell Disorders; **Admitting Hospital:** University of Arkansas for Medical Sciences; **Office Address:** Univ Hosp Arkansas Med Sci, Bone Marrow Clinic 4301 West Markham St - Slot 623 Little Rock, AR 72205; **Office Phone:** (501) 686-6000; **Medical School:** Germany 1969; **Fellowship:** Medical Oncology, MD Anderson Cancer Ctr, Houston, TX 1974-1976; **Faculty Appointment:** Prof Medicine, Univ Ark

Cobos, Everardo MD (Hematology) - *Special Expertise:* Bone Marrow Transplant; Bleeding/Coagulation Disorders; **Admitting Hospital:** University Medical Center; **Office Address:** Texas Tech Univ, HSC Dept Med 4th & Indiana Lubbock, TX 79408; **Office Phone:** (806) 743-3155; **Board Certifications:** Hematology 1988, Medical Oncology 1987; **Medical School:** Univ Tex, San Antonio 1981; **Residency:** Internal Medicine, Letterman Army Med Ctr, San Francisco, CA 1983-1985; **Fellowship:** Hematology and Oncology, Letterman Army Med Ctr, San Francisco, CA 1985-1988; **Faculty Appointment:** Assoc Prof Hematology, Texas Tech Univ

Kantarjian, Hagop M MD (Hematology) - *Special Expertise:* Leukemia; **Admitting Hospital:** University of Texas MD Anderson Cancer Center (Page 66); **Office Address:** 1515 Holcombe Blvd Houston, TX 77030-4009; **Office Phone:** (713) 792-7026; **Board Certifications:** Medical Oncology 1985, Hematology 1990; **Medical School:** Lebanon 1979; **Residency:** Internal Medicine, Univ Tex MD Anderson, Houston, TX 1981-1983; **Fellowship:** Univ Texas MD Anderson Cancer Ctr, Houston, TX 1981-1983; **Faculty Appointment:** Prof Medicine, Univ Tex, Houston

Miro-Quesada, Miguel MD (Hematology) - *Special Expertise:* Hematology - General; **Admitting Hospital:** St Luke's Episcopal Hospital - Houston (Page 76); **Office Address:** 920 Frostwood, Ste 780 Houston, TX 77030; **Office Phone:** (713) 827-9525; **Board Certifications:** Internal Medicine 1972, Hematology 1974; **Medical School:** Johns Hopkins Univ 1969; **Residencies:** Internal Medicine, Northwestern Univ Hosp, Chicago, IL 1970-1971; Internal Medicine, Rush-Presby-St Luke's Med Ctr, Chicago, IL 1971-1972; **Fellowship:** Hematology, Montefiore Hosp, New York, NY 1973-1974

West Coast and Pacific

Feinstein, Donald Ivan MD (Hematology) - *Special Expertise:* Bleeding/Coagulation Disorders; Bleeding/Coagulation Disorders; **Admitting Hospital:** USC Norris Cancer Comprehensive Center; **Office Address:** USC Keck School of Med 1355 San Pablo St, Bldg AHC 139, MC-9172 Los Angeles, CA 90033; **Office Phone:** (323) 442-5580; **Board Certifications:** Internal Medicine 1965, Hematology 1974; **Medical School:** Stanford Univ 1958; **Residency:** Internal Medicine, LAC & USC Med Ctr, Los Angeles, CA 1959-1962; **Fellowship:** Hematology, NYU, New York, NY 1964-1966; **Faculty Appointment:** Prof Medicine, USC Sch Med

Kaushansky, Kenneth MD (Hematology) - *Special Expertise:* Hematology - General; **Admitting Hospital:** University of Washington Medical Center; **Office Address:** Univ Wash Med Ctr, Dept Hematology 1959 NE Pacific St, HSB K-136, Box 357710 Seattle, WA 98195-7710; **Office Phone:** (206) 685-7868; **Board Certifications:** Internal Medicine 1982, Hematology 1984; **Medical School:** UCLA 1979; **Residency:** Internal Medicine, Univ Wash Med Ctr, Seattle, WA 1979-1982; **Fellowship:** Hematology, Univ Wash Med Ctr, Seattle, WA 1982-1986; **Faculty Appointment:** Prof Medicine, Univ Wash

Leung, Lawrence L MD (Hematology) - *Special Expertise:* Thrombotic Disorders; **Admitting Hospital:** Stanford Medical Center; **Office Address:** Stanford Univ Med Ctr, Dept Hem 269 Tempest Dr CCSR Bldg Rm 1155 Stanford, CA 94305; **Office Phone:** (650) 723-5007; **Board Certifications:** Hematology 1980, Medical Oncology 1981; **Medical School:** Columbia P&S 1975; **Residency:** Internal Medicine, NY Hosp/Cornell Med Ctr, New York, NY 1976-1978; **Fellowship:** Hematology, NY Hosp/Cornell Med Ctr, New York, NY 1978-1981; **Faculty Appointment:** Assoc Prof Medicine, Stanford Univ

Levine, Alexandra Mary MD (Hematology) - *Special Expertise:* Leukemia/Hematopoietic Malignancy; **Admitting Hospital:** USC Norris Cancer Comprehensive Center; **Office Address:** USC Kenneth Norris, Jr Cancer Hosp 1441 Eastlake Ave, rm 3468 Los Angeles, CA 90033; **Office Phone:** (323) 865-3913; **Medical School:** USC Sch Med 1971; **Residency:** Internal Medicine, LA CO-USC Med Ctr, Los Angeles, CA 1972-1974; **Fellowships:** Hematology, Grady Meml Hosp-Emory Univ, Atlanta, GA 1974-1975; Hematology, LA Co-USC Med Ctr, Los Angeles, CA 1975-1976; **Faculty Appointment:** Prof Medicine, USC Sch Med

Linenberger, Michael MD (Hematology) - *Special Expertise:* Hematology - General; **Admitting Hospital:** University of Washington Medical Center; **Office Address:** Univ Wash Med Ctr, Hematology 1959 NE Pacific St, Box 357710 Seattle, WA 98195; **Office Phone:** (206) 685-7873; **Board Certifications:** Internal Medicine 1985, Hematology 1988; **Medical School:** Univ Kans 1982; **Residency:** Internal Medicine, Rhode Island Hosp, Providence, RI 1983-1985; **Fellowship:** Hematology, Univ Wash Med Ctr, Seattle, WA 1986-1989; **Faculty Appointment:** Assoc Prof Medicine, Univ Wash

MEDICAL ONCOLOGY
New England

Antin, Joseph Harry MD (Medical Oncology) - *Special Expertise:* Bone Marrow Transplant; **Admitting Hospital:** Brigham & Women's Hospital; **Office Address:** Dana Farber Cancer Inst 44 Binney St Boston, MA 02115; **Office Phone:** (617) 632-2525; **Board Certifications:** Medical Oncology 1983, Hematology 1984; **Medical School:** Cornell Univ-Weil Med Coll 1978; **Residency:** Internal Medicine, Peter Bent Brigham Hosp., Boston, MA 1979-1981; **Fellowship:** Medical Oncology, Brigham-Womens, Boston, MA 1981-1984; **Faculty Appointment:** Assoc Prof Medicine, Harvard Med Sch

Canellos, George Peter MD (Medical Oncology) - *Special Expertise:* Lymphoma; Leukemia; Breast Cancer; **Admitting Hospital:** Dana Farber Cancer Institute; **Office Address:** Dana Farber Cancer Inst 44 Binney St Boston, MA 02115-6013; **Office Phone:** (617) 732-3470; **Board Certifications:** Medical Oncology 1973, Hematology 1972; **Medical School:** Columbia P&S 1960; **Residencies:** Internal Medicine, Mass Genl Hosp, Boston, MA 1962-1963; Internal Medicine, Mass Genl Hosp, Boston, MA 1965-1966; **Fellowships:** Medical Oncology, Natl Cancer Inst, Bethesda, MD 1963-1965; Hematology, Hammersmith Hosp, London, England 1966-1967; **Faculty Appointment:** Prof Medicine, Harvard Med Sch

Come, Steven Eliot MD (Medical Oncology) - *Special Expertise:* Breast Cancer; Hodgkin's Disease; **Admitting Hospital:** Beth Israel Deaconess Medical Center - Boston (Page 57); **Office Address:** Beth Israel Deaconess Med Ctr 330 Brookline Ave Boston, MA 02215-5491; **Office Phone:** (617) 667-4599; **Board Certifications:** Medical Oncology 1979, Internal Medicine 1975; **Medical School:** Harvard Med Sch 1972; **Residency:** Internal Medicine, Beth Israel Hosp, Boston, MA 1973-1977; **Fellowship:** Medical Oncology, Natl Cancer Inst, Bethesda, MD 1974-1976; **Faculty Appointment:** Prof Medicine, Harvard Med Sch

De Vita Jr, Vincent T MD (Medical Oncology) - *Special Expertise:* Lymphoma; Hodgkin's Disease; **Admitting Hospital:** Yale - New Haven Hospital; **Office Address:** Yale Univ Sch Med, Cancer Ctr 333 Cedar St, Ste 205, Box 208028 New Haven, CT 06520-8028; **Office Phone:** (203) 785-4371; **Board Certifications:** Hematology 1972, Medical Oncology 1973; **Medical School:** Geo Wash Univ 1961; **Residencies:** Internal Medicine, Geo Wash Hosp, Washington, DC 1962-1963; Internal Medicine, Yale-New Haven Med Ctr, New Haven, CT 1965-1966; **Fellowship:** Medical Oncology, Natl Cancer Inst, Bethesda, MD 1963-1965; **Faculty Appointment:** Prof Medicine, Yale Univ

Garber, Judy E MD (Medical Oncology) - *Special Expertise:* Breast Cancer; **Admitting Hospital:** Dana Farber Cancer Institute; **Office Address:** Dana Farber Cancer Inst 44 Binney St Boston, MA 02115; **Office Phone:** (617) 632-2282; **Board Certifications:** Hematology 1988, Medical Oncology 1987; **Medical School:** Yale Univ 1981; **Residency:** Internal Medicine, Brigham & Women's Hosp, Boston, MA 1982-1984; **Fellowships:** Medical Oncology, Dana Farber Canc Inst, Boston, MA 1985-1988; Epidemiology, Dana Farber Canc Inst, Boston, MA 1986-1990; **Faculty Appointment:** Asst Prof Medicine, Harvard Med Sch

Garnick, Marc Bennett MD (Medical Oncology) - *Special Expertise:* Prostate Cancer; Biotechnology; **Admitting Hospital:** Beth Israel Deaconess Medical Center - Boston (Page 57); **Office Address:** Beth Israel Deaconess Med Ctr 330 Brookline Ave Boston, MA 02215; **Office Phone:** (617) 667-5288; **Board Certifications:** Internal Medicine 1976, Medical Oncology 1979; **Medical School:** Univ Penn 1972; **Residency:** Internal Medicine, Univ Penn Hosp, Philadelphia, PA 1973-1974; **Fellowships:** Research, Natl Inst Hlth, Boston, MA 1974-1976; Medical Oncology, Dana-Farber Cancer Inst, Boston, MA 1976-1978; **Faculty Appointment:** Clin Prof Medicine, Harvard Med Sch

Johnson, Bruce Evan MD (Medical Oncology) - *Special Expertise:* Lung Cancer; **Admitting Hospital:** Dana Farber Cancer Institute; **Office Address:** Lowe Ctr. Thoracic Onc-Dana Farber Cancer Inst. 44 Binney St, Ste 1234 Boston, MA 02115; **Office Phone:** (617) 632-4790; **Board Certifications:** Medical Oncology 1985, Internal Medicine 1982; **Medical School:** Univ Minn 1979; **Residency:** Internal Medicine, U Chicago, Chicago, IL 1980-1982; **Fellowship:** Medical Oncology, Natl Cancer Inst., Bethesda, MD 1982-1985; **Faculty Appointment:** Assoc Prof Medical Oncology, Harvard Med Sch

Karp, Daniel David MD (Medical Oncology) - *Special Expertise:* Lung Cancer; **Admitting Hospital:** Beth Israel Deaconess Medical Center - Boston (Page 57); **Office Address:** Beth Israel Deaconess, Dept Hem/Onc 330 Brookline Ave Boston, MA 02111; **Office Phone:** (617) 667-1910; **Board Certifications:** Hand Surgery 1980, Medical Oncology 1981; **Medical School:** Duke Univ **Residency:** Internal Medicine, Dartmouth-Hitchcock Med Ctr., Hanover, NH 1974-1976; **Fellowships:** Hematology, Dartmouth-Hitchcock Med Ctr., Hanover, NH 1976-1978; Medical Oncology, Dana Farber Inst., Boston, MA 1978-1979; **Faculty Appointment:** Assoc Prof Medicine, Tufts Univ

Lynch, Thomas MD (Medical Oncology) - *Special Expertise:* Lung Cancer; **Admitting Hospital:** Massachusetts General Hospital; **Office Address:** Mass Genl Hosp Dept of Hem/Onc 55 Fruit Street Boston, MA 02114; **Office Phone:** (617) 724-1136; **Board Certifications:** Internal Medicine 1989, Medical Oncology 1991; **Medical School:** Yale Univ 1986; **Residency:** Internal Medicine, Mass Genl hosp., Boston, MA 1987-1989; **Fellowship:** Medical Oncology, Dana-Farber Cancer Inst., Boston, MA 1989-1991; **Faculty Appointment:** Asst Prof Medicine, Harvard Med Sch

Muss, Hyman MD (Medical Oncology) - *Special Expertise:* Breast Cancer; **Admitting Hospital:** Fletcher Allen Health Care Medical Center - Campus; **Office Address:** Fletcher Allen Hlth Care-Patrick 534 111 Colchester Ave Burlington, VT 05401-1429; **Office Phone:** (802) 656-3827; **Board Certifications:** Hematology 1974, Medical Oncology 1975; **Medical School:** SUNY Downstate 1968; **Residency:** Internal Medicine, Peter Bent Brigham Hosp, Boston, MA 1968-1970; **Fellowship:** Medical Oncology, Peter Bent Brigham Hosp, Boston, MA 1972-1974; **Faculty Appointment:** Prof Medicine, Univ VT Coll Med

Nadler, Lee Marshall MD (Medical Oncology) - *Special Expertise:* Lymphoma; **Admitting Hospital:** Dana Farber Cancer Institute; **Office Address:** Dana-Farber Cancer Inst 44 Binney St Boston, MA 02115; **Office Phone:** (617) 632-3331; **Board Certification:** Internal Medicine 1976; **Medical School:** Harvard Med Sch 1973; **Residency:** Internal Medicine, Columbia-Presby Hosp, New York, NY 1973-1975; **Fellowships:** Medical Oncology, Dana-Farber Cancer Inst, Boston, MA 1977-1978; Medical Oncology, Natl Cancer Inst, Bethesda, MD 1975-1977; **Faculty Appointment:** Prof Medicine, Harvard Med Sch

Winer, Eric P MD (Medical Oncology) - *Special Expertise:* Breast Cancer; **Admitting Hospital:** Dana Farber Cancer Institute; **Office Address:** Dana-Farber Cancer Inst 44 Binney St, rm 1210 Boston, MA 02115; **Office Phone:** (617) 632-3800; **Board Certifications:** Internal Medicine 1987, Medical Oncology 1989; **Medical School:** Yale Univ 1983; **Residency:** Internal Medicine, Yale-New Haven Hosp, New Haven, CT 1983-1987; **Fellowship:** Hematology and Oncology, Duke Univ, Durham, NC 1987-1989; **Faculty Appointment:** Assoc Clin Prof Medicine, Harvard Med Sch

Mid Atlantic

Abeloff, Martin MD (Medical Oncology) - *Special Expertise: Breast Cancer;* **Admitting Hospital:** Johns Hopkins Hospital - Baltimore (Page 65); **Office Address:** 401 N Broadway Baltimore, MD 21231; **Office Phone:** (410) 955-8822; **Board Certifications:** Medical Oncology 1973, Internal Medicine 1973; **Medical School:** Johns Hopkins Univ 1966; **Residency:** Internal Medicine, Beth Israel Hosp, Boston, MA 1969-1970; **Fellowship:** Hematology, New England Med Ctr, Boston, MA 1970-1971; **Faculty Appointment:** Prof Medicine, Johns Hopkins Univ

Ahlgren, James David MD (Medical Oncology) - *Special Expertise: Colon Cancer; Rectal Cancer;* **Admitting Hospital:** George Washington University Hospital; **Office Address:** Geo Wash Univ Med Ctr, Dept Hem & Onc 2150 Pennsylvania Ave NW, Ste 3-428 Washington, DC 20037; **Office Phone:** (202) 994-2746; **Board Certifications:** Medical Oncology 1989, Internal Medicine 1980; **Medical School:** Georgetown Univ 1977; **Residency:** Internal Medicine, Georgetown Univ Hosp, Washington, DC 1978-1979; **Fellowship:** Medical Oncology, Georgetown Univ Hosp, Washington, DC 1979-1981; **Faculty Appointment:** Prof Medicine, Geo Wash Univ

Aisner, Joseph MD (Medical Oncology) - *Special Expertise: Lung Cancer;* **Admitting Hospital:** Cancer Institute of New Jersey, The; **Office Address:** Cancer Inst of NJ 195 Little Albany St New Brunswick, NJ 08901-1914; **Office Phone:** (732) 235-2465; **Board Certifications:** Internal Medicine 1973, Medical Oncology 1975; **Medical School:** Wayne State Univ 1970; **Residency:** Internal Medicine, Georgetown Univ Hosp, Washington, DC 1971-1972; **Fellowship:** Medical Oncology, Natl Cancer Inst, Bethesda, MD 1972-1975

Antman, Karen MD (Medical Oncology) - *Special Expertise: Breast Cancer; Sarcoma;* **Admitting Hospital:** Columbia Presbyterian Medical Center (Page 72); **Office Address:** 177 Fort Washington Ave New York, NY 10032; **Office Phone:** (212) 305-8602; **Board Certification:** Internal Medicine 1977; **Medical School:** Columbia P&S 1974; **Residency:** Columbia-Presby, New York, NY 1974-1977; **Fellowship:** Medical Oncology, Dana-Farber Cancer Institute, Boston, MA; **Faculty Appointment:** Prof Medicine, Columbia P&S

Belani, Chandra MD (Medical Oncology) - *Special Expertise: Lung Cancer;* **Admitting Hospital:** UPMC - Presbyterian University Hospital; **Office Address:** Univ Pittsburgh Med Ctr - Montefiore 3459 Fifth Ave, 7 Main Pittsburgh, PA 15213; **Office Phone:** (412) 648-6619; **Board Certifications:** Internal Medicine 1986, Medical Oncology 1987; **Medical School:** India 1978; **Residencies:** Internal Medicine, SMS Med Hosp, Jaipur, India 1978-1981; Internal Medicine, Good Samaritan/Univ MD Hosp, Baltimore, MD 1983-1984; **Fellowship:** Hematology and Oncology, Univ MD Hosp, Baltimore, MD; **Faculty Appointment:** Prof Medicine, Univ Pittsburgh

Bosl, George MD (Medical Oncology) - *Special Expertise: Head & Neck Tumors;* **Admitting Hospital:** Memorial Sloan Kettering Cancer Center; **Office Address:** Meml Sloan-Kettering Cancer Ctr 1275 York Ave New York, NY 10021-6007; **Office Phone:** (212) 639-8473; **Board Certifications:** Internal Medicine 1976, Medical Oncology 1979; **Medical School:** Creighton Univ 1973; **Residencies:** Internal Medicine, NY Hosp, New York, NY 1974-1975; Internal Medicine, Memorial Sloan-Kettering Cancer Ctr, New York, NY 1974-1977; **Fellowship:** Medical Oncology, Univ Minn, Minneapolis, MN 1977-1979; **Faculty Appointment:** Prof Medicine, Cornell Univ-Weil Med Coll

Chapman, Paul MD (Medical Oncology) - *Special Expertise:* Melanoma; Immunology; **Admitting Hospital:** Memorial Sloan Kettering Cancer Center; **Office Address:** 1275 York Ave New York, NY 10021-6007; **Office Phone:** (212) 639-5015; **Board Certifications:** Internal Medicine 1984, Medical Oncology 1987; **Medical School:** Cornell Univ-Weil Med Coll 1981; **Residency:** Internal Medicine, Univ Chicago, Chicago, IL 1982-1984; **Fellowship:** Medical Oncology, Meml Sloan-Kettering Cancer Ctr, New York, NY 1984; **Faculty Appointment:** Assoc Prof Medicine, Cornell Univ-Weil Med Coll

Cohen, Seymour MD (Medical Oncology) - *Special Expertise:* Melanoma; Breast Cancer; Lung Cancer; **Admitting Hospital:** Mount Sinai Hospital (Page 70); **Office Address:** Oncology Consultants Inc 1045 5th Ave New York, NY 10028-0138; **Office Phone:** (212) 249-9141; **Board Certifications:** Internal Medicine 1971, Medical Oncology 1973; **Medical School:** Univ Pittsburgh 1962; **Residencies:** Internal Medicine, Montefiore Med Ctr, Bronx, NY 1963-1964; Internal Medicine, Mount Sinai Med Ctr, New York, NY 1964-1965; **Fellowships:** Hematology, Mount Sinai Med Ctr, New York, NY 1965-1967; Hematology and Oncology, LI Jewish Hosp, New Hyde Park, NY 1968-1969; **Faculty Appointment:** Assoc Clin Prof Medicine, Mount Sinai Sch Med

Coleman, Morton MD (Medical Oncology) - *Special Expertise:* Medical Oncology - General; **Admitting Hospital:** New York Weill Cornell Medical Center - NY Presbyterian Hospital (Page 72); **Office Address:** 407 E 70th St, FL 3 New York, NY 10021; **Office Phone:** (212) 517-5900; **Board Certifications:** Internal Medicine 1971, Hematology 1972; **Medical School:** Med Coll VA 1963; **Residencies:** NY Hosp, New York, NY 1967-1968; Grady Mem, Atlanta, GA 1963-1965; **Fellowship:** NY Hosp, New York, NY 1968-1970; **Faculty Appointment:** Clin Prof Medicine

Comis, Robert L MD (Medical Oncology) - *Special Expertise:* Lung Cancer; Oncology; **Admitting Hospital:** Hahnemann University Hospital; **Office Address:** Hahnemann Univ Hosp Broad & Vine Streets Philadelphia, PA 19102; **Office Phone:** (215) 789-3645; **Board Certifications:** Internal Medicine 1975, Medical Oncology 1977; **Medical School:** SUNY Syracuse 1971; **Residency:** Internal Medicine, SUNY Hlth Sci Ctr, Syracuse, NY 1971-1975

Davidson, Nancy E MD (Medical Oncology) - *Special Expertise:* Breast Cancer; Bone Marrow Transplant; **Admitting Hospital:** Johns Hopkins Hospital - Baltimore (Page 65); **Office Address:** Johns Hopkins Oncology Center 1650 Orleans St, Bldg CRB - rm 409 Baltimore, MD 21231-1000; **Office Phone:** (410) 955-8964; **Board Certifications:** Internal Medicine 1982, Medical Oncology 1985; **Medical School:** Harvard Med Sch 1979; **Residency:** Internal Medicine, John Hopkins Hosp, Baltimore, MD 1980-1982; **Fellowship:** Medical Oncology, Natl Cancer Inst, Bethesda, MD 1982-1986; **Faculty Appointment:** Prof Medical Oncology, Johns Hopkins Univ

Donehower, Ross Carl MD (Medical Oncology) - *Special Expertise:* Pancreatic Cancer; Colon Cancer; Prostate Cancer; **Admitting Hospital:** Johns Hopkins Hospital - Baltimore (Page 65); **Office Address:** 1650 Orleans St, Ste 187 Baltimore, MD 21287-0005; **Office Phone:** (410) 955-8838; **Board Certifications:** Internal Medicine 1977, Medical Oncology 1979; **Medical School:** Univ Minn 1974; **Residency:** Internal Medicine, Johns Hopkins Hosp, Baltimore, MD 1975-1976; **Fellowship:** Medical Oncology, Natl Inst Hlth, Bethesda, MD 1976-1980; **Faculty Appointment:** Prof Medicine, Johns Hopkins Univ

Ettinger, David Seymour MD (Medical Oncology) - *Special Expertise:* Lung Cancer; **Admitting Hospital:** Johns Hopkins Hospital - Baltimore (Page 65); **Office Address:** Johns Hopkins Onc Ctr 1650 Orleans St Baltimore, MD 21231-1000; **Office Phone:** (410) 955-8847; **Board Certifications:** Internal Medicine 1976, Medical Oncology 1977; **Medical School:** Univ Louisville Sch Med 1967; **Residency:** Internal Medicine, Mayo Grad Schl, Rochester, MN 1968-1971; **Fellowship:** Medical Oncology, Johns Hopkins Hosp, Baltimore, MD 1973-1975; **Faculty Appointment:** Prof Medicine, Johns Hopkins Univ

Gabrilove, Janice MD (Medical Oncology) - *Special Expertise:* Myelodysplastic Syndromes; Leukemia; **Admitting Hospital:** Mount Sinai Hospital (Page 70); **Office Address:** 5 E 98th St, Fl 14, Box 1129 New York, NY 10029; **Office Phone:** (212) 241-9650; **Board Certifications:** Internal Medicine 1980, Medical Oncology 1983; **Medical School:** Mount Sinai Sch Med 1977; **Residency:** Internal Medicine, Columbia-Presby Med Ctr, New York, NY 1978-1980; **Fellowship:** Hematology, Meml Sloan-Kettering, New York, NY 1984; **Faculty Appointment:** Prof Medicine, Mount Sinai Sch Med

Glick, John H MD (Medical Oncology) - *Special Expertise:* Breast Cancer; Hodgkin's Disease; Non-Hodgkins Lymphoma; **Admitting Hospital:** Hospital of the University of Pennsylvania; **Office Address:** Univ Penn Cancer Ctr 3400 Spruce St, Fl 16 Philadelphia, PA 19104; **Office Phone:** (215) 626-6334; **Board Certifications:** Internal Medicine 1973, Medical Oncology 1975; **Medical School:** Columbia P&S 1969; **Residency:** Internal Medicine, Presbyterian Hosp, New York, NY 1969-1971; **Fellowships:** Medical Oncology, Natl Cancer Inst, Bethesda, MD 1971-1973; Medical Oncology, Stanford Univ, Stanford, CA 1973-1974; **Faculty Appointment:** Prof Medicine, Univ Penn

Goldstein, Lori J MD (Medical Oncology) - *Special Expertise:* Breast Cancer; **Admitting Hospital:** Fox Chase Cancer Center; **Office Address:** Fox Chase Cancer Ctr, Dept Med Oncology 7701 Burholme Ave Philadelphia, PA 19111; **Office Phone:** (215) 728-2689; **Board Certifications:** Medical Oncology 1999, Internal Medicine 1985; **Medical School:** SUNY Syracuse 1982; **Residency:** Internal Medicine, Presby U Hosp, Pittsburgh, PA 1983-1985; **Fellowship:** Medical Oncology, NCI/NIH, Bethesda, MD 1986; **Faculty Appointment:** Assoc Prof Medical Oncology, Temple Univ

Grossbard, Michael Laurence MD (Medical Oncology) - *Special Expertise:* Lymphoma; Gastrointestinal Cancer; **Admitting Hospital:** St Luke's - Roosevelt Hospital Center - Roosevelt Division (Page 58); **Office Address:** 425 W 59th St, Ste 1A New York, NY 10019; **Office Phone:** (212) 523-5419; **Board Certifications:** Internal Medicine 1989, Medical Oncology 1991; **Medical School:** Yale Univ 1986; **Residency:** Internal Medicine, Mass Genl Hosp, Boston, MA 1986-1989; **Fellowship:** Medical Oncology, Dana Farber Cancer Inst, Boston, MA 1989; **Faculty Appointment:** Asst Clin Prof Medicine, Columbia P&S

Hait, William MD/PhD (Medical Oncology) - *Special Expertise:* Breast Cancer; Lung Cancer; **Admitting Hospital:** Robert Wood Johnson University Hospital @ New Brunswick; **Office Address:** Cancer Inst of NJ 195 Little Albany St New Brunswick, NJ 08901-1977; **Office Phone:** (732) 235-8064; **Board Certifications:** Medical Oncology 1987, Internal Medicine 1982; **Medical School:** Univ Penn 1978; **Residency:** Internal Medicine, Yale Univ Sch Med, New Haven, CT 1979-1982; **Fellowship:** Medical Oncology, Yale Univ Sch Med, New Haven, CT 1982-1983; **Faculty Appointment:** Prof Medicine, UMDNJ-NJ Med Sch, Newark

Haller, Daniel MD (Medical Oncology) - *Special Expertise:* Gastrointestinal Cancer; Colorectal Cancer; **Admitting Hospital:** Hospital of the University of Pennsylvania; **Office Address:** Hosp of the Univ PA, Dept Hem Onc 3400 Spruce St, Penn Tower Bldg, Fl 16 Philadelphia, PA 19104; **Office Phone:** (215) 662-7666; **Board Certifications:** Internal Medicine 1976, Medical Oncology 1979; **Medical School:** Univ Pittsburgh 1973; **Residency:** Internal Medicine, Georgetown Univ Hosp, Washington, DC 1974-1976; **Fellowship:** Medical Oncology, Georgetown Univ Hosp, Washington, DC 1976-1978

Hayes, Daniel Fleming MD (Medical Oncology) - *Special Expertise:* Breast Cancer; **Admitting Hospital:** Georgetown University Hospital; **Office Address:** Georgetown Univ Hosp, Dept Onc 3800 Resevoir Rd NW Washington, DC 20007; **Office Phone:** (202) 687-2103; **Board Certifications:** Medical Oncology 1985, Internal Medicine 1982; **Medical School:** Indiana Univ 1979; **Residency:** Internal Medicine, Parkland Meml Hosp, San Antonio, TX 1979-1982; **Fellowship:** Medical Oncology, Dana Farber Cancer Inst., Boston, MA 1982-1985; **Faculty Appointment:** Prof Medicine, Georgetown Univ

Holland, James F MD (Medical Oncology) - *Special Expertise:* Breast Cancer; **Admitting Hospital:** Mount Sinai Hospital (Page 70); **Office Address:** 5 E 98th St New York, NY 10029; **Office Phone:** (212) 241-4495; **Board Certification:** Internal Medicine 1955; **Medical School:** Columbia P&S 1947; **Residency:** Columbia-Presby, New York, NY 1947-1949; **Fellowship:** Medical Oncology, Francis Delafield Hosp, New York, NY 1951-1953; **Faculty Appointment:** Prof Medicine, Mount Sinai Sch Med

Hudes, Gary Robert MD (Medical Oncology) - *Special Expertise:* Prostate Cancer; Genitourinary Cancer; **Admitting Hospital:** Fox Chase Cancer Center; **Office Address:** Fox Chase Cancer Ctr 7701 Burholme Ave, rm W250 Philadelphia, PA 19111; **Office Phone:** (215) 728-3889; **Board Certifications:** Hematology 1984, Medical Oncology 1985; **Medical School:** SUNY Downstate 1979; **Residency:** Internal Medicine, Graduate Hosp-Tenet Hlth Sys, Philadelphia, PA 1979-1982; **Fellowship:** Hematology and Oncology, Presby-Univ Penn Med Ctr, Philadelphia, PA 1982-1985

Kemeny, Nancy MD (Medical Oncology) - *Special Expertise:* Colon Cancer; Rectal Cancer; **Admitting Hospital:** Memorial Sloan Kettering Cancer Center; **Office Address:** 1275 York Ave New York, NY 10021; **Office Phone:** (212) 639-8068; **Board Certifications:** Internal Medicine 1974, Medical Oncology 1982; **Medical School:** UMDNJ-NJ Med Sch, Newark 1971; **Residency:** Internal Medicine, St Luke's Roosevelt Hosp Ctr, New York, NY 1972-1974; **Fellowship:** Medical Oncology, Mem Sloan Kettering Cancer Ctr, New York, NY 1974-1976; **Faculty Appointment:** Prof Medicine, Cornell Univ-Weil Med Coll

Kirkwood, John Munn MD (Medical Oncology) - *Special Expertise:* Melanoma; Sentinel Node Assessment; **Admitting Hospital:** UPMC - Presbyterian University Hospital; **Office Address:** UPMC Montefiore 3459 Fifth Ave, rm N758 Pittsburgh, PA 15213; **Office Phone:** (412) 648-6570; **Board Certifications:** Internal Medicine 1976, Medical Oncology 1981; **Medical School:** Yale Univ 1973; **Residency:** Internal Medicine, Yale Univ Hosp, New Haven, CT 1973-1976; **Fellowships:** Medical Oncology, Dana Farber Cancer Inst., Boston, MA; Medical Oncology, Harvard Medical School, Boston, MA; **Faculty Appointment:** Prof Medicine, Univ Pittsburgh

Kris, Mark MD (Medical Oncology) - *Special Expertise:* Lung Cancer; Antiemetic Therapy; Mediastinal Tumors; **Admitting Hospital:** Memorial Sloan Kettering Cancer Center; **Office Address:** Meml Sloan Kettering Cancer Ctr 1275 York Ave, Bldg Howard - Fl 10 New York, NY 10021; **Office Phone:** (212) 639-7590; **Board Certifications:** Internal Medicine 1980, Medical Oncology 1983; **Medical School:** Cornell Univ-Weil Med Coll 1977; **Residency:** Internal Medicine, NY Hosp, New York, NY 1977-1980; **Fellowship:** Medical Oncology, Mem Sloan, New York, NY 1980-1983; **Faculty Appointment:** Prof Medicine, Cornell Univ-Weil Med Coll

Langer, Corey Jay MD (Medical Oncology) - *Special Expertise:* Lung Cancer; Head & Neck Cancer; **Admitting Hospital:** Fox Chase Cancer Center; **Office Address:** Fox Chase Cancer Center 7701 Burholme Ave, rm C307 Philadelphia, PA 19111; **Office Phone:** (215) 728-2985; **Board Certifications:** Medical Oncology 1986, Hematology 1986; **Medical School:** Boston Univ 1981; **Residencies:** Internal Medicine, Grad Hosp U Penn, Philadelphia, PA 1982-1984; Hematology and Oncology, Presby-Hosp U Penn, Philadelphia, PA 1984-1986; **Fellowship:** Medical Oncology, Fox Chase Cancer Ctr, Philadelphia, PA 1986-1987

Leichman, Lawrence Peter MD (Medical Oncology) - *Special Expertise:* Esophageal Cancer; Gastrointestinal Cancer; **Admitting Hospital:** Roswell Park Cancer Institute; **Office Address:** Roswell Park Canc Inst Elm & Carlton Buffalo, NY 14263; **Office Phone:** (716) 845-3511; **Board Certifications:** Internal Medicine 1977, Medical Oncology 1983; **Medical School:** Wayne State Univ 1973; **Residency:** Internal Medicine, Detroit Genl Hosp, Detroit, MI 1974-1977; **Fellowship:** Medical Oncology, Wayne Hospital, Wayne, MI 1977-1979; **Faculty Appointment:** Prof Medicine, SUNY Buffalo

Levine, Ellis MD (Medical Oncology) - *Special Expertise:* Breast Cancer; **Admitting Hospital:** Roswell Park Cancer Institute; **Office Address:** Rosewell Park Cancer Institute Elm & Carlton Sts Buffalo, NY 14263; **Office Phone:** (716) 845-8547; **Board Certifications:** Medical Oncology 1985, Internal Medicine 1982; **Medical School:** Univ Pittsburgh 1979; **Residency:** Internal Medicine, U Minn Hosps., MN 1980-1982; **Fellowship:** Medical Oncology, U Minn., MN 1982-1984

Livingston, Philip MD (Medical Oncology) - *Special Expertise:* Breast Cancer; **Admitting Hospital:** Memorial Sloan Kettering Cancer Center; **Office Address:** Memorial Sloan Kettering Cancer Ctr 1275 York Ave New York, NY 10021; **Office Phone:** (212) 639-7425; **Board Certifications:** Allergy & Immunology 1974, Medical Oncology 1981; **Medical School:** Harvard Med Sch 1969; **Residency:** Internal Medicine, N Shore Hosp-Cornell Med Ctr, New York, NY 1969-1970; **Fellowship:** Immunology, NYU Med Ctr, New York, NY 1971-1973; **Faculty Appointment:** Prof Medical Oncology, Cornell Univ-Weil Med Coll

MacDonald, John MD (Medical Oncology) - *Special Expertise:* Colon Cancer; **Admitting Hospital:** St Vincents Catholic Medical Center of New York; **Office Address:** St Vincents Cancer Ctr 325 W 15th St New York, NY 10011; **Office Phone:** (212) 604-6011; **Board Certifications:** Internal Medicine 1973, Medical Oncology 1975; **Medical School:** Harvard Med Sch 1969; **Residency:** Internal Medicine, Beth Israel Hosp, Boston, MA 1969-1971; **Fellowship:** Hematology and Oncology, Natl Cancer Inst, Bethesda, MD 1971-1974; **Faculty Appointment:** Prof Medicine, NY Med Coll

Marks, Stanley M MD (Medical Oncology) - *Special Expertise:* Medical Oncology - General; **Admitting Hospital:** University Hospital, Hahnemann; **Office Address:** 816 Middle St Pittsburg, PA 15212-4915; **Office Phone:** (412) 231-5400; **Board Certifications:** Internal Medicine 1976, Hematology 1978; **Medical School:** Univ Pittsburgh 1973; **Residency:** Internal Medicine, Presby Univ Hosp, Pittsburgh, PA 1974-1976; **Fellowship:** Hematology, Peter Bent Brigham Hosp, Boston, MA 1976-1978; **Faculty Appointment:** Assoc Prof Medicine, Hahnemann Univ

Moore, Anne MD (Medical Oncology) - *Special Expertise:* Breast Cancer; **Admitting Hospital:** New York Weill Cornell Medical Center - NY Presbyterian Hospital (Page 72); **Office Address:** New York Presbyterian Hospital 428 E 72nd St, Ste 300 New York, NY 10021-4873; **Office Phone:** (212) 746-2085; **Board Certifications:** Internal Medicine 1973, Medical Oncology 1977; **Medical School:** Columbia P&S 1969; **Residency:** Internal Medicine, Cornell Univ Med Ctr, New York, NY 1970-1973; **Fellowship:** Medical Oncology, Rockefeller Univ, New York, NY 1972-1973; **Faculty Appointment:** Prof Medical Oncology, Cornell Univ-Weil Med Coll

Motzer, Robert J MD (Medical Oncology) - *Special Expertise:* Kidney Cancer; Testicular Cancer; **Admitting Hospital:** Memorial Sloan Kettering Cancer Center; **Office Address:** Meml Sloan Kettering Cancer Ctr 1275 York Ave New York, NY 10021; **Office Phone:** (212) 639-6667; **Board Certifications:** Internal Medicine 1984, Medical Oncology 1987; **Medical School:** Univ Mich Med Sch 1981; **Residency:** Internal Medicine, Meml Sloan Kettering, New York, NY 1982-1984; **Fellowship:** Medical Oncology, Meml Sloan Kettering, New York, NY 1984-1987; **Faculty Appointment:** Assoc Prof Medicine, Cornell Univ-Weil Med Coll

Nissenblatt, Michael MD (Medical Oncology) - *Special Expertise:* Breast Cancer; Lung Cancer; Lymphoma; **Admitting Hospital:** Robert Wood Johnson University Hospital; **Office Address:** 205 Easton Ave New Brunswick, NJ 08901-1722; **Office Phone:** (732) 828-9570; **Board Certifications:** Internal Medicine 1976, Medical Oncology 1979; **Medical School:** Columbia P&S 1973; **Residency:** Internal Medicine, Johns Hopkins Hosp, Baltimore, MD 1973-1976; **Fellowship:** Medical Oncology, Johns Hopkins Hosp, Baltimore, MD 1976-1978; **Faculty Appointment:** Clin Prof Medicine, Robert W Johnson Med Sch

Norton, Larry MD (Medical Oncology) - *Special Expertise:* Breast Cancer; **Admitting Hospital:** Memorial Sloan Kettering Cancer Center; **Office Address:** 205 E 64th St, Concourse Level New York, NY 10021; **Office Phone:** (212) 639-5438; **Board Certifications:** Internal Medicine 1972, Medical Oncology 1977; **Medical School:** Columbia P&S 1972; **Residency:** Internal Medicine, Bronx Municipal Hosp Ctr-Albert Einstein Coll Med, Bronx, NY 1973-1974; **Faculty Appointment:** Prof Medicine, Cornell Univ-Weil Med Coll

Oster, Martin MD (Medical Oncology) - *Special Expertise:* Breast Cancer; Lung Cancer; Prostate Cancer; **Admitting Hospital:** Columbia Presbyterian Medical Center (Page 72); **Office Address:** 161 Fort Washington Ave New York, NY 10032-3713; **Office Phone:** (212) 305-8231; **Board Certifications:** Internal Medicine 1974, Medical Oncology 1975; **Medical School:** Columbia P&S 1971; **Residency:** Internal Medicine, Mass Genl Hosp, Boston, MA 1971-1973; **Fellowship:** Medical Oncology, Natl Cancer Inst/Natl Inst Hlth, Bethesda, MD 1973-1976; **Faculty Appointment:** Assoc Clin Prof Medical Oncology, Columbia P&S

Ozols, Robert Felix MD/PhD (Medical Oncology) - *Special Expertise:* Ovarian Cancer; **Admitting Hospital:** Fox Chase Cancer Center; **Office Address:** Fox Chase Cancer Ctr 7701 Burholme Ave, rm P 2050 Philadelphia, PA 19111; **Office Phone:** (215) 728-2673; **Board Certifications:** Internal Medicine 1977, Medical Oncology 1979; **Medical School:** Univ Rochester 1974; **Residency:** Internal Medicine, Dartmouth-Hitchcock Hosp, Lebanon, NH 1975-1976; **Fellowship:** Medical Oncology, Natl Cancer Inst, Bethesda, MD 1976-1979; **Faculty Appointment:** Assoc Prof Medicine, Temple Univ

Scheinberg, David MD/PhD (Medical Oncology) - *Special Expertise:* Leukemia; **Admitting Hospital:** Memorial Sloan Kettering Cancer Center; **Office Address:** Meml Sloan Kettering Cancer Ctr 1275 York Ave New York, NY 10021; **Office Phone:** (212) 639-5010; **Board Certifications:** Internal Medicine 1986, Medical Oncology 1995; **Medical School:** Johns Hopkins Univ 1983; **Residency:** Internal Medicine, NY Hosp Cornell, New York, NY 1984-1985; **Fellowship:** Medical Oncology, Meml Sloan Kettering Med Ctr, New York, NY 1985-1987; **Faculty Appointment:** Assoc Prof Medicine, Cornell Univ-Weil Med Coll

Scher, Howard MD (Medical Oncology) - *Special Expertise:* Genitourinary Cancer; Prostate Cancer; Bladder Cancer; **Admitting Hospital:** Memorial Sloan Kettering Cancer Center; **Office Address:** Meml Sloan Kettering Cancer Ctr 1275 York Ave New York, NY 10021; **Office Phone:** (212) 639-7585; **Board Certifications:** Internal Medicine 1979, Medical Oncology 1985; **Medical School:** NYU Sch Med 1976; **Residency:** Internal Medicine, Bellevue Hosp, New York, NY 1977-1980; **Fellowship:** Medical Oncology, Meml Sloan Kettering, New York, NY 1980-1983

Speyer, James MD (Medical Oncology) - *Special Expertise:* Ovarian Cancer; Breast Cancer; **Admitting Hospital:** NYU Medical Center (Page 70); **Office Address:** 160 E 32nd St, Fl 2 New York, NY 10016; **Office Phone:** (212) 652-1918; **Board Certifications:** Medical Oncology 1979, Hematology 1978; **Medical School:** Johns Hopkins Univ 1974; **Residency:** Internal Medicine, Columbia-Presby Med Ctr, New York, NY 1975-1976; **Fellowships:** Hematology, Columbia-Presby Med Ctr, New York, NY 1976-1977; Medical Oncology, Natl Cancer Inst, Bethesda, MD 1977-1979; **Faculty Appointment:** Clin Prof Medicine, NYU Sch Med

Treat, Joseph MD (Medical Oncology) - *Special Expertise:* Lung Cancer; **Admitting Hospital:** Fox Chase Cancer Center; **Office Address:** 3322 N Broad St Philadelphia, PA 19140; **Office Phone:** (215) 707-8030; **Board Certifications:** Internal Medicine 1982, Medical Oncology 1985; **Medical School:** Temple Univ 1979; **Residency:** Internal Medicine, Georgetown Univ Hosp, Washington, DC 1980-1982; **Fellowship:** Medical Oncology, Georgetown Univ Hosp, Washington, DC 1982-1984; **Faculty Appointment:** Prof Medical Oncology, Temple Univ

Weber, Barbara L MD (Medical Oncology) - *Special Expertise:* Breast Cancer; **Admitting Hospital:** Hospital of the University of Pennsylvania; **Office Address:** Univ Penn Cancer Ctr 3400 Spruce St, Bldg Penn Tower - Fl 14 Philadelphia, PA 19104; **Office Phone:** (215) 898-0247; **Board Certifications:** Internal Medicine 1985, Medical Oncology 1987; **Medical School:** Univ Wash 1982; **Residency:** Internal Medicine, Yale Univ, New Haven, CT 1983-1985; **Fellowship:** Medical Oncology, Dana-Farber Cancer Inst, Boston, MA 1985; **Faculty Appointment:** Prof Medical Oncology, Univ Penn

Weiner, Louis M MD (Medical Oncology) - *Special Expertise:* Gastrointestinal Cancer; Immunotherapy; **Admitting Hospital:** Fox Chase Cancer Center; **Office Address:** Fox Chase Cancer Ctr 7701 Burholme Ave Philadelphia, PA 19111; **Office Phone:** (215) 728-2480; **Board Certifications:** Internal Medicine 1980, Medical Oncology 1985; **Medical School:** Mount Sinai Sch Med 1977; **Residency:** Internal Medicine, Med Ctr Hosp of VT, VT; **Fellowship:** Hematology and Oncology, New England Med Ctr - Tufts Univ Sch Med, Boston, MA

Southeast

Balducci, Lodovico MD (Medical Oncology) - *Special Expertise:* Genitourinary Cancer; Breast Cancer; **Admitting Hospital:** H Lee Moffitt Cancer Center & Research Institute; **Office Address:** 12902 Magnolia Dr, rm 3157 Tampa, FL 33612-9416; **Office Phone:** (813) 979-3822; **Board Certifications:** Internal Medicine 1976, Medical Oncology 1979; **Medical School:** Italy 1968; **Residencies:** Internal Medicine, Univ Miss Med Ctr, Jackson, MS 1973-1976; Hematology and Oncology, Univ Miss Med Ctr, Jackson, MS 1976-1979; **Fellowship:** Internal Medicine, A Gemelli Genl Hosp, Rome, Italy 1968-1970; **Faculty Appointment:** Prof Medicine, Univ S Fla Coll Med

Crawford, Jeffrey MD (Medical Oncology) - *Special Expertise:* Lung Cancer; **Admitting Hospital:** Duke University Medical Center (Page 60); **Office Address:** Duke Med Ctr 25177 Morris Bldg, Box 3198 Durham, NC 27710; **Office Phone:** (919) 684-5621; **Board Certifications:** Hematology 1980, Medical Oncology 1981; **Medical School:** Ohio State Univ 1974; **Residencies:** Internal Medicine, Duke Med Ctr, Durham, NC 1975-1977; Internal Medicine, Duke Med Ctr, Durham, NC 1978-1979; **Fellowships:** Medical Oncology, Duke Med Ctr, Durham, NC 1977-1978; Hematology, Duke Med Ctr, Durham, NC 1979-1981; **Faculty Appointment:** Prof Medicine, Duke Univ

Gockerman, Jon Paul MD (Medical Oncology) - *Special Expertise:* Leukemia; Lymphoma; **Admitting Hospital:** Duke University Medical Center (Page 60); **Office Address:** Duke Univ Med Ctr Box 3872 Durham, NC 27710; **Office Phone:** (919) 684-8964; **Board Certifications:** Medical Oncology 1973, Hematology 1974; **Medical School:** Univ Chicago-Pritzker Sch Med 1967; **Residency:** Internal Medicine, Duke Univ Med Ctr, Durham, NC 1968-1969; **Fellowship:** Hematology and Oncology, Duke Univ Med Ctr, Durham, NC 1969-1971

Graham, Mark MD (Medical Oncology) - *Special Expertise:* Breast Cancer; **Admitting Hospital:** University of North Carolina Hospitals; **Office Address:** Univ NC Hlthcare - Cary Oncology 300 Ashville Ave Cary, NC 27511; **Office Phone:** (919) 859-6631; **Board Certification:** Internal Medicine 1989; **Medical School:** Mayo Med Sch 1982; **Residency:** Internal Medicine, Duke Univ Med Ctr, Durham, NC 1983-1985; **Fellowship:** Medical Oncology, Univ CO Hlth Sci Ctr, Denver, CO 1986-1990

Greco, F Anthony MD (Medical Oncology) - *Special Expertise:* Lung Cancer; **Admitting Hospital:** Centennial Medical Center; **Office Address:** Sarah Cannon - Minnie Pearl Cancer Center 250 25th Ave N, Ste 412 Nashville, TN 37203; **Office Phone:** (615) 342-1725; **Board Certifications:** Internal Medicine 1975, Medical Oncology 1977; **Medical School:** W VA Univ 1972; **Residency:** Internal Medicine, Univ West Virginia Hosp, Morgantown, WV 1973-1974; **Fellowship:** Medical Oncology, Natl Canc Inst, Bethesda, MD 1974-1976

Green, Mark MD (Medical Oncology) - *Special Expertise:* Lung Cancer; **Admitting Hospital:** MUSC Medical Center; **Office Address:** Med Univ SC - Hollings Cancer Ctr 96 Jonathan Lucas St, 903 Clin Serv Bldg Charleston, SC 29425; **Office Phone:** (843) 792-4179; **Board Certifications:** Internal Medicine 1973, Medical Oncology 1975; **Medical School:** Harvard Med Sch 1970; **Residencies:** Internal Medicine, Beth Israel Hosp, Boston, MA 1971-1972; Internal Medicine, Stanford Univ Hosp, Stanford, CA 1974-1975; **Fellowships:** Medical Oncology, Natl Canc Inst, Bethesda, MD 1972-1974; Medical Oncology, Stanford Univ Hosp, Stanford, CA 1975-1976; **Faculty Appointment:** Prof Medicine, Univ SC Sch Med

Grosh, William W MD (Medical Oncology) - *Special Expertise:* Melanoma & Sarcoma; Hepatoma; Carcinoid Tumors; **Admitting Hospital:** University of Virginia Health Systems; **Office Address:** Univ VA Cancer Ctr Box 800716 Charlottesville, VA 22908; **Office Phone:** (804) 924-1904; **Board Certifications:** Internal Medicine 1978, Medical Oncology 1985; **Medical School:** Columbia P&S 1974; **Residency:** Internal Medicine, Vanderbilt Univ Med Ctr, Nashville, TN 1975-1977; **Fellowship:** Medical Oncology, Vanderbilt Univ Med Ctr, Nashville, TN 1980-1983

Hande, Kenneth MD (Medical Oncology) - *Special Expertise:* Breast Cancer; **Admitting Hospital:** Vanderbilt University Medical Center; **Office Address:** Vanderbilt Univ Med Ctr 1956 The Vanderbilt Clinic Nashville, TN 37232-5536; **Office Phone:** (615) 322-4967; **Board Certifications:** Internal Medicine 1975, Medical Oncology 1977; **Medical School:** Johns Hopkins Univ 1972; **Residency:** Internal Medicine, Barnes Hosp, St Louis, MO 1973-1974; **Fellowship:** Medical Oncology, Natl Cancer Inst, Bethesda, MD 1974-1977; **Faculty Appointment:** Prof Medicine, Vanderbilt Univ

Horton, John MD (Medical Oncology) - *Special Expertise:* Breast Cancer; Gastrointestinal Cancer; **Admitting Hospital:** H Lee Moffitt Cancer Center & Research Institute; **Office Address:** 12902 Magnolia Dr, Ste 4035 Tampa, FL 33612-9416; **Office Phone:** (813) 972-8470; **Board Certifications:** Internal Medicine 1968, Medical Oncology 1973; **Medical School:** England 1957; **Residency:** Internal Medicine, Albany Med Ctr Hosp, Albany, NY 1957-1962; **Fellowship:** Medical Oncology, Albany Med Ctr Hosp, Albany, NY 1962-1963; **Faculty Appointment:** Prof Medical Oncology, Univ S Fla Coll Med

Jillella, Anand MD (Medical Oncology) - *Special Expertise:* Bone Marrow Transplant; Stem Cell Transplantation; **Admitting Hospital:** Medical College of Georgia Hospital; **Office Address:** Med Coll of GA, Comprehensive Cancer Ctr 1120 15th St Augusta, GA 30912; **Office Phone:** (706) 721-2505; **Board Certifications:** Internal Medicine 1992, Medical Oncology 1997; **Medical School:** India 1985; **Residencies:** Internal Medicine, Med Coll of GA, Augusta, GA; Medical Oncology, VA Med Ctr, West Haven, CT

Johnson, David MD (Medical Oncology) - *Special Expertise:* Lung Cancer; **Admitting Hospital:** Vanderbilt University Medical Center; **Office Address:** Vanderbilt Univ Med Ctr, Div Hem Onc 1956 Vanderbuilt Clinic Nashville, TN 37232-5536; **Office Phone:** (615) 322-4967; **Board Certifications:** Internal Medicine 1979, Medical Oncology 1983; **Medical School:** Med Coll GA 1976; **Residencies:** Internal Medicine, Univ South Alabama Med Ctr, Mobile, AL 1977-1979; Internal Medicine, Med Coll Georgia Hosps, Augusta, GA 1979-1980; **Fellowship:** Medical Oncology, Vanderbilt Univ Med Ctr, Nashville, TN 1981-1983; **Faculty Appointment:** Prof Medicine, Vanderbilt Univ

Lyckholm, Laurel Jean MD (Medical Oncology) - *Special Expertise:* Neuro-Onocology; **Admitting Hospital:** Medical College of Virginia Hospitals; **Office Address:** Med Coll Va-Div Hem Onc Box 980230 Richmond, VA 23298-0230; **Office Phone:** (804) 828-9723; **Board Certifications:** Medical Oncology 1993, Hematology 1994; **Medical School:** Creighton Univ 1985; **Residency:** Creighton U., NE 1986-1989; **Fellowships:** Medical Oncology, U IA Coll Med., IA 1989-1992; Hematology, Univ IA Coll Med, IA 1989-1992; **Faculty Appointment:** Asst Prof Medicine, Med Coll VA

McCarley, Dean L MD (Medical Oncology) - *Special Expertise:* Solid Tumors; Urologic Cancer; Lung Cancer; **Admitting Hospital:** Shands Healthcare at University Florida (Page 77); **Office Address:** Shands Healthcare-Univ Florida 2000 SW Archer Road Gainesville, FL 32608; **Office Phone:** (352) 395-0725; **Board Certifications:** Internal Medicine 1978, Medical Oncology 1985; **Medical School:** Duke Univ 1975; **Residency:** Internal Medicine, Univ Fla Affil. Hosp, Gainesville, FL 1976-1978; **Fellowship:** Hematology and Oncology, Shands Tchg Hosp, Gainesville, FL 1978-1981; **Faculty Appointment:** Assoc Prof Medical Oncology, Univ Fla Coll Med

Mitchell, Beverly MD (Medical Oncology) - *Special Expertise:* Leukemia/Hematopoietic Malignancy; Leukemia; Lymphoma; **Admitting Hospital:** University of North Carolina Hospitals; **Office Address:** Div Hematology 3009 Old Clinic Bldg, Box 7305 Chapel Hill, NC 27599-7305; **Office Phone:** (919) 966-4431; **Board Certifications:** Internal Medicine 1973, Hematology 1978; **Medical School:** Harvard Med Sch 1969; **Residency:** Internal Medicine, Univ Washington, Seattle, WA 1969-1972; **Fellowships:** Metabolism, Univ Zurich, Zurich, Switzerland 1973-1975; Hematology and Oncology, Univ Michigan, Ann Arbor, MI 1975-1977; **Faculty Appointment:** Prof Medicine, Univ NC Sch Med

Moores, Russell MD (Medical Oncology) - *Special Expertise:* Medical Oncology - General; **Admitting Hospital:** Medical College of Georgia Hospital; **Office Address:** Medical College of GA-Hemotology/Oncology Section 1120 15th St.-BAA6407 Augusta, GA 30912-3125; **Office Phone:** (706) 721-2505; **Board Certification:** Internal Medicine 1965; **Medical School:** Univ Ark 1958; **Residencies:** Internal Medicine, Strong Meml Hosp, Rochester, NY 1959-1960; Internal Medicine, Barnes Hosp, St. Louis, MO 1960-1961; **Fellowship:** Hematology, NIH, Bethesda, MD 1961-1963; **Faculty Appointment:** Prof Medical Oncology, Med Coll GA

Myers, Charles E MD (Medical Oncology) - *Special Expertise:* Prostate Cancer; **Admitting Hospital:** University of Virginia Health Systems; **Office Address:** Univ VA Cancer Ctr Jefferson Park Ave Charlottesville, VA 22908; **Office Phone:** (804) 982-4190; **Board Certifications:** Internal Medicine 1973, Medical Oncology 1975; **Medical School:** Univ Penn 1969; **Residency:** Internal Medicine, Univ Penn Hosp, Philadelphia, PA 1971; **Fellowship:** Medical Oncology, Natl Cancer Inst, Bethesada, MD 1971-1973

Nixon, Daniel MD (Medical Oncology) - *Special Expertise:* Medical Oncology - General; **Admitting Hospital:** Mount Sinai Medical Center; **Office Address:** Mount Sinai Comprehensive Ctr 4306 Alton Rd, Fl 3 Miami, FL 33140-2840; **Office Phone:** (305) 535-3300; **Board Certifications:** Internal Medicine 1967, Medical Oncology 1973; **Medical School:** Univ Pittsburgh 1959; **Residencies:** Internal Medicine, Univ Pittsburgh, Pittsburgh, PA 1960-1961; Internal Medicine, Mt Sinai Hosp, New York, NY 1961-1962; **Fellowships:** Hematology, Mt Sinai Hosp, New York, NY 1962-1963; Medical Oncology, Delafield-Columbia Univ, New York, NY 1968-1969; **Faculty Appointment:** Assoc Clin Prof Medical Oncology, Univ Miami Sch Med

Powell, Bayard Lowery MD (Medical Oncology) - *Special Expertise:* Leukemia; *Myelodysplastic Syndromes;* **Admitting Hospital:** Wake Forest University Baptist Medical Center; **Office Address:** Wake Forest Univ Baptist Med Ctr Medical Center Blvd - Cancer Center Winston-Salem, NC 27157; **Office Phone:** (336) 716-2946; **Board Certifications:** Medical Oncology 1985, Internal Medicine 1983; **Medical School:** Univ NC Sch Med 1980; **Residency:** Internal Medicine, NC Baptist Hospital, Winston Salem, NC 1981-1983; **Fellowship:** Medical Oncology, Wake Forest U Sch of Med, Winston Salem, NC 1983-1986; **Faculty Appointment:** Prof Hematology

Robert, Nicholas J MD (Medical Oncology) - *Special Expertise:* Breast Cancer; *Hematology;* **Admitting Hospital:** Inova Fairfax Hospital; **Office Address:** Inova Fairfax Hosp, Dept Hem/Onc 3289 Woodburn Rd, Ste 230 Annandale, VA 22003; **Office Phone:** (703) 280-5390; **Board Certifications:** Medical Oncology 1981, Hematology 1984; **Medical School:** McGill Univ 1974; **Residencies:** Internal Medicine, Royal Victoria Hosp, Montreal, Canada 1975-1976; Pathology, Mass Genl Hosp, Boston, MA 1976-1979; **Fellowship:** Hematology, Peter Bent Brigham Hosp, Boston, MA 1979-1984

Roth, Bruce Joseph MD (Medical Oncology) - *Special Expertise:* Prostate Cancer; Bladder Cancer; **Admitting Hospital:** Vanderbilt University Medical Center; **Office Address:** Vanderbilt Univ, Div Hem 1956 Vanderbilt Clinic Nashville, TN 37232-5532; **Office Phone:** (615) 322-4967; **Board Certifications:** Internal Medicine 1983, Medical Oncology 1985; **Medical School:** St Louis Univ 1980; **Residency:** Internal Medicine, Ind Univ Med Ctr, Indianapolis, IN 1981-1983; **Fellowship:** Medical Oncology, Ind Univ Med Ctr, Indianapolis, IN 1983-1986; **Faculty Appointment:** Assoc Prof Medical Oncology, Vanderbilt Univ

Rothenberg, Mace MD (Medical Oncology) - *Special Expertise:* Pancreatic Cancer; Colorectal Cancer; **Admitting Hospital:** Vanderbilt University Medical Center; **Office Address:** Vanderbilt Univ Med Ctr, Div Med Onc 1956 Vanderbilt Clinic Nashville, TN 37232-5536; **Office Phone:** (615) 322-4967; **Board Certifications:** Internal Medicine 1985, Medical Oncology 1987; **Medical School:** NYU Sch Med 1982; **Residency:** Internal Medicine, Vanderbilt Univ Med Ctr, Nashville, TN 1982-1985; **Fellowship:** Medical Oncology, Natl Cancer Inst, Bethesda, MD 1985-1988; **Faculty Appointment:** Assoc Prof Medical Oncology, Vanderbilt Univ

Ruckdeschel, John C MD (Medical Oncology) - *Special Expertise:* Lung Cancer; **Admitting Hospital:** H Lee Moffitt Cancer Center & Research Institute; **Office Address:** H Lee Moffitt Cancer Ctr 12908 Magnolia Dr Tampa, FL 33612-9497; **Office Phone:** (813) 979-7265; **Board Certifications:** Internal Medicine 1976, Medical Oncology 1977; **Medical School:** Albany Med Coll 1971; **Residency:** Internal Medicine, Beth Israel Hosp, Boston, MA 1975-1976; **Fellowship:** Medical Oncology, Natl Cancer Inst, Baltimore, MD 1972-1975; **Faculty Appointment:** Prof Medicine, Univ S Fla Coll Med

Shea, Thomas MD (Medical Oncology) - *Special Expertise:* Bone Marrow Transplant; **Admitting Hospital:** University of North Carolina Hospitals; **Office Address:** Univ North Carolina-Chapel Hill, Dept Medicine 3009 Old Clinic Bldg Chapel Hill, NC 27599; **Office Phone:** (919) 966-7746; **Board Certifications:** Clinical Genetics 1985, Hematology 1989; **Medical School:** Univ NC Sch Med 1980; **Residencies:** Internal Medicine, Univ North Carolina-Chapel Hill, Chapel Hill, NC 1980; Internal Medicine, Beth Israel Deaconess Med Ctr, Boston, MA 1981-1982; **Fellowships:** Hematology and Oncology, Beth Israel Deaconess Med Ctr, Boston, MA 1982-1985; Bone Marrow Transplant, Dana Farber Cancer Inst, Boston, MA 1985-1988; **Faculty Appointment:** Prof Medicine, Univ NC Sch Med

Smith, Thomas Joseph MD (Medical Oncology) - *Special Expertise:* Breast Cancer; Palliative Care; **Admitting Hospital:** Medical College of Virginia Hospitals; **Office Address:** Med Coll VA-Massey Cancer Ctr 401 College St, Box 980037 Richmond, VA 23298-0037; **Office Phone:** (804) 828-0450; **Board Certifications:** Medical Oncology 1987, Hematology 1990; **Medical School:** Yale Univ 1979; **Residencies:** Internal Medicine, Hosp Univ Penn, Philadelphia, PA 1980-1982; Medical Oncology, Med Coll VA, Richmond, VA 1984-1987; **Faculty Appointment:** Prof Medicine, Med Coll VA

Socinski, Mark A MD (Medical Oncology) - *Special Expertise:* Lung Cancer; **Admitting Hospital:** University of North Carolina Hospitals; **Office Address:** Univ North Carolina, Dept Hem Onc 3009 Old Clinic Bldg, CB 7305 Chapel Hill, NC 27599-7305; **Office Phone:** (919) 966-4431; **Board Certifications:** Internal Medicine 1988, Medical Oncology 1991; **Medical School:** Univ VT Coll Med 1984; **Residency:** Internal Medicine, Beth Israel Hosp, Boston, MA 1984-1986; **Fellowship:** Medical Oncology, Dana-Farber Cancer Inst, Boston, MA 1986-1989; **Faculty Appointment:** Asst Prof Medicine, Univ NC Sch Med

Stone, Joel MD (Medical Oncology) - *Special Expertise:* Lung Cancer; Breast Cancer; **Admitting Hospital:** St Vincent's Medical Center - Jacksonville; **Office Address:** 1801 Barrs St, Bldg 800 Jacksonville, FL 32204-4751; **Office Phone:** (904) 388-2619; **Board Certifications:** Internal Medicine 1977, Medical Oncology 1979; **Medical School:** Univ VA Sch Med 1974; **Residency:** Internal Medicine, Univ KY Med Ctr, Lexington, KY 1975-1977; **Fellowship:** Hematology, Emory Univ, Atlanta, GA 1977-1979

Torti, Frank M MD (Medical Oncology) - *Special Expertise:* Prostate Cancer; Urologic Cancer; **Admitting Hospital:** Wake Forest University Baptist Medical Center; **Office Address:** Wake Forest Univ Baptist Med Ctr-Comprehensive Cancer Ctr Medical Center Blvd Winston-Salem, NC 27157; **Office Phone:** (336) 716-7971; **Board Certifications:** Internal Medicine 1978, Medical Oncology 1979; **Medical School:** Harvard Med Sch 1974; **Residency:** Internal Medicine, Beth Israel Hosp, New York, NY 1975-1976; **Fellowship:** Medical Oncology, Stanford Univ Med Ctr, Stanford, CA 1977-1979; **Faculty Appointment:** Prof Medicine, Wake Forest Univ Sch Med

Troner, Michael MD (Medical Oncology) - *Special Expertise:* Medical Oncology - General; **Admitting Hospital:** Baptist Hospital - Miami; **Office Address:** 8950 N Kendall Dr, Ste 503 Miami, FL 33176-2132; **Office Phone:** (305) 271-6467; **Board Certifications:** Internal Medicine 1972, Medical Oncology 1973; **Medical School:** SUNY Downstate 1968; **Residency:** Internal Medicine, Univ Maryland Hosp, Baltimore, MD 1969-1971; **Fellowship:** Medical Oncology, Univ Miami Med Ctr, Miami, FL 1971-1973; **Faculty Appointment:** Assoc Clin Prof Medical Oncology, Univ Miami Sch Med

Williams, Michael MD (Medical Oncology) - *Special Expertise:* Lymphoma; Multiple Myeloma; Leukemia; **Admitting Hospital:** University of Virginia Health Systems; **Office Address:** Univ Virginia Hlth Sys, Dept Hematology, Rm 4275D, Box 800716 Charlottesville, VA 22908; **Office Phone:** (804) 924-9637; **Board Certifications:** Medical Oncology 1987, Hematology 1988; **Medical School:** Univ Cincinnati 1979; **Residency:** Internal Medicine, Univ Virginia Med Ctr, Charlottesville, VA 1980-1983; **Fellowship:** Medical Oncology, Univ Virginia Med Ctr, Charlottesville, VA 1983-1986; **Faculty Appointment:** Prof Medicine, Univ VA Sch Med

Wingard, John R MD (Medical Oncology) - *Special Expertise: Bone Marrow Transplant; Leukemia; Myeloma;* **Admitting Hospital:** Shands Healthcare at University Florida (Page 77); **Office Address:** 1600 SW Archer Rd rm 116, Box 27, MS 100277 Gainesville, FL 32610; **Office Phone:** (352) 846-2814; **Board Certifications:** Internal Medicine 1977, Medical Oncology 1981; **Medical School:** Johns Hopkins Univ 1973; **Residencies:** Internal Medicine, Memphis City Hosps, Memphis, TN 1974-1976; Internal Medicine, VA Hosp, Memphis, TN 1976-1977; **Fellowship:** Medical Oncology, Johns Hopkins Hosp, Baltimore, MD 1977-1979; **Faculty Appointment:** Prof Medicine, Univ Fla Coll Med

Midwest

Albain, Kathy MD (Medical Oncology) - *Special Expertise: Breast Cancer; Lung Cancer;* **Admitting Hospital:** Loyola University Health System; **Office Address:** Loyola Univ Med Ctr 2160 S First Ave, Ste 109 Maywood, IL 60153-3304; **Office Phone:** (708) 327-3102; **Board Certifications:** Internal Medicine 1981, Medical Oncology 1983; **Medical School:** Univ Mich Med Sch 1978; **Residency:** Internal Medicine, Univ Ill Med Ctr, Chicago, IL 1979-1981; **Fellowship:** Hematology and Oncology, Univ Chicago Med Ctr, Chicago, IL 1981-1984; **Faculty Appointment:** Prof Medicine, Loyola Univ-Stritch Sch Med

Anderson, Joseph MD (Medical Oncology) - *Special Expertise: Breast Cancer; Palliative Care;* **Admitting Hospital:** Henry Ford Health System (Page 62); **Office Address:** 2799 W Grand Blvd Detroit, MI 48202; **Office Phone:** (313) 916-1854; **Board Certifications:** Internal Medicine 1985, Medical Oncology 1989; **Medical School:** Univ Mich Med Sch 1982; **Residency:** Internal Medicine, Henry Ford Hosp, Detroit, MI 1982-1986; **Fellowship:** Medical Oncology, Henry Ford Hosp, Detroit, MI 1986-1988

Baker, Laurence H DO (Medical Oncology) - *Special Expertise: Sarcoma - Soft Tissue & Bone; Breast Cancer;* **Admitting Hospital:** University of Michigan Health Center; **Office Address:** Univ of Michigan Hosp, Comp Cancer Ctr 1500 E Med Ctr Drive, rm B1-371 CCGC, Recption C Ann Arbor, MI 48109-0912; **Office Phone:** (734) 647-8902; **Medical School:** Univ Hlth Sci, Coll Osteo Med 1966; **Residency:** Internal Medicine, Genesys Reg M C-W Flint Campus, Flint, MI 1966-1967; **Fellowship:** Medical Oncology, Wayne State Univ Affil Hosp, Detroit, MI 1970-1972; **Faculty Appointment:** Prof Medicine, Univ Mich Med Sch

Benson, Al B MD (Medical Oncology) - *Special Expertise: Colon Cancer; Rectal Cancer;* **Admitting Hospital:** Northwestern Memorial Hospital; **Office Address:** 676 N St Clair, Ste 850 Chicago, IL 60611; **Office Phone:** (312) 695-6180; **Board Certifications:** Internal Medicine 1979, Medical Oncology 1983; **Medical School:** SUNY Buffalo 1976; **Residency:** Internal Medicine, U Wisc Hosps, Madison, WI 1977-1979; **Fellowship:** Medical Oncology, U Wisc Hosps, Madison, WI 1981-1984; **Faculty Appointment:** Prof Medicine, Northwestern Univ

Bonomi, Philip MD (Medical Oncology) - *Special Expertise: Mesothelioma; Thymoma; Lung Cancer;* **Admitting Hospital:** Rush/Presbyterian - St Luke's Medical Center - Chicago (Page 74); **Office Address:** Rush Cancer Inst 1725 W Harrison St, Ste 809 Chicago, IL 60612; **Office Phone:** (312) 942-3312; **Board Certifications:** Internal Medicine 1975, Medical Oncology 1977; **Medical School:** Univ IL Coll Med 1970; **Residencies:** Internal Medicine, Geisinger, Danville, PA 1971-1972; Internal Medicine, Geisinger, Danville, PA 1974-1975; **Fellowship:** Medical Oncology, Rush Presby-St Luke's Med Ctr, Chicago, IL 1975-1977; **Faculty Appointment:** Prof Medicine, Rush Med Coll

Carbone, Paul MD (Medical Oncology) - *Special Expertise: Medical Oncology - General;* **Admitting Hospital:** University of Wisconsin Hospital & Clinics; **Office Address:** UW Comp Cancer Ctr 600 Highland Ave Madison, WI 53711; **Office Phone:** (608) 263-8090; **Board Certifications:** Internal Medicine 1963, Medical Oncology 1979; **Medical School:** Albany Med Coll 1956; **Residencies:** Internal Medicine, USPHS Hosp, San Francisco, CA 1958-1960; Medical Oncology, Natl Inst Hlth, Bethesda, MD 1961-1963; **Faculty Appointment:** Prof Medicine, Univ Wisc

Di Persio, John MD/PhD (Medical Oncology) - *Special Expertise: Bone Marrow Transplant; Hematology;* **Admitting Hospital:** Barnes - Jewish Hospital; **Office Address:** Washington Univ 660 S Euclid Ave, Box 8007 St Louis, MO 63110; **Office Phone:** (314) 454-8313; **Board Certifications:** Medical Oncology 1987, Hematology 1988; **Medical School:** Univ Rochester 1980; **Residency:** Internal Medicine, Parkland Meml Hosp, Dallas, TX 1981-1984; **Fellowship:** Hematology and Oncology, UCLA Sch Med, Los Angeles, CA 1984-1987; **Faculty Appointment:** Prof Medicine, Washington Univ, St Louis

Einhorn, Lawrence MD (Medical Oncology) - *Special Expertise: Testicular Cancer; Lung Cancer;* **Admitting Hospital:** Indiana University Hospital & Medical Center - Indianapolis; **Office Address:** 535 Barnhill Drive Indianapolis, IN 46202; **Office Phone:** (317) 274-0920; **Board Certifications:** Internal Medicine 1972, Medical Oncology 1975; **Medical School:** UCLA 1967; **Residency:** Internal Medicine, Indiana U Hosp, Indianapolis, IN 1968-1969; **Fellowship:** Medical Oncology, Indiana U Hosp, Indianapolis, IN 1971-1972

Fisher, Richard I MD (Medical Oncology) - *Special Expertise: Lymphoma; Hodgkin's Disease;* **Admitting Hospital:** Loyola University Health System; **Office Address:** 2160 S 1st Ave Maywood, IL 60153; **Office Phone:** (708) 327-1000; **Board Certifications:** Internal Medicine 1973, Medical Oncology 1977; **Medical School:** Harvard Med Sch 1970; **Residency:** Internal Medicine, Mass Genl Hosp, Boston, MA 1971-1972; **Faculty Appointment:** Prof Medical Oncology, Loyola Univ-Stritch Sch Med

Flynn, Patrick MD (Medical Oncology) - *Special Expertise: Medical Oncology - General;* **Admitting Hospital:** Fairview-University Medical Center - University Campus; **Office Address:** MN Oncl Hematology, PA 800 E 28th St, Piper Bldg, Ste 405 Minneapolis, MN 55407; **Office Phone:** (612) 863-8585; **Board Certifications:** Medical Oncology 1981, Hematology 1982; **Medical School:** Univ Minn 1975; **Residency:** Internal Medicine, Hennepin Co Med Ctr-Univ Minn, Minneapolis, MN 1976-1978; **Fellowship:** Hematology and Oncology, Univ Minn, Minneapolis, MN 1979-1981; **Faculty Appointment:** Asst Prof Medicine, Univ Minn

Gordon, Leo I MD (Medical Oncology) - *Special Expertise: Leukemia/Hematopoietic Malignancy; Hodgkin's Disease;* **Admitting Hospital:** Northwestern Memorial Hospital; **Office Address:** Northwestern Meml Hosp 676 N St Clair St, Ste 850 Chicago, IL 60611; **Office Phone:** (312) 695-4546; **Board Certifications:** Hematology 1978, Medical Oncology 1979; **Medical School:** Univ Cincinnati 1973; **Residency:** Internal Medicine, Univ Chicago Hosps, Chicago, IL 1974-1976; **Fellowships:** Hematology, Univ Minn Hosps, Minneapolis, MN 1976-1978; Hematology and Oncology, Univ Chicago Hosps, Chicago, IL 1978-1979; **Faculty Appointment:** Prof Medicine, Northwestern Univ

Ingle, James N MD (Medical Oncology) - *Special Expertise: Breast Cancer;* **Admitting Hospital:** Mayo Medical Center & Clinic - Rochester; **Office Address:** Mayo Clinic 200 First St SW, 12 Floor East Rochester, MN 55905; **Office Phone:** (507) 284-8432; **Board Certifications:** Infectious Disease 1974, Medical Oncology 1975; **Medical School:** Johns Hopkins Univ 1971; **Residencies:** Natl Cancer Inst, Bethesda, MD 1973-1975; John Hopkins Hosp, Baltimore, MD 1972-1976

Kosova, Leonard MD (Medical Oncology) - *Special Expertise:* Breast Cancer; Lymphoma; **Admitting Hospital:** Advocate Lutheran General Hospital; **Office Address:** 8915 W Golf Rd, Ste 3 Niles, IL 60714; **Office Phone:** (847) 827-9060; **Board Certifications:** Hematology 1972, Medical Oncology 1975; **Medical School:** Univ IL Coll Med 1961; **Residency:** Internal Medicine, Hines VA Hosp, Hines, IL 1962-1964; **Fellowship:** Hematology, Hektoen Inst-Cook Cty Hosp, Chicago, IL 1964-1965

Lippman, Marc E MD (Medical Oncology) - *Special Expertise:* Breast Cancer; **Admitting Hospital:** University of Michigan Health Center; **Office Address:** Univ Mich Med Ctr, Dept Internal Med 1500 E Medical Dr Ann Arbor, MI 48109-0368; **Office Phone:** (734) 647-8900; **Board Certifications:** Endocrinology, Diabetes & Metabolism 1975, Medical Oncology 1977; **Medical School:** Yale Univ 1968; **Residency:** Internal Medicine, Johns Hopkins Hosp, Baltimore, MD 1969-1970; **Fellowships:** Endocrinology, Diabetes & Metabolism, Yale, New Haven, CT 1973-1974; Medical Oncology, Natl Cancer Inst, Bethesda, MD 1970-1973; **Faculty Appointment:** Prof Medicine, Univ MD Sch Med

Markman, Maurie MD (Medical Oncology) - *Special Expertise:* Ovarian Cancer; **Admitting Hospital:** Cleveland Clinic Foundation; **Office Address:** Cleveland Clinic Foundation- Dept Hem/Onc 9500 Euclid Ave, MC-Desk R35 Cleveland, OH 44195; **Office Phone:** (216) 445-6888; **Board Certifications:** Medical Oncology 1981, Hematology 1982; **Medical School:** NYU Sch Med 1974; **Residency:** Internal Medicine, Bellevue Hosp Ctr, New York, NY 1975-1978; **Fellowship:** Medical Oncology, Johns Hopkins Hosp, Baltimore, MD 1980; **Faculty Appointment:** Prof Medicine, Ohio State Univ

Masters, Gregory MD (Medical Oncology) - *Special Expertise:* Lung Cancer; Esophageal Cancer; Thoracic Cancers; **Admitting Hospital:** Evanston Hospital; **Office Address:** Evanston Hosp 2650 Ridge Ave Evanston, IL 60201; **Office Phone:** (847) 570-2110; **Board Certifications:** Internal Medicine 1993, Medical Oncology 1996; **Medical School:** Northwestern Univ 1990; **Residency:** Internal Medicine, Hosp Univ PA, Philadelphia, PA 1991-1993; **Fellowship:** Medical Oncology, Univ Chicago, Chicago, IL 1993; **Faculty Appointment:** Asst Prof Medicine, Northwestern Univ

Mortimer, Joanne MD (Medical Oncology) - *Special Expertise:* Breast & Esophageal Cancer; **Admitting Hospital:** Barnes - Jewish Hospital; **Office Address:** 660 S Euclid, Box 8056 St Louis, MO 63110-1002; **Office Phone:** (314) 362-7502; **Board Certifications:** Internal Medicine 1980, Medical Oncology 1983; **Medical School:** Loyola Univ-Stritch Sch Med 1977; **Residency:** Internal Medicine, Cleveland Clin, Cleveland, OH 1978-1980; **Fellowship:** Medical Oncology, Cleveland Clin, Cleveland, OH 1980-1982; **Faculty Appointment:** Asst Prof Medical Oncology, Univ Wash

Olopade, Olufunmilayo I F MD (Medical Oncology) - *Special Expertise:* Breast Cancer; Lymphoma; **Admitting Hospital:** University of Chicago Hospitals (Page 78); **Office Address:** 5841 S Maryland Ave, MS 2115 Chicago, IL 60637; **Office Phone:** (773) 702-6149; **Board Certifications:** Medical Oncology 1989, Hematology 1990; **Medical School:** Nigeria 1980; **Residency:** Cook Co Hosp, Chicago, IL 1984-1986; **Fellowship:** Univ Chicago Med Ctr, Chicago, IL 1987-1991; **Faculty Appointment:** Asst Prof Medicine, Univ Chicago-Pritzker Sch Med

Perry, Michael MD (Medical Oncology) - *Special Expertise:* Lung Cancer; **Admitting Hospital:** University of Missouri Hospitals & Clinics; **Office Address:** Ellis Fischel Cancer Ctr. 115 Business Loop 70 W, rm 524 Columbia, MO 65203; **Office Phone:** (573) 882-4979; **Board Certifications:** Medical Oncology 1975, Hematology 1974; **Medical School:** Wayne State Univ 1970; **Residency:** Internal Medicine, Mayo Grad Sch., Rochester, MN 1971-1972; **Fellowship:** Medical Oncology, Mayo Grad. Sch., Rochester, MN 1972-1975; **Faculty Appointment:** Prof Medical Oncology, Univ Hlth Sci Coll -Osteo Med

Peters, William P MD/PhD (Medical Oncology) - *Special Expertise:* Breast Cancer; **Admitting Hospital:** Barbara Ann Karmanos Cancer Institute; **Office Address:** Barbara Ann Karmanos Cancer Inst 4100 John R St, Fl 2 Detroit, MI 48201; **Office Phone:** (313) 745-2754; **Board Certifications:** Internal Medicine 1981, Medical Oncology 1983; **Medical School:** Columbia P&S 1978; **Residency:** Internal Medicine, Brigham & Women's Hosp, Boston, MA 1978-1981; **Fellowship:** Medical Oncology, Dana-Farber Cancer Inst, Boston, MA 1981-1983

Piel, Ira MD (Medical Oncology) - *Special Expertise:* Medical Oncology - General; **Admitting Hospital:** Illinois Masonic Medical Center (Page 64); **Office Address:** 901 W Wellington Ave Medical Oncology & Hematology Chicago, IL 60657-4421; **Office Phone:** (773) 296-7089; **Board Certifications:** Medical Oncology 1975, Internal Medicine 1973; **Medical School:** Univ IL Coll Med 1967; **Residency:** Internal Medicine, St Lukes H, Chicago, IL 1970-1972; **Fellowship:** Medical Oncology, St Lukes H, Chicago, IL 1972-1974; **Faculty Appointment:** Rush Med Coll

Ratain, Mark J MD (Medical Oncology) - *Special Expertise:* Solid Tumors; **Admitting Hospital:** University of Chicago Hospitals (Page 78); **Office Address:** Center for Advanced Medicine 5758 S Maryland Ave, rm 6D Chicago, IL 60637; **Office Phone:** (773) 702-6149; **Board Certifications:** Hematology 1986, Medical Oncology 1985; **Medical School:** Yale Univ 1980; **Residency:** Internal Medicine, Johns Hopkins Hosp, Baltimore, MD 1981-1983; **Fellowship:** Hematology and Oncology, Univ Chicago, Chicago, IL 1983-1986; **Faculty Appointment:** Prof Medicine, Univ Chicago-Pritzker Sch Med

Richards, Jon MD/PhD (Medical Oncology) - *Special Expertise:* Testicular Cancer; Prostate Cancer; Melanoma; **Admitting Hospital:** Advocate Lutheran General Hospital; **Office Address:** Lutheran Genl Hosp-Cancer Care Ctr 1700 Luther Ln Park Ridge, IL 60068-1174; **Office Phone:** (847) 723-2500; **Board Certification:** Internal Medicine 1998; **Medical School:** Cornell Univ-Weil Med Coll 1983; **Residency:** Internal Medicine, Univ Chicago Hosps, Chicago, IL 1984-1985; **Fellowship:** Hematology, Univ Chicago, Chicago, IL 1985-1988; **Faculty Appointment:** Asst Prof Medicine, Univ IL Coll Med

Rosen, Steven T MD (Medical Oncology) - *Special Expertise:* Multiple Myeloma; Breast Cancer; **Admitting Hospital:** Northwestern Memorial Hospital; **Office Address:** Northwestern Univ 303 E Chicago Ave, Bldg Olsen Pavilion - Ste 8250 Chicago, IL 60611-3013; **Office Phone:** (312) 695-8697; **Board Certifications:** Medical Oncology 1981, Hematology 1984; **Medical School:** Northwestern Univ 1976; **Residency:** Internal Medicine, Northwestern Univ, Chicago, IL 1977-1979; **Fellowship:** Medical Oncology, Natl Cancer Ctr, Bethesda, MD 1979-1981; **Faculty Appointment:** Prof Medicine, Northwestern Univ

Samuels, Brian Louis MD (Medical Oncology) - *Special Expertise:* Medical Oncology - General; **Admitting Hospital:** Advocate Lutheran General Hospital; **Office Address:** Lutheran Genl Cancer Care Ctr 1700 Luther Ln Park Ridge, IL 60068; **Office Phone:** (847) 723-2500; **Board Certifications:** Internal Medicine 1984, Medical Oncology 1987; **Medical School:** Zimbabwe 1976; **Residencies:** Internal Medicine, Albert Einstein, Philadelphia, PA 1979-1981; Internal Medicine, Albert Einstein Med Ctr, Philadelphia, PA 1983-1984; **Fellowship:** Hematology and Oncology, Univ Chicago, Chicago, IL 1984-1988; **Faculty Appointment:** Assoc Prof Medicine, Univ IL Coll Med

Schiffer, Charles Alan MD (Medical Oncology) - *Special Expertise:* Leukemia; Lymphoma; **Admitting Hospital:** Harper Hospital - Detroit; **Office Address:** Harper Hosp, Dept Hematology/Oncology 3990 John R, 5 Hudson Detroit, MI 48201; **Office Phone:** (313) 745-8910; **Board Certifications:** Medical Oncology 1973, Internal Medicine 1972; **Medical School:** NYU Sch Med 1968; **Residency:** Internal Medicine, NYU, Bellevue-New York VA Hosp., New York, NY 1968-1972; **Faculty Appointment:** Prof Medical Oncology, Wayne State Univ

Schiller, Joan H (Medical Oncology) - *Special Expertise: Oncology; Lung Cancer;* **Admitting Hospital:** University of Wisconsin Hospital & Clinics; **Office Address:** 600 Highland Ave Madison, WI 53792; **Office Phone:** (608) 263-8090; **Board Certifications:** Internal Medicine 1983, Medical Oncology 1987; **Medical School:** Univ IL Coll Med 1980; **Residency:** Internal Medicine, Northwestern Meml Hosp, Chicago, IL 1981-1983; **Fellowship:** Medical Oncology, U Wisc Hosp, Madison, WI 1984-1986; **Faculty Appointment:** Prof Medicine, Univ Wisc

Schwartz, Burton MD (Medical Oncology) - *Special Expertise: Lymphoma; Breast Cancer;* **Admitting Hospital:** Abbott - Northwestern Hospital; **Office Address:** Abott - Northwestern Hosp 800 E 28th St Minn, MN 55417; **Office Phone:** (612) 863-8585; **Board Certifications:** Internal Medicine 1972, Medical Oncology 1977; **Medical School:** Meharry Med Coll 1968; **Residency:** Internal Medicine, Michael Reese Hospital, Chicago, IL 1969-1971; **Fellowship:** Hematology, U Minn Hosp, Minnesota, MN 1974-1976; **Faculty Appointment:** Clin Prof Hematology, Univ Minn

Shapiro, Charles L MD (Medical Oncology) - *Special Expertise: Breast Cancer;* **Admitting Hospital:** Arthur G. James Cancer Hospital & Research Institute; **Office Address:** Arthur G James Cancer Hosp, Dept Med Onc 300 W 10th Ave Columbus, OH 43210-1240; **Office Phone:** (614) 293-7530; **Board Certifications:** Internal Medicine 1987, Medical Oncology 1991; **Medical School:** SUNY Buffalo 1984; **Residency:** Internal Medicine, Temple Univ, Philadelphia, PA 1984-1987

Sledge Jr, George W MD (Medical Oncology) - *Special Expertise: Breast Cancer;* **Admitting Hospital:** Indiana University Hospital & Medical Center - Indianapolis; **Office Address:** Indiana Cancer Pavilion 535 Barnhill Indianapolis, IN 46202; **Office Phone:** (317) 274-0920; **Board Certifications:** Internal Medicine 1980, Medical Oncology 1983; **Medical School:** Tulane Univ 1977; **Residency:** Internal Medicine, St Louis Univ, St Louis, MO 1977-1980; **Fellowship:** Medical Oncology, Univ Texas, San Antonio, TX 1980-1983; **Faculty Appointment:** Prof Medicine, Indiana Univ

Todd III, Robert F MD/PhD (Medical Oncology) - *Special Expertise: Gastrointestinal Cancer; Lung Cancer;* **Admitting Hospital:** University of Michigan Health Center; **Office Address:** Univ Michigan Cancer Ctr B1371 1500 E Med Ctr Dr, Box 0913 Ann Arbor, MI 48109-0948; **Office Phone:** (734) 647-8903; **Board Certifications:** Internal Medicine 1979, Medical Oncology 1981; **Medical School:** Duke Univ 1976; **Residency:** Internal Medicine, Peter Bent Brigham Hosp, Boston, MA 1977-1978; **Fellowship:** Medical Oncology, Dana Farber Cancer Inst, Boston, MA 1978-1981; **Faculty Appointment:** Prof Medicine, Univ Mich Med Sch

Vogelzang, Nicholas MD (Medical Oncology) - *Special Expertise: Prostate Cancer; Mesothelioma; Gastrointestinal Cancer;* **Admitting Hospital:** University of Chicago Hospitals (Page 78); **Office Address:** Cancer Research Ctr 5841 S Maryland Ave, MS 1140 Chicago, IL 60637; **Office Phone:** (773) 702-6149; **Board Certifications:** Internal Medicine 1978, Medical Oncology 1981; **Medical School:** Univ IL Coll Med 1974; **Residency:** Internal Medicine, Rush-Presby St Lukes, Chicago, IL 1974-1978; **Fellowship:** Medical Oncology, Univ Minn, Minneapolis, MN 1978-1981; **Faculty Appointment:** Prof Medicine, Univ Chicago-Pritzker Sch Med

Vokes, Everett Emmett MD (Medical Oncology) - *Special Expertise: Lung Cancer; Head & Neck Cancer;* **Admitting Hospital:** University of Chicago Hospitals (Page 78); **Office Address:** Univ Chicago Med Ctr 5841 S Maryland Ave, MS 2115 Chicago, IL 60637-1470; **Office Phone:** (773) 834-3093; **Board Certifications:** Internal Medicine 1983, Medical Oncology 1985; **Medical School:** Germany 1980; **Residencies:** Internal Medicine, Ravenswood Hosp-U IL, Chicago, IL 1981-1982; Internal Medicine, USC Med Ctr, Los Angeles, CA 1982-1983; **Fellowship:** Medical Oncology, Univ Chicago, Chicago, IL 1983-1986; **Faculty Appointment:** Prof Medicine, Univ Chicago-Pritzker Sch Med

Wicha, Max S MD (Medical Oncology) - *Special Expertise:* Breast Cancer; **Admitting Hospital:** University of Michigan Health Center; **Office Address:** Univ Mich Comprehensive Cancer & Geriatric Ctr 1500 E Med Ctr Dr, rm 6302, Box 0942 Ann Arbor, MI 48109; **Office Phone:** (734) 647-8902; **Board Certifications:** Internal Medicine 1977, Medical Oncology 1983; **Medical School:** Stanford Univ 1974; **Residency:** Internal Medicine, Univ Chicago Hosp, Chicago, IL 1976-1977; **Fellowship:** Medical Oncology, Natl Inst Hlth, Bethesda, MD 1977-1980; **Faculty Appointment:** Prof Medicine, Univ Mich Med Sch

Great Plains and Mountains

Armitage, James MD (Medical Oncology) - *Special Expertise:* Lymphoma; Bone Marrow Transplant; **Admitting Hospital:** University of Nebraska Medical Center; **Office Address:** NHS-Univ Nebraska Med Ctr Emile at 42nd St Omaha, NE 68198; **Office Phone:** (402) 559-7290; **Board Certifications:** Internal Medicine 1976, Medical Oncology 1977; **Medical School:** Univ Nebr Coll Med 1973; **Residency:** Internal Medicine, Univ Nebr Med Ctr, Omaha, NE 1974-1975; **Fellowship:** Hematology and Oncology, Univ Iowa Hosp, Iowa City, IA 1975-1977; **Faculty Appointment:** Prof Medicine, Univ Nebr Coll Med

Bunn Jr, Paul MD (Medical Oncology) - *Special Expertise:* Lung Cancer; Lymphoma; **Admitting Hospital:** University of Colorado Health & Science Center; **Office Address:** Univ Colorado Cancer Ctr 4200 E Ninth Ave, Box B 188 Denver, CO 80262; **Office Phone:** (303) 315-3007; **Board Certifications:** Internal Medicine 1974, Medical Oncology 1975; **Medical School:** Cornell Univ-Weil Med Coll 1971; **Residency:** Internal Medicine, HC Moffitt/Univ California, San Francisco, CA 1972-1973; **Fellowship:** Medical Oncology, Natl Cancer Inst, Bethesda, MD 1973-1975; **Faculty Appointment:** Prof Medicine, Univ Colo

Fabian, Carol J MD (Medical Oncology) - *Special Expertise:* Breast Cancer; **Admitting Hospital:** University of Kansas Medical Center; **Office Address:** Univ Kansas Med Ctr, Div Clin Onc 3901 Rainbow Blvd Kansas City, KS 66160; **Office Phone:** (913) 588-7791; **Board Certifications:** Internal Medicine 1976, Medical Oncology 1977; **Medical School:** Univ Kans 1972; **Residency:** Internal Medicine, Wesley Med Ctr, Wichita, KS 1973-1975; **Fellowship:** Medical Oncology, Univ Kansas Med Ctr, Kansas City, KS 1975-1977; **Faculty Appointment:** Prof Medicine, Univ Kans

Ward, John Harris MD (Medical Oncology) - *Special Expertise:* Medical Oncology - General; **Admitting Hospital:** University of Utah Hospital and Clinics; **Office Address:** Huntsman Cancer Inst 2000 Circle of Hope, Ste 2100 Salt Lake City, UT 84112-5550; **Office Phone:** (801) 585-0255; **Board Certifications:** Internal Medicine 1979, Medical Oncology 1981; **Medical School:** Univ Utah 1976; **Residency:** Internal Medicine, Duke Univ, Durham, NC 1977-1979; **Fellowship:** Hematology and Oncology, Univ Utah, Salt Lake City, UT 1979-1981; **Faculty Appointment:** Prof Medicine, Univ Utah

Southwest

Abbruzzese, James L MD (Medical Oncology) - *Special Expertise:* Gastrointestinal Cancer; Pancreatic Cancer; **Admitting Hospital:** University of Texas MD Anderson Cancer Center (Page 66); **Office Address:** Univ Texas MD Anderson Cancer Ctr 1515 Holcombe Blvd Houston, TX 77030; **Office Phone:** (713) 792-2828; **Board Certifications:** Internal Medicine 1981, Medical Oncology 1983; **Medical School:** Univ Chicago-Pritzker Sch Med 1978; **Residency:** Internal Medicine, Johns Hopkins Hosp, Baltimore, MD 1979-1981; **Fellowship:** Medical Oncology, Dana-Farber Cancer Inst, Boston, MA 1981-1983; **Faculty Appointment:** Assoc Prof Medicine, Univ Tex, Houston

Benjamin, Robert S MD (Medical Oncology) - *Special Expertise:* Sarcoma - Soft Tissue; Sarcoma - Bone; **Admitting Hospital:** University of Texas MD Anderson Cancer Center (Page 66); **Office Address:** UT MD Anderson Cancer Ctr 1515 Holcombe Blvd, Box 0077 Houston, TX 77030; **Office Phone:** (713) 792-3626; **Board Certifications:** Internal Medicine 1973, Medical Oncology 1973; **Medical School:** NYU Sch Med 1968; **Residency:** Internal Medicine, Bellevue Hosp Ctr, New York, NY 1969-1970; **Fellowship:** Medical Oncology, Baltimore Cancer Rsrch Ctr, Baltimore, MD 1970-1972; **Faculty Appointment:** Prof Medicine, Univ Tex, Houston

Fossella, Frank V MD (Medical Oncology) - *Special Expertise:* Lung Cancer; **Admitting Hospital:** University of Texas MD Anderson Cancer Center (Page 66); **Office Address:** 1515 Holcomb Blvd, Box 80 Houston, TX 77030; **Office Phone:** (713) 792-6363; **Board Certifications:** Internal Medicine 1985, Medical Oncology 1987; **Medical School:** Baylor Coll Med 1982; **Residency:** Internal Medicine, Baylor Coll Med, Houston, TX 1983-1985; **Fellowship:** Medical Oncology, Baylor Coll Med, Houston, TX 1985-1987; **Faculty Appointment:** Clin Inst Medical Oncology, Univ Tex, Houston

Glisson, Bonnie S MD (Medical Oncology) - *Special Expertise:* Head & Neck Cancer; Lung Cancer; **Admitting Hospital:** University of Texas MD Anderson Cancer Center (Page 66); **Office Address:** Univ Texas - MD Anderson Cancer Ctr 1515 Holcombe Blvd, Box 80 Houston, TX 77030; **Office Phone:** (713) 792-6363; **Board Certifications:** Medical Oncology 1985, Internal Medicine 1982; **Medical School:** Ohio State Univ 1979; **Residency:** Internal Medicine, Univ Virginia, Charlottesville, VA 1979-1982; **Fellowship:** Medical Oncology, Univ Florida, Gainesville, FL 1982-1985; **Faculty Appointment:** Assoc Prof Medical Oncology

Hong, Waun Ki MD (Medical Oncology) - *Special Expertise:* Chemoprevention of Cancer; Lung Cancer; **Admitting Hospital:** University of Texas MD Anderson Cancer Center (Page 66); **Office Address:** MD Anderson Canc. Ctr/ Dept Thor-Heck-Neck Med Onc 1515 Holcombe, Box 80 Houston, TX 77030; **Office Phone:** (713) 792-6363; **Board Certifications:** Internal Medicine 1976, Medical Oncology 1979; **Medical School:** Other Foreign Country 1967; **Residency:** Internal Medicine, Boston VA Hosp., Boston, MA 1971-1973; **Fellowship:** Medical Oncology, Sloan-Kettering, New York, NY 1973-1975

Hutchins, Laura MD (Medical Oncology) - *Special Expertise:* Breast Cancer; Melanoma; **Admitting Hospital:** University of Arkansas for Medical Sciences; **Office Address:** Univ Hosp Arkansas 4301 W Markham St, Slot 508 Little Rock, AR 72205-7101; **Office Phone:** (501) 686-5222; **Board Certifications:** Hematology 1984, Medical Oncology 1987; **Medical School:** Univ Ark 1977; **Residency:** Internal Medicine, Univ Ark Med Scis, Little Rock, AR 1977-1980; **Fellowship:** Medical Oncology, Univ Ark Med Scis, Little Rock, AR 1980-1983; **Faculty Appointment:** Prof Medicine, Univ Ark

Jones, Stephen E MD (Medical Oncology) - *Special Expertise:* Breast Cancer; **Admitting Hospital:** Baylor University Medical Center; **Office Address:** Texas Oncology PA 3535 Worth St, Ste 600 Dallas, TX 75246; **Office Phone:** (214) 370-1000; **Board Certifications:** Internal Medicine 1972, Medical Oncology 1973; **Medical School:** Case West Res Univ 1966; **Residency:** Internal Medicine, Stanford Univ, Stanford, CA 1967-1968; **Fellowship:** Medical Oncology, Stanford Univ, Stanford, CA 1970-1972; **Faculty Appointment:** Prof Medical Oncology, Baylor Coll Med

Lee, Jin Soo MD (Medical Oncology) - *Special Expertise:* Lung Cancer; **Admitting Hospital:** University of Texas MD Anderson Cancer Center (Page 66); **Office Address:** Univ. Tex-MD Anderson Cancer Ctr. 1515 Holcombe Blvd. Box #80 Houston, TX 77030; **Office Phone:** (713) 792-6363; **Board Certifications:** Internal Medicine 1982, Medical Oncology 1985; **Medical School:** South Korea 1974; **Residency:** Internal Medicine, St Joseph Hosp., Chicago, IL 1980-1982; **Fellowship:** Medical Oncology, U Tex MD Anderson Hosp., Houston, TX 1982-1984; **Faculty Appointment:** Prof Medical Oncology, Univ Tex, Houston

MEDICAL ONCOLOGY

Legha, Sewa Singh MD (Medical Oncology) - *Special Expertise:* Melanoma; Breast CAncer; Tumors - Rare; **Admitting Hospital:** St Luke's Episcopal Hospital - Houston (Page 76); **Office Address:** 6624 Fannin, Box 1440 Houston, TX 77030; **Office Phone:** (713) 797-9711; **Board Certifications:** Internal Medicine 1987, Medical Oncology 1977; **Medical School:** India 1970; **Residencies:** Internal Medicine, Milwaukee Co Genl Hosp, Milwaukee, WI 1972-1974; Medical Oncology, Natl Cancer Inst, Bethesda, MD 1974-1976; **Fellowship:** Medical Oncology, MD Anderson Hosp, Houston, TX 1976-1977; **Faculty Appointment:** Prof Medical Oncology, Univ Tex, Houston

Osborne, Charles Kent MD (Medical Oncology) - *Special Expertise:* Breast Cancer; **Admitting Hospital:** University of Texas Health & Science Center; **Office Address:** 1 Baylor Plaza, rm N-500, MC-BCM-600 Baylor College of Medicine Houston, TX 77030; **Office Phone:** (713) 798-1600; **Board Certifications:** Medical Oncology 1977, Internal Medicine 1975; **Medical School:** Univ MO-Columbia Sch Med 1972; **Residency:** Internal Medicine, Johns Hopkins Hosp., Baltimore, MD 1973-1974; **Fellowship:** Medical Oncology, Natl Cancer Inst., Bethesda, MD 1974-1977; **Faculty Appointment:** Prof Medicine, Baylor Coll Med

Pisters, Katherine M W MD (Medical Oncology) - *Special Expertise:* Lung Cancer; **Admitting Hospital:** University of Texas MD Anderson Cancer Center (Page 66); **Office Address:** 1515 Holcombe Blvd Box #80 Houston, TX 77030; **Office Phone:** (713) 792-6363; **Board Certifications:** Internal Medicine 1988, Medical Oncology 1991; **Medical School:** Canada 1985; **Residency:** Internal Medicine, North Shore U Hosp, Manhasset, NY 1986-1988; **Fellowship:** Medical Oncology, Meml Sloan Kettering, New York, NY 1988-1991

Salem, Philip Adeeb MD (Medical Oncology) - *Special Expertise:* Breast Cancer; Lymphoma; **Admitting Hospital:** St Luke's Episcopal Hospital - Houston (Page 76); **Office Address:** 6624 Fannin St, Ste 1630 Houston, TX 77030; **Office Phone:** (713) 796-1221; **Medical School:** Lebanon 1965; **Residency:** Medical Oncology, Meml Sloan Kettering Cancer Ctr, New York, NY 1968-1970; **Fellowship:** Oncology Research, MD Anderson Cancer Ctr, Houston, TX 1971-1972; **Faculty Appointment:** Clin Prof Medicine, Univ Tex, Houston

Valero, Vicente MD (Medical Oncology) - *Special Expertise:* Breast Cancer; **Admitting Hospital:** University of Texas MD Anderson Cancer Center (Page 66); **Office Address:** Univ Texas MD Anderson Cancer Ctr 1515 Holcombe Blvd, Box 56 Houston, TX 77030; **Office Phone:** (713) 792-2817; **Board Certifications:** Medical Oncology 1987, Hematology 1988; **Medical School:** Mexico 1980; **Residencies:** Internal Medicine, Univ Cinn Coll Med, Cincinnati, OH 1982-1985; Hematology and Oncology, Univ Cinn Coll Med, Cincinnati, OH 1985-1987; **Fellowship:** Hematology and Oncology, Univ Texas Med Br, Galveston, TX 1987-1988

West Coast and Pacific

Abrams, Donald Ira MD (Medical Oncology) - *Special Expertise:* AIDS/HIV; **Admitting Hospital:** San Francisco General Hospital; **Office Address:** Positive Hlth Program Bldg 80, Ward 84 995 Potrero Ave San Francisco, CA 94110; **Office Phone:** (415) 476-4082; **Board Certifications:** Internal Medicine 1980, Medical Oncology 1983; **Medical School:** Stanford Univ 1977; **Residency:** Internal Medicine, Kaiser Fdn Hosp, San Francisco, CA 1978-1980; **Fellowship:** Medical Oncology, UCSF Cancer Rsch, San Francisco, CA 1980-1982; **Faculty Appointment:** Prof Medical Oncology, UCSF

Ball, Edward David MD (Medical Oncology) - *Special Expertise: Bone Marrow & Stem Cell Transplant; Leukemia/Lymphoma;* **Admitting Hospital:** University of California - San Diego Healthcare; **Office Address:** 9500 Gilman Dr, Box 0960 La Jolla, CA 92093-0960; **Office Phone:** (858) 657-7053; **Board Certifications:** Internal Medicine 1979, Medical Oncology 1983; **Medical School:** Case West Res Univ 1976; **Residency:** Internal Medicine, Hartford Hosp, Hartford, CT 1977-1979; **Fellowships:** Hematology, Univ Hosps, Cleveland, OH 1979-1981; Hematology and Oncology, Dartmouth-Hitchcock, Hanover, NH 1981-1982; **Faculty Appointment:** Prof Medicine, UCSD

Carlson, Robert Wells MD (Medical Oncology) - *Special Expertise: Breast Cancer;* **Admitting Hospital:** Stanford Medical Center; **Office Address:** Stanford Med Ctr, Onc Day Care Ctr 300 Pasteur Dr, MC-H0274 Stanford, CA 94305; **Office Phone:** (650) 723-7621; **Board Certifications:** Internal Medicine 1981, Medical Oncology 1983; **Medical School:** Stanford Univ 1978; **Residencies:** Internal Medicine, Barnes Hosp Group, St Louis, MO 1978-1980; Internal Medicine, Stanford Univ Hosp, Stanford, CA 1980-1981; **Fellowship:** Medical Oncology, Stanford Univ Med Ctr, Stanford, CA 1981-1983; **Faculty Appointment:** Prof Medicine, Stanford Univ

Chlebowski, Rowan Thomas MD/PhD (Medical Oncology) - *Special Expertise: Breast Cancer; Women's Health;* **Admitting Hospital:** LAC - Harbor - UCLA Medical Center; **Office Address:** Harbor UCLA Med Ctr 1000 W Carson St, Bldg J3 Torrance, CA 90509; **Office Phone:** (310) 222-2218; **Board Certifications:** Internal Medicine 1980, Medical Oncology 1981; **Medical School:** Case West Res Univ 1974; **Residencies:** Internal Medicine, MetroHealth Med Ctr, Cleveland, OH 1974-1976; Medical Oncology, LAC-USC Med Ctr, Los Angeles, CA 1978-1979; **Faculty Appointment:** Prof Medical Oncology, UCLA

Gandara, David R MD (Medical Oncology) - *Special Expertise: Lung Cancer;* **Admitting Hospital:** University of California - Davis Medical Center; **Office Address:** UC Davis Cancer Ctr 4510 X St, Ste 3016 Sacramento, CA 95817; **Office Phone:** (9167) 343-7719; **Board Certifications:** Internal Medicine 1976, Medical Oncology 1979; **Medical School:** Univ Tex Med Br, Galveston 1973; **Residency:** Internal Medicine, Madigan Med Ctr, Tacoma, WA 1974-1976; **Fellowship:** Medical Oncology, Letterman AMC, San Francisco, CA 1976-1978; **Faculty Appointment:** Asst Prof Medicine, UC Davis

Ganz, Patricia Anne MD (Medical Oncology) - *Special Expertise: Breast Cancer; Cancer Prevention;* **Admitting Hospital:** UCLA Medical Center; **Office Address:** UCLA, Div Cancer Prev & Control Rsch 950 Charles Young Dr S, PO Box 956900 Los Angeles, CA 90095-6900; **Office Phone:** (310) 206-1404; **Board Certifications:** Internal Medicine 1976, Medical Oncology 1979; **Medical School:** UCLA 1973; **Residency:** Internal Medicine, UCLA Med Ctr, Los Angeles, CA 1974-1976; **Fellowship:** Hematology, UCLA Med Ctr, Los Angeles, CA 1976-1978; **Faculty Appointment:** Prof Medicine, UCLA

Jacobs, Charlotte DeCroes MD (Medical Oncology) - *Special Expertise: Medical Oncology - General;* **Admitting Hospital:** Stanford Medical Center; **Office Address:** Stanford Med Ctr-Oncology Clinic Center 300 Pasteur Drive, rm H0274 Stanford, CA 94305; **Office Phone:** (650) 725-8738; **Board Certifications:** Internal Medicine 1975, Medical Oncology 1977; **Medical School:** Washington Univ, St Louis 1972; **Residencies:** Internal Medicine, Barnes, St Louis, MO 1974; Internal Medicine, UCSF, San Francisco, CA 1975; **Fellowship:** Medical Oncology, Stanford, Stanford, CA 1977; **Faculty Appointment:** Prof Medicine, Stanford Univ

MEDICAL ONCOLOGY West Coast and Pacific

Levy, Ronald MD (Medical Oncology) - *Special Expertise:* Medical Oncology - General; **Admitting Hospital:** Stanford Medical Center; **Office Address:** Stanford Med Ctr, Med Onc, Chief 300 Pasteur Drive, rm M207 Stanford, CA 94305; **Office Phone:** (650) 725-6452; **Board Certifications:** Internal Medicine 1973, Medical Oncology 1979; **Medical School:** Stanford Univ 1968; **Residency:** Internal Medicine, Mass Genl Hosp, Boston, MA 1969-1970; **Fellowship:** Medical Oncology, Standford Hosp, Stanford, CA 1972-1973; **Faculty Appointment:** Prof Medicine, Stanford Univ

Livingston, Robert B MD (Medical Oncology) - *Special Expertise:* Bone Marrow Transplant; Breast Cancer; Lung Cancer; **Admitting Hospital:** University of Washington Medical Center; **Office Address:** Univ Washington Cancer Center 1959 NE Pacific St, Box 356043 Seattle, WA 98195; **Office Phone:** (206) 598-4125; **Board Certifications:** Internal Medicine 1972, Medical Oncology 1973; **Medical School:** Univ Okla Coll Med 1965; **Residency:** Internal Medicine, U Oklahoma Med Ctr, Oklahoma City, OK 1969-1971; **Fellowship:** Medical Oncology, U Texas, Houston, TX 1971-1973; **Faculty Appointment:** Prof Medicine, Univ Wash

Natale, Ronald B MD (Medical Oncology) - *Special Expertise:* Lung Cancer; **Admitting Hospital:** Cedars-Sinai Medical Center; **Office Address:** Cedar Sinai Comprehensive Cancer Ctr 8700 Beverly Blvd Los Angeles, CA 90048; **Office Phone:** (310) 423-1101; **Board Certifications:** Internal Medicine 1977, Medical Oncology 1979; **Medical School:** Wayne State Univ 1974; **Residency:** Internal Medicine, Wayne State Univ. 1975-1977; **Fellowship:** Medical Oncology, Meml Sloan Kettering, New York, NY 1977-1980; **Faculty Appointment:** Prof Medical Oncology, Univ Mich Med Sch

Press, Oliver William MD/PhD (Medical Oncology) - *Special Expertise:* Lymphoma; Bone Marrow Transplant; **Admitting Hospital:** University of Washington Medical Center; **Office Address:** Cancer Center/University of Washington 1959 NE Pacific St, Box 356043 Seattle, WA 98195-6043; **Office Phone:** (206) 598-4207; **Board Certifications:** Medical Oncology 1985, Internal Medicine 1982; **Medical School:** Univ Wash 1979; **Residencies:** Internal Medicine, U Hosp., Seattle, WA 1982-1983; Internal Medicine, Mass Genl Hosp., Boston, MA 1980-1982; **Fellowship:** Medical Oncology, U Wash., Seattle, WA 1983-1985; **Faculty Appointment:** Prof Medicine, Univ Wash

Rosen, Peter J MD (Medical Oncology) - *Special Expertise:* Lymphoma; **Admitting Hospital:** UCLA Medical Center; **Office Address:** 10945 Le Conte Ave, Ste 2333 Los Angeles, CA 90095; **Office Phone:** (310) 794-1092; **Board Certifications:** Hematology 1974, Medical Oncology 1975; **Medical School:** USC Sch Med 1966; **Residency:** Internal Medicine, Johns Hopkins Hosp, Baltimore, MD 1966-1968; **Fellowship:** Hematology, USC, Los Angeles, CA 1970-1972

Volberding, Paul Arthur MD (Medical Oncology) - *Special Expertise:* AIDS/HIV; **Admitting Hospital:** University of California - San Francisco Medical Center; **Office Address:** AIDS Prog, Ward 84, San Francisco Genl Hosp 995 Potrero Ave, Bldg 80 San Francisco, CA 94110; **Office Phone:** (415) 476-4082; **Board Certifications:** Internal Medicine 1978, Medical Oncology 1981; **Medical School:** Univ Minn 1975; **Residency:** Internal Medicine, Univ Utah, Salt Lake City, UT 1976-1978; **Fellowship:** Medical Oncology, UCSF Med Ctr, San Francisco, CA 1978-1981; **Faculty Appointment:** Prof Medicine, UCSF

INFECTIOUS DISEASE

(a subspecialty of INTERNAL MEDICINE)

An internist who deals with infectious diseases of all types and in all organs. Conditions requiring selective use of antibiotics call for this special skill. This physician often diagnoses and treats AIDS patients and patients with fevers which have not been explained. Infectious disease specialists may also have expertise in preventive medicine and conditions associated with travel.

INTERNAL MEDICINE

An internist is a personal physician who provides long-term, comprehensive care in the office and the hospital, managing both common and complex illness of adolescents, adults and the elderly. Internists are trained in the diagnosis and treatment of cancer, infections and diseases affecting the heart, blood, kidneys, joints and digestive, respiratory and vascular systems. They are also trained in the essentials of primary care internal medicine which incorporates an understanding of disease prevention, wellness, substance abuse, mental health and effective treatment of common problems of the eyes, ears, skin, nervous system and reproductive organs.

Training required: Three years in internal medicine *plus* additional training and examination for certification in infectious disease

PHYSICIAN LISTINGS

New England

Craven, Donald Edward MD (Infectious Disease) - *Special Expertise: AIDS/HIV; Hepatitis C; Pneumonia;* **Admitting Hospital:** Lahey Clinic; **Office Address:** Lahey Clinic, Dept Infectious Disease 41 Mall Rd Burlington, MA 01805; **Office Phone:** (781) 744-8608; **Board Certifications:** Internal Medicine 1973, Infectious Disease 1982; **Medical School:** Albany Med Coll 1970; **Residencies:** Internal Medicine, Royal Victoria Hosp-McGill, Montreal, Canada 1971-1973; Infectious Disease, Boston Univ Hosp, Boston, MA 1974-1976; **Fellowship:** Internal Medicine, Royal Victoria Hosp, Montreal, Canada 1973-1974; **Faculty Appointment:** Prof Medicine, Boston Univ

Hirsch, Martin Stanley MD (Infectious Disease) - *Special Expertise: AIDS/HIV;* **Admitting Hospital:** Massachusetts General Hospital; **Office Address:** MA Genl Hosp - Inf Dis Unit 55 Fruit St Boston, MA 02114; **Office Phone:** (617) 726-3815; **Board Certifications:** Internal Medicine 1972, Infectious Disease 1976; **Medical School:** Johns Hopkins Univ 1964; **Residency:** Internal Medicine, Chicago Clins Hosps, Chicago, IL 1965-1966; **Fellowship:** Infectious Disease, Mass Genl Hosp, Boston, MA 1969-1971; **Faculty Appointment:** Prof Internal Medicine, Harvard Med Sch

Hopkins, Cyrus Clark MD (Infectious Disease) - *Special Expertise: Infections-Hospital Acquired;* **Admitting Hospital:** Massachusetts General Hospital; **Office Address:** Mass Genl Hosp, Inf Ctrl Unit 55 Fruit St Clinic 110 Boston, MA; **Office Phone:** (617) 726-2036; **Board Certifications:** Internal Medicine 1972, Infectious Disease 1972; **Medical School:** Harvard Med Sch 1964; **Residencies:** Internal Medicine, Mass Genl Hosp, Boston, MA 1965-1966; Internal Medicine, Mass Genl Hosp, Boston, MA 1968-1970; **Fellowship:** Infectious Disease, Mass Genl Hosp, Boston, MA 1969; **Faculty Appointment:** Assoc Prof Medicine, Harvard Med Sch

Karchmer, Adolph W MD (Infectious Disease) - *Special Expertise: Endocarditis;* **Admitting Hospital:** Beth Israel Deaconess Medical Center - Boston (Page 57); **Office Address:** Beth Israel Deaconess Med Ctr, Div Inf Dis One Deaconess Rd Boston, MA 02215; **Office Phone:** (617) 632-0760; **Board Certification:** Internal Medicine 1972; **Medical School:** Harvard Med Sch 1964; **Residencies:** Internal Medicine, Mass Genl Hosp, Boston, MA 1965-1966; Internal Medicine, Mass Genl Hosp, Boston, MA 1969-1970; **Fellowship:** Infectious Disease, Mass Genl Hosp, Boston, MA 1970-1971; **Faculty Appointment:** Prof Medicine, Harvard Med Sch

Maguire, James MD (Infectious Disease) - *Special Expertise: Tropical Diseases; Parasitic Infections;* **Admitting Hospital:** Brigham & Women's Hospital; **Office Address:** Brigham & Women's Hosp 75 Francis St Boston, MA 02115-6195; **Office Phone:** (617) 732-5885; **Board Certifications:** Infectious Disease 1978, Internal Medicine 1977; **Medical School:** Harvard Med Sch 1974; **Residency:** Internal Medicine, Peter Bent Brigham Hosp, Boston, MA 1975-1977; **Fellowship:** Infectious Disease, Peter Bent Brigham Hosp, Boston, MA 1976-1978; **Faculty Appointment:** Assoc Prof Medicine, Harvard Med Sch

Mid Atlantic

Auwaerter, Paul MD (Infectious Disease) - *Special Expertise: Ehrlichiosis; Tick-borne Diseases;* **Admitting Hospital:** Johns Hopkins Hospital - Baltimore (Page 65); **Office Address:** Johns Hopkins-Greenspring Stn 10755 Falls Rd, Fl 360 Lutherville, MD 21093; **Office Phone:** (410) 583-2774; **Board Certifications:** Internal Medicine 1992, Infectious Disease 1994; **Medical School:** Columbia P&S 1988; **Residencies:** Internal Medicine, Johns Hopkins Med Ctr, Baltimore, MD 1989-1991; Infectious Disease, Johns Hopkins Med Ctr, Baltimore, MD 1991-1992; **Fellowship:** Infectious Disease, Johns Hopkins Med Ctr, Baltimore, MD 1993-1996; **Faculty Appointment:** Asst Prof Medicine, Johns Hopkins Univ

Bartlett, John Gill MD (Infectious Disease) - *Special Expertise:* AIDS/HIV; Diarrhea; Pneumonia; **Admitting Hospital:** Johns Hopkins Hospital - Baltimore (Page 65); **Office Address:** 1830 E Monument St, Bldg Ross - Ste 439 Baltimore, MD 12287-0003; **Office Phone:** (410) 955-7634; **Board Certification:** Internal Medicine 1972; **Medical School:** SUNY Syracuse 1963; **Residencies:** Internal Medicine, Univ Hosp Birmingham, Birmingham, AL 1967-1968; Internal Medicine, Peter B Brigham Hosp., Boston, MA 1964-1965; **Fellowship:** Infectious Disease, Wadsworth VA Hosp., Los Angeles, CA 1968-1970

Berkowitz, Leonard B MD (Infectious Disease) - *Special Expertise:* Infectious Disease - General; **Admitting Hospital:** Brooklyn Hospital Center-Downtown; **Office Address:** 121 DeKalb Ave Brooklyn, NY 11201; **Office Phone:** (718) 250-6141; **Board Certifications:** Internal Medicine 1980, Infectious Disease 1984; **Medical School:** SUNY Hlth Sci Ctr 1977; **Residency:** Internal Medicine, Univ Hosp, Brooklyn, NY 1977-1981; **Fellowship:** Infectious Disease, Univ Hosp, Brooklyn, NY 1981-1983; **Faculty Appointment:** Asst Prof SUNY Hlth Sci Ctr

Blaser, Martin Jack MD (Infectious Disease) - *Special Expertise:* Helicobacter Pylori; **Admitting Hospital:** NYU Medical Center (Page 70); **Office Address:** 550 1st Avenue Rm 16North-I New York, NY 10016-6402; **Office Phone:** (212) 263-6394; **Board Certifications:** Internal Medicine 1977, Infectious Disease 1980; **Medical School:** NYU Sch Med 1973; **Residency:** Internal Medicine, U Colo Med Ctr, Denver, CO 1974-1977; **Fellowship:** Infectious Disease, U Colo Med Ctr, Denver, CO 1977-1979; **Faculty Appointment:** Prof Medicine, NYU Sch Med

Brause, Barry MD (Infectious Disease) - *Special Expertise:* Bone/Joint Infections; Lyme Disease; **Admitting Hospital:** New York Weill Cornell Medical Center - NY Presbyterian Hospital (Page 72); **Office Address:** 215 E 68th St New York, NY 10021-5718; **Office Phone:** (212) 570-6122; **Board Certifications:** Internal Medicine 1973, Infectious Disease 1976; **Medical School:** Univ Pittsburgh 1970; **Residency:** Internal Medicine, New York Hosp, New York, NY 1971-1973; **Fellowship:** Infectious Disease, New York Hosp, New York, NY 1973-1975; **Faculty Appointment:** Clin Prof Medicine, Cornell Univ-Weil Med Coll

Brennan, Patrick J MD (Infectious Disease) - *Special Expertise:* Tuberculosis; Infections in Immune Deficient; **Admitting Hospital:** Hospital of the University of Pennsylvania; **Office Address:** Univ of Pennsylvania Med Ctr 3400 Spruce St Philadelphia, PA 19104; **Office Phone:** (215) 662-6932; **Board Certifications:** Internal Medicine 1985, Infectious Disease 1990; **Medical School:** Temple Univ 1982; **Residency:** Internal Medicine, Temple Univ Hosp, Philadelphia, PA 1983-1985; **Fellowship:** Infectious Disease, Hosp Univ Penn, Philadelphia, PA 1985-1986; **Faculty Appointment:** Assoc Prof Medicine, Univ Penn

Chaisson, Richard Ernest MD (Infectious Disease) - *Special Expertise:* AIDS/HIV; Tuberculosis; **Admitting Hospital:** Johns Hopkins Hospital - Baltimore (Page 65); **Office Address:** 1830 E Monument St, rm 455 Baltimore, MD 21287; **Office Phone:** (410) 955-1755; **Board Certification:** Internal Medicine 1985; **Medical School:** Univ Mass Sch Med 1982; **Residency:** Internal Medicine, UCSF Med Ctr, San Francisco, CA 1983-1985; **Fellowship:** Infectious Disease, UCSF Med Ctr, San Francisco, CA 1985-1987; **Faculty Appointment:** Assoc Prof Medicine, Johns Hopkins Univ

Ellner, Jerrold Jay MD (Infectious Disease) - *Special Expertise:* AIDS/HIV; Tuberculosis in AIDS/HIV; **Admitting Hospital:** UMDNJ-University Hospital-Newark; **Office Address:** Med Sci Bldg 185 S Orange Ave, Fl 1 Newark, NJ 07103; **Office Phone:** (973) 972-7598; **Board Certifications:** Internal Medicine 1973, Infectious Disease 1978; **Medical School:** Johns Hopkins Univ 1970; **Residency:** Internal Medicine, Johns Hopkins Hosp, Baltimore, MD 1970-1972

Fauci, Anthony Stephen MD (Infectious Disease) - *Special Expertise:* *AIDS/HIV;* **Admitting Hospital:** National Institutes of Health - Clinical Center; **Office Address:** NIAID , Bldg 31 - rm 7A03 31 Center Drive MSC 2520 Bethesda, MD 20892-2520; **Office Phone:** (301) 496-2263; **Board Certifications:** Allergy & Immunology 1974, Infectious Disease 1974; **Medical School:** Cornell Univ-Weil Med Coll 1966; **Residencies:** Internal Medicine, NY Hosp Cornell Med Ctr, New York, NY 1967-1968; Internal Medicine, NY Hosp Cornell Med Ctr, New York, NY 1971-1972; **Fellowship:** Infectious Disease, Natl Inst Infectious Disease NIH, Bethesda, MD 1968-1971

Frank, Ian MD (Infectious Disease) - *Special Expertise:* *AIDS/HIV;* **Admitting Hospital:** Hospital of the University of Pennsylvania; **Office Address:** Univ Penn Medical Center-Infectious Disease 3400 Spruce St Philadelphia, PA 19104-6073; **Office Phone:** (215) 662-6932; **Board Certifications:** Internal Medicine 1983, Infectious Disease 1992; **Medical School:** Dartmouth Med Sch 1980; **Residency:** Internal Medicine, Graduate Hosp, Philadelphia, PA 1981-1983; **Fellowship:** Infectious Disease, Hosp Univ Penn, Philadelphia, PA 1983; **Faculty Appointment:** Assoc Prof Medicine, Univ Penn

Friedman, Harvey Michael MD (Infectious Disease) - *Special Expertise:* *AIDS/HIV; Herpes Simplex;* **Admitting Hospital:** Hospital of the University of Pennsylvania; **Office Address:** Univ Penn Med Ctr, Div Infectious Disease 3400 Spruce Street Philadelphia, PA 19104; **Office Phone:** (215) 662-3557; **Board Certifications:** Internal Medicine 1975, Infectious Disease 1976; **Medical School:** McGill Univ 1969; **Residencies:** Internal Medicine, Jewish Genl Hosp, Montreal, Canada 1970-1971; Virology, Wistar Inst, Philadelphia, PA 1971-1973; **Fellowship:** Infectious Disease, Hosp Univ Penn, Philadelphia, PA 1973-1975; **Faculty Appointment:** Prof Medicine, Univ Penn

Garvey, Glenda Josephine MD (Infectious Disease) - *Special Expertise:* *Endocarditis; Septic Shock;* **Admitting Hospital:** Columbia Presbyterian Medical Center (Page 72); **Office Address:** Columbia Presbyterian Med Ctr 622 W 168th St New York, NY 10032-3702; **Office Phone:** (212) 305-3272; **Board Certifications:** Infectious Disease 1976, Critical Care Medicine 1999; **Medical School:** Columbia P&S 1969; **Residency:** Internal Medicine, Columbia Presby Med Ctr, New York, NY 1969-1972; **Fellowship:** Infectious Disease, Columbia Presby Med Ctr, New York, NY 1972-1974; **Faculty Appointment:** Prof Medicine, Columbia P&S

Hammer, Glenn MD (Infectious Disease) - *Special Expertise:* *AIDS/HIV;* **Admitting Hospital:** Mount Sinai Hospital (Page 70); **Office Address:** 1100 Park Ave New York, NY 10128; **Office Phone:** (212) 427-9550; **Board Certifications:** Internal Medicine 1973, Infectious Disease 1974; **Medical School:** NYU Sch Med 1969; **Residency:** Internal Medicine, Mount Sinai Hosp, New York, NY 1970-1972; **Fellowship:** Infectious Disease, Mount Sinai Hosp, New York, NY 1972-1974; **Faculty Appointment:** Asst Clin Prof Medicine, Mount Sinai Sch Med

Hartman, Barry Jay MD (Infectious Disease) - *Special Expertise:* *Infectious Disease - General;* **Admitting Hospital:** New York Weill Cornell Medical Center - NY Presbyterian Hospital (Page 72); **Office Address:** 407 E 70th St, Fl 4 New York, NY 10021-5302; **Office Phone:** (212) 744-4882; **Board Certifications:** Internal Medicine 1976, Infectious Disease 1980; **Medical School:** Penn State Univ-Hershey Med Ctr 1973; **Residency:** Internal Medicine, NY Hosp /Cornell Med Ctr, New York, NY 1974-1976; **Fellowship:** Infectious Disease, NY Hosp/ Cornell Med Ctr, New York, NY 1978-1981; **Faculty Appointment:** Clin Prof Medicine, Cornell Univ-Weil Med Coll

INFECTIOUS DISEASE

Johnson, Warren MD (Infectious Disease) - *Special Expertise: Travel Medicine; Parasitic Infections; Toxoplasmosis, Amebiasis;* **Admitting Hospital:** New York Weill Cornell Medical Center - NY Presbyterian Hospital (Page 72); **Office Address:** 1300 York Ave Ste A421, Box 125 New York, NY 10021; **Office Phone:** (212) 746-6320; **Board Certifications:** Internal Medicine 1971, Infectious Disease 1974; **Medical School:** Columbia P&S 1962; **Residencies:** Internal Medicine, NY Hosp-Cornell Med Ctr, New York, NY 1963-1964; Internal Medicine, NY Hosp-Cornell Med Ctr, New York, NY 1968-1969; **Fellowship:** Infectious Disease, NY Hosp-Cornell Med Ctr, New York, NY 1966-1968; **Faculty Appointment:** Prof Medicine, Cornell Univ-Weil Med Coll

Kaplan, Mark H MD (Infectious Disease) - *Special Expertise: AIDS/HIV;* **Admitting Hospital:** North Shore University Hospital at Manhasset; **Office Address:** North Shore Univ Hosp 300 Community Dr Manhasset, NY 11030; **Office Phone:** (516) 562-4280; **Board Certifications:** Internal Medicine 1972, Infectious Disease 1974; **Medical School:** Cornell Univ-Weil Med Coll 1966; **Residencies:** Internal Medicine, Bellevue Hosp Ctr, New York, NY 1967-1968; Internal Medicine, Mem Sloan Kettering Cancer Ctr, New York, NY 1970-1971; **Fellowship:** Infectious Disease, Mem Sloan Kettering Cancer Ctr, New York, NY 1973-1974; **Faculty Appointment:** Clin Prof Medicine, NYU Sch Med

Mann, John MD (Infectious Disease) - *Special Expertise: Ehrlichiosis; Tick-borne Diseases;* **Admitting Hospital:** Johns Hopkins Hospital - Baltimore (Page 65); **Office Address:** 10755 Falls Rd Ste 200 Lutherville, MD 21093; **Office Phone:** (410) 583-7116; **Board Certifications:** Internal Medicine 1970, Infectious Disease 1972; **Medical School:** Georgetown Univ 1963; **Residency:** Internal Medicine, Johns Hopkins Med Ctr, Baltimore, MD 1964-1965; **Fellowship:** Infectious Disease, NIH, Bethesda, MD 1965-1967; **Faculty Appointment:** Assoc Prof Medicine, Johns Hopkins Univ

Masur, Henry MD (Infectious Disease) - *Special Expertise: Critical Care; AIDS/HIV;* **Admitting Hospital:** National Institutes of Health - Clinical Center; **Office Address:** National Institute of Health Clinical Center 7D43 Bethesda, MD 20892; **Office Phone:** (301) 496-9320; **Board Certifications:** Internal Medicine 1975, Infectious Disease 1978; **Medical School:** Cornell Univ-Weil Med Coll 1972; **Residencies:** Internal Medicine, New York Hosp, NewYork, NY 1973-1974; Internal Medicine, Johns Hopkins Hosp, Baltimore, MD 1974-1975; **Fellowship:** Infectious Disease, New York Hosp-Cornell Med Ctr, New York, NY 1975-1977

Mildvan, Donna MD (Infectious Disease) - *Special Expertise: AIDS/HIV;* **Admitting Hospital:** Beth Israel Medical Center - New York; **Office Address:** Div of Infectious Disease 1st Ave at 16th St New York, NY 10003; **Office Phone:** (212) 420-4005; **Board Certifications:** Internal Medicine 1972, Infectious Disease 1972; **Medical School:** Johns Hopkins Univ 1967; **Residency:** Internal Medicine, Mount Sinai Hosp, New York, NY 1968-1970; **Fellowship:** Infectious Disease, Mount Sinai Hosp, New York, NY 1970-1972; **Faculty Appointment:** Prof Medicine, Albert Einstein Coll Med

Perlman, David MD (Infectious Disease) - *Special Expertise: AIDS/HIV;* **Admitting Hospital:** Beth Israel Medical Center - New York; **Office Address:** Beth Israel Med Ctr 1st Ave at 16th St New York, NY 10003; **Office Phone:** (212) 420-4470; **Board Certifications:** Internal Medicine 1986, Infectious Disease 1988; **Medical School:** Albert Einstein Coll Med 1983; **Residency:** Internal Medicine, NY Hosp/Meml Sloan Kettering, New York, NY 1984-1986; **Fellowship:** Infectious Disease, Montefiore Hosp, Bronx, NY 1986-1988; **Faculty Appointment:** Assoc Prof Medicine, Albert Einstein Coll Med

Polsky, Bruce MD (Infectious Disease) - *Special Expertise: AIDS/HIV;* **Admitting Hospital:** St Luke's - Roosevelt Hospital Center - Roosevelt Division (Page 58); **Office Address:** Univ Med Practice 425 W 59th St New York, NY 10019; **Office Phone:** (212) 523-2525; **Board Certifications:** Internal Medicine 1983, Infectious Disease 2000; **Medical School:** Wayne State Univ 1980; **Residency:** Internal Medicine, Montefiore Hosp, Bronx, NY 1981-1983; **Fellowship:** Infectious Disease, Meml Sloan Kettering Hosp, New York, NY 1983-1986; **Faculty Appointment:** Prof Medicine, Columbia P&S

Rahal, James MD (Infectious Disease) - *Special Expertise: West Nile Virus;* **Admitting Hospital:** New York Hospital Medical Center of Queens; **Office Address:** New York Hospital - Queens Infectious Disease 56-45 Main St Flushing, NY 11355-5095; **Office Phone:** (718) 670-1525; **Board Certifications:** Internal Medicine 1967, Infectious Disease 1972; **Medical School:** Tufts Univ 1959; **Residency:** Internal Medicine, New England Ctr Hosp, Boston, MA 1961-1964; **Fellowship:** Infectious Disease, New England Ctr Hosp, Boston, MA 1962-1965; **Faculty Appointment:** Clin Prof Medicine, Cornell Univ-Weil Med Coll

Rao, Nalini MD (Infectious Disease) - *Special Expertise: Orthopaedic Infectious Disease; Tropical Diseases;* **Admitting Hospital:** UPMC - Presbyterian University Hospital; **Office Address:** Centre Commons, Suite 510 5750 Centre Ave Pittsburgh, PA 15206; **Office Phone:** (412) 661-1633; **Board Certifications:** Infectious Disease 1980, Internal Medicine 1975; **Medical School:** India 1970; **Residencies:** Internal Medicine, Geo Wash U Hosp., Washington, DC 1973-1974; Infectious Disease, Baylor College of Med, Houston, TX 1974-1975; **Fellowship:** Infectious Disease, U Pittsburgh Sch Med, Pittsburgh, PA 1975-1977; **Faculty Appointment:** Assoc Clin Prof Medicine, Univ Pittsburgh

Sepkowitz, Kent MD (Infectious Disease) - *Special Expertise: AIDS/HIV; Infections In Cancer Patients;* **Admitting Hospital:** Memorial Sloan Kettering Cancer Center; **Office Address:** Meml Sloan Kettering Cancer Ctr 1275 York Ave, rm 288 New York, NY 10021-0033; **Office Phone:** (212) 639-2441; **Board Certifications:** Internal Medicine 1983, Infectious Disease 2000; **Medical School:** Univ Okla Coll Med 1980; **Residency:** Internal Medicine, Roosevelt Hosp, New York, NY 1981-1984; **Fellowship:** Infectious Disease, Meml Sloan Kettering Cancer Ctr, New York, NY 1988-1991; **Faculty Appointment:** Assoc Prof Medicine, Cornell Univ-Weil Med Coll

Smith, Leon G MD (Infectious Disease) - *Special Expertise: AIDS/HIV;* **Admitting Hospital:** St Michael's Medical Center; **Office Address:** 268 Martin Luther King Jr Blvd Newark, NJ 07102; **Office Phone:** (973) 877-5481; **Board Certifications:** Internal Medicine 1963, Infectious Disease 1974; **Medical School:** Georgetown Univ 1956; **Residencies:** Infectious Disease, Nat Inst Health, Bethesda, MD 1957-1959; Internal Medicine, Yale-New Haven Hosp, New Haven, CT 1960-1962; **Fellowship:** Infectious Disease, Yale-New Haven Hosp, New Haven, CT 1959-1960 **Faculty Appointment:** Prof Medicine, UMDNJ-NJ Med Sch, Newark

Straus, Stephen MD (Infectious Disease) - *Special Expertise: Chronic Fatigue Syndrome;* **Admitting Hospital:** National Institutes of Health - Clinical Center; **Office Address:** NIH - Laboratory Clinical Investigation Bldg 10, Rm 11N228 Bethesda, MD 20892; **Office Phone:** (301) 496-5807; **Board Certifications:** Internal Medicine 1977, Infectious Disease 1980; **Medical School:** Columbia P&S 1972; **Residency:** Internal Medicine, Barnes Hosp, St Louis, MO 1975-1976; **Fellowship:** Infectious Disease, Barnes Hosp-Wash Univ, St Louis, MO 1976-1978

Welch, Peter MD (Infectious Disease) - *Special Expertise: Lyme Disease;* **Admitting Hospital:** Northern Westchester Hospital Center; **Office Address:** Medical Affairs Office 400 E Main St Mt Kisco, NY 10549-3446; **Office Phone:** (914) 666-1308; **Board Certifications:** Internal Medicine 1977, Infectious Disease 1980; **Medical School:** SUNY Buffalo 1974; **Residency:** Internal Medicine, NY Hosp, Westchester, NY 1974-1977; **Fellowship:** Infectious Disease, NY Hosp, New York, NY 1977-1979

Wormser, Gary MD (Infectious Disease) - *Special Expertise:* Lyme Disease; AIDS/HIV; **Admitting Hospital:** Westchester Medical Center; **Office Address:** Westchester Medical Center, Division of Infectious Disease Macy Pavillion, Rm 209SE Valhalla, NY 10595; **Office Phone:** (914) 493-8865; **Board Certifications:** Internal Medicine 1978, Infectious Disease 1982; **Medical School:** Johns Hopkins Univ 1972; **Residency:** Internal Medicine, Mount Sinai Hosp, New York, NY 1973-1975; **Fellowship:** Infectious Disease, Mount Sinai Hosp, New York, NY 1975-1977; **Faculty Appointment:** Prof Medicine, NY Med Coll

Yancovitz, Stanley MD (Infectious Disease) - *Special Expertise:* Lyme Disease; AIDS/HIV; **Admitting Hospital:** Beth Israel Medical Center - New York; **Office Address:** 10 Union Square East, Ste 3-F New York, NY 10003; **Office Phone:** (212) 420-2600; **Board Certifications:** Internal Medicine 1973, Infectious Disease 1976; **Medical School:** SUNY Downstate 1967; **Residencies:** Internal Medicine, Metropolitan Hosp, New York, NY 1968-1969; Internal Medicine, Beth Israel Med Ctr, New York, NY 1971-1972; **Fellowship:** Infectious Disease, Mount Sinai Hosp, New York, NY 1973-1975; **Faculty Appointment:** Assoc Prof Medicine, Albert Einstein Coll Med

Yu, Victor MD (Infectious Disease) - *Special Expertise:* Legionnaire's Disease; **Admitting Hospital:** VA Pittsburgh Health Care System; **Office Address:** VA Med Ctr Inf Disease Sec Univ Drive C Pittsburgh, PA 15240; **Office Phone:** (412) 688-6179; **Board Certifications:** Internal Medicine 1978, Infectious Disease 1982; **Medical School:** Univ Minn 1970; **Residencies:** Internal Medicine, Univ Colo Med Ctr, Denver, CO 1971-1972; Internal Medicine, Stanford Univ Med Ctr, Stanford, CA 1974-1975; **Fellowship:** Infectious Disease, Stanford Univ Med Ctr, Stanford, CA 1975-1977; **Faculty Appointment:** Prof Medicine, Univ Pittsburgh

Southeast

Archer, Gordon Lee MD (Infectious Disease) - *Special Expertise:* Staphylococcal Infections; **Admitting Hospital:** Medical College of Virginia Hospitals; **Office Address:** Med Coll VA Box 980049 Richmond, VA 23298-0049; **Office Phone:** (804) 828-9711; **Board Certifications:** Internal Medicine 1972, Infectious Disease 1976; **Medical School:** Univ VA Sch Med 1969; **Residency:** Internal Medicine, Univ Mich Hosps, Ann Arbor, MI 1970-1972; **Fellowship:** Infectious Disease, Univ Mich Hosps, Ann Arbor, MI 1972-1974; **Faculty Appointment:** Prof Internal Medicine, Med Coll VA

Bartlett, John A MD (Infectious Disease) - *Special Expertise:* AIDS/HIV; Anaerobic Infections; **Admitting Hospital:** Duke University Medical Center (Page 60); **Office Address:** Duke Univ Med Ctr 0212 Hospital South, Box 3238 Durham, NC 27710; **Office Phone:** (919) 684-6416; **Board Certifications:** Internal Medicine 1984, Infectious Disease 1988; **Medical School:** Univ VA Sch Med 1981; **Residency:** Internal Medicine, Duke Univ Med Ctr, Durham, NC 1982-1985; **Fellowship:** Infectious Disease, Duke Univ Med Ctr, Durham, NC 1985; **Faculty Appointment:** Assoc Prof Medicine, Duke Univ

Cancio, Margarita MD (Infectious Disease) - *Special Expertise:* AIDS/HIV; **Admitting Hospital:** Tampa General Hospital; **Office Address:** 4 Columbia Dr, Ste 820 Tampa, FL 33606-3568; **Office Phone:** (813) 251-8444; **Board Certifications:** Internal Medicine 1985, Infectious Disease 1988; **Medical School:** Univ S Fla Coll Med 1982; **Residencies:** Internal Medicine, Univ S Fla Coll Med, Tampa, FL 1982-1983; Internal Medicine, Univ S Fla Coll Med, Tampa, FL 1983-1985; **Fellowships:** Infectious Disease, Univ S Fla Coll Med, Tampa, FL 1986-1987; Infectious Disease, Univ S Fla Coll Med, Tampa, FL 1987-1988; **Faculty Appointment:** Assoc Prof Internal Medicine, Univ S Fla Coll Med

Chan, Joseph MD (Infectious Disease) - *Special Expertise:* AIDS/HIV; **Admitting Hospital:** Mount Sinai Medical Center; **Office Address:** Mt Sinai Medical Ctr 4300 Alton Rd, Ste G-23 Miami, FL 33140-2849; **Office Phone:** (305) 674-2766; **Board Certifications:** Internal Medicine 1980, Infectious Disease 1982; **Medical School:** UCSF 1977; **Residency:** Internal Medicine, Univ Miami Affil Hosps, Miami, FL 1978-1980; **Fellowship:** Infectious Disease, Univ Miami Affil Hosps, Miami, FL 1980-1982; **Faculty Appointment:** Assoc Prof Medicine, Univ Miami Sch Med

Corey, G Ralph MD (Infectious Disease) - *Special Expertise: Tropical Diseases; Travel Medicine;* **Admitting Hospital:** Duke University Medical Center (Page 60); **Office Address:** Duke North, Rm 8241 Durham, NC 27715; **Office Phone:** (919) 681-2458; **Board Certifications:** Internal Medicine 1977, Infectious Disease 1980; **Medical School:** Baylor Coll Med 1973; **Residency:** Internal Medicine, Duke Univ Med Ctr, Durham, NC 1975-1978; **Fellowship:** Infectious Disease, Duke Univ Med Ctr, Durham, NC 1978-1980; **Faculty Appointment:** Assoc Prof Medicine, Duke Univ

Dismukes, William Ernest MD (Infectious Disease) - *Special Expertise: Fungal Infections;* **Admitting Hospital:** University of Alabama Hospital at Birmingham; **Office Address:** 1900 Univ Blvd, rm 229THT Brimingham, AL 35294-0006; **Office Phone:** (205) 934-5191; **Board Certifications:** Internal Medicine 1977, Infectious Disease 1972; **Medical School:** Univ Ala 1964; **Residencies:** Internal Medicine, Peter Bent Brigham Hosp, Boston, MA 1965-1966; Internal Medicine, Peter Bent Brigham Hosp, Boston, MA 1968-1969; **Fellowship:** Infectious Disease, Mass Genl Hosp, Boston, MA 1969-1971; **Faculty Appointment:** Prof Medicine, Univ Ala

Droller, David G MD (Infectious Disease) - *Special Expertise:* AIDS/HIV; **Admitting Hospital:** Broward General Medical Center; **Office Address:** 5333 N Dixie Hwy, Ste 208 Fort Lauderdale, FL 33334-3454; **Office Phone:** (954) 771-7988; **Board Certifications:** Internal Medicine 1977, Infectious Disease 1980; **Medical School:** NYU Sch Med 1974; **Residency:** Internal Medicine, Univ of Miami Affil Hosps, Miami, FL 1974-1977; **Fellowship:** Infectious Disease, Univ of Miami Affil Hosps, Miami, FL 1977-1979; **Faculty Appointment:** Assoc Prof Medicine, Univ Miami Sch Med

Guerrant, Richard MD (Infectious Disease) - *Special Expertise: Tropical Diseases; Infectious Diarrhea; Travel Medicine;* **Admitting Hospital:** University of Virginia Health Systems; **Office Address:** Univ Virginia Med Ctr Jefferson Park Ave, Primary Care 4th Fl Charlottesville, VA 22903; **Office Phone:** (804) 924-5242; **Board Certifications:** Internal Medicine 1973, Infectious Disease 1976; **Medical School:** Univ VA Sch Med 1968; **Residencies:** Internal Medicine, Boston City Hosp, Boston, MA 1969-1970; Internal Medicine, Univ Virginia Hosp, Charlottesville, VA 1972-1973; **Fellowship:** Infectious Disease, Univ Virginia Hosp, Charlottesville, VA 1973-1974; **Faculty Appointment:** Prof Medicine, Univ VA Sch Med

Houston, Sally MD (Infectious Disease) - *Special Expertise: Infections-Transplant;* **Admitting Hospital:** Tampa General Hospital; **Office Address:** Tampa Genl Hosp, Inf Dis Ctr PO Box 1289 Tampa, FL 33601-1289; **Office Phone:** (813) 251-7670; **Board Certifications:** Internal Medicine 1990, Infectious Disease 1992; **Medical School:** Vanderbilt Univ 1987; **Residency:** Internal Medicine, Univ South Fla, Tampa, FL 1990; **Fellowship:** Infectious Disease, Univ South Fla, Tampa, FL 1992; **Faculty Appointment:** Assoc Prof Medicine, Univ S Fla Coll Med

Katner, Harold MD (Infectious Disease) - *Special Expertise:* AIDS/HIV; **Admitting Hospital:** Medical Center of Central Georgia; **Office Address:** Mercer Univ Sch of Med 1550 College St Macon, GA 31201; **Office Phone:** (478) 301-5851; **Board Certifications:** Internal Medicine 1983, Infectious Disease 1986; **Medical School:** Louisiana State Univ 1980; **Residency:** Internal Medicine, Univ Med Ctr, Lafayette, LA 1981-1983; **Fellowship:** Infectious Disease, Ochsner Fdn Hosp, New Orleans, LA 1983-1986; **Faculty Appointment:** Prof Medicine, Mercer Univ Sch Med

Mandell, Gerald MD (Infectious Disease) - *Special Expertise:* White Cell Defects(Agranulocytosis); **Admitting Hospital:** University of Virginia Health Systems; **Office Address:** Univ Virginia Med Sch Box 801341 Charlottesville, VA 22908; **Office Phone:** (804) 924-5942; **Board Certifications:** Internal Medicine 1968, Infectious Disease 1972; **Medical School:** Cornell Univ-Weil Med Coll 1962; **Residency:** Internal Medicine, NY Hosp-Cornell Med Ct, New York, NY 1965-1967; **Fellowship:** Infectious Disease, Cornell Med Ctr, New York, NY 1967-1969; **Faculty Appointment:** Prof Medicine, Univ VA Sch Med

McGowan Jr, John E MD (Infectious Disease) - *Special Expertise:* Infections-Hospital Acquired; Tuberculosis; **Admitting Hospital:** Emory University Hospital; **Office Address:** Emory Univ Hosp 1634 Clifton Rd NE Atlanta, GA 33032; **Office Phone:** (404) 727-9365; **Board Certifications:** Internal Medicine 1971, Infectious Disease 1978; **Medical School:** Harvard Med Sch 1967; **Residency:** Internal Medicine, Boston City Hosp, Boston, MA 1968-1969; **Fellowship:** Infectious Disease, Boston City Hosp, Boston, MA 1971-1973; **Faculty Appointment:** Prof Medicine, Emory Univ

Pearson, Richard Dale MD (Infectious Disease) - *Special Expertise:* Tropical Diseases; **Admitting Hospital:** University of Virginia Health Systems; **Office Address:** Box 800739 Charlottesville, VA 22908; **Office Phone:** (804) 924-5579; **Board Certifications:** Internal Medicine 1976, Infectious Disease 1980; **Medical School:** Univ Mich Med Sch 1973; **Residency:** Internal Medicine, Rochester- Strong Meml Hosp 1974-1976; **Fellowship:** Infectious Disease, Rochester-Strong Meml Hosp 1978-1979; **Faculty Appointment:** Prof Medicine, Univ VA Sch Med

Pegram Jr., Paul Samuel MD (Infectious Disease) - *Special Expertise:* AIDS/HIV; **Admitting Hospital:** Wake Forest University Baptist Medical Center; **Office Address:** Wake Forest Univ Baptist Med Ctr Med Ctr Blvd Winston Salem, NC 27157-1042; **Office Phone:** (336) 716-2700; **Board Certifications:** Infectious Disease 1978, Internal Medicine 1976; **Medical School:** Wake Forest Univ Sch Med 1970; **Residency:** Internal Medicine, NC Baptist Hosp, Winston Salem, NC 1973-1975; **Fellowship:** Infectious Disease, NC Baptist Hosp, Winston Salem, NC 1976-1978; **Faculty Appointment:** Prof Medicine, Wake Forest Univ Sch Med

Ratzan, Kenneth MD (Infectious Disease) - *Special Expertise:* AIDS/HIV; **Admitting Hospital:** Mount Sinai Medical Center; **Office Address:** 4300 Alton Rd Miami Beach, FL 33140-2800; **Office Phone:** (305) 673-5490; **Board Certifications:** Internal Medicine 1971, Infectious Disease 1974; **Medical School:** Harvard Med Sch 1965; **Residencies:** Internal Medicine, Columbia Presby Med Ctr, New York, NY 1966-1967; Infectious Disease, Tufts New Engl Med Ctr, Boston, MA 1971-1972; **Fellowship:** Infectious Disease, Tufts New England Med Ctr, Boston, MA 1969-1971; **Faculty Appointment:** Prof Medicine, Univ Miami Sch Med

Saag, Michael S MD (Infectious Disease) - *Special Expertise:* AIDS/HIV; **Admitting Hospital:** University of Alabama Hospital at Birmingham; **Office Address:** 908 20th St S, Bldg Community Care Birmingham, AL 35205; **Office Phone:** (205) 934-1917; **Board Certifications:** Internal Medicine 1985, Infectious Disease 1988; **Medical School:** Univ Louisville Sch Med 1981; **Residency:** Internal Medicine, Univ Ala Hosp, Birmingham, AL 1981-1984; **Fellowship:** Infectious Disease, Univ Ala Hosp, Birmingham, AL 1985-1987

Scheld, William Michael MD (Infectious Disease) - *Special Expertise:* Meningitis; **Admitting Hospital:** University of Virginia Health Systems; **Office Address:** Univ VA Hlth Sci Ctr PO Box 801342 Charlottesville, VA 22908; **Office Phone:** (804) 924-5241; **Board Certifications:** Internal Medicine 1976, Infectious Disease 1978; **Medical School:** Cornell Univ-Weil Med Coll 1973; **Residency:** Internal Medicine, Univ VA Med Ctr, Charlottesville, VA 1974-1976; **Fellowship:** Infectious Disease, Univ VA Med Ctr, Charlottesville, VA 1976-1979; **Faculty Appointment:** Prof Medicine, Univ VA Sch Med

Sexton, Daniel John MD (Infectious Disease) - *Special Expertise:* *Rocky Mountain Spotted Fever; Endocarditis;* **Admitting Hospital:** Duke University Medical Center (Page 60); **Office Address:** Duke Univ Med Ctr PO Box 3065 Durham, NC 27702-3605; **Office Phone:** (919) 684-4596; **Board Certifications:** Internal Medicine 1977, Infectious Disease 1978; **Medical School:** Northwestern Univ 1971; **Residency:** Internal Medicine, Univ Mo Med Ctr, Columbia, MO 1975-1977; **Fellowship:** Infectious Disease, Duke Univ Med Ctr, Durham, NC 1974-1975; **Faculty Appointment:** Prof Medicine, Duke Univ

Sparling, Philip Frederick MD (Infectious Disease) - *Special Expertise:* *Sexually Transmitted Diseases;* **Admitting Hospital:** University of North Carolina Hospitals; **Office Address:** Univ North Carolina Dept Medicine 547 Burnett-Womack, CB 7030 Chapel Hill, NC 27599; **Office Phone:** (919) 966-2536; **Board Certifications:** Internal Medicine 1970, Infectious Disease 1976; **Medical School:** Harvard Med Sch 1962; **Residency:** Internal Medicine, Mass Genl Hosp, Boston, MA 1963-1964; **Fellowship:** Infectious Disease, Mass Genl Hosp, Boston, MA 1968-1969; **Faculty Appointment:** Prof Medicine, Univ NC Sch Med

Van Der Horst, Charles MD (Infectious Disease) - *Special Expertise:* *AIDS/HIV; Fungal Infections; Viral Infections;* **Admitting Hospital:** University of North Carolina Hospitals; **Office Address:** Univ North Carolina, Dept Med AIDS Clinical Trials Unit Chapel Hill, NC 27599-7030; **Office Phone:** (919) 966-2536; **Board Certifications:** Internal Medicine 1982, Infectious Disease 1986; **Medical School:** Harvard Med Sch 1979; **Residency:** Internal Medicine, Monteifore Hosp, Bronx, NY 1980-1982; **Fellowship:** Infectious Disease, NC Meml Hosp, Chapel Hill, NC 1982-1985; **Faculty Appointment:** Prof Infectious Disease, Univ NC Sch Med

Midwest

Bakken, Johan Septimus MD (Infectious Disease) - *Special Expertise:* *Ehrlichiosis; Tick-borne Diseases;* **Admitting Hospital:** St Mary's Medical Center - Duluth; **Office Address:** St Mary's-Duluth Clin Hlth Sys/ Sec Inf Dis 400 E Third St Duluth, MN 55805; **Office Phone:** (218) 786-3737; **Board Certification:** Internal Medicine 1999; **Medical School:** Univ Wash 1972; **Residencies:** Internal Medicine, Univ Wash Hosp, Seattle, WA 1975-1977; Internal Medicine, Lillehammer Fylkessykehus, Lillehammer,Norway 1978-1981; **Fellowships:** Infectious Disease, Ulleval Hosp, Oslo,Norway 1981-1986; Microbiology, Creighton Univ, Omaha, NE 1986-1988; **Faculty Appointment:** Assoc Prof Family Practice, Univ Minn

Campbell, J William MD (Infectious Disease) - *Special Expertise:* *AIDS/HIV;* **Admitting Hospital:** Barnes - Jewish Hospital; **Office Address:** Grant Med Clin 114 N Taylor Ave St Louis, MO 63108-2102; **Office Phone:** (314) 534-8600; **Board Certifications:** Internal Medicine 1980, Infectious Disease 1982; **Medical School:** Washington Univ, St Louis 1977; **Residency:** Internal Medicine, Barnes Hosp-Wash U, St Louis, MO 1978-1980; **Fellowships:** Infectious Disease, U Texas Hlth Sci Ctr, San Antonio, TX 1980-1981; Infectious Disease, Wash Univ St Louis, St Louis, MO 1981-1982; **Faculty Appointment:** Assoc Clin Prof Medicine, Washington Univ, St Louis

Kazanjian Jr, Powel H MD (Infectious Disease) - *Special Expertise:* *AIDS/HIV;* **Admitting Hospital:** University of Michigan Health Center; **Office Address:** 1500 E Medical Ctr, rm 3120B, Box 0378 Taubman Health Care Ctr Ann Arbor, MI 48109-0378; **Office Phone:** (734) 647-5899; **Board Certifications:** Internal Medicine 1982, Infectious Disease 1986; **Medical School:** Tufts Univ 1979; **Residency:** Internal Medicine, Univ Chicago Hosp, Chicago, IL 1980-1982; **Fellowship:** Infectious Disease, Brigham-Womens Hosp, Boston, MA 1982-1984; **Faculty Appointment:** Assoc Prof Medicine, Univ Mich Med Sch

Maki, Dennis G MD (Infectious Disease) - *Special Expertise:* Urinary Tract Infections; **Admitting Hospital:** University of Wisconsin Hospital & Clinics; **Office Address:** 600 Highland Ave, rm H4, Box 57 Madison, WI 53792; **Office Phone:** (608) 263-0946; **Board Certifications:** Infectious Disease 1974, Critical Care Medicine 1987; **Medical School:** Univ Wisc 1967; **Residencies:** Infectious Disease, Mass Genl Hosp, Boston, MA 1971-1972; Internal Medicine, Harvard-Boston City Hosp, Boston, MA 1972-1973; **Fellowship:** Infectious Disease, Mass Genl Hosp, Boston, MA 1973-1974; **Faculty Appointment:** Prof Medicine, Univ Wisc

Paya, Carlos Vicente MD (Infectious Disease) - *Special Expertise:* AIDS/HIV; *Cytomegalovirus PTLD;* **Admitting Hospital:** Mayo Medical Center & Clinic - Rochester; **Office Address:** Mayo Clinic 200 1st St SW Rochester, MN 55905; **Office Phone:** (507) 284-3747; **Board Certifications:** Internal Medicine 1986, Infectious Disease 1988; **Medical School:** Spain 1981; **Residencies:** Internal Medicine, Hennepin Co Med Ctr, Minneapolis, MN 1983-1984; Internal Medicine, Mayo Grad Sch, Rochester, MN 1984-1986; **Fellowship:** Infectious Disease, Mayo Grad Sch, Rochester, MN 1986; **Faculty Appointment:** Prof Mayo Med Sch

Powderly, William MD (Infectious Disease) - *Special Expertise:* AIDS/HIV; **Admitting Hospital:** Barnes - Jewish Hospital; **Office Address:** 660 S Euclid Ave, Ste 8051 St Louis, MO 63110; **Office Phone:** (314) 362-7601; **Medical School:** Ireland 1979; **Fellowship:** Infectious Disease, Barnes Jewish Hosp, St Louis, MO 1983-1987; **Faculty Appointment:** Prof Medicine, Washington Univ, St Louis

Sobel, Jack MD (Infectious Disease) - *Special Expertise:* Sexually Transmitted Diseases; *Vaginitis;* **Admitting Hospital:** Harper Hospital (Page 59); **Office Address:** Harper Hosp, 4 Brush Ctr 3990 John R St, rm 4811 Detroit, MI 48201; **Office Phone:** (313) 745-7105; **Board Certifications:** Internal Medicine 1978, Infectious Disease 1982; **Medical School:** South Africa 1965; **Residency:** Internal Medicine, S Africa 1966-1970; **Fellowships:** Infectious Disease, Univ Penn Hosps, Philadelphia, PA 1976-1977; Research, Natl Inst Hlth, Bethesda, MD 1977-1978; **Faculty Appointment:** Prof Medicine, Wayne State Univ

Wilson, Walter Ray MD (Infectious Disease) - *Special Expertise:* Musculoskeletal Infections; **Admitting Hospital:** Mayo Medical Center & Clinic - Rochester; **Office Address:** Mayo Clinic 200 1st St SW Rochester, MN 55905; **Office Phone:** (507) 255-7761; **Board Certifications:** Internal Medicine 1973, Infectious Disease 1974; **Medical School:** Baylor Coll Med 1967; **Residencies:** Internal Medicine, Methodist Hosp, Houston, TX 1967-1968; Internal Medicine, Mayo Grad Sch Med, Rochester, MN 1972-1973; **Fellowships:** Infectious Disease, Mayo Grad Sch Med, Rochester, MN 1973-1974; Microbiology, Mayo Grad Sch Med, Rochester, MN 1974-1975; **Faculty Appointment:** Prof Medicine, Mayo Med Sch

Great Plains and Mountains

Cohn, David MD (Infectious Disease) - *Special Expertise:* Tuberculosis; AIDS/HIV; **Admitting Hospital:** Denver Health Medical Center; **Office Address:** Denver Public Health 605 Bannock Street Denver, CO 80204-4507; **Office Phone:** (303) 436-7204; **Board Certifications:** Internal Medicine 1978, Infectious Disease 1982; **Medical School:** Univ IL Coll Med 1975; **Residency:** Internal Medicine, Univ Wisc Hosp, Madison, WI 1976-1978; **Fellowship:** Infectious Disease, Univ Colo Hosp, Denver, CO 1979-1981; **Faculty Appointment:** Prof Medicine, Univ Colo

Southwest

DuPont, Herbert Lancashire MD (Infectious Disease) - *Special Expertise:* Tropical Diseases; Diarrhea; **Admitting Hospital:** St Luke's Episcopal Hospital - Houston (Page 76); **Office Address:** St Luke's Episcopal Hospital 6720 Bertner Ave Houston, TX 77030-1602; **Office Phone:** (713) 791-4122; **Board Certification:** Internal Medicine 1972; **Medical School:** Emory Univ 1965; **Residency:** Internal Medicine, Univ Minn Hosps, Minneapolis, MN 1966-1967; **Fellowship:** Infectious Disease, Univ MD Hosp, Baltimore, MD 1968-1969; **Faculty Appointment:** Prof Medicine, Baylor Coll Med

Keiser, Philip MD (Infectious Disease) - *Special Expertise:* AIDS/HIV; **Admitting Hospital:** Zale Lipshy University Hospital; **Office Address:** Univ TX SW Med Ctr 5323 Harry Hines Blvd, MC-9173 Dallas, TX 75390; **Office Phone:** (214) 648-8942; **Board Certifications:** Internal Medicine 1989, Infectious Disease 1992; **Medical School:** Univ MD Sch Med 1986; **Residency:** Internal Medicine, Francis Scott Key Med Ctr, Baltimore, MD 1986-1989; **Fellowship:** Infectious Disease, Univ Maryland, Baltimore, MD 1989; **Faculty Appointment:** Assoc Prof Medicine, Univ Tex SW, Dallas

Kimbrough, Robert MD (Infectious Disease) - *Special Expertise:* Infectious Disease - General; **Admitting Hospital:** University Medical Center; **Office Address:** Tex Tech U Hlth Scis Ctr Dept IM Div Inf Dis- 3601 4th Street Lubbock, TX 79430; **Office Phone:** (806) 743-3155; **Board Certifications:** Internal Medicine 1977, Infectious Disease 1978; **Medical School:** Univ Kans 1969; **Residency:** Internal Medicine, Baylor Affil Hosp, Houston, TX 1970-1973; **Fellowships:** Infectious Disease, Baylor Univ, Houston, TX 1973-1974; Infectious Disease, Oreg Hlth Sci Univ, Portland, OR 1974-1975; **Faculty Appointment:** Prof Medicine, Texas Tech Univ

Luby, James P MD (Infectious Disease) - *Special Expertise:* Viral Infections; **Admitting Hospital:** Parkland Memorial Hospital; **Office Address:** Univ Tex SW Med Ctr 5323 Hines Blvd Dallas, TX 75235-9113; **Office Phone:** (214) 648-3480; **Board Certifications:** Infectious Disease 1972, Internal Medicine 1968; **Medical School:** Northwestern Univ 1961; **Residency:** Internal Medicine, Northwestern Univ, Chicago, IL 1962-1964; **Faculty Appointment:** Prof Infectious Disease, Univ Tex SW, Dallas

Patterson, Jan E Evans MD (Infectious Disease) - *Special Expertise:* Hospital Infection Control; **Admitting Hospital:** University of Texas Health & Science Center; **Office Address:** Univ of TX, Dept Med 7703 Floyd Curl San Antonio, TX 78229-3900; **Office Phone:** (210) 616-2927; **Board Certifications:** Internal Medicine 1985, Infectious Disease 1988; **Medical School:** Univ Tex, Houston 1982; **Residency:** Internal Medicine, Vanderbilt Univ Hosp, Nashville, TN 1983-1985; **Fellowship:** Infectious Disease, Yale-New Haven Hosp, New Haven, CT 1985-1988; **Faculty Appointment:** Assoc Prof Medicine, Univ Tex, San Antonio

Patterson, Thomas F. MD (Infectious Disease) - *Special Expertise:* AIDS/HIV; **Admitting Hospital:** University of Texas Health & Science Center; **Office Address:** Dept of Medicine 7703 Floyd Curl Drive San Antonio, TX 78229-3900; **Office Phone:** (210) 567-4823; **Board Certifications:** Internal Medicine 1986, Infectious Disease 1988; **Medical School:** Univ Tex, Houston 1983; **Residencies:** Internal Medicine, Vanderbilt Univ Hosp, Nashville, TN 1984-1985; Internal Medicine, Yale-New Haven Hosp, New Haven, CT 1985-1986; **Fellowship:** Infectious Disease, Yale-New Haven Hosp., New Haven, CT 1986-1989; **Faculty Appointment:** Assoc Prof Medicine, Univ Tex, San Antonio

Wallace Jr, Richard James MD (Infectious Disease) - *Special Expertise: AIDS/HIV; Tuberculosis;* **Admitting Hospital:** University of Texas Health & Science Center; **Office Address:** Univ Tex Health Ctr 119 37 US Hwy 271 Tyler, TX 75708; **Office Phone:** (903) 877-7680; **Board Certifications:** Internal Medicine 1975, Infectious Disease 1976; **Medical School:** Baylor Coll Med 1972; **Residency:** Internal Medicine, Boston City Hosp, Boston, MA 1973-1974; **Fellowships:** Infectious Disease, Boston City Hosp, Boston, MA 1974-1975; Infectious Disease, Baylor Coll Med, Houston, TX 1975-1977

West Coast and Pacific

Ballon-Landa, Gonzalo MD (Infectious Disease) - *Special Expertise: Nosocomial Infections; AIDS/HIV;* **Admitting Hospital:** Mercy Hospital & Medical Center - San Diego; **Office Address:** 4136 Bachman Pl San Diego, CA 92103-2028; **Office Phone:** (619) 298-1443; **Board Certifications:** Internal Medicine 1980, Infectious Disease 1984; **Medical School:** Northwestern Univ 1977; **Residency:** Internal Medicine, Evanston Hosp, Evanston, IL 1978-1981; **Fellowship:** Infectious Disease, UCSD Med Ctr, San Diego, CA 1981-1983

Bayer, Arnold Sander MD (Infectious Disease) - *Special Expertise: Infective Endocarditis; Arthritis-Septic; Coccidioidomycosis;* **Admitting Hospital:** LAC - Harbor - UCLA Medical Center; **Office Address:** 1000 W Carson St, Bldg RB2 - Fl 2 Torrance, CA 90502; **Office Phone:** (310) 222-3813; **Board Certifications:** Internal Medicine 1973, Infectious Disease 1978; **Medical School:** Temple Univ 1970; **Residencies:** Internal Medicine, Thomas Jefferson Univ Hosp, Philadelphia, PA 1971-1972; Internal Medicine, LAC-Harbor UCLA Med Ctr, Torrance, CA 1973-1974; **Fellowships:** Infectious Disease, Veterans Affairs Med Ctr, Los Angeles, CA 1975-1976; Infectious Disease, LAC-Harbor UCLA Med Ctr, Torrance, CA 1974-1977; **Faculty Appointment:** Prof Medicine, UCLA

Edwards Jr., John Ellis MD (Infectious Disease) - *Special Expertise: Fungal Infections; Infections in Immune Deficient;* **Admitting Hospital:** LAC - Harbor - UCLA Medical Center; **Office Address:** Harbor-UCLA Med Ctr-Infectious Diseases 1124 W Carson St, Fl RB2 Torrance, CA 90509; **Office Phone:** (310) 222-3813; **Board Certifications:** Internal Medicine 1980, Infectious Disease 1974; **Medical School:** UC Irvine 1968; **Residency:** Internal Medicine, Harbor-UCLA Med Ctr, Los Angeles, CA 1969-1971; **Fellowship:** Infectious Disease, Harbor-UCLA Med Ctr, Los Angeles, CA 1971-1973; **Faculty Appointment:** Prof Medicine, UCLA

Hollander, Harry MD (Infectious Disease) - *Special Expertise: AIDS/HIV;* **Admitting Hospital:** University of California - San Francisco Medical Center; **Office Address:** 400 Parnassus Ave San Francisco, CA 94113; **Office Phone:** (415) 353-2119; **Board Certifications:** Internal Medicine 1983, Infectious Disease 1988; **Medical School:** Univ Penn 1980; **Residency:** Internal Medicine, UCSF Med Ctr, San Francisco, CA 1981-1983; **Faculty Appointment:** Clin Prof Medicine, UCSF

Holmes, King K MD (Infectious Disease) - *Special Expertise: AIDS/HIV; Sexually Transmitted Diseases;* **Admitting Hospital:** University of Washington Medical Center; **Office Address:** Harborview Medical Center 325 Ninth Ave Seattle, WA 98104; **Office Phone:** (206) 731-3000; **Board Certifications:** Internal Medicine 1971, Infectious Disease 1974; **Medical School:** Cornell Univ-Weil Med Coll 1963; **Residency:** Internal Medicine, Univ Wash Med Ctr, Seattle, WA 1967-1969; **Fellowship:** Infectious Disease, Univ Wash Med Ctr, Seattle, WA 1969-1970; **Faculty Appointment:** Prof Medicine, Univ Wash

Richman, Douglas MD (Infectious Disease) - *Special Expertise:* AIDS/HIV; **Admitting Hospital:** University of California - San Diego Healthcare; **Office Address:** UCSD, Dept Path & Med 9500 Gilman Dr La Jolla, CA 92093-0679; **Office Phone:** 858 5527439; **Board Certifications:** Internal Medicine 1973, Infectious Disease 1976; **Medical School:** Stanford Univ 1970; **Residency:** Infectious Disease, Stanford Univ Hosp, Stanford, CA 1971-1972; **Fellowships:** Infectious Disease, NIAID/NIH, Bethdesda, MD 1972-1975; Infectious Disease, Beth Israel Deaconess Med Ctr, Boston, MA 1975-1976; **Faculty Appointment:** Prof Medicine, UCSD

Wiviott, Lory David MD (Infectious Disease) - *Special Expertise:* AIDS/HIV; **Admitting Hospital:** California Pacific Medical Center; **Office Address:** Infectious Disease 2100 Webster St S, Ste 404 San Francisco, CA 94115; **Office Phone:** (415) 923-3883; **Board Certifications:** Internal Medicine 1986, Infectious Disease 1990; **Medical School:** Albert Einstein Coll Med 1982; **Residency:** Internal Medicine, Columbia Presby Med Ctr, New York, NY 1982-1985; **Fellowship:** Infectious Disease, UCSF Med Ctr, San Francisco, CA 1986-1989; **Faculty Appointment:** Asst Clin Prof Medicine, UCSF

Yoshikawa, Thomas T MD (Infectious Disease) - *Special Expertise:* Geriatric Infectious Disease; **Admitting Hospital:** LAC - King/Drew Medical Center; **Office Address:** 12021 S Wilmington Ave, rm MLK 4015 Los Angeles, CA 90059; **Office Phone:** (310) 668-4574; **Board Certifications:** Internal Medicine 1971, Infectious Disease 1974; **Medical School:** Univ Mich Med Sch 1966; **Residency:** Internal Medicine, Harbor Genl Hosp, Torrance, CA 1967-1970; **Fellowship:** Infectious Disease, Harbor Genl Hosp, Torrance, CA 1972; **Faculty Appointment:** Prof Medicine, Charles Drew Univ Med & Sci

INTERNAL MEDICINE

A personal physician who provides long-term, comprehensive care in the office and the hospital, managing both common and complex illness of adolescents, adults and the elderly. Internists are trained in the diagnosis and treatment of cancer, infections and diseases affecting the heart, blood, kidneys, joints and digestive, respiratory and vascular systems. They are also trained in the essentials of primary care internal medicine which incorporates an understanding of disease prevention, wellness, substance abuse, mental health and effective treatment of common problems of the eyes, ears, skin, nervous system and reproductive organs.

Training required: Three years

PHYSICIAN LISTINGS

Internal Medicine

New England

Barry, Michele MD (Internal Medicine) - *Special Expertise:* Travel Medicine; **Admitting Hospital:** Yale - New Haven Hospital; **Office Address:** 333 Cedar St PO BOX 208025 New Haven, CT 06520-8025; **Office Phone:** (203) 688-2476; **Board Certification:** Internal Medicine 1980; **Medical School:** Albert Einstein Coll Med 1977; **Residency:** Yale-New H, New Haven, CT 1978-1981; **Fellowships:** Rheumatology, Yale-New H, New Haven, CT 1980-1981; Walter Reed AMC, Washington, DC 1981; **Faculty Appointment:** Prof Medicine, Yale Univ

Beaser, Richard Seth MD (Internal Medicine) - *Special Expertise:* Diabetes; **Admitting Hospital:** Beth Israel Deaconess Medical Center - Boston (Page 57); **Office Address:** Joslin Diabetes Med Ctr 1 Joslin Pl Boston, MA 02215-5397; **Office Phone:** (617) 732-2665; **Board Certification:** Internal Medicine 1980; **Medical School:** Boston Univ 1977; **Residency:** Internal Medicine, Mass Med Ctr, Boston, MA 1978-1980; **Fellowship:** Endocrinology, Diabetes & Metabolism, Joslin Clinic, Boston, MA 1980-1981; **Faculty Appointment:** Asst Clin Prof Medicine, Harvard Med Sch

Horwitz, Ralph MD (Internal Medicine) - *Special Expertise:* Internal Medicine - General; **Admitting Hospital:** Yale - New Haven Hospital; **Office Address:** Yale Faculty Practice 333 Cedar St New Haven, CT 06520; **Office Phone:** (203) 785-4119; **Board Certification:** Internal Medicine 1976; **Medical School:** Penn State Univ-Hershey Med Ctr 1973; **Residencies:** Internal Medicine, Royal Victoria Hosp-McGill, Montreal, Canada 1974-1975; Internal Medicine, Mass Gen Hosp, Boston, MA 1977-1978; **Fellowship:** Epidemiology, Yale-New Haven Hosp, New Haven, CT 1975-1977; **Faculty Appointment:** Prof Medicine, Yale Univ

Robinson, Dwight R. MD (Internal Medicine) - *Special Expertise:* Arthritis; **Admitting Hospital:** Massachusetts General Hospital; **Office Address:** Mass Genl Hospital WACC 730 Boston, MA 02114; **Office Phone:** (617) 726-7938; **Board Certification:** Internal Medicine 1968; **Medical School:** Columbia P&S 1957; **Residencies:** Surgery, Mass Genl Hosp, Boston, MA 1958-1959; Internal Medicine, Mass Genl Hosp, Boston, MA 1960-1961; **Fellowships:** Research, Mass Genl Hosp, Boston, MA 1959-1960; Biochemistry, Brandeis Univ, Waltham, MA 1964; **Faculty Appointment:** Prof Medicine, Harvard Med Sch

Wood, Lawrence Crane MD (Internal Medicine) - *Special Expertise:* Thyroid Disorders; **Admitting Hospital:** Massachusetts General Hospital; **Office Address:** Massachusetts General Hospital 15 Parkman St, WACC 645 Boston, MA 02114; **Office Phone:** (617) 726-2377; **Board Certification:** Internal Medicine 1970; **Medical School:** Univ Penn 1961; **Residency:** Internal Medicine, Univ Va Hosp, Charlottesville, VA 1962-1964; **Fellowships:** Endocrinology, Univ Va Hosp, Charlottesville, VA 1964-1965; Endocrinology, Boston City Hosp, Charlottesville, MA 1968-1970; **Faculty Appointment:** Clin Inst Medicine, Harvard Med Sch

Mid Atlantic

Braunstein, Seth N MD/PhD (Internal Medicine) - *Special Expertise:* Diabetes; **Admitting Hospital:** Hospital of the University of Pennsylvania; **Office Address:** Hosp of Univ Penn, Diabetes Ctr 3400 Spuce St, Ste I Philadelphia, PA 19104-4219; **Office Phone:** (215) 662-7280; **Board Certification:** Internal Medicine 1975; **Medical School:** NYU Sch Med 1972; **Residency:** Internal Medicine, Univ Penn Hosp, Philadelphia, PA 1972-1975; **Faculty Appointment:** Assoc Prof Medicine, Univ Penn

Cirigliano, Michael MD (Internal Medicine) - *Special Expertise:* Alternative Medicine; **Admitting Hospital:** Hospital of the University of Pennsylvania; **Office Address:** Univ Pa Clinical Practices 3400 Sruce St, 9 Penn Tower Philadelphia, PA 19104; **Office Phone:** (215) 662-3400; **Board Certification:** Internal Medicine 1994; **Medical School:** Univ Penn 1990; **Residency:** Internal Medicine, Hosp Univ Penn, Philadelphia, PA 1990-1993; **Faculty Appointment:** Asst Prof Medicine, Univ Penn

Fisher, Laura MD (Internal Medicine) - *Special Expertise:* Lyme Disease; Travel Medicine; **Admitting Hospital:** New York Weill Cornell Medical Center - NY Presbyterian Hospital (Page 72); **Office Address:** 1385 York Ave New York, NY 10021-6305; **Office Phone:** (212) 717-5920; **Board Certifications:** Internal Medicine 1987, Infectious Disease 1990; **Medical School:** Brown Univ 1984; **Residency:** Internal Medicine, NY Hosp-Cornell Med Ctr, New York, NY 1984-1987; **Fellowship:** Infectious Disease, Mass Gen Hosp, Boston, MA 1987-1989; **Faculty Appointment:** Asst Clin Prof Medicine, Cornell Univ-Weil Med Coll

Gitlow, Stanley MD (Internal Medicine) - *Special Expertise:* Internal Medicine - General; **Admitting Hospital:** Mount Sinai Hospital (Page 70); **Office Address:** 1107 5th Ave New York, NY 10128; **Office Phone:** (212) 722-5731; **Board Certification:** Internal Medicine 1977; **Medical School:** SUNY Hlth Sci Ctr 1948; **Residencies:** Internal Medicine, Bronx VA Hosp, Bronx, NY 1949-1950; Internal Medicine, Mount Sinai Hosp, New York, NY 1951-1952; **Faculty Appointment:** Clin Prof Medicine, Mount Sinai Sch Med

Nash, Thomas MD (Internal Medicine) - *Special Expertise:* Asthma; **Admitting Hospital:** New York Weill Cornell Medical Center - NY Presbyterian Hospital (Page 72); **Office Address:** 310 E 72nd St New York, NY 10021; **Office Phone:** (212) 734-6612; **Board Certifications:** Pulmonary Disease 1985, Infectious Disease 1984; **Medical School:** NYU Sch Med 1978; **Residency:** Internal Medicine, NY Hosp-Cornell, New York, NY 1978-1981; **Fellowships:** Infectious Disease, NY Hosp-Cornell, New York, NY 1981-1985; Pulmonary Disease, Meml Sloan Kettering, New York, NY 1981-1985; **Faculty Appointment:** Assoc Clin Prof Medicine, NYU Sch Med

Selwyn, Peter MD (Internal Medicine) - *Special Expertise:* AIDS/HIV; Addiction; Palliative Care; **Admitting Hospital:** Montefiore Medical Center; **Office Address:** Montefiore Med Ctr 3544 Jerome Ave, Ste 2 Bronx, NY 10467; **Office Phone:** (718) 920-4678; **Board Certification:** Family Practice 1998; **Medical School:** Harvard Med Sch 1981; **Residency:** Family Practice, Montefiore Hosp, Bronx, NY 1981-1984; **Faculty Appointment:** Prof Medicine, NY Med Coll

Seremetis, Stephanie MD (Internal Medicine) - *Special Expertise:* Hemophilia/Bleeding Disorders; Women's Health; **Admitting Hospital:** Mount Sinai Hospital (Page 70); **Office Address:** Mt Sinai Medical Center 5 E 98th St New York, NY 10029; **Office Phone:** (212) 241-8818; **Board Certifications:** Internal Medicine 1982, Hematology 1988; **Medical School:** SUNY Hlth Sci Ctr 1978; **Residency:** Internal Medicine, Mount Sinai Med Ctr, New York, NY 1979-1981; **Fellowship:** Hematology, Mount Sinai Med Ctr, New York, NY 1981-1983; **Faculty Appointment:** Assoc Prof Medicine, Mount Sinai Sch Med

Yaffe, Bruce MD (Internal Medicine) - *Special Expertise:* Gastroscopy; Colonoscopy; **Admitting Hospital:** Lenox Hill Hospital; **Office Address:** 201 E 65th St New York, NY 10021; **Office Phone:** (212) 879-4700; **Board Certifications:** Internal Medicine 1979, Gastroenterology 1981; **Medical School:** Geo Wash Univ 1976; **Residencies:** Internal Medicine, Mount Sinai Hosp, New York, NY 1977-1979; Hepatology, Mount Sinai Hosp, New York, NY 1979-1980; **Fellowship:** Gastroenterology, Lenox Hill Hosp, New York, NY 1980-1982

Southeast

Carey, Timothy Stephen MD (Internal Medicine) - *Special Expertise:* Internal Medicine - General; **Admitting Hospital:** University of North Carolina Hospitals; **Office Address:** University of North Carolina 5039 Old Clinic Building, Box 7110 Chapel Hill, NC 27599; **Office Phone:** (919) 966-2276; **Board Certification:** Internal Medicine 1979; **Medical School:** Univ VT Coll Med 1976; **Residency:** Internal Medicine, Pacific Med Ctr, San Francisco, CA 1976-1979; **Fellowship:** Internal Medicine, Univ NC Hosp, Chapel Hill, NC 1983-1985; **Faculty Appointment:** Prof Medicine, Univ NC Sch Med

Corbett Jr, Eugene Charles MD (Internal Medicine) - *Special Expertise:* Nutrition; Diabetes; **Admitting Hospital:** University of Virginia Health Systems; **Office Address:** University of Virginia Health Sciences Center Box 800744 Charlottesville, VA 22908; **Office Phone:** (804) 924-1685; **Board Certification:** Internal Medicine 1987; **Medical School:** Univ Chicago-Pritzker Sch Med 1970; **Residency:** Internal Medicine, Baltimore City Hosp, Baltimore, MD 1973-1975; **Fellowship:** Johns Hopkins, Baltimore, MD 1973-1975; **Faculty Appointment:** Asst Prof Medicine, Univ VA Sch Med

Eustace, John C MD (Internal Medicine) - *Special Expertise:* Addiction; **Admitting Hospital:** Mount Sinai Medical Center; **Office Address:** 4300 Alton Rd, FL 6 Miami, FL 33140; **Office Phone:** (305) 674-2932; **Board Certification:** Internal Medicine 1978; **Medical School:** Univ Miami Sch Med 1974; **Residency:** Internal Medicine, Univ Miami-Jackson Meml Hosp, Miami, FL 1975-1978

Schaberg, Dennis Ray MD (Internal Medicine) - *Special Expertise:* Staphylococcal Infections; **Admitting Hospital:** University of Tennessee Bowld Hospital; **Office Address:** Univ Tenn 956 Court Ave, rm D334 Memphis, TN 38163; **Office Phone:** (901) 448-5752; **Board Certification:** Internal Medicine 1978; **Medical School:** Univ MO-Columbia Sch Med 1972; **Residencies:** Internal Medicine, Harborview Med Ctr, Seattle, WA 1972-1974; Preventive Medicine, Ctrs For Disease Ctrl, Atlanta, GA 1975-1977; **Fellowship:** Infectious Disease, Univ Wash, Seattle, WA 1978-1979; **Faculty Appointment:** Prof Medicine, Univ Tenn Coll Med, Memphis

Vance, Mary Lee MD (Internal Medicine) - *Special Expertise:* Pituitary Disorders; Adrenal Tumors; **Admitting Hospital:** University of Virginia Health Systems; **Office Address:** UVA Health Systems 5840 Hospital Drive, Box 800601 Charlottesville, VA 22908-0601; **Office Phone:** (804) 924-2284; **Board Certification:** Internal Medicine 1980; **Medical School:** Louisiana State Univ 1977; **Residency:** Internal Medicine, Baylor Univ Med Ctr, Dallas, TX 1978-1980; **Fellowship:** Endocrinology, Diabetes & Metabolism, Univ Virginia Med Ctr, Charlottesville, VA 1980-1983; **Faculty Appointment:** Prof Medicine, Univ VA Sch Med

Midwest

Esch, Peter MD (Internal Medicine) - *Special Expertise:* Geriatric Medicine; **Admitting Hospital:** Cleveland Clinic Foundation; **Office Address:** 5700 Cooper Foster Park Rd Lorain, OH 44053; **Office Phone:** (440) 366-8822; **Board Certifications:** Internal Medicine 1977, Geriatric Medicine 1994; **Medical School:** Case West Res Univ 1974; **Residency:** Internal Medicine, Hennepin Co Med Ctr, Minneapolis, MN 1974-1977

Messer, Joseph V MD (Internal Medicine) - *Special Expertise:* Coronary Artery Disease; Congestive Heart Failure; **Admitting Hospital:** Rush/Presbyterian - St Luke's Medical Center - Chicago (Page 74); **Office Address:** Associates in Cardioloy Ltd 1725 W Harrison St, Ste 1138 Chicago, IL 60612; **Office Phone:** (312) 243-6800; **Board Certification:** Internal Medicine 1972; **Medical School:** Harvard Med Sch 1956; **Residencies:** Internal Medicine, Peter Bent Brigham, Boston, MA 1957-1958; Internal Medicine, Peter Bent Brigham, Boston, MA 1960-1961; **Fellowships:** Cardiology (Cardiovascular Disease), Peter Bent Brigham, Boston, MA 1958-1960; Brandeis University 1963-1964; **Faculty Appointment:** Prof Medicine, Rush Med Coll

Pierach, Claus MD (Internal Medicine) - *Special Expertise:* Porphyria; **Admitting Hospital:** Abbott - Northwestern Hospital; **Office Address:** Abbott-Northwestern Hospital 800 E 28th St, MC-11135 Minneapolis, MN 55407; **Office Phone:** (612) 863-4342; **Medical School:** Germany 1959

Sarosi, George MD (Internal Medicine) - *Special Expertise:* Infection-Respiratory; Fungal Lung Disease; Diagnostic Problems; **Admitting Hospital:** Veterans Affairs Medical Center - Indianapolis; **Office Address:** Indiannapolis VA Med Ctr 1481 W 10th St, MC-111 Indianapolis, IN 46202; **Office Phone:** (317) 554-0181; **Board Certification:** Internal Medicine 1970; **Medical School:** Harvard Med Sch 1964; **Residency:** Internal Medicine, Univ. of Minn, Minneapolis, MN 1965-1968; **Faculty Appointment:** Prof Medicine, Indiana Univ

Schwartz, Gary Lee MD (Internal Medicine) - *Special Expertise:* Hypertension; Hypotension; **Admitting Hospital:** Mayo Medical Center & Clinic - Rochester; **Office Address:** Mayo Clinic 200 1st St SW Rochester, MN 55905; **Office Phone:** (507) 284-2511; **Board Certifications:** Internal Medicine 1980, Nephrology 1982; **Medical School:** Univ Wisc 1977; **Residencies:** Internal Medicine, Mayo Clinic, Rochester, MN 1977-1980; Nephrology, Mayo Clinic, Rochester, MN 1980-1982; **Faculty Appointment:** Asst Clin Prof Medicine, Mayo Med Sch

Shore, Bernard L MD (Internal Medicine) - *Special Expertise:* Pulmonary Disease; **Admitting Hospital:** Barnes - Jewish Hospital; **Office Address:** Maryland Med Group 4652 Maryland Ave St Louis, MO 63108-1913; **Office Phone:** (314) 367-3113; **Board Certifications:** Internal Medicine 1980, Pulmonary Disease 1982; **Medical School:** Washington Univ, St Louis 1977; **Residency:** Internal Medicine, Barnes Hosp, St Louis, MO 1978-1980; **Fellowship:** Pulmonary Disease, Wash Univ Med Ctr, St Louis, MO 1980-1982; **Faculty Appointment:** Assoc Clin Prof Medicine, Washington Univ, St Louis

Weder, Alan B MD (Internal Medicine) - *Special Expertise:* Hypertension; Vascular Medicine; **Admitting Hospital:** University of Michigan Health Center; **Office Address:** Taubman Hlth Care Ctr 1500 E Medical Ctr Dr Ann Arbor, MI 48109-0356; **Office Phone:** (734) 647-9342; **Board Certification:** Internal Medicine 1978; **Medical School:** Hahnemann Univ 1975; **Residency:** Internal Medicine, Univ of Chicago Hosp, Chicago, IL 1976-1978; **Faculty Appointment:** Prof Medicine, Univ Mich Med Sch

Great Plains and Mountains

Schooley, Robert Turner MD (Internal Medicine) - *Special Expertise:* AIDS/HIV; **Admitting Hospital:** University of Colorado Health & Science Center; **Office Address:** U Colo Hlth Scis Ctr 4200 E Ninth Ave Denver, CO 80262; **Office Phone:** (303) 372-0000; **Board Certification:** Internal Medicine 1977; **Medical School:** Johns Hopkins Univ 1974; **Residency:** Internal Medicine, Johns Hopkins Univ Hospital, Baltimore, MD 1975-1976; **Fellowship:** Infectious Disease, NIH/Mass. General Hospital, Boston, MA 1976-1981; **Faculty Appointment:** Prof Medicine, Univ Colo

Southwest

De Fronzo, Ralph Anthony MD (Internal Medicine) - *Special Expertise:* Diabetes; **Admitting Hospital:** University of Texas Health & Science Center; **Office Address:** U Tex Hlth Sci Ctr, Diabetes Div 7703 Floyd Curl Dr San Antonio, TX 78229-3900; **Office Phone:** (210) 567-6691; **Board Certifications:** Internal Medicine 1975, Nephrology 1976; **Medical School:** Harvard Med Sch 1969; **Residency:** Internal Medicine, Johns Hopkins Hosp, Baltimore, MD 1970-1971; **Fellowships:** Endocrinology, Diabetes & Metabolism, Baltimore City Hosp-NIH, Baltimore, MD 1971-1973; Renal Disease, Hosp Univ Penn, Philadelphia, PA 1973-1975; **Faculty Appointment:** Prof Medicine, Univ Tex, San Antonio

Graybill, John Richard MD (Internal Medicine) - *Special Expertise:* Fungal Infections; *Infectious Disease;* **Admitting Hospital:** University of Texas Health & Science Center; **Office Address:** VA Hosp rm E-703 San Antonio, TX 78284; **Office Phone:** (210) 617-5111; **Board Certification:** Internal Medicine 1972; **Medical School:** Cornell Univ-Weil Med Coll 1966; **Residency:** Internal Medicine, Vanderbilt Univ Hosp, Nashville, TN 1967-1969; **Fellowship:** Infectious Disease, Johns Hopkins Hosp, Baltimore, MD 1969-1970; **Faculty Appointment:** Prof Medicine, Univ Tex, San Antonio

West Coast and Pacific

Bissell Jr, Dwight Montgomery MD (Internal Medicine) - *Special Expertise:* Porphyria; **Admitting Hospital:** University of California - San Francisco Medical Center; **Office Address:** UCSF Med Ctr-Dept Gastroenterology 513 Parnassus Ave, rm S357 San Fransisco, CA 94143-0538; **Office Phone:** (415) 476-5072; **Board Certification:** Internal Medicine 1974; **Medical School:** Harvard Med Sch 1967; **Residency:** Internal Medicine, Boston City Hosp-Harvard, Boston, MA 1968-1970; **Fellowship:** Gastroenterology, UCSF Med Ctr, San Francisco, CA 1970-1973; **Faculty Appointment:** Prof Medicine, UCSF

Roth, Bennett E MD (Internal Medicine) - *Special Expertise:* Gastroesophageal Reflux; *Inflammatory Bowel Disease; Irritable Bowel Syndrome;* **Admitting Hospital:** UCLA Medical Center; **Office Address:** 2701 W Alameda Ave, Bldg 404 Burbank, CA 91505-4805; **Office Phone:** (310) 825-6618; **Board Certifications:** Internal Medicine 1972, Gastroenterology 1975; **Medical School:** Hahnemann Univ 1968; **Residency:** Internal Medicine, Univ Penn, Philadelphia, PA 1969-1971; **Fellowship:** Gastroenterology, UCLA Med Ctr, Los Angeles, CA 1973-1974; **Faculty Appointment:** Assoc Prof Medicine, UCLA

Maternal & Fetal Medicine

(a subspecialty of OBSTETRICS AND GYNECOLOGY)

An obstetrician/gynecologist possesses special knowledge, skills and professional capability in the medical and surgical care of the female reproductive system and associated disorders. This physician serves as a consultant to other physicians and as a primary physician for women.

OBSTETRICS & GYNECOLOGY

An obstetrician/gynecologist who cares for, or provides consultation on, patients with complications of pregnancy. This specialist has advanced knowledge of the obstetrical, medical and surgical complications of pregnancy and their effect on both the mother and the fetus. He/she also possesses expertise in the most current diagnostic and treatment modalities used in the care of patients with complicated pregnancies.

Training required: Four years plus two years in clinical practice before certification in obstetrics and gynecology is complete *plus* additional training and examination in maternal-fetal medicine

PHYSICIAN LISTINGS

New England

Acker, David B. MD (Maternal & Fetal Medicine) - *Special Expertise:* Multiple Gestation; Pregnancy-High Risk; **Admitting Hospital:** Brigham & Women's Hospital; **Office Address:** Department of Obstetics and Gynecology 75 Francis St Boston, MA 02115; **Office Phone:** (617) 732-5445; **Board Certifications:** Maternal & Fetal Medicine 1981, Obstetrics & Gynecology 1989; **Medical School:** NYU Sch Med 1968; **Residencies:** Vanderbilt U Affil Hosp., Nashville, TN 1973-1974; Einstein Affil Hosp., Bronx, NY 1969-1971; **Fellowship:** Boston Lying-In Hosp., Boston, MA 1977-1979; **Faculty Appointment:** Asst Prof Obstetrics & Gynecology, Harvard Med Sch

Copel, Joshua MD (Maternal & Fetal Medicine) - *Special Expertise:* Maternal & Fetal Medicine - General; **Admitting Hospital:** Yale - New Haven Hospital; **Office Address:** Yale Univ Sch Med Dept OB-GYN New Haven, CT 06520-8063; **Office Phone:** (203) 785-2671; **Board Certifications:** Obstetrics & Gynecology 1986, Maternal & Fetal Medicine 1988; **Medical School:** Tufts Univ 1979; **Residency:** Obstetrics & Gynecology, Penn Hosp, Philadelphia, PA 1980-1983; **Fellowship:** Maternal & Fetal Medicine, Yale-New Haven Hosp, New Haven, CT 1983-1985; **Faculty Appointment:** Prof Obstetrics & Gynecology, Yale Univ

Frigoletto Jr., Fredric D. MD (Maternal & Fetal Medicine) - *Special Expertise:* Maternal & Fetal Medicine - General; **Admitting Hospital:** Massachusetts General Hospital; **Office Address:** Mass General Hosp. 32 Fruit St Boston, MA 02114; **Office Phone:** (617) 724-3775; **Board Certifications:** Maternal & Fetal Medicine 1975, Obstetrics & Gynecology 1969; **Medical School:** Boston Univ 1962; **Residencies:** Obstetrics & Gynecology, Boston Womens Hosp., Boston, MA 1964-1967; Surgery, Boston City Hosp., Boston, MA 1963-1964; **Faculty Appointment:** Prof Obstetrics & Gynecology, Harvard Med Sch

Greene, Michael F. MD (Maternal & Fetal Medicine) - *Special Expertise:* Pregnancy-High Risk; Multiple Gestation; Seizure Disorders-Pregnancy; **Admitting Hospital:** Massachusetts General Hospital; **Office Address:** Mass General Hosp 32 Fruit St, Bldg Blake-10 Boston, MA 02114; **Office Phone:** (617) 724-2229; **Board Certifications:** Obstetrics & Gynecology 1997, Maternal & Fetal Medicine 1997; **Medical School:** SUNY Downstate 1976; **Residency:** Obstetrics & Gynecology, Boston Womens Hosp, Boston, MA 1977-1980; **Fellowship:** Maternal & Fetal Medicine, Brigham Womens Hosp, Boston, MA 1980-1982; **Faculty Appointment:** Assoc Prof Obstetrics & Gynecology, Harvard Med Sch

Heffner, Linda MD/PhD (Maternal & Fetal Medicine) - *Special Expertise:* Pregnancy-High Risk; **Admitting Hospital:** Brigham & Women's Hospital; **Office Address:** Brigham and Womens Hosp-Dept OB/GYN 75 Francis St. Boston, MA 02115; **Office Phone:** (617) 732-4840; **Board Certifications:** Maternal & Fetal Medicine 1998, Obstetrics & Gynecology 1998; **Medical School:** Johns Hopkins Univ 1977; **Residency:** Obstetrics & Gynecology, Hosp Univ Penn, Philadelphia, PA 1980-1983; **Fellowship:** Maternal & Fetal Medicine, Brigham-Womens Hosp., Boston, MA 1985; **Faculty Appointment:** Assoc Prof Obstetrics & Gynecology, Harvard Med Sch

Mid Atlantic

Bardeguez-Brown, Arlene D MD (Maternal & Fetal Medicine) - *Special Expertise:* AIDS/HIV in Pregnancy; **Admitting Hospital:** UMDNJ-University Hospital-Newark; **Office Address:** University OBGYN Associates 90 Bergen St, Ste 5100 Newark, NJ 07103; **Office Phone:** (973) 972-2700; **Board Certifications:** Obstetrics & Gynecology 1998, Maternal & Fetal Medicine 1998; **Medical School:** Univ Puerto Rico 1981; **Residency:** Obstetrics & Gynecology, Cath Med Ctr, Jamaica, NY 1981-1985; **Fellowship:** Maternal & Fetal Medicine, Nassau Co Med Ctr, East Meadow, NY 1985-1987; **Faculty Appointment:** Assoc Prof Obstetrics & Gynecology, UMDNJ-NJ Med Sch, Newark

Chervenak, Francis Anthony MD (Maternal & Fetal Medicine) - *Special Expertise:*
Ultrasound; Pregnancy-High Risk; **Admitting Hospital:** New York Weill Cornell Medical Center - NY
Presbyterian Hospital (Page 72); **Office Address:** Obstetrics and Gynecology 525 E 68th St, Ste J-
130 New York, NY 10021; **Office Phone:** (212) 746-3184; **Board Certifications:** Obstetrics &
Gynecology 1984, Maternal & Fetal Medicine 1985; **Medical School:** Jefferson Med Coll 1976;
Residencies: Obstetrics & Gynecology, NY Med Coll-Flower Fifth Ave Hosp, New York, NY 1977-
1979; Obstetrics & Gynecology, St Lukes Hosp, New York, NY 1979-1981; **Fellowship:** Maternal &
Fetal Medicine, Yale-New Haven Hosp, New Haven, CT 1981-1983; **Faculty Appointment:** Prof
Obstetrics & Gynecology, Cornell Univ-Weil Med Coll

Collea, Joseph Vincent MD (Maternal & Fetal Medicine) - *Special Expertise:* Breech Birth;
Multiple Gestation; **Admitting Hospital:** Georgetown University Hospital; **Office Address:** GUMC -
Pasquerilla Healthcare Center, 3rd Floor 3800 Reservoir Rd NW Washington, DC 20007-2194;
Office Phone: (202) 687-8531; **Board Certifications:** Obstetrics & Gynecology 1974, Maternal &
Fetal Medicine 1981; **Medical School:** SUNY Syracuse 1966; **Residency:** Obstetrics &
Gynecology, John Hopkins Hospital, Baltimore, MD 1967-1972; **Fellowship:** LA CO USC Medical
Center 1974-1976; **Faculty Appointment:** Prof Obstetrics & Gynecology, Georgetown Univ

D'Alton, Mary Elizabeth MD (Maternal & Fetal Medicine) - *Special Expertise:* Pregnancy-
High Risk; Multiple Gestation; **Admitting Hospital:** Columbia Presbyterian Medical Center (Page
72); **Office Address:** Columbia Presbyterian 622 W 168th St, Bldg PH16-64 New York, NY 10032;
Office Phone: (212) 305-6293; **Board Certifications:** Obstetrics & Gynecology 1997, Maternal &
Fetal Medicine 1997; **Medical School:** Ireland 1976; **Residency:** Obstetrics & Gynecology, Univ
Ottawa, Ontario, Canada 1977-1982; **Fellowship:** Obstetrics & Gynecology, Tufts-New England
Med Ctr, Boston, MA 1982-1984; **Faculty Appointment:** Clin Prof Obstetrics & Gynecology, Coll
Physicians & Surgeons

Fox, Harold E MD/PhD (Maternal & Fetal Medicine) - *Special Expertise:* Pregnancy-High
Risk; **Admitting Hospital:** Johns Hopkins Hospital - Baltimore (Page 65); **Office Address:** Johns
Hopkins Hosp, Dept ObGyn 600 N Wolfe St Baltimore, MD 21287; **Office Phone:** (410) 614-0178;
Board Certifications: Obstetrics & Gynecology 1994, Maternal & Fetal Medicine 1981; **Medical
School:** Univ Rochester 1972; **Residency:** Obstetrics & Gynecology, Strong Meml Hosp,
Rochester, NY 1973-1975; **Fellowship:** Maternal & Fetal Medicine, Univ Rochester Hosps,
Rochester, NY 1975-1977; **Faculty Appointment:** Prof Obstetrics & Gynecology, Johns Hopkins
Univ

Landers, Daniel V. MD (Maternal & Fetal Medicine) - *Special Expertise:* Reproductive
Infectious Disease; **Admitting Hospital:** Magee Women's Hospital; **Office Address:** Magee
Women's Hosp, Dept OB/GYN 300 Halket Street, rm 2336 Pittsburgh, PA 15213; **Office Phone:**
(412) 641-6253; **Board Certifications:** Obstetrics & Gynecology 1989, Maternal & Fetal Medicine
1991; **Medical School:** UCSF 1980; **Residency:** Obstetrics & Gynecology, UCSF Med Ctr, San
Francisco, CA 1980-1984; **Fellowships:** Maternal & Fetal Medicine, UCSF Med Ctr, San Francisco,
CA 1984-1986; Infectious Disease, San Francisco General Hospital, San Francisco, CA 1986-1988;
Faculty Appointment: Prof Obstetrics & Gynecology, Univ Pittsburgh

Landy, Helain Jody MD (Maternal & Fetal Medicine) - *Special Expertise:* Genetic
Disorders; Miscarriage-Recurrent; **Admitting Hospital:** Georgetown University Hospital; **Office
Address:** GUMC-Pasquerilla Healthcare Ctr 3800 Reservoir Rd NW, Bldg PHC - rm 3 Washington,
DC 20007; **Office Phone:** (202) 687-8531; **Board Certifications:** Obstetrics & Gynecology 1998,
Maternal & Fetal Medicine 1998; **Medical School:** Northwestern Univ 1982; **Residency:** Obstetrics
& Gynecology, Penn Hosp, Philadelphia, PA 1982-1986; **Fellowship:** Maternal & Fetal Medicine,
George Washington Univ Med Ctr, Washington, DC 1986-1988; **Faculty Appointment:** Assoc Prof
Obstetrics & Gynecology, Georgetown Univ

Lockwood, Charles MD (Maternal & Fetal Medicine) - *Special Expertise:* *Thrombosis/Hemostasis in Pregnancy; Pregnancy-High Risk;* **Admitting Hospital:** NYU Medical Center (Page 70); **Office Address:** 550 1st Ave, Ste 7N New York, NY 10016; **Office Phone:** (212) 263-8033; **Board Certifications:** Obstetrics & Gynecology 1988, Maternal & Fetal Medicine 1989; **Medical School:** Univ Penn 1981; **Residency:** Obstetrics & Gynecology, Hosp of Univ Penn, Philadelphia, PA 1981-1985; **Fellowship:** Maternal & Fetal Medicine, Yale-New Haven Hosp, New Haven, CT 1985-1987; **Faculty Appointment:** Prof Obstetrics & Gynecology, NYU Sch Med

Mennuti, Michael MD (Maternal & Fetal Medicine) - *Special Expertise:* *Congenital Abnormalities; Pregnancy-High Risk;* **Admitting Hospital:** Hospital of the University of Pennsylvania; **Office Address:** Univ Penn Hosp, Dept OB/GYN 3400 Spruce St Philadelphia, PA 19104-4204; **Office Phone:** (215) 662-3234; **Board Certifications:** Maternal & Fetal Medicine 1975, Clinical Genetics 1982; **Medical School:** Georgetown Univ 1968; **Residency:** Obstetrics & Gynecology, Hosp Univ Penn, Philadelphia, PA 1969-1973; **Fellowships:** Maternal & Fetal Medicine, Hosp Univ Penn, Philadelphia, PA 1975-1978; Clinical Genetics, Hosp Univ Penn, Philadelphia, PA; **Faculty Appointment:** Prof Obstetrics & Gynecology, Univ Penn

Nagey, David Augustus MD (Maternal & Fetal Medicine) - *Special Expertise:* *Maternal & Fetal Medicine - General;* **Admitting Hospital:** Johns Hopkins Hospital - Baltimore (Page 65); **Office Address:** Dept OB-GYN 600 N Wolfe St Baltimore, MD 21287-1228; **Office Phone:** (410) 955-6700; **Board Certifications:** Obstetrics & Gynecology 1991, Maternal & Fetal Medicine 1984; **Medical School:** Duke Univ 1975; **Residency:** Obstetrics & Gynecology, Duke Univ Med Ctr, Durham, NC 1975-1979; **Fellowship:** Maternal & Fetal Medicine, Duke Univ Med Ctr, Durham, NC 1979-1981; **Faculty Appointment:** Assoc Prof Obstetrics & Gynecology, Johns Hopkins Univ

Wapner, Ronald MD (Maternal & Fetal Medicine) - *Special Expertise:* *Perinatal Medicine;* **Admitting Hospital:** Thomas Jefferson University Hospital; **Office Address:** Thomas Jefferson Univ Hosp, Dept OB/GYN 834 Chestnut St, Ste 400 Philadelphia, PA 19107-5001; **Office Phone:** (215) 955-7996; **Board Certifications:** Obstetrics & Gynecology 1978, Maternal & Fetal Medicine 1981; **Medical School:** Jefferson Med Coll 1972; **Residency:** Obstetrics & Gynecology, Jefferson Med Coll, Philadelphia, PA 1972-1976; **Fellowship:** Maternal & Fetal Medicine, Jefferson Med Coll, Philadelphia, PA 1976-1978; **Faculty Appointment:** Prof Obstetrics & Gynecology, Jefferson Med Coll

Southeast

Boehm, Frank Henry MD (Maternal & Fetal Medicine) - *Special Expertise:* *Pregnancy-High Risk;* **Admitting Hospital:** Vanderbilt University Medical Center; **Office Address:** Vanderbilt Univ Med Ctr Dept ObGyn, rm B-1100 Nashville, TN 37232-2519; **Office Phone:** (615) 322-2071; **Board Certifications:** Obstetrics & Gynecology 1973, Maternal & Fetal Medicine 1976; **Medical School:** Vanderbilt Univ 1965; **Residency:** Obstetrics & Gynecology, Yale-New Haven Hosp, New Haven, CT 1966-1970; **Faculty Appointment:** Prof Obstetrics & Gynecology, Vanderbilt Univ

Cefalo, Robert Charles MD (Maternal & Fetal Medicine) - *Special Expertise:* *Maternal & Fetal Medicine - General;* **Admitting Hospital:** University of North Carolina Hospitals; **Office Address:** Univ NC Chapel Hill - Div of Ob/Gyn 214 MacNider Bldg - CB 7516 Chapel Hill, NC 27599-7516; **Office Phone:** (919) 966-1601; **Board Certifications:** Obstetrics & Gynecology 1967, Maternal & Fetal Medicine 1976; **Medical School:** Tufts Univ 1959; **Residency:** Obstetrics & Gynecology, US Naval Hosp, Oakland, CA 1961-1964; **Fellowships:** Maternal & Fetal Medicine, Duke Univ Med Ctr, Durham, NC 1967-1968; Maternal & Fetal Medicine, Georgetown Univ, Washington, DC 1971-1973; **Faculty Appointment:** Clin Prof Obstetrics & Gynecology, Univ NC Sch Med

Chescheir, Nancy Custer MD (Maternal & Fetal Medicine) - *Special Expertise: Ultrasound; Fetal Surgery;* **Admitting Hospital:** University of North Carolina Hospitals; **Office Address:** Univ North Carolina, Div Maternal-Fetal Med 214 MacNider Bldg Cb 7516 Chapel Hill, NC 27599-7516; **Office Phone:** (919) 966-1601; **Board Certifications:** Obstetrics & Gynecology 1989, Maternal & Fetal Medicine 1990; **Medical School:** Univ NC Sch Med 1982; **Residency:** Obstetrics & Gynecology, UNC Hosp, Chapel Hill, NC 1982-1986; **Fellowship:** Maternal & Fetal Medicine, NC Mem Hsp-UNC, Chapel Hill, NC 1986-1988; **Faculty Appointment:** Assoc Prof Obstetrics & Gynecology, Univ NC Sch Med

Ferguson II, James E MD (Maternal & Fetal Medicine) - *Special Expertise: Pregnancy-High Risk;* **Admitting Hospital:** University of Virginia Health Systems; **Office Address:** UVA Health System U Va Dept ObGyn Jefferson Park Ave, rm 5454, Box 800712 Charlottesville, VA 22908; **Office Phone:** (804) 924-2500; **Board Certifications:** Obstetrics & Gynecology 1995, Maternal & Fetal Medicine 1987; **Medical School:** Wake Forest Univ Sch Med 1977; **Residencies:** Obstetrics & Gynecology, Bowman Gray Sch Med., Winston-Salem, NC 1980-1981; Obstetrics & Gynecology, Stanford U Med Ctr., Stanford, CA 1978-1980; **Fellowship:** Maternal & Fetal Medicine, Stanford U Med Ctr., Standord, CA 1982-1984; **Faculty Appointment:** Asst Prof Univ VA Sch Med

McLaren, Rodney A MD (Maternal & Fetal Medicine) - *Special Expertise: Prenatal Diagnosis; Amniocentesis; Pregnancy-High Risk;* **Admitting Hospital:** Arlington Hospital; **Office Address:** 1701 N George Mason Drive, Fl 3rd Arlington, VA 22205; **Office Phone:** (703) 558-6077; **Board Certification:** Obstetrics & Gynecology 2001; **Medical School:** Tufts Univ 1983; **Residency:** Obstetrics & Gynecology, LI Coll Hosp, New York, NY 1983-1987; **Fellowship:** Maternal & Fetal Medicine, Georgetown Univ, Washington, DC 1989

O'Sullivan, Mary Jo MD (Maternal & Fetal Medicine) - *Special Expertise: Pregnancy-High Risk;* **Admitting Hospital:** University of Miami - Jackson Memorial Hospital; **Office Address:** 1611 NW 12th Ave, Bldg Holtz Center - rm 4070 Miami, FL 33136-1028; **Office Phone:** (305) 585-5610; **Board Certifications:** Obstetrics & Gynecology 1970, Maternal & Fetal Medicine 1976; **Medical School:** Med Coll PA Hahnemann 1963; **Residency:** Obstetrics & Gynecology, Womens Med Hosp, Philadelphia, PA 1964-1968

Thorp Jr, John Mercer MD (Maternal & Fetal Medicine) - *Special Expertise: Multiple Gestation; Premature Labor;* **Admitting Hospital:** University of North Carolina Hospitals; **Office Address:** Univ North Carolina, Dept ObGyn 214 MacNider Bldg, Box 7516 Chapel Hill, NC 27599; **Office Phone:** (919) 966-2496; **Board Certifications:** Obstetrics & Gynecology 1990, Maternal & Fetal Medicine 1991; **Medical School:** E Carolina Univ 1983; **Residency:** Obstetrics & Gynecology, Univ NC Hosp, Chapel Hill, NC 1983-1987; **Fellowship:** Maternal & Fetal Medicine, Univ NC Hosp, Chapel Hill, NC 1987-1989; **Faculty Appointment:** Assoc Prof Obstetrics & Gynecology, Univ NC Sch Med

Midwest

Bartelsmeyer, James MD (Maternal & Fetal Medicine) - *Special Expertise: Pregnancy-High Risk; Multiple Gestation;* **Admitting Hospital:** St John's Mercy Medical Center - St Louis; **Office Address:** 621 S New Ballas Rd, Bldg B - Ste 2009 St. Louis, MO 63141; **Office Phone:** (314) 569-6882; **Board Certifications:** Obstetrics & Gynecology 1992, Maternal & Fetal Medicine 1995; **Medical School:** Univ IL Coll Med 1985; **Residency:** Obstetrics & Gynecology, U Ill Coll Med. Hosps., Chicago, IL 1985-1989; **Fellowship:** Maternal & Fetal Medicine, Barnes Hosp.-U Wash., St. Louis, MO 1989-1991; **Faculty Appointment:** Assoc Prof Obstetrics & Gynecology, Washington Univ, St Louis

Dooley, Sharon L MD (Maternal & Fetal Medicine) - *Special Expertise: Fetal Anomaly; Pregnancy-High Risk; Multiple Gestation;* **Admitting Hospital:** Northwestern Memorial Hospital; **Office Address:** Prentice Women's Hosp 333 E Superior St, rm 410 Chicago, IL 60611-3095; **Office Phone:** (312) 926-7519; **Board Certifications:** Obstetrics & Gynecology 1989, Maternal & Fetal Medicine 1981; **Medical School:** Univ VA Sch Med 1973; **Residency:** Obstetrics & Gynecology, Northwestern Memorial Hosp, Chicago, IL 1974-1977; **Faculty Appointment:** Prof Obstetrics & Gynecology, Northwestern Univ

Gianopoulos, John MD (Maternal & Fetal Medicine) - *Special Expertise: Perinatal Medicine;* **Admitting Hospital:** Loyola University Health System; **Office Address:** Loyola Univ Med Ctr 2160 S 1st Ave, Bldg 103 - Ste 1019 Maywood, IL 60153; **Office Phone:** (708) 216-5423; **Board Certifications:** Obstetrics & Gynecology 1993, Maternal & Fetal Medicine 1985; **Medical School:** Loyola Univ-Stritch Sch Med 1977; **Residency:** Obstetrics & Gynecology, Loyola Univ Med Ctr, Maywood, IL 1977-1981; **Fellowship:** Maternal & Fetal Medicine, Loyola Univ Med Ctr, Maywood, IL 1981-1983; **Faculty Appointment:** Prof Obstetrics & Gynecology, Univ Chicago-Pritzker Sch Med

Hayashi, Robert H. MD (Maternal & Fetal Medicine) - *Special Expertise: Premature Labor; Labor-Abnormal; Pregnancy-High Risk;* **Admitting Hospital:** University of Michigan Health Center; **Office Address:** 1500 E Medical Ctr. Dr., rm F4882, Box 0264 C.S. Mott Children's Hospital Ann Arbor, MI 48109-0264; **Office Phone:** (734) 763-6295; **Board Certifications:** Obstetrics & Gynecology 1989, Maternal & Fetal Medicine 1976; **Medical School:** Temple Univ 1963; **Residency:** Obstetrics & Gynecology, U Mich Hosp., Ann Arbor, MI 1966-1970; **Fellowship:** U Pitt Hosp., Pittsburgh, PA 1970-1972; **Faculty Appointment:** Prof Obstetrics & Gynecology, Univ Mich Med Sch

Hibbard, Judith MD (Maternal & Fetal Medicine) - *Special Expertise: Lupus/SLE-Pregnancy; Cardiovascular Disease-Pregnancy;* **Admitting Hospital:** University of Chicago Hospitals (Page 78); **Office Address:** Univ Chicago Hosps, Dept OB-GYN 5841 N Maryland Ave, MC-2050 Chicago, IL 60637; **Office Phone:** (773) 702-5200; **Board Certifications:** Obstetrics & Gynecology 1999, Maternal & Fetal Medicine 1999; **Medical School:** Loyola Univ-Stritch Sch Med 1982; **Residency:** Obstetrics & Gynecology, Univ Chicago Hosp, Chicago, IL 1982-1986; **Fellowship:** Maternal & Fetal Medicine, Univ Chicago Hosp, Chicago, IL 1986-1988; **Faculty Appointment:** Assoc Prof Obstetrics & Gynecology, Univ Chicago-Pritzker Sch Med

Hussey, Michael J MD (Maternal & Fetal Medicine) - *Special Expertise: Perinatal Medicine; Tubal Ligation;* **Admitting Hospital:** Rush/Presbyterian - St Luke's Medical Center - Chicago (Page 74); **Office Address:** 1725 W Harrison St, Ste 408 Chicago, IL 60612; **Office Phone:** (312) 942-6611; **Board Certifications:** Obstetrics & Gynecology 1994, Maternal & Fetal Medicine 1998; **Medical School:** Univ IL Coll Med 1986; **Residency:** Obstetrics & Gynecology, Loyola Univ Med Ctr, Maywood, IL 1991-1993; **Fellowship:** Maternal & Fetal Medicine, Rush Presby, Chicago, IL 1993; **Faculty Appointment:** Asst Prof Obstetrics & Gynecology, Rush Med Coll

Ismail, Mahmoud MD (Maternal & Fetal Medicine) - *Special Expertise: Pregnancy-High Risk; Perinatal Medicine; Infections;* **Admitting Hospital:** University of Chicago Hospitals (Page 78); **Office Address:** Center for Advanced Medicine 5841 S Maryland Ave, MC-2050 Chicago, IL 60637; **Office Phone:** (773) 702-5200; **Board Certifications:** Obstetrics & Gynecology 1997, Maternal & Fetal Medicine 1997; **Medical School:** Egypt 1970; **Residency:** Obstetrics & Gynecology, Wayne St Univ Affil Hosp, Detroit, MI 1973-1977; **Fellowship:** Maternal & Fetal Medicine, Unic of Chicago Hosps, Chicago, IL 1980-1982; **Faculty Appointment:** Prof Obstetrics & Gynecology, Univ Chicago-Pritzker Sch Med

Philipson, Elliot MD (Maternal & Fetal Medicine) - *Special Expertise:* Pregnancy-High Risk; Amniocentesis; **Admitting Hospital:** Cleveland Clinic Foundation; **Office Address:** Cleveland Clinic 660 Euclid Ave, Box M62 Cleveland, OH 44195; **Office Phone:** (216) 445-3402; **Board Certifications:** Obstetrics & Gynecology 1984, Maternal & Fetal Medicine 1990; **Medical School:** Italy 1975; **Residency:** Obstetrics & Gynecology, Albany Med Ctr, Albany, NY 1977-1980; **Fellowship:** Maternal & Fetal Medicine, Metro Genl Hosp, Cleveland, OH 1980-1982

Pielet, Bruce MD (Maternal & Fetal Medicine) - *Special Expertise:* Ultrasound; Perinatal Medicine; **Admitting Hospital:** Advocate Lutheran General Hospital; **Office Address:** Advocate Medical Group-Parkside Ctr 1875 Dempster St, Ste 325 Park Ridge, IL 60068; **Office Phone:** (847) 723-8610; **Board Certifications:** Obstetrics & Gynecology 1990, Maternal & Fetal Medicine 1991; **Medical School:** Loyola Univ-Stritch Sch Med 1981; **Residency:** Obstetrics & Gynecology, U Chicago, Chicago, IL 1981-1985; **Fellowship:** Maternal & Fetal Medicine, Northwestern Univ Hosp, Chicago, IL 1985-1987

Strassner, Howard T MD (Maternal & Fetal Medicine) - *Special Expertise:* Fetal Transfusion; Amniocentesis; **Admitting Hospital:** Rush/Presbyterian - St Luke's Medical Center - Chicago (Page 74); **Office Address:** 1725 W Harrison St, Ste 408 Chicago, IL 60612; **Office Phone:** (312) 666-0285; **Board Certifications:** Maternal & Fetal Medicine 1982, Obstetrics & Gynecology 1998; **Medical School:** Univ Chicago-Pritzker Sch Med 1974; **Residency:** Obstetrics & Gynecology, Columbia Presby Med Ctr, New York, NY 1974-1978; **Fellowship:** Maternal & Fetal Medicine, LA Co-USC Med Ctr, Los Angeles, CA 1978-1980; **Faculty Appointment:** Assoc Prof Obstetrics & Gynecology, Rush Med Coll

Tomich, Paul MD (Maternal & Fetal Medicine) - *Special Expertise:* Pregnancy-High Risk; **Admitting Hospital:** Loyola University Health System; **Office Address:** Loyola University Phys Fdn 2160 S 1st Ave, Bldg 103 - rm 1013 Maywood, IL 60153-3304; **Office Phone:** (708) 216-8563; **Board Certifications:** Obstetrics & Gynecology 1999, Maternal & Fetal Medicine 1998; **Medical School:** Loyola Univ-Stritch Sch Med 1973; **Residency:** Obstetrics & Gynecology, Mayo Clinic, Rochester, MN 1974-1978; **Fellowship:** Maternal & Fetal Medicine, Barnes Hosp-Wash Univ, St Louis, MO 1978-1980; **Faculty Appointment:** Asst Prof Obstetrics & Gynecology, Loyola Univ-Stritch Sch Med

Treadwell, Marjorie Clarke MD (Maternal & Fetal Medicine) - *Special Expertise:* Obstetrical Ultrasound; Pregnancy-High Risk; **Admitting Hospital:** Harper Hospital (Page 59); **Office Address:** 4707 St Antoine, Ste 304 Detroit, MI 48201; **Office Phone:** (313) 745-0723; **Board Certifications:** Obstetrics & Gynecology 1991, Maternal & Fetal Medicine 1992; **Medical School:** Univ Mich Med Sch 1984; **Residency:** Obstetrics & Gynecology, Wayne State Univ, Detroit, MI 1984-1988; **Fellowship:** Obstetrics & Gynecology, Wayne State Univ, Detroit, MI 1989-1990; **Faculty Appointment:** Assoc Prof Obstetrics & Gynecology, Wayne State Univ

Winn, Hung MD (Maternal & Fetal Medicine) - *Special Expertise:* Multiple Gestation; Pregnancy-High Risk; **Admitting Hospital:** St Mary's Health Center - St Louis; **Office Address:** St Mary Hlth Ctr 6420 Clayton Rd St Louis, MO 63117; **Office Phone:** (314) 768-8873; **Board Certifications:** Obstetrics & Gynecology 1991, Maternal & Fetal Medicine 1992; **Medical School:** Univ IL Coll Med 1982; **Residency:** Obstetrics & Gynecology, Univ Illinois Hosp, Peoria, IL 1982-1986; **Fellowship:** Maternal & Fetal Medicine, Yale-New Haven Hosp, New Haven, CT 1986-1988; **Faculty Appointment:** Prof Obstetrics & Gynecology, St Louis Univ

Great Plains and Mountains

Gibbs, Ronald Steven MD (Maternal & Fetal Medicine) - *Special Expertise:* Maternal & Fetal Medicine - General; **Admitting Hospital:** University of Colorado Health & Science Center; **Office Address:** 101 University Denver, CO 80206; **Office Phone:** (303) 372-4444; **Board Certifications:** Obstetrics & Gynecology 1989, Maternal & Fetal Medicine 1981; **Medical School:** Univ Penn 1969; **Residency:** Obstetrics & Gynecology, Hosp Univ Penn, Philadelphia, PA 1970-1974; **Fellowship:** Maternal & Fetal Medicine, Univ Tex Hlth Sci Ctr, San Antonio, TX 1976-1978; **Faculty Appointment:** Prof Obstetrics & Gynecology, Univ Colo

Southwest

Wilkins, Isabelle MD (Maternal & Fetal Medicine) - *Special Expertise:* Multiple Gestation; Congenital Abnormalities; Prenatal Ultrasound; **Admitting Hospital:** St Luke's Episcopal Hospital - Houston (Page 76); **Office Address:** Univ Tex, Dept OB/GYN Reprod Sci 6550 Fannin, Ste 901 Houston, TX 77030-1501; **Office Phone:** (713) 798-7593; **Board Certifications:** Obstetrics & Gynecology 1987, Maternal & Fetal Medicine 1988; **Medical School:** Duke Univ 1980; **Residency:** Obstetrics & Gynecology, Mount Sinai Med Ctr, New York, NY 1980-1984; **Fellowship:** Maternal & Fetal Medicine, Mount Sinai Med Ctr, New York, NY 1984-1986; **Faculty Appointment:** Assoc Prof Obstetrics & Gynecology, Baylor Coll Med

West Coast and Pacific

Benedetti, Thomas J MD (Maternal & Fetal Medicine) - *Special Expertise:* Prematurity Prevention; Fetal Macrosomia; **Admitting Hospital:** University of Washington Medical Center; **Office Address:** Univ WA Med Ctr - Maternal & Infant Care Clinic 1959 NE Pacific St, Box 356460 Seattle, WA 98195-6127; **Office Phone:** (206) 543-3729; **Board Certifications:** Obstetrics & Gynecology 1980, Maternal & Fetal Medicine 1981; **Medical School:** Univ Wash 1973; **Residency:** Obstetrics & Gynecology, LAC-USC Med Ctr, Los Angeles, CA 1974-1977; **Fellowship:** Maternal & Fetal Medicine, LAC-USC Med Ctr, Los Angeles, CA 1977-1979; **Faculty Appointment:** Prof Obstetrics & Gynecology, Univ Wash

Druzin, Maurice L MD (Maternal & Fetal Medicine) - *Special Expertise:* Maternal & Fetal Medicine - General; **Admitting Hospital:** Stanford Medical Center; **Office Address:** 300 Pasteur Dr, Rm HH333 Stanford U Med Ctr-Dept OB/GYN Stanford, CA 94305; **Office Phone:** (650) 725-8617; **Board Certifications:** Obstetrics & Gynecology 1980, Maternal & Fetal Medicine 1981; **Medical School:** South Africa 1970; **Residency:** Obstetrics & Gynecology, Rose Med Ctr-U Colorado, CO 1974-1977; **Fellowship:** Maternal & Fetal Medicine, USC Med Ctr, Los Angelas, CA 1977-1979; **Faculty Appointment:** Prof Obstetrics & Gynecology

Gabbe, Steven G MD (Maternal & Fetal Medicine) - *Special Expertise:* Pregnancy-High Risk; Diabetes-Gestational; **Admitting Hospital:** University of Washington Medical Center; **Office Address:** Univ Wash Med Ctr 1959 NE Pacific St Seattle, WA 98195-6127; **Office Phone:** (206) 598-4070; **Board Certifications:** Obstetrics & Gynecology 1976, Maternal & Fetal Medicine 1977; **Medical School:** Cornell Univ-Weil Med Coll 1969; **Residency:** Obstetrics & Gynecology, Boston Hosp Women, Boston, MA 1972-1974; **Faculty Appointment:** Prof Obstetrics & Gynecology, Univ Wash

Goldberg, James David MD (Maternal & Fetal Medicine) - *Special Expertise: Prenatal Diagnosis; Fetal Therapy;* **Admitting Hospital:** California Pacific Medical Center; **Office Address:** California Pacific Med Ctr 3700 California St, Ste G330 San Francisco, CA 94118; **Office Phone:** (415) 750-6400; **Board Certifications:** Maternal & Fetal Medicine 1997, Clinical Genetics 1987; **Medical School:** Univ Minn 1979; **Residency:** Obstetrics & Gynecology, UCSF Med Ctr, San Francisco, CA 1979-1983; **Fellowships:** Maternal & Fetal Medicine, Mount Sinai Hosp, New York, NY 1983-1985; Clinical Genetics, Mount Sinai Hosp, New York, NY 1983-1985

Gravett, Michael Glen MD (Maternal & Fetal Medicine) - *Special Expertise: Maternal & Fetal Medicine - General;* **Admitting Hospital:** Oregon Health Science University Hospital and Clinics; **Office Address:** 3181 SW Sam Jackson Park Rd, MC-I458 Portland, OR 97201; **Office Phone:** (503) 494-2101; **Board Certifications:** Obstetrics & Gynecology 1985, Maternal & Fetal Medicine 1987; **Medical School:** UCLA 1977; **Residency:** Obstetrics & Gynecology, Univ Wash, Seattle, WA 1978-1981; **Fellowship:** Maternal & Fetal Medicine, Univ Wash, Seattle, WA 1981-1983

Hobel, Calvin John MD (Maternal & Fetal Medicine) - *Special Expertise: Prematurity Prevention; Fetal Stress;* **Admitting Hospital:** Cedars-Sinai Medical Center; **Office Address:** 8700 Beverly Blvd, Rm 160 Cedars Sinai Med Ctr Los Angeles, CA 90048-1804; **Office Phone:** (310) 423-3365; **Board Certifications:** Obstetrics & Gynecology 1971, Maternal & Fetal Medicine 1975; **Medical School:** Univ Nebr Coll Med 1963; **Residency:** Obstetrics & Gynecology, Harbor Genl Hosp, Torrance, CA 1964-1968; **Fellowship:** Maternal & Fetal Medicine, Natl Womens Hosp, Auckland, New Zealand 1966-1967; **Faculty Appointment:** Prof Obstetrics & Gynecology, UCLA

Koos, Brian John MD (Maternal & Fetal Medicine) - *Special Expertise: Pregnancy-High Risk; Fetal Diagnosis;* **Admitting Hospital:** UCLA Medical Center; **Office Address:** 10833 Le Conte Ave Los Angeles, CA 90095-3075; **Office Phone:** (310) 206-6404; **Board Certifications:** Obstetrics & Gynecology 1999, Maternal & Fetal Medicine 1999; **Medical School:** Loma Linda Univ 1974; **Residency:** Obstetrics & Gynecology, Brigham & Women's Hosp, Boston, MA 1976-1979; **Fellowship:** Maternal & Fetal Medicine, Women's Hosp, Los Angeles, CA 1982-1983; **Faculty Appointment:** Prof Obstetrics & Gynecology, UCLA

NEONATAL-PERINATAL MEDICINE

(a subspecialty of OBSTETRICS AND GYNECOLOGY)

A subspecialist in neonatal-perinatal medicine is a pediatrician who is the principal care provider for sick newborn infants. Clinical expertise is used for direct patient care and for consulting with obstetrical colleagues to plan for the care of mothers who have high-risk pregnancies.

PEDIATRICS

A pediatrician is concerned with the physical, emotional and social health of children from birth to young adulthood. Care encompasses a broad spectrum of health services ranging from preventive healthcare to the diagnosis and treatment of acute and chronic diseases. The pediatrician deals with biological, social and environmental influences on the developing child and with the impact of disease and dysfunction on development.

Training required: Three years in pediatrics *plus* additional training and examination

Physician Listings

Neonatal-Perinatal Medicine

New England

Cloherty, John (Neonatal-Perinatal Medicine) - *Special Expertise:* Neonatology; **Admitting Hospital:** Children's Hospital; **Office Address:** 319 Longwood Ave, Fl 4 Boston, MA 02115; **Office Phone:** (617) 355-7318; **Board Certifications:** Neonatal-Perinatal Medicine 1975, Pediatrics 1986; **Medical School:** Boston Univ 1962; **Residency:** Pediatrics, Mass Genl Hosp, Boston, MA 1967-1969; **Fellowship:** Neonatal-Perinatal Medicine, Chldns Hosp, Boston, MA 1969; **Faculty Appointment:** Assoc Prof Pediatrics, Harvard Med Sch

Ehrenkranz, Richard MD (Neonatal-Perinatal Medicine) - *Special Expertise:* Critical Care; Newborn Care; **Admitting Hospital:** Yale - New Haven Hospital; **Office Address:** Yale Univ-Dept Ped 333 Cedar St New Haven, CT 06520-8064; **Office Phone:** (203) 688-2320; **Board Certifications:** Neonatal-Perinatal Medicine 1979, Pediatrics 1977; **Medical School:** SUNY Downstate 1972; **Residency:** Pediatrics, Yale-New H, New Haven, CT 1973-1974; **Fellowship:** Neonatal-Perinatal Medicine, Yale Univ, New Haven, CT 1976-1978; **Faculty Appointment:** Prof Pediatrics, Yale Univ

Gross, Ian MD (Neonatal-Perinatal Medicine) - *Special Expertise:* Neonatal-Perinatal Medicine - General; **Admitting Hospital:** Yale - New Haven Hospital; **Office Address:** Yale Sch Med, Dept Pediatrics 333 Cedar St New Haven, CT 06520-8064; **Office Phone:** (203) 688-2320; **Board Certifications:** Pediatrics 1974, Neonatal-Perinatal Medicine 1977; **Medical School:** South Africa 1967; **Residencies:** Pediatrics, Childrens Hosp, Boston, MA 1971-1972; Pediatrics, Univ Witwatersrand Affil Hosps, Johannesburg, South Africa 1970-1971; **Fellowships:** Neonatal-Perinatal Medicine, Yale Univ Sch Med, New Haven, CT 1973-1974; Pediatrics, Harvard Med Sch, Boston, MA 1972-1973

Horbar, Jeffrey David MD (Neonatal-Perinatal Medicine) - *Special Expertise:* Neonatal-Perinatal Medicine - General; **Admitting Hospital:** Fletcher Allen Health Care Medical Center - Campus; **Office Address:** Fletcher Allen Healthcare 111 Colchester Ave, McClure Bldg, Rm 718 Burlington, VT 05401; **Office Phone:** (802) 656-2471; **Board Certifications:** Pediatrics 1982, Neonatal-Perinatal Medicine 1983; **Medical School:** SUNY Downstate 1977; **Residency:** Pediatrics, Med Ctr Hosp Vermont, Burlington, VT 1977-1979; **Fellowship:** Ocular Disease, Med Ctr Hosp Vermont, Burlington, VT 1979-1981

Mid Atlantic

Driscoll, John MD (Neonatal-Perinatal Medicine) - *Special Expertise:* Neonatal-Perinatal Medicine - General; **Admitting Hospital:** Columbia Presbyterian Medical Center (Page 72); **Office Address:** 3959 Broadway, Ste 114S New York, NY 10032; **Office Phone:** (212) 305-2934; **Board Certifications:** Pediatrics 1970, Neonatal-Perinatal Medicine 1975; **Medical School:** Wake Forest Univ Sch Med 1962; **Residencies:** Pediatrics, Children's Hosp, Pittsburgh, PA 1962-1963; Columbia-Presbyterian, New York, NY 1967-1969; **Fellowship:** Neonatal-Perinatal Medicine, Columbia-Presbyterian, New York, NY 1969-1971; **Faculty Appointment:** Prof Pediatrics, Columbia P&S

Hurt, Hallam MD (Neonatal-Perinatal Medicine) - *Special Expertise:* Neonatology; **Admitting Hospital:** Albert Einstein Medical Center; **Office Address:** Albert Einstein Med Ctr, Lifter Bldg 5501 Old York Rd, Fl 2nd - rm 2601 Philadelphia, PA 19140; **Office Phone:** (215) 456-6696; **Board Certifications:** Pediatrics 1976, Neonatal-Perinatal Medicine 1977; **Medical School:** Univ VA Sch Med 1971; **Residency:** Pediatrics, Univ Virginia Med Ctr, Charlottesville, VA 1972-1974; **Fellowship:** Neonatal-Perinatal Medicine, Univ Virginia Med Ctr, Charlottesville, VA 1974-1976; **Faculty Appointment:** Prof Pediatrics, Temple Univ

NEONATAL PERINATAL MEDICINE *Mid Atlantic*

Lawson, Edward Earle MD (Neonatal-Perinatal Medicine) - *Special Expertise:* Pregnancy-High Risk; Breathing Disorders; **Admitting Hospital:** Johns Hopkins Hospital - Baltimore (Page 65); **Office Address:** Johns Hopkins Chldns Ctr 600 N Wolfe St, Bldg CMSC - rm 210 Baltimore, MD 21287-3200; **Office Phone:** (410) 955-5259; **Board Certifications:** Neonatal-Perinatal Medicine 1997, Pediatrics 1997; **Medical School:** Northwestern Univ 1972; **Residency:** Pediatrics, Chldns Hosp Med Ctr, Boston, MA 1973-1975; **Fellowship:** Neonatal-Perinatal Medicine, Harvard Med Sch, Boston, MA 1975-1977; **Faculty Appointment:** Prof Pediatrics, Univ NC Sch Med

Polin, Richard MD (Neonatal-Perinatal Medicine) - *Special Expertise:* Neonatal Sepsis; **Admitting Hospital:** Columbia Presbyterian Medical Center (Page 72); **Office Address:** Columbia University 3959 Broadway, BHS 115 New York, NY 10032; **Office Phone:** (212) 305-5827; **Board Certifications:** Pediatrics 1975, Neonatal-Perinatal Medicine 1977; **Medical School:** Temple Univ 1970; **Residencies:** Pediatrics, Chldns Meml Hosp, Chicago, IL 1971-1972; Pediatrics, Babies Hosp-Columbia Presby, New York, NY 1972-1975; **Fellowship:** Neonatal-Perinatal Medicine, Babies Hosp-Columbia Presby, New York, NY 1973-1974; **Faculty Appointment:** Prof Pediatrics, Columbia P&S

Regan, Joan MD (Neonatal-Perinatal Medicine) - *Special Expertise:* Infection in Newborns; **Admitting Hospital:** Columbia Presbyterian Medical Center (Page 72); **Office Address:** 3959 Broadway New York, NY 10032-3702; **Office Phone:** (212) 305-5827; **Board Certification:** Pediatrics 1979; **Medical School:** Univ MO-Columbia Sch Med **Residency:** Pediatrics, Montefiore, New York, NY 1976; **Fellowship:** Neonatal-Perinatal Medicine, Columbia Univ, New York, NY 1976-1978; **Faculty Appointment:** Asst Prof Pediatrics, Columbia P&S

Southeast

Bancalari, Eduardo MD (Neonatal-Perinatal Medicine) - *Special Expertise:* Neonatology; **Admitting Hospital:** University of Miami - Jackson Memorial Hospital; **Office Address:** Univ Miami, Dept Pediatrics, rm R-131 Miami, FL 33101; **Office Phone:** (305) 585-2328; **Board Certifications:** Neonatal-Perinatal Medicine 1993, Pediatrics 1993; **Medical School:** Chile 1966; **Residency:** Pediatrics, Hosp Luis Calvo Mackenna, Santiago, Chile 1967-1969; **Fellowship:** Pediatric Cardiology, Univ Miami Med Ctr, Miami, FL 1971; **Faculty Appointment:** Prof Pediatrics, Univ Miami Sch Med

Boyle, Robert John MD (Neonatal-Perinatal Medicine) - *Special Expertise:* Neonatology; **Admitting Hospital:** University of Virginia Health Systems; **Office Address:** Univ VA, Hlth Sci Ctr. Box 800386 Charlottesville, VA 22908; **Office Phone:** (804) 295-1000; **Board Certifications:** Pediatrics 1978, Neonatal-Perinatal Medicine 1979; **Medical School:** Johns Hopkins Univ 1973; **Residency:** Pediatrics, Rainbow Babies Chldns Hosp 1973-1976; **Fellowship:** Neonatal-Perinatal Medicine, Women's Infants Hosp 1976-1978; **Faculty Appointment:** Assoc Prof Pediatrics, Univ VA Sch Med

Bucciarelli, Richard L MD (Neonatal-Perinatal Medicine) - *Special Expertise:* Neonatal Cardiology; **Admitting Hospital:** Shands Healthcare at University Florida (Page 77); **Office Address:** Shands Healthcare-Univ Fla 1600 SW Archer Rd, Ste M-100 Gainesville, FL 32610; **Office Phone:** (352) 392-9315; **Board Certifications:** Pediatric Cardiology 1977, Neonatal-Perinatal Medicine 1977; **Medical School:** Univ Mich Med Sch 1972; **Residency:** Pediatrics, Shands Hosp-Univ Fla, Gainesville, FL 1974-1975; **Fellowship:** Neonatal-Perinatal Medicine, Shands Hosp-Univ Fla, Gainesville, FL 1975-1977; **Faculty Appointment:** Prof Pediatrics, Univ Fla Coll Med

352

Neu, Josef MD (Neonatal-Perinatal Medicine) - *Special Expertise:* Neonatal Nutrition; **Admitting Hospital:** Shands Healthcare at University Florida (Page 77); **Office Address:** Shands Healthcare-Univ Fla 1600 SW Archer Rd Gainesville, FL 32610; **Office Phone:** (352) 392-3020; **Board Certifications:** Neonatal-Perinatal Medicine 1981, Pediatric Critical Care Medicine 1987; **Medical School:** Univ Wisc 1975; **Residency:** Pediatrics, Johns Hopkins Hosp, Baltimore, MD 1975-1975; **Fellowship:** Neonatal-Perinatal Medicine, Stanford Univ, Stanford, CA 1978-1980; **Faculty Appointment:** Prof Pediatrics, Univ Fla Coll Med

Stiles, Alan MD (Neonatal-Perinatal Medicine) - *Special Expertise:* Neonatology; **Admitting Hospital:** University of North Carolina Hospitals; **Office Address:** Univ North Carolina, Div Neonatalogy 509 Burnett Womack - CB7220 Chapel Hill, NC 27599; **Office Phone:** (919) 966-5063; **Board Certifications:** Pediatrics 1984, Neonatal-Perinatal Medicine 1985; **Medical School:** Univ NC Sch Med 1977; **Residency:** Pediatrics, North Carolina Meml Hosp, Chapel Hill, NC 1978-1982; **Fellowship:** Neonatal-Perinatal Medicine, Chldns Hosp/Brigham Hosp, Boston, MA 1982-1985; **Faculty Appointment:** Prof Pediatrics, Univ NC Sch Med

Midwest

Jobe, Alan Hall MD/PhD (Neonatal-Perinatal Medicine) - *Special Expertise:* Surfactant Biology; **Admitting Hospital:** Children's Hospital Medical Center; **Office Address:** Children's Hosp Med Ctr 3333 Burnett Cincinnati, OH 45229-3039; **Office Phone:** (513) 636-8563; **Board Certifications:** Pediatrics 1978, Neonatal-Perinatal Medicine 1979; **Medical School:** UCSD 1973; **Residency:** Pediatrics, UCSD, San Diego, CA 1974-1975; **Fellowship:** Neonatal-Perinatal Medicine, UCSD, San Diego, CA 1975-1977; **Faculty Appointment:** Prof Neonatal-Perinatal Medicine, Univ Cincinnati

Lemons, James A MD (Neonatal-Perinatal Medicine) - *Special Expertise:* Neonatology; Perinatal Medicine; **Admitting Hospital:** Riley Hospital for Children; **Office Address:** University Indiana Med Ctr. Dept.Neo Peri Medicine 699 West Drive RR 208 Indianapolis, IN 46202-5119; **Office Phone:** (317) 274-5000; **Board Certifications:** Pediatrics 1993, Neonatal-Perinatal Medicine 1993; **Medical School:** Northwestern Univ 1969; **Residency:** Neonatal-Perinatal Medicine, U Mich Med Sch, Ann Arbor, MI 1970-1972; **Fellowship:** Neonatal-Perinatal Medicine, U Colo Med Ctr 1973-1975; **Faculty Appointment:** Prof Pediatrics, Indiana Univ

Martin, Richard MD (Neonatal-Perinatal Medicine) - *Special Expertise:* Neonatology; Neonatal Respiratory Disease; **Admitting Hospital:** Rainbow Babies & Children's Hospital; **Office Address:** 11100 Euclid Ave Cleveland, OH 44106; **Office Phone:** (216) 844-3387; **Board Certifications:** Neonatal-Perinatal Medicine 1977, Pediatrics 1976; **Medical School:** Australia 1970; **Residency:** Pediatrics, Univ Missouri, Columbia, MO 1972-1973; **Fellowship:** Neonatal-Perinatal Medicine, Case West Res Univ, Cleveland, OH 1974-1975; **Faculty Appointment:** Prof Pediatrics, Case West Res Univ

Steinhorn, Robin MD (Neonatal-Perinatal Medicine) - *Special Expertise:* Pulmonary Hypertension; **Admitting Hospital:** Children's Memorial Hospital; **Office Address:** Children's Meml Hosp-Chicago 2300 Childrens Plaza, Box 45 Chicago, IL 60614; **Office Phone:** (773) 880-4142; **Board Certifications:** Neonatal-Perinatal Medicine 1997, Pediatrics 2000; **Medical School:** Washington Univ, St Louis 1980; **Residencies:** Obstetrics & Gynecology, Barnes Hosp, St Louis, MO 1980-1983; Pediatrics, Univ Minnesota, Minneapolis, MN 1983-1986; **Fellowship:** Neonatal-Perinatal Medicine, Univ Minnesota, Minneapolis, MN 1986-1988; **Faculty Appointment:** Assoc Prof Neonatal-Perinatal Medicine, Northwestern Univ

Southwest

Adams, James M MD (Neonatal-Perinatal Medicine) - *Special Expertise:* Lung Disease-Newborn; **Admitting Hospital:** Texas Children's Hospital - Houston; **Office Address:** 6621 Fannin St Houston, TX 77030; **Office Phone:** (832) 824-1380; **Board Certifications:** Pediatrics 1975, Neonatal-Perinatal Medicine 1975; **Medical School:** Baylor Coll Med 1969; **Residency:** Pediatrics, Baylor Affil Hosps, Houston, TX 1971-1973; **Fellowship:** Neonatal-Perinatal Medicine, Baylor, Houston, TX 1973-1975; **Faculty Appointment:** Asst Prof Pediatrics, Baylor Coll Med

Denson, Susan Ellen MD (Neonatal-Perinatal Medicine) - *Special Expertise:* Neonatology; **Admitting Hospital:** Memorial Hermann Healthcare System; **Office Address:** Univ Tex Med Sch - Peds 6431 Fannin St, Ste 3-256 Houston, TX 77030; **Office Phone:** (713) 500-5726; **Board Certifications:** Pediatrics 1978, Neonatal-Perinatal Medicine 1979; **Medical School:** Univ Tex SW, Dallas 1972; **Residency:** Pediatrics, Univ Ariz, Tucson, AZ 1973-1974; **Fellowships:** Neonatal-Perinatal Medicine, Univ Ariz, Tucson, AZ 1974-1975; Neonatal-Perinatal Medicine, Univ Tex Med Sch, Houston, TX 1975-1976; **Faculty Appointment:** Prof Pediatrics, Univ Tex, Houston

Escobedo, Marilyn Barnard MD (Neonatal-Perinatal Medicine) - *Special Expertise:* Newborn Critical Care; **Admitting Hospital:** University of Texas Health & Science Center; **Office Address:** 7703 Floyd Curl Dr San Antonio, TX 78229-3900; **Office Phone:** (210) 567-5225; **Board Certifications:** Neonatal-Perinatal Medicine 1986, Pediatrics 1986; **Medical School:** Washington Univ, St Louis 1970; **Residencies:** Pediatrics, Chldns Hosp, St Louis, MO 1971-1972; Pediatrics, Chldns Hosp, St Louis, MO 1972-1973; **Fellowship:** Neonatal-Perinatal Medicine, Vanderbilt Univ, Nashville, TN 1974-1976; **Faculty Appointment:** Prof Pediatrics, Univ Tex, San Antonio

Garcia-Prats, Joseph MD (Neonatal-Perinatal Medicine) - *Special Expertise:* Lung Disease-Newborn; **Admitting Hospital:** Texas Children's Hospital - Houston; **Office Address:** Harris County Hosp Dist - Ben Taub Genl Hosp, Dept Neonatalogy 1504 Taub Loop Houston, TX 77030; **Office Phone:** (713) 793-3515; **Board Certifications:** Pediatrics 1977, Neonatal-Perinatal Medicine 1977; **Medical School:** Tulane Univ 1972; **Residency:** Pediatrics, Baylor Affil Hosp, Houston, TX 1972-1975; **Fellowship:** Neonatal-Perinatal Medicine, Baylor Affil Hosp, Houston, TX 1975-1977; **Faculty Appointment:** Assoc Prof Pediatrics, Baylor Coll Med

Odom, Michael W MD (Neonatal-Perinatal Medicine) - *Special Expertise:* Neonatology; **Admitting Hospital:** University of Texas Health & Science Center; **Office Address:** 7703 Floyd Curl Dr, Dept Peds San Antonio, TX 78229; **Office Phone:** (210) 567-5225; **Board Certifications:** Pediatrics 1987, Neonatal-Perinatal Medicine 1997; **Medical School:** Univ Tex SW, Dallas 1983; **Residency:** Pediatrics, Vanderbilt Univ Affil Hosps, Nashville, TN 1983-1986; **Fellowship:** Neonatal-Perinatal Medicine, Mt Zion Med Ctr Rsch Inst, San Francisco, CA 1986-1989; **Faculty Appointment:** Assoc Prof Pediatrics, Univ Tex, San Antonio

Perlman, Jeffrey MD (Neonatal-Perinatal Medicine) - *Special Expertise:* Critically Ill Infants; Prematurity/Low Birth Weight Infants; **Admitting Hospital:** Parkland Memorial Hospital; **Office Address:** Univ of TX SW Med Ctr at Dallas, Dept Peds 5323 Harry Hines Blvd Dallas, TX 75390-9063; **Office Phone:** (214) 648-3903; **Board Certifications:** Pediatrics 1983, Neonatal-Perinatal Medicine 1983; **Medical School:** South Africa 1974; **Residencies:** Pediatrics, Johannesburg Chlds Hosp, South Africa 1977-1979; Pediatrics, St Louis Chldns Hosp, St Louis, MO 1979-1981; **Fellowship:** Neonatal-Perinatal Medicine, St Louis Chldns Hosp, St Louis, MO 1981-1983; **Faculty Appointment:** Asst Prof Pediatrics, Univ Texas SW, Dallas

Seidner, Steven Richard MD (Neonatal-Perinatal Medicine) - *Special Expertise:* Neonatal-Perinatal Medicine - General; **Admitting Hospital:** University of Texas Health & Science Center; **Office Address:** 7703 Floyd Curl Dr. Dept. of Pediatrics San Antonio, TX 78229-3900; **Office Phone:** (210) 567-5229; **Board Certifications:** Neonatal-Perinatal Medicine 1987, Pediatrics 1987; **Medical School:** Univ Ariz Coll Med 1982; **Residency:** Pediatrics, Harbor-UCLA Med Ctr., Torrance, CA 1983-1985; **Fellowship:** Neonatal-Perinatal Medicine, Harbor-UCLA Med Ctr., Torrance, CA 1985-1988; **Faculty Appointment:** Assoc Prof Pediatrics, Univ Tex, San Antonio

Tyson, Jon Edward MD (Neonatal-Perinatal Medicine) - *Special Expertise:* Neonatology; Epidemiology; **Admitting Hospital:** University of Texas Health & Science Center; **Office Address:** The Univ Tex Houston Med Sch, Dept Ped 6431 Fannin St Houston, TX 77030; **Office Phone:** (713) 500-5651; **Board Certifications:** Pediatrics 1973, Neonatal-Perinatal Medicine 1975; **Medical School:** Tulane Univ 1968; **Residency:** Pediatrics, Univ Tenn, Memphis, TN 1968-1971; **Fellowship:** Neonatology, McMaster Univ, Hamilton 1973-1975; **Faculty Appointment:** Prof Pediatrics, Univ Tex, Houston

West Coast and Pacific

Kitterman, Joseph A MD (Neonatal-Perinatal Medicine) - *Special Expertise:* Neonatal-Perinatal Medicine - General; **Admitting Hospital:** University of California - San Francisco Medical Center; **Office Address:** UCSF Sch Med, Dept Ped Room U-503, Box 0734 San Francisco, CA 94143-0734; **Office Phone:** (415) 476-7242; **Board Certifications:** Pediatrics 1969, Neonatal-Perinatal Medicine 1975; **Medical School:** McGill Univ 1962; **Residency:** Pediatrics, UCSF, San Francisco, CA 1965-1967; **Fellowship:** Neonatal-Perinatal Medicine, UCSF, San Francisco, CA 1967-1970; **Faculty Appointment:** Prof Pediatrics, UCSF

Sola, Augusto MD (Neonatal-Perinatal Medicine) - *Special Expertise:* Neonatal-Perinatal Medicine - General; **Admitting Hospital:** Cedars-Sinai Medical Center; **Office Address:** Cedars-Sinai Med Ctr, Dept Peds 8700 Beverly Blvd, rm 4310 Los Angeles, CA 90048; **Office Phone:** (310) 423-4434; **Board Certifications:** Neonatal-Perinatal Medicine 1979, Pediatrics 1979; **Medical School:** Argentina 1973; **Residencies:** Pediatrics, St Vincent's Hosp, Worchester, MA 1975-1976; Pediatrics, Univ Mass Meml Med Ctr, Worchester, MA 1976-1977; **Fellowship:** Neonatal-Perinatal Medicine, Univ Mass Meml Med Ctr, Worchester, MA 1977-1978; **Faculty Appointment:** Prof Pediatrics, UCLA

Stevenson, David K MD (Neonatal-Perinatal Medicine) - *Special Expertise:* Neonatology; **Admitting Hospital:** Stanford Medical Center; **Office Address:** Stanford Univ Med Ctr, Dept Peds 750 Welch Rd, Ste 315 Palo Alto, CA 94304; **Office Phone:** (650) 723-5711; **Board Certifications:** Pediatrics 1979, Neonatal-Perinatal Medicine 1997; **Medical School:** Univ Wash 1975; **Residency:** Pediatrics, Univ Washington, Seattle, WA 1976-1977; **Fellowship:** Neonatal-Perinatal Medicine, Stanford Univ, Stanford, CA 1977-1979; **Faculty Appointment:** Prof Pediatrics, Stanford Univ

NEPHROLOGY

(a subspecialty of INTERNAL MEDICINE)

An internist who treats disorders of the kidney, high blood pressure, fluid and mineral balance and dialysis of body wastes when the kidneys do not function. This specialist consults with surgeons about kidney transplantation.

INTERNAL MEDICINE

An internist is a personal physician who provides long-term, comprehensive care in the office and the hospital, managing both common and complex illness of adolescents, adults and the elderly. Internists are trained in the diagnosis and treatment of cancer, infections and diseases affecting the heart, blood, kidneys, joints and digestive, respiratory and vascular systems. They are also trained in the essentials of primary care internal medicine which incorporates an understanding of disease prevention, wellness, substance abuse, mental health and effective treatment of common problems of the eyes, ears, skin, nervous system and reproductive organs.

Training required: Three years in internal medicine *plus* additional training and examination for certification in nephrology

Physician Listings

New England

Aronson, Peter Samuel MD (Nephrology) - *Special Expertise:* Nephrology - General; **Admitting Hospital:** Yale - New Haven Hospital; **Office Address:** Yale Sch Med Dept IM Box 208029 New Haven, CT 06520-8029; **Office Phone:** (203) 785-4186; **Board Certifications:** Nephrology 1976, Internal Medicine 1973; **Medical School:** NYU Sch Med 1970; **Residency:** Internal Medicine, NC Meml Hosp- UNC, Chapel Hill, NC 1971-1972; **Fellowship:** Nephrology, Yale U. Sch Med, New Haven, CT 1974-1977; **Faculty Appointment:** Prof Medicine, Yale Univ

Brenner, Barry M MD (Nephrology) - *Special Expertise:* Hypertension; Diabetic Kidney Disease; Kidney Failure-Acute; **Admitting Hospital:** Brigham & Women's Hospital; **Office Address:** Brigham & Women's Hosp, Div Renal 75 Francis St Boston, MA 02115; **Office Phone:** (617) 732-5850; **Medical School:** Univ Pittsburgh 1962; **Residency:** Internal Medicine, Albert Einstein Coll Med, New York, NY 1966-1967; **Fellowship:** Nephrology, Nat Inst Health, Bethesda, MD 1967; **Faculty Appointment:** Prof Medicine, Harvard Med Sch

Carpenter, Charles B MD (Nephrology) - *Special Expertise:* Transplant Medicine-Kidney; Immunogenetics; **Admitting Hospital:** Brigham & Women's Hospital; **Office Address:** Brigham & Women's Hosp, Dept Nephr 75 Francis St Boston, MA 02115; **Office Phone:** (617) 732-5244; **Board Certification:** Internal Medicine 1966; **Medical School:** Harvard Med Sch 1958; **Residencies:** Internal Medicine, Meml Hosp, New York, NY 1959-1960; Internal Medicine, Bellevue Hosp, New York, NY 1959-1960; **Fellowships:** Nephrology, Peter Bent Brigham Hosp, Boston, MA 1962-1966; Pathology, Peter Bent Brigham Hosp, Boston, MA 1962-1966; **Faculty Appointment:** Prof Medicine, Harvard Med Sch

Coggins, Cecil MD (Nephrology) - *Special Expertise:* Kidney Disease; Hypertension; **Admitting Hospital:** Massachusetts General Hospital; **Office Address:** Mass Genl Hosp, Beacon Hill 100 Charles River Plaza, Fl 5th Boston, MA 02114; **Office Phone:** (617) 726-4900; **Board Certifications:** Nephrology 1975, Internal Medicine 1968; **Medical School:** Harvard Med Sch 1958; **Residencies:** Internal Medicine, Mass Genl, Boston, MA 1958-1959; Internal Medicine, Stanford Med Ctr, Palo Alto, CA 1961-1965; **Fellowships:** Nephrology, Stanford Med Ctr, Palo Alto, CA 1962-1963; Nephrology, Mass Genl, Boston, MA 1965-1967; **Faculty Appointment:** Assoc Prof Medicine, Harvard Med Sch

Fang, Leslie MD (Nephrology) - *Special Expertise:* Kidney Failure-Chronic; **Admitting Hospital:** Massachusetts General Hospital; **Office Address:** 100 Charles River Plaza, Ste 701 Boston, MA 02114-2724; **Office Phone:** (617) 726-2000; **Board Certifications:** Internal Medicine 1977, Nephrology 1980; **Medical School:** Harvard Med Sch 1974; **Residencies:** Internal Medicine, Mass Genl Hosp, Boston, MA 1975-1976; Internal Medicine, Mass Genl Hosp, Boston, MA 1979-1980; **Fellowship:** Nephrology, Mass Genl Hosp, Boston, MA 1976-1978

Kliger, Alan MD (Nephrology) - *Special Expertise:* Kidney Disease; Kidney Disease-Metabolic; **Admitting Hospital:** Yale - New Haven Hospital; **Office Address:** 136 Sherman Ave New Haven, CT 06511; **Office Phone:** (203) 787-0117; **Board Certifications:** Internal Medicine 1973, Nephrology 1976; **Medical School:** SUNY Syracuse 1970; **Residency:** Internal Medicine, SUNY Upstate, Syracuse, NY 1971-1973; **Fellowship:** Nephrology, Georgetown, Washington, DC 1973-1975; **Faculty Appointment:** Clin Prof Medicine, Yale Univ

Owen, William F. MD (Nephrology) - *Special Expertise:* Kidney Failure-Acute/Chronic; **Admitting Hospital:** Brigham & Women's Hospital; **Office Address:** Dialysis Office 75 Francis St Boston, MA 02115; **Office Phone:** (617) 732-6137; **Board Certifications:** Internal Medicine 1984, Neurology 1986; **Medical School:** Tufts Univ 1980; **Residency:** Internal Medicine, Brigham Womens Hosp, Boston, MA 1981-1983; **Fellowship:** Nephrology, Brigham Womens Hosp, Boston, MA 1983-1984; **Faculty Appointment:** Asst Prof Nephrology, Harvard Med Sch

359

Perrone, Ronald MD (Nephrology) - *Special Expertise:* Hypertension; **Admitting Hospital:** New England Medical Center; **Office Address:** New England Med Ctr 750 Washington St, Box 391 Boston, MA 02111; **Office Phone:** (617) 636-5866; **Board Certifications:** Internal Medicine 1979, Nephrology 1982; **Medical School:** Hahnemann Univ 1975; **Residency:** Internal Medicine, Grady Meml Hosp, Atlanta, Ga 1976-1978; **Fellowship:** Nephrology, Boston Med Ctr 1979-1982; **Faculty Appointment:** Assoc Prof Medicine, Tufts Univ

Salant, David MD (Nephrology) - *Special Expertise:* Kidney Disease-Glomerular; Kidney Disease-Immunologic; **Admitting Hospital:** Boston University Medical Center-East Newton Street Campus; **Office Address:** 1 Boston Med Ctr Pl Boston, MA 02118; **Office Phone:** (617) 638-7480; **Board Certifications:** Internal Medicine 1978, Nephrology 1980; **Medical School:** South Africa 1969; **Residency:** Johannesburg Genl Hosp, South Africa 1971-1973; **Fellowship:** Nephrology, Boston Univ Med Ctr., Boston, MA 1977-1978

Seifter, Julian L MD (Nephrology) - *Special Expertise:* Diabetic Kidney Disease; Kidney Failure-Chronic; Kidney stones; **Admitting Hospital:** Brigham & Women's Hospital; **Office Address:** Brigham & Women's Hosp, Div Renal 75 Francis St, Ste MRB4 Boston, MA 02115; **Office Phone:** (617) 732-7482; **Board Certification:** Nephrology 1980; **Medical School:** Albert Einstein Coll Med 1975; **Residency:** Internal Medicine, Bronx Muni Hosp Ctr, Bronx, NY 1978; **Fellowship:** Nephrology, Yale-New Haven Hosp, New Haven, CT 1982; **Faculty Appointment:** Assoc Prof Medicine, Harvard Med Sch

Tolkoff-Rubin, Nina MD (Nephrology) - *Special Expertise:* Transplant Medicine-Kidney; Hypertension; Kidney Failure-Acute; **Admitting Hospital:** Massachusetts General Hospital; **Office Address:** Mass Genl Hosp, Dept Nephrology 55 Fruit St, GRB Bldg, Ste 1003J Boston, MA 02114; **Office Phone:** (617) 726-3706; **Board Certifications:** Nephrology 1974, Internal Medicine 1972; **Medical School:** Harvard Med Sch 1968; **Residencies:** Internal Medicine, Mass Genl Hosp, Boston, MA 1969-1970; Internal Medicine, Mass Genl Hosp, Boston, MA 1971-1972; **Fellowship:** Nephrology, Mass Genl Hosp, Boston, MA 1970-1971; **Faculty Appointment:** Assoc Prof Medicine, Harvard Med Sch

Mid Atlantic

Appel, Gerald MD (Nephrology) - *Special Expertise:* Kidney Disease-Glomerular; Lupus Nephritis; **Admitting Hospital:** Columbia Presbyterian Medical Center (Page 72); **Office Address:** 622 W 168th St, Bldg Ste 4124 New York, NY 10032-3702; **Office Phone:** (212) 305-3273; **Board Certifications:** Internal Medicine 1975, Nephrology 1978; **Medical School:** Albert Einstein Coll Med 1972; **Residency:** Internal Medicine, Columbia Presby, New York, NY 1972-1975; **Fellowships:** Nephrology, Columbia Presby, New York, NY 1975-1976; Nephrology, Yale, New Haven, CT 1976-1978; **Faculty Appointment:** Clin Prof Medicine, Columbia P&S

Cohen, David MD (Nephrology) - *Special Expertise:* Transplant Medicine-Kidney; **Admitting Hospital:** Columbia Presbyterian Medical Center (Page 72); **Office Address:** 622 W 168th St, Ste PH4121 New York, NY 10032; **Office Phone:** (212) 305-3273; **Board Certifications:** Internal Medicine 1980, Nephrology 1984; **Medical School:** Albert Einstein Coll Med 1977; **Residencies:** Internal Medicine, Mount Sinai Med Ctr, New York, NY 1977-1978; Internal Medicine, Mount Sinai Med Ctr, New York, NY 1978-1980; **Fellowship:** Nephrology, Columbia Presby Med Ctr, New York, NY 1980-1981; **Faculty Appointment:** Assoc Prof Medicine, Columbia P&S

Dosa, Stefan MD (Nephrology) - *Special Expertise:* Transplant Medicine-Kidney; **Admitting Hospital:** Washington Hospital Center - DC (Page 79); **Office Address:** 730 24th St, Ste 17, Wash, DC 20037; **Office Phone:** (202) 337-7660; **Board Certifications:** Internal Medicine 1980, Nephrology 1982; **Medical School:** Czech Republic 1967; **Residency:** Maanchester Royal Infirmary, England, UK 1972-1977; **Fellowship:** Univ Cincinnati, Cincinnati, OH 1977-1979; **Faculty Appointment:** Assoc Clin Prof Medicine, Geo Wash Univ

Friedman, Eli A MD (Nephrology) - *Special Expertise:* Diabetic Kidney Disease; Transplant Medicine-Kidney; **Admitting Hospital:** University Hospital - Brooklyn; **Office Address:** 450 Clarkson Ave, Box 52 SUNY Health Science Ctr Brooklyn, NY 11203; **Office Phone:** (718) 270-1584; **Board Certifications:** Internal Medicine 1967, Nephrology 1974; **Medical School:** SUNY Downstate 1957; **Residency:** Internal Medicine, Peter Bent Brigham Hosp, Boston, MA 1957-1960; **Fellowship:** Nephrology, Peter Bent Brigham Hosp, Boston, MA 1960-1961; **Faculty Appointment:** Prof Medicine, SUNY Downstate

Johnston, James MD (Nephrology) - *Special Expertise:* Kidney Disease-Diabetic; Hypertension; **Admitting Hospital:** UPMC - Presbyterian University Hospital; **Office Address:** Univ of Pittsburgh Physicians, Div Renal 3550 Terrace St, Scaife Hall, rm A915 Pittsburgh, PA 15213; **Office Phone:** (412) 647-7157; **Board Certifications:** Internal Medicine 1982, Nephrology 1984; **Medical School:** Univ Pittsburgh 1979; **Residency:** Internal Medicine, Montefiore Hosp, Pittsburgh, PA 1980-1982; **Fellowships:** Nephrology, Brigham & Women's Hosp, Boston, MA 1983-1986; Nephrology, Univ Pittsburgh Med Ctr, Pittsburgh, PA 1982-1983; **Faculty Appointment:** Assoc Prof Nephrology, Univ Pittsburgh

Piraino, Beth Marie MD (Nephrology) - *Special Expertise:* Nephrology - General; **Admitting Hospital:** UPMC - Presbyterian University Hospital; **Office Address:** UPMC Montefiore-Univ Pittsburgh Phys, Div Renal 3459 Fifth Ave Pittsburgh, PA 15213; **Office Phone:** (412) 647-7157; **Board Certification:** Internal Medicine 1980; **Medical School:** Med Coll PA Hahnemann 1977; **Residency:** Internal Medicine, Presby Univ Hosp, Pittsburgh, PA 1978-1980; **Fellowship:** Nephrology, Presby Univ Hosp, Pittsburgh, PA 1980-1982; **Faculty Appointment:** Prof Medicine, Univ Pittsburgh

Rakowski, Thomas A MD (Nephrology) - *Special Expertise:* Polycystic Kidney Disease; Kidney Disease-Glomerular; **Admitting Hospital:** Georgetown University Hospital; **Office Address:** GUMC - Pasquerilla Healthcare Ctr 3800 Reservoir Rd NW, Fl 6 Washington, DC 20007; **Office Phone:** (202) 687-8539; **Board Certifications:** Nephrology 1974, Internal Medicine 1972; **Medical School:** Hahnemann Univ 1969; **Residency:** Internal Medicine, Georgetown Univ, Washington, DC 1970-1971; **Fellowship:** Nephrology, Georgetown Univ, Washington, DC 1971-1972

Sapir, Daniel Gustave MD (Nephrology) - *Special Expertise:* Kidney Disease; **Admitting Hospital:** Johns Hopkins Hospital - Baltimore (Page 65); **Office Address:** 10755 Falls Rd, Ste 320 Lutherville, MD 21093-4522; **Office Phone:** (410) 583-2660; **Board Certifications:** Internal Medicine 1967, Nephrology 1978; **Medical School:** Johns Hopkins Univ 1960; **Residency:** Internal Medicine, Johns Hopkins Hosp, Baltimore, MD 1961-1964; **Fellowship:** Renal Disease, Tufts Univ, Boston, MA 1964-1966; **Faculty Appointment:** Assoc Prof Medicine, Johns Hopkins Univ

Scheel Jr, Paul Joseph MD (Nephrology) - *Special Expertise:* Kidney Failure; **Admitting Hospital:** Johns Hopkins Hospital - Baltimore (Page 65); **Office Address:** 1830 E Monument St Ste 416 Baltimore, MD 21205; **Office Phone:** (410) 955-5268; **Board Certifications:** Internal Medicine 1990, Nephrology 1997; **Medical School:** Georgetown Univ 1987; **Residency:** Internal Medicine, John Hopkins, Baltimore, MD 1987-1990; **Fellowship:** Nephrology, John Hopkins, Baltimore, MD 1990-1992; **Faculty Appointment:** Assoc Prof Medicine, Johns Hopkins Univ

Umans, Jason MD/PhD (Nephrology) - *Special Expertise:* Hypertension; Kidney Disease; **Admitting Hospital:** Georgetown University Hospital; **Office Address:** Georgetown Univ Hosp, Div Nephr & Hyper 3800 Reservoir Rd NW, Bldg PHC - Fl 6 Washington, DC 20007; **Office Phone:** (202) 687-9183; **Board Certifications:** Internal Medicine 1988, Nephrology 1990; **Medical School:** Cornell Univ-Weil Med Coll 1984; **Residency:** Internal Medicine, Univ Chicago Hosps, Chicago, IL 1984-1987; **Fellowship:** Nephrology, Univ Chicago Hosps, Chicago, IL 1987-1988; **Faculty Appointment:** Assoc Prof Nephrology, Georgetown Univ

Wilcox, Christopher S MD (Nephrology) - *Special Expertise:* Hypertension-Renovascular/Adrenal; Hypertension-Drug Resistent; **Admitting Hospital:** Georgetown University Hospital; **Office Address:** Georgetown Univ Med Ctr - Pasquerilla Healthcare Center 3800 Reservoir Rd NW, Bldg PHC - Fl 6th Washington, DC 20007; **Office Phone:** (202) 687-8539; **Board Certifications:** Internal Medicine 1983, Nephrology 1986; **Medical School:** England 1968; **Residencies:** Internal Medicine, Middlesex Hosp, London, England 1970-1971; Nephrology, Middlesex Hosp, London, England 1971-1972; **Fellowship:** Nephrology, Middlesex Hosp, London, England 1972-1975; **Faculty Appointment:** Prof Nephrology, Georgetown Univ

Williams, Gail S MD (Nephrology) - *Special Expertise:* Kidney Failure-Chronic; **Admitting Hospital:** Columbia Presbyterian Medical Center (Page 72); **Office Address:** Atchley Pavilion 161 Fort Washington Ave, Ste 351 New York, NY 10032; **Office Phone:** (212) 305-5376; **Board Certifications:** Internal Medicine 1972, Nephrology 1974; **Medical School:** Columbia P&S 1968; **Residency:** Internal Medicine, Columbia Presby Hosp, New York, NY 1970-1972; **Fellowship:** Nephrology, Columbia Presby Hosp, New York, NY 1972-1973; **Faculty Appointment:** Assoc Clin Prof Medicine, Columbia P&S

Southeast

Bolton, Warren Kline MD (Nephrology) - *Special Expertise:* Kidney Disease-Glomerular; Kidney Disease; **Admitting Hospital:** University of Virginia Health Systems; **Office Address:** Univ of VA Hlth Scis Ctr Box 800 133 Charlottesville, VA 22908; **Office Phone:** (804) 924-5125; **Board Certifications:** Internal Medicine 1972, Nephrology 1974; **Medical School:** Univ VA Sch Med 1969; **Residency:** Internal Medicine, Boston City Hosp, Chicago, IL 1970-1971; **Fellowship:** Nephrology, Univ Chicago, Boston, MA 1971-1973; **Faculty Appointment:** Prof Medicine, Univ VA Sch Med

Bourgoignie, Jacques MD (Nephrology) - *Special Expertise:* Hypertension; Kidney Failure-Chronic; **Admitting Hospital:** University of Miami - Jackson Memorial Hospital; **Office Address:** Div Nephrology & Hypertension 1600 NW 10th Ave, Bldg R126 Miami, FL 33136; **Office Phone:** (305) 243-6251; **Medical School:** Belgium 1958; **Residency:** Internal Medicine, Catholic Univ- Louvain Hosp, Belgium 1958-1961; **Fellowships:** VA Med Ctr, St Louis, MO 1963-1965; Nephrology, Wash Univ, St Louis, MO 1965-1968; **Faculty Appointment:** Prof Medicine, Univ Miami Sch Med

Buckalew Jr., Vardaman Moore MD (Nephrology) - *Special Expertise:* Hypertension; Kidney Disease; **Admitting Hospital:** Wake Forest University Baptist Medical Center; **Office Address:** Wake Forest Univ Baptist Med Ctr Medical Center Blvd Winston Salem, NC 27157; **Office Phone:** (336) 716-2062; **Board Certification:** Internal Medicine 1966; **Medical School:** Univ Penn **Residency:** Internal Medicine, Hosp Univ Penn, Philadelphia, PA 1958-1962; **Fellowship:** Nephrology, Hosp Univ Penn, Philadelphia, PA 1964-1967; **Faculty Appointment:** Prof Nephrology, Wake Forest Univ Sch Med

Coffman, Thomas Myron MD (Nephrology) - *Special Expertise:* Transplant Medicine-Kidney; Hypertension; **Admitting Hospital:** Duke University Medical Center (Page 60); **Office Address:** Duke Univ Med Ctr Box 3014 Durham, NC 27710; **Office Phone:** (919) 286-6947; **Board Certifications:** Nephrology 1988, Internal Medicine 1983; **Medical School:** Ohio State Univ 1980; **Residency:** Internal Medicine, Duke Univ Med Ctr, Durham, NC 1980-1983; **Fellowship:** Nephrology, Duke Univ Med Ctr, Durham, NC 1983-1985; **Faculty Appointment:** Prof Medicine, Duke Univ

Falk, Ronald J MD (Nephrology) - *Special Expertise:* Kidney Disease-Glomerular; Lupus Nephritis; Vasculitis; **Admitting Hospital:** University of North Carolina Hospitals; **Office Address:** Univ NC Meml Hosp, Div Nephrology & Hypertension 349, Bldg MacNider Chapel Hill, NC 27599-7155; **Office Phone:** (919) 966-2561; **Board Certifications:** Internal Medicine 1980, Nephrology 1982; **Medical School:** Univ NC Sch Med 1977; **Residencies:** Internal Medicine, Univ NC Sch Med, Chapel Hill, NC 1978-1980; Nephrology, Univ NC Sch Med, Chapel Hill, NC 1980-1981; **Fellowship:** Research, Univ Minn, Minneapolis, MN 1981-1983; **Faculty Appointment:** Prof Medicine, Univ NC Sch Med

Gluck, Stephen MD (Nephrology) - *Special Expertise:* Kidney Disease-Glomerular; Hypertension; Transplant Medicine-Kidney; **Admitting Hospital:** Shands at Jacksonville; **Office Address:** Div Neph Hyperten & Trans-U FL Coll Med 1600 SW Archer Rd, Box 100224 Gainesville, FL 32610-0224; **Office Phone:** (352) 392-4008; **Board Certifications:** Internal Medicine 1980, Nephrology 1984; **Medical School:** UCLA 1977; **Residency:** Internal Medicine, Columbia Presby Med Ctr, New York, NY 1977-1980; **Fellowship:** Nephrology, Columbia Presby Med Ctr, New York, NY 1980-1983; **Faculty Appointment:** Prof Nephrology, Univ Fla Coll Med

Harris, Raymond C MD (Nephrology) - *Special Expertise:* Kidney Disease; Hypertension; **Admitting Hospital:** Vanderbilt University Medical Center; **Office Address:** Vanderbilt Univ Med Ctr Medical Center North, MS 3303 Nashville, TN 37232-2372; **Office Phone:** (615) 343-8496; **Board Certifications:** Nephrology 1986, Internal Medicine 1981; **Medical School:** Emory Univ 1978; **Residency:** UC San Francisco, San Francisco, CA 1979-1981; **Fellowship:** Nephrology, Brigham & Womens Hosp, Boston, MA 1982-1986; **Faculty Appointment:** Prof Medicine, Vanderbilt Univ

Hoffman, David MD (Nephrology) - *Special Expertise:* Kidney Stones; Renal Research; **Admitting Hospital:** Baptist Hospital - Miami; **Office Address:** Miami Kidney Group 7900 SW 57th Ave, Ste 21 South Miami, FL 33143-5546; **Office Phone:** (305) 662-3984; **Board Certifications:** Internal Medicine 1976, Nephrology 1978; **Medical School:** Univ Tenn Coll Med, Memphis 1975; **Residency:** Internal Medicine, Univ Miami, Miami, FL 1972-1973; **Fellowship:** Nephrology, Univ Miami, Miami, FL 1975-1977

Neylan, John Francis MD (Nephrology) - *Special Expertise:* Transplant Medicine-Kidney; Immunosuppression-Kidney Transplant; **Admitting Hospital:** Emory University Hospital; **Office Address:** Emory Univ Hosp 1364 Clifton Rd NE, Bldg EUH - Ste D240 Atlanta, GA 30322; **Office Phone:** (404) 712-5918; **Board Certifications:** Internal Medicine 1982, Nephrology 1988; **Medical School:** Rush Med Coll 1979; **Residency:** Internal Medicine, Vanderbilt Univ Hosp, Nashville, TN 1979-1982; **Fellowship:** Nephrology, Brigham&Women's Hosp, Boston, MA 1983-1986; **Faculty Appointment:** Prof Medicine, Emory Univ

Okusa, Mark D MD (Nephrology) - *Special Expertise:* Kidney Failure-Chronic; Nephrotic Syndrome; **Admitting Hospital:** University of Virginia Health Systems; **Office Address:** Univ of VA Hlth Sci Ctr, Div Nephrology Lee St, Box 800-133 Charlottesville, VA 22908-0133; **Office Phone:** (804) 924-5125; **Board Certifications:** Internal Medicine 1985, Nephrology 1988; **Medical School:** Med Coll VA 1982; **Residency:** Internal Medicine, Med Coll VA, Richmond, VA 1983-1985; **Fellowship:** Nephrology, Yale Univ Sch Med, New Haven, CT 1985-1988

Roth, David MD (Nephrology) - *Special Expertise: Transplant Medicine-Kidney; Kidney Failure-Chronic;* **Admitting Hospital:** University of Miami - Jackson Memorial Hospital; **Office Address:** Nephrology and Hypertension 1600 NW 10th Ave, Bldg RMSB - rm 7168 Miami, FL 33101; **Office Phone:** (305) 243-6251; **Board Certifications:** Internal Medicine 1980, Nephrology 1982; **Medical School:** SUNY Downstate 1977; **Residency:** Internal Medicine, Univ Miami-Jackson Meml Hosp, Miami, FL 1977-1980; **Fellowship:** Nephrology, Univ Miami-Jackson Meml Hosp, Miami, FL 1980-1982; **Faculty Appointment:** Prof Medicine, Univ Miami Sch Med

Schwab, Steve Joseph MD (Nephrology) - *Special Expertise: Polycystic Kidney Disease; Kidney Failure;* **Admitting Hospital:** Duke University Medical Center (Page 60); **Office Address:** Duke Univ Med Ctr Box 3014 Durham, NC 27710; **Office Phone:** (919) 684-3355; **Board Certifications:** Internal Medicine 1982, Nephrology 1986; **Medical School:** Univ MO-Columbia Sch Med 1979; **Residency:** Internal Medicine, Univ Kans Med Ctr, Kansas City 1980-1982; **Fellowship:** Nephrology, Wash Univ-Barnes Hosp, St Louis, MO 1982-1984

Weiner, Irving David MD (Nephrology) - *Special Expertise: Kidney Disease; Acid-Base Disorders; Kidney Stones;* **Admitting Hospital:** Shands Healthcare at University Florida (Page 77); **Office Address:** Shands at Univ Florida, Dept Neph 1600 SW Archer Rd, Box 100224 Gainesville, FL 32610-0224; **Office Phone:** (352) 392-4008; **Board Certifications:** Internal Medicine 1987, Nephrology 1990; **Medical School:** Vanderbilt Univ 1984; **Residency:** Internal Medicine, Univ Texas Hlth Sci Ctr, San Antonio, TX 1984-1987; **Faculty Appointment:** Assoc Prof Medicine, Univ Fla Coll Med

Midwest

Black, Henry R MD (Nephrology) - *Special Expertise: Hypertension; Nephrotic Syndrome;* **Admitting Hospital:** Rush/Presbyterian - St Luke's Medical Center - Chicago (Page 74); **Office Address:** 1700 W Van Buren, Ste 470 Chicago, IL 60612; **Office Phone:** (312) 942-3133; **Board Certifications:** Internal Medicine 1972, Nephrology 1974; **Medical School:** NYU Sch Med 1967; **Residencies:** Internal Medicine, Johns Hopkins, Baltimore, MD 1967-1968; Internal Medicine, Yale-New Haven, New Haven, CT 1971-1972; **Fellowship:** Nephrology, Yale-New Haven, New Haven, CT 1972-1974

Brazy, Peter C MD (Nephrology) - *Special Expertise: Kidney Disease; Kidney Disease-Metabolic; Phosphate Homeostasis;* **Admitting Hospital:** University of Wisconsin Hospital & Clinics; **Office Address:** Univ Wisconsin at Madison 600 Highland Ave Madison, WI 53705; **Office Phone:** (608) 263-6808; **Board Certifications:** Internal Medicine 1978, Nephrology 1984; **Medical School:** Washington Univ, St Louis 1972; **Residency:** Internal Medicine, Barnes Hosp, St Louis, MO 1973-1974; **Fellowship:** Nephrology, Duke Univ Med Ctr, Durham, NC 1976-1978; **Faculty Appointment:** Asst Prof Medicine, Duke Univ

Coe, Fredric MD (Nephrology) - *Special Expertise: Kidney Stones; Fluid/Electrolyte Balance; Kidney Stones;* **Admitting Hospital:** University of Chicago Hospitals (Page 78); **Office Address:** Center for Advanced Med 5758 S Maryland Ave S Chicago, IL 60637; **Office Phone:** (773) 702-1475; **Board Certification:** Internal Medicine 1968; **Medical School:** Univ Chicago-Pritzker Sch Med 1961; **Residency:** Internal Medicine, Michael Reese Hosp, Chicago, IL 1961-1965; **Fellowship:** Nephrology, Univ Texas SW, Dallas, TX 1967-1969; **Faculty Appointment:** Prof Medicine, Univ Chicago-Pritzker Sch Med

Delmez, James Albert MD (Nephrology) - *Special Expertise:* Kidney Disease; **Admitting Hospital:** Barnes - Jewish Hospital; **Office Address:** 4570 Children's Place St Louis, MO 63110; **Office Phone:** (314) 362-7603; **Board Certifications:** Internal Medicine 1976, Nephrology 1982; **Medical School:** Univ Rochester 1973; **Residency:** Internal Medicine, Barnes Hosp, St Louis, MO 1974-1976; **Fellowship:** Nephrology, Barnes Hosp, St Louis, MO 1976-1978; **Faculty Appointment:** Prof Medicine, Washington Univ, St Louis

Hruska, Keith Anthony MD (Nephrology) - *Special Expertise:* Kidney Disease; **Admitting Hospital:** Barnes - Jewish Hospital; **Office Address:** Barnes Jewish Hosp MS 9032-648 216 S Kings Hwy St Louis, MO 63110-1026; **Office Phone:** (314) 454-7771; **Board Certifications:** Internal Medicine 1972, Nephrology 1976; **Medical School:** Creighton Univ 1969; **Residencies:** Internal Medicine, NY Hosp-Cornell, New York, NY 1970-1971; Internal Medicine, Barnes Hosp-Wash U, St Louis, MO 1971-1972; **Fellowship:** Nephrology, Barnes Hosp-Wash Univ, St Louis, MO 1972-1974

Josephson, Michelle Ann MD (Nephrology) - *Special Expertise:* Transplant Medicine-Kidney; **Admitting Hospital:** University of Chicago Hospitals (Page 78); **Office Address:** 5841 S Maryland Ave Chicago, IL 60637; **Office Phone:** (773) 702-6134; **Board Certifications:** Internal Medicine 1986, Nephrology 1990; **Medical School:** Univ Penn 1983; **Residency:** Internal Medicine, Univ Chicago, Chicago, IL 1984-1986; **Fellowship:** Nephrology, Univ Chicago, Chicago, IL 1987-1991; **Faculty Appointment:** Asst Prof Medicine, Univ Chicago-Pritzker Sch Med

Kasiske, Bertram MD (Nephrology) - *Special Expertise:* Transplant Medicine-Kidney; Kidney Disease-Geriatric; **Admitting Hospital:** Hennepin County Medical Center; **Office Address:** Hennepin Co Med Ctr-Dept Nephrology 701 Park Ave S Minneapolis, MN 55415-1623; **Office Phone:** (612) 347-6088; **Board Certifications:** Internal Medicine 1980, Nephrology 1982; **Medical School:** Univ Iowa Coll Med 1976; **Residency:** Internal Medicine, Hennepin Co Med Ctr, Minneapolis, MN 1976-1980; **Fellowship:** Nephrology, Hennepin Co Med Ctr, Minneapolis, MN 1980-1983; **Faculty Appointment:** Prof Medicine, Univ Minn

Lewis, Edmund J MD (Nephrology) - *Special Expertise:* Lupus Nephritis; Diabetic Kidney Disease; **Admitting Hospital:** Rush/Presbyterian - St Luke's Medical Center - Chicago (Page 74); **Office Address:** 1426 W Washington St Chicago, IL 60607; **Office Phone:** (312) 850-8434; **Board Certification:** Nephrology 1969; **Medical School:** Univ British Columbia Fac Med 1962; **Residency:** Internal Medicine, Johns Hopkins Hosp, Baltimore, MD 1962-1965; **Fellowships:** Nephrology, Peter Bent Brigham Hosp, Boston, MA 1965-1966; Research, Peter Bent Brigham Hosp, Boston, MA 1968-1969; **Faculty Appointment:** Prof Medicine, Rush Med Coll

Paganini, Emil MD (Nephrology) - *Special Expertise:* Kidney Failure-Chronic; **Admitting Hospital:** Cleveland Clinic Foundation; **Office Address:** Cleveland Clinic Foundation 9500 Euclid Ave Cleveland, OH 44195; **Office Phone:** (216) 444-5792; **Board Certification:** Internal Medicine 1977; **Medical School:** Italy 1973; **Residency:** Internal Medicine, Winthrop Univ Hosp, Mineola, NY 1975-1977; **Fellowship:** Nephrology, Cleveland Clin Fdn, Cleveland, OH 1977-1979

Pohl, Marc MD (Nephrology) - *Special Expertise:* Hypertension; **Admitting Hospital:** Cleveland Clinic Foundation; **Office Address:** 9500 Euclid Ave Cleveland, OH 44195; **Office Phone:** (216) 444-6776; **Board Certifications:** Infectious Disease 1972, Nephrology 1978; **Medical School:** Case West Res Univ 1966; **Residencies:** Internal Medicine, Univ Hosps Cleveland 1967-1968; Internal Medicine, Mass Genl Hosp, Boston, MA 1970-1971

NEPHROLOGY

Roguska-Kyts, Jadwiga MD (Nephrology) - *Special Expertise:* Kidney Disease; **Admitting Hospital:** Northwestern Memorial Hospital; **Office Address:** 201 E Huron Street, Ste 11-205 Chicago, IL 60611; **Office Phone:** (312) 926-3626; **Board Certifications:** Nephrology 1976, Internal Medicine 1987; **Medical School:** Poland 1958; **Residency:** Internal Medicine, Northwestern Meml Hosp, Chicago, IL 1960-1962; **Fellowship:** Nephrology, Northwestern Meml Hosp, Chicago, IL 1963-1965; **Faculty Appointment:** Assoc Prof Medicine, Northwestern Univ

Somerville, James MD (Nephrology) - *Special Expertise:* Nephrology - General; **Admitting Hospital:** Fairview-University Medical Center - University Campus; **Office Address:** InterMed Consultants 6363 France Ave S, Ste 400 Edina, MN 55435; **Office Phone:** (612) 920-2070; **Board Certifications:** Nephrology 1982, Critical Care Medicine 1987; **Medical School:** Univ MD Sch Med 1975; **Residency:** Internal Medicine, Hennepin Co Med Ctr, Minneapolis, MN 1975-1978; **Fellowship:** Nephrology, Hennepin Co Med Ctr, Minneapolis, MN 1979-1980

Swartz, Richard D MD (Nephrology) - *Special Expertise:* Kidney Failure; Dialysis Care; **Admitting Hospital:** University of Michigan Health Center; **Office Address:** Univ Michigan Hlth System 3914 Taubman Ctr, Box 0364 Ann Arbor, MI 48109-0364; **Office Phone:** (734) 936-4890; **Board Certifications:** Internal Medicine 1975, Nephrology 1977; **Medical School:** Univ Mich Med Sch 1970; **Residencies:** Internal Medicine, Boston City Hosp, Boston, MA 1971-1975; Nephrology, Beth Israel Hosp, Boston, MA 1975-1977; **Faculty Appointment:** Prof Nephrology, Univ Mich Med Sch

Torres, Vincente Esbarranch MD (Nephrology) - *Special Expertise:* Polycystic Kidney Disease; **Admitting Hospital:** Mayo Medical Center & Clinic - Rochester; **Office Address:** Mayo Clinic 200 1st St SW Rochester, MN 55905; **Office Phone:** (507) 266-7093; **Board Certifications:** Internal Medicine 1977, Nephrology 1980; **Medical School:** Spain 1969; **Residency:** Internal Medicine, Mayo Grad Sch Med, Rochester, MN 1975-1977; **Fellowship:** Nephrology, Mayo Grad Sch Med, Rochester, MN 1977-1979; **Faculty Appointment:** Prof Medicine, Mayo Med Sch

Venkat, K K MD (Nephrology) - *Special Expertise:* Transplant Medicine-Kidney; **Admitting Hospital:** Henry Ford Health System (Page 62); **Office Address:** Henry Ford Hospital 2799 W Grand Blvd, rm CFP5 Detroit, MI 48202; **Office Phone:** (313) 876-2702; **Board Certifications:** Internal Medicine 1977, Nephrology 1978; **Medical School:** India 1970; **Residency:** Internal Medicine, Henry Ford Hosp, Detroit, MI 1975-1976; **Fellowship:** Nephrology, Henry Ford Hosp, Detroit, MI 1976-1978

Zimmerman, Stephen W MD (Nephrology) - *Special Expertise:* Transplant Medicine-Kidney; Kidney Failure-Chronic; **Admitting Hospital:** University of Wisconsin Hospital & Clinics; **Office Address:** VA Hosp, Univ Wisconsin, Dept Nephrology 2500 Overlook Terrace, Rm B3060 Madison, WI 53705; **Office Phone:** (608) 263-6808; **Board Certifications:** Nephrology 1972, Internal Medicine 1972; **Medical School:** Univ Wisc 1966; **Residency:** Internal Medicine, Univ Wisconsin, Madison, WI 1967-1969; **Fellowships:** Nephrology, Univ Wisconsin, Madison, WI 1969-1970; Research, Univ Wisconsin, Madison, WI 1972-1974; **Faculty Appointment:** Prof Nephrology, Univ Wisc

Great Plains and Mountains

Berl, Tomas MD (Nephrology) - *Special Expertise:* Fluid/Electrolyte Balance; **Admitting Hospital:** University of Colorado Health & Science Center; **Office Address:** Univ Colo Med Ctr, Dept Med Renal Div 4200 E 9th Ave, rm C281 Denver, CO 80220-3706; **Office Phone:** (303) 329-3066; **Board Certifications:** Internal Medicine 1972, Nephrology 1976; **Medical School:** NYU Sch Med 1968; **Residency:** Internal Medicine, Bronx Muni Hosp, Bronx, NY 1969-1970; **Fellowship:** Renal Disease, Moffit Hosp-UCSF, San Francisco, CA 1970-1971

Schrier, Robert William MD (Nephrology) - *Special Expertise:* Nephrology - General; **Admitting Hospital:** University of Colorado Health & Science Center; **Office Address:** U Colo Med Ctr 4200 E 9th Ave, Dept B 178 Denver, CO 80220; **Office Phone:** (303) 315-7765; **Board Certifications:** Nephrology, Internal Medicine; **Medical School:** Indiana Univ 1962; **Residencies:** Internal Medicine, Univ WA Med Ctr 1963-1965; Internal Medicine, Brigham & Women's Hospital 1965-1966; **Faculty Appointment:** Prof Medicine, Univ Colo

Southwest

Alpern, Robert MD (Nephrology) - *Special Expertise:* Nephrology - General; **Admitting Hospital:** Parkland Memorial Hospital; **Office Address:** Univ of TX SW Med Ctr, Dept Neph 5323 Harry Hines Blvd Dallas, TX 75390-8856; **Office Phone:** (214) 648-3442; **Board Certifications:** Internal Medicine 1979, Nephrology 1982; **Medical School:** Univ Chicago-Pritzker Sch Med 1976; **Residency:** Internal Medicine, Columbia Univ, New York, NY 1976-1977; **Fellowship:** Nephrology, UCSF, San Francisco, CA 1979-1982; **Faculty Appointment:** Prof Medicine, Univ Tex SW, Dallas

Barcenas, Camilo Gustavo MD (Nephrology) - *Special Expertise:* Transplant Medicine-Kidney; **Admitting Hospital:** St Luke's Episcopal Hospital - Houston (Page 76); **Office Address:** Renal Specs 6624 Fannin, Ste 2510 Houston, TX 77030; **Office Phone:** (713) 791-2648; **Board Certifications:** Internal Medicine 1973, Nephrology 1974; **Medical School:** Nicaragua 1968; **Residency:** Internal Medicine, Baylor Med Coll, Houston, TX 1970-1972; **Fellowship:** Nephrology, UTSW Hosps, Dallas, TX 1972-1974

Brennan, Thomas Stephen MD (Nephrology) - *Special Expertise:* Transplant Medicine-Kidney & Pancreas; Kidney Stones; Kidney Failure-Chronic; **Admitting Hospital:** Methodist Hospital - Houston (Page 69); **Office Address:** 2256 Holcombe Houston, TX 77030; **Office Phone:** (713) 790-9080; **Board Certifications:** Internal Medicine 1983, Nephrology 1988; **Medical School:** Loyola Univ-Stritch Sch Med 1979; **Residency:** Internal Medicine, Loyola Univ Med Ctr, Maywood, IL 1980-1983; **Fellowship:** Nephrology, Univ Wash-Barnes Hosp, St. Louis, MO 1983-1986; **Faculty Appointment:** Assoc Clin Prof Medicine, Baylor Coll Med

Kasinath, Balakuntalam S MD (Nephrology) - *Special Expertise:* Nephrology - General; **Admitting Hospital:** University of Texas Health & Science Center; **Office Address:** 7703 Floyd Curl Dr San Antonio, TX 78284; **Office Phone:** (210) 567-4700; **Board Certifications:** Internal Medicine 1980, Nephrology 1982; **Medical School:** India 1975; **Residency:** Internal Medicine, Ill Masonic Med Ctr, Chicago, IL 1977-1980; **Fellowship:** Nephrology, Univ Chicago Hosp, Chicago, IL 1980-1983; **Faculty Appointment:** Prof Medicine, Univ Tex, San Antonio

Olivero, Juan Jose MD (Nephrology) - *Special Expertise:* Kidney Failure; Fluid/Electrolyte Balance; **Admitting Hospital:** St Luke's Episcopal Hospital - Houston (Page 76); **Office Address:** 6560 Fannin, Bldg Scurlock - Ste 2206 Houston, TX 77030; **Office Phone:** (713) 790-4615; **Board Certifications:** Internal Medicine 1974, Nephrology 1976; **Medical School:** Guatemala 1970; **Residencies:** Internal Medicine, Baylor Affil Hosps, Houston, TX 1971-1973; Internal Medicine, Ben Taub Genl Hosp, Houston, TX 1973; **Fellowship:** Nephrology, Baylor Affil Hosps, Houston, TX 1974-1975

Suki, Wadi MD (Nephrology) - *Special Expertise:* Transplant Medicine-Kidney; **Admitting Hospital:** Methodist Hospital - Houston (Page 69); **Office Address:** 6550 Fannin St, Ste 1275 Houston, TX 77030-2742; **Office Phone:** (713) 790-3275; **Board Certifications:** Internal Medicine 1967, Nephrology 1972; **Medical School:** Sudan 1959; **Residency:** Internal Medicine, Parkland Meml Hosp, Dallas, TX 1961-1963; **Fellowships:** Nephrology, Univ Texas SW, Dallas, TX 1959-1961; Nephrology, Univ Texas SW, Dallas, TX 1963-1965; **Faculty Appointment:** Clin Prof Medicine, Baylor Coll Med

NEPHROLOGY

Southwest

Wesson, Donald MD (Nephrology) - *Special Expertise:* Nephrology - General; **Admitting Hospital:** University Medical Center; **Office Address:** Tex Tech Univ Hlth Sci Ctr, Dept Med, Div Nephrology 3601 4th St Lubbock, TX 79430; **Office Phone:** (806) 743-2521; **Board Certifications:** Internal Medicine 1981, Nephrology 1986; **Medical School:** Baylor Coll Med 1978; **Residency:** Internal Medicine, Baylor Coll Med Hosp, Houston, TX 1979-1981; **Fellowship:** Nephrology, University Illinois Med Ctr, Chicago, IL 1981-1983; **Faculty Appointment:** Prof Medicine, Texas Tech Univ

West Coast and Pacific

Ahmad, Suhail MD (Nephrology) - *Special Expertise:* Hypertension; Kidney Failure-Chronic; Kidney Stones; **Admitting Hospital:** University of Washington Medical Center; **Office Address:** Univ Washington - Scribner Kidney Ctr 2150 N 107th St, Ste 160 Seattle, WA 98133; **Office Phone:** (206) 363-5090; **Medical School:** India 1968; **Residency:** Internal Medicine, Univ Allahabad, Allahabad, India 1968-1971; **Fellowship:** Nephrology, Univ Washington, Seattle, WA 1976-1978; **Faculty Appointment:** Assoc Prof Medicine, Univ Wash

Amend Jr, William JC MD (Nephrology) - *Special Expertise:* Transplant-Kidney; **Admitting Hospital:** University of California - San Francisco Medical Center; **Office Address:** UCSF, Div Nephrology 513 Parnassus Ave, Box 0532 San Francisco, CA 94143; **Office Phone:** (415) 476-2172; **Board Certifications:** Internal Medicine 1972, Nephrology 1974; **Medical School:** Cornell Univ-Weil Med Coll 1967; **Residencies:** Internal Medicine, UCSF Hosp, San Francisco, CA 1968-1969; Internal Medicine, Mass Genl Hosp, Boston, MA 1971-1972; **Fellowship:** Nephrology, Peter Bent Brigham Hosp, Boston, MA 1972-1973; **Faculty Appointment:** Prof Nephrology, UCSF

Bennett, William M MD (Nephrology) - *Special Expertise:* Polycystic Kidney Disease; Transplant Medicine-Kidney; Drug Toxicity-Kidneys; **Admitting Hospital:** Legacy Good Samaritan Hospital and Medical Center; **Office Address:** Legacy Good Samaritan Hosp, Transplant Svcs NSC430 1040 NW 22nd Portland, OR 97210; **Office Phone:** (503) 413-7349; **Board Certifications:** Internal Medicine 1988, Nephrology 1972; **Medical School:** Nigeria 1963; **Residencies:** Internal Medicine, Northwestern Univ, Chicago, IL 1963-1965; Internal Medicine, Ore Hlth Sci Univ, Portland, OR 1965-1966; **Fellowship:** Nephrology, Mass Genl Hosp, Boston, MA 1968-1970; **Faculty Appointment:** Prof Medicine, Oregon Hlth Scis Univ

Couser, William MD (Nephrology) - *Special Expertise:* Kidney Disease-Glomerular; Nephrotic Syndrome; **Admitting Hospital:** University of Washington Medical Center; **Office Address:** UWMC, Div of Nep 1959 NE Pacific St, Fl 12th - rm 1265, Box 356521 Seattle, WA 98195; **Office Phone:** (206) 598-5068; **Board Certifications:** Internal Medicine 1971, Nephrology 1973; **Medical School:** Harvard Med Sch 1965; **Residencies:** Internal Medicine, Univ of CA Med Cter, San Francisco, CA 1965-1967; Internal Medicine, Boston City Hosp, Boston, MA 1969-1970; **Fellowships:** Nephrology, Boston City Hosp, Boston, MA 1970-1971; Nephrology, Univ of Chicago, Chicago, IL 1971-1973; **Faculty Appointment:** Prof Medicine, Univ Wash

Kaysen, George Alan MD/PhD (Nephrology) - *Special Expertise:* Kidney Disease-Metabolic; Kidney Failure-Chronic; **Admitting Hospital:** University of California - Davis Medical Center; **Office Address:** UC Davis Med Ctr, Div Nephr TB 136 Davis, CA 95616; **Office Phone:** (530) 752-4010; **Board Certifications:** Internal Medicine 1975, Nephrology 1980; **Medical School:** Albert Einstein Coll Med 1972; **Residency:** Internal Medicine, Bronx Muni Hosp, Bronx, NY 1973-1975; **Fellowship:** Renal Disease, Bronx Muni Hosp, Bronx, NY 1975-1977; **Faculty Appointment:** Prof Medicine, UC Davis

Kopple, Joel David MD (Nephrology) - *Special Expertise:* Kidney Disease-Nutrition; **Admitting Hospital:** LAC - Harbor - UCLA Medical Center; **Office Address:** UCLA Med Ctr 1000 W Carson St, Box 406 Torrance, CA 90509; **Office Phone:** (310) 222-3891; **Board Certifications:** Internal Medicine 1969, Nephrology 1974; **Medical School:** Univ IL Coll Med 1962; **Residency:** Internal Medicine, Wadsworth VA Hosp, Los Angeles, CA 1963-1966; **Fellowship:** Nephrology, Wadsworth VA Hosp Ctr, Los Angeles, CA 1966-1967; **Faculty Appointment:** Prof Medicine, UCLA

Massry, Shaul Gourgi MD (Nephrology) - *Special Expertise:* Hypertension; Parathyroid Disease; Kidney Disease-Metabolic; **Admitting Hospital:** LAC + USC Medical Center; **Office Address:** 1355 San Pablo St Dr, Ste 100 Los Angeles, CA 90033; **Office Phone:** (323) 442-5100; **Board Certifications:** Internal Medicine 1973, Nephrology 1974; **Medical School:** Israel 1954; **Residency:** Internal Medicine, Beilinson Med Ctr., Israel 1962-1965; **Fellowship:** Renal Disease, Cedars-Sinai Med Ctr., Los Angeles, CA 1966-1968; **Faculty Appointment:** Prof Medicine, Univ SC Sch Med

Myers, Bryan David MD (Nephrology) - *Special Expertise:* Kidney Disease; Hypertension; **Admitting Hospital:** Stanford Medical Center; **Office Address:** 900 Wilbur Dr, rm W-3045 Palo Alto, CA 94305; **Office Phone:** (650) 723-6961; **Medical School:** South Africa 1959

Omachi, Rodney S MD (Nephrology) - *Special Expertise:* Nephrology - General; **Admitting Hospital:** University of California - San Francisco Medical Center; **Office Address:** Nephrology Assocs Inc 400 Parnassus A-540 San Francisco, CA 94143; **Office Phone:** (415) 665-3400; **Board Certifications:** Internal Medicine 1973, Nephrology 1974; **Medical School:** Harvard Med Sch 1968; **Residency:** Internal Medicine, Mass Genl Hosp, Boston, MA 1969-1970; **Fellowships:** Nephrology, Natl Inst Hlth, Bethesda, MD 1970-1973; Nephrology, UCSF, San Franciscio, CA 1973-1974; **Faculty Appointment:** Clin Prof Nephrology, UCSF

Riordan, John William MD (Nephrology) - *Special Expertise:* Internal Medicine; **Admitting Hospital:** California Pacific Medical Center; **Office Address:** 2100 Webster St, Bldg 412 San Francisco, CA 94115; **Office Phone:** (415) 923-3815; **Board Certifications:** Internal Medicine 1990, Nephrology 1994; **Medical School:** Univ Tex Med Br, Galveston 1987; **Residency:** Internal Medicine, Univ TX Hlth Sci Ctr, San Antonio, TX 1988-1990; **Fellowship:** Nephrology, UCSF, San Francisco, CA 1991-1995

Saleh, Saleh MD (Nephrology) - *Special Expertise:* Kidney Stones; **Admitting Hospital:** UCLA Medical Center; **Office Address:** 100 UCLA Medical Plaza Pl Ste 690 Los Angeles, CA 90095; **Office Phone:** (310) 824-0088; **Board Certifications:** Internal Medicine 1983, Nephrology 1984; **Medical School:** McGill Univ 1977; **Residency:** Internal Medicine, Royal Victoria Hosp, Montreal, Canada 1978-1979; **Fellowship:** Nephrology, UCLA Ctr Hlth Scis, Los Angeles, CA 1981-1984; **Faculty Appointment:** Assoc Clin Prof Medicine, UCLA

Scandling Jr, John David MD (Nephrology) - *Special Expertise:* Transplant Medicine-Kidney; **Admitting Hospital:** Stanford Medical Center; **Office Address:** 750 Welch Rd, Ste 200 Stanford U Med Ctr, Med Dir Renal Trans Palo Alto, CA 94304; **Office Phone:** (650) 725-9891; **Board Certifications:** Internal Medicine 1981, Nephrology 1984; **Medical School:** Med Coll VA 1978; **Residency:** Internal Medicine, W Va U Hosp, Morgantown, VA 1979-1981; **Fellowship:** Nephrology, U Rochester, Rochester, NY 1981-1983; **Faculty Appointment:** Prof Medicine, Stanford Univ

NEUROLOGICAL SURGERY

A neurological surgeon provides the operative and non-operative management (i.e., prevention, diagnosis, evaluation, treatment, critical care and rehabilitation) of disorders of the central, peripheral and autonomic nervous systems, including their supporting structures and vascular supply; the evaluation and treatment of pathological processes which modify function or activity of the nervous system; and the operative and non-operative management of pain. A neurological surgeon treats patients with disorders of the nervous system; disorders of the brain, meninges, skull and their blood supply, including the extracranial carotid and vertebral arteries; disorders of the pituitary gland; disorders of the spinal cord, meninges and vertebral column, including those which may require treatment by spinal fusion or instrumentation; and disorders of the cranial and spinal nerves throughout their distribution.

Training required: Seven years (including general surgery)

PHYSICIAN LISTINGS

Neurological Surgery

New England

Awad, Issam A MD (Neurological Surgery) - *Special Expertise:* Neurovascular Surgery; Stroke; Cerebrovascular Disease; **Admitting Hospital:** Yale - New Haven Hospital; **Office Address:** Yale Univ Med Sch 333 Cedar St, Box TMP 405 New Haven, CT 06520; **Office Phone:** (203) 737-2096; **Board Certification:** Neurological Surgery 1988; **Medical School:** Loma Linda Univ 1980; **Residency:** Neurological Surgery, Cleveland Clin, Cleveland, OH 1981-1985; **Fellowship:** Neurological Vascular Surgery, Barrow Neur Inst, Pheonix, AZ 1985-1986; **Faculty Appointment:** Prof Neurological Surgery, Yale Univ

Black, Peter MD (Neurological Surgery) - *Special Expertise:* Seizure Surgery; Brain & Spinal Cord Tumors; Intra Operative MRI Surgery; **Admitting Hospital:** Brigham & Women's Hospital; **Office Address:** Brigham & Women's Hosp, Dept Neurosurg 75 Francis St Boston, MA 02115; **Office Phone:** (617) 355-7795; **Board Certification:** Neurological Surgery 1984; **Medical School:** McGill Univ 1970; **Residencies:** Surgery, Mass Genl Hosp, Boston, MA 1971-1972; Neurological Surgery, Mass Genl Hosp, Boston, MA 1975-1978; **Fellowship:** Neurological Oncology, Mass Genl Hosp, Boston, MA 1975-1976; **Faculty Appointment:** Prof Neurological Surgery, Harvard Med Sch

Borges, Lawrence F. MD (Neurological Surgery) - *Special Expertise:* Spinal Surgery; **Admitting Hospital:** Massachusetts General Hospital; **Office Address:** Mass Genl Hosp Div, Neuro Surg 32 Fruit St Boston, MA 02114-2620; **Office Phone:** (617) 726-6156; **Board Certification:** Neurological Surgery 1986; **Medical School:** Johns Hopkins Univ 1977; **Residency:** Neurological Surgery, Mass Genl Hosp, Boston, MA 1978-1983; **Faculty Appointment:** Assoc Prof Surgery, Harvard Med Sch

Chapman, Paul H. MD (Neurological Surgery) - *Special Expertise:* Neurosurgery-Pediatric; Stereotactic Radiosurgery; **Admitting Hospital:** Massachusetts General Hospital; **Office Address:** Mass Genl Hosp 55 Fruit St GRB 502 Boston, MA 02114-2698; **Office Phone:** (617) 726-3887; **Board Certification:** Neurological Surgery 1976; **Medical School:** Harvard Med Sch 1964; **Residencies:** Surgery, Mass Genl Hosp, Boston, MA 1965-1966; Neurological Surgery, Mass Genl Hosp, Boston, MA 1968-1972; **Fellowship:** Neurological Surgery, Hosp Sick Chldn, Tornto, Canada 1972; **Faculty Appointment:** Assoc Prof Surgery, Harvard Med Sch

Cosgrove, G. Rees MD (Neurological Surgery) - *Special Expertise:* Epilepsy/Seizure Disorders; Brain Tumors; **Admitting Hospital:** Massachusetts General Hospital; **Office Address:** Mass Gen Hosp, Dept of Neurosurgery 15 Parkman St, Ste 331 Boston, MA 02114; **Office Phone:** (617) 724-0357; **Board Certification:** Neurological Surgery 1989; **Medical School:** Queens Univ 1980; **Residency:** Neurological Surgery, Montreal Neur Inst, Canada 1981-1986

Nazzaro, Jules M. MD (Neurological Surgery) - *Special Expertise:* Parkinson's Disease; Movement Disorders; Stereotactic Radiosurgery; **Admitting Hospital:** Boston Medical Center; **Office Address:** Boston Medical Center 720 Harrison Ave, Ste 710 Boston, MA 02118; **Office Phone:** (617) 638-8993; **Board Certification:** Neurological Surgery 1996; **Medical School:** Albert Einstein Coll Med 1984; **Residency:** Neurology, NYU Med Ctr, New York, NY 1985-1991; **Fellowship:** Nephrology, Meml Sloan-Kettering Cancer Ctr, New York, NY 1991-1992; **Faculty Appointment:** Asst Prof Neurological Surgery, Boston Univ

Ojemann, Robert G. MD (Neurological Surgery) - *Special Expertise:* Brain Tumors; Spinal Cord Tumors; Acoustic Nerve Tumors; **Admitting Hospital:** Massachusetts General Hospital; **Office Address:** Mass Genl Dept of Neurosurgery 55 Fruit Street Boston, MA 02114-2621; **Office Phone:** (617) 726-2936; **Board Certification:** Nephrology 1964; **Residencies:** Sports Medicine, Baylor University, Houston, TX 1956-1957; Neurological Surgery, Mass Genl Hosp, Boston, MA 1957-1966; **Faculty Appointment:** Prof Surgery, Harvard Med Sch

NEUROLOGICAL SURGERY

Piepmeier, Joseph MD (Neurological Surgery) - *Special Expertise:* Neuro-Oncology; Brain & Spinal Cord Tumors; **Admitting Hospital:** Yale - New Haven Hospital; **Office Address:** Yale Univ Sch Med, Dept Neuro Surg 333 Cedar St New Haven, CT 06510-3289; **Office Phone:** (203) 785-2791; **Board Certification:** Neurological Surgery 1984; **Medical School:** Univ Tenn Coll Med, Memphis 1975; **Residency:** Neurological Surgery, Yale-New Haven Hosp, New Haven, CT 1977-1982; **Faculty Appointment:** Prof Neurological Surgery, Yale Univ

Scott, R. Michael MD (Neurological Surgery) - *Special Expertise:* Brain Tumors; *Cerebrovascular Surgery;* **Admitting Hospital:** Children's Hospital; **Office Address:** Children's Hosp, Dept Neurosurg 300 Longwood Ave, Bldg Bader - Ste 319 Boston, MA 02115-5724; **Office Phone:** (617) 355-6011; **Board Certification:** Neurological Surgery 1976; **Medical School:** Temple Univ 1966; **Residency:** Neurological Surgery, Massachusetts General Hospital, Boston, MA 1969-1973; **Faculty Appointment:** Prof Surgery, Harvard Med Sch

Shucart, William A MD (Neurological Surgery) - *Special Expertise:* Pituitary Surgery; **Admitting Hospital:** New England Medical Center; **Office Address:** New England Medical Center- Division of Neurosurgery 750 Washington St, Box 178 Boston, MA 02111; **Office Phone:** (617) 636-5858; **Board Certification:** Neurological Surgery 1973; **Medical School:** Univ MO-Columbia Sch Med 1961; **Residencies:** Neurological Surgery, Colum-Presby Hosp, New York, NY 1967-1970; Neurological Surgery, Hosp Sick Chldn, Toronto Canada 1970-1971

Spencer, Dennis D MD (Neurological Surgery) - *Special Expertise:* Epilepsy/Seizure *Disorders;* **Admitting Hospital:** Yale - New Haven Hospital; **Office Address:** Yale Neurosurgery Group 333 Cedar St, Bldg TMP4 New Haven, CT 06520; **Office Phone:** (203) 785-2811; **Board Certification:** Neurological Surgery 1980; **Medical School:** Washington Univ, St Louis 1971; **Residencies:** Surgery, Barnes Hosp, St Louis, MO 1971-1972; Neurological Surgery, Yale-New Haven Hosp, New Haven, CT 1972-1976; **Faculty Appointment:** Prof Neurological Surgery, Yale Univ

Mid Atlantic

Albright, Leland MD (Neurological Surgery) - *Special Expertise:* Neurosurgery-Pediatric; *Spasticity & Movement Disorders; Brain Tumors;* **Admitting Hospital:** Children's Hospital of Pittsburgh; **Office Address:** Children's Hosp- Pittsburgh, Dept Neurosurgery 3705 5th Ave Pittsburgh, PA 15213-2524; **Office Phone:** (412) 692-8142; **Board Certification:** Neurological Surgery 1981; **Medical School:** Louisiana State Univ 1969; **Residency:** Surgery, Barnes Hosp, St Louis, MO 1970-1971; **Fellowships:** Neurological Surgery, National Inst of Hlth, Bethesda, MD 1971-1974; Neurological Surgery, Univ Pittsburgh, Pittsburgh, PA 1974-1978; **Faculty Appointment:** Prof Neurological Surgery, Univ Pittsburgh

Baltuch, Gordon MD/PhD (Neurological Surgery) - *Special Expertise:* Movement Disorders; *Parkinson's Disease; Epilepsy/Seizure Disorders;* **Admitting Hospital:** Pennsylvania Hospital; **Office Address:** Penn Neurological Institute/Silverstein 5 3400 Spruce St Philadelphia, PA 19104; **Office Phone:** (215) 662-7788; **Board Certification:** Neurological Surgery 1998; **Medical School:** McGill Univ 1986; **Residency:** Neurological Surgery, Montreal Neuro Inst, Montreal, Canada; **Faculty Appointment:** Asst Prof Neurological Surgery, Univ Penn

Benjamin, Vallo MD (Neurological Surgery) - *Special Expertise:* Spinal Surgery; Skull Base *Surgery;* **Admitting Hospital:** NYU Medical Center (Page 70); **Office Address:** 530 First Ave, Ste 7W New York, NY 10016; **Office Phone:** (212) 263-5013; **Board Certification:** Neurological Surgery 1967; **Medical School:** Iran 1958; **Residency:** Neurological Surgery, Bellevue Hosp, New York, NY 1960-1964; **Fellowship:** Neurological Surgery, NYU Med Ctr, New York, NY 1965-1966; **Faculty Appointment:** Prof Neurological Surgery, NYU Sch Med

Camins, Martin B MD (Neurological Surgery) - *Special Expertise:* Spinal Surgery; **Admitting Hospital:** Mount Sinai Hospital (Page 70); **Office Address:** 205 E 68th St, Ste T1C New York, NY 10021-5735; **Office Phone:** (212) 570-0100; **Board Certification:** Neurological Surgery 1980; **Medical School:** Univ Hlth Sci/Chicago Med Sch 1969; **Residencies:** Neurology, Columbia-Presby, New York, NY 1970-1971; Neurological Surgery, Columbia-Presby, New York, NY 1971-1975; **Fellowships:** Neurological Surgery, Nat Hosp, London, England 1973; New York Univ Med Ctr, New York, NY 1976-1977; **Faculty Appointment:** Assoc Prof Neurological Surgery, Mount Sinai Sch Med

Caputy, Anthony J. MD (Neurological Surgery) - *Special Expertise:* Epilepsy/Seizure Disorders; Spinal Surgery; **Admitting Hospital:** Fairfax Hospital; **Office Address:** Geo Wash Univ, Dept Neuro Surg 2150 Pennsylvania Ave NW, Fl 7-420 Washington, DC 20037; **Office Phone:** (202) 994-9226; **Board Certification:** Neurological Surgery 1989; **Medical School:** Univ VA Sch Med 1980; **Residency:** Neurological Surgery, Georgetown Univ, Washington, DC 1981-1986; **Faculty Appointment:** Assoc Clin Prof Neurological Surgery, Univ MD Sch Med

Carmel, Peter MD (Neurological Surgery) - *Special Expertise:* Brain Tumors-Pediatric; Skull Base Surgery; **Admitting Hospital:** UMDNJ-University Hospital-Newark; **Office Address:** UMDNJ-NJ Med Sch 90 Bergen St, rm 1700 Newark, NJ 07103; **Office Phone:** (973) 972-2323; **Board Certification:** Neurological Surgery 1968; **Medical School:** NYU Sch Med 1960; **Residencies:** Neurological Surgery, Columbia Presby Med Ctr, New York, NY 1963-1967; Neurological Surgery, Neuro-Inst, New York, NY 1963-1967; **Faculty Appointment:** Prof Neurological Surgery, UMDNJ-NJ Med Sch, Newark

Carson, Benjamin S MD (Neurological Surgery) - *Special Expertise:* Brain Injury; Brain & Spinal Cord Tumors; **Admitting Hospital:** Johns Hopkins Hospital - Baltimore (Page 65); **Office Address:** John Hopkins Hosp, Dept Neuro-Surgery 600 N Wolfe St, Harvey 811 Baltimore, MD 21287-8811; **Office Phone:** (410) 955-7888; **Board Certification:** Neurological Surgery 1988; **Medical School:** Univ Mich Med Sch 1977; **Residency:** Neurological Surgery, Johns Hopkins Hosp, Baltimore, MD 1978-1983; **Fellowship:** Pediatric Neurological Surgery, Queen Elizabeth II Med Ctr, Western Australia 1983-1984; **Faculty Appointment:** Assoc Prof Neurological Surgery, Johns Hopkins Univ

Dennis, Gary Creed MD (Neurological Surgery) - *Special Expertise:* Brain & Spinal Surgery; Pain Management; Subarachnoid Hemorrhage; **Admitting Hospital:** Howard University Hospital; **Office Address:** Howard U Hosp 2041 Georgia Ave NW, Ste 5B-47 Washington, DC 20060; **Office Phone:** (202) 865-6681; **Board Certification:** Neurological Surgery 1983; **Medical School:** Howard Univ 1976; **Residency:** Neurological Surgery, Baylor Affil Hosps, Houston, TX 1977-1981; **Faculty Appointment:** Assoc Prof Surgery, Howard Univ

Eisenberg, Howard M MD (Neurological Surgery) - *Special Expertise:* Acoustic Nerve Tumors; Head & Spinal Cord Injury; Epilepsy/Seizure Disorders; **Admitting Hospital:** University of Maryland Medical System; **Office Address:** Univ MD Sch Med, Dept Neuro 22 S Greene St Baltimore, MD; **Office Phone:** (410) 328-3514; **Board Certification:** Neurological Surgery 1973; **Medical School:** SUNY Downstate 1964; **Residencies:** Surgery, NY Hosp, New York, NY 1965-1966; Neurological Surgery, Peter Bent Brigham Hosp, Boston, MA 1966-1970; **Fellowship:** Harvard Univ, Boston, MA 1969-1970; **Faculty Appointment:** Prof Neurological Surgery, Univ MD Sch Med

Epstein, Fred Jacob MD (Neurological Surgery) - *Special Expertise: Spinal Cord Tumors-Pediatric; Brain Stem Tumors-Pediatric;* **Admitting Hospital:** Beth Israel Medical Center - Herbert & Nell Singer Division (Page 58); **Office Address:** 170 East End Ave, rm 521 New York, NY 10128; **Office Phone:** (212) 870-9600; **Board Certification:** Neurological Surgery 1972; **Medical School:** NY Med Coll 1963; **Residencies:** Surgery, Montefiore Hosp, New York, NY 1964-1965; Neurological Surgery, NYU Med Ctr, New York, NY 1965-1970; **Faculty Appointment:** Prof Neurological Surgery, Albert Einstein Coll Med

Flamm, Eugene MD (Neurological Surgery) - *Special Expertise: Spinal Cord Tumors;* **Admitting Hospital:** Beth Israel Medical Center - Herbert & Nell Singer Division (Page 58); **Office Address:** Inst for Neurl & Neurosurg 170 E End Ave New York, NY 10128; **Office Phone:** (212) 870-7960; **Board Certification:** Neurological Surgery 1973; **Medical School:** SUNY Buffalo 1962; **Residencies:** Surgery, NY Hosp, New York, NY 1963-1964; Neurological Surgery, NYU Med C, New York, NY 1966-1970; **Fellowship:** Neurological Surgery, Univ Zurich, Zurich, Switzerland 1970-1971; **Faculty Appointment:** Prof Neurological Surgery, Albert Einstein Coll Med

Germano, Isabelle M MD (Neurological Surgery) - *Special Expertise: Brain Tumors; Movement Disorders;* **Admitting Hospital:** Mount Sinai Hospital (Page 70); **Office Address:** 5 E 98th St, Box 1136 New York, NY 10029-6504; **Office Phone:** (212) 241-9638; **Board Certification:** Neurological Surgery 1995; **Medical School:** Italy 1984; **Residencies:** Neurological Surgery, UCSF, San Francisco, CA 1988-1990; Neurological Surgery, Albert Einstein Coll Med, New York, NY 1990-1993; **Faculty Appointment:** Assoc Prof Neurological Surgery, Mount Sinai Sch Med

Grady, M Sean MD (Neurological Surgery) - *Special Expertise: Cerebrovascular Surgery; Stroke;* **Admitting Hospital:** Hospital of the University of Pennsylvania; **Office Address:** Hosp Univ Penn 3400 Spruce St Philadelphia, PA 19104; **Office Phone:** (215) 662-3487; **Board Certification:** Neurological Surgery 1990; **Medical School:** Georgetown Univ 1981; **Residency:** Neurological Surgery, Univ Virginia, Charlottesville, VA 1981-1987; **Faculty Appointment:** Assoc Prof Neurological Surgery, Univ Penn

Hodge Jr., Charles J. MD (Neurological Surgery) - *Special Expertise: Vascular Neurosurgery;* **Admitting Hospital:** Upstate University Medical Hospital; **Office Address:** 750 E Adams St Syracuse, NY; **Office Phone:** (315) 464-4470; **Board Certification:** Neurological Surgery 1977; **Medical School:** Columbia P&S 1967; **Residencies:** Neurological Surgery, SUNY Upstate Med Ctr, Syracuse, NY 1969-1974; Surgery, Yale-New Haven Hosp, New Haven, CT 1968-1969; **Faculty Appointment:** Prof Neurological Surgery, SUNY Syracuse

Hopkins, Leo Nelson MD (Neurological Surgery) - *Special Expertise: Cerebrovascular Surgery; Endovascular Surgery;* **Admitting Hospital:** Millard Fillmore Hospitals; **Office Address:** Millard Fillmore Hosp, Neurosurgery Dept 3 Gates Cir Buffalo, NY 14209; **Office Phone:** (716) 887-5210; **Board Certification:** Neurological Surgery 1977; **Medical School:** Albany Med Coll 1969; **Residency:** Neurological Surgery, SUNY Buffalo, Buffalo, NY 1971-1975; **Faculty Appointment:** Prof Neurological Surgery, SUNY Buffalo

Jacobson, Jeff MD (Neurological Surgery) - *Special Expertise: Acoustic Nerve Tumors;* **Admitting Hospital:** Washington Hospital Center - DC (Page 79); **Office Address:** 3 Washington Cir NW Ste 306 Washington, DC; **Office Phone:** (202) 223-1060; **Board Certification:** Neurological Surgery 1988; **Medical School:** Geo Wash Univ 1977; **Residencies:** Surgery, Geo Wash U, Washington, DC 1977-1978; Neurological Surgery, Geo Wash U, Washington, DC 1978-1983; **Faculty Appointment:** Clin Inst Neurological Surgery, Geo Wash Univ

Kelly, Patrick J. MD (Neurological Surgery) - *Special Expertise:* Brain Tumors; Stereotactic Radiosurgery; Movement Disorders; **Admitting Hospital:** NYU Medical Center (Page 70); **Office Address:** NYU Med Ctr, Dept Neurological Surgery 530 1st Ave, Ste 8R New York, NY 10016; **Office Phone:** (212) 263-8002; **Board Certification:** Neurological Surgery 1978; **Medical School:** SUNY Buffalo 1966; **Residencies:** Neurological Surgery, Northwestern, Chicago, IL 1970-1972; Neurological Surgery, Univ TX Med Hosp, Galveston, TX 1972-1974; **Fellowship:** Neurological Surgery, St Anne Hosp, Paris, France 1977; **Faculty Appointment:** Prof Neurological Surgery, NYU Sch Med

Khan, Agha S MD (Neurological Surgery) - *Special Expertise:* Skull Base Surgery; Spinal Surgery; **Admitting Hospital:** Maryland General Hospital; **Office Address:** 2435 W Belvedere Ave, Ste 41 Baltimore, MD 21201; **Office Phone:** (410) 601-8314; **Board Certification:** Neurological Surgery 1995; **Medical School:** Pakistan 1979; **Residencies:** Surgery, Washington Hosp Ctr, Washington, DC 1982-1983; Neurological Surgery, Univ Wisconsin Hosp & Clinic, Madison, WI 1983-1990

Kobrine, Arthur MD/PhD (Neurological Surgery) - *Special Expertise:* Spinal Cord Surgery; Brain & Spinal Cord Tumors; **Admitting Hospital:** Georgetown University Hospital; **Office Address:** 2440 M St NW, Ste 315 Washington, DC 20037-1404; **Office Phone:** (202) 293-7136; **Board Certification:** Neurological Surgery 1976; **Medical School:** Northwestern Univ **Residencies:** Neurological Surgery, Northwestern, Chicago, IL 1969-1970; Neurological Surgery, Walter Reed Genl Hosp, Washington, DC 1970-1973; **Fellowship:** Physiology, Geo Wash Univ, Washington, DC 1979; **Faculty Appointment:** Clin Prof Neurological Surgery, Georgetown Univ

Lavyne, Michael H MD (Neurological Surgery) - *Special Expertise:* Spinal Surgery; **Admitting Hospital:** New York Weill Cornell Medical Center - NY Presbyterian Hospital (Page 72); **Office Address:** 523 E 72nd St New York, NY 10021; **Office Phone:** (212) 717-0200; **Board Certification:** Neurological Surgery 1982; **Medical School:** Cornell Univ-Weill Med Coll 1972; **Residency:** Neurological Surgery, Mass Gen Hosp, Boston, MA 1974-1979; **Fellowship:** Neurology, Beth Israel, Boston, MA 1973-1974; **Faculty Appointment:** Assoc Prof Surgery

Long, Donlin M MD/PhD (Neurological Surgery) - *Special Expertise:* Skull Base Tumors; Acoustic Nerve Tumors; Spinal Diseases; **Admitting Hospital:** Johns Hopkins Hospital - Baltimore (Page 65); **Office Address:** Johns Hopkins Hospital 600 N Wolfe St, Bldg Meyer - rm 7-109 Baltimore, MD 21287-7709; **Office Phone:** (410) 955-2251; **Board Certification:** Neurological Surgery 1968; **Medical School:** Univ MO-Columbia Sch Med 1959; **Residencies:** Neurological Surgery, Univ Minnesota Hosp, Minneapolis, MN 1960-1964; Peter Bent Brigham Hosp, Boston, MA 1965; **Faculty Appointment:** Prof Neurological Surgery, Johns Hopkins Univ

Lunsford, L Dade MD (Neurological Surgery) - *Special Expertise:* Stereotactic Radiosurgery; Movement Disorders; **Admitting Hospital:** UPMC - Presbyterian University Hospital; **Office Address:** UPMC Presbyterian 200 Lothrop St, Ste B400 Pittsburgh, PA 15213; **Office Phone:** (412) 647-3685; **Board Certification:** Neurological Surgery 1983; **Medical School:** Columbia P&S 1974; **Residency:** Neurological Surgery, Univ Pittsburgh, Pittsburgh, PA 1975-1980; **Fellowship:** Stereo Neurological Surgery, Karolinska Hospital, Stockholm, Sweden 1980-1981; **Faculty Appointment:** Prof Neurological Surgery, Univ Pittsburgh

Mangiardi, John MD (Neurological Surgery) - *Special Expertise:* Brain Tumors; Spinal Surgery; **Admitting Hospital:** Lenox Hill Hospital; **Office Address:** 50 E 72 St New York, NY 10021; **Office Phone:** (212) 879-1919; **Board Certification:** Neurological Surgery 1987; **Medical School:** Wayne State Univ 1976; **Residencies:** Neurological Surgery, NYU Med Ctr, New York, NY 1978-1982; Neurological Surgery, NYU Med Ctr, New York, NY 1982-1983; **Faculty Appointment:** Prof Neurological Surgery, NYU Sch Med

NEUROLOGICAL SURGERY *Mid Atlantic*

Marion, Donald W. MD (Neurological Surgery) - *Special Expertise:* Trauma-Brain Injury; Spinal Surgery; Brain Tumors; **Admitting Hospital:** UPMC - Presbyterian University Hospital; **Office Address:** Presbyterian Univ Hosp 200 Lothrop St, Ste B400 Pittsburgh, PA 15213; **Office Phone:** (412) 647-0956; **Board Certification:** Surgery 1993; **Medical School:** UCSF 1982; **Residencies:** Surgery, Univ Pitts Med Ctr, Pittsburgh, PA 1982-1983; Neurological Surgery, Univ Pitts Med Ctr, Pittsburgh, PA 1983-1989; **Fellowship:** Neurological Trauma, Med Coll VA, Charlottesville, VA 1989-1990; **Faculty Appointment:** Prof Neurological Surgery, Univ Pittsburgh

McCormick, Paul MD (Neurological Surgery) - *Special Expertise:* Neurological Surgery - General; **Admitting Hospital:** Columbia Presbyterian Medical Center (Page 72); **Office Address:** 710 W 168th St, Ste 406 New York, NY 10032; **Office Phone:** (212) 305-7976; **Board Certification:** Neurological Surgery 1993; **Medical School:** Columbia P&S 1982; **Residency:** Neurological Surgery, Columbia Presby Med Ctr, New York, NY 1984-1989; **Fellowships:** Neurological Surgery, Natl Inst Hlth, Bethesda, MD 1982-1983; Spine Surgery, Med Coll Wisc, Milwaukee, WI 1989-1990; **Faculty Appointment:** Assoc Clin Prof Neurological Surgery, Columbia P&S

Milhorat, Thomas H MD (Neurological Surgery) - *Special Expertise:* Syringomyelia; Chiari's Deformity; Hydrocephalus; **Admitting Hospital:** Long Island College Hospital (Page 58); **Office Address:** Dept of Neurosurgery, SUNY Health Sciences Center-Brooklyn 450 Clarkson Ave, Box 1189 Brooklyn, NY 11203; **Office Phone:** (718) 270-2111; **Board Certification:** Neurological Surgery 1972; **Medical School:** Cornell Univ-Weil Med Coll 1961; **Residencies:** Surgery, NY Hosp-Cornel Med Ctr, New York, NY 1961-1963; Neurological Surgery, NY Hosp-Cornel Med Ctr, New York, NY 1965-1969; **Fellowship:** Neurological Surgery, Nat Inst Hlth, Bethesda, MD 1963-1965; **Faculty Appointment:** Prof Neurological Surgery, SUNY Downstate

Murali, Raj MD (Neurological Surgery) - *Special Expertise:* Neurological Surgery - General; **Admitting Hospital:** St Vincents Catholic Medical Center of New York; **Office Address:** 153 W 11th St, Ste NR 8 New York, NY 10011; **Office Phone:** (212) 604-7767; **Board Certification:** Neurological Surgery 1982; **Medical School:** India 1968; **Residencies:** Neurological Surgery, New York Univ Med Ctr, New York, NY 1975-1979; Surgery, Edinburgh University, United Kingdom; **Fellowship:** Neurological Surgery, Edinburgh University, United Kingdom; **Faculty Appointment:** Prof Neurological Surgery, NY Med Coll

Pollack, Ian MD (Neurological Surgery) - *Special Expertise:* Neurosurgery-Pediatric; Brain Tumors; Craniofacial Surgery; **Admitting Hospital:** Children's Hospital of Pittsburgh; **Office Address:** Children's Hosp of Pittsburgh, Dept of Neurosurgery 3705 Fifth Ave Pittsburgh, PA 15213; **Office Phone:** (412) 692-5881; **Board Certification:** Neurological Surgery 1996; **Medical School:** Johns Hopkins Univ 1984; **Residency:** Univ Pittsburgh Sch Med 1985-1991; **Fellowship:** Hosp Sick Chldn, Toronto, Canada 1991-1991; **Faculty Appointment:** Prof Neurological Surgery, Univ Pittsburgh

Post, Kalmon MD (Neurological Surgery) - *Special Expertise:* Pituitary Surgery; Acoustic Nerve Tumors; **Admitting Hospital:** Mount Sinai Hospital (Page 70); **Office Address:** 5 E 98th St, FL 7 New York, NY 10029-6501; **Office Phone:** (212) 241-0933; **Board Certification:** Neurological Surgery 1978; **Medical School:** NYU Sch Med 1967; **Residencies:** Surgery, Bellevue Hosp, New York, NY 1968-1969; Neurological Surgery, Bellevue Hosp, New York, NY 1971-1975; **Faculty Appointment:** Prof Neurological Surgery, Mount Sinai Sch Med

Solomon, Robert A MD (Neurological Surgery) - *Special Expertise:* Neurological Surgery - General; **Admitting Hospital:** Columbia Presbyterian Medical Center (Page 72); **Office Address:** Columbia Presbyterian Med Ctr, Dept NeuroSurg 710 W 168th St, Ste 439 New York, NY 10032; **Office Phone:** (212) 305-4118; **Board Certification:** Neurological Surgery 1988; **Medical School:** Johns Hopkins Univ 1980; **Residency:** Neurological Surgery, Neuro Inst-Columbia Univ, New York, NY 1981-1986; **Faculty Appointment:** Prof Neurological Surgery, Columbia P&S

Stieg, Philip E MD/PhD (Neurological Surgery) - *Special Expertise: Skull Base Surgery; Acoustic Nerve Tumors; Carotid Artery Surgery;* **Admitting Hospital:** New York Weill Cornell Medical Center - NY Presbyterian Hospital (Page 72); **Office Address:** Weil Cornell Med Ctr-NY Presby Hosp 520 E 70th St, STARR 651 New York, NY 10021; **Office Phone:** (212) 746-4684; **Board Certification:** Neurological Surgery 1992; **Medical School:** Med Coll Wisc 1983; **Residency:** Neurological Surgery, Dallas Chldns Hosp/Parkland Meml Hosp, Dallas, TX 1984-1988; **Fellowship:** Neurological Biology, Karolinska Inst, Stockholm, Sweden 1987-1988; **Faculty Appointment:** Prof Neurological Surgery, Cornell Univ-Weil Med Coll

Southeast

Branch Jr, Charles L MD (Neurological Surgery) - *Special Expertise: Spinal Surgery; Disc Disease; Stereotactic Radiosurgery;* **Admitting Hospital:** Wake Forest University Baptist Medical Center; **Office Address:** Wake Forest Univ Baptist Med Ctr Medical Center Blvd Winston Salem, NC 27157-0001; **Office Phone:** (336) 716-4038; **Board Certification:** Neurological Surgery 1991; **Medical School:** Univ Tex SW, Dallas 1981; **Residency:** Neurological Surgery, NC Bapt Hosp, Winston Salem, NC 1982-1987; **Faculty Appointment:** Assoc Prof Neurological Surgery, Wake Forest Univ Sch Med

Day, Arthur L MD (Neurological Surgery) - *Special Expertise: Cerebrovascular Surgery; Cranial/Orbital Tumors; Carotid Artery Disease;* **Admitting Hospital:** Shands Healthcare at University Florida (Page 77); **Office Address:** Shands Univ Florida, Dept Neuro Surg 1600 SW Archer Rd, Box 100265 Gainesville, FL 32610-0265; **Office Phone:** (352) 392-4331; **Board Certification:** Neurological Surgery 1980; **Medical School:** Louisiana State Univ 1972; **Residency:** Neurological Surgery, Shands-Univ Florida Hosp, Gainesville, FL 1973-1977; **Fellowship:** Neurological Pathology, Shands-Univ Florida Hosp, Gainesville, FL 1977-1978; **Faculty Appointment:** Prof Neurological Surgery, Univ Fla Coll Med

Faillace, Walter MD (Neurological Surgery) - *Special Expertise: Neurological Surgery - General;* **Admitting Hospital:** Shands Jacksonville Medical Center; **Office Address:** 653 W 8th St, Ste 1 Univ of FL/Dept Neurosurgery Jacksonville, FL 32209-6511; **Office Phone:** (909) 244-3950; **Board Certification:** Neurological Surgery 1991; **Medical School:** Italy 1980; **Residencies:** Surgery, Jewish Hosp Med Ctr, Brooklyn, NY 1981-1982; Neurological Surgery, U Rochester Sch Med Dent, Rochester, NY 1982-1987; **Fellowship:** Pediatrics, Chldns Hosp Mich Wayne State, Detroit, MI 1987-1988; **Faculty Appointment:** Neurological Surgery, Univ Fla Coll Med

Ferraz, Francisco M MD (Neurological Surgery) - *Special Expertise: Brain Tumors; Spinal Surgery; Cervical Spine Surgery;* **Admitting Hospital:** Arlington Hospital; **Office Address:** 611 S Carlin Springs Rd, Ste 105 Arlington, VA 22204-1064; **Office Phone:** (703) 845-1552; **Board Certification:** Neurological Surgery 1987; **Medical School:** Brazil 1975; **Residency:** Neurological Surgery, Georgetown Univ Affil Hosp, Washington, DC 1977-1982; **Faculty Appointment:** Clin Inst Neurological Surgery, Georgetown Univ

Freeman, Thomas B MD (Neurological Surgery) - *Special Expertise: Parkinson's Disease; Stereotactic Radiosurgery; Movement Disorders;* **Admitting Hospital:** Tampa General Hospital; **Office Address:** 4 Columbia Dr, Ste 730 Tampa, FL 33606; **Office Phone:** (813) 259-0889; **Board Certification:** Neurological Surgery 1993; **Medical School:** Johns Hopkins Univ 1981; **Residency:** Neurological Surgery, NYU Med Ctr, New York, NY 1982-1988; **Faculty Appointment:** Prof Neurological Surgery, Univ S Fla Coll Med

Friedman, William A MD (Neurological Surgery) - *Special Expertise:* Stereotactic *Radiosurgery; Brain Tumors; Parkinson's Disease;* **Admitting Hospital:** Shands Healthcare at University Florida (Page 77); **Office Address:** Shands- Univ Florida Hosp, Dept Surgery 1600 SW Archer Rd, Box 100265 Gainesville, FL 32610-0265; **Office Phone:** (352) 392-4331; **Board Certification:** Neurological Surgery 1984; **Medical School:** Ohio State Univ 1976; **Residency:** Neurological Surgery, Shands-Univ Florida Hosp, Gainesville, FL 1977-1982; **Faculty Appointment:** Prof Neurological Surgery, Univ Fla Coll Med

Green, Barth MD (Neurological Surgery) - *Special Expertise:* Spinal Surgery; **Admitting Hospital:** University of Miami - Jackson Memorial Hospital; **Office Address:** Univ Miami, Dept Neuro Surg 1611 NW 12th Ave, Ste 127 Miami, FL 33136; **Office Phone:** (305) 243-6946; **Board Certification:** Neurological Surgery 1978; **Medical School:** Indiana Univ 1969; **Residency:** Neurological Surgery, Northwestern Univ Sch Med, Chicago, IL 1970-1975; **Faculty Appointment:** Prof Neurological Surgery, Univ Miami Sch Med

Hadley, Mark MD (Neurological Surgery) - *Special Expertise:* Spinal Cord Surgery; **Admitting Hospital:** University of Alabama Hospital at Birmingham; **Office Address:** Univ Alabama-Birmingham Sch Med, Div Neurosurgery 1813 6th Ave S Birmingham, AL 35294; **Office Phone:** (205) 934-1439; **Board Certification:** Neurological Surgery 1992; **Medical School:** Albany Med Coll 1982; **Residency:** Neurology, St Josephs Hosp Med Ctr, Phoenix, AZ 1983-1988

Heros, Roberto MD (Neurological Surgery) - *Special Expertise:* Cerebrovascular Surgery; **Admitting Hospital:** Anne Bates Leach Eye Hosp; **Office Address:** 1501 NW 9th Ave, rm 2064 Miami, FL 33136; **Office Phone:** (305) 243-6672; **Board Certification:** Neurological Surgery 1978; **Medical School:** Univ Tenn Coll Med, Memphis 1968; **Residencies:** Surgery, Mass Genl Hosp, Boston, MA 1969-1970; Neurological Surgery, Mass Genl Hosp, Boston, MA 1972-1976; **Faculty Appointment:** Prof Neurological Surgery, Univ Miami Sch Med

Kelly Jr, David L MD (Neurological Surgery) - *Special Expertise:* Disc Disease; Spine Surgery-Degenerative; **Admitting Hospital:** Wake Forest University Baptist Medical Center; **Office Address:** Wake Forest Univ Baptist Med Ctr Med Ctr Blvd Winston Salem, NC 27157-1029; **Office Phone:** (336) 716-4049; **Board Certification:** Neurological Surgery 1967; **Medical School:** Univ NC Sch Med 1959; **Residencies:** Neurological Surgery, Chldns Hospital, Boston, MA 1962-1963; Neurological Surgery, NC Bapt Hosp, Winston Salem, NC 1960-1962; **Fellowship:** Neurological Physiology, Wash Univ, St Louis, MO 1963-1964; **Faculty Appointment:** Prof Neurological Surgery, Wake Forest Univ Sch Med

Laws Jr., Edward R MD (Neurological Surgery) - *Special Expertise:* Pituitary Surgery; *Epilepsy/Seizure Disorders;* **Admitting Hospital:** University of Virginia Health Systems; **Office Address:** Univ VA Hlth Scis Ctr, Dept Neurosurg Box 800212 Charlottesville, VA 22908-0212; **Office Phone:** (804) 924-2650; **Board Certification:** Neurological Surgery 1974; **Medical School:** Johns Hopkins Univ 1963; **Residency:** Neurological Surgery, Johns Hopkins Hosp, Baltimore, MD 1966-1971; **Faculty Appointment:** Prof Neurological Surgery, Univ VA Sch Med

Morrison, Glenn MD (Neurological Surgery) - *Special Expertise:* Neurosurgery-Pediatric; *Craniofacial Surgery; Hydrocephalus;* **Admitting Hospital:** Miami Children's Hospital; **Office Address:** Medical Arts Bldg 3200 SW 60th Ct, Ste 301 Miami, FL 33155-4071; **Office Phone:** (305) 662-8386; **Board Certification:** Neurological Surgery 1976; **Medical School:** Case West Res Univ 1967; **Residency:** Neurological Surgery, Case Western Univ Hosp, Cleveland, OH 1970-1974; **Faculty Appointment:** Prof Neurological Surgery, Univ Miami Sch Med

O'Brien, Mark S. MD (Neurological Surgery) - *Special Expertise:* Hydrocephalus-Pediatric; *Brain & Spinal Cord Tumors-Pediatric;* **Admitting Hospital:** Children's Healthcare of Atlanta; **Office Address:** 1900 Century Blvd NE, Ste 4 Atlanta, GA 30345-3307; **Office Phone:** (404) 321-9234; **Board Certification:** Neurological Surgery 1971; **Medical School:** St Louis Univ 1959; **Residencies:** Neurology, Charity Hosp, New Orleans, LA 1962-1963; Neurological Surgery, St Vincents hosp Med Ctr, New York, NY 1963-1965; **Fellowship:** Neuroradiology, Albert Einstein Sch of Med 1968-1969; **Faculty Appointment:** Prof Surgery, Emory Univ

Oakes, W. Jerry MD (Neurological Surgery) - *Special Expertise:* Neurosurgery-Pediatric; *Chiari's Deformity;* **Admitting Hospital:** Children's Hospital; **Office Address:** Children's Hospital of Alabama 1600 7th Ave S, Birmingham, AL 35233; **Office Phone:** (205) 939-9653; **Board Certification:** Neurological Surgery 1981; **Medical School:** Duke Univ 1972; **Residency:** Neurological Surgery, Duke Hosp, Durham, NC 1972-1978; **Fellowships:** Neurological Surgery, Hosp for Sick Chldn, Toronto, Canada 1975; Neurological Surgery, Great Ormond St Hosp, London, England 1978-1979; **Faculty Appointment:** Prof Neurological Surgery, Univ Ala

Rhoton Jr, Albert L MD (Neurological Surgery) - *Special Expertise:* Pituitary Surgery; *Acoustic Nerve Tumors; Trigeminal Neuralgia;* **Admitting Hospital:** Shands Healthcare at University Florida (Page 77); **Office Address:** Shands-Univ Florida Hosp, Dept Nero Surg 1600 SW Archer Blvd, Box 100265 Gainesville, FL 32610-0265; **Office Phone:** (352) 392-4331; **Board Certification:** Neurological Surgery 1968; **Medical School:** Univ Wash 1959; **Residencies:** Surgery, Columbia Presby Med Ctr, New York, NY 1960-1961; Neurological Surgery, Barnes Hosp, St Louis, MO 1962-1965; **Fellowship:** Neurological Anatomy, Natl Inst Neuro Disorder-NIH, Bethesda, MD 1965; **Faculty Appointment:** Prof Neurological Surgery, Univ Fla Coll Med

Rosomoff, Hubert L MD (Neurological Surgery) - *Special Expertise:* Pain Management; **Admitting Hospital:** South Shore Hospital - Miami Beach; **Office Address:** Univ Miami Compr Pain & Rehab Ctr 600 Alton Rd, Ste 932 Miami Beach, FL 33139; **Office Phone:** (305) 532-7246; **Board Certification:** Neurological Surgery 1961; **Medical School:** Hahnemann Univ 1952; **Residency:** Neurological Surgery, Neuro Inst, New York, NY 1953-1959; **Faculty Appointment:** Prof Neurological Surgery, Univ Miami Sch Med

Sekhar, Laligam N MD (Neurological Surgery) - *Special Expertise:* Aneurysm-Cerebral; *Brain/Skull Base Tumors; Arteriovenous Malformations;* **Admitting Hospital:** George Washington University Hospital; **Office Address:** 3301 Woodburn Rd, Ste 202 Annandale, VA 22003; **Office Phone:** (703) 641-5911; **Board Certification:** Neurological Surgery 1986; **Medical School:** India 1973; **Residency:** Neurological Surgery, Univ Pittsburgh Sch Med, Pittsburgh, PA 1976-1982; **Fellowships:** Neurological Surgery, Norstadt Krankenhaus, Germany 1982-1983; Neurological Surgery, Univ Zurich, Swittzerland 1983; **Faculty Appointment:** Clin Prof Neurological Surgery, Geo Wash Univ

Swaid, Swaid MD (Neurological Surgery) - *Special Expertise:* Neurological Surgery - General; **Admitting Hospital:** University of Alabama Hospital at Birmingham; **Office Address:** Neur Surg Assoc PC 1201 11th Ave S, Ste 500 Birmingham, AL 65205; **Office Phone:** (205) 930-8400; **Board Certification:** Neurological Surgery 1983; **Medical School:** Univ Ala 1976; **Residency:** Neurological Surgery, Univ Alabama Sch Med., Birmingham, AL 1977-1981

Atkinson, John MD (Neurological Surgery) - *Special Expertise: Pituitary Surgery; Brain Hemorrage; Cerebrovascular Surgery;* **Admitting Hospital:** Mayo Medical Center & Clinic - Rochester; **Office Address:** Mayo Clinic, Dept Neurosurgery 200 1st St SW Rochester, MN 55905; **Office Phone:** (507) 284-2376; **Board Certification:** Neurological Surgery 1992; **Medical School:** Univ Ala 1984; **Residency:** Neurological Surgery, Mayo Clinic, Rochester, MN 1985-1990; **Faculty Appointment:** Assoc Prof Neurological Surgery, Mayo Med Sch

Barnett, Gene H MD (Neurological Surgery) - *Special Expertise: Brain Tumors; Stereotactic Radiosurgery;* **Admitting Hospital:** Cleveland Clinic Foundation; **Office Address:** Cleveland Clinic, Dept Surgery 9500 Euclid Ave, rm S80 Cleveland, OH 44195-0001; **Office Phone:** (216) 444-5381; **Board Certification:** Neurological Surgery 1990; **Medical School:** Case West Res Univ 1980; **Residency:** Neurological Surgery, Cleveland Clinic, Cleveland, OH 1981-1986; **Fellowships:** Neurology, Cleveland Clinic, Cleveland, OH 1981-1982; Research, Mass Genl Hosp-Harvard, Boston, MA 1986-1987

Batjer, H. Hunt MD (Neurological Surgery) - *Special Expertise: Aneurysm-Cerebral; Arteriovenous Malformations;* **Admitting Hospital:** Northwestern Memorial Hospital; **Office Address:** Northwestern Univ Med Sch 233 E Erie - Ste 614 Chicago, IL 60611; **Office Phone:** (312) 695-8143; **Board Certification:** Neurological Surgery 1986; **Medical School:** Univ Tex SW, Dallas 1977; **Residency:** Neurological Surgery, Parkland Meml, Dallas, TX 1978-1981; **Fellowship:** Neurological Surgery, Univ West Ont, Ontario, Canada 1981-1982; **Faculty Appointment:** Prof Univ Tex SW, Dallas

Bauer, Jerry MD (Neurological Surgery) - *Special Expertise: Pain-Back & Neck; Brain Tumors;* **Admitting Hospital:** Advocate Lutheran General Hospital; **Office Address:** Ctr of Brain & Spine Surg-Parkside Ctr 1875 Dempster St, Ste 605 Park Ridge, IL 60068; **Office Phone:** (847) 698-1088; **Board Certification:** Neurological Surgery 1981; **Medical School:** Univ IL Coll Med 1974; **Residencies:** Neurological Surgery, Northwestern, Chicago, IL 1974-1975; Neurological Surgery, Univ IL Hosp, Chicago, IL 1975-1979; **Faculty Appointment:** Asst Clin Prof Neurological Surgery, Univ IL Coll Med

Brown, Frederick MD (Neurological Surgery) - *Special Expertise: Spinal Surgery; Pain-Chronic;* **Admitting Hospital:** University of Chicago Hospitals (Page 78); **Office Address:** 5841 S Maryland Ave, MS 3026 Chicago, IL 60637; **Office Phone:** (773) 702-2123; **Board Certifications:** Neurological Surgery 1982, Neurological Surgery; **Medical School:** Ohio State Univ 1972; **Residency:** Neurological Surgery, Univ Chicago, Chicago, IL 1974-1978; **Faculty Appointment:** Neurological Surgery, Univ Chicago-Pritzker Sch Med

Canady, Alexa I MD (Neurological Surgery) - *Special Expertise: Neurosurgery-Pediatric; Hydrocephalus;* **Admitting Hospital:** Children's Hospital of Michigan; **Office Address:** 3901 Beaubien St Detroit, MI 48201; **Office Phone:** (313) 833-4490; **Board Certification:** Neurological Surgery 1984; **Medical School:** Univ Mich Med Sch 1975; **Residency:** Neurological Surgery, Univ Minneapolis, Minneapolis, MN 1976-1981; **Fellowship:** Pediatric Surgery, Chldns Hosp, Philadelphia, PA 1981-1982; **Faculty Appointment:** Prof Neurological Surgery, Wayne State Univ

Chandler, William F MD (Neurological Surgery) - *Special Expertise: Pituitary Surgery; Brain Tumors;* **Admitting Hospital:** University of Michigan Health Center; **Office Address:** Univ Mich Taubman Ctr #2124 1500 E Med Ctr Ann Arbor, MI 48109; **Office Phone:** (734) 936-5020; **Board Certification:** Neurological Surgery 1980; **Medical School:** Univ Mich Med Sch 1971; **Residency:** Neurological Surgery, Michigan Hosp, Detroit, MI 1972-1977; **Faculty Appointment:** Prof Neurological Surgery, Univ Mich Med Sch

Dacey Jr., Ralph Gerald MD (Neurological Surgery) - *Special Expertise:* Vascular Neurosurgery; Aneurysm-Cerebral; **Admitting Hospital:** Barnes - Jewish Hospital; **Office Address:** Barnes-Jewish Hospital 660 S Euclid Ave, Box Campus - 8057 St. Louis, MO 63110; **Office Phone:** (314) 362-5039; **Board Certifications:** Neurological Surgery 1985, Internal Medicine 1978; **Medical School:** Univ VA Sch Med 1974; **Residencies:** Neurological Surgery, Univ VA, Charolettesville, VA 1977-1983; Internal Medicine, Strong Meml Hosp, Rochester 1975-1977; **Faculty Appointment:** Prof Neurological Surgery, Washington Univ, St Louis

Diaz, Fernando G MD (Neurological Surgery) - *Special Expertise:* Neck & Carotid Reconstruction; Carotid Artery Surgery; **Admitting Hospital:** Harper Hospital (Page 59); **Office Address:** Harper Professional Bldg 3750 Woodward, Ste C28 Detroit, MI 48201; **Office Phone:** (313) 745-4266; **Board Certification:** Neurological Surgery 1980; **Medical School:** Mexico 1968; **Residencies:** Neurological Surgery, Univ Minn, Minneapolis, MN 1973-1978; Surgery, Univ Kansas Med Ctr, Kansas City, MO 1971-1973; **Faculty Appointment:** Prof Wayne State Univ

Grubb, Robert MD (Neurological Surgery) - *Special Expertise:* Arteriovenous Malformations; Brain Tumors; **Admitting Hospital:** Barnes - Jewish Hospital; **Office Address:** One Barnes-Jewish Hospital Plz 517 S Euchlid , Bldg McMillan - Fl Ground St. Louis, MO 63110; **Office Phone:** (314) 362-3577; **Board Certification:** Neurological Surgery 1976; **Medical School:** Univ NC Sch Med 1965; **Residencies:** Surgery, Barnes Hosp, St Louis, MO 1966-1967; Neurological Surgery, Barnes Hosp, St Louis, MO 1969-1973; **Fellowship:** Neurological Surgery, Natl Inst Hlth, Bethesda, MD 1968-1969; **Faculty Appointment:** Prof Neurological Surgery, Univ Wash

Gutierrez, Francisco A MD (Neurological Surgery) - *Special Expertise:* Brain Tumors; Cerebrovascular Surgery; **Admitting Hospital:** Northwestern Memorial Hospital; **Office Address:** Northwestern Neurosurgeons Assocs 201 E Herron, Ste 9160 Chicago, IL 60611; **Office Phone:** (312) 926-3490; **Board Certification:** Neurological Surgery 1976; **Medical School:** Colombia 1965; **Residencies:** Neurological Surgery, San Juan de Dios Hosp, Bogota, Columbia 1967; Neurological Surgery, Northwestern Meml Hosp, Chicago, IL 1969-1973; **Faculty Appointment:** Asst Prof Neurological Surgery, Northwestern Univ

Hekmatpanah, Javad MD (Neurological Surgery) - *Special Expertise:* Brain Tumors; Spinal Stenosis; **Admitting Hospital:** University of Chicago Hospitals (Page 78); **Office Address:** Univ Chicago, Dept Neurosurgery 5758 S Maryland Ave, Fl 4 - Ste 4D Chicago, IL 60637; **Office Phone:** (773) 702-6157; **Board Certifications:** Neurological Surgery 1966, Neurology 1967; **Medical School:** Iran 1956; **Residencies:** Neurology, Wisconsin Genl Hosp-Univ Wisconsin, Milwaukee, WI 1958-1961; Neurological Surgery, Univ Chicago Hosp, Chicago, IL 1961-1964; **Faculty Appointment:** Prof Neurological Surgery, Univ Chicago-Pritzker Sch Med

Hoff, Julian T MD (Neurological Surgery) - *Special Expertise:* Brain & Spinal Surgery; Disc Disease-Lumbar; Neurofibromatosis; **Admitting Hospital:** University of Michigan Health Center; **Office Address:** Univ Mich Med Ctr, Dept NS 1500 N Med Ctr Drive, Ste 2128 Ann Arbor, MI 48109-0338; **Office Phone:** (734) 936-5015; **Board Certification:** Neurological Surgery 1973; **Medical School:** Cornell Univ-Weil Med Coll 1962; **Residencies:** Neurological Surgery, NY Hosp, New York, NY 1966-1970; Surgery, NY Hosp, New York, NY 1963-1964; **Fellowship:** Anesthesiology, Cardio Vascular Inst UCSF, San Francisco, CA 1970; **Faculty Appointment:** Prof Neurological Surgery, Univ Mich Med Sch

Kranzler, Leonard I MD (Neurological Surgery) - *Special Expertise:* Brain Tumors; **Admitting Hospital:** Illinois Masonic Medical Center (Page 64); **Office Address:** Neurosurgical Specialists Ltd 3000 N Halstead, Ste 701 Chicago, IL 60657; **Office Phone:** (773) 296-6666; **Board Certification:** Neurological Surgery 1974; **Medical School:** Northwestern Univ 1963; **Residencies:** Neurological Surgery, Northwestern Univ, Chicago, IL 1964-1969; Neurological Surgery, Chldns Meml Hosp, Chicago, IL 1966-1967; **Fellowship:** Neurological Surgery, Zurich, Switzerland 1971

NEUROLOGICAL SURGERY

Levy, Robert M MD (Neurological Surgery) - *Special Expertise:* Stereotactic Radiosurgery; Brain Tumors; Pain-Chronic; **Admitting Hospital:** Northwestern Memorial Hospital; **Office Address:** Northwestern Univ 233 E Erie St, Ste 614 Chicago, IL 60611-5935; **Office Phone:** (312) 695-8143; **Board Certification:** Neurological Surgery 1991; **Medical School:** Stanford Univ 1981; **Residency:** Neurological Surgery, UCSF, San Francisco, CA 1982-1987; **Fellowship:** Neurological Surgery, UCSF, San Francisco, CA 1983-1986; **Faculty Appointment:** Prof Neurological Surgery, Northwestern Univ

Luerssen, Thomas G. MD (Neurological Surgery) - *Special Expertise:* Neurosurgery-Pediatric; **Admitting Hospital:** Riley Hospital for Children; **Office Address:** J. W. Riley Hosp Chldn-Ind U Sch Med 702 Barnhill Dr, rm 2510 Indianapolis, IN 46202; **Office Phone:** (317) 274-5000; **Board Certification:** Neurological Surgery 1985; **Medical School:** Indiana Univ 1976; **Residency:** Neurological Surgery, Ind Univ Hosp, Indianapolis, IN 1977-1981; **Fellowship:** Childrens Hospital, Philadelphia, PA 1983-1984; **Faculty Appointment:** Prof Neurological Surgery, Indiana Univ

Luken, Martin MD (Neurological Surgery) - *Special Expertise:* Cervical Spine Surgery; Chiari's Deformity; **Admitting Hospital:** Rush/Presbyterian - St Luke's Medical Center - Chicago (Page 74); **Office Address:** Chicago Institue of Neurosurgery 71 W 156th St, Ste 208 Harvey, IL 60426; **Office Phone:** (708) 331-6669; **Board Certification:** Neurological Surgery 1983; **Medical School:** Columbia P&S 1973; **Residencies:** U IL Med Ctr, Chicago, NY 1975-1976; Neurological Surgery, Neuro Inst, Chicago, IL 1976-1980

Malik, Ghaus MD (Neurological Surgery) - *Special Expertise:* Cerebrovascular Surgery; Vascular Neurosurgery; **Admitting Hospital:** Henry Ford Health System (Page 62); **Office Address:** 2799 W Grand Blvd Detroit, MI 48202; **Office Phone:** (313) 876-2241; **Board Certification:** Neurological Surgery 1978; **Medical School:** Pakistan 1968; **Residencies:** Neurological Surgery, Henry Ford Hosp, Detroit, MI 1971-1975; Surgery, Henry Ford Hosp, Detroit, MI 1970-1971

Mayberg, Marc MD (Neurological Surgery) - *Special Expertise:* Pituitary Surgery; Stroke/Cerebrovascular Disease; Skull Base Tumors; **Admitting Hospital:** Cleveland Clinic Foundation; **Office Address:** Cleveland Clinic Foundation 9500 Euclid Ave, rm S80 Cleveland, OH 44195; **Office Phone:** (216) 445-4430; **Board Certification:** Neurological Surgery 1988; **Medical School:** Mayo Med Sch 1978; **Residency:** Neurological Surgery, Mass Genl Hosp, Boston, MA 1979-1984; **Fellowship:** Neurological Surgery, Natl Hosp for Vernous Disorders, London 1985; **Faculty Appointment:** Prof Surgery, Ohio State Univ

Menezes, Arnold MD (Neurological Surgery) - *Special Expertise:* Neurosurgery-Pediatric; Craniocervical Abnormalities; **Admitting Hospital:** University of Iowa Hospitals and Clinics; **Office Address:** 200 Hawkins, Bldg JPP - rm 1841 Iowa City, IA 52242; **Office Phone:** (319) 356-2768; **Board Certification:** Neurological Surgery 1976; **Medical School:** India 1967; **Residencies:** Surgery, Univ of Iowa Hosp, Iowa City, IA 1969-1970; Neurological Surgery, Univ of Iowa Hosp, Iowa City, IA 1970-1974; **Fellowship:** Child Neurology, Univ of Iowa Hosp, Iowa City, IA 1973; **Faculty Appointment:** Prof Neurological Surgery, Univ Iowa Coll Med

Nagib, Mahmoud MD (Neurological Surgery) - *Special Expertise:* Neurological Surgery - General; **Admitting Hospital:** Fairview-University Medical Center - University Campus; **Office Address:** 305 Piper Bldg 800 E 28th Street Minn, MN 55407-3723; **Office Phone:** (612) 871-7278; **Board Certification:** Neurological Surgery 1985; **Residency:** Neurological Surgery, University of Minn, Minneapolis, MN 1977-1982; **Faculty Appointment:** Clin Inst Neurological Surgery, Univ Minn

Papadopoulos, Stephen M. MD (Neurological Surgery) - *Special Expertise: Spinal Surgery; Stealth Guided Surgery; Stereotactic Radiosurgery;* **Admitting Hospital:** University of Michigan Health Center; **Office Address:** 1500 E Med Ctr Dr Univ Mich- 2128 Taubman Ctr Box 0338 Ann Arbor, MI 48109-0338; **Office Phone:** (734) 936-5024; **Board Certification:** Neurological Surgery 1991; **Medical School:** UCSD 1978; **Residency:** Neurological Surgery, U Mich., Ann Arbor, MI 1983-1988; **Fellowship:** Neurological Surgery, Barrow Neur. Inst., Phoenix, AZ 1989; **Faculty Appointment:** Assoc Prof Neurological Surgery, Univ Mich Med Sch

Piepgras, David MD (Neurological Surgery) - *Special Expertise: Vascular Neurosurgery;* **Admitting Hospital:** Mayo Medical Center & Clinic - Rochester; **Office Address:** Mayo Clin, Dept Neurosurgery 200 W First St SW Rochester, MN 55905; **Office Phone:** (507) 284-3331; **Board Certification:** Neurological Surgery 1977; **Medical School:** Univ Minn 1965; **Residencies:** Surgery, Hennipin Co Genl Hosp, Minneapolis, MN 1969-1970; Neurological Surgery, Mayo Grad Sch Med, Rochester, MN 1970-1974; **Faculty Appointment:** Prof Neurological Surgery, Mayo Med Sch

Rezai, Ali R MD (Neurological Surgery) - *Special Expertise: Parkinson's Disease; Pain-Chronic;* **Admitting Hospital:** Cleveland Clinic Foundation; **Office Address:** Cleveland Clin, Dept Neurosurgery 9500 Euclid S80 Ave Cleveland, OH 44195-0001; **Office Phone:** (216) 444-4720; **Board Certification:** Neurological Surgery 1992; **Medical School:** Univ SC Sch Med 1989; **Residency:** Neurological Surgery, NYU Med Ctr, New York, NY 1991-1997; **Fellowship:** Neurological Surgery, Univ Toronto Med Ctr, Canada 1997-1998

Rockswold, Gaylan MD (Neurological Surgery) - *Special Expertise: Spinal Surgery;* **Admitting Hospital:** Hennepin County Medical Center; **Office Address:** Hennepin County Med Ctr 701 Park Ave Minneapolis, MN 55415; **Office Phone:** (612) 871-7278; **Board Certification:** Neurological Surgery 1976; **Medical School:** Univ Minn 1966; **Residencies:** Surgery, USPHS Hosp, Baltimore, MD 1967; Neurological Surgery, Natl Cancer Inst-NIH, Bethesda, MD 1969; **Fellowship:** Neurological Surgery, Univ Minn, Minneapolis, MN 1969-1974; **Faculty Appointment:** Prof Neurological Surgery, Univ Minn

Rosenblum, Mark MD (Neurological Surgery) - *Special Expertise: Brain Tumors; Spinal Surgery;* **Admitting Hospital:** Henry Ford Health System (Page 62); **Office Address:** Henry Ford Hospital, K11 2799 W Grand Blvd Detroit, MI 48202; **Office Phone:** (313) 916-1340; **Board Certification:** Neurological Surgery 1982; **Residencies:** Surgery, UCLA, Los Angeles, CA 1972-1973; Neurological Surgery, UC San Francisco Med Ctr, San Francisco, CA 1973-1979; **Fellowship:** Natl Cancer Inst, Bethesda, MD 1970-1972

Ruge, John MD (Neurological Surgery) - *Special Expertise: Neurosurgery-Pediatric; Brain Tumors; Pain-Facial;* **Admitting Hospital:** Advocate Lutheran General Hospital; **Office Address:** Center of Brain & Spine Surg-Parkside Ctr 1875 Dempster St, Ste 605 Park Ridge, IL 60608; **Office Phone:** (847) 698-1088; **Board Certification:** Neurological Surgery 1993; **Medical School:** Northwestern Univ 1983; **Residency:** Neurological Surgery, Northwestern, Chicago, IL 1984-1989; **Fellowship:** Pediatric Neurological Surgery, Children's Hosp, Chicago, IL 1989-1990; **Faculty Appointment:** Asst Prof Surgery, Univ Chicago-Pritzker Sch Med

Selman, Warren R MD (Neurological Surgery) - *Special Expertise: Stroke-Microsurgery; Pituitary Surgery;* **Admitting Hospital:** University Hospital - Cleveland; **Office Address:** 11100 Euclid Ave, Ste 526 Cleveland, OH 44106; **Office Phone:** (216) 844-5745; **Board Certification:** Neurological Surgery 1986; **Medical School:** Case West Res Univ 1977; **Residency:** Neurological Surgery, Univ Hosp Cleveland, Cleveland, OH 1978-1984; **Fellowships:** Research, Univ Hosp Cleveland, Cleveland, OH 1978-1980; Neurological Surgery, Mayo Clin, Rochester, MN 1984; **Faculty Appointment:** Prof Neurological Surgery, Case West Res Univ

385

Whisler, Walter W MD (Neurological Surgery) - *Special Expertise:* Epilepsy/Seizure Disorders; **Admitting Hospital:** Rush/Presbyterian - St Luke's Medical Center - Chicago (Page 74); **Office Address:** 1725 W Harrison St, Ste 1117 Chicago, IL 60612; **Office Phone:** (312) 942-6628; **Board Certification:** Neurological Surgery 1967; **Medical School:** Univ IL Coll Med 1959; **Residencies:** Surgery, Rush Presb, Chicago, IL 1960-1961; Neurological Surgery, IL Rsch Ed Hosp, Chicago, IL 1961-1964; **Faculty Appointment:** Prof Neurological Surgery, Rush Med Coll

Great Plains and Mountains

Heilbrun, M Peter MD (Neurological Surgery) - *Special Expertise:* Stereotactic Radiosurgery; Movement Disorders; **Admitting Hospital:** University of Utah Hospital and Clinics; **Office Address:** Univ Utah Medical Center 50 N Medical Dr, MS 3B409 Salt Lake City, UT 84132; **Office Phone:** (801) 581-6908; **Board Certification:** Neurological Surgery 1973; **Medical School:** SUNY Buffalo 1962; **Residency:** Surgery, Barnes Hosp, St Louis, MO 1963-1964; **Fellowship:** Neurological Surgery, Univ Washington, St Louis, MO 1966-1967

Walker, Marion L. MD (Neurological Surgery) - *Special Expertise:* Neurosurgery-Pediatric; Hydrocephalus; Brain Tumors; **Admitting Hospital:** Primary Children's Medical Center; **Office Address:** Primary Chldns Med Ctr, Div Ped Neurosurg 100 N Medical Dr Salt Lake City, UT 84113-1103; **Office Phone:** (801) 588-3400; **Board Certifications:** Surgery 1979, Neurological Surgery 1996; **Medical School:** Univ Tenn Coll Med, Memphis 1969; **Residency:** Pediatrics, St Joseph's Hosp, Phoenix, AZ 1971-1976; **Fellowship:** Neurological Surgery, Hosp for Sick Chldn, Toronto, Ontario 1972-1973; **Faculty Appointment:** Prof Neurological Surgery, Univ Utah

Winston, Ken R. MD (Neurological Surgery) - *Special Expertise:* Neurosurgery-Pediatric; Craniosynostosis; Epilepsy/Seizure Disorders; **Admitting Hospital:** The Children's Hospital - Denver; **Office Address:** 1056 E 19th Ave, Box B330 Denver, CO 80218; **Office Phone:** (303) 861-6100; **Board Certification:** Neurological Surgery 1973; **Medical School:** Univ Tenn Coll Med, Memphis 1963; **Residencies:** Surgery, Colorado General Hosp, Denver, CO 1966-1967; Neurological Surgery, Colorado General Hospital, Denver, CO 1967-1971; **Faculty Appointment:** Prof Neurological Surgery, Univ Colo

Southwest

Al-Mefty, Ossama MD (Neurological Surgery) - *Special Expertise:* Skull Base Surgery; Neuro-Oncology; **Admitting Hospital:** University of Arkansas for Medical Sciences; **Office Address:** University Hospital of Arkansas for Medical Sciences 4301 W Markham Slot 507 Little Rock, AR 72205; **Office Phone:** (501) 686-8757; **Board Certification:** Neurological Surgery 1980; **Medical School:** Syria 1972; **Residencies:** Surgery, Med Coll Ohio, Toledo, OH 1973-1974; Neurological Surgery, West Va Med Ctr, WV 1974-1978; **Faculty Appointment:** Prof Univ Ark

Clifton, Guy MD (Neurological Surgery) - *Special Expertise:* Head Injury; Spinal Cord Surgery; **Admitting Hospital:** Memorial Hermann Healthcare System; **Office Address:** Univ Texas HSC-Houston, Dept Neuro Surg 6410 Fannin St, HPB, Ste 1020 Houston, TX 77030-1501; **Office Phone:** (713) 500-6135; **Board Certification:** Neurological Surgery 1983; **Medical School:** Univ Tex Med Br, Galveston 1975; **Residency:** Neurological Surgery, University of Texas Medical Branch, Galveston, TX 1976-1980; **Faculty Appointment:** Prof Neurological Surgery, Univ Tex, Houston

Hankinson, Hal L. MD (Neurological Surgery) - *Special Expertise:* Brain Tumors; **Admitting Hospital:** Presbyterian Hospital - Albuquerque; **Office Address:** New Mexico Neurosciences 522 Lomas Blvd NE Albuquerque, NM 87102-2454; **Office Phone:** (505) 247-4253; **Board Certification:** Neurological Surgery 1977; **Medical School:** Tulane Univ 1967; **Residency:** Neurological Surgery, UC San Francisco, San Francisco, CA 1970-1975; **Faculty Appointment:** Clin Prof Univ New Mexico

Harper, Richard L MD (Neurological Surgery) - *Special Expertise:* Spinal Surgery; Brain Tumors & Hemifacial Spasms; **Admitting Hospital:** Methodist Hospital - Houston (Page 69); **Office Address:** NeuroSurgical Group Texas 6560 Fannin, Ste 1200 Houston, TX 77030; **Office Phone:** (713) 790-1211; **Board Certification:** Neurological Surgery 1983; **Medical School:** Baylor Coll Med 1971; **Residency:** Baylor Hosps, Houston, TX 1974-1978

Hassenbusch, Samuel J MD/PhD (Neurological Surgery) - *Special Expertise:* Pain Management; Stereotactic Radiosurgery; Intratumoral Chemotherapy; **Admitting Hospital:** University of Texas MD Anderson Cancer Center (Page 66); **Office Address:** Univ Texas MD Anderson Cancer Ctr, Dept NeuroSurg 1515 Holcombe Blvd Houston, TX 77030; **Office Phone:** (713) 792-2400; **Board Certification:** Neurological Surgery 1992; **Medical School:** Johns Hopkins Univ 1978; **Residencies:** Surgery, Johns Hopkins Univ, Baltimore, MD 1979-1980; Neurological Surgery, Johns Hopkins Univ, Baltimore, MD 1980-1988; **Fellowship:** Research, Keck Foundation-UCSF, San Francisco, CA 1985-1986; **Faculty Appointment:** Assoc Prof Neurological Surgery, Univ Tex, Houston

Loftus, Christopher M. MD (Neurological Surgery) - *Special Expertise:* Cerebrovascular Surgery; Carotid Artery,Gamma Knife Surgery; **Admitting Hospital:** University Hospital; **Office Address:** Univ OK Hlth Sci Ctr, Dept Neurosurgery 711 Stanton L Young Blvd, Ste 206 Oklahoma City, OK 73104; **Office Phone:** (405) 271-4912; **Board Certification:** Neurological Surgery 1987; **Medical School:** SUNY Downstate 1979; **Residency:** Neurological Surgery, Columbia Presby Med Ctr, New York, NY 1980-1985; **Faculty Appointment:** Prof Neurological Surgery, Univ Okla Coll Med

Samson, Duke MD (Neurological Surgery) - *Special Expertise:* Vascular Neurosurgery; Cerebrovascular Surgery; **Admitting Hospital:** Zale Lipshy University Hospital; **Office Address:** U Tex SW Med Ctr @ Dallas, Dept Neuro Surg 5303 Harry Hines Blvd, MC-8855 Dallas, TX 75390-8855; **Office Phone:** (214) 648-3529; **Board Certification:** Neurological Surgery 1978; **Medical School:** Washington Univ, St Louis 1969; **Residency:** Neurological Surgery, Ctr Medico-Chirurgical Fech, Paris, France 1972-1973; **Fellowship:** Neurological Surgery, Univ Tex SW, Dallas, TX 1970-1975; **Faculty Appointment:** Prof Neurological Surgery, Univ Tex SW, Dallas

Sonntag, Volker MD (Neurological Surgery) - *Special Expertise:* Spinal Surgery; **Admitting Hospital:** St Joseph's Hospital & Medical Center - Phoenix; **Office Address:** Barrow Neurosurgical Assocs, Ltd 2910 N Third Ave Phoenix, AZ 85013; **Office Phone:** (602) 406-3458; **Board Certification:** Neurological Surgery 1980; **Medical School:** Univ Ariz Coll Med 1971; **Residency:** Neurological Surgery, Tufts-New England Med Ctr Hosp, Boston, MA 1972-1977; **Faculty Appointment:** Clin Prof Neurological Surgery, Univ Ariz Coll Med

Spetzler, Robert MD (Neurological Surgery) - *Special Expertise:* Vascular Neurosurgery; **Admitting Hospital:** St Joseph's Hospital & Medical Center - Phoenix; **Office Address:** Barrow Neurosurgical Assocs, Ltd 2910 N Third Ave Phoenix, AZ 85013; **Office Phone:** (602) 406-3489; **Board Certification:** Neurological Surgery 1979; **Medical School:** Northwestern Univ 1979; **Residency:** Neurological Surgery, UCSF Med Ctr, San Francisco, CA 1972-1976; **Faculty Appointment:** Prof Surgery, Univ Ariz Coll Med

West Coast and Pacific

Adler Jr, John R MD (Neurological Surgery) - *Special Expertise: Stereotactic Radiosurgery;* **Admitting Hospital:** Stanford Medical Center; **Office Address:** Stanford University Medical Ctr 300 Pastuer Drive #R155 Palo Alto, CA 94304-2203; **Office Phone:** (415) 723-5573; **Board Certification:** Neurological Surgery 1990; **Medical School:** Harvard Med Sch 1980; **Residencies:** Neurological Surgery, Children's Hosp, Boston, MA 1981-1987; Neurological Surgery, Massachuttes Genl Hosp, Boston, MA 1984-1985; **Fellowship:** Karolinka Inst, Stockholm, Sweden 1985-1986; **Faculty Appointment:** Prof Neurological Surgery, Stanford Univ

Apuzzo, Michael L J MD (Neurological Surgery) - *Special Expertise: Nervous System Tumors; Epilepsy/Seizure Disorders;* **Admitting Hospital:** LAC + USC Medical Center; **Office Address:** LA Co & USC Med Ctr 1200 N State St, rm 5046 Los Angeles, CA 90033-1029; **Office Phone:** (323) 226-7421; **Board Certification:** Neurological Surgery 1975; **Medical School:** Boston Univ 1965; **Residencies:** Neurological Surgery, Hartford Hosp, Hartford, CT 1966; Neurological Surgery, Hartford Hosp, Hartford, CT 1970-1973; **Fellowship:** Neurological Physiology, Yale Univ Hosp, New Haven, CT 1971; **Faculty Appointment:** Prof Neurological Surgery, USC Sch Med

Batzdorf, Ulrich MD (Neurological Surgery) - *Special Expertise: Chiari's Deformity; Syringomyelia; Spinal Cord Tumors;* **Admitting Hospital:** UCLA Medical Center; **Office Address:** 300 UCLA Medical Plaza, Fl B-1 - Ste B-200 Los Angeles, CA 90095-6901; **Office Phone:** (310) 825-5079; **Board Certification:** Neurological Surgery 1968; **Medical School:** NY Med Coll 1955; **Residencies:** Surgery, Univ Maryland Hosp, Baltimore, MD 1958-1960; Neurological Surgery, UCLA Ctr Hlth Sci, Los Angeles, CA 1963-1965; **Fellowship:** Pathology, UCSF-Moffit Hosp, San Francisco, CA 1961-1962; **Faculty Appointment:** Prof Neurological Surgery, UCLA

Berger, Mitchel Stuart MD (Neurological Surgery) - *Special Expertise: Brain Tumors-Adult & Pedatric;* **Admitting Hospital:** University of California - San Francisco Medical Center; **Office Address:** UCSF, Dept of Neurological Surgery 505 Parnassus Avenue, M-787 San Francisco, CA 94143-0350; **Office Phone:** (415) 502-7673; **Board Certification:** Neurological Surgery 1991; **Medical School:** Univ Miami Sch Med 1979; **Residency:** Neurological Surgery, Univ CA SF Sch Med, San Francisco, CA 1979-1985; **Fellowship:** Surgery, Univ CA SF Sch Med, San Francisco, CA 1985; **Faculty Appointment:** Neurological Surgery, UCSF

Black, Keith Lanier MD (Neurological Surgery) - *Special Expertise: Neurological Surgery - General;* **Admitting Hospital:** Cedars-Sinai Medical Center; **Office Address:** Maxine Dunitz Neurosurgical Institute 8631 W Third St, Fl E800 Los Angeles, CA 90048; **Office Phone:** (310) 423-7900; **Board Certification:** Neurological Surgery 1990; **Medical School:** Univ Mich Med Sch 1981; **Residency:** Neurological Surgery, Univ Mich Med Ctr, Ann Arbor 1982-1987; **Faculty Appointment:** Prof Neurological Surgery, UC Irvine

Burchiel, Kim James MD (Neurological Surgery) - *Special Expertise: Pain Management; Stereotactic Radiosurgery; Epilepsy/Seizure Disorders;* **Admitting Hospital:** Oregon Health Science University Hospital and Clinics; **Office Address:** 3181 SW Sam Jackson Park Rd Portland, OR 97201; **Office Phone:** (503) 494-4314; **Board Certification:** Neurological Surgery 1984; **Medical School:** UCSD 1976; **Residency:** Neurological Surgery, Univ Washington, Seattle, WA 1977-1982; **Faculty Appointment:** Assoc Prof Neurological Surgery, Oregon Hlth Scis Univ

Dogali, Michael MD (Neurological Surgery) - *Special Expertise:* Parkinson's Disease; Pain/Seizures; **Admitting Hospital:** USC University Hospital - Richard K. Eamer Medical Plaza; **Office Address:** USC Univ Hosp- USC Health Care Consultation Ctr 1510 San Pablo St, Ste 268 Los Angeles, CA 90033; **Office Phone:** (323) 443-1799; **Board Certification:** Neurological Surgery 1980; **Medical School:** McGill Univ 1970; **Residencies:** Surgery, Duke University, Durham, NC 1970-1971; Neurological Surgery, Montreal Neuro Inst, Monteal, Quebec 1971-1976; **Faculty Appointment:** Prof Neurological Surgery, USC Sch Med

Ellenbogen, Richard MD (Neurological Surgery) - *Special Expertise:* Neurosurgery-Pediatric; Chiari's Deformity; **Admitting Hospital:** Children's Hospital and Regional Medical Center - Seattle; **Office Address:** 4800 Sand Point Way NE Seattle, WA 98105; **Office Phone:** (206) 526-2544; **Board Certification:** Neurological Surgery 1992; **Medical School:** Brown Univ 1983; **Residency:** Neurological Surgery, Brigham&Womens Hosp, Boston, MA 1984-1989; **Faculty Appointment:** Asst Prof Neurological Surgery, Univ MD Sch Med

Giannotta, Steven L MD (Neurological Surgery) - *Special Expertise:* Aneurysm-Cerebral; Skull Base Tumors; **Admitting Hospital:** USC University Hospital - Richard K. Eamer Medical Plaza; **Office Address:** 1510 San Pablo St, Ste 268 Los Angeles, CA 90033; **Office Phone:** (323) 442-5757; **Board Certification:** Neurological Surgery 1980; **Medical School:** Univ Mich Med Sch 1972; **Residency:** Neurological Surgery, Univ Michigan, Ann Arbor, MI 1973-1978; **Faculty Appointment:** Prof Neurological Surgery, USC Sch Med

Greene Jr, Clarence S MD (Neurological Surgery) - *Special Expertise:* Neurosurgery-Pediatric; **Admitting Hospital:** Long Beach Memorial Medical Center; **Office Address:** 2650 Elm Ave, Ste 218 Long Beach, CA 90806; **Office Phone:** (562) 426-4121; **Board Certification:** Neurological Surgery 1984; **Medical School:** Howard Univ 1974; **Residencies:** Neurological Surgery, Childrens Hosp, Boston, MA 1977-1981; Neurological Surgery, Peter Bent Brigham Hosp, Boston, MA 1977-1981; **Fellowship:** Child Neurology, Childrens Hosp, Boston, MA 1984

Loeser, John D MD (Neurological Surgery) - *Special Expertise:* Pain Management; **Admitting Hospital:** University of Washington Medical Center; **Office Address:** Univ Wash, Dept NeuroSurg 1959 NE Pacific St Seattle, WA 98195; **Office Phone:** (206) 543-3570; **Board Certification:** Neurological Surgery 1970; **Medical School:** NYU Sch Med 1961; **Residency:** Neurological Surgery, Univ Wash, Seattle, WA 1962-1967; **Faculty Appointment:** Prof Anesthesiology, Univ Wash

McComb, J Gordon MD (Neurological Surgery) - *Special Expertise:* Neurosurgery-Pediatric; **Admitting Hospital:** Children's Hospital - Los Angeles; **Office Address:** Children's Hosp, Queen of Angels Bldg 1300 N Vermont Ave, Ste 906 Los Angeles, CA 90027-6005; **Office Phone:** (323) 663-8128; **Board Certification:** Neurological Surgery 1976; **Medical School:** Univ Miami Sch Med 1965; **Residencies:** Neurological Surgery, Chldns Hosp/Brigham Hosp, Boston, MA 1969-1973; Pediatrics, Chldns Hosp, Los Angeles, CA 1966-1967; **Fellowship:** Physiology, Univ Coll London, London, UK 1973-1974; **Faculty Appointment:** Prof Neurological Surgery, USC Sch Med

Pitts, Lawrence H MD (Neurological Surgery) - *Special Expertise:* Acoustic Nerve Tumors; Skull Base Surgery; Spinal Surgery; **Admitting Hospital:** University of California - San Francisco Medical Center; **Office Address:** UCSF, Div Neurosurg M708C, Box 0112 San Francisco, CA 94143-0112; **Office Phone:** (415) 353-2071; **Board Certification:** Neurological Surgery 1978; **Medical School:** Case West Res Univ 1969; **Residency:** Neurological Surgery, UCSF, SanFrancisco, CA 1969-1975; **Faculty Appointment:** Prof Neurological Surgery, UCSF

Shaffrey, Christopher I. MD (Neurological Surgery) - *Special Expertise:* Neurological Surgery - General; **Admitting Hospital:** University of Washington Medical Center; **Office Address:** 1959 NE Pacific St Seattle, WA 98195; **Office Phone:** (206) 543-3570; **Board Certifications:** Neurological Surgery 1997, Orthopaedic Surgery 1997; **Medical School:** Univ VA Sch Med 1986; **Residency:** Neurological Surgery, Univ Virginia Med Ctr, Charlottesville, VA 1987-1995; **Faculty Appointment:** Assoc Prof Neurological Surgery, Univ Wash

Steinberg, Gary K MD (Neurological Surgery) - *Special Expertise:* Aneurysm-Cerebral; Moyamoya Syndrome-Adult; Arteriovenous Malformations; **Admitting Hospital:** Stanford Medical Center; **Office Address:** Stanford University Hospital, Dept Neurosurg 300 Pasteur Dr, Fl 2 - rm 200 Stanford, CA 94305-5327; **Office Phone:** (650) 723-5575; **Board Certification:** Neurological Surgery 1989; **Medical School:** Stanford Univ 1980; **Residencies:** Neuropathology, Stanford Univ, Palto Alto, CA 1981-1982; Neurological Surgery, Stanford Univ, Palto Alto, CA 1982-1987; **Fellowship:** Cerebrovascular Neurosurgery, Univ West Ontario, Canada 1984-1985; **Faculty Appointment:** Assoc Prof Neurological Surgery, Stanford Univ

Weiss, Martin Harvey MD (Neurological Surgery) - *Special Expertise:* Brain Tumors; Spinal Cord Tumors; **Admitting Hospital:** USC University Hospital - Richard K. Eamer Medical Plaza; **Office Address:** LAC-USC Med Ctr 1200 N State St, Ste 5046 Los Angeles, CA 90033-1029; **Office Phone:** (323) 226-7421; **Board Certification:** Neurological Surgery 1972; **Medical School:** Cornell Univ-Weil Med Coll 1963; **Residencies:** Surgery, US Army Hosp, West Point, NY 1964-1966; Neurological Surgery, Univ Hosp, Cleveland, OH 1966-1970; **Fellowship:** Neurological Surgery, NIH, Cleveland, OH 1969-1970; **Faculty Appointment:** Prof Neurological Surgery, USC Sch Med

Wilson, Charles B MD (Neurological Surgery) - *Special Expertise:* Pituitary Surgery; Brain Tumors; Spinal Cord Tumors; **Admitting Hospital:** University of California - San Francisco Medical Center; **Office Address:** UCSF, Dept Neurological Surg 533 Parnassus Ave, rm U125 San Francisco, CA 94143-0350; **Office Phone:** (415) 353-7500; **Board Certification:** Neurological Surgery 1963; **Medical School:** Tulane Univ 1954; **Residencies:** Pathology, Charity Hosp, New Orleans, LA 1955-1956; Neurological Surgery, Ochsner Fdn Hosp, New Orleans, LA 1956-1960; **Faculty Appointment:** Prof Neurological Surgery, UCSF

Winn, H Richard MD (Neurological Surgery) - *Special Expertise:* Cerebrovascular Surgery; Arteriovenous Malformations; **Admitting Hospital:** University of Washington Medical Center; **Office Address:** Univ Wash Med Ctr, Dept Neuro Surg 700 Ninth Ave, Fl 311 Seattle, WA 98104; **Office Phone:** (206) 521-1833; **Board Certification:** Neurological Surgery 1979; **Medical School:** Univ Penn 1968; **Residencies:** Surgery, Univ Hosp, Cleveland, OH 1969-1970; Neurological Surgery, Univ VA, Charlottesville, VA 1970-1974; **Faculty Appointment:** Prof Neurological Surgery, Univ Wash

NEUROLOGY

A neurologist specializes in the diagnosis and treatment of all types of disease or impaired function of the brain, spinal cord, peripheral nerves, muscles and autonomic nervous system, as well as the blood vessels that relate to these structures. A child neurologist has special skills in the diagnosis and management of neurologic disorders of the neonatal period, infancy, early childhood and adolescence.

Training required: Four years

Certification in the following subspecialty requires additional training and examination.

Spinal Cord Injury Medicine: A physician who addresses the prevention, diagnosis, treatment and management of traumatic spinal cord injury and non-traumatic etiologies of spinal cord dysfunction by working in an interdisciplinary manner. Care is provided to patients of all ages on a lifelong basis and covers related medical, physical, psychological and vocational disabilities and complications.

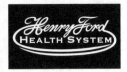

HENRY FORD HOSPITAL
DEPARTMENTS OF
NEUROLOGY & NEUROSURGERY

The Departments of Neurology and Neurosurgery offer a broad spectrum of medical and surgical services, each backed by strong teaching and research programs. For the past two years the departments have been ranked among the top 25 neurology and neurosurgery programs in the nation by *U.S. News & World Report*.

Spinal Care
The neurology EMG laboratory is the second busiest in the country and more spine surgery is performed at Henry Ford than any other neurosurgery department in Michigan. The departments offer a full range of spine care services, including spinal complex surgery, spinal cord stimulators and rehabilitative medicine.

Epilepsy
The Epilepsy Program is one of the largest medical-surgical programs in Michigan. It includes the Midwest's only MEG for pre-surgery tests and the newest experimental anti-seizure medications and surgical options.

Parkinson's Disease
Henry Ford offers state-of-the-art clinical and surgical programs, including comprehensive diagnostic and therapeutic services and the most active surgical program in Michigan using brain stimulators to treat Parkinson's and other movement disorders with excellent results.

Amyotrophic Lateral Sclerosis (ALS)
The Harry J. Hoenselaar ALS Clinic at Henry Ford Hospital is one of only 13 clinics in the country recognized by the national ALS Association.

Stroke
The Henry Ford Stroke Program is one of only 14 stroke centers in the United States funded by the National Institutes of Health and one of 10 nationally to rapidly assess, triage and treat hyperacute stroke within 90 minutes. The program has one of the best outcomes in the country for aneurysm and AVM surgery.

www.HenryFord.com
1-888-291-8304

LEADING EDGE PATIENT CARE

The Hermelin Brain Tumor Center is one of the largest neuro-oncology centers in the nation.

The Center has access to advanced clinical protocols from the New Approaches to Brain Tumor Therapy (NABTT) consortium, which is selected by the National Cancer Institute, to study new treatments and therapies, including gene therapy, for patients with brain tumors.

The Center also handles brain and spinal cord tumors of all types, especially complex ones and those in critically important brain regions. It also has a comprehensive radiation oncology program for adjunctive treatment of residual or recurrent benign and malignant brain tumors. The brain tumor team is developing one of the largest and most comprehensive research laboratories in the country studying gene therapy, tumor invasion, angiogenesis and other molecular targets.

New York's Neurology and Neurosurgery Leaders

The Department of Neurology at **The Mount Sinai Hospital** continues to build on its 100-year history of excellence in neurological care. In 1900 it established the first neurological ward in New York City and in 1910, the Neurosurgery Program it supports today. It offers surgeons known for their work in skull-base, cerebrovascular, pituitary, acoustic, epilepsy, radiosurgery, stereotactic and primary brain tumor surgery and neuroendoscopy among others.

NYU Hospitals Center is one of the premiere centers for adult and pediatric neurosurgery in the United States and the world. Physicians at NYU Hospitals Center pioneered steriotactic volumetric brain tumor surgery, and new methods for spinal surgery. With a clinical program that focuses on the surgical treatment of movement disorders, epilepsy, facial pain, and deep brain tumors among other disorders, the neurosurgery department at NYU Hospitals Center is proud to be the first in New York City to offer bloodless brain surgery with its revolutionary Gamma Knife.

The Neurologists of **NYU Hospitals Center** are also dedicated to exceptional patient care and advanced scientific research. Close cooperation with physicians from Neurosurgery, Neuroradiology, Psychiatry, and the Rusk Institute of Rehabilitation Medicine assure all patients of integrated care for problems of the central and peripheral nervous systems. Its neurologists offer unparalleled expertise in the diagnosis and treatments of Epilepsy, developmental disorders, Stroke, Neuromuscular disease, Neuroradiology, degenerative disorders, brain tumors and infection, and movement disorders.

The Neurosciences Program at the **Hospital for Joint Diseases** offers a full array of diagnostic and specialized treatment services for neurological disorders:

• Orthopaedic Neurology
• Multiple Sclerosis Comprehensive Care Center
• Comprehensive Pain Management Center
• Initiative for Women with Disabilities (gynecologic and primary care for women with physical and sensory disabilities)
• Clinical Neurophysiology
• Neuroimmunology
• Comprehensive Center for Adults with Cerebral Palsy
• Attention Deficit Disorder Clinic
• Functional Neurosurgery and Neurostimulation for Parkinson's disease and Movement Disorders, Neurorehabilitation and traumatic brain injury

The University of Chicago Hospitals
Neurology Program

5841 S. Maryland Avenue
Chicago, IL 60637-1470
For help finding a physician: 1-888-UCH-0200

AT THE FOREFRONT OF NEUROLOGY

The University of Chicago Hospitals' neurology program ranks among the top in the nation and first in Illinois, according to *U.S. News & World Report*. Here, neurologists combine clinical expertise with state-of-the-art therapies and groundbreaking research. With more than 20 physicians and PhD psychologists on staff, the department of neurology provides extraordinary care for patients with all types of neurological diseases.

Behind the scenes, physicians and basic scientists delve into the causes and workings of specific neurologic disorders as they aim to find more effective treatments for these chronic conditions. Medical science is truly interwoven with patient care as physicians here are able to bring new understanding of the disease processes and the very newest therapies to the treatment of these challenging diseases. Patients at the University of Chicago Hospitals have access to the newest, most promising solutions for complex neurological disorders.

TREATING CHALLENGING
NEUROLOGICAL DISORDERS

Specialists at the University of Chicago Hospitals offer innovative solutions for diseases of the nervous system including Parkinson's disease, ALS, multiple sclerosis, epilepsy, stroke and brain tumors. The University of Chicago is one of only three in the world offering electrical source imaging for the treatment of epilepsy. This remarkable non-invasive technique identifies the source of the seizure with pinpoint accuracy, leading to more effective treatment.

To Find a University of Chicago Specialist in Neurology, call 1-888-UCH-0200

COMPASSIONATE, EXPERT CARE FOR A WIDE RANGE OF NEUROLOGICAL CONDITIONS

Experts in all facets of neurology provide compassionate care to patiens and families, using the most advanced and promising approaches to manage diseases of the nervous system.

PHYSICIAN LISTINGS

New England

Caplan, Louis Robert MD (Neurology) - *Special Expertise:* Stroke; **Admitting Hospital:** Beth Israel Deaconess Medical Center - Boston (Page 57); **Office Address:** Beth Israel Deaconess, Dept Neuro 330 Brookline Ave Boston, MA 02111-1854; **Office Phone:** (617) 667-0571; **Board Certification:** Neurology 1972; **Medical School:** Univ MD Sch Med 1962; **Residencies:** Neurology, Boston City Hosp., Boston, MA 1966-1967; Neurology, Boston City Hosp., Boston, MA 1967-1969; **Fellowship:** Neurology, Harvard, Boston, MA 1966-1970; **Faculty Appointment:** Prof Neurology, Tufts Univ

Cole, Andrew J. MD (Neurology) - *Special Expertise:* Epilepsy/Seizure Disorders; **Admitting Hospital:** Massachusetts General Hospital; **Office Address:** 32 Fruit St, MS VBK830 Boston, MA 02114; **Office Phone:** (617) 726-3311; **Board Certifications:** Neurology 1987, Clinical Neurophysiology 1992; **Medical School:** Dartmouth Med Sch 1982; **Residency:** Neurology, Neuro Inst-McGill, Montreal, Canada 1983-1986; **Fellowships:** Electroencephalography, Neuro Inst-McGill, Montreal, Canada 1986-1987; Neurological Surgery, Johns Hopkins Hospital, Baltimore, MD 1987-1988; **Faculty Appointment:** Asst Prof Neurology, Harvard Med Sch

Easton, J Donald MD (Neurology) - *Special Expertise:* Stroke; **Admitting Hospital:** Rhode Island Hospital; **Office Address:** 2 Dudley, Ste 555 Providence, RI 02905; **Office Phone:** (401) 444-8795; **Board Certification:** Neurology 1971; **Medical School:** Univ Wash 1964; **Residency:** Neurology, NY Hosp-Cornell Med Ctr, New York, NY 1965-1968; **Faculty Appointment:** Prof Neurology, Brown Univ

Feldman, Robert G MD (Neurology) - *Special Expertise:* Movement Disorders; Parkinson's Disease; **Admitting Hospital:** Boston Medical Center; **Office Address:** Boston Univ Neurological Associates 720 Harrison Ave, Ste 707 Boston, MA 02118; **Office Phone:** (617) 638-8456; **Board Certification:** Neurology 1965; **Medical School:** Univ Cincinnati 1958; **Residency:** Neurology, Yale New Haven Med Ctr, New Haven, CT 1959-1962; **Fellowship:** Neurology, Yale Univ, New Haven, CT 1962-1963; **Faculty Appointment:** Prof Neurology, Boston Univ

Feldmann, Edward MD (Neurology) - *Special Expertise:* Cerebrovascular Disease; Stroke; **Admitting Hospital:** Rhode Island Hospital; **Office Address:** 110 Lockwood St, Ste 322 Providence, RI 02903-4801; **Office Phone:** (401) 444-8806; **Board Certification:** Neurology 1988; **Medical School:** Harvard Med Sch 1983; **Residency:** Neurology, NY Hosp, Cornell Med Ctr, New York, NY 1984-1987; **Fellowship:** Neurology, Tufts New Eng Med Ctr, Boston, MA 1987-1988; **Faculty Appointment:** Assoc Prof Neurology, Brown Univ

Fink, J. Stephen MD (Neurology) - *Special Expertise:* Parkinson's Disease; Movement Disorders; **Admitting Hospital:** Boston Medical Center; **Office Address:** 720 Harrison Ave, Ste 707 Boston, MA 02118; **Office Phone:** (617) 638-8456; **Board Certification:** Neurology 1985; **Medical School:** Cornell Univ-Weil Med Coll 1980; **Residency:** Neurology, Mass Genl Hosp, Boston, MA 1981-1984; **Faculty Appointment:** Prof Neurology, Harvard Med Sch

Hafler, David A. MD (Neurology) - *Special Expertise:* Multiple Sclerosis; **Admitting Hospital:** Brigham & Women's Hospital; **Office Address:** Center for Neurologic Diseases 77 Louis Pasteur Ave, - rm 786 Boston, MA 02115; **Office Phone:** (617) 525-5330; **Board Certification:** Neurology 1987; **Medical School:** Univ Miami Sch Med 1978; **Residency:** Neurology, NY Hosp-Cornell Med Ctr, New York, NY 1979-1982; **Fellowship:** Neurological Immunology, Harvard Med Sch, Boston, MA 1982-1984; **Faculty Appointment:** Assoc Prof Neurology, Harvard Med Sch

Hochberg, Fred MD (Neurology) - *Special Expertise: Brain Tumors; Occupational Movement Disorders;* **Admitting Hospital:** Massachusetts General Hospital; **Office Address:** One Hawthorne Pl, Ste 105 Boston, MA 02114-2698; **Office Phone:** (617) 726-8657; **Board Certification:** Neurology 1976; **Medical School:** Case West Res Univ 1967; **Residencies:** Neurology, Cleveland Metro Genl Hosp, Cleveland, OH 1968-1970; Neuropathology, Mass Genl Hosp, Boston, MA 1972-1974; **Faculty Appointment:** Assoc Prof Neurology, Harvard Med Sch

Kase, Carlos S. MD (Neurology) - *Special Expertise: Stroke; Seizure Disorders;* **Admitting Hospital:** Boston University Medical Center-East Newton Street Campus; **Office Address:** 720 Harrison Ave Roxbury, MA 02018; **Office Phone:** (617) 638-8456; **Board Certification:** Neurology 1980; **Medical School:** Chile 1967; **Residencies:** Neurology, Mass Genl Hospital, Boston, MA 1972-1973; Neurology, Mass Genl Hospital, Boston, MA 1977-1978; **Faculty Appointment:** Prof Neurology, Boston Univ

Kistler, John Philip MD (Neurology) - *Special Expertise: Stroke;* **Admitting Hospital:** Massachusetts General Hospital; **Office Address:** Mass Genl Hosp, Stroke Service 55 Fruit St, Bldg VBK - rm 802 Boston, MA 02114; **Office Phone:** (617) 726-8459; **Board Certifications:** Internal Medicine 1970, Neurology 1976; **Medical School:** Columbia P&S 1964; **Residencies:** Internal Medicine, Columbia Presby Hosp, New York, NY 1966-1968; Neurology, Mass Genl Hosp-Harvard Med Sch, New York, NY 1972-1975; **Fellowship:** Neurology, Mass Genl Hosp, Boston, MA 1971-1972; **Faculty Appointment:** Prof Neurology, Harvard Med Sch

Koroshetz, Walter J. MD (Neurology) - *Special Expertise: Stroke; Huntington's Disease; Movement Disorders;* **Admitting Hospital:** Massachusetts General Hospital; **Office Address:** Mass Genl Hosp, Dept Neuro 32 Fruit Street Ste VBK 915 Boston, MA 02114; **Office Phone:** (617) 726-1067; **Board Certifications:** Internal Medicine 1982, Neurology 1986; **Medical School:** Univ Chicago-Pritzker Sch Med 1979; **Residencies:** Internal Medicine, Univ Chicago, Chicago, IL 1980-1981; Internal Medicine, Mass Genl Hosp, Boston, MA 1981-1982; **Fellowships:** Neurology, Mass Genl Hosp, Boston, MA 1985-1987; Research, Mass Genl Hosp, Boston, MA 1989; **Faculty Appointment:** Asst Prof Medicine, Harvard Med Sch

Ropper, Allan MD (Neurology) - *Special Expertise: Trauma Neurology; Guillain-Barre Syndrome;* **Admitting Hospital:** St Elizabeth's Medical Center; **Office Address:** St Elizabeth Hosp, Dept of Neurology 736 Cambridge St Boston, MA 02135; **Office Phone:** (617) 789-3300; **Board Certifications:** Neurology 1980, Critical Care Medicine 1987; **Medical School:** Cornell Univ-Weil Med Coll 1974; **Residencies:** Neurology, Mass Genl Hosp, Boston, MA 1976-1979; Internal Medicine, Univ California- San Francisco, San Francisco, CA 1975-1976; **Faculty Appointment:** Prof Neurology, Tufts Univ

Samuels, Martin Allen MD (Neurology) - *Special Expertise: Neurological Aspects of Systemic Disease;* **Admitting Hospital:** Brigham & Women's Hospital; **Office Address:** BWH, Dept Neurology 75 Francis St, Bldg Armory 2 Boston, MA 02115; **Office Phone:** (617) 732-5355; **Board Certifications:** Neurology 1978, Internal Medicine 1974; **Medical School:** Univ Cincinnati 1971; **Residencies:** Internal Medicine, Boston City Hosp, Boston, MA 1972-1975; Neurology, Mass Genl Hosp, Boston, MA 1973-1977; **Fellowship:** Neurological Pathology, Mass Genl Hosp, Boston, MA 1975-1976; **Faculty Appointment:** Prof Neurology, Harvard Med Sch

Selkoe, Dennis MD (Neurology) - *Special Expertise: Alzheimer's Disease; Neurobiology;* **Admitting Hospital:** Brigham & Women's Hospital; **Office Address:** Brigham & Women's Hosp, Ctr for Neuro Dis 77 Louis Pasteur Ave, MC-HIM 730 Boston, MA 02115-5716; **Office Phone:** (617) 525-5200; **Board Certification:** Neurology 1977; **Medical School:** Univ VA Sch Med 1969; **Residency:** Neurology, Peter Bent Brigham, Boston, MA 1972-1975; **Fellowship:** Neurological Biology, Chldns Hosp Med Ctr, Boston, MA 1975-1978; **Faculty Appointment:** Prof Neurology, Harvard Med Sch

Spencer, Susan S MD (Neurology) - *Special Expertise:* *Epilepsy/Seizure Disorders;* **Admitting Hospital:** Yale - New Haven Hospital; **Office Address:** Yale Univ Sch Med, Dept Neurology 333 Cedar St New Haven, CT 06520-8018; **Office Phone:** (203) 785-3865; **Board Certification:** Neurology 1980; **Medical School:** Univ Rochester 1974; **Residency:** Neurology, Yale Univ-New Haven Hosp, New Haven, CT 1975-1978; **Faculty Appointment:** Prof Neurology, Yale Univ

Vollmer, Timothy Lee MD (Neurology) - *Special Expertise:* *Multiple Sclerosis;* **Admitting Hospital:** Yale - New Haven Hospital; **Office Address:** 15 York St New Haven, CT 06510; **Office Phone:** (203) 785-4085; **Board Certification:** Neurology 1991; **Medical School:** Stanford Univ 1983; **Residency:** Neurology, Stanford Univ Sch Med, CA 1984-1987; **Fellowship:** Neurological Immunology, Stanford Univ Sch Med, CA 1985-1986; **Faculty Appointment:** Assoc Prof Yale Univ

Waxman, Stephen G. MD/PhD (Neurology) - *Special Expertise:* *Multiple Sclerosis; Spinal Cord Injury;* **Admitting Hospital:** Yale - New Haven Hospital; **Office Address:** Yale Univ Sch of Med 15 York St, Bldg LCI - rm 708, Box 20818 New Haven, CT 06520-8018; **Office Phone:** (203) 785-5947; **Board Certification:** Neurology 1977; **Medical School:** Albert Einstein Coll Med 1972; **Residency:** Neurology, Boston City Hosp, Boston, MA 1972-1975; **Fellowship:** Neurology, Harvard Univ, Boston, MA 1972-1975; **Faculty Appointment:** Prof Neurology, Yale Univ

Weiner, Howard MD (Neurology) - *Special Expertise:* *Multiple Sclerosis; Autoimmune Disease;* **Admitting Hospital:** Brigham & Women's Hospital; **Office Address:** 77 Ave, Louis Pasteur, HIM 730 Boston, MA 02115; **Office Phone:** (617) 732-7432; **Board Certification:** Neurology 1978; **Medical School:** Univ Colo 1969; **Residencies:** Internal Medicine, Beth Israel, Boston, MA 1970-1971; Neurology, Longwood Prog, Boston, MA 1971-1974; **Fellowship:** Immunology, Univ Colo, Denver, CO 1974-1976; **Faculty Appointment:** Prof Neurology, Harvard Med Sch

Young, Anne MD (Neurology) - *Special Expertise:* *Huntington's Disease; Parkinson's Disease; Movement Disorders;* **Admitting Hospital:** Massachusetts General Hospital; **Office Address:** Mass Genl Hlth, Dept of Neurology 32 Fruit Street, VBK 915 Boston, MA 02114; **Office Phone:** (617) 726-5532; **Board Certification:** Neurology 1981; **Medical School:** Johns Hopkins Univ 1973; **Residency:** Neurology, UCSF, San Francisco, CA 1975-1978; **Faculty Appointment:** Prof Neurology, Harvard Med Sch

Mid Atlantic

Apatoff, Brian R MD/PhD (Neurology) - *Special Expertise:* *Multiple Sclerosis; Neuro-Immunology;* **Admitting Hospital:** New York Weill Cornell Medical Center - NY Presbyterian Hospital (Page 72); **Office Address:** 520 E 70th St New York, NY 10021; **Office Phone:** (212) 746-4504; **Board Certification:** Neurology 1991; **Medical School:** Univ Chicago-Pritzker Sch Med 1984; **Residency:** Neurology, Columbia Presby, New York, NY 1987-1990; **Fellowship:** Multiple Sclerosis, Neuro Inst-Columbia Univ, New York, NY 1990-1992; **Faculty Appointment:** Assoc Prof Neurology, Cornell Univ-Weil Med Coll

Asbury, Arthur K MD (Neurology) - *Special Expertise:* *Peripheral Neuropathy; Guillain-Barre Syndrome;* **Admitting Hospital:** Hospital of the University of Pennsylvania; **Office Address:** Univ Penn Hosp, Dept Neurology 3400 Spruce St Philadelphia, PA 19104; **Office Phone:** (215) 662-2629; **Board Certification:** Neurology 1967; **Medical School:** Univ Cincinnati 1958; **Residencies:** Neurology, Mass Genl Hosp, Boston, MA 1960-1963; Internal Medicine, Mass Genl Hosp, Boston, MA 1959-1960; **Fellowship:** Neurology, Mass Genl Hosp, Boston, MA 1963-1965; **Faculty Appointment:** Prof Emeritus Neurology, Univ Penn

Beal, Myron Flint MD (Neurology) - *Special Expertise:* Huntington's Disease; Alzheimer's Disease; Neurodegenerative Disease; **Admitting Hospital:** New York Weill Cornell Medical Center - NY Presbyterian Hospital (Page 72); **Office Address:** 520 E 70th St New York, NY 10021; **Office Phone:** (212) 746-6575; **Board Certifications:** Internal Medicine 1979, Neurology 1982; **Medical School:** Univ VA Sch Med 1976; **Residencies:** Internal Medicine, NY Hosp-Cornell Med Ctr, New York, NY 1977-1978; Neurology, Mass Genl Hosp, Boston, MA 1978-1981; **Faculty Appointment:** Prof Neurology, Cornell Univ-Weil Med Coll

Bernad, Peter MD (Neurology) - *Special Expertise:* Stroke; Headache-Migraine; Head Injury; **Admitting Hospital:** Fairfax Hospital; **Office Address:** 2616 Sherwood Hall Ln, Ste 201 Washington, DC 20037; **Office Phone:** (202) 728-0099; **Board Certifications:** Internal Medicine 1979, Neurology 1981; **Medical School:** McGill Univ 1974; **Residencies:** Internal Medicine, USC, Los Angeles, CA 1975-1976; Neurology, Mass Genl Hosp-Harvard, Boston, MA 1976-1979; **Fellowship:** Neurological Muscular Disease, Natl Inst Hlth, Bethesda, MD 1979-1981; **Faculty Appointment:** Assoc Clin Prof Neurology, Geo Wash Univ

Braun, Carl MD (Neurology) - *Special Expertise:* Cerebrovascular Disease; Neuromuscular Disorders; **Admitting Hospital:** St Luke's - Roosevelt Hospital Center - Roosevelt Division (Page 58); **Office Address:** 1090 Amsterdam Ave, Ste 5F New York, NY 10025; **Office Phone:** (212) 523-3650; **Board Certification:** Neurology 1970; **Medical School:** Univ Penn 1962; **Residencies:** Internal Medicine, St Lukes Hosp, New York, NY 1963-1964; Neurology, Colum-Presby Med, New York, NY 1964-1967; **Faculty Appointment:** Clin Prof Neurology, Columbia P&S

Brust, John C MD (Neurology) - *Special Expertise:* Stroke; **Admitting Hospital:** Harlem Hospital Center; **Office Address:** 506 Lenox Ave, rm 16-101 New York, NY 10037-1802; **Office Phone:** (212) 939-4244; **Board Certification:** Neurology 1971; **Medical School:** Columbia P&S 1962; **Residencies:** Internal Medicine, Columbia Presby, New York, NY 1965-1966; Neurology, Columbia Presby, New York, NY 1966-1969; **Faculty Appointment:** Clin Prof Neurology, Columbia P&S

Caronna, John J MD (Neurology) - *Special Expertise:* Stroke; Cerebrovascular Disease; **Admitting Hospital:** New York Weill Cornell Medical Center - NY Presbyterian Hospital (Page 72); **Office Address:** Cornell Univ, Dept Neurology 520 E 70th St, Ste 607 New York, NY 10021; **Office Phone:** (212) 746-2304; **Board Certification:** Neurology 1974; **Medical School:** Cornell Univ-Weil Med Coll 1965; **Residencies:** Internal Medicine, NY Hosp, New York, NY 1965-1967; Neurology, NY Hosp, New York, NY 1969-1971; **Fellowship:** Neurology, NY Hosp, New York, NY 1972-1973; **Faculty Appointment:** Prof Neurology, Cornell Univ-Weill Med Coll

Charney, Jonathan MD (Neurology) - *Special Expertise:* Neurology - General; **Admitting Hospital:** Mount Sinai Hospital (Page 70); **Office Address:** 1111 Park Ave, Ste 1A New York, NY 10128-1234; **Office Phone:** (212) 831-2886; **Board Certification:** Neurology 1977; **Medical School:** NY Med Coll 1969; **Residencies:** Neurology, Meth Hosp-Baylor, Dallas, TX 1970-1971; Neurology, Columbia-Presby Med Ctr, New York, NY 1971-1973; **Faculty Appointment:** Asst Prof Neurology, Mount Sinai Sch Med

Cook, Stuart MD (Neurology) - *Special Expertise:* Infectious & Demyelinating Diseases; **Admitting Hospital:** UMDNJ-University Hospital-Newark; **Office Address:** 65 Bergen St, Ste 1535 Newark, NJ 07107; **Office Phone:** (973) 972-4400; **Board Certification:** Neurology 1970; **Medical School:** Univ VT Coll Med 1962; **Residency:** Neurology, Albert Einstein Coll Meded Ctr, Bronx, NY 1965-1968; **Faculty Appointment:** Prof Neurology, UMDNJ-NJ Med Sch, Newark

Cornblath, David R. MD (Neurology) - *Special Expertise:* Peripheral Neuropathy; **Admitting Hospital:** Johns Hopkins Hospital - Baltimore (Page 65); **Office Address:** Johns Hopkins Hosp, Dept Neurology 600 N Wolfe St Baltimore, MD 21287-6965; **Office Phone:** (410) 955-2229; **Board Certifications:** Neurology 1982, Clinical Neurophysiology 1994; **Medical School:** Case West Res Univ 1977; **Residency:** Neurology, Hosp Univ Penn, Philadelphia, PA 1978-1981; **Fellowship:** Neurology, Hosp Univ Penn, Philadelphia, PA 1981-1982; **Faculty Appointment:** Prof Neurology, Johns Hopkins Univ

Coyle, Patricia K MD (Neurology) - *Special Expertise:* Multiple Sclerosis; Neuro-Immunology; Lyme Disease; **Admitting Hospital:** University Hospital & Medical Center at Stony Brook; **Office Address:** SUNY Stony Brook Dept Neurology, HSC T12-020 Stony Brook, NY 11794-8121; **Office Phone:** (631) 444-2599; **Board Certification:** Neurology 1978; **Medical School:** Johns Hopkins Univ 1974; **Residency:** Neurology, Johns Hopkins, Baltimore, MD 1975-1978; **Fellowship:** Neurological Immunology, Johns Hopkins, Blatimore, MD 1978-1980; **Faculty Appointment:** Prof Neurology, SUNY Stony Brook

De Angelis, Lisa MD (Neurology) - *Special Expertise:* Neuro-Oncology; **Admitting Hospital:** Memorial Sloan Kettering Cancer Center; **Office Address:** 1275 York Ave New York, NY 10021-6007; **Office Phone:** (212) 639-7123; **Board Certification:** Neurology 1986; **Medical School:** Columbia P&S 1980; **Residency:** Neurology, Columbia Presby, New York, NY 1981-1984; **Fellowships:** Neurological Oncology, Neuro Inst Presby Hosp, New York, NY 1984-1985; Neurological Oncology, Meml Sloan-Kettering Cancer Ctr, New York, Ny 1985-1986; **Faculty Appointment:** Prof Emeritus Neurology, Cornell Univ-Weill Med Coll

DeKosky, Steven T. MD (Neurology) - *Special Expertise:* Alzheimer's Disease; **Admitting Hospital:** UPMC - Presbyterian University Hospital; **Office Address:** Univ Pittsburgh 3811 O'Hara St Pittsburgh, PA 15213; **Office Phone:** (412) 624-6889; **Board Certification:** Neurology 1979; **Medical School:** Univ Fla Coll Med 1974; **Residency:** Neurology, Univ Florida, Gainesville, FL 1975-1978; **Fellowship:** Neurology, Univ Virginia, Charlottesville, VA 1978-1979; **Faculty Appointment:** Prof Neurology, Univ Pittsburgh

Dewberry, Robert Gerard MD (Neurology) - *Special Expertise:* Neurology - General; **Admitting Hospital:** Maryland General Hospital; **Office Address:** Maryland Gen Hosp, Div Neurology 827 Linden Ave Baltimore, MD 21201; **Office Phone:** (410) 225-8290; **Board Certification:** Neurology 1982; **Medical School:** Univ MD Sch Med 1987; **Residency:** Neurology, Barnes Hospital, St. Louis, MO 1988-1991; **Fellowship:** Neurological Muscular Disease, Univ VA Hosp, Charlottesville, VA 1991-1993

Dichter, Marc Allen MD (Neurology) - *Special Expertise:* Epilepsy/Seizure Disorders; **Admitting Hospital:** Hospital of the University of Pennsylvania; **Office Address:** 3400 Spruce St Dept Neurology 3 Westgate Bldg, Philadelphia, PA 19104; **Office Phone:** (215) 349-5166; **Board Certification:** Neurology 1978; **Medical School:** NYU Sch Med 1969; **Residencies:** Neurology, Beth Israel Hosp, Boston, MA 1972-1975; Neurology, Children's Hosp/PB Brgham Hosp-Harvard, Boston, MA 1972-1975; **Faculty Appointment:** Prof Neurology, Univ Penn

Drachman, Daniel Bruce MD (Neurology) - *Special Expertise:* Muscular Dystrophy; Neuromuscular Disorders; **Admitting Hospital:** Johns Hopkins Hospital - Baltimore (Page 65); **Office Address:** Johns Hopkins Med Ctr 600 N Wolfe St, Bldg Meyer - Fl 5119 Baltimore, MD 21287; **Office Phone:** (410) 955-5406; **Board Certification:** Neurology 1963; **Medical School:** NYU Sch Med 1956; **Residency:** Neuropathology, Mallory Inst Path/Boston City Hosp., Boston, MA 1959-1960; **Fellowship:** Neurology, Harvard Med Sch, Boston, MA 1957-1960; **Faculty Appointment:** Prof Neurology

Fahn, Stanley MD (Neurology) - *Special Expertise:* Movement Disorders; Parkinson's Disease; **Admitting Hospital:** Columbia Presbyterian Medical Center (Page 72); **Office Address:** 710 W 168th St, 3rd Fl - rm 350 New York, NY 10032; **Office Phone:** (212) 305-5277; **Board Certification:** Neurology 1958; **Medical School:** UCSF 1958; **Residency:** Neurology, Columbia Presby, New York, NY 1959-1962; **Faculty Appointment:** Prof Neurology, Columbia P&S

Frankel, Jeffrey MD (Neurology) - *Special Expertise:* Neurology - General; **Admitting Hospital:** St Barnabas Medical Center; **Office Address:** Essex Neurological Assoc 340 E Northfield Rd, Ste 2A Livingston, NJ 07039-4812; **Office Phone:** (973) 994-3322; **Board Certification:** Neurology 1972; **Medical School:** Univ Chicago-Pritzker Sch Med 1966; **Residency:** Neurology, Albert Einstein, Bronx, NY 1967-1970; **Faculty Appointment:** Assoc Clin Prof Neurology, UMDNJ Sch Osteo Med

French, Jacqueline MD (Neurology) - *Special Expertise:* Epilepsy/Seizure Disorders; **Admitting Hospital:** Hospital of the University of Pennsylvania; **Office Address:** Hosp Univ Penn, Dept Neuro 3400 Spruce St Philadelphia, PA 19104; **Office Phone:** (215) 662-3381; **Board Certification:** Neurology 1987; **Medical School:** Brown Univ 1982; **Residency:** Neurological Surgery, Mount Sinai Hosp, New York, NY 1982-1986; **Fellowships:** Epilepsy, Mount Sinai Hosp, New York, NY 1986-1988; Epilepsy, Yale Univ, New Haven, CT 1988-1989; **Faculty Appointment:** Assoc Prof Neurology, Univ Penn

Galetta, Steven MD (Neurology) - *Special Expertise:* Neuro-Ophthalmology; **Admitting Hospital:** Hospital of the University of Pennsylvania; **Office Address:** Hosp Univ Penn, Dept Neurology 3400 Spruce St Philadelphia, PA 19104; **Office Phone:** (215) 662-8100; **Board Certification:** Neurology 1988; **Medical School:** Cornell Univ-Weill Med Coll 1983; **Residency:** Neurology, Univ Penn Med Ctr, Philadelphia, PA 1984-1987; **Fellowship:** Neurological Ophthalmology, Bascom Palmer Eye Inst, Miami, FL 1987-1988; **Faculty Appointment:** Assoc Prof Neurology, Univ Penn

Gendelman, Seymour MD (Neurology) - *Special Expertise:* Parkinson's Disease; Dementia; **Admitting Hospital:** Mount Sinai Hospital (Page 70); **Office Address:** 5 E 98th St, Fl 7 New York, NY 10029; **Office Phone:** (212) 241-8172; **Board Certification:** Neurology 1971; **Medical School:** Geo Wash Univ 1964; **Residency:** Neurology, Mount Sinai, New York, NY 1965-1968; **Faculty Appointment:** Clin Prof Neurology, Mount Sinai Sch Med

Goodgold, Albert MD (Neurology) - *Special Expertise:* Parkinson's Disease; Movement Disorders; **Admitting Hospital:** NYU Medical Center (Page 70); **Office Address:** NYU Medical Center 530 First Ave, Ste 5A New York, NY 10016; **Office Phone:** (212) 263-7205; **Medical School:** Switzerland 1955; **Residency:** Neurology, Bellevue Hosp, New York, NY 1957-1960; **Faculty Appointment:** Neurology, NYU Sch Med

Griffin, John Wesley MD (Neurology) - *Special Expertise:* Neuropathy; **Admitting Hospital:** Johns Hopkins Hospital - Baltimore (Page 65); **Office Address:** Johns Hopkins Hosp, Dept Neurology 600 N Wolfe St, Meyer Bldg 6-113 Baltimore, MD 21287-7613; **Office Phone:** (410) 955-2227; **Board Certifications:** Neurology 1976, Internal Medicine 1974; **Medical School:** Stanford Univ 1968; **Residencies:** Neurology, Johns Hopkins Hosp, Baltimore, MD 1970-1973; Internal Medicine, Johns Hopkins Hosp, Baltimore, MD 1969-1970; **Faculty Appointment:** Prof Neurology, Johns Hopkins Univ

Hiesiger, Emile MD (Neurology) - *Special Expertise:* Pain Management; Neuro-Oncology; **Admitting Hospital:** NYU Medical Center (Page 70); **Office Address:** 530 1st Ave, Ste 5A New York, NY 10016-6402; **Office Phone:** (212) 263-6123; **Board Certification:** Neurology 1983; **Medical School:** NY Med Coll 1978; **Residency:** Neurology, New York Univ, New York, NY 1979-1982; **Fellowship:** Neurology, Mem Sloan-Kettering Cancer Ctr, New York, NY 1982-1984; **Faculty Appointment:** Assoc Clin Prof Neurology, NYU Sch Med

Hurtig, Howard MD (Neurology) - *Special Expertise:* Parkinson's Disease; Movement Disorders; **Admitting Hospital:** Pennsylvania Hospital; **Office Address:** 330 S 9th St Philadelphia, PA 19107; **Office Phone:** (215) 829-6500; **Board Certification:** Neurology 1976; **Medical School:** Tulane Univ 1966; **Residencies:** Internal Medicine, New York Hosp- Cornell Med Ctr., New York, NY 1966-1968; Neurology, Hosp Univ Penn, Philadelphia, PA 1970-1973; **Faculty Appointment:** Prof Neurology, Univ Penn

Johnson, Kenneth P MD (Neurology) - *Special Expertise:* Multiple Sclerosis; **Admitting Hospital:** University of Maryland Medical System; **Office Address:** Univ Maryland Med Ctr 22 S Greene St, rm N4W46 Baltimore, MD 21201-1544; **Office Phone:** (410) 328-6484; **Board Certification:** Neurology 1968; **Medical School:** Jefferson Med Coll 1959; **Residencies:** Neurology, Buffalo Genl Hosp, Buffalo, NY 1960-1961; Neurology, Univ Hosp, Cleveland, OH 1963-1965; **Fellowship:** Neurology, Univ Case West Res, Cleveland, OH 1965-1968; **Faculty Appointment:** Prof Neurology, Univ Maryland Sch Med

Kolodny, Edwin H MD (Neurology) - *Special Expertise:* Neurology - General; **Admitting Hospital:** NYU Medical Center (Page 70); **Office Address:** 403 East 34st Ave, Fl 2 New York, NY 10016-6402; **Office Phone:** (212) 263-7755; **Board Certifications:** Clinical Genetics 1987, Neurology 1971; **Medical School:** NYU Sch Med 1962; **Residencies:** Internal Medicine, Bellevue Hosp, New York, NY 1962-1964; Neurology, Mass Gen Hosp, Boston, MA 1964-1967; **Fellowship:** Nat Inst Neurol Dis & Stroke, Bethesda, MD 1967-1970; **Faculty Appointment:** Prof Neurology, NYU Sch Med

Krumholz, Allan MD (Neurology) - *Special Expertise:* Epilepsy/Seizure Disorders; **Admitting Hospital:** University of Maryland Medical System; **Office Address:** 22 S Greene St Baltimore, MD 21201-1544; **Office Phone:** (410) 328-6266; **Board Certifications:** Neurology 1977, Clinical Neurophysiology 1996; **Medical School:** Univ Hlth Sci/Chicago Med Sch 1970; **Residencies:** Neurology, Johns Hopkins Hosp, Baltimore, MD 1972-1975; Internal Medicine, Baltimore City Hospital, Baltimore, MD 1971-1972; **Fellowship:** Electroencephalography, Johns Hopkins Hosp, Baltimore, MD 1980; **Faculty Appointment:** Prof Neurology, Univ Maryland Sch Med

Levine, David MD (Neurology) - *Special Expertise:* Dementia; Stroke; **Admitting Hospital:** NYU Medical Center (Page 70); **Office Address:** 400 E 34th St, Ste RIRM- 311 New York, NY 10016; **Office Phone:** (212) 263-7744; **Board Certification:** Neurology 1976; **Medical School:** Harvard Med Sch 1968; **Residency:** Mass Gen Hosp, Boston, MA 1971-1974; **Fellowship:** Neurology, Mass Gen Hosp, Boston, MA 1974-1976; **Faculty Appointment:** Prof Neurology, NYU Sch Med

Logigian, Eric L MD (Neurology) - *Special Expertise:* Lyme Disease; Sleep Disorders/Apnea; **Admitting Hospital:** Strong Memorial Hospital - Medical Center; **Office Address:** Univ Rochester, Dept of Neurology 601 Elmwood Ave, Box 673 Rochester, NY 14642; **Office Phone:** (716) 275-4568; **Board Certifications:** Neurology 1985, Clinical Neurophysiology 1999; **Medical School:** Boston Univ 1978; **Residencies:** Internal Medicine, Beth Israel Hosp, Boston, MA 1979-1981; Neurology, Mass Genl Hosp, Boston, MA 1981-1984; **Fellowship:** Clinical Neurophysiology, Mass General Hosp, Boston, MA 1984-1985; **Faculty Appointment:** Assoc Prof Neurology, Univ Rochester

Lublin, Fred MD (Neurology) - *Special Expertise:* Multiple Sclerosis; **Admitting Hospital:** Mount Sinai Hospital (Page 70); **Office Address:** Mount Sinai Hospital Dept of Neurology 1 Gustaue L. Levy Pl New York, NY 10029; **Office Phone:** (212) 241-7317; **Board Certification:** Neurology 1977; **Medical School:** Jefferson Med Coll 1972; **Residency:** Neurology, NY Hosp.-Cornell, New York, NY 1973-1976; **Faculty Appointment:** Prof Neurology, Mount Sinai Sch Med

Max, Mitchell Bruce MD (Neurology) - *Special Expertise:* Pain Management; **Admitting Hospital:** National Institutes of Health - Clinical Center; **Office Address:** Natl Inst of Hlth, Bldg 10 Bethesda, MD 20892; **Office Phone:** (301) 496-5483; **Board Certifications:** Neurology 1982, Internal Medicine 1978; **Medical School:** Harvard Med Sch 1974; **Residencies:** Internal Medicine, Univ Chicago Hosp, Chicago, IL 1974-1976; Neurology, NY Presby- Cornell Med Ctr, New York, NY 1979-1982; **Fellowship:** Neurology, Meml Sloan Kettering Cancer Ctr, New York, NY

Mohr, Jay Preston MD (Neurology) - *Special Expertise:* Aphasia; Stroke; **Admitting Hospital:** Columbia Presbyterian Medical Center (Page 72); **Office Address:** Columbia Presbyterian, Dept Neuro-Neuro Inst 710 W 168 Street New York, NY 10032-2603; **Office Phone:** (212) 305-8033; **Board Certification:** Neurology 1971; **Medical School:** Univ VA Sch Med 1963; **Residencies:** Neurology, Columbia Presby Med Ctr, New York, NY 1965-1966; Neurology, Mass Genl Hosp, Boston, MA 1966-1968; **Fellowship:** Neurology, Mass Genl Hosp, Boston, MA 1967-1969; **Faculty Appointment:** Clin Prof Neurology, Columbia P&S

Morrell, Martha MD (Neurology) - *Special Expertise:* Epilepsy; Epilepsy-Women's Issues; **Admitting Hospital:** Columbia Presbyterian Medical Center (Page 72); **Office Address:** 710 W 168th St, Fl 7 New York, NY 10032; **Office Phone:** (212) 305-1742; **Board Certifications:** Neurology 1989, Clinical Neurophysiology 1992; **Medical School:** Stanford Univ 1984; **Residency:** Neurology, Univ Penn Hosp, Philadelphia, PA 1985-1988; **Fellowship:** Epilepsy, Univ Penn Hosp, Philadelphia, PA 1988-1990; **Faculty Appointment:** Prof Neurology, Columbia P&S

Olanow, C Warren MD (Neurology) - *Special Expertise:* Parkinson's Disease; Movement Disorders; **Admitting Hospital:** Mount Sinai Hospital (Page 70); **Office Address:** 5 E 98th St New York, NY 10029; **Office Phone:** (212) 241-4623; **Board Certification:** Neurology 1970; **Medical School:** Univ Toronto 1965; **Residencies:** Neurology, Toronto Genl Hosp, Toronto, Canada 1967-1968; Neurology, Columbia Presby, New York, NY 1968-1970; **Fellowship:** Neurological Anatomy, Columbia Presby, New York, NY 1970-1971; **Faculty Appointment:** Neurology, Mount Sinai Sch Med

Pedley, Timothy A. MD (Neurology) - *Special Expertise:* Epilepsy/Seizure Disorders; **Admitting Hospital:** Columbia Presbyterian Medical Center (Page 72); **Office Address:** The Neurological Institute 710 W 168th St, Fl 14 - rm 1401 New York, NY 10032; **Office Phone:** (212) 305-6489; **Board Certifications:** Neurology 1975, Clinical Neurophysiology 1993; **Medical School:** Yale Univ 1969; **Residency:** Neurology, Stanford Hosp & Cln, Stanford, CA 1970-1973; **Fellowship:** Clinical Neurophysiology, Stanford Hosp & Cln, Stanford, CA 1973-1975; **Faculty Appointment:** Prof Neurology, Columbia P&S

Petito, Frank MD (Neurology) - *Special Expertise:* Multiple Sclerosis; Headache; Lyme Disease; **Admitting Hospital:** New York Weill Cornell Medical Center - NY Presbyterian Hospital (Page 72); **Office Address:** 525 E 70th St, Ste 607 New York, NY 10021-9800; **Office Phone:** (212) 746-2309; **Board Certification:** Neurology 1972; **Medical School:** Columbia P&S 1967; **Residency:** Neurology, NY Hosp-Cornell Univ, New York, NY 1967-1971; **Faculty Appointment:** Prof Neurology, Cornell Univ-Weill Med Coll

Plum, Fred MD (Neurology) - *Special Expertise: Coma; Stroke;* **Admitting Hospital:** New York Weill Cornell Medical Center - NY Presbyterian Hospital (Page 72); **Office Address:** 525 E 70th St, Ste 607 New York, NY 10021; **Office Phone:** (212) 746-6141; **Board Certification:** Neurology 1956; **Medical School:** Cornell Univ-Weill Med Coll 1947; **Residencies:** Internal Medicine, NY Hosp-Cornell Univ, New York, NY 1948-1949; Neurology, NY Hosp-Cornell Univ, New York, NY 1949-1950; **Fellowship:** Neurology, Bellevue Psyc Inst, New York, NY 1950-1951; **Faculty Appointment:** Prof Neurology, Cornell Univ-Weil Med Coll

Posner, Jerome MD (Neurology) - *Special Expertise: Neuro-Oncology; Brain Tumors;* **Admitting Hospital:** Memorial Sloan Kettering Cancer Center; **Office Address:** Meml Sloan Kettering Cancer Ctr, Dept Neuro 1275 York Ave New York, NY 10021-6007; **Office Phone:** (212) 639-7047; **Board Certification:** Neurology 1962; **Medical School:** Univ Wash 1955; **Residency:** Neurology, Univ WA Affil Hosp, Seattle, WA 1955-1959; **Fellowship:** Neurology, Univ WA Affil Hosp, Seattle, WA 1961-1963; **Faculty Appointment:** Prof Neurology, Cornell Univ-Weil Med Coll

Pula, Thaddeus MD (Neurology) - *Special Expertise: Neurophysiology; Electromyography & Nerve Conduction;* **Admitting Hospital:** Maryland General Hospital; **Office Address:** Maryland Genl Hosp Div Neur 827 Linden Ave Baltimore, MD 21201-4606; **Office Phone:** (410) 225-8290; **Board Certifications:** Neurology 1981, Clinical Neurophysiology 1994; **Medical School:** Univ Maryland Sch Med 1976; **Residency:** Internal Medicine, Mercy Hosp Med Ctr

Richert, John R MD (Neurology) - *Special Expertise: Multiple Sclerosis; Neuro-Immunology;* **Admitting Hospital:** Georgetown University Hospital; **Office Address:** Georgetown Univ Med Ctr 3800 Reservoir Rd NW Washington, DC 20007-2196; **Office Phone:** (202) 878-8525; **Board Certification:** Neurology 1978; **Medical School:** Univ Rochester 1970; **Residencies:** Internal Medicine, Rochester-Strong Meml Hosp, Rochester, NY 1971-1972; Neurology, Mayo Clinic, Rochester, MN 1974-1977; **Fellowship:** Multiple Sclerosis, NIH, Bethesda, MD 1977-1980; **Faculty Appointment:** Prof Neurology, Georgetown Univ

Sage, Jacob MD (Neurology) - *Special Expertise: Neurology - General;* **Admitting Hospital:** Robert Wood Johnson University Hospital @ New Brunswick; **Office Address:** UMDNJ, Dept Neurology 125 Paterson St New Brunswick, NJ 08903; **Office Phone:** (732) 235-7731; **Board Certification:** Neurology 1979; **Medical School:** Univ Pittsburgh 1972; **Residency:** Neurology, Pittsburgh Hosp, Pittsburgh, PA 1978; **Fellowship:** Neurological Chemistry, New York Hosp-Cornell Univ, New York, NY 1978-1980; **Faculty Appointment:** Prof Neurology, UMDNJ-RW Johnson Med Sch

Schold Jr., S. Clifford MD (Neurology) - *Special Expertise: Brain Tumors;* **Admitting Hospital:** UPMC - Presbyterian University Hospital; **Office Address:** Univ Pitts Cancer Inst 3471 5th Ave Pittsburgh, PA 15213; **Office Phone:** (412) 692-2600; **Board Certification:** Neurology 1980; **Medical School:** Univ Ariz Coll Med 1973; **Residency:** Neurology, Colo Med Ctr, Denver, CO 1974-1977; **Fellowship:** Neurological Oncology, Sloan-Kettering Cancer Ctr, New York, NY 1977-1978

Shoulson, Ira MD (Neurology) - *Special Expertise: Parkinson's Disease; Movement Disorders; Huntington's Disease;* **Admitting Hospital:** Strong Memorial Hospital - Medical Center; **Office Address:** 919 Westfall Rd, Bldg C - Ste 220 Rochester, NY 14618; **Office Phone:** (716) 275-2585; **Board Certifications:** Internal Medicine 1974, Neurology 1980; **Medical School:** Univ Rochester 1971; **Residencies:** Internal Medicine, Strong Meml Hospital, Rochester, MN 1972-1973; Neurology, Strong Meml Hosp, Rochester, MN 1975-1977; **Fellowship:** Neurology, Natl Inst Hlth, Bethesda, MD 1973-1975; **Faculty Appointment:** Prof Neurology, Univ Rochester

NEUROLOGY

Sirdofsky, Michael D MD (Neurology) - *Special Expertise:* Neuromuscular Disorders; Electrodiagnosis-EEG, EMG; **Admitting Hospital:** Georgetown University Hospital; **Office Address:** Georgetown Univ Hosp, Dept Neurology 3800 Reservior Rd NW Washington, DC 20007; **Office Phone:** (202) 687-8525; **Board Certification:** Neurology 1981; **Medical School:** Georgetown Univ 1976; **Residency:** Neurology, Georgetown Univ Hosp, Washington, DC 1977-1980; **Faculty Appointment:** Assoc Prof Neurology, Georgetown Univ

Stern, Matthew MD (Neurology) - *Special Expertise:* Parkinson's Disease; Movement Disorders; Botox Therapy; **Admitting Hospital:** Pennsylvania Hospital; **Office Address:** Penn Hosp, Dept Neurology 330 S 9th St, Fl 4 Philadelphia, PA 19107; **Office Phone:** (215) 829-6500; **Board Certification:** Neurology 1983; **Medical School:** Duke Univ 1970; **Residency:** Neurology, Hosp Univ Penn, Philadelphia, PA 1979-1982

Swerdlow, Michael MD (Neurology) - *Special Expertise:* Myasthenia Gravis; **Admitting Hospital:** Montefiore Medical Center; **Office Address:** Neurological Assoc 3400 Bainbridge Ave, Ste 5A Bronx, NY 10467; **Office Phone:** (718) 920-4178; **Board Certification:** Neurology 1975; **Medical School:** Univ Penn 1967; **Residencies:** Internal Medicine, Mount Sinai Hosp, New York, NY 1967-1969; Neurology, Albert Einstein Coll, Bronx, NY 1969-1972; **Faculty Appointment:** Clin Prof Neurology, Albert Einstein Coll Med

Vas, George A MD (Neurology) - *Special Expertise:* Stroke; **Admitting Hospital:** University Hospital - Brooklyn; **Office Address:** 450 Clarkson Ave, Ste A Brooklyn, NY 11203; **Office Phone:** (718) 270-1950; **Board Certifications:** Internal Medicine 1973, Neurology 1977; **Medical School:** Univ Pittsburgh 1970; **Residencies:** Internal Medicine, New York Hosp-Cornell Univ, New York, NY 1971-1972; Neurology, New York Hosp-Cornell Univ, New York, NY 1972-1975; **Faculty Appointment:** Prof SUNY Downstate

Wechsler, Lawrence Richard MD (Neurology) - *Special Expertise:* Neurophysiology; Stroke; Transcranial Doppler; **Admitting Hospital:** UPMC - Presbyterian University Hospital; **Office Address:** 220 Meyran Ave Pittsburgh, PA 15213; **Office Phone:** (412) 692-4920; **Board Certifications:** Neurology 1984, Clinical Neurophysiology 1994; **Medical School:** Univ Penn 1978; **Residencies:** Internal Medicine, Univ Hosp - Presby, Pittsburgh, PA 1979-1980; Neurology, MA Genl Hosp, Boston, MA 1980-1983; **Fellowships:** Neurological Physiology, MA Genl Hosp, Boston, MA 1983-1984; Cerebrovascular Disease, MA Genl Hosp, Boston, MA 1984-1985; **Faculty Appointment:** Asst Clin Prof Neurology, Univ Pittsburgh

Weinberg, Harold MD (Neurology) - *Special Expertise:* Headache; Muscular Dystrophy; **Admitting Hospital:** NYU Medical Center (Page 70); **Office Address:** 650 1st Ave, Fl 4 New York, NY 10016-3292; **Office Phone:** (212) 139-9339; **Board Certification:** Neurology 1979; **Medical School:** Albert Einstein Coll Med 1978; **Residency:** Neurology, Columbia-Presby Med Ctr, New York, NY 1979-1982; **Fellowship:** Neurological Muscular Disease, Columbia-Presby Med Ctr, New York, NY 1982; **Faculty Appointment:** Assoc Prof Neurology, NYU Sch Med

Zimmerman, Earl Abram MD (Neurology) - *Special Expertise:* Movement Disorders; Alzheimer's Disease; **Admitting Hospital:** Albany Medical Center; **Office Address:** Albany Med Ctr, 47 New Scotland Ave, MC-342 Albany, NY 12208; **Office Phone:** (518) 262-5226; **Board Certifications:** Neurology 1970, Internal Medicine 1970; **Medical School:** Univ Penn 1963; **Residencies:** Internal Medicine, Columbia Presby Hosp, New York, NY 1964-1965; Neurology, Presby Hosp., New York, NY 1965-1968; **Fellowship:** Endocrinology, Diabetes & Metabolism, Columbia Presby Hosp, New York, NY 1970-1972

Southeast

Adams, Robert Joseph MD (Neurology) - *Special Expertise:* Stroke; **Admitting Hospital:** Medical College of Georgia Hospital; **Office Address:** Med Coll of Georgia, Dept Neuro 1467 Harper St-HB2060 Augusta, GA 30912; **Office Phone:** (706) 721-4670; **Board Certification:** Neurology 1987; **Medical School:** Univ Ark 1980; **Residency:** Neurology, Med Coll GA, Augusta, GA 1982-1985; **Faculty Appointment:** Assoc Prof Med Coll GA

Berger, Joseph MD (Neurology) - *Special Expertise:* Multiple Sclerosis; AIDS/HIV; Infectious & Demyelinating Diseases; **Admitting Hospital:** University of Kentucky Medical Center; **Office Address:** Kentucky Clinic rm L445 Lexington, KY 40536-0284; **Office Phone:** (606) 323-1279; **Board Certifications:** Internal Medicine 1977, Neurology 1983; **Medical School:** Jefferson Med Coll 1974; **Residencies:** Internal Medicine, Georgetown Univ Hosp, Washington, DC 1975-1977; Neurology, Jackson Meml Hosp, Miami, FL 1978-1981; **Faculty Appointment:** Prof Emeritus Neurology, Univ KY Coll Med

Corbett, James MD (Neurology) - *Special Expertise:* Neuro-Ophthalmology; Optic Nerve Diseases; Multiple Sclerosis; **Admitting Hospital:** University Hospital & Clinics- Mississippi; **Office Address:** Univ Mississippi Med Ctr Neuro Grp 2500 N State St Jackson, MS 39216; **Office Phone:** (601) 984-5501; **Board Certification:** Neurology 1974; **Medical School:** Univ Hlth Sci/Chicago Med Sch 1966; **Residencies:** Internal Medicine, Rhode Island Hosp, Providence, RI 1967-1968; Neurology, Univ Hosp-CWRU, Cleveland, OH 1968-1971; **Faculty Appointment:** Prof Neurology, Univ Miss

De Long, Mahlon R. MD (Neurology) - *Special Expertise:* Parkinson's Disease; Movement Disorders; **Admitting Hospital:** Emory University Hospital; **Office Address:** 1639 Pierce, Ste 6000 Atlanta, GA 30322; **Office Phone:** (404) 727-3818; **Board Certification:** Neurology 1980; **Medical School:** Harvard Med Sch 1966; **Residencies:** Neurology, Johns Hopkins Hosp, Baltimore, MD 1973-1976; Internal Medicine, Boston City Hosp, Boston, MA 1967-1968; **Fellowship:** Neurology, NIMH, Bethesda, MD 1968-1973; **Faculty Appointment:** Prof Neurology, Johns Hopkins Univ

Dokson, Joel MD (Neurology) - *Special Expertise:* Neurology - General; **Admitting Hospital:** Mount Sinai Medical Center; **Office Address:** 4302 Alton Rd, Ste 680 Miami Beach, FL 33140-2877; **Office Phone:** (305) 538-1877; **Board Certification:** Neurology 1973; **Medical School:** Univ Miami Sch Med 1967; **Residency:** Neurology, Mount Sinai Hosp, New York, NY 1968-1971

Finkel, Michael MD (Neurology) - *Special Expertise:* Lyme Disease; ADHD/Headaches; **Admitting Hospital:** Cleveland Clinic Florida; **Office Address:** Cleveland Clinic-Florida Naples 6101 Pine Ridge Rd Naples, FL 34119; **Office Phone:** (941) 348-4000; **Board Certification:** Neurology 1979; **Medical School:** Washington Univ, St Louis 1973; **Residency:** Neurology, Strong Meml Hosp, Rochester, NY 1974-1977; **Faculty Appointment:** Asst Prof Neurology, Mayo Med Sch

Glass, Jonathan MD (Neurology) - *Special Expertise:* Neuropathology; **Admitting Hospital:** Emory University Hospital; **Office Address:** Emory Univ Sch Med, Dept Neurology 1639 Pierce Dr, WMRB Bldg, Ste 6000 Atlanta, GA 30322; **Office Phone:** (404) 727-3507; **Board Certifications:** Clinical Neurophysiology 1996, Neuropathology 1997; **Medical School:** Univ VT Coll Med 1985; **Residency:** Neurology, John Hopkins Univ, Baltimore, MD 1986-1989; **Fellowship:** Neuropathology, John Hopkins Univ, Baltimore, MD 1989-1991

NEUROLOGY *Southeast*

Goldstein, Larry Bruce MD (Neurology) - *Special Expertise:* Stroke; Carotid Artery Disease; **Admitting Hospital:** Duke University Medical Center (Page 60); **Office Address:** Duke University Medical Center Box 3651 Durham, NC 27710; **Office Phone:** (919) 684-3801; **Board Certification:** Neurology 1987; **Medical School:** Mount Sinai Sch Med 1981; **Residency:** Neurology, Mt Sinai Hosp, New York, NY 1982-1985; **Fellowship:** Cerebrovascular Disease, Duke Univ Med Ctr, Durham, NC 1985-1986; **Faculty Appointment:** Assoc Prof Neurology, Duke Univ

Haley Jr, Elliott Clarke MD (Neurology) - *Special Expertise:* Stroke; **Admitting Hospital:** University of Virginia Health Systems; **Office Address:** Univ Virginia Health Sciences Center PO Box 800394 Charlottesville, VA 22908; **Office Phone:** (804) 924-8041; **Board Certifications:** Neurology 1985, Internal Medicine 1978; **Medical School:** Tulane Univ 1974; **Residencies:** Internal Medicine, Univ Virginia Hosp, Charlottesville, VA 1976-1978; Neurology, Univ Virginia Hosp, Charlottesville, VA 1979-1982; **Fellowship:** Cerebrovascular Disease, Mass Genl Hosp, Boston, MA 1983-1984

Heilman, Kenneth MD (Neurology) - *Special Expertise:* Behavioral Neurology; Memory Disorders; **Admitting Hospital:** Shands Healthcare at University Florida (Page 77); **Office Address:** Hlth Ctr Univ Fla Coll Med, Dept Neuro Box 100236 Gainesville, FL 32610-0236; **Office Phone:** (352) 392-3491; **Board Certification:** Neurology 1973; **Medical School:** Univ VA Sch Med 1963; **Residencies:** Bellevue Hosp Ctr, New York, NY 1964-1965; Neurology, Boston City Hosp, Boston, MA 1967-1970; **Faculty Appointment:** Prof Neurology, Univ Fla Coll Med

Hess, David Charles MD (Neurology) - *Special Expertise:* Stroke; **Admitting Hospital:** Medical College of Georgia Hospital; **Office Address:** Med Coll Georgia, Dept Neurology One Freedom Way Augusta, GA 30904; **Office Phone:** (706) 721-5494; **Board Certifications:** Internal Medicine 1986, Neurology 1990; **Medical School:** Univ MD Sch Med 1983; **Residencies:** Internal Medicine, Allegheny Genl Hosp, Pittsburgh, PA 1984-1985; Neurology, Med Coll Georgia, Augusta, GA 1986-1989; **Fellowship:** Cerebrovascular Disease, Med Coll Georgia, Augusta, GA 1989-1990; **Faculty Appointment:** Assoc Prof Neurology, Med Coll GA

Hurwitz, Barrie MD (Neurology) - *Special Expertise:* Multiple Sclerosis; **Admitting Hospital:** Duke University Medical Center (Page 60); **Office Address:** 122 Baker House Box 3184 Durham, NC 27710; **Office Phone:** (919) 684-4126; **Board Certification:** Neurology 1979; **Medical School:** Africa 1968; **Residencies:** Internal Medicine, Johannesburg Genl, Johannesburg 1971-1973; Neurology, Sloan Kettering hosp, New York, NY 1974-1977; **Fellowship:** Neurology, Cornell, New York, NY 1974-1976; **Faculty Appointment:** Assoc Prof Duke Univ

Kirshner, Howard S MD (Neurology) - *Special Expertise:* Stroke; Aphasia; **Admitting Hospital:** Vanderbilt University Medical Center; **Office Address:** Med Ctr South 2100 Pierce Ave, Fl 362 Nashville, TN 37212; **Office Phone:** (615) 936-0060; **Board Certification:** Neurology 1980; **Medical School:** Harvard Med Sch 1972; **Residencies:** Internal Medicine, Mass Genl Hosp, Boston, MA 1972-1973; Neurology, Mass Genl Hosp, Boston, MA 1975-1978; **Fellowship:** Neurological Science, Natl Inst of Hlth, Bethesda, MD 1973-1975; **Faculty Appointment:** Prof Neurology, Vanderbilt Univ

Koller, William C MD (Neurology) - *Special Expertise:* Movement Disorders; Parkinson's Disease; **Admitting Hospital:** University of Miami - Jackson Memorial Hospital; **Office Address:** Univ Miami, Dept Neuro, Fl 2, 1501 NW Ninth Ave Miami, FL 33136; **Office Phone:** (305) 243-2235; **Board Certification:** Neurology 1982; **Medical School:** Northwestern Univ 1976; **Residency:** Neurology, Rush-Presby-St Lukes Med Ctr, Chicago, IL 1977-1980; **Faculty Appointment:** Prof Neurology, Univ Miami Sch Med

Kurtzke, Robert MD (Neurology) - *Special Expertise:* Neurology - General; **Admitting Hospital:** Fairfax Hospital; **Office Address:** Neuro Ctr Fairfax Ltd 3020 Hamaker Ct Ste 400 Fairfax, VA 22031-2220; **Office Phone:** (703) 876-0800; **Board Certifications:** Clinical Neurophysiology 1994, Neurology 1990; **Medical School:** Georgetown Univ 1985; **Residencies:** Neurology, Neuro Inst, New York, NY 1988-1989; Neurology, Neur Inst, New York, NY 1986-1989; **Fellowship:** Neurological Muscular Disease, Duke Med Ctr, Durham, NC 1989-1990; **Faculty Appointment:** Clin Inst Neurology, Georgetown Univ

Lopez, Raul MD (Neurology) - *Special Expertise:* Headache; **Admitting Hospital:** Mercy Hospital - Miami; **Office Address:** 3661 S Miami Ave, Ste 209 Miami, FL 33133-4206; **Office Phone:** (305) 856-8942; **Board Certification:** Neurology 1970; **Medical School:** Univ Fla Coll Med 1963; **Residencies:** Internal Medicine, Univ Florida Med Ctr, Gainesville, FL 1963-1965; Neurology, Univ Florida Med Ctr, Gainesville, FL 1967-1968; **Fellowship:** Neurology, Univ Florida Med Ctr, Gainesville, FL 1965-1967

Morgenlander, Joel Charles MD (Neurology) - *Special Expertise:* Neurology - General; **Admitting Hospital:** Duke University Medical Center (Page 60); **Office Address:** Duke Univ Med Ctr Box 3394 Durham, NC 27710-0001; **Office Phone:** (919) 684-6887; **Board Certification:** Neurology 1992; **Medical School:** Univ Pittsburgh 1986; **Residencies:** Neurology, Duke Univ, Durham, NC 1987-1990; Duke Univ, Durham, NC 1990-1991; **Faculty Appointment:** Assoc Prof Neurology, Univ Pittsburgh

Nadeau, Stephen E MD (Neurology) - *Special Expertise:* Dementia; Cerebrovascular Disease; Collagen Vascular Disease; **Admitting Hospital:** Shands Healthcare at University Florida (Page 77); **Office Address:** The Brain Inst 100 S Newell Dr, rm L3-100 Gainesville, FL 32610; **Office Phone:** (352) 392-3491; **Board Certification:** Neurology 1984; **Medical School:** Univ Fla Coll Med 1977; **Residency:** Neurology, Shands Teaching Hosp, Gainesville, FL 1978-1981; **Fellowship:** Behavioral Neurology, Shands Teaching Hosp, Gainesville, FL 1981-1982; **Faculty Appointment:** Prof Neurology, Univ Fla Coll Med

Newman, Nancy Jean MD (Neurology) - *Special Expertise:* Neuro-Ophthalmology; **Admitting Hospital:** Emory University Hospital; **Office Address:** Emory Eye Center 1365-B Clifton RD NE Atlanta, GA 30322; **Office Phone:** (404) 778-5360; **Board Certification:** Neurology 1989; **Medical School:** Harvard Med Sch 1984; **Residency:** Neurology, Mass Genl Hosp, Boston, MA 1985-1988; **Fellowship:** Neurological Ophthalmology, Mass EE Infirm, Boston, MA 1988-1989; **Faculty Appointment:** Prof Neurology, Emory Univ

Nolan, Bruce A MD (Neurology) - *Special Expertise:* Sleep Disorders/Apnea; **Admitting Hospital:** University of Miami - Jackson Memorial Hospital; **Office Address:** Univ Miami Sleep Disorder Ctr 1201 NW 16th St, rm A212 Miami, FL 33101-6960; **Office Phone:** (305) 324-3371; **Board Certification:** Neurology 1974; **Medical School:** Wayne State Univ 1966; **Residency:** Neurology, Univ Miami Med Ctr, Miami, FL 1967-1970; **Faculty Appointment:** Assoc Prof Neurology, Univ Miami Sch Med

Rothrock, John MD (Neurology) - *Special Expertise:* Aneurysm; Headache; **Admitting Hospital:** University of South Alabama Medical Center; **Office Address:** Univ S Alabama Med Ctr 3401 Medical Park Dr, Bldg 3 - Ste 205 Mobile, AL 36693; **Office Phone:** (334) 660-5108; **Board Certification:** Neurology 1984; **Medical School:** Univ VA Sch Med 1977; **Residency:** Neurology, Univ Ariz Med Ctr, Tucson, AZ 1978-1981; **Faculty Appointment:** Prof Neurology, Univ S Ala Coll Med

Sadowsky, Carl Howard MD (Neurology) - *Special Expertise:* Memory Disorders; **Admitting Hospital:** St Mary's Medical Center - West Palm Beach; **Office Address:** 5205 Greenwood Ave, Ste 200 West Palm Beach, FL 33407-2493; **Office Phone:** (561) 845-0500; **Board Certification:** Neurology 1977; **Medical School:** Cornell Univ-Weil Med Coll 1971; **Residencies:** Internal Medicine, Dartmouth-Hitchcock Med Ctr, Hanover, NH 1972-1973; Neurology, Dartmouth-Hitchcock Med Ctr, Hanover, NH 1973-1976

Schatz, Norman Joseph MD (Neurology) - *Special Expertise:* Neuro-Ophthalmology; **Admitting Hospital:** Mercy Hospital - Miami; **Office Address:** 325 Alhambra Cir Coral Gable, FL 33134; **Office Phone:** (305) 442-3355; **Board Certification:** Neurology 1969; **Medical School:** Hahnemann Univ 1961; **Residency:** Neurology, Jefferson Hosp, Philadelphia, PA 1962-1965; **Fellowship:** Neurological Ophthalmology, Univ Miami, Miami, FL 1965-1966; **Faculty Appointment:** Clin Prof Neurology, Univ Penn

Sethi, Kapil MD (Neurology) - *Special Expertise:* Parkinson's Disease; Movement Disorders; Botox Therapy; **Admitting Hospital:** Medical College of Georgia Hospital; **Office Address:** Neurology Dept 1120 15th St, rm BIW 3078 Augusta, GA 30912; **Office Phone:** (706) 721-2798; **Board Certification:** Neurology 1987; **Medical School:** India 1976; **Residencies:** Neurology, Pgimer, Chandigarh, India 1979-1981; Neurology, Med Coll Georgia, Augusta, GA 1983-1985; **Faculty Appointment:** Prof Neurology, Med Coll GA

Troost, Bradley Todd MD (Neurology) - *Special Expertise:* Headache; Neuro-Ophthalmology; Dizziness; **Admitting Hospital:** Wake Forest University Baptist Medical Center; **Office Address:** Wake Forest Univ Baptist Med Ctr Medical Center Blvd Winston Salem, NC 27157-0001; **Office Phone:** (336) 716-3429; **Board Certification:** Neurology 1972; **Medical School:** Harvard Med Sch 1963; **Residency:** Neurology, Univ Colo Med Ctr, Denver, CO 1966-1969; **Fellowship:** Ophthalmology, UCSF Med Ctr, San Francisco, CA 1969-1970; **Faculty Appointment:** Prof Neurology, Wake Forest Univ Sch Med

Valenstein, Edward MD (Neurology) - *Special Expertise:* Nerve and Muscle Diseases; Amyotrophic Lateral Sclerosis(ALS); **Admitting Hospital:** Shands Healthcare at University Florida (Page 77); **Office Address:** 1600 SW Archer Rd, Box 100236 Gainesville, FL 32610-0236; **Office Phone:** (352) 392-3491; **Board Certifications:** Neurology 1974, Clinical Neurophysiology 1996; **Medical School:** Albert Einstein Coll Med 1967; **Residency:** Neurology, Boston City Hosp, Boston, MA 1968-1971; **Faculty Appointment:** Prof Neurology, Univ Fla Coll Med

Vitek, Jerrold Lee MD (Neurology) - *Special Expertise:* Movement Disorders; **Admitting Hospital:** Emory University Hospital; **Office Address:** Emory Univ Sch Med, Dept Neurology 1639 Pierce Dr, Ste 6000 Atlanta, GA 30322; **Office Phone:** (404) 727-7177; **Board Certification:** Neurology 1992; **Medical School:** Univ Minn 1984; **Residency:** Neurology, Johns Hopkins Univ, Baltimore, MD 1985-1988; **Faculty Appointment:** Assoc Prof Neurology, Emory Univ

Watts, Ray Lannon MD (Neurology) - *Special Expertise:* Parkinson's Disease; Movement Disorders; **Admitting Hospital:** Emory University Hospital; **Office Address:** Emory Univ Sch Med, Dept Neuro 1639 Pierce Drive, Ste 6000 Atlanta, GA 30322; **Office Phone:** (404) 727-5002; **Board Certification:** Neurology 1985; **Medical School:** Washington Univ, St Louis 1980; **Residency:** Neurology, Mass Genl Hosp, Boston, MA 1981-1984; **Fellowship:** Electromyography, Mass Genl Hosp, Boston, MA 1982-1983; **Faculty Appointment:** Neurology, Emory Univ

Weiner, William J. MD (Neurology) - *Special Expertise:* Movement Disorders; Parkinson's Disease; Huntington's Disease; **Admitting Hospital:** University of Miami - Jackson Memorial Hospital; **Office Address:** Univ Miami Sch Med, Dept Neur 1501 NW 9th Ave Miami, FL 33136; **Office Phone:** (305) 243-6332; **Board Certification:** Neurology 1975; **Medical School:** Univ IL Coll Med 1969; **Residencies:** Neurology, Univ Minn, Minneapolis, MN 1970-1971; Neurology, Rush-Presby Med Ctr, Chicago, IL 1971-1973; **Faculty Appointment:** Prof Neurology, Univ Miami Sch Med

Whitaker, John N MD (Neurology) - *Special Expertise:* Multiple Sclerosis; **Admitting Hospital:** University of Alabama Hospital at Birmingham; **Office Address:** Univ Alabama Med Ctr, Dept Neurology 619 19th St S, Ste JT120 Birmingham, AL 35249-7340; **Office Phone:** (205) 934-2402; **Board Certification:** Neurology 1972; **Medical School:** Univ Tenn Coll Med, Memphis 1965; **Residency:** Neurology, Albert Einstein Coll Med, Bronx, NY 1967-1970; **Faculty Appointment:** Prof Neurology, Univ Ala

Wooten, George Frederick MD (Neurology) - *Special Expertise:* Movement Disorders; Parkinson's Disease; **Admitting Hospital:** University of Virginia Health Systems; **Office Address:** Univ Virginia Med Ctr, Dept Neurology The McKim Hall, Box 394 Charlottesville, VA 22908; **Office Phone:** (804) 924-8369; **Board Certification:** Neurology; **Medical School:** Cornell Univ-Weil Med Coll 1970; **Residency:** Neurology, NY Hosp-Cornell Med, New York, NY 1974-1977; **Fellowship:** Pharmacology, Natl Inst Mental Hlth, Bethesda, MD 1971-1974; **Faculty Appointment:** Prof Neurology, Univ VA Sch Med

Midwest

Adams Jr., Harlold Pomeroy MD (Neurology) - *Special Expertise:* Stroke; **Admitting Hospital:** University of Iowa Hospitals and Clinics; **Office Address:** 200 Hawkins Dr. Univ Iowa Hosps-Dept. of Neurology Iowa City, IA 52242; **Office Phone:** (319) 356-4110; **Board Certification:** Neurology 1977; **Medical School:** Northwestern Univ 1970; **Residency:** Neurology, Iowa Hosp., Iowa City, IA 1971-1974; **Faculty Appointment:** Prof Neurology, Univ Iowa Coll Med

Ahlskog, J. Eric MD (Neurology) - *Special Expertise:* Parkinson's Disease; Movement Disorders; **Admitting Hospital:** Mayo Medical Center & Clinic - Rochester; **Office Address:** Mayo Clinic, Dept Neuro 200 First St SW Rochester, MN 55905; **Office Phone:** (507) 284-4409; **Board Certification:** Neurology 1984; **Medical School:** Dartmouth Med Sch 1976; **Residencies:** Internal Medicine, Univ Chicago Hosps, Chicago, IL 1977-1978; Neurology, Mayo Grad Sch Med, Rochester, MN 1978-1981; **Faculty Appointment:** Prof Neurology, Mayo Med Sch

Arnason, Barry G W MD (Neurology) - *Special Expertise:* Multiple Sclerosis; Guillain-Barre Syndrome; Myasthenia Gravis; **Admitting Hospital:** University of Chicago Hospitals (Page 78); **Office Address:** 5758 S Maryland Ave MC-2030 Chicago, IL 60637; **Office Phone:** (773) 702-6386; **Board Certification:** Neurology 1971; **Medical School:** Univ Manitoba 1957; **Residencies:** Neurology, Mass Genl Hosp, Boston, MA 1958-1959; Neurology, Mass Genl Hosp, Boston, MA 1961-1962; **Faculty Appointment:** Prof Neurology, Univ Chicago-Pritzker Sch Med

Brooks, Benjamin MD (Neurology) - *Special Expertise:* Neuromuscular Disorders; Multiple Sclerosis; **Admitting Hospital:** University of Wisconsin Hospital & Clinics; **Office Address:** Univ Wisc Hosp, Dept Neurology 600 Highland Ave, MC-H6 558 Madison, WI 53792; **Office Phone:** (608) 263-5422; **Board Certifications:** Internal Medicine 1974, Neurology 1978; **Medical School:** Harvard Med Sch 1970; **Residencies:** Neurology, Mass Genl Hosp, Bethesda, MD 1972-1974; Neurology, Natl Inst Neuro Disorders & Stroke-NIH, Boston, MA 1974-1976; **Fellowship:** Neurological Virus, Johns Hopkins, Baltimore, MD 1976-1978; **Faculty Appointment:** Prof Neurology, Univ Wisc

Burke, Allan M MD (Neurology) - *Special Expertise:* Cerebrovascular Disease; **Admitting Hospital:** Northwestern Memorial Hospital; **Office Address:** Neurology Associates Ltd 150 E Huron St, Ste 803 Chicago, IL 60611-2912; **Office Phone:** (312) 944-0063; **Board Certification:** Neurology 1982; **Medical School:** Columbia P&S 1976; **Residencies:** Internal Medicine, NY Hosp, New York, NY 1977-1978; Neurology, Columbia Presby Med Ctr, New York, NY 1978-1981; **Fellowship:** Cerebrovascular Disease, Univ Penn, Philadelphia, PA 1981-1983; **Faculty Appointment:** Assoc Clin Prof Neurology, Northwestern Univ

Burns, R Stanley MD (Neurology) - *Special Expertise:* Movement Disorders; Ataxia; *Neurodegenerative Disease;* **Admitting Hospital:** Cleveland Clinic Foundation; **Office Address:** 9500 Euclid Ave, MS S90 Cleveland, OH 44195; **Office Phone:** (216) 444-6467; **Board Certification:** Neurology 1985; **Medical School:** Univ Minn 1969; **Residencies:** Internal Medicine, Huntington Meml Hosp, Pasadena, CA 1970-1971; Neurology, UC Irvine Med Ctr, Irvine, CA 1975-1978; **Fellowship:** Clinical Pharmacology, Natl Inst Genl Med Sci, Bethesda, MD 1978-1980; **Faculty Appointment:** Asst Prof Neurology, Vanderbilt Univ

Choi, Dennis W MD (Neurology) - *Special Expertise:* Neurology - General; **Admitting Hospital:** Barnes - Jewish Hospital; **Office Address:** Wash Univ Neuro Clinic 517 S Euclid Ave St Louis, MO 63110-1010; **Office Phone:** (314) 362-5262; **Board Certification:** Neurology 1983; **Medical School:** Harvard Med Sch 1974; **Residency:** Neurology, Brigham & Women's Hosp, Boston, MA 1979-1982; **Fellowship:** Electroencephalography, Mass Genl Hosp, Boston, MA 1982-1983; **Faculty Appointment:** Assoc Prof Neurology, Washington Univ, St Louis

Cohen, Jeffrey Alan MD (Neurology) - *Special Expertise:* Multiple Sclerosis; Neuro-Immunology; **Admitting Hospital:** Cleveland Clinic Foundation; **Office Address:** The Cleveland Clin, Mellen Ctr, 9500 Euclid Ave Cleveland, OH 44195; **Office Phone:** (216) 445-8110; **Board Certification:** Neurology 1985; **Medical School:** Univ Chicago-Pritzker Sch Med 1980; **Residency:** Neurology, Hosp Univ Penn, Philadelphia, PA 1981-1984; **Fellowship:** Neurological Immunology, Hosp Univ Penn, Philadelphia, PA 1984-1987

Elias, Stanton B MD (Neurology) - *Special Expertise:* Multiple Sclerosis; Myasthenia Gravis; **Admitting Hospital:** Henry Ford Health System (Page 62); **Office Address:** Henry Ford Hosp, Dept Neuro 2799 W Grand Blvd, Fl K-11 Detroit, MI 48202-2608; **Office Phone:** (313) 876-7207; **Board Certification:** Neurology 1979; **Medical School:** Univ Pittsburgh 1972; **Residency:** Neurology, Duke Univ, Durham, NC 1976-1977; **Fellowship:** Neurology, Duke Univ, Durham, NC 1973-1976

Feldman, Eva L. MD/PhD (Neurology) - *Special Expertise:* Neuromuscular Disorders; *Amyotrophic Lateral Sclerosis(ALS); Neuropathy;* **Admitting Hospital:** University of Michigan Health Center; **Office Address:** Taubman Health Care Center 1500 E Medical Drive, rm 1324, Box 0322 Ann Arbor, MI 48109-0322; **Office Phone:** (734) 936-9020; **Board Certification:** Neurology 1988; **Medical School:** Univ Mich Med Sch 1983; **Residency:** Neurology, Johns Hopkins Hosp, Baltimore, MD 1984-1987; **Fellowship:** Neurology, Univ Mich, Ann Arbor, MI 1987-1988; **Faculty Appointment:** Prof Neurology, Univ Mich Med Sch

Fox, Jacob H MD (Neurology) - *Special Expertise:* Alzheimer's Disease; Dementia; **Admitting Hospital:** Rush/Presbyterian - St Luke's Medical Center - Chicago (Page 74); **Office Address:** Rush Presby - St Luke's Med Ctr, Dept Neurology 710 S Paulina St, 8 North JRB Chicago, IL 60612; **Office Phone:** (312) 942-4463; **Board Certification:** Neurology 1974; **Medical School:** Univ IL Coll Med 1967; **Residency:** Neurology, Washington-Barnes Hosp, St Louis, MO 1968-1971

Furlan, Anthony J MD (Neurology) - *Special Expertise:* Stroke; Thrombolytic Therapy-Stroke; **Admitting Hospital:** Cleveland Clinic Foundation; **Office Address:** Cleveland Clinic Fdtn, Dept Neurology 9500 Euclid Ave, Ste S91 Cleveland, OH 44195-0001; **Office Phone:** (216) 444-5535; **Board Certification:** Neurology 1979; **Medical School:** Loyola Univ-Stritch Sch Med 1973; **Residency:** Neurology, Cleveland Clinic, Cleveland, OH 1974-1977; **Fellowship:** Cerebrovascular Disease, Mayo Clinic, Rochester, MN 1977-1978; **Faculty Appointment:** Assoc Prof Neurology, Ohio State Univ

Gilman, Sid MD (Neurology) - *Special Expertise:* Movement & Cognitive Disorders; Alzheimer's Disease; Ataxia; **Admitting Hospital:** University of Michigan Health Center; **Office Address:** Univ Michigan Med Ctr, Dept Neur 1500 E Med Ctr Dr, 1914 Taubman Ctr Ann Arbor, MI 48109-0316; **Office Phone:** (734) 936-9020; **Board Certification:** Neurology 1966; **Medical School:** UCLA 1957; **Residency:** Neurology, Boston City Hosp-Harvard, Boston, MA 1960-1963; **Fellowship:** Neurological Physiology, Boston City Hosp-Harvard, Boston, MA 1963-1965

Goetz, Christopher MD (Neurology) - *Special Expertise:* Movement Disorders; Parkinson's Disease; **Admitting Hospital:** Rush/Presbyterian - St Luke's Medical Center - Chicago (Page 74); **Office Address:** Rush Presby - St Luke's Med Ctr 1725 W Harrison St, Ste 1118 Chicago, IL 60612-3835; **Office Phone:** (312) 942-4500; **Board Certification:** Neurology 1982; **Medical School:** Rush Med Coll 1975; **Residency:** Neurology, Rush Presby-St Luke's Med Ctr, Chicago, IL; **Faculty Appointment:** Assoc Prof Neurology, Rush Med Coll

Greenberg, Harry S. MD (Neurology) - *Special Expertise:* Neuro-Oncology; Brain Tumors; **Admitting Hospital:** University of Michigan Health Center; **Office Address:** Taubman Hlth Care Ctr 1500 E Med Ctr Dr Ann Arbor, MI 48109-0316; **Office Phone:** (734) 936-9055; **Board Certification:** Neurology 1980; **Medical School:** SUNY Syracuse 1973; **Residency:** Neurology, Stanford Hosp, Stanford, CA 1974-1977; **Fellowship:** Medical Oncology, Sloan Kettering Cancer Ctr, New York, NY 1979; **Faculty Appointment:** Prof Neurology, Univ Mich Med Sch

Hubble, Jean Pintar MD (Neurology) - *Special Expertise:* Movement Disorders; Parkinson's Disease; Neuro-Pharmacology; **Admitting Hospital:** Ohio State University Medical Center; **Office Address:** 1581 Dodd, Ste 371 Columbus, OH 43210; **Office Phone:** (614) 688-4048; **Board Certification:** Neurology 1988; **Medical School:** Univ Kans 1983; **Residency:** Neurology, Ohio State Univ, Columbus, OH 1984-1988; **Fellowship:** Neuropharmacology, Ohio State Univ, Columbus, OH 1987-1989; **Faculty Appointment:** Assoc Clin Prof Neurology, Ohio State Univ

Levine, Steven R MD (Neurology) - *Special Expertise:* Stroke; **Admitting Hospital:** Harper Hospital (Page 59); **Office Address:** Waye St Univ Sch Med, Univ Hlth Ctr 4201 St Antoine, Ste 8A Detroit, MI 48201; **Office Phone:** (313) 745-4275; **Board Certification:** Neurology 1986; **Medical School:** Med Coll Wisc 1981; **Residency:** Neurology, Univ Mich Hosp, Ann Arbor, MI 1982-1985; **Fellowship:** Cerebrovascular Disease, Henry Ford Hosp, Detroit, MI 1985-1987; **Faculty Appointment:** Prof Neurology, Wayne State Univ

Lisak, Robert Philip MD (Neurology) - *Special Expertise:* Multiple Sclerosis; Myasthenia Gravis; **Admitting Hospital:** Harper Hospital (Page 59); **Office Address:** Wayne State Univ Sch Med 4201 St Antoine, Hlth Ctr 6E Detroit, MI 48201-2194; **Office Phone:** (313) 745-4275; **Board Certification:** Neurology 1975; **Medical School:** Columbia P&S 1965; **Residencies:** Internal Medicine, Bronx Muni Hosp-Einstein, Bronx, NY 1968-1969; Neurology, Hosp Penn, Philadelphia, PA 1969-1972; **Faculty Appointment:** Prof Neurology, Wayne State Univ

Mahowald, Mark W MD (Neurology) - *Special Expertise:* Sleep Disorders/Apnea; **Admitting Hospital:** Hennepin County Medical Center; **Office Address:** Hennepin Co Med Ctr, Sleep Disorders Ctr 701 Park Ave S Minneapolis, MN 55415-1829; **Office Phone:** (612) 347-6288; **Board Certification:** Neurology 1976; **Medical School:** Univ Minn 1968; **Residency:** Neurology, Univ Minn Hosp, Minneapolis, MN 1971-1974; **Fellowship:** Hennepin Co Med Ctr, Minneapolis, MN 1974-1975; **Faculty Appointment:** Prof Neurology, Univ Minn

Mendell, Jerry R MD (Neurology) - *Special Expertise:* Neuromuscular Disorders; **Admitting Hospital:** Ohio State University Medical Center; **Office Address:** 410 W 10th Ave Columbus, OH 43210; **Office Phone:** (614) 293-4962; **Board Certification:** Neurology 1972; **Medical School:** Univ Tex SW, Dallas 1966; **Residencies:** Neurology, NY Neur Inst, New York, NY 1967-1969; Neurology, Natl Inst Hlth, Bethesda, MD 1969-1970; **Fellowship:** Neurological Muscular Disease, Natl Inst Hlth, Bethesda, MD 1970-1972; **Faculty Appointment:** Prof Neurology, Ohio State Univ

Mesulam, Marek Marsel MD (Neurology) - *Special Expertise:* Alzheimer's Disease; Tourette's Syndrome; Dementia; **Admitting Hospital:** Northwestern Memorial Hospital; **Office Address:** Neuro Behavior & Memory Hlth Service 675 N St Claire, Chicago,, IL 60611; **Office Phone:** (312) 695-9627; **Board Certification:** Neurology 1977; **Medical School:** Harvard Med Sch 1972; **Residency:** Neurology, Boston City Hosp, Boston, MA 1973-1976; **Faculty Appointment:** Prof Harvard Med Sch

Morris, John MD (Neurology) - *Special Expertise:* Alzheimer's Disease; **Admitting Hospital:** Barnes - Jewish Hospital; **Office Address:** Memory Diagnostic Ctr. 4488 Forest Park, Ste 160 St Louis, MO 63108; **Office Phone:** (314) 286-1967; **Board Certifications:** Internal Medicine 1979, Neurology 1985; **Medical School:** Univ Rochester 1974; **Residencies:** Internal Medicine, Akron Genl Med Ctr, Akron, OH 1977-1979; Neurology, Cleveland Metro Genl Hosp, Cleveland, OH 1979-1982; **Fellowship:** Neuropharmacology, Washington Univ, St Louis, MO 1982-1985; **Faculty Appointment:** Prof Neurology, Washington Univ, St Louis

Perlmutter, Joel S MD (Neurology) - *Special Expertise:* Parkinson's Disease; Movement Disorders; **Admitting Hospital:** Barnes - Jewish Hospital; **Office Address:** Washington Univ, Movement Disorders Ctr 660 S Euclid Ave, Box 8111 St Louis, MO 63110; **Office Phone:** (314) 362-6908; **Board Certification:** Neurology 1985; **Medical School:** Univ MO-Columbia Sch Med 1979; **Residency:** Neurology, Banres Hosp-Wash Univ, St Louis, MO 1980-1983; **Fellowship:** Neurology, Barnes Hosp-Wash Univ, St Louis, MO 1983-1984; **Faculty Appointment:** Assoc Prof Neurology, Washington Univ, St Louis

Porth, Karen MD (Neurology) - *Special Expertise:* Muscular Dystrophy; Electromyography; **Admitting Hospital:** Fairview-University Medical Center - University Campus; **Office Address:** 6363 France Ave, Ste 200 Edina, MN 55345; **Office Phone:** (952) 920-7200; **Board Certification:** Neurology 1988; **Medical School:** Univ Cincinnati 1983; **Residency:** Neurology, Univ Chicago, Chicago, IL 1984-1987

Reder, Anthony T MD (Neurology) - *Special Expertise:* Multiple Sclerosis; Dementia; Myasthenia Gravis; **Admitting Hospital:** University of Chicago Hospitals (Page 78); **Office Address:** Center for Advanced Medicine 5758 S Maryland Ave Chicago, IL 60637-1470; **Office Phone:** (773) 702-6204; **Board Certification:** Neurology 1984; **Medical School:** Univ Mich Med Sch 1978; **Residency:** Neurology, Univ Minn Hosps, Minneapolis, MN 1979-1982; **Fellowship:** Neurological Immunology, Univ Chicago, Chicago, IL 1982-1984; **Faculty Appointment:** Assoc Prof Neurology, Univ Chicago-Pritzker Sch Med

Reed, Robert L MD (Neurology) - *Special Expertise:* Multiple Sclerosis; Stroke; **Admitting Hospital:** Good Samaritan Hosp - Cincinnati; **Office Address:** 111 Wellington Pl Cincinnati, OH 45219; **Office Phone:** (513) 241-2370; **Board Certification:** Neurology 1975; **Medical School:** Univ Cincinnati 1966; **Residencies:** Internal Medicine, Mayo Grad Sch Med, Rochester, MN 1969-1970; Neurology, Mayo Grad Sch Med, Rochester, MN 1970-1973

Rogers, Lisa R DO (Neurology) - *Special Expertise:* Neuro-Oncology; **Admitting Hospital:** Henry Ford Health System (Page 62); **Office Address:** 2799 W Grand Blvd Detroit, MI 48202; **Office Phone:** 313 9162648; **Board Certification:** Neurology 1982; **Medical School:** Kirksville Coll Osteo Med 1976; **Residency:** Neurology, Cleveland Clinic Fdn, Cleveland, OH 1977-1980; **Fellowship:** Neurological Oncology, Meml-Sloan Kettering Cancer Ctr, New York, NY 1980-1982

Roos, Raymond MD (Neurology) - *Special Expertise:* Amyotrophic Lateral Sclerosis(ALS); Multiple Sclerosis; **Admitting Hospital:** University of Chicago Hospitals (Page 78); **Office Address:** Univ of Chicago Med Ctr, Dept of Neurology 5841 S Maryland Ave, MC-2030 Chicago, IL 60637; **Office Phone:** (773) 702-6390; **Board Certification:** Neurology 1976; **Medical School:** SUNY Downstate 1968; **Residency:** Neurology, Johns Hopkins Hosp, Baltimore, MD 1971-1974; **Fellowships:** Neurology, Natl Inst of Neuro Dis & Stroke, Bethesda, MD 1969-1971; Neurology, Johns Hospkins Hosp, Baltimore, MD 1974-1976; **Faculty Appointment:** Prof Neurology, Univ Chicago-Pritzker Sch Med

Rubin, Susan MD (Neurology) - *Special Expertise:* Multiple Sclerosis; Parkinson's Disease; Seizure Disorders; **Admitting Hospital:** Advocate Lutheran General Hospital; **Office Address:** Lake Cook Neurological Consultants 8780 W Golf Rd, Ste 202 Niles, IL 60714; **Office Phone:** (847) 298-4590; **Board Certification:** Neurology 1996; **Medical School:** Univ IL Coll Med 1988; **Residency:** Neurology, Northwestern Meml Hosp, Chicago, IL 1990-1993; **Fellowship:** Neurology, Northwestern Meml Hosp, Chicago, IL 1993-1994

Schapiro, Randall MD (Neurology) - *Special Expertise:* Multiple Sclerosis; **Admitting Hospital:** Fairview-University Medical Center - University Campus; **Office Address:** 701 25th Ave S, Ste 200 Minneapolis, MN 55454; **Office Phone:** (612) 672-6100; **Board Certification:** Neurology 1976; **Medical School:** Univ Minn 1970; **Residencies:** Internal Medicine, Wadsworth VA Hosp, Los Angeles, CA 1971-1972; Neurology, Univ Minn Hosp, Minneapolis, MN 1972-1975; **Faculty Appointment:** Clin Prof Neurology, Univ Minn

Siddique, Teepu MD (Neurology) - *Special Expertise:* Amyotrophic Lateral Sclerosis(ALS); Muscular Dystrophy; **Admitting Hospital:** Northwestern Memorial Hospital; **Office Address:** Dept of Neurology 233 E Erie St, Ste 500 Chicago, IL 60611-5935; **Office Phone:** (312) 503-4737; **Board Certification:** Neurology 1980; **Medical School:** Pakistan 1973; **Residency:** Neurology, UMDNJ-RW Johnson Med Sch, Plainfield, NJ 1976-1979; **Fellowships:** Electromyography, Hosp for Special Surg- Cornell MC, New York, NY 1979-1980; Neurological Muscular Disease, Natl Inst Hlth, Bethesda, MD 1980-1981; **Faculty Appointment:** Prof Neurology, Northwestern Univ

Wright, Robert B MD (Neurology) - *Special Expertise:* Myasthenia Gravis; Trigeminal Neuralgia; **Admitting Hospital:** Rush/Presbyterian - St Luke's Medical Center - Chicago (Page 74); **Office Address:** 1725 W Harrison St, Ste 1106 Chicago, IL 60612; **Office Phone:** (312) 942-5936; **Board Certification:** Neurology 1988; **Medical School:** Univ IL Coll Med 1982; **Residency:** Neurology, Rush Presby-St Luke's Med Ctr, Chicago, IL 1983-1986; **Fellowship:** Neurological Muscular Disease, Rush Presby-St Luke's Med Ctr, Chicago, IL 1986-1987

Great Plains and Mountains

Cilo, Mark P MD (Neurology) - *Special Expertise:* Brain Injury; **Admitting Hospital:** Craig Hospital; **Office Address:** Craig Hosp 3425 S Clarkson St Englewood, CO 80110-2811; **Office Phone:** (303) 789-8220; **Board Certification:** Neurology 1979; **Medical School:** Mount Sinai Sch Med 1972; **Residency:** Neurology, Mount Sinai Hosp, New York, NY 1973-1976; **Fellowship:** Spinal Cord & Brain Injury Rehab, Craig Hosp, Englewood, NJ 1977-1978; **Faculty Appointment:** Asst Clin Prof Medicine, Univ Colo

O'Brien, Christopher Flint MD (Neurology) - *Special Expertise:* Movement Disorders; **Admitting Hospital:** Swedish Medical Center - Englewood; **Office Address:** Colo Neuro Inst 701 E Hampden Ave Englewood, CO 80110; **Office Phone:** (303) 788-4600; **Board Certification:** Neurology 1991; **Medical School:** Univ Minn 1985; **Residency:** Neurology, Univ Minn, Minneapolis, MN 1986-1989

Ringel, Steven MD (Neurology) - *Special Expertise:* Neuromuscular Disorders; **Admitting Hospital:** University of Colorado Health & Science Center; **Office Address:** Univ Colo Hlth Scis Ctr, Dept Neur 4200 E Ninth Ave, Box 185 Denver, CO 80262; **Office Phone:** 303 3157221; **Board Certification:** Neurology 1974; **Medical School:** Univ Mich Med Sch 1968; **Residency:** Neurology, Rush-Presby-St Lukes Med Hosp, Denver, CO 1968-1972; **Fellowship:** Neurology, Natl Inst Neuro Disease-NIH, Bethesda, MD 1974-1976; **Faculty Appointment:** Prof Neurology, Univ Colo

Southwest

Carter, John E MD (Neurology) - *Special Expertise:* Neuro-Ophthalmology; **Admitting Hospital:** University of Texas Health & Science Center; **Office Address:** Univ Texas Hlth & Sci Ctr, Dept Med 7703 Floyd Curl Dr San Antonio, TX 78229-3900; **Office Phone:** (210) 567-4615; **Board Certification:** Neurology 1978; **Medical School:** Univ Ark 1969; **Residencies:** Neurology, Boston Univ, Boston, MA 1974-1978; Neurological Ophthalmology, Tufts Univ, Boston, MA 1978-1979; **Faculty Appointment:** Assoc Prof Neurology, Univ Tex, San Antonio

Coull, Bruce MD (Neurology) - *Special Expertise:* Stroke; Cerebrovascular Disease; **Admitting Hospital:** University Medical Center; **Office Address:** 707 N Alvernon, Ste 201 Tuscon, AZ 85711; **Office Phone:** (520) 694-1450; **Board Certification:** Neurology 1979; **Medical School:** Univ Pittsburgh 1972; **Residency:** Neurology, Stanford Univ 1973-1976

Ferrendelli, James A MD (Neurology) - *Special Expertise:* Epilepsy/Seizure Disorders; Neuropharmacology; Geriatric Medicine; **Admitting Hospital:** Memorial Hermann Healthcare System; **Office Address:** Univ Tex-Houston, Dept Neuro 6431 Fannin St, Ste 7044 Houston, TX 77030; **Office Phone:** (713) 500-7100; **Board Certification:** Neurology 1973; **Medical School:** Univ Colo 1962; **Residency:** Neurology, Cleveland Metro Genl Hosp, Cleveland, OH 1965-1968; **Fellowship:** Neuropharmacology, Washington Univ Med Sch, St Louis, MO 1968-1971; **Faculty Appointment:** Prof Neurology, Univ Tex, Houston

Fox, Peter Thornton MD (Neurology) - *Special Expertise:* PET Scans; **Admitting Hospital:** University of Texas Health & Science Center; **Office Address:** Univ Texas Hlth Sci Ctr, Dept Rad 7703 Floyd Curl Dr San Antonio, TX 78229-3900; **Office Phone:** (210) 567-8150; **Board Certification:** Neurology 1985; **Medical School:** Georgetown Univ 1979; **Residency:** Neurology, Washington Univ, St Louis, MO 1980-1983; **Fellowship:** Radiotracer Imaging, Washington Univ, St Louis, MO 1983-1984; **Faculty Appointment:** Prof Neurology, Univ Tex, San Antonio

Garcia, Carlos MD (Neurology) - *Special Expertise:* Muscular Dystrophy; Myasthenia Gravis; **Admitting Hospital:** Tulane University Medical Center Hospital & Clinic; **Office Address:** Tulane Univ Med Ctr 1430 Tulane Ave New Orleans, LA 70112-2699; **Office Phone:** (504) 588-5231; **Board Certifications:** Neuropathology 1974, Neurology 1976; **Medical School:** Colombia 1961; **Residencies:** Pathology, Univ Hosp - Cali, Cali, Colombia 1960-1962; Neurology, Louisiana Med Ctr, New Orleans, LA 1965-1967; **Fellowship:** Neuropathology, Louisiana Med Ctr, New Orleans, LA 1962-1965; **Faculty Appointment:** Prof Neurology, Tulane Univ

Grotta, James MD (Neurology) - *Special Expertise:* Stroke; **Admitting Hospital:** Memorial Hermann Healthcare System; **Office Address:** Univ Tex Med Sch 6410 Fannin St Houston, TX 77030-1501; **Office Phone:** (713) 704-0780; **Board Certification:** Neurology 1978; **Medical School:** Univ VA Sch Med 1971; **Residency:** Neurology, Univ Colorado Hlth Sci Ctr, Denver, CO 1974-1977; **Fellowship:** Diagnostic Radiology, Mass Genl Hosp, Boston, MA 1978-1979; **Faculty Appointment:** Prof Neurology, Univ Tex, Houston

Hart, Robert G. MD (Neurology) - *Special Expertise:* Stroke; **Admitting Hospital:** University of Texas Health & Science Center; **Office Address:** Univ Texas Hlth & Sci Ctr, Dept Neurology 7703 Floyd Curl Dr San Antonio, TX 78229-3900; **Office Phone:** (210) 617-5161; **Board Certification:** Neurology 1985; **Medical School:** Univ MO-Columbia Sch Med 1977; **Residency:** Neurology, Univ Hosp & Clinic, Columbia, MO 1978-1981; **Faculty Appointment:** Prof Neurology, Univ Tex, San Antonio

Infante, Ernesto MD (Neurology) - *Special Expertise:* Amyotrophic Lateral Sclerosis(ALS); Cervical Disc Disease; **Admitting Hospital:** Methodist Hospital - Houston (Page 69); **Office Address:** Diagnostic Clinic of Houston 6448 Fannin, Fl 12 Houston, TX 77030; **Office Phone:** (713) 797-9191; **Board Certification:** Neurology 1973; **Medical School:** Spain 1964; **Residency:** Neurology, Univ Minn Hosps, Minneapolis, MN 1966-1969; **Fellowship:** Electromyography, Mayo Clinic, Rochester, MN 1969-1970; **Faculty Appointment:** Assoc Clin Prof Neurology, Univ Tex, Houston

Jackson, John Kevin MD (Neurology) - *Special Expertise:* Neuro-Psychiatry; Neuro-Behavioral Disorder; **Admitting Hospital:** Tulane University Medical Center Hospital & Clinic; **Office Address:** Tulane Medical Center 1415 Tulane Ave New Orleans, LA; **Office Phone:** (504) 588-5231; **Board Certification:** Neurology; **Medical School:** Tulane Univ 1990; **Residency:** Neurology, Tulane Univ Sch of Med, New Orleans, LA

Jankovic, Joseph MD (Neurology) - *Special Expertise:* Movement Disorders; Parkinson's Disease; Tourette's Syndrome; **Admitting Hospital:** Methodist Hospital - Houston (Page 69); **Office Address:** Baylor Coll Med, Dept Neur, Smith Twr #1801 6550 Fannin St Houston, TX 77030-2717; **Office Phone:** (713) 798-5998; **Board Certification:** Neurology 1979; **Medical School:** Univ Ariz Coll Med 1973; **Residency:** Neurology, Columbia-Presby Med Ctr, New York, NY 1974-1977; **Faculty Appointment:** Prof Neurology, Baylor Coll Med

Knoefel, Janice E MD (Neurology) - *Special Expertise:* Neurology-Geriatric; **Admitting Hospital:** University of New Mexico Hospital; **Office Address:** New Mexico VA Hlth Care Sys 1501 San Pedro Dr SE Albuquerque, NM 87108-5128; **Office Phone:** (505) 256-2795; **Board Certification:** Neurology 1983; **Medical School:** Ohio State Univ 1977; **Residencies:** Internal Medicine, Univ Cinn Med Ctr, Cincinnati, OH 1978-1979; Neurology, Boston Univ Med Ctr, Boston, MA 1979-1982; **Fellowship:** Geriatric Medicine, Boston Univ Med Ctr, Boston, MA 1982-1983; **Faculty Appointment:** Assoc Prof Neurology, Univ New Mexico

NEUROLOGY

Southwest

Levin, Victor Alan MD (Neurology) - *Special Expertise:* Brain Tumors; **Admitting Hospital:** University of Texas MD Anderson Cancer Center (Page 66); **Office Address:** UT MD Anderson Cancer Ctr 1515 Holcombe Blvd, Box 100 Houston, TX 77030-4009; **Office Phone:** (713) 792-8297; **Board Certification:** Neurology 1976; **Medical School:** Univ Wisc 1966; **Residency:** Neurology, Mass Genl Hosp, Boston, MA 1969-1972; **Faculty Appointment:** Prof Neurology, Univ Tex, Houston

Shapiro, William R. MD (Neurology) - *Special Expertise:* Neuro-Oncology; **Admitting Hospital:** St Joseph's Hospital & Medical Center - Phoenix; **Office Address:** Barrow Neurological Group 500 W Thomas Ste 300 Rd Phoenix, AZ 85013; **Office Phone:** (602) 279-7300; **Board Certification:** Neurology 1969; **Medical School:** UCSF 1961; **Residencies:** Internal Medicine, Univ Wash, Seattle, WA 1962-1963; Neurology, NY Hosp-Cornell Med Ctr, New York, NY 1963-1966; **Fellowship:** Neurological Oncology, National Inst Hlth, Bethesda, MD 1966-1969; **Faculty Appointment:** Prof Clinical Neurophysiology, Univ Ariz Coll Med

Sherman, David MD (Neurology) - *Special Expertise:* Cerebrovascular Disease; Stroke; **Admitting Hospital:** University of Texas Health & Science Center; **Office Address:** Univ TX Hlth Scis Ctr, Dept Med 7703 Floyd Curl Dr San Antonio, TX 78229-3900; **Office Phone:** (210) 617-5161; **Board Certification:** Neurology 1976; **Medical School:** Univ Okla Coll Med 1967; **Residencies:** Internal Medicine, Baylor Affil Hosp, Houston, TX 1968-1969; Neurology, UCSD Med Ctr, San Diego, CA 1971-1974; **Faculty Appointment:** Prof Neurology, Univ Tex, San Antonio

Weisberg, Leon MD (Neurology) - *Special Expertise:* Stroke; **Admitting Hospital:** Tulane University Medical Center Hospital & Clinic; **Office Address:** Tulane Medical Center 1415 Tulane Ave New Orleans, LA 70112-2605; **Office Phone:** (504) 588-5231; **Board Certification:** Neurology 1975; **Medical School:** Columbia P&S 1968; **Residency:** Neurology, NY Hosp, New York, NY 1969-1972

Wolinsky, Jerry MD (Neurology) - *Special Expertise:* Multiple Sclerosis; **Admitting Hospital:** Memorial Hermann Healthcare System; **Office Address:** Univ Texas Med Sch 6431 Fannin St, Ste 7044 Houston, TX 77225-0708; **Office Phone:** (715) 500-7135; **Board Certification:** Neurology 1975; **Medical School:** Univ IL Coll Med 1975; **Residency:** Neurology, UCSF, San Francisco, CA 1970-1973; **Fellowship:** Neurology, VA Hosp, San Francisco, CA 1973-1975; **Faculty Appointment:** Prof Neurology, Univ Tex, Houston

West Coast and Pacific

Adornato, Bruce T. MD (Neurology) - *Special Expertise:* Sleep Disorders/Apnea; Neuropathy; Stroke; **Admitting Hospital:** Stanford Medical Center; **Office Address:** 1101 Welch Road, C5 Palo Alto, CA 94304; **Office Phone:** (650) 324-4300; **Board Certifications:** Internal Medicine 1975, Neurology 1978; **Medical School:** UCSD 1972; **Residencies:** Internal Medicine, UCSF-Moffitt Hosp, San Francisco, CA 1973-1974; Neurology, UCSF-Moffitt Hosp, San Francisco, CA 1974-1976; **Fellowship:** Neurology, Natl Inst Hlth, Bethesda, MD 1976-1978; **Faculty Appointment:** Clin Prof Neurology, Stanford Univ

Albers, Gregory William MD (Neurology) - *Special Expertise:* Cerebrovascular Disease; Stroke; **Admitting Hospital:** Stanford Medical Center; **Office Address:** Stanford Stroke Ctr 701 Welch Rd, Ste 325 Palo Alto, CA 94304; **Office Phone:** (650) 723-4448; **Board Certification:** Neurology 1990; **Medical School:** UCSD 1984; **Residency:** Neurology, Standford Univ Med Ctr, Stanford, CA 1984-1988; **Fellowship:** Stroke, Standford Univ Med Ctr, Stanford, CA 1988-1989; **Faculty Appointment:** Assoc Prof Neurology, Stanford Univ

418

Aminoff, Michael J MD (Neurology) - *Special Expertise:* *Neurology - General;* **Admitting Hospital:** University of California - San Francisco Medical Center; **Office Address:** 505 Parnassus Ave, Fl 3 - rm M348 San Francisco, CA 94143; **Office Phone:** (415) 353-1986; **Board Certifications:** Neurology 1982, Clinical Neurophysiology 1992; **Medical School:** England 1965; **Residencies:** Neurology, Middlesex Hosp, London, England 1970-1971; Neurology, Natl Hosp Queen Sq, London, England 1971-1972; **Faculty Appointment:** Prof Neurology, UCSF

Armon, Carmel MD (Neurology) - *Special Expertise:* *Epilepsy/Seizure Disorders; Amyotrophic Lateral Sclerosis(ALS);* **Admitting Hospital:** Loma Linda University Behavioral Medical Center - Redlands; **Office Address:** Loma Linda Univ, Dept Neuro 11370 Anderson St, Ste 2400 Loma Linda, CA 92354; **Office Phone:** (909) 799-5037; **Board Certifications:** Neurology 1990, Clinical Neurophysiology 1992; **Medical School:** Israel 1980; **Residency:** Neurology, Mayo Clinic, Rochester 1984-1988; **Fellowships:** Neurology, Mayo Clinic, Rochester 1988-1989; Clinical Neurophysiology, Duke Univ Med Ctr, Durham, NC 1989-1991; **Faculty Appointment:** Assoc Prof Neurology, Loma Linda Univ

Bourdette, Dennis MD (Neurology) - *Special Expertise:* *Multiple Sclerosis;* **Admitting Hospital:** Oregon Health Science University Hospital and Clinics; **Office Address:** Oregon Health Science Univ Hosp 3181 Sam Jackson Park Rd Portland, OR 97201; **Office Phone:** (503) 494-5759; **Board Certification:** Neurology 1985; **Medical School:** UC Davis 1978; **Residency:** Neurology, Oregon Hlth Sci Univ, Portland, OR 1979-1982; **Fellowship:** Neurological Immunology, VA Med Ctr, Portland, OR 1982-1985; **Faculty Appointment:** Assoc Prof Neurology, Oregon Hlth Scis Univ

Bowen, James MD (Neurology) - *Special Expertise:* *Neurology - General;* **Admitting Hospital:** University of Washington Medical Center; **Office Address:** UWMC - Neurology Clinic 1959 NE Pacific St Seattle, WA 98195; **Office Phone:** (206) 598-7688; **Board Certifications:** Psychiatry 1990, Neurology 1990; **Medical School:** Johns Hopkins Univ 1982; **Residencies:** Internal Medicine, Univ Washington Med Ctr, Seattle, WA 1983-1984; Neurology, Univ Washington Med Ctr, Seattle, WA 1984-1987; **Faculty Appointment:** Asst Prof Neurology, Univ Wash

Chui, Helena Chang MD (Neurology) - *Special Expertise:* *Stroke; Dementia/Alzheimer's;* **Admitting Hospital:** LAC - Rancho Los Amigos Medical Center; **Office Address:** Rancho Los Amigos Med Ctr-JPI Building 7601 E Imperial Hwy, Ste 3 - rm 3135 Downey, CA 90242; **Office Phone:** (562) 401-7713; **Board Certification:** Neurology 1984; **Medical School:** Johns Hopkins Univ 1977; **Residency:** Neurology, Univ Iowa Med Ctr, Iowa City, IA 1979-1981; **Fellowship:** Behavioral Neurology, Univ Iowa Med Ctr, Iowa City, IA 1978-1979; **Faculty Appointment:** Prof Neurology, USC Sch Med

Cloughesy, Timothy Francis MD (Neurology) - *Special Expertise:* *Neuro-Oncology; Seizure Disorders;* **Admitting Hospital:** UCLA Medical Center; **Office Address:** UCLA Neurological Services 300 UCLA Medical Plaza , Ste B200 Los Angeles, CA 90095; **Office Phone:** (310) 825-5321; **Board Certification:** Neurology 1993; **Medical School:** Tulane Univ 1987; **Residency:** Neurology, UCLA, Los Angeles, CA 1986-1991; **Fellowship:** Neurological Oncology, Meml Sloan-Kettering Cancer Ctr, New York, NY 1992; **Faculty Appointment:** Asst Clin Prof Neurology, UCLA

Cummings, Jeffrey Lee MD (Neurology) - *Special Expertise:* *Neuro-Psychiatry; Parkinson's Disease;* **Admitting Hospital:** UCLA Medical Center; **Office Address:** UCLA- Reed Neuro Rsch Ctr 710 Westwood Plaza, rm 2-232 Los Angeles, CA 90095-1769; **Office Phone:** (310) 206-5238; **Board Certification:** Neurology 1979; **Medical School:** Univ Wash 1974; **Residency:** Neurology, Boston, MA 1975-1978; **Fellowship:** Behavioral Neurology & Psychiatry, Boston, MA 1978-1979; **Faculty Appointment:** Assoc Prof Neurology, UCLA

419

Dobkin, Bruce H MD (Neurology) - *Special Expertise:* Stroke; Spinal Cord Injury; **Admitting Hospital:** UCLA Medical Center; **Office Address:** UCLA-RNRC, Dept Neuro 710 Westwood Plaza, Ste 1129 Los Angeles, CA 90095-1769; **Office Phone:** (310) 206-6500; **Board Certification:** Neurology 1979; **Medical School:** Temple Univ 1973; **Residency:** Neurology, UCLA Med Ctr, Los Angeles, CA 1973-1977; **Faculty Appointment:** Prof Neurology, UCLA

Engel, William King MD (Neurology) - *Special Expertise:* Neurology - General; **Admitting Hospital:** Good Samaritan Hospital - Los Angeles; **Office Address:** USC Neuromuscular Ctr-Good Samaritan Hospital 637 S Lucas Ave Los Angeles, CA 90017-1912; **Office Phone:** (213) 743-1612; **Board Certification:** Neurology 1962; **Medical School:** McGill Univ 1955; **Residencies:** Neurology, Natl Inst Hlth, Bethesda, MD 1956-1959; Neurology, Natl Hosp, London, England 1959-1960; **Fellowship:** Neurology, Natl Inst Hlth, Bethesda, MD 1960-1961; **Faculty Appointment:** Prof Neuropathology, USC Sch Med

Engstrom, John Walter MD (Neurology) - *Special Expertise:* Neurology - General; **Admitting Hospital:** University of California - San Francisco Medical Center; **Office Address:** UCSF, Dept of Neurology 400 Parnassus Ave, Bldg ACC - Fl 8 - rm A887, Box 0348, MC-0348 San Francisco, CA 94143-0348; **Office Phone:** (415) 353-2273; **Board Certifications:** Neurology 1991, Clinical Neurophysiology 1992; **Medical School:** Stanford Univ 1981; **Residencies:** Internal Medicine, Johns Hopkins, Baltimore, MD 1981-1984; Neurology, UCSF, San Francisco, CA 1984-1988; **Fellowship:** Neurology, UCSF, San Francisco, CA 1988-1989; **Faculty Appointment:** Assoc Prof Neurology, UCSF

Fisher, Mark MD (Neurology) - *Special Expertise:* Neurology - General; **Admitting Hospital:** University of California - Irvine Medical Center; **Office Address:** UC Irvine Med Ctr, Dept Neuro 101 The City Los Angeles, CA 92868; **Office Phone:** (714) 456-6808; **Board Certification:** Neurology 1981; **Medical School:** Univ Cincinnati 1975; **Residencies:** Neurology, UCLA VA Wadsworth Medical Ctr, Los Angeles, CA 1979-1980; Neurology, UCLA VA Wadsworth Med Ctr, Los Angeles, CA 1976-1979; **Faculty Appointment:** Prof Neurology, UC Irvine

Fisher, Robert MD (Neurology) - *Special Expertise:* Epilepsy/Seizure Disorders; **Admitting Hospital:** Stanford Medical Center; **Office Address:** Stanford Univ Med Ctr, Dept Neuro 300 Pasteur Dr, rm A343 Stanford, CA 94305; **Office Phone:** (650) 498-6648; **Board Certifications:** Neurology 1983, Clinical Neurophysiology 1992; **Medical School:** Stanford Univ 1977; **Residencies:** Internal Medicine, Stanford Univ, Stanford, CA 1977-1979; Neurology, Johns Hopkins, Baltimore, MD 1979-1982

Goodin, Douglas MD (Neurology) - *Special Expertise:* Multiple Sclerosis; **Admitting Hospital:** University of California - San Francisco Medical Center; **Office Address:** University of California, Neurology Dept. M794 San Francisco, CA 94143-0001; **Office Phone:** (415) 476-5459; **Board Certifications:** Neurology 1985, Clinical Neurophysiology 1992; **Medical School:** UC Irvine 1978; **Residency:** Neurology, Univ CA Hosps., San Francisco, CA 1979-1981; **Faculty Appointment:** Assoc Prof Neurology, UCSF

Graves, Michael Clark MD (Neurology) - *Special Expertise:* Amyotrophic Lateral Sclerosis(ALS); **Admitting Hospital:** UCLA Medical Center; **Office Address:** UCLA Med Ctr, Dept Neuro 300 Medical Plaza, Ste B200 Los Angeles, CA 90095; **Office Phone:** (310) 825-7266; **Board Certification:** Neurology 1977; **Medical School:** Stanford Univ 1970; **Residencies:** Internal Medicine, UC San Diego, San Diego, CA 1971-1972; Neurology, Johns Hopkins Hosp, Baltimore, MD 1972-1975; **Fellowship:** Rockefeller Univ Hosp, New York, NY; **Faculty Appointment:** Assoc Prof Neurology, UCLA

Gress, Daryl Ray MD (Neurology) - *Special Expertise:* Critical Care; Stroke; **Admitting Hospital:** University of California - San Francisco Medical Center; **Office Address:** UC San Francisco Med Ctr, Dept Neurology 505 Parnassus Ave, rm 830 San Francisco, CA 94143-0348; **Office Phone:** (415) 476-7489; **Board Certifications:** Neurology 1989, Neurological Surgery; **Medical School:** Washington Univ, St Louis 1982; **Residencies:** Internal Medicine, Johns Hopskins Hosp, Baltimore, MD 1983-1984; Neurology, Mass Genl Hsop, Boston, MA 1984-1987; **Fellowship:** Neurological Surgery, Mass Genl Hosp, Boston, MA 1987-1988; **Faculty Appointment:** Assoc Prof Neurology, UCSF

Hauser, Stephen Lawrence MD (Neurology) - *Special Expertise:* Multiple Sclerosis; **Admitting Hospital:** UCSF - Mount Zion Medical Center; **Office Address:** Multiple Sclerosis Ctr 1701 Divisadeo St, Ste 480 San Francisco, CA 94115-1642; **Office Phone:** (415) 885-7844; **Board Certification:** Neurology 1981; **Medical School:** Harvard Med Sch 1975; **Residencies:** Neurology, Mass Genl Hosp, Boston, MA 1977-1980; Internal Medicine, NY Presby - Cornell, New York, NY 1976-1977; **Fellowship:** Neurology, Harvard, Boston, MA 1977-1980; **Faculty Appointment:** Prof Neurology, UCSF

Langston, J William MD (Neurology) - *Special Expertise:* Parkinson's Disease; Movement Disorders; Tremor; **Admitting Hospital:** *The Parkinson's Institute/Movement Disorders Treament Center; **Office Address:** The Parkinsons Institute 1170 Morse Ave Sunnyvale, CA 94089; **Office Phone:** (408) 734-2800; **Board Certification:** Neurology 1986; **Medical School:** Univ MO-Kansas City 1967; **Residency:** Neurology, Stanford Univ, Stanford, CA 1971-1974; **Fellowship:** Neurological Muscular Disease, Stanford Univ, Stanford, CA 1974

Nutt Jr, John G. MD (Neurology) - *Special Expertise:* Movement Disorders; Parkinson's Disease; **Admitting Hospital:** Oregon Health Science University Hospital and Clinics; **Office Address:** Oregon Hlth Sciences Univ, Dept Neuro 3181 SW Sam Jackson Park Rd, MC-OP-32 Portland, OR 97201-3098; **Office Phone:** (503) 494-7772; **Board Certification:** Neurology 1978; **Medical School:** Baylor Coll Med 1970; **Residency:** Neurology, Univ Wash, Seattle, WA 1973-1976; **Fellowship:** Pharmacology, Nuero Inst Neuro Disorders Stroke, Bethesda, MD 1976-1978 **Faculty Appointment:** Prof Neurology, Oregon Hlth Scis Univ

Olney, Richard Koch MD (Neurology) - *Special Expertise:* Amyotrophic Lateral Sclerosis(ALS); Peripheral Neuropathy; **Admitting Hospital:** University of California - San Francisco Medical Center; **Office Address:** UCSF, Dept Neurology 400 Parnassus Ave, Ste 8, Box 0114 San Francisco, CA 94143-0114; **Office Phone:** (415) 476-4173; **Board Certifications:** Neurology 1980, Clinical Neurophysiology 1994; **Medical School:** Baylor Coll Med 1973; **Residencies:** Psychiatry, UCLA, Los Angeles, CA 1974-1976; Neurology, Oregon Hlth Scis Univ, Portland, OR 1976-1979; **Faculty Appointment:** Prof Neurology, UCSF

Selby, Richard N MD (Neurology) - *Special Expertise:* Neurology - General; **Admitting Hospital:** USC University Hospital - Richard K. Eamer Medical Plaza; **Office Address:** 801 N Tustin Ave, Ste 706 Santa Ana, CA 92705-3611; **Office Phone:** (714) 558-1126; **Board Certification:** Neurology 1975; **Medical School:** SUNY Downstate 1966; **Residency:** Neurology, Mt Sinai Hosp, New York, NY 1967-1970

Seybold, Marjorie MD (Neurology) - *Special Expertise:* Myasthenia Gravis; Neuromuscular Disorders; Neuro-Ophthalmology; **Admitting Hospital:** VA Medical Affairs - San Diego HealthCare Center; **Office Address:** 3350 La Jolla Village Dr., Ste 127, San Diego, CA 92161; **Office Phone:** (858) 552-8585; **Board Certification:** Neurology 1971; **Medical School:** Temple Univ 1965; **Residency:** Neurology, Mayo Grad School, Rochester, MN 1966-1969; **Fellowship:** Neurology, Johns Hopkins Hosp, Baltimore, MD 1970-1971; **Faculty Appointment:** Adjct Prof Neurology, UCSD

Shults, Clifford Walter MD (Neurology) - *Special Expertise:* Parkinson's Disease; Movement Disorders; **Admitting Hospital:** University of California - San Diego Healthcare; **Office Address:** VA Med Ctr-V 127 3350 La Jolla Vlg Drive San Diego, CA 92161; **Office Phone:** (858) 552-8585; **Board Certification:** Neurology 1985; **Medical School:** Univ Tenn Coll Med, Memphis 1977; **Residencies:** Internal Medicine, Univ Calif, San Francisco, CA 1977-1979; Neurology, Albert Einstein Coll Med, Bronx, NY 1979-1982; **Fellowship:** Movement Disorders, Natl Inst Hlth, Bethesda, MD 1982-1985; **Faculty Appointment:** Prof Neurology, UCSD

Smith, Wade S MD/PhD (Neurology) - *Special Expertise:* Stroke; **Admitting Hospital:** University of California - San Francisco Medical Center; **Office Address:** UCSF, Dept Neurology 505 Parnassus Ave, Box 0114 San Francisco, CA 94143; **Office Phone:** (415) 476-7489; **Board Certification:** Neurology 1996; **Medical School:** Univ Wash 1989; **Residency:** Neurology, UCSF-Moffitt Hosp, San Francisco, CA 1990-1993; **Fellowship:** Critical Care Medicine, UCSF-Moffitt Hosp, San Francisco, CA 1993-1994; **Faculty Appointment:** Asst Clin Prof Neurology, UCSF

Spence, Alexander Morton MD (Neurology) - *Special Expertise:* Neuro-Oncology; **Admitting Hospital:** University of Washington Medical Center; **Office Address:** Univ Wash, Dept Neur 1959 NE Pacific St, MS 356465 Seattle, WA 98195; **Office Phone:** (206) 543-2342; **Board Certification:** Neurology 1971; **Medical School:** Univ Chicago-Pritzker Sch Med 1965; **Residencies:** Neurology, Chldns Hosp, Boston, MA 1966-1969; Neuropathology, Stanford Univ Med Ctr, Standford, CA 1971-1974; **Faculty Appointment:** Prof Neurology, Univ Wash

Tanner, Caroline M MD/PhD (Neurology) - *Special Expertise:* Parkinson's Disease; **Admitting Hospital:** *The Parkinson's Institute/Movement Disorders Treament Center; **Office Address:** The Parkinsons Institute 1170 Morse Ave Sunnyvale, CA 94089; **Office Phone:** (408) 734-2800; **Board Certification:** Neurology 1982; **Medical School:** Loyola Univ-Stritch Sch Med 1976; **Residency:** Neurology, Rush-Presby, Chicago, IL 1977-1980; **Fellowship:** Neurological Pharmacology, Rush-Presby, Chicago, IL 1980-1982

Tetrud, James W MD (Neurology) - *Special Expertise:* Movement Disorders; Parkinson's Disease; Tremor; **Admitting Hospital:** *The Parkinson's Institute/Movement Disorders Treament Center; **Office Address:** The Parkinson's Inst 1170 Morse Ave Sunnyvale, CA 94089; **Office Phone:** (408) 734-2800; **Board Certification:** Neurology 1981; **Medical School:** NYU Sch Med 1973; **Residencies:** Internal Medicine, Vet Affairs Med Ctr-West Los Angeles, Los Angeles 1973-1974; Neurology, Vet Affairs Med Ctr-West Los Angeles, Los Angeles 1974-1978

Weiner, Leslie P MD (Neurology) - *Special Expertise:* Multiple Sclerosis; Amyotrophic Lateral Sclerosis(ALS); **Admitting Hospital:** USC University Hospital - Richard K. Eamer Medical Plaza; **Office Address:** USC Sch Med, Dept Neur 1975 Zonal Ave, Bldg KAM - rm 410, MS 9031 Los Angeles, CA 90033; **Office Phone:** (323) 442-3020; **Board Certification:** Neurology 1969; **Medical School:** Univ Cincinnati 1961; **Residencies:** Neurology, Baltimore City Hosp, Baltimore, MD 1962-1963; Neurology, Johns Hopkins Hosp, Baltimore, MD 1963-1965; **Fellowship:** Neurology, Johns Hopkins Univ, Baltimore, MD 1967-1969; **Faculty Appointment:** Prof Neurology, Univ SC Sch Med

NUCLEAR MEDICINE

A nuclear medicine specialist employs the properties of radioactive atoms and molecules in the diagnosis and treatment of disease, and in research. Radiation detection and imaging instrument systems are used to detect disease as it changes the function and metabolism of normal cells, tissues and organs. A wide variety of diseases can be found in this way, usually before the structure of the organ involved by the disease can be seen to be abnormal by any other techniques. Early detection of coronary artery disease (including acute heart attack); early cancer detection and evaluation of the effect of tumor treatment; diagnosis of infection and inflammation anywhere in the body; and early detection of blood clot in the lungs, are all possible with these techniques. Unique forms of radioactive molecules can attack and kill cancer cells (e.g., lymphoma, thyroid cancer) or can relieve the severe pain of cancer that has spread to bone.

The nuclear medicine specialist has special knowledge in the biologic effects of radiation exposure, the fundamentals of the physical sciences and the principles and operation of radiation detection and imaging instrumentation systems.

Training required: Three years

Physician Listings

Nuclear Medicine

Mid Atlantic

Alavi, Abass MD (Nuclear Medicine) - *Special Expertise:* Brain Cancer; Pulmonary Imaging; **Admitting Hospital:** Hospital of the University of Pennsylvania; **Office Address:** Univ of PA Med Ctr, Div of Nuclear Med, Donner Bldg 3400 Spruce St, rm 110 Philadelphia, PA 19104; **Office Phone:** (215) 662-3014; **Board Certifications:** Nuclear Medicine 1973, Internal Medicine 1972; **Medical School:** Iran 1964; **Residencies:** Internal Medicine, Albert Einstein Med Ctr, Philadelphia, PA 1967-1968; Hematology, Univ of PA Hlth Syst, Philadelphia, PA 1969-1970; **Fellowship:** Nuclear Medicine, Hosp of Univ of PA, Philadelphia, PA 1971-1973; **Faculty Appointment:** Prof Radiology, Univ Penn

Carrasquillo, Jorge Amilcar MD (Nuclear Medicine) - *Special Expertise:* Nuclear Medicine - General; **Admitting Hospital:** National Institutes of Health - Clinical Center; **Office Address:** 9000 Rockville Pike #10 Bethesda, MD 20892-0001; **Office Phone:** (301) 496-5675; **Board Certifications:** Nuclear Medicine 1982, Internal Medicine 1977; **Medical School:** Univ Puerto Rico 1974; **Residencies:** Internal Medicine, Univ Dist Hosp, San Juan, Puerto Rico 1976-1977; Nuclear Medicine, Univ Wash Hosp, Seattle, WA 1980-1982

Goldsmith, Stanley J MD (Nuclear Medicine) - *Special Expertise:* Nuclear Medicine - General; **Admitting Hospital:** New York Weill Cornell Medical Center - NY Presbyterian Hospital (Page 72); **Office Address:** 525 E 68th St, Bldg Starr 221 New York, NY 10021; **Office Phone:** (212) 746-4588; **Board Certifications:** Internal Medicine 1969, Nuclear Medicine 1972; **Medical School:** SUNY Downstate 1962; **Residency:** Internal Medicine, Kings Co Hosp, Brooklyn, NY 1965-1967; **Fellowship:** Endocrinology, Diabetes & Metabolism, Mt Sinai Hosp, New York, NY 1967-1968; **Faculty Appointment:** Prof Radiology, Cornell Univ-Weil Med Coll

Larson, Steven MD (Nuclear Medicine) - *Special Expertise:* Thyroid Cancer; PET Imaging; **Admitting Hospital:** Memorial Sloan Kettering Cancer Center; **Office Address:** Meml Sloan Kettering Cancer Ctr 1275 York Ave, Ste S212 New York, NY 10021; **Office Phone:** (212) 639-7373; **Board Certifications:** Nuclear Medicine 1972, Internal Medicine 1973; **Medical School:** Univ Wash 1965; **Residencies:** Internal Medicine, Virginia Mason Hosp, Seattle, WA 1968-1970; Nuclear Medicine, Natl Inst Hlth, Bethesda, MD 1970-1972; **Faculty Appointment:** Prof Nuclear Medicine, Cornell Univ-Weil Med Coll

Majd, Massoud MD (Nuclear Medicine) - *Special Expertise:* Nuclear Medicine-Pediatric; **Admitting Hospital:** Children's National Medical Center - DC; **Office Address:** Chldns Natl Med Ctr 111 Michigan Ave NW Washington, DC 20010-2916; **Office Phone:** (202) 884-5088; **Board Certifications:** Radiology 1972, Nuclear Medicine 1973; **Medical School:** Iran 1960; **Residency:** Radiology, Georgetown Hosp, Washington, DC 1962-1965; **Faculty Appointment:** Prof Radiology, Geo Wash Univ

Neumann, Ronald D MD (Nuclear Medicine) - *Special Expertise:* Nuclear Medicine - General; **Admitting Hospital:** National Institutes of Health - Clinical Center; **Office Address:** Natl Inst Hlth Clin Ctr, Dept NuM, Bldg 10 - rm 1C-453 10 Center Dr, MSC 1180 Bethesda, MD 20892-1180; **Office Phone:** (301) 496-6455; **Board Certification:** Nuclear Medicine 1979; **Medical School:** Yale Univ 1974; **Residencies:** Pathology, Yale-New Haven Hosp, New Haven, CT 1974-1977; Nuclear Medicine, Yale-New Haven Hosp, New Haven, CT 1977-1979

Strashun, Arnold M MD (Nuclear Medicine) - *Special Expertise:* Neurologic Imaging; Nuclear Cardiology; **Admitting Hospital:** University Hospital - Brooklyn; **Office Address:** 450 Clarkson Ave, Fl 2nd Brooklyn, NY 11203; **Office Phone:** (718) 245-3692; **Board Certifications:** Internal Medicine 1977, Nuclear Medicine 1979; **Medical School:** Baylor Coll Med 1974; **Residencies:** Internal Medicine, Baylor Med Ctr, Dallas, TX 1974-1975; Internal Medicine, Texas Med, Houston, TX 1975- 1977; **Fellowships:** Nuclear Medicine, VA Med Ctr/NYU/Bellevue, Bronx, NY; Nuclear Medicine, Mount Sinai, New York, NY; **Faculty Appointment:** Prof Radiology, SUNY Downstate

Van Heertum, Ronald Lanny MD (Nuclear Medicine) - *Special Expertise:* Nuclear Medicine - General; **Admitting Hospital:** Columbia Presbyterian Medical Center (Page 72); **Office Address:** Columbia Presby Med Ctr, Dept Rad 177 Fort Washington Ave, rm MHB2131 New York, NY 10032; **Office Phone:** (212) 305-7132; **Board Certifications:** Radiology 1971, Nuclear Medicine 1973; **Medical School:** UMDNJ-NJ Med Sch, Newark 1966; **Residency:** Radiology, St Vincents Hosp Med Ctr, New York, NY 1967-1970; **Fellowships:** Neuroradiology, St Vincents Hosp Med Ctr, New York, NY 1970-1971; Nuclear Medicine, SUNY-Upstate Med Ctr, Syracuse, NY 1974-1975; **Faculty Appointment:** Prof Radiology, Columbia P&S

Southeast

Alazraki, Naomi Parver MD (Nuclear Medicine) - *Special Expertise:* Nuclear Oncology; **Admitting Hospital:** Emory University Hospital; **Office Address:** VAMC Atlanta 1670 Clairmont Rd Decatur, GA 30033; **Office Phone:** (404) 728-7629; **Board Certifications:** Nuclear Medicine 1972, Diagnostic Radiology 1972; **Medical School:** Albert Einstein Coll Med 1966; **Residency:** Radiology, Univ Hospital, San Diego, CA 1968-1971; **Faculty Appointment:** Prof Radiology, Emory Univ

Coleman, Ralph Edward MD (Nuclear Medicine) - *Special Expertise:* PET Imaging; Tumors; **Admitting Hospital:** Duke University Medical Center (Page 60); **Office Address:** Duke Univ Med Ctr Erwin Rd, Box 3949 Durham, NC 27710; **Office Phone:** (919) 684-7244; **Board Certifications:** Nuclear Medicine 1974, Internal Medicine 1973; **Medical School:** Washington Univ, St Louis 1968; **Residency:** Internal Medicine, Royal Victoria, Montreal, Canada 1969-1970; **Fellowship:** Nuclear Medicine, Mallinckrodt Institute of Radiology, St Louis, MO 1972-1974; **Faculty Appointment:** Prof Radiology, Duke Univ

Dubovsky, Eva V MD/PhD (Nuclear Medicine) - *Special Expertise:* Renal Nuclear Medicine; Thyroid Disease; **Admitting Hospital:** University of Alabama Hospital at Birmingham; **Office Address:** Univ Ala Hosp, Div NuM 619 19th St S Birmingham, AL 35233; **Office Phone:** (205) 934-2140; **Board Certification:** Nuclear Medicine 1973; **Medical School:** Czech Republic 1957; **Residencies:** Internal Medicine, Univ Hosp-Charles Univ, Prague, Czech Republic 1957-1963; Nuclear Medicine, VA Med Ctr, Birmingham, AL 1970-1972; **Fellowships:** Endocrinology, Diabetes & Metabolism, Univ Hosp-Charles Univ, Prague, Czech Republic 1963-1965; Endocrinology, Diabetes & Metabolism, Univ Hosp-Univ Ala Sch Med, Birmingham, AL 1968-1970; **Faculty Appointment:** Prof Radiology, Univ Ala

Partain, Clarence Leon MD (Nuclear Medicine) - *Special Expertise:* MRI; Nuclear Radiology; **Admitting Hospital:** Vanderbilt University Medical Center; **Office Address:** Vanderbilt University Med Ctr Rad Dept Rm RR1223 MCN Nashville, TN 37232-2675; **Office Phone:** (615) 343-3588; **Board Certifications:** Nuclear Medicine 1979, Diagnostic Radiology 1980; **Medical School:** Washington Univ, St Louis 1975; **Residencies:** Diagnostic Radiology, Univ North Carolina, Chapel Hill, NC 1975-1979; Nuclear Medicine, Univ North Carolina, Chapel Hill, NC 1975-1979; **Faculty Appointment:** Prof Radiology, Vanderbilt Univ

Sandler, Martin P MD (Nuclear Medicine) - *Special Expertise: Nuclear Endocrinology; Cardiac Imaging;* **Admitting Hospital:** Vanderbilt University Medical Center; **Office Address:** Vanderbilt Univ Med Ctr, Dept Rad & Rad Scis 1161 21st Ave S Nashville, TN 37232; **Office Phone:** (615) 343-3585; **Board Certification:** Nuclear Medicine 1983; **Medical School:** South Africa 1972; **Residency:** Groote Schur Hosp, Cape Town, Johannesburg; **Fellowships:** Endocrinology, Diabetes & Metabolism, Vanderbilt Univ, Nashville, TN; Nuclear Medicine, Vanderbilt Univ, Nashville, TN; **Faculty Appointment:** Prof Radiology, Vanderbilt Univ

Midwest

Siegel, Barry MD (Nuclear Medicine) - *Special Expertise: Cancer Detection & Staging; PET Imaging;* **Admitting Hospital:** Barnes - Jewish Hospital; **Office Address:** Mallinckrodt Inst of Rad 510 S Kingshighway Blvd, West Pavilion St Louis, MO 63110-1016; **Office Phone:** (314) 362-2809; **Board Certifications:** Diagnostic Radiology 1977, Nuclear Medicine 1973; **Medical School:** Washington Univ, St Louis 1969; **Residency:** Diagnostic Radiology, Mallinckrodt Inst of Rad, St Louis, MO 1970-1973; **Fellowship:** Nuclear Medicine, Mallinckrodt Inst of Rad, St Louis, MO 1973; **Faculty Appointment:** Prof Radiology, Washington Univ, St Louis

Wahl, Richard MD (Nuclear Medicine) - *Special Expertise: Radioimmunotherapy of Cancer; Positron Emission Tomography (PET) scans;* **Admitting Hospital:** University of Michigan Health Center; **Office Address:** Univ MI Med Ctr, Dept of Rad, Div Nucl Med 1500 E Medical Center Dr, rm B1G50, Box 0028 Ann Arbor, MI 48109-0028; **Office Phone:** (734) 936-5384; **Board Certifications:** Nuclear Medicine 1985, Diagnostic Radiology 1982; **Medical School:** Washington Univ, St Louis 1978; **Residency:** Diagnostic Radiology, Mallinckrodt Inst., St. Louis, MO 1979-1982; **Fellowship:** Nuclear Radiology, Mallinckrodt Inst., St. Louis, MO 1982-1983; **Faculty Appointment:** Prof Radiology, Univ Mich Med Sch

Southwest

Podoloff, Donald MD (Nuclear Medicine) - *Special Expertise: Prostate Cancer; Breast Cancer;* **Admitting Hospital:** University of Texas MD Anderson Cancer Center (Page 66); **Office Address:** UT MD Anderson Cancer Ctr 1515 Holcombe Blvd, Box 83 Houston, TX 77030; **Office Phone:** (713) 792-6535; **Board Certifications:** Diagnostic Radiology 1973, Nuclear Medicine 1975; **Medical School:** SUNY Downstate 1964; **Residencies:** Internal Medicine, Beth Israel Med Ctr, New York, NY 1965-1968; Radiology, Wilford Hall USAF Med Ctr, Lackland AFB, TX 1970-1973; **Faculty Appointment:** Prof Nuclear Radiology, Univ Tex, Houston

West Coast and Pacific

Scheff, Alice M MD (Nuclear Medicine) - *Special Expertise: Breast Imaging; Thyroid Imaging; Neurologic Imaging;* **Admitting Hospital:** Santa Clara Valley Medical Center; **Office Address:** Santa Clara Valley Med Ctr 751 S Bascom Ave San Jose, CA 95128; **Office Phone:** (408) 885-6970; **Board Certifications:** Nuclear Medicine 1982, Nuclear Radiology 1983; **Medical School:** Penn State Univ-Hershey Med Ctr 1978; **Residencies:** Diagnostic Radiology, Penn State-Hershey Med Ctr, Hershey, PA 1978-1982; Nuclear Medicine, Penn State-Hershey Med Ctr, Hershey, PA 1978-1982; **Fellowship:** Magnetic Resonance Imaging, Long Beach Meml Med Ctr, Long Beach, CA 1993

NUCLEAR MEDICINE

Schelbert, Heinrich R MD/PhD (Nuclear Medicine) - *Special Expertise:* Cardiology;
Admitting Hospital: UCLA Medical Center; **Office Address:** UCLA Sch Med , Dept Molecular &
Med Pharm 23-148 CHS Los Angeles, CA 90095-1735; **Office Phone:** (310) 825-3076; **Board
Certification:** Nuclear Medicine 1976; **Medical School:** Germany 1964; **Residencies:** Internal
Medicine, Mercy Med Ctr, Philadelphia, PA 1967-1968; Cardiology (Cardiovascular Disease),
Univ of Duesseldorf Sch of Med, Germany 1971-1972; **Fellowships:** Nuclear Medicine, UC San
Diego Sch of Med, San Diego, CA 1972-1973; Cardiology (Cardiovascular Disease), UC San
Diego Sch of Med, San Diego, CA 1968-1969; **Faculty Appointment:** Prof Radiology, UCLA

Strauss, H William MD (Nuclear Medicine) - *Special Expertise:* Nuclear Medicine - General;
Admitting Hospital: Stanford Medical Center; **Office Address:** Stanford Univ Sch Med, Div Nuc
Med 300 Pasteur Drive, rm H-010, MS 5281 Stanford, CA 94305; **Office Phone:** (650) 725-7441;
Board Certification: Nuclear Medicine 1972; **Medical School:** SUNY Downstate 1965;
Residencies: Internal Medicine, Downstate Med Ctr, Brooklyn, NY 1966-1967; Internal Medicine,
Bellevue Hosp, New York, NY 1967-1968; **Fellowship:** Nuclear Medicine, Johns Hopkins Hosp,
Baltimore, MD 1968-1970; **Faculty Appointment:** Prof Radiology, Stanford Univ

Waxman, Alan D MD (Nuclear Medicine) - *Special Expertise:* Nuclear Medicine - General;
Admitting Hospital: Cedars-Sinai Medical Center; **Office Address:** Cedars-Sinai Med Ctr 8700
Beverly Blvd, rm A041 Los Angeles, CA 90048-1804; **Office Phone:** (310) 423-4216; **Board
Certification:** Nuclear Medicine 1972; **Medical School:** USC Sch Med 1963; **Residency:** Nuclear
Medicine, Wadsworth VA Hosp, Los Angeles, CA 1964-1965; **Fellowship:** Internal Medicine, Natl
Inst Hlth, Bethesda, MD 1965-1967; **Faculty Appointment:** Clin Prof Radiology, USC Sch Med

OBSTETRICS & GYNECOLOGY

An obstetrician/gynecologist possesses special knowledge, skills and professional capability in the medical and surgical care of the female reproductive system and associated disorders. This physician serves as a consultant to other physicians and as a primary physician for women.

Training required: Four years *plus* two years in clinical practice before certification is complete

PHYSICIAN LISTINGS

Obstetrics & Gynecology

New England

Hunt, Robert Bridger MD (Obstetrics & Gynecology) - *Special Expertise:* Pelvic Reconstruction; **Admitting Hospital:** New England Baptist Hospital (Page 57); **Office Address:** 319 Longwood Ave Boston, MA 02115-5728; **Office Phone:** (617) 731-6111; **Board Certification:** Obstetrics & Gynecology 1975; **Medical School:** Med Univ SC 1964; **Residencies:** Obstetrics & Gynecology, Brigham & Womens Hosp, Boston, MA 1969-1971; Surgery, Mary Imogene Bassett Hosp, Cooperstown, NY 1967-1968; **Faculty Appointment:** Clin Inst Obstetrics & Gynecology, Harvard Med Sch

Jackson, Neil MD (Obstetrics & Gynecology) - *Special Expertise:* Uro-Gynecology; **Admitting Hospital:** Women & Infants Hospital - Rhode Island; **Office Address:** Center for Womens Surg.-Dir. Uro-Gyn 100 Dudley St Providence, RI 02905-3233; **Office Phone:** (401) 453-7560; **Board Certification:** Obstetrics & Gynecology 1972; **Medical School:** Boston Univ 1962; **Residency:** Natl Naval Med Ctr, Bethesda, MD 1966-1969; **Faculty Appointment:** Clin Prof Obstetrics & Gynecology, Brown Univ

Naftolin, Frederick MD (Obstetrics & Gynecology) - *Special Expertise:* Neuro-Endocrinology; Reproductive Endocrinology; **Admitting Hospital:** Yale - New Haven Hospital; **Office Address:** 20 York St, rm 335FMB New Haven, CT 06504; **Office Phone:** (203) 785-4003; **Board Certification:** Obstetrics & Gynecology 1972; **Medical School:** UCSF 1961; **Residency:** Obstetrics & Gynecology, UCLA, Los Angeles, CA 1962-1966; **Fellowships:** Reproductive Endocrinology, Univ Wash, Seattle, WA 1966-1968; Obstetrics & Gynecology, UCLA, Los Angeles, CA 1968-1970; **Faculty Appointment:** Prof Obstetrics & Gynecology, Yale Univ

Reilly, Raymond J MD (Obstetrics & Gynecology) - *Special Expertise:* Gynecologic Surgery; **Admitting Hospital:** Brigham & Women's Hospital; **Office Address:** New England OB/GYN Assocs One Brookline Pl, Ste 522 Brookline, MA 02440; **Office Phone:** (617) 731-3400; **Board Certification:** Obstetrics & Gynecology 1969; **Medical School:** Ireland 1958; **Residency:** Obstetrics & Gynecology, Johns Hopkins Hosp., Baltimore, MD 1962-1964; **Faculty Appointment:** Assoc Prof Obstetrics & Gynecology, Harvard Med Sch

Mid Atlantic

Amstey, Marvin S. MD (Obstetrics & Gynecology) - *Special Expertise:* Infectious Disease in Pregnancy; Vulva Disease/Neoplasia; **Admitting Hospital:** Via Health System-Genesee Hospital; **Office Address:** 220 Alexander St, Ste 604 Rochester, NY 14607; **Office Phone:** (716) 922-8390; **Board Certification:** Obstetrics & Gynecology 1989; **Medical School:** Duke Univ 1964; **Residency:** Internal Medicine, Strong Meml Hosp, Rochester, NY 1967-1971; **Fellowship:** Virology, Natl Inst of Hlth, Bethesda, MD 1965-1967; **Faculty Appointment:** Prof Emeritus Obstetrics & Gynecology, Univ Rochester

Baxi, Laxmi V MD (Obstetrics & Gynecology) - *Special Expertise:* Pregnancy-High Risk; Miscarriage-Recurrent; Multiple Gestation; **Admitting Hospital:** Columbia Presbyterian Medical Center (Page 72); **Office Address:** Columbia Presby Med Ctr, Dept OB/GYN 161 Ft Washington Ave, Fl 3 - Ste 336 New York, NY 10032-3713; **Office Phone:** (212) 305-5899; **Board Certifications:** Obstetrics & Gynecology 1995, Maternal & Fetal Medicine 1997; **Medical School:** India 1962; **Residencies:** Obstetrics & Gynecology, Bombay, India 1963-1969; Obstetrics & Gynecology, St Peter's Med Ctr-Rutgers Univ NJ, New Brunswick, NJ 1976-1977; **Fellowship:** Maternal & Fetal Medicine, Columbia-Presbyterian Med Ctr, New York, NY 1977-1979; **Faculty Appointment:** Prof Obstetrics & Gynecology, Columbia P&S

Berkowitz, Richard MD (Obstetrics & Gynecology) - *Special Expertise: Obstetrics & Gynecology - General;* **Admitting Hospital:** Mount Sinai Hospital (Page 70); **Office Address:** 5 E 98th St, Fl 2 New York, NY 10029; **Office Phone:** (212) 241-5681; **Board Certifications:** Obstetrics & Gynecology 1974, Maternal & Fetal Medicine 1979; **Medical School:** NYU Sch Med 1965; **Residency:** Obstetrics & Gynecology, NY Hosp-Cornell Univ, New York, NY 1968-1972; **Faculty Appointment:** Prof Obstetrics & Gynecology, Mount Sinai Sch Med

Boyce, John G MD (Obstetrics & Gynecology) - *Special Expertise: Gynecologic Cancer;* **Admitting Hospital:** University Hospital - Brooklyn; **Office Address:** 450 Clarkson Ave, Box 24 Brooklyn, NY 11203; **Office Phone:** (718) 270-2081; **Board Certifications:** Obstetrics & Gynecology 1969, Gynecologic Oncology 1974; **Medical School:** Univ British Columbia Fac Med 1962; **Residency:** Obstetrics & Gynecology, Kings Co Hosp, Brooklyn, NY 1963-1967; **Fellowship:** Gynecologic Oncology, Kings Co Hosp, Brooklyn, NY 1967-1969; **Faculty Appointment:** Prof Obstetrics & Gynecology, SUNY Hlth Sci Ctr

Cundiff, Geoffrey Williams DO (Obstetrics & Gynecology) - *Special Expertise: Pelvic Reconstruction;* **Admitting Hospital:** Johns Hopkins Hospital - Baltimore (Page 65); **Office Address:** 600 N Wolfe, Bldg Harve - rm 319 Baltimore, MD 21287; **Office Phone:** (410) 614-2870; **Board Certification:** Obstetrics & Gynecology 1996; **Medical School:** Univ Tex SW, Dallas 1989; **Residency:** Obstetrics & Gynecology, Parkland Memorial Hospital/ Univ Tex SW Med Ctr, Dallas, TX 1990-1993; **Fellowships:** Reconstructive Pelvic Surgery, Duke Med Ctr, Durham, NC 1994-1995; Urogynecology, Greater Baltimore Medical Center, Baltimore, MD 1993-1994; **Faculty Appointment:** Asst Prof Duke Univ

Divon, Michael Y MD (Obstetrics & Gynecology) - *Special Expertise: Maternal & Fetal Medicine; Pregnancy-High Risk;* **Admitting Hospital:** Lenox Hill Hospital; **Office Address:** Lenox Hill Hosp, Dept OB/GYN 130 E 77th St, Bldg Black Hall - Fl 2 New York, NY 10021; **Office Phone:** (212) 434-2160; **Board Certification:** Obstetrics & Gynecology 1993; **Medical School:** Israel 1982; **Residency:** Obstetrics & Gynecology, Rambam Med Ctr, Israel 1979-1983; **Fellowships:** Perinatal Medicine, USC, Los Angeles, CA 1983-1985; Perinatal Medicine, Albert Einstein, Bronx, NY 1987-1989; **Faculty Appointment:** Clin Prof Maternal & Fetal Medicine, Albert Einstein Coll Med

Ledger, William MD (Obstetrics & Gynecology) - *Special Expertise: AIDS/HIV in Pregnancy; Infectious Disease in Pregnancy;* **Admitting Hospital:** New York Weill Cornell Medical Center - NY Presbyterian Hospital (Page 72); **Office Address:** New York Weil Cornell Med Ctr 525 E 68th St, Bldg J130 New York, NY 10021; **Office Phone:** (212) 746-3009; **Board Certification:** Obstetrics & Gynecology 1967; **Medical School:** Univ Penn 1958; **Residency:** Obstetrics & Gynecology, Temple Univ Hosp, Philadelphia, PA 1961-1964; **Faculty Appointment:** Prof Obstetrics & Gynecology, Cornell Univ-Weil Med Coll

Minkoff, Howard L MD (Obstetrics & Gynecology) - *Special Expertise: AIDS/HIV in Pregnancy;* **Admitting Hospital:** Maimonides Medical Center (Page 67); **Office Address:** Maimonides Med Ctr 4802 Tenth Ave Brooklyn, NY 11219; **Office Phone:** (718) 283-7048; **Board Certifications:** Obstetrics & Gynecology 1995, Maternal & Fetal Medicine 1983; **Medical School:** Penn State Univ-Hershey Med Ctr 1975; **Residencies:** Obstetrics & Gynecology, Kings Co Hosp Ctr, Brooklyn, NY 1976-1979; Obstetrics & Gynecology, SUNY Hlth Sci Ctr, Brooklyn, NY 1979-1981; **Fellowship:** Maternal & Fetal Medicine, Kings Co Hosp Ctr, Brooklyn, NY 1979-1981; **Faculty Appointment:** Prof Obstetrics & Gynecology, SUNY Hlth Sci Ctr

Sanz, Luis E MD (Obstetrics & Gynecology) - *Special Expertise:* Uro-Gynecology; Hysteroscopic Surgery; Laparoscopic Surgery; **Admitting Hospital:** Georgetown University Hospital; **Office Address:** GUMC - Pasquerilla Healthcare Ctr, 3rd Floor 3800 Reservoir Rd NW Washington, DC 20007; **Office Phone:** (301) 652-7679; **Board Certification:** Obstetrics & Gynecology 1982; **Medical School:** Georgetown Univ 1976; **Residency:** Obstetrics & Gynecology, Georgetown Univ, Washington, DC 1977-1980; **Fellowship:** Advanced Pelvic Surgery, Georgetown Univ, Washington, DC 1980-1982; **Faculty Appointment:** Prof Obstetrics & Gynecology, Georgetown Univ

Scialli, Anthony R MD (Obstetrics & Gynecology) - *Special Expertise:* Reproductive Toxicology; Menopause Problems; Bone Densitometry; **Admitting Hospital:** Georgetown University Hospital; **Office Address:** Georetown Univ Med Ctr - Pasquerilla Hlthcare Ctr 3800 Reservoir Rd NW, Fl 3 Washington, DC 20007; **Office Phone:** (202) 687-8531; **Board Certification:** Obstetrics & Gynecology 1981; **Medical School:** Albany Med Coll 1975; **Residency:** Obstetrics & Gynecology, Geo Wash Univ Hosp, Washington, DC 1975-1979; **Fellowship:** Reproductive Medicine, Repro Toxic Ctr, Washington, DC 1982-1984; **Faculty Appointment:** Prof Obstetrics & Gynecology, Georgetown Univ

Sweet, Richard Lance MD (Obstetrics & Gynecology) - *Special Expertise:* Sexually Transmitted Diseases; **Admitting Hospital:** UPMC - Presbyterian University Hospital; **Office Address:** Magee-Women's Hosp 300 Halket St Pittsburgh, PA 15213; **Office Phone:** (412) 641-4200; **Board Certification:** Obstetrics & Gynecology 1975; **Medical School:** Univ Mich Med Sch 1966; **Residency:** Obstetrics & Gynecology, Univ Mich, Ann Arbor 1969-1973; **Faculty Appointment:** Prof Obstetrics & Gynecology

Witter, Frank Robert MD (Obstetrics & Gynecology) - *Special Expertise:* Pregnancy-High Risk; Multiple Gestation; **Admitting Hospital:** Johns Hopkins Hospital - Baltimore (Page 65); **Office Address:** Johns Hopkins Univ Sch Med 600 N Wolfe St Baltimore, MD 21205; **Office Phone:** (410) 955-6700; **Board Certifications:** Maternal & Fetal Medicine 1987, Obstetrics & Gynecology 1985; **Medical School:** Univ Chicago-Pritzker Sch Med 1976; **Residency:** Obstetrics & Gynecology, Johns Hopkins Hosp, Baltimore, MD 1977-1980; **Fellowships:** Clinical Pharmacology, Johns Hopkins Hosp, Baltimore, MD 1982-1984; Maternal & Fetal Medicine, Johns Hopkins Hosp, Baltimore, MD 1980-1982; **Faculty Appointment:** Assoc Prof Obstetrics & Gynecology, Johns Hopkins Univ

Wylen, Michele MD (Obstetrics & Gynecology) - *Special Expertise:* Gynecology-Adolescent; Menopause Problems; **Admitting Hospital:** Georgetown University Hospital; **Office Address:** Georetown Univ Med Ctr - Pasquerilla Hlthcare Ctr, 3rd Floor 3800 Reservoir Rd NW Washington, DC 20007; **Office Phone:** (202) 687-8531; **Board Certification:** Obstetrics & Gynecology 1999; **Medical School:** Georgetown Univ 1988; **Residency:** Obstetrics & Gynecology, Georgetown Univ, Washington, DC 1990-1992

Southeast

Duff, W Patrick MD (Obstetrics & Gynecology) - *Special Expertise:* Pregnancy-High Risk; Infectious Disease in Pregnancy; **Admitting Hospital:** Shands Healthcare at University Florida (Page 77); **Office Address:** Park Avenue Clinic 807 NW 57th St Gainesville, FL 32605; **Office Phone:** (352) 392-6200; **Board Certifications:** Obstetrics & Gynecology 1999, Maternal & Fetal Medicine 1999; **Medical School:** Georgetown Univ 1974; **Residency:** Obstetrics & Gynecology, Walter Reed Med Ctr, Washington, DC 1974-1978; **Fellowship:** Maternal & Fetal Medicine, UT - San Antonio, San Antonio, TX 1981-1983; **Faculty Appointment:** Prof Obstetrics & Gynecology, Univ S Fla Coll Med

Filip, Stanley John MD (Obstetrics & Gynecology) - *Special Expertise:* Obstetrics & Gynecology - General; **Admitting Hospital:** Duke University Medical Center (Page 60); **Office Address:** Duke Univ Med Ctr Box 3840 Durham, NC 27710; **Office Phone:** (919) 684-9696; **Board Certification:** Obstetrics & Gynecology 1985; **Medical School:** Mount Sinai Sch Med 1979; **Residency:** Obstetrics & Gynecology, Univ Colo Hlth Scis Ctr, Denver, CO 1980-1983

Gluck, Paul MD (Obstetrics & Gynecology) - *Special Expertise:* Gynecology; **Admitting Hospital:** Baptist Hospital - Miami; **Office Address:** Salkind Gluck & Chavoustie 8950 N Kendall Dr, Ste 507 Miami, FL 33176-2132; **Office Phone:** (305) 279-3773; **Board Certification:** Obstetrics & Gynecology 1978; **Medical School:** NYU Sch Med 1972; **Residency:** Obstetrics & Gynecology, Univ of Miami Jackson Meml Hosp, Miami, FL 1972-1976; **Faculty Appointment:** Assoc Clin Prof Obstetrics & Gynecology, Univ Miami Sch Med

Hager, William David MD (Obstetrics & Gynecology) - *Special Expertise:* Yeast Infection-Chronic; Salpingitis; Infectious Disease; **Admitting Hospital:** University of Kentucky Medical Center; **Office Address:** Womens Care Ctr. 2620 Wilhite Lexington, KY 40503-3385; **Office Phone:** (606) 278-0363; **Board Certification:** Obstetrics & Gynecology 1993; **Medical School:** Univ KY Coll Med 1972; **Residency:** Obstetrics & Gynecology, KY Med Ctr - Univ Hosp, Lexingtin, KY 1976; **Faculty Appointment:** Prof Obstetrics & Gynecology, Univ KY Coll Med

McLeod, Allan G W MD (Obstetrics & Gynecology) - *Special Expertise:* Pelvic Reconstruction; Pelvic Prolapse Repair; **Admitting Hospital:** University of Miami - Jackson Memorial Hospital; **Office Address:** 1611 NW 12th Ave, Bldg Holtz - rm 7007 Miami, FL 33136; **Office Phone:** (305) 585-5160; **Board Certification:** Obstetrics & Gynecology 1981; **Medical School:** Scotland 1952; **Residencies:** Obstetrics & Gynecology, Western Hosp, Doncaster, England 1956-1957; Obstetrics & Gynecology, Southern Genl Hosp, Glasgow, Scotland 1957-1959; **Faculty Appointment:** Prof Obstetrics & Gynecology, Univ Miami Sch Med

Morgan, Linda S MD (Obstetrics & Gynecology) - *Special Expertise:* Gynecologic Cancer; **Admitting Hospital:** Shands Healthcare at University Florida (Page 77); **Office Address:** Univ Florida, Dept of OB, MS 0 PO Box 100294 Gainesville, FL 32610; **Office Phone:** (352) 392-2893; **Board Certifications:** Obstetrics & Gynecology 1982, Gynecologic Oncology 1983; **Medical School:** Med Coll PA Hahnemann 1975; **Residency:** Obstetrics & Gynecology, Shands Hosp, Gainesville, FL 1975-1979; **Fellowship:** Gynecologic Oncology, Mass Genl Hosp, Boston, MA 1979-1981; **Faculty Appointment:** Prof Obstetrics & Gynecology, Univ Fla Coll Med

Nahmias, Jaime Pablo MD (Obstetrics & Gynecology) - *Special Expertise:* Reproductive Endocrinology; Infertility-Female; **Admitting Hospital:** University of Miami Hosp & Clinics/Sylvestor Comp Cancer Cntr; **Office Address:** Univ of Miami Med Group, Dept of OB/GYN 1611 NW 12th Ave Maimi, FL 33136; **Office Phone:** (305) 585-5160; **Board Certification:** Obstetrics & Gynecology 1996; **Medical School:** Chile 1978; **Residency:** Obstetrics & Gynecology, Jackson Meml Hosp Univ Miami, Miami, Fl 1986-1988; **Fellowship:** Reproductive Endocrinology, Jackson Meml Hosp Univ Miami, Miami, Fl 1991-1994; **Faculty Appointment:** Asst Prof Obstetrics & Gynecology, Univ Miami Sch Med

Steege, John Francis MD (Obstetrics & Gynecology) - *Special Expertise:* Laparoscopic Surgery (Advanced); Gynecologic Surgery-Benign; **Admitting Hospital:** University of North Carolina Hospitals; **Office Address:** Univ NC Chapel Hill, Dept OB/GYN MacNider CB 7570 Chapel Hill, NC 27599-7570; **Office Phone:** (919) 966-7764; **Board Certification:** Obstetrics & Gynecology 1978; **Medical School:** Yale Univ 1972; **Residency:** Obstetrics & Gynecology, Yale - New Haven Hosp, New Haven, CT 1973-1976; **Faculty Appointment:** Prof Obstetrics & Gynecology, Univ NC Sch Med

Midwest

Beer, Alan Earl MD (Obstetrics & Gynecology) - *Special Expertise:* *Infertility-Female; Reproductive Immunology;* **Admitting Hospital:** University of Chicago Hospitals (Page 78); **Office Address:** Chicago Medical School 3333 Green Bay Rd North Chicago, IL 60064; **Office Phone:** (847) 578-3233; **Board Certification:** Obstetrics & Gynecology 1971; **Medical School:** Indiana Univ 1962; **Residency:** Obstetrics & Gynecology, Hosp Univ Penn, Philadelphia, PA 1965-1969; **Fellowship:** Obstetrics & Gynecology, Univ Penn, Philadelphia, PA 1968-1970; **Faculty Appointment:** Prof Obstetrics & Gynecology, Univ Chicago-Pritzker Sch Med

Elias, Sherman MD (Obstetrics & Gynecology) - *Special Expertise:* *Prenatal Diagnosis;* **Admitting Hospital:** University of Illinois at Chicago Medical Center; **Office Address:** Univ of IL, Dept of Ob/Gyn 820 S Wood St, MC-808 Chicago, IL 60612; **Office Phone:** (312) 413-2040; **Board Certifications:** Clinical Genetics 1982, Obstetrics & Gynecology 1996; **Medical School:** Univ KY Coll Med 1976; **Residencies:** Obstetrics & Gynecology, Michael Reese Hosp, Chicago, IL 1972-1973; Obstetrics & Gynecology, Univ Louisville, Louisville, KY 1973-1976; **Fellowships:** Clinical Genetics, Yale, New Haven, CT 1974-1975; Clinical Genetics, Northwestern Univ, Chicigo, IL 1976-1978; **Faculty Appointment:** Prof Obstetrics & Gynecology, Univ IL Coll Med

Evans, Mark Ira MD (Obstetrics & Gynecology) - *Special Expertise:* *Reproductive Genetics;* **Admitting Hospital:** Hutzel Hospital - Detroit; **Office Address:** Hutzel Hosp, Dept OB/GYN 4707 St Antione Blvd, Fl 5th Detroit, MI 48201-1498; **Office Phone:** (313) 745-7067; **Board Certifications:** Obstetrics & Gynecology 1999, Clinical Genetics 1984; **Medical School:** SUNY Downstate 1978; **Residency:** Obstetrics & Gynecology, Lying-In Hosp/U Chicago, Chicago, IL 1979-1982; **Fellowship:** Clinical Genetics, Natl Inst Hlth Bethesda, Bethesada, MD 1982-1984; **Faculty Appointment:** Prof Obstetrics & Gynecology, Wayne State Univ

Galask, Rudolph P. MD (Obstetrics & Gynecology) - *Special Expertise:* *Vulva Disease/Neoplasia; Infectious Disease in Pregnancy;* **Admitting Hospital:** University of Iowa Hospitals and Clinics; **Office Address:** Univ Iowa Coll Med, Univ Hosp OG Fl 2nd - rm BT 2004J Iowa City, IA 52242; **Office Phone:** (319) 353-6323; **Board Certification:** Obstetrics & Gynecology 1972; **Medical School:** Univ Iowa Coll Med 1964; **Residency:** Obstetrics & Gynecology, Univ Iowa, Iowa City, IA 1967-1970

Gonik, Bernard MD (Obstetrics & Gynecology) - *Special Expertise:* *Maternal & Fetal Medicine;* **Admitting Hospital:** Sinai-Grace Hospital - Detroit; **Office Address:** Sinai-Grace Hosp, Dept Ob/Gyn 6071 W Outer Dr Detroit, MI 48235; **Office Phone:** (313) 966-1880; **Board Certifications:** Obstetrics & Gynecology 1995, Maternal & Fetal Medicine 1987; **Medical School:** Mich State Univ 1978; **Residency:** Obstetrics & Gynecology, Univ Texas Med Sch, Houston, TX 1978-1982; **Fellowship:** Maternal & Fetal Medicine, Univ Texas Med Sch, Houston, TX 1982-1985; **Faculty Appointment:** Asst Prof Univ Tex, Houston

Gonzalez-Loya, Juan MD (Obstetrics & Gynecology) - *Special Expertise:* *Obstetrics & Gynecology - General;* **Admitting Hospital:** Loyola University Health System; **Office Address:** 154 N Broadway Ave Melrose Park, IL 60160; **Office Phone:** (708) 681-3535; **Board Certification:** Obstetrics & Gynecology 1999; **Medical School:** Mexico 1959; **Residency:** Internal Medicine, Metropolitan HospCtr, New York, NY

Johnson, Timothy R.B. MD (Obstetrics & Gynecology) - *Special Expertise:* *Fetal Assessment; Prenatal Diagnosis;* **Admitting Hospital:** University of Michigan Health Center; **Office Address:** Women's Hospital 1500 E Med Ctr Dr, rm L4000, Box 0276 Ann Arbor, MI 48109-0276; **Office Phone:** (734) 764-8123; **Board Certifications:** Obstetrics & Gynecology 1991, Maternal & Fetal Medicine 1983; **Medical School:** Univ VA Sch Med 1975; **Residency:** Obstetrics & Gynecology, Univ Michigan Med Ctr, Ann Arbor, MI 1976-1979; **Fellowship:** Maternal & Fetal Medicine, Johns Hopkins Hosp, Baltimore, MD 1979-1981; **Faculty Appointment:** Prof Obstetrics & Gynecology, Univ Mich Med Sch

Levine, Elliot Mark MD (Obstetrics & Gynecology) - *Special Expertise:* *Obstetrics & Gynecology - General;* **Admitting Hospital:** Illinois Masonic Medical Center (Page 64); **Office Address:** 3000 N Halsted St, Ste 209B Chicago, IL 60657-5190; **Office Phone:** (773) 296-3300; **Board Certification:** Obstetrics & Gynecology 1984; **Medical School:** Univ Hlth Sci/Chicago Med Sch 1978; **Residency:** Obstetrics & Gynecology, Illinois Masonic Med Ctr, Chicago, IL 1978-1982

Linn, Edward S MD (Obstetrics & Gynecology) - *Special Expertise:* *Menopause Problems; Infectious Disease in Pregnancy;* **Admitting Hospital:** Advocate Lutheran General Hospital; **Office Address:** Advocate Medical Group-Parkside Ctr 1875 Dempster St, Ste 665 Park Ridge, IL 60068; **Office Phone:** (847) 825-1590; **Board Certification:** Obstetrics & Gynecology 1994; **Medical School:** Univ Chicago-Pritzker Sch Med 1974; **Residency:** Obstetrics & Gynecology, Michael Reese Hosp, Chicago, IL 1974-1978; **Faculty Appointment:** Assoc Prof Obstetrics & Gynecology, Rush Med Coll

Merrick, Frank W MD (Obstetrics & Gynecology) - *Special Expertise:* *Gynecologic Surgery; Menstrual Disorders;* **Admitting Hospital:** Rush/Presbyterian - St Luke's Medical Center - Chicago (Page 74); **Office Address:** 1725 W Harrison St, Ste 738 Chicago, IL 60612; **Office Phone:** (312) 829-4405; **Board Certification:** Obstetrics & Gynecology 1996; **Medical School:** Univ Mich Med Sch 1958; **Residency:** Obstetrics & Gynecology, Chicago Lying-In Hosp, Chicago, IL 1959-1962

Merritt, Diane MD (Obstetrics & Gynecology) - *Special Expertise:* *Gynecology-Adolescent;* **Admitting Hospital:** Barnes - Jewish Hospital; **Office Address:** 2 Maternity 4911 Barnes Jewish Plaza, Fl 2 St. Louis, MO 63110; **Office Phone:** (314) 747-1454; **Board Certification:** Obstetrics & Gynecology 1984; **Medical School:** NYU Sch Med 1975; **Residencies:** Obstetrics & Gynecology, Barnes Hospital University Washington, St. Louis, MO 1977-1980; Surgery, Barnes Hospital University Washington, St. Louis, MO 1976-1977; **Faculty Appointment:** Prof Obstetrics & Gynecology, Washington Univ, St Louis

Moawad, Atef H MD (Obstetrics & Gynecology) - *Special Expertise:* *Pregnancy-High Risk; Premature Labor;* **Admitting Hospital:** University of Chicago Hospitals (Page 78); **Office Address:** Univ Chicago Hosp, Dept OB/GYN 5841 S Maryland Ave, MC-2050 Chicago, IL 60637; **Office Phone:** (773) 702-5200; **Board Certification:** Obstetrics & Gynecology 1989; **Medical School:** Egypt 1957; **Residency:** Obstetrics & Gynecology, Thomas Jefferson, Philadelphia, PA 1961-1964; **Fellowships:** Obstetrics & Gynecology, Univ Lund Hosp, Sweden 1966-1967; Case Western, Cleveland, OH 1965-1966; **Faculty Appointment:** Prof Obstetrics & Gynecology, Univ Chicago-Pritzker Sch Med

Muraskas, Erik MD (Obstetrics & Gynecology) - *Special Expertise:* *Obstetrics & Gynecology - General;* **Admitting Hospital:** Loyola University Health System; **Office Address:** Loyola Univ Med Ctr 2160 S First S Avenue Maywood, IL 60153; **Office Phone:** (708) 327-1000; **Board Certification:** Obstetrics & Gynecology 1990; **Medical School:** Loyola Univ-Stritch Sch Med 1981; **Residency:** Obstetrics & Gynecology, Loyola U-Stritch Sch Med, Maywood, IL 1981-1985; **Faculty Appointment:** Asst Prof Obstetrics & Gynecology, Loyola Univ-Stritch Sch Med

Sciarra, John J MD (Obstetrics & Gynecology) - *Special Expertise: Gynecologic Surgery;* **Admitting Hospital:** Northwestern Memorial Hospital; **Office Address:** Northwestern Med Faculty Foundation 675 N St Clair St, Fl 14 - Ste 20 Chicago, IL 60611-4407; **Office Phone:** (312) 695-5656; **Board Certification:** Obstetrics & Gynecology 1967; **Medical School:** Columbia P&S 1957; **Residency:** Obstetrics & Gynecology, Columbia-Presby Hosp, New York, NY 1958-1964; **Faculty Appointment:** Prof Obstetrics & Gynecology, Northwestern Univ

Socol, Michael MD (Obstetrics & Gynecology) - *Special Expertise: Diabetes in Pregnancy; Multiple Gestation; Premature Labor;* **Admitting Hospital:** Northwestern Memorial Hospital; **Office Address:** Northwestern Univ Hosp 333 E Superior St, Ste 410 Chicago, IL 60611-3056; **Office Phone:** (312) 695-7542; **Board Certifications:** Obstetrics & Gynecology 1979, Maternal & Fetal Medicine 1981; **Medical School:** Univ IL Coll Med 1974; **Residency:** Obstetrics & Gynecology, Univ Illinois Med Ctr, Chicago, IL 1974-1977; **Fellowship:** Maternal & Fetal Medicine, USC Med Ctr, Los Angeles, CA 1977-1979; **Faculty Appointment:** Prof Obstetrics & Gynecology, Northwestern Univ

Tan, Merita R.C. MD (Obstetrics & Gynecology) - *Special Expertise: Menstrual Disorders; Laser Surgery;* **Admitting Hospital:** Northwestern Memorial Hospital; **Office Address:** 680 N Lake Shore Dr, Ste 1424 Chicago, IL 60611-8700; **Office Phone:** (312) 482-8484; **Board Certification:** Obstetrics & Gynecology 1995; **Medical School:** Univ Hlth Sci/Chicago Med Sch 1989; **Residency:** Obstetrics & Gynecology, Cook Co Hosp, Chicago, IL 1989-203; **Faculty Appointment:** Clin Inst Obstetrics & Gynecology, Northwestern Univ

Toig, Randall MD (Obstetrics & Gynecology) - *Special Expertise: Advanced Maternal Age; Osteoporosis;* **Admitting Hospital:** Northwestern Memorial Hospital; **Office Address:** Northwestern Meml Hosp, Dept Ob/Gyn 680 N Lake Shore Dr, Ste 830 Chicago, IL 60611-4449; **Office Phone:** (312) 440-1600; **Board Certification:** Obstetrics & Gynecology 1985; **Medical School:** Univ Pittsburgh 1977; **Residency:** Obstetrics & Gynecology, Northwestern Meml Hosp, Chicago, IL 1978-1982; **Faculty Appointment:** Assoc Prof Northwestern Univ

Walters, Mark MD (Obstetrics & Gynecology) - *Special Expertise: Uro-Gynecology; Vaginal Reconstructive surgery;* **Admitting Hospital:** Cleveland Clinic Foundation; **Office Address:** Cleveland Clinic Fdn Cleveland Clinic, Ste A81 Cleveland, OH 44195; **Office Phone:** (216) 445-6586; **Board Certification:** Obstetrics & Gynecology 1996; **Medical School:** Ohio State Univ 1980; **Residency:** Obstetrics & Gynecology, New England Med Ctr, Boston, MA 1980-1984

Southwest

Carr, Bruce MD (Obstetrics & Gynecology) - *Special Expertise: Infertility-Female;* **Admitting Hospital:** Zale Lipshy University Hospital; **Office Address:** 5323 Harry Hines Blvd, rm J6-114 Dallas, TX 75390-9032; **Office Phone:** (214) 648-2784; **Board Certifications:** Obstetrics & Gynecology 1989, Reproductive Endocrinology 1982; **Medical School:** Univ Mich Med Sch 1971; **Residency:** Obstetrics & Gynecology, Parkland Meml Hosp, Dallas, TX 1972-1975; **Fellowship:** Reproductive Endocrinology, Univ TX SW Med Ctr, Dallas, TX 1978-1980; **Faculty Appointment:** Prof Obstetrics & Gynecology, Univ Tex SW, Dallas

Faro, Sebastian MD (Obstetrics & Gynecology) - *Special Expertise: Infectious Disease in Pregnancy;* **Admitting Hospital:** The Woman's Hospital of Texas; **Office Address:** Assocs Infectious Disease 7400 Fannin, Ste 1160 Houston, TX 77054; **Office Phone:** (713) 799-8994; **Board Certification:** Obstetrics & Gynecology 1991; **Medical School:** Creighton Univ 1975; **Residency:** Obstetrics & Gynecology, Creighton Univ, Omaha, NE 1975-1978

Huff, Robert Whitley MD (Obstetrics & Gynecology) - *Special Expertise: Genetic Disorders;* **Admitting Hospital:** University of Texas Health & Science Center; **Office Address:** UT Hlth Scis, Dept OB/GYN 7703 Floyd Curl San Antonio, TX 78229-3900; **Office Phone:** (210) 567-4999; **Board Certifications:** Maternal & Fetal Medicine 1979, Clinical Genetics 1990; **Medical School:** Baylor Coll Med 1966; **Residency:** Obstetrics & Gynecology, Bexar Co Hosp, San Antonio, TX 1969-1972; **Faculty Appointment:** Prof Obstetrics & Gynecology, Univ Tex, San Antonio

Simpson, Joe Leigh MD (Obstetrics & Gynecology) - *Special Expertise: Prenatal Diagnosis; Ovarian Failure-Recurrent; Spontaneous Abortion;* **Admitting Hospital:** Methodist Hospital - Houston (Page 69); **Office Address:** Baylor Coll Med 6550 Fannin St, Ste 729A Houston, TX 77030-2717; **Office Phone:** (713) 798-8360; **Board Certifications:** Clinical Genetics 1982, Obstetrics & Gynecology 1989; **Medical School:** Duke Univ 1968; **Residency:** Obstetrics & Gynecology, NY Hosp, New York, NY 1969-1973; **Faculty Appointment:** Prof Obstetrics & Gynecology, Baylor Coll Med

West Coast and Pacific

Berman, Michael Leonard MD (Obstetrics & Gynecology) - *Special Expertise: Gynecologic Cancer;* **Admitting Hospital:** University of California - Irvine Medical Center; **Office Address:** UCI Med Ctr, Div of Gyn/Onc 101 The City Drive S, Bldg 23 - rm 107 Orange, CA 92868-3298; **Office Phone:** (714) 456-6570; **Board Certifications:** Obstetrics & Gynecology 1999, Gynecologic Oncology 1999; **Medical School:** Geo Wash Univ 1967; **Residencies:** Obstetrics & Gynecology, GW Univ Hosp, Washington, DC 1968-1969; Obstetrics & Gynecology, Los Angeles Co-Harbor, Torrence, CA 1971-1974; **Fellowship:** Gynecologic Oncology, UCLA Med Ctr, Los Angeles, CA 1974-1976; **Faculty Appointment:** Prof Obstetrics & Gynecology, UC Irvine

DeCherney, Alan Hersh MD (Obstetrics & Gynecology) - *Special Expertise: Infertility-Female; Reproductive Endocrinology;* **Admitting Hospital:** UCLA Medical Center; **Office Address:** UCLA Sch of Med 10833 Le Conte Ave, Bldg 27-117 CHS Los Angeles, CA 90095; **Office Phone:** (310) 794-1884; **Board Certifications:** Obstetrics & Gynecology 1989, Reproductive Endocrinology 1979; **Medical School:** Temple Univ 1967; **Residency:** Obstetrics & Gynecology, Hosp Univ Penn, Philadelphia, PA 1968-1972

Eschenbach, David Arthur MD (Obstetrics & Gynecology) - *Special Expertise: Gynecologic Surgery; Infectious Disease in Pregnancy; Vaginal Disorders;* **Admitting Hospital:** University of Washington Medical Center; **Office Address:** Univ Washington Med Ctr Box 356460 Seattle, WA 98195; **Office Phone:** (206) 543-2444; **Board Certification:** Obstetrics & Gynecology 1975; **Medical School:** Univ Wisc 1968; **Residency:** Obstetrics & Gynecology, Univ Wash Hosp, Seattle, WA 1969-1973; **Fellowship:** Infectious Disease, Univ Wash Hosp, Seattle, WA 1972-1974; **Faculty Appointment:** Prof Obstetrics & Gynecology, Univ Wash

Novy, Miles MD (Obstetrics & Gynecology) - *Special Expertise: Transabdominal Cervical Cerclage (TCIC); Reproductive Endocrinology;* **Admitting Hospital:** Oregon Health Science University Hospital and Clinics; **Office Address:** OHSU, Dept Ob/Gyn 3181 SW Sam Jackson Park Rd, MC-L466 Portland, OR 97201-3098; **Office Phone:** (503) 494-8311; **Board Certifications:** Obstetrics & Gynecology 1972, Maternal & Fetal Medicine 1975; **Medical School:** Harvard Med Sch 1963; **Residency:** Obstetrics & Gynecology, Boston Hosp Women, Boston, MA 1964-1965; **Fellowship:** Maternal & Fetal Medicine, Univ Oregon, Portland, OR 1965-1967; **Faculty Appointment:** Prof Obstetrics & Gynecology, Oregon Hlth Scis Univ

Olive, David MD (Obstetrics & Gynecology) - *Special Expertise:* Infertility-IVF; Endometriosis; **Admitting Hospital:** Mills - Peninsula Health Center Hospital; **Office Address:** 230 Lake Merced Hills Rd N, Ste 4A San Francisco, CA 94132; **Office Phone:** (415) 239-5391; **Board Certifications:** Obstetrics & Gynecology 1995, Reproductive Endocrinology 1995; **Medical School:** Baylor Coll Med 1979; **Residency:** Obstetrics & Gynecology, Northwestern Univ, Chicago, IL 1980-1983; **Fellowship:** Reproductive Endocrinology, Duke Univ, Durham, NC 1983-1985; **Faculty Appointment:** Asst Prof Obstetrics & Gynecology, Univ N Tex Hlth Sci Ctr, Coll Osteo Med

Platt, Lawrence David MD (Obstetrics & Gynecology) - *Special Expertise:* Maternal & Fetal Medicine; Ultrasound; **Admitting Hospital:** Cedars-Sinai Medical Center; **Office Address:** 8635 W 3rd St, Ste 160 Los Angeles, CA 90048; **Office Phone:** (310) 423-7433; **Board Certifications:** Obstetrics & Gynecology 1979, Maternal & Fetal Medicine 1981; **Medical School:** Wayne State Univ 1972; **Residencies:** Obstetrics & Gynecology, Sinai Hosp, Detroit, MI 1973-1975; Obstetrics & Gynecology, Sinai Hosp, Detroit, MI 1975-1976; **Fellowship:** Maternal & Fetal Medicine, USC Med Ctr, Los Angeles, CA 1976-1978

OPHTHALMOLOGY

An ophthalmologist has the knowledge and professional skills needed to provide comprehensive eye and vision care. Ophthalmologists are medically trained to diagnose, monitor and medically or surgically treat all ocular and visual disorders. This includes problems affecting the eye and its component structures, the eyelids, the orbit and the visual pathways. In so doing, an ophthalmologist prescribes vision services, including glasses and contact lenses.

Training required: Four years

Physician Listings

Ophthalmology

New England

Aiello, Lloyd MD (Ophthalmology) - *Special Expertise:* Diabetic Eye Disease/Retinopathy; **Admitting Hospital:** Beth Israel Deaconess Medical Center - Boston (Page 57); **Office Address:** Beetham Eye Inst-Joslin Diabetes Ctr 1 Joslin Pl Boston, MA 02215-5397; **Office Phone:** (617) 732-2520; **Board Certification:** Ophthalmology 1966; **Medical School:** Boston Univ 1960; **Residency:** Ophthalmology, Mass Genl Hosp, Boston, MA 1962-1964; **Faculty Appointment:** Assoc Prof Ophthalmology, Harvard Med Sch

Foster, Charles Stephen MD (Ophthalmology) - *Special Expertise:* Uveitis; Corneal Disease; Cataract Surgery; **Admitting Hospital:** Massachusetts Eye & Ear Infirmary (Page 68); **Office Address:** Mass Eye and Ear 243 Charles St Boston, MA 02114-3002; **Office Phone:** (617) 573-3591; **Board Certification:** Ophthalmology 1976; **Medical School:** Duke Univ 1969; **Residency:** Ophthalmology, Wash Univ - Barnes Hosp, St Louis, MO 1972-1975; **Fellowships:** Cornea, Mass EE Infirm - Harvard, Boston, MA 1975-1976; Ocular Immunology, Mass EE Infirm - Harvard, Boston, MA 1976-1977; **Faculty Appointment:** Prof Ophthalmology, Harvard Med Sch

Jakobiec, Frederick A. MD (Ophthalmology) - *Special Expertise:* Eye & Orbital Tumors/Cancer; Eyelid & Conjunctival Tumors; **Admitting Hospital:** Massachusetts Eye & Ear Infirmary (Page 68); **Office Address:** Mass EE Infirm-Chairman Oph. 243 Charles St Boston, MA 02114-3002; **Office Phone:** (617) 573-3526; **Board Certifications:** Ophthalmology 1975, Anatomic Pathology 1978; **Medical School:** Harvard Med Sch 1971; **Residencies:** Ophthalmology, Harkness Eye Inst, New York, NY 1969-1973; Pathology, Columbia P&S, New York, NY 1969-1973; **Fellowship:** Columbia P&S, New York, NY 1969-1970

McKeown, Craig A MD (Ophthalmology) - *Special Expertise:* Ophthalmology - General; **Admitting Hospital:** New England Medical Center; **Office Address:** New England Med Ctr 750 Washington St, Box 450 Boston, MA 02111; **Office Phone:** (617) 636-7293; **Board Certification:** Ophthalmology 1982; **Medical School:** Northwestern Univ 1971; **Residency:** Ophthalmology, Walter Reed Med Ctr, Washington, DC 1977-1980; **Fellowships:** Pediatric Ophthalmology, Chldns Hosp Natl Med Ctr, Washington, DC 1983-1984; Pediatric Ophthalmology, Wilmer Inst-Johns Hospkins, Baltimore, MD 1984-1985

Mitchell, Paul Ralph MD (Ophthalmology) - *Special Expertise:* Ophthalmology-Pediatric; **Admitting Hospital:** Hartford Hospital; **Office Address:** Chldns Eye Care PC 100 Retreat Ave, Ste 700 Hartford, CT 06106-2528; **Office Phone:** (860) 525-2673; **Board Certification:** Ophthalmology 1977; **Medical School:** Geo Wash Univ 1970; **Residency:** Ophthalmology, Wills Eye Hosp, Philadelphia, PA 1973-1976; **Fellowship:** Ophthalmology, Chldns Hosp MC/Geo Wash, Washington, DC 1976-1977; **Faculty Appointment:** Asst Clin Prof Ophthalmology, Univ Conn

Petersen, Robert Allen MD (Ophthalmology) - *Special Expertise:* Ophthalmology-Pediatric; **Admitting Hospital:** Children's Hospital; **Office Address:** Children's Hosp, Dept of Oph 300 Longwood Ave Boston, MA 02115; **Office Phone:** (617) 355-6415; **Board Certification:** Ophthalmology 1967; **Medical School:** Columbia P&S 1959; **Residencies:** Internal Medicine, Presby Hosp, New York, NY 1960-1961; Ophthalmology, Mass EE Infirm, Boston, MA 1962-1966; **Fellowships:** Ophthalmology, Columbia Presby Hosp, New York, NY 1961-1962; Research, MAss EE Infirm, Boston, MA 1962-1963

Robb, Richard M MD (Ophthalmology) - *Special Expertise:* Strabismus; Cataract-Congenital; Lacrimal Gland Disorders; **Admitting Hospital:** Children's Hospital; **Office Address:** Chldns Hosp, Dept Oph 300 Longwood Ave Boston, MA 02115; **Office Phone:** (617) 355-6412; **Board Certification:** Ophthalmology 1967; **Medical School:** Univ Penn 1960; **Residency:** Ophthalmology, Mass EE Infirm, Boston, MA 1961-1965; **Faculty Appointment:** Prof Emeritus Ophthalmology, Harvard Med Sch

443

Steinert, Roger F MD (Ophthalmology) - *Special Expertise:* Refractive, Cataract Surgery; Cornea Transplant; **Admitting Hospital:** Massachusetts Eye & Ear Infirmary (Page 68); **Office Address:** Oph Consults Boston 50 Staniford St, Ste 600 Boston, MA 02114-2517; **Office Phone:** (617) 367-4800; **Board Certification:** Ophthalmology 1982; **Medical School:** Harvard Med Sch 1977; **Residency:** Ophthalmology, Mass EE Infirm., Boston, MA 1978-1981; **Faculty Appointment:** Asst Clin Prof Ophthalmology, Harvard Med Sch

Walton, David S MD (Ophthalmology) - *Special Expertise:* Glaucoma-Pediatric; Cataract-Pediatric; Neuro-Ophthalmology; **Admitting Hospital:** Massachusetts Eye & Ear Infirmary (Page 68); **Office Address:** MA Eye and Ear Infirm 2 Longfellow Pl, Fl 201 Boston, MA 02114; **Office Phone:** (617) 227-3011; **Board Certifications:** Ophthalmology 1969, Pediatrics 1983; **Medical School:** Duke Univ 1961; **Residency:** Ophthalmology, MA EE Infirm, Boston, MA 1964-1967; **Faculty Appointment:** Asst Prof Ophthalmology, Harvard Med Sch

Mid Atlantic

Abramson, David Harold MD (Ophthalmology) - *Special Expertise:* Eye Tumors; Eye Tumors/Cancer; **Admitting Hospital:** New York Eye & Ear Infirmary (Page 71); **Office Address:** 70 E 66th St New York, NY 10021; **Office Phone:** (212) 744-1700; **Board Certification:** Ophthalmology 1975; **Medical School:** Albert Einstein Coll Med 1969; **Residency:** Ophthalmology, Edward S Harkness Eye Inst, New York, NY 1970-1974; **Fellowships:** Ocular Oncology, Columbia Presby Med Ctr, New York, NY 1974-1975; **Faculty Appointment:** Clin Prof Ophthalmology, Cornell Univ-Weil Med Coll

Aronian, Dianne D MD (Ophthalmology) - *Special Expertise:* Ophthalmology-Pediatric; Retinopathy of Prematurity; **Admitting Hospital:** New York Weill Cornell Medical Center - NY Presbyterian Hospital (Page 72); **Office Address:** 438 E 87th St New York, NY 10128; **Office Phone:** (212) 534-4404; **Board Certification:** Ophthalmology 1977; **Medical School:** Cornell Univ-Weil Med Coll 1972; **Residency:** Ophthalmology, New York Hosp, New York 1973-1976; **Faculty Appointment:** Assoc Prof Ophthalmology, Cornell Univ-Weil Med Coll

Behrens, Myles MD (Ophthalmology) - *Special Expertise:* Neuro-Ophthalmology; **Admitting Hospital:** Columbia Presbyterian Medical Center (Page 72); **Office Address:** 635 W 165th St New York, NY 10032; **Office Phone:** (212) 305-5415; **Board Certification:** Ophthalmology 1971; **Medical School:** Columbia P&S 1962; **Residencies:** Internal Medicine, Columbia Presby Hosp, New York, NY 1963-1964; Ophthalmology, Columbia Presby Hosp, New York, NY 1967-1970; **Fellowship:** Neurological Ophthalmology, UCSF, San Francisco, CA 1970-1971; **Faculty Appointment:** Prof Ophthalmology, Columbia P&S

Biglan, Albert William MD (Ophthalmology) - *Special Expertise:* Ophthalmology-Pediatric; **Admitting Hospital:** Children's Hospital of Pittsburgh; **Office Address:** 20397 Route 19, Ste 232 Cranberry, PA 16066; **Office Phone:** (724) 772-3388; **Board Certification:** Ophthalmology 1977; **Medical School:** SUNY Buffalo 1968; **Residency:** Ophthalmology, EE Hosp - Univ Pitt, Pittsburgh, PA 1973-1976; **Fellowship:** Pediatric Ophthalmology, Indiana Univ Med Ctr, Indianapolis, IN 1977; **Faculty Appointment:** Assoc Prof Ophthalmology, Univ Pittsburgh

Burde, Ronald MD (Ophthalmology) - *Special Expertise:* Ischemic/Optic/Neuropathy; Glaucoma; Pseudotumor Cerebri; **Admitting Hospital:** Montefiore Medical Center; **Office Address:** 111 E 210th St Bronx, NY 10467-2401; **Office Phone:** (718) 920-6665; **Board Certification:** Ophthalmology 1970; **Medical School:** Jefferson Med Coll 1964; **Residency:** Ophthalmology, Washington Univ Hosp, St Louis, MO 1965-1968; **Fellowship:** Neurological Ophthalmology, Washington Hosp, St Louis, MO 1968-1970; **Faculty Appointment:** Prof Ophthalmology, Albert Einstein Coll Med

Caputo, Anthony R MD (Ophthalmology) - *Special Expertise: Ophthalmology-Pediatric; Strabismus;* **Admitting Hospital:** Columbus Community Hospital; **Office Address:** 556 Eagle Rock Ave, Fl 203 Roseland, NJ 07068-1500; **Office Phone:** (973) 228-3111; **Board Certification:** Ophthalmology 1976; **Medical School:** Italy 1969; **Residency:** Ophthalmology, UMDNJ, Newark, NJ 1971-1974; **Fellowship:** Ophthalmology, Wills Eye Hosp, Philadelphia, PA 1974-1975; **Faculty Appointment:** Prof Ophthalmology, UMDNJ-NJ Med Sch, Newark

Chang, Stanley MD (Ophthalmology) - *Special Expertise: Retina/Vitreous Surgery;* **Admitting Hospital:** Columbia Presbyterian Medical Center (Page 72); **Office Address:** 635 W 165th St New York, NY 10032; **Office Phone:** (212) 305-9535; **Board Certification:** Ophthalmology 1979; **Medical School:** Columbia P&S 1974; **Residency:** Ophthalmology, Mass Eye & Ear Infirmary, Boston, MA 1976-1978; **Fellowship:** Vitreoretinal Surgery, Bascom Palmer Eye Institute, Miami, FL 1978-1979; **Faculty Appointment:** Prof Ophthalmology, Columbia P&S

De Juan Jr, Eugene MD (Ophthalmology) - *Special Expertise: Retina/Vitreous Surgery;* **Admitting Hospital:** Johns Hopkins Hospital - Baltimore (Page 65); **Office Address:** John Hopkins Hosp 600 N Wolfe St, Bldg Maumenee - rm 721 Baltimore, MD 21287-9277; **Office Phone:** (410) 955-2159; **Board Certification:** Ophthalmology 1985; **Medical School:** Univ S Ala Coll Med 1979; **Residency:** Ophthalmology, Johns Hopkins Hosp, Baltimore, DC 1980-1983; **Fellowship:** Vitreoretinal Surgery, Duke Univ Eye Ctr, Durham, NC 1983-1984; **Faculty Appointment:** Prof Ophthalmology, Johns Hopkins Univ

Della Rocca, Robert MD (Ophthalmology) - *Special Expertise: Eyelid Reconstruction; Cosmetic Surgery-Eyelid;* **Admitting Hospital:** New York Eye & Ear Infirmary (Page 71); **Office Address:** 310 E 14th St, Bldg South - rm 319 New York, NY 10003; **Office Phone:** (212) 979-4575; **Board Certification:** Ophthalmology 1975; **Medical School:** Creighton Univ 1967; **Residency:** Ophthalmology, NY Eye & Ear Infirm, New York, NY 1970-1973; **Fellowship:** Ophthalmology, Albany Med Ctr, New York, NY 1973

Diamond, Gary Richard MD (Ophthalmology) - *Special Expertise: Eye Diseases-Pediatric; Crossed Eyes; Amblyopia;* **Admitting Hospital:** St Christopher's Hospital for Children; **Office Address:** St. Christopher's Hosp for Chldn, Div Oph Front Street at Erie Ave Philadelphia, PA 19134-1095; **Office Phone:** (215) 427-8120; **Board Certification:** Ophthalmology 1979; **Medical School:** Johns Hopkins Univ 1974; **Residencies:** Ophthalmology, Wilmer Inst-Johns Hopkins, Baltimore, MD 1975-1979; Ophthalmology, Chldns Hosp Med Ctr, Washington, DC 1978-1979; **Fellowship:** Pediatric Ophthalmology, Harkness Eye Inst, Baltimore, MD 1978-1979; **Faculty Appointment:** Prof Ophthalmology, Hahnemann Univ

Dodick, Jack M MD (Ophthalmology) - *Special Expertise: Ophthalmology - General;* **Admitting Hospital:** Manhattan Eye, Ear & Throat Hospital; **Office Address:** 535 Park Ave New York, NY 10021; **Office Phone:** (212) 288-7638; **Board Certification:** Ophthalmology 1969; **Medical School:** Univ Toronto 1963; **Residency:** Ophthalmology, Manhattan Eye & Ear, New York, NY 1964-1967; **Fellowship:** Surgery, NY Med Coll, New York, NY 1967-1968; **Faculty Appointment:** Clin Prof Ophthalmology, Columbia P&S

Eggers, Howard M MD (Ophthalmology) - *Special Expertise: Ophthalmology-Pediatric; Strabismus;* **Admitting Hospital:** Columbia Presbyterian Medical Center (Page 72); **Office Address:** 635 W 165th St New York, NY 10032; **Office Phone:** (212) 305-5409; **Board Certification:** Ophthalmology 1978; **Medical School:** Columbia P&S 1971; **Residency:** Ophthalmology, Harkness Inst - Presby Hosp, New York, NY 1972-1975; **Faculty Appointment:** Prof Ophthalmology, Columbia P&S

Fuchs, Wayne MD (Ophthalmology) - *Special Expertise: Diabetic Eye Disease/Retinopathy; Macular Disease/Degeneration;* **Admitting Hospital:** Mount Sinai Hospital (Page 70); **Office Address:** 121 E 60th St, Fl 5 New York, NY 10022; **Office Phone:** (212) 319-8205; **Board Certification:** Ophthalmology 1985; **Medical School:** Mount Sinai Sch Med 1979; **Residency:** Ophthalmology, Mount Sinai Hosp, New York, NY 1980-1983; **Fellowship:** Ophthalmology, NY Cornell Med Ctr, New York, NY 1983-1984; **Faculty Appointment:** Assoc Clin Prof Ophthalmology, Mount Sinai Sch Med

Gentile, Ronald MD (Ophthalmology) - *Special Expertise: Retina/Vitreous Surgery; Diabetic Eye Disease; Macular Degeneration;* **Admitting Hospital:** New York Eye & Ear Infirmary (Page 71); **Office Address:** New York Eye and Ear Infirmary Second Ave at Fourteenth Street, Bldg South - Ste 319 New York, NY 10003-4201; **Office Phone:** (212) 794-4120; **Board Certification:** Ophthalmology 1997; **Medical School:** SUNY Downstate 1991; **Residency:** Ophthalmology, NY Eye & Ear Infirm, New York, NY 1992-1995; **Fellowship:** Vitreoretinal Surgery & Disease, Kresge Eye Inst, Detroit, MI 1996-1998; **Faculty Appointment:** Asst Prof Ophthalmology, NY Med Coll

Goldberg, Morton MD (Ophthalmology) - *Special Expertise: Macular Disease/Degeneration; Diabetic Eye Disease/Retinopathy;* **Admitting Hospital:** Johns Hopkins Hospital - Baltimore (Page 65); **Office Address:** Johns Hopkins Hosp, Maumenee Bldg 727 600 N Wolfe St Baltimore, MD 21287-9278; **Office Phone:** (410) 955-6846; **Board Certification:** Ophthalmology 1968; **Medical School:** Harvard Med Sch 1962; **Residency:** Ophthalmology, Wilmer Oph Inst, Baltimore, MD 1963-1966; **Fellowships:** Ophthalmology, Wilmer Oph Inst, Baltimore, MD 1966-1967; Research, Johns Jopkins Hosp, Baltimore, MD 1966-1967; **Faculty Appointment:** Prof Ophthalmology, Johns Hopkins Univ

Guyer, David MD (Ophthalmology) - *Special Expertise: Macular Disease/Degeneration; Diabetic Eye Disease/Retinopathy;* **Admitting Hospital:** Manhattan Eye, Ear & Throat Hospital; **Office Address:** 519 E 72nd St, rm 203 New York, NY 10021-4028; **Office Phone:** (212) 861-9797; **Board Certification:** Ophthalmology 1991; **Medical School:** Johns Hopkins Univ 1986; **Residency:** Ophthalmology, Wilmer Eye Inst/ Johns Hopkins, Baltimore, MS 1987-1990; **Fellowship:** Vitreoretinal Surgery, Mass EE Infirm/Harvard Med Sch, Boston, MA 1990-1992; **Faculty Appointment:** Assoc Clin Prof Ophthalmology, Cornell Univ-Weil Med Coll

Guyton, David Lee MD (Ophthalmology) - *Special Expertise: Optics; Strabismus;* **Admitting Hospital:** Johns Hopkins Hospital - Baltimore (Page 65); **Office Address:** Wilmer Eye Inst 233, Johns Hopkins Hosp 600 N Wolff St Baltimore City, MD 21287-9028; **Office Phone:** (410) 955-8314; **Board Certification:** Ophthalmology 1977; **Medical School:** Harvard Med Sch 1969; **Residency:** Ophthalmology, Johns Hopkins Hospital, Baltimore, MD 1973-1976; **Fellowship:** Pediatric Ophthalmology, Baylor College of Medicine, Houston, TX 1976-1977; **Faculty Appointment:** Prof Ophthalmology, Johns Hopkins Univ

Hall, Lisabeth MD (Ophthalmology) - *Special Expertise: Ophthalmology-Pediatric; Lazy Eye; Double Vision;* **Admitting Hospital:** New York Eye & Ear Infirmary (Page 71); **Office Address:** 310 E 14th St, Bldg South - Fl 2nd New York, NY 10003; **Office Phone:** (212) 979-4375; **Board Certification:** Ophthalmology 1998; **Medical School:** SUNY Stony Brook 1992; **Residency:** Ophthalmology, Manhattan Eye Ear & Throat, New York City, NY 1993-1996; **Fellowship:** Ophthalmology, Jules Stein Eye Institute, Loas Angeles, LA 1996-1997; **Faculty Appointment:** Asst Prof Ophthalmology, NY Med Coll

Hersh, Peter MD (Ophthalmology) - *Special Expertise: Corneal Disease; Laser Vision Correction; Cataract Surgery;* **Admitting Hospital:** Hackensack University Medical Center; **Office Address:** Cornea and Laser Eye Inst 300 Frank W Burr Blvd Teaneck, NJ 07666; **Office Phone:** (201) 883-0505; **Board Certification:** Ophthalmology 1987; **Medical School:** Johns Hopkins Univ 1982; **Residencies:** Ophthalmology, Lenox Hill Hosp, New York, NY 1982-1983; Ophthalmology, Mass Eye & Ear Infirm, Boston, MA 1983-1986; **Fellowship:** Ophthalmology, Mass Eye & Ear Infirm, Boston, MA 1986-1987; **Faculty Appointment:** Prof Ophthalmology, UMDNJ-NJ Med Sch, Newark

Hornblass, Albert MD (Ophthalmology) - *Special Expertise: Orbital Tumors; Lacrimal Gland Disorders; Laser Eyebrow Surgery;* **Admitting Hospital:** Manhattan Eye, Ear & Throat Hospital; **Office Address:** Occuloplastic Surgery 130 E 67th St New York, NY 10021; **Office Phone:** (212) 879-6824; **Board Certifications:** Ophthalmology 1970, Plastic Surgery 1972; **Medical School:** Univ Cincinnati 1964; **Residency:** Ophthalmology, SUNY Health Science Center, Brooklyn, NY 1965-1969; **Fellowship:** Plastic Surgery, Manhattan Eye, Ear, & Throat, New York, NY 1971-1972; **Faculty Appointment:** Clin Prof Ophthalmology, SUNY Downstate

Jaafar, Mohamad S MD (Ophthalmology) - *Special Expertise: Glaucoma & Strabismus-Pediatric; Retinopathy of Prematurity; Marcus Gunn Syndrome;* **Admitting Hospital:** Children's National Medical Center - DC; **Office Address:** Chldns Natl Med Ctr, Dept of Oph 111 Michigan Ave NW Washington, DC 20010; **Office Phone:** (202) 884-3017; **Board Certification:** Ophthalmology 1997; **Medical School:** Other Foreign Country 1978; **Residencies:** Ophthalmology, Am U Beirut Med Ctr, Beirut Lebanon 1978-1981; Ophthalmology, Washington Hosp Ctr, Washington, DC 1989-1994; **Fellowships:** Pediatric Ophthalmology, Chldns Hosp, Boston, MA 1981-1982; Pediatric Ophthalmology, Baylor Coll Med, Houston, TX 1982-1983; **Faculty Appointment:** Prof Ophthalmology, Geo Wash Univ

Katowitz, James A MD (Ophthalmology) - *Special Expertise: Oculoplastic & Orbital Surgery; Ophthalmology-Pediatric; Cornea Plastic Surgery;* **Admitting Hospital:** The Children's Hospital of Philadelphia; **Office Address:** Chldn's Hosp, Div Oph Wood Bldg 1st FL 34th St & Civic Center Blvd Philadelphia, PA 19104; **Office Phone:** (215) 590-2791; **Board Certification:** Ophthalmology 1969; **Medical School:** Univ Penn 1963; **Residency:** Ophthalmology, Hosp Penn, Philadelphia, PA 1964-1967; **Fellowships:** Oculoplatic Surgery, Queen Victoria Hosp, London, England 1967-1968; Oculoplatic Surgery, Moorfield Eye Hosp, London, England 1967-1968; **Faculty Appointment:** Prof Ophthalmology, Univ Penn

Kupersmith, Mark MD (Ophthalmology) - *Special Expertise: Neuro-Ophthalmology;* **Admitting Hospital:** New York Eye & Ear Infirmary (Page 71); **Office Address:** 170 East End Ave Ste 535 New York, NY 10128; **Office Phone:** (212) 870-9418; **Board Certifications:** Ophthalmology 1981, Neurology 1981; **Medical School:** Northwestern Univ 1974; **Residencies:** Neurology, NYU Med Ctr, New York, NY 1974-1978; Ophthalmology, NYU Med Ctr, New York, NY 1976-1980

Laibson, Peter R MD (Ophthalmology) - *Special Expertise: Corneal Disease;* **Admitting Hospital:** Wills Eye Hospital; **Office Address:** Wills Eye Hospital 900 Walnut St, Fl 3rd Philadelphia, PA 19107; **Office Phone:** (215) 928-3180; **Board Certification:** Ophthalmology 1965; **Medical School:** SUNY Downstate 1959; **Residency:** Ophthalmology, Wills Eye Hosp, Philadelphia, PA 1961-1964; **Fellowship:** Mass EE Infirm, Boston, MA 1964-1965; **Faculty Appointment:** Prof Emeritus Ophthalmology, Jefferson Med Coll

Liebmann, Jeffrey MD (Ophthalmology) - *Special Expertise: Glaucoma;* **Admitting Hospital:** St Luke's - Roosevelt Hospital Center - Roosevelt Division (Page 58); **Office Address:** Glaucoma Associates 310 E 14th St, Ste 3 New York, NY 10003-4201; **Office Phone:** (212) 477-7540; **Board Certification:** Ophthalmology 1989; **Medical School:** Boston Univ 1983; **Residency:** Ophthalmology, SUNY Downstate, Brooklyn, NY 1984-1987; **Fellowship:** Glaucoma, NY EE Infirm, New York, NY 1988; **Faculty Appointment:** Assoc Clin Prof Ophthalmology, NY Med Coll

OPHTHALMOLOGY

Lisman, Richard MD (Ophthalmology) - *Special Expertise:* Oculoplastic Surgery; **Admitting Hospital:** NYU Medical Center (Page 70); **Office Address:** 635 Park Ave New York, NY 10021; **Office Phone:** (212) 585-1405; **Board Certification:** Ophthalmology 1981; **Medical School:** NYU Sch Med 1976; **Residency:** Ophthalmology, Manhattan EE Hosp, New York, NY 1977-1980; **Fellowship:** Oculoplatic Surgery, NY Eye and Ear-Cornell, New York, NY 1980-1981; **Faculty Appointment:** Clin Prof Ophthalmology, NYU Sch Med

Mackool, Richard MD (Ophthalmology) - *Special Expertise:* Cataract Surgery; *Refractive Surgery-LASIK;* **Admitting Hospital:** New York Eye & Ear Infirmary (Page 71); **Office Address:** Mackool Eye Inst & Laser Ctr 31-27 41st St Astoria, NY 11103; **Office Phone:** (718) 728-3400; **Board Certification:** Ophthalmology 1975; **Medical School:** Boston Univ 1968; **Residency:** Ophthalmology, New York EE Infirm, New York, NY 1970-1973; **Faculty Appointment:** Asst Clin Prof Ophthalmology, NY Med Coll

Magramm, Irene MD (Ophthalmology) - *Special Expertise:* Ophthalmology-Pediatric; *Strabismus; Cataract Surgery;* **Admitting Hospital:** Manhattan Eye, Ear & Throat Hospital; **Office Address:** 225 E 64th St New York, NY 10021; **Office Phone:** (212) 644-5100; **Board Certification:** Ophthalmology 1987; **Medical School:** Cornell Univ-Weil Med Coll 1981; **Residency:** Ophthalmology, North Shore Univ Hosp, Manhasset, NY 1982-1985; **Fellowship:** Pediatric Ophthalmology, Manhattan Ear, Eye & Throat Hosp, New York, NY 1985-1986; **Faculty Appointment:** Clin Inst Ophthalmology, Cornell Univ-Weil Med Coll

Medow, Norman MD (Ophthalmology) - *Special Expertise:* Cataract-Pediatric; Glaucoma; *Corneal Disease-Pediatric;* **Admitting Hospital:** Manhattan Eye, Ear & Throat Hospital; **Office Address:** 225 E 64th St, Ste 6 New York, NY 10021; **Office Phone:** (212) 644-5100; **Board Certification:** Ophthalmology 1975; **Medical School:** SUNY Hlth Sci Ctr 1966; **Residency:** Ophthalmology, Manhattan Eye, Ear & Throat Hosp, New York, NY 1969-1972; **Faculty Appointment:** Assoc Clin Prof Ophthalmology, Cornell Univ-Weil Med Coll

Metz, Henry MD (Ophthalmology) - *Special Expertise:* Ophthalmology-Pediatric; **Admitting Hospital:** Rochester General Hospital; **Office Address:** 1425 Portland Ave Rochester, NY 14621-3001; **Office Phone:** (716) 338-4787; **Board Certification:** Ophthalmology 1967; **Medical School:** SUNY Downstate 1961; **Residency:** Ophthalmology, Strong Meml Hosp, Rochester, NY 1962-1966; **Fellowship:** Strabismus, Smith-Kettlewell Inst Vis, San Franscico, CA 1968-1969

Miller, Neil MD (Ophthalmology) - *Special Expertise:* Neuro-Ophthalmology; **Admitting Hospital:** Johns Hopkins Hospital - Baltimore (Page 65); **Office Address:** Johns Hopkins - Wilmer Eye Inst 600 N Wolfe , Fl 109, MS 0 Baltimore, MD 21287-0001; **Office Phone:** (410) 955-8679; **Board Certification:** Ophthalmology 1976; **Medical School:** Johns Hopkins Univ 1971; **Residency:** Ophthalmology, Johns Hopkins Hosp, Baltimore, MD 1972-1975; **Fellowship:** Neurological Ophthalmology, UC San Francisco, San Francisco, CA 1975; **Faculty Appointment:** Prof Ophthalmology, Johns Hopkins Univ

Muldoon, Thomas O MD (Ophthalmology) - *Special Expertise:* Retina/Vitreous Surgery; *Macular Disease/Degeneration;* **Admitting Hospital:** New York Eye & Ear Infirmary (Page 71); **Office Address:** 310 E 14th St New York, NY 10003-4201; **Office Phone:** (212) 979-4595; **Board Certification:** Ophthalmology 1971; **Medical School:** Univ Rochester 1962; **Residencies:** Surgery, St Lukes Hosp, New York, NY 1965-1966; Ophthalmology, New York EE Infirm, New York, NY 1966-1969; **Fellowship:** Strabismus, New York EE Infirm, New York, NY 1969-1970; **Faculty Appointment:** Assoc Clin Prof Ophthalmology, NY Med Coll

Olitsky, Scott Eric MD (Ophthalmology) - *Special Expertise: Ophthalmology-Pediatric; Strabismus;* **Admitting Hospital:** The Children's Hospital of Buffalo; **Office Address:** Chldns Hosp, Dept Oph 219 Bryant, Ste 2C Buffalo, NY 14222; **Office Phone:** (716) 878-7567; **Board Certification:** Ophthalmology 1993; **Medical School:** Jefferson Med Coll 1988; **Residency:** Ophthalmology, SUNY Buffalo, Buffalo, NY 1989-1992; **Fellowship:** Pediatric Ophthalmology, Wills Eye Hosp, Philadelphia, PA 1992-1993; **Faculty Appointment:** Assoc Prof Ophthalmology, SUNY Buffalo

Parks, Marshall M MD (Ophthalmology) - *Special Expertise: Ophthalmology - General;* **Admitting Hospital:** Children's National Medical Center - DC; **Office Address:** 3400 Massachusettes Ave NW Washington, DC 20007-1445; **Office Phone:** (202) 338-3680; **Board Certification:** Ophthalmology 1951; **Medical School:** St Louis Univ 1943; **Residency:** Ophthalmology, Naval Med Ctr, San Diego, CA; **Faculty Appointment:** Clin Prof Ophthalmology, Geo Wash Univ

Podos, Steven M MD (Ophthalmology) - *Special Expertise: Glaucoma;* **Admitting Hospital:** Mount Sinai Hospital (Page 70); **Office Address:** 5 E 98th St New York, NY 10029-6501; **Office Phone:** (212) 241-6752; **Board Certification:** Ophthalmology 1968; **Medical School:** Harvard Med Sch 1962; **Residency:** Ophthalmology, Washington Univ-Barnes Hosp, St Louis, MO 1963-1967; **Faculty Appointment:** Prof Ophthalmology, Mount Sinai Sch Med

Quigley, Harry Alan MD (Ophthalmology) - *Special Expertise: Glaucoma;* **Admitting Hospital:** Johns Hopkins Hospital - Baltimore (Page 65); **Office Address:** Johns Hopkins-Wilmer Inst. 601 N Broadway St Baltimore, MD 21287-0001; **Office Phone:** (410) 955-6052; **Board Certification:** Ophthalmology 1976; **Medical School:** Johns Hopkins Univ 1971; **Residency:** Ophthalmology, Wilmer Inst-Johns Hopkins, Baltimore, MD 1972-1975; **Fellowship:** Ophthalmology, Bascom Palmer Eye Inst., Miami, FL 1975-1977; **Faculty Appointment:** Prof Ophthalmology, Johns Hopkins Univ

Quinn, Graham Earl MD (Ophthalmology) - *Special Expertise: Ophthalmology-Pediatric; Eye Growth/Development;* **Admitting Hospital:** The Children's Hospital of Philadelphia; **Office Address:** Children's Hospital of Philadelphia - Division of Ophthalmology 34th st & civiv center blvrd Philadelphia, PA 19104; **Office Phone:** (215) 590-4594; **Board Certification:** Ophthalmology 1979; **Medical School:** Duke Univ 1973; **Residencies:** Pathology, Cleveland Metro Genl Hosp 1974-1975; Ophthalmology, Univ Penn 1975-1978; **Fellowship:** Chldns Hosp Philadelphia, PA 1978-1979

Raab, Edward MD (Ophthalmology) - *Special Expertise: Ophthalmology-Pediatric; Strabismus; Glaucoma;* **Admitting Hospital:** Mount Sinai Hospital (Page 70); **Office Address:** 5 E 98th St, Fl 7 New York, NY 10029; **Office Phone:** (212) 369-0988; **Board Certification:** Ophthalmology 1966; **Medical School:** NYU Sch Med 1958; **Residency:** Mount Sinai, New York, NY 1964; **Fellowship:** Pediatric Ophthalmology, Children's Hosp, Washington, DC 1966-1967; **Faculty Appointment:** Prof Ophthalmology, Mount Sinai Sch Med

Reynolds, James D. MD (Ophthalmology) - *Special Expertise: Ophthalmology-Pediatric; Strabismus;* **Admitting Hospital:** The Children's Hospital of Buffalo; **Office Address:** Children's Hospital - Department of Ophthalmology 219 Bryant St Buffalo, NY 14222; **Office Phone:** (716) 878-7567; **Board Certification:** Ophthalmology; **Medical School:** SUNY Buffalo 1978; **Residency:** Erie CO Medical Center, Buffalo, NY 1978-1981; **Fellowship:** Ophthalmology, Pittsburgh EE Hospital 1981-1982; **Faculty Appointment:** Prof Ophthalmology, SUNY Buffalo

Ritch, Robert MD (Ophthalmology) - *Special Expertise:* Glaucoma; **Admitting Hospital:** New York Eye & Ear Infirmary (Page 71); **Office Address:** 310 E 14th St, Ste 304 New York, NY 10003-4201; **Office Phone:** (212) 477-7540; **Board Certification:** Ophthalmology 1977; **Medical School:** Albert Einstein Coll Med 1972; **Residency:** Ophthalmology, Mount Sinai Hosp, New York, NY 1973-1976; **Fellowship:** Glaucoma, Mount Sinai Hosp, New York, NY 1976-1978; **Faculty Appointment:** Clin Prof Ophthalmology, NY Med Coll

Rosen, Richard MD (Ophthalmology) - *Special Expertise:* Diabetic Eye Disease/Retinopathy; Macular Disease/Degeneration; **Admitting Hospital:** New York Eye & Ear Infirmary (Page 71); **Office Address:** NY Eye and Ear Infirm Fac Prac 310 E 14th St, Fl 3 - Ste 319 New York, NY 10003-4201; **Office Phone:** (212) 979-4288; **Board Certification:** Ophthalmology 1991; **Medical School:** Univ Miami Sch Med 1985; **Residency:** Ophthalmology, New York EE Infirm, New York, NY 1986-1989; **Fellowship:** Ophthalmology, New York EE Infirm, New York, NY 1989-1991

Savino, Peter MD (Ophthalmology) - *Special Expertise:* Neuro-Ophthalmology; **Admitting Hospital:** Wills Eye Hospital; **Office Address:** Wills Eye Hosp 900 Walnut St, Fl 2nd Philadelphia, PA 19107; **Office Phone:** (215) 928-3130; **Board Certification:** Ophthalmology 1975; **Medical School:** Italy 1968; **Residency:** Ophthalmology, Georgetown Med Ctr, Washington, DC 1970-1973; **Fellowship:** Neurological Ophthalmology, Bascom Palmer Eye Inst, Miami, FL 1973-1974

Sergott, Robert C MD (Ophthalmology) - *Special Expertise:* Neuro-Ophthalmology; **Admitting Hospital:** Wills Eye Hospital; **Office Address:** Wills Eye Hosp 900 Walnut St Philadelphia, PA 19107; **Office Phone:** (215) 928-3130; **Board Certification:** Ophthalmology 1982; **Medical School:** Johns Hopkins Univ 1975; **Residencies:** Internal Medicine, Mary Imogene Bassett Hospital, Cooperstown, NY 1975-1976; Ophthalmology, Jackson Memorial Hospital, Miami, FL 1979-1980; **Fellowship:** Ophthalmology, Jackson Memorial Hospital, Miami, FL 1979-1980

Shields, Jerry MD (Ophthalmology) - *Special Expertise:* Eye Tumors/Cancer; Ophthalmology-Pediatric; **Admitting Hospital:** Wills Eye Hospital; **Office Address:** 9th & Walnut Sts Philadelphia, PA 19107; **Office Phone:** (215) 928-3105; **Board Certification:** Ophthalmology 1972; **Medical School:** Univ Mich Med Sch 1964; **Residency:** Ophthalmology, Wills Eye Hosp, Philadelphia, PA 1967-1970; **Fellowship:** Ophthalmology, Wills Eye Hosp, Philadelphia, PA 1970-1972

Simon, John W MD (Ophthalmology) - *Special Expertise:* Ophthalmology-Pediatric; Strabismus; **Admitting Hospital:** Albany Medical Center; **Office Address:** Albany Med Ctr, Dept Ped Opth 35 Hackett Blvd Albany, NY 12208; **Office Phone:** (518) 262-2500; **Board Certification:** Ophthalmology 1981; **Medical School:** Mount Sinai Sch Med 1976; **Residency:** Ophthalmology, Mt Sinai Hosp, New York, NY 1977-1980; **Fellowship:** Pediatric Ophthalmology, Wills Eye Hosp, Philadelphia, PA 1980-1981; **Faculty Appointment:** Prof Ophthalmology, Albany Med Coll

Stark, Walter J MD (Ophthalmology) - *Special Expertise:* Corneal Disease & Transplant; Cataract Surgery; Refractive Surgery; **Admitting Hospital:** Johns Hopkins Hospital - Baltimore (Page 65); **Office Address:** Johns Hopkins Sch Med-Wilmer Opth Inst 600 N Wolfe St, Maumenee 327 Baltimore, MD 21287-9238; **Office Phone:** (410) 955-5490; **Board Certification:** Ophthalmology 1973; **Medical School:** Univ Okla Coll Med 1967; **Residency:** Ophthalmology, Wilmer Inst-Johns Hopkins, Baltimore, MD 1968-1971; **Faculty Appointment:** Prof Ophthalmology, Johns Hopkins Univ

Stern, Kathleen MD (Ophthalmology) - *Special Expertise:* Strabismus; Ophthalmology-Pediatric; **Admitting Hospital:** New York Methodist Hospital (Page 72); **Office Address:** 485 Park Ave New York, NY 10022-1228; **Office Phone:** (212) 753-6464; **Board Certification:** Ophthalmology 1983; **Medical School:** Harvard Med Sch 1978; **Residency:** Ophthalmology, Manhattan Eye, Ear & Throat Hosp, New York, NY 1979-1982; **Fellowship:** Neuropathology, NY Hosp, New York, NY 1982-1983; **Faculty Appointment:** Asst Clin Prof Ophthalmology, Cornell Univ-Weil Med Coll

Walsh, Joseph MD (Ophthalmology) - *Special Expertise:* Ophthalmology - General; **Admitting Hospital:** New York Eye & Ear Infirmary (Page 71); **Office Address:** 310 E 14th St, Bldg S - Fl 3 New York, NY 10003; **Office Phone:** (212) 979-4447; **Board Certification:** Ophthalmology 1976; **Medical School:** Georgetown Univ 1966; **Residencies:** New York Eye and Ear Infirmary, New York, NY 1970-1973; **Fellowship:** Montefiore Hosp Med Ctr, Bronx, NY 1973-1974; **Faculty Appointment:** Prof NY Med Coll

Wang, Frederick MD (Ophthalmology) - *Special Expertise:* Ophthalmology - General; **Admitting Hospital:** New York Eye & Ear Infirmary (Page 71); **Office Address:** 30 E 40th St, Ste 405 New York, NY 10016; **Office Phone:** (212) 684-3980; **Board Certification:** Ophthalmology 1980; **Residencies:** Pediatrics, Jacobi Med Ctr, Bronx, NY 1974; Ophthalmology, Albert Einstein, Bronx, NY 1979; **Fellowship:** Children's Hosp, Washington, DC 1980; **Faculty Appointment:** Clin Prof Albert Einstein Coll Med

Yannuzzi, Lawrence MD (Ophthalmology) - *Special Expertise:* Retina/Vitreous Surgery; Macular Disease/Degeneration; **Admitting Hospital:** Manhattan Eye, Ear & Throat Hospital; **Office Address:** Vitreous Retina Macula Consultants Of NY 519 E 72nd St, Ste 203 New York, NY 10021-4028; **Office Phone:** (212) 861-9797; **Board Certification:** Ophthalmology 1970; **Medical School:** Boston Univ 1964; **Residency:** Ophthalmology, Manhattan Eye, Ear & Throat Hosp, New York, NY 1965-1968; **Faculty Appointment:** Prof Ophthalmology, Columbia P&S

Zaidman, Gerald MD (Ophthalmology) - *Special Expertise:* Laser Vision Surgery; Cornea Transplant; **Admitting Hospital:** Westchester Medical Center; **Office Address:** Westchester Med Ctr Dept Opth, Rm 1100 - Macy Pavilion Valhalla, NY 10595; **Office Phone:** (914) 493-1599; **Board Certification:** Ophthalmology 1981; **Medical School:** Albert Einstein Coll Med 1975; **Residencies:** Geriatric Medicine, Beth Abraham Hosp, Westchester, NY 1976-1977; Ophthalmology, Lenox Hill Hosp, New York, NY 1977-1980; **Fellowship:** Univ of Pittsburgh, Pittsburgh, PA 1980-1982; **Faculty Appointment:** Assoc Prof Ophthalmology, NY Med Coll

Southeast

Aaberg Sr, Thomas Marshall MD (Ophthalmology) - *Special Expertise:* Retina/Vitreous Surgery; **Admitting Hospital:** Emory University Hospital; **Office Address:** Emory Eye Clinic, Dept Opth Clifton Rd NE, Ste 1365B Atlanta, GA 30322; **Office Phone:** (404) 778-4456; **Board Certification:** Ophthalmology 1967; **Medical School:** Harvard Med Sch 1961; **Residency:** Ophthalmology, Mass EE Infirm, Boston, MA 1962-1966; **Fellowship:** Bascom-Palmer Eye Inst Med, Miami, FL 1968-1969; **Faculty Appointment:** Prof Ophthalmology, Emory Univ

Alfonso, Eduardo MD (Ophthalmology) - *Special Expertise:* Corneal and External Eye Disease; **Admitting Hospital:** Anne Bates Leach Eye Hosp; **Office Address:** Bascom Palmer Eye Inst 900 NW 17th St Miami, FL 33136-1119; **Office Phone:** (305) 326-6366; **Board Certification:** Ophthalmology 1985; **Medical School:** Yale Univ 1980; **Residency:** Ophthalmology, Bascom Palmer Eye Inst-U Miami, Miami, FL 1981-1984; **Fellowships:** Ophthalmology, Mass Eye & Ear Hosp, Boston, MA 1984-1986; **Faculty Appointment:** Prof Ophthalmology, Univ Miami Sch Med

Anderson, Douglas R MD (Ophthalmology) - *Special Expertise:* Ophthalmology - General; **Admitting Hospital:** Anne Bates Leach Eye Hosp; **Office Address:** Bascom Palmer Eye Inst 900 NW 17th St Miami, FL 33136-1119; **Office Phone:** (305) 326-6146; **Board Certification:** Ophthalmology 1970; **Medical School:** Washington Univ, St Louis 1962; **Residency:** Ophthalmology, UCSF Hosp, San Francisco, CA 1965-1968; **Fellowship:** Ophthalmology, Mass Eye & Ear Infirm-Howe Lab, Boston, MA 1968-1969; **Faculty Appointment:** Prof Ophthalmology, Univ Miami Sch Med

Buckley, Edward G MD (Ophthalmology) - *Special Expertise:* Eye Diseases-Pediatric; *Strabismus;* **Admitting Hospital:** Duke University Medical Center (Page 60); **Office Address:** Duke Univ Med Ctr - Eye Ctr PO Box 3802 DUEC Durham, NC 27710; **Office Phone:** (919) 684-6084; **Board Certification:** Ophthalmology 1982; **Medical School:** Duke Univ 1977; **Residency:** Ophthalmology, Duke Univ Eye Ctr, Durham, NC 1978-1981; **Fellowship:** Ophthalmology, Bascom Palmer Eye Inst, Miami, FL 1981-1983; **Faculty Appointment:** Prof Ophthalmology, Duke Univ

Capo, Hilda MD (Ophthalmology) - *Special Expertise:* Ophthalmology-Pediatric; *Strabismus; Neuro-Ophthalmology;* **Admitting Hospital:** Anne Bates Leach Eye Hosp; **Office Address:** Bascom Plamer Eye Inst 900 NW 17th St Miami, FL 33136; **Office Phone:** (305) 326-6555; **Board Certification:** Ophthalmology 1989; **Medical School:** Puerto Rico 1982; **Residency:** Ophthalmology, Univ PR Med Sch, San Juan, Puerto Rico 1984-1987; **Fellowships:** Neurological Ophthalmology, NYU Med Ctr, New York, NY 1988-1989; Pediatric Ophthalmology, Johns Hopkins Hosp, Baltimore, MD 1987-1988; **Faculty Appointment:** Asst Clin Prof Ophthalmology, Univ Miami Sch Med

Culbertson, William MD (Ophthalmology) - *Special Expertise:* Refractive Surgery-LASIK; *Corneal Disease;* **Admitting Hospital:** Anne Bates Leach Eye Hosp; **Office Address:** Bascom Palmer Eye Inst 900 NW 17th St Miami, FL 33136-1119; **Office Phone:** (305) 326-6364; **Board Certification:** Ophthalmology 1976; **Medical School:** Emory Univ 1970; **Residency:** Ophthalmology, Vanderbilt Univ Hosp, Nashville, TN 1971-1974; **Fellowship:** Ophthalmology, Bascom Palmer Eye Inst, Miami, FL 1978-1979; **Faculty Appointment:** Prof Ophthalmology, Univ Miami Sch Med

Driebe Jr, William T MD (Ophthalmology) - *Special Expertise:* Cornea Transplant; Lens *Implant Complications;* **Admitting Hospital:** Shands Healthcare at University Florida (Page 77); **Office Address:** Shands Hlthcare Univ FL 1600 SW Archer Rd Gainesville, FL 32610-0284; **Office Phone:** (352) 392-3451; **Board Certification:** Ophthalmology 1984; **Medical School:** Univ VA Sch Med 1979; **Residency:** Ophthalmology, Shands Hlthcare Univ FL, Gainesville, FL 1980-1983; **Fellowship:** Bascom Palmer Eye Inst, Miami, FL 1983-1984; **Faculty Appointment:** Prof Ophthalmology, Univ Fla Coll Med

Fagien, Steven MD (Ophthalmology) - *Special Expertise:* Oculoplastic Surgery; **Admitting Hospital:** Boca Raton Community Hosp; **Office Address:** Boca Raton Ctr for Oph 1000 NW 9th Ct, Ste 104 Boca Raton, FL 33486-2268; **Office Phone:** (561) 393-9898; **Board Certification:** Ophthalmology 1988; **Medical School:** Univ Fla Coll Med 1983; **Residency:** Ophthalmology, Univ IL Michael Reese Hosp, Chicago, IL 1987-1988; **Fellowship:** Ophthalmology, Shands Hosp - Univ FL, Gainesville, FL 1984-1987; **Faculty Appointment:** Assoc Clin Prof Ophthalmology, Univ Fla Coll Med

Flynn, Harry W MD (Ophthalmology) - *Special Expertise: Retina/Vitreous Surgery; Diabetic Eye Disease/Retinopathy;* **Admitting Hospital:** Anne Bates Leach Eye Hosp; **Office Address:** 900 NW 17th St Miami, FL 33136-1119; **Office Phone:** (305) 326-6118; **Board Certification:** Ophthalmology 1976; **Medical School:** Univ VA Sch Med 1971; **Residency:** Ophthalmology, Univ VA Hosp, Charlottesville, VA 1972-1975; **Fellowship:** Retina, Pacific Med Ctr, San Francisco, CA 1975-1976; **Faculty Appointment:** Prof Ophthalmology, Univ Miami Sch Med

Forster, Richard K MD (Ophthalmology) - *Special Expertise: Cornea Transplant; Cataract Surgery;* **Admitting Hospital:** Anne Bates Leach Eye Hosp; **Office Address:** 900 NW 17th St Miami, FL 33125; **Office Phone:** (305) 326-6373; **Board Certification:** Ophthalmology 1971; **Medical School:** Boston Univ 1963; **Residency:** Ophthalmology, Bascom Palmer Eye Inst, Miami, FL 1966-1969; **Faculty Appointment:** Prof Ophthalmology, Univ Miami Sch Med

Freedman, Sharon MD (Ophthalmology) - *Special Expertise: Ophthalmology-Pediatric; Glaucoma-Congenital/Pediatric;* **Admitting Hospital:** Duke University Medical Center (Page 60); **Office Address:** Duke Eye Center Erwin Rd Durham, NC 27710; **Office Phone:** (919) 684-4584; **Board Certification:** Ophthalmology 1991; **Medical School:** Harvard Med Sch 1985; **Residency:** Ophthalmology, Chldns Hosp., Boston, MA 1986-1989; **Fellowships:** Duke Eye Ctr., Durham, NC 1990-1992; Chldns Hosp., Boston, MA 1989-1990; **Faculty Appointment:** Asst Prof Ophthalmology, Duke Univ

Gass, James Donald MD (Ophthalmology) - *Special Expertise: Retinal Disorders;* **Admitting Hospital:** Vanderbilt University Medical Center; **Office Address:** Vanderbilt Univ, Dept Oph, MC-E 2115 21st Ave S Nashville, TN 37232-8808; **Office Phone:** (615) 936-2100; **Board Certification:** Ophthalmology 1963; **Medical School:** Vanderbilt Univ 1957; **Residencies:** Ophthalmology, Wilmer Inst-Johns Hopkins, Baltimore, MD 1962-1963; Ophthalmology, Wilmer Inst-Johns Hopkins, Baltimore, MD 1958-1961; **Fellowship:** Ophthalmic Pathology, Armed Forces Institute 1961-1962; **Faculty Appointment:** Prof Ophthalmology, Vanderbilt Univ

Gills Jr, James P MD (Ophthalmology) - *Special Expertise: Ophthalmology - General;* **Admitting Hospital:** Helen Ellis Memorial Hospital, Fl; **Office Address:** St Luke's Cataract and Laser Inst 43309 US Highway 19 N Tarpon Springs, FL 34689-6221; **Office Phone:** (727) 938-2020; **Board Certification:** Ophthalmology 1967; **Medical School:** Duke Univ 1959; **Residency:** Ophthalmology, Johns Hopkins Hosp, Baltimore, MD 1962-1965

Glaser, Joel MD (Ophthalmology) - *Special Expertise: Neuro-Ophthalmology; Orbital Diseases;* **Admitting Hospital:** Mercy Hospital - Miami; **Office Address:** 4121 Crawford Ave Miami, FL 33133-6160; **Office Phone:** (305) 661-2147; **Board Certification:** Ophthalmology 1968; **Medical School:** Duke Univ 1963; **Residency:** Ophthalmology, Univ Miami, Miami, FL 1964-1967; **Fellowship:** Neurological Ophthalmology, UC San Francisco, San Francisco, CA 1969; **Faculty Appointment:** Prof Ophthalmology, Univ Miami Sch Med

Haik, Barrett MD (Ophthalmology) - *Special Expertise: Eye Tumors/Cancer;* **Admitting Hospital:** St Jude Children's Research Hospital; **Office Address:** 920 Madison Ave, Ste 915 Memphis, TN 38103; **Office Phone:** (901) 448-6650; **Board Certification:** Ophthalmology 1981; **Medical School:** Louisiana State Univ 1976; **Residency:** Ophthalmology, Columbia-Presby Harkness Eye Inst, New York, NY 1977-1980; **Faculty Appointment:** Prof Ophthalmology, Univ Tenn Coll Med, Memphis

Hess, J Bruce MD (Ophthalmology) - *Special Expertise: Ophthalmology-Pediatric; Strabismus;* **Admitting Hospital:** All Children's Hospital; **Office Address:** 880 6th St S, Ste 350 St Petersburg, FL 33701; **Office Phone:** (727) 892-4393; **Board Certification:** Ophthalmology 1978; **Medical School:** Baylor Coll Med 1971; **Residencies:** Ophthalmology, Geisinger Med Ctr, Danville, PA 1974-1977; Ophthalmology, Wills Eye Hosp, Philadelphia, PA 1977-1978

Holliday, James N MD/PhD (Ophthalmology) - *Special Expertise: Corneal Disease;* **Admitting Hospital:** Methodist Healthcare Central - Memphis Hospital; **Office Address:** Holliday Vision Ctr 1795 N Germantown Pkwy Cordova, TN 38018; **Office Phone:** (901) 759-9757; **Board Certification:** Ophthalmology 1994; **Medical School:** Duke Univ 1987; **Residency:** Ophthalmology, UC Irvine, Orange, CA 1989-1992; **Fellowship:** Anterior Segment - External Disease, Mayo Clinic, Rochester, MN 1992-1993

Lambert, Scott MD (Ophthalmology) - *Special Expertise: Ophthalmology-Pediatric; Retinal Disorders;* **Admitting Hospital:** Emory University Hospital; **Office Address:** Emory Eye Ctr, Dept Ped Opth 1365B Clifton Rd Ste 4500 Atlanta, GA 30322; **Office Phone:** (404) 778-7777; **Board Certification:** Ophthalmology 1989; **Medical School:** Yale Univ 1983; **Residency:** Ophthalmology, UCSF, San Francisco, CA 1984-1987; **Fellowship:** Pediatric Ophthalmology, Hosp Sick Chldn, London, UK 1987-1988; **Faculty Appointment:** Assoc Prof Ophthalmology, Emory Univ

Lee, Paul P MD (Ophthalmology) - *Special Expertise: Glaucoma;* **Admitting Hospital:** Duke University Medical Center (Page 60); **Office Address:** Duke Univ Eye Ctr, Erwin Rd, Wadsworth Bldg, Box 3802, Durham, NC 27710; **Office Phone:** (919) 681-2793; **Board Certification:** Ophthalmology 1991; **Medical School:** Univ Mich Med Sch 1986; **Residency:** Ophthalmology, Wilmer Eye Inst/Johns Hopkins, Baltimore, MD 1987-1990; **Fellowship:** Glaucoma, Mass EE Infirm., Boston, MA 1990-1991; **Faculty Appointment:** Prof Ophthalmology, Duke Univ

McCord, Clinton MD (Ophthalmology) - *Special Expertise: Eyelid Surgery; Oculoplastic Surgery;* **Admitting Hospital:** Piedmont Hospital; **Office Address:** 3200 Dunwoody Cir, Ste 640 Atlanta, GA 30327; **Office Phone:** (404) 351-0051; **Board Certification:** Ophthalmology 1968; **Medical School:** Emory Univ 1961; **Fellowship:** Oculoplatic Surgery, Man Eye&Ear Inst, New York, NY 1966-1967

Palmberg, Paul MD/PhD (Ophthalmology) - *Special Expertise: Glaucoma;* **Admitting Hospital:** Anne Bates Leach Eye Hosp; **Office Address:** Bascom Palmer Eye Inst 900 NW 17th St Miami, FL 33101-6880; **Office Phone:** (305) 326-6386; **Board Certification:** Ophthalmology 1976; **Medical School:** Northwestern Univ 1970; **Residencies:** Ophthalmology, Washington Univ, St Louis, MO 1971-1974; Ophthalmology, Barnes Hosp, St Louis, MO 1976-1977; **Fellowship:** Glaucoma, Univ Washington, St Louis, MO 1974-1976; **Faculty Appointment:** Prof Ophthalmology, Univ Miami Sch Med

Parrish, Richard K MD (Ophthalmology) - *Special Expertise: Glaucoma;* **Admitting Hospital:** Anne Bates Leach Eye Hosp; **Office Address:** 900 NW 17th St, Fl 4th Miami, FL 33136; **Office Phone:** (305) 326-6389; **Board Certification:** Ophthalmology 1981; **Medical School:** Indiana Univ 1976; **Residency:** Ophthalmology, Wills Eye Hosp, Philadelphia, PA 1977-1980; **Fellowship:** Ophthalmology, Bascom Palmer Eye Inst, Miami, FL 1980-1982; **Faculty Appointment:** Prof Ophthalmology, Univ Miami Sch Med

Pollard, Zane F MD (Ophthalmology) - *Special Expertise: Ophthalmology-Pediatric; Strabismus;* **Admitting Hospital:** Children's Healthcare of Atlanta at Scottish Rite; **Office Address:** Eye Consultants of Atlanta 5455 Meridian Mark Rd, Ste 220 Atlanta, GA 30342; **Office Phone:** (404) 255-2419; **Board Certification:** Ophthalmology 1975; **Medical School:** Tufts Univ 1966; **Residencies:** Surgery, UC San Francisco, San Francisco, CA 1967-1968; Ophthalmology, USC, Los Angeles, CA 1970-1973; **Fellowship:** Pediatric Ophthalmology, Wills Eye Hosp, Philadelphia, PA 1974-1975

Pollock, Stephen MD (Ophthalmology) - *Special Expertise: Neuro-Ophthalmology; Optic Nerve Disorders;* **Admitting Hospital:** Duke University Medical Center (Page 60); **Office Address:** Duke University Eye Center Box 3802 Durham, NC 27710-3802; **Office Phone:** (919) 684-4417; **Board Certification:** Ophthalmology 1986; **Medical School:** Univ IL Coll Med 1981; **Residency:** Ophthalmology, U Ill EE Infirm., Chicago, IL 1982-1987; **Fellowship:** Ophthalmology, Wilmer Inst./Johns Hopkins, Baltimore, MD 1985-1986; **Faculty Appointment:** Assoc Prof Ophthalmology, Duke Univ

Sternberg Jr, Paul MD (Ophthalmology) - *Special Expertise: Retina/Vitreous Surgery; Macular Disease/Degeneration;* **Admitting Hospital:** Emory University Hospital; **Office Address:** Thomas Eye Group 5671 Peachtree Dunwoody Rd NE, rm 400 Atlanta, GA 30342; **Office Phone:** (404) 256-1507; **Board Certification:** Ophthalmology 1985; **Medical School:** Univ Chicago-Pritzker Sch Med 1979; **Residency:** Ophthalmology, Johns Hopkins Hosp, Baltimore, MD 1980-1983; **Fellowship:** Vitreoretinal Surgery, Duke Univ, Durham, NC 1983-1984; **Faculty Appointment:** Prof Ophthalmology, Emory Univ

Stulting, R. Doyle MD (Ophthalmology) - *Special Expertise: Corneal Disease & Transplant; Refractive Surgery-Laser; Cataract Surgery;* **Admitting Hospital:** Emory University Hospital; **Office Address:** Emory Eye Clinic 1365B Clifton Rd NE Atlanta, GA 30322; **Office Phone:** (404) 778-5818; **Board Certification:** Ophthalmology 1982; **Medical School:** Duke Univ 1976; **Residencies:** Internal Medicine, Barnes Hosp, St Louis, MO 1976-1978; Ophthalmology, Bascom Palmer Eye Inst, Miami, FL 1978-1981; **Fellowship:** Cornea, Emory Univ Clinic, Atlanta, GA 1981-1982; **Faculty Appointment:** Prof Ophthalmology, Emory Univ

Tse, David MD (Ophthalmology) - *Special Expertise: Oculoplastic & Orbital Surgery; Eye Lid Repair; Lacrimal Gland Disorders;* **Admitting Hospital:** Anne Bates Leach Eye Hosp; **Office Address:** Bascom Palmer Eye Inst 900 NW 17th St Miami, FL 33136-1119; **Office Phone:** (305) 326-6086; **Board Certification:** Ophthalmology 1983; **Medical School:** Univ Miami Sch Med 1976; **Residency:** Ophthalmology, LAC/USC Med Ctr, Los Angeles, CA 1979-1981; **Fellowship:** Oculoplatic Surgery, Univ Iowa, Iowa City, IA 1981-1982

Waring III, George Oral MD (Ophthalmology) - *Special Expertise: Cataract Surgery; Cornea Transplant; Refractive Surgery-LASIK;* **Admitting Hospital:** Emory University Hospital; **Office Address:** Emory Eye Clinic, Dept Oph 1365-B Clifton Rd NE Atlanta, GA 30322; **Office Phone:** (404) 778-4190; **Board Certification:** Ophthalmology 1975; **Medical School:** Baylor Coll Med 1967; **Residency:** Ophthalmology, Wills Eye Hosp, Philadelphia, PA 1970-1973; **Fellowship:** Cornea External Disease, Wills Eye Hosp, Philadelphia, PA 1972-1974; **Faculty Appointment:** Prof Ophthalmology, Emory Univ

Midwest

Abrams, Gary W MD (Ophthalmology) - *Special Expertise: Retina/Vitreous Surgery;* **Admitting Hospital:** Harper Hospital (Page 59); **Office Address:** Kresge Eye Institute 4717 St Antoine St Detroit, MI 48201; **Office Phone:** (313) 577-8900; **Board Certification:** Ophthalmology 1977; **Medical School:** Univ Okla Coll Med 1965; **Residency:** Ophthalmology, Med Coll Wisc, Milwaukee, WI 1973-1976; **Fellowship:** Vitreoretinal Surgery, Bascom Palmer Eye Inst, Miami, FL 1976-1978; **Faculty Appointment:** Prof Ophthalmology, Wayne State Univ

OPHTHALMOLOGY

Albert, Daniel M. MD (Ophthalmology) - *Special Expertise:* Eye Tumors/Cancer; Ophthalmic Pathology; **Admitting Hospital:** University of Wisconsin Hospital & Clinics; **Office Address:** U Wisc Med Sch-Dept. Ophthalmology and Visual Sciences 600 Highland Ave, Bldg CSC - Ste F4 - rm 336 Madison, WI 53792; **Office Phone:** (608) 636-6070; **Board Certification:** Ophthalmology 1969; **Medical School:** Penn State Univ-Hershey Med Ctr 1962; **Residencies:** Ophthalmology, University of Penn, Philadelphia, PA 1963-1966; Neurological Ophthalmology, Natl Inst Hlth, Bethesda, MD 1966-1968; **Fellowship:** Pathology, Natl Inst Hlth, Bethesda, MD 1968-1969; **Faculty Appointment:** Prof Ophthalmology, Univ Wisc

Alward, Wallace MD (Ophthalmology) - *Special Expertise:* Glaucoma; **Admitting Hospital:** University of Iowa Hospitals and Clinics; **Office Address:** 200 Hawkins Drive Iowa City, IA 52242; **Office Phone:** (319) 356-3938; **Board Certification:** Ophthalmology 1987; **Medical School:** Ohio State Univ 1976; **Residency:** Ophthalmology, Univ Louisville, Louisville, KY 1983-1986; **Fellowship:** Ophthalmology, Univ Miami-Bascom Palmer Eye, Miami, FL 1986-1987; **Faculty Appointment:** Prof Ophthalmology, Univ Iowa Coll Med

Archer, Steven M MD (Ophthalmology) - *Special Expertise:* Ophthalmology-Pediatric; **Admitting Hospital:** University of Michigan Health Center; **Office Address:** Univ Mich-W K Kellog Eye Ctr 1000 Wall St Ann Arbor, MI 48105-1912; **Office Phone:** (734) 764-7558; **Board Certification:** Ophthalmology 1986; **Medical School:** Univ Chicago-Pritzker Sch Med 1978; **Residency:** Ophthalmology, Univ Chicago, Chicago, IL 1981-1984; **Fellowship:** Pediatric Ophthalmology, Indiana Univ, Indianapolis, IN 1984-1986; **Faculty Appointment:** Asst Prof Ophthalmology, Univ Mich Med Sch

Baker, John D MD (Ophthalmology) - *Special Expertise:* Ophthalmology-Pediatric; **Admitting Hospital:** Children's Hospital of Michigan; **Office Address:** 2355 Monroe Blvd Dearborn, MI 48124; **Office Phone:** (313) 561-1777; **Board Certification:** Ophthalmology 1974; **Medical School:** Wayne State Univ 1967; **Residency:** Detroit General Hospital, Detroit, MI 1968-1971; **Fellowship:** Pediatrics, Childrens Hospital DC, Washington, DC 1972; **Faculty Appointment:** Assoc Clin Prof Medicine, Wayne State Univ

Burke, Miles Joseph MD (Ophthalmology) - *Special Expertise:* Ophthalmology-Pediatric; Eye Muscle Disorders-Adult; Amblyopia; **Admitting Hospital:** Children's Hospital Medical Center; **Office Address:** 10475 Montgomery Rd, Ste 4F Cincinnati, OH 45242-5200; **Office Phone:** (513) 984-4949; **Board Certification:** Ophthalmology 1979; **Medical School:** Univ Ariz Coll Med 1974; **Residency:** Ophthalmology, U Michigan, Ann Arbor, MI 1975-1978; **Fellowship:** Wills Eye Hosp, Philadelphia, PA 1978-1979; **Faculty Appointment:** Assoc Prof Ophthalmology, Univ Cincinnati

Cibis, Gerhard W MD (Ophthalmology) - *Special Expertise:* Ophthalmology-Pediatric; Strabismus; **Admitting Hospital:** Children's Mercy Hospital & Clinics; **Office Address:** 4620 J C Nichols Pkwy, Ste 421 Kansas, MO 64112; **Office Phone:** (816) 561-0306; **Board Certification:** Ophthalmology 1976; **Medical School:** Washington Univ, St Louis 1968; **Residencies:** Ophthalmology, Univ Iowa, Iowa City, IA 1972-1975; Ophthalmology, Univ Iowa, Iowa City, IA 1969-1970; **Fellowship:** Pediatric Ophthalmology, Univ Miami 1976-1977; **Faculty Appointment:** Clin Prof Ophthalmology, Univ Kans

Del Monte, Monte A MD (Ophthalmology) - *Special Expertise:* Ophthalmology-Pediatric; **Admitting Hospital:** University of Michigan Health Center; **Office Address:** Univ Mich Hosp-W K Kellogg Eye Ctr 1000 Wall St Ann Arbor, MI 48105-1912; **Office Phone:** (734) 764-3111; **Board Certification:** Ophthalmology 1982; **Medical School:** Johns Hopkins Univ 1974; **Residencies:** Pediatrics, Chldns Hosp Med Ctr, Boston, MA 1975-1977; Ophthalmology, Wilmer Eye Inst, Baltimore, MD 1978-1981; **Fellowships:** Ophthalmology, Wilmer Eye Inst, Baltimore, MD 1977-1978; Pediatric Ophthalmology, Chldns Hosp, Washington, DC 1981

Farrell, Thomas A. MD (Ophthalmology) - *Special Expertise: Cataract Surgery;* **Admitting Hospital:** University of Wisconsin Hospital & Clinics; **Office Address:** 2870 University Ave, Ste 102 Madison, WI 53705; **Office Phone:** (608) 263-7171; **Board Certification:** Ophthalmology 1972; **Medical School:** McGill Univ 1961; **Residency:** Ophthalmology, Mass EE infirm, Boston, MA 1967-1970; **Faculty Appointment:** Assoc Prof Ophthalmology, Univ Wisc

Feder, Robert S MD (Ophthalmology) - *Special Expertise: Corneal Disease; Refractive Surgery-LASIK; Cataract Surgery;* **Admitting Hospital:** Northwestern Memorial Hospital; **Office Address:** 675 N St Clair, Fl 15 Chicago, IL 60611; **Office Phone:** (312) 695-8150; **Board Certification:** Ophthalmology 1983; **Medical School:** Northwestern Univ 1978; **Residency:** Ophthalmology, Barnes Hosp-Wash Univ, St Louis, MO 1979-1982; **Fellowship:** Cornea, Univ IA, Iowa City, IA 1982-1983; **Faculty Appointment:** Assoc Prof Ophthalmology, Northwestern Univ

France, Thomas D MD (Ophthalmology) - *Special Expertise: Ophthalmology-Pediatric; Strabismus; Vision Development;* **Admitting Hospital:** University of Wisconsin Hospital & Clinics; **Office Address:** Univ Station Clinics, Dept Oph 2880 University Ave Madison, WI 53705; **Office Phone:** (608) 263-6414; **Board Certification:** Ophthalmology 1971; **Medical School:** Northwestern Univ 1962; **Residency:** Ophthalmology, UCSF, San Francisco, CA 1966-1969; **Fellowships:** Pediatric Ophthalmology, DC Chldns Hosp, Washington, DC 1969-1970; Pediatric Ophthalmology, Hosp for Sick Chldn, London, England 1970; **Faculty Appointment:** Prof Ophthalmology, Univ Wisc

Holland, Edward J. MD (Ophthalmology) - *Special Expertise: Corneal Disease; Refractive Surgery; Cataract Surgery;* **Admitting Hospital:** University Hospital - Cincinnati; **Office Address:** Cincinnati Eye Inst 10494 Montgomery Rd Cincinnati, OH 55455-0501; **Office Phone:** (800) 544-5133; **Board Certification:** Ophthalmology 1986; **Medical School:** Loyola Univ-Stritch Sch Med 1981; **Residencies:** Ophthalmology, Univ Minn Med Ctr, Minneapolis, MN 1982-1985; Ophthalmology, Univ Iowa, Iowa City, IA 1985-1986; **Fellowship:** Ocular Immunology, Natl Eye Inst, Bethesda, MD 1986-1987; **Faculty Appointment:** Clin Prof Ophthalmology, Univ Cincinnati

Kass, Michael A MD (Ophthalmology) - *Special Expertise: Glaucoma;* **Admitting Hospital:** Barnes - Jewish Hospital; **Office Address:** 660 S Euclid Ave St Louis, MO 63110-1010; **Office Phone:** (314) 362-3937; **Board Certification:** Ophthalmology 1974; **Medical School:** Northwestern Univ 1966; **Residency:** Ophthalmology, Washington Univ Med Ctr, St Louis, MO 1969-1972; **Fellowship:** Glaucoma, Washington Univ Med Ctr, St Louis, MO 1972-1973; **Faculty Appointment:** Prof Ophthalmology, Washington Univ, St Louis

Krachmer, Jay H. MD (Ophthalmology) - *Special Expertise: Corneal Disease;* **Admitting Hospital:** Fairview-University Medical Center - University Campus; **Office Address:** Univ Minn Med Sch, Dept Oph 420 Delaware St SE, Box 493 Minneapolis, MN 55455; **Office Phone:** (612) 625-4400; **Board Certification:** Ophthalmology 1972; **Medical School:** Tulane Univ 1966; **Residency:** Ophthalmology, Univ Hosp, Iowa City, IA 1967-1970; **Faculty Appointment:** Prof Ophthalmology, Univ Minn

Krueger, Ronald MD (Ophthalmology) - *Special Expertise: Corneal Disease; Refractive Surgery;* **Admitting Hospital:** Cleveland Clinic Foundation; **Office Address:** Cole Eye Institute,Cleveland Clinic Foundation 9500 Euclid Ave, Ste i-32 Cleveland, OH 44195; **Office Phone:** (216) 444-8158; **Board Certification:** Ophthalmology 1992; **Medical School:** UMDNJ-NJ Med Sch, Newark 1987; **Residency:** Colombia Presby Med Ctr, New York, NY 1988-1991; **Fellowships:** U So. Calif Dohery Eye Inst, Los Angeles, CA 1992-1993; U Okla Hlth Sci Ctr Dean A. McGee Eye Ins., Oklahoma City, OK 1991; **Faculty Appointment:** Asst Prof Ophthalmology, St Louis Univ

Kushner, Burton J MD (Ophthalmology) - *Special Expertise: Ophthalmology-Pediatric; Optics;* **Admitting Hospital:** University of Wisconsin Hospital & Clinics; **Office Address:** Univ Wisc, Dept Ped Oph 2870 University Ave, Ste 206 Madison, WI 53705-3611; **Office Phone:** (608) 263-6414; **Board Certification:** Ophthalmology 1975; **Medical School:** Northwestern Univ 1969; **Residency:** Ophthalmology, Univ Wisc Hosp, Madison, WI 1970-1973; **Fellowship:** Ophthalmology, Bascom Palmer Eye Inst, Miami, FL 1973-1974; **Faculty Appointment:** Prof Ophthalmology, Univ Wisc

Lewis, Hilel MD (Ophthalmology) - *Special Expertise: Retina/Vitreous Surgery;* **Admitting Hospital:** Cleveland Clinic Foundation; **Office Address:** Cleveland Clinic Fdn 9500 Euclid Ave Cleveland, OH 44195-0001; **Office Phone:** (216) 444-0430; **Board Certification:** Ophthalmology 1990; **Medical School:** Mexico 1980; **Residency:** Ophthalmology, Jules Stein Eye Inst-UCLA, Los Angeles, CA 1983-1986; **Fellowships:** Ocular Pathology, Jules Stein Eye Inst-UCLA, Los Angeles, CA 1982-1983; Vitreoretinal Surgery, Med Coll Wisc, Milwaukee, WI 1986-1987; **Faculty Appointment:** Assoc Prof Ophthalmology, UCLA

Lichter, Paul R. MD (Ophthalmology) - *Special Expertise: Cataract Surgery; Glaucoma;* **Admitting Hospital:** University of Michigan Health Center; **Office Address:** 1000 Wall St, rm 740, Box 0714 W.K Kellogg Eye Ctr. Ann Arbor, MI 48105-1912; **Office Phone:** (734) 763-5874; **Board Certification:** Ophthalmology 1970; **Medical School:** Univ Mich Med Sch 1964; **Residency:** Ophthalmology, U Mich. Med Ctr., Ann Arbor, MI 1965-1968; **Fellowship:** Ophthalmology, UC San Francisco, San Francisco, CA 1968-1969; **Faculty Appointment:** Prof Ophthalmology, Univ Mich Med Sch

Lindstrom, Richard Lyndon MD (Ophthalmology) - *Special Expertise: Corneal Disease; Cataract Surgery; Refractive Surgery;* **Admitting Hospital:** Phillips Eye Institute; **Office Address:** 710 E 24th St, Ste 106 Minneapolis, MN 55404-3810; **Office Phone:** (800) 526-7632; **Board Certification:** Ophthalmology 1978; **Medical School:** Univ Minn 1972; **Residencies:** Ophthalmology, U Minn, Minneapolis, MN 1978-1979; U Minn, Minneapolis, MN 1974-1978; **Fellowships:** Univ Hosp, Salt Lake City, UT; Mary Shields Eye Hosp, Dallas, TX; **Faculty Appointment:** Prof Ophthalmology, Univ Minn

Meredith, Travis MD (Ophthalmology) - *Special Expertise: Retina/Vitreous Surgery;* **Admitting Hospital:** Barnes - Jewish Hospital; **Office Address:** One Barnes Hosp Plaza, Fl 17413 St. Louis, MO 63110-1036; **Office Phone:** (314) 367-1181; **Board Certification:** Ophthalmology 1976; **Medical School:** Johns Hopkins Univ 1969; **Residencies:** Wilmer Inst-Johns Hopkins, Baltimore, MD 1970-1971; Wilmer Inst-Johns Hopkins, Baltimore, MD 1973-1975; **Fellowship:** Med Coll Wisc, Milwaukee, WI 1975-1976; **Faculty Appointment:** Clin Prof Ophthalmology, Univ Wash

Mets, Marilyn MD (Ophthalmology) - *Special Expertise: Ophthalmology-Pediatric; Ophthalmology-Genetics;* **Admitting Hospital:** Children's Memorial Hospital; **Office Address:** Chldns Meml Hosp 2300 Children's Plaza Chicago, IL 60614; **Office Phone:** (773) 880-4000; **Board Certification:** Ophthalmology 1981; **Medical School:** Geo Wash Univ 1976; **Residency:** Ophthalmology, Cleveland Clinic Fdn, Cleveland, OH 1977-1980; **Fellowship:** Ophthalmology, Natl Chldns Hosp, Washington, DC 1980-1981; **Faculty Appointment:** Assoc Prof Ophthalmology, Northwestern Univ

Miller, Marilyn T MD (Ophthalmology) - *Special Expertise: Eye Diseases-Hereditary; Ophthalmology-Pediatric;* **Admitting Hospital:** University of Illinois @ Chicago Eye & Ear; **Office Address:** University-Illinois At Chicago 1855 W Taylor St, rm 205 Chicago, IL 60612-7242; **Office Phone:** (312) 996-7445; **Board Certification:** Ophthalmology 1966; **Medical School:** Univ IL Coll Med 1959; **Residencies:** Ophthalmology, U IL Hosps, Chicago, IL 1961-1964; IL Eye & E, Chicago, IL 1964; **Fellowship:** Ophthalmology, IL Eye & E, Chicago, IL 1965-1967; **Faculty Appointment:** Prof Ophthalmology, Univ IL Coll Med

Nussbaum, Julian MD (Ophthalmology) - *Special Expertise: Diabetic Eye Disease/Retinopathy; Macular Degeneration;* **Admitting Hospital:** Henry Ford Health System (Page 62); **Office Address:** 2799 W Grand Blvd Detroit, MI 48202; **Office Phone:** (313) 916-8695; **Board Certification:** Ophthalmology 1981; **Medical School:** Univ Miami Sch Med 1976; **Residencies:** Internal Medicine, Jackson Memorial, Miami, FL 1976-1977; Ophthalmology, Medical College Of Georgia, Augusta, GA 1977-1980; **Fellowships:** Ophthalmology, Retina Foundation, Boston, MA 1980-1982; Ophthalmology, Mass Eye & Ear, Boston, MA 1980-1982

Pepose, Jay MD (Ophthalmology) - *Special Expertise: Refractive Surgery-LASIK; Glaucoma; Corneal and External Eye Disease;* **Admitting Hospital:** Barnes - Jewish Hospital; **Office Address:** 16216 Baxter Rd, Ste 205 Chesterfield, MO 63017; **Office Phone:** (636) 728-0111; **Board Certification:** Ophthalmology 1989; **Medical School:** UCLA 1982; **Residency:** Ophthalmology, Johns Hopkins Hospital, Baltimore, MD 1984-1987; **Fellowship:** Georgetown U Med Ctr, Washington, DC 1987-1988; **Faculty Appointment:** Prof Ophthalmology, Washington Univ, St Louis

Price, Ronald MD (Ophthalmology) - *Special Expertise: Ophthalmology-Pediatric; Eye Muscle Disorders (Strabismus);* **Admitting Hospital:** University Hospital - Cleveland; **Office Address:** Univ Ophth Assocs 1611 S Green Rd, Ste 306-C Cleveland, OH 44121; **Office Phone:** (216) 382-8022; **Board Certification:** Ophthalmology 1971; **Medical School:** Columbia P&S 1965; **Residency:** Internal Medicine, Univ Louisville Hosps, Louisville, KY 1966-1970; **Fellowship:** Pediatric Ophthalmology, DC Chldns Hosp, Washington, DC 1970-1971; **Faculty Appointment:** Asst Clin Prof Ophthalmology, Case West Res Univ

Putterman, Allen M. MD (Ophthalmology) - *Special Expertise: Oculoplastic Surgery;* **Admitting Hospital:** Michael Reese Hospital & Medical Center; **Office Address:** 111 N Wabash Ave, Ste 1722 Chicago, IL 60602-2002; **Office Phone:** (312) 372-2256; **Board Certification:** Ophthalmology 1971; **Medical School:** Univ Wisc 1963; **Residency:** Ophthalmology, Michael reese Hosp, Chicago, IL 1966-1969; **Fellowship:** Oculoplatic Surgery, Manhattan EE infirm., New York, NY 1969-1970; **Faculty Appointment:** Prof Ophthalmology, Univ IL Coll Med

Rogers, Gary L MD (Ophthalmology) - *Special Expertise: Strabismus (Adult & Pediatric);* **Admitting Hospital:** Children's Hospital; **Office Address:** 555 S 18th St, Ste 4C Columbus, OH 43205-2654; **Office Phone:** (614) 224-6222; **Board Certification:** Ophthalmology 1974; **Medical School:** Ohio State Univ 1968; **Residency:** Ophthalmology, Mt Sinai Hosp, Cleveland, OH 1969-1972; **Fellowship:** Pediatric Ophthalmology, Chldns Natl Med Ctr, Washington, DC 1973-1974

Rosenberg, Michael A MD (Ophthalmology) - *Special Expertise: Neuro-Ophthalmology; Refractive Surgery;* **Admitting Hospital:** Northwestern Memorial Hospital; **Office Address:** Northwestern Med Faculty Foundation 675 N St Clair, Ste 15-150 Chicago, IL 60611; **Office Phone:** (312) 695-8150; **Board Certification:** Ophthalmology 1975; **Medical School:** Northwestern Univ 1967; **Residency:** Ophthalmology, Bascom Palmer Eye Inst, Miami, FL 1970-1973; **Fellowship:** Neurological Ophthalmology, U Calif, San Franicsco, CA 1973-1974; **Faculty Appointment:** Assoc Prof Neonatal-Perinatal Medicine, Northwestern Univ

OPHTHALMOLOGY

Samuelson, Thomas (Ophthalmology) - *Special Expertise:* Glaucoma; **Admitting Hospital:** Phillips Eye Institute; **Office Address:** 710 E 24th St, Ste 106 Minneapolis, MN 55404; **Office Phone:** (612) 874-9982; **Board Certification:** Ophthalmology 1991; **Medical School:** Univ Minn 1985; **Residency:** Ophthalmology, Univ South Fla, Tampa, FL 1987-1990; **Fellowship:** Glaucoma, Wills Eye Hosp, Philadelphia, PA 1990-1991; **Faculty Appointment:** Assoc Clin Prof Ophthalmology, Univ Minn

Scott, William MD (Ophthalmology) - *Special Expertise:* Ophthalmology-Pediatric; **Admitting Hospital:** University of Iowa Hospitals and Clinics; **Office Address:** Univ Iowa Hosps, Dept Ophthalmology 200 Hawkins Drive, Ste 11290 PFP Iowa City, IA 52242-1091; **Office Phone:** (319) 356-0382; **Board Certification:** Ophthalmology 1972; **Medical School:** Univ Iowa Coll Med 1964; **Residency:** Ophthalmology, Univ Iowa Hosps, Iowa City, IA 1967-1970; **Fellowship:** Smith-Kettlewell Inst Vision, San Francisco, CA 1971

Stone, Edwin MD (Ophthalmology) - *Special Expertise:* Retinal Disorders; Eye Diseases-Hereditary; **Admitting Hospital:** University of Iowa Hospitals and Clinics; **Office Address:** 200 Hawkins Dr Iowa City, IA 52242; **Office Phone:** (319) 356-2864; **Board Certification:** Ophthalmology 1990; **Medical School:** Baylor Coll Med 1985; **Residency:** Ophthalmology, Univ Iowa Hosps & Clins, Iowa City, IA 1986-1989; **Fellowship:** Retina, Univ Iowa Hosps & Clins, Iowa City, IA 1990-1992; **Faculty Appointment:** Assoc Prof Ophthalmology, Univ Iowa Coll Med

Traboulsi, Elias Iskan MD (Ophthalmology) - *Special Expertise:* Ophthalmology-Pediatric; Eye Diseases; Glaucoma-Pediatric; **Admitting Hospital:** Cleveland Clinic Foundation; **Office Address:** Cleveland Clinic Fdn 9500 Euclid Ave, Ste I32 Cleveland, OH 44195; **Office Phone:** (216) 444-4363; **Board Certifications:** Clinical Genetics 1987, Ophthalmology 1991; **Medical School:** American Univ of Beirut 1982; **Residencies:** Ophthalmology, American Univ Beirut Hosp, Beirut, Lebanon 1982-1985; Ophthalmology, Georgetown Hosp, Washington, DC 1986-1989; **Fellowships:** Ophthalmology, Johns Hopkins Hosp, Baltimore, MD 1985-1986; Pediatric Ophthalmology, Chldns Hosp, Washington, DC 1989-1990

Trese, Michael T MD (Ophthalmology) - *Special Expertise:* Retina/Vitreous Surgery; **Admitting Hospital:** William Beaumont Hospital; **Office Address:** Assoc Retinal Cons PC 3535 W 13 Mile Rd, Ste 632 Royal Oak, MI 48073-6704; **Office Phone:** (248) 288-2280; **Board Certification:** Ophthalmology 1981; **Medical School:** Geo Wash Univ 1976; **Residency:** Ophthalmology, Jules Stein Eye Inst-UCLA, Los Angeles, CA 1977-1980; **Fellowship:** Retina, Duke Univ Med Ctr, Durham, NC 1980-1981; **Faculty Appointment:** Assoc Clin Prof Ophthalmology, Wayne State Univ

Tychsen, Lawrence MD (Ophthalmology) - *Special Expertise:* Ophthalmology-Pediatric; **Admitting Hospital:** St Louis Children's Hospital; **Office Address:** St Louis Chldns Hosp 1 Chldns Pl, rm 2S89 St. Louis, MO 63110; **Office Phone:** (314) 454-6026; **Board Certification:** Ophthalmology 1984; **Medical School:** Georgetown Univ 1979; **Residency:** Ophthalmology, Univ Iowa Hosp, Iowa City, IA 1980-1983; **Fellowship:** Pediatric Ophthalmology, Univ Calif Med Ctr, San Francisco, CA 1984-1985

Younge, Brian R MD (Ophthalmology) - *Special Expertise:* Neuro-Ophthalmology; Temporal Arteritis; Ocular Palsies; **Admitting Hospital:** Mayo Medical Center & Clinic - Rochester; **Office Address:** Mayo Clinic 200 First St SW Rochester, MN 55905-0001; **Office Phone:** (507) 284-4567; **Board Certification:** Ophthalmology 1974; **Medical School:** Univ Alberta 1965; **Residency:** Ophthalmology, Montreal Genl Hosp, Montreal, Canada 1969-1972; **Fellowship:** Neurological Ophthalmology, Mayo Clinic, Rochester, MN 1973-1974; **Faculty Appointment:** Assoc Prof Ophthalmology, Mayo Med Sch

Great Plains and Mountains

Bateman, Jane Bronwyn MD (Ophthalmology) - *Special Expertise: Ophthalmology-Pediatric; Family Genetics;* **Admitting Hospital:** The Children's Hospital - Denver; **Office Address:** 1056 E 19th Ave, Box B-430 Denver, CO 80218; **Office Phone:** (303) 861-6062; **Board Certifications:** Ophthalmology 1979, Clinical Genetics 1982; **Medical School:** Coll Physicians & Surgeons 1974; **Residencies:** Internal Medicine, UCLA Med Ctr, Los Angeles, CA 1975-1978; Ophthalmology, Chldns Natl Med Ctr, Washington DC 1979; **Fellowships:** Ophthalmology, UCLA Med Ctr, Los Angeles, CA 1978; Pediatric Ophthalmology, Chldns Natl Med Ctr, Washington DC 1979

Crandall, Alan Slade MD (Ophthalmology) - *Special Expertise: Glaucoma; Cataract Surgery;* **Admitting Hospital:** University of Utah Hospital and Clinics; **Office Address:** Univ Utah Hosp, Moran Eye Ctr 50 N Medical Dr Salt Lake City, UT 84132; **Office Phone:** (801) 581-2769; **Board Certification:** Ophthalmology 1977; **Medical School:** Univ Utah 1973; **Residency:** Ophthalmology, Univ Penn, Philadelphia, PA 1973-1976; **Fellowship:** Glaucoma, Scheie Eye Inst, Philadelphia, PA 1981; **Faculty Appointment:** Prof Ophthalmology, Univ Utah

Durrie, Daniel MD (Ophthalmology) - *Special Expertise: Refractive Surgery-LASIK; Corneal Disease;* **Admitting Hospital:** St Luke's Hospital; **Office Address:** 5520 College Blvd, Fl 2 Overland Park, KS 66211; **Office Phone:** (913) 491-3737; **Board Certification:** Ophthalmology 1979; **Medical School:** Univ Nebr Coll Med 1975; **Residency:** Ophthalmology, Univ Nebr Med Coll, Omaha, NE 1976-1979; **Faculty Appointment:** Asst Clin Prof Ophthalmology, Univ Nebr Coll Med

Southwest

Boniuk, Milton MD (Ophthalmology) - *Special Expertise: Cornea Transplant; Eye Tomors/Cancer;* **Admitting Hospital:** Methodist Hospital - Houston (Page 69); **Office Address:** 6560 Fannin St, Ste 902 Houston, TX 77030; **Office Phone:** (713) 798-5955; **Board Certification:** Ophthalmology 1960; **Medical School:** Dalhousie Univ 1956; **Residency:** Ophthalmology, Wills Eye Hosp, Philadelphia, PA 1957-1959; **Fellowship:** Pathology, AFIP, Washington, DC 1959-1961

Ellis Jr, George S MD (Ophthalmology) - *Special Expertise: Ophthalmology-Pediatric; Eye & Muscle Motility;* **Admitting Hospital:** Children's Hospital - New Orleans; **Office Address:** Chldns Hosp 200 Henry Clay Ave New Orleans, LA 70118; **Office Phone:** (504) 896-9426; **Board Certification:** Ophthalmology 1982; **Medical School:** Tulane Univ 1977; **Residencies:** Pediatric Ophthalmology, Hall Eye Clin, Atlanta, GA; Ophthalmology, Duke Univ Med Ctr-Eye Ctr, Durham, NC 1979-1982; **Fellowship:** Pediatric Ophthalmology, Chldns Hosp, Washington, DC; **Faculty Appointment:** Clin Prof Ophthalmology, Tulane Univ

Eustis, Horatio Sprague MD (Ophthalmology) - *Special Expertise: Ophthalmology-Pediatric;* **Admitting Hospital:** Ochsner Foundation Hospital; **Office Address:** Ochsner Clinic 1514 Jefferson Hwy New Orleans, LA 70121; **Office Phone:** (504) 842-3995; **Board Certification:** Ophthalmology 1985; **Medical School:** Louisiana State Univ 1980; **Residency:** Ophthalmology, La State Univ Eye Ctr, New Orleans, LA 1981-1984; **Fellowships:** Hosp Sick Chldn, Toronto, Canada 1984-1985; Chldns Hosp, Washington, DC 1985

Holladay, Jack T. MD (Ophthalmology) - *Special Expertise: Refractive Surgery-LASIK; Cataract Surgery; Eye Surgery-Lens;* **Admitting Hospital:** Memorial Hermann Healthcare System; **Office Address:** 926 N Wilcrest St Houston, TX 77025; **Office Phone:** (713) 668-7337; **Board Certification:** Ophthalmology 1979; **Medical School:** Univ Tex, Houston 1974; **Residency:** Ophthalmology, Univ Tex Hlth Sci Ctr, Houston, TX 1974-1975; **Faculty Appointment:** Assoc Prof Ophthalmology, Univ Tex, Houston

Koch, Douglas D MD (Ophthalmology) - *Special Expertise: Cataract Surgery; Refractive Surgery; Corneal Disease;* **Admitting Hospital:** Methodist Hospital - Houston (Page 69); **Office Address:** 6565 Fannin, MC-NC205 Houston, TX 77030; **Office Phone:** (713) 798-6443; **Board Certification:** Ophthalmology 1982; **Medical School:** Harvard Med Sch 1977; **Residency:** Baylor Coll Med, Houston, TX 1978-1981; **Fellowships:** Moorfields Eye Hosp., London, UK 1981-1982; Baylor Coll of Med 1982; **Faculty Appointment:** Prof Ophthalmology, Baylor Coll Med

Lambert, H. Michael MD (Ophthalmology) - *Special Expertise: Retina/Vitrous Surgery; Macular Disease/Degeneration; Diabetic Eye Disease/Retinopathy;* **Admitting Hospital:** Methodist Hospital - Houston (Page 69); **Office Address:** Retina and Vitreous of Texas 6500 Fannin, Ste 1100 Houston, TX 77030; **Office Phone:** (713) 799-9975; **Board Certification:** Ophthalmology 1983; **Medical School:** Baylor Coll Med 1977; **Residency:** Ophthalmology, Wilford Hall USAF Med Ctr, San Antonio, TX 1979-1982; **Fellowship:** Vitreoretinal Surgery, Duke Univ Eye Ctr, Durham, NC 1982-1983; **Faculty Appointment:** Assoc Clin Prof Ophthalmology, Baylor Coll Med

Mazow, Malcolm L. MD (Ophthalmology) - *Special Expertise: Ophthalmology - General;* **Admitting Hospital:** Memorial Hermann Healthcare System; **Office Address:** 2855 Gramercy St Houston, TX 77025; **Office Phone:** (713) 668-6828; **Board Certification:** Ophthalmology 1967; **Medical School:** Univ Iowa Coll Med **Residency:** Ophthalmology, Univ Iowa Hosp, Iowa City, IA 1962-1965; **Faculty Appointment:** Asst Clin Prof Ophthalmology, Univ Tex, Houston

McCulley, James P MD (Ophthalmology) - *Special Expertise: Corneal & External Eye Disease; Refractive Surgery-Laser; Cataract Surgery;* **Admitting Hospital:** Zale Lipshy University Hospital; **Office Address:** U Texas SW Med School 5323 Harry Hines Blvd Dallas, TX 75390-9057; **Office Phone:** (214) 648-2020; **Board Certification:** Ophthalmology 1974; **Medical School:** Washington Univ, St Louis 1968; **Residency:** Ophthalmology, Mass EE Infirmary, Boston, MA 1969-1973; **Fellowships:** Cornea, t CDepornea Rsch-Retina Fdtn, Boston, MA 1973-1974; Cornea, Mass EE Infirmary, Boston, MA 1973-1974; **Faculty Appointment:** Prof Ophthalmology, Univ Tex SW, Dallas

McDonald, Marguerite B. MD (Ophthalmology) - *Special Expertise: Refractive Surgery;* **Admitting Hospital:** Memorial Medical Center - Baptist Campus; **Office Address:** Southern Vision Ins 2820 Napleon Ave, Ste 750 New Orleans, LA 70115; **Office Phone:** (504) 896-1240; **Board Certification:** Ophthalmology 1981; **Medical School:** Columbia P&S 1976; **Residency:** Ophthalmology, Manhattan EET Hosp., New York, NY 1977-1980; **Fellowship:** LSU Eye Ctr., New Orleans, LA 1980-1981; **Faculty Appointment:** Clin Prof Ophthalmology, Tulane Univ

Mims III, James Luther MD (Ophthalmology) - *Special Expertise: Ophthalmology-Pediatric; Strabismus;* **Admitting Hospital:** Baptist Medical Center; **Office Address:** 311 Camden, Ste 511 San Antonio, TX 78215; **Office Phone:** (210) 225-0084; **Board Certification:** Ophthalmology 1977; **Medical School:** Tulane Univ 1968; **Residency:** Ophthalmology, Wills Eye Hosp, Philadelphia, PA 1973-1976; **Fellowship:** Pediatric Ophthalmology, Wills Eye Hosp, Philadelphia, PA 1976-1977; **Faculty Appointment:** Clin Prof Ophthalmology, Univ Tex, San Antonio

Piest, Kenneth L MD (Ophthalmology) - *Special Expertise: Ophthalmologic Plastic Surgery;* **Admitting Hospital:** North Central Baptist Hospital; **Office Address:** 540 Madison Oak, Ste 450 San Antonio, TX 78258; **Office Phone:** (210) 494-8859; **Board Certification:** Ophthalmology 1991; **Medical School:** Univ IL Coll Med 1984; **Residency:** Ophthalmology, Univ Tex Hlth Scis Ctr, San Antonio, TX 1985-1986; **Fellowships:** Ophthalmological Pathology, Univ Utah, Salt Lake City, UT 1985-1986; Oculoplatic Surgery, Chldns Hosp/Sheie Eye Inst/UPenn, Philadelphia, PA 1989-1990; **Faculty Appointment:** Assoc Clin Prof Ophthalmology, Univ Tex, San Antonio

Richard, James Marshall MD (Ophthalmology) - *Special Expertise: Ophthalmology-Pediatric;* **Admitting Hospital:** Children's Hospital of Oklahoma; **Office Address:** Chldns Eye Care 11013 Hefner Pointe Dr Oklahoma City, OK 73120-5050; **Office Phone:** (405) 751-2020; **Board Certification:** Ophthalmology 1979; **Medical School:** Univ Okla Coll Med 1974; **Residency:** Obstetrics & Gynecology, Baylor Coll Med, Houston, TX 1975-1978; **Fellowships:** Pediatric Ophthalmology, Childns Hosp, Washington, DC 1978-1979; Ophthalmology, Johns Hopkins Hosp, Baltimore, MD 1970-1980; **Faculty Appointment:** Clin Prof Ophthalmology, Univ Okla Coll Med

Wilhelmus, Kirk R MD (Ophthalmology) - *Special Expertise: Cornea Transplant; Corneal and External Eye Disease;* **Admitting Hospital:** Methodist Hospital - Houston (Page 69); **Office Address:** Cullen Eye Inst 6500 Fannin St, Ste 1501 Houston, TX 77030; **Office Phone:** (713) 798-6100; **Board Certification:** Ophthalmology 1981; **Medical School:** Vanderbilt Univ 1975; **Residency:** Ophthalmology, Baylor Coll Med, Houston, TX 1976-1979; **Fellowship:** Cornea External Disease, Moorfields Eye Hosp, London, England 1979-1981; **Faculty Appointment:** Prof Ophthalmology, Baylor Coll Med

West Coast and Pacific

Arnold, Anthony C MD (Ophthalmology) - *Special Expertise: Neuro-Ophthalmology;* **Admitting Hospital:** UCLA Medical Center; **Office Address:** 100 Stein Plaza Los Angeles, CA 90095-7065; **Office Phone:** (310) 825-4344; **Board Certification:** Ophthalmology 1980; **Medical School:** UCLA 1975; **Residency:** Ophthalmology, Jules Stein Eye Inst. UCLA, Los Angeles, CA 1976-1979; **Fellowship:** Ophthalmology, Jules Stein Eye Inst UCLA, Los Angeles, CA 1982-1983; **Faculty Appointment:** Clin Prof Ophthalmology, UCLA

Baylis, Henry I MD (Ophthalmology) - *Special Expertise: Oculoplastic Surgery;* **Office Address:** 1551 Ocean Ave, Ste 200 Santa Monica, CA 90401; **Office Phone:** (310) 207-0300; **Board Certification:** Ophthalmology 1969; **Medical School:** Univ Mich Med Sch 1960; **Residency:** Ophthalmology, UCLA Med Ctr, Los Angeles, CA 1963-1966; **Fellowship:** Oculoplatic Surgery, Manhattan EET Hosp, New York, NY 1966-1967; **Faculty Appointment:** Clin Prof Ophthalmology, UCLA

Binder, Perry Scott MD (Ophthalmology) - *Special Expertise: Refractive Surgery;* **Admitting Hospital:** Sharp Memorial Hospital; **Office Address:** 8910 Univ Center Lane, Ste 800 San Diego, CA 92122; **Office Phone:** (858) 455-6800; **Board Certification:** Ophthalmology 1975; **Medical School:** Northwestern Univ 1969; **Residency:** USC Med Ctr, Los Angeles, CA 1970-1973; **Fellowship:** U Fla Hosp, Gainesville, FL 1973-1974; **Faculty Appointment:** Assoc Clin Prof Ophthalmology, UCSD

Borchert, Mark S MD (Ophthalmology) - *Special Expertise: Ophthalmology-Pediatric; Vision-Unexplained Loss; Optic Nerve Disorders;* **Admitting Hospital:** Children's Hospital - Los Angeles; **Office Address:** Childrens Hospital - Division of Ophthalmology 4650 Sunset Blvd, MC-88 Los Angeles, CA 90027-6062; **Office Phone:** (323) 669-2344; **Board Certification:** Ophthalmology 1989; **Medical School:** Baylor Coll Med 1983; **Residency:** Ophthalmology, USC, Los Angeles, CA 1984-1987; **Fellowship:** Ophthalmology, Harvard, Boston, MA 1987-1988; **Faculty Appointment:** Asst Prof Ophthalmology, USC Sch Med

Boxrud, Cynthia Ann MD (Ophthalmology) - *Special Expertise: Oculoplastic Surgery; Ophthalmologic Plastic Surgery;* **Admitting Hospital:** UCLA Medical Center; **Office Address:** 2021 Santa Monica Blvd, Ste 700E Santa Monica, CA 90404; **Office Phone:** (310) 914-3440; **Board Certification:** Ophthalmology 1997; **Medical School:** Case West Res Univ 1986; **Residency:** Ophthalmology, NYU-Bellevue Hosp Ctr, New York, NY 1987-1990

Caprioli, Joseph MD (Ophthalmology) - *Special Expertise:* Glaucoma; **Admitting Hospital:** UCLA-Sepulveda VA Greater LA Health Care System; **Office Address:** UCLA- Jules Stein 100 Stein Plaza Los Angeles, CA 90095-7006; **Office Phone:** (310) 794-9442; **Board Certification:** Ophthalmology 1985; **Medical School:** SUNY Buffalo 1979; **Residency:** Ophthalmology, Yale-New Haven Hosp., New Haven, CT 1980-1983; **Fellowship:** Ophthalmology, Wills Eye Hosp., Philadelphia, PA 1983-1984; **Faculty Appointment:** Prof Ophthalmology, UCLA

Char, Devron H MD (Ophthalmology) - *Special Expertise:* Eye Tumors/Cancer; Thyroid Eye Disease; **Admitting Hospital:** California Pacific Medical Center; **Office Address:** 45 Castro St, Ste 309 San Francisco, CA 94114; **Office Phone:** (415) 522-0700; **Board Certification:** Ophthalmology 1978; **Medical School:** Univ Minn 1970; **Residencies:** Internal Medicine, Mass Genl Hosp, Boston, MA 1970-1972; Medical Oncology, Natl Cancer Inst, Bethesda, MD 1972-1974; **Fellowships:** Ophthalmology, UCSF, San Francisco, CA 1974-1977; Ophthalmology, UCSF, San Francisco, CA 1977-1978; **Faculty Appointment:** Prof Ophthalmology, Stanford Univ

Choy, Andrew Eng MD (Ophthalmology) - *Special Expertise:* Eye Motility-Pediatric; Oculoplastic & Orbital Surgery; **Admitting Hospital:** Long Beach Memorial Medical Center; **Office Address:** Long Beach Meml Med Ctr, 4100 Long Beach Blvd, Ste 108, Long Beach, CA 90807-2619; **Office Phone:** (562) 426-3925; **Board Certification:** Ophthalmology 1976; **Medical School:** USC Sch Med 1969; **Residencies:** Neurology, Los Angeles Co-USC Med Ctr, Los Angeles, CA 1970-1971; Ophthalmology, Bellevue Hosp Ctr-NYU, New York, NY 1971-1974; **Fellowship:** Columbia-Presby Med Ctr, New York, NY 1974-1975; **Faculty Appointment:** Assoc Clin Prof Ophthalmology, UCLA

Day, Susan H MD (Ophthalmology) - *Special Expertise:* Ophthalmology-Pediatric; **Admitting Hospital:** California Pacific Medical Center; **Office Address:** 2340 Clay St, Ste 100 San Francisco, CA 94115-1932; **Office Phone:** (415) 202-1500; **Board Certification:** Ophthalmology 1980; **Medical School:** Louisiana State Univ 1975; **Residency:** Ophthalmology, Pacific Med Ctr, San Francisco, CA 1976-1979; **Fellowship:** Sick Chldns Hosp, London, England 1979-1980

Demer, Joseph L MD/PhD (Ophthalmology) - *Special Expertise:* Ophthalmology-Pediatric; **Admitting Hospital:** UCLA Medical Center; **Office Address:** Jules Stein Eye Inst-UCLA - Div Comprehensive Oph, 100 Stein Plaza, MC-700219 Los Angeles, CA 90095-7002; **Office Phone:** (310) 825-5931; **Board Certification:** Ophthalmology 1988; **Medical School:** Johns Hopkins Univ 1983; **Residency:** Ophthalmology, Baylor Coll Med, Houston, TX 1984-1987; **Fellowship:** Pediatric Ophthalmology, TX Chldns Hosp, Houston, TX 1987-1988; **Faculty Appointment:** Prof Ophthalmology, UCLA

Fein, William MD (Ophthalmology) - *Special Expertise:* Oculoplastic Surgery; Lacrimal Gland Disorders; **Admitting Hospital:** Cedars-Sinai Medical Center; **Office Address:** 415 N Crescent Drive, Ste 200 Beverly Hills, CA 90210-4860; **Office Phone:** (310) 859-0760; **Board Certification:** Ophthalmology 1969; **Medical School:** UC Irvine 1960; **Residency:** Ophthalmology, Los Angeles Co General Hospital, Los Angeles, CA 1963-1966; **Fellowship:** Ophthalmology, Manhattan Eye, Ear & Throat Infirmiry 1966-1967; **Faculty Appointment:** Assoc Clin Prof Ophthalmology, USC Sch Med

Feldon, Steven E MD (Ophthalmology) - *Special Expertise:* Neuro-Ophthalmology; Orbital Surgery; Strabismus; **Admitting Hospital:** USC University Hospital - Richard K. Eamer Medical Plaza; **Office Address:** Doheny Eye Institute 1450 San Pablo St Los Angeles, CA 90033; **Office Phone:** (323) 342-6488; **Board Certification:** Ophthalmology 1979; **Medical School:** Albert Einstein Coll Med 1973; **Residency:** Ophthalmology, Mass Eye & Ear, Boston, MA 1975-1978; **Fellowship:** Ophthalmology, UCSF Med Ctr, San Francisco, CA 1978-1979; **Faculty Appointment:** Prof Ophthalmology, USC Sch Med

Granet, David Bruce MD (Ophthalmology) - *Special Expertise:* *Ophthalmology-Pediatric; Sports Vision;* **Admitting Hospital:** University of California - San Diego Healthcare; **Office Address:** UCSD-Ratner Chldns Eye Ctr 9415 Campus Point Dr La Jolla, CA 92093-0946; **Office Phone:** (858) 534-7440; **Board Certification:** Ophthalmology 1994; **Medical School:** Yale Univ 1987; **Residency:** Ophthalmology, Bellevue Hosp-NYU, New York, NY 1988-1991; **Fellowship:** Pediatric Ophthalmology, Chldns Hosp, Philadelphia, PA 1991-1993; **Faculty Appointment:** Asst Prof Ophthalmology, UCSD

Hoyt, Creig S MD (Ophthalmology) - *Special Expertise:* *Ophthalmology - General;* **Admitting Hospital:** University of California - San Francisco Medical Center; **Office Address:** UCSF Med Ctr 400 Parnassus Ave, rm 702A, Box 0344 San Francisco, CA 94143; **Office Phone:** (415) 353-2289; **Board Certifications:** Ophthalmology 1978; **Medical School:** Cornell Univ-Weil Med Coll 1968; **Residencies:** Neurology, UCSF, San Francisco, CA 1969-1970; Ophthalmology, UCSF, San Francisco 1970; **Fellowship:** Pediatric Ophthalmology, Chldns Hosp, Melbourne 1977-1977; **Faculty Appointment:** Prof Ophthalmology, UCSF

Hoyt, William Fletcher MD (Ophthalmology) - *Special Expertise:* *Neuro-Ophthalmology;* **Admitting Hospital:** University of California - San Francisco Medical Center; **Office Address:** UCSF, Dept Neuro Oph U-521 505-533 Parnassus Ave San Fransisco, CA 94143; **Office Phone:** (415) 476-1130; **Board Certification:** Ophthalmology 1958; **Medical School:** UCSF 1950; **Residency:** Ophthalmology, UCSF Hosp, San Francisco, CA 1953-1956; **Fellowship:** Neurological Ophthalmology, Johns Hopkins Hosp, Baltimore, MD 1958-1958; **Faculty Appointment:** Prof Ophthalmology, UCSF

Irvine, John Alexander MD (Ophthalmology) - *Special Expertise:* *Corneal & External Eye Disease;* **Admitting Hospital:** USC University Hospital - Richard K. Eamer Medical Plaza; **Office Address:** Doheny Eye Institute 1450 San Pablo St Los Angeles, CA 90033-4684; **Office Phone:** (323) 442-6335; **Board Certification:** Ophthalmology 1989; **Medical School:** USC Sch Med 1982; **Residency:** Ophthalmology, Mass EE Infirm/Harvard, Boston, MA 1983-1986; **Fellowship:** Cornea External Disease, Mass EE Infirm, Boston, MA 1986-1987; **Faculty Appointment:** Prof Ophthalmology, USC Sch Med

Isenberg, Sherwin Jay MD (Ophthalmology) - *Special Expertise:* *Strabismus; Ophthalmology-Pediatric;* **Admitting Hospital:** LAC - Harbor - UCLA Medical Center; **Office Address:** Jules Stein Eye Inst 100 Stein Plaza Los Angeles, CA 90095-7000; **Office Phone:** (310) 825-8840; **Board Certification:** Ophthalmology 1978; **Medical School:** UCLA 1973; **Residency:** Ophthalmology, Illinois Ear & Eye Infirmary, Chicago, IL 1974-1977; **Fellowship:** Pediatric Ophthalmology, Chldns Hosp Natl Med Ctr, Washington, DC 1977-1978; **Faculty Appointment:** Prof Ophthalmology, UCLA

Kramer, Steven G MD (Ophthalmology) - *Special Expertise:* *Corneal Disease;* **Admitting Hospital:** University of California - San Francisco Medical Center; **Office Address:** University of California San Francisco 10 Kirkham St San Francisco, CA 94143-0730; **Office Phone:** (415) 476-1921; **Board Certification:** Ophthalmology 1971; **Medical School:** Case West Res Univ 1965; **Residency:** Ophthalmology, U Chicago Hosps, Chicago, IL 1966-1969; **Fellowship:** USPHS, Chicago, IL 1970-1971; **Faculty Appointment:** Prof Ophthalmology, UCSF

Mahon, Kathleen MK MD (Ophthalmology) - *Special Expertise:* *Ophthalmology-Pediatric;* **Admitting Hospital:** Sunrise Hospital & Medical Center; **Office Address:** Mahon Eye Ctr 3201 S Maryland Pkwy, Ste 400 Las Vegas, NV 89109-2426; **Office Phone:** (702) 731-3333; **Board Certification:** Ophthalmology 1980; **Medical School:** Univ New Mexico 1975; **Residency:** Ophthalmology, Univ FL Med Ctr, Gainsville, FL 1976-1979; **Fellowship:** Pediatric Ophthalmology, Univ Tex Hlth Sci Ctr, Houston, TX 1979-1980; **Faculty Appointment:** Clin Prof Ophthalmology, Univ Nevada

Maloney, Robert Keller MD (Ophthalmology) - *Special Expertise:* Refractive Surgery; Refractive Surgery-LASIK; **Admitting Hospital:** UCLA Medical Center; **Office Address:** 10921 Wilshire Blvd, Ste 900 Maloney Vision Inst. Los Angeles, CA 90024; **Office Phone:** (310) 208-3937; **Board Certification:** Ophthalmology 1991; **Medical School:** UCSF 1985; **Residency:** Ophthalmology, Johns Hopkins Hosp, MD 1986-1989; **Fellowship:** Emory Univ, GA 1989-1991; **Faculty Appointment:** Assoc Clin Prof Ophthalmology, UCLA

Manche, Edward Emanuel MD (Ophthalmology) - *Special Expertise:* Refractive Surgery; Corneal Disease; **Admitting Hospital:** Stanford Medical Center; **Office Address:** 900 Blake Wilbur Dr rm W3002 Stanford, CA 94305; **Office Phone:** (650) 498-7020; **Board Certification:** Ophthalmology 1996; **Medical School:** Albert Einstein Coll Med 1990; **Residency:** Ophthalmology, New Jersey Medical school, Newark, NJ 1991-1994; **Fellowship:** Cornea External Disease, Jules Stein Eye Inst-UCLA, Los Angeles, CA 1994-1996; **Faculty Appointment:** Assoc Prof Ophthalmology, Stanford Univ

Marmor, Michael F MD (Ophthalmology) - *Special Expertise:* Eye Diseases-Neurophysiologic; **Admitting Hospital:** Stanford Medical Center; **Office Address:** Stanford Med Ctr, Dept Oph 300 Pasteur Rd, rm A157 Stanford, CA 94305-5308; **Office Phone:** (650) 723-5517; **Board Certification:** Ophthalmology 1974; **Medical School:** Harvard Med Sch 1966; **Residency:** Ophthalmology, Mass EE Infirm, Boston, MA 1970-1973; **Fellowship:** Neurological Physiology, Natl Inst Mental Hlth, Bethesda, MD 1967-1970; **Faculty Appointment:** Assoc Prof Ophthalmology, Stanford Univ

Masket, Samuel MD (Ophthalmology) - *Special Expertise:* Cataract Surgery; **Admitting Hospital:** West Hills Medical Center; **Office Address:** 2080 Century Park E, Ste 911 Los Angeles, CA 90067; **Office Phone:** (310) 229-1220; **Board Certification:** Ophthalmology 1974; **Medical School:** NY Med Coll 1968; **Residency:** Ophthalmology, Metro Hosp Ctr, New York, NY 1969-1973; **Fellowship:** Ophthalmology, Columbia Presby Med Ctr, NewYork, NY; **Faculty Appointment:** Asst Clin Prof Ophthalmology, UCLA

Minckler, Donald Saier MD (Ophthalmology) - *Special Expertise:* Glaucoma; **Admitting Hospital:** LAC + USC Medical Center; **Office Address:** Doheny Eye Inst 1450 San Pablo St, Fl 4 Los Angeles, CA 90033-4507; **Office Phone:** (323) 442-6415; **Board Certifications:** Ophthalmology 1975, Pathology 1978; **Medical School:** Oregon Hlth Scis Univ 1964; **Residencies:** Anatomic Pathology, Univ Wash Med Ctr, Seattle, WA 1968-1970; Ophthalmology, Univ Wash Med Ctr, Seattle, Wa 1970-1973; **Fellowships:** Pathology, Armed Forces Inst Path, Washington, DC 1973-1975; Glaucoma, Shaffer Assocs-UCSF, San Francisco, CA 1981-1982; **Faculty Appointment:** Prof Ophthalmology, Univ SC Sch Med

Mondino, Bartly John MD (Ophthalmology) - *Special Expertise:* Corneal & External Eye Disease; **Admitting Hospital:** UCLA Medical Center; **Office Address:** 100 Stein Plaza, MC-70019 Los Angeles, CA 90095; **Office Phone:** (310) 825-5053; **Board Certification:** Ophthalmology 1976; **Medical School:** Stanford Univ 1971; **Residency:** Ophthalmology, NY Hosp/Cornell Univ, New York, NY 1972-1975; **Fellowship:** Univ Pittsburgh Eye & Ear Hosp, Pittsburgh, PA 1975-1976; **Faculty Appointment:** Prof Ophthalmology, UCLA

Murphree, A. Linn MD (Ophthalmology) - *Special Expertise:* Ophthalmology-Pediatric; Eye Diseases-Hereditary; **Admitting Hospital:** Children's Hospital - Los Angeles; **Office Address:** Childrens Hospital - Div Oph 4650 W Sunset Blvd, MS 88 Los Angeles, CA 90027-6016; **Office Phone:** (323) 669-5603; **Board Certification:** Ophthalmology 1978; **Medical School:** Baylor Coll Med 1972; **Residencies:** Clinical Genetics, Baylor Heed, Houston, TX 1972-1973; Ophthalmology, Baylor College Medicine, Houston, TX 1973-1976; **Fellowship:** Ophthalmology, Wilmer Institute/Johns Hopkins, Baltimore, MD 1976-1977; **Faculty Appointment:** Prof Ophthalmology, USC Sch Med

Nesburn, Anthony B MD (Ophthalmology) - *Special Expertise:* Corneal Disease; Refractive Surgery-Laser; Herpes; **Admitting Hospital:** Cedars-Sinai Medical Center; **Office Address:** Cedars-Sinai Med Ctr, Dept Opthalmology 8635 W 3rd St, Ste 390W Los Angeles, CA 90048; **Office Phone:** (310) 652-1133; **Board Certification:** Ophthalmology 1969; **Medical School:** Harvard Med Sch 1960; **Residency:** Ophthalmology, Mass Eye & Ear Infirm, Boston, MA 1966-1968; **Fellowship:** Virology, Harvard, Boston, MA 1964-1965; **Faculty Appointment:** Clin Prof Ophthalmology, UCLA

Palmer, Earl A. MD (Ophthalmology) - *Special Expertise:* Ophthalmology-Pediatric; **Admitting Hospital:** Oregon Health Science University Hospital and Clinics; **Office Address:** Casey Eye Institute 3375 SW Terwilliger Blvd Portland, OR 97201-4197; **Office Phone:** (503) 494-7675; **Board Certifications:** Pediatrics 1975, Ophthalmology 1976; **Medical School:** Duke Univ 1966; **Residencies:** Pediatrics, Univ Colo Med Ctr, Denver, CO 1967-1968; Ophthalmology, Oreg Hlth Scis Univ, Portland, OR 1971-1974; **Fellowship:** Pediatric Ophthalmology, Univ Colo Med Ctr, Denver, CO 1966-1967; **Faculty Appointment:** Prof Ophthalmology, Oregon Hlth Scis Univ

Paul, Theodore Otis MD (Ophthalmology) - *Special Expertise:* Ophthalmology-Pediatric; Strabismus; **Admitting Hospital:** California Pacific Medical Center; **Office Address:** Pediat Ophthalmology and Strabismus 2100 Webster St, Ste 214 San Francisco, CA 94115; **Office Phone:** (415) 923-3007; **Board Certification:** Ophthalmology 1974; **Medical School:** UCLA 1967; **Residency:** Ophthalmology, Naval Hospital, San Diego, CA 1969-1972; **Fellowship:** Ophthalmology, California Pacific Medical Center, San Francisco, CA 1973-1974

Rao, Narsing Adupa MD (Ophthalmology) - *Special Expertise:* Uveitis/AIDS; Eye Pathology; **Admitting Hospital:** USC University Hospital - Richard K. Eamer Medical Plaza; **Office Address:** Doheny Eye Inst 1450 San Pablo St, Fl 210 Los Angeles, CA 90033-4581; **Office Phone:** (323) 342-6645; **Board Certifications:** Ophthalmology 1977, Pathology 1974; **Medical School:** India 1967; **Residencies:** Ophthalmology, Georgetown Hosp, Washington, DC 1972-1975; Pathology, Georgetown Hosp, Washington, DC 1969-1972; **Faculty Appointment:** Prof Ophthalmology, USC Sch Med

Salz, James Joseph MD (Ophthalmology) - *Special Expertise:* Eye Laser Surgery (LASIK); Cataract Surgery; **Admitting Hospital:** Cedars-Sinai Medical Center; **Office Address:** Laser Vision Med Assoc Inc 444 S San Vicente Blvd, Ste 704 Los Angeles, CA 90048-5901; **Office Phone:** (323) 653-3800; **Board Certification:** Ophthalmology 1971; **Medical School:** Duke Univ 1965; **Residency:** Ophthalmology, Los Angeles Co-USC Med Ctr., Los Angeles, CA 1966-1969; **Faculty Appointment:** Clin Prof Ophthalmology, USC Sch Med

Serafano, Donald Natale MD (Ophthalmology) - *Special Expertise:* Laser Vision Correction; Cataract Surgery; Lens Implants; **Admitting Hospital:** Los Alamitos Medical Center; **Office Address:** 10861 Cherry St, Ste 204 Box 250 Los Alamitos, CA 90720; **Office Phone:** (562) 598-3160; **Board Certification:** Ophthalmology 1978; **Medical School:** Wayne State Univ 1971; **Residency:** Ophthalmology, Mayo Clinic, Rochester, MN 1975-1978; **Faculty Appointment:** Assoc Clin Prof Ophthalmology, USC Sch Med

Shorr, Norman MD (Ophthalmology) - *Special Expertise:* Oculoplastic Surgery; **Admitting Hospital:** UCLA Medical Center; **Office Address:** 435 N Roxbury Dr, Ste 104 Beverly Hills, CA 90210-5003; **Office Phone:** (310) 278-1839; **Board Certification:** Ophthalmology 1976; **Medical School:** Univ Miami Sch Med 1969; **Residency:** Ophthalmology, Jules Stein Eye Inst-UCLA, Los Angeles, CA 1972-1975; **Fellowship:** UCLA Med Ctr, Los Angeles, CA 1975-1976; **Faculty Appointment:** Clin Prof Ophthalmology, UCLA

OPHTHALMOLOGY

Smith, Ronald E MD (Ophthalmology) - *Special Expertise:* Ophthalmology - General; **Admitting Hospital:** USC University Hospital - Richard K. Eamer Medical Plaza; **Office Address:** Doheny Eye Medical Group 1450 San Pablo Los Angeles, CA 90033; **Office Phone:** (323) 442-6440; **Board Certification:** Ophthalmology 1974; **Medical School:** Johns Hopkins Univ 1967; **Residency:** Wilmer Oph. Inst./Johns Hopkins, Baltimore, MD; **Fellowship:** Francis I Proctor Fdn/UCSF, San Francisco, CA; **Faculty Appointment:** Ophthalmology, USC Sch Med

Stout, J Timothy MD/PhD (Ophthalmology) - *Special Expertise:* Retinal Disorders-Pediatric; Retina/Vitreous Surgery; Retinopathy of Prematurity; **Admitting Hospital:** Oregon Health Science University Hospital and Clinics; **Office Address:** Casey Eye Institute 3375 SW Terwilliger Blvd Portland, OR 97201; **Office Phone:** (503) 494-2435; **Board Certification:** Ophthalmology 1999; **Medical School:** Baylor Coll Med 1989; **Residency:** Ophthalmology, Doheny Eye Inst, Los Angeles, CA 1990-1993; **Fellowships:** Moorfields Eye Hosp, London, England 1993-1994; Doheny Eye Inst, Los Angeles, CA 1994-1995; **Faculty Appointment:** Assoc Clin Prof Ophthalmology, Oregon Hlth Scis Univ

Teplick, Stanley MD (Ophthalmology) - *Special Expertise:* Refractive Surgery; Cataract Surgery; **Office Address:** 9989 SW Nimbus Ave Beaverton, OR 97008; **Office Phone:** (503) 520-0800; **Board Certification:** Ophthalmology 1983; **Medical School:** Hahnemann Univ 1977; **Residency:** Ophthalmology, Mayo Clinic, Rochester, MN 1979-1981;

Turner, Stephen Gordon MD (Ophthalmology) - *Special Expertise:* Refractive Surgery; **Admitting Hospital:** Eden Medical Center; **Office Address:** Turner Eye Inst Med Grp 420 Estudillo Ave San Leandro, CA 94577; **Office Phone:** (510) 614-1515; **Board Certification:** Ophthalmology 1977; **Medical School:** Baylor Coll Med 1968; **Residency:** Ophthalmology, UCSF, San Francisco, CA 1971-1974; **Fellowship:** Ophthalmology, St John Oph Hosp, Jerusalem, Israel 1974-1975; **Faculty Appointment:** Assoc Clin Prof Ophthalmology, UCSF

Weiss, Avery MD (Ophthalmology) - *Special Expertise:* Ophthalmology-Pediatric; Strabismus and Amblyopia; **Admitting Hospital:** Children's Hospital and Regional Medical Center - Seattle; **Office Address:** Chldns Hosp & Med Ctr - Dept Oph, 4800 Sand Point Way NE, MS CH-61 Seattle, WA 98105; **Office Phone:** (206) 526-2100; **Board Certification:** Ophthalmology 1981; **Medical School:** Univ Miami Sch Med 1974; **Residencies:** Internal Medicine, Barnes Hospital, St Louis, MO 1974-1976; Ophthalmology, Barnes Hospital, St Louis, MO 1977-1980; **Fellowships:** Research, Barnes Hospital, St Louis, MO 1976-1977; Pediatric Ophthalmology, Chldns Hosp National Med Ctr, Washington, DC 1980-1981; **Faculty Appointment:** Assoc Prof Ophthalmology, Univ Wash

Wright, Kenneth W MD (Ophthalmology) - *Special Expertise:* Ophthalmology-Pediatric; **Admitting Hospital:** University of California - Irvine Medical Center; **Office Address:** Cedars Sinai Med Ctr Twr 8631 W 3rd St, Ste 304-E Los Angeles, CA 90048; **Office Phone:** (310) 652-6420; **Board Certification:** Ophthalmology 1983; **Medical School:** Boston Univ **Residency:** Ophthalmology, USC Med Ctr, Los Angeles, CA 1978-1981; **Fellowship:** Pediatric Ophthalmology, Johns Hopkins, Baltimore, MD 1981; **Faculty Appointment:** Asst Prof Ophthalmology, UC Irvine

Yoshizumi, Marc Osamu MD (Ophthalmology) - *Special Expertise:* Retinal Disorders; Eye Trauma; **Admitting Hospital:** UCLA Medical Center; **Office Address:** Jules Stein Eye Inst 200 Stein Plaza Los Angeles, CA 90095-7000; **Office Phone:** (310) 825-4749; **Board Certification:** Ophthalmology 1978; **Medical School:** Yale Univ 1970; **Residencies:** Ophthalmology, Mass EE Infirm/Harvard, Boston, MA 1974-1977; Neuropathology, Oxford Univ, Oxford, England 1970-1971; **Fellowship:** Retina, Harvard Med Sch, Boston, MA 1977-1978; **Faculty Appointment:** Prof Ophthalmology, UCLA

Orthopaedic Surgery

An orthopaedic surgeon is trained in the preservation, investigation and restoration of the form and function of the extremities, spine and associated structures by medical, surgical and physical means.

An orthopaedic surgeon is involved with the care of patients whose musculoskeletal problems include congenital deformities, trauma, infections, tumors, metabolic disturbances of the musculoskeletal system, deformities, injuries and degenerative diseases of the spine, hands, feet, knee, hip, shoulder and elbow in children and adults. An orthopaedic surgeon is also concerned with primary and secondary muscular problems and the effects of central or peripheral nervous system lesions of the musculoskeletal system.

Training required: Five years (including general surgery training) plus two years in clinical practice before final certification is achieved

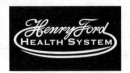

HENRY FORD HOSPITAL
BONE & JOINT CENTER

Henry Ford's Bone and Joint Center treats patients with a variety of bone and joint ailments, including osteoporosis and provides the latest advancements in joint replacement. The multidisciplinary center is comprised of the divisions of Athletic Medicine, Bone and Mineral, Orthopaedics and Rheumatology.

Orthopaedics
Henry Ford is consistently ranked by *U.S. News & World Report* as one of the top orthopaedic departments in the country. More than 25,000 patients throughout the Midwest are treated each year.

Where the Pros Go
Henry Ford physicians are the team doctors for the Detroit Red Wings, Lions and Tigers.

Trauma
In cases of severe injury, the orthopaedic trauma team is available around the clock. Henry Ford experts specialize in treating complex bond infections, including Osteymyelitis.

Pediatrics
Henry Ford offers comprehensive care for developmental dyplasia of the hip, congenital clubfeet, Leg-Calve-Perthes disease, cerebral palsy, spina bifida, Blount's disease, fractures, bone and joint infections and benign bone tumors.

Specialty Care
Services are offered through the Center for Joint Replacement, Foot and Ankle Surgery and Hand Surgery.

Research
Henry Ford scientists are conducting DNA research to develop strategies for enhancing repair of damaged cartilage. Researchers also are developing tools to predict bone strength and identify osteoporosis patients who are at high risk for fractures, and the underlying reasons responsible for degeneration of bone quality.

www.HenryFord.com
1-888-291-8304

LEADING-EDGE PATIENT CARE

The William Clay Ford Center for Athletic Medicine (CAM), which opened in 1980, was one of Detroit's first comprehensive facilities specializing in sports medicine.

Physicians trained in orthopaedic surgery and sports medicine work with physical therapists and athletic trainers to provide the highest quality care to athletes at all levels, including recreational, high school, college and professional.

The patient clinic at CAM is designed to provide diagnosis and treatment for acute and chronic athletic injuries. Rehabilitation and pre- and post-sseason biomechanical evaluations are also offered at the center.

The Athletic Trainers Outreach Program provides on-site certified athletic trainers and team physician services to a variety of high school, college and professional teams.

Orthopaedics and Orthopaedic Surgery
A Heritage of Excellence

Mount Sinai NYU Health offers patients the largest and most accomplished network of orthopaedists and orthopaedic surgeons in the region, with three major centers for orthopaedic care in Manhattan alone. Our orthopaedic surgeons are respected throughout the world for their expertise, scientific contributions, and for their dedication to providing individualized, compassionate care for all orthopaedic patients.

Together, **The Mount Sinai Hospital, NYU Hospitals Center** and the **Hospital for Joint Diseases** provide state-of-the-art diagnosis and treatment for all conditions of the musculoskeletal system, with specialties in:

- Adult and Pediatric Orthopaedics (including diagnosis and treatment for Scoliosis)

- Orthopaedic Oncology

- Joint Replacement (with specialized expertise in Hip, Shoulder and Knee Replacement)

- Arthroscopic Surgery

- Bone Tumor Service

- Podiatric Medicine and Surgery (including Foot and Ankle Surgery)

- Hand and Upper Extremity/Microvascular Surgery

- Limb Lengthening and Bone Growth

- Occupational and Industrial Orthopaedic Care

- Sports Medicine

- Shoulder Surgery

- Neuromuscular and Developmental Disorders

- Geriatric Hip Fracture

- Spine Surgery

- Dance Injuries

- 24-Hour Immediate Orthopaedic Care

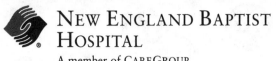

NEW ENGLAND BAPTIST HOSPITAL
A member of CAREGROUP

125 Parker Hill Avenue
Boston, MA 02120
Tel. 617.754.5800 Main number
Tel. 617.754.5477 Physician Referral Line
www.nebh.caregroup.org

GENERAL OVERVIEW

New England Baptist Hospital is a 141-bed adult medical/surgical hospital, in Boston, with specialty services in musculoskeletal care, sports medicine, occupational medicine and cardiology. New England Baptist Hospital is the flagship hospital of the New England Baptist Bone & Joint Institute, the region's leading resource for musculoskeletal treatment, education and research.

WORLD-CLASS MUSCULOSKELETAL CARE

New England Baptist Hospital was the site of one of the first artificial hip replacements in the country. Today, the Baptist ranks among the nation's foremost providers of hip and knee replacement surgery and complex spine surgery and continues to pioneer new methods of diagnosis and treatment of musculosketal conditions.

FULL RANGE OF SERVICES

Through the hospital's physicians, a full range of prevention and education, diagnostic, treatment and rehabilitation services are available in orthopedics and rheumatology, joint replacement, spine care, foot and ankle care, hand surgery, occupational medicine and sports medicine. NEBH is the sports medicine hospital of the Boston Celtics and has cared for elite athletes for many years. To schedule an appointment or for more information call 617-754-5477.

INTERNATIONAL SERVICES

Patients from around the world come to New England Baptist Hospital for world-renowned orthopedic and medical care. In order to meet the individual needs of international patients and families, the hospital established the International Services program. The program offers a wide array of administrative and hospitality services to ensure a positive healthcare experience while at New England Baptist Hospital.

LEADER IN PATIENT SATISFACTION

Since its inception, New England Baptist Hospital has continually taken patient care to new levels and today is recognized for its exceptional blend of caring and commitment.

In each of the past five years, the Press, Ganey survey has ranked New England Baptist Hospital in at least the top 5% of its nationwide hospital survey on patient satisfaction.

PHYSICIAN LISTINGS

New England

Bierbaum, Benjamin MD (Orthopaedic Surgery) - *Special Expertise: Hip Replacement; Knee Surgery;* **Admitting Hospital:** New England Baptist Hospital (Page 57); **Office Address:** New England Baptist Hosp- Main Bldg 125 Parker Hill Ave, Ste 490 Boston, MA 02120-2847; **Office Phone:** (617) 277-1205; **Board Certification:** Orthopaedic Surgery 1993; **Medical School:** Univ Iowa Coll Med 1960; **Residencies:** Orthopaedic Surgery, Philadelphia Gen Hosp, PA 1960-1961; Surgery, Univ Hosp, IA 1961-1962; **Fellowship:** Mass Gen Hosp, MA 1967-1968; **Faculty Appointment:** Clin Prof Orthopaedic Surgery, Tufts Univ

Boland Jr., Arthur L MD (Orthopaedic Surgery) - *Special Expertise: Knee Surgery; Sports Medicine;* **Admitting Hospital:** Massachusetts General Hospital; **Office Address:** 10 Hawthorne Pl, Ste 114 Boston, MA 02114-2336; **Office Phone:** (617) 726-2000; **Board Certification:** Orthopaedic Surgery 1971; **Medical School:** Cornell Univ-Weil Med Coll 1961; **Residencies:** Surgery, NY Hosp-Cornell Med Ctr, New York, NY 1962-1963; Orthopaedic Surgery, Chldns Hosp Med Ctr, Boston, MA 1965-1969

Brick, Gregory MD (Orthopaedic Surgery) - *Special Expertise: Hip & Knee Replacement; Spinal Surgery; Hip & Knee Replacement;* **Admitting Hospital:** Brigham & Women's Hospital; **Office Address:** Brigham and Womens-Dept. Ortho 75 Francis St Boston, MA; **Office Phone:** (617) 732-5386; **Board Certification:** Orthopaedic Surgery 1984; **Medical School:** New Zealand 1976; **Fellowships:** Brigham & Women's Hospital, Boston, MA 1985-1986; Orthopaedic Surgery, Vanderbuilt University Medical Center, Nashville, TN 1986-1987; **Faculty Appointment:** Asst Clin Prof Orthopaedic Surgery, Harvard Med Sch

Browner, Bruce D MD (Orthopaedic Surgery) - *Special Expertise: Fractures-Complex; Osteomyelitis;* **Admitting Hospital:** John Dempsey Hospital - University Connecticut Health Center; **Office Address:** Univ of CT Hlth Ctr 10 Talcott Notch Rd Farmington, CT 06034-4037; **Office Phone:** (860) 679-6655; **Board Certification:** Orthopaedic Surgery 1997; **Medical School:** SUNY Downstate 1973; **Residency:** Orthopaedic Surgery, Albany Med Ctr, Albany, NY 1973-1978; **Fellowship:** Trauma, Albany Med Ctr, Albany, NY 1974-1975

Friedlaender, Gary MD (Orthopaedic Surgery) - *Special Expertise: Bone Tumors;* **Admitting Hospital:** Yale - New Haven Hospital; **Office Address:** Yale Univ Sch Med, Dept Ortho Surg Box 208071 New Haven, CT 06520; **Office Phone:** (203) 785-2579; **Board Certification:** Orthopaedic Surgery 1975; **Medical School:** Univ Mich Med Sch 1969; **Residencies:** Orthopaedic Surgery, Michigan Med Ctr, Ann Arbor, MI 1970-1971; Orthopaedic Surgery, Newington Chldns Hosp, CT 1971-1972; **Fellowship:** Muscular Skel Onc, Mass Genl Hosp, Boston, MA 1983; **Faculty Appointment:** Prof Orthopaedic Surgery, Yale Univ

Gebhardt, Mark MD (Orthopaedic Surgery) - *Special Expertise: Musculoskeletal Tumors; Bone Tmors;* **Admitting Hospital:** Massachusetts General Hospital; **Office Address:** Mass Genl Hosp 55 Fruit St, Gray Bldg-rm 606 Boston, MA 02114; **Office Phone:** (617) 726-5234; **Board Certification:** Orthopaedic Surgery 1992; **Medical School:** Univ Cincinnati 1975; **Residencies:** Surgery, Univ Pitts Hlth Ctr, Pittsburgh, PA 1976-1977; Orthopaedic Surgery, Harvard Med Sch, Boston, MA 1978-1982; **Fellowship:** Pediatric Orthopedic Surgery, Mass Genl Hosp-Boston Chldns Hosp, Boston, MA 1982-1983; **Faculty Appointment:** Assoc Prof Orthopaedic Surgery, Harvard Med Sch

Goldberg, Michael Jay MD (Orthopaedic Surgery) - *Special Expertise: Orthopaedic Surgery-Pediatric; Congenital Malformations & Syndromes; Cerebral Palsy;* **Admitting Hospital:** New England Medical Center; **Office Address:** Tufts-New Eng Med Ctr 750 Washington St, Box 202 Boston, MA 02111-1533; **Office Phone:** (617) 636-7922; **Board Certification:** Orthopaedic Surgery 1992; **Medical School:** SUNY Downstate 1964; **Residencies:** Surgery, Presby Hosp, New York, NY 1965-1966; Orthopaedic Surgery, Boston Hosps, Boston, MA 1967-1970; **Faculty Appointment:** Prof Orthopaedic Surgery, Tufts Univ

Jokl, Peter MD (Orthopaedic Surgery) - *Special Expertise: Knee Surgery;* **Admitting Hospital:** Yale - New Haven Hospital; **Office Address:** 1 Longwharf Dr, Ste 600 New Haven, CT 06511; **Office Phone:** (203) 764-9771; **Board Certification:** Orthopaedic Surgery 1974; **Medical School:** Yale Univ 1968; **Residency:** Orthopaedic Surgery, Yale-New Haven Hosp, New Haven, CT 1969-1972; **Faculty Appointment:** Prof Orthopaedic Surgery, Yale Univ

Jupiter, Jesse B MD (Orthopaedic Surgery) - *Special Expertise: Upper Extremity Trauma; Hand Surgery;* **Admitting Hospital:** Massachusetts General Hospital; **Office Address:** 15 Parkman St, Ste 527, WAC Building Boston, MA 02114-2698; **Office Phone:** (617) 726-8530; **Board Certification:** Orthopaedic Surgery 1982; **Medical School:** Yale Univ 1972; **Residencies:** Surgery, Mass Genl Hosp, Boston, MA 1975-1976; Orthopaedic Surgery, Mass Genl Hosp, Boston, MA 1976-1979; **Fellowship:** Hand Surgery, Univ Louisville, Louisville, KY 1981; **Faculty Appointment:** Assoc Prof Orthopaedic Surgery, Harvard Med Sch

Kasser, James MD (Orthopaedic Surgery) - *Special Expertise: Orthopaedic Surgery-Pediatric;* **Admitting Hospital:** Children's Hospital; **Office Address:** 300 Longwood Avenue Children's Hospital- Orthopaedic Patient Office Boston, MA 02115-5737; **Office Phone:** (617) 355-6021; **Board Certification:** Orthopaedic Surgery 1984; **Medical School:** Tufts Univ 1976; **Residency:** Orthopaedic Surgery, Tufts, Boston, MA 1978-1981; **Fellowship:** Pediatric Orthopedic Surgery, Dupont Institute, Wilmington, DE; **Faculty Appointment:** Orthopaedic Surgery, Harvard Med Sch

Leffert, Robert D. MD (Orthopaedic Surgery) - *Special Expertise: Hand Surgery;* **Admitting Hospital:** Massachusetts General Hospital; **Office Address:** Mass Genl Hosp. Fruit St Boston, MA 02114-2620; **Office Phone:** (617) 726-2954; **Board Certification:** Orthopaedic Surgery 1983; **Medical School:** Tufts Univ 1958; **Residencies:** Orthopaedic Surgery, Hosp. Joint Disease, New York, NY 1960-1963; Surgery, Bellevue Hosp-Cornell U, New York, NY 1959-1960; **Fellowship:** Hand Surgery, Royal Natl Ortho Hosp, London, England 1977-1990; **Faculty Appointment:** Prof Orthopaedic Surgery, Harvard Med Sch

Lipson, Stephen Jay MD (Orthopaedic Surgery) - *Special Expertise: Spinal Surgery;* **Admitting Hospital:** Beth Israel Deaconess Medical Center - Boston (Page 57); **Office Address:** Beth Israel Deaconess Med Ctr 330 Brookline Ave Boston, MA 02215-5400; **Office Phone:** (617) 667-3939; **Board Certification:** Orthopaedic Surgery 1980; **Medical School:** Harvard Med Sch 1972; **Residencies:** Surgery, Mass General Hosp, Boston, MA 1973-1974; Orthopaedic Surgery, Harvard Med Sch, Boston, MA 1974-1977; **Faculty Appointment:** Assoc Prof Orthopaedic Surgery, Harvard Med Sch

Micheli, Lyle J MD (Orthopaedic Surgery) - *Special Expertise: Sports Medicine; Dance/Ballet Injuries;* **Admitting Hospital:** Beth Israel Deaconess Medical Center - Boston (Page 57); **Office Address:** 300 Longwood Ave Boston, MA 02115-5737; **Office Phone:** (617) 355-6028; **Board Certification:** Orthopaedic Surgery 1973; **Medical School:** Harvard Med Sch 1966; **Residencies:** Surgery, U Hospitals, Cleveland, OH 1967; Orthopaedic Surgery, Mass Genl Hospital, Boston, MA 1968-1972; **Faculty Appointment:** Assoc Clin Prof Orthopaedic Surgery, Harvard Med Sch

Poss, Robert MD (Orthopaedic Surgery) - *Special Expertise: Reconstructive Surgery-Hip/Knee;* **Admitting Hospital:** Brigham & Women's Hospital; **Office Address:** Brigham & Women's Hosp, Dept Ortho 75 Francis St Boston, MA 02115; **Office Phone:** (617) 732-5380; **Board Certification:** Orthopaedic Surgery 1992; **Medical School:** SUNY Syracuse 1962; **Residencies:** Surgery, Univ Hosps, Cleveland, OH 1963-1964; Orthopaedic Surgery, Boston Hosps, Boston, MA 1966-1970; **Fellowship:** Research, MIT, Dept Biology, Cambridge, MA 1970-1974; **Faculty Appointment:** Prof Orthopaedic Surgery, Harvard Med Sch

Reilly, Donald T. MD (Orthopaedic Surgery) - *Special Expertise: Hip & Knee Replacement;* **Admitting Hospital:** Beth Israel Deaconess Medical Center - Boston (Page 57); **Office Address:** 330 Brookline Ave Boston, MA; **Office Phone:** (617) 667-3935; **Board Certification:** Orthopaedic Surgery 1984; **Medical School:** Case West Res Univ 1975; **Residency:** Orthopaedic Surgery, Harvard 1977-1981

Scheller, Arnold MD (Orthopaedic Surgery) - *Special Expertise: Sports Medicine;* **Admitting Hospital:** New England Baptist Hospital (Page 57); **Office Address:** Pro Sports Orthopedics 840 Winter St Waltham, MA 02451; **Office Phone:** (781) 487-9444; **Board Certification:** Orthopaedic Surgery 1980; **Medical School:** Rush Med Coll 1980; **Residency:** Orthopaedic Surgery, New England Hosp, Boston, MA 1981-1983; **Faculty Appointment:** Asst Clin Prof Orthopaedic Surgery, Tufts Univ

Scott, Richard David MD (Orthopaedic Surgery) - *Special Expertise: Orthopaedic Surgery - General;* **Admitting Hospital:** Brigham & Women's Hospital; **Office Address:** 125 Parker Hill Ave Boston, MA 02120-2847; **Office Phone:** (617) 738-9151; **Board Certification:** Orthopaedic Surgery 1975; **Medical School:** Temple Univ 1968; **Residency:** Orthopaedic Surgery, Mass General Hosp, Boston, MA 1971-1974; **Fellowships:** Orthopaedic Surgery, Mass General Hosp, Boston, MA 1974; Robert B Brigham Hosp 1975; **Faculty Appointment:** Prof Orthopaedic Surgery, Harvard Med Sch

Thornhill, Thomas S MD (Orthopaedic Surgery) - *Special Expertise: Hip & Knee Replacement; Arthritis;* **Admitting Hospital:** Brigham & Women's Hospital; **Office Address:** Brigham Ortho Assoc 75 Francis St Boston, MA 02115; **Office Phone:** (617) 732-5383; **Board Certifications:** Internal Medicine 1973, Orthopaedic Surgery 1978; **Medical School:** Cornell Univ-Weil Med Coll 1970; **Residencies:** Internal Medicine, Peter Brent Brigham Hosp, Boston, MA 1970-1972; Orthopaedic Surgery, Harvard Combined Prog, Boston, MA 1975-1978; **Faculty Appointment:** Prof Orthopaedic Surgery, Harvard Med Sch

Zarins, Bertram MD (Orthopaedic Surgery) - *Special Expertise: Knee Injuries; Arthroscopic Surgery; Sports Medicine;* **Admitting Hospital:** Massachusetts General Hospital; **Office Address:** Mass Genl Hosp 55 Fruit St, WAC 514 Boston, MA 02114; **Office Phone:** (617) 726-3421; **Board Certification:** Orthopaedic Surgery 1994; **Medical School:** SUNY Syracuse 1967; **Residencies:** Surgery, Johns Hopkins Hosp, Baltimore, MD 1968-1969; Orthopaedic Surgery, Boston Hosp, Boston, MA 1970-1973; **Fellowship:** Sports Medicine, Mass Genl Hosp, Boston, MA 1976; **Faculty Appointment:** Assoc Clin Prof Orthopaedic Surgery, Harvard Med Sch

Mid Atlantic

Balderston, Richard MD (Orthopaedic Surgery) - *Special Expertise: Scoliosis;* **Admitting Hospital:** Pennsylvania Hospital; **Office Address:** Booth Bartolozzi Balderston Orthopedics 800 Spruce St, Fl 1 Philadelphia, PA 19107; **Office Phone:** (215) 829-2222; **Board Certification:** Orthopaedic Surgery 1985; **Medical School:** Univ Penn 1977; **Residency:** Orthopaedic Surgery, Hosp Univ Penn, Philadelphia, PA 1978-1982; **Fellowship:** Spine Surgery, Univ Minn Affil Hosp, Minneapolis, MN 1982-1983; **Faculty Appointment:** Assoc Prof Orthopaedic Surgery, Univ Penn

ORTHOPAEDIC SURGERY *Mid Atlantic*

Baratz, Mark E MD (Orthopaedic Surgery) - *Special Expertise:* Hand Surgery; Upper Extremity Surgery; **Admitting Hospital:** Allegheny General Hospital; **Office Address:** Allegheny Profl Bldg 490 E North Ave, Ste 500 Pittsburgh, PA 15212; **Office Phone:** (412) 359-5196; **Board Certifications:** Orthopaedic Surgery 1993, Hand Surgery 1994; **Medical School:** Univ Pittsburgh 1984; **Residency:** Orthopaedic Surgery, Univ Hlth Ctr PA, Pittsburgh, PA 1987-1990; **Fellowships:** Orthopaedic Surgery, Univ Hlth Ctr PA, Pittsburgh, PA 1985-1987; Hand Surgery, Med Coll of PA, Pittsburgh, PA 1990-1991; **Faculty Appointment:** Assoc Prof Orthopaedic Surgery, Med Coll PA Hahnemann

Bartolozzi, Arthur R. MD (Orthopaedic Surgery) - *Special Expertise:* Sports Medicine; **Admitting Hospital:** Pennsylvania Hospital; **Office Address:** Booth Bartolozzi Balderston Orthopedics 800 Spruce St, Fl 1 Philadelphia, PA; **Office Phone:** (215) 829-2222; **Board Certification:** Orthopaedic Surgery 2000; **Medical School:** UCSD 1981; **Residency:** Orthopaedic Surgery, Hosp Univ Penn, Philadelphia, PA 1982-1986; **Fellowship:** Sports Medicine, UCLA Med Ctr, Los Angeles, CA 1986-1987; **Faculty Appointment:** Assoc Prof Orthopaedic Surgery, Univ Penn

Bauman, Phillip MD (Orthopaedic Surgery) - *Special Expertise:* Sports/Dance Medicine; Arthroscopy of Knee/Foot, Ankle Surgery; **Admitting Hospital:** St Luke's - Roosevelt Hospital Center - Roosevelt Division (Page 58); **Office Address:** 343 W 58th St Orthopaedic Associates of New York New York, NY 10019; **Office Phone:** (212) 765-2260; **Board Certification:** Orthopaedic Surgery 1990; **Medical School:** Columbia P&S 1981; **Residencies:** St Luke's, New York, NY 1981-1983; Orthopaedic Surgery, Columbia-Presby, New York, NY 1984-1987; **Faculty Appointment:** Asst Prof Orthopaedic Surgery, Columbia P&S

Benevenia, Joseph MD (Orthopaedic Surgery) - *Special Expertise:* Musculoskeletal Tumors; **Admitting Hospital:** UMDNJ-University Hospital-Newark; **Office Address:** Doctors Office Ctr 90 Bergen St, Ste 200 Newark, NJ 07103; **Office Phone:** (973) 972-2150; **Board Certification:** Orthopaedic Surgery 1992; **Medical School:** UMDNJ-NJ Med Sch, Newark 1984; **Residency:** Orthopaedic Surgery, UMDNJ-NJ Med Sch., Newark, NJ 1985-1988; **Fellowship:** Orthopedic Oncology, Case Western Reserve Univ, Cleveland, OH 1990-1991; **Faculty Appointment:** Asst Prof Orthopaedic Surgery, UMDNJ-NJ Med Sch, Newark

Bigliani, Louis MD (Orthopaedic Surgery) - *Special Expertise:* Shoulder Surgery; Sports Medicine; **Admitting Hospital:** Columbia Presbyterian Medical Center (Page 72); **Office Address:** 161 Fort Washington Ave New York, NY 10032; **Office Phone:** (212) 305-5564; **Board Certification:** Orthopaedic Surgery 1979; **Medical School:** Loyola Univ-Stritch Sch Med 1973; **Residencies:** Surgery, St Lukes Hosp, New York, NY 1972-1974; Orthopaedic Surgery, Columbia Presby Med Ctr, New York, NY 1974-1977; **Fellowship:** Columbia Presby Med Ctr, New York, NY 1978; **Faculty Appointment:** Prof Orthopaedic Surgery

Blaha, J David MD (Orthopaedic Surgery) - *Special Expertise:* Hip & Knee Replacement; **Admitting Hospital:** West Virginia University Hospital - Ruby Memorial; **Office Address:** West Virginia Univ Hosp PO Box 782 Morgantown, WV 26506-9196; **Office Phone:** (304) 598-4830; **Board Certification:** Orthopaedic Surgery 1979; **Medical School:** Univ Mich Med Sch 1973; **Residencies:** Surgery, Univ Mich, Ann Arbor, MI 1974-1975; Orthopaedic Surgery, Univ Mich, Ann Arbor, MI 1975-1978; **Fellowship:** Joint Replacement Surgery, Univ London, London, England 1979-1980; **Faculty Appointment:** Prof Orthopaedic Surgery, W VA Univ

Boachie, Oheneba MD (Orthopaedic Surgery) - *Special Expertise:* Spinal Surgery; Scoliosis; **Admitting Hospital:** Hospital for Special Surgery (Page 63); **Office Address:** Hosp Spec Surg, Dept Orth 535 E 70th St New York, NY 10021; **Office Phone:** (212) 606-1948; **Board Certification:** Orthopaedic Surgery 2000; **Medical School:** Columbia P&S 1980; **Residencies:** Surgery, St Vincents Hosp, New York, NY 1981-1982; Orthopaedic Surgery, Hosp Spec Surg, New York, NY 1983-1986; **Fellowships:** Orthopaedic Pathology, Hosp Spec Surg, New York, NY 1982-1983; Spine Surgery, Twin Cities Scol Ctr, Minneapolis, MN 1986-1987; **Faculty Appointment:** Assoc Clin Prof Surgery, Cornell Univ-Weil Med Coll

Booth, Robert MD (Orthopaedic Surgery) - *Special Expertise:* Knee Replacement; **Admitting Hospital:** Pennsylvania Hospital; **Office Address:** Booth Bartolozzi Balderston Orthopedics 800 Spruce St, Fl 1 Philadelphia, PA 19107; **Office Phone:** (215) 829-2214; **Board Certification:** Orthopaedic Surgery 1978; **Medical School:** Univ Penn 1971; **Residencies:** Surgery, Penn Hosp, Philadelphia, PA 1972-1973; Orthopaedic Surgery, Penn Hosp, Philadelphia, PA 1973-1977; **Faculty Appointment:** Clin Prof Orthopaedic Surgery, Jefferson Med Coll

Bradley, James P. MD (Orthopaedic Surgery) - *Special Expertise:* Sports Medicine; **Admitting Hospital:** UPMC - Presbyterian University Hospital; **Office Address:** Med Arts Bldg 200 Delafield Ave, Ste 4010 Pittsburgh, PA 15215; **Office Phone:** (412) 784-5770; **Board Certification:** Orthopaedic Surgery 1990; **Medical School:** Georgetown Univ 1982; **Residencies:** Orthopaedic Surgery, Univ Hlth Ctr of Pitts, Pittsburgh, PA 1984-1987; Surgery, Univ TN, Chattanooga, TN 1982-1984; **Fellowship:** Sports Medicine, Kerlan-Jobe Orth Clinic, Inglewood, CA 1987-1988; **Faculty Appointment:** Asst Clin Prof Orthopaedic Surgery, Univ Pittsburgh

Brushart, Thomas M MD (Orthopaedic Surgery) - *Special Expertise:* Hand Surgery; **Admitting Hospital:** Johns Hopkins Hospital - Baltimore (Page 65); **Office Address:** Johns Hopkins Outpatient, Dept Orth Surg 601 N Caroline St Baltimore, MD 21287-0882; **Office Phone:** (410) 955-9663; **Board Certifications:** Orthopaedic Surgery 1985, Hand Surgery 1989; **Medical School:** Harvard Med Sch 1978; **Residency:** Orthopaedic Surgery, Harvard Univ, Boston, MA 1978-1981; **Fellowship:** Hand Surgery, Curtis Hand Ctr, Baltimore, MD 1982-1983; **Faculty Appointment:** Prof Orthopaedic Surgery, Johns Hopkins Univ

Burgess, Andrew MD (Orthopaedic Surgery) - *Special Expertise:* Trauma; **Admitting Hospital:** University of Maryland Medical System; **Office Address:** Univ MD, Dept Orth Surg 22 S Greene St, Ste S11B Baltimore, MD 21201; **Office Phone:** (410) 328-6040; **Board Certification:** Orthopaedic Surgery 1980; **Medical School:** Albany Med Coll 1975; **Residency:** Orthopaedic Surgery, Albany Med Coll, Albany, NY 1976-1979; **Fellowship:** Trauma, MD Inst Emer Med, Baltimore, MD 1981-1982; **Faculty Appointment:** Asst Prof Surgery, Univ MD Sch Med

Crossett, Lawrence MD (Orthopaedic Surgery) - *Special Expertise:* Shoulder Surgery; **Admitting Hospital:** UPMC - Presbyterian University Hospital; **Office Address:** Univ Orth 3471 Fifth Ave Ste 1010 Pittsburgh, PA 15213; **Office Phone:** (412) 687-3900; **Board Certification:** Orthopaedic Surgery 2000; **Medical School:** Temple Univ 1981; **Residencies:** Orthopaedic Surgery, Shriners Hosp Crippled Chldn 1983-1984; Orthopaedic Surgery, Temple Univ, Philadelphia, PA 1984-1986; **Faculty Appointment:** Asst Prof Orthopaedic Surgery, Univ Pittsburgh

Delahay, John Norris MD (Orthopaedic Surgery) - *Special Expertise:* Trauma; Orthopaedic Surgery-Pediatric; **Admitting Hospital:** Georgetown University Hospital; **Office Address:** 3800 Reservoir Rd NW PHC Bldg, Ground FL Washington, DC 20007; **Office Phone:** (202) 687-1438; **Board Certification:** Orthopaedic Surgery 1975; **Medical School:** Georgetown Univ 1969; **Residency:** Orthopaedic Surgery, Georgetown Univ Hosp, Washington, DC 1970-1974; **Faculty Appointment:** Prof Orthopaedic Surgery, Georgetown Univ

ORTHOPAEDIC SURGERY

Mid Atlantic

Deland, Jonathan T MD (Orthopaedic Surgery) - *Special Expertise:* Foot & Ankle Surgery; Sports Medicine; Rheumatoid Arthritis-Reconstruction; **Admitting Hospital:** Hospital for Special Surgery (Page 63); **Office Address:** 523 E 72nd St, Ste 516 New York, NY 10021; **Office Phone:** (212) 606-1665; **Board Certification:** Orthopaedic Surgery 1992; **Medical School:** Columbia P&S 1980; **Residencies:** Orthopaedic Surgery, St Luke's-Roosevelt Hosp Ctr, Boston, MA 1980-1982; Orthopaedic Surgery, Mass Genl Hosp, Boston, MA 1982-1987; **Faculty Appointment:** Asst Prof Surgery, Cornell Univ-Weil Med Coll

Dines, David Michael MD (Orthopaedic Surgery) - *Special Expertise:* Shoulder Surgery; **Admitting Hospital:** North Shore University Hospital at Manhasset; **Office Address:** 935 Northern Blvd, Ste 201 Great Neck, NY 11021; **Office Phone:** (516) 482-1037; **Board Certification:** Orthopaedic Surgery 1980; **Medical School:** UMDNJ-NJ Med Sch, Newark 1974; **Residencies:** Surgery, NY Hosp-Cornell Med Ctr, New York, NY 1975-1976; Orthopaedic Surgery, Hosp for Special Surg, New York, NY 1976-1979; **Faculty Appointment:** Assoc Clin Prof Orthopaedic Surgery, Albert Einstein Coll Med

Donaldson III, William F MD (Orthopaedic Surgery) - *Special Expertise:* Spinal Surgery; **Admitting Hospital:** UPMC - Presbyterian University Hospital; **Office Address:** Univ Pitts Med Ctr, Dept Orth 3471 5th Ave, Ste 1010 Pittsburgh, PA 15213; **Office Phone:** (412) 605-3218; **Board Certification:** Orthopaedic Surgery 1998; **Medical School:** Rush Med Coll 1980; **Residencies:** Surgery, Rush Presby-St Luke's Med Ctr, Chicago, IL 1980-1981; Orthopaedic Surgery, Hosp Special Surg, New York, NY 1981-1985; **Fellowship:** Spine Surgery, Hosp Special Surg, New York, NY 1985-1986; **Faculty Appointment:** Asst Prof Orthopaedic Surgery, Univ Pittsburgh

Farcy, Jean-Pierre MD (Orthopaedic Surgery) - *Special Expertise:* Spinal Surgery; **Admitting Hospital:** Maimonides Medical Center (Page 67); **Office Address:** 927 49th St Brooklyn, NY 11219; **Office Phone:** (718) 283-6520; **Medical School:** France 1967; **Residency:** Orthopaedic Surgery, Univ Marseilles Med Ctr, France 1961-1967; **Fellowship:** Orthopaedic Surgery, Columbia Presby Med Ctr, New York, NY 1981-1983; **Faculty Appointment:** Assoc Clin Prof Orthopaedic Surgery, NYU Sch Med

Flatow, Evan MD (Orthopaedic Surgery) - *Special Expertise:* Shoulder Surgery; **Admitting Hospital:** Mount Sinai Hospital (Page 70); **Office Address:** 5 E 98th St, FL 9 Box 1188 New York, NY 10029; **Office Phone:** (212) 2411663; **Board Certification:** Orthopaedic Surgery 1989; **Medical School:** Columbia P&S 1981; **Residencies:** Surgery, St Luke's, New York, NY 1982-1983; Orthopaedic Surgery, Columbia-Presby, New York, NY 1983-1985; **Fellowship:** Columbia-Presby, New York, NY 1986-1987; **Faculty Appointment:** Prof Orthopaedic Surgery, Columbia P&S

Frassica, Frank John MD (Orthopaedic Surgery) - *Special Expertise:* Orthopaedic Surgery - General; **Admitting Hospital:** Johns Hopkins Hospital - Baltimore (Page 65); **Office Address:** JHOC Dept. of Oncology 601 N Caroline St, Ste 5215 Baltimore, MD 21287-0882; **Office Phone:** (410) 955-9414; **Board Certification:** Orthopaedic Surgery 1990; **Medical School:** Univ SC Sch Med 1982; **Residency:** Orthopaedic Surgery, Mayo Clinic, Rochester, MN 1983-1987; **Fellowship:** Orthopaedic Surgery, Mayo Clinic, Rochester, MN 1987-1988; **Faculty Appointment:** Prof Orthopaedic Surgery, Johns Hopkins Univ

Fu, Freddie MD (Orthopaedic Surgery) - *Special Expertise:* Sports Medicine; **Admitting Hospital:** UPMC - Presbyterian University Hospital; **Office Address:** Dept. of Orthoapedic Surgery 3471 5th Ave, Ste 1011 Pittsburgh, PA 15213; **Office Phone:** (412) 605-3265; **Board Certification:** Orthopaedic Surgery 1984; **Medical School:** Dartmouth Med Sch 1977; **Residency:** Orthopaedic Surgery, U Pittsburgh, Pittsburgh, PA 1979-1982; **Fellowship:** Orthopaedic Surgery, U Pittsburgh, Pittsburgh, PA 1978-1979; **Faculty Appointment:** Prof Orthopaedic Surgery, Univ Pittsburgh

Grant, Richard E MD (Orthopaedic Surgery) - *Special Expertise:* Hip & Knee Replacement; Spine Surgery-Low Back; **Admitting Hospital:** Howard University Hospital; **Office Address:** Howard Univ Hosp, Dept Ortho Surg 2041 Georgia Ave NW, Towers Bldg, Ste 4300 Washington, DC 20060; **Office Phone:** (202) 865-1183; **Board Certification:** Orthopaedic Surgery 1992; **Medical School:** Howard Univ 1976; **Residency:** Orthopaedic Surgery, Wilford Hall Med Ctr-Lackland, San Antonio, TX 1980-1984; **Fellowships:** Joint Arthroplasty, Ohio State Univ Hosp, Columbus, OH 1985; Spinal Cord Injury Medicine, St Lukes/Baylor Univ, Houston, TX 1986; **Faculty Appointment:** Assoc Prof Surgery, Howard Univ

Grelsamer, Ronald MD (Orthopaedic Surgery) - *Special Expertise:* Patella Problems; Sports Medicine; Hip & Knee Replacement; **Admitting Hospital:** Hospital for Joint Diseases; **Office Address:** The Knee Center 345 E 37th St, Fl 317A New York, NY 10016; **Office Phone:** (212) 535-4848; **Board Certification:** Orthopaedic Surgery 1987; **Medical School:** Columbia P&S 1979; **Residency:** Surgery, Columbia Presby Med Ctr, New York, NY 1981-1984; **Fellowship:** Orthopaedic Surgery, Columbia Presby Med Ctr, New York, NY 1984-1985

Hannafin, Jo MD/PhD (Orthopaedic Surgery) - *Special Expertise:* Sports Medicine-Women; **Admitting Hospital:** Hospital for Special Surgery (Page 63); **Office Address:** 523 E 72nd St, Fl 3rd New York, NY 10021; **Office Phone:** (212) 606-1469; **Board Certification:** Orthopaedic Surgery 1994; **Medical School:** Albert Einstein Coll Med 1985; **Residencies:** Surgery, Montefiore Hosp Med Ctr, Bronx, NY 1986-1990; Orthopaedic Surgery, Montefiore Hosp Med Ctr, Bronx, NY 1990-1991; **Fellowship:** Sports Medicine, Hosp Special Surg-Cornell Med Coll, New York, NY 1990-1992; **Faculty Appointment:** Asst Prof Surgery, Cornell Univ-Weil Med Coll

Healey, John MD (Orthopaedic Surgery) - *Special Expertise:* Bone Tumors; **Admitting Hospital:** Memorial Sloan Kettering Cancer Center; **Office Address:** Meml Sloan-Kettering Cancer Ctr, Dept Orth Surg 1275 York Ave, Ste A675 New York, NY 10021-6007; **Office Phone:** (212) 639-7610; **Board Certification:** Orthopaedic Surgery 1986; **Medical School:** Univ VT Coll Med 1978; **Residency:** Orthopaedic Surgery, Hosp for Spec Surg, New York, NY 1979-1983; **Fellowships:** Orthopaedic Surgery, Meml Sloan Kettering Cancer Ctr, New York, NY 1983-1984; Orthopaedic Surgery, Hosp For Spec Surg, New York, NY 1983-1984; **Faculty Appointment:** Assoc Prof Orthopaedic Surgery, Cornell Univ-Weil Med Coll

Helfet, David L MD (Orthopaedic Surgery) - *Special Expertise:* Fractures-Complex; Trauma; **Admitting Hospital:** Hospital for Special Surgery (Page 63); **Office Address:** 535 E 70th St New York, NY 10021; **Office Phone:** (212) 606-1888; **Board Certification:** Orthopaedic Surgery 1984; **Medical School:** South Africa 1975; **Residencies:** Surgery, Edendale Hosp, Pietermaritzburg, South Africa 1975-1977; Orthopaedic Surgery, Johns Hopkins, Baltimore, MD 1977-1981; **Fellowships:** Orthopaedic Surgery, Inselspita Hosp, Bern, Switzerland 1981; Orthopaedic Surgery, UCLA Med Ctr, Los Angeles, CA 1981-1982; **Faculty Appointment:** Prof Orthopaedic Surgery, Cornell Univ-Weil Med Coll

Hotchkiss, Robert MD (Orthopaedic Surgery) - *Special Expertise:* Hand Surgery; **Admitting Hospital:** Hospital for Special Surgery (Page 63); **Office Address:** 523 E 72nd St New York, NY 10021; **Office Phone:** (212) 606-1964; **Board Certifications:** Orthopaedic Surgery 1989, Hand Surgery 2000; **Medical School:** Johns Hopkins Univ 1980; **Residencies:** Surgery, Johns Hopkins Hosp, Baltimore, MD 1981-1982; Orthopaedic Surgery, Johns Hopkins Hosp, Baltimore, MD 1982-1985; **Fellowship:** Hand Surgery, Union Meml Hosp, Baltimore, MD 1986-1987; **Faculty Appointment:** Assoc Prof Orthopaedic Surgery, Cornell Univ-Weil Med Coll

ORTHOPAEDIC SURGERY

Mid Atlantic

Johnson, Carl A MD (Orthopaedic Surgery) - *Special Expertise:* Knee Surgery; **Admitting Hospital:** Johns Hopkins Hospital - Baltimore (Page 65); **Office Address:** Johns Hopkins Univ, Dept Orth Surg 601 N Caroline St Baltimore, MD 21287-0881; **Office Phone:** (410) 955-7084; **Board Certification:** Orthopaedic Surgery 1983; **Medical School:** Johns Hopkins Univ 1976; **Residencies:** Surgery, Johns Hopkins Hosp, Baltimore, MD 1977-1978; Orthopaedic Surgery, Johns Hopkins Hosp, Baltimore, MD 1978-1981; **Faculty Appointment:** Assoc Prof Orthopaedic Surgery, Johns Hopkins Univ

Lauerman, William MD (Orthopaedic Surgery) - *Special Expertise:* Spinal Deformities-Adult & Pediatric; Spinal Surgery; **Admitting Hospital:** Georgetown University Hospital; **Office Address:** GUMC-Spine Surgery Office, 1 Gorman Bldg 3800 Reservoir Rd NW Washington, DC 20007; **Office Phone:** (202) 687-0655; **Board Certification:** Orthopaedic Surgery 1990; **Medical School:** Georgetown Univ 1982; **Residency:** Orthopaedic Surgery, Georgetown Univ Med Ctr, Washington, DC 1982-1987; **Fellowship:** Orthopaedic Surgery, Univ Minn-Twin Cities Scoliosis Ctr, Minneapolis, MN 1987-1988; **Faculty Appointment:** Assoc Prof Orthopaedic Surgery, Georgetown Univ

Myerson, Mark MD (Orthopaedic Surgery) - *Special Expertise:* Foot & Ankle Surgery; **Admitting Hospital:** Union Memorial Hospital - Baltimore; **Office Address:** 3333 N Calvert St, Ste 400 Baltimore, MD 21218-6501; **Office Phone:** (410) 554-2866; **Board Certification:** Orthopaedic Surgery 1999; **Medical School:** South Africa 1979; **Residencies:** John Hopkins Hospital University MD, Baltimore, MD 1982-1985; Sinai Hospital, Baltimore, MD 1980-1981; **Fellowship:** Hospital Joint Disease, New York, NY 1986

O'Leary, Patrick MD (Orthopaedic Surgery) - *Special Expertise:* Spinal Surgery; **Admitting Hospital:** Lenox Hill Hospital; **Office Address:** 1160 Park Ave New York, NY 10128; **Office Phone:** (212) 249-8100; **Board Certification:** Orthopaedic Surgery 1976; **Medical School:** Ireland 1968; **Residencies:** Surgery, Roosevelt Hosp., New York, NY 1969-1972; Orthopaedic Surgery, Hosp Spec Surg-Cornell, New York, NY 1972-1975; **Fellowship:** Spine Surgery, Univ Toronto Genl Hosp, Toronto, Canada 1975-1976; **Faculty Appointment:** Assoc Clin Prof Orthopaedic Surgery, Cornell Univ-Weil Med Coll

Osterman Jr, Arthur Lee MD (Orthopaedic Surgery) - *Special Expertise:* Hand Surgery; Wrist Arthroscopy; Nerve and Muscle Diseases; **Admitting Hospital:** Thomas Jefferson University Hospital; **Office Address:** Philadelphia Hand Center 700 S Henderson Rd, Ste 200 King of Prussia, PA 19406; **Office Phone:** (610) 768-4467; **Board Certifications:** Orthopaedic Surgery 1980, Hand Surgery 1990; **Medical School:** Univ Penn 1973; **Residencies:** Orthopaedic Surgery, Hosp Univ Penn, Philadelphia, PA 1974-1978; Orthopaedic Surgery, Hos Univ Penn, Philadelphia, PA 1977-1978; **Fellowship:** Hand Surgery, Hos Univ Penn, Philadelphia, PA 1978-1979; **Faculty Appointment:** Prof Surgery, Jefferson Med Coll

Palmer, Andrew MD (Orthopaedic Surgery) - *Special Expertise:* Hand Surgery; **Admitting Hospital:** University Hospital - SUNY Upstate Medical University; **Office Address:** SUNY Hlth Sci Ctr, Dept Orth 550 Harrison Street Syracuse, NY 13202-3096; **Office Phone:** (315) 472-2015; **Board Certifications:** Orthopaedic Surgery 1978, Hand Surgery 1998; **Medical School:** SUNY Syracuse 1972; **Residency:** Orthopaedic Surgery, Univ Mich, Ann Arbor, MI 1973-1976; **Fellowship:** Hand Surgery, Mayo Clinic, Rochester, MN 1976; **Faculty Appointment:** Prof Orthopaedic Surgery, SUNY Syracuse

Ranawat, Chitranjan MD (Orthopaedic Surgery) - *Special Expertise: Hip Surgery; Knee Surgery;* **Admitting Hospital:** Lenox Hill Hospital; **Office Address:** 130 E 77th St, FL 11 New York, NY 10021; **Office Phone:** (212) 434-4700; **Board Certification:** Orthopaedic Surgery 1969; **Medical School:** India 1962; **Residencies:** Surgery, MY Hosp. Indore, India 1959-1963; Orthopaedic Surgery, Albany Med Ctr, Albany, NY 1964-1965; **Fellowship:** Orthopaedic Surgery, Hospital Special Surgery, New York, NY 1967-1969; **Faculty Appointment:** Prof Orthopaedic Surgery, Cornell Univ-Weil Med Coll

Rosenwasser, Melvin MD (Orthopaedic Surgery) - *Special Expertise: Carpal Tunnel Syndrome; Hand Surgery;* **Admitting Hospital:** Columbia Presbyterian Medical Center (Page 72); **Office Address:** Columbia Presby Med Ctr, Dept Orth 161 Fort Washington Ave, rm 251 New York, NY 10032; **Office Phone:** (212) 305-8036; **Board Certifications:** Orthopaedic Surgery 1985, Hand Surgery 1989; **Medical School:** Columbia P&S 1976; **Residencies:** Surgery, St Lukes Roosevelt, New York, NY 1976-1979; Orthopaedic Surgery, Columbia Presby Med Ctr, New York, NY 1979-1982; **Fellowship:** Hand Surgery, Columbia Presby Med Ctr, New York, NY 1982-1983; **Faculty Appointment:** Asst Prof Orthopaedic Surgery, Columbia P&S

Rosier, Randy MD/PhD (Orthopaedic Surgery) - *Special Expertise: Bone Disorders-Metabolic;* **Admitting Hospital:** Strong Memorial Hospital - Medical Center; **Office Address:** 601 Elmwood Ave, Box 655 Rochester, NY 14642; **Office Phone:** (716) 275-3100; **Board Certification:** Orthopaedic Surgery 2007; **Medical School:** Univ Rochester 1978; **Residency:** Univ Iowa, Iowa City, IA 1979-1981; **Fellowship:** Univ Iowa, Iowa City, IA 1982-1983

Rothman, Richard MD (Orthopaedic Surgery) - *Special Expertise: Hip & Knee Replacement;* **Admitting Hospital:** Thomas Jefferson University Hospital; **Office Address:** 925 Chesnut St, Fl 5 Philadelphia, PA 19107; **Office Phone:** (215) 955-3458; **Board Certification:** Orthopaedic Surgery 1970; **Medical School:** Univ Penn 1962; **Residency:** Orthopaedic Surgery, Jefferson Hosp, Philadelphia, PA 1963-1968; **Faculty Appointment:** Prof Orthopaedic Surgery, Jefferson Med Coll

Roye, David MD (Orthopaedic Surgery) - *Special Expertise: Orthopaedic Surgery-Pediatric; Scoliosis;* **Admitting Hospital:** Columbia Presbyterian Medical Center (Page 72); **Office Address:** Columbia Presby, Dept Ped Surg 3959 Broadway New York, NY 10032; **Office Phone:** (212) 305-5475; **Board Certification:** Orthopaedic Surgery 1981; **Medical School:** Columbia P&S 1975; **Residency:** Orthopaedic Surgery, Columbia P&S, New York, NY 1976-1979; **Fellowship:** Orthopaedic Surgery, Hosp For Sick Chldrn, Toronto, Canada 1979-1980; **Faculty Appointment:** Prof Orthopaedic Surgery, Columbia P&S

Salvati, Eduardo Augustin MD (Orthopaedic Surgery) - *Special Expertise: Hip Surgery; Hip & Knee Replacement;* **Admitting Hospital:** Hospital for Special Surgery (Page 63); **Office Address:** Hosp for Spec Surg 535 E 70th Street New York, NY 10021-4872; **Office Phone:** (212) 606-1472; **Board Certification:** Orthopaedic Surgery 1972; **Medical School:** Argentina 1963; **Residencies:** Orthopaedic Surgery, Univ of Florence Orth Clinic, Florence, Italy 1963-1965; Orthopaedic Surgery, Hosp Buenos Aires, Buenos Aires, Argentina 1966-1969; **Fellowship:** Hip Surgery, Hosp For Spec Surg, New York, NY 1969-1972; **Faculty Appointment:** Clin Prof Orthopaedic Surgery, Cornell Univ-Weil Med Coll

Scott, W Norman MD (Orthopaedic Surgery) - *Special Expertise: Knee Injuries; Knee Replacement;* **Admitting Hospital:** Beth Israel Medical Center - Herbert & Nell Singer Division (Page 58); **Office Address:** 170 East End Ave, Fl 4 Bet 87th & 88th Sts New York, NY 10128-7603; **Office Phone:** (212) 870-9740; **Board Certification:** Orthopaedic Surgery 1978; **Medical School:** Cornell Univ-Weil Med Coll 1972; **Residencies:** Orthopaedic Surgery, Hosp For Special Surgery, New York, NY 1974-1977; Surgery, St Luke's-Roosevelt Hosp Ctr, New York, NY 1973-1974; **Faculty Appointment:** Assoc Clin Prof Orthopaedic Surgery, Cornell Univ-Weil Med Coll

Sculco, Thomas Peter MD (Orthopaedic Surgery) - *Special Expertise: Hip & Knee Replacement;* **Admitting Hospital:** Hospital for Special Surgery (Page 63); **Office Address:** 535 E 70TH St, Fl 238 New York, NY 10021; **Office Phone:** (212) 606-1475; **Board Certification:** Orthopaedic Surgery 1976; **Medical School:** Columbia P&S 1969; **Residencies:** Surgery, St Luke's Roosevelt, New York, NY 1970-1971; Orthopaedic Surgery, Hosp For Spec Surg, New York, NY 1971-1974; **Fellowship:** Orthopaedic Surgery, London Hosp, London, England 1974-1975; **Faculty Appointment:** Prof Surgery, Cornell Univ-Weil Med Coll

Sherman, Orrin MD (Orthopaedic Surgery) - *Special Expertise: Knee Injuries/Ligament Surgery; Shoulder Surgery; Arthroscopic Surgery;* **Admitting Hospital:** NYU Downtown Hospital; **Office Address:** 530 1st Ave, Fl 8U New York, NY 10016; **Office Phone:** (212) 263-8961; **Board Certification:** Orthopaedic Surgery 1997; **Medical School:** Geo Wash Univ 1978; **Residency:** Orthopaedic Surgery, NYU Med Ctr, New York, NY 1979-1983; **Fellowship:** Sports Medicine, So Cal Med Ctr, Van Nuys, CA 1983-1984; **Faculty Appointment:** Asst Prof Orthopaedic Surgery, NYU Sch Med

Sponseller, Paul D MD (Orthopaedic Surgery) - *Special Expertise: Cerebral Palsy; Scoliosis; Orthopaedic Surgery-Pediatric;* **Admitting Hospital:** Johns Hopkins Hospital - Baltimore (Page 65); **Office Address:** Johns Hopkins Med Ctr 601 N Caroline St, rm 5253 Baltimore, MD 21287-0006; **Office Phone:** (410) 955-1795; **Board Certification:** Orthopaedic Surgery 2000; **Medical School:** Univ Mich Med Sch 1980; **Residency:** Orthopaedic Surgery, Univ Wisc Hosp, Madison, WI 1980-1985; **Fellowship:** Pediatric Orthopedic Surgery, Chldns Hosp, Boston, MA 1985-1986; **Faculty Appointment:** Prof Orthopaedic Surgery, Johns Hopkins Univ

Springfield, Dempsey MD (Orthopaedic Surgery) - *Special Expertise: Bone Tumors;* **Admitting Hospital:** Mount Sinai Hospital (Page 70); **Office Address:** Mt Sinai Med Ctr, Dept Ortho 5 E 98th St, Fl 9, Box 1188 New York, NY 10029; **Office Phone:** (212) 241-8311; **Board Certification:** Orthopaedic Surgery 1992; **Medical School:** Univ Fla Coll Med 1971; **Residency:** Orthopaedic Surgery, Univ Florida/Shands, Gainesville, FL 1972-1978; **Fellowship:** Orthopaedic Surgery, Univ Florida/Shands, Gainesville, FL 1978-1979; **Faculty Appointment:** Prof Orthopaedic Surgery, Mount Sinai Sch Med

Strongwater, Allan MD (Orthopaedic Surgery) - *Special Expertise: Orthopaedic Surgery-Pediatric;* **Admitting Hospital:** Maimonides Medical Center (Page 67); **Office Address:** Maimonides Med Ctr 927 49th St Brooklyn, NY 11219-2923; **Office Phone:** (718) 283-7400; **Board Certification:** Orthopaedic Surgery 1986; **Medical School:** Rush Med Coll 1978; **Residencies:** Orthopaedic Surgery, Yale-New Haven Hosp, New Haven, CT 1978-1983; Orthopaedic Surgery, Hosp Joint Diseases, New York, NY 1983-1984; **Faculty Appointment:** Clin Prof Orthopaedic Surgery, SUNY Hlth Sci Ctr

Tischler, Henry MD (Orthopaedic Surgery) - *Special Expertise: Hip Replacement;* **Admitting Hospital:** University Hospital - Brooklyn; **Office Address:** Brooklyn Spine and Arthritis Ctr 519 6th St Brooklyn, NY 11203; **Office Phone:** (718) 780-3104; **Board Certification:** Orthopaedic Surgery 1995; **Medical School:** SUNY Downstate 1985; **Residencies:** Surgery, Univ Hosp, Brooklyn, NY 1985-1986; Orthopaedic Surgery, Univ Hosp, Brooklyn, NY 1986-1990; **Fellowship:** Orthopaedic Surgery, Tampa Gen, Tampa, FL 1990-1991; **Faculty Appointment:** Asst Prof Orthopaedic Surgery, SUNY Hlth Sci Ctr

Waller, John F MD (Orthopaedic Surgery) - *Special Expertise: Foot Surgery; Ankle Surgery;* **Admitting Hospital:** Lenox Hill Hospital; **Office Address:** 133 E 58th St, Fl 14 New York, NY 10022; **Office Phone:** (212) 583-2920; **Board Certification:** Orthopaedic Surgery 1979; **Medical School:** NY Med Coll 1971; **Residency:** Orthopaedic Surgery, Lenox Hill Hosp, New York, NY 1974-1977; **Fellowship:** Orthopaedic Surgery, Hosp For Special Surgery, New York, NY 1978-1979

Wapner, Keith Leslie MD (Orthopaedic Surgery) - *Special Expertise:* Foot Surgery; **Admitting Hospital:** Hahnemann University Hospital; **Office Address:** The Farm Journal Bldg 5th FL. 230 W Washington Square Philadelphia, PA 19106; **Office Phone:** (215) 829-3668; **Board Certification:** Orthopaedic Surgery 1999; **Medical School:** Temple Univ 1980; **Residencies:** Surgery, Hosp Univ Penn, Philadelphia, PA 1980-1981; Orthopaedic Surgery, Hosp Univ Penn, Philadelphia, PA 1981-1985; **Fellowships:** Joint Reconstruction, Ohio St Univ Med Ctr, Columbus, OH 1985; Foot/Ankle Reconstruction, UCSF Med Ctr, San Francisco, CA 1986; **Faculty Appointment:** Prof Orthopaedic Surgery, Hahnemann Univ

Warren, Russell MD (Orthopaedic Surgery) - *Special Expertise:* Knee Surgery; Shoulder Reconstruction; **Admitting Hospital:** Hospital for Special Surgery (Page 63); **Office Address:** 535 E 70th St New York, NY 10021-4892; **Office Phone:** (212) 606-1178; **Board Certification:** Orthopaedic Surgery 1974; **Medical School:** SUNY Syracuse 1966; **Residencies:** Surgery, St Luke's Hosp, New York, NY 1966-1968; Orthopaedic Surgery, Hosp For Special Surgery, New York, NY 1970-1973; **Fellowship:** Sports Medicine, Columbia-Presby Med Ctr, New York, NY 1976; **Faculty Appointment:** Prof Orthopaedic Surgery, Cornell Univ-Weil Med Coll

Wickiewicz, Thomas MD (Orthopaedic Surgery) - *Special Expertise:* Shoulder Surgery; Sports Medicine; **Admitting Hospital:** Hospital for Special Surgery (Page 63); **Office Address:** 525 E 70th St New York, NY 10021; **Office Phone:** (212) 606-1450; **Board Certification:** Orthopaedic Surgery 1984; **Medical School:** UMDNJ-NJ Med Sch, Newark 1976; **Residency:** Orthopaedic Surgery, Hosp for Special Surg, New York, NY 1977-1981; **Fellowship:** Sports Medicine, UCLA, Los Angeles, CA 1981-1982; **Faculty Appointment:** Prof Orthopaedic Surgery, Cornell Univ-Weil Med Coll

Wiesel, Sam W MD (Orthopaedic Surgery) - *Special Expertise:* Spinal Surgery; **Admitting Hospital:** Georgetown University Hospital; **Office Address:** Georgetown Univ Hosp, Dept Ortho Surg 3800 Reservoir Rd Washington, DC 20007-2113; **Office Phone:** (202) 687-7803; **Board Certification:** Orthopaedic Surgery 1977; **Medical School:** Univ Penn 1971; **Residency:** Orthopaedic Surgery, Univ Penn, Philadelphia, PA 1972-1973; **Fellowship:** Orthopaedic Surgery, Univ Penn, Philadelphia, PA 1973-1976

Zuckerman, Joseph MD (Orthopaedic Surgery) - *Special Expertise:* Shoulder Surgery; Hip & Knee Replacement; **Admitting Hospital:** Hospital for Joint Diseases; **Office Address:** Hosp for Joint Dis, Dept of Orth 301 E 17th St, Fl 14 New York, NY 10003-3804; **Office Phone:** (212) 598-6674; **Board Certifications:** Orthopaedic Surgery 1986, Orthopaedic Surgery 1992; **Medical School:** Med Coll Wisc 1978; **Residency:** Orthopaedic Surgery, Univ WA Med Ctr, Seattle, WA 1979-1983; **Fellowships:** Arthritis Surgery, Brigham & Woman's Hosp, Boston, MA 1983-1984; Shoulder Surgery, Mayo Clin, Rochester, MN 1984; **Faculty Appointment:** Prof Orthopaedic Surgery, NYU Sch Med

Southeast

Beaty, James Harold MD (Orthopaedic Surgery) - *Special Expertise:* Trauma; Orthopaedic Surgery-Pediatric; **Admitting Hospital:** Campbell Clinic; **Office Address:** Cambell Clinic 910 Madison Ave Memphis, TN 38103; **Office Phone:** (901) 759-3125; **Board Certification:** Orthopaedic Surgery 1995; **Medical School:** Univ Tenn Coll Med, Memphis 1976; **Residencies:** Surgery, Baptist Meml Hosp, Memphis, TN 1978-1979; Orthopaedic Surgery, Campbell Clin Fdn, Memphis, TN 1979-1982; **Fellowship:** Orthopaedic Surgery, Alfred I Dupont Inst, Wilmington, TN 1982; **Faculty Appointment:** Prof Orthopaedic Surgery, Univ Tenn Coll Med, Memphis

ORTHOPAEDIC SURGERY

Cuckler, John MD (Orthopaedic Surgery) - *Special Expertise:* Hip & Knee Replacement; **Admitting Hospital:** University of Alabama Hospital at Birmingham; **Office Address:** 2000 6TH Ave South Birmingham, AL; **Office Phone:** (205) 975-2663; **Board Certification:** Orthopaedic Surgery 1981; **Medical School:** NYU Sch Med 1975; **Residency:** Orthopaedic Surgery, Hosp Univ Penn, Philadelphia, PA; **Faculty Appointment:** Prof Orthopaedic Surgery, Univ Ala

Curl, Walton Wright MD (Orthopaedic Surgery) - *Special Expertise:* Sports Medicine; **Admitting Hospital:** Wake Forest University Baptist Medical Center; **Office Address:** Comp-Rehab Assoc 131 Miller Winston Salem, NC 27157; **Office Phone:** (336) 716-8091; **Board Certification:** Orthopaedic Surgery 1980; **Medical School:** Duke Univ 1973; **Residency:** Orthopaedic Surgery, Letterman Army Med Ctr, San Francisco, CA 1975-1978; **Fellowship:** Sports Medicine, Keller Army Hosp, West Point, NY 1978-1979; **Faculty Appointment:** Asst Prof Orthopaedic Surgery, Wake Forest Univ Sch Med

Eismont, Frank MD (Orthopaedic Surgery) - *Special Expertise:* Spinal Surgery; **Admitting Hospital:** University of Miami - Jackson Memorial Hospital; **Office Address:** Univ Miami, Dept Orth Surg 1475 NW 12th Ave Miami, FL 33136; **Office Phone:** (305) 243-3000; **Board Certification:** Orthopaedic Surgery 1994; **Medical School:** Univ Rochester 1973; **Residency:** Orthopaedic Surgery, Case Western Res Univ Hosp, Cleveland, OH 1975-1978; **Fellowships:** Spine Surgery, Case Western Res Univ Hosp, Cleveland, OH 1978-1979; Spine Surgery, PA Hosp, Philadelphia, PA 1979-1980

Garrett, William MD (Orthopaedic Surgery) - *Special Expertise:* Sports Medicine; Shoulder & Knee Surgery; Shoulder & Knee Reconstruction; **Admitting Hospital:** University of North Carolina Hospitals; **Office Address:** Univ NC Sch Med, Dept Orthopaedics Burnett Womack Bldg Rm 236 - CB 7055 Chapel Hill, NC 27599-7055; **Office Phone:** (919) 966-6637; **Board Certification:** Orthopaedic Surgery 1985; **Medical School:** Duke Univ 1976; **Residency:** Orthopaedic Surgery, Duke Univ Med Ctr, Durham, NC 1976-1982; **Faculty Appointment:** Prof Orthopaedic Surgery, Univ NC Sch Med

Goldner, Richard MD (Orthopaedic Surgery) - *Special Expertise:* Orthopaedic Surgery - General; **Admitting Hospital:** Duke University Medical Center (Page 60); **Office Address:** Duke Univ Med Ctr, Dept Orth Surg Box 3480 Durham, NC 27710; **Office Phone:** (919) 684-6461; **Board Certifications:** Orthopaedic Surgery 1982, Hand Surgery 2000; **Medical School:** Duke Univ 1974; **Residencies:** Orthopaedic Surgery, Univ Virginia, Charlottesville, VA 1976-1980; Surgery, Duke Univ Med Ctr, Durham, NC 1975-1976; **Fellowship:** Hand Surgery, Duke Univ Med Ctr, Durham, NC 1980-1981; **Faculty Appointment:** Assoc Prof Orthopaedic Surgery, Duke Univ

Green, Neil Edward MD (Orthopaedic Surgery) - *Special Expertise:* Orthopaedic Surgery-Pediatric; Scoliosis & Kyphosis; **Admitting Hospital:** Vanderbilt University Medical Center; **Office Address:** Vanderbilt Univ Medical Center Medical Center North, rm D4207 Nashville, TN 37232; **Office Phone:** (615) 322-7133; **Board Certification:** Orthopaedic Surgery 1992; **Medical School:** Albany Med Coll 1968; **Residencies:** Surgery, Duke Univ Med Ctr, Durham, NC 1969-1970; Orthopaedic Surgery, Duke Univ Med Ctr, Durham, NC 1970-1974

Johnson, Darren Lee MD (Orthopaedic Surgery) - *Special Expertise:* Knee Injuries; Sports Medicine; **Admitting Hospital:** University of Kentucky Medical Center; **Office Address:** Univ of Kentucky 740 S Limestone, Ste K401 Lexington, KY 40536-0284; **Office Phone:** (859) 257-4969; **Board Certification:** Orthopaedic Surgery 1995; **Medical School:** UCLA 1987; **Residency:** Orthopaedic Surgery, LA Co-USC Med Ctr, Los Angeles, CA 1988-1992; **Fellowship:** Sports Medicine, Univ Pittsburgh, Pittsburgh, PA 1992-1993; **Faculty Appointment:** Assoc Prof Orthopaedic Surgery, Univ KY Coll Med

Minkoff, Jeffrey MD (Orthopaedic Surgery) - *Special Expertise:* Sports Medicine; **Admitting Hospital:** Cleveland Clinic Florida; **Office Address:** Cleveland Clinic, Dept Ortho Surgery 3000 W Cypress Creek Rd Ft Lauderdale, FL 33309; **Office Phone:** (954) 978-7425; **Board Certification:** Orthopaedic Surgery 1973; **Medical School:** SUNY Downstate 1967; **Residencies:** Orthopaedic Surgery, Bronx Muni Hosp, New York, NY 1968-1969; Orthopaedic Surgery, Lenox Hill Hosp, New York, NY 1969-1972

Perry, James MD (Orthopaedic Surgery) - *Special Expertise:* Hip & Knee Replacement; **Admitting Hospital:** Mayo/St Luke's Hospital; **Office Address:** 4555 Emerson Expressway Ste 100 Jacksonville, FL 32207; **Office Phone:** (904) 346-1772; **Board Certification:** Orthopaedic Surgery 1982; **Medical School:** Univ Fla Coll Med 1975; **Residency:** Orthopaedic Surgery, Dartmouth Affil Hosps, Hanover, NH 1976-1979; **Fellowship:** Sports Medicine, Boston Chldns Hosp, Boston, MA; **Faculty Appointment:** Asst Prof Orthopaedic Surgery, Univ Fla Coll Med

Pettrone, Frank A MD (Orthopaedic Surgery) - *Special Expertise:* Sports Medicine; Shoulder & Knee Surgery; **Admitting Hospital:** Arlington Hospital; **Office Address:** 1635 N George Mason Dr, Ste 310 Arlington, VA 22205; **Office Phone:** 703 5256100; **Board Certification:** Orthopaedic Surgery 1975; **Medical School:** Georgetown Univ 1969; **Residency:** Orthopaedic Surgery, Georgetown Hosp, Washington, DC 1970-1974

Poehling, Gary G. MD (Orthopaedic Surgery) - *Special Expertise:* Orthopaedic Surgery - General; **Admitting Hospital:** Wake Forest University Baptist Medical Center; **Office Address:** 131 Miller St. Comp-Rehab Assoc. Winston Salem, NC 27157; **Office Phone:** (336) 716-8091; **Board Certifications:** Orthopaedic Surgery 1977, Hand Surgery 1989; **Medical School:** Marquette Sch Med 1968; **Residencies:** Orthopaedic Surgery, Duke Med Ctr., Durham, NC 1972-1976; Surgery, Duke Med Ctr., Durham, NC 1969-1970; **Faculty Appointment:** Prof Medicine, Wake Forest Univ Sch Med

Rechtine, Glenn MD (Orthopaedic Surgery) - *Special Expertise:* Spinal Surgery; **Admitting Hospital:** Shands Healthcare at University Florida (Page 77); **Office Address:** Shands Hlthcare Univ FL 1600 Archer Rd, Box 100246 Gainesville, FL 32610; **Office Phone:** (813) 978-9700; **Board Certification:** Orthopaedic Surgery 1982; **Medical School:** Univ S Fla Coll Med 1975; **Residency:** Orthopaedic Surgery, NRMC, Portsmouth, NH 1977-1980; **Fellowship:** Spine Surgery, Case West Res U, Cleveland, OH 1980-1981; **Faculty Appointment:** Assoc Clin Prof Orthopaedic Surgery, Univ S Fla Coll Med

Scarborough, Mark MD (Orthopaedic Surgery) - *Special Expertise:* Bone Tumors; Sarcoma; **Admitting Hospital:** Shands Healthcare at University Florida (Page 77); **Office Address:** Shands Hlthcare Univ FL 1600 SW Archer Rd, Box 100246 Gainesville, FL 32610-0246; **Office Phone:** (352) 392-4251; **Board Certification:** Orthopaedic Surgery 1993; **Medical School:** Univ Fla Coll Med 1985; **Residency:** Orthopaedic Surgery, UT Med Ctr, Galveston, TX 1985-1990; **Fellowship:** Orthopaedic Surgery, Mass Genl Hosp, Boston, MA 1990-1991; **Faculty Appointment:** Assoc Prof Orthopaedic Surgery, Univ Fla Coll Med

Spengler, Dan M MD (Orthopaedic Surgery) - *Special Expertise:* Spinal Surgery; **Admitting Hospital:** Vanderbilt University Medical Center; **Office Address:** Vanderbilt Univ Med Ctr, Med Ctr North 1161 21st Ave S, rm D4221 Nashville, TN 37232-2550; **Office Phone:** (615) 343-6364; **Board Certification:** Orthopaedic Surgery 1974; **Medical School:** Univ Mich Med Sch 1966; **Residency:** Orthopaedic Surgery, Univ Mich Med Ctr, Ann Arbor, MI 1967-1973; **Fellowship:** Orthopaedic Surgery, Case West Res Hosp, Cleveland, OH 1973-1974; **Faculty Appointment:** Prof Orthopaedic Surgery, Vanderbilt Univ

Spindler, Kurt Paul MD (Orthopaedic Surgery) - *Special Expertise: Sports Medicine; Arthroscopic Surgery;* **Admitting Hospital:** Vanderbilt University Medical Center; **Office Address:** Vanderbilt Sports Med Ctr 2601 Jess Neely Dr, McGugin Ctr Nashville, TN 37212; **Office Phone:** (615) 343-1685; **Board Certification:** Orthopaedic Surgery 1993; **Medical School:** Univ Penn 1985; **Residency:** Orthopaedic Surgery, Univ Penn, Philadelphia, PA 1986-1990; **Fellowship:** Sports Medicine, Cleveland Clinic Fdn, Cleveland, OH 1990-1991; **Faculty Appointment:** Assoc Prof Orthopaedic Surgery, Vanderbilt Univ

Taft, Timothy MD (Orthopaedic Surgery) - *Special Expertise: Sports Medicine; Ligament Injuries; Shoulder Impingement Syndrome;* **Admitting Hospital:** University of North Carolina Hospitals; **Office Address:** Univ North Carolina Hosp, Dept Ortho 101 Manning Dr, Burnett Womack Bldg Chapel Hill, NC 27514; **Office Phone:** (919) 962-6637; **Board Certification:** Orthopaedic Surgery 1976; **Medical School:** Univ MO-Columbia Sch Med 1969; **Residencies:** Orthopaedic Surgery, Univ N Carolina Hosps, Chapel Hill, NC 1970-1974; Orthopaedic Surgery, N Carolina Ortho Hosp, Gastonia, NC 1972; **Faculty Appointment:** Prof Sports Medicine, Univ NC Sch Med

Uribe, John MD (Orthopaedic Surgery) - *Special Expertise: Shoulder & Elbow Surgery;* **Admitting Hospital:** Healthsouth Doctor's Hospital; **Office Address:** 1150 Campo Sano Ave, Ste 200 Coral Gables, FL 33146-6960; **Office Phone:** (305) 669-3320; **Board Certification:** Orthopaedic Surgery 1982; **Medical School:** Univ NC Sch Med 1976; **Residency:** Orthopaedic Surgery, Jackson Meml Hosp-Univ Miami, Miami, FL 1977-1981; **Fellowship:** Orthopaedic Surgery, Hughston Sports Med Hosp, Columbus, OH 1984-1985; **Faculty Appointment:** Assoc Prof Orthopaedic Surgery, Univ Miami Sch Med

Vail, Thomas Parker MD (Orthopaedic Surgery) - *Special Expertise: Hip & Knee Replacement; Arthritis;* **Admitting Hospital:** Duke University Medical Center (Page 60); **Office Address:** Duke Univ Med Ctr PO Box 3332 Durham, NC 27710; **Office Phone:** (919) 684-6166; **Board Certification:** Orthopaedic Surgery 1994; **Medical School:** Loyola Univ-Stritch Sch Med 1985; **Residencies:** Thoracic Surgery, Duke Univ Med Ctr, Durham, NC 1986-1987; Orthopaedic Surgery, Duke Univ Med Ctr, Durham, NC 1987-1991; **Fellowship:** Sports Medicine, North Amer/Euro Trav Prgm 1991-1992; **Faculty Appointment:** Assoc Prof Orthopaedic Surgery, Duke Univ

Webb, Lawrence MD (Orthopaedic Surgery) - *Special Expertise: Trauma; Foot & Ankle Surgery;* **Admitting Hospital:** Wake Forest University Baptist Medical Center; **Office Address:** Wake Forest Univ Baptist Med Ctr Medical Center Blvd Winston Salem, NC 27157-1070; **Office Phone:** (336) 716-3606; **Board Certification:** Orthopaedic Surgery 1997; **Medical School:** Temple Univ 1978; **Residency:** Orthopaedic Surgery, Bowman Gray Sch Med Ctr, Winston-Salem, NC 1979-1983; **Fellowship:** Trauma, Harborview Med Ctr, Seattle, WA 1983-1984; **Faculty Appointment:** Assoc Prof Medicine, Wake Forest Univ Sch Med

Weiner, Richard MD (Orthopaedic Surgery) - *Special Expertise: Orthopaedic Surgery - General;* **Admitting Hospital:** St Mary's Medical Center - West Palm Beach; **Office Address:** 733 US Highway 1 North Palm Beach, FL 33408-3833; **Office Phone:** (561) 840-1090; **Board Certification:** Orthopaedic Surgery 1993; **Medical School:** Univ Penn 1986; **Residency:** Orthopaedic Surgery, UMDNJ Hosp, Newark, NJ 1987-1991

Midwest

Aamoth, Gordon MD (Orthopaedic Surgery) - *Special Expertise:* Limb Surgery; **Admitting Hospital:** Abbott - Northwestern Hospital; **Office Address:** Minneapolis Ortho & Arth Inst 825 S 8th St, Ste 550 Minneapolis, MN 55404; **Office Phone:** (612) 333-5000; **Board Certification:** Orthopaedic Surgery 1992; **Medical School:** Northwestern Univ 1966; **Residency:** Orthopaedic Surgery, Moffitt Hosp-UCSF, San Francisco, CA 1973; **Faculty Appointment:** Clin Prof Surgery, Univ Minn

Alander, Dirk Huntley MD (Orthopaedic Surgery) - *Special Expertise:* Spinal Surgery; Spinal Cord Injury; **Admitting Hospital:** Truman Medical Center; **Office Address:** Truman Medical Center, Dept of Orthopedic Surgery 2301 Holmes Kansas City, MO 64108; **Office Phone:** (816) 556-3476; **Board Certifications:** Orthopaedic Surgery 1992, Spinal Cord Injury Medicine 1999; **Medical School:** Univ IL Coll Med 1984; **Residency:** Orthopaedic Surgery, Grand Rapids Orth Progrm-Meml Med Ctr, Grand Rapids, MI 1985-1990; **Fellowship:** Spinal Cord Injury Medicine, Southern Ill Univ, Springfield, IL 1992-1993; **Faculty Appointment:** Assoc Prof Surgery, Univ MO-Kansas City

Bach Jr, Bernard R MD (Orthopaedic Surgery) - *Special Expertise:* Sports Medicine; Knee Surgery; **Admitting Hospital:** Rush/Presbyterian - St Luke's Medical Center - Chicago (Page 74); **Office Address:** 1725 W Harrison St, Ste 1063 Chicago, IL 60612; **Office Phone:** (312) 243-4244; **Board Certification:** Orthopaedic Surgery 2009; **Medical School:** Univ Cincinnati 1979; **Residencies:** Surgery, New England Deaconess Hosp, Boston, MA 1980-1981; Orthopaedic Surgery, Combined Harvard Orth, Boston, MA 1981-1985; **Fellowship:** Sports Medicine, Hosp Special Surg 1985-1986

Bergfeld, John MD (Orthopaedic Surgery) - *Special Expertise:* Sports Medicine; **Admitting Hospital:** Cleveland Clinic Foundation; **Office Address:** Cleveland Clinic Foundation A41 9500 Euclid Ave Cleveland, OH 44195-5027; **Office Phone:** (216) 444-2618; **Board Certification:** Orthopaedic Surgery 1972; **Medical School:** Temple Univ 1964; **Residencies:** Orthopaedic Surgery, Cleveland Clinic, Cleveland, OH 1966-1970; Surgery, Cleveland Clinic, Cleveland, OH 1966

Bohlman, Henry H MD (Orthopaedic Surgery) - *Special Expertise:* Spinal Surgery; **Admitting Hospital:** University Hospital - Cleveland; **Office Address:** Univ Hosp-Cleveland-Case West Res 11100 Euclid Ave Cleveland, OH 44106-1736; **Office Phone:** (216) 844-1025; **Board Certification:** Orthopaedic Surgery 1972; **Medical School:** Univ MD Sch Med 1964; **Residencies:** Surgery, Baltimore U Hosp, Baltimore, MD 1964-1966; Orthopaedic Surgery, Johns Hopkins Hosp, Baltimore, MD 1966-1970; **Fellowship:** Spine Surgery, Johns Hopkins Hosp, Baltimore, MD 1967-1968; **Faculty Appointment:** Prof Orthopaedic Surgery, Case West Res Univ

Bridwell, Keith MD (Orthopaedic Surgery) - *Special Expertise:* Scoliosis; Spinal Surgery; **Admitting Hospital:** Barnes - Jewish Hospital; **Office Address:** Barnes-Jewish Hosp One W Pavilion Plaza St. Louis, MO 63110; **Office Phone:** (314) 362-4080; **Board Certification:** Orthopaedic Surgery 1985; **Medical School:** Washington Univ, St Louis 1977; **Residencies:** Orthopaedic Surgery, Barnes Hosptial, St. Louis, MO 1978-1981; Rush Med Coll, Chicago, IL 1982; **Faculty Appointment:** Prof Medicine, Washington Univ, St Louis

Callaghan, John J MD (Orthopaedic Surgery) - *Special Expertise:* Hip & Knee *Replacement; Sports Medicine;* **Admitting Hospital:** University of Iowa Hospitals and Clinics; **Office Address:** 200 Hawkins Dr Iowa City, IA 52242; **Office Phone:** (319) 356-3110; **Board Certification:** Orthopaedic Surgery 1985; **Medical School:** Loyola Univ-Stritch Sch Med 1978; **Residency:** Orthopaedic Surgery, Univ IA Hosp Clin, Iowa City, IA 1979-1983; **Fellowship:** Orthopaedic Surgery, Hosp Special Surg, New York, NY 1983-1984; **Faculty Appointment:** Prof Orthopaedic Surgery, Univ Iowa Coll Med

Cofield, Robert H MD (Orthopaedic Surgery) - *Special Expertise:* Shoulder Surgery; **Admitting Hospital:** Mayo Medical Center & Clinic - Rochester; **Office Address:** Mayo Clinic 200 1st St SW Rochester, MN 55905; **Office Phone:** (507) 284-2511; **Board Certification:** Orthopaedic Surgery 1976; **Medical School:** Univ KY Coll Med 1969; **Residencies:** Surgery, Charity Hosp - Tulane Div, New Orleans, LA 1969-1971; Orthopaedic Surgery, Mayo Grad Sch Med, Rochester, MN 1971-1975; **Faculty Appointment:** Prof Orthopaedic Surgery, Mayo Med Sch

Gage, James (Orthopaedic Surgery) - *Special Expertise:* Orthopaedic Surgery-Pediatric; **Admitting Hospital:** Gillette Children's Specialty Healthcare; **Office Address:** Gillette Chldns Hosp, Orth Assocs 200 E University Ave St Paul, MN 55101-2507; **Office Phone:** (651) 290-8707; **Board Certification:** Orthopaedic Surgery 1983; **Medical School:** Northwestern Univ 1964; **Residency:** Orthopaedic Surgery, Minneapolis VA Hosp, Minneapolis, MN 1967-1971; **Faculty Appointment:** Prof Orthopaedic Surgery, Univ Minn

Galante, Jorge O MD (Orthopaedic Surgery) - *Special Expertise:* Knee & Hip Surgery; Hip & Knee Replacement; **Admitting Hospital:** Rush/Presbyterian - St Luke's Medical Center - Chicago (Page 74); **Office Address:** 1725 W Harrison St, Ste 1063 Chicago, IL 60612; **Office Phone:** (312) 243-4244; **Board Certification:** Orthopaedic Surgery 1968; **Medical School:** Argentina 1958; **Residency:** Orthopaedic Surgery, Michael Reese Hosp, Chicago, IL 1959-1961; **Fellowship:** Orthopaedic Surgery, Univ Goteborg, Sweden 1964-1967; **Faculty Appointment:** Prof Orthopaedic Surgery, Rush Med Coll

Goitz, Henry MD (Orthopaedic Surgery) - *Special Expertise:* Sports Medicine; Arthroscopic Surgery; **Admitting Hospital:** Henry Ford Health System (Page 62); **Office Address:** 14500 Hall Rd 14500 Hall Rd Detroit, MI 48313; **Office Phone:** (810) 247-3765; **Board Certification:** Orthopaedic Surgery 1995; **Medical School:** Rutgers Univ 1985; **Residencies:** Surgery, Univ Virginia, Charlottesville, VA 1986-1987; Orthopaedic Surgery, Univ Virginia, Charlottesville, VA 1987-1991; **Fellowships:** Hand Surgery, Univ Virginia, Charlottesville, VA 1991; Sports Medicine, Am Sports Med Inst, Birmingham, AL 1992; **Faculty Appointment:** Asst Prof Orthopaedic Surgery

Goldberg, Victor M MD (Orthopaedic Surgery) - *Special Expertise:* Hip & Knee *Replacement; Arthritis;* **Admitting Hospital:** University Hospital - Cleveland; **Office Address:** Case Western Res Univ, Dept Ortho Surg 11100 Euclid Ave Cleveland, OH 44106-2602; **Office Phone:** (216) 844-3044; **Board Certification:** Orthopaedic Surgery 1973; **Medical School:** SUNY Downstate 1964; **Residencies:** Surgery, Univ Hosp, Cleveland, OH 1965-1966; Orthopaedic Surgery, Spl Surg Hosp, New York, NY 1968-1971; **Faculty Appointment:** Prof Orthopaedic Surgery, Case West Res Univ

Goldstein, Wayne MD (Orthopaedic Surgery) - *Special Expertise:* Hip Replacement; Knee *Replacement;* **Admitting Hospital:** Advocate Lutheran General Hospital; **Office Address:** Illinois Bone & Joint Inst-Parkside Ctr 1875 W Dempster St, Ste 301 Park Ridge, IL 60068; **Office Phone:** (847) 375-3000; **Board Certification:** Orthopaedic Surgery 1986; **Medical School:** Univ IL Coll Med 1978; **Residency:** Orthopaedic Surgery, Univ IL Med Ctr, Chicago, IL 1979-1983; **Fellowship:** Orthopaedic Surgery, Harvard Med Ctr, Cambridge, MA 1983-1984; **Faculty Appointment:** Asst Clin Prof Orthopaedic Surgery, Univ Chicago-Pritzker Sch Med

Graf, Ben K MD (Orthopaedic Surgery) - *Special Expertise:* Sports Medicine; **Admitting Hospital:** University of Wisconsin Hospital & Clinics; **Office Address:** Univ Hosp 600 Highland Ave Madison, WI 53792; **Office Phone:** (608) 263-8850; **Board Certification:** Orthopaedic Surgery 1998; **Medical School:** Univ Wisc 1979; **Residency:** Univ Wisconsin Hosps, Madison, WI 1980-1984; **Fellowship:** Sports Medicine, Long Beach Meml Hosp 1984-1985; **Faculty Appointment:** Assoc Prof Surgery, Univ Wisc

Hensinger, Robert MD (Orthopaedic Surgery) - *Special Expertise:* Orthopaedic Surgery-Pediatric; Spine Surgery-Pediatric; **Admitting Hospital:** University of Michigan Health Center; **Office Address:** Univ Michigan Med Ctr, Dept Ortho Surg 2912 Taubman Ctr, 1500 E Medical Ctr Dr Ann Arbor, MI 48109; **Office Phone:** (734) 936-5780; **Board Certification:** Orthopaedic Surgery 1992; **Medical School:** Univ Mich Med Sch 1964; **Residencies:** Orthopaedic Surgery, Univ Michigan, Ann Arbor, MI 1965-1966; Orthopaedic Surgery, Univ Michigan, Ann Arbor, MI 1968-1971; **Fellowship:** Pediatric Orthopedic Surgery, Al DuPont Inst, Wilmington, NC 1971-1972

Iannotti, Joseph MD (Orthopaedic Surgery) - *Special Expertise:* Shoulder Surgery; **Admitting Hospital:** Cleveland Clinic Foundation; **Office Address:** Cleveland Clinic Foundation, Dept Ors Desk 4A 9500 Euclid Ave Cleveland, OH; **Office Phone:** (216) 445-5151; **Board Certification:** Orthopaedic Surgery 1987; **Medical School:** Northwestern Univ 1979; **Residency:** Orthopaedic Surgery, Hosp U Penn, Philadelphia, PA 1980-1984; **Fellowship:** Orthopaedic Surgery, Hosp U Penn, Philadelphia, PA 1984-1985

Lock, Terrence Ralph MD (Orthopaedic Surgery) - *Special Expertise:* Sports Medicine; **Admitting Hospital:** Henry Ford Health System (Page 62); **Office Address:** 6525 2nd Ave Detroit, MI 48202; **Office Phone:** (313) 972-4065; **Board Certification:** Orthopaedic Surgery 1991; **Medical School:** Wayne State Univ 1983; **Residency:** Orthopaedic Surgery, Wayne St Univ Sch Med, Detroit, MI 1984-1988; **Fellowship:** Sports Medicine, Mass Genl Hosp, Boston, MA 1988-1989

Mallory, Thomas MD (Orthopaedic Surgery) - *Special Expertise:* Hip & Knee Replacement; **Admitting Hospital:** Ohio State University Medical Center; **Office Address:** 720 E Broad St Columbus, OH 43210-3947; **Office Phone:** (614) 221-6331; **Board Certification:** Orthopaedic Surgery 1972; **Medical School:** Ohio State Univ 1965; **Residency:** Orthopaedic Surgery, Ohio State Univ Hosp, Colombus, OH 1966-1970; **Fellowship:** Hip Surgery, Harvard Med Sch, Boston, MA 1970-1971; **Faculty Appointment:** Asst Clin Prof Orthopaedic Surgery, Ohio State Univ

Manoli II, Arthur MD (Orthopaedic Surgery) - *Special Expertise:* Foot Surgery; **Admitting Hospital:** St Joseph's Mercy - Oakland; **Office Address:** 44555 Woodward Ave Ste 105 Pontiac, MI 48341; **Office Phone:** (248) 858-6773; **Board Certification:** Orthopaedic Surgery 1992; **Medical School:** Univ Mich Med Sch 1970; **Residencies:** Surgery, Oakwood Hosp, Dearborn, MI 1971-1972; Orthopaedic Surgery, Wayne St Univ Affil Hosps, Detroit, MI 1972-1975; **Fellowship:** Ankle and Foot Surgery, Univ Wash/Vanderbilt, Seattle, WA 1989-1990; **Faculty Appointment:** Assoc Prof Univ Pittsburgh

Martell, John Mark MD (Orthopaedic Surgery) - *Special Expertise:* Hip & Knee Replacement; Knee Surgery; **Admitting Hospital:** University of Chicago Hospitals (Page 78); **Office Address:** Univ of Chicago Hosp 5841 S Maryland Ave, rm E309, MC-3079 Chicago, IL 60637; **Office Phone:** (773) 702-7297; **Board Certification:** Orthopaedic Surgery 1991; **Medical School:** Univ Chicago-Pritzker Sch Med 1983; **Residency:** U Chicago, Chicago, IL 1987-1988; **Fellowship:** Orthopaedic Surgery, Rush Presb, Chicago, IL 1988-1989; **Faculty Appointment:** Orthopaedic Surgery, Univ Chicago-Pritzker Sch Med

Nagle, Daniel J MD (Orthopaedic Surgery) - *Special Expertise:* Hand Surgery; **Admitting Hospital:** Northwestern Memorial Hospital; **Office Address:** Bell, Stromberg, Harris & Nagle 448 E Ontario St, Ste 500 Chicago, IL 60611-7108; **Office Phone:** (312) 908-3366; **Board Certifications:** Orthopaedic Surgery 1986, Hand Surgery 1989; **Medical School:** Belgium 1978; **Residency:** Orthopaedic Surgery, Northwestern Univ Med Sch, Chicago, IL 1979-1983; **Fellowship:** Hand Surgery, Christine Kleinhart, Louisville, KY 1983-1984; **Faculty Appointment:** Asst Prof Surgery, Northwestern Univ

Nuber, Gordon MD (Orthopaedic Surgery) - *Special Expertise:* Arthroscopic Surgery; *Cartilage Problems;* **Admitting Hospital:** Northwestern Memorial Hospital; **Office Address:** Northwestern Orth Inst 680 N Lakeshore Dr, Ste 1028 Chicago, IL 60611; **Office Phone:** (312) 664-6848; **Board Certification:** Orthopaedic Surgery 1986; **Medical School:** Wayne State Univ 1978; **Residency:** Orthopaedic Surgery, Northwestern Meml Hosp, Chicago, IL 1978-1983; **Fellowship:** Sports Medicine, Natl Alth Hlth inst, Ingelwood, CA 1983-1984; **Faculty Appointment:** Assoc Clin Prof Orthopaedic Surgery, Northwestern Univ

Riew, K Daniel MD (Orthopaedic Surgery) - *Special Expertise:* Cervical Spine Surgery; *Neuro-Rehabilitation; Pain-Back;* **Admitting Hospital:** Barnes - Jewish Hospital; **Office Address:** 1 Barnes-Jewish Hosp Plaza West Pavilion, Ste 11300 St. Louis, MO 63110; **Office Phone:** (314) 747-2500; **Board Certifications:** Internal Medicine 1987, Orthopaedic Surgery 1997; **Medical School:** Case West Res Univ 1984; **Residencies:** Internal Medicine, NY Hosp - Cornell Med Ctr, New York, NY 1984-1987; Orthopaedic Surgery, George Wash Univ Med Ctr, Washington, DC 1990-1994; **Fellowship:** Spine Surgery, Case Western, Cleveland, OH 1994-1995; **Faculty Appointment:** Asst Prof Orthopaedic Surgery, Washington Univ, St Louis

Saltzman, Charles Louis MD (Orthopaedic Surgery) - *Special Expertise:* Foot & Ankle Surgery; **Admitting Hospital:** University of Iowa Hospitals and Clinics; **Office Address:** Univ. of Iowa Hosp-Dept. Ortho 200 Hawkins Dr, MS 01017JPP Iowa City, IA 52242-1009; **Office Phone:** (319) 356-7149; **Board Certification:** Orthopaedic Surgery; **Medical School:** Univ NC Sch Med 1985; **Faculty Appointment:** Assoc Prof Orthopaedic Surgery

Schafer, Michael F MD (Orthopaedic Surgery) - *Special Expertise:* Sports Medicine; Spinal Surgery; **Admitting Hospital:** Northwestern Memorial Hospital; **Office Address:** 675 N St. Clair, Ste 17-100 Chicago, IL 60611; **Office Phone:** (312) 695-6800; **Board Certification:** Orthopaedic Surgery 1983; **Medical School:** Univ Iowa Coll Med 1967; **Residency:** Orthopaedic Surgery, Northwestern U Hospitals, Chicago, IL 1968-1972; **Fellowship:** Natl Foundation Traveling Fellowship, Sydney, Australia 1972; **Faculty Appointment:** Prof Orthopaedic Surgery, Northwestern Univ

Shelbourne, K Donald MD (Orthopaedic Surgery) - *Special Expertise:* Sports Medicine; *Knee Surgery;* **Admitting Hospital:** Methodist Hospital - Indianapolis; **Office Address:** 1815 N Capitol Ave, Ste 530 Indianapolis, IN 46202-1288; **Office Phone:** (317) 924-8636; **Board Certification:** Orthopaedic Surgery 1984; **Medical School:** Indiana Univ 1976; **Residency:** Orthopaedic Surgery, Indiana Univ Hosp, Indianapolis, IN 1977-1981; **Fellowship:** Sports Medicine, Univ of WI, Madison, WI 1981-1982; **Faculty Appointment:** Assoc Clin Prof Orthopaedic Surgery, Indiana Univ

Simon, Michael MD (Orthopaedic Surgery) - *Special Expertise:* Bone Tumors; Soft Tissue Tumors; Sarcoma; **Admitting Hospital:** University of Chicago Hospitals (Page 78); **Office Address:** Univ of Chicago Hosp 5841 S Maryland Ave, MC-3079 Chicago, IL 60637; **Office Phone:** (773) 702-6144; **Board Certification:** Orthopaedic Surgery 1983; **Medical School:** Univ Mich Med Sch 1967; **Residencies:** Surgery, U Mich Med Ctr, Ann Arbor, MI 1968-1969; Orthopaedic Surgery, U Mich Med Ctr, Ann Arbor, MI 1971-1974; **Fellowship:** Orthopedic Oncology, U Fla, Gainesville, FL 1974-1975; **Faculty Appointment:** Prof Surgery, Univ Chicago-Pritzker Sch Med

Stulberg, Samuel David MD (Orthopaedic Surgery) - *Special Expertise:* Arthritis; Hip & Knee Replacement; **Admitting Hospital:** Northwestern Memorial Hospital; **Office Address:** Northwestern Orth Inst 680 N Lakeshore Dr, Ste 1028 Chicago, IL 60611; **Office Phone:** (312) 664-6848; **Board Certification:** Orthopaedic Surgery 1977; **Medical School:** Univ Mich Med Sch 1969; **Residencies:** Orthopaedic Surgery, Mass Genl Hosp, Boston, MA 1970-1971; Orthopaedic Surgery, Harvard Med Ctr, Boston, MA 1972-1974; **Fellowship:** Research, Sick Childrens Hosp, Toronto, Canada 1975-1976; **Faculty Appointment:** Prof Orthopaedic Surgery, Northwestern Univ

Swiontkowski, Marc F MD (Orthopaedic Surgery) - *Special Expertise:* Osteomyelitis; Fractures-Non Union; Trauma; **Admitting Hospital:** Fairview-University Medical Center - University Campus; **Office Address:** Univ Minn Med Sch, Mayo Meml Bldg 420 Delaware St SE, MC-492 Minneapolis, MN 55455; **Office Phone:** (612) 625-1177; **Board Certification:** Orthopaedic Surgery 1998; **Medical School:** USC Sch Med 1979; **Residency:** Orthopaedic Surgery, Univ Wash, Seattle, WA 1980-1984; **Faculty Appointment:** Prof Orthopaedic Surgery, Univ Minn

Weinstein, Stuart L MD (Orthopaedic Surgery) - *Special Expertise:* Scoliosis; Developmental Hip Dysplasia; **Admitting Hospital:** University of Iowa Hospitals and Clinics; **Office Address:** 200 Hawkins Drive, rm 01026 Iowa City, IA 52242; **Office Phone:** (319) 356-1872; **Board Certification:** Orthopaedic Surgery 1995; **Medical School:** Univ Iowa Coll Med 1972; **Residency:** Orthopaedic Surgery, Univ Iowa Coll Med, Iowa City, IA 1973-1976; **Faculty Appointment:** Prof Orthopaedic Surgery, Univ Iowa Coll Med

Wixson, Richard L MD (Orthopaedic Surgery) - *Special Expertise:* Hip & Knee Replacement; **Admitting Hospital:** Northwestern Memorial Hospital; **Office Address:** NW Ctr Orthopaedic Assocs - Chicago 676 N Saint Clair St, Ste 450 Chicago, IL 60611-2983; **Office Phone:** (312) 943-7850; **Board Certification:** Orthopaedic Surgery 1979; **Medical School:** Univ Wisc 1972; **Residencies:** Orthopaedic Surgery, Henry Ford Hosp, Boston, MA 1974-1977; Orthopaedic Surgery, New Eng Bapt Hosp, Boston, MA 1978-1979; **Fellowship:** Orthopaedic Surgery, Mass Genl Hosp, Boston, MA 1977; **Faculty Appointment:** Clin Prof Orthopaedic Surgery, Northwestern Univ

Zdeblick, Thomas MD (Orthopaedic Surgery) - *Special Expertise:* Spinal Surgery; **Admitting Hospital:** University of Wisconsin Hospital & Clinics; **Office Address:** 600 Highland Ave, Ste 315 G5 Madison, WI 53792-0001; **Office Phone:** (608) 265-3207; **Board Certification:** Orthopaedic Surgery 1991; **Medical School:** Tufts Univ 1982; **Residency:** Orthopaedic Surgery, Case West Res Univ, Cleveland, OH 1984-1988; **Fellowship:** Spine Surgery, Johns Hopkins Univ, Baltimore, MD 1988-1989; **Faculty Appointment:** Assoc Prof Orthopaedic Surgery, Univ Wisc

Great Plains and Mountains

Coughlin, Michael MD (Orthopaedic Surgery) - *Special Expertise:* Foot & Ankle Surgery; **Admitting Hospital:** St Alphonsus Regional Medical Center; **Office Address:** 901 N Curtis, Ste 503 Boise, ID 83706-1343; **Office Phone:** (208) 377-1000; **Board Certification:** Orthopaedic Surgery 1980

Dunn, Harold Kenneth MD (Orthopaedic Surgery) - *Special Expertise:* Hip Surgery; Spinal Surgery; **Admitting Hospital:** University of Utah Hospital and Clinics; **Office Address:** 50 N Medical Dr Salt Lake City, UT 84132-0001; **Office Phone:** (801) 581-7601; **Board Certification:** Orthopaedic Surgery 1983; **Medical School:** Baylor Coll Med 1963; **Residencies:** Orthopaedic Surgery, U NM Affil Hosp, Alberquerque, NM 1966-1967; Orthopaedic Surgery, Baylor Coll Med, Houston, TX 1967-1969; **Faculty Appointment:** Prof Orthopaedic Surgery, Univ Utah

Neff, James R MD (Orthopaedic Surgery) - *Special Expertise: Musculoskeletal Tumors;* **Admitting Hospital:** Nebraska Health System - Clarkson; **Office Address:** Dept Orth Surg 981080 Nebraska Med Ctr. Omaha, NE 68198-1080; **Office Phone:** (402) 559-8000; **Board Certification:** Orthopaedic Surgery 1974; **Medical School:** Univ Kans 1966; **Residencies:** Surgery, U Mich Hosp, Ann Arbor, MI 1967-1968; Orthopaedic Surgery, U Mich Hosp, Ann Arbor, MI 1970-1973; **Fellowship:** Fla Univ 1973-1974; **Faculty Appointment:** Prof Orthopaedic Surgery, Univ Nebr Coll Med

Paulos, Leon MD (Orthopaedic Surgery) - *Special Expertise: Sports Medicine; Shoulder & Knee Surgery;* **Admitting Hospital:** Orthopedic Specialty Hospital, The; **Office Address:** 5848 S 300 E Salt Lake City, UT 84107-6121; **Office Phone:** (801) 269-4100; **Board Certification:** Orthopaedic Surgery 1980; **Medical School:** Univ Utah 1973; **Residency:** Orthopaedic Surgery, Univ Utah Sch Med, Salt Lake City, UT 1974-1978; **Fellowships:** Sports Medicine, Atlanta Sports Med Fdn, Atlanta, GA 1978; Sports Medicine, Univ Hosp - Cincinatti, Cincinatti, OH 1979; **Faculty Appointment:** Asst Clin Prof Orthopaedic Surgery, Univ Utah

Rosenberg, Thomas D MD (Orthopaedic Surgery) - *Special Expertise: Knee Surgery; Sports Medicine;* **Admitting Hospital:** Orthopedic Specialty Hospital, The; **Office Address:** Ortho Spec Hosp 5848 S 300 E Salt Lake City, UT 84107-6121; **Office Phone:** 435 6556601; **Board Certification:** Orthopaedic Surgery 1979; **Medical School:** Univ Utah 1973; **Residencies:** Orthopaedic Surgery, Univ Utah Affil Hosps, Salt Lake City, UT 1973-1978; Sports Medicine, Univ WI Hosp & Clinics, Madison, WI 1977-1978

Wiedel, Jerome D MD (Orthopaedic Surgery) - *Special Expertise: Orthopaedic Surgery - General;* **Admitting Hospital:** University of Colorado Health & Science Center; **Office Address:** Orthopaedics 4701 E 9th Ave, MC-E203 Denver, CO 80262-0001; **Office Phone:** (303) 372-1254; **Board Certification:** Orthopaedic Surgery 1993; **Medical School:** Univ Nebr Coll Med 1964; **Residency:** Orthopaedic Surgery, Univ Colorado Med Ctr, Denver, CO 1967-1971; **Fellowship:** Adult Reconstruction, Robert Jones-A Hunt Ortho Hosp, Oswestry, England 1971-1972; **Faculty Appointment:** Prof Orthopaedic Surgery, Univ Colo

Southwest

Aronson, James MD (Orthopaedic Surgery) - *Special Expertise: Ilizarov Procedure; Hip Disorders; Clubfoot;* **Admitting Hospital:** Arkansas Children's Hospital; **Office Address:** Arkansas Children's Hospital 800 Marshall St, Slot 653 Little Rock, AR 72202; **Office Phone:** (501) 320-1468; **Board Certification:** Orthopaedic Surgery 1997; **Medical School:** Univ Pittsburgh 1975; **Residencies:** Surgery, Maine Med Ctr, Portland, ME 1976-1977; Orthopaedic Surgery, Duke U Med Ctr, Durham, NC 1978-1982; **Fellowship:** Pediatric Orthopedic Surgery, Alfred I DuPont Inst, Wilmington, DE 1983; **Faculty Appointment:** Prof Orthopaedic Surgery, Univ Ark

Brodsky, James White MD (Orthopaedic Surgery) - *Special Expertise: Foot Surgery;* **Admitting Hospital:** Baylor University Medical Center; **Office Address:** 411 N Washington #7000 LB14 Dallas, TX 75246-1777; **Office Phone:** (214) 823-7090; **Board Certification:** Orthopaedic Surgery 1998; **Medical School:** Case West Res Univ 1979; **Residencies:** Orthopaedic Surgery, Baylor Coll Med, Houston, TX 1981-1984; Orthopaedic Surgery, Bellevue-NYU, New York, NY 1980-1981; **Fellowship:** Ankle and Foot Surgery, USC/LAC Hosp, Los Angeles, CA 1984-1985

Bucholz, Robert MD (Orthopaedic Surgery) - *Special Expertise: Trauma;* **Admitting Hospital:** Parkland Memorial Hospital; **Office Address:** Parkland Meml Hosp 5323 Harry Hines Blvd Dallas, TX 75390-7208; **Office Phone:** (214) 648-3870; **Board Certification:** Orthopaedic Surgery 1994; **Medical School:** Yale Univ 1973; **Residency:** Orthopaedic Surgery, Yale - New Haven Hosp, New Haven, CT 1974-1977; **Faculty Appointment:** Prof Orthopaedic Surgery, Univ Tex SW, Dallas

Dabezies, Eugene MD (Orthopaedic Surgery) - *Special Expertise:* Hand Surgery; **Admitting Hospital:** University Medical Center; **Office Address:** 3601 4TH St Ste 4A-138 Lubbock, TX 79430; **Office Phone:** (806) 743-4263; **Board Certification:** Orthopaedic Surgery 1968; **Medical School:** Tulane Univ 1960; **Residency:** Orthopaedic Surgery, Charity Hosp, New Orleans, LA 1961-1965; **Faculty Appointment:** Prof Orthopaedic Surgery, Louisiana State Univ

Mabrey, Jay D MD (Orthopaedic Surgery) - *Special Expertise:* Knee Surgery; **Admitting Hospital:** University of Texas Health & Science Center; **Office Address:** Univ TX Hlth Sci Ctr. Dept of Orthopaedics 7703 Floyd Curl Drive San Antonio, TX 78229-3900; **Office Phone:** (210) 567-5125; **Board Certification:** Orthopaedic Surgery 2000; **Medical School:** Cornell Univ-Weil Med Coll 1981; **Residencies:** Orthopaedic Surgery, Duke U MC, Durham, NC 1983-1987; Surgery, Duke U MC, Durham, NC 1982-1983; **Fellowship:** Hosp Special Surg., New York, NY 1990-1991; **Faculty Appointment:** Assoc Prof Orthopaedic Surgery, Univ Tex, San Antonio

Nelson, Carl MD (Orthopaedic Surgery) - *Special Expertise:* Hip Surgery; *Hip & Knee Replacement;* **Admitting Hospital:** University of Arkansas for Medical Sciences; **Office Address:** Univ Hosp AR for Med Scis 4301 West Markham Slot-531 Little Rock, AR 72205; **Office Phone:** (501) 686-5505; **Board Certification:** Orthopaedic Surgery 1969; **Medical School:** Indiana Univ 1959; **Residencies:** Internal Medicine, Los Angeles Co Genl Hosp, Los Angeles, CA 1960-1961; Surgery, Cleveland Clin Fdn, Cleveland, OH 1962-1963; **Fellowship:** Orthopaedic Surgery, Cleveland Clin Fdn, Cleveland, OH 1963-1966; **Faculty Appointment:** Prof Orthopaedic Surgery, Univ Ark

Rockwood Jr, Charles A MD (Orthopaedic Surgery) - *Special Expertise:* Shoulder Surgery; **Admitting Hospital:** University Hospital; **Office Address:** Univ Hosp, Dept Orth Surg 7703 Floyd Curl Dr San Antonio, TX 78229-3900; **Office Phone:** (210) 567-5125; **Board Certification:** Orthopaedic Surgery 1994; **Medical School:** Univ Okla Coll Med 1956; **Residency:** Orthopaedic Surgery, Univ Oklahoma Med Ctr, Oklahoma City, OK 1957-1961; **Fellowship:** Shoulder Surgery, Columbia Presby Med Ctr, New York, NY; **Faculty Appointment:** Prof Orthopaedic Surgery, Univ Tex, San Antonio

Trick, Lorence Wain MD (Orthopaedic Surgery) - *Special Expertise:* Hip & Knee Replacement; Joint Revision; **Admitting Hospital:** Southwest Texas Methodist Hospital; **Office Address:** 414 Navarro St, Ste 1128 San Antonio, TX 78205; **Office Phone:** (210) 351-6500; **Board Certification:** Orthopaedic Surgery 1973; **Medical School:** Geo Wash Univ 1967; **Residency:** Orthopaedic Surgery, Wilford Hall USAF Med Ctr, San Antonio, TX 1968-1972; **Fellowship:** Orthopaedic Surgery, New England Baptist Med Ctr, Boston, MA 1973; **Faculty Appointment:** Clin Prof Orthopaedic Surgery, Univ Tex, San Antonio

Wirth, Michael A MD (Orthopaedic Surgery) - *Special Expertise:* Shoulder Surgery; **Admitting Hospital:** University of Texas Health & Science Center; **Office Address:** UT Hlth & Sci Ctr, Dept Orth 7703 Floyd Curl Dr San Antonio, TX 78229-3900; **Office Phone:** (210) 567-5135; **Board Certification:** Orthopaedic Surgery 1993; **Medical School:** Oregon Hlth Scis Univ 1985; **Residency:** Orthopaedic Surgery, UT Hlth Sci Ctr, San Antonio, TX 1986-1990; **Fellowship:** Shoulder Surgery, Charles Rockwood Jr MD, San Antonio, TX 1990-1991; **Faculty Appointment:** Prof Orthopaedic Surgery, Univ Tex, San Antonio

West Coast and Pacific

Anderson, Lesley J MD (Orthopaedic Surgery) - *Special Expertise: Knee Injuries-Women; Sports Medicine;* **Admitting Hospital:** California Pacific Medical Center; **Office Address:** 2100 Webster St, Ste 309 San Francisco, CA 94115; **Office Phone:** (415) 923-3029; **Board Certification:** Orthopaedic Surgery 1997; **Medical School:** Penn State Univ-Hershey Med Ctr 1976; **Residency:** Orthopaedic Surgery, UCLA, Los Angeles, CA 1979-1983; **Fellowship:** Sports Medicine, Precept ME Blazina, Sherman Oaks, CA 1983-1984

Bradford, David S MD (Orthopaedic Surgery) - *Special Expertise: Scoliosis/Spine Deformities; Spinal Surgery;* **Admitting Hospital:** University of California - San Francisco Medical Center; **Office Address:** UCSF, Dept Orthopaedics 400 Parnassus Ave, Fl 3, Box 0728 San Francisco, CA 94143-0728; **Office Phone:** (415) 476-2280; **Board Certification:** Orthopaedic Surgery 1988; **Medical School:** Univ Penn 1962; **Residency:** Orthopaedic Surgery, Columbia-Presbyterian Med Ctr, New York, NY 1966-1968; **Fellowship:** Orthopaedic Surgery, Columbia-Presbyterian Med Ctr, New York, NY 1968-1969; **Faculty Appointment:** Prof Orthopaedic Surgery, UCSF

Brage, Michael MD (Orthopaedic Surgery) - *Special Expertise: Foot & Ankle Surgery;* **Admitting Hospital:** University of California - San Diego Healthcare; **Office Address:** Univ CA San Diego, Dept Ortho 200 W Arbor Rd, MS 8894 San Diego, CA 92103-8894; **Office Phone:** (619) 543-7456; **Board Certification:** Orthopaedic Surgery 1994; **Medical School:** Univ IL Coll Med 1986; **Residency:** University Chicago, Chicago, IL 1986-1991; **Fellowship:** University Washington, Seattle, WA 1991-1992; **Faculty Appointment:** Asst Clin Prof Surgery, UCSD

Cannon Jr, W Dilworth MD (Orthopaedic Surgery) - *Special Expertise: Sports Medicine; Knee Surgery;* **Admitting Hospital:** University of California - San Francisco Medical Center; **Office Address:** 1701 Divisadero St, Ste 240 San Francisco, CA 94115-1351; **Office Phone:** (415) 353-7566; **Board Certification:** Orthopaedic Surgery 1972; **Medical School:** Columbia P&S 1963; **Residencies:** Surgery, St Vincents Hosp, New York, NY 1963-1965; Orthopaedic Surgery, NY Ortho Hosp, New York, NY 1967-1970; **Fellowship:** Orthopaedic Surgery, Royal Nat Ortho Hosp, London England 1970-1971; **Faculty Appointment:** Clin Prof Orthopaedic Surgery, UCSF

Chambers, Richard Byron MD (Orthopaedic Surgery) - *Special Expertise: Diabetes-Amputation;* **Admitting Hospital:** LAC - Rancho Los Amigos Medical Center; **Office Address:** Rancho Los Amigos Med Ctr 7601 E Imperial Hwy, rm 145-HB Downey, CA 90242; **Office Phone:** (562) 401-7225; **Board Certification:** Orthopaedic Surgery 1977; **Medical School:** Columbia P&S 1971; **Residencies:** Orthopaedic Surgery, Hosp for Special Surgery, New York, NY; Surgery, Harlem Hosp, New York, NY

Dillingham, Michael Francis MD (Orthopaedic Surgery) - *Special Expertise: Orthopaedic Surgery - General;* **Admitting Hospital:** Stanford Medical Center; **Office Address:** 2884 Sand Hill Rd, Ste 110 Menlo Park, CA 94025; **Office Phone:** (650) 851-4900; **Board Certifications:** Physical Medicine & Rehabilitation 1979, Orthopaedic Surgery 1977; **Medical School:** Stanford Univ 1971; **Residencies:** Internal Medicine, Santa Clara Valley Med Ctr, San Jose, CA 1975-1977; Orthopaedic Surgery, Standford, Stanford, CA 1972-1975; **Fellowship:** Orthopaedic Surgery, Santa Clara Valley Med Ctr, San Jose, CA 1975-1976; **Faculty Appointment:** Clin Prof Orthopaedic Surgery, Stanford Univ

Dorr, Lawrence Douglas MD (Orthopaedic Surgery) - *Special Expertise: Hip & Knee Replacement;* **Admitting Hospital:** Good Samaritan Hospital - Los Angeles; **Office Address:** Bone & Joint Inst 1245 Wilshire Blvd, Fl 2 Los Angeles, CA 90017; **Office Phone:** (213) 202-2800; **Board Certification:** Orthopaedic Surgery 1978; **Medical School:** Univ Iowa Coll Med 1967; **Residency:** Orthopaedic Surgery, LA Co-USC Sch Med, Los Angeles, CA 1974-1976; **Fellowship:** Joint Replacement Surgery, Hosp Spec Surg, New York, NY 1976-1977; **Faculty Appointment:** Prof Orthopaedic Surgery, USC Sch Med

Eckardt, Jeffrey J MD (Orthopaedic Surgery) - *Special Expertise: Bone Tumors;* **Admitting Hospital:** UCLA Medical Center; **Office Address:** UCLA Med Ctr, Dept OrS 10833 LeConte Ave Los Angeles, CA 90095-6902; **Office Phone:** (310) 206-6503; **Board Certification:** Orthopaedic Surgery 1981; **Medical School:** Cornell Univ-Weil Med Coll 1971; **Residency:** Orthopaedic Surgery, UCLA, Los Angeles, CA 1975-1979; **Fellowship:** Orthopedic Oncology, Mayo Clinic, Rochester, MN 1979-1980; **Faculty Appointment:** Prof Orthopaedic Surgery, UCLA

Finerman, Gerald MD (Orthopaedic Surgery) - *Special Expertise: Sports Medicine; Hip & Knee Replacement;* **Admitting Hospital:** UCLA Medical Center; **Office Address:** UCLA Med Ctr, Dep Orth Surg 10833 Le Conte Ave, rm 76-13 Los Angeles, CA 90095-1301; **Office Phone:** (310) 825-6019; **Board Certification:** Orthopaedic Surgery 1971; **Medical School:** Johns Hopkins Univ 1962; **Residencies:** Surgery, John Hopkins Hosp, Baltimore, MD 1963-1964; Orthopaedic Surgery, John Hopkins Hosp, Baltimore, MD 1966-1969; **Faculty Appointment:** Prof Orthopaedic Surgery, UCLA

Goodman, Stuart Barry MD/PhD (Orthopaedic Surgery) - *Special Expertise: Orthopaedic Surgery - General;* **Admitting Hospital:** Stanford Medical Center; **Office Address:** Stanford Univ Med Ctr, Dept Orth Surg 300 Pasteur Dr, rm RI44 Stanford, CA 94305; **Office Phone:** (650) 723-7072; **Board Certification:** Orthopaedic Surgery 1998; **Medical School:** Univ Toronto 1978; **Residency:** Orthopaedic Surgery, Univ of Toronto, Toronto, Canada 1979-1984; **Fellowship:** Orthopaedic Surgery, Univ of Toronto, Toronto, Canada 1984-1985; **Faculty Appointment:** Prof Orthopaedic Surgery, Stanford Univ

Hansen Jr., Sigvard MD (Orthopaedic Surgery) - *Special Expertise: Foot/Ankle;* **Admitting Hospital:** University of Washington Medical Center; **Office Address:** Harborview Medical Ctr, Dept Ortho 325 9th Ave, Box 359798 Seattle, WA 98104-2499; **Office Phone:** (206) 731-4487; **Board Certification:** Orthopaedic Surgery 1993; **Medical School:** Univ Wash 1961; **Residency:** Orthopaedic Surgery, Univ Washington Affiliation Hosp, Seattle, WA 1965-1969; **Fellowship:** Orthopaedic Surgery, Sheffield Chldrns Hosp, England 1970; **Faculty Appointment:** Prof Orthopaedic Surgery, Univ Wash

Lowenberg, David W MD (Orthopaedic Surgery) - *Special Expertise: Osteomyelitis; Ilizarov Procedure;* **Admitting Hospital:** California Pacific Medical Center; **Office Address:** 2351 Clay St, Ste 134 San Francisco, CA 94115; **Office Phone:** (415) 600-3835; **Board Certification:** Orthopaedic Surgery 1992; **Medical School:** UCLA 1985; **Residency:** Orthopaedic Surgery, UCSF, San Francisco, CA 1986-1990; **Faculty Appointment:** Prof Orthopaedic Surgery, UCSF

Luck Jr, James Vernon MD (Orthopaedic Surgery) - *Special Expertise: Hemophilia Related Disease; Hip & Knee Replacement; Musculoskeletal Tumors;* **Admitting Hospital:** Orthopaedic Hospital; **Office Address:** 2300 S Flower St, Ste 200 Los Angeles, CA 90007-2660; **Office Phone:** (213) 749-8255; **Board Certification:** Orthopaedic Surgery 1975; **Medical School:** USC Sch Med 1967; **Residency:** Orthopaedic Surgery, Orthopaedic Hosp, Los Angeles, CA 1968-1973; **Fellowships:** Orthopedic Oncology, Orthopaedic Hosp, Los Angeles, CA 1973-1974; Reconstructive Surgery, Rancho Los Amigos, Downey, CA 1973-1974

Patzakis, Michael J MD (Orthopaedic Surgery) - *Special Expertise: Rheumatological Surgery;* **Admitting Hospital:** USC University Hospital - Richard K. Eamer Medical Plaza; **Office Address:** 1200 N State St GNH3900 Los Angeles, CA 90033-4525; **Office Phone:** (213) 226-7201; **Board Certification:** Orthopaedic Surgery 1983; **Medical School:** Ohio State Univ **Residency:** Orthopaedic Surgery, Los Angeles Co-USC Med Ctr, Los Angeles, CA 1964-1968; **Fellowship:** Rheumatology, Univ CO Med Ctr, Denver, CO 1968-1969; **Faculty Appointment:** Prof Orthopaedic Surgery, USC Sch Med

Sangeorzan, Bruce J. MD (Orthopaedic Surgery) - *Special Expertise: Fott & Ankle Surgery;* **Admitting Hospital:** University of Washington Medical Center; **Office Address:** Harborview Med Ctr-U of W 325 9th Ave, Box 359798 Seattle, WA 98104-2499; **Office Phone:** (206) 731-3466; **Board Certification:** Orthopaedic Surgery 1997; **Medical School:** Wayne State Univ 1981; **Residency:** Orthopaedic Surgery, Wayne State U, Detroit, MI 1982-1986; **Fellowship:** U Wash, Seattle, WA 1986-1987; **Faculty Appointment:** Prof Orthopaedic Surgery, Univ Wash

Schmalzried, Thomas P MD (Orthopaedic Surgery) - *Special Expertise: Hip Replacement;* **Admitting Hospital:** Orthopaedic Hospital; **Office Address:** 2400 S Flower St Los Angeles, CA 90007-2629; **Office Phone:** (213) 742-1075; **Board Certification:** Orthopaedic Surgery 1993; **Medical School:** UCLA 1984; **Residency:** Orthopaedic Surgery, UCLA Med Ctr, Los Angeles, CA 1985-1990; **Fellowships:** Orthopaedic Surgery, UCLA Med Ctr, Los Angeles, CA 1986-1987; Hip Surgery, Mass Genl Hosp - Harvard U, Boston, MA 1990-1991; **Faculty Appointment:** Asst Prof Orthopaedic Surgery, UCLA

Schurman, David J MD (Orthopaedic Surgery) - *Special Expertise: Orthopaedic Surgery - General;* **Admitting Hospital:** Stanford Medical Center; **Office Address:** Stanford Univ Med Ctr, Dept Ortho Surg 300 Pasteur Dr, rm R144 Stanford, CA 94305; **Office Phone:** (415) 723-7608; **Board Certification:** Orthopaedic Surgery 1994; **Medical School:** Columbia P&S 1965; **Residencies:** Surgery, Mount Sinai Hosp, New York, NY 1966-1967; Orthopaedic Surgery, UCLA Med Ctr, Los Angeles, CA 1967-1972; **Fellowship:** Orthopaedic Surgery, UCLA Med Ctr, Los Angeles, CA 1972-1973; **Faculty Appointment:** Prof Orthopaedic Surgery, Stanford Univ

Tolo, Vernon Thorpe MD (Orthopaedic Surgery) - *Special Expertise: Spinal Deformity-Pediatric; Skeletal Dysplasias;* **Admitting Hospital:** Children's Hospital - Los Angeles; **Office Address:** Chldns Hosp LA 4650 W Sunset Blvd, MC-69 Los Angeles, CA 90027-6062; **Office Phone:** (323) 669-4658; **Board Certification:** Orthopaedic Surgery 1977; **Medical School:** Johns Hopkins Univ 1968; **Residency:** Orthopaedic Surgery, Johns Hopkins Hosp, Baltimore, MD 1972-1975; **Fellowship:** Pediatrics, Hosp Sick Chldn, Toronto, Canada 1975-1976; **Faculty Appointment:** Prof Orthopaedic Surgery, USC Sch Med

Watkins, Robert Green MD (Orthopaedic Surgery) - *Special Expertise: Spinal Surgery;* **Admitting Hospital:** USC University Hospital - Richard K. Eamer Medical Plaza; **Office Address:** 1510 San Pablo St, Ste 700 Los Angeles, CA 90033; **Office Phone:** (323) 442-5300; **Board Certification:** Orthopaedic Surgery 1982; **Medical School:** Univ Tenn Coll Med, Memphis 1969; **Residency:** Orthopaedic Surgery, LAC-USC Med Ctr, Los Angeles, CA; **Fellowship:** Spine Surgery, Jones-Hunt Orth Hosp, Oswestry, UK; **Faculty Appointment:** Assoc Prof Orthopaedic Surgery, USC Sch Med

OTOLARYNGOLOGY

An otolaryngologist-head and neck surgeon provides comprehensive medical and surgical care for patients with diseases and disorders that affect the ears, nose, throat, the respiratory and upper alimentary systems and related structures of the head and neck.

An otolaryngologist diagnoses and provides medical and/or surgical therapy or prevention of diseases, allergies, neoplasms, deformities, disorders and/or injuries of the ears, nose, sinuses, throat, respiratory and upper alimentary systems, face, jaws and the other head and neck systems. Head and neck oncology, facial plastic and reconstructive surgery and the treatment of disorders of hearing and voice are fundamental areas of expertise.

Certification in the following subspecialty requires additional training and examination.

Plastic Surgery within the Head and Neck: An otolaryngologist with additional training in plastic and reconstructive procedures within the head, face, neck and associated structures, including cutaneous head and neck oncology and reconstruction, management of maxillofacial trauma, soft tissue repair and neural surgery.

This field is diverse and involved a wide age range of patients, from the newborn to the aged. While both cosmetic and reconstructive surgeries are practiced, there are many additional procedures which interface with them.

Training required: Five years

PHYSICIAN LISTINGS

500

New England

Cheney, Mack Lowell MD (Otolaryngology) - *Special Expertise:* Facial Reconstruction; Cosmetic Surgery-Face; Facial Paralysis; **Admitting Hospital:** Massachusetts Eye & Ear Infirmary (Page 68); **Office Address:** Mass EEI- Facial Plastic Surg Unit 243 Charles St Boston, MA 02114; **Office Phone:** (617) 573-3709; **Board Certification:** Otolaryngology 1987; **Medical School:** Univ Miss 1982; **Residency:** Surgery, Tulane Univ, New Orleans, LA 1983-1987; **Fellowship:** Plastic Surgery, Harvard Med Sch, Boston, MA 1987; **Faculty Appointment:** Assoc Prof Otolaryngology, Harvard Med Sch

Fabian, Richard MD (Otolaryngology) - *Special Expertise:* Head & Neck Cancer; **Admitting Hospital:** Massachusetts Eye & Ear Infirmary (Page 68); **Office Address:** 243 Charles St Boston, MA 02114; **Office Phone:** (617) 573-4084; **Board Certification:** Otolaryngology 1972; **Medical School:** Tufts Univ 1966; **Residencies:** Otolaryngological Rhinoplasty, Mass Genl Hosp, Boston, MA 1968-1971; Surgery, Kings Co Hosp - SUNY Brooklyn, Brooklyn, NY 1967-1968; **Faculty Appointment:** Assoc Prof Otolaryngology, Harvard Med Sch

Kveton, John MD (Otolaryngology) - *Special Expertise:* Sinus Disorders/Surgery; **Admitting Hospital:** Yale - New Haven Hospital; **Office Address:** 46 Prince St, Ste 601 New Haven, CT 06519; **Office Phone:** (203) 752-1726; **Board Certification:** Otolaryngology 1982; **Medical School:** St Louis Univ 1978; **Residency:** Otolaryngology, Yale-New Haven Hosp, New Haven, CT 1978-1982; **Fellowship:** Otolaryngology, The Otology Group, Nashville, TN 1982-1983; **Faculty Appointment:** Prof Otolaryngology, Yale Univ

Nadol, Joseph MD (Otolaryngology) - *Special Expertise:* Ear Disorders/Surgery; Hearing Disorders; **Admitting Hospital:** Massachusetts Eye & Ear Infirmary (Page 68); **Office Address:** Mass Eye & Ear 243 Charles St Boston, MA 02114; **Office Phone:** (617) 573-3632; **Board Certification:** Otolaryngology 1975; **Medical School:** Johns Hopkins Univ 1970; **Residencies:** Surgery, Beth Israel Hosp, Boston, MA 1971-1972; Otolaryngology, Mass EE Infirm, Boston, MA 1972-1975; **Faculty Appointment:** Prof Otolaryngology, Harvard Med Sch

Poe, Dennis MD (Otolaryngology) - *Special Expertise:* Neuro-Otolaryngology; Cochlear Implants; Skull Base Surgery; **Admitting Hospital:** Massachusetts Eye & Ear Infirmary (Page 68); **Office Address:** Zero Emerson Pl Boston, MA 02114; **Office Phone:** (617) 636-5498; **Board Certification:** Otolaryngology 1987; **Medical School:** SUNY Syracuse 1982; **Residencies:** Surgery, Univ Mass Med Ctr, Worcester 1982-1983; Otolaryngology, Univ Chicago Med Ctr 1983-1987; **Fellowship:** Neurological Otology, Otology Grp, Nashville, TN 1987-1988; **Faculty Appointment:** Clin Prof Otolaryngology, Harvard Med Sch

Sasaki, Clarence T MD (Otolaryngology) - *Special Expertise:* Head & Neck Cancer; Voice/Swallowing Disorders; **Admitting Hospital:** Yale - New Haven Hospital; **Office Address:** Yale Sch of Medicine 337 Cedar St, Bldg FL4, Box 20804 New Haven, CT 06520-8041; **Office Phone:** (203) 785-2592; **Board Certification:** Otolaryngology 1973; **Medical School:** Yale Univ 1966; **Residencies:** Surgery, Dartmouth, Hanover, NH 1967-1968; Otolaryngology, Yale, New Haven, CT 1970-1973; **Fellowships:** Surgery, Univ Milan, Italy 1978; Surgery, Univ Zurich, Switzerland 1982; **Faculty Appointment:** Prof Otolaryngology, Yale Univ

Vining, Eugenia MD (Otolaryngology) - *Special Expertise:* Sinus Disorders/Surgery; **Admitting Hospital:** Yale - New Haven Hospital; **Office Address:** ENT Med & Surg Group 46 Prince St, Fl 6 New Haven, CT 06519; **Office Phone:** (203) 752-1726; **Board Certification:** Otolaryngology 1993; **Medical School:** Yale Univ 1987; **Residencies:** Otolaryngology, Yale-New Haven Hosp, New Haven, CT 1988-1991; Otolaryngology, Yale-New Haven Hosp, New Haven, CT 1991-1992; **Fellowship:** Sinus Surgery, Univ Penn Med Ctr, Philadelphia, PA 1992-1993; **Faculty Appointment:** Clin Inst Otolaryngology, Yale Univ

OTOLARYNGOLOGY *New England*

Zeitels, Steven MD (Otolaryngology) - *Special Expertise:* Laryngeal Disorders; Voice Disorders; Head & Neck Surgery; **Admitting Hospital:** Massachusetts Eye & Ear Infirmary (Page 68); **Office Address:** Mass Eye & Ear Infirm, Dept Oto 243 Charles St Boston, MA 02114; **Office Phone:** (617) 573-3557; **Board Certification:** Otolaryngology 1988; **Medical School:** Boston Univ 1982; **Residencies:** Surgery, Univ Hosp-Boston City Hosp, Boston, MA 1982-1983; Otolaryngology, Boston Univ-Tufts Univ, Boston, MA 1983-1987; **Fellowship:** Head and Neck Surgery, Boston VA Med Ctr-Boston Univ, Boston, MA 1987-1988; **Faculty Appointment:** Assoc Prof Otolaryngology, Harvard Med Sch

Mid Atlantic

Abramson, Allan MD (Otolaryngology) - *Special Expertise:* Throat Tumors; Head & Neck Surgery; **Admitting Hospital:** Long Island Jewish Medical Center; **Office Address:** Long Island Jewish Med Ctr, Dept Oto 270-05 76th Ave New Hyde Park, NY 11040; **Office Phone:** (516) 470-7555; **Board Certification:** Otolaryngology 1972; **Medical School:** SUNY Downstate 1967; **Residencies:** Surgery, Long Island Jewish Med Ctr, New Hyde Park, NY 1968-1969; Otolaryngology, Mount Sinai Med Ctr, New York, NY 1969-1972; **Faculty Appointment:** Prof Otolaryngology, Albert Einstein Coll Med

Arriaga, Moises Alberto MD (Otolaryngology) - *Special Expertise:* Neuro-Otolaryngology; **Admitting Hospital:** Allegheny General Hospital; **Office Address:** Pittsburgh Ear Assoc 420 E North Ave, Ste 402 Pittsburgh, PA 15212; **Office Phone:** (412) 359-6690; **Board Certification:** Otolaryngology 1990; **Medical School:** Brown Univ 1985; **Residency:** Otolaryngology, Univ Pittsburgh, Pittsburgh, PA 1986-1990; **Fellowship:** Neurological Otology, House Ear Clin, Los Angeles, CA 1990-1991

Aviv, Jonathan MD (Otolaryngology) - *Special Expertise:* Voice Disorders; Swallowing Disorders; **Admitting Hospital:** Columbia Presbyterian Medical Center (Page 72); **Office Address:** Columbia Presbyterian Assoc 16 E 60th St, Ste 360 New York, NY 10022-1002; **Office Phone:** (212) 326-8475; **Board Certification:** Otolaryngology 1990; **Medical School:** Columbia P&S 1985; **Residencies:** Surgery, Mount Sinai Med Ctr, New York, NY 1986-1987; Otolaryngology, Mount Sinai Med Ctr, New York, NY 1987-1990; **Fellowship:** Otolaryngology, Mount Sinai Med Ctr, New York, NY 1990-1991; **Faculty Appointment:** Assoc Prof Otolaryngology, Columbia P&S

Blitzer, Andrew MD (Otolaryngology) - *Special Expertise:* Pain-Orofacial; Oromandibular Dystonia; **Admitting Hospital:** St Luke's - Roosevelt Hospital Center - Roosevelt Division (Page 58); **Office Address:** Head & Neck Surgical Group 425 W 59th St, Fl 10 New York, NY 10019-1128; **Office Phone:** (212) 262-9500; **Board Certification:** Otolaryngology 1977; **Medical School:** Mount Sinai Sch Med 1973; **Residencies:** Surgery, Beth Israel, New York, NY 1973-1974; Otolaryngology, Mount Sinai, New York, NY 1974-1977; **Faculty Appointment:** Prof Otolaryngology, Columbia P&S

Brookler, Kenneth MD (Otolaryngology) - *Special Expertise:* Dizziness; Hearing Loss/Tinnitus; **Admitting Hospital:** Lenox Hill Hospital; **Office Address:** 111 E 77th St Neurotologic Associates, PC New York, NY 10021; **Office Phone:** (212) 861-6900; **Board Certification:** Otolaryngology 1968; **Medical School:** Canada 1962; **Residencies:** Surgery, Deer Lodge Hospital, Winnipeg, Canada 1963-1964; Otolaryngology, Mayo Clinic, Rochester, MN 1964-1967; **Fellowship:** Neurology, Mayo Clinic, Rochester, MN 1968

Carrau, Ricardo L. MD (Otolaryngology) - *Special Expertise:* Skull Base Surgery; Swallowing Disorders; **Admitting Hospital:** UPMC - Presbyterian University Hospital; **Office Address:** Univ Pittsburgh Med Ctr 200 Lothrop St, Ste 300 Pittsburg, PA 15213-2546; **Office Phone:** (412) 647-2100; **Board Certification:** Otolaryngology 1987; **Medical School:** Univ Puerto Rico 1981; **Residencies:** Surgery, University Hosp, San Juan, Puerto Rico 1984-1987; Head and Neck Surgery, University Hosp, San Juan, Puerto Rico 1982-1984; **Fellowship:** Head and Neck Surgery, University Pittsburgh, Pittsburgh, PA 1989-1990; **Faculty Appointment:** Asst Prof Otolaryngology, Univ Pittsburgh

Close, Lanny Garth MD (Otolaryngology) - *Special Expertise:* Skull Base Surgery; Head & Neck Cancer; Sinus Disorders/Surgery; **Admitting Hospital:** Columbia Presbyterian Medical Center (Page 72); **Office Address:** Columbia Presbyterian Eastside 16 E 60th St, Ste 360 New York, NY 10022-1002; **Office Phone:** (212) 326-8475; **Board Certification:** Otolaryngology 1977; **Medical School:** Baylor Coll Med 1972; **Residencies:** Surgery, Johns Hopkins, Baltimore, MD 1972-1974; Otolaryngology, Baylor Affil Hosp, Houston, TX 1974-1977; **Fellowship:** Otolaryngology, MD Anderson, Houston, TX 1978-1979; **Faculty Appointment:** Prof Otolaryngology, Columbia P&S

Cohen, Noel L MD (Otolaryngology) - *Special Expertise:* Cochlear Implants; Acoustic Nerve Tumors; **Admitting Hospital:** NYU Medical Center (Page 70); **Office Address:** 530 1st Ave, Fl 3C New York, NY 10016; **Office Phone:** (212) 263-7373; **Board Certification:** Otolaryngology 1963; **Medical School:** Other Foreign Country 1957; **Residency:** Otolaryngology, NYU Med Ctr, New York, NY 1959-1962; **Faculty Appointment:** Clin Prof Otolaryngology, NYU Sch Med

Cummings, Charles MD (Otolaryngology) - *Special Expertise:* Head & Neck Surgery; Laryngeal Disorders; **Admitting Hospital:** Johns Hopkins Hospital - Baltimore (Page 65); **Office Address:** Johns Hopkins U-Dept. Oto HNS 601 N Caroline St Baltimore, MD 21282; **Office Phone:** (410) 955-7400; **Board Certification:** Otolaryngology 1968; **Medical School:** Univ VA Sch Med 1961; **Residencies:** Surgery, U VA Hosp, Charlottesville, VA 1962-1963; Otolaryngology, Mass Genl, Boston, MA 1965-1968; **Faculty Appointment:** Otolaryngology, Johns Hopkins Univ

Davidson, Bruce J MD (Otolaryngology) - *Special Expertise:* Head & Neck Cancer; Thyroid Disorders; **Admitting Hospital:** Georgetown University Hospital; **Office Address:** Georgetown University Hospital, Dept Oto/HNS 3800 Reservoir Rd NW, Bldg 1 Gorman Washington, DC 20007; **Office Phone:** (202) 687-8186; **Board Certification:** Otolaryngology 1993; **Medical School:** W VA Univ 1987; **Residency:** Otolaryngology, Georgetown, Washington, DC 1988-1992; **Fellowship:** Otolaryngology, Memorial Sloan Kettering, New York, NY 1992-1994; **Faculty Appointment:** Asst Prof Otolaryngology, Georgetown Univ

Eisele, David MD (Otolaryngology) - *Special Expertise:* Salivary Gland Tumors; Head & Neck Cancer; **Admitting Hospital:** Johns Hopkins Hospital - Baltimore (Page 65); **Office Address:** Johns Hopkins Outpatient Center 601 N Caroline St, rm 6221 Baltimore, MD 21287; **Office Phone:** (410) 955-9772; **Board Certification:** Otolaryngology 1988; **Medical School:** Cornell Univ-Weil Med Coll **Residencies:** Surgery, Univ Wash, Seattle, WA 1982-1984; Otolaryngology, Univ Wash, Seattle, WA 1984-1988; **Faculty Appointment:** Prof Otolaryngology, Johns Hopkins Univ

Glasgold, Alvin MD (Otolaryngology) - *Special Expertise:* Cosmetic Surgery-Face; **Admitting Hospital:** Robert Wood Johnson University Hospital @ New Brunswick; **Office Address:** Ctr for Facial Plastic Surg 31 River Rd Highland Park, NJ 08904; **Office Phone:** (732) 846-6540; **Board Certification:** Otolaryngology 1967; **Medical School:** NY Med Coll 1961; **Residencies:** Surgery, Bronx VA Hosp, Bronx, NY 1962-1963; Otolaryngology, Bronx VA Hosp, Bronx, NY 1963-1966; **Faculty Appointment:** Clin Prof Otolaryngology, UMDNJ-RW Johnson Med Sch

Har-El, Gady MD (Otolaryngology) - *Special Expertise:* Head & Neck Cancer; Sinus & Skull Base Surgery; **Admitting Hospital:** Long Island College Hospital (Page 58); **Office Address:** University Otolaryngologists 134 Atlantic Ave Brooklyn, NY 11201; **Office Phone:** (718) 780-1498; **Board Certification:** Otolaryngology 1992; **Medical School:** Israel 1982; **Residency:** Otolaryngology, SUNY Hosp, Brooklyn, NY 1986-1991; **Faculty Appointment:** Prof Otolaryngology, SUNY Hlth Sci Ctr

Hayden, Richard Earle MD (Otolaryngology) - *Special Expertise:* Head & Neck Surgery; **Admitting Hospital:** Hahnemann University Hospital; **Office Address:** Med Coll Penn - Hahnemann Univ 2 Logan Sq, Ste 1815 Philadelphia, PA 19103-2722; **Office Phone:** (215) 665-8140; **Board Certification:** Otolaryngology 1978; **Medical School:** McGill Univ 1974; **Residency:** Otolaryngology, Univ Toronto, Toronto, Canada 1975-1978; **Fellowships:** Head and Neck Surgery, MD Anderson Hosp, Houston, TX 1978-1979; Radiation Oncology, Princess Margaret Hosp, Toronto, Canada 1979-1980; **Faculty Appointment:** Prof Otolaryngology, Hahnemann Univ

Hurst, Michael K MD (Otolaryngology) - *Special Expertise:* Nasal Allergy; **Admitting Hospital:** West Virginia University Hospital - Ruby Memorial; **Office Address:** Morgantown ENT Clinic 1188 Pineview Dr Morgantown, WV 26505; **Office Phone:** (304) 599-3959; **Board Certification:** Otolaryngology 1994; **Medical School:** Marshall Univ 1988; **Residency:** Otolaryngology, W Va Sch Med Hosps, Morgantown, WV 1989-1993; **Faculty Appointment:** Asst Prof Otolaryngology, W VA Sch Osteo Med

Johnson, Jonas Talmadge MD (Otolaryngology) - *Special Expertise:* Head & Neck Surgery; Head & Neck Cancer; **Admitting Hospital:** UPMC - Presbyterian University Hospital; **Office Address:** Eye and Ear Inst 200 Lothrop St, Ste 300 Pittsburgh, PA 15213; **Office Phone:** (412) 647-2100; **Board Certification:** Otolaryngology 1977; **Medical School:** SUNY Syracuse 1972; **Residencies:** Surgery, Med Ctr VA, Richmond, VA 1973-1974; Otolaryngology, SUNY Hlth Sci Ctr, Syracuse, NY 1974-1977; **Faculty Appointment:** Prof Otolaryngology, Univ Pittsburgh

Josephson, Jordan S MD (Otolaryngology) - *Special Expertise:* Nasal & Sinus Disorders; **Admitting Hospital:** Manhattan Eye, Ear & Throat Hospital; **Office Address:** 111 E 77th St New York, NY 10021; **Office Phone:** (212) 717-1773; **Board Certification:** Otolaryngology 1988; **Medical School:** SUNY Hlth Sci Ctr 1983; **Residency:** Otolaryngology, Long Island Jewish Med Ctr, New Hyde Park, NY 1984-1988; **Fellowship:** Sinus Surgery, Johns Hopkins, Baltimore, MD 1988-1989

Kennedy, David MD (Otolaryngology) - *Special Expertise:* Endoscopic Sinus Surgery; **Admitting Hospital:** Hospital of the University of Pennsylvania; **Office Address:** Univ Penn, Dept Oto/HNS 3400 Spruce St Philadelphia, PA 19104; **Office Phone:** (215) 662-2777; **Board Certification:** Otolaryngology 1978; **Medical School:** Ireland 1972; **Residencies:** Surgery, Johns Hopkins Hosp, Baltimore, MD 1973-1974; Otolaryngology, Johns Hopkins Hosp, Baltimore, MD 1974-1978; **Faculty Appointment:** Prof Otolaryngology, Univ Penn

Lawson, William MD (Otolaryngology) - *Special Expertise:* Sinus Disorders/Surgery; **Admitting Hospital:** Mount Sinai Hospital (Page 70); **Office Address:** Mount Sinai Hosp 5 E 98th St, Fl 8 New York, NY 10029-6501; **Office Phone:** (212) 241-9410; **Board Certification:** Otolaryngology 1974; **Medical School:** NYU Sch Med 1965; **Residencies:** Surgery, Bronx VA Hosp, Bronx, NY 1966-1967; Otolaryngology, Mount Sinai Hosp, New York, NY 1970-1973; **Fellowship:** Otolaryngology, Mount Sinai Hosp, New York, NY 1969-1970; **Faculty Appointment:** Prof Otolaryngology, Mount Sinai Sch Med

Myers, Eugene MD (Otolaryngology) - *Special Expertise:* Head/Neck Surgery; Head & Neck Cancer; **Admitting Hospital:** UPMC - Presbyterian University Hospital; **Office Address:** Otolaryngology 200 Lothrop St, Bldg EEI - Fl 3rd - Ste 300 Pittsburgh, PA 15213; **Office Phone:** (412) 647-2100; **Board Certification:** Otolaryngology 1966; **Medical School:** Temple Univ 1960; **Residencies:** Surgery, VA Hosp, Boston, MA 1961-1962; Otolaryngology, Mass EE Infirm, Boston, MA 1962-1965; **Fellowships:** Otolaryngology, Harvard Med School, Boston, MA 1964-1965; Otolaryngology, St Vincents Hosp, New York, NY 1967-1968; **Faculty Appointment:** Prof Otolaryngology, Univ Pittsburgh

Niparko, John MD (Otolaryngology) - *Special Expertise:* Ear Disorders/Surgery; Neuro-Otology; **Admitting Hospital:** Johns Hopkins Hospital - Baltimore (Page 65); **Office Address:** Johns Hopkins Hosp, Dept Oto 601 N Caroline St, Ste 6223 Baltimore, MD 21287-6214; **Office Phone:** (410) 955-2689; **Board Certification:** Otolaryngology 1986; **Medical School:** Univ Mich Med Sch 1980; **Residencies:** Otolaryngology, Univ Mich, Ann Arbor, MI 1982-1986; Surgery, William Beaumont Hosp., Royal Oak, MI 1980-1982; **Fellowship:** Otolaryngology, Univ Mich, Ann Arbor, MI 1986; **Faculty Appointment:** Prof Otolaryngology, Johns Hopkins Univ

Papel, Ira David MD (Otolaryngology) - *Special Expertise:* Cosmetic Surgery-Face; **Admitting Hospital:** Johns Hopkins Hospital - Baltimore (Page 65); **Office Address:** Facial Plastic Surgicenter 21 Crossroads Dr Owing Mills, MD 21117-5441; **Office Phone:** (410) 363-6677; **Board Certification:** Otolaryngology 1986; **Medical School:** Boston Univ 1981; **Residency:** Otolaryngology, John Hopkins Hosp, Baltimore, MD 1982-1986; **Fellowship:** Facial Plastic Surgery, UCSF, San Francisco, CA 1986-1987; **Faculty Appointment:** Asst Prof Otolaryngology, Johns Hopkins Univ

Parisier, Simon MD (Otolaryngology) - *Special Expertise:* Cochlear Implants; **Admitting Hospital:** Lenox Hill Hospital; **Office Address:** 186 E 76th St New York, NY 10021-7400; **Office Phone:** (212) 535-6400; **Board Certification:** Otolaryngology 1967; **Medical School:** Boston Univ 1961; **Residency:** Otolaryngology, Mount Sinai, New York, NY 1962-1966; **Faculty Appointment:** Clin Prof Otolaryngology, NY Coll Osteo Med

Pastorek, Norman MD (Otolaryngology) - *Special Expertise:* Otolaryngology - General; **Admitting Hospital:** New York Weill Cornell Medical Center - NY Presbyterian Hospital (Page 72); **Office Address:** 12 E 88th St New York, NY 10128-0535; **Office Phone:** (212) 987-4700; **Board Certification:** Otolaryngology 1970; **Medical School:** Univ IL Coll Med 1964; **Residencies:** Surgery, VA Hosp, Hines, IL 1966-1967; Otolaryngology, U IL Med Ctr, Chicago, IL 1967-1969

Persky, Mark MD (Otolaryngology) - *Special Expertise:* Head & Neck Cancer; **Admitting Hospital:** Beth Israel Medical Center - Herbert & Nell Singer Division (Page 58); **Office Address:** 10 Union Square East Pl, Ste 4J Beth Israel Medical Center New York, NY 10003; **Office Phone:** (212) 844-8648; **Board Certification:** Otolaryngology 1976; **Medical School:** SUNY Syracuse 1972; **Residency:** Otolaryngology, Bellevue Hosp, New York, NY 1973-1976; **Fellowship:** Beth Israel Med Ctr, New York, NY 1976-1977; **Faculty Appointment:** Clin Prof Otolaryngology, Albert Einstein Coll Med

Picken, Catherine A MD (Otolaryngology) - *Special Expertise:* Head & Neck Reconstruction; Thyroid Disorders; Sinus Disorders/Surgery; **Admitting Hospital:** Georgetown University Hospital; **Office Address:** GUMC, First Floor, Gorman Building 3800 Reservoir Rd NW Washington, DC 20007; **Office Phone:** (202) 687-8186; **Board Certification:** Otolaryngology 1989; **Medical School:** Northwestern Univ 1979; **Residencies:** Surgery, Northwestern Meml Hosp, Chicago, IL 1980-1981; Otolaryngology, Georgetown Univ, Washington, DC 1985-1989; **Fellowship:** Surgery, Natl Heart Lung Blood Inst, Bethesda, MD 1981-1983; **Faculty Appointment:** Assoc Prof Otolaryngology, Georgetown Univ

Quatela, Vito Charles MD (Otolaryngology) - *Special Expertise:* Cosmetic Surgery-Face; Rhinoplasty; Forehead Lift-Endoscpic; **Admitting Hospital:** Strong Memorial Hospital - Medical Center; **Office Address:** University of Rochester 973 East Ave, Box 629 Rochester, NY 14607; **Office Phone:** 716 2441000; **Board Certification:** Otolaryngology 1985; **Medical School:** Northwestern Univ 1979; **Residencies:** Surgery, Med Ctr Hosp Vermont, Burlington 1980-1981; Orthopaedic Surgery, Northwestern Univ, Chicago, IL 1982-1985; **Fellowships:** Facial Plastic Surgery, Tulane Univ, New Orleans, LA 1985-1986; Facial Plastic Surgery, Oregon Hlth Science Univ, Portland 1986-1987; **Faculty Appointment:** Assoc Clin Prof Otolaryngology, Univ Rochester

Romo III, Thomas MD (Otolaryngology) - *Special Expertise:* Cosmetic Surgery-Face; **Admitting Hospital:** New York Eye & Ear Infirmary (Page 71); **Office Address:** 150 Broadway, Ste 616 New York, NY 10038-4311; **Office Phone:** (212) 619-3501; **Board Certification:** Otolaryngology 1985; **Medical School:** Baylor Coll Med 1979; **Residencies:** Plastic Surgery, New York Eye & Ear, New York, NY 1984-1985; Otolaryngology, New York Eye & Ear, New York, NY 1982-1984; **Fellowship:** Plastic Surgery, Tampa General, Tampa, FL 1985

Sataloff, Robert MD (Otolaryngology) - *Special Expertise:* Laryngeal Disorders; **Admitting Hospital:** Thomas Jefferson University Hospital; **Office Address:** 1721 Pine Street Philadelphia, PA 19103-6701; **Office Phone:** (215) 545-3322; **Board Certification:** Otolaryngology 1980; **Medical School:** Jefferson Med Coll 1975; **Residency:** Otolaryngology, Unvi Mich Hosp, Ann Harbor, MI 1976-1980; **Fellowship:** Otolaryngology, Univ Mich Hosp, Ann Harbor, MI 1980-1981; **Faculty Appointment:** Prof Otolaryngology, Jefferson Med Coll

Schaefer, Steven MD (Otolaryngology) - *Special Expertise:* Sinus Disorders/Surgery; Head & Neck Surgery; **Admitting Hospital:** New York Eye & Ear Infirmary (Page 71); **Office Address:** NY Eye and Eye Infirm, Dept Oto 310 E 14th St New York, NY 10003; **Office Phone:** (212) 979-4200; **Board Certification:** Otolaryngology 1978; **Medical School:** UC Irvine 1972; **Residencies:** Surgery, UCLA Med Ctr, Los Angeles, CA 1972-1974; Otolaryngology, Stanford Med Ctr, Stanford, CA 1973-1974; **Faculty Appointment:** Prof Otolaryngology, NY Med Coll

Urken, Mark MD (Otolaryngology) - *Special Expertise:* Microvascular Reconstruction; Head & Neck Surgery; **Admitting Hospital:** Mount Sinai Hospital (Page 70); **Office Address:** Otolaryngology Associates 5 E 98th St, Fl 8th - Ste 8th New York, NY 10029-6501; **Office Phone:** (212) 241-9410; **Board Certification:** Otolaryngology 1986; **Medical School:** Univ VA Sch Med 1981; **Residency:** Otolaryngology, Mount Sinai Hosp, New York, NY 1983-1986; **Fellowship:** Plastic Surgery, Mercy Hospital, Pittsburgh, PA 1986-1987; **Faculty Appointment:** Assoc Prof Otolaryngology, Mount Sinai Sch Med

Ward, Robert MD (Otolaryngology) - *Special Expertise:* Ophthalmology-Pediatric; Sinus Disorders/Surgery; **Admitting Hospital:** Lenox Hill Hospital; **Office Address:** 186 E 76th St New York, NY 10021; **Office Phone:** (212) 327-3000; **Board Certification:** Otolaryngology 1986; **Medical School:** Cornell Univ-Weil Med Coll 1981; **Residencies:** Surgery, NY Hosp, New York, NY 1982-1983; Otolaryngology, NY Hosp, New York, NY 1983-1986; **Fellowship:** Pediatric Otolaryngology, Chldns Hosp, Boston, MA 1986; **Faculty Appointment:** Assoc Clin Prof Otolaryngology, Cornell Univ-Weil Med Coll

Wazen, Jack MD (Otolaryngology) - *Special Expertise:* Skull Base Surgery; Meniere's Disease; Acoustic Nerve Tumors; **Admitting Hospital:** Columbia Presbyterian Medical Center (Page 72); **Office Address:** 111 E 77th St New York, NY 10021-1802; **Office Phone:** (212) 249-3232; **Board Certification:** Otolaryngology 1983; **Medical School:** Lebanon 1978; **Residencies:** Surgery, St Lukes Hosp, New York, NY 1979-1980; Otolaryngology, Columbia Presby Hosp, New York, NY 1980-1983; **Fellowship:** Neurological Otology, Ear Rsch Fdn, Sarasota, FL 1983-1984; **Faculty Appointment:** Assoc Clin Prof Otolaryngology, Columbia P&S

Weber, Randal Scott MD (Otolaryngology) - *Special Expertise:* Thyroid Tumors; Thyroid & Parathyroid Surgery; Skull Base Tumors; **Admitting Hospital:** Hospital of the University of Pennsylvania; **Office Address:** Hosp of Univ Penn, Dept Oto 3400 Spruce St Philadelphia, PA 19104; **Office Phone:** (215) 662-2777; **Board Certification:** Otolaryngology 1985; **Medical School:** Univ Tenn Coll Med, Memphis 1976; **Residencies:** Surgery, Baylor Coll Med, Houston, TX 1981-1982; Otolaryngology, Baylor Coll Med, Houston, TX 1982-1985; **Fellowship:** Head and Neck Surgery, Univ TX MD Anderson Cancer Ctr, Houston, TX 1985-1986; **Faculty Appointment:** Prof Otolaryngology, Univ Penn

Weinstein, Gregory MD (Otolaryngology) - *Special Expertise:* Head & Neck Cancer; **Admitting Hospital:** Hospital of the University of Pennsylvania; **Office Address:** Hosp of Univ Penn, Dept Oto 3400 Spruce St, Bldg Ravdin 5 Philadelphia, PA 19104; **Office Phone:** (215) 349-5390; **Board Certification:** Otolaryngology 1990; **Medical School:** NY Med Coll 1985; **Residencies:** Otolaryngology, St Vincent's Hosp, New York, NY 1985-1986; Otolaryngology, Univ Iowa Hosp, Iowa City, IA 1986-1990; **Faculty Appointment:** Assoc Prof Otolaryngology, Univ Penn

Woo, Peak MD (Otolaryngology) - *Special Expertise:* Voice Disorders; Laryngology; **Admitting Hospital:** Mount Sinai Hospital (Page 70); **Office Address:** Mount Sinai Hosp 5 E 98th St, Fl 1 New York, NY 10029; **Office Phone:** (212) 241-9425; **Board Certification:** Otolaryngology 1983; **Medical School:** Boston Univ 1978; **Residency:** Otolaryngology, Boston Univ - Tuft Univ, Boston, MA 1979-1983

Zalzal, George MD (Otolaryngology) - *Special Expertise:* Airway Disorders; Laryngeal & Tracheal Disorders; Ear Disorders; **Admitting Hospital:** Children's National Medical Center - DC; **Office Address:** 111 Michigan Ave NW Washington, DC 20010; **Office Phone:** (202) 884-3455; **Board Certification:** Otolaryngology 1996; **Medical School:** Lebanon 1979; **Residency:** American Univ Hosp, Beirut, Lebanon 1979-1983; **Fellowship:** Pediatric Otolaryngology, Univ Cincinnati, Cincinnati, OH 1983-1985; **Faculty Appointment:** Prof Pediatric Otolaryngology, Geo Wash Univ

Southeast

Antonelli, Patrick MD (Otolaryngology) - *Special Expertise:* Hearing Disorders; Ear Disorders/Surgery; **Admitting Hospital:** Shands Healthcare at University Florida (Page 77); **Office Address:** Shands Hlthcare at Univ of FL 1600 SW Archer Rd, Box 100264 Gainesville, FL 32610; **Office Phone:** (352) 392-4061; **Board Certification:** Otolaryngology 1994; **Medical School:** Univ Minn 1988; **Residencies:** Surgery, Hannepin Co Med Ctr, Minneapolis, MN 1986-1989; Otolaryngology, Univ of Minnesota, Minneapolis, MN 1989-1993; **Fellowship:** Neurological Otology, Michigan Ear Inst, Farmington, MI 1993-1994; **Faculty Appointment:** Assoc Prof Otolaryngology, Univ Fla Coll Med

Balkany, Thomas Jay MD (Otolaryngology) - *Special Expertise:* Deafness & Ear Disorders; Neuro-Otology; **Admitting Hospital:** University of Miami - Jackson Memorial Hospital; **Office Address:** Univ of Miami Ear Inst 1666 NW 10th Ave, Ste 306 Miami, FL 33136-1015; **Office Phone:** (305) 585-7129; **Board Certification:** Otolaryngology 1977; **Medical School:** Univ Miami Sch Med 1972; **Residencies:** Surgery, St Joseph Hosp, Denver, CO 1973-1974; Otolaryngology, Colo Med Ctr, Denver, CO 1974-1977; **Fellowship:** Otolaryngology, House Ear Inst, Los Angeles, CA 1978; **Faculty Appointment:** Clin Prof Otolaryngology, Univ Miami Sch Med

Burkey, Brian MD (Otolaryngology) - *Special Expertise:* Parotid Gland Tumors; Head & Neck Cancer; **Admitting Hospital:** Vanderbilt University Medical Center; **Office Address:** Vanderbilt Univ, Dept Oto S-2100 MCN Nashville, TN 37232-2559; **Office Phone:** (615) 322-7267; **Board Certification:** Otolaryngology 1992; **Medical School:** Univ VA Sch Med 1986; **Residency:** Otolaryngology, Univ Mich, Ann Arbor, MI 1987-1991; **Fellowship:** Microsurgery, Ohio State Univ, Columbus, OH 1991; **Faculty Appointment:** Assoc Prof Otolaryngology, Vanderbilt Univ

Cassisi, Nicholas J MD (Otolaryngology) - *Special Expertise:* Head & Neck Cancer; Voice Disorders; **Admitting Hospital:** Shands Healthcare at University Florida (Page 77); **Office Address:** Shands Healthcare at Univ FL 1600 SW Archer Rd, Box 100264 Gainesville, FL 32610; **Office Phone:** (352) 392-4461; **Board Certification:** Otolaryngology 1971; **Medical School:** Univ Miami Sch Med 1965; **Residencies:** Surgery, Jackson Memorial Hosp, Miami, FL 1966-1967; Otolaryngology, Barnes Hosp - Washington U, Seattle, WA 1968-1971; **Faculty Appointment:** Prof Otolaryngology, Univ Fla Coll Med

Courey, Mark Sam MD (Otolaryngology) - *Special Expertise:* Laryngeal Disorders; **Admitting Hospital:** Vanderbilt University Medical Center; **Office Address:** Vanderbilt Voice Ctr 1500 21st Ave S Nashville, TN 37212; **Office Phone:** (615) 343-7464; **Board Certification:** Otolaryngology 1993; **Medical School:** SUNY Buffalo 1987; **Residency:** Otolaryngology, SUNY, Buffalo, NY 1989-1992; **Fellowship:** Otolaryngology, Vanderbilt Univ, Nashville, TN 1992-1993; **Faculty Appointment:** Assoc Prof Otolaryngology, Vanderbilt Univ

Farmer, Joseph MD (Otolaryngology) - *Special Expertise:* Ear Disorders/Surgery; Hearing Disorders; Balance Disorders; **Admitting Hospital:** Duke University Medical Center (Page 60); **Office Address:** Duke Univ Med Ctr Box 3805 Durham, NC 27710; **Office Phone:** (919) 684-6357; **Board Certification:** Otolaryngology 1971; **Medical School:** Duke Univ 1962; **Residencies:** Surgical Oncology, Natl Cancer Inst, Bethesda, MD 1965-1967; Otolaryngology, Duke Univ Med Ctr, Durham, NC 1967-1970; **Fellowship:** Thoracic Surgery, Duke Univ Med Ctr, Durham, NC 1964; **Faculty Appointment:** Prof Otolaryngology, Duke Univ

Farrior, Edward MD (Otolaryngology) - *Special Expertise:* Cosmetic Surgery-Face; **Admitting Hospital:** Tampa General Hospital; **Office Address:** 2909 W Azeele St Tampa, FL 33609-3109; **Office Phone:** (813) 875-3223; **Board Certification:** Otolaryngology 1987; **Medical School:** Univ VA Sch Med 1982; **Residency:** Otolaryngology, Univ Mich Hosps, Ann Arbor, MI 1983-1987; **Fellowship:** Facial Plastic Surgery, Tampa Genl Hosp, Tampa, Fl 1987-1988; **Faculty Appointment:** Assoc Clin Prof Surgery, Univ Fla Coll Med

Farrior, Joseph Brown MD (Otolaryngology) - *Special Expertise:* Ear Disorders/Surgery; **Admitting Hospital:** St Joseph's Hospital - Tampa; **Office Address:** 509 W Bay St Tampa, FL 33606; **Office Phone:** (800) 342-3277; **Board Certification:** Otolaryngology 1981; **Medical School:** Emory Univ 1975; **Residencies:** Surgery, Johns Hopkins Hosp, Baltimore, MD 1976-1977; Otolaryngology, Johns Hopkins HOsp, Baltimore, MD 1977-1981; **Fellowship:** Otolaryngology, Farrior Clin/St Josephs Hosp, Tampa, FL 1979-1980; **Faculty Appointment:** Assoc Clin Prof Otolaryngology, Univ S Fla Coll Med

Goodwin, Jerry MD (Otolaryngology) - *Special Expertise:* Head & Neck Cancer; Skull Base Surgery; **Admitting Hospital:** University of Miami Hosp & Clinics/Sylvestor Comp Cancer Cntr; **Office Address:** Univ Miami/Sylvester Comprehensive Cancer Center 1475 NW 12th Ave, rm 4023 Miami, FL 33136; **Office Phone:** (305) 243-4387; **Board Certification:** Otolaryngology 1978; **Medical School:** Albany Med Coll 1972; **Residencies:** Surgery, U of MIami, FL 1972-1973; Otolaryngology, U of Miami, FL 1974-1977; **Fellowship:** Hand Surgery, MD Anderson, TX 1979-1980; **Faculty Appointment:** Prof Otolaryngology, Univ Miami Sch Med

Goodwin, W Jarrard MD (Otolaryngology) - *Special Expertise:* Head & Neck Tumors; **Admitting Hospital:** University of Miami Hosp & Clinics/Sylvestor Comp Cancer Cntr; **Office Address:** Univ Miami, Dept Oto 1475 NW 12th Ave, Ste 4037 Miami, FL 33136-1015; **Office Phone:** (305) 243-4387; **Board Certification:** Otolaryngology 1978; **Medical School:** Albany Med Coll 1972; **Residencies:** Surgery, Univ Miami/Jackson Hosp Meml Hosp, Miami, FL 1973-1979; Otolaryngology, Univ Miami/Jackson Hosp, Miami, FL 1974-1977; **Fellowship:** Surgery, MD Anderson Hosp, Houston, TX 1979-1980; **Faculty Appointment:** Prof Otolaryngology, Univ Miami Sch Med

Grobman, Lawrence R MD (Otolaryngology) - *Special Expertise:* Otolaryngology - General; **Admitting Hospital:** Mercy Hospital - Miami; **Office Address:** 3661 S Miami Ave, Ste 409 Miami, FL 33133-4236; **Office Phone:** (305) 854-5971; **Board Certification:** Otolaryngology 1986; **Medical School:** Univ Miami Sch Med 1980; **Residencies:** Surgery, U Miami Med Ctr, Miami, FL 1981-1982; Otolaryngology, U Miami Med Ctr, Miami, FL 1982-1985; **Fellowship:** Otolaryngology, U Zurich Med Ctr, Zurich, Switzerland 1985-1986; **Faculty Appointment:** Assoc Prof Otolaryngology, Univ Miami Sch Med

Koufman, James Alan MD (Otolaryngology) - *Special Expertise:* Voice Disorders; Laryngeal Disorders; **Admitting Hospital:** Wake Forest University Baptist Medical Center; **Office Address:** Wake Forest Univ Baptist Med Ctr Medical Center Blvd Winston Salem, NC 27157; **Office Phone:** (336) 716-4161; **Board Certification:** Otolaryngology 1978; **Medical School:** Boston Univ 1973; **Residencies:** Surgery, Hartford Hosp, Hartford, CT 1974-1975; Otolaryngology, Boston Univ Med Ctr, Boston, MA 1975-1978; **Faculty Appointment:** Prof Surgery, Wake Forest Univ Sch Med

Kuhn, Frederick MD (Otolaryngology) - *Special Expertise:* Nasal & Sinus Disorders; Sinus Disorders/Surgery; **Admitting Hospital:** Memorial Medical Center - Savannah; **Office Address:** Georgia Nasal & Sinus Inst 4750 Waters Ave, Ste 112 Savannah, GA 31404; **Office Phone:** (912) 355-1070; **Board Certification:** Otolaryngology 1972; **Medical School:** Univ Okla Coll Med 1966; **Residencies:** Surgery, Univ Oklahoma Teaching Hosp, Oklahoma City, OK 1966-1967; Surgery, St Luke's Hosp, St Louis, MO 1967-1968; **Fellowship:** Otolaryngology, Barnes Hosp/Wash Univ, St Louis, MO 1968-1972

Lambert, Paul R MD (Otolaryngology) - *Special Expertise:* Neuro-Otology; **Admitting Hospital:** MUSC Medical Center; **Office Address:** MUSC, Dep OTO/Head & Neck Surg 150 Ashley Ave, Box 250582 Charleston, SC 29425; **Office Phone:** (843) 792-3531; **Board Certification:** Otolaryngology 1981; **Medical School:** Duke Univ 1976; **Residencies:** Surgery, UCLA Med Ctr, Los Angeles, CA 1977-1978; Otolaryngology, UCLA Med Ctr, Los Angeles, CA 1978-1981; **Fellowship:** Neurological Otology, Otologic Med Group, Los Angeles, CA 1981-1982; **Faculty Appointment:** Prof Otolaryngology, Med Univ SC

Levine, Paul MD (Otolaryngology) - *Special Expertise:* Head & Neck Cancer; Head & Neck Reconstruction; **Admitting Hospital:** University of Virginia Health Systems; **Office Address:** Univ VA Hlth Scis Ctr, Dept Oto/HNS Box 430 Charlottesville, VA 22908-0430; **Office Phone:** (804) 924-5593; **Board Certification:** Otolaryngology 1978; **Medical School:** Albany Med Coll 1973; **Residency:** Otolaryngology, Yale-New Haven Hosp, New Haven, CT 1974-1977; **Fellowship:** Head and Neck Surgery, Stanford Med Ctr, Stanford, CA 1977-1978; **Faculty Appointment:** Prof Otolaryngology, Univ VA Sch Med

Mattox, Douglas MD (Otolaryngology) - *Special Expertise:* Neuro-Otology; **Admitting Hospital:** Emory University Hospital; **Office Address:** Emory Clinic , Dept. Otolaryngology 1365 Clifton Rd Atlanta, GA 30322; **Office Phone:** (404) 778-3381; **Board Certification:** Otolaryngology 1977; **Medical School:** Yale Univ 1973; **Residency:** Otolaryngology, Stanford Univ Hosp, Stanford, CA 1974-1977; **Faculty Appointment:** Prof Otolaryngology, Emory Univ

McGuirt, W Fredrick MD (Otolaryngology) - *Special Expertise:* Head & Neck Cancer; Laryngeal Disorders; **Admitting Hospital:** Wake Forest University Baptist Medical Center; **Office Address:** Wake Forest Univ Baptist Med Ctr Medical Center Blvd Winston Salem, NC 27157; **Office Phone:** (336) 716-4161; **Board Certification:** Otolaryngology 1976; **Medical School:** Wake Forest Univ Sch Med 1968; **Residencies:** Otolaryngology, Iowa Hosp, Iowa City, IA 1972-1976; Surgery, NC Bapt Hosp, Winston Salem, NC 1969-1970

Netterville, James MD (Otolaryngology) - *Special Expertise:* Head & Neck Surgery; **Admitting Hospital:** Vanderbilt University Medical Center; **Office Address:** Vanderbilt Univ Med Ctr S 2100 Medl Ctr N Nashville, TN 37232-2559; **Office Phone:** (615) 322-6180; **Board Certification:** Otolaryngology 1985; **Medical School:** Univ Tenn Coll Med, Memphis 1980; **Residencies:** Surgery, Meth Hosp, Memphis, TN 1981-1982; Otolaryngology, Univ Tenn, Memphis, TN 1982-1985; **Fellowship:** Surgical Oncology, Univ Iowa, Iowa City, IA 1985-1986; **Faculty Appointment:** Assoc Prof Otolaryngology, Vanderbilt Univ

Orobello Jr, Peter W MD (Otolaryngology) - *Special Expertise:* Otolaryngology-Pediatric; **Admitting Hospital:** All Children's Hospital; **Office Address:** Otolaryngology-Head and Neck Surgery 801 6th St S St Petersburg, FL 33701-4816; **Office Phone:** (727) 892-4305; **Board Certification:** Otolaryngology 1988; **Medical School:** Univ Cincinnati 1983; **Residencies:** Surgery, Univ Cincinnati, Cincinnati, OH 1984; Otolaryngology, Univ Cincinnati, Cincinnati, OH 1984-1988; **Fellowship:** Pediatric Otolaryngology, Johns Hopkins Univ, Baltimore, MD 1989; **Faculty Appointment:** Asst Clin Prof Pediatrics, Univ S Fla Coll Med

Pearson, Bruce MD (Otolaryngology) - *Special Expertise:* Laryngeal Cancer; Head & Neck Surgery; **Admitting Hospital:** Mayo/St Luke's Hospital; **Office Address:** 4500 San Pablo Rd Jacksonville, FL 32224; **Office Phone:** (904) 953-2217; **Board Certification:** Otolaryngology 1975; **Medical School:** Univ Toronto 1966; **Residencies:** Otolaryngology, Univ Toronto, Toronto, Canada 1967-1971; Head and Neck Surgery, Royal National, London, England 1972; **Fellowship:** Head and Neck Surgery, Mayo Clinic, Rochester, MN 1973; **Faculty Appointment:** Prof Otolaryngology, Mayo Med Sch

Peters, Glenn Eidson MD (Otolaryngology) - *Special Expertise:* Head & Neck Cancer; Skull Base Surgery; **Admitting Hospital:** University of Alabama Hospital at Birmingham; **Office Address:** UAB Medical Center, Head and Neck Surgery Clinic 1501 S Fifth Ave Birmingham, AL 35233; **Office Phone:** (205) 934-9766; **Board Certification:** Otolaryngology 1985; **Medical School:** Louisiana State Univ 1980; **Residencies:** Surgery, Bapt Med Ctr, Birmingham, AL 1981-1982; Otolaryngology, Univ Ala, Birmingham, AL 1982-1984; **Fellowship:** Medical Oncology, Johns Hopkins Hosp, Baltimore, MD 1986-1987

Pillsbury, Harold Crockett MD (Otolaryngology) - *Special Expertise:* Cochlear Implants; **Admitting Hospital:** University of North Carolina Hospitals; **Office Address:** U NC CB 7070 610 Burnett Womack Bldg Chapel Hill, NC 27599-7070; **Office Phone:** (919) 966-8926; **Board Certification:** Otolaryngology 1978; **Medical School:** Geo Wash Univ 1972; **Residencies:** Surgery, Univ NC, Chapel Hill, NC 1973-1976; Otolaryngology, NC Meml Hosp, Chapel Hill, NC 1973-1976; **Faculty Appointment:** Prof Otolaryngology, Univ NC Sch Med

Postma, Gregory N MD (Otolaryngology) - *Special Expertise:* Voice Disorders; **Admitting Hospital:** Wake Forest University Baptist Medical Center; **Office Address:** Wake Forest Univ Sch Med, Dept Oto Med Ctr Blvd Winston Salem, NC 27157; **Office Phone:** (336) 716-4161; **Board Certification:** Otolaryngology 1994; **Medical School:** Hahnemann Univ 1984; **Residencies:** Otolaryngology, Oakland Naval Hosp, Oakland, CA 1989-1992; Otolaryngology, Univ NC, Chapel Hill, NC 1992-1993; **Fellowship:** Otolaryngology, Vanderbilt Univ, Nashvile, TN 1995-1996; **Faculty Appointment:** Asst Prof Otolaryngology, Wake Forest Univ Sch Med

Robbins, Thomas MD (Otolaryngology) - *Special Expertise:* Head & Neck Surgery; **Admitting Hospital:** Shands Healthcare at University Florida (Page 77); **Office Address:** Univ Florida, Dept Oto 1600 SW Archer Rd, Bldg M - rm 228, Box 100264 Gainesville, FL 32610; **Office Phone:** (352) 392-4461; **Board Certification:** Otolaryngology 1981; **Medical School:** Dalhousie Univ 1973; **Residencies:** Surgery, Dalhousie Univ, Halifax, Canada 1978-1979; Otolaryngology, Univ Toronto, Toronto, Canada 1979-1981; **Fellowships:** Head and Neck Surgery, Inst Laryngology & Otology, London, England 1981-1982; Head and Neck Surgery, MD Anderson, Houston, TX 1982-1982; **Faculty Appointment:** Prof Otolaryngology, Univ Fla Coll Med

Sillers, Michael MD (Otolaryngology) - *Special Expertise:* Nasal & Sinus Disorders; Sinus Disorders/Surgery; **Admitting Hospital:** University of Alabama Hospital at Birmingham; **Office Address:** UAB Med Ctr, Head and Neck Surg Clin 1501 5th Ave S Birmingham, AL 35249-6889; **Office Phone:** (205) 934-9779; **Board Certification:** Otolaryngology 1994; **Medical School:** Univ Ala 1988; **Residency:** Otolaryngology, Univ of Alabama, Birmingham, AL 1989-1993; **Fellowship:** Sinus Surgery, Med Coll Ga, Augusta, GA 1993-1994; **Faculty Appointment:** Asst Prof Surgery, Univ Ala

Silverstein, Herbert MD (Otolaryngology) - *Special Expertise:* Ear Disorders/Surgery; Meniere's Disease; **Admitting Hospital:** Sarasota Memorial Hospital; **Office Address:** Florida Ear & Sinus Center 1961 Floyd St, Ste A Sarasota, FL 34239-2931; **Office Phone:** (941) 366-9222; **Board Certification:** Otolaryngology 1967; **Medical School:** Temple Univ 1961; **Residencies:** Surgery, Univ Penn, Philadelphia, PA 1961-1963; Otolaryngology, Mass EE Infirm, Boston, MA 1963-1966; **Faculty Appointment:** Clin Prof Surgery, Univ S Fla Coll Med

Spektor, Zorik MD (Otolaryngology) - *Special Expertise:* Otolaryngology - General; **Admitting Hospital:** St Mary's Medical Center - West Palm Beach; **Office Address:** Ranes Pavilion 5325 Greenwood Ave West Palm Beach, FL 33407; **Office Phone:** (561) 736-8141; **Board Certification:** Otolaryngology 1995; **Medical School:** Albany Med Coll 1986; **Residency:** Otolaryngology, Univ Conn Hlth Ctr, Farmington, CT 1987-1991; **Fellowship:** Surgery, Le Bonheur Chldns Med Ctr, Memphis, TN 1994-1995

Stringer, Scott Pearson MD (Otolaryngology) - *Special Expertise:* Head & Neck Cancer; Nasal & Sinus Disorders; Maxillofacial Surgery; **Admitting Hospital:** Shands Healthcare at University Florida (Page 77); **Office Address:** Shands Healthcare - Univ Florida 1600 SW Archer Rd, Box 100264 Gainesville, FL 32610-4480; **Office Phone:** (352) 392-4461; **Board Certification:** Otolaryngology 1987; **Medical School:** Univ Tex SW, Dallas 1982; **Residencies:** Otolaryngology, Univ Tex SW Med Ctr, Dallas, TX 1984-1987; Surgery, Univ Tex SW Med Ctr, Dallas, TX 1982-1984; **Faculty Appointment:** Prof Otolaryngology, Univ Fla Coll Med

Tucci, Debara Lyn MD (Otolaryngology) - *Special Expertise:* Skull Base Surgery; Middle Ear Disease; **Admitting Hospital:** Duke University Medical Center (Page 60); **Office Address:** Duke Univ Med Ctr, Dept Surg, Div Oto Box 3805 Durham, NC 27710; **Office Phone:** (919) 684-6968; **Board Certification:** Otolaryngology 1990; **Medical School:** Univ VA Sch Med 1985; **Residency:** Otolaryngology, Univ Va Hlth Sci Ctr, Charlottesville, VA 1986-1990; **Fellowship:** Otology & Neurotology, Univ Mich Med Ctr, Ann Arbor, MI 1990-1992; **Faculty Appointment:** Assoc Prof Surgery, Duke Univ

Valentino, Joseph MD (Otolaryngology) - *Special Expertise:* Head & Neck Cancer; **Admitting Hospital:** University of Kentucky Medical Center; **Office Address:** Kentucky Clinic 740 S Limestone St, rm B317 Lexington, KY 40536-0284; **Office Phone:** (859) 257-5405; **Board Certification:** Otolaryngology 1993; **Medical School:** UMDNJ-RW Johnson Med Sch 1987; **Residency:** Otolaryngology, Univ Minn, Minneapolis, MN 1988-1992; **Fellowship:** Otolaryngology, Univ Iowa Coll Med, Iowa City, IA 1992-1993; **Faculty Appointment:** Asst Prof Otolaryngology, Univ KY Coll Med

Weissler, Mark Christian MD (Otolaryngology) - *Special Expertise:* Head & Neck Cancer; *Voice Disorders;* **Admitting Hospital:** University of North Carolina Hospitals; **Office Address:** Otolaryngology, Univ NC 610 Burnett-Womack Building Chapel Hill, NC 27599-7070; **Office Phone:** (919) 966-3341; **Board Certification:** Otolaryngology 1985; **Medical School:** Boston Univ 1980; **Residencies:** Surgery, Mass Genl Hosp, Boston, MA 1980-1982; Otolaryngology, Mass Eye & Ear Infirm, Boston, MA 1982-1985; **Fellowship:** Otolaryngology, Univ Cincinnati, Cincinnati, OH 1985-1986; **Faculty Appointment:** Prof Surgery, Univ NC Sch Med

Woodson, Gayle Ellen MD (Otolaryngology) - *Special Expertise:* Voice Disorders; **Admitting Hospital:** Shands Healthcare at University Florida (Page 77); **Office Address:** Shands Healthcare at Univ Florida 1600 SW Archer Rd, rm A 191, Box 100264 Gainesville, FL 32610; **Office Phone:** (352) 392-4461; **Board Certification:** Otolaryngology 1981; **Medical School:** Baylor Coll Med **Residencies:** Surgery, Johns Hopkins Hosp, Baltimore, MD 1977-1978; Otolaryngology, Baylor Coll Med, Houston, TX 1978-1981; **Fellowship:** Otolaryngology, London, Engalnd, London, England 1981-1982; **Faculty Appointment:** Prof Otolaryngology, Univ Fla Coll Med

Midwest

Baim, Howard MD (Otolaryngology) - *Special Expertise:* Head & Neck Surgery; **Admitting Hospital:** Illinois Masonic Medical Center (Page 64); **Office Address:** 2532 W Lincoln Ave Chicago, IL 60614-1712; **Office Phone:** (773) 883-1177; **Board Certification:** Otolaryngology 1978; **Medical School:** Univ IL Coll Med 1973; **Residencies:** Otolaryngology, IL Met Grp Hosps, Chicago, IL 1973-1975; Surgery, IL EE Infirmary, Chicago, IL 1975-1978; **Faculty Appointment:** Asst Clin Prof Otolaryngology, Univ IL Coll Med

Baker, Shan Ray MD (Otolaryngology) - *Special Expertise:* Cosmetic Surgery-Face; **Admitting Hospital:** University of Michigan Health Center; **Office Address:** Ctr for Facial Cosmetic Surg 19900 Haggerty Rd, Ste 103 Livonia, MI 48152; **Office Phone:** (734) 432-7823; **Board Certification:** Otolaryngology 1977; **Medical School:** Univ Iowa Coll Med 1971; **Residencies:** Plastic Surgery, Univ Iowa Hosps, Iowa City, IA 1973-1977; Surgery, UCSD Med Ctr, San Diego, CA 1971-1973; **Faculty Appointment:** Prof Plastic Surgery, Univ Mich Med Sch

Benninger, Michael S MD (Otolaryngology) - *Special Expertise:* Vocal Cord Disorders; *Nasal & Sinus Disorders;* **Admitting Hospital:** Henry Ford Health System (Page 62); **Office Address:** 2799 W Grand Blvd , Fl 8 - rm k807 Detroit, MI 48202; **Office Phone:** (313) 916-3275; **Board Certification:** Otolaryngology 1988; **Medical School:** Case West Res Univ 1983; **Residencies:** Surgery, Cleveland Clin Fdn, Cleveland, OH 1983-1985; Otolaryngology, Cleveland Clin Fdn, Cleveland, OH 1985-1988

Caldarelli, David D MD (Otolaryngology) - *Special Expertise:* Larynx & Vocal Cord Surgery; *Meniere's Disease;* **Admitting Hospital:** Rush/Presbyterian - St Luke's Medical Center - Chicago (Page 74); **Office Address:** 1725 W Harrison St, Bldg 308 Chicago, IL 60612-3814; **Office Phone:** (312) 733-4341; **Board Certification:** Otolaryngology 1970; **Medical School:** Univ Hlth Sci/Chicago Med Sch 1965; **Residencies:** Surgery, Presby-St Lukes Hosp, Chicago, IL 1966-1967; Otolaryngology, Univ III EE Infirm, Chicago, IL 1967-1970; **Faculty Appointment:** Prof Otolaryngology, Rush Med Coll

Chernoff, William Gregory MD (Otolaryngology) - *Special Expertise:* Facial *Plastic/Reconstructive Surgery; Ear, Nose, & Throat; Laser Surgery;* **Admitting Hospital:** Methodist Hospital - Indianapolis; **Office Address:** Chernoff Plastic Surgery & Laser 9002 N Meridian St, Ste 205 Indianapolis, IN 46260; **Office Phone:** (317) 573-8899; **Board Certification:** Otolaryngology 1994; **Medical School:** Canada 1986; **Residency:** Otolaryngology, Univ of Western Ontario, London, Canada 1987-1992; **Fellowship:** Head and Neck Surgery, Methodist Hosp of Indiana, Indianapolis, ID 1992-1993; **Faculty Appointment:** Asst Prof Otolaryngology, Indiana Univ

Christiansen, Thomas MD (Otolaryngology) - *Special Expertise:* Ear, Nose & Throat; **Admitting Hospital:** Fairview-University Medical Center - University Campus; **Office Address:** Ear, Nose, and Throat Specialty Care 2211 Park Ave S Minneapolis, MN 55404; **Office Phone:** (612) 871-1144; **Board Certification:** Otolaryngology 1973; **Medical School:** Univ IL Coll Med 1968; **Residency:** Otolaryngology, Univ of MN Hosp, Minneapolis, MN 1969-1974; **Faculty Appointment:** Asst Clin Prof Otolaryngology, Univ Minn

Corey, Jacquelynne P MD (Otolaryngology) - *Special Expertise:* Nasal Disorders; Allergy; **Admitting Hospital:** University of Chicago Hospitals (Page 78); **Office Address:** Univ of Chicago Hosps 5841 S Maryland St, MC-1035 Chicago, IL 60637; **Office Phone:** (773) 702-0978; **Board Certification:** Otolaryngology 1985; **Medical School:** Univ IL Coll Med 1979; **Residency:** Otolaryngology, Rush Presby Saint Lukes, Chicago, IL 1979-1984; **Faculty Appointment:** Assoc Prof Surgery, Univ Chicago-Pritzker Sch Med

Ford, Charles N MD (Otolaryngology) - *Special Expertise:* Voice Disorders; **Admitting Hospital:** University of Wisconsin Hospital & Clinics; **Office Address:** Univ of WI Hosp & Clinics 600 Highland Avenue-K4-714 Madison, WI 53792; **Office Phone:** (608) 263-0192; **Board Certification:** Otolaryngology 1971; **Medical School:** Univ Louisville Sch Med 1965; **Residency:** Otolaryngology, Henry Ford Hosp, Detroit, MI 1966-1970

Friedman, Michael MD (Otolaryngology) - *Special Expertise:* Sleep Disorders/Apnea; Snoring-Surgery; Sinus Disorders/Surgery; **Admitting Hospital:** Rush/Presbyterian - St Luke's Medical Center - Chicago (Page 74); **Office Address:** 30 N Michigan St, Ste 1107 Chicago, IL 60602; **Office Phone:** (312) 236-3642; **Board Certification:** Otolaryngology 1977; **Medical School:** Univ IL Coll Med 1972; **Residencies:** Surgery, Illinois Med Ctr, Chicago, IL 1973-1974; Otolaryngology, Univ IL Med Ctr, Chicago, IL 1974-1977; **Faculty Appointment:** Prof Otolaryngology, Rush Med Coll

Funk, Gerry Franklin MD (Otolaryngology) - *Special Expertise:* Head & Neck Trauma; **Admitting Hospital:** University of Iowa Hospitals and Clinics; **Office Address:** Univ Iowa Hosps, Dept Oto - Div Head & Neck Surg 200 Hawkins Dr Iowa City, IA 52242; **Office Phone:** (319) 356-2201; **Board Certification:** Otolaryngology 1992; **Medical School:** Univ Chicago-Pritzker Sch Med 1986; **Residency:** Otolaryngology, LAC - USC Med Ctr, Los Angeles, CA; **Fellowship:** Head and Neck Surgery, Univ Iowa Hosp, Iowa City, IA; **Faculty Appointment:** Asst Prof Otolaryngology, Univ Iowa Coll Med

Gantz, Bruce MD (Otolaryngology) - *Special Expertise:* Ear Disorders/Surgery; Neuro-Otology; **Admitting Hospital:** University of Iowa Hospitals and Clinics; **Office Address:** Univ Iowa Hosps & Clinics, Dept Oto 21200 PFP 200 Hawkins Dr Iowa City, IA 52242; **Office Phone:** (319) 356-2173; **Board Certification:** Otolaryngology 1980; **Medical School:** Univ Iowa Coll Med 1974; **Residency:** Otolaryngology, Univ Iowa Hosps, Iowa City, IA 1976-1980; **Fellowships:** Otolaryngology, Univ Iowa Hosps, Iowa City, IA 1975-1976; Neurology, Univ Zurich, Zurich, Switzerland 1981-1982

Gluckman, Jack L MD (Otolaryngology) - *Special Expertise:* Head & Neck Cancer; Head & Neck Surgery; **Admitting Hospital:** University Hospital - Cincinnati; **Office Address:** Univ Cincinnati Med Ctr Box 670528 Cincinnati, OH 45267-0528; **Office Phone:** (513) 558-4152; **Board Certification:** Otolaryngology 1990; **Medical School:** South Africa 1967; **Residencies:** Surgery, St James Hosp, Balham, England 1969-1971; Otolaryngology, Cape Town, South Africa 1971-1974; **Fellowship:** Otolaryngology, Univ Cincinnati Med Ctr, Cincinnati, OH 1977-1979; **Faculty Appointment:** Prof Otolaryngology, Univ Cincinnati

OTOLARYNGOLOGY

Midwest

Goebel, Joel Alan MD (Otolaryngology) - *Special Expertise:* Dizziness; Hearing Disorders; **Admitting Hospital:** Barnes - Jewish Hospital; **Office Address:** Barnes Jewish Hosp South 517 S Euclid, Fl 8th St. Louis, MO 63110; **Office Phone:** (314) 362-7509; **Board Certification:** Otolaryngology 1985; **Medical School:** Washington Univ, St Louis 1980; **Residency:** Otolaryngology, Barnes Hosp/Wash Univ, St Louis, MO 1981-1985; **Faculty Appointment:** Assoc Prof Otolaryngology, Washington Univ, St Louis

Hamaker, Ronald MD (Otolaryngology) - *Special Expertise:* Head & Neck Cancer; Ear, Nose & Throat; **Admitting Hospital:** Methodist Hospital - Indianapolis; **Office Address:** Head & Neck Surg Assocs 7440 N Shadeland Ave, Ste 107 Indianapolis, IN 46250; **Office Phone:** (317) 926-1056; **Board Certification:** Otolaryngology 1971; **Medical School:** Wayne State Univ 1965; **Residencies:** Surgery, Butterworth Hosp, Grand Rapids, MI 1966-1967; Otolaryngology, Wayne St Univ, Detroit, MI 1967-1970; **Fellowship:** Head and Neck Surgery, New York, NY 1972-1973; **Faculty Appointment:** Assoc Clin Prof Orthopaedic Surgery, Indiana Univ

Haughey, Bruce MD (Otolaryngology) - *Special Expertise:* Cosmetic Surgery-Face; Head & Neck Cancer; **Admitting Hospital:** Barnes - Jewish Hospital; **Office Address:** Barnes Jewish Hospital South, 8th Fl - Maternity Dept 660 S Euclid Ave, Box 8115 St Louis, MO 63110; **Office Phone:** (314) 362-7509; **Board Certification:** Otolaryngology 1984; **Medical School:** New Zealand 1976; **Residencies:** Surgery, Univ Auckland, Auckland, NZ 1977-1980; Otolaryngology, Univ Iowa, Iowa City, IA 1981-1984; **Faculty Appointment:** Assoc Prof Otolaryngology, St Louis Univ

Hilger, Peter A. MD (Otolaryngology) - *Special Expertise:* Cosmetic Surgery-Face; **Admitting Hospital:** Regions Hospital - St Paul; **Office Address:** 7373 France Ave S Ste 410 Edina, MN 55435-4538; **Office Phone:** (952) 844-0404; **Board Certification:** Otolaryngology 1979; **Medical School:** Univ Minn 1974; **Residencies:** Surgery, Univ Minnesota Hosp, Minneapolis, MN 1974-1975; Otolaryngology, Univ Minnesota Hosp, Minneapolis, MN 1975-1979; **Fellowship:** Plastic Surgery, Mass EE Infirm, Boston, MA 1979-1980; **Faculty Appointment:** Asst Prof Otolaryngology, Univ Minn

Jones, Paul John MD (Otolaryngology) - *Special Expertise:* Otolaryngology - General; **Admitting Hospital:** Rush/Presbyterian - St Luke's Medical Center - Chicago (Page 74); **Office Address:** 25 E Washington St, Fl 820 Chicago, IL 60602-1708; **Office Phone:** (312) 553-0152; **Board Certification:** Otolaryngology 1989; **Medical School:** Rush Med Coll 1983; **Residency:** Otolaryngology, Rush Presby St Lukes Med Ctr, Chicago, IL 1984-1988; **Faculty Appointment:** Asst Prof Otolaryngology, Rush Med Coll

Kartush, Jack MD (Otolaryngology) - *Special Expertise:* Ear Disorders/Surgery; **Admitting Hospital:** Providence Hospital - Southfield; **Office Address:** Mich Ear Inst 27555 Middlebelt Rd Farmington, MI 48334-5011; **Office Phone:** (248) 476-4622; **Board Certification:** Otolaryngology 1984; **Medical School:** Univ Mich Med Sch 1978; **Residency:** Otolaryngology, U Mich., Ann Arbor, MI 1980-1984; **Fellowship:** Otolaryngology, U Mich., Ann Arbor, MI 1984-1985; **Faculty Appointment:** Assoc Clin Prof Otolaryngology, Wayne State Univ

Kern, Robert MD (Otolaryngology) - *Special Expertise:* Head & Neck Cancer; Smell/Taste Disorders; **Admitting Hospital:** Northwestern Memorial Hospital; **Office Address:** 675 N St Clair, 15-200 Chicago, IL 60611; **Office Phone:** (312) 695-8182; **Board Certification:** Otolaryngology 1990; **Medical School:** Jefferson Med Coll 1985; **Residency:** Otolaryngology, Wayne St Affil Hosp, Detroit, MI 1986-1990; **Fellowship:** Research, Natl Inst of Hlth, Bethesda, MD 1990-1991; **Faculty Appointment:** Asst Prof Otolaryngology, Northwestern Univ

514

Lanza, Donald MD (Otolaryngology) - *Special Expertise: Skull Base Tumors; Sinus Disorders/Surgery; Rhinitis;* **Admitting Hospital:** Cleveland Clinic Foundation; **Office Address:** Cleveland Clinic-Dept Otolaryngology 9500 Euclid Ave, rm A71 Cleveland, OH 44195-0001; **Office Phone:** (216) 444-4939; **Board Certification:** Otolaryngology 1990; **Medical School:** SUNY Hlth Sci Ctr 1985; **Residencies:** Surgery, Albany Med Ctr 1986-1987; Otolaryngology, Albany Med Ctr 1987-1990; **Fellowships:** Johns Hopkins Univ 1990-1991; Univ Of Penn 1991

Leonetti, John MD (Otolaryngology) - *Special Expertise: Skull Base Surgery;* **Admitting Hospital:** Loyola University Health System; **Office Address:** 2160 S First Ave Maywood, IL 60153; **Office Phone:** (708) 327-1000; **Board Certification:** Otolaryngology 1987; **Medical School:** Loyola Univ-Stritch Sch Med 1982; **Residencies:** Otolaryngology, Fell-House Ear Inst, Los Angeles, CA 1987; Otolaryngology, Loyola U-Stritch Sch Med., Maywood, IL 1983-1987; **Fellowship:** Neurological Otology, Barnes Hosp, St Louis, MO 1987-1988; **Faculty Appointment:** Assoc Prof Otolaryngology, Loyola Univ-Stritch Sch Med

Mangat, Devinder Singh MD (Otolaryngology) - *Special Expertise: Cosmetic Surgery-Face;* **Admitting Hospital:** Christ Hospital, The; **Office Address:** Facial Pl Cosmetic Surg Ctr 8044 Montgomery rd, Ste 230 Cincinnati, OH 45236; **Office Phone:** (513) 984-3223; **Board Certification:** Otolaryngology 1978; **Medical School:** Univ KY Coll Med 1973; **Residency:** Otolaryngology, U Okla Hlth Scis Ctr, OKL city, OK 1975-1978; **Faculty Appointment:** Assoc Prof Otolaryngology, Univ Cincinnati

Miyamoto, Richard MD (Otolaryngology) - *Special Expertise: Neuro-Otology; Acoustic Nerve Tumors; Middle Ear Disorders;* **Admitting Hospital:** Indiana University Hospital & Medical Center - Indianapolis; **Office Address:** Ind University School Medical Riley Hospital, Ste 0860 702 Barnhill Dr. Indianapolis, IN 46202-5128; **Office Phone:** (317) 274-3556; **Board Certification:** Otolaryngology 1975; **Medical School:** Univ Mich Med Sch 1970; **Residencies:** Surgery, Butterworth Hosp, Grand Rapids, MI 1971-1972; Otolarynological Rhinoplasty, Indiana Univ Hosps, Indianapolis, IN 1972-1975; **Fellowship:** Otolaryngology, Otologic Med Grp, Los Angeles, CA 1977-1978; **Faculty Appointment:** Prof Otolaryngology, Indiana Univ

Naclerio, Robert MD (Otolaryngology) - *Special Expertise: Allergy; Otolaryngology-Pediatric;* **Admitting Hospital:** University of Chicago Hospitals (Page 78); **Office Address:** Univ Chicago Hosps 5841 S Maryland Ave , MC-1035 Chicago, IL 60637; **Office Phone:** (773) 702-0080; **Board Certification:** Otolaryngology 1983; **Medical School:** Baylor Coll Med 1976; **Residencies:** Surgery, Johns Hopkins Hosp, Baltimore, MD 1977-1978; Otolaryngology, Baylor Coll Med, Houston, TX 1978-1980; **Fellowship:** Clinical Immunology, Johns Hopkins Hosp, Baltimore, MD 1980-1982; **Faculty Appointment:** Prof Otolaryngology, Univ Chicago-Pritzker Sch Med

Paparella, Michael MD (Otolaryngology) - *Special Expertise: Ear, Neck & Throat;* **Admitting Hospital:** Fairview-University Medical Center - University Campus; **Office Address:** MN EH&N Clinic 701 25th Avenue S #200 Minneapolis, MN 55454-1443; **Office Phone:** (612) 339-2836; **Board Certification:** Otolaryngology 1963; **Medical School:** Univ Mich Med Sch 1957; **Residency:** Otolaryngology, Hnery Ford Hosp, Detroit, MI 1958-1961; **Faculty Appointment:** Clin Prof Otolaryngology, Univ Minn

Pelzer, Harold J MD/DDS (Otolaryngology) - *Special Expertise: Head & Neck Cancer; Swallowing Disorders;* **Admitting Hospital:** Northwestern Memorial Hospital; **Office Address:** Ambulatory Care Center 675 N St. Claire, Ste 15-200 Chicago, IL 60611; **Office Phone:** (312) 695-8182; **Board Certification:** Otolaryngology 1985; **Medical School:** Northwestern Univ 1979; **Residency:** Surgery, Northwestern Meml Hosp, Chicago, IL 1981-1983; **Fellowship:** Otolaryngology, Northwestern Meml Hosp, Chicago, IL 1984-1985; **Faculty Appointment:** Asst Prof Otolaryngology, Northwestern Univ

Pensak, Myles MD (Otolaryngology) - *Special Expertise:* Skull Base Tumors; Facial Paralysis; Vertigo; **Admitting Hospital:** University Hospital - Cincinnati; **Office Address:** Univ Cincinnati Dept Oto/HNS PO Box 670528 Cincinnati, OH 45267-0528; **Office Phone:** (513) 475-8427; **Board Certification:** Otolaryngology 1983; **Medical School:** NY Med Coll 1978; **Residencies:** Surgery, Upstate Med Ctr, Syracuse, NY 1978-1980; Otolaryngology, Yale Univ, New Haven, CT 1980-1983; **Fellowship:** Otolaryngology, Ear Foundation, Nashville, TN 1983-1984; **Faculty Appointment:** Prof Otolaryngology, Univ Cincinnati

Piccirillo, Jay MD (Otolaryngology) - *Special Expertise:* Sleep Disorders/Apnea; Sinus Disorders/Surgery; **Admitting Hospital:** Barnes - Jewish Hospital; **Office Address:** Wash Univ, Dept Oto 517 S Euclid, Box 8115 St Louis, MO 63110; **Office Phone:** (314) 362-7509; **Board Certification:** Otolaryngology 1990; **Medical School:** Univ VT Coll Med 1985; **Residency:** Otolaryngology, Albany Med Ctr, Albany, NY 1987-1990; **Fellowship:** Yale Univ, New Haven, CT 1990-1992; **Faculty Appointment:** Asst Prof Washington Univ, St Louis

Schuller, David MD (Otolaryngology) - *Special Expertise:* Head & Neck Cancer; Head & Neck Surgery; **Admitting Hospital:** Arthur G. James Cancer Hospital & Research Institute; **Office Address:** Univ Otolaryngologsit Inc 456 W Tenth Ave, Ste 4110 Columbus, OH 43210-1240; **Office Phone:** (614) 293-8074; **Board Certification:** Otolaryngology 1975; **Medical School:** Ohio State Univ 1970; **Residencies:** Otolaryngology, OH State Univ Affil Hosps, Columbus, OH 1971-1975; Surgery, Univ Hosps, Cleveland, OH 1972-1973; **Fellowships:** Head and Neck Surgery, Pack Med Fdn; Head and Neck Oncology, Univ Iowa, Iowa City, IA 1975-1976

Siegel, Gordon J MD (Otolaryngology) - *Special Expertise:* Head & Neck Cancer; Nasal & Sinus Disorders; **Admitting Hospital:** Northwestern Memorial Hospital; **Office Address:** Midwest Ear Nose & Throat 55 E Washington St, Ste 2600 Chicago, IL 60602-2216; **Office Phone:** (312) 332-4242; **Board Certification:** Otolaryngology 1984; **Medical School:** Univ Hlth Sci/Chicago Med Sch 1978; **Residency:** Otolaryngology, Northwestern Univ, Chicago, IL 1979-1982

Stankiewicz, James MD (Otolaryngology) - *Special Expertise:* Endoscopic Sinus Surgery; Rhinosinusitis; **Admitting Hospital:** Loyola University Health System; **Office Address:** Loyola Univ Med Ctr, Dept Oto 2160 S First Ave Maywood, IL 60153; **Office Phone:** (708) 327-1000; **Board Certification:** Otolaryngology 1978; **Medical School:** Univ Chicago-Pritzker Sch Med 1974; **Residency:** Otolaryngology, Univ Chicago Hosp, Chicago, IL 1975-1978; **Faculty Appointment:** Prof Otolaryngology, Loyola Univ-Stritch Sch Med

Strome, Marshall MD (Otolaryngology) - *Special Expertise:* Sleep Disorders/Apnea; **Admitting Hospital:** Cleveland Clinic Foundation; **Office Address:** Cleveland Clinic Fdn 9500 Euclid Ave, Ste A71 Cleveland, OH 44195; **Office Phone:** (216) 444-6686; **Board Certification:** Otolaryngology 1970; **Medical School:** Univ Mich Med Sch 1964; **Residencies:** Otolarynological Rhinoplasty, Univ Mich, Ann Arbor, MI 1966-1970; Surgery, Harper Hosp, Detroit, MI 1965-1966

Szachowicz II, Edward H MD (Otolaryngology) - *Special Expertise:* Cosmetic Surgery-Face; Rhinoplasty; **Admitting Hospital:** Abbott - Northwestern Hospital; **Office Address:** 7373 France Ave S, Ste 310 Edina, MN 55435-4538; **Office Phone:** (952) 835-5665; **Board Certification:** Otolaryngology 1984; **Medical School:** Univ IL Coll Med 1979; **Residencies:** Surgery, Univ Minn, Minneapolis, MN 1979-1980; Otolaryngology, Univ Minn, Minneapolis, MN 1980-1984; **Fellowship:** Facial Plastic Surgery, Univ Minn, Minneapolis, MN 1985-1986; **Faculty Appointment:** Asst Clin Prof Otolaryngology, Univ Minn

Telian, Steven Allen MD (Otolaryngology) - *Special Expertise:* Cochlear Implants; Ear Disorders/Surgery; **Admitting Hospital:** University of Michigan Health Center; **Office Address:** Univ Mich Med Ctr, Dept Oto-HNS 1500 E Med Ctr Dr, Taubman Hall Ann Arbor, MI 48109-0312; **Office Phone:** (734) 936-8006; **Board Certification:** Otolaryngology 1985; **Medical School:** Univ Penn 1980; **Residency:** Otolaryngology, Univ Penn, Philadelphia, PA 1982-1985; **Fellowship:** Otolaryngology, Univ Mich Med Ctr, Ann Arbor, MI 1985-1986; **Faculty Appointment:** Prof Otolaryngology, Univ Mich Med Sch

Toriumi, Dean MD (Otolaryngology) - *Special Expertise:* Rhinoplasty; Cosmetic Surgery-Face; **Admitting Hospital:** University of Illinois at Chicago Medical Center; **Office Address:** Univ Illinois at Chicago Med Ctr 1855 W Taylor St, rm 242 Chicago, IL 60612-7242; **Office Phone:** (312) 996-8897; **Board Certification:** Otolaryngology 1988; **Medical School:** Rush Med Coll 1981; **Residencies:** Surgery, Univ Illinois Med Ctr, Chicago, IL 1983-1985; Otolaryngology, Northwestern Univ Med Sch, Chicago, IL 1985-1987; **Fellowships:** Facial Plastic Surgery, Tulane Med Sch, New Orleans, LA 1988; Facial Plastic Surgery, Virginia Mason Med Ctr, Seattle, WA 1989; **Faculty Appointment:** Assoc Prof Otolaryngology, Univ IL Coll Med

Wackym, Phillip MD (Otolaryngology) - *Special Expertise:* Cochlear Implant Surgery; Acoustic Nerve Tumors; Head & Neck Surgery; **Admitting Hospital:** Children's Hospital of Wisconsin; **Office Address:** Med Coll of WI, Dept Oto 9200 W Wisconsin Ave Milwaukee, WI 53226; **Office Phone:** (414) 055-5582; **Board Certification:** Otolaryngology 1992; **Medical School:** Vanderbilt Univ 1985; **Residencies:** Neurological Surgery, UCLA Med Ctr, Los Angeles, CA 1985-1987; Head and Neck Surgery, UCLA Med Ctr, Los Angeles, CA 1987-1991; **Fellowships:** Otology & Neurotology, Univ Iowa, Iowa City, IA 1991-1992; Neurological Science, UCLA Medical Center, Los Angeles, CA 1992-1995; **Faculty Appointment:** Prof Otolaryngology, Med Coll Wisc

Wiet, Richard James MD (Otolaryngology) - *Special Expertise:* Otolaryngology - General; **Admitting Hospital:** Northwestern Memorial Hospital; **Office Address:** 1000 Central St, Ste 610 Chicago, IL 60201; **Office Phone:** (847) 570-1360; **Board Certification:** Otolaryngology 1976; **Medical School:** Loyola Univ-Stritch Sch Med 1971; **Residency:** Otolaryngology, Cincinnati Med Ctr, Cincinnati, OH 1972-1976; **Fellowship:** Otolaryngology, Univ Zurich Ed Rsch Hosp, Nashville, TN 1978-1979; **Faculty Appointment:** Clin Prof Otolaryngology, Northwestern Univ

Wolf, Gregory MD (Otolaryngology) - *Special Expertise:* Cosmetic Surgery-Face; Laryngeal Cancer; **Admitting Hospital:** University of Michigan Health Center; **Office Address:** Univ Mich, Dept Oto 1500 E Med Ctr Dr, Bldg Taubman Ctr - rm 1904 Ann Arbor, MI 48109; **Office Phone:** (734) 936-8029; **Board Certification:** Otolaryngology 1978; **Medical School:** Univ Mich Med Sch 1973; **Residencies:** Otolaryngology, SUNY Upstate, Syracuse, NY 1975-1978; Surgery, Georgetown, Washington, DC 1973-1975; **Faculty Appointment:** Prof Otolaryngology, Univ Mich Med Sch

Great Plains and Mountains

Davis, Roy Kim MD (Otolaryngology) - *Special Expertise:* Laser Surgery-Larynx; Thyroid & Parathyroid Surgery; **Admitting Hospital:** University of Utah Hospital and Clinics; **Office Address:** 50 N Medical Center Dr, rm 3C 134 Salt Lake City, UT 84132; **Office Phone:** (801) 581-7514; **Board Certification:** Otolaryngology 1979; **Medical School:** Univ Utah 1975; **Residencies:** Otolaryngology, Madigan AMC 1976-1979; Surgery, Madigan AMC 1975-1976; **Fellowship:** Medical Oncology, Boston Univ, Boston, MA 1979-1980; **Faculty Appointment:** Prof Surgery, Univ Utah

Denenberg, Steven M MD (Otolaryngology) - *Special Expertise:* *Cosmetic Surgery-Face;* *Reconstructive Surgery;* **Admitting Hospital:** Nebraska Methodist Hospital; **Office Address:** 7640 Pacific St Omaha, NE 68114-5421; **Office Phone:** (402) 391-7640; **Board Certification:** Otolaryngology 1984; **Medical School:** Univ Nebr Coll Med 1980; **Residency:** Otolaryngology, Stanford univ, Palo Alto, CA 1981-1984; **Faculty Appointment:** Asst Clin Prof Surgery, Univ Nebr Coll Med

Leopold, Donald Arthur MD (Otolaryngology) - *Special Expertise:* *Olfactory Disorders; Sinus Disorders/Surgery;* **Admitting Hospital:** University of Nebraska Medical Center; **Office Address:** Univ Nebr, Dept Oto-Head & Neck Surg 981225 Nebraska Med Ctr Omaha, NE 68198-1225; **Office Phone:** (402) 559-8007; **Board Certification:** Otolaryngology 1978; **Medical School:** Ohio State Univ 1973; **Residencies:** Surgery, St Luke's Med Ctr, New York, NY 1973-1974; Otolaryngology, Univ Iowa, Iowa City, IA 1974-1978; **Faculty Appointment:** Prof Otolaryngology, Univ Nebr Coll Med

Southwest

Alford, Bobby R MD (Otolaryngology) - *Special Expertise:* *Neurovestibular Disease; Thyroid Surgery;* **Admitting Hospital:** Methodist Hospital - Houston (Page 69); **Office Address:** Neurosensory Ctr 6501 Fannin, Ste NA-102 Houston, TX 77030; **Office Phone:** (713) 798-5906; **Board Certification:** Otolaryngology 1962; **Medical School:** Baylor Coll Med 1956; **Residency:** Otolaryngology, Baylor Univ, Houston, TX 1957-1960; **Fellowship:** Neurological Physiology, Johns Hopkins Med Sch, Baltimore, MD; **Faculty Appointment:** Prof Otolaryngology, Baylor Coll Med

Bailey, Byron J MD (Otolaryngology) - *Special Expertise:* *Head & Neck Surgery;* **Admitting Hospital:** University of Texas Medical Branch Hospitals at Galveston; **Office Address:** Univ of Tex Medical Branch, Dept Oto 301 University Blvd Galveston, TX 77555-0521; **Office Phone:** (409) 772-2704; **Board Certification:** Otolaryngology 1965; **Medical School:** Univ Okla Coll Med 1959; **Residency:** Surgery, UCLA Med Ctr, Los Angeles, CA 1960-1964

Bower, Charles MD (Otolaryngology) - *Special Expertise:* *Airway Disorders; Otolaryngology-Pediatric; Sinus Disorders/Surgery;* **Admitting Hospital:** University of Arkansas for Medical Sciences; **Office Address:** Ark Chldns Hosp, Dept Ped Oto 800 Marshall ST Little Rock, AR 72202; **Office Phone:** (501) 320-1047; **Board Certification:** Otolaryngology 1990; **Medical School:** Univ Ark 1985; **Residency:** Otolaryngology, Univ Arkansas, Little Rock, AR 1986-1991; **Fellowship:** Pediatric Otolaryngology, Chldns Hosp, Cincinnati, OH 1991-1992

Clayman, Gary Lee MD (Otolaryngology) - *Special Expertise:* *Thyroid Surgery; Salivary Gland Surgery; Head & Neck Cancer;* **Admitting Hospital:** University of Texas MD Anderson Cancer Center (Page 66); **Office Address:** Univ TX/MD Andeson Cancer Center 1515 Holcombe Blvd, Box 069 Houston, TX 77030-4009; **Office Phone:** (713) 792-8837; **Board Certification:** Otolaryngology 1992; **Medical School:** NE Ohio Univ 1986; **Residencies:** Surgery, Hennepin County Med Ctr, Minneapolis, MN 1986-1987; Otolaryngology, Univ Minn, Minneapolis, MN; **Faculty Appointment:** Prof Otolaryngology, Univ Tex, Houston

Daspit, C Phillip MD (Otolaryngology) - *Special Expertise:* *Hearing Disorders; Balance Disorders; Skull Base Surgery;* **Admitting Hospital:** St Joseph's Hospital & Medical Center - Phoenix; **Office Address:** 222 W Thomas Rd, Ste 114 Phoenix, AZ 85013; **Office Phone:** (602) 279-5444; **Board Certification:** Otolaryngology 1977; **Medical School:** Louisiana State Univ 1968; **Residencies:** Surgery, UCSF, San Francisco, CA 1972-1973; Otolaryngology, Ft Miley VA Hosp, San Francisco, CA 1974-1977; **Fellowship:** Otolaryngology, House Ear Inst/St Vincents Med Ctr, Los Angeles, CA 1977-1978; **Faculty Appointment:** Clin Prof Surgery, Univ Ariz Coll Med

Donovan, Donald Thomas MD (Otolaryngology) - *Special Expertise:* Head & Neck Cancer; Nasal Injuries; Cosmetic Surgery-Face; **Admitting Hospital:** Methodist Hospital - Houston (Page 69); **Office Address:** 6550 Fannin St, Ste 1701 Houston, TX 77030; **Office Phone:** (713) 798-3232; **Board Certification:** Otolaryngology 1981; **Medical School:** Baylor Coll Med 1976; **Residencies:** Surgery, Baylor Affil Hosps, Houston, TX 1977-1978; Otolaryngology, Baylor Affil Hosps, Houston, TX 1978-1981; **Fellowship:** Head and Neck Surgery, Colum-Presby Med Ctr, New York, NY 1981-1982; **Faculty Appointment:** Assoc Prof Otolaryngology, Baylor Coll Med

Friedman, Ellen MD (Otolaryngology) - *Special Expertise:* Ophthalmology-Pediatric; **Admitting Hospital:** Texas Children's Hospital - Houston; **Office Address:** Texas Chldns Hosp 1102 Bates, Ste 340 Houston, TX 77030; **Office Phone:** (832) 824-3250; **Board Certification:** Otolaryngology 1981; **Medical School:** Albert Einstein Coll Med 1975; **Residencies:** Surgery, Montefiore Hosp, New York, NY 1975-1976; Otolaryngology, Wash Hosp Ctr, Washington, DC 1976-1979; **Fellowship:** Pediatric Otolaryngology, Boston Chldns Hosp, Boston, MA; **Faculty Appointment:** Prof Otolaryngology, Baylor Coll Med

Gianoli, Gerard MD (Otolaryngology) - *Special Expertise:* Otolaryngology - General; **Admitting Hospital:** North Oaks Medical Center; **Office Address:** 3636 S Sherwood Forest, Ste 600 Baton Rouge, LA 70816; **Office Phone:** (225) 293-6973; **Board Certification:** Otolaryngology 1993; **Medical School:** Tulane Univ 1986; **Residencies:** Pediatrics, Tulane Univ, New Orleans, LA 1987-1988; Tulane Univ, New Orleans, LA 1988-1992; **Fellowship:** Otolaryngology, Michigan Ear Inst, Farmington Hills, MI

Goepfert, Helmuth MD (Otolaryngology) - *Special Expertise:* Head & Neck Surgery; Head & Neck Cancer; **Admitting Hospital:** University of Texas MD Anderson Cancer Center (Page 66); **Office Address:** 1515 Holcombe Blvd, Box 69 Houston, TX 77030-4009; **Office Phone:** (713) 792-6925; **Board Certification:** Otolaryngology 1974; **Medical School:** Chile 1961; **Residencies:** Otolaryngology, Baylor Coll Med, Houston, TX 1971-1974; Medical Oncology, UCLA, Los Angeles, CA 1964-1966; **Fellowship:** Surgery, Univ Tex MD Anderson, Houston, TX 1966-1968; **Faculty Appointment:** Prof Otolaryngology, Univ Tex, Houston

Hanna, Ehab MD (Otolaryngology) - *Special Expertise:* Skull Base Surgery; Head & Neck Cancer; **Admitting Hospital:** University of Arkansas for Medical Sciences; **Office Address:** Univ Arkansas for Medical Sciences 4301 W Markham St, S543 Little Rock, AR 72205-7199; **Office Phone:** (501) 686-5140; **Board Certification:** Otolaryngology 1994; **Medical School:** Egypt 1982; **Residencies:** Otolaryngology, Cleveland Clinic, Cleveland, OH 1988-1989; Otolaryngology, Cleveland Clinic, Cleveland, OH 1990-1993; **Fellowship:** Otolaryngology, Univ Pittsburgh Med Ctr, Pittsburgh, PA 1993-1994

Hansen, Lori Eldean MD (Otolaryngology) - *Special Expertise:* Cosmetic Surgery-Face; **Admitting Hospital:** Mercy Health Center - Oklahoma City; **Office Address:** 11011 Hefner Point Dr Oklahoma City, OK 73120; **Office Phone:** (405) 752-0606; **Board Certification:** Otolaryngology 1985; **Medical School:** Univ Okla Coll Med 1979; **Residencies:** Otolaryngology, Univ Ala Hosp, Birmingham, AL 1980-1981; Otolaryngology, Univ Ok Hlth Scis Ctr, Oklahoma City, OK 1981-1984; **Fellowship:** Plastic Surgery, Lasky Clinic, Beverly Hills, CA 1984-1985

Jenkins, Herman A. MD (Otolaryngology) - *Special Expertise:* Ear Disorders/Surgery; Neuro-Otology; Acoustic Nerve Tumors; **Admitting Hospital:** Methodist Hospital - Houston (Page 69); **Office Address:** Smith Tower 6550 Fannin, Ste 1701 Houston, TX 77030; **Office Phone:** (713) 798-7211; **Board Certification:** Otolaryngology 1977; **Medical School:** Vanderbilt Univ 1970; **Residencies:** Surgery, UCLA, Los Angeles, CA 1971-1972; Otolaryngology, UCLA, Los Angeles, CA 1974-1977; **Fellowship:** Neurology, U Hosp, Zurich Switzerland 1979-1980; **Faculty Appointment:** Prof Baylor Coll Med

519

OTOLARYNGOLOGY

Southwest

Johnson Jr, Calvin M MD (Otolaryngology) - *Special Expertise:* Ear & Nasal *Disorders/Surgery; Cosmetic Surgery-Face;* **Admitting Hospital:** Memorial Medical Center - Baptist Campus; **Office Address:** Hedgewood Surg Ctr 2427 St Charles Ave New Orleans, LA 70130; **Office Phone:** (504) 895-7642; **Board Certifications:** Otolaryngology 1974, Plastic Surgery 1989; **Medical School:** Tulane Univ 1967; **Residencies:** Surgery, Tulane Univ Sch Med, New Orleans, LA 1970-1971; Otolaryngology, Tulane Univ Sch Med, New Orleans, LA 1971-1974; **Fellowship:** Facial Plastic Surgery, Amer Academy Facial Plastic & Recon Surg, Los Angeles, CA 1974-1975

Medina, Jesus MD (Otolaryngology) - *Special Expertise:* Head & Neck Cancer; **Admitting Hospital:** University Hospital; **Office Address:** Univ OK Hlth Sci Ctr 920 Stanton L Young WP 1360 Oklahoma City, OK 73104-5041; **Office Phone:** (405) 271-5504; **Board Certification:** Otolaryngology 1980; **Medical School:** Peru 1973; **Residencies:** Surgery, Wayne St Univ Affil Hosp, Detroit, MI 1975-1977; Otolaryngology, Wayne St Univ Affil Hosp, Detroit, MI 1977-1980; **Fellowship:** Surgery, Univ Tex Sys Cancer Ctrs, Houston, TX 1980-1981; **Faculty Appointment:** Prof Otolaryngology, Univ Okla Coll Med

Otto, Randal A MD (Otolaryngology) - *Special Expertise:* Head & Neck Cancer; **Admitting Hospital:** University of Texas Health & Science Center; **Office Address:** 7979 Warzbach Rd San Antonio, TX 78240; **Office Phone:** (210) 567-6488; **Board Certification:** Otolaryngology 1987; **Medical School:** Univ MO-Columbia Sch Med 1981; **Residencies:** Pathology, Queens Med Ctr, Honolulu, HI 1981-1982; Otolaryngology, Univ Missouri, Colombia, MO 1982-1987; **Faculty Appointment:** Prof Otolaryngology, Univ Tex, San Antonio

Roland, Peter S MD (Otolaryngology) - *Special Expertise:* Ear Disorders/Surgery; Skull Base *Surgery; Neuro-Otolaryngology;* **Admitting Hospital:** Parkland Memorial Hospital; **Office Address:** Univ Tex Med Ctr 5323 Harry Hines Blvd Dallas, TX 75390-9035; **Office Phone:** (214) 648-3071; **Board Certification:** Otolaryngology 1981; **Medical School:** Univ Tex Med Br, Galveston 1976; **Residency:** Otolaryngology, Hershey Med Ctr, Hershey, PA 1976-1979; **Fellowship:** Skull Base Surgery, E.A.R. Institute, Nashville, TN 1984-1985; **Faculty Appointment:** Prof Otolaryngology, Univ Tex SW, Dallas

Suen, James MD (Otolaryngology) - *Special Expertise:* Head & Neck Cancer; Vascular *Lesions-Head & Neck; Laryngeal Disorders;* **Admitting Hospital:** University of Arkansas for Medical Sciences; **Office Address:** Univ Hosp Arkansas Med Scis 4301 W Markham St, Bldg 543 Little Rock, AR 72205; **Office Phone:** (501) 686-5140; **Board Certification:** Otolaryngology 1973; **Medical School:** Univ Ark 1966; **Residencies:** Surgery, Univ Arkansas Med Ctr, Little Rock, AR 1969-1970; Otolaryngology, Univ Arkansas Med Ctr, Little Rock, AR 1970-1973; **Fellowship:** Surgery, Univ Texas-M D Anderson Hosp, Houston, TX 1973-1974; **Faculty Appointment:** Prof Otolaryngology, Univ Ark

Waner, Milton MD (Otolaryngology) - *Special Expertise:* Vascular Malformations; *Hemangioma;* **Admitting Hospital:** Arkansas Children's Hospital; **Office Address:** 800 Marshall St Little Rock, AR 72202; **Office Phone:** (501) 320-7546; **Medical School:** South Africa 1977; **Residency:** Otolaryngology, Univ Witwatersrand, Johannesburg, South Africa; **Fellowship:** Otolaryngology, Univ Cincinnatti Med Ctr, Cincinnatti, OH 1984-1985; **Faculty Appointment:** Prof Otolaryngology, Univ Ark

520

West Coast and Pacific

Berke, Gerald Spencer MD (Otolaryngology) - *Special Expertise:* Head & Neck Surgery; Voice Disorders; **Admitting Hospital:** UCLA Medical Center; **Office Address:** UCLA Med Ctr 200 UCLA Medical Plaza, Ste 550 Los Angeles, CA 90095; **Office Phone:** (310) 825-5179; **Board Certification:** Otolaryngology 1984; **Medical School:** USC Sch Med 1978; **Residency:** Otolaryngology, LAC-Univ So CA Med Ctr, Los Angeles, CA 1978-1979; **Fellowship:** Head and Neck Surgery, UCLA Med Ctr, Los Angeles, CA 1980-1984

Brackmann, Derald E MD (Otolaryngology) - *Special Expertise:* Neuro-Otology; **Admitting Hospital:** St Vincent's Medical Center - Los Angeles; **Office Address:** House Ear Clin Inc 2100 W 3rd St, Fl 1st Los Angeles, CA 90057-1902; **Office Phone:** (213) 483-9930; **Board Certification:** Otolaryngology 1971; **Medical School:** Univ IL Coll Med 1962; **Residency:** Otolaryngology, Los Angeles Co USC Med Ctr, Los Angeles, CA 1966-1970; **Fellowship:** Otolaryngology, House Ear Clinic, Los Angeles, CA 1970-1971; **Faculty Appointment:** Clin Prof Otolaryngology, USC Sch Med

Calcaterra, Thomas Charles MD (Otolaryngology) - *Special Expertise:* Head & Neck Cancer; Sinus Disorders/Surgery; **Admitting Hospital:** UCLA Medical Center; **Office Address:** UCLA Med Ctr, Div HNS 10833 Le Conte Ave, rm 62-158 CHS, Box 951624 Los Angeles, CA 90095-1624; **Office Phone:** (310) 825-6740; **Board Certification:** Otolaryngology 1969; **Medical School:** Univ Mich Med Sch 1962; **Residencies:** Surgery, VA Hosp Wadsworth, Los Angeles, CA 1965-1966; Otolaryngology, Washington Univ, St Louis, MO 1966-1969; **Faculty Appointment:** Prof Otolaryngology, UCLA

Cook, Ted MD (Otolaryngology) - *Special Expertise:* Cosmetic Surgery-Face; **Admitting Hospital:** Oregon Health Science University Hospital and Clinics; **Office Address:** Oregon Hlth and Sci Univ 3181 SW Sam Jackson Park Rd Portland, OR 97201; **Office Phone:** (503) 494-5678; **Board Certification:** Otolaryngology 1973; **Medical School:** Baylor Coll Med 1964; **Residencies:** Surgery, Baylor Hosp, Houston, TX 1969-1970; Otolarynological Rhinoplasty, Baylor Hosp, Houston, TX 1970-1973; **Fellowships:** Facial Plastic Surgery, Tampa General Hosp, Tampa, FL 1973; Facial Plastic Surgery, Melrose-Wakefield Hosp, Boston, MA 1975; **Faculty Appointment:** Assoc Prof Otolaryngology, Oregon Hlth Scis Univ

De la Cruz, Antonio MD (Otolaryngology) - *Special Expertise:* Head & Neck Surgery; Acoustic Nerve Tumors; Otosclerosis/Stapedotomy; **Admitting Hospital:** St Vincent's Medical Center - Los Angeles; **Office Address:** House Ear Clinic Inc 2100 W 3rd St, Fl 1 Los Angeles, CA 90057-1922; **Office Phone:** (213) 483-9930; **Board Certification:** Otolaryngology 1973; **Medical School:** Costa Rica 1967; **Residencies:** Otolaryngology, Univ Miami Med Ctr, Miami, FL 1970-1973; Surgery, Univ Costa Rica Hosp, Costa Rica 1968; **Fellowship:** Otolaryngology, House Ear Clinic, Los Angeles, CA 1974; **Faculty Appointment:** Clin Prof Otolaryngology, USC Sch Med

Donald, Paul MD (Otolaryngology) - *Special Expertise:* Skull Base Surgery; Head & Neck Cancer; Ear, Nose & Throat; **Admitting Hospital:** University of California - Davis Medical Center; **Office Address:** 2521 Stockton Blvd, rm 7200 Sacramento, CA 95817; **Office Phone:** (916) 734-2832; **Board Certification:** Otolaryngology 1973; **Medical School:** Univ British Columbia Fac Med 1964; **Residencies:** Surgery, St Pauls Hosp, Vancouver 1968-1969; Otolaryngology, Univ Iowa Hosp, Iowa City, IA 1969-1973; **Faculty Appointment:** Prof Otolaryngology, UC Davis

Fee Jr, Willard E MD (Otolaryngology) - *Special Expertise:* Otolaryngology - General; **Admitting Hospital:** Stanford Medical Center; **Office Address:** Stanford Univ Med Ctr rm 135 Stanford, CA 94305-5328; **Office Phone:** (650) 723-5281; **Board Certification:** Otolaryngology 1974; **Medical School:** Univ Colo 1969; **Residencies:** Surgery, UCLA Med Ctr, Los Angeles, CA 1971-1974; Surgery, Wadsworth VA Hosp, Los Angeles, CA 1970-1971

521

OTOLARYNGOLOGY

West Coast and Pacific

Geller, Kenneth Allen MD (Otolaryngology) - *Special Expertise: Otolaryngology - General;* **Admitting Hospital:** Children's Hospital - Los Angeles; **Office Address:** Chldns Hosp, Dept Oto 4650 Sunset Blvd, Bldg CHLA, MC-58 Los Angeles, CA 90027; **Office Phone:** (323) 669-4145; **Board Certification:** Otolaryngology 1978; **Medical School:** USC Sch Med 1972; **Residencies:** Surgery, Wadsworth VA Hospital, Los Angeles, CA 1973-1975; Otolaryngology, UCLA Hlth Scis Ctr, Los Angeles, CA 1975-1978; **Fellowships:** Otolaryngology, UCLA Hlth Scis Ctr, Los Angeles, CA 1975-1978; Pediatric Otolaryngology, Chldns Hosp, Los Angeles, CA 1978-1979; **Faculty Appointment:** Assoc Clin Prof Otolaryngology, USC Sch Med

Jackler, Robert K MD (Otolaryngology) - *Special Expertise: Neuro-Otology; Skull Base Surgery; Ear Tumors;* **Admitting Hospital:** University of California - San Francisco Medical Center; **Office Address:** UCSF, Dept Oto-Head & Neck Surg 400 Parnassus Ave, A-717 San Francisco, CA 94143-0342; **Office Phone:** (415) 353-2757; **Board Certification:** Otolaryngology 1984; **Medical School:** Boston Univ 1979; **Residency:** Otolaryngology, UCSF, San Francisco, CA 1980-1984; **Fellowship:** Otolaryngology, Oto Med Grp, Los Angeles, CA 1985; **Faculty Appointment:** Prof Otolaryngology, UCSF

Kamer, Frank M MD (Otolaryngology) - *Special Expertise: Rhinoplasty; Cosmetic Surgery-Face;* **Admitting Hospital:** St John's Regional Medical Center; **Office Address:** 201 S Lasky Dr Beverly Hills, CA 90212-3647; **Office Phone:** (310) 556-8155; **Board Certification:** Otolaryngology 1971; **Medical School:** Albert Einstein Coll Med 1963; **Residencies:** Surgery, Long Is Jewish Hosp, Long Island, NY 1964-1965; Otolaryngology, Mt Sinai Hosp, New York, NY 1968-1970; **Faculty Appointment:** Prof Otolaryngology, UCLA

Keller, Gregory Steele MD (Otolaryngology) - *Special Expertise: Cosmetic Surgery-Face;* **Admitting Hospital:** Goleta Valley Cottage Hospital; **Office Address:** 222 W Pueblo Santa Barbara, CA 93105-3878; **Office Phone:** (805) 687-6408; **Board Certification:** Otolaryngology 1976; **Medical School:** Univ IL Coll Med 1971; **Residencies:** Otolaryngology, Univ IL, Chicago, IL 1973-1976; Surgery, Cottage Hosp, Santa Barbara, CA 1972-1973; **Faculty Appointment:** Asst Clin Prof Surgery, UCLA

Larrabee Jr., Wayne F. MD (Otolaryngology) - *Special Expertise: Cosmetic Surgery-Face; Eyelid Surgery;* **Admitting Hospital:** Swedish Medical Center; **Office Address:** Facial Plas Surg 600 Broadway Ste 280 Seattle, WA 98122; **Office Phone:** (206) 386-3550; **Board Certification:** Otolaryngology 1979; **Medical School:** Tulane Univ 1971; **Residencies:** Surgery, Charity Hosp, New Orleans, LA 1975-1976; Otolaryngology, Tulane Univ, New Orleans, LA 1976-1979; **Faculty Appointment:** Clin Prof Otolaryngology, Univ Wash

Perkins, Rodney MD (Otolaryngology) - *Special Expertise: Neuro-Otology;* **Admitting Hospital:** Stanford Medical Center; **Office Address:** Calif Ear Inst at Stanford 801 Welch Rd Palo Alto, CA 94304; **Office Phone:** (650) 494-1000; **Board Certification:** Otolaryngology; **Medical School:** Indiana Univ 1961; **Residencies:** Otolaryngology, Parkland Meml Hosp, Dallas, TX 1961-1962; Otolaryngology, Stanford Univ Hosp, Stanford, CA 1963-1967; **Fellowship:** Otolaryngology, Natl Inst Hlth, Bethesda, MD; **Faculty Appointment:** Clin Prof Surgery, Stanford Univ

Powell, Nelson Bert MD/DDS (Otolaryngology) - *Special Expertise: Sleep Disorders/Apnea; Maxillofacial Surgery;* **Admitting Hospital:** Stanford Medical Center; **Office Address:** 750 Welch Rd, Ste 317 Palo Alto, CA 94304; **Office Phone:** (650) 328-0511; **Board Certification:** Otolaryngology 1984; **Medical School:** Univ Wash 1979; **Residency:** Otolaryngology, Stanford Univ Hosp & Clinics, Stanford, CA

522

Rice, Dale MD (Otolaryngology) - *Special Expertise:* Head & Neck Cancer; Sinus Disorders/Surgery; **Admitting Hospital:** USC University Hospital - Richard K. Eamer Medical Plaza; **Office Address:** USC Keck School of Medicine 1200 N State St, Box 795 Los Angeles, CA 90033; **Office Phone:** (323) 442-5790; **Board Certification:** Otolaryngology 1976; **Medical School:** Univ Mich Med Sch 1968; **Residencies:** Otolaryngology, Univ Mich Med Ctr, Ann Arbor, MI 1972-1976; Surgery, Univ Mich Med Ctr, Ann Arbor, MI 1969-1970; **Faculty Appointment:** Prof Otolaryngology, USC Sch Med

Schindler, Robert Allen MD (Otolaryngology) - *Special Expertise:* Cochlear Implants; **Admitting Hospital:** University of California - San Francisco Medical Center; **Office Address:** 350 Parnassus Ave, Ste 210 San Francisco, CA 94117; **Office Phone:** (415) 476-0757; **Board Certification:** Otolaryngology 1972; **Medical School:** UCSF 1967; **Residency:** Otolaryngology, Univ Calif, San Francisco, CA 1968-1972; **Fellowship:** Karolinska Inst Hosp, Sweden 1973-1974; **Faculty Appointment:** Prof Otolaryngology, UCSF

Sinha, Uttam Kumar MD (Otolaryngology) - *Special Expertise:* Head & Neck Cancer; Voice Disorders; **Admitting Hospital:** USC University Hospital - Richard K. Eamer Medical Plaza; **Office Address:** USC - Keck Sch Med, Dept Oto GNH 4136 Bldg, MC-9300 Los Angeles, CA 90033; **Office Phone:** (323) 226-7315; **Board Certification:** Otolaryngology 1998; **Medical School:** India 1985; **Residency:** LAC+USC Med Ctr, Los Angeles, CA 1991-1995; **Fellowships:** Mount Sinai Med Sch, New York, NY 1986-1988; LAC+USC Med Ctr, Los Angeles, CA 1988-1990; **Faculty Appointment:** Asst Prof Otolaryngology, USC Sch Med

Weymuller, Ernest MD (Otolaryngology) - *Special Expertise:* Head & Neck Cancer; Sinus Disorders/Surgery; **Admitting Hospital:** University of Washington Medical Center; **Office Address:** Univ of Wash 1959 NE Pacific St, Box 356515 Seattle, WA 98195; **Office Phone:** (206) 543-5230; **Board Certification:** Otolaryngology 1973; **Medical School:** Harvard Med Sch 1966; **Residencies:** Otolaryngology, Mass Eye and Ear Infirm, Boston, MA 1970-1973; Surgery, Vanderbilt Univ Hosp, Nashville, TN 1967-1968; **Faculty Appointment:** Prof Otolaryngology, Univ Wash

PAIN MANAGEMENT

(Subspecialty of ANESTHESIOLOGY, NEUROLOGY, PHYSICAL MEDICINE AND REHABILITATION or PSYCHIATRY)

Some physicians who have their primary board certification in anesthesiology, neurology, physical medicine and rehabilitation, or psychiatry have completed additional training and passed an examination in the subspecialty called pain management. These doctors provide a high level of care, either as a primary physician or consultant, for patients experiencing problems with acute, chronic and/or cancer pain in both hospital and ambulatory settings.

For more information about the main specialties of these physicians, see **Anesthesiology** *(see page 873)*, **Neurology** *(see page 391)*, **Physical Medicine and Rehabilitation** *(see page 621)* or **Pyschiatry** *(see page 657)*.

Training required: Number of years required for primary specialty *plus* additional training and examination

PHYSICIAN LISTINGS

Pain Management

New England

Berde, Charles Benjamin MD (Pain Management) - *Special Expertise:* Pain Management-Pediatric; *Critical Care;* **Admitting Hospital:** Children's Hospital; **Office Address:** Chldns Hosp, Pain Treatment Srv, Dept Anes 333 Longwood Ave, Fl 5 Boston, MA 02115-5724; **Office Phone:** (617) 355-5015; **Board Certifications:** Pain Management 1993, Pediatric Critical Care Medicine 1999; **Medical School:** Stanford Univ 1980; **Residencies:** Pediatrics, Chldns Hosp, Boston, MA 1981-1983; Anesthesiology, Mass Genl Hosp, Boston, MA 1983-1985; **Fellowship:** Pediatric Anesthesiology, Chldns Hosp, Boston, MA 1985; **Faculty Appointment:** Prof Pediatrics, Harvard Med Sch

Mid Atlantic

Ferrante, F Michael MD (Pain Management) - *Special Expertise:* Pain Management - General; **Admitting Hospital:** Hospital of the University of Pennsylvania; **Office Address:** Univ Penn Hlth Sys - Pain Med Prog 39th & Market St, Med Office 140 Philadelphia, PA 19104-2699; **Office Phone:** (215) 662-8650; **Board Certifications:** Anesthesiology 1987, Pain Management 1993; **Medical School:** NY Med Coll 1980; **Residencies:** Internal Medicine, Emroy Univ Affil Hosp, Atlanta, GA 1981-1983; Anesthesiology, Emroy Univ Affil Hosp, Atlanta, GA 1984-1986; **Fellowships:** Infectious Disease, Barnes Hosp-Wash Univ, St Louis, MO 1983-1984; Pain Management, Brigham-Women's Hosp, Boston, MA 1986-1987

Foley, Kathleen M MD (Pain Management) - *Special Expertise:* Pain Management - General; **Admitting Hospital:** Memorial Sloan Kettering Cancer Center; **Office Address:** 1275 York Ave, Box 52 New York, NY 10021-6007; **Office Phone:** (212) 639-7050; **Board Certification:** Neurology 1977; **Medical School:** Cornell Univ-Weil Med Coll 1969; **Residency:** Neurology, NY Hosp-Cornell, New York, NY 1969-1970; **Fellowship:** Clinical Genetics, NY Hosp-Cornell, New York, NY 1970-1971; **Faculty Appointment:** Prof Neurology, Cornell Univ-Weil Med Coll

Jain, Subhash MD (Pain Management) - *Special Expertise:* Pain-Cancer; **Admitting Hospital:** Memorial Sloan Kettering Cancer Center; **Office Address:** Meml Sloan Kettering Hosp 1275 York Ave New York, NY 10021; **Office Phone:** (212) 639-6851; **Board Certifications:** Anesthesiology 1994, Pain Management 1998; **Medical School:** India 1968; **Residencies:** Surgery, St Vincent Med Ctr, Staten Island, NY 1976-1977; Anesthesiology, NY Hosp-Cornell Med Ctr, New York, NY 1977-1979; **Fellowship:** Pain Management, NY Hosp-Cornell Med Ctr, New York, NY 1979-1980; **Faculty Appointment:** Asst Prof Pain Management, Cornell Univ-Weil Med Coll

Kreitzer, Joel MD (Pain Management) - *Special Expertise:* Pain-Back; Pain-Cancer; **Admitting Hospital:** Mount Sinai Hospital (Page 70); **Office Address:** Pain Management Service 5 E 98th St, Fl 6, Box 1192 New York, NY 10029; **Office Phone:** (212) 241-6372; **Board Certifications:** Anesthesiology 1990, Pain Management 1993; **Medical School:** Albert Einstein Coll Med 1985; **Residency:** Anesthesiology, Mount Sinai, New York, NY 1986-1989; **Fellowship:** Pain Management, Mount Sinai, New York, NY 1988-1989; **Faculty Appointment:** Assoc Clin Prof Anesthesiology, Mount Sinai Sch Med

Lema, Mark J MD (Pain Management) - *Special Expertise:* Pain Management; **Admitting Hospital:** Roswell Park Cancer Institute; **Office Address:** Roswell Park Cancer Inst Carlton & Elm Streets Buffalo, NY 14263-0001; **Office Phone:** (716) 845-3240; **Board Certifications:** Anesthesiology 1987, Pain Management 1994; **Medical School:** SUNY Downstate 1982; **Residency:** Anesthesiology, Brigham-Womens/Harvard, Boston, MA 1983-1984; **Fellowship:** Physiology, SUNY, Buffalo, NY 1974-1978; **Faculty Appointment:** Prof Anesthesiology, SUNY Buffalo

Ngeow, Jeffrey MD (Pain Management) - *Special Expertise:* Pain-Musculoskeletal; Acupuncture; **Admitting Hospital:** Hospital for Special Surgery (Page 63); **Office Address:** 535 E 70th St New York, NY 10021; **Office Phone:** (212) 606-1059; **Board Certifications:** Anesthesiology 1980, Pain Management 1994; **Medical School:** England 1971; **Residency:** Anesthesiology, Peter Bent Brigham Hosp., Boston, MA 1975-1977; **Fellowship:** Pain Management, Tufts NE Med Ctr, Boston, MA 1977-1978; **Faculty Appointment:** Assoc Clin Prof Anesthesiology, Cornell Univ-Weil Med Coll

Payne, Richard MD (Pain Management) - *Special Expertise:* Palliative Care; **Admitting Hospital:** Memorial Sloan Kettering Cancer Center; **Office Address:** Meml Sloan Kettering Cancer Ctr, Dept Neuro 1275 York Ave, Ste C723 New York, NY 10021; **Office Phone:** (212) 639-8031; **Board Certification:** Neurology 1984; **Medical School:** Harvard Med Sch 1977; **Residency:** Neurology, NY Hosp-Cornell Med Ctr, New York, NY 1979-1982; **Fellowship:** Medical Oncology, Meml Sloan Kettering Cancer Ctr, New York, NY 1982-1984; **Faculty Appointment:** Prof Neurology, Cornell Univ-Weil Med Coll

Portenoy, Russell MD (Pain Management) - *Special Expertise:* Pain Management; Palliative Care; **Admitting Hospital:** Beth Israel Medical Center - New York; **Office Address:** Beth Israel Med Ctr, Dept Pain Med & Palliative Care First Ave at 16th St New York, NY 10003; **Office Phone:** (212) 844-1505; **Board Certification:** Neurology 1985; **Medical School:** Univ MD Sch Med 1980; **Residency:** Neurology, Albert Einstein, Bronx, NY 1981-1984; **Fellowship:** Pain Management, Meml Sloan-Kettering, New York, NY 1984-1985; **Faculty Appointment:** Prof Neurology, Albert Einstein Coll Med

Raja, Srinivasa MD (Pain Management) - *Special Expertise:* Pain-Sympathetic; **Admitting Hospital:** Johns Hopkins Hospital - Baltimore (Page 65); **Office Address:** Johns Hopkins Hosp 600 N Wolfe St, Bldg Osler - Ste 292 Baltimore, MD 21287; **Office Phone:** (410) 955-1822; **Board Certifications:** Anesthesiology 1982, Pain Management 1993; **Medical School:** India 1974; **Residency:** Anesthesiology, Univ of Washington, Seattle, WA 1977-1979; **Fellowship:** Pain Management, Univ of Virginia, Charlottesville, VA 1979-1981; **Faculty Appointment:** Prof Anesthesiology, Johns Hopkins Univ

Rosner, Howard L MD (Pain Management) - *Special Expertise:* Reflex Sympathetic Dystrophy; **Admitting Hospital:** New York Weill Cornell Medical Center - NY Presbyterian Hospital (Page 72); **Office Address:** 525 E 68th St Fl Sub Bsmnt - Ste M0026 New York, NY 10021; **Office Phone:** (212) 746-2960; **Board Certifications:** Anesthesiology 1989, Pain Management 1993; **Medical School:** Univ Miami Sch Med 1980; **Residency:** Anesthesiology, Mass General Hosp, Boston, MA 1980-1983; **Fellowship:** Pain Management, Columbia-Presbyterian Medical Center, New York, NY; **Faculty Appointment:** Assoc Prof Anesthesiology, Cornell Univ-Weil Med Coll

Staats, Peter MD (Pain Management) - *Special Expertise:* Pain-Cancer; **Admitting Hospital:** Johns Hopkins Hospital - Baltimore (Page 65); **Office Address:** Johns Hopkins Univ 550 N Broadway, Ste 301 Baltimore, MD 21205; **Office Phone:** (410) 955-1818; **Board Certifications:** Pain Management 1994, Anesthesiology 1994; **Medical School:** Univ Mich Med Sch 1989; **Residency:** Anesthesiology, Johns Hopkins Hosp, Baltimore, MD 1990-1993; **Fellowship:** Anesthesiology, Johns Hopkins Hosp, Baltimore, MD 1993-1994; **Faculty Appointment:** Asst Prof Anesthesiology, Johns Hopkins Univ

Weinberger, Michael MD (Pain Management) - *Special Expertise:* Pain-Cancer; Pain-Back; **Admitting Hospital:** St Vincents Catholic Medical Center of New York; **Office Address:** University Pain Center 95 University Pl, Ste 8 New York, NY 10003; **Office Phone:** (212) 604-1300; **Board Certifications:** Anesthesiology 1990, Pain Management 1991; **Medical School:** Columbia P&S 1983; **Residencies:** Internal Medicine, St Vincent's Hosp & Med Ctr, New York, NY 1983-1986; Anesthesiology, Columbia-Presby, New York, NY 1986-1989; **Fellowship:** Pain Management, Memorial Sloan Kettering, New York, NY 1990

Southeast

Berger, Jerry MD (Pain Management) - *Special Expertise:* Pain Management - General; **Admitting Hospital:** Shands Healthcare at University Florida (Page 77); **Office Address:** 1600 S Archer Rd Gainesville, FL 32610; **Office Phone:** (800) 749-7424; **Board Certifications:** Anesthesiology 1981, Pain Management 1993; **Medical School:** Duke Univ 1977; **Residency:** Anesthesiology, Shands-Univ Florida, Gainesville, FL 1978-1980; **Fellowship:** Pain Management, Shands-Univ Florida, Gainesville, FL 1980-1981; **Faculty Appointment:** Asst Prof Anesthesiology, Univ Fla Coll Med

Gorchesky, Mark MD (Pain Management) - *Special Expertise:* Pain Management - General; **Admitting Hospital:** Shands Jacksonville Medical Center; **Office Address:** 655 W 8th St Jacksonville, FL 32209-6511; **Office Phone:** (904) 244-7246; **Board Certifications:** Anesthesiology 1992, Pain Management 1998; **Medical School:** France 1985; **Residencies:** Anesthesiology, Western Penn Hosp, Pittsburgh, PA 1986-1989; Pain Management, Western Penn Hosp, Pittsburgh, PA 1989

Midwest

Benzon, Honorio T MD (Pain Management) - *Special Expertise:* Pain-Back; **Admitting Hospital:** Northwestern Memorial Hospital; **Office Address:** 675 N St.Clair St, Fl 20 Ste 20-100 Chicago, IL 60611-3015; **Office Phone:** (312) 695-2500; **Board Certifications:** Anesthesiology 1995, Pain Management 1993; **Medical School:** Philippines 1971; **Residencies:** Anesthesiology, Cincinnati Med Ctr, Cincinnati, OH 1973-1975; Anesthesiology, Northwestern Meml Hosp, Chicago, IL 1975-1976; **Fellowship:** Pain Management, Brigham & Womens, Boston, MA 1985-1986; **Faculty Appointment:** Prof Anesthesiology, Northwestern Univ

Green, Carmen R MD (Pain Management) - *Special Expertise:* Pain Management; **Admitting Hospital:** University of Michigan Health Center; **Office Address:** Univ Mich Med Ctr, Multidisciplinary Pain Ctr 1500 E Medical Center Dr, rm 1G323 Ann Arbor, MI 48109; **Office Phone:** (734) 763-5459; **Board Certifications:** Anesthesiology 1996, Pain Management 1998; **Medical School:** Mich State Univ 1988; **Fellowship:** Anesthesiology, U Mich Medical Ctr, Ann Haror, MI 1993; **Faculty Appointment:** Clin Inst Anesthesiology, Univ Mich Med Sch

Harden, Norman MD (Pain Management) - *Special Expertise:* Pain Management-Back & Headache; Reflex Sympathetic Dystrophy; **Admitting Hospital:** Rehabilitation Institute - Chicago; **Office Address:** 1030 North Clark Ste 320 Chicago, IL 60610; **Office Phone:** (312) 238-7800; **Medical School:** Med Coll GA 1984; **Residency:** Neurology, Univ South Carolina, Columbia, SC 1984-1985; **Fellowship:** Pain Management, Rehab Inst - Georgia, Atlanta, GA 1989; **Faculty Appointment:** Asst Prof Physical Medicine & Rehabilitation, Northwestern Univ

Mullin, Vildan MD (Pain Management) - *Special Expertise:* Pain Management; **Admitting Hospital:** University of Michigan Health Center; **Office Address:** Med Inn - Pain Center 1500 East Med Ctr Dr, Bldg C - Ste 213, Box 0824 Ann Arbor, MI 48109-0824; **Office Phone:** (734) 936-4280; **Board Certifications:** Anesthesiology 1987, Pain Management 1993; **Medical School:** Turkey 1972; **Residencies:** Anesthesiology, Univ Michigan, Ann Arbor, MI 1976-1978; Surgery, Sinai Hosp, Detroit, MI 1975-1976; **Fellowship:** Pain Management, Univ Virginia, Charlottesville, VA 1978-1979; **Faculty Appointment:** Assoc Prof Pain Management, Univ Mich Med Sch

Smith, Joanne MD (Pain Management) - *Special Expertise:* Women's Medicine; Pain-Back; Pain-Musculoskeletal; **Admitting Hospital:** Rehabilitation Institute - Chicago; **Office Address:** Rehab Inst - Chicago 345 E Superior St Chicago, IL 60611; **Office Phone:** (312) 238-0185; **Board Certification:** Physical Medicine & Rehabilitation 1993; **Medical School:** Mich State Univ 1988; **Residency:** Physical Medicine & Rehabilitation, Northwestern Univ Med Sch, Chicago, IL 1989-1992; **Faculty Appointment:** Asst Prof Physical Medicine & Rehabilitation, Northwestern Univ

Swarm, Robert A MD (Pain Management) - *Special Expertise:* Pain Management - General; **Admitting Hospital:** Barnes - Jewish Hospital; **Office Address:** Pain Mngmt Ctr - Barnes Jewish Hosp South #1 Barnes Jewish Hosp Plaza St Louis, MO 63110; **Office Phone:** (314) 362-8820; **Board Certifications:** Anesthesiology 1990, Pain Management 1993; **Medical School:** Washington Univ, St Louis 1983; **Residencies:** Surgery, Barnes Hosp-Washington Univ, St Louis, MO 1983-1986; Anesthesiology, Washington Univ, St Louis, MO 1986-1989; **Fellowship:** Pain Management, Univ Sydney, Sydney, Australia 1991; **Faculty Appointment:** Assoc Prof Anesthesiology, Washington Univ, St Louis

Weisman, Steven Jay MD (Pain Management) - *Special Expertise:* Pain Management-Pediatric Acute/Chronic; Palliative Care-Pediatric; **Admitting Hospital:** Children's Hospital of Wisconsin; **Office Address:** Children's Hosp - Wisc 9000 W Wisconsin Ave Milwaukee, WI 53226; **Office Phone:** (414) 266-2775; **Board Certifications:** Pediatric Hematology-Oncology 1984, Anesthesiology 1996; **Medical School:** Albert Einstein Coll Med 1978; **Residency:** Pediatrics, Chldns Hosp, Philadelphia, PA 1978-1981; **Fellowship:** Pediatric Hematology-Oncology, Indiana Univ Sch Med, Indianapolis, IN 1981-1984; **Faculty Appointment:** Prof Anesthesiology, Med Coll Wisc

Great Plains and Mountains

Ashburn, Michael MD (Pain Management) - *Special Expertise:* Pain Management; **Admitting Hospital:** University of Utah Hospital and Clinics; **Office Address:** U Utah Hosps & Clinics-Pain Mgmt Ctr 546 Chipeta Way , Ste G-200 Salt Lake City, UT; **Office Phone:** (801) 581-7246; **Board Certifications:** Anesthesiology 1988, Pain Management 1993; **Medical School:** Univ S Ala Coll Med 1984; **Residency:** Anesthesiology, U South Ala, Mobile, AL 1984-1987; **Fellowship:** Pain Management, U Utah, Salt Lake City, UT 1987-1988; **Faculty Appointment:** Prof Pain Management, Univ Utah

Southwest

Abram, Stephen Edward MD (Pain Management) - *Special Expertise:* Critical Care; **Admitting Hospital:** University of New Mexico Hospital; **Office Address:** Dept Anes & Critical Care Univ New Mexico Sch of Med Albuquerque, NM 87131-5216; **Office Phone:** (505) 272-2730; **Board Certifications:** Pain Management 1993, Anesthesiology 1976; **Medical School:** Jefferson Med Coll 1970; **Residency:** Anesthesiology, Mary Hitchcock Meml Hosp, Lebanon, NH 1971-1973; **Faculty Appointment:** Prof Anesthesiology, Univ New Mexico

Racz, Gabor MD (Pain Management) - *Special Expertise:* Pain Management; **Admitting Hospital:** University Medical Center; **Office Address:** 3601 4th St, rm 1C282 Lubbock, TX 79430; **Office Phone:** (806) 743-3112; **Board Certifications:** Anesthesiology 1993, Pain Management 1993; **Medical School:** England 1962; **Residency:** Anesthesiology, SUNY Upstate Med Ctr, Syracuse, NY 1966; **Faculty Appointment:** Prof Anesthesiology, Texas Tech Univ

Ramamurthy, Somayaji MD (Pain Management) - *Special Expertise:* Pain-Back; Pain-Chronic; **Admitting Hospital:** University of Texas Health & Science Center; **Office Address:** Univ TX Hlth Sci Ctr, Dept Anes 7703 Floyd Curl, MC-7838 San Antonio, TX 78229-3900; **Office Phone:** (210) 567-4543; **Board Certifications:** Pain Management 1993, Anesthesiology 1972; **Medical School:** India 1965; **Residency:** Anesthesiology, Cook Co Hosp, San Antonio, TX 1968-1970; **Faculty Appointment:** Prof Anesthesiology, Univ Tex, San Antonio

Rogers, James N MD (Pain Management) - *Special Expertise:* Pain-Chronic; Pain-Acute; **Admitting Hospital:** University of Texas Health & Science Center; **Office Address:** Dept Anes 7703 Floyd Curl Dr San Antonio, TX 78229-3900; **Office Phone:** (210) 567-4543; **Board Certifications:** Pain Management 1994, Anesthesiology 1993; **Medical School:** Univ Ariz Coll Med 1987; **Residency:** Anesthesiology, Bexar Co Hosp, San Antonio, TX 1988-1991; **Fellowship:** Pain Management, Bexar Co Hosp, San Antonio, TX 1991-1992; **Faculty Appointment:** Prof Anesthesiology, Univ Tex, San Antonio

West Coast and Pacific

Du Pen, Stuart L MD (Pain Management) - *Special Expertise:* Pain Management; **Admitting Hospital:** Swedish Medical Center; **Office Address:** Pain Consultation Service 1221 Madison St, Ste 410 Seattle, WA 98104-3537; **Office Phone:** (206) 386-2013; **Board Certifications:** Anesthesiology 1972, Pain Management 1993; **Medical School:** St Louis Univ 1967; **Residency:** VA Mason Clin, Seattle, WA 1968-1971; **Faculty Appointment:** Asst Clin Prof Anesthesiology, Univ Wash

Fitzgibbon, Dermot Richard MD (Pain Management) - *Special Expertise:* Pain Management-Pre Operative; Pain-Cancer; **Admitting Hospital:** University of Washington Medical Center; **Office Address:** Univ Wash, Dept Anes 1959 NE Pacific St, Box 356540 Seattle, WA 98195; **Office Phone:** (206) 598-4260; **Board Certifications:** Anesthesiology 1996, Pain Management 1998; **Medical School:** Ireland 1983; **Residencies:** Anesthesiology, St Vincent's Hosp, Dublin, Ireland 1985-1992; Anesthesiology, Univ Wash, Seattle, WA 1994-1995; **Fellowship:** Pain Management, Univ Wash-Pain Mngmt Clinic, Seattle, WA 1992

Prager, Joshua Philip MD (Pain Management) - *Special Expertise:* Pain Management - General; **Admitting Hospital:** UCLA Medical Center; **Office Address:** Calif Pain Med Ctrs 100 UCLA Medical Plaza, Ste 760 Los Angeles, CA 90095; **Office Phone:** (310) 264-7246; **Board Certifications:** Anesthesiology 1987, Pain Management 1993; **Medical School:** Stanford Univ 1981; **Residencies:** Internal Medicine, UCLA Med Ctr, Los Angeles, CA 1982-1984; Anesthesiology, Mass Genl Hosp, Boston, MA 1984-1986; **Faculty Appointment:** Assoc Prof Anesthesiology, UCLA

Ready, L Brian MD (Pain Management) - *Special Expertise:* Pain Management-Cancer; **Admitting Hospital:** University of Washington Medical Center; **Office Address:** UWMC, Pain Service 1959 NE Pacific St, Box 356540 Seattle, WA 98195; **Office Phone:** (206) 598-4260; **Board Certification:** Anesthesiology; **Medical School:** Canada 1967; **Residency:** Anesthesiology, Univ WA Med Ctr, Seattle, WA 1973-1975

Rowbotham, Michael Charles MD (Pain Management) - *Special Expertise:* *Reflex Sympathetic Dystrophy; Pain-Shoulder/Hand Syndrome; Herpetic Neuralgia;* **Admitting Hospital:** UCSF - Mount Zion Medical Center; **Office Address:** 2255 Post St San Francisco, CA 94115; **Office Phone:** (415) 885-7246; **Board Certification:** Neurology 1989; **Medical School:** UCSF 1979; **Residencies:** Neurology, Boston Univ, Boston, MD 1984-1986; Neurology, UCSF, San Francisco, CA 1986-1987; **Fellowships:** Neurological Pharmacology, UCSF, San Francisco, CA 1979-1980; Pain Management, UCSF, San Francisco, CA 1987-1989; **Faculty Appointment:** Assoc Prof Neurology, UCSF

PATHOLOGY

A pathologist deals with the causes and nature of disease and contributes to diagnosis, prognosis and treatment through knowledge gained by the laboratory application of the biologic, chemical and physical sciences.

A pathologist uses information gathered from the microscopic examination of tissue specimens, cells and body fluids, and from clinical laboratory tests on body fluids and secretions for the diagnosis, exclusion and monitoring of disease.

Training required: Five to seven years

Certification in the following subspecialty requires additional training and examination.

Dermatopathology: A dermatopathologist has the expertise to diagnose and monitor diseases of the skin including infectious, immunologic, degenerative and neoplastic diseases. This entails the examination and interpretation of specially prepared tissue sections, cellular scrapings and smears of skin lesions by means of routine and special (electron and flourescent) microscopes.

Physician Listings

New England

Bhan, Atul Kumar MD (Pathology) - *Special Expertise:* Immunopathology; Liver Disease; **Admitting Hospital:** Massachusetts General Hospital; **Office Address:** Mass Genl Hosp 55 Fruit St, Bldg Cox 502 Boston, MA 02114-2620; **Office Phone:** (617) 726-2588; **Board Certifications:** Anatomic Pathology 1976, Immunopathology 1985; **Medical School:** India 1965; **Residencies:** Pathology, Boston Univ Hosp, Boston, MA 1970-1971; Pathology, Chldns Univ Hosp, Boston, MA 1971-1974; **Faculty Appointment:** Assoc Prof Pathology, Harvard Med Sch

Carter, Darryl MD (Pathology) - *Special Expertise:* Breast Cancer; **Admitting Hospital:** Yale - New Haven Hospital; **Office Address:** Yale Univ Sch Med, Dept Path Box 208070 New Haven, CT 06520-8070; **Office Phone:** (203) 785-2786; **Board Certification:** Anatomic Pathology 1969; **Medical School:** Johns Hopkins Univ 1961; **Residencies:** Pathology, Johns Hopkins Hosp, Baltimore, MD 1965-1968; Surgery, Ohio State Univ, Columbus, OH 1962-1963; **Fellowship:** Pathology, Meml Hosp Cancer, New York, NY 1968-1969; **Faculty Appointment:** Prof Pathology, Yale Univ

Cole, Solon R MD (Pathology) - *Special Expertise:* Lung Disease; **Admitting Hospital:** Hartford Hospital; **Office Address:** Hartford Hosp, Dept Pathology 80 Seymour St Hartford, CT 06102; **Office Phone:** (860) 545-2866; **Board Certification:** Anatomic Pathology 1971; **Medical School:** Tulane Univ 1962; **Residency:** Anatomic Pathology, Boston City Hosp, Boston, MA 1964-1967; **Fellowships:** Pulmonary Pathology, AFIP, Washington, DC 1970-1972; Electron Microscopy, Harvard Med Sch, Boston, MA 1967-1969; **Faculty Appointment:** Assoc Prof Pathology, Univ Conn

Connolly, James Leo MD (Pathology) - *Special Expertise:* Breast Pathology; **Admitting Hospital:** Beth Israel Deaconess Medical Center - Boston (Page 57); **Office Address:** Beth Israel, Dept Pathology 330 Brookline Ave, rm ES 112 Boston, MA 02215-5400; **Office Phone:** (617) 667-4344; **Board Certification:** Anatomic Pathology 1980; **Medical School:** Vanderbilt Univ 1974; **Residency:** Anatomic Pathology, Beth Israel Hospital, Boston, MA 1974-1978; **Faculty Appointment:** Assoc Prof Pathology, Harvard Med Sch

Fletcher, Christopher MD (Pathology) - *Special Expertise:* Soft-Tissue Tumors/Sarcomas; Surgical Pathology; **Admitting Hospital:** Brigham & Women's Hospital; **Office Address:** Brigham & Womens Hosp, Dept Path 75 Francis St Boston, MA 02115; **Office Phone:** (617) 732-8558; **Board Certification:** Pathology 1988; **Medical School:** England 1981; **Residency:** Pathology, St Thomas Hosp, London, England 1982-1985; **Fellowship:** Pathology, St Thomas Hosp, London, England 1985; **Faculty Appointment:** Prof Pathology, Harvard Med Sch

Harris, Nancy L MD (Pathology) - *Special Expertise:* Lymphoma; Hematopathology; **Admitting Hospital:** Massachusetts General Hospital; **Office Address:** Mass Genl Hosp, Dept Pathology 55 Fruit St, Warren 2 Bldg Boston, MA 02114; **Office Phone:** (617) 726-5155; **Board Certifications:** Anatomic Pathology 1978, Clinical Pathology 1978; **Medical School:** Stanford Univ 1970; **Residency:** Pathology, Beth Israel Hosp, Boston, MA 1974-1978; **Fellowship:** Hematology, Mass Genl Hosp, Boston, MA 1978-1980; **Faculty Appointment:** Prof Pathology, Harvard Med Sch

Mark, Eugene J. MD (Pathology) - *Special Expertise:* Lung Disease; Cardiac Pathology; **Admitting Hospital:** Massachusetts General Hospital; **Office Address:** Mass Genl Hospital 55 Fruit St, Bldg Warren 246 Boston, MA 02114; **Office Phone:** (617) 726-8891; **Board Certifications:** Anatomic Pathology 1973, Dermatopathology 1975; **Medical School:** Harvard Med Sch 1967; **Residencies:** Pathology, Mass Genl Hosp., Boston, MA 1968-1972; Pathology, Mass Genl Hosp., Boston, MA 1974-1979; **Fellowship:** Pathology, Dantonsspital, Winterhur 1965-1966; **Faculty Appointment:** Assoc Prof Pathology, Harvard Med Sch

Schnitt, Stuart MD (Pathology) - *Special Expertise:* Breast Pathology; **Admitting Hospital:** Beth Israel Deaconess Medical Center - Boston (Page 57); **Office Address:** Beth Israel Hosp-Dept Pathology 330 Brookline Ave Boston, MA 02215-5400; **Office Phone:** (617) 667-4344; **Medical School:** Albany Med Coll 1979

Young, Robert Henry MD (Pathology) - *Special Expertise:* Breast Pathology; **Admitting Hospital:** Massachusetts General Hospital; **Office Address:** Mass Genl Hosp 55 Fruit St, Fl WRN 215 Boston, MA 02114; **Office Phone:** (617) 726-8892; **Board Certifications:** Anatomic Pathology 1980; **Medical School:** Ireland 1974; **Residencies:** Pathology, Mas Genl Hosp, Boston, MA 1977-1979; Pathology, Dublin Univ, Dublin, Ireland 1975-1977; **Faculty Appointment:** Assoc Prof Pathology, Harvard Med Sch

Mid Atlantic

Burger, Peter MD (Pathology) - *Special Expertise:* Brain Tumors; **Admitting Hospital:** Johns Hopkins Hospital - Baltimore (Page 65); **Office Address:** 600 N Wolfe St, Bldg Carnegie 484 Johns Hopkins Hosp-Dept Path Baltimore, MD 21287; **Office Phone:** (410) 955-8378; **Board Certifications:** Anatomic Pathology 1976, Neuropathology 1976; **Medical School:** Northwestern Univ 1966; **Residency:** Anatomic Pathology, Duke U Med Ctr, Durham, NC 1969-1973; **Fellowship:** Neuropathology, Duke U Med Ctr, Durham, NC 1969-1973

Dorfman, Howard MD (Pathology) - *Special Expertise:* Bone Tumor Pathology; Soft Tissue Tumors; Joint Pathology; **Admitting Hospital:** Montefiore Medical Center - Weiler/Einstein Division; **Office Address:** Montefior Med Ctr, Div Orthopaedic Path 111 E 210th St Bronx, NY 10467; **Office Phone:** (718) 920-5622; **Board Certification:** Pathology 1958; **Medical School:** SUNY Downstate 1951; **Residencies:** Pathology, Mt Sinai Hosp, New York, NY 1952-1953; Pathology, Columbia-Presby Med Ctr, New York, NY 1956-1958; **Fellowship:** Pathology, Mt Sinai Med Ctr, New York, NY 1953-1954; **Faculty Appointment:** Prof Pathology, Albert Einstein Coll Med

Epstein, Jonathan MD (Pathology) - *Special Expertise:* Urologic Pathology; **Admitting Hospital:** Johns Hopkins Hospital - Baltimore (Page 65); **Office Address:** Johns Hopkins Hosp, Dept Path 600 N Wolfe St Baltimore, MD 21287-0005; **Office Phone:** (410) 955-3580; **Board Certification:** Pathology 1986; **Medical School:** Boston Univ 1981; **Residency:** Pathology, Johns Hopkins, Baltimore, MD 1984-1985; **Fellowship:** Pathology, Meml Sloan Kettering Canc. C., New York, NY 1983-1984; **Faculty Appointment:** Prof Pathology, Johns Hopkins Univ

Frizzera, Glauco MD (Pathology) - *Special Expertise:* Hematopathology; **Admitting Hospital:** New York Weill Cornell Medical Center - NY Presbyterian Hospital (Page 72); **Office Address:** NY Weill Cornell Univ, Dept Path 525 E 70th St, Bldg Starr Pavillion - Ste 737A New York, NY 10021; **Office Phone:** (212) 746-6401; **Board Certification:** Pathology 1997; **Medical School:** Italy 1964; **Residency:** Pathology, Univ Bologna, Bologna, Italy 1965-1969; **Fellowship:** Hematology, Univ Chicago, Chicago, IL 1972-1974; **Faculty Appointment:** Prof Pathology, Cornell Univ-Weil Med Coll

Huvos, Andrew MD (Pathology) - *Special Expertise:* Bone/Bone Marrow Pathology; **Admitting Hospital:** Memorial Sloan Kettering Cancer Center; **Office Address:** Meml Sloan Kettering Cancer Ctr, Dept Path 1275 York Ave, Ste 6 New York, NY 10021; **Office Phone:** (212) 639-5905; **Board Certification:** Anatomic Pathology 1998; **Medical School:** Hungary 1963; **Residency:** Pathology, Meml Sloan Kettering Cancer Ctr, New York, NY 1967-1969; **Fellowship:** Surgical Pathology, Columbia Presby Med Ctr, New York, NY 1966-1967; **Faculty Appointment:** Prof Pathology, Cornell Univ-Weil Med Coll

Ishak, Kamal G. MD (Pathology) - *Special Expertise:* Liver Pathology; **Admitting Hospital:** Armed Forces Institute of Pathology; **Office Address:** Armed Forces Institute of Pathology 6825 16th St NW, Bldg 54 - rm 3107 Washington, DC 20306-6000; **Office Phone:** (202) 782-1707; **Board Certifications:** Anatomic Pathology 1961, Clinical Pathology 1962; **Medical School:** Egypt 1951; **Residencies:** Anatomic Pathology, Baptist Meml Hosp, San Antonio, TX 1957-1959; Clinical Pathology, Baylor Univ Med Ctr, Dallas, TX 1959-1961; **Fellowship:** Pathology, US Naval Rsch Unit, Cairo, Egypt 1955-1956

Jaffe, Elaine Sarkin MD (Pathology) - *Special Expertise:* Lymphoma; **Admitting Hospital:** National Institutes of Health - Clinical Center; **Office Address:** Natl Cancer Inst. NIH-Lab Path. Bldg 10 - rm 2N202 MSC 1500 Bethesda, MD 20892; **Office Phone:** (301) 496-0183; **Board Certification:** Anatomic Pathology 1974; **Medical School:** Univ Penn 1969; **Residency:** Pathology, Clin Ctr/NIH, Bethesda, MD 1970-1972; **Fellowships:** Hematology, Natl Cancer Inst, Bethesda, MD 1972-1974; Pathology, Natl Cancer Inst, Bethesda, MD 1972-1974; **Faculty Appointment:** Clin Prof Geo Wash Univ

Katzenstein, Anna-Luise A. MD (Pathology) - *Special Expertise:* Pulmonary Pathology; Interstitial Lung Disease; Surgical Pathology; **Admitting Hospital:** Crouse Hospital; **Office Address:** Crouse Hosp 736 Irving Ave, Fl 9 Syracuse, NY 13210; **Office Phone:** (315) 470-7396; **Board Certification:** Anatomic Pathology 1976; **Medical School:** Johns Hopkins Univ 1971; **Residency:** Pathology, Univ Hospital, San Diego, CA 1972-1975; **Fellowship:** Surgical Pathology, Barnes Hosp-Wash U, St Louis, MO 1976-1977; **Faculty Appointment:** Prof Pathology, SUNY Syracuse

Knowles, Daniel MD (Pathology) - *Special Expertise:* Lymph Node Pathology; Bone/Bone Marrow Pathology; **Admitting Hospital:** New York Weill Cornell Medical Center - NY Presbyterian Hospital (Page 72); **Office Address:** New York Presbyterian Hosp, Dept Pathology 525 E 68th St New York, NY 10021; **Office Phone:** (212) 746-6464; **Board Certifications:** Pathology 1978, Immunopathology 1984; **Medical School:** Univ Chicago-Pritzker Sch Med 1973; **Residencies:** Anatomic Pathology, Columbia-Presby Med Ctr, New York, NY 1974-1975; Anatomic Pathology, Columbia-Presby Med Ctr, New York, NY 1977-1978; **Fellowship:** Immunopathology, Rockefeller Univ, New York, NY 1975-1977; **Faculty Appointment:** Prof Pathology, Cornell Univ-Weil Med Coll

Kurman, Robert J MD (Pathology) - *Special Expertise:* Gynecologic Pathology; **Admitting Hospital:** Johns Hopkins Hospital - Baltimore (Page 65); **Office Address:** Johns Hopkins Univ Sch of Med 401 N Broadway, rm 2242 Baltimore, MD 21231-2410; **Office Phone:** (410) 955-0471; **Board Certifications:** Anatomic Pathology 1972, Obstetrics & Gynecology 1980; **Medical School:** SUNY Syracuse 1968; **Residencies:** Pathology, Peter Bent Brigham Hosp, Boston, MA 1969-1971; Pathology, Mass Genl Hosp, Boston, MA 1971-1972; **Fellowship:** Obstetrics & Gynecology, Harvard Univ Hosp, Boston, MA 1972-1973; **Faculty Appointment:** Prof Pathology, Johns Hopkins Univ

McCormick, Steven MD (Pathology) - *Special Expertise:* Ophthalmologic Pathology; **Admitting Hospital:** New York Eye & Ear Infirmary (Page 71); **Office Address:** New York Eye & Ear Infirm 310 E 14th St New York, NY 10003; **Office Phone:** (212) 979-4156; **Board Certification:** Anatomic Pathology 1988; **Medical School:** W VA Univ 1984; **Residency:** Anatomic Pathology, W VA Univ Hosp, Morgantown, WV 1984-1988; **Fellowship:** Ophthalmological Pathology, W Va Univ Hosp, Morgantown, WV 1987-1988; **Faculty Appointment:** Assoc Prof Pathology, NY Med Coll

McNutt, N Scott MD (Pathology) - *Special Expertise:* Skin Pathology; **Admitting Hospital:** New York Weill Cornell Medical Center - NY Presbyterian Hospital (Page 72); **Office Address:** NY Presbyterian Hosp 525 E 68th St, rm F309 New York, NY 10021-4873; **Office Phone:** (212) 746-6434; **Board Certifications:** Anatomic Pathology 1973, Dermatopathology 1979; **Medical School:** Harvard Med Sch 1966; **Residency:** Pathology, Mass Genl Hosp, Boston, MA 1968-1970; **Fellowship:** Pathology, Mass Genl Hosp, Boston, MA 1970-1972; **Faculty Appointment:** Prof Pathology, Cornell Univ-Weil Med Coll

Rosen, Paul Peter MD (Pathology) - *Special Expertise:* Breast Pathology; **Admitting Hospital:** New York Weill Cornell Medical Center - NY Presbyterian Hospital (Page 72); **Office Address:** New York Presbyterian, Dept Pathology 525 E 68th St, Ste C410 New York, NY 10021; **Office Phone:** (212) 746-6482; **Board Certification:** Anatomic Pathology 1998; **Medical School:** Columbia P&S 1964; **Residencies:** Pathology, Presby Hosp, New York, NY 1965-1966; Pathology, VA Hosp, New York, NY 1966-1968; **Fellowship:** Pathology, Meml Hosp Cancer, New York, NY 1968-1970; **Faculty Appointment:** Prof Pathology, Cornell Univ-Weil Med Coll

Sanchez, Miguel MD (Pathology) - *Special Expertise:* Breast Cancer; **Admitting Hospital:** Englewood Hospital & Medical Center; **Office Address:** Englewood Hosp & Med Ctr, Dept Pathology 350 Engle St Englewood, NJ 07631-1808; **Office Phone:** (201) 894-3423; **Board Certifications:** Clinical Pathology 1979, Cytopathology 1991; **Medical School:** Spain 1969; **Residencies:** Pathology, Englewood Hosp, Englewood, NJ 1971-1973; Pathology, St Vincents Hosp, New York, NY 1973-1974; **Fellowship:** Pathology, Meml Sloan Kettering Cancer Ctr, New York, NY 1974-1975; **Faculty Appointment:** Assoc Prof Pathology, Mount Sinai Sch Med

Schiller, Alan MD (Pathology) - *Special Expertise:* Bone/Bone Marrow Pathology; **Admitting Hospital:** Mount Sinai Hospital (Page 70); **Office Address:** Mount Sinai Med Ctr, Dept Pathology 1 Gustave Levy Pl, Box 1194 New York, NY 10029; **Office Phone:** (212) 241-8014; **Board Certification:** Anatomic Pathology 1973; **Medical School:** Univ Hlth Sci/Chicago Med Sch 1967; **Residency:** Pathology, Mass Genl Hosp, Boston, MA 1968-1972; **Faculty Appointment:** Prof Pathology, Mount Sinai Sch Med

Schlaepfer, William W MD (Pathology) - *Special Expertise:* Neurofilament Metabolism; Neuro-Pathology; **Admitting Hospital:** Hospital of the University of Pennsylvania; **Office Address:** 609 Stellar Chance Lab 422 Curie Blvd Philadelphia, PA 19104-6100; **Office Phone:** (215) 662-7372; **Board Certifications:** Anatomic Pathology 1964, Neuropathology 1964; **Medical School:** Yale Univ 1958; **Residency:** Pathology, Grace-New Haven Comm Hosp, New Haven, CT 1959-1961

Swerdlow, Steven Howard MD (Pathology) - *Special Expertise:* Lymphoma; **Admitting Hospital:** UPMC - Presbyterian University Hospital; **Office Address:** UPMC-Presby, Div Hematopathology 200 Lothrop St, rm C606, Box PUH Pittsburgh, PA 15213; **Office Phone:** (412) 647-5191; **Board Certification:** Anatomic Pathology 1979; **Medical School:** Harvard Med Sch 1975; **Residency:** Pathology, Beth Israel Hosp., Boston, MA 1976-1979; **Fellowships:** Pathology, Vanderbilt Univ, Nashville, TN 1979-1981; Hand Surgery, St Bartholmew's Hosp, London, UK 1981-1983; **Faculty Appointment:** Prof Pathology, Univ Pittsburgh

Woodruff, James M. MD (Pathology) - *Special Expertise:* Breast Cancer; **Admitting Hospital:** Memorial Sloan Kettering Cancer Center; **Office Address:** Memorial Sloan Kettering Cancer Ctr 1275 York Ave, Fl 6 New York, NY 10021; **Office Phone:** (212) 639-5905; **Board Certification:** Anatomic Pathology 1970; **Medical School:** Temple Univ 1963; **Residencies:** Anatomic Pathology, Cornell Med Ctr, New York, NY 1964-1966; Clinical Pathology, Colorado Med Ctr, Dencer, CO 1968-1970; **Fellowship:** Surgical Pathology, NY Meml Cancer Ctr, New York, NY 1970-1971; **Faculty Appointment:** Prof Pathology, Cornell Univ-Weil Med Coll

Yousem, Samuel A. MD (Pathology) - *Special Expertise:* Lung Disease; Inflammatory Lung Disease; **Admitting Hospital:** UPMC - Presbyterian University Hospital; **Office Address:** UPMC-Presbyterian, Dept Pathology 200 Lothrop St, rm A610 Pittsburgh, PA 15213; **Office Phone:** (412) 647-6193; **Board Certification:** Anatomic Pathology 1985; **Medical School:** Univ MD Sch Med 1981; **Residency:** Pathology, Stanford Univ Med Ctr, Palo Alto, CA 1982-1983; **Fellowship:** Pathology, Stanford Univ Med Ctr, Palo Alto, CA 1983-1984; **Faculty Appointment:** Prof Pathology, Univ Pittsburgh

Southeast

Banks, Peter MD (Pathology) - *Special Expertise:* Hematopathology; Lymphoma; **Admitting Hospital:** Carolinas Medical Center; **Office Address:** Carolinas Medical Center 1000 Blythe Blvd, Box 32861 Charlotte, NC 28203; **Office Phone:** (704) 355-3467; **Board Certification:** Anatomic Pathology 1997; **Medical School:** Harvard Med Sch 1971; **Residencies:** Pathology, Natl Cancer Inst, Bethesda, MD 1972-1974; Duke U Med Ctr, Durham, NC 1974-1975; **Fellowship:** Anatomic Pathology, U Minn Med Ctr, Minneapolis, MN 1975-1976; **Faculty Appointment:** Prof Pathology, Univ NC Sch Med

Bostwick, David MD (Pathology) - *Special Expertise:* Urologic Pathology; Gastrointestinal Pathology; **Admitting Hospital:** University of Maryland Medical System; **Office Address:** Pathology 9351 W Broad St Richmond, VA 23294; **Office Phone:** (804) 288-6564; **Board Certification:** Pathology 1985; **Medical School:** Univ MD Sch Med 1979; **Residency:** Pathology, Stanford Univ, Stanford, CA 1979-1981; **Fellowship:** Pathology, Stanford Univ, Stanford, CA 1981-1984; **Faculty Appointment:** Clin Prof Pathology, Univ VA Sch Med

Braylan, Raul MD (Pathology) - *Special Expertise:* Lymphoma; Leukemia-Pathology; **Admitting Hospital:** Shands Healthcare at University Florida (Page 77); **Office Address:** Univ of Florida, Dept of Pathology Box 100275 Gainesville, FL 32610; **Office Phone:** (352) 392-3477; **Board Certification:** Pathology 1972; **Medical School:** Argentina 1960; **Residencies:** Pathology, Meml Hosp Cancer, New York, NY 1967-1968; Pathology, Einstein Affil Hosps, New York, NY 1965-1967; **Fellowships:** Pathology, Natl Cancer Ctr, Bethesda, MD 1973-1977; Pathology, Univ Chicago, Chicago, IL 1971-1973; **Faculty Appointment:** Prof Pathology, Univ Fla Coll Med

Kao, Kuo-Jang MD/PhD (Pathology) - *Special Expertise:* Blood Disorders; Transfusion Medicine; Paternity Testing; **Admitting Hospital:** Shands Healthcare at University Florida (Page 77); **Office Address:** Dept Pathology Box 100275 Gainesville, FL 32610-0275; **Office Phone:** (352) 392-7841; **Board Certification:** Pathology 1983; **Medical School:** Taiwan 1974; **Residency:** Pathology, Duke Univ Med Ctr, Durham, NC 1981-1983; **Faculty Appointment:** Prof Pathology, Univ Fla Coll Med

Mills, Stacey E MD (Pathology) - *Special Expertise:* Breast Pathology; Otolaryngologic Pathology; **Admitting Hospital:** University of Virginia Health Systems; **Office Address:** Univ VA Health Sciences System Dept Path, Box 800214, Bldg OMS - Fl 3 - rm 3874 Charlottesville, VA 22908; **Office Phone:** (804) 982-4406; **Board Certification:** Pathology 1981; **Medical School:** Univ VA Sch Med 1977; **Residency:** Pathology, Univ VA, Charlottesville, VA 1977-1980; **Faculty Appointment:** Prof Pathology, Univ VA Sch Med

Norenberg, Michael D MD (Pathology) - *Special Expertise:* Liver Metabolic Disorders; Parkinson's Disease; **Admitting Hospital:** University of Miami - Jackson Memorial Hospital; **Office Address:** Jackson Meml Hosp, Dept Pathology 1611 Northwest 12th Ave Miami, FL 33136; **Office Phone:** (305) 585-7049; **Board Certifications:** Pathology 1972, Neuropathology 1974; **Medical School:** Univ Rochester 1965; **Residency:** Pathology, Strong Meml Hosp, Rochester, MN 1966-1970; **Fellowship:** Neuropathology, Strong Meml Hosp, Rochester, MN 1970-1972; **Faculty Appointment:** Prof Pathology, Univ Miami Sch Med

PATHOLOGY

Southeast

Page, David L MD (Pathology) - *Special Expertise:* Breast Cancer; Skin Cancer; **Admitting Hospital:** Vanderbilt University Medical Center; **Office Address:** Vanderbilt Univ Med Ctr 1161 S 21st Ave Nashville, TN 37232; **Office Phone:** (615) 322-3759; **Board Certifications:** Anatomic Pathology 1972, Dermatopathology 1974; **Medical School:** Johns Hopkins Univ 1966; **Residencies:** Pathology, Johns Hopkins Hosp, Baltimore, MD 1971-1972; Pathology, Mass Genl Hosp, Boston, MA 1967-1969; **Faculty Appointment:** Prof Pathology, Vanderbilt Univ

Petito, Carol MD (Pathology) - *Special Expertise:* Neuro-Pathology; **Admitting Hospital:** University of Miami - Jackson Memorial Hospital; **Office Address:** 1550 NW 10th Ave, rm 417, MS Locator Code R-5 Dept. Pathology-PAP Bldg Miami, FL 33136; **Office Phone:** (305) 243-3584; **Board Certifications:** Anatomic Pathology 1973, Neuropathology 1973; **Medical School:** Columbia P&S 1967; **Residencies:** Pathology, NY Hosp-Cornell Med Ctr, New York, NY 1968-1970; Neuropathology, Armed Forces Inst, Washington, DC 1971; **Faculty Appointment:** Prof Pathology, Cornell Univ-Weil Med Coll

Weiss, Sharon MD (Pathology) - *Special Expertise:* Soft Tissue Pathology; **Admitting Hospital:** Emory - Adventist Hospital; **Office Address:** Emory-Adventist Hosp, Dept Path 1364 Clifton Rd NE, Fl H180 Atlanta, GA 30322; **Office Phone:** (404) 712-0707; **Board Certification:** Anatomic Pathology 1974; **Medical School:** Johns Hopkins Univ 1971; **Residency:** Pathology, Johns Hopkins Hosp, Baltimore, MD 1972-1975; **Faculty Appointment:** Prof Pathology, Emory Univ

Midwest

Appelman, Henry MD (Pathology) - *Special Expertise:* Gastrointestinal Pathology; **Admitting Hospital:** University of Michigan Health Center; **Office Address:** U Hosp- Dept. Path 1500 E Med Ctr Dr Ann Arbor, MI 48109; **Office Phone:** (734) 936-6770; **Board Certification:** Anatomic Pathology 1966; **Medical School:** Univ Mich Med Sch 1961; **Residency:** Pathology, U Mich, Ann Arbor, MI 1962-1966; **Faculty Appointment:** Prof Pathology, Univ Mich Med Sch

Hart, William MD (Pathology) - *Special Expertise:* Gynecologic Pathology; **Admitting Hospital:** Cleveland Clinic Foundation; **Office Address:** Cleveland Clinic Foundation/ Div Path & Laboratory Med 9500 Euclid Ave, MS L21 Cleveland, OH 44195; **Office Phone:** (216) 444-2840; **Board Certification:** Anatomic Pathology 1970; **Medical School:** Univ Mich Med Sch 1965; **Residency:** Anatomic Pathology, Univ Mich Med Ctr, Ann Arbor, MI 1966-1970; **Faculty Appointment:** Prof Pathology, Ohio State Univ

Scheithauer, Bernd MD (Pathology) - *Special Expertise:* Brain Tumors; Pituitary Disorders; Neuro-Pathology; **Admitting Hospital:** Mayo Medical Center & Clinic - Rochester; **Office Address:** 200 1st St SW Rochester, MN 55905-0001; **Office Phone:** (507) 284-8350; **Board Certifications:** Anatomic Pathology 1979, Neuropathology 1979; **Medical School:** Loma Linda Univ 1973; **Residencies:** Anatomic Pathology, Stanford Med Ctr, CA 1974-1976; Neuropathology, Stanford Med Ctr, CA 1976-1978; **Faculty Appointment:** Prof Pathology, Mayo Med Sch

Unni, K Krishnan MD (Pathology) - *Special Expertise:* Bone Tumor Pathology; Surgical Pathology; **Admitting Hospital:** Mayo Medical Center & Clinic - Rochester; **Office Address:** Mayo Clinic, Dept Pathology 200 1st St SW Rochester, MN 55905; **Office Phone:** (507) 284-1193; **Board Certification:** Anatomic Pathology 1969; **Medical School:** India 1962; **Residency:** Pathology, Mayo Grad Sch, Rochester, MN 1967-1970; **Fellowship:** Pathology, Mayo Clinic, Rochester, MN 1973-1974; **Faculty Appointment:** Prof Pathology, Mayo Med Sch

540

Great Plains and Mountains

Weisenburger, Dennis (Pathology) - *Special Expertise:* Hematopathology; Lymphoma; **Admitting Hospital:** University of Nebraska Medical Center; **Office Address:** Univ Nebr Med Ctr, Dept Path 600 S 42nd St Omaha, NE 68198-3135; **Office Phone:** (402) 559-7688; **Board Certification:** Pathology 1979; **Medical School:** Univ Minn 1974; **Residency:** Anatomic Pathology, Iowa Hosp, Iowa City, IA 1975-1978; **Fellowship:** Hematology, City of Hope Natl Med Ctr, Duarte, CA 1979-1980; **Faculty Appointment:** Prof Pathology, Univ Nebr Coll Med

Southwest

Colby, Thomas V MD (Pathology) - *Special Expertise:* Pulmonary Pathology; Surgical Pathology; **Admitting Hospital:** Mayo Medical Center & Clinic - Scottsdale; **Office Address:** Mayo Med Ctr & Clinic 13400 E Shea Blvd Scottsdale, AZ 85259; **Office Phone:** (480) 301-6550; **Board Certification:** Anatomic Pathology 1978; **Medical School:** Univ Mich Med Sch 1974; **Residency:** Anatomic Pathology, Stanford Univ Hosp, Stanford, CA; **Fellowship:** Surgical Pathology, Stanford Univ Hosp, Stanford, CA; **Faculty Appointment:** Prof Pathology, Mayo Med Sch

Grogan, Thomas MD (Pathology) - *Special Expertise:* Immunopathology; Lymphoma; **Admitting Hospital:** University Medical Center; **Office Address:** Arizona Hlth Sci Ctr, Dept Pathology 1501 N Campbell Ave, rm 5212 Tucson, AZ 85724; **Office Phone:** (520) 626-2212; **Board Certification:** Anatomic Pathology 1976; **Medical School:** Geo Wash Univ 1971; **Residency:** Pathology, Letterman Army Med Ctr, San Francisco, CA 1972-1976; **Fellowship:** Immunopathology, Stanford Univ Sch Med, Stanford, CA 1990; **Faculty Appointment:** Prof Pathology, Univ Ariz Coll Med

Reed, Richard J MD (Pathology) - *Special Expertise:* Dermatopathology; **Admitting Hospital:** Touro Infirmary; **Office Address:** 234 Loyola Ave, Ste 302 New Orleans, LA 70115; **Office Phone:** (504) 897-8754; **Board Certifications:** Anatomic Pathology 1961, Dermatology 1974; **Medical School:** Tulane Univ 1952; **Residency:** Anatomic Pathology, Tulane Univ Sch Med, New Orleans, LA 1957-1960; **Fellowship:** Surgical Pathology, Barnes Hosp, St Louis, MO 1960-1961

Roberts, William MD (Pathology) - *Special Expertise:* Phen/Fen Heart Valve Pathology; Cardiac Pathology; **Admitting Hospital:** Baylor University Medical Center; **Office Address:** Cardiovascular Inst 3500 Gaston Ave Dallas, TX 75246; **Office Phone:** (214) 820-7500; **Board Certification:** Anatomic Pathology 1965; **Medical School:** Emory Univ 1958; **Residencies:** Anatomic Pathology, Natl Inst Hlth, Bethesda, MD 1959-1962; Internal Medicine, Johns Hopkins Hosp, Baltimore, MD 1962-1963; **Fellowship:** Cardiology (Cardiovascular Disease), Natl Heart Inst-NIH, Bethesda, MD 1963-1964

Walker, David H MD (Pathology) - *Special Expertise:* Infectious Disease; Tropical Diseases; Ehrlichiosis; **Admitting Hospital:** University of Texas Medical Branch Hospitals at Galveston; **Office Address:** UT Med Br Galveston, Dept Path 301 University Blvd, MC-0609 Galveston, TX 77555-0609; **Office Phone:** (409) 772-9998; **Board Certifications:** Pathology 1974, Clinical Pathology 1974; **Medical School:** Vanderbilt Univ 1969; **Residency:** Anatomic Pathology, Peter Bent Brigham Hosp, Boston, MA 1970-1973; **Fellowship:** Pathology, Harvard/Boston Hosps, Boston, MA 1971-1973; **Faculty Appointment:** Prof Pathology, Univ Tex Med Br, Galveston

Wheeler, Thomas M MD (Pathology) - *Special Expertise:* Thyroid Disorders; **Admitting Hospital:** Methodist Hospital - Houston (Page 69); **Office Address:** Methodist Hosp MS-205 6565 Fannin St, rm M227A Houston, TX 77030; **Office Phone:** (713) 394-6475; **Board Certifications:** Anatomic Pathology 1999, Cytopathology 1990; **Medical School:** Baylor Coll Med 1977; **Residency:** Anatomic Pathology, Baylor Hosps, Houston, TX 1977-1981; **Faculty Appointment:** Prof Pathology, Baylor Coll Med

West Coast and Pacific

Bollen, Andrew W MD (Pathology) - *Special Expertise:* Brain Tumors; Brain Infections; **Admitting Hospital:** University of California - San Francisco Medical Center; **Office Address:** UCSF Med Ctr, Dept Path, NeuroPath Unit 513 Parnassus Ave San Francisco, CA 94143-0506; **Office Phone:** (415) 476-5236; **Board Certifications:** Clinical Pathology 1993, Neuropathology 1992; **Medical School:** UCSD 1985; **Residency:** Anatomic Pathology, UCSF, San Francisco, CA 1985-1991; **Fellowship:** Neuropathology, UCSF, San Francisco, CA 1988-1989; **Faculty Appointment:** Assoc Prof Pathology, UCSF

Chandrasoma, Parakrama T MD (Pathology) - *Special Expertise:* Gastrointestinal Pathology; Neuro-Pathology; **Admitting Hospital:** LAC + USC Medical Center; **Office Address:** LAC-USC Med Ctr, Dept Pathology 1200 N State St, Fl 16 - rm 905 Los Angeles, CA 90033; **Office Phone:** (323) 226-4600; **Board Certification:** Anatomic Pathology 1982; **Medical School:** Sri Lanka 1971; **Residencies:** Anatomic Pathology, Univ Sri Lanka, Colombo, Sri Lanka 1973-1978; Anatomic Pathology, Los Angeles County-USC Med Ctr, Los Angeles, CA 1978-1982; **Faculty Appointment:** Prof Pathology, USC Sch Med

Cochran, Alistair J MD (Pathology) - *Special Expertise:* Melanoma-Sentinel Node; Dermatopathology; **Admitting Hospital:** UCLA Medical Center; **Office Address:** UCLA Med Ctr, Dept Path & Med 10833 Le Conte Ave, rm 13-145CHS, Box 951732 Los Angeles, CA 90095-1713; **Office Phone:** (310) 825-8182; **Board Certification:** Pathology 1968; **Medical School:** Scotland 1966; **Residencies:** Pathology, Western Infirmary, Glasgow, UK 1962-1968; Pathology, Karolinska Inst, Stockholm,Sweden 1969-1970; **Faculty Appointment:** Prof Pathology, UCLA

Cote, Richard MD (Pathology) - *Special Expertise:* Sentinel Node Pathology; Bladder Cancer; **Admitting Hospital:** USC Norris Cancer Comprehensive Center; **Office Address:** USC Kenneth Norris Cancer Hosp 1441 Eastlake Ave Los Angeles, CA 90033; **Office Phone:** (323) 865-3270; **Medical School:** Univ Chicago-Pritzker Sch Med 1980; **Residency:** Pathology, NY Hosp-Cornell Med Ctr, New York, NY 1985-1987; **Fellowship:** Pathology, Meml Sloan-Kettering Cancer Ctr, New York, NY 1987-1989; **Faculty Appointment:** Prof Pathology, USC Sch Med

Davis, Richard L MD (Pathology) - *Special Expertise:* Neuro-Pathology; Brain Tumors; **Admitting Hospital:** University of California - San Francisco Medical Center; **Office Address:** UCSF Med Ctr, Dept Neuropathology 513 Parnassus Ave, rm HSW430 San Francisco, CA 94143-0506; **Office Phone:** (415) 476-5236; **Board Certifications:** Pathology 1961, Neuropathology 1962; **Medical School:** Univ Minn 1956; **Fellowships:** Pathology, Univ Minn, Minneapolis, MN 1958-1960; Neuropathology, AFIP, Washington, DC; **Faculty Appointment:** Prof Emeritus Pathology, UCSF

Ferrell, Linda MD (Pathology) - *Special Expertise:* Pathology - General; **Admitting Hospital:** University of California - San Francisco Medical Center; **Office Address:** UCSF Med Ctr, Dept Pathology 505 Parnassus Ave, rm M590 San Francisco, CA 94143-0102; **Office Phone:** (415) 353-1090; **Board Certification:** Anatomic Pathology 1982; **Medical School:** Univ Kans 1977; **Residencies:** Anatomic Pathology, UCSF, San Francisco, CA 1980-1981; Anatomic Pathology, Univ Kansas Med Ctr, Kansas City, KS 1978-1979; **Faculty Appointment:** Prof Anatomic Pathology, UCSF

Govindarajan, Sugantha MD (Pathology) - *Special Expertise:* Liver Pathology; **Admitting Hospital:** LAC - Rancho Los Amigos Medical Center; **Office Address:** Rancho Los Amigos Med Ctr - Natl Rehab Ctr, Dept Path 7601 E Imperial Hwy, Bldg JPI - rm B170 Downey, CA 90242; **Office Phone:** (562) 401-8994; **Board Certification:** Anatomic Pathology 1976; **Medical School:** India 1969; **Residency:** Pathology, St Lukes Hosp, Cleveland, OH 1972-1976; **Fellowship:** Pathology, Cleveland Clinic, Cleveland, OH 1976-1977; **Faculty Appointment:** Prof Pathology, USC Sch Med

Hendrickson, Michael MD (Pathology) - *Special Expertise:* Gynecologic Pathology; **Admitting Hospital:** Stanford Medical Center; **Office Address:** Stanford Med Ctr, Dept Pathology 300 Pasteur Dr Stanford, CA 94305; **Office Phone:** (650) 723-4000; **Board Certification:** Anatomic Pathology 1975; **Medical School:** Stanford Univ 1971; **Residency:** Anatomic Pathology, Stanford Univ Med Sch, Stanford, CA 1972-1974; **Faculty Appointment:** Prof Pathology, Stanford Univ

Kanel, Gary Craig MD (Pathology) - *Special Expertise:* Liver Disease; **Admitting Hospital:** LAC - Rancho Los Amigos Medical Center; **Office Address:** Natl Rehab Ctr, Dept Pathology 7601 E Imperial Hwy, Bldg JPI - rm B134 Downey, CA 90242; **Office Phone:** (562) 401-8994; **Board Certification:** Pathology 1979; **Medical School:** Tufts Univ 1974; **Residencies:** Pathology, Tufts-New England Med Ctr, Boston, MA 1975-1976; Pathology, Univ Chicago Hosp, Chicago, IL 1976-1977; **Fellowship:** Pathology, Tufts-New England Med Ctr, Boston, MA 1977-1979; **Faculty Appointment:** Prof Pathology, USC Sch Med

Kempson, Richard MD (Pathology) - *Special Expertise:* Breast Pathology; Gynecologic Pathology; **Admitting Hospital:** Stanford Medical Center; **Office Address:** Stanford Univ, Dept Path 300 Pasteur Dr Stanford, CA 94305; **Office Phone:** (650) 723-7211; **Board Certification:** Anatomic Pathology 1963; **Medical School:** Tulane Univ 1955; **Residency:** Surgical Pathology, Barnes Hosp, St Louis, MO 1962-1963; **Fellowship:** Anatomic Pathology, Tulane Univ Med Ctr, New Orleans, LA 1959-1962

Lewin, Klaus J MD (Pathology) - *Special Expertise:* Liver Disease; Gastrointestinal Pathology; **Admitting Hospital:** UCLA Medical Center; **Office Address:** UCLA Hlth Scis Ctr- Dept. Path 10833 Le Conte Ave Los Angeles, CA 90095-1732; **Office Phone:** (310) 825-9377; **Board Certification:** Anatomic Pathology 1973; **Medical School:** England 1959; **Residency:** Pathology, Westminister Med Sch, London, England 1962-1968; **Faculty Appointment:** Prof Pathology, UCLA

Nathwani, Bharat N MD (Pathology) - *Special Expertise:* Lymphoma; **Admitting Hospital:** LAC + USC Medical Center; **Office Address:** Dept Pathology 1200 N State St Los Angeles, CA 90033-4526; **Office Phone:** (323) 226-7064; **Board Certification:** Pathology 1977; **Medical School:** India 1969; **Residencies:** Pathology, JJ Group-Grant Med Ctr, Columbus, OH 1969-1972; Pathology, Rush-Presbyterian-St Luke's Med Ctr, Chicago, IL 1974; **Fellowship:** Hematopathology, City Hope Natl Med Ctr, Duarte, CA 1975; **Faculty Appointment:** Prof Pathology, Univ SC Sch Med

Turner, Roderick Randolph MD (Pathology) - *Special Expertise:* Sentinel Node Pathology; *Breast Cancer;* **Admitting Hospital:** St John's Health Center; **Office Address:** St John's Health Center, Dept Pathology 1328 22nd St Santa Monica, CA 90404-2032; **Office Phone:** (310) 829-8101; **Board Certifications:** Hematology 1991, Anatomic Pathology 1985; **Medical School:** UCLA 1979; **Residencies:** Anatomic Pathology, UCLA, Los Angeles, CA 1983-1985; Anatomic Pathology, Stanford Univ, Stanford, CA 1979-1982; **Fellowship:** Pathology, Stanford Univ, Stanford, CA 1982-1983; **Faculty Appointment:** Asst Clin Prof Pathology, USC Sch Med

Warnke, Roger Allen MD (Pathology) - *Special Expertise: Lymphoma;* **Admitting Hospital:** Stanford Medical Center; **Office Address:** Stanford Univ, Dept Pathology 300 Pasteur Dr Stanford, CA 94304; **Office Phone:** (415) 723-5303; **Board Certification:** Anatomic Pathology 1975; **Medical School:** Washington Univ, St Louis 1971; **Residency:** Pathology, Stanford Med Ctr, Stanford, CA 1972-1973; **Fellowship:** Surgical Pathology, Stanford Med Ctr, Stanford, CA 1973-1975; **Faculty Appointment:** Prof Pathology, Stanford Univ

Weiss, Lawrence M MD (Pathology) - *Special Expertise: Lymphoma; Surgical Pathology;* **Admitting Hospital:** City of Hope National Medical Center; **Office Address:** City of Hope Natl Med Ctr, Div Path 1500 E Duarte Rd Duarte, CA 91010-0269; **Office Phone:** (626) 359-8111; **Board Certification:** Anatomic Pathology 1985; **Medical School:** Univ MD Sch Med 1981; **Residency:** Pathology, Brigham & Women's Hosp, Boston, MA 1981-1983; **Fellowship:** Pathology, Stanford Univ Hosp, Stanford, CA 1983-1984

PEDIATRICS

A pediatrician is concerned with the physical, emotional and social health of children from birth to young adulthood. Care encompasses a broad spectrum of health services ranging from preventive healthcare to the diagnosis and treatment of acute and chronic diseases.

A pediatrician deals with biological, social and environmental influences on the developing child, and with the impact of disease and dysfunction on development.

Training required: Three years

Pediatric Allergy and Immunology: An allergist-immunologist is trained in evaluation, physical and laboratory diagnosis and management of disorders involving the immune system. Selected examples of such conditions include asthma, anaphylaxis, rhinitis, eczema and adverse reactions to drugs, foods and insect stings as well as immune deficiency diseases (both acquired and congenital), defects in host defense and problems related to autoimmune disease, organ transplantation or malignancies of the immune system. As our understanding of the immune system develops, the scope of this specialty is widening.

Training programs are available at some medical centers to provide individuals with expertise in both allergy/immunology and pediatric pulmonology. Such individuals are candidates for dual certification.

Training required: Prior certification in pediatrics *plus* two years in allergy/immunology

Certification in one of the following subspecialties requires additional training and examination.

Pediatric Cardiology: A pediatric cardiologist provides comprehensive care to patients with cardiovascular problems. This specialist is skilled in selecting, performing and evaluating the structural and functional assessment of the heart and blood vessels and the clinical evaluation of cardiovascular disease.

Pediatric Endocrinology: A pediatrician who provides expert care to infants, children and adolescents who have diseases that result from an abnormality in the endocrine glands (glands which secrete hormones). These diseases include diabetes mellitus, growth failure, unusual size for age, early or late pubertal development, birth defects, the genital region and disorders of the thyroid, the adrenal and pituitary glands.

Pediatric Gastroenterology: A pediatrician who specializes in the diagnosis and treatment of diseases of the digestive systems of infants, children and adolescents. This specialist treats conditions such as abdominal pain, ulcers, diarrhea, cancer and jaundice and performs complex diagnostic and therapeutic procedures using lighted scopes to see internal organs.

Pediatric Hematology-Oncology: A pediatrician trained in the combination of pediatrics, hematology and oncology to recognize and manage pediatric blood disorders and cancerous diseases.

Pediatric Infectious Diseases: A pediatrician trained to care for children in the diagnosis, treatment and prevention of infectious diseases. This specialist can apply specific knowledge to affect a better outcome for pediatric infections with complicated courses, underlying diseases that predispose to unusual or severe

546

infections, unclear diagnoses, uncommon diseases and complex or investigational treatments.

Pediatric Nephrology: A pediatrician who deals with the normal and abnormal development and maturation of the kidney and urinary tract, the mechanisms by which the kidney can be damaged, the evaluation and treatment of renal diseases, fluid and electrolyte abnormalities, hypertension and renal replacement therapy.

Pediatric Otolaryngology: A pediatric otolaryngologist has special expertise in the management of infants and children with disorders that include congenital and acquired conditions involving the aerodigestive tract, nose and paranasal sinuses, the ear and other areas of the head and neck. The pediatric otolaryngologist has special skills in the diagnosis, treatment and management of childhood disorders of voice, speech, language and hearing.

Pediatric Pulmonology: A pediatrician dedicated to the prevention and treatment of all respiratory diseases affecting infants, children and young adults. This specialist is knowledgeable about the growth and development of the lung, assessment of respiratory function in infants and children and experienced in a variety of invasive and noninvasive diagnostic techniques.

Pediatric Rheumatology: A pediatrician who treats diseases of joints, muscle, bones and tendons. A pediatric rheumatologist diagnoses and treats arthritis, back pain, muscle strains, common athletic injuries and ìcollagenî diseases.

Pediatric Surgery: A surgeon with expertise in the management of surgical conditions in premature and newborn infants, children and adolescents.

CHILDREN'S HOSPITAL OF MICHIGAN

3901 Beaubien   Detroit, Michigan 48201
Tel. 1-888-DMC-2500   www.chmkids.org

We treat your children like our own.™

THE ONLY PEDIATRIC HOSPITAL IN SOUTHEAST MICHIGAN

Children's Hospital of Michigan, one of the oldest and largest pediatric facilities in the nation, is the only hospital in Michigan dedicated exclusively to caring for children, and has been since its founding in 1886. The 228-bed non-profit hospital has the most kid-friendly emergency room in the state, treating over 60,000 kids a year. Equipped with 18 exam rooms, a 10-bed observation room, and a three-bed trauma bay, the emergency department has a 24-hour advanced RN triage. In addition, Children's has the only trauma center in the state dedicated exclusively to treating children.

CHILDREN'S STAFF

This free-standing facility is staffed by more than 200 pediatricians, 600 pediatric nurses, 125 pediatric specialists and over 1,000 specially trained employees. In fact, more Michigan pediatricians are trained at Children's Hospital than at any other hospital in the state.

A LEADER IN MEDICAL RESEARCH & TREATMENT

Children's Hospital of Michigan is an international leader in pediatric neurosurgery, and a national leader in pediatric heart, kidney and bone marrow transplantation. It is the state leader in the treatment and education of children with asthma, and is home of the only burn center in Michigan dedicated exclusively to children.

CHILDREN'S RESEARCH CENTER OF MICHIGAN

The Children's Research Center of Michigan is focused on treatments and cures for devastating pediatric diseases like HIV, sickle cell anemia, cerebral palsy and cancer. Staffed by internationally recognized researchers and scientists, the center is equipped with state-of-the-art laboratories and draws upon the research-rich environment of Wayne State University School of Medicine.

THE RONALD MCDONALD HOUSE

The Ronald McDonald House of Detroit is adjacent to Children's and provides a home-away-from-home and support services to parents with hospitalized children. The House is owned and operated by a non-profit board comprised of leaders of the community and residents. Eighty-five percent of its funding depends on continued generosity of individuals and businesses.

SPECIAL PROGRAMS AND SERVICES

• The Children's Hospital of Michigan Neonatal Intensive Care Transport Team, comprised of nurses and respiratory therapists, operates as a mobile intensive care unit, transferring infants and pediatric patients from community hospitals for specialized pediatric care.

• Children's provides PPAL, the Pediatric Physician Access Line, 877-CHM-PEDS, which connects physicians from around the country with pediatric specialists and gives them an instant resource for a second opinion.

• Children's Regional Poison Control Center is one of two centers in the state focused on poison prevention, education, triage and treatment.

• Children's Hospital is the lead agency for the Metro Detroit Safe Kids Coalition, a grassroots organization dedicated to eliminating preventable injuries.

• Child life specialists at Children's offer developmental play as a way for children to express fears or concerns and understand the hospital environment.

CHILDREN'S HOSPITAL OF NEW YORK
NEWYORK-PRESBYTERIAN

Morgan Stanley Dean Witter
Children's Hospital of New York
3959 Broadway
New York, NY 10032

NewYork Weill Cornell
Children's Hospital of New York
525 East 68th Street
New York, NY 10021

OVERVIEW:

The Children's Hospital of New York brings together the outstanding pediatric services and resources of Columbia Presbyterian and NewYork Weill Cornell to create one of the largest, most comprehensive children's hospitals in the world. This major academic center is supported by affiliations with two of the most prestigious medical schools in the nation: Columbia University College of Physicians & Surgeons and the Joan and Sanford I. Weill Medical College of Cornell University.

With more than 1,000 pediatricians, medical and surgical subspecialists on staff, and teams of specially trained pediatric health professionals, the Children's Hospital of New York provides the highest level of care from infancy to adolescence. The Hospital's expertise in addressing simple and complex medical conditions and the psychological and emotional issues that accompany them is unparalleled, with particular focus on:

allergy, burn treatment, cardiology, critical care medicine, endocrinology and diabetes, gastroenterology and nutrition, hematology, human genetics, immunology, nephrology, neurology, oncology, ophthalmology, otolaryngology, psychiatry, pulmonary, rheumatology, surgery , transplant, trauma

The Hospital's facilities are designed to deliver state-of-the-art care while providing comfort to children and parents alike. Its Child Life Program helps with adjustment to hospital life through play and support groups.

Physician Referral: For a physician referral or to learn more about the Children's Hospital of New York, call 1-800-245-KIDS (1-800-245-5437) or visit our Web site at www.chony.org.

THE COMPREHENSIVE SERVICES INCLUDE:

The Hospital has:

- the largest pediatric cardiology and cardiac surgery programs in the country, including corrective open-heart surgery in the first days of life.

- the nation's only pediatric pulmonary hypertension center.

- the only provider in the region to offer four major transplant surgeries — heart, liver, kidney and lung.

- one of only three Level 1-designated Pediatric Trauma Centers in New York State.

- recognition for highly specialized treatment in pediatric oncology, such as bone marrow transplantation or stereotactic gamma radiation for brain tumors.

- a sophisticated neonatal intensive care, with units for very sick newborns that set standards nationwide.

- critical care teams which transport critically ill and injured children to the Hospital's state-of-the-art neonatal intensive care units or pediatric intensive care units.

- one of the largest Sickle Cell Centers in the country.

INFANTS AND CHILDREN'S HOSPITAL
MAIMONIDES MEDICAL CENTER

4802 Tenth Avenue   Brooklyn, NY 11219
Tel. 718.283.7500   Fax. 718.283.7005   www.maimonidesmed.org

Led by Steven Shelov MD—author of several best-selling books on child-rearing—Maimonides Medical Center's Infants and Children's Hospital provides the best care a child could ever need. Serving one of the largest pediatric populations in New York City, Maimonides has made a major commitment to caring for babies, children, adolescents and their families. It is a commitment that often begins before a baby is born and continues well into the teenage years.

For many young patients, this commitment is simply a matter of preventing illness, facilitating healthy growth or addressing common childhood diseases. For others, however, the problems are more complicated. It is for the benefit of these children that Maimonides now provides a full complement of specialists specifically trained to deal with nearly every manner of childhood affliction, no matter how rare or how complex.

Dr. Shelov has helped recruit well-respected physicians in the following pediatric specialties:

- Adolescent Medicine
- Allergy/Pulmonology
- Anesthesiology
- Behavioral and Developmental Pediatrics
- Cardiology
- Critical Care Medicine
- Dental Surgery
- Emergency Medicine
- Endocrinology
- Gastroenterology
- Genetics
- Hematology/Oncology
- Infectious Diseases
- Neonatology
- Nephrology
- Neurology
- Ophthalmology
- Orthopaedic Surgery
- Otolaryngology
- Primary Care
- Psychiatry/Psychology
- Radiology
- Surgery
- Urology

INFANTS AND CHILDREN'S HOSPITAL

The physicians at Infants and Children's Hospital work in some of the most advanced medical environments in the New York region. In recent years, Maimonides Medical Center has renovated and expanded its pediatric emergency room, opened the Norma Sutton Center for Neonatology, and dedicated a new pediatric critical care unit. Pediatric services also are available at 12 primary care sites throughout Brooklyn.

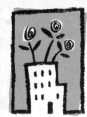

PHYSICIAN LISTINGS

PHYSICIAN LISTINGS

Mid Atlantic

Eggleston, Peyton Archer MD (Pediatric Allergy & Immunology) - *Special Expertise:* *Allergy;* **Admitting Hospital:** Johns Hopkins Hospital - Baltimore (Page 65); **Office Address:** Johns Hopkins Hosp, Div Immun-Ped 600 N Wolfe St, Ste CMSC Baltimore, MD 21287; **Office Phone:** (410) 955-5883; **Board Certifications:** Allergy & Immunology 1974, Pediatrics 1992; **Medical School:** Univ VA Sch Med 1965; **Residency:** Pediatrics, Univ Wash, Seattle, WA 1968-1970; **Fellowship:** Allergy & Immunology, Univ Wash, Seattle, WA 1970-1972; **Faculty Appointment:** Prof Pediatrics, Johns Hopkins Univ

Sampson, Hugh MD (Pediatric Allergy & Immunology) - *Special Expertise:* *Pediatric* *Allergy & Immunology - General;* **Admitting Hospital:** Mount Sinai Hospital (Page 70); **Office Address:** Mt Sinai Sch Med, Dept Peds 1 Gustave Levy Pl, Box 1198 New York, NY 10029; **Office Phone:** (212) 241-5548; **Board Certifications:** Pediatrics 1980, Allergy & Immunology 1981; **Medical School:** SUNY Buffalo 1975; **Residency:** Pediatrics, Childns Meml Hosp-NW Univ, Chicago, IL 1976-1979; **Fellowship:** Allergy & Immunology, Duke Univ Med Ctr, Durham, NC 1978-1980; **Faculty Appointment:** Prof Pediatrics, Mount Sinai Sch Med

Schuberth, Kenneth Charles MD (Pediatric Allergy & Immunology) - *Special Expertise:* *Allergy;* **Admitting Hospital:** Johns Hopkins Hospital - Baltimore (Page 65); **Office Address:** 10807 Falls Rd Lutherville, MD 21093-4502; **Office Phone:** (410) 427-1604; **Board Certifications:** Allergy & Immunology 1983, Pediatrics 1979; **Medical School:** Johns Hopkins Univ 1973; **Residency:** Pediatrics, Johns Hopkins, Baltimore, MD 1974-1978; **Fellowship:** Allergy & Immunology, Johns Hopkins, Baltimore, MD 1978-1980; **Faculty Appointment:** Assoc Prof Pediatrics, Johns Hopkins Univ

Skoner, David Peter MD (Pediatric Allergy & Immunology) - *Special Expertise:* *Rhinitis;* *Asthma; Allergy;* **Admitting Hospital:** Children's Hospital of Pittsburgh; **Office Address:** Children's Hospital, Allergy and Immunology 3705 5th Ave, MC-4B 320 Pittsburgh, PA 15213; **Office Phone:** (412) 692-6850; **Board Certifications:** Pediatrics 1985, Allergy & Immunology 1985; **Medical School:** Temple Univ 1980; **Residency:** Pediatrics, Chldns Hosp, Cincinnati, OH 1981-1983; **Fellowship:** Allergy & Immunology, Chldns Hosp, Pittsburgh, PA 1983-1985

Sly, Ridge Michael MD (Pediatric Allergy & Immunology) - *Special Expertise:* *Asthma;* *Allergy;* **Admitting Hospital:** Children's National Medical Center - DC; **Office Address:** Children's Natl Med Ctr 111 Michigan Ave NW Washington, DC 20010-2970; **Office Phone:** (202) 884-2033; **Board Certifications:** Pediatroics 1980; Allergy & Immunology 1987; **Medical School:** Washington Univ, St Louis 1960; **Residencies:** Pediatrics, St Louis Chldns Hosp, St Louis, MI 1960-1962; Pediatrics, Univ KY Med Ctr, Lexington, KY 1962-1963; **Fellowship:** Pediatric Allergy & Immunology, UCLA, Los Angeles, CA 1965-1967; **Faculty Appointment:** Prof Medicine, Washington Univ, St Louis

Winkelstein, Jerry Allen MD (Pediatric Allergy & Immunology) - *Special Expertise:* *Immune Deficiency;* **Admitting Hospital:** Johns Hopkins Hospital - Baltimore (Page 65); **Office Address:** Johns Hopkins Hosp, Dept Ped 600 N Wolfe St Baltimore, MD 21287-0001; **Office Phone:** (410) 955-5883; **Board Certification:** Pediatrics 1972; **Medical School:** Albert Einstein Coll Med 1965; **Residencies:** Pediatrics, Johns Hopkins Hosp, Baltimore, MD 1966-1968; Pediatrics, Johns Hopkins Hosp, Baltimore, MD 1971-1972; **Fellowship:** Immunology, Johns Hopkins Hosp, Baltimore, MD 1970-1973; **Faculty Appointment:** Prof Pediatrics, Johns Hopkins Univ

Wood, Robert Alan MD (Pediatric Allergy & Immunology) - *Special Expertise:* Food Allergy; Asthma; **Admitting Hospital:** Johns Hopkins Hospital - Baltimore (Page 65); **Office Address:** Johns Hopkins Univ 10807 Falls Rd Baltimore, MD 21287; **Office Phone:** (410) 955-5883; **Board Certifications:** Pediatrics 1987, Allergy & Immunology 1997; **Medical School:** Univ Rochester 1982; **Residency:** Pediatrics, Johns Hopkins Hosp, Baltimore, MD 1983-1985; **Fellowship:** Allergy & Immunology, Johns Hopkins Hosp, Baltimore, MD 1986-1988; **Faculty Appointment:** Assoc Prof Pediatrics, Johns Hopkins Univ

Southeast

Bahna, Sami Labib MD (Pediatric Allergy & Immunology) - *Special Expertise:* Food Allergy; Asthma; **Admitting Hospital:** All Children's Hospital; **Office Address:** 801 6th St S, Box 6990 St Petersburg, FL 33701-4816; **Office Phone:** (727) 892-8688; **Board Certifications:** Pediatrics 1980, Allergy & Immunology 1981; **Medical School:** Egypt 1964; **Residency:** Pediatrics, Univ Maryland, Baltimore, MD 1974-1975; **Fellowship:** Allergy & Immunology, Harbor-UCLA Med Ctr, Torrance, CA 1976-1978; **Faculty Appointment:** Prof Pediatrics, Univ S Fla Coll Med

Barrett, Douglas John MD (Pediatric Allergy & Immunology) - *Special Expertise:* IVIG Infusion; Immune Deficiency; **Admitting Hospital:** Shands Healthcare at University Florida (Page 77); **Office Address:** 1600 SW Archer Rd, Fl 4 Gainesville, FL 32610; **Office Phone:** (352) 265-8250; **Board Certifications:** Pediatrics 1979, Allergy & Immunology 1981; **Medical School:** Univ S Fla Coll Med 1974; **Residency:** Pediatrics, SUNY, Syracuse, NY 1975-1977; **Faculty Appointment:** Prof Pediatric Allergy & Immunology, Univ Fla Coll Med

Buckley, Rebecca Hatcher MD (Pediatric Allergy & Immunology) - *Special Expertise:* Immune Deficiency; Allergy; **Admitting Hospital:** Duke University Medical Center (Page 60); **Office Address:** Duke Univ Sch of Med Box 2898 Durham, NC 27710-2898; **Office Phone:** (919) 684-2922; **Board Certification:** Allergy & Immunology 1977; **Medical School:** Univ NC Sch Med 1958; **Residency:** Pediatrics, Duke Univ Med Ctr, Durham, NC 1959-1961; **Fellowship:** Pediatric Allergy & Immunology, Duke Univ Med Ctr, Durham, NC 1961-1963; **Faculty Appointment:** Prof Pediatric Allergy & Immunology, Duke Univ

Midwest

Berger, Melvin MD/PhD (Pediatric Allergy & Immunology) - *Special Expertise:* Immune Deficiency; Asthma & Allergy; **Admitting Hospital:** Rainbow Babies & Children's Hospital; **Office Address:** Pediatrics 11100 Euclid Ave, Bldg RB&C - rm 586 Cleveland, OH 44106; **Office Phone:** (216) 844-3237; **Board Certifications:** Pediatrics 1981, Allergy & Immunology 1981; **Medical School:** Case West Res Univ 1976; **Residency:** Pediatrics, Children's Hosp Med Ctr, Boston, MA 1976-1978; **Fellowship:** Allergy & Immunology, Natl Inst Allergy & Infect Dis (NIH), Bethesda, MD 1978-1981; **Faculty Appointment:** Prof Pediatrics, Case West Res Univ

Blum, Paul MD (Pediatric Allergy & Immunology) - *Special Expertise:* Asthma; **Admitting Hospital:** Fairview-University Medical Center - University Campus; **Office Address:** Southdale Pediatric-Edina 3955 Park Lawn Ave, Ste 120 Edina, MN 55435; **Office Phone:** (612) 831-4454; **Board Certifications:** Pediatrics 1973, Allergy & Immunology 1981; **Medical School:** Univ Minn 1968; **Residency:** Pediatrics, Univ Minn Hosp, Minneapolis, MN 1969-1971; **Fellowship:** Allergy & Immunology, UCLA, Los Angeles, CA 1978-1980; **Faculty Appointment:** Assoc Prof Pediatrics, Univ Minn

Evans III, Richard MD (Pediatric Allergy & Immunology) - *Special Expertise:* Asthma; Allergy; **Admitting Hospital:** Children's Memorial Hospital; **Office Address:** Children's Memorial Medical Ctr 2300 N Childrens Plaza, Box 60 Chicago, IL 60614-3318; **Office Phone:** (773) 880-3562; **Board Certifications:** Allergy & Immunology 1972, Pediatrics 1967; **Medical School:** Univ Minn 1958; **Residencies:** Allergy & Immunology, Walter Reed Med Ctr, Washington, DC 1969-1970; Buffalo Children's Hosp, Buffalo, NY 1970-1971; **Faculty Appointment:** Prof Pediatric Allergy & Immunology, Northwestern Univ

Gewurz, Anita MD (Pediatric Allergy & Immunology) - *Special Expertise:* Pediatric Allergy & Immunology - General; **Admitting Hospital:** Rush/Presbyterian - St Luke's Medical Center - Chicago (Page 74); **Office Address:** Univ Consultants in A&I 1725 W Harrison St, Ste 207 Chicago, IL 60612; **Office Phone:** (312) 942-6296; **Board Certifications:** Pediatrics 1976, Allergy & Immunology 1977; **Medical School:** Albany Med Coll 1970; **Residency:** Pediatrics, Univ III, Chicago, IL 1972-1973; **Fellowships:** Allergy & Immunology, Grant Hosp, Chicago, IL 1974-1977; Allergy & Immunology, Northwestern Univ Med Sch, Chicago, IL 1983-1985; **Faculty Appointment:** Assoc Prof Allergy & Immunology, Rush Med Coll

Lemanske Jr, Robert F MD (Pediatric Allergy & Immunology) - *Special Expertise:* Asthma; **Admitting Hospital:** University of Wisconsin Hospital & Clinics; **Office Address:** 600 Highland Ave, rm TA4916/916-998 Madison, WI 53792; **Office Phone:** (608) 263-6180; **Board Certifications:** Allergy & Immunology 1981, Pediatrics 1980; **Medical School:** Univ Wisc 1975; **Residency:** Pediatrics, Univ Wisc Hosp, Madison, WI 1976-1978; **Faculty Appointment:** Prof Medicine, Univ Wisc

Pongracic, Jacqueline MD (Pediatric Allergy & Immunology) - *Special Expertise:* Latex Allergy; Asthma; **Admitting Hospital:** Children's Memorial Hospital; **Office Address:** Children's Memorial Hosp 2300 Children's Plaza Chicago, IL 60614; **Office Phone:** (773) 880-4920; **Board Certifications:** Allergy & Immunology 1991, Internal Medicine 1988; **Medical School:** Northwestern Univ 1985; **Residency:** North Shore Univ Hosp, Manhasset, NY 1985-1988; **Fellowship:** Johns Hopkins Univ Med Sch, Baltimore, MD 1988-1991; **Faculty Appointment:** Asst Prof Pediatrics, Northwestern Univ

Strunk, Robert MD (Pediatric Allergy & Immunology) - *Special Expertise:* Asthma; **Admitting Hospital:** St Louis Children's Hospital; **Office Address:** One Children's Place, rm 5S30 St Louis, MO 63110; **Office Phone:** (314) 454-2694; **Board Certifications:** Pediatric Allergy & Immunology 1987, Pediatrics 1974; **Medical School:** Northwestern Univ 1968; **Residency:** Pediatrics, Cincinnati Chldns Hosp, Cincinnati, OH 1969-1970; **Fellowship:** Pediatric Allergy & Immunology, Boston Chldns Hosp, Boston, MA 1972-1974; **Faculty Appointment:** Prof Pediatrics, Washington Univ, St Louis

Wolf, Raoul MD (Pediatric Allergy & Immunology) - *Special Expertise:* Asthma; Allergy; **Admitting Hospital:** University of Chicago Hospitals (Page 78); **Office Address:** Univ Chicago Chldns Hosp 5839 S Maryland Ave Chicago, IL 60637; **Office Phone:** (773) 753-8637; **Board Certifications:** Allergy & Immunology 1983, Pediatrics 1980; **Medical School:** South Africa 1969; **Residencies:** Pediatrics, Baragwanath Hosp, Johannesburg, South Africa 1970-1973; Pediatrics, Transvaal Meml Hosp Chldn, Johannesburg, South Africa 1973-1976; **Fellowship:** Allergy & Immunology, Chldns Hosp Med Ctr, Boston, MA 1976-1979; **Faculty Appointment:** Assoc Clin Prof Pediatrics, Univ Chicago-Pritzker Sch Med

Great Plains and Mountains

Gelfand, Erwin MD (Pediatric Allergy & Immunology) - *Special Expertise:* Immune *Deficiency; Asthma;* **Admitting Hospital:** National Jewish Medical & Research Center; **Office Address:** National Jewish Med & Research Ctr 1400 Jackson St Denver, CO 80206; **Office Phone:** (303) 981-1196; **Board Certifications:** Pediatrics 1972, Allergy & Immunology 1979; **Medical School:** McGill Univ 1966; **Residencies:** Pediatrics, Montreal Children's Hosp, Montreal, Canada 1967-1968; Pediatrics, Children's Hosp Med Ctr, Boston, MA 1968-1969; **Fellowship:** Allergy & Immunology, Children's Hosp Med Ctr, Boston, MA 1969-1971; **Faculty Appointment:** Prof Pediatrics, Univ Colo

Leung, Donald MD/PhD (Pediatric Allergy & Immunology) - *Special Expertise:* Atopic *Dermatitis; Kawasaki Disease;* **Admitting Hospital:** National Jewish Medical & Research Center; **Office Address:** 1400 Jackson St Bldg K - Fl 926I Denver, CO 80206; **Office Phone:** (303) 398-1186; **Board Certifications:** Pediatrics 1982, Allergy & Immunology 1983; **Medical School:** Univ Chicago-Pritzker Sch Med 1977; **Residency:** Pediatrics, Chldns Hosp, Boston, MA 1978-1979; **Fellowships:** Pediatrics, Harvard Med Sch, Boston, MA 1977-1979; Allergy & Immunology, Chldns Hosp, Boston, MA 1979-1981; **Faculty Appointment:** Prof Pediatrics, Univ Colo

Southwest

Mazow, Jack Bernard MD (Pediatric Allergy & Immunology) - *Special Expertise:* Pediatric *Allergy & Immunology - General;* **Admitting Hospital:** Texas Children's Hospital - Houston; **Office Address:** Texas Chldrns Hosp, Allergy & Immunology Service 6621 Fannin, MC-1-3291 Houston, TX 77030; **Office Phone:** (832) 824-1319; **Board Certifications:** Internal Medicine 1974, Allergy & Immunology 1989; **Medical School:** Univ Tex, Houston 1947; **Residencies:** Internal Medicine, Jefferson Davis Hosp, Houston, TX 1948-1949; Internal Medicine, VA Hosp-Baylor, Houston, TX 1949-1954; **Fellowship:** Allergy & Immunology, SUNY Affil Hosp, Buffalo, NY 1962-1964; **Faculty Appointment:** Clin Prof Medicine, Univ Tex, Houston

Shearer, William T MD (Pediatric Allergy & Immunology) - *Special Expertise:* AIDS/HIV; *Immune Deficiency;* **Admitting Hospital:** Texas Children's Hospital - Houston; **Office Address:** Texas Chldns Hosp-Allergy and Immunology Service 6621 Fannin, MC-1-3291 Houston, TX 77030-3291; **Office Phone:** (832) 824-1274; **Board Certifications:** Pediatrics 1986, Allergy & Immunology 1989; **Medical School:** Washington Univ, St Louis 1970; **Residency:** Pediatrics, Chldns Hosp-Wash Univ, St Louis, MO 1971-1972; **Fellowship:** Allergy & Immunology, Barnes Hosp-Wash Univ, St Louis, MO 1972-1974; **Faculty Appointment:** Prof Pediatric Allergy & Immunology, Baylor Coll Med

West Coast and Pacific

Church, Joseph August MD (Pediatric Allergy & Immunology) - *Special Expertise:* AIDS/HIV; Immune Deficiency; **Admitting Hospital:** Children's Hospital - Los Angeles; **Office Address:** Children's Hosp LA MS 54700 Los Angeles, CA 90027; **Office Phone:** (323) 669-2501; **Board Certifications:** Pediatrics 1977, Allergy & Immunology 1977; **Medical School:** UMDNJ-NJ Med Sch, Newark 1972; **Residency:** Pediatrics, Chldns Hosp/Natl Med Ctr, Washington, DC 1973-1974; **Fellowship:** Allergy & Immunology, Georgetown Med Ctr, Washington, DC 1974-1976; **Faculty Appointment:** Prof Pediatrics, USC Sch Med

Epstein, Stuart Zane MD (Pediatric Allergy & Immunology) - *Special Expertise: Asthma; Allergy/Food Allergy;* **Admitting Hospital:** Cedars-Sinai Medical Center; **Office Address:** 9735 Wilshire Blvd, Bldg 121 Beverly Hills, CA 90212-2101; **Office Phone:** (310) 274-6853; **Board Certifications:** Allergy & Immunology 1991, Pediatrics 1998; **Medical School:** Univ IL Coll Med 1978; **Residency:** Pediatrics, Cedars Sinai Med Ctr, Los Angeles, CA 1979-1980; **Fellowships:** Pediatrics, USC Med Ctr, Los Angeles, CA 1981-1982; Pediatrics, Univ CA Irvine, Orange, CA 1980-1981; **Faculty Appointment:** Asst Clin Prof Pediatrics, UCLA

Fanous, Yvonne F MD (Pediatric Allergy & Immunology) - *Special Expertise: Asthma & Allergy; Cystic Fibrosis; Immune Deficiency;* **Admitting Hospital:** Loma Linda University Medical Center; **Office Address:** Loma Linda Univ Med Ctr 11370 Anderson Rd, Fl B100 Loma Linda, CA 92354; **Office Phone:** (909) 799-3387; **Board Certifications:** Allergy & Immunology 1985, Pediatrics 1981; **Medical School:** Egypt 1973; **Residencies:** Pediatrics, Loma Linda Univ, Loma Linda, CA 1980-1981; Pediatrics, Texas Tech Hosp, El Paso, TX 1978-1980; **Fellowship:** Allergy & Immunology, Univ CA, Irvine, CA 1981-1983; **Faculty Appointment:** Assoc Prof Pediatric Allergy & Immunology, Loma Linda Univ

Ostrom, Nancy Kay MD (Pediatric Allergy & Immunology) - *Special Expertise: Asthma & Allergy;* **Admitting Hospital:** Children's Hospital and Health Center; **Office Address:** Asthma & Allergy Medical Group & Research 9610 Granite Ridge DR, Ste B San Diego, CA 92123; **Office Phone:** (858) 268-2368; **Board Certifications:** Pediatrics 1984, Allergy & Immunology 1987; **Medical School:** Mayo Med Sch 1980; **Residency:** Pediatrics, Mayo Grad Sch Med, Rochester 1981-1983; **Fellowship:** Allergy & Immunology, Mayo Grad Sch Med, Rochester 1983-1985; **Faculty Appointment:** Asst Clin Prof Pediatric Allergy & Immunology, UCSD

Shapiro, Gail Greenberg MD (Pediatric Allergy & Immunology) - *Special Expertise: Asthma & Allergy;* **Admitting Hospital:** Children's Hospital and Regional Medical Center - Seattle; **Office Address:** NW Asthma & Allergy 4540 Sand Point Way NE, Ste 200 Seattle, WA 98105-3941; **Office Phone:** (206) 527-1200; **Board Certifications:** Allergy & Immunology 1975, Pediatrics 1975; **Medical School:** Johns Hopkins Univ 1970; **Residency:** Pediatrics, Univ Wash, Seattle, WA 1971-1972; **Fellowship:** Allergy & Immunology, Univ Wash, Seattle, WA 1972-1974; **Faculty Appointment:** Clin Prof Pediatrics, Univ Wash

Stiehm, E Richard MD (Pediatric Allergy & Immunology) - *Special Expertise: AIDS/HIV; Immune Deficiency;* **Admitting Hospital:** UCLA Medical Center; **Office Address:** UCLA Children's Hosp, 22-387 MDCC 10833 Le Conte Ave Los Angeles, CA 90095; **Office Phone:** (310) 825-6481; **Board Certifications:** Pediatrics 1964, Allergy & Immunology 1974; **Medical School:** Univ Wisc 1957; **Residency:** Pediatrics, Babies Hosp, New York, NY 1961-1963; **Fellowships:** Allergy & Immunology, Univ Wisc, Madison, WI 1958-1959; Allergy & Immunology, Univ CA, San Francisco, CA 1963-1965; **Faculty Appointment:** Prof Pediatrics, UCLA

Umetsu, Dale T MD/PhD (Pediatric Allergy & Immunology) - *Special Expertise: Asthma; Immune Deficiency;* **Admitting Hospital:** Stanford Medical Center; **Office Address:** Stanford Hospital and Clinics - Division of Allergy and Immunology Department of Pediatrics, rm H309 Stanford, CA 94305-5208; **Office Phone:** (650) 723-5227; **Board Certifications:** Allergy & Immunology 1985, Pediatrics 1984; **Medical School:** NYU Sch Med 1979; **Residency:** Pediatrics, Children's Hosp/Harvard Med Sch, Boston, MA 1980-1982; **Fellowship:** Allergy & Immunology, Children;s Hosp/Harvard Med Sch, Boston, MA 1982-1984; **Faculty Appointment:** Prof Pediatrics, Stanford Univ

Wara, Diane Wickizer MD (Pediatric Allergy & Immunology) - *Special Expertise:* AIDS/HIV; **Admitting Hospital:** University of California - San Francisco Medical Center; **Office Address:** 505 Parnassus Ave, Box 0105 San Francisco, CA 94143; **Office Phone:** (415) 353-2725; **Board Certifications:** Pediatrics 1974, Allergy & Immunology 1975; **Medical School:** UC Irvine 1969; **Residency:** Pediatrics, UCSF Med Ctr, San Francisco, CA 1970-1972; **Fellowship:** Immunology, UCSF Med Ctr, San Francisco, CA 1972-1975; **Faculty Appointment:** Prof Pediatrics, UCSF

PEDIATRIC CARDIOLOGY

New England

Lock, James E MD (Pediatric Cardiology) - *Special Expertise: Interventional Cardiology; Angioplasty-Pulmonary Artery;* **Admitting Hospital:** Children's Hospital; **Office Address:** Chldns Hosp, Dept Cardiology 300 Longwood Ave, Bader Building, Fl 2 Boston, MA 02115; **Office Phone:** (617) 355-7313; **Board Certifications:** Pediatrics 1978, Pediatric Cardiology 1981; **Medical School:** Stanford Univ 1973; **Residencies:** Pediatrics, Univ Minn Hosp, Minneapolis, MN 1974-1975; Pediatric Cardiology, Univ Minn Hosp, Minneapolis, MN 1975-1977; **Fellowship:** Cardiology (Cardiovascular Disease), Hosp Sick Chldn, Toronto,Canada 1977-1979; **Faculty Appointment:** Prof Pediatrics, Harvard Med Sch

Newburger, Jane MD (Pediatric Cardiology) - *Special Expertise: Cholesterol/Lipid Disorders; Heart Disease-Congenital; Kawasaki Disease;* **Admitting Hospital:** Children's Hospital; **Office Address:** Children's Hospital - Pediatric Cardiology - Bader Building 300 Longwood Ave Boston, MA 02115; **Office Phone:** (617) 355-5427; **Board Certifications:** Pediatrics 1979, Pediatric Cardiology 1983; **Medical School:** Harvard Med Sch 1974; **Residency:** Pediatrics, Chldns Hosp Med Ctr, Boston, MA 1975-1976; **Fellowship:** Pediatric Cardiology, Chldns Hosp Med Ctr, Boston, MA 1976-1979; **Faculty Appointment:** Assoc Prof Pediatrics, Harvard Med Sch

Perry, Stanton Bruce MD (Pediatric Cardiology) - *Special Expertise: Interventional Cardiology;* **Admitting Hospital:** Children's Hospital; **Office Address:** 300 Longwood Ave Boston, MA 02115; **Office Phone:** (617) 355-4278; **Board Certifications:** Pediatrics 1986, Pediatric Cardiology 1988; **Medical School:** Iceland 1978; **Residency:** Pediatrics, St Louis Chldns Hosp, St Louis, MO 1980-1983; **Fellowship:** Pediatric Cardiology, Chldns Hosp, Boston, MA 1983-1984; **Faculty Appointment:** Asst Prof Pediatrics, Harvard Med Sch

Walsh, Edward Patrick MD (Pediatric Cardiology) - *Special Expertise: Cardiac Electrophysiology; Arrhythmias;* **Admitting Hospital:** Children's Hospital; **Office Address:** Chldns Hosp, Dept Card 300 Longwood Ave Boston, MA 02115; **Office Phone:** (617) 355-6328; **Board Certifications:** Pediatric Cardiology 1985, Pediatrics 1985; **Medical School:** Univ Penn 1979; **Residency:** Pediatrics, Chldns Hosp, Philadelphia, PA 1980-1982; **Fellowship:** Pediatric Cardiology, Chldns Hosp, Boston, MA 1982-1985; **Faculty Appointment:** Assoc Prof Pediatrics, Harvard Med Sch

Mid Atlantic

Beerman, Lee MD (Pediatric Cardiology) - *Special Expertise: Transplant Medicine-Heart;* **Admitting Hospital:** Children's Hospital of Pittsburgh; **Office Address:** Chldns Hosp Pittsburgh - Heart Ctr 3705 5th Ave Pittsburgh, PA 15213; **Office Phone:** (412) 692-5540; **Board Certifications:** Pediatrics 1979, Pediatric Cardiology 1979; **Medical School:** Univ Pittsburgh 1974; **Residency:** Pediatrics, Chldns Hosp, Philadelphia, PA 1974-1977; **Fellowship:** Pediatric Cardiology, Chldns Hosp, Pittsburgh, PA 1977-1979; **Faculty Appointment:** Prof Pediatrics, Univ Pittsburgh

Brenner, Joel I MD (Pediatric Cardiology) - *Special Expertise: Heart Disease-Congenital;* **Admitting Hospital:** Johns Hopkins Hospital - Baltimore (Page 65); **Office Address:** Johns Hopkins Hosp. 600 N Wolfe St Baltimore, MD 21287; **Office Phone:** (410) 614-6746; **Board Certifications:** Pediatrics 1975, Pediatric Cardiology 1977; **Medical School:** NY Med Coll 1970; **Residency:** Pediatrics, New York Hospital, New York, NY 1971-1972; **Fellowship:** Pediatric Cardiology, Yale New Haven 1972-1974; **Faculty Appointment:** Assoc Prof Pediatrics, Johns Hopkins Univ

Gersony, Welton Mark MD (Pediatric Cardiology) - *Special Expertise:* Heart Disease-Congenital; **Admitting Hospital:** Columbia Presbyterian Medical Center (Page 72); **Office Address:** Babies and Children Hosp of New York 3959 Broadway, Fl 2nd - Ste 2 North - rm 263 New York, NY 10032; **Office Phone:** (212) 305-3262; **Board Certifications:** Pediatrics 1963, Pediatric Cardiology; **Medical School:** SUNY Hlth Sci Ctr 1958; **Residency:** Pediatrics, Babies Chldns, Cleveland, OH 1959-1961; **Fellowship:** Pediatric Cardiology, Harvard Chldns, Boston, MA 1963-1963; **Faculty Appointment:** Prof Pediatrics, Columbia P&S

Gewitz, Michael MD (Pediatric Cardiology) - *Special Expertise:* Pediatric Cardiology - General; **Admitting Hospital:** Westchester Medical Center; **Office Address:** New York Medical College/Westchester Med Ctr Rte 100, Munger Pavillion, Ste 618 Valhalla, NY 10595; **Office Phone:** (914) 594-4370; **Board Certifications:** Pediatrics 1979, Pediatric Cardiology 1981; **Medical School:** Hahnemann Univ 1974; **Residencies:** Pediatrics, Children's Hosp, Philadelphia, PA 1974-1976; Pediatrics, Hosp Sick Children, London England 1976-1977; **Fellowship:** Pediatric Cardiology, Yale-New Haven, New Haven, CT 1977-1979; **Faculty Appointment:** Prof Pediatric Cardiology, NY Med Coll

Hellenbrand, William E MD (Pediatric Cardiology) - *Special Expertise:* Interventional Cardiology; **Admitting Hospital:** Columbia Presbyterian Medical Center (Page 72); **Office Address:** 3959 Broadway New York, NY 10032-1537; **Office Phone:** (212) 305-8509; **Board Certifications:** Pediatrics 1975, Pediatric Cardiology 1977; **Medical School:** SUNY Downstate 1970; **Residency:** Pediatrics, Yale-New Haven, New Haven, CT 1970-1972; **Fellowships:** Pediatric Cardiology, Yale-New Haven, New Haven, CT 1972-1973; Pediatric Cardiology, Yale-New Haven, New Haven, CT 1975-1976; **Faculty Appointment:** Prof Pediatrics, Yale Univ

Kan, Jean MD (Pediatric Cardiology) - *Special Expertise:* Angioplasty; **Admitting Hospital:** Johns Hopkins Hospital - Baltimore (Page 65); **Office Address:** Johns Hopkins Hosp, Ped Dept 600 N Wolfe St, Bldg Brady 5 Baltimore, MD 21205; **Office Phone:** (410) 955-3665; **Board Certifications:** Pediatrics 1974, Pediatric Cardiology 1977; **Medical School:** Case West Res Univ 1969; **Residencies:** Pediatrics, Johns Hopkins Hosp, Baltimore, MD 1976; Pediatrics, Yale New Haven Hosp, New Haven, CT

Parness, Ira MD (Pediatric Cardiology) - *Special Expertise:* Echocardiography; **Admitting Hospital:** Mount Sinai Hospital (Page 70); **Office Address:** Mount Sinai Med Ctr 1 Gustave Levy Pl, Box 1201 New York, NY 10029-6504; **Office Phone:** (212) 241-8662; **Board Certifications:** Pediatrics 1982, Pediatric Cardiology 1985; **Medical School:** SUNY Hlth Sci Ctr 1979; **Residency:** Pediatrics, Brookdale Hosp, Brooklyn, NY 1979-1982; **Fellowship:** Pediatric Cardiology, Children's Hosp, Boston, MA 1982-1985; **Faculty Appointment:** Assoc Prof Pediatrics, Mount Sinai Sch Med

Southeast

Bayron, Harry MD (Pediatric Cardiology) - *Special Expertise:* Heart Murmurs; Heart Failure; **Admitting Hospital:** St Mary's Medical Center - West Palm Beach; **Office Address:** 5325 Greenwood Ave, Ste 302 West Palm Beach, FL 33407-2452; **Office Phone:** (561) 844-9858; **Board Certifications:** Pediatrics 1986, Pediatric Cardiology 1992; **Medical School:** Univ Puerto Rico 1978; **Residency:** Pediatrics, Univ Conn, Farmington, CT 1979-1982; **Fellowship:** Pediatric Cardiology, Univ Miami Jackson Meml Hosp, Miami, FL 1982-1985

Boucek, Robert MD (Pediatric Cardiology) - *Special Expertise:* Heart Disease-Congenital; Cardiomyopathy; Transplant Medicine-Heart; **Admitting Hospital:** All Children's Hospital; **Office Address:** 880 6th St S, Ste 280 St Petersburg, FL 33701-4823; **Office Phone:** (727) 892-4200; **Board Certification:** Pediatrics 1975; **Medical School:** Tulane Univ 1969; **Residency:** Pediatrics, Duke Univ, Durham, NC 1969-1971; **Fellowship:** Pediatric Cardiology, Vanderbilt Med Ctr, Nashville, TN 1973-1976; **Faculty Appointment:** Prof Pediatrics, Univ S Fla Coll Med

Colvin, Edward V MD (Pediatric Cardiology) - *Special Expertise:* Heart Disease-Congenital; Fetal Echogram; Transplant Medicine-Heart; **Admitting Hospital:** University of Alabama Hospital at Birmingham; **Office Address:** Hillman Bldg 320 620 20th St S Birmingham, AL 35233; **Office Phone:** (201) 934-3460; **Board Certifications:** Pediatrics 1982, Pediatric Cardiology 1985; **Medical School:** Univ Ala 1977; **Residency:** Pediatrics, Chldns Hosp, Birmingham, AL 1977-1980; **Fellowship:** Pediatric Cardiology, Baylor Coll Med, Houston, TX 1980-1983; **Faculty Appointment:** Prof Pediatrics, Univ Ala

Fricker, Frederick Jay MD (Pediatric Cardiology) - *Special Expertise:* Transplant Medicine-Heart; **Admitting Hospital:** Shands Healthcare at University Florida (Page 77); **Office Address:** 1600 SW Archer Rd, Box 100296 Gainesville, FL 32610-0296; **Office Phone:** (352) 392-6431; **Board Certifications:** Pediatrics 1975, Pediatric Cardiology 1981; **Medical School:** Loyola Univ-Stritch Sch Med 1970; **Residency:** Pediatrics, Children's Hosp, Pittsburgh, PA 1971-1973; **Fellowship:** Pediatric Cardiology, Children's Hosp, Pittsburgh, PA 1975-1977; **Faculty Appointment:** Prof Pediatrics, Univ Fla Coll Med

O'Laughlin, Martin P MD (Pediatric Cardiology) - *Special Expertise:* Cardiac Catheterization; **Admitting Hospital:** Duke University Medical Center (Page 60); **Office Address:** Duke Univ Med Ctr rm 7607 DHN, Box 3090 Durham, NC 27710; **Office Phone:** (919) 684-3574; **Board Certifications:** Pediatrics 1985, Pediatric Cardiology 1996; **Medical School:** Columbia P&S 1980; **Residencies:** Pediatrics, Baylor Coll Med, Houston, TX 1980-1983; Pediatrics, Baylor Coll Med, Houston, TX 1983-1984; **Fellowship:** Pediatric Cardiology, Baylor Coll Med, Houston, TX 1984-1987; **Faculty Appointment:** Assoc Prof Pediatrics, Duke Univ

Sanders, Stephen Pruett MD (Pediatric Cardiology) - *Special Expertise:* Echocardiography; Fetal Cardiology; **Admitting Hospital:** Duke University Medical Center (Page 60); **Office Address:** Duke Univ Med Ctr Box 3090, Bldg DHN - rm 7617 Durham, NC 27710; **Office Phone:** (919) 681-2916; **Board Certifications:** Pediatrics 1980, Pediatric Cardiology 1981; **Medical School:** Univ Louisville Sch Med 1975; **Residencies:** Pediatrics, Univ Oregon Hlth Sci Ctr, Portland, OR 1976-1978; Pediatrics; **Fellowship:** Pediatric Cardiology, Children's Hosp, Boston, MA 1978-1981; **Faculty Appointment:** Prof Pediatrics, Duke Univ

Tamer, Dolores MD (Pediatric Cardiology) - *Special Expertise:* Kawasaki Disease; **Admitting Hospital:** University of Miami - Jackson Memorial Hospital; **Office Address:** Univ Miami-Jackson Mem Hosp Box 016960 (R76) Miami, FL 33101; **Office Phone:** (305) 585-6683; **Board Certifications:** Pediatrics 1966, Pediatric Cardiology 1967; **Medical School:** SUNY Buffalo 1961; **Residencies:** Pediatrics, Chldns Hosp, Philadelphia, PA 1962-1963; Pediatrics, Chldns Hosp, Buffalo, NY 1963-1964; **Fellowship:** Pediatrics, Chldns Hosp, Buffalo, NY 1964-1965; **Faculty Appointment:** Prof Pediatrics, Univ Miami Sch Med

Wolff, Grace Susan MD (Pediatric Cardiology) - *Special Expertise:* Arrhythmias; Cardiac Electrophysiology; **Admitting Hospital:** University of Miami - Jackson Memorial Hospital; **Office Address:** 1475 NW 12th Ave Miami, FL 33101; **Office Phone:** (305) 585-6683; **Board Certifications:** Pediatrics 1971, Pediatric Cardiology 1973; **Medical School:** Med Coll Wisc 1965; **Residency:** Pediatrics, Colum-Presby Med Ctr, New York, NY 1967-1969; **Fellowship:** Pediatric Cardiology, Children's Hosp, Boston, MA 1969-1971; **Faculty Appointment:** Prof Pediatric Cardiology, Univ Miami Sch Med

Young, Ming-Lon MD (Pediatric Cardiology) - *Special Expertise: Cardiac Electrophysiology; Arrhythmias;* **Admitting Hospital:** University of Miami - Jackson Memorial Hospital; **Office Address:** Univ Miami, Dept Ped Box 016960 (R-76) Miami, FL 33101; **Office Phone:** (305) 585-6683; **Board Certifications:** Pediatric Cardiology 1985, Pediatrics 1985; **Medical School:** Taiwan 1976; **Residencies:** Pediatrics, St Agnes Hosp, Baltimore, MD 1979-1981; Preventive Medicine, Johns Hopkins Univ, Baltimore, MD 1978-1979; **Fellowship:** Pediatric Cardiology, Univ Miami, Miami, FL 1981-1985; **Faculty Appointment:** Prof Pediatrics, Univ Miami Sch Med

Midwest

Agarwala, Brojendra MD (Pediatric Cardiology) - *Special Expertise: Pediatric Cardiology - General;* **Admitting Hospital:** University of Chicago Hospitals (Page 78); **Office Address:** 5841 S Maryland St, MC-4051 Chicago, IL 60637; **Office Phone:** (773) 702-6172; **Board Certifications:** Pediatrics 1970, Pediatric Cardiology 1978; **Medical School:** India 1965; **Residency:** Pediatrics, St Vincent Hosp Med Ctr, New York, NY 1967-1969; **Fellowship:** Pediatric Cardiology, NYU Med Ctr, New York, NY 1969-1972; **Faculty Appointment:** Prof Pediatrics, Univ Chicago-Pritzker Sch Med

Caldwell, Randall MD (Pediatric Cardiology) - *Special Expertise: Transplant Medicine-Heart; Echocardiography;* **Admitting Hospital:** Riley Hospital for Children; **Office Address:** Ind Univ Med Ctr 702 Barnhill Drive Indianapolis, IN 46202; **Office Phone:** (317) 274-8906; **Board Certifications:** Pediatric Cardiology 1978, Pediatrics 1976; **Medical School:** Indiana Univ 1971; **Residency:** Pediatrics, Ind Med Ctr, Indianapolis, IN 1972-1975; **Fellowship:** Pediatric Cardiology, Ind Med Ctr, Indianapolis, IN 1975-1978; **Faculty Appointment:** Prof Pediatric Cardiology, Indiana Univ

Cutilletta, Anthony F MD (Pediatric Cardiology) - *Special Expertise: Angioplasty; Cardiomyopathy;* **Admitting Hospital:** Rush/Presbyterian - St Luke's Medical Center - Chicago (Page 74); **Office Address:** 1725 W Harrison, Ste 710 Chicago, IL 60612; **Office Phone:** (312) 942-6003; **Board Certifications:** Pediatrics 1973, Pediatric Cardiology 1973; **Medical School:** Univ Chicago-Pritzker Sch Med 1968; **Residency:** Pediatrics, Wyler Chldns Hosp, Chicago, IL 1969-1970; **Fellowship:** Pediatric Cardiology, Wyler Chldns Hosp, Chicago, IL 1970-1972; **Faculty Appointment:** Prof Pediatrics, Rush Med Coll

Driscoll, David J MD (Pediatric Cardiology) - *Special Expertise: Exercise Physiology; Klippel-Trenaunay Syndrome; Cardiomyopathy;* **Admitting Hospital:** Mayo Medical Center & Clinic - Rochester; **Office Address:** Mayo Clinic - Pediatric Cardiology 200 1st St SW Rochester, MN 55905; **Office Phone:** (507) 284-1270; **Board Certifications:** Pediatrics 1976, Pediatric Cardiology 1991; **Medical School:** Marquette Sch Med 1970; **Residencies:** Pediatrics, Milwaukee Chldns Hosp, Milwaukee, WI 1971-1972; Milwaukee Chldns Hosp, Milwaukee, WI 1974-1975; **Fellowship:** Pediatric Cardiology, Baylor 1975-1978; **Faculty Appointment:** Prof Pediatrics, Mayo Med Sch

Epstein, Michael MD (Pediatric Cardiology) - *Special Expertise: Heart Disease-Congenital;* **Admitting Hospital:** Children's Hospital of Michigan; **Office Address:** Chldns Hosp Mich, Dept Cardiology 3901 Beaubien Blvd, Fl 2nd Detroit, MI 48201; **Office Phone:** (313) 745-5956; **Board Certifications:** Pediatrics 1976, Pediatric Cardiology 1981; **Medical School:** Univ Tex Med Br, Galveston 1971; **Residency:** Pediatrics, Univ Ariz Hlth Sci Ctr, Tucson, AZ 1971-1974; **Fellowship:** Pediatric Cardiology, Univ MN Hosp, Minneapolis, MN 1976-1979; **Faculty Appointment:** Prof Pediatrics, Wayne State Univ

Hijazi, Ziyad M MD (Pediatric Cardiology) - *Special Expertise: Interventional Cardiology; Heart Disease-Congenital;* **Admitting Hospital:** University of Chicago Hospitals (Page 78); **Office Address:** Univ Chicago Chldns Hosp 5841 S Maryland Ave, rm C104, MC-4051 Chicago, IL 60637; **Office Phone:** (773) 702-6172; **Board Certifications:** Pediatrics 1991, Pediatric Cardiology 1992; **Medical School:** Jordan 1982; **Residency:** Pediatrics, Yale-New Haven Hosp, New Haven, CT 1987-1988; **Fellowship:** Pediatric Cardiology, Yale Univ Sch Med, New Haven, CT 1988-1991; **Faculty Appointment:** Prof Pediatrics, Univ Chicago-Pritzker Sch Med

Liebman, Jerome MD (Pediatric Cardiology) - *Special Expertise: Cholesterol/Lipid Disorders; Heart Disease-Congenital;* **Admitting Hospital:** Rainbow Babies & Children's Hospital; **Office Address:** Rainbow Baby & Chldns Hosp 11100 Euclid Ave, Ste 3400 Cleveland, OH 44106-2624; **Office Phone:** (216) 844-7700; **Board Certifications:** Pediatric Cardiology 1962, Pediatrics 1959; **Medical School:** Harvard Med Sch 1955; **Residency:** Pediatrics, Babies & Chldns Hosp, Cleveland, OH 1955-1957; **Fellowship:** Pediatric Cardiology, Harvard Med Sch, Boston, MA 1957-1959; **Faculty Appointment:** Prof Pediatrics, Case West Res Univ

Moodie, Douglas MD (Pediatric Cardiology) - *Special Expertise: Cholesterol/Lipid Disorders; Heart Disease Imaging-Congenital;* **Admitting Hospital:** Cleveland Clinic Foundation; **Office Address:** Cleveland Clinic Foundation 9500 Euclid Ave, MC-A120 Cleveland, OH 44195; **Office Phone:** (216) 444-6717; **Board Certifications:** Pediatrics 1977, Pediatric Cardiology 1977; **Medical School:** Med Coll Wisc 1972; **Residency:** Pediatrics, Mayo Med Clinic, Rochester, MN 1974-1977; **Fellowship:** Pediatric Cardiology, Mayo Med Clinic, Rochester, MN 1973-1974

Porter, Co-burn Joseph MD (Pediatric Cardiology) - *Special Expertise: Arrhythmias; Arrhythmias-Fetal; Transplant Medicine-Heart;* **Admitting Hospital:** Mayo Medical Center & Clinic - Rochester; **Office Address:** Mayo Med Ctr, Dept Ped Cardiology 200 1st St SW Rochester, MN 55905; **Office Phone:** (507) 284-3297; **Board Certifications:** Pediatrics 1977, Pediatric Cardiology 1983; **Medical School:** Creighton Univ 1972; **Residency:** Pediatrics, Univ Colo Hlth Sci Ctr, Denver, CO 1973-1975; **Fellowships:** Pediatric Cardiology, Baylor Coll Med, Houston, TX 1975-1977; Pediatric Cardiology, Baylor Coll Med, Houston, TX 1980-1981; **Faculty Appointment:** Assoc Prof Pediatrics, Mayo Med Sch

Rocchini, Albert P MD (Pediatric Cardiology) - *Special Expertise: Interventional Cardiology; Heart Disease-Congenital;* **Admitting Hospital:** University of Michigan Health Center; **Office Address:** Univ of Michigan 1500 Medical Ctr Dr Ann Arbor, MI 48109; **Office Phone:** (734) 764-5176; **Board Certifications:** Pediatric Cardiology 1989, Pediatrics 1989; **Medical School:** Univ Pittsburgh 1972; **Residency:** Pediatrics, Univ Mich Med, Ann Arbor, MI 1973-1974; **Fellowship:** Pediatric Cardiology, Children's Hosp, Boston, MA 1974-1977; **Faculty Appointment:** Prof Pediatric Cardiology, Northwestern Univ

Rosenthal, Amnon MD (Pediatric Cardiology) - *Special Expertise: Heart Disease-Congenital;* **Admitting Hospital:** University of Michigan Health Center; **Office Address:** Univ Mich-Mott Children's Hosp 1500 E Medical Ctr Dr Ann Arbor, MI 48109-0204; **Office Phone:** (734) 764-5176; **Board Certifications:** Pediatric Cardiology 1986, Pediatrics 1986; **Medical School:** Albany Med Coll 1959; **Residency:** Pediatrics, Boston Chldns Hosp., Boston, MA 1960-1962; **Fellowship:** Cardiology (Cardiovascular Disease), Boston Chldns Hosp., Boston, MA 1965-1968; **Faculty Appointment:** Prof Pediatrics, Univ Mich Med Sch

Sodt, Peter MD (Pediatric Cardiology) - *Special Expertise: Birth Defects-Cardiac; Arrhythmias;* **Admitting Hospital:** Rush/Presbyterian - St Luke's Medical Center - Chicago (Page 74); **Office Address:** 1575 N Barrington Rd, Ste 430 Hoffman Estates, IL 60194; **Office Phone:** (847) 884-1212; **Board Certifications:** Pediatrics 1986, Pediatric Cardiology 1995; **Medical School:** Northwestern Univ 1980; **Residency:** Pediatrics, Doernbecker Meml Hosp/OHSU, Portland, OR 1981-1984; **Fellowship:** Pediatric Cardiology, Wyler Chldns Hosp/Univ Chicago, Chicago, IL 1984-1986; **Faculty Appointment:** Asst Prof Pediatrics, Rush Med Coll

Great Plains and Mountains

Boucek, Mark M. MD (Pediatric Cardiology) - *Special Expertise: Transplant Medicine-Heart; Cardiac Catheterization;* **Admitting Hospital:** The Children's Hospital - Denver; **Office Address:** The Children's Hosp, Dept Ped Cardiology 1056 E 19th Ave Denver, CO 80218; **Office Phone:** (303) 837-2940; **Board Certifications:** Pediatrics 1982, Pediatric Cardiology 1983; **Medical School:** Univ Miami Sch Med 1977; **Residency:** Pediatrics, Vanderbilt Univ Hosp, Nashville, TN 1978-1979; **Fellowship:** Pediatric Cardiology, Univ Utah, Salt Lake City, UT 1979-1981; **Faculty Appointment:** Prof Pediatrics, Loma Linda Univ

Southwest

Bricker, John Timothy MD (Pediatric Cardiology) - *Special Expertise: Preventive Cardiology; Transplant Medicine-Heart;* **Admitting Hospital:** Texas Children's Hospital - Houston; **Office Address:** Texas Chldns Med Ctr 6621 Fannin St, MC-2-2280 Houston, TX 77030; **Office Phone:** (832) 824-5677; **Board Certifications:** Pediatric Cardiology 1997, Pediatric Critical Care Medicine 1998; **Medical School:** Ohio State Univ 1976; **Residency:** Pediatrics, Texas Chlds Hosp, Houston, TX 1976-1980; **Fellowship:** Pediatric Cardiology, Texas Chlds Hosp, Houston, TX 1980-1983; **Faculty Appointment:** Prof Pediatrics, Baylor Coll Med

Dreyer, William Jeffrey MD (Pediatric Cardiology) - *Special Expertise: Heart Disease-Congenital;* **Admitting Hospital:** St Luke's Episcopal Hospital - Houston (Page 76); **Office Address:** Texas Children's Hosp 6621 Fannin St, Ste A-260, MC-2-2280 Houston, TX 77030; **Office Phone:** (713) 770-5600; **Board Certifications:** Pediatrics 1987, Pediatric Cardiology 2005; **Medical School:** Univ Fla Coll Med 1981; **Residency:** Pediatrics, Univ CA, San Francisco, CA 1982-1984; **Fellowship:** Pediatric Cardiology, Baylor Coll Med, Houston, TX 1984-1988; **Faculty Appointment:** Assoc Prof Pediatrics, Baylor Coll Med

Gillette, Paul Crawford MD (Pediatric Cardiology) - *Special Expertise: Arrhythmias;* **Admitting Hospital:** Cook Children's Medical Center; **Office Address:** Pediatric Cardiology 901 7th Ave, Ste 310 Fort Worth, TX 76104; **Office Phone:** (817) 810-2140; **Board Certifications:** Pediatrics 1974, Pediatric Cardiology 1975; **Medical School:** Med Univ SC 1969; **Residency:** Pediatrics, Baylor Coll Med, Houston, TX 1971-1972; **Fellowship:** Pediatric Cardiology, Baylor Coll Med, Houston, TX 1972-1974

Mahony, Lynn MD (Pediatric Cardiology) - *Special Expertise: Heart Disease-Congenital;* **Admitting Hospital:** Children's Medical Center of Dallas; **Office Address:** Children's Med Ctr-Cardiology 1935 Motor St Dallas, TX 75235; **Office Phone:** (214) 456-2333; **Board Certifications:** Pediatrics 1979, Pediatric Cardiology 1987; **Medical School:** Stanford Univ 1975; **Residency:** Pediatrics, Stanford Univ, Stanford, CA 1976-1978; **Fellowship:** Pediatric Cardiology, UCSF, San Francisco, CA 1978; **Faculty Appointment:** Assoc Prof Pediatrics, Univ Tex SW, Dallas

Mullins, Charles MD (Pediatric Cardiology) - *Special Expertise:* Heart Disease-Congenital; **Admitting Hospital:** Texas Children's Hospital - Houston; **Office Address:** Texas Children's Hospital 6621 Fannin St, MC-2-2280 Houston, TX 77030; **Office Phone:** (832) 824-5600; **Board Certifications:** Pediatric Surgery 1963, Pediatric Cardiology 1968; **Medical School:** France 1958; **Residencies:** Pediatrics, Walter Reed Genl Hosp 1959-1961; Cardiology (Cardiovascular Disease), Walter Reed Genl Hosp 1961-1962; **Fellowship:** Cardiology (Cardiovascular Disease), Walter Reed Genl Hosp 1962-1963; **Faculty Appointment:** Prof Pediatrics, Baylor Coll Med

Rogers Jr, James Henry MD (Pediatric Cardiology) - *Special Expertise:* Heart Disease-Congenital; **Admitting Hospital:** University of Texas Health & Science Center; **Office Address:** Univ Tex Hlth Sci Ctr, Dept Ped 7730 Floyd Curl Dr San Antonio, TX 78229-3900; **Office Phone:** (210) 341-7722; **Board Certifications:** Pediatrics 1976, Pediatric Cardiology 1977; **Medical School:** Med Coll GA 1971; **Residency:** Pediatrics, Wilford Hall USAF Med Ctr, San Antonio, TX 1972-1974; **Fellowship:** Pediatric Cardiology, Med Coll GA, Augusta, GA 1974-1976; **Faculty Appointment:** Assoc Prof Pediatrics, Univ Tex, San Antonio

West Coast and Pacific

Bernstein, Daniel MD (Pediatric Cardiology) - *Special Expertise:* Transplant Medicine-Heart; Cardiomyopathy; **Admitting Hospital:** Stanford Medical Center; **Office Address:** Pediatric Cardiology Division 750 Welch Rd, Ste 305 Palo Alto, CA 94304; **Office Phone:** (650) 723-7913; **Board Certifications:** Pediatrics 1984, Pediatric Cardiology 1985; **Medical School:** NYU Sch Med 1978; **Residency:** Pediatrics, Montefiore Hosp, Bronx, NY 1978-1982; **Fellowships:** Albert Einstein Coll, Bronx, NY 1982-1983; Pediatric Cardiology, UCSF, San Francisco, CA 1983-1986; **Faculty Appointment:** Assoc Prof Pediatric Cardiology, Stanford Univ

Hohn, Arno R MD (Pediatric Cardiology) - *Special Expertise:* Hypertension; Preventive Cardiology; **Admitting Hospital:** Children's Hospital - Los Angeles; **Office Address:** Childrens Hospital LA 4650 Sunset Blvd, MS 34 Los Angeles, CA 90027; **Office Phone:** (323) 669-2535; **Board Certifications:** Pediatrics 1963, Pediatric Cardiology 1965; **Medical School:** NY Med Coll 1956; **Residencies:** Pediatrics, Buffalo Childrens Hosp, Buffalo, NY 1957-1958; Pediatrics, Childrens Hosp, Philadelphia, PA 1961-1962; **Fellowships:** Pediatric Cardiology, Buffalo Childrens Hosp, Buffalo, NY 1962-1963; Pediatric Cardiology, Buffalo Childrens Hosp, Buffalo, NY 1958-1959; **Faculty Appointment:** Prof Pediatrics, USC Sch Med

Pitlick, Paul T MD (Pediatric Cardiology) - *Special Expertise:* Interventional Cardiology; **Admitting Hospital:** Stanford Medical Center; **Office Address:** Pediatric Cardiology 725 Welch Rd Palo Alto, CA 94304; **Office Phone:** (650) 723-7913; **Board Certifications:** Pediatrics 1975, Pediatric Cardiology 1978; **Medical School:** St Louis Univ 1970; **Residency:** Pediatrics, Univ Hosp, San Diego, CA 1971-1972; **Fellowship:** Pediatric Cardiology, Univ Hosp, San Diego, CA 1972-1976; **Faculty Appointment:** Assoc Prof Pediatrics, Stanford Univ

Takahashi, Masato MD (Pediatric Cardiology) - *Special Expertise:* Kawasaki Disease; Cardiac Catheterization; **Admitting Hospital:** Children's Hospital - Los Angeles; **Office Address:** Children's Hosp-LA, Dept Cardiology 4650 Sunset Blvd, MS 34 Los Angeles, CA 90027; **Office Phone:** (323) 669-4634; **Board Certifications:** Pediatrics 1966, Pediatric Cardiology 1992; **Medical School:** Indiana Univ 1960; **Residency:** Pediatrics, Ind Med Ctr, Indianapolis, IN 1961-1963; **Fellowship:** Pediatric Cardiology, UCLA Med Ctr, Los Angeles, CA 1964-1967; **Faculty Appointment:** Prof Pediatrics, Univ SC Sch Med

Teitel, David F MD (Pediatric Cardiology) - *Special Expertise: Cardiac Disease;* **Admitting Hospital:** University of California - San Francisco Medical Center; **Office Address:** UCSF, Dept Ped Cardiology 521 Parnassus, Rm C344 San Francisco, CA 94143; **Office Phone:** (415) 476-1040; **Board Certifications:** Pediatrics 1980, Pediatric Cardiology 1997; **Medical School:** Univ Toronto 1975; **Residency:** Pediatrics, Children's Hosp, Montreal, Canada 1980; **Fellowship:** Pediatric Cardiology, UCSF, San Francisco, CA 1980-1982; **Faculty Appointment:** Prof Pediatrics, UCSF

PEDIATRIC CRITICAL CARE MEDICINE

New England

Fleisher, Gary Robert MD (Pediatric Critical Care Medicine) - *Special Expertise: Trauma;* **Admitting Hospital:** Children's Hospital; **Office Address:** Chldns Hosp Boston-Emergency Med 300 Longwood Ave Boston, MA 02115-5724; **Office Phone:** (617) 355-6000; **Board Certifications:** Pediatric Emergency Medicine 1999, Pediatric Infectious Disease 1999; **Medical School:** Jefferson Med Coll 1973; **Residencies:** Pediatrics, Chldns Hosp, Philadelphia, PA 1974-1976; Pediatrics, Chldns Hosp, Philadelphia, PA 1976-1977; **Fellowship:** Infectious Disease, Chldns Hosp, Philadelphia, PA 1977-1979; **Faculty Appointment:** Prof Pediatrics, Harvard Med Sch

Lister, George MD (Pediatric Critical Care Medicine) - *Special Expertise: Pediatric Critical Care Medicine - General;* **Admitting Hospital:** Yale - New Haven Hospital; **Office Address:** Yale Univ. Sch Med-Peds 333 Cedar St. New Haven, CT 06520-8064; **Office Phone:** (203) 785-4651; **Board Certifications:** Pediatric Critical Care Medicine 1996, Pediatrics 1992; **Medical School:** Yale Univ 1973; **Residency:** Pediatrics, Yale-New Haven Hosp., New Haven, CT 1974-1975; **Fellowship:** Pediatric Critical Care Medicine, University California, CA 1975-1978; **Faculty Appointment:** Prof Pediatrics, Yale Univ

Mid Atlantic

Fuhrman, Bradley P MD (Pediatric Critical Care Medicine) - *Special Expertise: Liquid Ventilation;* **Admitting Hospital:** The Children's Hospital of Buffalo; **Office Address:** Chldns Hosp Buffalo, Dept Ped Critical Care 219 Bryant St Buffalo, NY 14222-2006; **Office Phone:** (716) 878-7442; **Board Certifications:** Pediatric Cardiology 1979, Pediatric Critical Care Medicine 1996; **Medical School:** NYU Sch Med 1971; **Residency:** Pediatrics, Univ Minnesota, Minneapolis, MN 1972-1973; **Fellowships:** Pediatric Cardiology, Univ Minnesota, Minneapolis, MN 1973-1974; Pediatric Cardiology, Univ Minnesota, Minneapolis, MN 1976-1979; **Faculty Appointment:** Prof Pediatrics, SUNY Buffalo

Holbrook, Peter MD (Pediatric Critical Care Medicine) - *Special Expertise: Pediatric Critical Care Medicine - General;* **Admitting Hospital:** Children's National Medical Center - DC; **Office Address:** Chldns Natl Med Ctr 111 Michigan Ave NW Washington, DC 20010-2916; **Office Phone:** (202) 884-3256; **Board Certifications:** Pediatrics 1975, Pediatric Critical Care Medicine 1987; **Medical School:** Penn State Univ-Hershey Med Ctr 1970; **Residency:** Pediatrics, Johns Hopkins Hosp, Baltimore, MD 1971-1972; **Fellowship:** Pediatric Critical Care Medicine, Univ Pittsburgh, Pittsburgh, PA 1972-1973; **Faculty Appointment:** Prof Pediatrics, Geo Wash Univ

Kochanek, Patrick MD (Pediatric Critical Care Medicine) - *Special Expertise: Head Injury;* **Admitting Hospital:** Children's Hospital of Pittsburgh; **Office Address:** 3434 5TH Ave Ste 201 Pittsburgh, PA 15260; **Office Phone:** (412) 383-1900; **Board Certifications:** Pediatrics 1985, Pediatric Critical Care Medicine 1987; **Medical School:** Univ Chicago-Pritzker Sch Med 1980; **Residency:** Pediatrics, UC San Diego, San Diego, CA 1981-1983; **Fellowship:** Pediatric Critical Care Medicine, Chldns Hosp, Washington, DC 1983-1986; **Faculty Appointment:** Assoc Prof Critical Care Medicine, Univ Pittsburgh

Nichols, David Gregory MD (Pediatric Critical Care Medicine) - *Special Expertise:*
Respiratory Failure; Mechanical Ventilation; **Admitting Hospital:** Johns Hopkins Hospital -
Baltimore (Page 65); **Office Address:** Johns Hopkins Univ Hosp 600 N Wolfe St, Bldg Blalock - rm
912 Baltimore, MD 21287-4912; **Office Phone:** (410) 955-6412; **Board Certifications:** Pediatrics
1982, Pediatric Critical Care Medicine 1996; **Medical School:** Mount Sinai Sch Med 1977;
Residencies: Pediatrics, Chldns Hosp, Philadelphia, PA 1978-1980; Anesthesiology, Hosp Univ
Penn, Philadelphia, PA 1981-1983; **Fellowship:** Anesthesiology, Chldns Hosp, Philadelphia, PA
1983; **Faculty Appointment:** Prof Pediatrics, Johns Hopkins Univ

Thompson, Ann Ellen MD (Pediatric Critical Care Medicine) - *Special Expertise:*
Mechanical Ventilation; Critical Care; Respiratory Failure; **Admitting Hospital:** Children's Hospital
of Pittsburgh; **Office Address:** Chldns Hosp Pittsburgh, Dept Ped Critical Care 3705 Fifth Ave
Pittsburgh, PA 15213-2524; **Office Phone:** (412) 692-5164; **Board Certifications:** Pediatrics 1979,
Anesthesiology 1980; **Medical School:** Tufts Univ 1974; **Residencies:** Pediatrics, Chldns Hosp,
Philadelphia, PA 1976-1977; Anesthesiology, Hosp Penn, Philadelphia, PA 1977-1980; **Fellowship:**
Pediatric Anatomy, Chldns Hosp, Philadelphia, PA 1979; **Faculty Appointment:** Prof
Anesthesiology, Univ Pittsburgh

Midwest

Latson, Larry Allen MD (Pediatric Critical Care Medicine) - *Special Expertise:* Heart
Disease-Congenital; Interventional Cardiology; **Admitting Hospital:** Cleveland Clinic Foundation;
Office Address: Clevland Clin Fdn 9500 Euclid Ave M41 Cleveland, OH 44195; **Office Phone:**
(216) 445-6532; **Board Certifications:** Pediatric Cardiology 1983, Pediatric Critical Care Medicine
1992; **Medical School:** Baylor Coll Med 1976; **Residency:** Pediatrics, Baylor Coll Med, Houston, TX
1976-1978; **Fellowship:** Pediatric Cardiology, Baylor Coll Med, Houston, TX 1978-1981

Perez Fontan, J Julio MD (Pediatric Critical Care Medicine) - *Special Expertise:*
Respiratory Failure; **Admitting Hospital:** St Louis Children's Hospital; **Office Address:** St Louis
Chldns Hosp 1 Children's Pl, Ste 5-S20 St Louis, MO 63110; **Office Phone:** (314) 454-2527; **Board
Certifications:** Pediatrics 1987, Pediatric Critical Care Medicine 1996; **Medical School:** Spain
1977; **Residency:** Pediatrics, Chldns Hosp/Univ Barcelona 1979-1981; **Fellowship:** Critical Care
Medicine, UCSF, San Francisco, CA 1981-1984; **Faculty Appointment:** Prof Pediatrics, Washington
Univ, St Louis

Sarnaik, Ashok P MD (Pediatric Critical Care Medicine) - *Special Expertise: Critical Care;
Perinatal Medicine;* **Admitting Hospital:** Children's Hospital of Michigan; **Office Address:** Chldns
Hosp, Intensive Care Unit 3901 Beaubien Street Detroit, MI 48201-2119; **Office Phone:** (313) 745-
5629; **Board Certifications:** Pediatric Critical Care Medicine 1996, Neonatal-Perinatal Medicine
1979; **Medical School:** India 1969; **Residencies:** Pediatrics, Chldns Hosp Mich, Detroit, MI 1971-
1974; Critical Care Medicine, JJ Hosp-Bombay Univ, Bombay, India 1970-1971; **Fellowship:**
Neonatal-Perinatal Medicine, Childns Hosp Mich, Detroit, MI 1974-1975; **Faculty Appointment:**
Prof Pediatrics, Wayne State Univ

Southwest

Anand, Kanwaljeet Singh MD/PhD (Pediatric Critical Care Medicine) - *Special Expertise:* *Pain Management; Critical Care;* **Admitting Hospital:** Arkansas Children's Hospital; **Office Address:** Arkansas Childrens Hosp, Div CCM 800 Marshall Street, Bldg Sturg - rm 431 Little Rock, AR 72202; **Office Phone:** (501) 320-1008; **Board Certifications:** Pediatrics 1991, Critical Care Medicine 1994; **Medical School:** India 1981; **Residencies:** Pediatrics, Children's Hosp, Boston, MA 1988-1991; Pediatric Critical Care Medicine, Mass Genl Hosp, Boston, MA 1991-1993; **Fellowships:** Neonatal-Perinatal Medicine, John Radcliffe Hosp, Headington, Oxford, U.K. 1982-1985; Anesthesiology, Children's Hosp, Boston, MA 1985-1988; **Faculty Appointment:** Prof Pediatrics, Univ Ark

West Coast and Pacific

Brill, Judith Eileen MD (Pediatric Critical Care Medicine) - *Special Expertise:* Pediatric Critical Care Medicine - General; **Admitting Hospital:** UCLA Medical Center; **Office Address:** UCLA Med Ctr, Dept Peds 10833 Le Conte Ave Los Angeles, CA 90095; **Office Phone:** (310) 825-9124; **Board Certifications:** Anesthesiology 1986, Pediatrics 1982; **Medical School:** Harvard Med Sch 1977; **Residencies:** Pediatrics, Chldns Hosp Med Ctr, Boston, MA 1978-1979; Pediatrics, UCLA, Los Angeles, CA 1980-1981; **Fellowship:** Anesthesiology, Mass Genl Hosp, Boston, MA 1979-1982; **Faculty Appointment:** Prof Emeritus UCLA

Yeh, Timothy S MD (Pediatric Critical Care Medicine) - *Special Expertise:* Pediatric Critical Care Medicine - General; **Admitting Hospital:** Children's Medical Center - Oakland; **Office Address:** Childrens Hosp-Oakland 747 52nd St Oakland, CA 94609-1809; **Office Phone:** (510) 428-3714; **Board Certifications:** Pediatrics 1982, Pediatric Critical Care Medicine 1996; **Medical School:** UC Davis 1976; **Residency:** Pediatrics, Univ CA - Davis, Sacramento, CA 1977-1979; **Fellowship:** Pediatric Critical Care Medicine, Chldns Hosp Natl Med Ctr, Oakland, CA 1979-1981; **Faculty Appointment:** Clin Prof Pediatrics

Zimmerman, Jerry John MD (Pediatric Critical Care Medicine) - *Special Expertise:* Lung Injury; Sepsis & Septic Shock; **Admitting Hospital:** Children's Hospital and Regional Medical Center - Seattle; **Office Address:** Children's Hosp & Regl Med Ctr, G-906 CH-05 4800 Sandpoint Way NE Seattle, WA 98105; **Office Phone:** (206) 527-3862; **Board Certifications:** Pediatrics 1984, Pediatric Critical Care Medicine 1987; **Medical School:** Univ Wisc 1979; **Residency:** Pediatrics, Univ Wisc, Madison, WI 1980-1982; **Fellowship:** Pediatric Critical Care Medicine, Chldns Natl Med Ctr, Washintgon, DC 1982-1984; **Faculty Appointment:** Prof Pediatrics, Univ Wash

PEDIATRIC ENDOCRINOLOGY
New England

Levitsky, Lynne Lipton MD (Pediatric Endocrinology) - *Special Expertise: Diabetes; Growth/Development Disorders; Cushing's Syndrome;* **Admitting Hospital:** Massachusetts General Hospital; **Office Address:** Mass Genl Hosp, Dept Endo 55 Fruit St Boston, MA 02114; **Office Phone:** (617) 726-2909; **Board Certifications:** Pediatrics 1971, Pediatric Endocrinology 1978; **Medical School:** Yale Univ 1966; **Residencies:** Pediatrics, Albert Einstein Coll Med, Bronx, NY 1966-1967; Pediatrics, Children's Hosp, Philadelphia, PA 1967-1968; **Fellowship:** Pediatric Endocrinology, Univ Maryland Hosp, Baltimore, MD 1968-1970; **Faculty Appointment:** Assoc Prof Pediatrics, Harvard Med Sch

Tamborlane, William V MD (Pediatric Endocrinology) - *Special Expertise: Diabetes;* **Admitting Hospital:** Yale - New Haven Hospital; **Office Address:** Yale Sch Med 333 Cedar St New Haven, CT 06510-3289; **Office Phone:** (203) 785-4648; **Board Certifications:** Pediatrics 1978, Pediatric Endocrinology 1986; **Medical School:** Georgetown Univ 1972; **Residency:** Pediatrics, Georgetown U Hosp, Washington, DC 1972-1975; **Fellowship:** Pediatric Endocrinology, Yale U Sch Med, New Haven, CT 1975-1977

Mid Atlantic

Becker, Dorothy Joan MD (Pediatric Endocrinology) - *Special Expertise: Diabetes;* **Admitting Hospital:** Children's Hospital of Pittsburgh; **Office Address:** Children's Hosp-Pitts, Div EDM 3705 5th Ave Pittsburgh, PA 15213; **Office Phone:** (412) 692-5172; **Board Certifications:** Pediatrics 1978, Pediatric Endocrinology 1978; **Medical School:** Univ Pittsburgh 1964; **Residencies:** Endocrinology, Diabetes & Metabolism, Univ Capetown, South Africa 1972-1974; Pediatrics, Univ Capetown, South Africa 1970-1972; **Fellowship:** Pediatric Endocrinology, Univ Pitts, Pittsburgh, PA 1974-1976; **Faculty Appointment:** Prof Pediatrics, Univ Pittsburgh

Casella, Samuel Joseph MD (Pediatric Endocrinology) - *Special Expertise: Thyroid Disorders; Growth/Development Disorders;* **Admitting Hospital:** Johns Hopkins Hospital - Baltimore (Page 65); **Office Address:** Johns Hopkins Hosp 600 N Wolfe St, Bldg Park - Fl 2 - rm 211 Baltimore, MD 21287; **Office Phone:** (410) 955-3533; **Board Certifications:** Pediatric Endocrinology 1986, Pediatrics 1985; **Medical School:** SUNY Syracuse 1981; **Residency:** Pediatrics, Upstate Med Ctr, Syracuse, NY 1981-1984; **Fellowship:** Pediatric Endocrinology, NC Meml Hosp-Univ NC, Chapel Hill, NC 1984-1986; **Faculty Appointment:** Assoc Prof Pediatrics, Johns Hopkins Univ

Chrousos, George MD (Pediatric Endocrinology) - *Special Expertise: Stress Disorders;* **Admitting Hospital:** National Institutes of Health - Clinical Center; **Office Address:** Natl Hlth Inst 10 Centre Dr, Bldg 10 - rm 9D42 Bethesda, MD 20892-1583; **Office Phone:** (301) 496-5800; **Board Certifications:** Pediatrics 1980, Pediatric Endocrinology 1980; **Medical School:** Greece 1975; **Residency:** Pediatrics, NYU Med Ctr, New York, NY 1976-1978; **Fellowship:** Endocrinology, Natl Inst Hlth, Bethesda, MD 1978-1980

Levine, Lenore S. MD (Pediatric Endocrinology) - *Special Expertise: Sexual Development;* **Admitting Hospital:** Columbia Presbyterian Medical Center (Page 72); **Office Address:** 630 W 168th St, rm PHE52 New York, NY 10032; **Office Phone:** (212) 305-6559; **Board Certifications:** Pediatrics 1964, Pediatric Endocrinology 1978; **Medical School:** NYU Sch Med 1958; **Residencies:** Pediatric Endocrinology, NY Hosp, New York, NY 1967-1969; Pediatrics, Bellevue Hosp Ctr, New York, NY 1959-1960; **Fellowship:** Pediatrics, NY Hosp, New York, NY 1960-1961; **Faculty Appointment:** Prof Pediatrics, Columbia P&S

Moshang Jr., Thomas MD (Pediatric Endocrinology) - *Special Expertise:* *Growth/Development Disorders;* **Admitting Hospital:** The Children's Hospital of Philadelphia; **Office Address:** Children's Hospital of Philadelphia - Div Endocrinology 34th St and Civic Center Blvd Philadelphia, PA 19104; **Office Phone:** (215) 590-3173; **Board Certifications:** Pediatrics 1967, Pediatric Endocrinology 1978; **Medical School:** Univ MD Sch Med 1962; **Residency:** Pediatrics, Childrens Hosp, Philadelphia, PA 1963-1965; **Fellowship:** Pediatric Endocrinology, Childrens Hosp, Philadelphia, PA 1967-1970; **Faculty Appointment:** Prof Pediatrics, Univ Penn

New, Maria Iandolo MD (Pediatric Endocrinology) - *Special Expertise:* *Diabetes; Adrenal Disorders; Growth/Development Disorders;* **Admitting Hospital:** New York Weill Cornell Medical Center - NY Presbyterian Hospital (Page 72); **Office Address:** NY Weill Cornell Med Ctr- NY Presby 525 E 68th St, rm M622 New York, NY 10021; **Office Phone:** (212) 746-3450; **Board Certification:** Pediatrics 1960; **Medical School:** Univ Penn 1954; **Residency:** Pediatrics, NY Hosp, New York, NY 1955-1957; **Fellowships:** Pediatric Endocrinology, NY Hosp, New York, NY 1957-1958; Endocrinology, Diabetes & Metabolism, NY Hosp, New York, NY 1961-1964; **Faculty Appointment:** Prof Pediatrics, Cornell Univ-Weil Med Coll

Oberfield, Sharon MD (Pediatric Endocrinology) - *Special Expertise:* *Adrenal Disorders; Thyroid Disorders;* **Admitting Hospital:** Columbia Presbyterian Medical Center (Page 72); **Office Address:** Columbia Presby Med Ctr 630 W 168th St, Bldg PH - Fl 5E New York, NY 10032; **Office Phone:** (212) 305-6559; **Board Certifications:** Pediatrics 1979, Pediatric Endocrinology 1981; **Medical School:** Cornell Univ-Weil Med Coll 1974; **Residency:** Pediatrics, NY Hosp-Cornell, New York, NY 1974-1976; **Fellowship:** Pediatric Endocrinology, NY Hosp-Cornell, New York, NY 1976-1979; **Faculty Appointment:** Prof Pediatric Endocrinology, Columbia P&S

Plotnick, Leslie Parker MD (Pediatric Endocrinology) - *Special Expertise:* *Diabetes;* **Admitting Hospital:** Johns Hopkins Hospital - Baltimore (Page 65); **Office Address:** Johns Hopkins Hosp 600 N Wolfe St, Bldg Park - rm 211 Baltimore, MD 21287-2520; **Office Phone:** (410) 955-6463; **Board Certifications:** Pediatrics 1975, Pediatric Endocrinology 1978; **Medical School:** Univ MD Sch Med 1970; **Residency:** Pediatrics, Johns Hopkins Hosp, Baltimore, MD 1971-1972; **Fellowship:** Pediatric Endocrinology, Johns Hopkins Hosp, Baltimore, MD 1972-1974; **Faculty Appointment:** Assoc Prof Pediatrics, Johns Hopkins Univ

Slonim, Alfred MD (Pediatric Endocrinology) - *Special Expertise:* *Muscular Disorders-Metabolic;* **Admitting Hospital:** North Shore University Hospital at Manhasset; **Office Address:** North Shore Univ Hosp, Div Metabolism 300 Community Manhasset, NY 11030-3801; **Office Phone:** (516) 869-3390; **Board Certifications:** Pediatrics 1978, Pediatric Endocrinology 1986; **Medical School:** Australia 1958; **Residency:** Pediatrics, Royal Chlds Hosp, Melbourne, Australia 1961-1963; **Fellowship:** Pediatrics, Royal Chlds Hosp, Melbourne, Australia 1964-1965; **Faculty Appointment:** Assoc Prof Pediatrics, NYU Sch Med

Sperling, Mark Alexander MD (Pediatric Endocrinology) - *Special Expertise:* *Diabetes;* **Admitting Hospital:** Children's Hospital of Pittsburgh; **Office Address:** Chldns Hosp-Pittsburgh, Dept Endo 3705 Fifth Ave, DeSot Bldg, Fl 4A - Ste 400 Pittsburgh, PA 15213-2583; **Office Phone:** (412) 692-5172; **Board Certifications:** Pediatrics 1986, Pediatric Endocrinology 1986; **Medical School:** Australia 1962; **Residencies:** Internal Medicine, Prince Henry Hosp, Melbourne, Australia 1963-1964; Pediatrics, Royal Chldns Hosp, Melbourne, Australia 1964-1968; **Fellowship:** Pediatric Endocrinology, Chldns Hosp, Pittsburgh, PA 1968-1970; **Faculty Appointment:** Prof Pediatrics, Univ Pittsburgh

Southeast

Cleveland, William MD (Pediatric Endocrinology) - *Special Expertise:* Pediatric Endocrinology - General; **Admitting Hospital:** University of Miami - Jackson Memorial Hospital; **Office Address:** 1601 NW 12th Ave Miami, FL 33101; **Office Phone:** (305) 243-6936; **Board Certifications:** Pediatrics 1957, Pediatric Endocrinology 1978; **Medical School:** Meharry Med Coll 1950; **Residencies:** Pediatrics, Vanderbilt Univ, Nashville, TN 1951-1952; Pediatrics, Childrens Hosp, St Louis, MO 1955-1956; **Fellowship:** Pediatric Endocrinology, Johns Hopkins Hosp, Baltimore, MD 1958-1960; **Faculty Appointment:** Prof Pediatric Endocrinology, Univ Miami Sch Med

Diamond, Frank MD (Pediatric Endocrinology) - *Special Expertise:* Pediatric Endocrinology - General; **Admitting Hospital:** All Children's Hospital; **Office Address:** 880 6th St South, Ste 120 St Petersburg, FL 33701; **Office Phone:** (727) 892-4237; **Board Certifications:** Pediatrics 1979, Pediatric Endocrinology 1980; **Medical School:** Penn State Univ-Hershey Med Ctr 1974; **Residency:** Pediatrics, Childrens Hosp-Univ Alabama, Birmingham, AL 1975-1976; **Fellowship:** Pediatric Endocrinology, Childrens Hosp-Univ Penn, Philadelphia, PA 1976-1978; **Faculty Appointment:** Asst Clin Prof Pediatrics, Univ S Fla Coll Med

Freemark, Michael Scott MD (Pediatric Endocrinology) - *Special Expertise:* Thyroid Disorders; Growth/Development Disorders; Diabetes; **Admitting Hospital:** Duke University Medical Center (Page 60); **Office Address:** Duke Univ Med Ctr Erwin Rd, Bldg Bell - rm 314, Box 3080 Durham, NC 27710; **Office Phone:** (919) 684-3772; **Board Certifications:** Pediatric Endocrinology 1984, Pediatrics 1980; **Medical School:** Duke Univ 1976; **Residency:** Pediatrics, Duke Univ Med Ctr, Durham, NC 1976-1979; **Fellowships:** Pediatric Endocrinology, Duke Univ Med Ctr, Durham, NC 1980-1984; Pediatric Endocrinology, Hospital Necker Enfants Malades, Paris, France 1993-1993; **Faculty Appointment:** Assoc Prof Pediatrics, Duke Univ

Friedman, Nancy Eisenberg MD (Pediatric Endocrinology) - *Special Expertise:* Calcium Disorders; Bone Disorders-Metabolic; Growth/Development Disorders; **Admitting Hospital:** Duke University Medical Center (Page 60); **Office Address:** Duke Univ Med Ctr, Div Endocrinology PO Box 3080 Durham, NC 27710; **Office Phone:** (919) 684-3772; **Board Certifications:** Pediatrics 1979, Pediatric Endocrinology 1995; **Medical School:** Med Coll VA 1975; **Residencies:** Pediatrics, Chldns Hosp Med Ctr, Cincinnati, OH 1975-1977; Pediatrics, Chldns Meml Hosp, Chicago, IL 1977-1978; **Fellowship:** Endocrinology, Diabetes & Metabolism, Michael Reese Hosp, Chicago, IL 1978-1980; **Faculty Appointment:** Asst Clin Prof Pediatrics, Duke Univ

Schwartz, Robert P MD (Pediatric Endocrinology) - *Special Expertise:* Pediatric Endocrinology - General; **Admitting Hospital:** Wake Forest University Baptist Medical Center; **Office Address:** Wake Forest Univ Sch of Med - Dept Ped Med Ctr Blvd Winston Salem, NC 27157; **Office Phone:** (800) 277-7654; **Board Certifications:** Pediatric Endocrinology 1986, Pediatrics 1994; **Medical School:** Univ Fla Coll Med 1968; **Residencies:** Pediatrics, Charlotte Meml Hosp, Charlotte, NC 1969-1970; Pediatrics, Duke Med Ctr, Durham, NC 1971; **Fellowships:** Pediatric Endocrinology, Duke Med Ctr, Durham, NC 1970-1971; Pediatric Endocrinology, Duke Med Ctr, Durham, NC 1973-1974; **Faculty Appointment:** Assoc Prof Pediatrics, Wake Forest Univ Sch Med

Silverstein, Janet H MD (Pediatric Endocrinology) - *Special Expertise: Diabetes; Growth/Development Disorders;* **Admitting Hospital:** Shands Healthcare at University Florida (Page 77); **Office Address:** Univ Florida - Shands Hlthcare 1600 SW Archer Rd, Box 100296 Gainesville, FL 32610; **Office Phone:** (352) 334-1390; **Board Certifications:** Pediatrics 1975, Pediatric Endocrinology 1978; **Medical School:** Univ Penn 1970; **Residencies:** Pediatrics, Children's Hosp, Philadelphia, PA 1970-1972; Pediatrics, Children's Hosp, Philadelphia, PA 1974-1975; **Fellowship:** Pediatric Endocrinology, Duke Univ Med Ctr, Durham, NC 1975-1977; **Faculty Appointment:** Prof Pediatric Endocrinology, Univ Fla Coll Med

Midwest

Allen, David Bruce MD (Pediatric Endocrinology) - *Special Expertise: Diabetes;* **Admitting Hospital:** University of Wisconsin Hospital & Clinics; **Office Address:** 600 Highland Ave, rm H4-4 Madison, WI 53792; **Office Phone:** (608) 263-6420; **Board Certifications:** Pediatrics 1986, Pediatric Endocrinology 2003; **Medical School:** Duke Univ 1980; **Residency:** Pediatrics, Univ Wisc Hosp, Madison, WI 1982-1985; **Fellowship:** Pediatric Endocrinology, Univ Wisc Hosp, Madison, WI 1985-1988; **Faculty Appointment:** Assoc Prof Pediatrics, Univ Wisc

Dahms, William MD (Pediatric Endocrinology) - *Special Expertise: Diabetes; Growth/Development Disorders;* **Admitting Hospital:** Rainbow Babies & Children's Hospital; **Office Address:** 11100 Euclid Ave Ste 737 Cleveland, OH 44106; **Office Phone:** (216) 844-3661; **Board Certifications:** Pediatrics 1974, Pediatric Endocrinology 1983; **Medical School:** Univ Wash 1969; **Residency:** Pediatrics, Cornell Med Ctr, New York, NY 1969-1973; **Fellowship:** Pediatric Endocrinology, ULCA-Harbor Genl Hosp, Los Angeles, CA 1973-1975; **Faculty Appointment:** Prof Pediatrics, Case West Res Univ

Foster, Carol M MD (Pediatric Endocrinology) - *Special Expertise: Diabetes; Growth/Development Disorders; Pubertal Disorders;* **Admitting Hospital:** Motts Children's Hospital; **Office Address:** Univ Michigan Med Ctr - Endocrinology D1205 MPB 0718, Box 0718 Ann Arbor, MI 48109; **Office Phone:** (734) 764-5175; **Board Certifications:** Pediatrics 1983, Pediatric Endocrinology 1983; **Medical School:** Washington Univ, St Louis 1978; **Residency:** Pediatrics, Univ Utah, Salt Lake City, UT 1979-1981; **Fellowship:** Pediatric Endocrinology, NIH, Bethesda, MD 1981-1984; **Faculty Appointment:** Prof Pediatrics, Univ Mich Med Sch

Gutai, James MD (Pediatric Endocrinology) - *Special Expertise: Pediatric Endocrinology - General;* **Admitting Hospital:** Children's Hospital of Michigan; **Office Address:** Children's Hospital of Michigan 3901 Beaubien Blvd Detroit, MI 48201; **Office Phone:** (313) 745-5531; **Board Certifications:** Pediatrics 1977, Pediatric Endocrinology 1980; **Medical School:** Temple Univ 1970; **Residency:** Pediatrics, Johns Hopkins Hosp, Baltimore, MD 1975-1976; **Fellowship:** Pediatric Endocrinology, Johns Hopkins Hosp, Baltimore, MD 1973-1976; **Faculty Appointment:** Prof Pediatrics, Wayne State Univ

Levy, Richard Alshuler MD (Pediatric Endocrinology) - *Special Expertise: Adrenal Disorders; Pituitary Disorders; Thyroid Disorders;* **Admitting Hospital:** Rush/Presbyterian - St Luke's Medical Center - Chicago (Page 74); **Office Address:** 1725 W Harrison St, Ste 938 Chicago, IL 60612-3863; **Office Phone:** (312) 942-8989; **Board Certifications:** Pediatric Endocrinology 1986, Endocrinology, Diabetes & Metabolism 1985; **Medical School:** Louisiana State Univ 1971; **Residencies:** Internal Medicine, Univ Mass Med, Worchester, MA 1975-1977; Pediatrics, Beth Israel, New York, NY 1977-1978; **Fellowship:** Endocrinology, Diabetes & Metabolism, Barnes Hosp, St Louis, MO 1979-1982; **Faculty Appointment:** Asst Prof Medicine, Rush Med Coll

Maurer, William MD (Pediatric Endocrinology) - *Special Expertise: Growth/Development Disorders; Thyroid Disorders;* **Admitting Hospital:** Advocate Lutheran General Hospital; **Office Address:** Yacktman Pavilion 1675 Dempster St, Fl 3 Park Ridge, IL 60068; **Office Phone:** (847) 318-9330; **Board Certifications:** Pediatrics 1971, Pediatric Endocrinology 1978; **Medical School:** Ohio State Univ 1966; **Residency:** Pediatrics, Columbus Children's Hosp, Columbus, OH 1966-1968; **Fellowships:** Pediatric Endocrinology, Columbus Children's Hosp, Columbus, OH 1968-1970; Pediatric Endocrinology, Duke Univ Med Ctr, Durham, NC 1972-1975

Rogers, Douglas G MD (Pediatric Endocrinology) - *Special Expertise: Diabetes; Growth/Development Disorders; Thyroid Disorders;* **Admitting Hospital:** Cleveland Clinic Foundation; **Office Address:** Cleveland Clinic - Pediatric Endocrinology 9500 Euclid Ave, Box A120 Cleveland, OH 44195; **Office Phone:** (216) 445-8048; **Board Certifications:** Pediatrics 1984, Pediatric Endocrinology 1986; **Medical School:** Univ Hlth Sci/Chicago Med Sch 1978; **Residency:** Pediatrics, St Louis Univ Sch Med, St Louis, MO 1978-1981; **Fellowship:** Endocrinology, Diabetes & Metabolism, Wash Univ Sch Med, St Louis, MO 1983-1985

Rosenfield, Robert MD (Pediatric Endocrinology) - *Special Expertise: Acne; Pubertal Disorders; Menstrual Disorders-Hyperandrogenic;* **Admitting Hospital:** University of Chicago Hospitals (Page 78); **Office Address:** 5841 S Maryland Ave Univ of Chicago Hospital-Dept of Ped.Endocrin. Chicago, IL 60637; **Office Phone:** (773) 702-6169; **Board Certifications:** Pediatrics 1986, Pediatric Endocrinology 1986; **Medical School:** Northwestern Univ 1960; **Residency:** Pediatrics, Children's Hospital, Philadelphia, PA 1961-1963; **Fellowship:** Pediatric Endocrinology, Children's Hospital, Philadelphia, PA 1965-1968; **Faculty Appointment:** Prof Pediatrics, Univ Chicago-Pritzker Sch Med

White, Neil H MD (Pediatric Endocrinology) - *Special Expertise: Pediatric Endocrinology - General;* **Admitting Hospital:** St Louis Children's Hospital; **Office Address:** One Chldns Pl, rm 4S30 St Louis, MO 63110; **Office Phone:** (314) 454-6051; **Board Certifications:** Pediatrics 1981, Pediatric Endocrinology 1983; **Medical School:** Albert Einstein Coll Med 1975; **Residency:** Pediatrics, St Louis Chldns Hosp, St Louis, MO 1976-1977; **Fellowship:** Endocrinology, Diabetes & Metabolism, Washington Univ, St Louis, MO 1977-1979; **Faculty Appointment:** Assoc Prof Pediatrics, Univ Mich Med Sch

Zimmerman, Donald MD (Pediatric Endocrinology) - *Special Expertise: Growth/Development Disorders; Thyroid Cancer; Hyperthyroidism;* **Admitting Hospital:** Mayo Medical Center & Clinic - Rochester; **Office Address:** Mayo Clinic, Dept Peds 200 1st St SW Rochester, MN 55905; **Office Phone:** (507) 284-2091; **Board Certifications:** Pediatrics 1983, Pediatric Endocrinology 1983; **Residencies:** Internal Medicine, Johns Hopkins Hosp, Baltimore, MD 1975-1977; Pediatrics, Mayo Grad Sch Med, Rochester, MN 1980-1981; **Fellowship:** Endocrinology, Diabetes & Metabolism, Mayo Grad Sch Med, Rochester, MN 1977-1980

Great Plains and Mountains

Kappy, Michael Steven MD/PhD (Pediatric Endocrinology) - *Special Expertise: Growth/Development Disorders; Thyroid Disorders; Pubertal Disorders;* **Admitting Hospital:** The Children's Hospital - Denver; **Office Address:** Children's Hospital, Dept Ped Endocrinology 1056 E 19th Ave, Box 265 Denver, CO 80218; **Office Phone:** (303) 861-6061; **Board Certifications:** Pediatrics 1973, Pediatric Endocrinology 1980; **Medical School:** Univ Wisc 1967; **Residencies:** Pediatrics, Univ Colorado Med Ctr, Boulder, CO 1967-1968; Pediatrics, Univ Colorado Med Ctr, Boulder, CO 1970-1972; **Fellowship:** Pediatric Endocrinology, Johns Hopkins Hosp, Baltimore, MD 1978-1980; **Faculty Appointment:** Prof Pediatrics, Univ Colo

Klingensmith, Georgeanna MD (Pediatric Endocrinology) - *Special Expertise: Diabetes;* **Admitting Hospital:** University of Colorado Health & Science Center; **Office Address:** Barbara Davis Ctr for Childhood Diabetes 4200 E Ninth Ave, Box B-140 Denver, CO 80262; **Office Phone:** (303) 315-8796; **Board Certifications:** Pediatrics 1976, Pediatric Endocrinology 1978; **Medical School:** Duke Univ 1971; **Residency:** Pediatrics, Chldns Hosp, St Louis, MO 1972-1973; **Fellowship:** Pediatric Endocrinology, John Hopkins, Batimore, MD 1974-1976; **Faculty Appointment:** Prof Pediatrics, Univ Colo

Southwest

Kirkland III, John Lindsey MD (Pediatric Endocrinology) - *Special Expertise: Pediatric Endocrinology - General;* **Admitting Hospital:** Texas Children's Hospital - Houston; **Office Address:** Texas Chldns Hosp, Endo Clinic 6621 Fannin St Houston, TX 77030; **Office Phone:** (832) 824-3676; **Board Certifications:** Pediatrics 1973, Pediatric Endocrinology 1978; **Medical School:** Univ NC Sch Med 1968; **Residencies:** Pediatrics, Baylor, Houston, TX 1969-1970; Pediatrics, Guys Hosp, London,England 1970; **Fellowship:** Pediatric Endocrinology, Baylor, Houston, TX 1971-1973; **Faculty Appointment:** Prof Pediatrics, Baylor Coll Med

West Coast and Pacific

Geffner, Mitchell Eugene MD (Pediatric Endocrinology) - *Special Expertise: Growth/Development Disorders; Pubertal Disorders;* **Admitting Hospital:** UCLA Medical Center; **Office Address:** Mattel Children's Hosp at UCLA - Div Endocrinology 10833 Le Conte Ave, Bldg MDCC - rm 22-315 Los Angeles, CA 90095-1752; **Office Phone:** (310) 825-6496; **Board Certifications:** Pediatrics 1980, Pediatric Endocrinology 1983; **Medical School:** Albert Einstein Coll Med 1975; **Residency:** Pediatrics, LAC-USC Med Ctr, Los Angeles, CA 1975-1979; **Fellowship:** Pediatric Endocrinology, UCLA, Los Angeles, CA 1979; **Faculty Appointment:** Prof Pediatric Endocrinology, UCLA

Kaufman, Francine R MD (Pediatric Endocrinology) - *Special Expertise: Diabetes; Growth/Development Disorders;* **Admitting Hospital:** Children's Hospital - Los Angeles; **Office Address:** Children's Hospital - Div of Endocrinology 4650 W Sunset Blvd Los Angeles, CA 90027; **Office Phone:** (323) 669-4606; **Board Certifications:** Pediatrics 1980, Pediatric Endocrinology 1983; **Medical School:** Univ Hlth Sci/Chicago Med Sch 1976; **Residency:** Pediatrics, Chldn's Hosp, Los Angeles, CA 1976-1978; **Fellowship:** Pediatric Endocrinology, Chldn's Hosp, Los Angeles, CA 1978-1980; **Faculty Appointment:** Prof Pediatrics, USC Sch Med

Mahoney, Charles Patrick MD (Pediatric Endocrinology) - *Special Expertise: Diabetes; Growth/Development Disorders;* **Admitting Hospital:** Children's Hospital and Regional Medical Center - Seattle; **Office Address:** Children's Hospital - Dept. of Endocrinology 4800 Sand Point Way NE Seattle, WA 98105; **Office Phone:** (206) 528-2616; **Board Certifications:** Pediatric Endocrinology 1978, Pediatrics 1962; **Medical School:** Univ Colo 1955; **Residencies:** University Washington, Seattle, WA 1959-1960; Standford Hospitals, Stanford, CA 1958-1959; **Fellowship:** Pediatric Endocrinology, University Washington, Seattle, WA 1960-1963; **Faculty Appointment:** Clin Prof Pediatrics, Univ Wash

Wilson, Darrell Mealer MD (Pediatric Endocrinology) - *Special Expertise: Endocrinology;* **Admitting Hospital:** Stanford Medical Center; **Office Address:** Stanford Med Ctr, S-302 Stanford, CA 94305-5208; **Office Phone:** (650) 723-5791; **Board Certifications:** Pediatrics 1982, Pediatric Endocrinology 1995; **Medical School:** UCSD 1977; **Residency:** Pediatrics, Stanford, Stanford, CA 1978-1980; **Fellowship:** Endocrinology, Diabetes & Metabolism, Stanford, Stanford, CA 1980-1984; **Faculty Appointment:** Assoc Prof Pediatric Endocrinology, Stanford Univ

PEDIATRIC GASTROENTEROLOGY

New England

Kleinman, Ronald Ellis MD (Pediatric Gastroenterology) - *Special Expertise:* Transplant Medicine-Liver; Nutrition; **Admitting Hospital:** Massachusetts General Hospital; **Office Address:** Mass Genl Hosp 55 Fruit St, Vincent 107 Boston, MA; **Office Phone:** (617) 726-2930; **Board Certifications:** Pediatrics 1992, Pediatric Gastroenterology 2004; **Medical School:** NY Med Coll 1972; **Residency:** Pediatrics, Albert Einstein Coll Med, Bronx, NY 1973-1977; **Fellowship:** Pediatric Gastroenterology, Mass Genl Hosp, Boston, MA 1977-1980

Mid Atlantic

Levy, Joseph MD (Pediatric Gastroenterology) - *Special Expertise:* Gastroenterology; **Admitting Hospital:** Columbia Presbyterian Medical Center (Page 72); **Office Address:** Children's Digestive Hlth Ctr 3959 Broadway, Bldg BHN - rm 726 New York, NY 10032; **Office Phone:** (212) 305-5693; **Board Certifications:** Pediatrics 1979, Pediatric Gastroenterology 1990; **Medical School:** Israel 1973; **Residency:** Pediatrics, Beth Israel Med Ctr, New York, NY 1975-1977; **Fellowship:** Pediatric Gastroenterology, Columbia-Presby Med Ctr, New York, NY 1977-1979; **Faculty Appointment:** Clin Prof Pediatrics, Columbia P&S

Mones, Richard MD (Pediatric Gastroenterology) - *Special Expertise:* Pediatric Gastroenterology - General; **Admitting Hospital:** Columbia Presbyterian Medical Center (Page 72); **Office Address:** 401 W 118th St, Ste 2 New York, NY 10027; **Office Phone:** (212) 666-4610; **Board Certifications:** Pediatrics 1977, Pediatric Gastroenterology 1997; **Medical School:** NY Med Coll 1971; **Residencies:** Pediatrics, Columbia-Presby, New York, NY 1971-1973; Pediatrics, Columbia-Presby, New York, NY 1975-1977; **Fellowship:** Pediatrics, Columbia-Presby, New York, NY; **Faculty Appointment:** Columbia P&S

Newman, Leonard MD (Pediatric Gastroenterology) - *Special Expertise:* Pediatric Gastroenterology - General; **Admitting Hospital:** Westchester Medical Center; **Office Address:** NY Med College, Dept Ped Munger Pavillion - rm 123 Valhalla, NY 10595; **Office Phone:** (914) 594-4280; **Board Certifications:** Pediatrics 1975, Pediatric Gastroenterology 1990; **Medical School:** NY Med Coll 1970; **Residencies:** Pediatrics, Univ of Calif, San Diego, CA 1971-1972; Pediatrics, NY Med Coll, New York, NY 1972-1973; **Fellowship:** Gastroenterology, Albert Einstein, Bronx, NY 1973-1974; **Faculty Appointment:** Prof Pediatrics, NY Med Coll

Oliva-Hemker, Maria Magdalena MD (Pediatric Gastroenterology) - *Special Expertise:* Inflammatory Bowel Disease; **Admitting Hospital:** Johns Hopkins Hospital - Baltimore (Page 65); **Office Address:** Johns Hopkins Hosp 600 N Wolfe St, Bldg Brady - Fl 320 Baltimore, MD 21287-2631; **Office Phone:** (410) 955-8769; **Board Certifications:** Pediatric Gastroenterology 2000, Pediatrics 1990; **Medical School:** Johns Hopkins Univ 1986; **Residency:** Pediatrics, Johns Hopkins Hosp, Baltimore, MD 1986-1989; **Fellowship:** Gastroenterology, Johns Hopkins Hosp, Baltimore, MD 1989-1992

Schwarz, Kathleen MD (Pediatric Gastroenterology) - *Special Expertise:* Hepatitis C; Hepatitis B; **Admitting Hospital:** Johns Hopkins Hospital - Baltimore (Page 65); **Office Address:** Johns Hopkins Hosp, Div Ped Gastro & Nutrition 600 N Wolfe St N Brady 320 Baltimore, MD 21287; **Office Phone:** (410) 955-8769; **Board Certifications:** Pediatrics 1977, Pediatric Gastroenterology 1998; **Medical School:** Washington Univ, St Louis 1972; **Residency:** Pediatric Surgery, St Louis Chldrns Hosp, St Louis, MO 1972-1974; **Faculty Appointment:** Assoc Prof Pediatrics, Johns Hopkins Univ

578

Schwarz, Steven M MD (Pediatric Gastroenterology) - *Special Expertise:* Inflammatory Bowel Disease; Nutritional Disorders; Gastroesophageal Reflux; **Admitting Hospital:** Long Island College Hospital (Page 58); **Office Address:** LI Coll Hosp, Dept of Pediatrics 339 Hicks St Brooklyn, NY 11201-5514; **Office Phone:** (718) 780-1146; **Board Certifications:** Pediatrics 1979, Pediatric Gastroenterology 1997; **Medical School:** Columbia P&S 1974; **Residency:** Pediatrics, Columbia-Presby Med Ctr, New York, NY 1974-1977; **Fellowships:** Pediatric Gastroenterology, Stanford Med Ctr, Stanford, CA 1977-1978; Pediatric Gastroenterology, Columbia-Presby Med Ctr, New York, NY 1978-1980; **Faculty Appointment:** Prof Pediatrics, SUNY Hlth Sci Ctr

Southeast

Novak, Donald A MD (Pediatric Gastroenterology) - *Special Expertise:* Liver Disease; **Admitting Hospital:** Shands Healthcare at University Florida (Page 77); **Office Address:** Shands Healthcare at Univ Florida 1600 SW Archer Rd Gainesville, FL 32610-0296; **Office Phone:** (352) 392-6410; **Board Certifications:** Pediatrics 1987, Pediatric Gastroenterology 1990; **Medical School:** Univ S Fla Coll Med 1981; **Residency:** Pediatrics, Univ South Fla, Tampa, FL 1982-1984; **Fellowship:** Pediatric Gastroenterology, Childrens Hosp, Cincinnati, OH 1984-1987; **Faculty Appointment:** Prof Pediatrics, Univ Fla Coll Med

Rhoads, Jon Marc MD (Pediatric Gastroenterology) - *Special Expertise:* Pediatric Gastroenterology - General; **Admitting Hospital:** University of North Carolina Hospitals; **Office Address:** Univ of NC, Dept Ped CB 7220 Chapel Hill, NC 27599-7220; **Office Phone:** (919) 966-1343; **Board Certifications:** Pediatrics 1986, Pediatric Gastroenterology 1998; **Medical School:** Johns Hopkins Univ 1980; **Residency:** Pediatric Surgery, UCLA Med Ctr, Los Angeles, CA 1981-1983; **Fellowship:** Pediatrics, Hosp for Sick Chldn, Toronto, Canada 1983-1986; **Faculty Appointment:** Prof Pediatrics, Univ NC Sch Med

Thompson, John MD (Pediatric Gastroenterology) - *Special Expertise:* Crohn's Disease; Short Bowel Syndrome; Ulcerative Colitis; **Admitting Hospital:** University of Miami - Jackson Memorial Hospital; **Office Address:** Jackson Meml Hosp, Dept Ped, Div GE & Nutrition 1601 NW 12th Ave, rm 3005A, MC-CD 6001 Miami, FL 33136; **Office Phone:** (305) 243-6426; **Board Certifications:** Pediatric Gastroenterology 1998, Pediatrics 1983; **Medical School:** Loyola Univ-Stritch Sch Med 1977; **Residency:** Pediatrics, Wylers Chldns Hosp-Univ Chicago, Chicago, IL 1978-1980; **Fellowship:** Pediatric Gastroenterology, Babies Hosp-Columbia Univ, New York, NY 1982-1984; **Faculty Appointment:** Assoc Prof Pediatrics, Univ Miami Sch Med

Treem, William R MD (Pediatric Gastroenterology) - *Special Expertise:* Liver Disease; Inflammatory Bowel Disease; **Admitting Hospital:** Duke University Medical Center (Page 60); **Office Address:** Duke Univ Med Ctr Box 3009 Durham, NC 27710; **Office Phone:** (919) 684-5068; **Board Certifications:** Pediatrics 1981, Pediatric Gastroenterology 1997; **Medical School:** Stanford Univ 1977; **Residency:** Pediatrics, Children's Hosp, Boston, MA 1977-1980; **Fellowship:** Pediatric Gastroenterology, Children's Hosp, Philadelphia, PA 1982-1985; **Faculty Appointment:** Prof Pediatrics, Duke Univ

Ulshen, Martin H MD (Pediatric Gastroenterology) - *Special Expertise:* Intestinal Disease; Liver Disease; **Admitting Hospital:** Duke University Medical Center (Page 60); **Office Address:** Duke Univ Med Ctr Box 3009 Durham, NC 27710; **Office Phone:** (919) 684-5068; **Board Certifications:** Pediatrics 1993, Pediatric Gastroenterology 1997; **Medical School:** Univ Rochester 1969; **Residencies:** Pediatrics, Univ North Carolina Hosps, Chapel Hill, NC 1969-1970; Pediatrics, Univ Colorado, Denver, CO 1972-1974; **Fellowships:** Pediatric Gastroenterology, Univ Colorado, Denver, CO 1974-1975; Pediatric Gastroenterology, Chldns Hosp, Boston, MA 1975-1977; **Faculty Appointment:** Prof Pediatrics, Duke Univ

Midwest

Berman, James MD (Pediatric Gastroenterology) - *Special Expertise:* Inflammatory Bowel Disease; Feeding & Nutrition; **Admitting Hospital:** Loyola University Health System; **Office Address:** 2160 S First Ave Maywood, IL 60153; **Office Phone:** (708) 279-9073; **Board Certifications:** Pediatrics 1986, Pediatric Gastroenterology 1997; **Medical School:** Univ Pittsburgh 1981; **Residency:** Pediatrics, Chldns Hosp, Pittsburgh, PA 1981-1984; **Fellowship:** Pediatric Gastroenterology, Chldns Hosp, Boston, MA 1984-1987; **Faculty Appointment:** Asst Clin Prof Pediatrics, Loyola Univ-Stritch Sch Med

Boyle, John T MD (Pediatric Gastroenterology) - *Special Expertise:* Gastrointestinal Motility Disorders; Liver Disease; **Admitting Hospital:** Rainbow Babies & Children's Hospital; **Office Address:** 5850 Landerbrook Dr Mayfield Heights, OH 44124; **Office Phone:** (216) 844-1765; **Board Certifications:** Pediatrics 1993, Pediatric Gastroenterology 1998; **Medical School:** Cornell Univ-Weil Med Coll 1972; **Residency:** Pediatrics, Tufts-New England Med Ctr, Boston, MA 1973-1975; **Fellowship:** Pediatric Gastroenterology, Penn-Chldrns Hosp, Philadelphia, PA 1977-1979; **Faculty Appointment:** Assoc Prof Pediatrics, Case West Res Univ

El-Youssef, Mounif MD (Pediatric Gastroenterology) - *Special Expertise:* Liver Disease; **Admitting Hospital:** Mayo Medical Center & Clinic - Rochester; **Office Address:** Mayo Clinic-Peds Gastro 41402 200 1st St SW Rochester, MN 55905; **Office Phone:** (507) 284-2141; **Board Certifications:** Pediatric Gastroenterology 1990, Pediatrics 1989; **Medical School:** Belgium 1982; **Residency:** Pediatrics, Cleveland Clinic, Cleveland, OH 1985-1987; **Fellowship:** Pediatric Gastroenterology, Harvard Med Sch, Cambridge, MA 1987-1990

Gunasekaran, T S MD (Pediatric Gastroenterology) - *Special Expertise:* Pediatric Gastroenterology - General; **Admitting Hospital:** Advocate Lutheran General Hospital; **Office Address:** Lutheran Genl Chldns Hosp, Dept Ped Gastro 1675 Dempster St Park Ridge, IL 60068; **Office Phone:** (847) 318-9330; **Board Certifications:** Pediatrics 2000, Pediatric Gastroenterology 2000; **Medical School:** India 1977; **Residencies:** Pediatrics, Hosps, India 1977-1982; Pediatrics, Hosps, United Kingdom 1983-1987; **Fellowship:** Pediatric Gastroenterology, BC Childrens Hosp, Vancouver, Canada 1991-1992; **Faculty Appointment:** Asst Clin Prof Pediatrics, Univ Chicago-Pritzker Sch Med

Hillemeier, A Craig MD (Pediatric Gastroenterology) - *Special Expertise:* Gastroesophageal Reflux; Inflammatory Bowel Disease; **Admitting Hospital:** University of Michigan Health Center; **Office Address:** C S Mott Childrens Hospital 1500 E Medical Center Dr Ann Arbor, MI 48109-0200; **Office Phone:** (734) 936-4185; **Board Certifications:** Pediatrics 1981, Pediatric Gastroenterology 1998; **Medical School:** Loyola Univ-Stritch Sch Med 1976; **Residency:** Pediatrics, Loyola Univ Stritch, Maywood, IL 1976-1978; **Fellowship:** Pediatric Gastroenterology, Yale New Haven Med Ctr, New Haven, CT 1978-1982; **Faculty Appointment:** Prof Pediatrics, Univ Mich Med Sch

Kirschner, Barbara S MD (Pediatric Gastroenterology) - *Special Expertise:* Ulcerative Colitis; Abdominal Pain-Recurrent; Crohn's Disease; **Admitting Hospital:** University of Chicago Hospitals (Page 78); **Office Address:** Univ Chicago 5839 S Maryland Ave, rm C-474, MS 40-65 Chicago, IL 60637; **Office Phone:** (773) 702-6418; **Board Certifications:** Pediatrics 1977, Pediatric Gastroenterology 1999; **Medical School:** Med Coll PA Hahnemann 1967; **Residency:** Pediatrics, Univ of Chicago, Chicago, IL 1967-1970; **Fellowship:** Pediatric Gastroenterology, Univ of Chicago, Chicago, IL 1975-1977; **Faculty Appointment:** Prof Pediatrics, Univ Chicago-Pritzker Sch Med

Rothbaum, Robert Jay MD (Pediatric Gastroenterology) - *Special Expertise:* Inflammatory *Bowel Disease;* **Admitting Hospital:** St Louis Children's Hospital; **Office Address:** St Louis Chldns Hosp One Chldn Pl St Louis, MO 63110; **Office Phone:** (314) 454-6173; **Board Certifications:** Pediatrics 1981, Pediatric Gastroenterology 2004; **Medical School:** Univ Chicago-Pritzker Sch Med 1976; **Residency:** Pediatrics, Chldns Hosp Med Ctr, St Louis, MO 1977-1978; **Fellowships:** Ambulatory Pediatrics, Chldns Hosp Med Ctr, St Louis, MO 1978-1979; Pediatric Gastroenterology, Chldns Hosp Med Ctr, Cincinnati, OH 1979-1982; **Faculty Appointment:** Prof Pediatrics, Washington Univ, St Louis

Whitington, Peter MD (Pediatric Gastroenterology) - *Special Expertise:* Transplant *Medicine-Liver; Liver Disease;* **Admitting Hospital:** Children's Memorial Hospital; **Office Address:** Ped Gastroenterology, Hepatology and Nutrition 2300 Children's Plaza, Box 57 Chicago, IL 60614-3394; **Office Phone:** (773) 880-4643; **Board Certifications:** Pediatrics 1977, Pediatric Gastroenterology 1998; **Medical School:** Univ Tenn Coll Med, Memphis 1971; **Residency:** Pediatrics, Univ Tenn Hosp, Memphis, TN 1971-1974; **Fellowships:** Gastroenterology, Johns Hopkins, Baltimore, MD 1975-1977; Gastroenterology, Univ Wisconsin, Madison, WI 1977-1978; **Faculty Appointment:** Prof Pediatrics, Northwestern Univ

Wyllie, Robert MD (Pediatric Gastroenterology) - *Special Expertise:* Inflammatory Bowel *Disease; Esophageal Disorders;* **Admitting Hospital:** Cleveland Clinic Foundation; **Office Address:** 9500 Euclid Ave, #A120 Cleveland, OH 44195; **Office Phone:** (216) 444-2237; **Board Certifications:** Pediatrics 1982, Pediatric Gastroenterology 1997; **Medical School:** Indiana Univ 1976; **Residency:** Pediatrics, Indiana Univ Med Ctr, Indianapolis, IN 1977-1979; **Fellowship:** Pediatric Gastroenterology, Indiana Univ Med Ctr, Indianapolis, IN 1979-1980

Southwest

Klish, William John MD (Pediatric Gastroenterology) - *Special Expertise:* Pediatric *Gastroenterology - General;* **Admitting Hospital:** Texas Children's Hospital - Houston; **Office Address:** Baylor Coll Med Nutr & Gastro 3-3391 6621 Fannin St Houston, TX 77030-2303; **Office Phone:** (832) 824-3600; **Board Certifications:** Pediatrics 1992, Pediatric Gastroenterology 1998; **Medical School:** Univ Wisc 1967; **Residency:** Pediatrics, Baylor Sch Med, Houston, TX 1970-1972; **Fellowship:** Nutrition, Baylor Sch Med, Houston, TX 1972-1974; **Faculty Appointment:** Prof Pediatrics, Baylor Coll Med

West Coast and Pacific

Christie, Dennis MD (Pediatric Gastroenterology) - *Special Expertise:* Gastroenterology; **Admitting Hospital:** Children's Hospital and Regional Medical Center - Seattle; **Office Address:** Chldns Hosp Med Ctr, Div GE 4800 Sand Pointn Way, Box C 5371 Seattle, WA 98105-0371; **Office Phone:** (206) 526-2521; **Board Certifications:** Pediatrics 1992, Pediatric Gastroenterology 1998; **Medical School:** Northwestern Univ 1968; **Residency:** Pediatrics, Univ Washington, Seattle, WA 1969-1971; **Fellowship:** Pediatric Gastroenterology, UCLA Ctr Hlth & Sci, Los Angeles, CA 1974-1976; **Faculty Appointment:** Assoc Prof Pediatrics, Univ Wash

Heyman, Melvin Bernard MD (Pediatric Gastroenterology) - *Special Expertise:* Inflammatory Bowel Disease; Short Bowel Syndrome; **Admitting Hospital:** University of California - San Francisco Medical Center; **Office Address:** UCSF, Ped Ge Nutrition 500 Parnassus Ave, Box 0136 San Francisco, CA 94143-0136; **Office Phone:** (415) 476-5892; **Board Certifications:** Pediatrics 1981, Pediatric Gastroenterology 1998; **Medical School:** UCLA 1976; **Residency:** Pediatrics, LA Co-USC Med Ctr, Loa Angeles, CA 1976-1979; **Fellowship:** Gastroenterology, UCLA Med Ctr, Los Angeles, CA 1979-1981; **Faculty Appointment:** Prof Pediatrics, UCSF

McDiarmid, Suzanne V MD (Pediatric Gastroenterology) - *Special Expertise:* Transplant *Medicine-Liver; Transpant Medicine-Intestine; Transplant Immunology;* **Admitting Hospital:** UCLA Medical Center; **Office Address:** UCLA Med Ctr 200 Medical Plaza, Ste 265 Los Angeles, CA 90024; **Office Phone:** (310) 206-6134; **Board Certifications:** Pediatrics 1984, Pediatric Gastroenterology 2000; **Medical School:** New Zealand 1976; **Residencies:** Pediatrics, UCLA Med Center, Los Angeles, CA; Pediatrics, Univ Med Ctr; **Faculty Appointment:** Clin Prof Pediatric Surgery, UCLA

PEDIATRIC HEMATOLOGY-ONCOLOGY

New England

Weinstein, Howard MD (Pediatric Hematology-Oncology) - *Special Expertise:* Bone Marrow Transplant; Leukemia; Lymphoma; **Admitting Hospital:** Massachusetts General Hospital; **Office Address:** Mass General Hospital 55 Fruit Street WAC-712 Boston, MA 02114-2696; **Office Phone:** (617) 724-3315; **Board Certification:** Pediatrics 1977; **Medical School:** Univ MD Sch Med 1972; **Residency:** Pediatrics, Mass Genl Hosp, Boston, MA 1974

Mid Atlantic

Brodeur, Garrett MD (Pediatric Hematology-Oncology) - *Special Expertise:* Neuroblastoma; **Admitting Hospital:** The Children's Hospital of Philadelphia; **Office Address:** Children's Hospital of Philadelphia 34th & Civic Center Rd Philadelphia, PA 19104; **Office Phone:** (215) 590-3925; **Board Certifications:** Pediatrics 1980, Pediatric Hematology-Oncology 1980; **Medical School:** Washington Univ, St Louis 1975; **Residency:** Pediatrics, St Louis Childrns Hosp, St Louis, MO 1976-1977; **Fellowship:** Pediatric Hematology-Oncology, St Jude Childrns Rsch Hosp, Memphis, TN 1977-1979; **Faculty Appointment:** Prof Pediatrics, Univ Penn

Bussel, James MD (Pediatric Hematology-Oncology) - *Special Expertise:* Platelet Disorders; Immune Deficiency; Bleeding/Coagulation Disorders; **Admitting Hospital:** New York Weill Cornell Medical Center - NY Presbyterian Hospital (Page 72); **Office Address:** NYPH - Weill Med Coll of Cornell Univ 525 E 68th St, P-695 New York, NY 10021; **Office Phone:** (212) 746-3474; **Board Certifications:** Pediatric Surgery 1980, Pediatric Hematology-Oncology 1979; **Medical School:** Columbia P&S 1975; **Residency:** Pediatrics, Chldrns Hosp, Cincinnati, OH 1975-1978; **Fellowship:** Pediatric Hematology-Oncology, New York Hosp, New York, NY 1979-1981; **Faculty Appointment:** Assoc Prof Pediatric Hematology-Oncology, Cornell Univ-Weil Med Coll

Cairo, Mitchell MD (Pediatric Hematology-Oncology) - *Special Expertise:* Bone Marrow Transplant; Leukemia; **Admitting Hospital:** Columbia Presbyterian Medical Center (Page 72); **Office Address:** Babies and Children's Hospital, Columbia 3959 Broadway, Bldg BHN-8 - rm 801D New York, NY 10032; **Office Phone:** (212) 305-8316; **Board Certifications:** Pediatrics 1980, Pediatric Hematology-Oncology 1982; **Medical School:** UCSF 1976; **Residency:** Pediatrics, UCLA, Los Angeles, CA 1976-1978

Civin, Curt Ingraham MD (Pediatric Hematology-Oncology) - *Special Expertise:* Pediatric Hematology-Oncology - General; **Admitting Hospital:** Johns Hopkins Hospital - Baltimore (Page 65); **Office Address:** Johns Hopkins Hospital 1650 Orleans St, rm 2M44 Baltimore, MD 21231; **Office Phone:** (410) 955-8816; **Board Certifications:** Pediatrics 1979, Pediatric Hematology-Oncology 1980; **Medical School:** Harvard Med Sch 1974; **Residencies:** Pediatrics, Chldns Hosp, Boston, MA 1974-1975; Pediatrics, Chldns Hosp, Boston, MA 1975-1976; **Fellowship:** Pediatric Hematology-Oncology, Natl Cancer Inst, Bethesda, MD 1976-1979; **Faculty Appointment:** Prof Medical Oncology, Johns Hopkins Univ

Dover, George Joseph MD (Pediatric Hematology-Oncology) - *Special Expertise:* Sickle Cell Disease; **Admitting Hospital:** Johns Hopkins Hospital - Baltimore (Page 65); **Office Address:** Johns Hopkins Hosp 600 N Wolfe St, Ste CMSC - rm 2-116 Baltimore, MD 21287; **Office Phone:** (410) 955-5976; **Board Certifications:** Pediatric Hematology-Oncology 1978, Pediatrics 1976; **Medical School:** Louisiana State Univ 1972; **Residency:** Pediatrics, Johns Hopkins Hosp, Baltimore, MD 1973-1975; **Fellowship:** Pediatric Hematology-Oncology, Johns Hopkins Hosp, Baltimore, MD 1975-1977; **Faculty Appointment:** Prof Medicine, Johns Hopkins Univ

Garvin, James MD/PhD (Pediatric Hematology-Oncology) - *Special Expertise:* Pediatric Hematology-Oncology - General; **Admitting Hospital:** Columbia Presbyterian Medical Center (Page 72); **Office Address:** Div Ped Onc, Bldg HP - Fl 5 180 Fort Washington Ave, rm 539 New York, NY 10032; **Office Phone:** (212) 305-9770; **Board Certifications:** Pediatrics 1982, Pediatric Hematology-Oncology 1984; **Medical School:** Jefferson Med Coll 1976; **Residencies:** Pediatrics, Chldns Hosp, Philadelphia, PA 1976-1978; Pediatrics, Middlesex Hosp, London, England 1978-1979; **Fellowship:** Pediatric Hematology-Oncology, Chldns Hosp, Boston, MA 1979-1982; **Faculty Appointment:** Clin Prof Pediatrics, Columbia P&S

Keller Jr, Frank G MD (Pediatric Hematology-Oncology) - *Special Expertise:* Pediatric Hematology-Oncology - General; **Admitting Hospital:** West Virginia University Hospital - Ruby Memorial; **Office Address:** WVA Hlth Sci Ctr North Box 9214 Morgantown, WV 26506; **Office Phone:** (304) 293-1217; **Board Certifications:** Pediatrics 1990, Pediatric Hematology-Oncology 1994; **Medical School:** Univ NC Sch Med 1986; **Residency:** Pediatrics, Vanderbilt Univ Med Ctr, Nashville, TN 1986-1990; **Fellowship:** Pediatric Hematology-Oncology, Duke Univ Med Ctr, Durham, NC 1990-1993

Kushner, Brian MD (Pediatric Hematology-Oncology) - *Special Expertise:* Neuroblastoma; Bone Marrow Transplant; **Admitting Hospital:** Memorial Sloan Kettering Cancer Center; **Office Address:** 1275 York Ave, rm H1113 New York, NY 10021-6007; **Office Phone:** (212) 639-6793; **Board Certification:** Pediatrics 1983; **Medical School:** Johns Hopkins Univ 1976; **Residencies:** Pediatrics, NY Hosp, New York 1978-1979; Pediatrics, Colum-Presby Med Ctr, New York, NY 1977-1978; **Fellowship:** Pediatric Hematology-Oncology, Meml Sloan Kettering Cancer Ctr, New York, NY 1983-1986

Meek, Rita MD (Pediatric Hematology-Oncology) - *Special Expertise:* Pediatric Hematology-Oncology - General; **Admitting Hospital:** Alfred I Dupont Hospital for Children; **Office Address:** Alfred I Dupont Institute for Chilldren - Div of Hematology Oncology 1600 Rockland Rd Wilmington, DE 19899; **Office Phone:** (302) 651-5500; **Board Certifications:** Pediatrics 1979, Pediatric Hematology-Oncology 1980; **Medical School:** Geo Wash Univ 1974; **Residency:** Pediatrics, Childns Hosp Natl Med Ctr, Washington, DC 1975-1977; **Fellowship:** Pediatric Hematology-Oncology, Chldns Hosp Natl Med Ctr, Washington, DC 1977-1979; **Faculty Appointment:** Assoc Clin Prof Pediatrics, Jefferson Med Coll

Meyers, Paul MD (Pediatric Hematology-Oncology) - *Special Expertise:* Solid Tumors; Bone Tumors; **Admitting Hospital:** Memorial Sloan Kettering Cancer Center; **Office Address:** 1275 York Ave New York, NY 10021-6007; **Office Phone:** (212) 639-5952; **Board Certifications:** Pediatrics 1978, Pediatric Hematology-Oncology 1978; **Medical School:** Mount Sinai Sch Med 1973; **Residency:** Pediatrics, Mount Sinai, New York, NY 1973-1976; **Fellowship:** Pediatric Hematology-Oncology, NY Hosp-Cornell, New York, NY 1976-1979; **Faculty Appointment:** Assoc Clin Prof Pediatrics, Cornell Univ-Weil Med Coll

O'Reilly, Richard MD (Pediatric Hematology-Oncology) - *Special Expertise:* Bone Marrow Transplant; **Admitting Hospital:** Memorial Sloan Kettering Cancer Center; **Office Address:** Memorial Sloan Kettering Cancer Ctr 1275 York Ave, rm H1409 New York, NY 10021; **Office Phone:** (212) 639-5957; **Board Certifications:** Pediatric Hematology-Oncology 1973, Pediatrics 1974; **Medical School:** Univ Rochester 1968; **Residency:** Pediatrics, Chldrns Hosp, Boston, MA 1971-1972; **Fellowship:** Infectious Disease, Chldrns Hosp, Boston, MA 1972-1973

Reaman, Gregory MD (Pediatric Hematology-Oncology) - *Special Expertise: Leukemia; Oncology;* **Admitting Hospital:** Children's National Medical Center - DC; **Office Address:** Chldns Natl Med Ctr 111 Michigan Ave NW Washington, DC 20010-2916; **Office Phone:** (202) 884-2147; **Board Certifications:** Pediatric Hematology-Oncology, Pediatrics; **Medical School:** Loyola Univ-Stritch Sch Med 1973; **Residencies:** Hematology, Montreal Chldrns Hosp-McGill, Montreal, Canada 1974-1975; Pediatrics, Montreal Chldrns Hosp-McGill, Montreal, Canada 1975-1976; **Fellowship:** Pediatric Neuro-Oncology, Natl Cancer Inst, Bethesda, MD 1976-1979; **Faculty Appointment:** Prof Pediatrics, Geo Wash Univ

Schwartz, Cindy Lee MD (Pediatric Hematology-Oncology) - *Special Expertise: Osteosarcoma; Hodgkin's Disease;* **Admitting Hospital:** Johns Hopkins Hospital - Baltimore (Page 65); **Office Address:** Johns Hopkins Hosp 601 N Wolfe St, rm CMSC-800 Baltimore, MD 21287; **Office Phone:** (410) 955-2457; **Board Certifications:** Pediatrics 1985, Pediatric Hematology-Oncology 1994; **Medical School:** Brown Univ 1979; **Residency:** Pediatrics, Johns Hopkins, Baltimore, MD 1979-1982; **Faculty Appointment:** Assoc Prof Medical Oncology, Johns Hopkins Univ

Steinherz, Peter G MD (Pediatric Hematology-Oncology) - *Special Expertise: Burkett's Lymphoma; Leukemia;* **Admitting Hospital:** Memorial Sloan Kettering Cancer Center; **Office Address:** Memorial Sloan Kettering Cancer Ctr 1275 York Ave, Box 411 New York, NY 10021; **Office Phone:** (212) 639-7951; **Board Certifications:** Pediatrics 1973, Pediatric Hematology-Oncology 1978; **Medical School:** Albert Einstein Coll Med 1968; **Residency:** Pediatrics, NY Cornell Med Ctr, New York, NY 1969-1971; **Fellowship:** Pediatric Hematology-Oncology, NY Cornell Med Ctr, New York, NY 1973-1975; **Faculty Appointment:** Prof Pediatrics, Cornell Univ-Weil Med Coll

Weiner, Michael MD (Pediatric Hematology-Oncology) - *Special Expertise: Pediatric Hematology-Oncology - General;* **Admitting Hospital:** Columbia Presbyterian Medical Center (Page 72); **Office Address:** 180 Fort Washington Ave New York, NY 10032; **Office Phone:** (212) 305-9770; **Board Certifications:** Pediatrics 1980, Pediatric Hematology-Oncology 1980; **Medical School:** SUNY Hlth Sci Ctr 1972; **Residency:** Pediatrics, Montefiore Med Ctr, Bronx, NY 1973-1974; **Fellowships:** Pediatric Hematology-Oncology, NYU, New York, NY 1974-1976; Pediatric Hematology-Oncology, Johns Hopkins Univ, Baltimore, MD 1977-1977; **Faculty Appointment:** Prof Pediatrics, Columbia P&S

Southeast

Barbosa, Jerry L MD (Pediatric Hematology-Oncology) - *Special Expertise: Oncology;* **Admitting Hospital:** All Children's Hospital; **Office Address:** 880 6th St S, Ste 140 St Petersburg, FL 33701-4823; **Office Phone:** (727) 892-4175; **Board Certifications:** Pediatrics 1976, Pediatric Hematology-Oncology 1978; **Medical School:** Spain 1969; **Residency:** Pediatrics, RI Hosp-Brown Univ, Providence, RI 1972-1974; **Fellowship:** Pediatric Hematology-Oncology, Med Coll VA, Richmond, VA 1974-1976; **Faculty Appointment:** Assoc Clin Prof Pediatric Hematology-Oncology, Univ S Fla Coll Med

Falletta, John MD (Pediatric Hematology-Oncology) - *Special Expertise: Hematology;* **Admitting Hospital:** Duke University Medical Center (Page 60); **Office Address:** Duke Univ Med Ctr Box 2916 Durham, NC 27710-2916; **Office Phone:** (919) 684-3401; **Board Certifications:** Pediatrics 1972, Pediatric Hematology-Oncology 1974; **Medical School:** Univ Kans 1966; **Residencies:** Pediatrics, Baylor, Houston, TX 1969-1971; Pediatrics, Texas Childns Hosp, Houston, TX 1971; **Fellowship:** Pediatric Hematology-Oncology, Baylor, Houston, TX 1971-1973; **Faculty Appointment:** Prof Pediatric Hematology-Oncology, Duke Univ

Graham-Pole, John R MD (Pediatric Hematology-Oncology) - *Special Expertise:* *Pediatric Hematology-Oncology - General;* **Admitting Hospital:** Shands Healthcare at University Florida (Page 77); **Office Address:** Dept Ped Hematology-Oncology 2000 Archer Rd Gainesville, FL 32610-0296; **Office Phone:** (352) 392-5633; **Board Certifications:** Pediatrics 1983, Pediatric Hematology-Oncology 1987; **Medical School:** England 1966; **Residencies:** Pediatrics, Hosp Sick Chldn, London, England 1968; Pediatrics, Royal Hosp Sick Chldn, London, England 1970; **Fellowship:** Pediatric Hematology-Oncology, Royal Hosp for Sick Chldn, Glasgow, England 1971; **Faculty Appointment:** Prof Pediatrics, Univ Fla Coll Med

Pegelow Jr, Charles Henry MD (Pediatric Hematology-Oncology) - *Special Expertise:* *Sickle Cell Disease; Bleeding/Coagulation Disorders;* **Admitting Hospital:** University of Miami - Jackson Memorial Hospital; **Office Address:** Univ Miami Sch of Med - Dept Ped (R131) 1611 NW 12th East Tower Ave, rm 6006 Miami, FL 33136; **Office Phone:** (305) 585-6042; **Board Certifications:** Pediatrics 1975, Pediatric Hematology-Oncology 1976; **Medical School:** Univ Minn 1970; **Residency:** Pediatrics, LA County - USC Med Ctr, Los Angeles, CA; **Fellowship:** Pediatric Hematology-Oncology, LA County - USC Med Ctr, Los Angeles, CA; **Faculty Appointment:** Prof Pediatrics, Univ Miami Sch Med

Rosoff, Phillip Martin MD (Pediatric Hematology-Oncology) - *Special Expertise:* *Cancer Survivors; Down Syndrome; Leukemia;* **Admitting Hospital:** Duke University Medical Center (Page 60); **Office Address:** 750 Washington St, Ste 245 Durham, NC 02111; **Office Phone:** (919) 684-6946; **Board Certifications:** Pediatrics 1984, Pediatric Hematology-Oncology 1994; **Medical School:** Case West Res Univ 1978; **Residency:** Pediatrics, Children's Hosp, Boston, MA 1978-1980; **Fellowship:** Pediatric Hematology-Oncology, Children's Hosp, Boston, MA 1980-1984; **Faculty Appointment:** Assoc Prof Pediatric Hematology-Oncology, Duke Univ

Midwest

Abella, Esteban MD (Pediatric Hematology-Oncology) - *Special Expertise:* *Bone Marrow Transplant;* **Admitting Hospital:** Children's Hospital of Michigan; **Office Address:** Chldrns Hosp, Div Ped/Hem 3901 Beaubien Blvd, Ste 2 Detroit, MI 48201; **Office Phone:** (313) 745-5515; **Board Certifications:** Pediatric Hematology-Oncology 1994, Pediatrics 1998; **Medical School:** Dominican Republic 1985; **Residency:** Pediatrics, Chldrns Hosp, Detroit, MI 1985-1988; **Fellowship:** Pediatric Hematology-Oncology, Chldrns Hosp, Detroit, MI 1988-1991; **Faculty Appointment:** Assoc Clin Prof Pediatric Hematology-Oncology, Wayne State Univ

Castle, Valerie MD (Pediatric Hematology-Oncology) - *Special Expertise:* *Neuroblastoma; Bleeding/Coagulation Disorders;* **Admitting Hospital:** University of Michigan Health Center; **Office Address:** Univ Mich Comp Cancer & Ger Ctrs, Box 0938 1500 E Medical Ctr, rm 4303 Ann Arbor, MI 48109; **Office Phone:** (734) 936-9814; **Board Certifications:** Pediatrics 1992, Pediatric Hematology-Oncology 1998; **Medical School:** McMaster Univ 1983; **Residency:** Pediatrics, McMaster Univ Med Ctr, Hamilton, ON 1984-1986; **Fellowship:** Pediatric Hematology-Oncology, Univ Mich Hosp, Ann Arbor, MI 1986-1989; **Faculty Appointment:** Assoc Prof Pediatrics, Univ Mich Med Sch

Crist, William MD (Pediatric Hematology-Oncology) - *Special Expertise:* *Leukemia-Acute Lymphcytic; Rhabdomyosarcoma;* **Admitting Hospital:** Mayo Medical Center & Clinic - Rochester; **Office Address:** Mayo Clinic 200 First St SW Rochester, MN 55905; **Office Phone:** (507) 284-3300; **Board Certifications:** Pediatrics 1975, Pediatric Hematology-Oncology 1976; **Medical School:** Univ MO-Columbia Sch Med 1969; **Residency:** Pediatric Hematology-Oncology, Washington Univ, St Louis, MO 1970-1972; **Faculty Appointment:** Prof Pediatrics, Univ Rochester

Ferrara, James MD (Pediatric Hematology-Oncology) - *Special Expertise:* Bone Marrow Transplant; Graft vs Host Disease; **Admitting Hospital:** University of Michigan Health Center; **Office Address:** Bone Marrow Transplant Ctr 1500 E Med Ctr Dr, rm 6308 Ann Arbor, MI 48109-0942; **Office Phone:** (734) 936-4015; **Board Certification:** Pediatrics 1997; **Medical School:** Georgetown Univ 1980; **Residency:** Pediatrics, Chldns Hosp, Boston, MA; **Fellowship:** Pediatric Hematology-Oncology, Chldns Hosp, Boston, MA; **Faculty Appointment:** Prof Pediatrics, Univ Mich Med Sch

Nachman, James MD (Pediatric Hematology-Oncology) - *Special Expertise:* Leukemia; Osteogenic Sarcomas; **Admitting Hospital:** University of Chicago Hospitals (Page 78); **Office Address:** 5841 S Maryland Ave, MC-4060 Chicago, IL 60637; **Office Phone:** (773) 702-6808; **Board Certifications:** Pediatrics 1979, Pediatric Hematology-Oncology 1980; **Medical School:** Johns Hopkins Univ 1974; **Residencies:** Pediatrics, Chldns Meml Hosp, Chicago, IL 1975-1977; Pediatrics, Fell-Wylers Chldns Hosp, Chicago, IL 1979-1980; **Fellowship:** Pediatric Hematology-Oncology, Chldns Meml Hosp, Chicago, IL 1977-1979; **Faculty Appointment:** Prof Pediatric Surgery, Univ Chicago-Pritzker Sch Med

Puccetti, Diane MD (Pediatric Hematology-Oncology) - *Special Expertise:* Brain Tumors; Neuro-Oncology; **Admitting Hospital:** University of Wisconsin Hospital & Clinics; **Office Address:** Univ Wisc Chldns Hosp 600 Highland Ave, rm K4/430 Madison, WI 53706; **Office Phone:** (608) 263-6420; **Board Certifications:** Pediatrics 1989, Pediatric Hematology-Oncology 2000; **Medical School:** Med Coll OH 1985; **Residencies:** Pediatrics, UC-Irvine, Orange, CA 1985-1986; Pediatrics, Med Coll Ohio, Toledo, OH 1986-1988; **Fellowship:** Pediatric Hematology-Oncology, Riley Hosp for Chldn, Indianapolis, IN 1988-1991; **Faculty Appointment:** Asst Clin Prof Pediatrics, Univ Wisc

Sondel, Paul M MD (Pediatric Hematology-Oncology) - *Special Expertise:* Pediatric Hematology-Oncology - General; **Admitting Hospital:** University of Wisconsin Hospital & Clinics; **Office Address:** Univ Wisc Clinics 600 Highland Ave, K4/448 Clinical Sci Ctr Madison, WI 53792; **Office Phone:** (608) 263-6420; **Board Certification:** Pediatrics 1981; **Medical School:** Harvard Med Sch 1977; **Residency:** Pediatrics, Univ Wisc Hosp, Madison, WI 1978-1980; **Fellowships:** Research, Sidney Farber Cancer Inst/Harvard, Boston, MA 1975-1977; Pediatric Hematology-Oncology, Midwest Chldns Cancer Ctr, Milwaukee, WI 1980; **Faculty Appointment:** Prof Pediatrics, Univ Wisc

Suarez, Carlos MD (Pediatric Hematology-Oncology) - *Special Expertise:* Hematology; **Admitting Hospital:** Loyola University Health System; **Office Address:** 2160 S First Ave Maywood, IL 60153; **Office Phone:** (708) 216-9200; **Board Certifications:** Pediatrics 1978, Pediatric Hematology-Oncology 1984; **Medical School:** Puerto Rico 1972; **Residency:** Pediatrics, Mayo Clinic, Rochester, MN 1973-1975; **Fellowship:** Hematology and Oncology, Meml Sloan-Kettering Cancer Ctr, New York, NY 1979-1981; **Faculty Appointment:** Assoc Prof Pediatrics, Loyola Univ-Stritch Sch Med

Valentino, Leonard A MD (Pediatric Hematology-Oncology) - *Special Expertise:* Hematology; Bleeding/Coagulation Disorders; **Admitting Hospital:** Rush/Presbyterian - St Luke's Medical Center - Chicago (Page 74); **Office Address:** 1725 W Harrison St, Ste 710 Chicago, IL 60612-3828; **Office Phone:** (312) 942-5983; **Board Certification:** Pediatrics 1988; **Medical School:** Creighton Univ 1984; **Residency:** Pediatrics, Univ Illinios Med Ctr, Chicago, IL 1984-1987; **Fellowship:** Pediatric Hematology-Oncology, UCLA Med Ctr, Los Angeles, CA 1987-1990; **Faculty Appointment:** Asst Prof Pediatrics, Rush Med Coll

Great Plains and Mountains

Carroll, William L MD (Pediatric Hematology-Oncology) - *Special Expertise:* Pediatric Hematology-Oncology - General; **Admitting Hospital:** Primary Children's Medical Center; **Office Address:** Primary Chldn's Med Ctr, Dept Hem/Onc 100 N Medical Dr Salt Lake City, UT 84113; **Office Phone:** (801) 588-2680; **Board Certifications:** Pediatrics 1984, Pediatric Hematology-Oncology 1987; **Medical School:** UC Irvine 1978; **Residencies:** Pediatrics, Chldns Hosp, Cincinnati, OH 1978-1979; Pediatrics, Chldns Hosp, Cincinnati, OH 1979-1981; **Fellowships:** Pediatric Hematology-Oncology, Stanford Univ, Stanford, CA 1982-1984; Pediatric Hematology-Oncology, Stanford Univ, Stanford, CA 1984-1987; **Faculty Appointment:** Prof Pediatrics, Univ Utah

Odom, Lorrie Furman MD (Pediatric Hematology-Oncology) - *Special Expertise:* Leukemia; Solid Tumors; **Admitting Hospital:** The Children's Hospital - Denver; **Office Address:** Children's Hosp Cancer Ctr 1056 E 19th Ave Denver, CO 80218-1007; **Office Phone:** (303) 861-6740; **Board Certifications:** Pediatrics 1974, Pediatric Hematology-Oncology 1976; **Medical School:** Univ Colo 1969; **Residencies:** Pediatrics, Chldns Hosp, Boston, MA 1969-1970; Pediatrics, Chldrns Hosp, Boston, MA 1970-1972; **Fellowships:** Pediatric Hematology-Oncology, Dana-Farber Cancer Inst, Boston, MA 1972-1974; Pediatric Hematology-Oncology, Univ Colo Med Ctr, Denver, CO 1974-1975; **Faculty Appointment:** Prof Pediatrics, Univ Colo

Southwest

Berg, Stacy MD (Pediatric Hematology-Oncology) - *Special Expertise:* Pediatric Hematology-Oncology - General; **Admitting Hospital:** Texas Children's Hospital - Houston; **Office Address:** Pediatric Hematology-Oncology 6621 Fannin St Houston, TX 77030; **Office Phone:** (832) 824-4588; **Board Certifications:** Pediatrics 2000, Pediatric Hematology-Oncology 2000; **Medical School:** Univ Pittsburgh 1985; **Residency:** Pediatrics, Chldns Hosp, Pittsburgh, PA 1985-1988; **Fellowship:** Pediatric Hematology-Oncology, NIH, Bethesda, MD 1988-1991

Bleyer, W Archie MD (Pediatric Hematology-Oncology) - *Special Expertise:* Leukemia; Brain & Spinal Cord Tumors; **Admitting Hospital:** University of Texas MD Anderson Cancer Center (Page 66); **Office Address:** Univ Texas/MD Anderson Cancer Ctr 1515 Holcombe Blvd Houston, TX 77030-4009; **Office Phone:** (713) 792-6603; **Board Certifications:** Pediatrics 1986, Pediatric Hematology-Oncology 1986; **Medical School:** Univ Rochester 1969; **Residencies:** Pediatric Hematology-Oncology, NCI, Bethesda, MA 1971-1974; Pediatrics, Univ Washington, Seattle, WA 1970-1971; **Fellowship:** Pediatric Hematology-Oncology, Univ Washington, Seattle, WA 1974-1975

West Coast and Pacific

Feig, Stephen A MD (Pediatric Hematology-Oncology) - *Special Expertise:* Pediatric Hematology-Oncology - General; **Admitting Hospital:** UCLA Medical Center; **Office Address:** UCLA Medical Center - Department of Pediatrics Los Angeles, CA 90024; **Office Phone:** (310) 825-6708; **Board Certifications:** Pediatrics 1968, Pediatric Hematology-Oncology 1974; **Medical School:** Columbia P&S 1963; **Residency:** Pediatrics, Mt Sinai Hospital, New York, NY 1963-1966; **Fellowship:** Pediatric Hematology-Oncology, Children's Hospital, Boston, MA 1968-1972; **Faculty Appointment:** Prof Pediatrics, UCLA

Glader, Bertil E MD (Pediatric Hematology-Oncology) - *Special Expertise:* Pediatric Hematology-Oncology - General; **Admitting Hospital:** Stanford Medical Center; **Office Address:** Stanford Univ Medical Center, Dept Ped Hem-Onc 300 Pasteur Dr Stanford, CA 94305-5208; **Office Phone:** (650) 723-5535; **Board Certifications:** Hematology 1983, Pediatric Hematology-Oncology 1994; **Medical School:** Northwestern Univ 1968; **Residency:** Pediatrics, Chldns Hosp Med Ctr, Boston, MA 1972-1973; **Fellowship:** Hematology, Chldns Hosp Med Ctr, Boston, MA 1973-1975

Matthay, Katherine Kurshan MD (Pediatric Hematology-Oncology) - *Special Expertise:* Hematology/Oncology; Neuroblastoma/Solid Tumors; Retinoblastoma; **Admitting Hospital:** University of California - San Francisco Medical Center; **Office Address:** UCSF, Dept Ped Onc 505 Parnassus Ave, Box 0106 San Francisco, CA 94143; **Office Phone:** (415) 476-0603; **Board Certifications:** Pediatrics 1979, Pediatric Hematology-Oncology 1980; **Medical School:** Univ Penn 1973; **Residency:** Pediatrics, Univ of CO, Denver, CO 1974-1976; **Fellowship:** Pediatric Hematology-Oncology, UCSF, San Francisco, CA 1977-1979; **Faculty Appointment:** Prof Pediatrics, UCSF

Siegel, Stuart E MD (Pediatric Hematology-Oncology) - *Special Expertise:* Brain Tumors; Cancer & Infections; **Admitting Hospital:** Children's Hospital - Los Angeles; **Office Address:** Children's Hospital 4650 Sunset Blvd, MS 54 Los Angeles, CA 90027-6016; **Office Phone:** (323) 669-2205; **Board Certifications:** Pediatrics 1973, Pediatric Hematology-Oncology 1976; **Medical School:** Boston Univ 1967; **Residency:** Pediatrics, U Minnesota Hosps, MN 1968-1969; **Fellowship:** Pediatric Hematology-Oncology, Natl Cancer Inst, Bethesda, MD 1969-1972; **Faculty Appointment:** Prof Pediatrics, USC Sch Med

PEDIATRIC INFECTIOUS DISEASE

New England

Andiman, Warren A. MD (Pediatric Infectious Disease) - *Special Expertise:* AIDS/HIV; **Admitting Hospital:** Yale - New Haven Hospital; **Office Address:** Yale University School of Medicine 333 Cedar St, rm 418 LSOG New Haven, CT 06520; **Office Phone:** (203) 785-4730; **Board Certifications:** Pediatric Infectious Disease 1975, Pediatric Infectious Disease; **Medical School:** Albert Einstein Coll Med 1969; **Residency:** Pediatrics, Babies Hosp-Col Presby, New York, NY 1969-1971; **Fellowship:** Pediatric Infectious Disease, Yale Univ Sch Med, New Haven, CT 1971-1973; **Faculty Appointment:** Prof Pediatrics, Yale Univ

Durbin, William Applebee MD (Pediatric Infectious Disease) - *Special Expertise:* Pediatric Infectious Disease - General; **Admitting Hospital:** UMASS Memorial Health Care - Worcester; **Office Address:** UMASS Memorial Health Care 55 Lake Ave N Worcester, MA; **Office Phone:** (508) 856-2650; **Board Certifications:** Pediatrics 1978, Pediatric Infectious Disease 2001; **Medical School:** Columbia P&S 1972; **Residency:** Pediatrics, Boston Chlns Hosp, Boston, MA 1975-1977; **Fellowship:** Infectious Disease, Boston Chldns Hosp/beth Israel, Boston, MA 1977-1979; **Faculty Appointment:** Prof Pediatrics, Univ Mass Sch Med

Shapiro, Eugene D MD (Pediatric Infectious Disease) - *Special Expertise:* Lyme Disease; **Admitting Hospital:** Yale - New Haven Hospital; **Office Address:** Yale Sch Med, Dept Ped 333 Cedars St New Haven, CT 06520; **Office Phone:** (203) 688-4518; **Board Certifications:** Pediatrics 1980, Pediatric Infectious Disease 1994; **Medical School:** UCSF 1976; **Residency:** Pediatrics, Chldns Hosp, Pittsburgh, PA 1976-1979; **Fellowships:** Pediatric Infectious Disease, Chldns Hosp, Pittsburgh, PA 1979-1981; Research, Yale Univ, New Haven, CT 1981-1983; **Faculty Appointment:** Assoc Prof Pediatrics, Yale Univ

Mid Atlantic

Borkowsky, William MD (Pediatric Infectious Disease) - *Special Expertise:* AIDS/HIV; **Admitting Hospital:** NYU Medical Center (Page 70); **Office Address:** 550 1st Ave New York, NY 10016; **Office Phone:** (212) 263-6513; **Board Certifications:** Pediatrics 1979, Infectious Disease 1979; **Medical School:** NYU Sch Med 1979; **Residency:** Pediatrics, Bellevue Hosp, New York, NY 1972-1975; **Fellowship:** Infectious Disease, NYU Sch of Med, New York, NY 1975-1978; **Faculty Appointment:** Prof Pediatrics, NYU Sch Med

Gershon, Anne MD (Pediatric Infectious Disease) - *Special Expertise:* Herpes; Meningitis; **Admitting Hospital:** Columbia Presbyterian Medical Center (Page 72); **Office Address:** 650 W 168th St, Ste BD4 - rm 427 New York, NY 10032-3702; **Office Phone:** (212) 305-9445; **Board Certifications:** Pediatrics 1969, Infectious Disease 1994; **Medical School:** Cornell Univ-Weil Med Coll 1964; **Residency:** Pediatrics, NY Hosp-Cornell, New York, NY 1966-1968; **Fellowships:** Infectious Disease, New York Univ, New York, NY 1968-1970; Infectious Disease, Oxford Univ, Oxford, England; **Faculty Appointment:** Prof Pediatrics, Columbia P&S

Long, Sarah S MD (Pediatric Infectious Disease) - *Special Expertise:* Pediatric Infectious Disease - General; **Admitting Hospital:** St Christopher's Hospital for Children; **Office Address:** St Christopher's Hosp for Chldrn 1112 Erie Ave @ Front St Philadelphia, PA 19134; **Office Phone:** (215) 427-5204; **Board Certifications:** Pediatrics 1993, Pediatric Infectious Disease 2001; **Medical School:** Jefferson Med Coll 1970; **Residency:** Pediatrics, St Chris Hosp Chldn, Philadelphia, PA 1971-1973; **Fellowship:** Pediatric Infectious Disease, Temple Univ Sch Med, Philadelphia, PA 1973-1975; **Faculty Appointment:** Prof Pediatrics, Hahnemann Univ

Rennels, Margaret MD (Pediatric Infectious Disease) - *Special Expertise:* Pediatric
Infectious Disease - General; **Admitting Hospital:** University of Maryland Medical System; **Office
Address:** Univ Maryland Sch of Med 22 S Greene St Baltimore, MD 21201-1554; **Office Phone:**
(410) 328-6919; **Board Certifications:** Pediatrics 1979, Pediatric Infectious Disease 1994; **Medical
School:** Univ MD Sch Med 1973; **Residency:** Pediatrics, Univ MD Hosp, Baltimore, MD 1974-1977;
Fellowship: Infectious Disease, Univ MD Hosp, Baltimore, MD 1977-1979; **Faculty Appointment:**
Prof Pediatrics, Univ MD Sch Med

Saiman, Lisa MD (Pediatric Infectious Disease) - *Special Expertise:* Cystic Fibrosis Infection;
Fungal Infection; Hospital Epidemiology; **Admitting Hospital:** Columbia Presbyterian Medical
Center (Page 72); **Office Address:** 650 W 168th St, Ste 427 New York, NY 10032-3702; **Office
Phone:** (212) 305-7935; **Board Certification:** Pediatrics 1987; **Medical School:** Albert Einstein Coll
Med 1983; **Residency:** Pediatrics, Babies Hosp, New York, NY 1983-1986; **Fellowship:** Infectious
Disease, Babies Hosp, New York, NY

Singh, Nalini MD (Pediatric Infectious Disease) - *Special Expertise:* Infectious Disease;
Admitting Hospital: Children's National Medical Center - DC; **Office Address:** Chldns Hosp Natl
Med Ctr, Dept Inf Disease 111 Michigan Ave NW Washington, DC 20010; **Office Phone:** (202)
884-5051; **Board Certifications:** Pediatrics 1982, Pediatric Infectious Disease 1997; **Medical
School:** India 1973; **Residency:** Pediatrics, Univ Mass Med Ctr, Worcester, MA 1976-1979;
Fellowship: Infectious Disease, Natl Inst Med Sci, Bethesda, MD 1979-1981; **Faculty Appointment:**
Assoc Prof Infectious Disease, Geo Wash Univ

Wald, Ellen MD (Pediatric Infectious Disease) - *Special Expertise:* Urinary Tract Infections;
Infection-Respiratory; **Admitting Hospital:** Children's Hospital of Pittsburgh; **Office Address:**
Chldns Hosp of Pittsburgh 3705 Fifth Ave Pittsburgh, PA 15213; **Office Phone:** (412) 692-5105;
Board Certifications: Pediatrics 1973, Pediatric Infectious Disease 1994; **Medical School:** SUNY
Downstate 1968; **Residency:** Pediatrics, Kings Co Hosp, Brooklyn, NY 1969-1971; **Fellowship:**
Infectious Disease, Univ MD Hosp, Baltimore, MD 1973; **Faculty Appointment:** Prof Pediatrics, Univ
Pittsburgh

Southeast

Clements III, Dennis Alfred MD/PhD (Pediatric Infectious Disease) - *Special Expertise:*
Vaccine Preventable Diseases; **Admitting Hospital:** Duke University Medical Center (Page 60);
Office Address: Duke Univ Med Ctr Box 3810 Durham, NC 27710; **Office Phone:** (919) 613-7651;
Board Certifications: Pediatrics 1978, Pediatric Infectious Disease 2004; **Medical School:** Univ
Rochester 1973; **Residency:** Pediatrics, Duke Univ Med Ctr, Durham, NC 1974-1976; **Fellowship:**
Pediatric Infectious Disease, Duke Univ Med Ctr, Durham, NC 1986-1988; **Faculty Appointment:**
Assoc Prof Pediatrics, Duke Univ

Emmanuel, Patricia MD (Pediatric Infectious Disease) - *Special Expertise:* Infections in
Immune Deficient; **Admitting Hospital:** Tampa General Hospital; **Office Address:** Pediatric Clinic
17 Davis Blvd Tampa, FL 33606; **Office Phone:** (813) 259-8800; **Board Certifications:** Pediatrics
1998, Pediatric Infectious Disease 1994; **Medical School:** Univ Fla Coll Med 1986; **Residency:**
Pediatrics, Univ So Fla, Tampa, FL 1986-1989; **Fellowship:** Infectious Disease, Univ So Fla, Tampa,
FL 1990-1993; **Faculty Appointment:** Asst Prof Pediatrics, Univ S Fla Coll Med

Givner, Laurence Bruce MD (Pediatric Infectious Disease) - *Special Expertise:* AIDS/HIV; *Fevers-Unknown Origin;* **Admitting Hospital:** Wake Forest University Baptist Medical Center; **Office Address:** Wake Forest University School of Medicine,Dept. Pediatrics 1 Medical Center Blvd Winston Salem, NC 27157-0001; **Office Phone:** (336) 716-9661; **Board Certifications:** Pediatrics 1984, Pediatric Infectious Disease 2001; **Medical School:** Univ MD Sch Med 1978; **Residency:** Pediatrics, Univ Maryland, Baltimore, MD 1979-1982; **Fellowship:** Infectious Disease, Baylor Coll Med, Houston, TX 1982-1984

Gorensek, Margaret MD (Pediatric Infectious Disease) - *Special Expertise:* Infectious Disease; AIDS/HIV; Chronic Fatigue Syndrome; **Admitting Hospital:** Cleveland Clinic Florida; **Office Address:** Cleveland Clinic Florida 3000 W Cypress Creek Rd Fort Lauderdale, FL 33309-1743; **Office Phone:** (954) 978-5165; **Board Certifications:** Pediatrics 1986, Infectious Disease 1988; **Medical School:** Case West Res Univ 1981; **Residency:** Pediatrics, Cleveland Clinic, Cleveland, OH 1981-1985; **Fellowship:** Infectious Disease, Cleveland Clinic, Cleveland, OH 1985-1987; **Faculty Appointment:** Asst Clin Prof Medicine, Univ Miami Sch Med

Ingram, David MD (Pediatric Infectious Disease) - *Special Expertise:* Infectious Disease; **Admitting Hospital:** WakeMed New Bern Avenue Campus; **Office Address:** Wake Med Ctr, Med Education Inst 3024 New Bern Ave, Ste 307 Raleigh, NC 27610-1215; **Office Phone:** (919) 350-7846; **Board Certifications:** Pediatrics 1980, Pediatric Infectious Disease 1994; **Medical School:** Yale Univ 1967; **Residency:** Pediatrics, Yale-New Haven Hosp, New Haven, Ct 1968-1971; **Fellowship:** Pediatric Infectious Disease, Chldns Hosp Med Ctr, Boston, MA 1971-1973; **Faculty Appointment:** Prof Pediatrics, Univ NC Sch Med

McKinney Jr, Ross E MD (Pediatric Infectious Disease) - *Special Expertise:* Infections in Immune Deficient; **Admitting Hospital:** Duke University Medical Center (Page 60); **Office Address:** Duke Univ Med Ctr PO Box 3499 Durham, NC, 27710; **Office Phone:** (919) 684-6335; **Board Certification:** Pediatrics 1983; **Medical School:** Univ Rochester 1979; **Residency:** Pediatrics, Duke Univ Med Ctr, Durham, NC 1982-1985; **Fellowship:** Pediatrics, Duke Univ Med Ctr, Durham, NC 1979-1982; **Faculty Appointment:** Assoc Prof Pediatrics, Duke Univ

Mitchell, Charles MD (Pediatric Infectious Disease) - *Special Expertise:* AIDS/HIV; Infections-Viral; **Admitting Hospital:** University of Miami - Jackson Memorial Hospital; **Office Address:** Jackson Meml, Dept Ped Inf Disease 1550 NW 10th Ave, Ste 201 Miami, FL 33136; **Office Phone:** (305) 243-2755; **Board Certifications:** Pediatric Infectious Disease 1994, Pediatrics 1986; **Medical School:** Univ Tex Med Br, Galveston 1977; **Residency:** Pediatrics, Univ Minn Hosp, Minneapolis, MN; **Fellowship:** Pediatric Infectious Disease, Univ Minn Hosp, Minneapolis, MN; **Faculty Appointment:** Asst Prof Pediatrics, Univ Miami Sch Med

Scott, Gwendolyn MD (Pediatric Infectious Disease) - *Special Expertise:* AIDS/HIV; **Admitting Hospital:** University of Miami - Jackson Memorial Hospital; **Office Address:** Univ Miami Sch Med, Dept Ped Div Inf Dis/Immun, Box 016960 (D4-4) Miami, FL 33101; **Office Phone:** (305) 243-6676; **Board Certifications:** Pediatrics 1978, Pediatric Infectious Disease 1994; **Medical School:** UCSF 1972; **Residencies:** Pediatrics, San Fran Genl Hosp, San Francisco, CA 1972-1973; Pediatrics, Univ MD Hosp, Baltimore, MD 1974-1975; **Fellowship:** Pediatric Infectious Disease, Univ Miami, Miami, FL 1976-1978; **Faculty Appointment:** Prof Pediatrics, Univ Miami Sch Med

Midwest

Kleiman, Martin MD (Pediatric Infectious Disease) - *Special Expertise: Pediatric Infectious Disease - General;* **Admitting Hospital:** Riley Hospital for Children; **Office Address:** Riley Hospital for Children 702 Barnhill Drive Indianapolis, IN 46202; **Office Phone:** (317) 274-5000; **Board Certifications:** Pediatrics 1973, Pediatric Infectious Disease 1994; **Medical School:** SUNY Syracuse 1968; **Residency:** Pediatrics, Upstate Med Ctr, Syracuse, NY 1969-1971; **Fellowship:** Infectious Disease, Johns Hopkins Hosp, Baltimore, MD 1973-1976; **Faculty Appointment:** Prof Pediatrics, Indiana Univ

Shackelford, Penelope Greta MD (Pediatric Infectious Disease) - *Special Expertise: Pediatric Infectious Disease - General;* **Admitting Hospital:** St Louis Children's Hospital; **Office Address:** St Louis Chldrns Hosp One Chldrns Pl rm 2S26 St Louis, MO 63110; **Office Phone:** (314) 454-6050; **Board Certifications:** Pediatric Infectious Disease 2001, Pediatrics 1973; **Medical School:** Washington Univ, St Louis 1968; **Residency:** Pediatrics, St Louis Chldns Hosp, St Louis, MO 1969-1971; **Fellowship:** Infectious Disease, St Louis Chldns Hosp, St Louis, MO 1970-1972; **Faculty Appointment:** Prof Pediatrics, Washington Univ, St Louis

Southwest

Baker, Carol MD (Pediatric Infectious Disease) - *Special Expertise: Infection-B Strep; Neonatal Infections;* **Admitting Hospital:** Texas Children's Hospital - Houston; **Office Address:** Texas Children's Hospital 6621 Fannin, MC-3-2371 Houston, TX 77030; **Office Phone:** (713) 798-4790; **Board Certifications:** Pediatrics 1973, Pediatric Infectious Disease 1994; **Medical School:** Baylor Coll Med 1968; **Residency:** Pediatrics, Baylor Coll of Med, Houston, TX 1969-1971; **Fellowships:** Infectious Disease, Baylor Coll of Med, Houston, TX 1971-1973; Harvard Med Sch, Boston, MA 1973-1974; **Faculty Appointment:** Prof Pediatrics, Baylor Coll Med

Jacobs, Richard MD (Pediatric Infectious Disease) - *Special Expertise: Tuberculosis;* **Admitting Hospital:** Arkansas Children's Hospital; **Office Address:** Ark Children's Hospital 800 Marshall St Little Rock, AR; **Office Phone:** (501) 320-1202; **Board Certifications:** Pediatrics 1982, Pediatric Infectious Disease 1994; **Medical School:** Univ Ark 1977; **Residency:** Pediatrics, Ark Chldns Hosp, Little Rock, AR 1977-1980; **Fellowship:** Infectious Disease, Univ Wash, Seattle, WA 1980-1982; **Faculty Appointment:** Prof Pediatrics, Univ Ark

Jenson, Hal B MD (Pediatric Infectious Disease) - *Special Expertise: Epstein-Barr Virus;* **Admitting Hospital:** University of Texas Health & Science Center; **Office Address:** 7703 Floyd Curl Dept. of Pediatrics San Antonio, TX 78229-3900; **Office Phone:** (210) 567-5301; **Board Certifications:** Pediatric Infectious Disease 1994, Pediatrics 1985; **Medical School:** Geo Wash Univ 1979; **Residency:** Pediatrics, Rainbow Babies-Chldns Hosp., Cleveland, OH 1979-1983; **Fellowship:** Pediatric Infectious Disease, Yale U. Sch. Med., New Haven, CT 1983-1985; **Faculty Appointment:** Prof Pediatrics, Univ Tex, San Antonio

Kaplan, Sheldon MD (Pediatric Infectious Disease) - *Special Expertise: Pediatric Infectious Disease - General;* **Admitting Hospital:** Texas Children's Hospital - Houston; **Office Address:** Texas Chldrns Hosp, Div Ped Inf Dis 6621 Fannin St, Ste 1150, MC-3-2371 Houston, TX 77030; **Office Phone:** (832) 824-4330; **Board Certifications:** Pediatrics 1978, Pediatric Infectious Disease 1994; **Medical School:** Univ MO-Columbia Sch Med 1973; **Residency:** Pediatrics, St Louis Chldns Hosp, St Louis, MO 1979-1981; **Faculty Appointment:** Prof Pediatrics, Baylor Coll Med

PEDIATRIC INFECTIOUS DISEASE Southwest

Kline, Mark MD (Pediatric Infectious Disease) - *Special Expertise: AIDS/HIV;* **Admitting Hospital:** Texas Children's Hospital - Houston; **Office Address:** Baylor Coll of Med, Dept Peds 1 Baylor Plaza, MC-1-4000 Houston, TX 77030-3411; **Office Phone:** (832) 824-1038; **Board Certifications:** Pediatrics 1987, Pediatric Infectious Disease 1994; **Medical School:** Baylor Coll Med 1981; **Residency:** Pediatrics, Baylor Coll Med, Houston, TX 1981-1985; **Fellowship:** Pediatric Infectious Disease, Baylor Coll Med, Houston, TX 1985-1987; **Faculty Appointment:** Prof Pediatrics, Baylor Coll Med

Waagner, David MD (Pediatric Infectious Disease) - *Special Expertise: Pediatric Infectious Disease - General;* **Admitting Hospital:** University Medical Center; **Office Address:** 3601 4th St, rm 4b104 Lubbock, TX 79430-0001; **Office Phone:** (806) 743-7337; **Board Certifications:** Pediatrics 1998, Pediatric Infectious Disease 1994; **Medical School:** Texas Tech Univ 1984; **Residency:** Pediatrics, Lubbock Genl Hosp/Tex Tech, Lubbock, TX 1984-1987; **Fellowship:** Pediatric Infectious Disease, Univ Tex Med Ctr, Dallas, TX 1987-1989; **Faculty Appointment:** Assoc Prof Pediatrics, Texas Tech Univ

West Coast and Pacific

Bradley, John S MD (Pediatric Infectious Disease) - *Special Expertise: Meningococcemia; Brain Infections; Meningitis;* **Admitting Hospital:** Children's Hospital and Health Center; **Office Address:** Children's Hosp and Hlth Ctr 3020 Children Way, MC-5041 San Diego, CA 92123; **Office Phone:** (858) 495-7785; **Board Certifications:** Pediatrics 1981, Pediatric Infectious Disease 1994; **Medical School:** UC Davis 1976; **Residency:** Pediatrics, UC - Davis, Sacramento, CA; **Fellowship:** Pediatric Infectious Disease, Stanford Univ, Stanford, CA; **Faculty Appointment:** Assoc Clin Prof Pediatrics, UCSD

Bryson, Yvonne Joyce MD (Pediatric Infectious Disease) - *Special Expertise: AIDS/HIV;* **Admitting Hospital:** UCLA Medical Center; **Office Address:** UCLA Sch Med, Dept Ped 10833 Le Conte Ave Los Angeles, CA 90095-1752; **Office Phone:** (310) 825-5235; **Board Certification:** Pediatrics 1976; **Medical School:** Univ Tex SW, Dallas 1970; **Residencies:** Pediatrics, UCSD Med Ctr, San Diego, CA 1971-1974; Pediatrics, UCSD Med Ctr, San Diego, CA 1974-1974; **Fellowship:** Infectious Disease, UCSD Med Ctr, San Diego, CA 1974-1976; **Faculty Appointment:** Prof Pediatric Infectious Disease, UCLA

Cherry, James Donald MD (Pediatric Infectious Disease) - *Special Expertise: Pediatric Infectious Disease - General;* **Admitting Hospital:** Children's Hospital - Los Angeles; **Office Address:** UCLA, Dept Ped rm 22-442 MDCC 10833 Le Conte Ave Los Angeles, CA 90095-1752; **Office Phone:** (310) 825-5226; **Board Certifications:** Pediatrics 1962, Pediatric Infectious Disease 2001; **Medical School:** Univ VT Coll Med 1957; **Residencies:** Pediatrics, Boston City Hosp, Boston, MA 1958-1959; Pediatrics, Kings Co Hosp, Brooklyn, NY 1959-1960; **Fellowship:** Internal Medicine, Boston, Boston, MA 1961-1962; **Faculty Appointment:** Prof Pediatrics, UCLA

Mason, Wilbert Henry MD (Pediatric Infectious Disease) - *Special Expertise: Kawasaki Disease;* **Admitting Hospital:** Children's Hospital - Los Angeles; **Office Address:** 4650 W Sunset Blvd Los Angeles, CA 90027-6062; **Office Phone:** (310) 669-2509; **Board Certifications:** Pediatrics 1975, Pediatric Infectious Disease 1994; **Medical School:** UC Irvine 1970; **Residency:** Childrens Hosp, Los Angeles, CA 1971-1973; **Fellowship:** Infectious Disease, Childrens Hospital, Los Angeles, CA 1973-1974; **Faculty Appointment:** Assoc Clin Prof Pediatrics, USC Sch Med

PEDIATRIC NEPHROLOGY

New England

Harmon, William E MD (Pediatric Nephrology) - *Special Expertise: Pediatric Nephrology - General;* **Admitting Hospital:** Children's Hospital; **Office Address:** 300 Longwood Ave Boston, MA 02115-5737; **Office Phone:** (617) 355-6129; **Board Certifications:** Pediatrics 1976, Pediatric Critical Care Medicine 1998; **Medical School:** Case West Res Univ 1971; **Residency:** Pediatrics, Childrens Hosp Med Ctr, Boston, MA 1972-1976; **Fellowship:** Pediatric Nephrology, Childrens Hosp Med Ctr, Boston, MA 1976-1979; **Faculty Appointment:** Assoc Prof Pediatrics, Harvard Med Sch

Mid Atlantic

Fivush, Barbara A MD (Pediatric Nephrology) - *Special Expertise: Pediatric Nephrology - General;* **Admitting Hospital:** Johns Hopkins Hospital - Baltimore (Page 65); **Office Address:** Johns Hopkins Hosp-Div. Nephrology 600 N Wolfe St, Bldg Park - rm 327 Baltimore, MD 21205-2104; **Office Phone:** (410) 955-2467; **Medical School:** Boston Univ 1978; **Residency:** Pediatrics, Johns Hopkins Hosp, Baltimore, MD 1979-1981; **Fellowships:** Pediatric Nephrology, Johns Hopkins Hosp, Baltimore, MD 1981-1983; Pediatric Nephrology, Childns Hosp-Natl Med Ctr, Washington, DC 1983-1984; **Faculty Appointment:** Assoc Prof Pediatrics, Johns Hopkins Univ

Kaplan, Bernard S MD (Pediatric Nephrology) - *Special Expertise: Hemolytic Uremic Syndrome; Polycystic Kidney Disease;* **Admitting Hospital:** The Children's Hospital of Philadelphia; **Office Address:** Children's Hosp-Philadelphia, Dept Nephrology 34th St & Civic Blvd, rm 2143 Philadelphia, PA 19104; **Office Phone:** (215) 590-2449; **Board Certifications:** Pediatrics 1972, Pediatric Nephrology 1974; **Medical School:** South Africa 1964; **Residency:** Pediatrics, South Africa 1967-1970; **Fellowship:** Nephrology, Montreal Chldns Hosp, Canada 1970-1972; **Faculty Appointment:** Prof Pediatrics, Univ Penn

Nash, Martin MD (Pediatric Nephrology) - *Special Expertise: Pediatric Nephrology - General;* **Admitting Hospital:** Columbia Presbyterian Medical Center (Page 72); **Office Address:** Babies & Childrens Hosp of New York 3959 Broadway, rm 701 New York, NY 10032-1537; **Office Phone:** (212) 305-5825; **Board Certifications:** Pediatrics 1969, Nephrology 1974; **Medical School:** Duke Univ 1964; **Residencies:** Internal Medicine, Georgetown Univ Hosp, Washington, DC 1964-1965; Pediatrics, Columbia-Presbyterian, New York, NY 1965-1967; **Fellowship:** Pediatric Nephrology, Albert Einstein Coll of Med, Bronx, NY 1969-1971; **Faculty Appointment:** Clin Prof Pediatrics, Columbia P&S

Roskes, Saul David MD (Pediatric Nephrology) - *Special Expertise: Pediatric Nephrology - General;* **Admitting Hospital:** Johns Hopkins Hospital - Baltimore (Page 65); **Office Address:** Maryland Pediatric 10807 Falls Rd, Ste 200 Lutherville, MD 21093-4502; **Office Phone:** (410) 321-9393; **Board Certifications:** Pediatrics 1970, Pediatric Nephrology 1976; **Medical School:** Johns Hopkins Univ 1963; **Residencies:** Pediatrics, Bronx Muni Hosp Ctr., New York, NY 1964-1965; Pediatrics, Johns Hopkins Hosp, Baltimore, MD 1967-1968; **Faculty Appointment:** Assoc Prof Pediatrics, Johns Hopkins Univ

Southeast

Bunchman, Timothy E MD (Pediatric Nephrology) - *Special Expertise:* Lupus Nephritis; **Admitting Hospital:** University of Alabama Hospital at Birmingham; **Office Address:** Univ Alabama-Birmingham 1600 Seventh Ave S Birmingham, AL 35233-0011; **Office Phone:** (205) 939-9141; **Board Certifications:** Pediatrics 1986, Pediatric Nephrology 1996; **Medical School:** Loyola Univ-Stritch Sch Med 1981; **Residencies:** Pediatrics, St Louis Univ, St Louis, MO 1982-1984; Internal Medicine, St Louis Univ, St Louis, MO; **Fellowships:** Pediatric Nephrology, Mayo Clinic, Rochester, MN 1985-1986; Pediatric Nephrology, Univ Minn, Minneapolis, MN 1986-1987; **Faculty Appointment:** Prof Pediatrics, Univ Ala

Chandar, Jayanthi MD (Pediatric Nephrology) - *Special Expertise:* Pediatric Nephrology - General; **Admitting Hospital:** University of Miami - Jackson Memorial Hospital; **Office Address:** Jackson Memorial Hosp, Div Ped Nephrology Box 016960, MS M714 Miami, FL 33163; **Office Phone:** (305) 585-6726; **Board Certifications:** Pediatric Nephrology 1995, Pediatrics 1998; **Medical School:** India 1983; **Residency:** Pediatrics, Jackson Memorial Hosp, Miami, FL 1985-1987; **Fellowship:** Pediatric Nephrology, Jackson Memorial Hosp, Miami, FL 1991; **Faculty Appointment:** Asst Prof Pediatrics, India

Fennell III, Robert Samuel MD (Pediatric Nephrology) - *Special Expertise:* Transplant Medicine-Kidney; Kidney Failure-Chronic; **Admitting Hospital:** Shands Healthcare at University Florida (Page 77); **Office Address:** Shands Healthcare at Univ Florida 1600 SW Archer Rd, Box 100296 Gainesville, FL 32610-0296; **Office Phone:** (352) 392-8250; **Board Certifications:** Pediatrics 1974, Pediatric Nephrology 2000; **Medical School:** Univ Fla Coll Med 1964; **Residency:** Pediatrics, Shands Teaching Hosp, Gainesville, FL 1969-1971; **Fellowship:** Pediatric Nephrology, Shands Teaching Hosp, Gainesville, FL 1972-1973; **Faculty Appointment:** Prof Pediatrics, Univ Fla Coll Med

Garin, Eduardo Humberto MD (Pediatric Nephrology) - *Special Expertise:* Pediatric Nephrology - General; **Admitting Hospital:** Tampa General Hospital; **Office Address:** 17 Davis Blvd, Ste 200 Tampa, FL 33606-3438; **Office Phone:** (813) 272-2345; **Board Certifications:** Pediatrics 1976, Pediatric Nephrology 1976; **Medical School:** Chile 1970; **Residency:** Pediatrics, Univ Hosp and Clinics, Colombia, MO 1972-1973; **Fellowship:** Pediatric Nephrology, Shands at Univ FL, Gainesville, FL 1973-1975; **Faculty Appointment:** Prof Pediatrics, Univ S Fla Coll Med

Richard, George MD (Pediatric Nephrology) - *Special Expertise:* Hypertension; Hematuria; Kidney Disease; **Admitting Hospital:** Shands Healthcare at University Florida (Page 77); **Office Address:** Shands Healthcare at Univ Fla 1600 SW Archer Rd, rm HD214, Box 100296 Gainesville, FL 32610-0296; **Office Phone:** (352) 392-4434; **Board Certifications:** Pediatrics 1967, Pediatric Nephrology 1974; **Medical School:** Univ Pittsburgh 1961; **Residencies:** Nephrology, Univ Florida, Gainesville, FL 1967-1968; Pediatrics, Chldns Hosp, Pittsburgh, PA 1964-1967; **Fellowship:** Nephrology, Univ Florida, Gainesville, FL 1967-1968; **Faculty Appointment:** Prof Pediatrics, Univ Fla Coll Med

Midwest

Andreoli, Sharon MD (Pediatric Nephrology) - *Special Expertise:* Kidney Disease; **Admitting Hospital:** Riley Hospital for Children; **Office Address:** Barnhill Wells Research Ctr 2626 Indianapolis, IN 46202-5225; **Office Phone:** (317) 274-2563; **Board Certifications:** Pediatrics 1981, Pediatric Nephrology 1983; **Medical School:** Indiana Univ 1978; **Residency:** Pediatrics, James W Riley Hosp, Indianapolis, IN 1978-1981; **Fellowships:** Pediatric Nephrology, U Minnesota, Minneapolis, MN 1981; Pediatric Nephrology, James W Riley Hosp, Indianapolis, IN 1982-1984; **Faculty Appointment:** Prof Pediatrics, Indiana Univ

Avner, Ellis D MD (Pediatric Nephrology) - *Special Expertise: Polycystic Kidney Disease;* **Admitting Hospital:** Rainbow Babies & Children's Hospital; **Office Address:** Rainbow Babies & Chldrn's Hosp 1100 Euclid Cleveland, OH 44106-6003; **Office Phone:** (216) 844-3884; **Board Certifications:** Pediatrics 1980, Pediatric Nephrology 1982; **Medical School:** Univ Penn 1975; **Residency:** Pediatrics, Chldrn's Hosp, Boston, MA 1976-1978; **Fellowship:** Pediatric Nephrology, Chldrn's Hosp, Boston, MA 1978-1980; **Faculty Appointment:** Prof Pediatrics, Case West Res Univ

Bergstein, Jerry MD (Pediatric Nephrology) - *Special Expertise: Dialysis-Peritoneal; Kidney Disease; Hypertension;* **Admitting Hospital:** Riley Hospital for Children; **Office Address:** Riley Hospital for Children 702 Barnhill Drive Indianapolis, IN 46202; **Office Phone:** (317) 274-2563; **Board Certifications:** Pediatrics 1971, Pediatric Nephrology 1974; **Medical School:** Univ Minn 1965; **Residencies:** Pediatrics, U Minn, Minneapolis, MN 1966-1967; Pediatrics, U Mlnn, Minneapolis, MN 1969-1970; **Fellowship:** Pediatric Nephrology, U Minn, Minneapolis, MN 1970-1973; **Faculty Appointment:** Prof Pediatric Nephrology, Indiana Univ

Cohn, Richard MD (Pediatric Nephrology) - *Special Expertise: Transplant Medicine-Kidney;* **Admitting Hospital:** Children's Memorial Hospital; **Office Address:** Children's Meml Hosp 2300 Children's Plaza, Box 37 Chicago, IL 60614-3394; **Office Phone:** (773) 880-4326; **Board Certifications:** Pediatrics 1978, Pediatric Nephrology 1979; **Medical School:** Albert Einstein Coll Med 1972; **Residencies:** Pediatrics, Johns Hopkins, Baltimore, MD 1973-1975; Pediatric Nephrology, Univ Minn, Minneapolis, MN 1975-1978; **Faculty Appointment:** Assoc Prof Pediatrics, Northwestern Univ

Cole, Barbara R MD (Pediatric Nephrology) - *Special Expertise: Pediatric Nephrology - General;* **Admitting Hospital:** St Louis Children's Hospital; **Office Address:** St Louis Chldrns Hosp, Dept Nephrology One Chldrns Pl St Louis, MO 63110; **Office Phone:** (314) 454-6043; **Board Certifications:** Pediatrics 1972, Pediatric Nephrology 1995; **Medical School:** Univ Kans 1967; **Residency:** Pediatrics, Kansas Med Ctr 1968-1970; **Fellowship:** Pediatric Nephrology, Washington Univ, St. Louis, MO 1970-1972; **Faculty Appointment:** Assoc Prof Pediatrics, Washington Univ, St Louis

Dabbagh, Shermine MD (Pediatric Nephrology) - *Special Expertise: Kidney Disease; Kidney Failure-Chronic;* **Admitting Hospital:** Children's Hospital of Michigan; **Office Address:** Chldns Hosp Michigan, Dept Ped Nephrology 3901 Beaubien Blvd Detroit, MI 48201; **Office Phone:** (313) 745-5604; **Board Certifications:** Pediatrics 1985, Pediatric Nephrology 1985; **Medical School:** Lebanon 1979; **Residency:** Pediatrics, Univ Virginia, Charlottesville, VA 1979-1981; **Fellowship:** Pediatric Nephrology, Univ Wisconsin, Madison, WI 1981-1984; **Faculty Appointment:** Prof Pediatrics, Wayne State Univ

Davis, Ira D MD (Pediatric Nephrology) - *Special Expertise: Kidney Development; Kidney Failure-Chronic;* **Admitting Hospital:** Rainbow Babies & Children's Hospital; **Office Address:** 5850 Landerbrook Dr Mayfield Heights, OH 44124; **Office Phone:** (216) 844-1389; **Board Certifications:** Pediatrics 1999, Pediatric Nephrology 1999; **Medical School:** Univ Minn 1980; **Residency:** Pediatrics, Univ Hosps, Cleveland, OH 1984-1987; **Fellowship:** Pediatric Nephrology, Univ Minn Hosps, Minneapolis, MN 1987-1990; **Faculty Appointment:** Asst Prof Pediatrics, Case West Res Univ

Friedman, Aaron MD (Pediatric Nephrology) - *Special Expertise: Pediatric Nephrology - General;* **Admitting Hospital:** University of Wisconsin Hospital & Clinics; **Office Address:** Univ Wisconsin Chldns Hosp 600 Highland Ave, H4-458 CSC Madison, WI 53792; **Office Phone:** (608) 263-6420; **Board Certifications:** Pediatrics 1979, Pediatric Nephrology 1996; **Medical School:** SUNY Syracuse 1974; **Residency:** Pediatrics, Univ Wisconsin, Madison, WI 1975-1976; **Fellowship:** Pediatric Nephrology, Univ Wisconsin, Madison, WI 1976-1980; **Faculty Appointment:** Prof Pediatrics, Univ Wisc

Kashtan, Clifford MD (Pediatric Nephrology) - *Special Expertise: Transplant Medicine-Kidney; Genetic Kidney Disease;* **Admitting Hospital:** Fairview-University Medical Center - University Campus; **Office Address:** U Minn Med Sch- Dept of Ped-MMC491 420 Delaware St SE Minneapolis, MN 55455-0348; **Office Phone:** (612) 624-9193; **Board Certifications:** Pediatrics 1983, Pediatric Nephrology 1996; **Medical School:** Wayne State Univ 1978; **Residency:** Pediatrics, City Hospital, Boston, MA 1979-1981; **Fellowships:** Pediatric Nephrology, Mass Genl Hosp, Boston, MA 1983-1984; Pediatric Nephrology, Univ of Minn, Minneapolis, MN 1984-1987; **Faculty Appointment:** Prof Pediatric Nephrology, Univ Minn

Langman, Craig MD (Pediatric Nephrology) - *Special Expertise: Kidney Stones; Osteoporosis-Juvenile;* **Admitting Hospital:** Children's Memorial Hospital; **Office Address:** Children's Meml Hosp 2300 N Children's Plaza, Box 37 Chicago, IL 60614-3394; **Office Phone:** (773) 880-4326; **Board Certifications:** Pediatrics 1982, Pediatric Nephrology 1992; **Medical School:** Hahnemann Univ 1977; **Residency:** Pediatrics, Children's Hosp, Philadelphia, PA 1977-1979; **Fellowship:** Pediatric Nephrology, Children's Hosp, Philadelphia, PA 1979-1981; **Faculty Appointment:** Prof Pediatrics, Northwestern Univ

Nevins, Thomas E MD (Pediatric Nephrology) - *Special Expertise: Kidney Failure-Chronic; Transplant Medicine-Kidney;* **Admitting Hospital:** Fairview-University Medical Center - University Campus; **Office Address:** Fairview Univ Med Ctr, Dept Peds 420 Delaware St SE Minneapolis, MN 55455-0374; **Office Phone:** (612) 624-3995; **Board Certifications:** Pediatrics 1975, Pediatric Nephrology 1979; **Medical School:** Washington Univ, St Louis 1969; **Residency:** Pediatrics, Minnesota Hosps, Minneapolis, MN 1970-1972; **Fellowship:** Nephrology, Minnesota Hosps, Minneapolis, MN 1974-1978; **Faculty Appointment:** Prof Pediatrics, Univ Minn

Warady, Bradley MD (Pediatric Nephrology) - *Special Expertise: Peritoneal Dialysis; Transplant Medicine-Kidney;* **Admitting Hospital:** Children's Mercy Hospital & Clinics; **Office Address:** Children's Mercy Hosp, Dept Pediatric Nephrology 2401 Gillham Rd Kansas City, MO 64108; **Office Phone:** (816) 234-3010; **Board Certifications:** Pediatrics 1984, Pediatric Nephrology 1985; **Medical School:** Univ IL Coll Med **Residency:** Pediatrics, Chldns Mercy Hosp, Kansas City, MO 1979-1982; **Fellowship:** Pediatric Nephrology, Colorado Univ Med Ctr, Denver, CO 1982-1984

West Coast and Pacific

Alexander, Steven R MD (Pediatric Nephrology) - *Special Expertise: Kidney Failure; Transplant Medicine-Kidney;* **Admitting Hospital:** Stanford Medical Center; **Office Address:** Pediatric Renal Center 770 Welch Road Palo Alto, CA 94324; **Office Phone:** (650) 498-5480; **Board Certifications:** Pediatrics 1986, Pediatric Nephrology 1986; **Medical School:** Baylor Coll Med 1971; **Residency:** Pediatrics, Baylor Affil Hosp, Houston, TX 1974-1976; **Fellowship:** Pediatric Nephrology, Baylor Affil Hosp, Houston, TX 1976-1978; **Faculty Appointment:** Prof Pediatrics, Stanford Univ

Ettenger, Robert Bruce MD (Pediatric Nephrology) - *Special Expertise: Transplant Medicine-Kidney;* **Admitting Hospital:** UCLA Medical Center; **Office Address:** Childrens Health Center 200 UCLA Medical Plaza Los Angeles, CA 90024; **Office Phone:** (310) 206-6987; **Board Certifications:** Pediatrics 1986, Pediatric Nephrology 1986; **Medical School:** Univ Penn 1968; **Residency:** Pediatrics, St Christophers Hosp Chldn, Philadelphia, PA 1969-1971; **Fellowship:** Pediatric Nephrology, Chldns Hosp, Los Angeles, CA 1973-1975; **Faculty Appointment:** Prof Pediatrics, UCLA

McDonald, Ruth A MD (Pediatric Nephrology) - *Special Expertise:* Transplant Medicine-Kidney; **Admitting Hospital:** Children's Hospital and Regional Medical Center - Seattle; **Office Address:** Chldrns Hosp, Div Neph CH-46 4800 Sand Point Way NE Seattle, WA 98105; **Office Phone:** (206) 526-2524; **Board Certifications:** Pediatrics 1997, Pediatric Nephrology 2004; **Medical School:** Univ Minn 1987; **Residency:** Pediatrics, Chldns Hosp & Med Ctr, Seattle, WA 1988-1990; **Fellowship:** Pediatric Nephrology, Chldns Hosp & Med Ctr, Seattle, WA 1990-1993; **Faculty Appointment:** Assoc Prof Pediatrics, Univ Wash

Stapleton, F Bruder MD (Pediatric Nephrology) - *Special Expertise:* Kidney Stones; **Admitting Hospital:** Children's Hospital and Regional Medical Center - Seattle; **Office Address:** Children's Hosp & Reg Med Ctr, Dept Pediatrics 4800 Sand Point Way NE, MS CH-65 Seattle, WA 98105-0371; **Office Phone:** (206) 526-2150; **Board Certifications:** Pediatrics 1989, Pediatric Nephrology 1997; **Medical School:** Univ Kans 1972; **Residency:** Pediatrics, Univ Washington Med Ctr 1972-1974; **Fellowship:** Pediatric Nephrology, Univ Kansas Med Ctr, Kansas City, KS 1975-1977; **Faculty Appointment:** Prof Pediatrics, Univ Wash

Watkins, Sandra MD (Pediatric Nephrology) - *Special Expertise:* Kidney Failure-Chronic; Hemolytic Uremic Syndrome; **Admitting Hospital:** Children's Hospital and Regional Medical Center - Seattle; **Office Address:** Chldns Hosp and Regl Med Ctr 4800 Sand Point Way NE, MC-CH46 Seattle, WA 98105; **Office Phone:** (206) 526-2524; **Board Certifications:** Pediatrics 1987, Pediatric Nephrology 1988; **Medical School:** Univ Tex, Houston 1981; **Residency:** Pediatrics, Univ WA Chldns Hosp, Seattle, WA 1982-1984; **Fellowship:** Nephrology, Univ WA Sch Med, Seattle, WA 1984-1986; **Faculty Appointment:** Asst Prof Pediatric Nephrology, Univ Wash

PEDIATRIC OTOLARYNGOLOGY

New England

Eavey, Roland Douglas MD (Pediatric Otolaryngology) - *Special Expertise:* Microtia Reconstruction; Ear Disorders/Surgery; **Admitting Hospital:** Massachusetts Eye & Ear Infirmary (Page 68); **Office Address:** 243 Charles St Boston, MA 02114; **Office Phone:** (617) 573-3190; **Board Certifications:** Pediatrics 1982, Otolaryngology 1981; **Medical School:** Univ Penn 1975; **Residencies:** Pediatrics, Chldns Hoso, Los Angeles, CA 1976-1977; Surgery, Kaiser Hosp, San Francisco, CA 1977-1978; **Fellowship:** Otolaryngology, Mass EE Infirm, Boston, MA 1978-1981; **Faculty Appointment:** Assoc Prof Otolaryngology, Harvard Med Sch

Grundfast, Kenneth MD (Pediatric Otolaryngology) - *Special Expertise:* Pediatric Otolaryngology - General; **Admitting Hospital:** Boston Medical Center; **Office Address:** Boston Med Ctr, Dept Oto 720 Harrison Ave, Ste 601 Boston, MA 02118; **Office Phone:** (617) 638-7933; **Board Certification:** Otolaryngology 1977; **Medical School:** SUNY Syracuse 1969; **Residencies:** Surgery, Sibley Meml Hosp, Washington, DC 1973-1974; Otolaryngology, Boston-Affil Hosps, Boston, MA 1974-1977; **Fellowship:** Pediatric Otolaryngology, Chldns Hosp, Pittsburgh, PA 1977-1978

Healy, Gerald MD (Pediatric Otolaryngology) - *Special Expertise:* Pediatric Otolaryngology - General; **Admitting Hospital:** Children's Hospital; **Office Address:** Chldns Hosp, Dept Oto 300 Longwood Ave Boston, MA 02115; **Office Phone:** (617) 355-6417; **Board Certification:** Otolaryngology 1972; **Medical School:** Boston Univ 1967; **Residencies:** Surgery, Univ Boston Hosps, Boston, MA 1968-1969; Otolaryngology, Univ Boston Hosps, Boston, MA 1969-1972; **Faculty Appointment:** Prof Otolaryngology, Harvard Med Sch

Mid Atlantic

Bluestone, Charles D MD (Pediatric Otolaryngology) - *Special Expertise:* Pediatric Otolaryngology - General; **Admitting Hospital:** Children's Hospital of Pittsburgh; **Office Address:** Chldn Hosp Pitts-Oto 3705 5th Ave Pittsburgh, PA 15213; **Office Phone:** (412) 692-5902; **Board Certification:** Otolaryngology 1963; **Medical School:** Univ Pittsburgh 1958; **Residency:** Otolaryngology, Eye and Ear Infirmary, Chicago, IL 1959-1962; **Faculty Appointment:** Prof Otolaryngology, Univ Pittsburgh

Goldsmith, Ari MD (Pediatric Otolaryngology) - *Special Expertise:* Pediatric Otolaryngology - General; **Admitting Hospital:** Long Island College Hospital (Page 58); **Office Address:** University Otolaryngologists 134 Atlantic Ave Brooklyn, NY 11201; **Office Phone:** (718) 780-1498; **Board Certifications:** Pediatrics 1994, Otolaryngology 1993; **Medical School:** Albert Einstein Coll Med 1988; **Residency:** Otolaryngology, Long Island Jewish, New Hyde Park, NY 1993-1993; **Fellowship:** Pediatric Otolaryngology, Children's Hospital, Boston, MA 1993-1994; **Faculty Appointment:** Prof Otolaryngology, SUNY Hlth Sci Ctr

Jones, Jacqueline MD (Pediatric Otolaryngology) - *Special Expertise:* Pediatric Otolaryngology - General; **Admitting Hospital:** New York Weill Cornell Medical Center - NY Presbyterian Hospital (Page 72); **Office Address:** 520 E 70th St, Ste 541 New York, NY 10021-4873; **Office Phone:** (212) 746-2236; **Board Certification:** Otolaryngology 1989; **Medical School:** Cornell Univ-Weil Med Coll 1984; **Residency:** Otolaryngology, Hosp-Univ of Penn, Philadelphia, PA 1984-1989; **Fellowship:** Children's Hosp, Boston, MA 1989-1990; **Faculty Appointment:** Assoc Prof Cornell Univ-Weil Med Coll

Milmoe, Gregory J MD (Pediatric Otolaryngology) - *Special Expertise:* Sinus Disorders/Surgery; Airway Disorders; **Admitting Hospital:** Georgetown University Hospital; **Office Address:** Georgetown Univ Med Ctr 3800 Reservoir Rd, Bldg Gorman - Fl 1 Washington, DC; **Office Phone:** (202) 687-8186; **Board Certification:** Otolaryngology 1981; **Medical School:** Univ Chicago-Pritzker Sch Med 1973; **Residencies:** Surgery, Hosp of Univ Penn, Philadelphia, PA 1975-1976; Otolaryngology, Yale Univ Hosp, Philadelphia, PA 1976-1979; **Fellowship:** Pediatric Otolaryngology, Chldrns Hosp, Pittsburgh, PA 1979-1980; **Faculty Appointment:** Assoc Prof Otolaryngology, Georgetown Univ

Potsic, William Paul MD (Pediatric Otolaryngology) - *Special Expertise:* Ear Disorders; Ear Tumors; Hearing Disorders; **Admitting Hospital:** The Children's Hospital of Philadelphia; **Office Address:** Childrens Hosp-Philadelphia 34 Civic Center Blvd, Bldg Wood - Fl 1 Philadelphia, PA 19104-4303; **Office Phone:** (215) 590-3450; **Board Certification:** Otolaryngology 1974; **Medical School:** Emory Univ 1969; **Residency:** Otolaryngology, Univ Chicago, Chicago, IL 1969-1974; **Faculty Appointment:** Prof Otolaryngology, Univ Penn

Richardson, Mark A. MD (Pediatric Otolaryngology) - *Special Expertise:* Pediatric Otolaryngology - General; **Admitting Hospital:** Johns Hopkins Hospital - Baltimore (Page 65); **Office Address:** Johns Hopkins Outpatient Ctr, Dept Oto/HNS 601 N Caroline St, rm 6215 Baltimore, MD 21287; **Office Phone:** (410) 955-7400; **Board Certification:** Otolaryngology 1979; **Medical School:** Med Univ SC 1975; **Residency:** Otolaryngology, Med Univ Hosp, Charleston, SC 1976-1979; **Fellowship:** Pediatric Otolaryngology, Chldns Hosp Med Ctr, Cincinnati, OH 1979-1980; **Faculty Appointment:** Prof Otolaryngology, Johns Hopkins Univ

Rosenfeld, Richard M MD (Pediatric Otolaryngology) - *Special Expertise:* Sinus Disorders/Surgery; Head & Neck Surgery; **Admitting Hospital:** Long Island College Hospital (Page 58); **Office Address:** Univ Otolaryngologists 134 Atlantic Ave Brooklyn, NY 11201; **Office Phone:** (718) 780-1498; **Board Certification:** Otolaryngology 1989; **Medical School:** SUNY Buffalo 1984; **Residency:** Otolaryngology, Mount Sinai Med Ctr, New York, NY 1984-1989; **Fellowship:** Pediatric Otolaryngology, Chldrn's Hosp, Pittsburgh, PA 1989-1991; **Faculty Appointment:** Prof Otolaryngology, SUNY Downstate

Tunkel, David Eric MD (Pediatric Otolaryngology) - *Special Expertise:* Head & Neck Surgery; **Admitting Hospital:** Johns Hopkins Hospital - Baltimore (Page 65); **Office Address:** Johns Hopkins Outpatient Ctr 601 N Caroline St, rm 6231 Baltimore, MD 21287; **Office Phone:** (410) 955-1559; **Board Certification:** Otolaryngology 1990; **Medical School:** Johns Hopkins Univ 1984; **Residencies:** Surgery, Johns Hopkins Hosp, Baltimore, MD 1984-1986; Otolaryngology, Johns Hopkins Hosp, Baltimore, MD 1986-1990; **Fellowship:** Pediatric Otolaryngology, Chldns Natl Med Ctr, Washington, DC 1990-1991; **Faculty Appointment:** Assoc Prof Otolaryngology, Johns Hopkins Univ

Southeast

Drake, Amelia MD (Pediatric Otolaryngology) - *Special Expertise:* Pediatric Surgery; Head & Neck Surgery; **Admitting Hospital:** University of North Carolina Hospitals; **Office Address:** Univ NC at Chapel Hill - Div Otolaryngology 610 Burnett Wolmack Bldg CB# 7070 , MC-7070 Chapel Hill, NC 27599; **Office Phone:** (919) 966-8926; **Board Certification:** Otolaryngology 1987; **Medical School:** Univ NC Sch Med 1981; **Residencies:** Otolaryngology, Univ MI Hosps; Surgery, Univ MI Hosps

Gross, Charles MD (Pediatric Otolaryngology) - *Special Expertise:* Sinus Disorders/Surgery; **Admitting Hospital:** University of Virginia Health Systems; **Office Address:** UVA Health System P. O. Box 800713 Charlottesville, VA 22908-0713; **Office Phone:** (804) 924-5934; **Board Certification:** Pediatric Otolaryngology 1967; **Medical School:** Univ VA Sch Med 1961; **Residencies:** Otolaryngology, Mass EE Infirm, Boston, MA 1963-1966; Surgery, Beckley Meml Hosp 1962-1963; **Faculty Appointment:** Prof Emeritus Univ VA Sch Med

Midwest

Belenky, Walter MD (Pediatric Otolaryngology) - *Special Expertise:* Otolaryngology; Cochlear Implants; **Admitting Hospital:** Children's Hospital of Michigan; **Office Address:** 3901 Beaubien Detroit, MI 48201; **Office Phone:** (313) 745-9048; **Board Certification:** Otolaryngology 1970; **Medical School:** Univ Mich Med Sch 1963; **Residencies:** Surgery, WM Beaumont Hosp, Royal Oak, MI 1964-1965; Otolaryngology, Wayne Affil Hosp, Detroit, MI 1965-1968; **Faculty Appointment:** Assoc Prof Otolaryngology, Wayne State Univ

Cotton, Robin MD (Pediatric Otolaryngology) - *Special Expertise:* Tracheal Reconstruction; Head & Neck Surgery; **Admitting Hospital:** Children's Hospital Medical Center; **Office Address:** Chldns Hosp Med Ctr, Dept Oto 3333 Burnet Ave Cincinnati, OH 45229-2883; **Office Phone:** (513) 636-4355; **Board Certification:** Otolaryngology 1972; **Medical School:** England 1965; **Residencies:** Otolaryngology, Univ Birmingham, Birmingham, AL 1966-1968; Otolaryngology, Univ Toronto, Toronto, Canada 1968-1972; **Fellowship:** Otolaryngology, Univ Toronto, Toronto, Canada 1971-1973; **Faculty Appointment:** Prof Otolaryngology, Univ Cincinnati

Holinger, Lauren MD (Pediatric Otolaryngology) - *Special Expertise:* Airway Disorders; Swallowing Disorders; Aspiration; **Admitting Hospital:** Children's Memorial Hospital; **Office Address:** Childrens Meml Hosp 2300 N Childrens Plaza, Box 25 Chicago, IL 60614-3394; **Office Phone:** (773) 880-4457; **Board Certification:** Otolaryngology 1976; **Medical School:** Univ Hlth Sci/Chicago Med Sch 1971; **Residencies:** Surgery, Univ CO Affil Hosp, Denver, CO 1971-1972; Otolaryngology, Univ CO Affil Hosp, Denver, CO 1972-1975; **Fellowship:** Pediatrics, Univ of IL Eye & Ear Infirm, Chicago, IL 1975-1976; **Faculty Appointment:** Prof Otolaryngology, Northwestern Univ

Katz, Robert L MD (Pediatric Otolaryngology) - *Special Expertise:* Ear Infections & Hearing Problems; Sinus Disorders/Surgery; Voice Disorders; **Admitting Hospital:** Cleveland Clinic Foundation; **Office Address:** 29800 Bainbridge Rd Solon, OH 44139; **Office Phone:** (440) 519-6950; **Board Certification:** Otolaryngology 1968; **Medical School:** Case West Res Univ 1963; **Residencies:** Surgery, Mount Sinai Hosp, Cleveland, OH 1963-1965; Otolaryngology, Mass EE Infirm, Boston, MA 1965-1968; **Faculty Appointment:** Clin Prof Otolaryngology, Ohio State Univ

Lusk, Rodney MD (Pediatric Otolaryngology) - *Special Expertise:* Cochlear Implants; Sinus Disorders/Surgery; Sleep Disorders/Apnea; **Admitting Hospital:** St Louis Children's Hospital; **Office Address:** St. Louis Childrens Hospital 1 Children's Place, Fl 3 St. Louis, MO 63110-1077; **Office Phone:** (314) 454-6162; **Board Certification:** Otolaryngology 1982; **Medical School:** Univ MO-Columbia Sch Med 1977; **Residency:** Univ. Iowa Hosp/Clinic, Iowa City, IA 1978-1982; **Fellowship:** Otolaryngology, Childrens hospital, Pittsburgh, PA 1982-1983; **Faculty Appointment:** Assoc Prof Pediatrics, Washington Univ, St Louis

Miller, Robert MD (Pediatric Otolaryngology) - *Special Expertise:* Ear Disorders/Surgery; Airway Disorders; **Admitting Hospital:** Advocate Lutheran General Hospital; **Office Address:** 64 Old Orchard Ctr, Ste 630 Skokie, IL 60077; **Office Phone:** (847) 674-5585; **Board Certification:** Otolaryngology 1978; **Medical School:** Northwestern Univ 1946; **Residency:** Otolaryngology, Univ Ill, Chicago, IL 1975-1978; **Fellowship:** Pediatric Otolaryngology, Chldns Med Ctr- Univ Cincinnati, Cincinnati, OH 1986-1987; **Faculty Appointment:** Asst Clin Prof Otolaryngology, Univ IL Coll Med

Southwest

Duncan III, Newton Oran MD (Pediatric Otolaryngology) - *Special Expertise:* *Ear, Nose & Throat; Head & Neck Surgery;* **Admitting Hospital:** Texas Children's Hospital - Houston; **Office Address:** 6550 Fannin St, Ste 2001 Houston, TX 77030; **Office Phone:** (713) 796-2001; **Board Certification:** Otolaryngology 1986; **Medical School:** Baylor Coll Med 1978; **Residencies:** Surgery, Baylor Coll Med, Houston, TX 1982-1983; Otolaryngology, Baylor Coll Med, Houston, TX 1983-1986; **Fellowships:** Pediatric Otolaryngology, Univ Wash, Seattle, WA 1990-1991; Pediatric Otolaryngology, Royal Alexandra Hosp Chld, Sydney, Australia 1991; **Faculty Appointment:** Asst Prof Otolaryngology, Baylor Coll Med

West Coast and Pacific

Crockett, Dennis M MD (Pediatric Otolaryngology) - *Special Expertise:* *Airway Disorders;* **Admitting Hospital:** Children's Hospital - Los Angeles; **Office Address:** Childrens Hospital, Div Otolaryngology 4650 Sunset Blvd, MC-58 Los Angeles, CA 90027; **Office Phone:** (323) 669-2145; **Board Certification:** Otolaryngology 1985; **Medical School:** USC Sch Med 1979; **Residency:** Otolaryngology, LA Co-USC Med Ctr, Los Angeles, CA 1980-1984; **Fellowship:** Pediatrics, Boston Chldns Hosp, Boston, MA 1984-1985; **Faculty Appointment:** Assoc Prof Otolaryngology, USC Sch Med

Inglis, Andrew MD (Pediatric Otolaryngology) - *Special Expertise:* *Airway Disorders; Voice Problems;* **Admitting Hospital:** Children's Hospital and Regional Medical Center - Seattle; **Office Address:** Children's Hospital & Regional Medical Center 4800 Sand Point Way NE Seattle, WA 98105; **Office Phone:** (206) 526-2105; **Board Certification:** Otolaryngology 1987; **Medical School:** Med Coll PA Hahnemann 1981; **Residencies:** Surgery, U Washington, Seattle, WA 1981-1983; Otolaryngology, Virginia Mason Hosp, Seattle, WA 1983-1987; **Fellowship:** Pediatric Otolaryngology, Alexandria Hosp-Chldn 1982-1987; **Faculty Appointment:** Assoc Prof Otolaryngology, Univ Wash

PEDIATRIC PULMONOLOGY

New England

Lapey, Allen MD (Pediatric Pulmonology) - *Special Expertise:* Cystic Fibrosis; Asthma; Food Allergy; **Admitting Hospital:** Massachusetts General Hospital; **Office Address:** Mass Genl Hosp 55 Fruit St, Bldg ACC-709 Boston, MA 02114; **Office Phone:** (617) 726-8707; **Board Certifications:** Pediatric Pulmonology 1996, Allergy & Immunology 1978; **Medical School:** Univ Rochester 1966; **Residency:** Pediatrics, Chldns Hosp Med Ctr., Boston, MA 1967-1968; **Fellowships:** Pediatric Pulmonology, Mass Genl Hosp., Boston, MA 1970-1972; Allergy & Immunology, Mass Genl Hosp., Boston, MA 1970-1972; **Faculty Appointment:** Asst Clin Prof Pediatrics, Harvard Med Sch

Mid Atlantic

Loughlin, Gerald M MD (Pediatric Pulmonology) - *Special Expertise:* Asthma; Sleep & Breathing Disorders; **Admitting Hospital:** Johns Hopkins Hospital - Baltimore (Page 65); **Office Address:** Johns Hopkins Hosp- Dept. Ped 600 N Wolfe St, Bldg Park - rm 316 Baltimore, MD 21287-2533; **Office Phone:** (410) 955-2035; **Board Certifications:** Pediatric Pulmonology 1996, Pediatrics 1993; **Medical School:** Univ Rochester 1973; **Residency:** Pediatrics, U Ariz Med Ctr, Tucson, AZ 1973-1975; **Fellowship:** Pediatric Pulmonology, U Ariz Med Ctr, Tucson, AZ 1975-1977; **Faculty Appointment:** Prof Pediatrics, Johns Hopkins Univ

Mellins, Robert MD (Pediatric Pulmonology) - *Special Expertise:* Asthma; **Admitting Hospital:** Columbia Presbyterian Medical Center (Page 72); **Office Address:** Pediatric Pulmonary Dept 3959 Broadway, Ste BHS746 New York, NY 10032-1537; **Office Phone:** (212) 305-5122; **Board Certifications:** Pediatrics 1958, Pediatric Pulmonology 1995; **Medical School:** Johns Hopkins Univ 1952; **Residencies:** Pediatrics, NY Hosp, New York, NY 1955-1956; Pediatrics, Columbia Presby Med Ctr, New York, NY 1956-1957; **Fellowship:** Pulmonary Disease, Columbia Presby Med Ctr, New York, NY 1961-1964; **Faculty Appointment:** Prof Pediatrics, Columbia P&S

Quittell, Lynne MD (Pediatric Pulmonology) - *Special Expertise:* Cystic Fibrosis; **Admitting Hospital:** Columbia Presbyterian Medical Center (Page 72); **Office Address:** 3959 Broadway, rm 7 South New York, NY 10032-1537; **Office Phone:** (212) 305-5122; **Board Certifications:** Pediatrics 1986, Pediatric Pulmonology 1996; **Medical School:** Israel 1981; **Residency:** Pediatrics, Schneider Chldn's Hosp, New Hyde Park, NY 1981-1984; **Fellowship:** Pediatric Pulmonology, St Christopher Med Ctr, Philadelphia, PA 1984-1988

Zeitlin, Pamela Leslie MD (Pediatric Pulmonology) - *Special Expertise:* Cystic Fibrosis; **Admitting Hospital:** Johns Hopkins Hospital - Baltimore (Page 65); **Office Address:** Johns Hopkins Hosp, Dept Ped 600 N Wolfe St, Bldg Park - rm 316 Baltimore, MD 21287-2533; **Office Phone:** (410) 955-2035; **Board Certifications:** Pediatrics 1988, Pediatric Pulmonology 2000; **Medical School:** Yale Univ 1983; **Residency:** Pediatrics, Johns Hopkins Hosp, Baltimore, MD 1983-1986; **Fellowship:** Pediatric Pulmonology, Johns Hopkins Hosp, Baltimore, MD 1986-1989; **Faculty Appointment:** Assoc Prof Pediatrics, Johns Hopkins Univ

Southeast

Murphy, Thomas M MD (Pediatric Pulmonology) - *Special Expertise:* Cystic Fibrosis; Bronchopulmonary Dysplasia; Pneumonia-Chronic; **Admitting Hospital:** Duke University Medical Center (Page 60); **Office Address:** Duke Univ Med Ctr Box 2994 Durham, NC 27710; **Office Phone:** (919) 684-3364; **Board Certifications:** Internal Medicine 1976, Pediatric Pulmonology 1989; **Medical School:** Univ Rochester 1973; **Residency:** Internal Medicine, Georgetown Univ Hosp, Washington, DC 1973-1976; **Fellowship:** Pediatric Pulmonology, Georgetown Univ Hosp, Washington, DC 1976-1978; **Faculty Appointment:** Assoc Prof Pediatrics, Duke Univ

Sallent, Jorge MD (Pediatric Pulmonology) - *Special Expertise:* Pediatric Pulmonology - General; **Admitting Hospital:** St Mary's Medical Center - West Palm Beach; **Office Address:** Pediatric Respiratory Ctr 5325 Greenwood Avenue Ste 301 West Palm Beach, FL 33407-2452; **Office Phone:** (561) 863-0105; **Board Certifications:** Pediatrics 1984, Pediatric Pulmonology 1996; **Medical School:** Dominican Republic 1978; **Residency:** Pediatrics, Orlando Regional Med Ctr, Orlando, FL 1980-1983; **Fellowship:** Pediatric Pulmonology, Univ Florida, Gainesville, FL 1985-1986; **Faculty Appointment:** Asst Prof Pediatrics, Univ Fla Coll Med

Sherman, James MD (Pediatric Pulmonology) - *Special Expertise:* Cystic Fibrosis; **Admitting Hospital:** Shands Healthcare at University Florida (Page 77); **Office Address:** Medical Plaza 2000 SW Archer Rd, Fl 2 Gainesville, FL 32608; **Office Phone:** (352) 392-4458; **Board Certifications:** Pediatrics 1981, Pediatric Pulmonology 1996; **Medical School:** Univ S Fla Coll Med 1975; **Residencies:** Pediatrics, SUNY Upstate Med Ctr, Syracuse, NY 1976-1977; Pediatrics, Tampa Genl Hosp- Univ So Florida, Tampa, FL 1977-1978; **Fellowship:** Pediatric Pulmonology, Rainbow Babies & Children's Hosp, Cleveland, OH 1978-1981; **Faculty Appointment:** Prof Pediatrics, Univ Fla Coll Med

Midwest

Kim, Young-Jee MD (Pediatric Pulmonology) - *Special Expertise:* Asthma; Sleep Disorders/Apnea; Bronchopulmonary Dysplasia; **Admitting Hospital:** University of Chicago Hospitals (Page 78); **Office Address:** 5841 South Maryland Ave MC-4064 Chicago, IL 60637; **Office Phone:** (773) 702-6178; **Board Certifications:** Pediatrics 1995, Pediatric Pulmonology 1998; **Medical School:** South Korea 1986; **Residency:** Pediatrics, Duke Univ Med Ctr, Durham, NC 1992-1995; **Fellowships:** Pediatric Pulmonology, Yale U Med Sch, New Haven, CT 1988-1991; Pediatric Pulmonology, Riley Hospital Children, Indianapolis, IN 1995

Kurachek, Stephen Charles MD (Pediatric Pulmonology) - *Special Expertise:* Critical Care; Asthma; **Admitting Hospital:** Children's Hospital and Clinics; **Office Address:** 2545 Chicago Ave S, Fl 617 Minneapolis, MN 55404; **Office Phone:** (612) 863-3226; **Board Certifications:** Pediatric Pulmonology 1995, Pediatric Critical Care Medicine 1995; **Medical School:** Univ Miami Sch Med 1978; **Residency:** Pediatrics, Univ Hosp, Ann Arbor, MI 1979-1981; **Fellowship:** Pulmonary Disease, Boston Chldns Hosp., Boston, MA 1981-1984; **Faculty Appointment:** Asst Clin Prof Pediatrics, Univ Minn

Stern, Robert C MD (Pediatric Pulmonology) - *Special Expertise:* Cystic Fibrosis; Lung Disease; **Admitting Hospital:** Rainbow Babies & Children's Hospital; **Office Address:** Rainbow Babies & Chldns Hosp 11100 Euclid Ave, rm 3001 Cleveland, OH 44106; **Office Phone:** (216) 844-3267; **Board Certifications:** Pediatrics 1968, Pediatric Pulmonology 1994; **Medical School:** Albert Einstein Coll Med 1963; **Residencies:** Pediatrics, Univ Hosp, Cleveland, OH 1964-1965; Pediatrics, Municipal Hosp Ctr, Bronx, NY 1965-1966; **Fellowship:** Pediatric Pulmonology, Univ Hosp, Cleveland, OH 1968; **Faculty Appointment:** Prof Pediatrics, Case West Res Univ

Great Plains and Mountains

Accurso, Frank J MD (Pediatric Pulmonology) - *Special Expertise:* Cystic Fibrosis; **Admitting Hospital:** The Children's Hospital - Denver; **Office Address:** Chldns Hosp 1056 E 19th Ave, rm B-395 Denver, CO 80218-1007; **Office Phone:** (303) 837-2522; **Board Certifications:** Pediatrics 1980, Pediatric Critical Care Medicine 1996; **Medical School:** Albert Einstein Coll Med 1974; **Residency:** Pediatrics, Univ Colo Hlth Sci Ctr, Denver, CO 1978-1980; **Fellowship:** Pulmonary Disease, Univ Colo Hlth Sci Ctr, Denver, CO 1975-1977; **Faculty Appointment:** Prof Pediatrics, Univ Colo

Larsen, Gary MD (Pediatric Pulmonology) - *Special Expertise:* Lung Disease; **Admitting Hospital:** National Jewish Medical & Research Center; **Office Address:** Natl Jewish Med & Research Ctr 1400 Jackson St Denver, CO 80206-2761; **Office Phone:** (303) 398-1617; **Board Certifications:** Pediatric Pulmonology 1996, Pediatrics 1976; **Medical School:** Columbia P&S 1971; **Residency:** Pediatrics, Univ Colorado, Denver, CO 1972-1974; **Fellowship:** Pediatric Pulmonology, Univ Colorado, Denver, CO 1976-1978; **Faculty Appointment:** Prof Pediatrics, Univ Colo

Southwest

Fan, Leland Lane MD (Pediatric Pulmonology) - *Special Expertise:* Interstitial Lung Disease; **Admitting Hospital:** Texas Children's Hospital - Houston; **Office Address:** Tex Chldns Hosp Feigin Ctr 6621 Fannin MC 3-2571 Houston, TX 77030; **Office Phone:** (832) 824-3300; **Board Certifications:** Pediatric Critical Care Medicine 1996, Pediatric Pulmonology 1996; **Medical School:** Baylor Coll Med 1973; **Residencies:** Pediatrics, UCSF, San Francisco, CA 1974-1975; Pediatrics, Univ Colo Hlth Sci Ctr, Denver, CO 1975-1976; **Fellowship:** Pediatric Critical Care Medicine, Univ Colo Hlth Sci Ctr, Denver, CO 1976-1978; **Faculty Appointment:** Prof Pediatrics, Baylor Coll Med

Morgan, Wayne J. MD (Pediatric Pulmonology) - *Special Expertise:* Cystic Fibrosis; **Admitting Hospital:** University Medical Center; **Office Address:** U Ariz Hlth Sci Ctr-Ped Pulm 1501 N Campbell Ave Tucson, AZ 85724; **Office Phone:** (520) 626-6412; **Board Certifications:** Pediatrics 1982, Pediatric Pulmonology 1996; **Medical School:** McGill Univ 1976; **Residency:** Pediatrics, Montreal Chldns Hosp., Montreal, CN 1977-1980; **Fellowship:** Pediatric Pulmonology, U Ariz, Tucson, AZ 1980-1982; **Faculty Appointment:** Assoc Prof Pediatric Pulmonology, Univ Ariz Coll Med

Warren, Robert Hughes MD (Pediatric Pulmonology) - *Special Expertise:* Assisted Breathing; Muscular Dystrophy; **Admitting Hospital:** Arkansas Children's Hospital; **Office Address:** Arkansas Chldns Hosp, Dept Pul 800 Marshall St, Slot 900 Little Rock, AR 72202; **Office Phone:** (501) 320-1006; **Board Certifications:** Pediatrics 1973, Pediatric Pulmonology 1996; **Medical School:** Univ Ark 1967; **Residency:** Pediatrics, LSU Med Ctr, Shreveport, LA 1968-1971; **Fellowship:** Pediatric Pulmonology, Tulane Univ Sch Med, New Orleans, LA 1973; **Faculty Appointment:** Assoc Prof Pediatrics, Univ Ark

West Coast and Pacific

Platzker, Arnold CG MD (Pediatric Pulmonology) - *Special Expertise:* Pediatric Pulmonology - General; **Admitting Hospital:** Children's Hospital - Los Angeles; **Office Address:** Univ Childrens Med Grp 4650 Sunset Blvd, Box 83 Los Angeles, CA 90027; **Office Phone:** (213) 669-2101; **Board Certifications:** Pediatrics 1967, Neonatal-Perinatal Medicine 1975; **Medical School:** Tufts Univ 1962; **Residencies:** Pediatrics, City Hosp, Boston, MA 1962-1964; Pediatrics, Stanford Univ, Palo Alto, CA 1964-1966; **Fellowship:** Pediatric Pulmonology, Univ Calif Med Ctr, San Francisco, CA 1968-1971; **Faculty Appointment:** Prof Pediatrics, UCLA

Ramsey, Bonnie W MD (Pediatric Pulmonology) - *Special Expertise:* Cystic Fibrosis; **Admitting Hospital:** Children's Hospital and Regional Medical Center - Seattle; **Office Address:** Chldrn's Hosp 4800 Sand Point Way NE Seattle, WA 98105; **Office Phone:** (206) 527-5725; **Board Certifications:** Pediatrics 1981, Pediatric Pulmonology 2006; **Medical School:** Harvard Med Sch 1976; **Residencies:** Pediatrics, Chldns Hosp, Boston, MA 1977-1978; Pediatrics, Chldns Hosp, Boston, MA 1978-1979; **Fellowship:** Pediatric Critical Care Medicine, Chldns Hosp, Seattle, WA 1979-1981; **Faculty Appointment:** Prof Pediatrics, Univ Wash

Redding, Gregory MD (Pediatric Pulmonology) - *Special Expertise:* Asthma; Ventilator Dependent Children; Infection-Respiratory; **Admitting Hospital:** Children's Hospital and Regional Medical Center - Seattle; **Office Address:** Chldrns Hosp & Regional Med Ctr/Pulmonary Medicine 4800 Sand Point Way NE, MS CH-68 Seattle, WA 98105; **Office Phone:** (206) 526-2174; **Board Certifications:** Pediatrics 1993, Pediatric Pulmonology 1993; **Medical School:** Stanford Univ 1974; **Residency:** Pediatrics, Harbor-UCLA Affil Hosps, Los Angeles, CA 1974-1977; **Fellowship:** Pediatric Pulmonology, Univ Colo Affil Hosps, Denver, CO 1977-1980; **Faculty Appointment:** Prof Pediatrics, Univ Wash

PEDIATRIC RHEUMATOLOGY

New England

McCarthy, Paul L MD (Pediatric Rheumatology) - *Special Expertise: Arthritis;* **Admitting Hospital:** Yale - New Haven Hospital; **Office Address:** Yale School of Medicine 333 Cedar St, Box 208064 New Haven, CT 06520; **Office Phone:** (203) 785-2475; **Board Certifications:** Pediatric Rheumatology 1992, Rheumatology 1974; **Medical School:** Georgetown Univ 1969; **Residency:** Pediatrics, Children's Hosp, Buffalo, NY 1970-1972; **Fellowship:** Pediatrics, Children's Hosp, Boston, MA 1972-1974; **Faculty Appointment:** Prof Pediatrics, Yale Univ

Mid Atlantic

Haines, Kathleen MD (Pediatric Rheumatology) - *Special Expertise: Pediatric Rheumatology - General;* **Admitting Hospital:** Hospital for Joint Diseases; **Office Address:** 305 2nd Ave at 17th St Ste 16 New York, NY 10003; **Office Phone:** (212) 598-6516; **Board Certifications:** Allergy & Immunology 1981, Pediatric Rheumatology 1999; **Medical School:** Albert Einstein Coll Med 1975; **Residency:** Pediatrics, NY Hosp, New York, NY 1975-1977; **Fellowships:** Allergy & Immunology, NY Hosp, New York, NY 1977-1980; Rheumatology, NYU Med Sch, New York, NY 1980-1982; **Faculty Appointment:** Assoc Prof Pediatrics, NYU Sch Med

Ilowite, Norman T MD (Pediatric Rheumatology) - *Special Expertise: Rheumatoid Arthritis-Juvenile; Lyme Disease;* **Admitting Hospital:** Schneider Children's Hospital; **Office Address:** 269-01 76th Ave New Hyde Park, NY 11040; **Office Phone:** (718) 470-3530; **Board Certifications:** Pediatrics 1985, Rheumatology 1992; **Medical School:** SUNY Downstate 1979; **Residency:** Pediatrics, Children's Hosp Natl Med Ctr, Washington, DC 1979-1982; **Fellowship:** Pediatric Rheumatology, U WA Med C, Seattle, WA 1982-1984; **Faculty Appointment:** Assoc Prof Pediatrics, Albert Einstein Coll Med

Lehman, Thomas MD (Pediatric Rheumatology) - *Special Expertise: Arthritis; Kawasaki's Disease; Lupus/SLE;* **Admitting Hospital:** Hospital for Special Surgery (Page 63); **Office Address:** 535 E 70th St New York, NY 10021-4872; **Office Phone:** (212) 606-1151; **Board Certifications:** Pediatrics 1979, Pediatric Rheumatology 1999; **Medical School:** Jefferson Med Coll 1974; **Residencies:** Pediatrics, Chldns Hosp, Los Angeles, CA 1974-1976; Pediatrics, UCSF Med Ctr, San Francisco, CA 1976-1977; **Fellowships:** Pediatric Rheumatology, Chldns Hosp, Los Angeles, CA 1977-1979; Rheumatology, Nat Inst Hlth, Bethesda, MD 1981-1983; **Faculty Appointment:** Clin Prof Pediatrics, Cornell Univ-Weil Med Coll

Sills, Edward M MD (Pediatric Rheumatology) - *Special Expertise: Juvenile Arthritis; Lupus/SLE;* **Admitting Hospital:** Johns Hopkins Hospital - Baltimore (Page 65); **Office Address:** 600 N Wolfe St Baltimore, MD 21287-2534; **Office Phone:** (410) 556-6145; **Board Certifications:** Pediatric Rheumatology 1999, Pediatrics 1968; **Medical School:** NYU Sch Med 1963; **Residency:** Pediatrics, Bronx Muni Hosp, New York, NY 1963-1967; **Faculty Appointment:** Assoc Prof Pediatrics, Johns Hopkins Univ

Southeast

Kredich, Deborah Welt MD (Pediatric Rheumatology) - *Special Expertise: Connective Tissue Disorders;* **Admitting Hospital:** Duke University Medical Center (Page 60); **Office Address:** Duke Univ Med Ctr Box 3212 Durham, NC 27710; **Office Phone:** (919) 684-6575; **Board Certifications:** Pediatrics 1992, Pediatric Rheumatology 2000; **Medical School:** Univ Mich Med Sch 1962; **Residencies:** Pediatrics, Duke Univ Med Ctr, Durham, NC 1969-1971; Pediatrics, Duke Univ Med Ctr, Durham, NC 1963-1964; **Faculty Appointment:** Assoc Prof Pediatrics, Duke Univ

Schanberg, Laura Eve MD (Pediatric Rheumatology) - *Special Expertise:* Rrheumatic *Diseases of Childhood; Fibromyalgia;* **Admitting Hospital:** Duke University Medical Center (Page 60); **Office Address:** Duke Univ Med Ctr, Div Ped Rhu Erwin Rd, Box 3212 Durham, NC 27710; **Office Phone:** (919) 684-6575; **Board Certifications:** Pediatric Rheumatology 2000, Pediatrics 2000; **Medical School:** Duke Univ 1984; **Residency:** Pediatrics, Duke Univ Med Ctr, Durham, NC 1984-1987; **Fellowship:** Pediatric Rheumatology, Duke Univ Med Ctr, Durham, NC 1987-1991; **Faculty Appointment:** Asst Prof Pediatrics, Duke Univ

Sleasman, John W MD (Pediatric Allery & Immunology) - *Special Expertise:* Infectious *Disease;* **Admitting Hospital:** Shands Healthcare at University Florida (Page 77); **Office Address:** Univ FL Sch Med, Dept Peds-Immunology/Inf Dis 1600 SW Archer Rd Gainesville, FL 32610; **Office Phone:** (352) 392-2961; **Board Certifications:** Pediatrics 1988, Pediatric Rheumatology 1994; **Medical School:** Univ Tenn Coll Med, Memphis 1981; **Residency:** Pediatrics, Shands Hosp, Gainesville, FL 1982-1984; **Fellowships:** Pediatric Infectious Disease, Shands Hosp, Gainesville, FL 1985-1987; Immunology, Dana Farber Cancer Inst, Boston, MA 1987-1988; **Faculty Appointment:** Assoc Prof Pediatrics, Univ Fla Coll Med

Midwest

Passo, Murray Howard MD (Pediatric Rheumatology) - *Special Expertise:* Pediatric *Rheumatology - General;* **Admitting Hospital:** Children's Hospital Medical Center; **Office Address:** Chldns Hosp & Med Ctr 3333 Burnett Ave Cincinnati, OH 45229; **Office Phone:** (513) 636-4676; **Board Certifications:** Pediatrics 1979, Pediatric Rheumatology 2000; **Medical School:** Indiana Univ 1974; **Residency:** Pediatrics, Riley Chldns Hosp, Indianapolis, IN 1975-1977; **Fellowship:** Rheumatology, Ind Univ Hosps, Indianapolis, IN 1977-1979

Wagner-Weiner, Linda MD (Pediatric Rheumatology) - *Special Expertise:* Lupus/SLE; *Arthritis-Juvenile;* **Admitting Hospital:** University of Chicago Hospitals (Page 78); **Office Address:** La Rabida Chldns Hosp East 65th Street at Lake Michigan Chicago, IL 60649; **Office Phone:** (773) 753-8644; **Board Certifications:** Pediatrics 1984, Pediatric Rheumatology 1999; **Medical School:** Rush Med Coll 1979; **Residency:** Pediatrics, Univ Chicago Hosps, Chicago, IL 1979-1982; **Fellowship:** Pediatric Rheumatology, Univ Chicago/La Rabida Chldns Hosp, Chicago, IL 1982-1984; **Faculty Appointment:** Asst Prof Pediatrics, Univ Chicago-Pritzker Sch Med

Southwest

Myones, Barry Lee MD (Pediatric Rheumatology) - *Special Expertise:* Vasculitis; Kawasaki *Disease; Juvenile Dermatomyositis, Sclerdoma;* **Admitting Hospital:** Texas Children's Hospital - Houston; **Office Address:** Texas Chldns Hosp, Ped Rheum Ctr 6621 Fannin St, MS 3-2290 Houston, TX 77030; **Office Phone:** (832) 824-3830; **Board Certifications:** Pediatrics 1983, Pediatric Rheumatology 2000; **Medical School:** Albany Med Coll 1977; **Residency:** Pediatrics, Duke University Med Ctr, Durham, NC 1978-1980; **Fellowships:** Pediatric Rheumatology, Chldns Hosp-Stanford, Palo Alto, CA 1981-1983; Rheumatology, Univ North Carolina, Chapel Hill, NC 1983-1988; **Faculty Appointment:** Assoc Clin Prof Pediatrics, Baylor Coll Med

Warren, Robert Wells MD (Pediatric Rheumatology) - *Special Expertise:* Pediatric *Rheumatology - General;* **Admitting Hospital:** Texas Children's Hospital - Houston; **Office Address:** TX Chldns Hosp, MC-3-2290 6621 Fannin St, Ste 940 Houston, TX 77030; **Office Phone:** (713) 770-3830; **Board Certifications:** Pediatric Rheumatology 1992, Allergy & Immunology 1983; **Medical School:** Washington Univ, St Louis 1978; **Residency:** Pediatrics, Duke Univ, Durham, NC 1978-1979; **Fellowships:** Rheumatology, Duke Univ, Durham, NC 1980-1982; Rheumatology, Duke Univ, Durham, NC 1982-1983; **Faculty Appointment:** Assoc Prof Pediatric Rheumatology, Baylor Coll Med

Wilking, Andrew MD (Pediatric Rheumatology) - *Special Expertise:* Pediatric Rheumatology - General; **Admitting Hospital:** Texas Children's Hospital - Houston; **Office Address:** 6621 Fannin St, Ste 940 Houston, TX 77030; **Office Phone:** (832) 824-3830; **Board Certification:** Pediatrics 1985; **Medical School:** Columbia P&S 1978; **Residency:** Pediatrics, Babies Hosp, New York, NY 1979-1981; **Fellowship:** Pediatric Rheumatology, Tex Chldns Hosp, Houston, TX 1981-1983; **Faculty Appointment:** Assoc Prof Pediatrics, Baylor Coll Med

West Coast and Pacific

Bernstein, Bram Henry MD (Pediatric Rheumatology) - *Special Expertise:* Reheumatic Diseases of Childhood; **Admitting Hospital:** Children's Hospital - Los Angeles; **Office Address:** 4650 W Sunset Blvd Chldns Hosp Los Angeles M/S 60 Los Angeles, CA 90027-6062; **Office Phone:** (323) 669-2119; **Board Certifications:** Pediatrics 1969, Pediatric Rheumatology 1992; **Medical School:** McGill Univ 1964; **Residencies:** Pediatrics, Chldns Hosp, Los Angeles, CA 1965-1967; Rheumatology, Chldns Hosp, Los Angeles, CA 1967-1968; **Fellowship:** Rheumatology, Vancouver Genl Hosp, Canada 1968-1970; **Faculty Appointment:** Clin Prof Pediatrics, Univ SC Sch Med

Emery, Helen Margaret MD (Pediatric Rheumatology) - *Special Expertise:* Rheumatoid Diseases of Childhood; **Admitting Hospital:** University of California - San Francisco Medical Center; **Office Address:** 533 Parnassus Ave UC San Francisco-Ped Rheum San Francisco, CA 94143; **Office Phone:** (415) 476-1736; **Board Certifications:** Pediatrics 1992, Pediatric Rheumatology 1992; **Medical School:** Australia 1971; **Residency:** Pediatrics, Chldns Or Hosp-U Wash, Washington, DC 1973-1975; **Fellowship:** Pediatric Rheumatology, Chldns Or Hosp-U Wash, Washington, DC 1975-1977; **Faculty Appointment:** Clin Prof Pediatrics, UCSF

Sherry, David MD (Pediatric Rheumatology) - *Special Expertise:* Reflex Sympathetic Dystrophy; **Admitting Hospital:** Children's Hospital and Regional Medical Center - Seattle; **Office Address:** Chldns Hosp Med Ctr, Ped Rheum 4800 Sand Point Way NE Seattle, WA 98105-3901; **Office Phone:** (206) 526-2057; **Board Certifications:** Pediatrics 1981, Pediatric Rheumatology 1992; **Medical School:** Texas Tech Univ 1977; **Residency:** Pediatrics, Duke Univ Med Ctr, Durham, NC 1977-1980; **Fellowship:** Pediatric Rheumatology, Univ British Columbia, Vancouver, Canada 1980-1982; **Faculty Appointment:** Assoc Prof Pediatrics, Univ Wash

PEDIATRIC SURGERY
New England

Mayer, John MD (Pediatric Surgery) - *Special Expertise:* Cardiac Surgery; **Admitting Hospital:** Children's Hospital; **Office Address:** Children's Hospital Dept. Cardiac Surgery 300 Longwood Ave Boston, MA 02115; **Office Phone:** (617) 355-7930; **Board Certification:** Thoracic Surgery 1994; **Medical School:** Yale Univ 1972; **Residency:** Surgery, University Minn, Minneapolis, MN 1973-1979; **Fellowship:** Cardiothoracic Surgery, University Minn, Minnepolis, MN 1979-1981; **Faculty Appointment:** Prof Surgery, Harvard Med Sch

Ziegler, Moritz M MD (Pediatric Surgery) - *Special Expertise:* Cancer & General Surgery; **Admitting Hospital:** Children's Hospital; **Office Address:** Chldns Hosp, Dept Surgery 300 Longwood Ave Boston, MA 02115; **Office Phone:** (617) 355-2469; **Board Certifications:** Pediatric Surgery 1995, Surgical Critical Care 1990; **Medical School:** Univ Mich Med Sch 1968; **Residencies:** Surgery, Univ Penn Hosp, Philadelphia, PA 1969-1975; Pediatric Surgery, Chldns Hosp, Philadelphia, PA 1975-1977; **Fellowship:** Medical Oncology, Amer Oncologic Hosp, Philadelphia, PA 1975; **Faculty Appointment:** Prof Surgery, Harvard Med Sch

Mid Atlantic

Adkins, John Crawford MD (Pediatric Surgery) - *Special Expertise:* Neonatal Surgery-Gastrointestinal; **Admitting Hospital:** Children's Hospital of Pittsburgh; **Office Address:** Children's Hospital - Pittsburgh 3705 5th Ave Pittsburgh, PA 15213; **Office Phone:** (412) 359-5222; **Board Certifications:** Surgery 1974, Pediatric Surgery 1993; **Medical School:** Johns Hopkins Univ 1965; **Residencies:** Surgery, Duke Med Ctr, Durham, NC 1966-1967; Surgery, Pittsburgh Med Ctr, Pittsburgh, PA 1970-1973; **Fellowship:** Pediatric Surgery, Chldns Hosp, Pittsburgh, PA 1973-1974; **Faculty Appointment:** Asst Prof Pediatrics, Univ Pittsburgh

Adzick, Nick Scott MD (Pediatric Surgery) - *Special Expertise:* Fetal Surgery; **Admitting Hospital:** The Children's Hospital of Philadelphia; **Office Address:** Chldns Hosp-Philadelphia, Wood Bldg 34th and Civic Ctr Blvd, Fl 5 Philadelphia, PA 19104-4399; **Office Phone:** (215) 590-2727; **Board Certifications:** Pediatric Surgery 1999, Surgical Critical Care 1991; **Medical School:** Harvard Med Sch 1979; **Residencies:** Surgery, Mass Genl Hosp, Boston, MA 1985-1986; Pediatric Surgery, Chldns Hosp, Boston, MA 1986-1988; **Faculty Appointment:** Assoc Prof Surgery, UCSF

Colombani, Paul M MD (Pediatric Surgery) - *Special Expertise:* Pediatric Surgery - General; **Admitting Hospital:** Johns Hopkins Hospital - Baltimore (Page 65); **Office Address:** Johns Hopkins Hosp, Box CMSC 7-1130 600 N Wolfe St, CMSC 7-113 Baltimore, MD 21287; **Office Phone:** (410) 955-2717; **Board Certifications:** Surgery 1993, Pediatric Surgery 1993; **Medical School:** Univ KY Coll Med 1976; **Residency:** Surgery, Geo Wash Univ Hosp, Washington, DC 1977-1981; **Fellowship:** Pediatric Surgery, Johns Hopkins Hosp, Baltimore, MD 1981-1983; **Faculty Appointment:** Prof Surgery, Johns Hopkins Univ

Ginsburg, Howard MD (Pediatric Surgery) - *Special Expertise:* Neonatal Surgery; **Admitting Hospital:** NYU Medical Center (Page 70); **Office Address:** NYU Med Ctr 530 1st Ave, Ste 10W New York, NY 10016-6402; **Office Phone:** 212 2637391; **Board Certifications:** Surgery 1978, Pediatric Surgery 1984; **Medical School:** Univ Cincinnati 1972; **Residencies:** Surgery, NYU-Bellvue Hosp, New York, NY 1972-1977; Pediatric Surgery, Colum-Presby Med Ctr, New York, NY 1977-1979; **Fellowship:** Pediatric Surgery, Mass General Hosp, Boston, MA 1979-1980; **Faculty Appointment:** Assoc Prof Surgery, NYU Sch Med

LaQuaglia, Michael MD (Pediatric Surgery) - *Special Expertise:* Cancer Surgery; Neuroblastoma; Liver Tumors; **Admitting Hospital:** Memorial Sloan Kettering Cancer Center; **Office Address:** Meml Sloan Kettering Cancer Ctr 1275 York Ave New York, NY 10021-6007; **Office Phone:** (212) 639-7002; **Board Certifications:** Surgery 1994, Pediatric Surgery 1997; **Medical School:** UMDNJ-NJ Med Sch, Newark 1976; **Residencies:** Surgery, Mass General Hosp, Boston, MA 1976-1983; Transplant Surgery, Mass General Hosp, Boston, MA 1980-1981; **Fellowships:** Thoracic Surgery, Broadgreen Regl Ctr, Liverpool, England 1982; Pediatric Surgery, Childrens Hospital, Boston, MA 1985; **Faculty Appointment:** Assoc Prof Surgery, Cornell Univ-Weil Med Coll

Lehman, Wallace B MD (Pediatric Surgery) - *Special Expertise:* Orthopaedic Surgery; **Admitting Hospital:** Hospital for Joint Diseases; **Office Address:** Hosp for Joint Diseases, Ped Orth Surgery 301 E 17th St, rm A800 New York, NY 10003; **Office Phone:** (212) 598-6403; **Board Certification:** Orthopaedic Surgery 1966; **Medical School:** SUNY Hlth Sci Ctr 1958; **Residency:** Orthopaedic Surgery, Hosp Joint Diseases, New York, NY 1958-1963; **Faculty Appointment:** Clin Prof Orthopaedic Surgery, NYU Sch Med

Paidas, Charles Nicholas MD (Pediatric Surgery) - *Special Expertise:* Tumor Surgery; Chest Wall Deformities; **Admitting Hospital:** Johns Hopkins Hospital - Baltimore (Page 65); **Office Address:** Johns Hopkins Hosp, Dept Ped Surg 600 N Wolfe St, Bldg CMSC - rm 7-116 Baltimore, MD 21287; **Office Phone:** (410) 955-2960; **Board Certifications:** Pediatric Surgery 1992, Surgical Critical Care 1992; **Medical School:** NY Med Coll 1981; **Residency:** Surgery, NY Med Coll Affil Hosps, Westchester, NY 1982-1987; **Fellowship:** Pediatric Surgery, Johns Hopkins Hosp, Baltimore, MD 1987-1991; **Faculty Appointment:** Assoc Prof Surgery, Johns Hopkins Univ

Quaegebeur, Jan Modest MD (Pediatric Surgery) - *Special Expertise:* Arterial Switch; Heart Valve Surgery; Cardiac Surgery; **Admitting Hospital:** Columbia Presbyterian Medical Center (Page 72); **Office Address:** Babies & Chldns Hosp of NY 3959 Broadway, Ste BN 276 New York, NY 10032; **Office Phone:** (212) 305-5975; **Medical School:** Belgium 1969; **Residency:** Surgery, St Michel Clinic, Brussels, Belgium 1969-1973; **Fellowships:** Thoracic Surgery, Baylor Coll Med, Houston, TX 1973-1974; Thoracic Surgery, Univ Hosp, Leiden, Belgium 1974-1978; **Faculty Appointment:** Prof Surgery, Columbia P&S

Ramenofsky, Max MD (Pediatric Surgery) - *Special Expertise:* Pediatric Surgery - General; **Admitting Hospital:** University Hospital - Brooklyn; **Office Address:** Brooklyn Pediatric Surgical Assoc, PC 450 Clarkson Ave, Box 40 Brooklyn, NY 11203-2012; **Office Phone:** (718) 270-1386; **Board Certifications:** Surgery 1972, Pediatric Surgery 1995; **Medical School:** Univ Tenn Coll Med, Memphis 1965; **Residencies:** Surgery, Michael Reese Hosp, Chicago, IL 1966-1967; Surgery, Cook County Hosp, Chicago, IL 1967-1971; **Fellowship:** Pediatric Surgery, Children's Hosp, Pittsburgh, PA 1972-1974; **Faculty Appointment:** Prof Pediatric Surgery, SUNY Downstate

Spray, Thomas L MD (Pediatric Surgery) - *Special Expertise:* Cardiac Surgery; Transplant-Heart & Lung; Ross Procedure; **Admitting Hospital:** The Children's Hospital of Philadelphia; **Office Address:** Chldns Hosp Philadelphia 34th & Civic Ctr Blvd, Ste 8527 Philadelphia, PA 19104; **Office Phone:** (215) 590-2708; **Board Certifications:** Surgery 1983, Thoracic Surgery 1985; **Medical School:** Duke Univ 1973; **Residencies:** Surgery, Duke Univ Med Ctr, Durham, NC 1973-1975; Thoracic Surgery, Duke Univ Med Ctr, Durham, NC 1977-1980; **Faculty Appointment:** Prof Surgery, Univ Penn

Stylianos, Steven MD (Pediatric Surgery) - *Special Expertise: Trauma; Plastic Surgery;* **Admitting Hospital:** Columbia Presbyterian Medical Center (Page 72); **Office Address:** Babies & Chldns Hosp of NY 3959 Broadway, rm 205 New York, NY 10032; **Office Phone:** (212) 305-8861; **Board Certifications:** Surgery 1989, Pediatric Surgery 1994; **Medical School:** NYU Sch Med 1983; **Residencies:** Surgery, Columbia Presby Med Ctr, New York, NY 1983-1988; Pediatric Surgery, Chldns Hosp, Boston, MA 1990-1992; **Fellowship:** Pediatric Trauma, New England Med Ctr, Boston, MA 1988-1990; **Faculty Appointment:** Asst Prof Pediatric Surgery, Columbia P&S

Velcek, Francisca MD (Pediatric Surgery) - *Special Expertise: Pediatric Surgery - General;* **Admitting Hospital:** Lenox Hill Hospital; **Office Address:** Ped Surgery & Urology Associates 965 5th Ave New York, NY 10021; **Office Phone:** (212) 744-9396; **Board Certifications:** Surgery 1974, Pediatric Surgery 1997; **Medical School:** Philippines 1966; **Residency:** Surgery, St Clare's Hosp, New York, NY 1966-1971; **Fellowships:** Pediatric Surgery, SUNY Hosp, Brooklyn, NY 1973-1975; SUNY Hosp, Brooklyn, NY 1972-1973; **Faculty Appointment:** Prof Surgery, SUNY Hlth Sci Ctr

Wiener, Eugene MD (Pediatric Surgery) - *Special Expertise: Cancer Surgery;* **Admitting Hospital:** Children's Hospital of Pittsburgh; **Office Address:** Chldns Hosp, Dept Ped Surgery 3705 5th Ave, Ste 4A - rm 485 Pittsburgh, PA 15213; **Office Phone:** (412) 692-7280; **Board Certifications:** Surgery 1973, Pediatric Surgery 1995; **Medical School:** Med Coll VA 1964; **Residency:** Surgery, Med Coll VA Hosps, Richmond, VA 1965-1971; **Faculty Appointment:** Prof Surgery, Univ Pittsburgh

Southeast

Drucker, David E MD (Pediatric Surgery) - *Special Expertise: Pediatric Surgery - General;* **Admitting Hospital:** Memorial Regional Hospital- Hollywood; **Office Address:** S FL Ped Surgeons 1150 N 35th Ave, Ste 555 Hollywood, FL 33021-5431; **Office Phone:** (954) 981-0072; **Board Certifications:** Pediatric Surgery 1999, Surgical Critical Care 1992; **Medical School:** Univ Hlth Sci/Chicago Med Sch 1978; **Residency:** Surgery, Med Coll VA Hosps, Richmond, VA 1983-1988; **Fellowship:** Pediatric Surgery, Chldns Hosp, Detroit, MI 1988-1990

Georgeson, Keith E MD (Pediatric Surgery) - *Special Expertise: Hirschsprung's Disease; Laparoscopic Surgery;* **Admitting Hospital:** Children's Hospital; **Office Address:** Chldns Hosp of Alabama, Dept Ped Surgery 1600 7th Ave S, Ste ACC300 Birmingham, AL 35233; **Office Phone:** (205) 939-9688; **Board Certifications:** Pediatric Surgery 1995, Surgery 1992; **Medical School:** Loma Linda Univ 1969; **Residencies:** Surgery, Loma Linda Univ Med Ctr, Loma Linda, CA 1970-1973; Pediatric Surgery, Chldns Hosp, Detroit, MI 1973-1975; **Faculty Appointment:** Assoc Prof Surgery, Univ Ala

Nakayama, Don Ken MD (Pediatric Surgery) - *Special Expertise: Neonatal Surgery; Minimally Invasive Surgery;* **Admitting Hospital:** University of North Carolina Hospitals; **Office Address:** Univ North Carolina, Dept Gen Surg 3010 Old Clinic Bldg - CB 7210 Chapel Hill, NC 27599-7210; **Office Phone:** (919) 966-4643; **Board Certifications:** Pediatric Surgery 1998, Surgery 1994; **Medical School:** UCSF 1978; **Residency:** Surgery, UCSF Hosps, San Francisco, CA 1978-1984; **Fellowship:** Pediatric Surgery, Chldns Hosp, Philadelphia, PA 1984-1986; **Faculty Appointment:** Prof Surgery, Univ NC Sch Med

Neblett, Wallace W MD (Pediatric Surgery) - *Special Expertise: Thyroid Surgery; Pancreatic Disease; Inflammatory Bowel Disease;* **Admitting Hospital:** Vanderbilt University Medical Center; **Office Address:** Vanderbilt Univ Med Ctr, Dept Ped Surg 1211 21st Ave S, Ste 338 Nashville, TN 37212-2712; **Office Phone:** (615) 936-1050; **Board Certification:** Pediatric Surgery 1991; **Medical School:** Vanderbilt Univ **Residencies:** Surgery, Vanderbilt Univ Med Ctr, Nashville, TN 1973-1977; Pediatric Surgery, Chldns Hosp Med Ctr, Cincinnati, OH 1978-1980; **Faculty Appointment:** Prof Surgery, Vanderbilt Univ

Othersen, H Biemann MD (Pediatric Surgery) - *Special Expertise:* Lung Surgery; Tracheal Surgery; Esophageal Surgery; **Admitting Hospital:** MUSC Medical Center; **Office Address:** 171 Ashley Avenue Medical University of South Carolina Charleston, SC 29425; **Office Phone:** (803) 792-3851; **Board Certifications:** Thoracic Surgery 1966, Pediatric Surgery 1975; **Medical School:** Med Univ SC 1953; **Residencies:** Thoracic Surgery, Med U SC, Charleston, SC 1957-1962; Pediatric Surgery, Columbus Childrens, Columbus, OH 1962-1964; **Fellowship:** Surgery, Mass Genl Hosp, Boston, MA 1964-1965; **Faculty Appointment:** Prof Surgery, Med Univ SC

Rodgers, Bradley Moreland MD (Pediatric Surgery) - *Special Expertise:* Thoracic Surgery; **Admitting Hospital:** University of Virginia Health Systems; **Office Address:** Univ VA Hlth Scis Ctr, Dept Surgery Box 800709 Charlottesville, VA 22908-0709; **Office Phone:** (804) 924-2673; **Board Certifications:** Pediatric Surgery 1995, Surgery 1997; **Medical School:** Johns Hopkins Univ 1966; **Residencies:** Surgery, Duke Univ Med Ctr, Durham, NC 1967-1968; Surgery, Duke Univ Med Ctr, Durham, NC 1970-1973; **Fellowship:** Pediatric Surgery, Chldns Hosp, Montreal, CN 1973-1974; **Faculty Appointment:** Prof Pediatric Surgery, Univ VA Sch Med

Toufanian, Ahmad MD (Pediatric Surgery) - *Special Expertise:* Hernia; **Admitting Hospital:** St Mary's Medical Center - West Palm Beach; **Office Address:** 1500 N Dixie Hwy, Ste 202 West Palm Beach, FL 33401-2716; **Office Phone:** (561) 655-6800; **Board Certification:** Surgery 1983; **Medical School:** Iran 1971; **Residencies:** Pediatric Surgery, Chldns Hosp, Columbus, OH 1977-1978; Pediatric Surgery, Univ Miami, Miami, FL 1978-1980; **Fellowship:** Pediatric Surgery, Univ Miami, Miami, FL 1978-1980

Weinberger, Malvin MD (Pediatric Surgery) - *Special Expertise:* Pediatric Surgery - General; **Admitting Hospital:** Miami Children's Hospital; **Office Address:** Nahmad Lankau Weinberger 3200 SW 60th Ct Miami, FL 33155-4070; **Office Phone:** (305) 662-8320; **Board Certifications:** Surgery 1970, Pediatric Surgery 1995; **Medical School:** Temple Univ 1962; **Residencies:** Surgery, Temple Univ Hlth Scis Ctr, Philadelphia, PA 1965-1969; Pediatric Surgery, Columbus Chldns Hosp, Columbus, OH 1969-1971; **Faculty Appointment:** Assoc Clin Prof Surgery, Univ Miami Sch Med

Midwest

Bove, Edward MD (Pediatric Surgery) - *Special Expertise:* Cardiothoracic Surgery; Hypoplastic Left Heart Syndrome; **Admitting Hospital:** University of Michigan Health Center; **Office Address:** Univ Mich Med Ctr, Dept Surg, Ped Cardiac Surg 1500 E Medical Ctr Drive Ann Arbor, MI 48109; **Office Phone:** (734) 763-7354; **Board Certifications:** Thoracic Surgery 1998, Surgery 1978; **Medical School:** Albany Med Coll 1972; **Residencies:** Surgery, Univ Mich Med Ctr, Ann Arbor, MI 1973-1976; Thoracic Surgery, Univ Mich Med Ctr, Ann Arbor, MI 1977-1979; **Fellowship:** Pediatric Cardiac Surgery, Hosp Sick Chldn, London, England 1979-1980; **Faculty Appointment:** Prof Surgery, Univ Mich Med Sch

Cohen, Roger David MD (Pediatric Surgery) - *Special Expertise:* Thoracic Surgery; Laparoscopic Surgery; **Admitting Hospital:** Children's Hospital of Wisconsin; **Office Address:** Chldns Hosp - Wisc 9000 W Wisconsin Ave, Ste 403 Milwaukee, WI 53226; **Office Phone:** (414) 266-6550; **Board Certifications:** Thoracic Surgery 1972, Pediatric Surgery 1995; **Medical School:** Columbia P&S 1963; **Residencies:** Surgery, Presby Hosp, New York, NY 1964-1969; Surgery, Chldns Meml Hosp, Chicago, IL 1969-1971; **Faculty Appointment:** Prof Surgery, Med Coll Wisc

Coran, Arnold G MD (Pediatric Surgery) - *Special Expertise:* Ulcerative Colitis; Hirschsprung's Disease; **Admitting Hospital:** Motts Children's Hospital; **Office Address:** Motts Chldns Hosp-F3970 Box 0245 Ann Arbor, MI 48109-0245; **Office Phone:** (734) 764-4151; **Board Certifications:** Surgery 1969, Thoracic Surgery 1970; **Medical School:** Harvard Med Sch 1963; **Residencies:** Surgery, Peter Bent Brigham Hosp, Boston, MA 1964-1968; Surgery, Children's Hosp, Boston, MA 1964-1968; **Fellowship:** Neonatal Metabolism, Univ of Oslo, Oslo, Norway 1969; **Faculty Appointment:** Prof Surgery, Univ Mich Med Sch

Grosfeld, Jay L MD (Pediatric Surgery) - *Special Expertise:* Cancer Surgery; **Admitting Hospital:** Riley Hospital for Children; **Office Address:** Indiana Univ - JW Riley Hosp for Chldn, Dept Ped Surg 702 Barnhill Dr, Ste 2500 Indianapolis, IN 46202-5200; **Office Phone:** (317) 274-4682; **Board Certifications:** Surgery 1967, Pediatric Surgery 1975; **Medical School:** NYU Sch Med 1961; **Residencies:** Surgery, Bellevue-NYU Hosp, New York, NY 1962-1966; Pediatric Surgery, Ohio State Univ, Columbus, OH 1968-1970; **Fellowship:** Pediatric Hematology-Oncology, Childrens Hosp, Columbus, OH 1968-1970; **Faculty Appointment:** Prof Surgery, Indiana Univ

Oldham, Keith T MD (Pediatric Surgery) - *Special Expertise:* Neonatal Surgery; Cardiothoracic Surgery; **Admitting Hospital:** Children's Hospital of Wisconsin; **Office Address:** Chldns Hosp of WI 9000 W Wisconsin Ave Milwaukee, WI 53226; **Office Phone:** (414) 266-6557; **Board Certifications:** Pediatric Surgery 1991, Surgical Critical Care 1995; **Medical School:** Med Coll VA 1976; **Residency:** Surgery, Univ Wash Med Ctr, Seattle, WA 1977-1981; **Fellowship:** Pediatric Surgery, Univ Cincinnati Chldns Hosp, Cincinnati, OH 1981-1983; **Faculty Appointment:** Prof Pediatric Surgery, Med Coll Wisc

Reynolds, Marleta MD (Pediatric Surgery) - *Special Expertise:* Critical Care; Trauma; **Admitting Hospital:** Children's Memorial Hospital; **Office Address:** Chldns Meml Hosp, Dept Peds 2300 Children's Plaza Chicago, IL 60614; **Office Phone:** (773) 880-4292; **Board Certifications:** Pediatric Surgery 1986, Thoracic Surgery 1995; **Medical School:** Tulane Univ 1976; **Residencies:** Surgery, Tulane Univ Affil Hosp, New Orleans, LA 1977-1981; Pediatric Surgery, Chldns Meml Hosp, Chicago, IL 1981-1983; **Fellowship:** Cardiothoracic Surgery, Northwestern Univ, Chicago, IL 1983-1985

Sato, Thomas Tad MD (Pediatric Surgery) - *Special Expertise:* Neonatal Surgery; Congenital Defect Repair; Laparoscopy & Thoracostomy; **Admitting Hospital:** Children's Hospital of Wisconsin; **Office Address:** Chldns Hosp - Wisc 9000 W Wisconsin Ave Milwaukee, WI 53226; **Office Phone:** (414) 266-6550; **Board Certifications:** Surgery 1996, Pediatric Surgery 1998; **Medical School:** USC Sch Med 1988; **Residency:** Surgery, Univ Wash Med Ctr, Seattle, WA 1988-1995; **Fellowships:** Surgery, Harborview Med Ctr, Seattle, WA 1991-1993; Pediatric Surgery, Chldns Natl Med Ctr, Washington, DC 1995-1997; **Faculty Appointment:** Asst Prof Pediatric Surgery, Med Coll Wisc

West Coast and Pacific

Anderson, Kathryn D MD (Pediatric Surgery) - *Special Expertise:* Pediatric Surgery - General; **Admitting Hospital:** Children's Hospital - Los Angeles; **Office Address:** Chldns Hosp - Los Angeles 4650 Sunset Blvd, MS 72 Los Angeles, CA 90027; **Office Phone:** (323) 669-2104; **Board Certifications:** Surgery 1971, Pediatric Surgery 1993; **Medical School:** Harvard Med Sch 1964; **Residency:** Surgery, Georgetown Univ Hosp, Washington, DC 1965-1969; **Fellowship:** Pediatric Surgery, Chldns Natl Med Ctr, Washington, DC 1970-1972; **Faculty Appointment:** Prof Surgery, USC Sch Med

PEDIATRIC SURGERY *West Coast and Pacific*

Atkinson, James B MD (Pediatric Surgery) - *Special Expertise:* Pediatric Surgery - General; **Admitting Hospital:** UCLA Medical Center; **Office Address:** UCLA Med Ctr 10833 LeConte Ave, Bldg 200 - Ste 542, Box 951749 Los Angeles, CA 90095-1749; **Office Phone:** (310) 206-2429; **Board Certifications:** Surgery 1989, Pediatric Surgery 1993; **Medical School:** Wake Forest Univ Sch Med 1976; **Residency:** Surgery, UCLA Med Ctr, Los Angeles, CA 1977-1981; **Fellowship:** Pediatric Surgery, Chldns Hosp, Los Angeles, CA 1981-1983; **Faculty Appointment:** Prof Surgery, UCLA

Fonkalsrud, Eric W MD (Pediatric Surgery) - *Special Expertise:* Thoracic Surgery; *Gastroesophageal Reflux; Colorectal Surgery;* **Admitting Hospital:** UCLA Medical Center; **Office Address:** UCLA Med Ctr, Dept Surg 72-126CHS 10833 Le Conte Ave Los Angeles, CA 90095-1749; **Office Phone:** (310) 825-6712; **Board Certifications:** Pediatric Surgery 1984, Thoracic Surgery 1966; **Medical School:** Johns Hopkins Univ 1957; **Residencies:** Surgery, Johns Hopkins Hosp, Baltimore, MD 1957-1959; Thoracic Surgery, UCLA Med Ctr, Los Angeles, CA 1959-1963; **Fellowship:** Pediatric Surgery, Columbus Chldns Hosp, Columbus, OH 1963-1965; **Faculty Appointment:** Prof Emeritus Surgery, UCLA

Harrison, Michael R MD (Pediatric Surgery) - *Special Expertise:* Fetal Surgery; **Admitting Hospital:** University of California - San Francisco Medical Center; **Office Address:** Bay Area Pediatric Surgeons 533 Parnassus Ave, rm U-149, Box 0712 San Francisco, CA 94143; **Office Phone:** (415) 476-2538; **Board Certifications:** Surgery 1986, Pediatric Surgery 1999; **Medical School:** Harvard Med Sch 1969; **Residencies:** Surgery, Mass Genl Hosp, Boston, MA 1969-1971; Surgery, Mass Genl Hosp, Boston, MA 1973-1975; **Fellowships:** Pediatric Surgery, Rikshospitalet, Oslo, Norway 1975-1976; Pediatric Surgery, Chldns Hosp, Los Angeles, CA 1976-1978; **Faculty Appointment:** Prof Surgery, UCSF

Krummel, Thomas M. MD (Pediatric Surgery) - *Special Expertise:* Minimally Invasive Surgery; **Admitting Hospital:** Stanford Medical Center; **Office Address:** 701B Welch Rd, Ste 225, MC-5784 Stanford, CA 94305-5784; **Office Phone:** (650) 498-4292; **Board Certifications:** Surgery 1994, Pediatric Surgery 1997; **Medical School:** Univ Wisc 1977; **Residencies:** Surgery, Med Coll Va Hosp, Richmond, VA 1978-1983; Pediatric Surgery, Chldns Hosp, Pittsburgh, PA 1983-1985; **Fellowships:** Surgery, Med Coll Va Hosp, Richmond, VA 1979-1980; Fetal Surgery, UCSF, San Francisco, CA 1985; **Faculty Appointment:** Prof Surgery, Stanford Univ

Tapper, David MD (Pediatric Surgery) - *Special Expertise:* Critical Care; **Admitting Hospital:** Children's Hospital and Regional Medical Center - Seattle; **Office Address:** Chldns Hosp Med Ctr 4800 NE Sand Point Way, Box C5371 Seattle, WA 98105-0371; **Office Phone:** (206) 526-2039; **Board Certifications:** Surgery 1978, Surgical Critical Care 1987; **Medical School:** Univ MD Sch Med 1970; **Residency:** Surgery, Moffitt Hosp, San Francisco, CA 1971-1977; **Fellowship:** Pediatric Surgery, Chldns Hosp Med Ctr, Boston, MA 1977-1979; **Faculty Appointment:** Prof Surgery, Univ Wash

PEDIATRICS
New England

Pizzo, Philip Anthony MD (Pediatrics) - *Special Expertise: Infections-Cancer Patients; AIDS/HIV;* **Admitting Hospital:** Children's Hospital; **Office Address:** Children's Hospital- Dept. Med 300 Longwood Ave Honeywell Bldg Rm 350 Boston, MA 02115; **Office Phone:** (617) 355-7681; **Board Certifications:** Pediatrics 1975, Pediatric Hematology-Oncology 1976; **Medical School:** Univ Rochester 1970; **Residency:** Chldns Hosp Med Ctr, Boston, MA 1971-1973; **Fellowship:** Hematology, Natl Cancer Inst, Bethesda, MD 1973-1976; **Faculty Appointment:** Prof Pediatrics, Uniformed Srvs Univ, Bethesda

Rappaport, Leonard MD (Pediatrics) - *Special Expertise: Development/Behavioral Pediatrics;* **Admitting Hospital:** Children's Hospital; **Office Address:** Longwood Pediatrics 319 Longwood Ave Boston, MA; **Office Phone:** (617) 277-7320; **Board Certification:** Pediatrics 1983; **Medical School:** Yale Univ 1977; **Residency:** Pediatrics, Chldns Hosp, Boston, MA 1978-1980; **Fellowship:** Developmental Pediatrics, Chldns Hosp, Boston, MA 1980-1982; **Faculty Appointment:** Asst Prof Pediatrics, Harvard Med Sch

Shaywitz, Sally Epstein MD (Pediatrics) - *Special Expertise: Learning Disorders; Dyslexia;* **Admitting Hospital:** Yale - New Haven Hospital; **Office Address:** Yale U School of Med-Dept. Ped 333 Cedar St, rm LMP3089 New Haven, CT 06520; **Office Phone:** (203) 785-4641; **Board Certification:** Pediatrics 1971; **Medical School:** Albert Einstein Coll Med 1966; **Residency:** Pediatrics, Bronx Municipal Hosp, NY, NY 1967-1968; **Fellowships:** Pediatrics, Albert Einstein Coll Med, NY, NY 1968-1970; Pediatrics, Albert Einstein Coll Med, NY, NY 1968-1970; **Faculty Appointment:** Prof Pediatrics, Yale Univ

Mid Atlantic

Cohen, Herbert J MD (Pediatrics) - *Special Expertise: Development/Behavioral Pediatrics;* **Admitting Hospital:** Montefiore Medical Center - Weiler/Einstein Division; **Office Address:** Children's Evaluation Rehab Ctr 1410 Pelham Pkwy S Bronx, NY 10461; **Office Phone:** (718) 430-8522; **Board Certification:** Pediatrics 1964; **Medical School:** SUNY Hlth Sci Ctr 1959; **Residency:** Pediatrics, NY Hosp-Cornell Med Ctr, New York, NY 1960-1962; **Fellowship:** Albert Einstein, Bronx, NY 1964-1966; **Faculty Appointment:** Prof Pediatrics, Albert Einstein Coll Med

Hofkosh, Dena MD (Pediatrics) - *Special Expertise: Pediatrics - General;* **Admitting Hospital:** Children's Hospital of Pittsburgh; **Office Address:** Chldns Hosp - Child Development Unit 3705 Fifth Ave Pittsburgh, PA 15213; **Office Phone:** (412) 692-5560; **Board Certification:** Pediatrics 1984; **Medical School:** NYU Sch Med 1979; **Residency:** Pediatrics, Univ Pitts Med Ctr, Pittsburgh, PA 1979-1984

Ludwig, Stephen MD (Pediatrics) - *Special Expertise: Child Abuse & Neglect; Emergency Medicine;* **Admitting Hospital:** The Children's Hospital of Philadelphia; **Office Address:** Chldns Hosp - Philadelphia 34th St and Civic Center Blvd Philadelhia, PA 19104; **Office Phone:** (215) 590-2162; **Board Certifications:** Pediatrics 1992, Pediatric Emergency Medicine 2000; **Medical School:** Temple Univ 1971; **Residency:** Pediatrics, Chldns Hosp Natl Med Ctr, Washington, DC 1972-1974; **Faculty Appointment:** Prof Pediatrics, Univ Penn

Pasquariello Jr, Patrick S MD (Pediatrics) - *Special Expertise: Chronic Fatigue Syndrome; Failure to Thrive;* **Admitting Hospital:** The Children's Hospital of Philadelphia; **Office Address:** Chldns Hosp - Philadelphia 3400 Civic Center Blvd Philadelphia, PA 19104; **Office Phone:** (215) 590-2164; **Board Certification:** Pediatrics 1963; **Medical School:** Jefferson Med Coll 1956; **Residency:** Pediatrics, Chldns Hosp, Philadelphia, PA 1961-1963

PEDIATRICS   *Southeast*

Southeast

Levine, Melvin David MD (Pediatrics) - *Special Expertise:* Learning Disorders; Child Development; **Admitting Hospital:** University of North Carolina Hospitals; **Office Address:** Ctr for Stdy of Dev & Lrng 400 Roberson St Carrboro, NC 27510; **Office Phone:** (919) 966-1020; **Board Certification:** Pediatrics 1971; **Medical School:** Harvard Med Sch 1966; **Residency:** Pediatrics, Chldns Hosp, Boston, MA 1967-1969; **Faculty Appointment:** Prof Pediatrics, Univ NC Sch Med

Lohr, Jacob MD (Pediatrics) - *Special Expertise:* Infectious Disease; Urinary Tract Infection; **Admitting Hospital:** University of North Carolina Hospitals; **Office Address:** 50021 Brogden Rd Chapel Hill, NC 27514; **Office Phone:** (919) 966-2085; **Board Certification:** Pediatrics 1999; **Medical School:** Univ NC Sch Med 1967; **Residency:** Pediatrics, University of VA, VA 1968-1970; **Faculty Appointment:** Prof Pediatrics, Univ NC Sch Med

Underwood, Louis MD (Pediatrics) - *Special Expertise:* Endocrinology; Growth/Development Disorders; **Admitting Hospital:** University of North Carolina Hospitals; **Office Address:** Univ North Carolina Hosps - Dept Peds 101 Manning Dr, CB 7220 Chapel Hill, NC 27514; **Office Phone:** (919) 966-7890; **Board Certifications:** Pediatrics 1993, Pediatric Endocrinology 1993; **Medical School:** Vanderbilt Univ 1961; **Residencies:** Pediatrics, Vanderbilt Univ Hosp, Nashville, TN 1962-1963; Pediatrics, North Carolina Mem Hosp, Chapel Hill, NC 1963-1964; **Fellowship:** Pediatric Endocrinology, Univ North Carolina, Chapel Hill, NC 1967-1970; **Faculty Appointment:** Prof Pediatrics, Univ NC Sch Med

Zilleruelo, Gaston E MD (Pediatrics) - *Special Expertise:* Transplant Medicine-Kidney; Nephrotic Syndrome; Genitourinary-Congenital Anomaly; **Admitting Hospital:** University of Miami - Jackson Memorial Hospital; **Office Address:** Jackson Meml Hosp, Dept Ped Neph Box 16960 Miami, FL 33101-6960; **Office Phone:** (305) 585-6726; **Board Certifications:** Pediatrics 1979, Pediatric Nephrology 1979; **Medical School:** Chile 1969; **Residencies:** Pediatrics, L Calvo-Mackenna Chldns Hosp, Santiago, Chile 1969-1972; Pediatrics, Jackson Meml Hosp, Miami, FL 1976-1977; **Fellowship:** Pediatric Nephrology, Jackson Meml Hosp, Miami, FL 1976-1978; **Faculty Appointment:** Prof Pediatrics, Univ Miami Sch Med

Midwest

Berman, Brian MD (Pediatrics) - *Special Expertise:* Sickle Cell Disease; Thrombocytopenia; **Admitting Hospital:** Rainbow Babies & Children's Hospital; **Office Address:** 11100 Euclid Ave Cleveland, OH 44106; **Office Phone:** (216) 844-8260; **Board Certifications:** Pediatrics 1989, Pediatric Hematology-Oncology 1989; **Medical School:** Temple Univ 1975; **Residency:** Pediatrics, St Chris Hosp Chldn, Philadelphia, PA 1976-1978; **Fellowship:** Pediatric Hematology-Oncology, Yale, New Haven, CT 1978-1980; **Faculty Appointment:** Assoc Prof Pediatrics, Case West Res Univ

Jacob, Molly MD (Pediatrics) - *Special Expertise:* Pediatrics - General; **Admitting Hospital:** Illinois Masonic Medical Center (Page 64); **Office Address:** 4315 N Lincoln Ave, Fl 1 Chicago, IL 60618-1711; **Office Phone:** (773) 528-3403; **Board Certification:** Pediatrics 1980; **Medical School:** India 1968; **Residency:** Pediatrics, Ill Masonic Med Ctr, Chicago, IL 1975-1979; **Fellowship:** Ambulatory Pediatrics, Ill Masonic Med Ctr, Chicago, IL 1978-1979

Lantos, John MD (Pediatrics) - *Special Expertise:* Chronic Disease; **Admitting Hospital:** University of Chicago Hospitals (Page 78); **Office Address:** East 65th Street at Lake Michigan Chicago, IL 60649; **Office Phone:** (773) 363-6700; **Board Certification:** Pediatrics 1986; **Medical School:** Univ Pittsburgh 1981; **Residency:** Pediatrics, Chldrns Natl Med Ctr, Washington, DC 1982-1984; **Fellowship:** Clinical Ethics, Univ Chicago, Chicago, IL 1986; **Faculty Appointment:** Assoc Prof Pediatrics, Univ Chicago-Pritzker Sch Med

Mendelsohn, Janis MD (Pediatrics) - *Special Expertise:* *Pediatrics - General;* **Admitting Hospital:** University of Chicago Hospitals (Page 78); **Office Address:** 800 E 55th St Chicago, IL 60615; **Office Phone:** (773) 702-0660; **Board Certification:** Pediatrics 1973; **Medical School:** Univ Tenn Coll Med, Memphis 1967; **Residency:** Pediatrics, Chldns Meml Hosp, Chicago, IL 1969-1971; **Fellowship:** Geriatric Medicine, Chldns Meml Hosp, Chicago, IL 1970-1971; **Faculty Appointment:** Assoc Prof Clinical Genetics, Univ Chicago-Pritzker Sch Med

Southwest

Boyd, Robert MD (Pediatrics) - *Special Expertise:* *Pediatrics - General;* **Admitting Hospital:** Texas Children's Hospital - Houston; **Office Address:** Houston Pediatric Associates 4110 Bellaire Blvd Houston, TX 77025-1007; **Office Phone:** (713) 666-1953; **Board Certification:** Pediatrics 1987; **Medical School:** Univ Kans 1969; **Residency:** Pediatrics, Baylor Coll Med, Houston, TX 1970-1972; **Faculty Appointment:** Assoc Clin Prof Pediatrics, Baylor Coll Med

Drutz, Jan Edwin MD (Pediatrics) - *Special Expertise:* *Pediatrics - General;* **Admitting Hospital:** Texas Children's Hospital - Houston; **Office Address:** 1102 Bates Ave, Ste 550 Houston, TX 77030; **Office Phone:** (832) 842-3436; **Board Certification:** Pediatrics 1989; **Medical School:** Univ Louisville Sch Med 1968; **Residency:** Baylor Affil Hosps, Houston, TX 1969-1971; **Faculty Appointment:** Assoc Prof Pediatrics, Baylor Coll Med

West Coast and Pacific

McCabe, Edward MD (Pediatrics) - *Special Expertise:* *Neonatal Genetics;* **Admitting Hospital:** UCLA Medical Center; **Office Address:** UCLA Sch Med-Dept Ped—22-412 MDCC 10833 LeConte Ave Los Angeles, CA 90095-1752; **Office Phone:** (310) 825-5095; **Board Certifications:** Pediatrics 1979, Clinical Genetics 1982; **Medical School:** USC Sch Med 1974; **Residency:** Pediatrics, Univ Minn Hosp, Minneapolis, MN 1975-1976; **Fellowship:** Pediatric Metabolism, Univ Colo Hosp, Denver, CO 1976-1978; **Faculty Appointment:** Prof Pediatrics, UCLA

Miller, Carol A MD (Pediatrics) - *Special Expertise:* *Pediatrics - General;* **Admitting Hospital:** University of California - San Francisco Medical Center; **Office Address:** Univ Calif Med Ctr 400 Parnassus Ave San Francisco, CA 94122; **Office Phone:** (415) 353-2000; **Board Certification:** Pediatrics 1981; **Medical School:** Stanford Univ 1975; **Residency:** Pediatrics, Mt Zion Hosp, San Francisco, CA 1976-1977; **Fellowship:** Neonatal-Perinatal Medicine, Mt Zion Hosp, San Francisco, CA 1977-1979; **Faculty Appointment:** Clin Prof Pediatrics, UCSF

Pantell, Robert Howard MD (Pediatrics) - *Special Expertise:* *Febrile Infants;* **Admitting Hospital:** University of California - San Francisco Medical Center; **Office Address:** UCSF Med Ctr 400 Parnassus Ave San Francisco, CA 94143-0503; **Office Phone:** (415) 476-5473; **Board Certification:** Pediatrics 1974; **Medical School:** Boston Univ 1969; **Residency:** Pediatrics, NC Meml Hosp, Chapel Hill, NC 1970-1972; **Fellowship:** Pediatrics, Stanford Univ Hosp, Stanford, CA 1974-1977; **Faculty Appointment:** Prof Pediatrics, UCSF

Zeltzer, Lonnie Kaye MD (Pediatrics) - *Special Expertise:* *Pain Management; Adolescent Medicine;* **Admitting Hospital:** UCLA Medical Center; **Office Address:** UCLA Sch Med, Dept Ped Pain Prog 10833 Le Conte Ave, 22-464 MDCC Los Angeles, CA 90095-1752; **Office Phone:** (310) 825-0731; **Board Certification:** Pediatrics 1976; **Medical School:** Univ Cincinnati 1970; **Residency:** Pediatrics, Univ Ariz Hosp, Tucson, AZ 1971-1973; **Fellowship:** Adolescent Medicine, Chldns Hosp, Los Angeles, CA 1975-1976; **Faculty Appointment:** Prof Pediatrics, UCLA

PHYSICAL MEDICINE & REHABILITATION

Physical medicine and rehabilitation, also referred to as rehabilitation medicine, is the medical specialty concerned with diagnosing, evaluating and treating patients with physical disabilities. These disabilities may arise from conditions affecting the musculoskeletal system such as neck and back pain, sports injuries, or other painful conditions affecting the limbs, for example carpal tunnel syndrome. Alternatively, the disabilities may result from neurological trauma or disease such as spinal cord injury, head injury or stroke.

A physician certified in physical medicine and rehabilitation is often called a physiatrist. The primary goal of the physiatrist is to achieve maximal restoration of physical, psychological, social and vocational function through comprehensive rehabilitation. Pain management is often an important part of the role of the physiatrist. For diagnosis and evaluation, a physiatrist may include the techniques of electromyography to supplement the standard history, physical, X-ray and laboratory examinations. The physiatrist has expertise in the appropriate use of therapeutic exercise, prosthetics (artificial limbs), orthotics and mechanical and electrical devices.

Training required: Four years *plus* one year clinical practice

Physician Listings

Physical Medicine & Rehabilitation

Mid Atlantic

Ahn, Jung Hwan MD (Physical Medicine & Rehabilitation) - *Special Expertise: Spinal Cord Injury; Stroke Rehabilitation;* **Admitting Hospital:** NYU Medical Center (Page 70); **Office Address:** NYU Medical Center 400 E 34th St, rm 421 New York, NY 10016; **Office Phone:** (212) 263-6122; **Board Certifications:** Physical Medicine & Rehabilitation 1980, Spinal Cord Injury Medicine 2008; **Medical School:** South Korea 1970; **Residencies:** Obstetrics & Gynecology, Elmhurst City Hosp - Mt Sinai, New York, NY 1975-1976; Physical Medicine & Rehabilitation, NYU Med Ctr, New York, NY 1976-1979; **Fellowship:** Spinal Cord Injury Medicine, NYU Med Ctr, New York, NY 1979-1980; **Faculty Appointment:** Assoc Clin Prof NYU Sch Med

Aseff, John Namer MD (Physical Medicine & Rehabilitation) - *Special Expertise: Electrodiagnosis; Pain-Soft Tissue;* **Admitting Hospital:** National Rehabilitation Hospital; **Office Address:** Wahington Hosp Ctr, Dept PM&R 110 Irving St NW Washington, DC 20010; **Office Phone:** (202) 877-1916; **Board Certification:** Physical Medicine & Rehabilitation 1978; **Medical School:** Ohio State Univ 1973; **Residencies:** Surgery, Case Western Reserve Univ Hosps, Cleveland, OH 1973-1975; Physical Medicine & Rehabilitation, Ohio State Univ Hosps, Columbus, OH 1975-1977; **Faculty Appointment:** Assoc Clin Prof Physical Medicine & Rehabilitation, Georgetown Univ

Bach, John MD (Physical Medicine & Rehabilitation) - *Special Expertise: Pulmonary Rehabilitation; Spinal Cord Injury;* **Admitting Hospital:** UMDNJ-University Hospital-Newark; **Office Address:** Univ. Hosp-Dept. PMR 150 Bergen St, Ste B403 Newark, NJ 07103-2425; **Office Phone:** (973) 972-7195; **Board Certification:** Physical Medicine & Rehabilitation 1986; **Medical School:** UMDNJ-NJ Med Sch, Newark 1976; **Residency:** Physical Medicine & Rehabilitation, NYU Med Ctr, New York, NY 1977-1980; **Fellowship:** Univ Hosp, Poitiers France 1981-1983; **Faculty Appointment:** Prof Physical Medicine & Rehabilitation, UMDNJ-NJ Med Sch, Newark

Ballard, Pamela H MD (Physical Medicine & Rehabilitation) - *Special Expertise: Spasticity Management; Infertility-Male; Neuromuscular Rehabilitation;* **Admitting Hospital:** National Rehabilitation Hospital; **Office Address:** 102 Irving St NW, rm 2164 Washington, DC 20010; **Office Phone:** (202) 877-1750; **Board Certifications:** Physical Medicine & Rehabilitation 1991, Spinal Cord Injury Medicine 1999; **Medical School:** Howard Univ 1986; **Residency:** Physical Medicine & Rehabilitation, Sinai Hosp, Baltimore, MD 1987-1990

De Lateur, Barbara J MD (Physical Medicine & Rehabilitation) - *Special Expertise: Frailty;* **Admitting Hospital:** Johns Hopkins Hospital - Baltimore (Page 65); **Office Address:** Good Samaritan Prof Bldg 5601 Loch Raven Blvd, Ste 406 Baltimore, MD 21239-2905; **Office Phone:** (410) 532-4717; **Board Certification:** Physical Medicine & Rehabilitation 1970; **Medical School:** Univ Wash 1963; **Residency:** Physical Medicine & Rehabilitation, Univ Wash Hosp, Seattle, WA 1964-1968; **Faculty Appointment:** Prof Physical Medicine & Rehabilitation, Johns Hopkins Univ

Dillingham, Timothy R MD (Physical Medicine & Rehabilitation) - *Special Expertise: Physical Medicine & Rehabilitation - General;* **Admitting Hospital:** Johns Hopkins Hospital - Baltimore (Page 65); **Office Address:** Good Samaritan Profl 5601 Loch Raven Blvd, Ste 406 Baltimore, MD 21239; **Office Phone:** (410) 532-4576; **Board Certification:** Physical Medicine & Rehabilitation 1991; **Medical School:** Univ Wash 1986; **Residency:** Physical Medicine & Rehabilitation, Univ Wash Affil, Seattle, WA 1987-1990

Ditunno, John Francis MD (Physical Medicine & Rehabilitation) - *Special Expertise: Spinal Cord Injury;* **Admitting Hospital:** Thomas Jefferson University Hospital; **Office Address:** 111 S 11th St, rm 9604 Philadelphia, PA 19107; **Office Phone:** (215) 955-5580; **Board Certifications:** Physical Medicine & Rehabilitation 1968, Spinal Cord Injury Medicine 1998; **Medical School:** Hahnemann Univ 1958; **Residencies:** Physical Medicine & Rehabilitation, Abraham Jacobi Hosp, New York, NY 1963; Physical Medicine & Rehabilitation, U Penn Hospital, Philadelphia, PA 1964-1965; **Faculty Appointment:** Prof Physical Medicine & Rehabilitation, Jefferson Med Coll

Esquenazi, Alberto MD (Physical Medicine & Rehabilitation) - *Special Expertise: Amputee Rehabilitation; Mobility Evaluation & Treatment; Polio Rehabilitation;* **Admitting Hospital:** Moss Rehab Hospital; **Office Address:** Moss Rehab Hosp 1200 W Tabor Rd Philadelphia, PA 19141-3019; **Office Phone:** (215) 456-9470; **Board Certification:** Physical Medicine & Rehabilitation 1986; **Medical School:** Mexico 1981; **Residency:** Physical Medicine & Rehabilitation, Temple Univ, Philadelphia, PA 1982-1985; **Fellowship:** Gait Prostheses, Moss Rehab Hosp, Philadelphia, PA 1985-1986; **Faculty Appointment:** Assoc Prof Physical Medicine & Rehabilitation, Temple Univ

Feinberg, Joseph Hunt MD (Physical Medicine & Rehabilitation) - *Special Expertise: Sports-Orthopedic Related Injuries; Spine & Nerve Injuries;* **Admitting Hospital:** Hospital for Special Surgery (Page 63); **Office Address:** Hosp Special Surg 523 E 72nd St New York, NY 10021; **Office Phone:** (212) 606-1568; **Board Certification:** Physical Medicine & Rehabilitation 1991; **Medical School:** Albany Med Coll 1983; **Residencies:** Surgery, Mt Sinai Hosp, New York, NY 1984-1985; Physical Medicine & Rehabilitation, Rusk Inst Rehab, New York, NY 1987-1990; **Fellowships:** Orthopaedic Pathology, Hosp Spec Surg, New York, NY 1985-1986; Orthopedic Biomechanics, Univ Iowa Hosp & Clins, Iowa City, IA 1986-1987; **Faculty Appointment:** Asst Prof Medicine, UMDNJ Sch Osteo Med

Francis, Kathleen MD (Physical Medicine & Rehabilitation) - *Special Expertise: Lymphedema; Amyotrophic Lateral Sclerosis(ALS); Neurodegenerative Disease;* **Admitting Hospital:** Kessler Institute for Rehabilitation - East Orange; **Office Address:** Kessler Inst for Rehab 1199 Pleasant Valley Way West Orange, NJ 07052; **Office Phone:** (973) 731-3600; **Board Certification:** Physical Medicine & Rehabilitation 1994; **Medical School:** UMDNJ-NJ Med Sch, Newark 1989; **Residency:** Physical Medicine & Rehabilitation, UMDNJ-Kessler Inst Rehab, Newark, NJ 1990-1993; **Faculty Appointment:** Asst Clin Prof Physical Medicine & Rehabilitation, UMDNJ-NJ Med Sch, Newark

Kirshblum, Steven C MD (Physical Medicine & Rehabilitation) - *Special Expertise: Spinal Cord Injury;* **Admitting Hospital:** Kessler Institute for Rehabilitation - East Orange; **Office Address:** 1199 Pleasant Valley Way West Orange, NJ 07052; **Office Phone:** (973) 731-3600; **Board Certifications:** Physical Medicine & Rehabilitation 1991, Spinal Cord Injury Medicine 1998; **Medical School:** Univ Hlth Sci/Chicago Med Sch 1986; **Residency:** Physical Medicine & Rehabilitation, Mount Sinai Med Ctr, New York, NY 1987-1990; **Faculty Appointment:** Asst Prof Physical Medicine & Rehabilitation, UMDNJ-NJ Med Sch, Newark

Lieberman, James MD (Physical Medicine & Rehabilitation) - *Special Expertise: Physical Medicine & Rehabilitation - General;* **Admitting Hospital:** Columbia Presbyterian Medical Center (Page 72); **Office Address:** Rehabilitation Med Assoc 630 W 168th St, Box 38 New York, NY 10032; **Office Phone:** (212) 305-4818; **Board Certifications:** Neurology 1971, Physical Medicine & Rehabilitation 1981; **Medical School:** UCSF 1963; **Residencies:** Neurology, Univ Mich Med Ctr, Ann Arbor, MI 1964-1965; Neurology, Yale-New Haven Hosp, New Haven, CT 1965-1967; **Fellowship:** Physical Medicine & Rehabilitation, UC Davis, Sacramento, CA 1978-1980; **Faculty Appointment:** Prof Physical Medicine & Rehabilitation, Columbia P&S

Ma, Dong M MD (Physical Medicine & Rehabilitation) - *Special Expertise:*
Electrodiagnosis; Musculoskeletal Disease; **Admitting Hospital:** NYU Medical Center (Page 70);
Office Address: 400 E 34th St New York, NY 10016; **Office Phone:** (212) 263-6338; **Board
Certification:** Physical Medicine & Rehabilitation 1979; **Medical School:** South Korea 1968;
Residency: Physical Medicine & Rehabilitation, NYU Med Ctr, New York, NY 1973-1975;
Fellowship: Physical Medicine & Rehabilitation, NYU Med Ctr, New York, NY 1976-1977; **Faculty
Appointment:** Assoc Clin Prof Physical Medicine & Rehabilitation, NYU Sch Med

Mayer, Nathaniel MD (Physical Medicine & Rehabilitation) - *Special Expertise:* Motor
Control Analysis; Spasticity Management; **Admitting Hospital:** Moss Rehab Hospital; **Office
Address:** Moss Rehab 1200 W Tabor Rd Philadelphia, PA 19141; **Office Phone:** (215) 456-9560;
Board Certification: Physical Medicine & Rehabilitation 1976; **Medical School:** Albert Einstein Coll
Med 1968; **Residency:** Physical Medicine & Rehabilitation, Temple Hospital, Philadelphia, PA
1969-1973; **Faculty Appointment:** Prof Physical Medicine & Rehabilitation, Temple Univ

Munin, Michael Craig MD (Physical Medicine & Rehabilitation) - *Special Expertise:*
Spasticity Management; Amputee Rehabilitation; Hip Surgery Rehabilitation; **Admitting Hospital:**
UPMC - Presbyterian University Hospital; **Office Address:** Univ Pittsburgh Physicians- PM&R Assoc
3471 Fifth Ave Lilliane S Kaufman Bldg Ste 1103 Pittsburgh, PA 15213; **Office Phone:** (412) 692-
4400; **Board Certification:** Physical Medicine & Rehabilitation 1993; **Medical School:** Jefferson
Med Coll 1988; **Residency:** Physical Medicine & Rehabilitation, Thomas Jefferson Univ Hosp,
Philadelphia, PA 1989-1992; **Faculty Appointment:** Assoc Prof Physical Medicine & Rehabilitation,
Univ Pittsburgh

Ragnarsson, Kristjan MD (Physical Medicine & Rehabilitation) - *Special Expertise:* Spinal
Cord Injury; **Admitting Hospital:** Mount Sinai Hospital (Page 70); **Office Address:** 5 E 98th St New
York, NY 10029; **Office Phone:** (212) 659-9360; **Board Certification:** Physical Medicine &
Rehabilitation 1976; **Medical School:** Iceland 1969; **Residency:** Physical Medicine &
Rehabilitation, NYU, New York, NY 1971-1974; **Fellowship:** Physical Medicine & Rehabilitation,
NYU, New York, NY 1974-1975; **Faculty Appointment:** Prof Physical Medicine & Rehabilitation,
Mount Sinai Sch Med

Staas Jr, William E MD (Physical Medicine & Rehabilitation) - *Special Expertise:* Spinal
Cord Injury; **Admitting Hospital:** Magee Rehabilitation Hospital; **Office Address:** Magee Rehab
Hosp Six Franklin Plaza Philadelphia, PA 19102; **Office Phone:** (215) 587-3099; **Board
Certifications:** Physical Medicine & Rehabilitation 1970, Spinal Cord Injury Medicine 1998;
Medical School: Jefferson Med Coll 1962; **Residency:** Physical Medicine & Rehabilitation, Univ
Penn Hosp, Philadelphia, PA 1965-1968; **Faculty Appointment:** Prof Physical Medicine &
Rehabilitation, Jefferson Med Coll

Zafonte, Ross DO (Physical Medicine & Rehabilitation) - *Special Expertise:* Brain Injury
Rehabilitation; Spinal Cord Injury; **Admitting Hospital:** UPMC - Presbyterian University Hospital;
Office Address: Lillian Kaufman Bldg 3471 Fifth Ave, Ste 901 Pittsburgh, PA 15213-3221; **Office
Phone:** (412) 648-6979; **Board Certification:** Physical Medicine & Rehabilitation 1990; **Medical
School:** Nova SE Univ, Coll Osteo Med 1985; **Residency:** Physical Medicine & Rehabilitation, Mt
Sinai Sch Med, New York, NY 1986-1989; **Faculty Appointment:** Prof Physical Medicine &
Rehabilitation, Univ Pittsburgh

Southeast

Creamer, Michael DO (Physical Medicine & Rehabilitation) - *Special Expertise:* Spinal Cord Injury; **Admitting Hospital:** Florida Hospital; **Office Address:** 100 W Gore St, Ste 203 Orlando, FL 32806-1041; **Office Phone:** (407) 649-8707; **Board Certifications:** Physical Medicine & Rehabilitation 1992, Spinal Cord Injury Medicine 1998; **Medical School:** Chicago Coll Osteo Med 1987; **Residency:** Physical Medicine & Rehabilitation, Rehab Inst Chicago, Chicago, IL 1988-1991; **Faculty Appointment:** Asst Prof Physical Medicine & Rehabilitation, Southeastern Univ Coll Osteo Med

Jackson, Amie Brown MD (Physical Medicine & Rehabilitation) - *Special Expertise:* Spinal Cord Injury; **Admitting Hospital:** University of Alabama Hospital at Birmingham; **Office Address:** 1717 6th Ave S Birmingham, AL 35233-1801; **Office Phone:** (205) 934-4131; **Board Certification:** Physical Medicine & Rehabilitation 1990; **Medical School:** Univ Ala 1984; **Residency:** Physical Medicine & Rehabilitation, U Alabama, Birmingham, AL 1984-1987; **Faculty Appointment:** Assoc Prof Univ Ala

Lipkin, David L MD (Physical Medicine & Rehabilitation) - *Special Expertise:* Sports Medicine; Pain-Back; **Admitting Hospital:** Mount Sinai Medical Center; **Office Address:** Assocs Rehab, Lowenstein Bldg 4300 Alton Rd, Ste 137 Miami Beach, FL 33140-2800; **Office Phone:** (305) 674-2171; **Board Certification:** Physical Medicine & Rehabilitation 1971; **Medical School:** Belgium 1964; **Residencies:** Pediatrics, Jersey City Med Ctr, Jersey City, NJ 1964-1966; Physical Medicine & Rehabilitation, Bronx Muni Hosp, New York, NY 1966-1969; **Fellowship:** Research, Natl Inst Hlth-Eins Coll Med, Bronx, NY 1966-1969; **Faculty Appointment:** Asst Prof Physical Medicine & Rehabilitation, Univ Miami Sch Med

Peppard, Terrence Richard MD (Physical Medicine & Rehabilitation) - *Special Expertise:* Physical Medicine & Rehabilitation - General; **Admitting Hospital:** Mercy Hospital - Miami; **Office Address:** Mercy Outpatient Care 3663 S Miami Ave Miami, FL 33133-4206; **Office Phone:** (305) 285-2966; **Board Certification:** Physical Medicine & Rehabilitation 1989; **Medical School:** Univ Miami Sch Med 1984; **Residency:** Physical Medicine & Rehabilitation, NYU Med Ctr, New York, NY 1984-1987; **Fellowship:** Neurological Muscular Disease, NYU Med Ctr, New York, NY 1987-1988

Midwest

Chen, David MD (Physical Medicine & Rehabilitation) - *Special Expertise:* Spinal Cord Injury; **Admitting Hospital:** Rehabilitation Institute - Chicago; **Office Address:** Rehab Inst Chicago 345 E Superior St Chicago, IL 60611; **Office Phone:** (312) 238-0764; **Board Certifications:** Physical Medicine & Rehabilitation 1992, Spinal Cord Injury Medicine 1998; **Medical School:** Univ IL Coll Med 1987; **Residency:** Physical Medicine & Rehabilitation, Norhthwestern Med Sch, Chicago, IL 1988-1991; **Faculty Appointment:** Asst Prof Physical Medicine & Rehabilitation, Northwestern Univ

Clairmont, Albert MD (Physical Medicine & Rehabilitation) - *Special Expertise:* Pain Management; **Admitting Hospital:** Ohio State University Medical Center; **Office Address:** 480 W 9th Ave Columbus, OH 43210; **Office Phone:** (614) 293-4837; **Board Certifications:** Physical Medicine & Rehabilitation 1985, Pediatrics 1985; **Medical School:** Jamaica 1974; **Residencies:** Pediatric Surgery, Columbus Chldns Hosp, Columbus, OH 1980-1981; Physical Medicine & Rehabilitation, Ohio St Univ Hosps, Columbus, OH 1981-1983

Colachis III, Samuel C MD (Physical Medicine & Rehabilitation) - *Special Expertise:* Spinal Cord Injury; Electrodiagnosis; **Admitting Hospital:** Ohio State University Medical Center; **Office Address:** 1025 Dodd Hall Columbus, OH 43210; **Office Phone:** (614) 293-4837; **Board Certification:** Physical Medicine & Rehabilitation 1988; **Medical School:** USC Sch Med 1984; **Residency:** Physical Medicine & Rehabilitation, Ohio State Univ Hosps, Columbus, OH 1985-1987; **Fellowship:** Electrodiagnosis, Ohio State Univ Hosps, Columbus, OH 1987-1988; **Faculty Appointment:** Asst Prof Physical Medicine & Rehabilitation, Ohio State Univ

Gittler, Michelle MD (Physical Medicine & Rehabilitation) - *Special Expertise:* Spinal Cord Injury; Amputee Rehabilitation; **Admitting Hospital:** University of Chicago Hospitals (Page 78); **Office Address:** 1401 S California Chicago, IL 60640; **Office Phone:** (773) 522-5856; **Board Certifications:** Physical Medicine & Rehabilitation 1993, Spinal Cord Injury Medicine 1998; **Medical School:** Univ IL Coll Med 1988; **Residency:** Physical Medicine & Rehabilitation, Rehab Inst Chicago, Chicago, IL 1989-1992; **Faculty Appointment:** Asst Clin Prof Physical Medicine & Rehabilitation, Univ Chicago-Pritzker Sch Med

Haig, Andrew MD (Physical Medicine & Rehabilitation) - *Special Expertise:* Sports Medicine; Pain-Back & Neck; **Admitting Hospital:** University of Michigan Health Center; **Office Address:** University Hosp 325 E Eisenhower Pkwy, Fl 2 - Ste 202 Ann Artbor, MI 48108; **Office Phone:** (888) 254-2225; **Board Certification:** Physical Medicine & Rehabilitation 1987; **Medical School:** Med Coll Wisc 1983; **Residency:** Physical Medicine & Rehabilitation, Northwestern University, Chicago, IL 1984-1986; **Faculty Appointment:** Asst Prof Orthopaedic Surgery, Univ VT Coll Med

Leonard Jr., James A. MD (Physical Medicine & Rehabilitation) - *Special Expertise:* Amputee Rehabilitation; Electrodiagnosis; **Admitting Hospital:** University of Michigan Health Center; **Office Address:** Univ Hosp Dept. Physical Medicine & Rehabilitation 1500 E Medical Center Drive Ann Arbor, MI 48109-0718; **Office Phone:** (734) 936-7190; **Board Certification:** Physical Medicine & Rehabilitation 1977; **Medical School:** Univ Mich Med Sch 1972; **Residency:** U Mich Med Ctr, Ann Arbor, MI 1972-1975; **Faculty Appointment:** Clin Prof Physical Medicine & Rehabilitation, Univ Mich Med Sch

Mason, Kristin Denise MD (Physical Medicine & Rehabilitation) - *Special Expertise:* Stroke; Electrodiagnosis of Muscle/Nerve Disease; **Admitting Hospital:** Swedish Covenant Hospital; **Office Address:** 5145 N California Ave Chicago, IL 60625; **Office Phone:** (773) 989-1696; **Board Certification:** Physical Medicine & Rehabilitation 1993; **Medical School:** Baylor Coll Med 1988; **Residency:** Physical Medicine & Rehabilitation, Rehab Inst of Chicago, Chicago, IL 1989-1992; **Faculty Appointment:** Clin Inst Physical Medicine & Rehabilitation, Northwestern Univ

Nobunaga, Austin MD (Physical Medicine & Rehabilitation) - *Special Expertise:* Spinal Cord Injury; Electrodiagnosis; **Admitting Hospital:** University of Michigan Health Center; **Office Address:** Univ Mich Med Ctr, Dept PM&R 1500 E Medical Center Dr Ann Arbor, MI 48109-0718; **Office Phone:** (734) 647-6954; **Board Certifications:** Physical Medicine & Rehabilitation 1990, Spinal Cord Injury Medicine 1999; **Medical School:** Univ Mich Med Sch 1985; **Residency:** Physical Medicine & Rehabilitation, Rehab Inst Chicago, Chicago, IL 1986-1989; **Faculty Appointment:** Asst Prof Physical Medicine & Rehabilitation, Univ Mich Med Sch

Press, Joel MD (Physical Medicine & Rehabilitation) - *Special Expertise:* Sports Medicine; Pain-Back; Musculoskeletal Injuries; **Admitting Hospital:** Rehabilitation Institute - Chicago; **Office Address:** 1030 N Clark St, Ste 500 Rehabilitation Institute-Dept of Spine & Sport Chicago, IL 60610; **Office Phone:** (312) 238-7767; **Board Certification:** Physical Medicine & Rehabilitation 1988; **Medical School:** Univ IL Coll Med 1984; **Residency:** Physical Medicine & Rehabilitation, Northwestern Med Hosp, Chicago, IL 1984-1988; **Faculty Appointment:** Assoc Clin Prof Medicine, Northwestern Univ

Roth, Elliot MD (Physical Medicine & Rehabilitation) - *Special Expertise:* Stroke *Rehabilitation; Neuro-Rehabilitation;* **Admitting Hospital:** Rehabilitation Institute - Chicago; **Office Address:** Rehab Inst - Chicago 345 E Superior St, Ste 1572 Chicago, IL 60611-3015; **Office Phone:** (312) 238-4637; **Board Certification:** Physical Medicine & Rehabilitation 1987; **Medical School:** Northwestern Univ 1982; **Residency:** Physical Medicine & Rehabilitation, Northwestern Univ, Chicago, IL 1983-1985; **Fellowship:** Physical Medicine & Rehabilitation, Rehab Inst-Chicago, Chicago, IL 1986; **Faculty Appointment:** Prof Physical Medicine & Rehabilitation, Northwestern Univ

Sisung, Charles MD (Physical Medicine & Rehabilitation) - *Special Expertise:* Rheumatoid *Diseases of Childhood; Trauma; Burns;* **Admitting Hospital:** Rehabilitation Institute - Chicago; **Office Address:** Rehab Inst Chicago 345 E Superior St, rm 1158 Chicago, IL 60611; **Office Phone:** (312) 238-1246; **Board Certifications:** Pediatrics 1989, Physical Medicine & Rehabilitation 1991; **Medical School:** Univ Mich Med Sch 1981; **Residencies:** Pediatrics, Univ Mich Med Ctr, Ann Arbor, MI 1981-1984; Physical Medicine & Rehabilitation, Schwab Rehab Hosp, Chicago, IL 1986-1989; **Fellowship:** Pediatric Rheumatology, Univ Chicago Hosp, Chicago, IL 1989-1991; **Faculty Appointment:** Asst Prof Physical Medicine & Rehabilitation, Northwestern Univ

Sliwa, James DO (Physical Medicine & Rehabilitation) - *Special Expertise:* Pain-Back; *Multiple Sclerosis;* **Admitting Hospital:** Rehabilitation Institute - Chicago; **Office Address:** 345 E Superior St Chicago, IL 60611; **Office Phone:** (312) 238-4093; **Board Certification:** Physical Medicine & Rehabilitation 1985; **Medical School:** Chicago Coll Osteo Med 1980; **Residency:** Physical Medicine & Rehabilitation, Rehab Inst Chicago, Chicago, IL 1981-1984; **Faculty Appointment:** Assoc Clin Prof Northwestern Univ

Volshteyn, Oksana MD (Physical Medicine & Rehabilitation) - *Special Expertise:* Spinal *Cord Injury;* **Admitting Hospital:** Barnes - Jewish Hospital; **Office Address:** 216 S Kingshighway, rm 2133 St Louis, MO 63110; **Office Phone:** (314) 454-7757; **Board Certifications:** Physical Medicine & Rehabilitation 1986, Spinal Cord Injury Medicine 1999; **Medical School:** Russia 1976; **Residency:** Physical Medicine & Rehabilitation, Barnes Jewish Hosp, St Louis, MO 1982-1985; **Faculty Appointment:** Asst Prof Neurology, Washington Univ, St Louis

Great Plains and Mountains

Lammertse, Daniel MD (Physical Medicine & Rehabilitation) - *Special Expertise:* Spinal *Cord Injury;* **Admitting Hospital:** Craig Hospital; **Office Address:** Craig Hosp 3425 S Clarkson St Engelwood, CO 80110-2811; **Office Phone:** (303) 789-8220; **Board Certifications:** Physical Medicine & Rehabilitation 1980, Spinal Cord Injury Medicine 1998; **Medical School:** Ohio State Univ 1976; **Residency:** Physical Medicine & Rehabilitation, Ohio State Univ Hosp, Columbus, OH 1976-1979; **Faculty Appointment:** Asst Clin Prof Physical Medicine & Rehabilitation, Univ Colo

Matthews, Dennis Jerome MD (Physical Medicine & Rehabilitation) - *Special Expertise:* Brain Injury Rehabilitation; Musculoskeletal Disease; Cerebral Palsy; **Admitting Hospital:** The Children's Hospital - Denver; **Office Address:** Chldns Hosp - Denver 1056 E 19th Ave Denver, CO 80218-1007; **Office Phone:** (303) 861-6633; **Board Certification:** Physical Medicine & Rehabilitation 1979; **Medical School:** Univ Colo 1975; **Residency:** Physical Medicine & Rehabilitation, Minn Hosps, Minneapolis, MN 1975-1978; **Fellowship:** Research, Minn Hosps, Minneapolis, MN 1978; **Faculty Appointment:** Assoc Prof Physical Medicine & Rehabilitation, Univ Colo

Barber, Douglas Byron MD (Physical Medicine & Rehabilitation) - *Special Expertise:*
Spinal Cord Injury; **Admitting Hospital:** University Health System; **Office Address:** Univ Hlth Sci Ctr,
Dept of Rehab Med 7703 Floyd Curl Drive San Antonio, TX 78229-3900; **Office Phone:** (210) 567-
5351; **Board Certifications:** Physical Medicine & Rehabilitation 1992, Spinal Cord Injury Medicine
1999; **Medical School:** Univ Tex, Houston 1987; **Residency:** Physical Medicine & Rehabilitation,
Univ TX Hlth Scis Ctr, San Antonio, TX 1988-1991; **Faculty Appointment:** Assoc Prof Physical
Medicine & Rehabilitation, Univ Tex, San Antonio

Donovan, William Henry MD (Physical Medicine & Rehabilitation) - *Special Expertise:*
Spinal Cord Injury; Amputee Rehabilitation; **Admitting Hospital:** TIRR LifeBridge Hospital; **Office
Address:** TIRR 1333 Moursund St, Ste D-107 Houston, TX 77030-3405; **Office Phone:** (713) 797-5912;
Board Certification: Physical Medicine & Rehabilitation 1975; **Medical School:** Albany Med Coll
1966; **Residencies:** Internal Medicine, Marquette Univ, Milwaukee, WI 1967-1968; Physical
Medicine & Rehabilitation, Univ Wash, Seattle, WA 1970-1972; **Faculty Appointment:** Prof
Physical Medicine & Rehabilitation, Univ Tex, Houston

Dumitru, Daniel MD (Physical Medicine & Rehabilitation) - *Special Expertise:*
Electrodiagnosis; Electrodiagnosis; **Admitting Hospital:** University of Texas Health & Science
Center; **Office Address:** Univ. of Texas Health Science Center-Dept. of Rehab Medicine 7703
Floyd Curl St San Antonio, TX 78229-3900; **Office Phone:** (210) 567-5347; **Board Certification:**
Physical Medicine & Rehabilitation 1984; **Medical School:** Univ Cincinnati 1980; **Residency:**
Physical Medicine & Rehabilitation, VA Hosp., San Antonio, TX 1980-1983; **Faculty Appointment:**
Prof Physical Medicine & Rehabilitation, Univ Tex, San Antonio

Francisco, Gerard E MD (Physical Medicine & Rehabilitation) - *Special Expertise:* Physical
Medicine & Rehabilitation - General; **Admitting Hospital:** TIRR LifeBridge Hospital; **Office Address:**
The Inst Rehab & Rsch 1333 Moursund St Houston, TX 77030-3405; **Office Phone:** (713) 797-5246;
Board Certification: Physical Medicine & Rehabilitation 1995; **Medical School:** Philippines 1989;
Residency: Physical Medicine & Rehabilitation, UMDNJ-Univ Hosp, Newark, NJ 1991-1994;
Fellowship: Physical Medicine & Rehabilitation, Baylor Coll Med, Houston, TX 1994-1995

Ivanhoe, Cindy MD (Physical Medicine & Rehabilitation) - *Special Expertise:* Brain Injury
Rehabilitation; **Admitting Hospital:** TIRR LifeBridge Hospital; **Office Address:** TIRR 1333 Moursund
Rd Houston, TX 77030-3405; **Office Phone:** (713) 797-5236; **Board Certification:** Physical Medicine
& Rehabilitation 1993; **Medical School:** Mexico 1984; **Residency:** Physical Medicine &
Rehabilitation, U ILL Coll Med, Chicago, IL 1989-1992; **Fellowship:** Baylor Coll Of Med, Houston,
TX 1992-1993; **Faculty Appointment:** Asst Clin Prof Univ Tex, Houston

Kevorkian, Charles George MD (Physical Medicine & Rehabilitation) - *Special Expertise:*
Stroke; Neuromuscular Rehabilitation; **Admitting Hospital:** St Luke's Episcopal Hospital - Houston
(Page 76); **Office Address:** Baylor Coll Med 6624 Fannin St, Ste 2330 Houston, TX 77030; **Office
Phone:** (713) 798-4061; **Board Certification:** Physical Medicine & Rehabilitation 1980; **Medical
School:** England 1972; **Residencies:** Physical Medicine & Rehabilitation, Prince Henry Hosp,
Sydney, Australia 1975-1976; Physical Medicine & Rehabilitation, Mayo Clin, Rochester 1976-
1979; **Faculty Appointment:** Physical Medicine & Rehabilitation, Baylor Coll Med

King, John Chandler MD (Physical Medicine & Rehabilitation) - *Special Expertise:* Stroke *Rehabilitation;* **Admitting Hospital:** University of Texas Health & Science Center; **Office Address:** Univ Tx Hlth Sci Ctr, Dept Rehab Med 7703 Floyd Curl Dr, rm 615E San Antonio, TX 78229-3900; **Office Phone:** (210) 567-5345; **Board Certification:** Physical Medicine & Rehabilitation 1987; **Medical School:** Oral Roberts Sch Med 1983; **Residency:** Physical Medicine & Rehabilitation, Baylor Coll Med, Houston, TX 1984-1986; **Faculty Appointment:** Assoc Prof Physical Medicine & Rehabilitation, Univ Tex, San Antonio

Nelson, Maureen R MD (Physical Medicine & Rehabilitation) - *Special Expertise:* Rehabilitation-Pediatric; **Admitting Hospital:** Texas Children's Hospital - Houston; **Office Address:** 6620 Fannin St, W Tower B130, MC-2-2590 Houston, TX 77030-2399; **Office Phone:** (832) 824-5205; **Board Certification:** Physical Medicine & Rehabilitation 1990; **Medical School:** Univ IL Coll Med 1985; **Residency:** Physical Medicine & Rehabilitation, Univ Tex Hlth Scis Ctr, San Antonio, TX 1986-1989; **Fellowship:** Pediatric Sports Medicine, Alfred I Dupont Inst, Wilmington, DE 1989-1990; **Faculty Appointment:** Assoc Prof Physical Medicine & Rehabilitation, Baylor Coll Med

Parsons, Kenneth C. MD (Physical Medicine & Rehabilitation) - *Special Expertise:* Spinal Cord Injury; **Admitting Hospital:** TIRR LifeBridge Hospital; **Office Address:** TIRR 1333 Moursund Ave Houston, TX 77030-3405; **Office Phone:** (713) 797-5252; **Board Certifications:** Physical Medicine & Rehabilitation 1977, Spinal Cord Injury Medicine 1998; **Medical School:** Univ Mich Med Sch 1970; **Residency:** Physical Medicine & Rehabilitation, Univ Hosp, Ann Arbor, MI 1971-1976; **Faculty Appointment:** Asst Clin Prof Physical Medicine & Rehabilitation, Baylor Coll Med

Walsh, Nicolas Eugene MD (Physical Medicine & Rehabilitation) - *Special Expertise:* Pain Management; **Admitting Hospital:** University of Texas Health & Science Center; **Office Address:** UT Hlth Sci Ctr, Dept Rehab Med 7703 Floyd Curl San Antonio, TX 78229-3900; **Office Phone:** (210) 567-5350; **Board Certification:** Physical Medicine & Rehabilitation 1983; **Medical School:** Univ Colo 1979; **Residency:** Physical Medicine & Rehabilitation, Univ Tex Hlth Sci Ctr, San Antonio, TX 1979-1982; **Faculty Appointment:** Prof Physical Medicine & Rehabilitation, Univ Tex, San Antonio

West Coast and Pacific

Cardenas, Diana MD (Physical Medicine & Rehabilitation) - *Special Expertise:* Spinal Cord Injury; **Admitting Hospital:** University of Washington Medical Center; **Office Address:** Univ Wash, Dept Rehab Med Box 356490 Seattle, WA 98195; **Office Phone:** (206) 543-8171; **Board Certification:** Physical Medicine & Rehabilitation 1977; **Medical School:** Univ Tex SW, Dallas 1973; **Residency:** Physical Medicine & Rehabilitation, Univ Wash Affil Hosp, Seattle, WA 1973-1976; **Faculty Appointment:** Prof Physical Medicine & Rehabilitation, Univ Wash

Jaffe, Kenneth M MD (Physical Medicine & Rehabilitation) - *Special Expertise:* Arthrogryposis-Limb Deficiency; Muscular Dystrophy; Brain/Spinal Cord Injury; **Admitting Hospital:** Children's Hospital and Regional Medical Center - Seattle; **Office Address:** Chldns Hosp & Regl MC, Dept Rehabilitation 4800 Sand Point Way NE Seattle, WA 98105; **Office Phone:** (206) 526-2114; **Board Certifications:** Pediatrics 1980, Physical Medicine & Rehabilitation 1983; **Medical School:** Harvard Med Sch 1975; **Residencies:** Pediatrics, Univ Wash-Chldns Hosp, Seattle, WA 1975-1980; Physical Medicine & Rehabilitation, Univ Wash-Affil Hosp, Seattle, WA 1980-1982; **Faculty Appointment:** Prof Physical Medicine & Rehabilitation, Univ Wash

Kraft, George Howard MD (Physical Medicine & Rehabilitation) - *Special Expertise:* *Multiple Sclerosis; Spinal Cord Injury;* **Admitting Hospital:** University of Washington Medical Center; **Office Address:** Univ Wash Med Ctr-Rehab Med Clin 1959 NE Pacific St Seattle, WA 98195; **Office Phone:** (206) 598-4295; **Board Certifications:** Physical Medicine & Rehabilitation 1969, Spinal Cord Injury Medicine 2008; **Medical School:** Ohio State Univ 1963; **Residencies:** Physical Medicine & Rehabilitation, UCSF-Moffitt Hosp, San Francisco, CA 1964-1965; Physical Medicine & Rehabilitation, Ohio State Univ Med Ctr, Columbus, OH 1965-1967; **Faculty Appointment:** Prof Physical Medicine & Rehabilitation, Univ Wash

Massagli, Teresa Luisa MD (Physical Medicine & Rehabilitation) - *Special Expertise:* *Spinal Cord Injury-Pediatric; Cerebral Palsy;* **Admitting Hospital:** Children's Hospital and Regional Medical Center - Seattle; **Office Address:** Chlds Hosp & Med Ctr 4800 Sand Point Way NE, Box 5371 Seattle, WA 98105; **Office Phone:** (206) 526-2114; **Board Certifications:** Physical Medicine & Rehabilitation 1989, Spinal Cord Injury Medicine 1998; **Medical School:** Yale Univ 1982; **Residency:** Pediatrics, Yale New Haven Hosp, New Haven, CT 1983-1985; **Fellowship:** Physical Medicine & Rehabilitation, Univ. Washington, Seattle, WA 1985-1988; **Faculty Appointment:** Assoc Prof Medicine, Univ Wash

Robinson, Lawrence MD (Physical Medicine & Rehabilitation) - *Special Expertise:* *Electrodiagnosis; Electromyography; Botulinum Toxin Injections;* **Admitting Hospital:** Harbor Hospital; **Office Address:** Univ Washington Med Ctr-Haborview, Dept Rehab Med 325 9th Ave, Box 359740 Seattle, WA 98104; **Office Phone:** (206) 731-3167; **Board Certification:** Physical Medicine & Rehabilitation 1987; **Medical School:** Baylor Coll Med 1982; **Residency:** Physical Medicine & Rehabilitation, Northwestern Univ, Chicago, IL 1982-1985; **Faculty Appointment:** Prof Physical Medicine & Rehabilitation, Univ Wash

PLASTIC SURGERY

A plastic surgeon deals with the repair, reconstruction or replacement of physical defects of form or function involving the skin, musculoskeletal system, craniomaxillofacial structures, hand, extremities, breast and trunk and external genitalia. He/she uses aesthetic surgical principles not only to improve undesirable qualities of normal structures (commonly called "cosmetic surgery") but in all reconstructive procedures as well.

A plastic surgeon possesses special knowledge and skill in the design and surgery of grafts, flaps, free tissue transfer and replantation. Competence in the management of complex wounds, the use of implantable materials, and in tumor surgery is required.

Training required: Five to seven years

Certification in one of the following subspecialties requires additional training and examination.

Plastic Surgery within the Head and Neck: A plastic surgeon with additional training in plastic and reconstructive procedures within the head, face, neck and associated structures, including cutaneous head and neck oncology and reconstruction, management of maxillofacial trauma, soft tissue repair and neural surgery.

The field is diverse and involves a wide age range of patients, from the newborn to the aged. While both cosmetic and reconstructive surgery are practiced, there are many additional procedures which interface with them.

Surgery of the Hand *(see Hand Surgery page 265)*

Physician Listings

New England

Ariyan, Stephan MD (Plastic Surgery) - *Special Expertise: Melanoma; Head & Neck Surgery; Reconstructive Surgery;* **Admitting Hospital:** Yale - New Haven Hospital; **Office Address:** 60 Temple St, Ste 7C New Haven, CT 06511; **Office Phone:** (203) 786-3000; **Board Certifications:** Plastic Surgery 1977, Surgery 1978; **Medical School:** NY Med Coll 1966; **Residencies:** Surgery, Yale Univ Hosp, New Haven, CT 1971-1975; Plastic Surgery, Yale Univ Hosp, New Haven, CT 1973-1976; **Fellowship:** Surgical Oncology, Yale Univ Hosp, New Haven, CT 1970-1971; **Faculty Appointment:** Clin Prof Plastic Surgery, Yale Univ

Constantian, Mark B MD (Plastic Surgery) - *Special Expertise: Nasal Reconstruction;* **Admitting Hospital:** Southern New Hampshire Medical Center; **Office Address:** 19 Tyler St, Ste 302 Nashua, NH 03060-2951; **Office Phone:** (603) 880-7700; **Board Certification:** Plastic Surgery 1979; **Medical School:** Univ VA Sch Med 1972; **Residencies:** Surgery, Boston Med Ctr, Boston, MA 1972-1976; Surgery, NIGMS Academy Surg, Boston, MA 1975-1976; **Fellowship:** Reconstructive Surgery, Medical Coll VA, Richmond, VA 1976-1978; **Faculty Appointment:** Asst Prof Surgery, Dartmouth Med Sch

Eriksson, Elof MD (Plastic Surgery) - *Special Expertise: Abdominal Plasty; Breast Reconstruction & Augmentation; Skin Laser Surgery;* **Admitting Hospital:** Brigham & Women's Hospital; **Office Address:** 75 Francis St Boston, MA 02115; **Office Phone:** (617) 732-5093; **Board Certifications:** Plastic Surgery 1980, Surgery 1989; **Medical School:** Sweden 1969; **Residency:** Surgery, Chicago Affil Hosps, Chicago, IL 1972-1977; **Fellowship:** Plastic Surgery, Med Ctr Va, Charlottesville, VA 1977-1979; **Faculty Appointment:** Prof Plastic Surgery, Harvard Med Sch

Feldman, Joel MD (Plastic Surgery) - *Special Expertise: Cosmetic Surgery-Face; Reconstructive Surgery;* **Admitting Hospital:** Mount Auburn Hospital; **Office Address:** 300 Mt Auburn St, Ste 304 Cambridge, MA 02138-5600; **Office Phone:** (617) 661-5998; **Board Certifications:** Surgery 1975, Plastic Surgery 1977; **Medical School:** Harvard Med Sch 1969; **Residencies:** Surgery, Mass Genl Hosp, Boston, MA 1970-1974; Plastic Surgery, Johns Hopkins Hosp, Baltimore, MD 1974-1976; **Faculty Appointment:** Asst Clin Prof Plastic Surgery, Harvard Med Sch

Gallico, G Gregory MD (Plastic Surgery) - *Special Expertise: Plastic Surgery - General;* **Admitting Hospital:** Massachusetts General Hospital; **Office Address:** Mass Genl Hosp, Prof Office Bldg 275 Cambridge St, Ste 502 Boston, MA 02114; **Office Phone:** (617) 726-3440; **Board Certifications:** Plastic Surgery 1982, Surgery 1981; **Medical School:** Harvard Med Sch 1973; **Residencies:** Surgery, Mass Genl Hosp, Boston, MA 1974-1980; Plastic Surgery, Mass Genl Hosp, Boston, MA 1980-1981; **Fellowship:** Immunology, Oxford Univ Med Sch, Oxford, England 1975-1977; **Faculty Appointment:** Asst Prof Surgery, Harvard Med Sch

May Jr, James W MD (Plastic Surgery) - *Special Expertise: Cosmetic Surgery; Breast Reconstruction; Hand Surgery;* **Admitting Hospital:** Massachusetts General Hospital; **Office Address:** 15 Parkman St, Fl 5 - rm 453 Boston, MA 02114; **Office Phone:** (617) 726-8220; **Board Certifications:** Surgery 1975, Plastic Surgery 1977; **Medical School:** Northwestern Univ 1969; **Residency:** Plastic Surgery, Mass Genl Hosp, Boston, MA 1970-1975; **Fellowship:** Hand Surgery, Univ Louisville, Louisville, KY 1975; **Faculty Appointment:** Prof Surgery, Harvard Med Sch

Mulliken, John B. MD (Plastic Surgery) - *Special Expertise: Plastic Surgery-Pediatric; Cleft Palate/Lip; Vascular Malformations;* **Admitting Hospital:** Children's Hospital; **Office Address:** 300 Longwood Ave Boston, MA 02115-5724; **Office Phone:** (617) 355-7686; **Board Certifications:** Surgery 1972, Plastic Surgery 1975; **Medical School:** Columbia P&S 1964; **Residencies:** Surgery, Mass Genl Hosp, Baltimorem, MD 1965-1970; Plastic Surgery, Johns Hopkins Hosp, Baltimore, MD 1972-1974

PLASTIC SURGERY *New England*

Pribaz, Julian MD (Plastic Surgery) - *Special Expertise:* Microsurgery; **Admitting Hospital:** Brigham & Women's Hospital; **Office Address:** Brigham & Women's Hosp, Dept Plastic Surg 75 Francis St Boston, MA 02115; **Office Phone:** (617) 732-6390; **Board Certifications:** Plastic Surgery 1986, Hand Surgery 1990; **Medical School:** Australia 1972; **Residencies:** Surgery, St Vincent's Hosp, Melbourne, Australia 1974-1976; Surgery, Geelong Hosp, Victoria, Australia 1976-1977; **Fellowship:** Plastic Surgery, Southern Ill Univ Sch Med, Springfield, IL 1980-1982; **Faculty Appointment:** Assoc Prof Surgery, Harvard Med Sch

Sullivan, Patrick Kevin MD (Plastic Surgery) - *Special Expertise:* Craniofacial Surgery/Reconstruction; **Admitting Hospital:** Rhode Island Hospital; **Office Address:** Rhode Island Hospital 235 Plain St, Ste 502 Providence, RI 02905-3240; **Office Phone:** (401) 831-8300; **Board Certifications:** Otolaryngology 1985, Plastic Surgery 1989; **Medical School:** Mayo Med Sch 1979; **Residencies:** Otolaryngology, Univ Colo Hlth Scis Ctr, Denver, CO 1981-1984; Plastic Surgery, Rhode Island Hosp, Providence, RI 1984-1986; **Fellowship:** Craniofacial Surgery, Dr Paul Tessier & Dr Hugo Obwegeser, Paris-Zurich 1986-1987; **Faculty Appointment:** Plastic Surgery, Brown Univ

Mid Atlantic

Aston, Sherrell MD (Plastic Surgery) - *Special Expertise:* Cosmetic Surgery-Face; Rhinoplasty; **Admitting Hospital:** Manhattan Eye, Ear & Throat Hospital; **Office Address:** 728 Park Ave New York, NY 10021; **Office Phone:** (212) 249-6000; **Board Certifications:** Surgery 1974, Plastic Surgery 1978; **Medical School:** Univ VA Sch Med 1968; **Residencies:** Surgery, UCLA Med Ctr, Los Angeles, CA 1969-1973; Plastic Surgery, New York Univ, New York, NY 1973-1975; **Fellowship:** Surgery, Johns Hopkins Hosp, Baltimore, MD 1970; **Faculty Appointment:** Assoc Prof Plastic Surgery, NYU Sch Med

Attinger, Chris MD (Plastic Surgery) - *Special Expertise:* Lower Extremities Reconstruction; Diabetic Leg Reconstruction; **Admitting Hospital:** Georgetown University Hospital; **Office Address:** 3800 Reservoir Rd NW 1 Wound Ctr Washington, DC 20007; **Office Phone:** (202) 784-5462; **Board Certification:** Plastic Surgery 1992; **Medical School:** Yale Univ 1981; **Residencies:** Surgery, Brigham & Women's Hosp, Boston, MA 1982-1986; Plastic Surgery, NYU Med Sch, New York, NY 1987-1989; **Fellowships:** Vascular Surgery (General), Brigham & Women's Hosp, Boston, MA 1986-1987; Hand Surgery, NYU Med Sch, New York, NY 1989-1990; **Faculty Appointment:** Assoc Prof Surgery, Geo Wash Univ

Baker, Daniel MD (Plastic Surgery) - *Special Expertise:* Cosmetic Surgery-Face; Reconstructive Plastic Surgery Face; **Admitting Hospital:** Manhattan Eye, Ear & Throat Hospital; **Office Address:** 65 E 66th St New York, NY 10021; **Office Phone:** (212) 734-9695; **Board Certification:** Plastic Surgery 1978; **Medical School:** Columbia P&S 1968; **Residencies:** Surgery, UC-San Francisco, San Francisco, CA 1973-1975; Plastic Surgery, NYU Med Ctr, New York, NY 1975-1977; **Fellowship:** Head and Neck Surgery, NYU Med Ctr, New York, NY 1977-1978; **Faculty Appointment:** Assoc Prof Plastic Surgery, NYU Sch Med

Bartlett, Scott P MD (Plastic Surgery) - *Special Expertise:* Craniofacial Surgery/Reconstruction; **Admitting Hospital:** Hospital of the University of Pennsylvania; **Office Address:** Children's Hospital of Philadelphia-10 Penn Tower 34th and Spruce St Philadelphia, PA 19118-4221; **Office Phone:** (215) 590-2209; **Board Certification:** Plastic Surgery 1987; **Medical School:** Washington Univ, St Louis 1975; **Residencies:** Surgery, Mass Genl Hosp, Boston, MA 1976-1983; Plastic Surgery, Mass Genl Hosp, Boston, MA 1983-1985; **Fellowship:** Craniofacial Surgery, Univ Penn, Philadelphia, PA 1985-1986; **Faculty Appointment:** Assoc Prof Plastic Surgery, Univ Penn

Boyajian, Michael MD (Plastic Surgery) - *Special Expertise:* Plastic Surgery-Pediatric; **Admitting Hospital:** Children's National Medical Center - DC; **Office Address:** Chldns Natl Med Ctr 111 Michigan Ave NW Washington, DC 20010; **Office Phone:** (202) 884-2150; **Board Certifications:** Surgery 1982, Plastic Surgery 1984; **Medical School:** NYU Sch Med 1976; **Residencies:** Surgery, Univ Colo Med Ctr, Denver, CO 1977-1979; Surgery, Univ Cincinnati Hosp, Cincinnati, OH 1979-1981; **Fellowships:** Plastic Surgery, Brigham & Women's Hosp, Boston, MA 1981-1983; Craniofacial Surgery, Chldns Hosp, Boston, MA 1983; **Faculty Appointment:** Asst Prof Plastic Surgery, Geo Wash Univ

Bucky, Louis P MD (Plastic Surgery) - *Special Expertise:* Breast Reconstruction; **Admitting Hospital:** Hospital of the University of Pennsylvania; **Office Address:** Univ Penn Med Ctr, Div Plastic Surg 3400 Spruce Street, 10 Penn Tower Philadelphia, PA 19104; **Office Phone:** (215) 662-4286; **Board Certifications:** Surgery 1993, Plastic Surgery 1997; **Medical School:** Harvard Med Sch 1986; **Residencies:** Surgery, Mass Genl Hosp, Boston, MA 1987-1992; Plastic Surgery, Mass Genl Hosp, Boston, MA 1992-1994; **Fellowships:** Microsurgery, Meml Sloan Kettering, New York, NY 1994-1995; Craniofacial Surgery, Miami Chldns Hosp, Miami, FL 1995; **Faculty Appointment:** Asst Prof Surgery, Univ Penn

Cutting, Court MD (Plastic Surgery) - *Special Expertise:* Cleft Palate/Lip; Craniofacial Surgery/Reconstruction; **Admitting Hospital:** NYU Medical Center (Page 70); **Office Address:** NYU Med Ctr 550 1St Ave New York, NY; **Office Phone:** (212) 263-5502; **Board Certifications:** Otolaryngology 1980, Plastic Surgery 1986; **Medical School:** Univ Chicago-Pritzker Sch Med 1975; **Residencies:** Otolaryngology, Univ IA Hosps, Iowa City, IA 1976-1980; Plastic Surgery, NYU Med Ctr, New York, NY 1980-1983; **Fellowship:** Craniofacial Surgery, NYU Med Ctr, New York, NY 1983-1984; **Faculty Appointment:** Assoc Prof Plastic Surgery, NYU Sch Med

Di Spaltro, Franklin MD (Plastic Surgery) - *Special Expertise:* Plastic Surgery - General; **Admitting Hospital:** St Barnabas Medical Center; **Office Address:** 101 Old Short Hills Rd, Ste 510 West Orange, NJ 07052-1023; **Office Phone:** (973) 736-5907; **Board Certification:** Plastic Surgery 1975; **Medical School:** NY Med Coll 1965; **Residency:** Surgery, Metropolitan Hosp Ctr, New York, NY 1966-1970; **Fellowships:** Plastic Surgery, St Barnabas Med Ctr, Livingston, NJ 1970-1972; Plastic Surgery, Bellevue Hosp, New York, NY 1972-1973

Gold, Alan MD (Plastic Surgery) - *Special Expertise:* Cosmetic Surgery; Reconstructive Surgery; **Admitting Hospital:** North Shore University Hospital at Manhasset; **Office Address:** 833 Northern Blvd, Ste 240 Great Neck, NY 11021; **Office Phone:** (516) 498-2800; **Board Certification:** Plastic Surgery 1979; **Medical School:** SUNY Hlth Sci Ctr 1971; **Residencies:** Surgery, North Shore Univ Hosp, Manhasset, NY 1972-1975; Plastic Surgery, Kings County-Suny Med Ctr, Brooklyn, NY 1976-1978; **Fellowship:** Hand Surgery, Nassau County Med Ctr, East Meadow, NY 1975-1976; **Faculty Appointment:** Assoc Clin Prof Surgery, Cornell Univ-Weil Med Coll

Hidalgo, David MD (Plastic Surgery) - *Special Expertise:* Breast Reconstruction; Microsurgery Reconstruction; Cosmetic Surgery-Face & Breast; **Admitting Hospital:** Manhattan Eye, Ear & Throat Hospital; **Office Address:** 655 Park Ave, Fl 1 New York, NY 10021; **Office Phone:** (212) 517-9777; **Board Certification:** Plastic Surgery 1987; **Medical School:** Georgetown Univ 1978; **Residencies:** Surgery, NYU, New York, NY 1978-1983; Plastic Surgery, NYU, New York, NY 1983-1985; **Fellowship:** Surgery, NYU, New York, NY 1985-1986; **Faculty Appointment:** Assoc Prof Surgery, Cornell Univ-Weil Med Coll

Hoffman, Lloyd MD (Plastic Surgery) - *Special Expertise:* Burns; Breast Reconstruction; **Admitting Hospital:** New York Weill Cornell Medical Center - NY Presbyterian Hospital (Page 72); **Office Address:** Cornell Univ-Weill Med Coll 525 E 68th St, Box 115 New York, NY 10021-4873; **Office Phone:** (212) 452-5125; **Board Certifications:** Plastic Surgery 1989, Hand Surgery 1992; **Medical School:** Northwestern Univ 1978; **Residencies:** Surgery, NY Hosp-Cornell Med Ctr, New York, NY 1978-1983; Plastic Surgery, NYU Med Ctr, New York, NY 1983-1986; **Fellowship:** Hand Surgery, NYU Med Ctr, New York, NY 1986-1987; **Faculty Appointment:** Assoc Prof Plastic Surgery, Cornell Univ-Weil Med Coll

Hurwitz, Dennis MD (Plastic Surgery) - *Special Expertise:* Reconstructive Surgery; **Admitting Hospital:** Magee Women's Hospital; **Office Address:** Magee Women's Hosp 300 Halket St, rm 5104 Pittsburgh, PA 15213; **Office Phone:** (412) 641-3600; **Board Certifications:** Surgery 1976, Plastic Surgery 1979; **Medical School:** Univ MD Sch Med 1970; **Residencies:** Surgery, Dartmouth Med Ctr, Lebannon, NH 1972-1975; Plastic Surgery, Univ Pitts Med Ctr, Pittsburgh, PA 1975-1977; **Faculty Appointment:** Prof Surgery, Univ Pittsburgh

Jelks, Glenn MD (Plastic Surgery) - *Special Expertise:* Cosmetic Surgery-Body; Cosmetic Surgery-Face; **Admitting Hospital:** NYU Medical Center (Page 70); **Office Address:** 875 Park Ave New York, NY 10021; **Office Phone:** (212) 988-3303; **Board Certifications:** Ophthalmology 1979, Plastic Surgery 1982; **Medical School:** Mich State Univ 1973; **Residency:** Ophthalmology, UCLA Med Ctr, Los Angeles, CA 1975-1978; **Fellowship:** Plastic Surgery, New York Univ, New York, NY 1978-1980; **Faculty Appointment:** Assoc Prof Plastic Surgery, NYU Sch Med

Klatsky, Stanley A MD (Plastic Surgery) - *Special Expertise:* Cosmetic Surgery-Face; Eyelid Surgery; Cosmetic Surgery-Body; **Admitting Hospital:** Johns Hopkins Hospital - Baltimore (Page 65); **Office Address:** 122 Slade Ave, Ste 100 Baltimore, MD 21208-4917; **Office Phone:** (410) 484-0400; **Board Certification:** Plastic Surgery 1970; **Medical School:** Univ MD Sch Med 1962; **Residencies:** Surgery, Sinai Hosp, Baltimore, MD 1962-1966; Plastic Surgery, Columbia-Presby Med Ctr, New York, NY 1966-1968; **Faculty Appointment:** Assoc Prof Surgery, Johns Hopkins Univ

Leipziger, Lyle S MD (Plastic Surgery) - *Special Expertise:* Cosmetic Surgery-Face; **Admitting Hospital:** Long Island Jewish Medical Center; **Office Address:** Long Island Jewish Med Ctr, Dept Plastic Surg 825 Northern Blvd, Fl 3 Great Neck, NY 11021; **Office Phone:** (516) 465-8787; **Board Certification:** Plastic Surgery 1994; **Medical School:** Cornell Univ-Weil Med Coll 1985; **Residency:** Plastic Surgery, NY Hosp-Cornell Med Ctr, New York, NY 1988-1990; **Fellowship:** Craniofacial Surgery, Johns Hopkins Hosp, Baltimore, MD 1990-1991; **Faculty Appointment:** Asst Prof Surgery, Albert Einstein Coll Med

Little, John W MD (Plastic Surgery) - *Special Expertise:* Cosmetic Surgery-Face; **Admitting Hospital:** Georgetown University Hospital; **Office Address:** 1145 19th St NW, Ste 802 Washington, DC 20036; **Office Phone:** (202) 467-6700; **Board Certifications:** Surgery 1975, Plastic Surgery 1977; **Medical School:** Harvard Med Sch 1969; **Residencies:** Surgery, Univ Hosps-Case West Res, Cleveland, OH 1969-1974; Plastic Surgery, Univ Hosps-Case West Res, Cleveland, OH 1974-1975; **Fellowship:** Plastic Surgery, Jackson Meml Hosp, Miami, FL 1976-1977; **Faculty Appointment:** Clin Prof Plastic Surgery, Georgetown Univ

Manson, Paul MD (Plastic Surgery) - *Special Expertise:* Maxillofacial Surgery; Facial Trauma/Fractures; **Admitting Hospital:** Johns Hopkins Hospital - Baltimore (Page 65); **Office Address:** 601 N Caroline St Baltimore, MD 21287-0980; **Office Phone:** (410) 955-9470; **Board Certification:** Plastic Surgery 1979; **Medical School:** Northwestern Univ 1968; **Residencies:** Surgery, New Eng Deaconess, Boston, MA 1968-1974; Plastic Surgery, Johns Hopkins Hosp, Baltimore, MD 1976-1978; **Fellowship:** Surgery, Lahey Clinic, Boston, MA 1974-1975; **Faculty Appointment:** Prof Plastic Surgery, Johns Hopkins Univ

Matarasso, Alan MD (Plastic Surgery) - *Special Expertise: Rhinoplasty; Eyelid Surgery;* **Admitting Hospital:** Manhattan Eye, Ear & Throat Hospital; **Office Address:** 1009 Park Ave New York, NY 10028-0936; **Office Phone:** (212) 249-7500; **Board Certification:** Plastic Surgery 1986; **Medical School:** Univ Miami Sch Med 1979; **Residencies:** Surgery, Montefiore Med Ctr, Bronx, NY 1979-1983; Plastic Surgery, Montefiore Med Ctr, Bronx, NY 1983-1985; **Fellowship:** Plastic Surgery, Manhattan EET Hosp, New York, NY 1985; **Faculty Appointment:** Assoc Clin Prof Plastic Surgery, Albert Einstein Coll Med

McCarthy, Joseph MD (Plastic Surgery) - *Special Expertise: Cosmetic Surgery-Face; Craniofacial Surgery/Reconstruction;* **Admitting Hospital:** NYU Medical Center (Page 70); **Office Address:** 722 Park Ave New York, NY 10021; **Office Phone:** (212) 628-4420; **Board Certification:** Plastic Surgery 1974; **Medical School:** Columbia P&S 1964; **Residencies:** Surgery, Columbia-Presby, New York, NY 1964-1971; Plastic Surgery, NYU Med Ctr, New YOrk, NY 1971-1973; **Faculty Appointment:** Prof Plastic Surgery, NYU Sch Med

Pitman, Gerald MD (Plastic Surgery) - *Special Expertise: Cosmetic Surgery-Face; Cosmetic Surgery-Liposuction;* **Admitting Hospital:** Manhattan Eye, Ear & Throat Hospital; **Office Address:** 170 E 73rd St New York, NY 10021; **Office Phone:** (212) 517-2600; **Board Certifications:** Plastic Surgery 1978, Surgery 1976; **Medical School:** Univ Penn 1968; **Residencies:** Surgery, Columbia-Presby Hosp, New York, NY 1971-1975; Plastic Surgery, NYU Med Ctr, New York, NY 1975-1977; **Fellowship:** Microsurgery, NYU Med Ctr, New York, NY 1980-1981; **Faculty Appointment:** Assoc Clin Prof Plastic Surgery, NYU Sch Med

Posnick, Jeffrey Craig MD/DMD (Plastic Surgery) - *Special Expertise: Cosmetic Surgery-Face; Craniofacial Surgery/Reconstruction; Maxillofacial Surgery;* **Admitting Hospital:** Georgetown University Hospital; **Office Address:** Posnick Ctr for Plastic Surgery 5530 Wisconsin Ave, Ste 1250 Chevy Chase, MD 20815; **Office Phone:** (301) 986-9475; **Board Certification:** Plastic Surgery 1988; **Medical School:** Vanderbilt Univ 1979; **Residencies:** Surgery, Eastern VA Med Sch, Norfolk, VA 1984-1986; Plastic Surgery, Mass Genl Hosp, Boston, MA 1981-1983; **Fellowships:** Craniofacial Surgery, Univ Penn, Philadephia, PA 1983; Craniofacial Surgery, Vanderbilt Med Ctr, Nashville, TN 1979-1981; **Faculty Appointment:** Clin Prof Plastic Surgery, Georgetown Univ

Ramirez, Oscar M MD (Plastic Surgery) - *Special Expertise: Endoscopic Facelift (Scarless);* **Admitting Hospital:** Greater Baltimore Medical Center; **Office Address:** 2219 York Rd, Ste 100 Timonium, MD 21093; **Office Phone:** (410) 560-7090; **Board Certification:** Plastic Surgery 1985; **Medical School:** Peru 1976; **Residencies:** Surgery, Franklin Sq Hosp, Baltimore, MD 1977-1982; Plastic Surgery, Univ Pitts Affil Hosps, Pittsburgh, PA 1982-1984; **Fellowship:** Craniofacial Surgery, Manuel Gea Gonzalez, Mexico City, Mexico 1984; **Faculty Appointment:** Asst Clin Prof Surgery, Johns Hopkins Univ

Spear, Scott L MD (Plastic Surgery) - *Special Expertise: Breast Reconstruction; Cosmetic Surgery-Face;* **Admitting Hospital:** Georgetown University Hospital; **Office Address:** Georgetown Univ Med Ctr, Div Plas Surg 3800 Reservoir Rd NW Washington, DC 20007; **Office Phone:** (202) 687-8612; **Board Certifications:** Surgery 1979, Plastic Surgery 1981; **Medical School:** Univ Chicago-Pritzker Sch Med 1972; **Residencies:** Surgery, Beth Israel Hosp, Boston, MA 1973-1978; Plastic Surgery, Univ Miami Hosps, Miami, FL 1978-1980; **Faculty Appointment:** Prof Plastic Surgery, Georgetown Univ

Spinelli, Henry M MD (Plastic Surgery) - *Special Expertise:* Craniofacial Surgery/Reconstruction; Orbital Surgery; **Admitting Hospital:** New York Weill Cornell Medical Center - NY Presbyterian Hospital (Page 72); **Office Address:** Cornell Univ Med School 875 Fifth Ave New York, NY 10021; **Office Phone:** (212) 570-6235; **Board Certifications:** Ophthalmology 1987, Plastic Surgery 1993; **Medical School:** NYU Sch Med 1981; **Residencies:** Surgery, Columbia-Presby, New York, NY 1985-1988; Plastic Surgery, NYU-Bellevue Hosp, New York, NY 1988-1990; **Fellowships:** NYU Med Ctr, New York, NY 1990-1991; Ophthalmology, Manhattan EET Hosp, New York, NY 1982-1985; **Faculty Appointment:** Assoc Prof Plastic Surgery, Cornell Univ-Weil Med Coll

Sultan, Mark MD (Plastic Surgery) - *Special Expertise:* Breast Reconstruction; Cosmetic Surgery; **Admitting Hospital:** St Luke's - Roosevelt Hospital Center - Roosevelt Division (Page 58); **Office Address:** 425 W 59th St, Ste 7a New York, NY 10019; **Office Phone:** (212) 523-7277; **Board Certifications:** Surgery 1988, Plastic Surgery 1992; **Medical School:** Columbia P&S 1982; **Residencies:** Surgery, Columbia-Presby Hosp, New York, NY 1982-1987; Plastic Surgery, Columbia-Presby Hosp, New York, NY 1987-1990; **Fellowship:** Head and Neck Surgery, Emory Univ Hosp, Atlanta, GA 1988-1989; **Faculty Appointment:** Assoc Prof Surgery, Columbia P&S

Tabbal, Nicolas MD (Plastic Surgery) - *Special Expertise:* Rhinoplasty; Prosthetic Nose; **Admitting Hospital:** Manhattan Eye, Ear & Throat Hospital; **Office Address:** 521 Park Ave New York, NY 10021-8140; **Office Phone:** (212) 644-5800; **Board Certifications:** Surgery 1977, Plastic Surgery 1980; **Medical School:** Lebanon 1972; **Residencies:** Surgery, Am Univ Med Ctr, Beirut, Lebanon 1972-1976; Plastic Surgery, Akron City Hosp, Akron, OH 1977-1979; **Fellowships:** Surgery, Upstate Med Ctr, Syracuse, NY 1976-1977; Reconstructive Surgery, NYU Med Ctr, New York, NY 1979-1980; **Faculty Appointment:** Clin Inst Plastic Surgery, NYU Sch Med

Thorne, Charles MD (Plastic Surgery) - *Special Expertise:* Ear Disorders/Surgery; Cosmetic Surgery-Face; Cranial Plastic Surgery; **Admitting Hospital:** Manhattan Eye, Ear & Throat Hospital; **Office Address:** 812 Park Ave New York, NY 10021; **Office Phone:** (212) 794-0044; **Board Certifications:** Surgery 1987, Plastic Surgery 1991; **Medical School:** UCLA 1981; **Residencies:** Surgery, Mass Genl Hosp, Boston, MA 1981-1986; Plastic Surgery, NYU Med Ctr, New York, NY 1986-1988; **Fellowship:** Craniofacial Surgery, NYU Med Ctr, New York, NY 1988-1989; **Faculty Appointment:** Assoc Prof Plastic Surgery, NYU Sch Med

Vander Kolk, Craig Alan MD (Plastic Surgery) - *Special Expertise:* Craniofacial Surgery/Reconstruction; Cleft Palate/Lip; **Admitting Hospital:** Johns Hopkins Hospital - Baltimore (Page 65); **Office Address:** Johns Hopkins Outpatient Ctr 601 N Caroline St, rm 8152D Baltimore, MD 21287-0981; **Office Phone:** (410) 955-6897; **Board Certification:** Plastic Surgery 1989; **Medical School:** Univ Mich Med Sch 1980; **Residencies:** Surgery, Univ Mich Med Ctr, Ann Arbor, MI 1980-1983; Plastic Surgery, Univ Mich Med Ctr, Ann Arbor, MI 1983-1986; **Fellowships:** Hand Surgery, St Vincents Hosp, Melbourne, Australia 1984-1985; Craniofacial Surgery, Chldns Hosp, Philadelphia, PA 1986-1987; **Faculty Appointment:** Assoc Prof Plastic Surgery, Johns Hopkins Univ

Whitaker, Linton A MD (Plastic Surgery) - *Special Expertise:* Craniofacial Surgery/Reconstruction; Cosmetic Surgery-Face; **Admitting Hospital:** Hospital of the University of Pennsylvania; **Office Address:** Univ Med Ctr-10 Penn Tower 3400 Spruce St Philadelphia, PA 19104; **Office Phone:** (215) 662-2048; **Board Certifications:** Surgery 1970, Plastic Surgery 1978; **Medical School:** Tulane Univ 1962; **Residencies:** Surgery, Dartmouth Affl Hosp, Lebanon, NH 1965-1969; Plastic Surgery, Hosp Univ Penn, Philadelphia, PA 1969-1971; **Faculty Appointment:** Prof Plastic Surgery, Univ Penn

Wood-Smith, Donald MD (Plastic Surgery) - *Special Expertise:* Plastic Surgery - General; **Admitting Hospital:** New York Eye & Ear Infirmary (Page 71); **Office Address:** 830 Park Ave New York, NY 10021-2757; **Office Phone:** (212) 744-2224; **Board Certification:** Plastic Surgery 1970; **Medical School:** Australia 1954; **Residencies:** Plastic Surgery, NYU Med Ctr, New York, NY 1961-1963; Surgery, Stanford Univ, Stanford, CA 1967-1968; **Faculty Appointment:** Prof Surgery, Columbia P&S

Southeast

Argenta, Louis Charles MD (Plastic Surgery) - *Special Expertise:* Plastic Reconstructive Surgery; **Admitting Hospital:** Wake Forest University Baptist Medical Center; **Office Address:** Wake Forest Univ Baptist Med Ctr Medical Center Blvd Winston Salem, NC 27157; **Office Phone:** (336) 716-4416; **Board Certification:** Plastic Surgery 1982; **Medical School:** Univ Mich Med Sch 1969; **Residencies:** Surgery, Univ Mich, Ann Arbor, MI 1973-1977; Plastic Surgery, Univ Mich, Ann Arbor, MI 1977-1979; **Fellowship:** Craniofacial Surgery, Hosp Foch, Paris, France 1982; **Faculty Appointment:** Prof Plastic Surgery, Wake Forest Univ Sch Med

Baker Jr, James L MD (Plastic Surgery) - *Special Expertise:* Plastic Surgery - General; **Admitting Hospital:** Winter Park Memorial Hospital; **Office Address:** 400 W Morse Blvd, Ste 203 Winter Park, FL 32789; **Office Phone:** (407) 644-5242; **Board Certification:** Plastic Surgery 1973; **Medical School:** Holland 1964; **Residencies:** Surgery, Monmouth Med Ctr, Long Branch, NJ 1965-1969; Plastic Surgery, Orlando Regl Med Ctr, Orlando, FL 1969-1971; **Fellowship:** Hand Surgery, Dr Harold Klinert-Univ Louisvi, KY 1971; **Faculty Appointment:** Clin Prof Surgery, Univ S Fla Coll Med

Baker Jr, Thomas J MD (Plastic Surgery) - *Special Expertise:* Cosmetic Surgery; Skin Laser Surgery; Breast Surgery; **Admitting Hospital:** Mercy Hospital - Miami; **Office Address:** Plastic Surgery Assoc 1501 S Miami Ave Miami, FL 33129-1102; **Office Phone:** (305) 854-2424; **Board Certifications:** Plastic Surgery 1959, Surgery 1958; **Medical School:** Indiana Univ 1949; **Residencies:** Plastic Surgery, Univ Tex Med Branch, Galveston, TX 1955-1957; Surgery, Jackson Mem Hosp, Miami, FL 1951-1955; **Faculty Appointment:** Prof Plastic Surgery, Univ Miami Sch Med

Beasley, Michael MD (Plastic Surgery) - *Special Expertise:* Breast Surgery; **Admitting Hospital:** Carolinas Medical Center; **Office Address:** 2215 Randolph Rd 2215 Randolph Rd Charlotte, NC 28207; **Office Phone:** (704) 372-6846; **Board Certification:** Plastic Surgery 1989; **Medical School:** Univ NC Sch Med 1980; **Residencies:** Surgery, NC Meml Hosp, Chapel Hill, NC 1981-1985; Plastic Surgery, Emory Univ Hosp, Atlanta, GA 1985-1987; **Faculty Appointment:** Assoc Clin Prof Plastic Surgery, Univ NC Sch Med

Becker, Ferdinand Francis MD (Plastic Surgery) - *Special Expertise:* Cosmetic Surgery-Face; **Admitting Hospital:** Indian River Memorial Hosp; **Office Address:** 5070 N A1a, Ste A Vero Beach, FL 32963-1229; **Office Phone:** (561) 234-3700; **Board Certification:** Otolaryngology 1972; Plastic Surgery 1991; **Medical School:** Tulane Univ 1965; **Residencies:** Surgery, Charity Hosp, New Orleans, LA 1968-1969; Otolaryngology, Charity Hosp, New Orleans, LA 1969-1972; **Faculty Appointment:** Asst Clin Prof Plastic Surgery, Univ Fla Coll Med

Bostwick III, John J MD (Plastic Surgery) - *Special Expertise:* Cosmetic Surgery-Face; Breast Reconstruction; **Admitting Hospital:** Emory University Hospital; **Office Address:** Emory Plastic Surgery 1365 Clifton Rd NE, Bldg B - Ste 2100 Atlanta, GA 30322-1013; **Office Phone:** (404) 778-3832; **Board Certifications:** Surgery 1974, Plastic Surgery 1976; **Medical School:** Univ Tenn Coll Med, Memphis 1966; **Residencies:** Surgery, Emory Univ Hosp, Atlanta, GA 1970-1973; Plastic Surgery, Emory Univ Hosp, Atlanta, GA 1973-1974; **Faculty Appointment:** Prof Surgery, Emory Univ

Caffee, Henry Hollis MD (Plastic Surgery) - *Special Expertise:* Plastic Surgery - General; **Admitting Hospital:** Shands Healthcare at University Florida (Page 77); **Office Address:** Shands Hlthcare at Univ FL 1600 SW Archer Rd Gainesville, FL 32610; **Office Phone:** (352) 395-6810; **Board Certifications:** Plastic Surgery 1979, Hand Surgery 1997; **Medical School:** Univ Fla Coll Med 1968; **Residencies:** Surgery, Harbor Genl Hosp, Torrance, CA 1969-1975; Plastic Surgery, UCLA Med Ctr, Los Angeles, CA 1975-1977; **Faculty Appointment:** Prof Plastic Surgery, Univ Fla Coll Med

Carraway, James Howard MD (Plastic Surgery) - *Special Expertise:* Oculoplastic Surgery; *Cosmetic Surgery-Face; Eyelid Surgery;* **Admitting Hospital:** Sentara Norfolk General Hospital; **Office Address:** Eastern VA Med Sch, Dept Plas Surg 5589 Greenwich Rd, Ste 100 Virginia Beach, VA 23462; **Office Phone:** (757) 557-0300; **Board Certifications:** Surgery 1972, Plastic Surgery 1974; **Medical School:** Univ VA Sch Med 1962; **Residencies:** Surgery, Norfolk Med Ctr, Norfolk, VA 1966-1970; Plastic Surgery, Eastern VA Med Ctr, Norfolk, VA 1971-1973; **Fellowship:** Plastic Surgery, Glasgow Royal Infirmary, Glasgow,Scotland 1970; **Faculty Appointment:** Prof Plastic Surgery, Eastern VA Med Sch

Cole, Norman M MD (Plastic Surgery) - *Special Expertise:* Plastic Surgery - General; **Admitting Hospital:** Norton Hospital; **Office Address:** Alliant Med Pavilion 315 E Broadway, Box 1027 Louisville, KY 40201-1027; **Office Phone:** (502) 589-5544; **Board Certifications:** Surgery 1969, Plastic Surgery 1974; **Medical School:** Loma Linda Univ 1962; **Residencies:** Surgery, LA Co Genl Hosp, Los Angeles, CA 1963-1967; Plastic Surgery, Duke Univ Med Ctr, Durham, NC; **Fellowship:** Hand Surgery, Univ Louisville Med Ctr, Louisville, KY 1971; **Faculty Appointment:** Clin Prof Surgery, Univ Louisville Sch Med

Cruse, C Wayne MD (Plastic Surgery) - *Special Expertise:* Burns; **Admitting Hospital:** Tampa General Hospital; **Office Address:** 12902 Magnolia Dr, Ste 4035 Tampa, FL 33612-9416; **Office Phone:** (813) 972-8410; **Board Certifications:** Surgery 1978, Plastic Surgery 1981; **Medical School:** Univ Louisville Sch Med 1972; **Residencies:** Surgery, Univ S Fla Hosp, Tampa, FL 1973-1977; Plastic Surgery, Univ KY Hosp-Chandler Med Ctr, Lexington, KY 1977; **Faculty Appointment:** Prof Surgery, Univ S Fla Coll Med

Fisher, Jack MD (Plastic Surgery) - *Special Expertise:* Breast Reconstruction; **Admitting Hospital:** Baptist Hospital; **Office Address:** Nashville Plas Surg Ltd 2021 Church St, Ste 806 Nashville, TN 37203; **Office Phone:** (615) 340-4500; **Board Certifications:** Surgery 1979, Plastic Surgery 1981; **Medical School:** Emory Univ 1973; **Residencies:** Surgery, Geo Wash Univ Hosp, Washington, DC 1974-1978; Plastic Surgery, Emory Univ Hosp, Atlanta, GA 1978-1980; **Faculty Appointment:** Asst Clin Prof Plastic Surgery, Vanderbilt Univ

Fix, R Jobe MD (Plastic Surgery) - *Special Expertise:* Breast Reconstruction; Hand Surgery; **Admitting Hospital:** University of Alabama Hospital at Birmingham; **Office Address:** Univ AL, Div Plas Surg 1813 6th Ave S, #Meb524 Birmingham, AL 35294-3295; **Office Phone:** (205) 934-3358; **Board Certifications:** Plastic Surgery 1991, Hand Surgery 1992; **Medical School:** Univ Nebr Coll Med 1982; **Residencies:** Surgery, Valley Med Ctr, Fresno, CA 1982-1987; Plastic Surgery, Univ Ala Hosp, Birmingham, AL 1987-1989; **Faculty Appointment:** Assoc Prof Plastic Surgery, Univ Ala

Georgiade, Gregory MD (Plastic Surgery) - *Special Expertise:* Breast Reconstruction; Cleft Palate/Lip; **Admitting Hospital:** Duke University Medical Center (Page 60); **Office Address:** Duke Univ Med Ctr 141 Baker House, Box 3960 Durham, NC 27710-0001; **Office Phone:** (919) 684-3039; **Board Certifications:** Plastic Surgery 1981, Surgery 1990; **Medical School:** Duke Univ 1973; **Residencies:** Surgery, Duke Univ Med Ctr, Durham, NC 1974-1978; Plastic Surgery, Duke Univ Med Ctr, Durham, NC 1979-1980; **Faculty Appointment:** Prof Surgery, Duke Univ

Gregory, Richard MD (Plastic Surgery) - *Special Expertise:* Skin Laser Surgery; Cosmetic Surgery-Face; **Admitting Hospital:** Florida Hospital; **Office Address:** 400 Celebration Pl, Ste A320 Celebration, FL 34747; **Office Phone:** (407) 303-4250; **Board Certifications:** Plastic Surgery 1981, Surgery 1979; **Medical School:** Indiana Univ 1971; **Residencies:** Surgery, Duke Univ Med Ctr, Durham, NC 1972-1977; Plastic Surgery, Duke Univ Med Ctr, Durham, NC 1977-1979; **Fellowship:** Hand Surgery, Univ Louisville, Louisville, KY 1978-1979; **Faculty Appointment:** Assoc Clin Prof Plastic Surgery, Univ S Fla Coll Med

Grotting, James MD (Plastic Surgery) - *Special Expertise:* Cosmetic Surgery; **Admitting Hospital:** Healthsouth Medical Center - Birmingham; **Office Address:** Grotting, Core, Wolfley & Clinton Plastic Surg Clinic One Inverness Center Pkwy, Ste 100 Birmingham, AL 35242; **Office Phone:** (205) 930-1800; **Board Certifications:** Plastic Surgery 1986, Hand Surgery 1989; **Medical School:** Univ Minn 1978; **Residencies:** Surgery, Univ Wash Affil Hosp, Seattle, WA 1979-1983; Plastic Surgery, UC-San Francisco, San Francisco, CA 1983-1985; **Faculty Appointment:** Asst Prof Plastic Surgery, Univ Ala

Hagan, Kevin Francis MD (Plastic Surgery) - *Special Expertise:* Reconstructive Surgery; **Admitting Hospital:** Vanderbilt University Medical Center; **Office Address:** Vanderbilt Univ Med Ctr South 2100 Pierce Ave, Ste 230 Nashville, TN 37232-3631; **Office Phone:** (615) 936-0160; **Board Certifications:** Plastic Surgery 1983, Hand Surgery 1993; **Medical School:** Johns Hopkins Univ 1974; **Residencies:** Surgery, Med Coll VA Hosps, Richmond, VA 1975-1979; Plastic Surgery, UCSF Med Ctr, San Francisco, CA 1980-1982; **Fellowship:** Microsurgery, Dr Harry Buncke Med Clinic, San Francisco, CA 1980

Hester Jr, Thomas R MD (Plastic Surgery) - *Special Expertise:* Cosmetic Surgery-Face; **Admitting Hospital:** Emory University Hospital; **Office Address:** Paces Pl Surg 3200 Downwood Cir, Ste 640 Atlanta, GA 30327; **Office Phone:** (404) 351-0051; **Board Certifications:** Plastic Surgery 1980, Surgery 1973; **Medical School:** Emory Univ 1967; **Residency:** Surgery, Emory Affil Hosps, Atlanta, GA 1968-1972

Hunstad, Joseph P. MD (Plastic Surgery) - *Special Expertise:* Cosmetic Surgery-Face & Body; **Admitting Hospital:** University Hospital - Charlotte; **Office Address:** The Hunstad Ctr 8220 Univ Exec Park, Ste 100 Charlotte, NC 28262; **Office Phone:** (704) 549-0500; **Board Certification:** Plastic Surgery 1989; **Medical School:** Mich State Univ 1981; **Residencies:** Surgery, Butterworth Hosp, Grand Rapids, MI 1982-1984; Plastic Surgery, Grand Rapids Area Med Ed Ct, Grand Rapids, MI 1984-1986; **Fellowship:** Reconstructive Microsurgery, MECOM MicSurg Inst., Houston, TX 1986-1987

Krizek, Thomas MD (Plastic Surgery) - *Special Expertise:* Cosmetic Surgery-Face; Burns; **Admitting Hospital:** Tampa General Hospital; **Office Address:** 4 Columbia Dr, Ste 730 Tampa, FL 33606; **Office Phone:** (813) 974-7560; **Board Certifications:** Surgery 1965, Plastic Surgery 1968; **Medical School:** Marquette Sch Med 1957; **Residencies:** Surgery, Univ Hosp, Cleveland, OH 1961-1964; Plastic Surgery, Univ Hosp, Cleveland, OH 1964-1966; **Faculty Appointment:** Prof Surgery, Univ S FL Coll Med

Levin, L Scott MD (Plastic Surgery) - *Special Expertise:* Transplant-Toe to Hand; Reconstructive Microvascular Surgery; **Admitting Hospital:** Duke University Medical Center (Page 60); **Office Address:** Duke Univ Med Ctr Box 3945 Durham, NC 27707; **Office Phone:** (919) 681-5079; **Board Certifications:** Orthopaedic Surgery 1993, Hand Surgery 1994; **Medical School:** Temple Univ 1982; **Residencies:** Orthopaedic Surgery, Duke Univ Med Ctr, Durham, NC 1984-1988; Plastic Surgery, Duke Univ Med Ctr, Durham, NC 1988-1989; **Faculty Appointment:** Assoc Prof Surgery, Duke Univ

643

Matthews, David MD (Plastic Surgery) - *Special Expertise:* Craniofacial Surgery/Reconstruction; **Admitting Hospital:** Carolinas Medical Center; **Office Address:** 2215 Randolph Rd Charolette, NC 28207-0752; **Office Phone:** (703) 372-6846; **Board Certifications:** Plastic Surgery 1983, Surgery 1981; **Medical School:** Univ Cincinnati 1974; **Residencies:** Plastic Surgery, Univ of Penn Hosp, Philadelphia, PA 1980-1982; Surgery, Univ of Penn Hosp, Philadelphia, PA 1979-1980; **Fellowship:** Royal Melbourne, Australia; **Faculty Appointment:** Assoc Clin Prof Plastic Surgery, Univ NC Sch Med

Maxwell, G Patrick MD (Plastic Surgery) - *Special Expertise:* Breast Reconstruction; **Admitting Hospital:** Baptist Hospital; **Office Address:** Baptist Med Plaza II 2021 Church St, Ste 806 Nashville, TN 37203; **Office Phone:** (615) 340-4500; **Board Certification:** Plastic Surgery 1981; **Medical School:** Vanderbilt Univ 1972; **Residencies:** Plastic Surgery, John Hopkins Hosp, Baltimore, MD 1976-1979; Surgery, John Hopkins Hosp, Baltimore, MD 1973-1976; **Fellowship:** Microsurgery, Davies Med Ctr, San Francisco, CA 1975; **Faculty Appointment:** Asst Clin Prof Plastic Surgery, Vanderbilt Univ

Mladick, Richard MD (Plastic Surgery) - *Special Expertise:* Cosmetic Surgery-Liposuction; Hand Surgery; Breast Surgery; **Admitting Hospital:** Virginia Beach General Hospital; **Office Address:** Mladick Ctr Cosmetic Surg 1037 First Colonial Rd Virginia Beach, VA 23454; **Office Phone:** (757) 481-5151; **Board Certifications:** Surgery 1965, Plastic Surgery 1969; **Medical School:** Northwestern Univ 1959; **Residencies:** Surgery, Cook Co Hosp, Chicago, IL 1960-1964; Plastic Surgery, Duke Med Ctr, Durham, NC 1964-1967; **Faculty Appointment:** Prof Plastic Surgery, Eastern VA Med Sch

Molnar, Joseph MD (Plastic Surgery) - *Special Expertise:* Burns; Burns; Microvascular Surgery; **Admitting Hospital:** Wake Forest University Baptist Medical Center; **Office Address:** Wake Forest Univ Med Ctr Medical Ctr Blvd Winston Salem, NC 27157-1075; **Office Phone:** (336) 716-0432; **Board Certification:** Plastic Surgery 1996; **Medical School:** Ohio State Univ 1977; **Residencies:** Surgery, Univ Wash Med Ctr, Seattle, WA 1985-1989; Plastic Surgery, Med Coll VA, Richmond, VA 1990-1992; **Fellowships:** Trauma, Mass Genl Hosp, Boston, MA 1979-1985; Hand Surgery, Med Coll Wisc, Milwaukee, WI 1992-1994; **Faculty Appointment:** Asst Prof Plastic Surgery, Wake Forest Univ Sch Med

Morgan, Raymond MD (Plastic Surgery) - *Special Expertise:* Hand Surgery; **Admitting Hospital:** University of Virginia Health Systems; **Office Address:** University of Virginia, Dept of Plas Surg Charlottesville, VA 22908-0376; **Office Phone:** (804) 924-1234; **Board Certifications:** Plastic Surgery 1983, Hand Surgery 1990; **Medical School:** W VA Univ 1976; **Residencies:** Surgery, Johns Hopkins Hosp, Baltimore, MD 1977-1980; Plastic Surgery, John Hopkins Hosp, Baltimore, MD 1980-1982; **Fellowship:** Hand Surgery, Union Meml Hosp, Baltimore, MD; **Faculty Appointment:** Prof Plastic Surgery, Univ VA Sch Med

Mullin, Walter MD (Plastic Surgery) - *Special Expertise:* Breast Reconstruction; Ear Reconstruction; **Admitting Hospital:** Cedars Medical Center - Miami; **Office Address:** Plastic Surgery Ctr 1444 NW 14th Ave Miami, FL 33125-1645; **Office Phone:** (305) 325-1441; **Board Certification:** Plastic Surgery 1977; **Medical School:** Univ Miami Sch Med 1969; **Residencies:** Surgery, Jackson Meml Hosp, Miami, FL 1970-1973; Plastic Surgery, Jackson Meml Hosp, Miami, FL 1974-1976; **Fellowship:** Plastic Surgery, Bangour Genl Hosp, Edinburgh, Scotland 1973-1974; **Faculty Appointment:** Assoc Clin Prof Plastic Surgery, Univ Miami Sch Med

Nahai, Foad MD (Plastic Surgery) - *Special Expertise:* Cosmetic Surgery; Cosmetic Surgery-Face; Cosmetic Surgery-Liposuction; **Admitting Hospital:** St Joseph's Hospital - Atlanta; **Office Address:** 3200 Downwood, Ste 640 Atlanta, GA 30327; **Office Phone:** (404) 351-0051; **Board Certification:** Surgery 1980; **Medical School:** England 1969; **Residencies:** Surgery, Johns Hopkins Affil Hosps, Baltimore, MD 1970-1972; Surgery, Emory Univ Affil Hosps, Atlanta, GA 1972-1975; **Fellowship:** Plastic Surgery, Emory Univ Affil Hosps, Atlanta, GA 1975-1978

Stuzin, James M MD (Plastic Surgery) - *Special Expertise:* Cosmetic Surgery-Body; Breast Surgery; **Admitting Hospital:** Mercy Hospital - Miami; **Office Address:** Plastic Surgery Ctr 1501 S Miami Ave Miami, FL 33129-1102; **Office Phone:** (305) 854-2424; **Board Certification:** Plastic Surgery 1989; **Medical School:** Univ Fla Coll Med 1978; **Residencies:** Surgery, Univ Wash Affil Hosp, Seattle, WA 1979-1983; Plastic Surgery, NYU Med Ctr, New York, NY 1984-1986; **Fellowship:** Craniofacial Surgery, UCLA Med Ctr, Los Angeles, CA 1987; **Faculty Appointment:** Asst Clin Prof Plastic Surgery, Univ Miami Sch Med

Vasconez, Luis O MD (Plastic Surgery) - *Special Expertise:* Cosmetic Surgery-Face; Breast Reconstruction; **Admitting Hospital:** University of Alabama Hospital at Birmingham; **Office Address:** Kirkland Clinic 2000 20th St Birmingham, AL 35294; **Office Phone:** (205) 934-3245; **Board Certifications:** Surgery 1970, Plastic Surgery 1971; **Medical School:** Washington Univ, St Louis 1962; **Residencies:** Surgery, Strong Meml Hosp, Rochester, NY 1963-1970; Plastic Surgery, Shands Hosp-Univ FL, Gainsville, FL 1966-1969; **Faculty Appointment:** Prof Surgery, Univ Ala

Wolfe, S Anthony MD (Plastic Surgery) - *Special Expertise:* Craniofacial Surgery/Reconstruction; Maxillofacial Surgery; **Admitting Hospital:** Cedars Medical Center - Miami; **Office Address:** Plastic Surgery Ctr 1444 NW 14th Ave, Ste 2 Miami, FL 33125; **Office Phone:** (305) 325-1300; **Board Certifications:** Surgery 1973, Plastic Surgery 1976; **Medical School:** Harvard Med Sch 1965; **Residencies:** Surgery, Peter Bent Brigham Hosp, Boston, MA 1968-1972; Plastic Surgery, Jackson Meml Hosp, Miami, FL 1972-1974; **Faculty Appointment:** Clin Prof Plastic Surgery, Univ Miami Sch Med

Midwest

Arnold, Phillip MD (Plastic Surgery) - *Special Expertise:* Cosmetic Surgery-Face; Chemical Peel; **Admitting Hospital:** Mayo Medical Center & Clinic - Rochester; **Office Address:** 200 SW First St Rochester, MN 55905-0001; **Office Phone:** (507) 284-3214; **Board Certification:** Plastic Surgery 1977; **Medical School:** Univ NC Sch Med 1967; **Residencies:** Surgery, Univ NC Meml Hosp, Chapel Hill, NC 1968-1974; Plastic Surgery, Emory Univ Hosp, Atlanta, GA 1974-1976; **Faculty Appointment:** Prof Plastic Surgery, Mayo Med Sch

Bauer, Bruce MD (Plastic Surgery) - *Special Expertise:* Cleft Palate/Lip; Congenital birth defects; Vascular Malformations; **Admitting Hospital:** Children's Memorial Hospital; **Office Address:** Childrens Memorial Hospital 2300 Childrens Plaza Chicago, IL 60614-3394; **Office Phone:** (773) 880-4094; **Board Certification:** Plastic Surgery 1980; **Medical School:** Northwestern Univ 1974; **Residencies:** Surgery, Northwest Meml Hosp, Chicago, IL 1975-1977; Plastic Surgery, Northwest Meml Hosp, Chicago, IL 1977-1979; **Faculty Appointment:** Prof Surgery, Northwestern Univ

Burget, Gary C MD (Plastic Surgery) - *Special Expertise:* Nasal Reconstruction; Cosmetic Surgery-Face; Reconstructive Surgery; **Admitting Hospital:** St Joseph's Hospital - Chicago; **Office Address:** 2913 N Commonwealth Ave, Ste 400 Chicago, IL 60657-6238; **Office Phone:** (773) 880-0062; **Board Certification:** Plastic Surgery 1980; **Medical School:** Yale Univ 1967; **Residencies:** Surgery, Jackson Meml Med Ctr, Miami, FL 1969-1972; Plastic Surgery, Jackson Meml Med Ctr, Miami, FL 1972-1974; **Fellowship:** Pediatric Plastic Surgery, Chldns Meml Hosp, Chicago, IL 1985-1986; **Faculty Appointment:** Asst Clin Prof Surgery, Univ Chicago-Pritzker Sch Med

Coleman, John MD (Plastic Surgery) - *Special Expertise: Cancer Reconstruction; Melanoma-Head & Neck;* **Admitting Hospital:** Indiana University Hospital & Medical Center - Indianapolis; **Office Address:** Univ Plas Surg Assoc 545 Barnhill Drive, Emerson Hall 235 Indianapolis, IN 46202-8106; **Office Phone:** (317) 274-8106; **Board Certifications:** Surgery 1979, Plastic Surgery 1981; **Medical School:** Harvard Med Sch 1973; **Residencies:** Surgery, Emory Univ Affil Hosp, Atlanta, GA 1974-1978; Plastic Surgery, Emory Univ Affil Hosp, Atlanta, GA 1978-1979; **Fellowship:** Surgical Oncology, Univ MD Med Ctr, Baltimore, MD 1980; **Faculty Appointment:** Prof Surgery, Indiana Univ

Hammond, Dennis MD (Plastic Surgery) - *Special Expertise: Breast Surgery;* **Admitting Hospital:** St Mary's Mercy Medical Center; **Office Address:** Hand & Plastic Surgery Center 245 Cherry St, Ste 302 Grand Rapids, MI 49503; **Office Phone:** (616) 459-4994; **Board Certification:** Plastic Surgery 1994; **Medical School:** Univ Mich Med Sch 1985; **Residency:** Plastic Surgery, Grand Rapids Med Edu & Res Ctr, Grand Rapids, MI

Luce, Edward MD (Plastic Surgery) - *Special Expertise: Reconstructive Surgery;* **Admitting Hospital:** Rainbow Babies & Children's Hospital; **Office Address:** 11100 Euclid Avenue University Hospital of Cleveland Div of Plastic Surgery Cleveland, OH; **Office Phone:** (216) 844-4780; **Board Certifications:** Surgery 1972, Plastic Surgery 1974; **Medical School:** Univ KY Coll Med 1965; **Residencies:** Surgery, Barnes Hosp-Wash U, St Louis, MO 1966-1971; Plastic Surgery, John Hopkins Hosp, Baltimore, MD 1971-1973; **Faculty Appointment:** Prof Plastic Surgery, Univ KY Coll Med

Mackinnon, Susan MD (Plastic Surgery) - *Special Expertise: Peripheral Nerve Surgery; Nerve Transplantation;* **Admitting Hospital:** Barnes - Jewish Hospital; **Office Address:** One Barnes-Jewish Hospital Plaza St Louis, MO 63110; **Office Phone:** (314) 362-4587; **Board Certification:** Plastic Surgery 1980; **Medical School:** Canada 1975; **Residencies:** Surgery, Queens Univ-Kingston, Ontario, Canada 1975-1978; Plastic Surgery, Univ Toronto, Toronto, Canada 1978-1980; **Fellowships:** Neurological Surgery, Univ Toronto, Toronto, Canada 1980-1981; Hand Surgery, Union Meml Hosp, Baltimore, MD 1981-1982; **Faculty Appointment:** Prof Surgery, Washington Univ, St Louis

Marsh, Jeffrey L MD (Plastic Surgery) - *Special Expertise: Cleft Palate/Lip; Craniofacial Surgery/Reconstruction;* **Admitting Hospital:** St Louis Children's Hospital; **Office Address:** St Louis Chldns Hosp One S Children's Pl, Box 8238, MS 2S86 St Louis, MO 63110-1077; **Office Phone:** (314) 454-6020; **Board Certifications:** Plastic Surgery 1979, Surgery 1987; **Medical School:** Johns Hopkins Univ 1970; **Residencies:** Surgery, UCLA Med Ctr, Los Angeles, CA 1971-1975; Plastic Surgery, Univ Va Hosp, Charlottesville, VA 1975-1977; **Fellowships:** Craniofacial Surgery, Cannisburn Hosp, Glasgow, Scotland 1977; Craniofacial Surgery, Clinic Belvedere Hosp, Foch, Paris 1977; **Faculty Appointment:** Prof Surgery, Washington Univ, St Louis

McKinney, Peter W. MD (Plastic Surgery) - *Special Expertise: Plastic Surgery - General;* **Admitting Hospital:** Northwestern Memorial Hospital; **Office Address:** 60 E Delaware Pl, Ste 1400 Chicago, IL 60611-1425; **Office Phone:** (312) 266-0300; **Board Certification:** Plastic Surgery 1968; **Medical School:** McGill Univ 1960; **Residencies:** Surgery, Bellevue Hosp Ctr, New York, NY 1961-1964; Plastic Surgery, NY Hosp-Cornell Med Ctr, New York, NY 1964-1967; **Faculty Appointment:** Prof Plastic Surgery, Northwestern Univ

Mustoe, Thomas MD (Plastic Surgery) - *Special Expertise: Breast Cosmetic Surgery; Wound Healing/Care; Cosmetic Surgery-Face;* **Admitting Hospital:** Northwestern Memorial Hospital; **Office Address:** NW Med Fac Fdn, Dept Plastic Surg 675 N St Clair St, Ste 19-250 Chicago, IL 60611; **Office Phone:** (312) 695-6022; **Board Certifications:** Otolaryngology 1983, Plastic Surgery 1987; **Medical School:** Harvard Med Sch 1978; **Residencies:** Otolaryngology, Mass Eye & Ear Infirm, Boston, MA 1980-1983; Plastic Surgery, Brigham-Womens, Boston, MA 1983-1985; **Faculty Appointment:** Prof Surgery, Northwestern Univ

Newman, M Haskell MD (Plastic Surgery) - *Special Expertise:* Craniofacial Surgery/Reconstruction; **Admitting Hospital:** University of Michigan Health Center; **Office Address:** Mott Chldns Hosp 1500 E Medical Center Drive, rm F7859 Ann Arbor, MI 48109-0340; **Office Phone:** (734) 763-8063; **Board Certifications:** Otolaryngology 1969, Plastic Surgery 1978; **Medical School:** Univ Tenn Coll Med, Memphis 1962; **Residencies:** Otolaryngology, Univ Mich Hosps, Ann Arbor, MI 1963-1968; Plastic Surgery, Univ Mich Hosp, Ann Arbor, MI 1975-1977; **Fellowship:** Craniofacial Surgery, Toronto Genl Hosp, Toronto, CN 1977; **Faculty Appointment:** Assoc Clin Prof Surgery, Univ Mich Med Sch

Puckett, Charles Linwood MD (Plastic Surgery) - *Special Expertise:* Cosmetic & Reconstructive Surgery; Breast Surgery; **Admitting Hospital:** University of Missouri Hospitals & Clinics; **Office Address:** Univ MO-Columbia Hlth Scis Ctr, Div Plas Surg One Hospital Dr, rm M349 Columbia, MO 65212-5276; **Office Phone:** (573) 882-2275; **Board Certifications:** Plastic Surgery 1977, Hand Surgery 1990; **Medical School:** Wake Forest Univ Sch Med 1966; **Residencies:** Surgery, Duke Univ Med Ctr, Durham, NC 1967-1971; Plastic Surgery, Duke Univ Med Ctr, Durham, NC 1973-1976; **Faculty Appointment:** Prof Plastic Surgery, Univ MO-Columbia Sch Med

Sanger, James MD (Plastic Surgery) - *Special Expertise:* Reconstructive Surgery; Hand Surgery; **Admitting Hospital:** Froedtert Memorial Lutheran Hospital; **Office Address:** Med Coll Wisc-CF, Dept Plas & Reconstr Surg 9200 W Wisconsin Ave Milwaukee, WI 53226-3522; **Office Phone:** (414) 805-3666; **Board Certifications:** Plastic Surgery 1982, Hand Surgery 1999; **Medical School:** Univ Wisc 1974; **Residencies:** Surgery, LAC-Harbor UCLA Med Ctr, Torrance, CA 1974-1979; Plastic Surgery, Med Coll Wisc Affil Hosps, Milwaukee, WI 1979-1981; **Fellowship:** Hand Surgery, Med Coll Wisc Affil Hosps, Milwaukee, WI 1981-1982; **Faculty Appointment:** Prof Surgery, Med Coll Wisc

Vogt, Peter MD (Plastic Surgery) - *Special Expertise:* Cosmetic Surgery; **Admitting Hospital:** Mercy Hospital - Coon Rapids; **Office Address:** 4825 Olson Meml Hwy, Ste 200 Minneapolis, MN 55422-5156; **Office Phone:** (763) 545-0443; **Board Certification:** Plastic Surgery 1974; **Medical School:** Canada 1965; **Residencies:** Surgery, Montreal Genl Hosp, Montreal, Canada 1968-1970; Plastic Surgery, Winnipeg Hlth Scis Ctr, Mantoba, Canada 1971-1973

Walton, Robert Lee MD (Plastic Surgery) - *Special Expertise:* Cosmetic Surgery-Face; Nasal Reconstruction; Breast Reconstruction; **Admitting Hospital:** University of Chicago Hospitals (Page 78); **Office Address:** Univ Chicago, Dept Plas Surg 5841 S Maryland Ave, MC-6035 Chicago, IL 60637-1463; **Office Phone:** (773) 702-6302; **Board Certifications:** Surgery 1989, Plastic Surgery 1980; **Medical School:** Univ Kans 1972; **Residencies:** Surgery, Johns Hopkins Hosp, Baltimore, MD 1972-1974; Plastic Surgery, Yale-New Haven Hosp, New Haven, CT 1974-1978; **Faculty Appointment:** Prof Plastic Surgery, Univ Chicago-Pritzker Sch Med

Young, Vernon Leroy MD (Plastic Surgery) - *Special Expertise:* Breast Augmentation; Skin Laser Surgery-Resurfacing; **Admitting Hospital:** Barnes - Jewish Hospital; **Office Address:** Washington Univ Sch Med 1040 N Mason, Ste 206 St Louis, MO 63141-6366; **Office Phone:** (314) 996-8050; **Board Certifications:** Plastic Surgery 1981, Surgery 1988; **Medical School:** Univ KY Coll Med 1970; **Residencies:** Surgery, Univ KY Med Ctr, Lexington, KY 1973-1977; Plastic Surgery, Barnes Hosp-Wash Univ, St Louis, MO 1977-1979; **Faculty Appointment:** Prof Plastic Surgery, Washington Univ, St Louis

Zins, James MD (Plastic Surgery) - *Special Expertise:* Cosmetic Surgery-Face; **Admitting Hospital:** Cleveland Clinic Foundation; **Office Address:** Cleveland Clin 9500 Euclid Ave, Desk A60 Cleveland, OH 44195; **Office Phone:** (216) 444-6901; **Board Certifications:** Surgery 1981, Plastic Surgery 1985; **Medical School:** Univ Penn 1974; **Residencies:** Surgery, Hosp Univ Penn, Philadelphia, PA 1975-1980; Plastic Surgery, Hosp Univ Penn, Philadelphia, PA 1980-1982; **Fellowships:** Craniofacial Surgery, Hosp Univ Penn, Philadelphia, PA 1977-1978; Maxillofacial Surgery, Hosp Sick Chldn, London, England 1982-1983

Great Plains and Mountains

Ketch, Lawrence Levant MD (Plastic Surgery) - *Special Expertise:* Cosmetic Surgery-Face; *Head & Neck Reconstruction; Cleft Palate/Lip;* **Admitting Hospital:** University of Colorado Health & Science Center; **Office Address:** 4200 E 9th Ave, Box C309 Denver, CO 80262; **Office Phone:** (303) 315-6668; **Board Certifications:** Plastic Surgery 1982, Surgery 1980; **Medical School:** Univ Colo 1974; **Residency:** Surgery, Univ Colo Affil Hosp, Baltimore, MD 1975-1979; **Fellowship:** Plastic Surgery, Univ Miami, Miami, FL 1980-1981; **Faculty Appointment:** Assoc Prof Plastic Surgery, Univ Colo

Knize, David Maurice MD (Plastic Surgery) - *Special Expertise:* Cosmetic Surgery-Face; **Admitting Hospital:** Swedish Medical Center - Englewood; **Office Address:** Knize Clin Plas Surg 3555 S Clarkson St Englewood, CO 80110-3916; **Office Phone:** (303) 761-9990; **Board Certifications:** Surgery 1971, Plastic Surgery 1975; **Medical School:** Univ Tex SW, Dallas 1963; **Residencies:** Surgery, Univ Colo Med Ctr, Denver, CO 1966-1969; Plastic Surgery, NYU Med Ctr, New York, NY 1971-1974; **Faculty Appointment:** Assoc Clin Prof Plastic Surgery, Univ Colo

Lockwood, Ted MD (Plastic Surgery) - *Special Expertise:* Cosmetic Surgery-Body; **Admitting Hospital:** Overland Park Regional Medical Center; **Office Address:** 10600 Quivira Rd, Ste 470 Overland Park, KS 66215-2377; **Office Phone:** (913) 894-1070; **Board Certification:** Plastic Surgery 1981; **Medical School:** Univ Kans 1971; **Residencies:** Surgery, Univ Texas Hlth Sci Ctrn, Dallas, TX 1972-1976; Plastic Surgery, Univ Penn, Philadelphia, PA 1978-1980; **Faculty Appointment:** Asst Clin Prof Surgery, Univ MO-Kansas City

Southwest

Barton Jr, Fritz MD (Plastic Surgery) - *Special Expertise:* Cosmetic Surgery-Face; **Admitting Hospital:** Baylor University Medical Center; **Office Address:** Dallas Day Surgery Ctr 411 N Washington Ave, Ste 5000 Dallas, TX 75246-1713; **Office Phone:** (214) 821-9355; **Board Certifications:** Surgery 1975, Plastic Surgery 1977; **Medical School:** Univ Tex SW, Dallas 1967; **Residencies:** Surgery, Parkland Meml Hosp, Dallas, TX 1970-1974; Plastic Surgery, NYU Med Ctr, New York, NY 1974-1976; **Faculty Appointment:** Prof Plastic Surgery, Univ Tex SW, Dallas

Biggs Jr, Thomas M MD (Plastic Surgery) - *Special Expertise:* Cosmetic Surgery-Face; **Admitting Hospital:** Christus St Joseph's Hospital; **Office Address:** 1315 St Joseph Pkwy Houston, TX 77002-8231; **Office Phone:** (713) 650-0800; **Board Certification:** Plastic Surgery 1978; **Medical School:** Baylor Coll Med 1958; **Residencies:** Surgery, Baylor Univ Affil Hosp, Houston, TX 1959-1962; Plastic Surgery, Baylor Univ Affil Hosp, Houston, TX 1963-1964; **Faculty Appointment:** Clin Prof Plastic Surgery, Baylor Coll Med

Burns, Alton Jay MD (Plastic Surgery) - *Special Expertise:* Cosmetic Surgery; Skin Laser Surgery; **Admitting Hospital:** Baylor University Medical Center; **Office Address:** 411 N Washington St, Ste 6000 Dallas, TX 75246; **Office Phone:** (214) 823-1978; **Board Certifications:** Surgery 1987, Plastic Surgery 1990; **Medical School:** Univ Tex SW, Dallas 1981; **Residencies:** Surgery, Univ Utah Hosp, Salt Lake City, UT 1982-1986; Plastic Surgery, Univ TX SW Med Ctr, Dallas, TX 1986-1988; **Fellowship:** Vascular Anomalies, Chldns Hosp, Boston, MA 1988; **Faculty Appointment:** Asst Prof Plastic Surgery, Univ Tex SW, Dallas

Byrd, Henry S MD (Plastic Surgery) - *Special Expertise:* Cosmetic Surgery-Face; **Admitting Hospital:** Baylor University Medical Center; **Office Address:** 411 N Washington Ave, Ste 6000 - rm LD13 Dallas, TX 75246-1713; **Office Phone:** (214) 821-9662; **Board Certifications:** Surgery 1978, Plastic Surgery 1980; **Medical School:** Univ Tex Med Br, Galveston 1972; **Residencies:** Surgery, Univ Utah Med Ctr, Salt Lake City, UT 1973-1977; Plastic Surgery, Dallas Co Hosp-Parkland Meml, Dallas, TX 1977-1979; **Faculty Appointment:** Clin Prof Plastic Surgery, Univ Tex SW, Dallas

Colon, Gustavo MD (Plastic Surgery) - *Special Expertise:* Cosmetic Surgery; **Admitting Hospital:** East Jefferson General Hospital; **Office Address:** 4204 Tueton St Metaririe, LA 70006; **Office Phone:** (504) 888-4297; **Board Certification:** Plastic Surgery 1972; **Medical School:** Univ MD Sch Med 1964; **Residencies:** Surgery, US Public Hlth Svc Hosp, New Orleans, LA 1965-1969; Plastic Surgery, Tulane Affil Prog, New Orleans, LA 1969-1971; **Faculty Appointment:** Prof Surgery, Tulane Univ

Gunter, Jack MD (Plastic Surgery) - *Special Expertise:* Rhinoplasty; Rhinoplasty-Secondary Surgery; **Admitting Hospital:** Presbyterian Hospital of Dallas; **Office Address:** 8315 Wallnut Hill Lane, Ste 225 Dallas, TX 75231-4218; **Office Phone:** (214) 369-8123; **Board Certifications:** Otolaryngology 1969, Plastic Surgery 1981; **Medical School:** Okla State Univ, Coll Osteo Med 1963; **Residencies:** Surgery, U Ark Med Ctr, Little Rock, AR 1964-1965; Otolaryngology, Tulane U Hospital, New Orleans, LA 1965-1968; **Fellowships:** Mercy Hospital, Pittsburgh, PA 1968-1969; Plastic Surgery, U Mich Hospital, Ann Arbor, MI 1978-1980; **Faculty Appointment:** Clin Prof Otolaryngology, Texas Tech Univ

Hamra, Sameer T MD (Plastic Surgery) - *Special Expertise:* Cosmetic Surgery-Face; Rhinoplasty; **Admitting Hospital:** Mary Shiels Hospital; **Office Address:** 2731 Lemmon Ave E, Ste 304 Dallas, TX 75204; **Office Phone:** (214) 823-9080; **Board Certifications:** Surgery 1970, Plastic Surgery 1977; **Medical School:** Univ Okla Coll Med 1963; **Residencies:** Plastic Surgery, NYU Med Ctr, New York, NY 1970-1973; Surgery, Univ Okla, Oklahoma City, OK 1964-1968; **Fellowship:** Surgery, Univ Lausanne 1965-1966; **Faculty Appointment:** Asst Clin Prof Surgery, Univ N Tex Hlth Sci Ctr, Coll Osteo Med

Kelly, John Michael MD (Plastic Surgery) - *Special Expertise:* Cosmetic Surgery-Face; Breast Surgery; **Admitting Hospital:** Intergris Baptist Medical Center - Oklahoma; **Office Address:** 3301 NW 63rd St Oklahoma City, OK 73116-3705; **Office Phone:** (405) 842-9732; **Board Certifications:** Surgery 1970, Plastic Surgery 1978; **Medical School:** Univ Ark 1963; **Residencies:** Surgery, Univ VA Hosp, Charlottesville, VA 1964-1969; Plastic Surgery, Johns Hopkins Hosp, Baltimore, MD 1969-1971; **Faculty Appointment:** Clin Prof Surgery, Univ Okla Coll Med

Kroll, Stephen S MD (Plastic Surgery) - *Special Expertise:* Cancer Reconstruction; Breast Reconstruction; **Admitting Hospital:** University of Texas MD Anderson Cancer Center (Page 66); **Office Address:** Univ Tex MD Anderson Cancer Ctr, Plastic Surg 1515 Holcombe Blvd, Box 62 Houston, TX 77030; **Office Phone:** (713) 794-1247; **Board Certifications:** Plastic Surgery 1986, Otolaryngology 1977; **Medical School:** Harvard Med Sch 1969; **Residencies:** Plastic Surgery, Georgetown Univ, Washington, DC 1982-1984; Otolaryngology, Case West Res., Cleveland, OH 1976; **Fellowship:** MD Anderson Hosp, Houston, TX 1984; **Faculty Appointment:** Prof Plastic Surgery, Univ Tex, Houston

Nath, Rahul Kamur MD (Plastic Surgery) - *Special Expertise:* Brachial Plexus-Pediatric; **Admitting Hospital:** Texas Children's Hospital - Houston; **Office Address:** 1102 Bates Street, Ste 330 Houston, TX 77030; **Office Phone:** (832) 824-3193; **Board Certification:** Plastic Surgery 1998; **Medical School:** Northwestern Univ 1988; **Residencies:** Surgery, Northwestern Med Ctr., Chicago, IL 1989-1991; Plastic Surgery, Washington University, St. Louis, MO 1991-1994; **Fellowship:** Washington University, St. Louis, MO 1995-1996; **Faculty Appointment:** Asst Prof Plastic Surgery, Baylor Coll Med

Rohrich, Rodney James MD (Plastic Surgery) - *Special Expertise:* Nasal Surgery; Cosmetic Surgery-Face & Breast; Cosmetic Surgery-Liposuction; **Admitting Hospital:** Zale Lipshy University Hospital; **Office Address:** Univ Texas SW Med Ctr, Plastic & Recon Surg 5323 Harry Hines Blvd Dallas, TX 75390-9132; **Office Phone:** (214) 648-3571; **Board Certifications:** Plastic Surgery 1987, Hand Surgery 1990; **Medical School:** Baylor Coll Med 1979; **Residencies:** Plastic Surgery, Univ Mich Hosp, Ann Arbor, MI 1982-1985; Plastic Surgery, Radcliffe Infirm/Oxford, Oxford, England 1983; **Fellowship:** Hand Surgery, Mass Genl Hosp-Harvard, Boston, MA 1986-1987; **Faculty Appointment:** Prof Plastic Surgery, Univ Tex SW, Dallas

Schnur, Paul MD (Plastic Surgery) - *Special Expertise:* Hand Surgery; **Admitting Hospital:** Mayo Medical Center & Clinic - Scottsdale; **Office Address:** Mayo Clinic Scottsdale 13400 E Shea Blvd Scottsdale, AZ 85259-5404; **Office Phone:** (480) 301-8139; **Board Certifications:** Surgery 1971, Plastic Surgery 1973; **Medical School:** Baylor Coll Med 1962; **Residencies:** Surgery, Mayo Clin, Rochester, MN 1966-1970; Plastic Surgery, Mayo Clin, Rochester, MN 1970-1972; **Faculty Appointment:** Assoc Prof Plastic Surgery, Mayo Med Sch

Schusterman, Mark A MD (Plastic Surgery) - *Special Expertise:* Breast Reconstruction; Cosmetic Surgery-Face; **Admitting Hospital:** St Luke's Episcopal Hospital - Houston (Page 76); **Office Address:** 7505 S Main St, Ste 200 Houston, TX 77030; **Office Phone:** (713) 794-0368; **Board Certifications:** Surgery 1986, Plastic Surgery 1989; **Medical School:** Univ Louisville Sch Med 1980; **Residencies:** Surgery, Univ Hosp, Cincinnati, OH 1981-1985; Pediatric Surgery, Univ Pitts Med Ctr, Pittsburgh, PA 1985-1987; **Fellowship:** Microsurgery, Univ Pitts Med Ctr, Pittsburgh, PA 1987-1988; **Faculty Appointment:** Asst Prof Surgery, Univ Tex SW, Dallas

Shenaq, Saleh MD (Plastic Surgery) - *Special Expertise:* Microsurgery; Hand Surgery; **Admitting Hospital:** Methodist Hospital - Houston (Page 69); **Office Address:** Baylor Coll Med 6560 Fannin St, Scurlock Tower, Ste 800 Houston, TX 77030-2706; **Office Phone:** (713) 798-6141; **Board Certifications:** Plastic Surgery 1983, Hand Surgery 1990; **Medical School:** Egypt 1972; **Residencies:** Surgery, Med Coll Ohio Hosp, Toledo, OH 1974-1979; Plastic Surgery, Univ Pitts Med Ctr, Pittsburgh, PA 1979-1981; **Fellowship:** Hand Surgery, Univ Louisville Hosp, Louisville, KY 1981; **Faculty Appointment:** Prof Plastic Surgery, Baylor Coll Med

Tebbetts, John B MD (Plastic Surgery) - *Special Expertise:* Cosmetic Surgery-Liposuction; Breast Augmentation; Rhinoplasty; **Admitting Hospital:** Mary Shiels Hospital; **Office Address:** 2801 Lemmon Ave, Ste 300 Dallas, TX 75204-2398; **Office Phone:** (214) 220-2712; **Board Certifications:** Surgery 1978, Plastic Surgery 1980; **Medical School:** Univ Tex Med Br, Galveston 1972; **Residencies:** Surgery, Univ Utah Med Ctr, Salt Lake City, UT 1973-1977; Plastic Surgery, Dallas Co Hospital-Parkland Meml Hosp, Dallas, TX 1977-1979; **Faculty Appointment:** Asst Clin Prof Plastic Surgery, Other Texas School

West Coast and Pacific

Berner, Carl Frederick MD (Plastic Surgery) - *Special Expertise:* Cosmetic Surgery; **Admitting Hospital:** Overlake Hospital Medical Center; **Office Address:** Bellevue Plas Surg 1551 116th St NE Bellevue, WA 98004-3814; **Office Phone:** (425) 453-2161; **Board Certifications:** Surgery 1967, Plastic Surgery 1974; **Medical School:** Univ MD Sch Med 1961; **Residencies:** Surgery, Univ MD Hosp, Baltimore, MD 1963-1966; Plastic Surgery, Univ Mich Med Ctr, Ann Arbor, MI 1969-1971; **Faculty Appointment:** Asst Clin Prof Surgery, Univ Wash

Brink, Robert Ross MD (Plastic Surgery) - *Special Expertise:* Cosmetic Surgery; **Admitting Hospital:** Mills - Peninsula Health Center Hospital; **Office Address:** 66 Bovet Rd, Ste 101 San Mateo, CA 94402; **Office Phone:** (650) 570-6066; **Board Certifications:** Plastic Surgery 1980, Surgery 1980; **Medical School:** Univ Mich Med Sch 1970; **Residencies:** Surgery, UC Davis Med Ctr, Sacramento, CA 1973-1977; Plastic Surgery, UCSF Med Ctr, San Francisco, CA 1977-1979

Brody, Garry S MD (Plastic Surgery) - *Special Expertise:* Hand Surgery; **Admitting Hospital:** USC University Hospital - Richard K. Eamer Medical Plaza; **Office Address:** 1450 San Pablo St, Ste 2000 Los Angeles, CA 90033-1042; **Office Phone:** (323) 442-6462; **Board Certifications:** Surgery 1963, Plastic Surgery 1967; **Medical School:** Univ Alberta 1956; **Residencies:** Surgery, Georetown Univ Hosp, Washington, DC 1959-1961; Plastic Surgery, Univ Pittsburgh, Pittsburgh, PA 1962-1964; **Fellowship:** Surgery, McGill Univ, Montreal, Canada 1958-1959; **Faculty Appointment:** Clin Prof Plastic Surgery, USC Sch Med

Buncke Jr, Harry J MD (Plastic Surgery) - *Special Expertise:* Microsurgery; **Admitting Hospital:** Davies Medical Center; **Office Address:** Buncke Med Clin Inc, MOB Annex Ste 140 45 Castro St San Francisco, CA 94114; **Office Phone:** (415) 565-6136; **Board Certification:** Plastic Surgery 1978; **Medical School:** NY Med Coll 1951; **Residencies:** Surgery, Flower Fifth Ave Hosp, New York, NY 1952-1954; Plastic Surgery, Bronx VA Med Ctr, New York, NY 1954-1956; **Fellowship:** Plastic Surgery, Queen Victoria Hosp, E Grinstead, England 1956-1957; **Faculty Appointment:** Assoc Clin Prof Plastic Surgery, Stanford Univ

Daniel, Rollin K MD (Plastic Surgery) - *Special Expertise:* Cosmetic Surgery-Face; **Admitting Hospital:** Hoag Memorial Hospital Presbyterian; **Office Address:** 1441 Avocado Ave, Ste 308 Newport Beach, CA 92660-7704; **Office Phone:** (949) 721-0494; **Board Certification:** Plastic Surgery 1977; **Medical School:** Columbia P&S **Residencies:** Plastic Surgery, McGill Univ Affil Hosps, Montreal, Canada 1973-1975; Hand Surgery, Univ Louisville Hosp, Louisville, KY 1975-1976; **Fellowship:** Craniofacial Surgery, Toronto Genl Hosp, Toronto, Canada 1984

Flowers, Robert MD (Plastic Surgery) - *Special Expertise:* Coronal Canthopexy; **Admitting Hospital:** Queen's Medical Center - Honolulu; **Office Address:** Plastic Surgery Center of the Pacific 677 Ala Moana Blvd, Ste 1101 Honolulu, HI 96813; **Office Phone:** (808) 521-1999; **Board Certification:** Plastic Surgery 1971; **Medical School:** Univ Ala 1960; **Residencies:** Surgery, Cleveland Clinic, Cleveland, OH 1963-1966; Plastic Surgery, Cleveland Clinic, Cleveland, OH 1966-1968; **Faculty Appointment:** Asst Clin Prof Surgery, Univ Hawaii JA Burns Sch Med

Fodor, Peter Bela MD (Plastic Surgery) - *Special Expertise:* Cosmetic Surgery; **Admitting Hospital:** Century City Hospital; **Office Address:** 2080 Century Park E, Ste 710 Los Angeles, CA 90067; **Office Phone:** (310) 203-9818; **Board Certifications:** Surgery 1976, Plastic Surgery 1977; **Medical School:** Univ Wisc 1966; **Residencies:** Surgery, Columbia-Presby Med Ctr, New York, NY 1967-1968; Plastic Surgery, St Luke's Hosp, New York, NY 1974-1976; **Faculty Appointment:** Asst Clin Prof Surgery, UCLA

Grossman, John A MD (Plastic Surgery) - *Special Expertise: Cosmetic Surgery;* **Admitting Hospital:** Century City Hospital; **Office Address:** 435 N Bedford Dr, Ste 300 Beverly Hills, CA 90210; **Office Phone:** (310) 557-2307; **Board Certifications:** Plastic Surgery 1976, Surgery 1974; **Medical School:** Cornell Univ-Weil Med Coll 1967; **Residencies:** Surgery, Boston City Hosp, Boston, MA 1968-1973; Plastic Surgery, Univ Colo Hlth Scis Ctr, Denver, CO 1973-1975; **Fellowship:** Surgery, Harvard Med Sch, Boston, MA 1971-1973; **Faculty Appointment:** Clin Inst Plastic Surgery, Univ Colo

Gruss, Joseph MD (Plastic Surgery) - *Special Expertise: Maxillofacial & Craniofacial Surgery; Facial Trauma/Fractures;* **Admitting Hospital:** Children's Hospital and Regional Medical Center - Seattle; **Office Address:** Childrens Hosp & Regional Med Ctr 4800 Sand Point Way NE, Box 5371, MS CH-78 Seattle, WA 98105-3901; **Office Phone:** (206) 526-2039; **Medical School:** South Africa 1969; **Residencies:** Plastic Surgery, Toronto Western Hosp, Toronto, Canada 1976; Plastic Surgery, Hosp for Sick Children, Totonto, Canada 1976; **Fellowships:** Surgical Oncology, Princess Margaret Hosp, Toronto, Canada 1977; Head and Neck Surgery, Princess Margaret Hosp, Toronto, Canada 1977; **Faculty Appointment:** Prof Plastic Surgery, Univ Wash

Hardesty, Robert MD (Plastic Surgery) - *Special Expertise: Facial Reconstruction;* **Admitting Hospital:** Loma Linda University Medical Center; **Office Address:** Loma Linda Univ Health Care 11370 Anderson St, Ste 2100 Loma Linda, CA 92354-3450; **Office Phone:** (909) 796-4822; **Board Certifications:** Surgery 1984, Plastic Surgery 1989; **Medical School:** Loma Linda Univ 1978; **Residencies:** Surgery, Loma Linda Univ Med Ctr, Loma Linda, CA 1979-1983; Plastic Surgery, Univ Pittsburgh, Pittsburgh, PA 1984-1986; **Fellowship:** Pediatric Plastic Surgery, Washington Univ Chldns Hosp, St Louis, MO 1986-1987

Hoefflin, Steven M MD (Plastic Surgery) - *Special Expertise: Cosmetic Surgery-Face; Reconstructive Surgery;* **Admitting Hospital:** St John's Health Center; **Office Address:** 1530 Arizona Ave Santa Monica, CA 90404-1208; **Office Phone:** (310) 451-4733; **Board Certification:** Plastic Surgery 1978; **Medical School:** UCLA 1972; **Residencies:** Surgery, UCLA Med Ctr, Los Angeles, CA 1973-1974; Plastic Surgery, UCLA Med Ctr, Los Angeles, CA 1976-1977; **Faculty Appointment:** Assoc Clin Prof Plastic Surgery, UCLA

Horowitz, Jed H MD (Plastic Surgery) - *Special Expertise: Breast Augmentation; Cosmetic Surgery-Face;* **Admitting Hospital:** Long Beach Memorial Medical Center; **Office Address:** Plasticos Inst for Plas Surg 7677 Center Ave, Ste 401 Huntington Beach, CA 92647; **Office Phone:** (714) 902-1100; **Board Certification:** Plastic Surgery 1986; **Medical School:** SUNY Buffalo 1977; **Residencies:** Univ Of VA, Charlottesville, VA 1983-1984; Univ Of VA, Charlottesville, VA 1984-1985; **Fellowship:** Univ Of VA, Charlottesville, VA 1982-1983; **Faculty Appointment:** Clin Inst Plastic Surgery, UCSF

Jewell, Mark L MD (Plastic Surgery) - *Special Expertise: Hand Surgery; Burns;* **Admitting Hospital:** Sacred Heart Hospital; **Office Address:** 630 E 13th St Eugene, OR 97401-8610; **Office Phone:** (541) 683-3234; **Board Certification:** Plastic Surgery 1981; **Medical School:** Univ Kans 1973; **Residencies:** Surgery, Los Angeles Co, Torrance, CA 1973-1976; Plastic Surgery, Erlanger Hosp, Chattanooga, TN 1977-1979; **Fellowship:** Burn Surgery, USC med Ctr, Los Angeles, CA 1976-1977

Kawamoto Jr, Henry K MD (Plastic Surgery) - *Special Expertise: Cosmetic Surgery; Craniofacial Surgery/Reconstruction; Maxilofacial Surgery;* **Admitting Hospital:** UCLA Medical Center; **Office Address:** 1301 20th St, Ste 460 Santa Monica, CA 90404-2054; **Office Phone:** (310) 829-0391; **Board Certifications:** Surgery 1972, Plastic Surgery 1976; **Medical School:** USC Sch Med 1964; **Residencies:** Surgery, Columbia-Presby Med Ctr, New York, NY 1965-1971; Plastic Surgery, NYU Med Ctr, New York, NY 1971-1973; **Fellowship:** Craniofacial Surgery, Dr Paul Tessier, Paris, France 1973-1974; **Faculty Appointment:** Assoc Clin Prof Plastic Surgery, UCLA

Koplin, Lawrence Mark MD (Plastic Surgery) - *Special Expertise:* Cosmetic Surgery-Face; **Admitting Hospital:** Cedars-Sinai Medical Center; **Office Address:** 436 N Bedford Dr, Ste 103 Beverly Hills, CA 90210-4310; **Office Phone:** (310) 277-3223; **Board Certifications:** Surgery 1982, Plastic Surgery 1983; **Medical School:** Baylor Coll Med 1976; **Residencies:** Surgery, Kaiser Foundation Hosp, Los Angeles, CA 1978-1981; Plastic Surgery, St Joseph Hosp, Houston, TX 1981-1983

Leaf, Norman MD (Plastic Surgery) - *Special Expertise:* Plastic Surgery - General; **Admitting Hospital:** Cedars-Sinai Medical Center; **Office Address:** 436 N Bedford Dr Beverly Hills, CA 90210-4310; **Office Phone:** (310) 274-8001; **Board Certifications:** Surgery 1973, Plastic Surgery 1974; **Medical School:** Univ Chicago-Pritzker Sch Med 1966; **Residencies:** Surgery, Univ Chicago Hosps, Chicago, IL 1967-1972; Plastic Surgery, Univ Chicago Hosps, Chicago, IL 1972-1973; **Fellowship:** Research, Univ Chicago Hosp-US Pub Hlth Svc-NIH, Chicago, IL 1968-1969; **Faculty Appointment:** Asst Clin Prof Plastic Surgery, UCLA

Lesavoy, Malcolm A MD (Plastic Surgery) - *Special Expertise:* Reconstructive Surgery; **Admitting Hospital:** UCLA Medical Center; **Office Address:** 16311 Ventura Blvd, Ste 550 Encino, CA 91436; **Office Phone:** (818) 986-8270; **Board Certification:** Plastic Surgery 1977; **Medical School:** Univ Hlth Sci/Chicago Med Sch 1969; **Residencies:** Surgery, Univ Chicago Hosps, Chicago, IL 1969-1974; Plastic Surgery, Univ Miami Hosp/Clins, Miami, FL 1974-1976; **Faculty Appointment:** Clin Prof Plastic Surgery, UCLA

Markowitz, Bernard Lloyd MD (Plastic Surgery) - *Special Expertise:* Microvascular Surgery; Cranial Facial Surgery; Cosmetic Surgery; **Admitting Hospital:** UCLA Medical Center; **Office Address:** 200 UCLA Med Plaza, Ste 465 Los Angeles, CA 90095-8344; **Office Phone:** (310) 206-3759; **Board Certification:** Plastic Surgery 1989; **Medical School:** NYU Sch Med 1979; **Residencies:** Surgery, NYU Med Ctr, New York, NY 1979-1984; Plastic Surgery, NYU Med Ctr, New York, NY 1984-1986; **Fellowship:** Maxillofacial Surgery, John Hopkins Hosp, Baltimore, MD 1986-1987; **Faculty Appointment:** Assoc Prof Plastic Surgery, UCLA

Marten, Timothy James MD (Plastic Surgery) - *Special Expertise:* Cosmetic Surgery; Cosmetic Surgery-Face; Cosmetic Surgery-Face; **Admitting Hospital:** California Pacific Medical Center; **Office Address:** Marten Clinic of Plastic Surgery 450 Sutter St, rm 826 San Francisco, CA 94108; **Office Phone:** (415) 677-9937; **Board Certification:** Plastic Surgery 1993; **Medical School:** UC Davis 1982; **Residencies:** Surgery, Kaiser Fdn Hosp, San Francisco, CA 1982-1987; Plastic Surgery, Univ IL Hosp, Chicago, IL 1987-1989

Mathes, Stephen MD (Plastic Surgery) - *Special Expertise:* Breast Reconstruction; **Admitting Hospital:** University of California - San Francisco Medical Center; **Office Address:** University of California Dept. Plastic Surgery 359 Parnassus San Francisco, CA 94143-0001; **Office Phone:** (415) 476-3061; **Board Certifications:** Plastic Surgery 1979, Surgery 1993; **Medical School:** Louisiana State Univ 1968; **Residencies:** Plastic Surgery, Emory Affil Hosp., Atlanta, GA 1975-1977; Surgery, Emory Affil Hosp, Atlanta, GA 1972-1975; **Faculty Appointment:** Prof Plastic Surgery, UCSF

Meltzer, Toby R MD (Plastic Surgery) - *Special Expertise:* Transgender Surgery; Penile Inversion Technique; Breast Augmentation; **Admitting Hospital:** Eastmoreland Hospital; **Office Address:** Crown Plaza 1500 SW First Ave, Ste 1120 Portland, OR 97201; **Office Phone:** (800) 525-9323; **Board Certifications:** Surgery 1989, Plastic Surgery 1992; **Medical School:** Louisiana State Univ 1983; **Residencies:** Surgery, Charity Hosp of Louisiana, New Orleans, LA 1984-1988; Plastic Surgery, Univ Michigan, Ann Arbor, MI 1988-1990; **Fellowship:** Burn Surgery, Wayne State Univ, Detroit, MI 1986-1987; **Faculty Appointment:** Asst Clin Prof Surgery, Oregon Hlth Scis Univ

Miller, Timothy Alden MD (Plastic Surgery) - *Special Expertise: Plastic Surgery - General;* **Admitting Hospital:** UCLA Medical Center; **Office Address:** UCLA Plastic Surgery 200 UCLA Med Plaza, Ste 465 Los Angeles, CA 90095; **Office Phone:** (310) 825-5644; **Board Certifications:** Surgery 1971, Plastic Surgery 1973; **Medical School:** UCLA 1963; **Residencies:** Surgery, Johns Hopkins Hosp, Baltimore, MD 1967; Thoracic Surgery, UCLA, Los Angeles, CA 1967-1969; **Fellowship:** Plastic Surgery, Univ Pittsburgh, Pittsburgh, PA 1970-1971; **Faculty Appointment:** Prof Surgery, UCLA

Owsley, John Q MD (Plastic Surgery) - *Special Expertise: Plastic Surgery - General;* **Admitting Hospital:** California Pacific Medical Center; **Office Address:** California Pacific Med Ctr-Davies Campus 45 Castro St, Ste 111 San Francisco, CA 94114; **Office Phone:** (415) 861-8040; **Board Certification:** Plastic Surgery 1978; **Medical School:** Vanderbilt Univ 1953; **Residencies:** Surgery, UCSF Med Ctr, San Francisco, CA 1953-1958; Plastic Surgery, UCSF Med Ctr, San Francisco, CA 1958-1959; **Faculty Appointment:** Clin Prof Surgery, UCSF

Paul, Malcolm D MD (Plastic Surgery) - *Special Expertise: Cosmetic Surgery-Face;* **Admitting Hospital:** Hoag Memorial Hospital Presbyterian; **Office Address:** 1401 Avocado Ave, Ste 810 Newport Beach, CA 92660-7717; **Office Phone:** (949) 760-5047; **Board Certification:** Plastic Surgery 1976; **Medical School:** Univ MD Sch Med 1969; **Residencies:** Surgery, Geo Wash Med Ctr, Washington, DC 1971-1973; Plastic Surgery, Geo Wash Med Ctr, Washington, DC 1973-1975; **Faculty Appointment:** Asst Clin Prof Surgery, UC Irvine

Rand, Richard Pierce MD (Plastic Surgery) - *Special Expertise: Cosmetic Surgery; Breast Surgery;* **Admitting Hospital:** Overlake Hospital Medical Center; **Office Address:** 1135 116th Ave NE, Ste 630 Bellevue, WA 98004; **Office Phone:** (425) 688-8828; **Board Certifications:** Surgery 1998, Plastic Surgery 1991; **Medical School:** Univ Mich Med Sch 1981; **Residencies:** Surgery, New Eng Med Ctr, Boston, MA 1981-1986; Plastic Surgery, Emory Univ Hosp, Atlanta, GA 1986-1988; **Fellowship:** Craniofacial Surgery, Univ Miami, Miami, FL 1989; **Faculty Appointment:** Assoc Prof Surgery, Univ Wash

Reinisch, John F MD (Plastic Surgery) - *Special Expertise: Ear Reconstruction; Cleft Palate/Lip; Craniofacial Surgery/Reconstruction;* **Admitting Hospital:** Children's Hospital - Los Angeles; **Office Address:** Chldns Hosp Los Angeles 4650 Sunset Blvd, Box 96 Los Angeles, CA 90027; **Office Phone:** (323) 669-4544; **Board Certification:** Plastic Surgery 1980; **Medical School:** Harvard Med Sch 1970; **Residencies:** Plastic Surgery, Univ VA Hosp, Richmond, VA 1976-1978; Surgery, Univ Mich Med Ctr, Ann Arbor, MI 1970-1975; **Faculty Appointment:** Prof Surgery, USC Sch Med

Ristow, Brunno MD (Plastic Surgery) - *Special Expertise: Cosmetic Surgery-Face;* **Admitting Hospital:** California Pacific Medical Center; **Office Address:** Pan Med Bldg 2100 Webster St, Ste 501 San Francisco, CA 94115; **Office Phone:** (415) 202-1507; **Board Certification:** Plastic Surgery 1975; **Medical School:** Brazil 1966; **Residencies:** Surgery, NY Hosp-Cornell Med Ctr, New York, NY 1968-1971; Plastic Surgery, NYU Med Ctr, NY, NY 1970-1973; **Fellowship:** Plastic Surgery, NYU Med Ctr, New York City, NY 1967-1968

Seyfer, Alan MD (Plastic Surgery) - *Special Expertise: Chest Wall Reconstruction; Cleft Palate/Lip; Hand Surgery;* **Admitting Hospital:** Oregon Health Science University Hospital and Clinics; **Office Address:** Oreg Hlth Scis Univ. Div PLS L352A 3181 Sam Jackson PK RD Portland, OR 97201; **Office Phone:** (503) 494-7824; **Board Certifications:** Plastic Surgery 1982, Hand Surgery 1989; **Medical School:** Louisiana State Univ 1973; **Residencies:** Surgery, Fitzsimons AMC, Denver, CO 1974-1978; Plastic Surgery, Walter Reed AMC, Washington, DC 1978-1981; **Fellowship:** Hand Surgery, Duke U Med Ctr, Durham, NC 1980; **Faculty Appointment:** Prof Surgery

654

Shaw, William Wei-Lien MD (Plastic Surgery) - *Special Expertise:* Microsurgery; Breast Surgery; Cosmetic Surgery-Face; **Admitting Hospital:** UCLA Medical Center; **Office Address:** 200 UCLA Medical Plaza, Ste 465 Los Angeles, CA 90095; **Office Phone:** (310) 206-7520; **Board Certification:** Plastic Surgery 1978; **Medical School:** UCLA 1968; **Residencies:** Surgery, UCLA Med Ctr, Los Angeles, CA 1969-1974; Plastic Surgery, NYU Med Ctr, New York, NY 1975-1977; **Faculty Appointment:** Prof Plastic Surgery, UCLA

Sheen, Jack MD (Plastic Surgery) - *Special Expertise:* Rhinoplasty; **Admitting Hospital:** St Francis Medical Center of Santa Barbara; **Office Address:** 216 W Pueblo St., Ste A Santa Barbara, CA 93105-3855; **Office Phone:** (805) 898-8888; **Board Certification:** Plastic Surgery 1968; **Medical School:** Stanford Univ 1955; **Residencies:** Surgery, Newton Wellesly Hosp, Newton Lwr Fls 1960-1962; Plastic Surgery, Cook Co Hosp, Chicago, IL 1962-1964; **Faculty Appointment:** Clin Prof Plastic Surgery, UCLA

Sherman, Randolph MD (Plastic Surgery) - *Special Expertise:* Breast Reconstruction; Limb Surgery/Reconstruction; **Admitting Hospital:** USC University Hospital - Richard K. Eamer Medical Plaza; **Office Address:** Univ for Plastic Surgeons 1450 San Pablo St Ste 2000 Los Angeles, CA 90033-4680; **Office Phone:** (323) 442-6482; **Board Certifications:** Plastic Surgery 1986, Hand Surgery 1989; **Medical School:** Univ MO-Kansas City 1977; **Residencies:** Surgery, NY Upstate Med Ctr, Syracuse, NY 1981-1983; Surgery, State Univ of New York, Syracuse, NY 1981-1983; **Fellowship:** Plastic Surgery, USC Med Ctr, Los Angeles, CA 1983-1985; **Faculty Appointment:** Prof Surgery, USC Sch Med

Singer, Robert MD (Plastic Surgery) - *Special Expertise:* Reconstructive Surgery; **Admitting Hospital:** Scripps Hospital - La Jolla; **Office Address:** Scripps Meml Hosp-La Jolla 9834 Genesee Ave #100 La Jolla, CA 92037-1214; **Office Phone:** (858) 455-0290; **Board Certification:** Plastic Surgery 1977; **Medical School:** SUNY Buffalo 1967; **Residencies:** Surgery, Stanford Med Ctr, Palo Alto, CA 1968-1969; Physical Medicine & Rehabilitation, Vanderbilt Univ Hosp, Nashville, TN 1974-1976; **Fellowship:** Neurological Surgery, Rigs Hosp-Kommunes Hosp, Copenhagen, Denmark; **Faculty Appointment:** Asst Clin Prof Plastic Surgery, UCSD

Stevenson, Thomas Ray MD (Plastic Surgery) - *Special Expertise:* Reconstructive Surgery; Cosmetic Surgery; **Admitting Hospital:** University of California - Davis Medical Center; **Office Address:** Univ Surg Assocs 2825 J St, Ste 400 Sacramento, CA 95816; **Office Phone:** (916) 734-0779; **Board Certifications:** Plastic Surgery 1983, Hand Surgery 1994; **Medical School:** Univ Kans 1972; **Residencies:** Surgery, Univ VA Hosp, Charlottesville, VA 1973-1978; Plastic Surgery, Emory Univ Hosp, Atlanta, GA 1980-1982; **Faculty Appointment:** Prof Plastic Surgery, UC Davis

Wells, James H MD (Plastic Surgery) - *Special Expertise:* Cleft Palate/Lip; Breast Surgery; **Admitting Hospital:** Long Beach Memorial Medical Center; **Office Address:** 2880 Atlantic Ave, Ste 290 Long Beach, CA 90806-1716; **Office Phone:** (562) 595-6543; **Board Certification:** Plastic Surgery 1978; **Medical School:** Univ Tex Med Br, Galveston 1966; **Residencies:** Surgery, Ochsner Fdn Hosp, New Orleans, LA 1967-1971; Plastic Surgery, Univ VA Hosp, Charlottesville, VA 1973-1975

Zarem, Harvey Alan MD (Plastic Surgery) - *Special Expertise:* Breast Surgery; Cosmetic Surgery-Face; **Admitting Hospital:** St John's Health Center; **Office Address:** Pacific Surgicenter Inc 1301 20th St, Ste 470 Santa Monica, CA 90404-2054; **Office Phone:** (310) 315-0222; **Board Certifications:** Plastic Surgery 1978, Surgery 1964; **Medical School:** Columbia P&S 1957; **Residencies:** Surgery, Peter Bent Brigham Hosp, Boston, MA 1958-1961; Plastic Surgery, Johns Hopkins Hosp, Boston, MA 1964-1966; **Fellowship:** Pathology, NYU Med Ctr, New York, NY 1963-1964; **Faculty Appointment:** Prof Emeritus Plastic Surgery, UCLA

PSYCHIATRY

A psychiatrist specializes in the prevention, diagnosis and treatment of mental, addictive and emotional disorders such as schizophrenia and other psychotic disorders, mood disorders, anxiety disorders, substance-related disorders, sexual and gender identity disorders and adjustment disorders. The psychiatrist is able to understand the biologic, psychologic and social components of illness, and therefore is uniquely prepared to treat the whole person. A psychiatrist is qualified to order diagnostic laboratory tests and to prescribe medications, evaluate and treat psychologic and interpersonal problems and to intervene with families who are coping with stress, crises and other problems in living.

Training required: Four years

Certification in one of the following subspecialties requires additional training and examination.

Addiction Psychiatry: A psychiatrist who focuses on the evaluation and treatment of individuals with alcohol, drug, or other substance-related disorders and of individuals with the dual diagnosis of substance-related and other psychiatric disorders.

Child and Adolescent Psychiatry: A psychiatrist with additional training in the diagnosis and treatment of developmental, behavioral, emotional and mental disorders of childhood and adolescence.

Geriatric Psychiatry: A psychiatrist with expertise in the prevention, evaluation, diagnosis and treatment of mental and emotional disorders in the elderly. The geriatric psychiatrist seeks to improve the psychiatric care of the elderly both in health and in disease.

FOUR WINDS HOSPITAL

800 Cross River Road   Katonah, New York 10536
Tel. 914-763-8151   Fax. 914-763-9598   www.fourwindshospital.com

LEADING MENTAL HEALTH TREATMENT PROVIDER

Four Winds Hospital, located in Westchester (914-763-8151), is the leading provider of child and adolescent mental health treatment services in the Northeast. In addition to providing a comprehensive range of inpatient and outpatient services for children and adolescents, the Four Winds Adult Program includes an intensive psychiatric service, a dual diagnosis service and an outpatient Partial Hospitalization Program. Triage (evaluation and referral) Services are provided 24 hours a day, 7 days a week. Child and Adolescent Partial Hospitalization Programs are also provided. Four Winds operates two other sites in Saratoga Springs, NY (518-584-3600) and Syracuse, NY (315-476-2161).

ADMISSION AND REFERRAL INFORMATION

Four Winds Hospital accepts patients 24 hours a day, 7 days a week with 24 hour triage services. It is Four Winds' philosophy that quality treatment, delivered at the appropriate level of care, is not only clinically effective, but cost effective as well. Our goal is to ensure that every individual receives the exact services that they require during the course of their treatment.

PROFESSIONAL CONTINUING EDUCATION SERIES

In the Spring and Fall of each year, Four Winds provides community and professional education lectures and clinical grand rounds to the community-at-large. To be placed on the mailing list, or to receive a free listing of the current grand rounds calendar of events, call 1-914-763-8151, ext. 2413.

CLINICAL OUTCOME STUDIES

Four Winds Hospital, for over 10 years, has continuously evaluated the effectiveness of our treatment. We have studied how well our treatment works and have used this research to make clinical improvements to our programs. This clinical outcome research, conducted by clinical psychologists, the patient, the therapist and the Four Winds research staff is ongoing. We are committed to continue to use research to improve the quality of our treatment. Four Winds begins each study with an extensive assessment of each patient chosen for the study. With a specialized staff collecting data, and with ratings for over 5,000 persons at this time, Four Winds is able to dynamically change treatment services, where necessary, while continuing to provide intensive inpatient and outpatient mental health treatment programs.

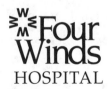

PHYSICIAN LISTINGS

New England

Kosten, Thomas MD (Addiction Psychiatry) - *Special Expertise: Cocaine Addiction; Alcoholism;* **Admitting Hospital:** VA New England Healthcare System; **Office Address:** VA Connecticit Hlth Care System, Bldg 35 950 Campbell Ave, rm 41, MC-Psych 151D West Haven, CT 06516; **Office Phone:** (203) 932-5711; **Board Certifications:** Psychiatry 1984, Addiction Psychiatry 1993; **Medical School:** Cornell Univ-Weil Med Coll 1977; **Residency:** Psychiatry, Yale-New Haven Hosp, New Haven, CT 1978-1981; **Fellowship:** Epidemiology, Yale-New Haven Hosp, New Haven, CT 1981-1983; **Faculty Appointment:** Assoc Prof Medicine, Yale Univ

Schottenfeld, Richard MD (Addiction Psychiatry) - *Special Expertise: Addiction Psychiatry - General;* **Admitting Hospital:** Yale - New Haven Hospital; **Office Address:** 34 Park St, rm SS New Haven, CT 06519-1109; **Office Phone:** (203) 974-7349; **Board Certifications:** Psychiatry 1984, Addiction Psychiatry 1994; **Medical School:** Yale Univ 1976; **Residency:** Psychiatry, Yale Psych Inst, New Haven, CT 1979-1982; **Fellowship:** Epidemiology, Yale, New Haven, CT 1982-1984; **Faculty Appointment:** Assoc Prof Psychiatry, Yale Univ

Mid Atlantic

Galanter, Marc MD (Addiction Psychiatry) - *Special Expertise: Alcoholism; Drug Abuse;* **Admitting Hospital:** NYU Medical Center (Page 70); **Office Address:** 285 Central Park West New York, NY 10024-3006; **Office Phone:** (212) 877-4093; **Board Certifications:** Psychiatry 1974, Addiction Psychiatry 1993; **Medical School:** Albert Einstein Coll Med 1967; **Residencies:** Psychiatry, UCLA Med Ctr, Los Angeles, CA 1967-1968; Psychiatry, Albert Einstein Med Ctr, Bronx, NY 1968-1971; **Faculty Appointment:** Prof Addiction Psychiatry, NYU Sch Med

Gorelick, David Alan MD (Addiction Psychiatry) - *Special Expertise: Addiction;* **Admitting Hospital:** National Institutes of Health - Clinical Center; **Office Address:** Natl Inst on Drug Abuse 5500 Nathan Shock Dr Baltimore, MD 21224; **Office Phone:** (410) 550-1478; **Board Certifications:** Psychiatry 1982, Addiction Psychiatry 1993; **Medical School:** Albert Einstein Coll Med 1976; **Residencies:** Psychiatry, UCLA-Neuropsyh Hosp, Los Angeles, CA 1977-1980; Brentwood VA Med Ctr, Los Angeles, CA 1980-1983; **Faculty Appointment:** Prof Psychiatry, Univ MD Sch Med

Kleber, Herbert MD (Addiction Psychiatry) - *Special Expertise: Addiction Psychiatry - General;* **Admitting Hospital:** Columbia Presbyterian Medical Center (Page 72); **Office Address:** CASA 633 Ave, Fl 19 New York, NY 10019; **Office Phone:** (212) 841-5220; **Board Certifications:** Psychiatry, Addiction Psychiatry; **Medical School:** Jefferson Med Coll 1960; **Residency:** Psychiatry, Yale-New Haven, New Haven, CT 1961-1964

Midwest

Compton III, Wilson M MD (Addiction Psychiatry) - *Special Expertise: Addiction Psychiatry - General;* **Admitting Hospital:** Barnes - Jewish Hospital; **Office Address:** Washington Univ Sch Med 40 N Kings Hwy, Ste 4 St Louis, MO 63108; **Office Phone:** (314) 286-2261; **Board Certifications:** Psychiatry 1992, Addiction Psychiatry 1993; **Medical School:** Washington Univ, St Louis 1986; **Residency:** Psychiatry, Barnes Hosp, St Louis, MO 1986-1990; **Faculty Appointment:** Assoc Prof Psychiatry, Washington Univ, St Louis

Miller, Sheldon I MD (Addiction Psychiatry) - *Special Expertise: Addiction Psychiatry - General;* **Admitting Hospital:** Northwestern Memorial Hospital; **Office Address:** Northwest Univ Med, Passavant 561 303 E Superior St Chicago, IL 60611-3015; **Office Phone:** (312) 908-2323; **Board Certifications:** Psychiatry 1972, Addiction Psychiatry 1993; **Medical School:** Tufts Univ 1964; **Residency:** Psychiatry, Univ Hosp Cleveland, Cleveland, OH 1965-1968; **Faculty Appointment:** Prof Psychiatry, Northwestern Univ

Great Plains and Mountains

Crowley, Thomas J. MD (Addiction Psychiatry) - *Special Expertise:* *Inhalant Addiction;* **Admitting Hospital:** University of Colorado Health & Science Center; **Office Address:** 4200 E 9th Ave Box C268-35 Denver, CO 80220-3706; **Office Phone:** (303) 315-7573; **Board Certification:** Psychiatry 1971; **Medical School:** Univ Minn 1962; **Residency:** Psychiatry, Univ Minn, Minneapolis, MN 1963-1966; **Faculty Appointment:** Prof Psychiatry, Univ Conn

West Coast and Pacific

Schuckit, Marc A MD (Addiction Psychiatry) - *Special Expertise:* *Alcoholism;* *Psychopharmacology;* **Admitting Hospital:** VA Medical Affairs - San Diego HealthCare Center; **Office Address:** VA San Diego Healthcare System, Dept Psyc (116A) 3350 La Jolla Village Dr San Diego, CA 92161; **Office Phone:** (858) 552-8585; **Board Certification:** Psychiatry 1974; **Medical School:** Washington Univ, St Louis 1968; **Residencies:** Psychiatry, Washington Univ, St Louis, MO 1969-1971; Psychiatry, UC San Diego, San Diego, CA 1971-1972; **Faculty Appointment:** Prof Psychiatry, UCSD

Weinstock, Robert MD (Addiction Psychiatry) - *Special Expertise:* *Addiction Psychiatry - General;* **Admitting Hospital:** Cedars-Sinai Medical Center; **Office Address:** 1100 Glendon Ave, Ste 2005 Los Angeles, CA 90024-3524; **Office Phone:** (310) 208-7200; **Board Certifications:** Geriatric Psychiatry 1995, Addiction Psychiatry 1996; **Medical School:** NYU Sch Med 1966; **Residencies:** Psychiatry, McLean Hosp, Belmont, MA 1967-1970; Child & Adolescent Psychiatry, McLean Hosp, Belmont, MA 1970-1972; **Fellowship:** Psychiatric Research, Boston Univ, Boston, MA 1972-1974; **Faculty Appointment:** Clin Prof Psychiatry, UCLA

CHILD & ADOLESCENT PSYCHIATRY
New England

Biederman, Joseph MD (Child & Adolescent Psychiatry) - *Special Expertise:* ADD/ADHD; *Anxiety & Mood Disorders;* **Admitting Hospital:** Massachusetts General Hospital; **Office Address:** 15 Parkman St, WACC 725 Boston, MA 02114; **Office Phone:** (617) 726-1743; **Board Certifications:** Psychiatry 1983, Child & Adolescent Psychiatry 1984; **Medical School:** Brazil 1971; **Residencies:** Psychiatry, Hadassah Univ Hosp, Jerusalem, Israel 1972-1977; Child & Adolescent Psychiatry, Harvard Chldns Hosp, Boston, MA 1977-1979; **Faculty Appointment:** Clin Prof Child & Adolescent Psychiatry, Harvard Med Sch

Cohen, Donald MD (Child & Adolescent Psychiatry) - *Special Expertise:* Autism; Tourette's Syndrome; **Admitting Hospital:** Yale - New Haven Hospital; **Office Address:** Yale Child Study Ctr 230 S Frontage Rd New Haven, CT 06520-7900; **Office Phone:** (203) 785-5759; **Board Certifications:** Psychiatry 1972, Child & Adolescent Psychiatry 1976; **Medical School:** Yale Univ 1966; **Residencies:** Psychiatry, Mass Mental Health Ctr, Boston, MA 1967-1969; Child & Adolescent Psychiatry, Children's Hosp, Boston, MA 1969-1970; **Fellowship:** Psychiatry, Harvard, Boston, MA 1969-1970; **Faculty Appointment:** Prof Pediatrics, Yale Univ

Coyle, Joseph MD (Child & Adolescent Psychiatry) - *Special Expertise:* Mental Retardation; **Admitting Hospital:** McLean Hospital; **Office Address:** McLean Hosp 15 Mill St Belmont, MA 02478-1048; **Office Phone:** (617) 855-2101; **Board Certification:** Psychiatry 1980; **Medical School:** Johns Hopkins Univ 1969; **Residency:** Psychiatry, Johns Hopkins Hosp, Baltimore, MD 1973-1976; **Fellowship:** Psychiatry, NIMH, Bethesda, MD 1970-1973; **Faculty Appointment:** Prof Psychiatry, Harvard Med Sch

Herzog, David B MD (Child & Adolescent Psychiatry) - *Special Expertise:* Eating Disorders; **Admitting Hospital:** Massachusetts General Hospital; **Office Address:** Mass Genl Hosp-ACC 725 15 Parkman St Boston, MA 02114; **Office Phone:** (617) 724-0799; **Board Certifications:** Pediatrics 1980, Child & Adolescent Psychiatry 1986; **Medical School:** Mexico 1973; **Residencies:** Pediatrics, Univ Wisc, Madison, WI 1974-1975; Pediatrics, Boston City Hosp, Boston, MA 1975-1976; **Fellowships:** Child & Adolescent Psychiatry, Chldns Hosp, Boston, MA 1976-1978; Psychiatry, Mass Genl Hosp, Boston, MA 1978-1980; **Faculty Appointment:** Prof Child & Adolescent Psychiatry, Harvard Med Sch

King, Bryan Harry MD (Child & Adolescent Psychiatry) - *Special Expertise:* Mental Retardation; **Admitting Hospital:** Dartmouth - Hitchcock Medical Center; **Office Address:** Dartmouth Hitchcock Psychiatry Association One Medical Center Lebanon, NH 03756; **Office Phone:** (603) 650-7520; **Board Certifications:** Psychiatry 1991, Child & Adolescent Psychiatry 1992; **Medical School:** Med Coll Wisc 1983; **Residency:** Psychiatry, UCLA Neuro Inst, Los Angeles, CA 1984-1987; **Fellowship:** Child & Adolescent Psychiatry, UCLA Neuropsyc Inst, Los Angeles, CA 1987-1990

Leonard, Henrietta MD (Child & Adolescent Psychiatry) - *Special Expertise:* Neuro-Psychiatry; Movement Disorders; **Admitting Hospital:** Rhode Island Hospital; **Office Address:** Rhode Island Hosp, Dept Child Psyc 593 Eddy St Providence, RI 02903; **Office Phone:** (401) 444-3762; **Board Certifications:** Psychiatry 1987, Child & Adolescent Psychiatry 1988; **Medical School:** Geo Wash Univ 1982; **Residency:** Psychiatry, Geo Wash Med Ctr, Washington, DC 1982-1985; **Fellowship:** Child & Adolescent Psychiatry, Chldns Hosp, Washington, DC 1985-1987; **Faculty Appointment:** Prof Psychiatry, Brown Univ

Nickman, Steven L. MD (Child & Adolescent Psychiatry) - *Special Expertise: Adoption;* **Admitting Hospital:** Massachusetts General Hospital; **Office Address:** Mass Genl Hosp 15 Parkman St, WACC 725 Boston, MA 02114; **Office Phone:** (617) 726-2724; **Board Certifications:** Pediatrics 1971, Psychiatry 1977; **Medical School:** Duke Univ 1964; **Residencies:** Pediatrics, Montefiore Hosp, New York, NY 1965-1966; Psychiatry, Mass Genl Hosp, Boston, MA 1969-1971; **Fellowship:** Child & Adolescent Psychiatry, Mass Genl Hosp, Boston, MA 1969-1973; **Faculty Appointment:** Asst Clin Prof Psychiatry, Harvard Med Sch

Spencer, Thomas MD (Child & Adolescent Psychiatry) - *Special Expertise: ADD/ADHD;* **Admitting Hospital:** Massachusetts General Hospital; **Office Address:** Mass Genl Hosp 15 Parkman St, WACC 725 Boston, MA 02114; **Office Phone:** (617) 726-1731; **Board Certifications:** Psychiatry 1984, Child & Adolescent Psychiatry 1993; **Medical School:** Univ Wisc 1978; **Residencies:** Psychiatry, New Eng Med Ctr, Boston, MA; Child & Adolescent Psychiatry, Mass Genl Hosp, Boston, MA; **Faculty Appointment:** Assoc Prof Psychiatry, Harvard Med Sch

Volkmar, Fred R MD (Child & Adolescent Psychiatry) - *Special Expertise: Autism; Asperger's Syndrome;* **Admitting Hospital:** Yale - New Haven Hospital; **Office Address:** Yale Child Study Ctr 230 Frontage Rd S, Box 207900 New Haven, CT 06520; **Office Phone:** (203) 785-2510; **Board Certifications:** Psychiatry 1981, Child & Adolescent Psychiatry 1988; **Medical School:** Stanford Univ 1976; **Residencies:** Psychiatry, Stanford Univ, Stanford, CA 1978-1980; Child & Adolescent Psychiatry, Yale Univ Child Study Ctr, New Haven, CT 1980-1982; **Faculty Appointment:** Prof Child & Adolescent Psychiatry, Yale Univ

Wilens, Timothy MD (Child & Adolescent Psychiatry) - *Special Expertise: ADD/ADHD;* **Admitting Hospital:** Massachusetts General Hospital; **Office Address:** Mass Genl Hosp 15 Parkman St, WACC 725 Boston, MA 02114; **Office Phone:** (617) 726-1731; **Board Certifications:** Psychiatry 1990, Child & Adolescent Psychiatry 1991; **Medical School:** Univ Mich Med Sch 1985; **Residencies:** Internal Medicine, Henry Ford Hosp, Detroit, MI 1985-1986; Psychiatry, Mass Genl Hosp, Boston, MA 1986-1988; **Fellowship:** Child & Adolescent Psychiatry, Mass Genl Hosp, Boston, MA 1988-1990; **Faculty Appointment:** Assoc Prof Psychiatry, Harvard Med Sch

Mid Atlantic

Abright, Arthur Reese MD (Child & Adolescent Psychiatry) - *Special Expertise: Depression and Bipolar Disorder; Attention Deficit Hyperactivity Disorder;* **Admitting Hospital:** St Vincents Catholic Medical Center of New York; **Office Address:** 203 W 12th St New York, NY 10011; **Office Phone:** (212) 604-8213; **Board Certifications:** Psychiatry 1978, Child & Adolescent Psychiatry 1981; **Medical School:** Univ Tex SW, Dallas 1973; **Residencies:** Psychiatry, St Vincent's Hosp, New York, NY 1973-1974; Psychiatry, NY Hosp-Cornell Med Ctr, New York, NY 1974-1977; **Fellowship:** Child & Adolescent Psychiatry, NY Hosp-Cornell Med Ctr, New York, NY 1977-1979; **Faculty Appointment:** Assoc Prof Psychiatry, NY Med Coll

Bird, Hector MD (Child & Adolescent Psychiatry) - *Special Expertise: Child & Adolescent Psychiatry - General;* **Admitting Hospital:** Columbia Presbyterian Medical Center (Page 72); **Office Address:** 145 Central Park West, Ste 1C New York, NY 10023; **Office Phone:** (212) 874-5311; **Board Certifications:** Psychiatry 1975, Child & Adolescent Psychiatry 1977; **Medical School:** Yale Univ 1965; **Residencies:** Psychiatry, Columbia-Presbyterian, New York, NY 1968-1971; Child & Adolescent Psychiatry, Columbia-Presbyterian, New York, NY 1970-1972; **Fellowship:** Psychiatry, WA White Institute, New York, NY 1972-1977; **Faculty Appointment:** Prof Psychiatry, Columbia P&S

Bogrov, Michael MD (Child & Adolescent Psychiatry) - *Special Expertise: ADD/ADHD; Mood Disorders;* **Admitting Hospital:** Sheppard Pratt Healthsystem; **Office Address:** 6501 N Charles St Baltimore, MD 21204-6819; **Office Phone:** (410) 938-4913; **Board Certifications:** Psychiatry 1993, Child & Adolescent Psychiatry 1994; **Medical School:** Emory Univ 1987; **Residencies:** Psychiatry, Univ of Maryland, Baltimore, MD 1987-1990; Child & Adolescent Psychiatry, Johns Hopkins Hosp, Baltimore, MD 1990-1992; **Faculty Appointment:** Asst Prof Psychiatry, Johns Hopkins Univ

Egan, James Harold MD (Child & Adolescent Psychiatry) - *Special Expertise: Psychopharmocology; Psychotherapy;* **Admitting Hospital:** Children's National Medical Center - DC; **Office Address:** 5480 Wisconsin Ave Chevy Chase, MD 20815; **Office Phone:** (301) 913-5953; **Board Certifications:** Psychiatry 1973, Child & Adolescent Psychiatry 1975; **Medical School:** Columbia P&S 1964; **Residencies:** Psychiatry, St Vincents Hosp, New York, NY 1967-1969; Child & Adolescent Psychiatry, St Lukes Hosp, New York, NY 1969-1971; **Faculty Appointment:** Clin Prof Pediatrics, Geo Wash Univ

Foley, Carmel MD (Child & Adolescent Psychiatry) - *Special Expertise: Mood Disorders;* **Admitting Hospital:** Schneider Children's Hospital; **Office Address:** Schneider Chldns Hosp, Div Child & Adolescent Psych 269-01 76th Ave New Hyde Park, NY 11040; **Office Phone:** (718) 470-3510; **Board Certifications:** Psychiatry 1979, Child & Adolescent Psychiatry 1981; **Medical School:** Ireland 1972; **Residencies:** Psychiatry, St Patrick's Hosp, Dublin, Ireland 1975-1976; Psychiatry, Lafayette Clinic, Detroit, MI 1976-1978; **Fellowship:** Child & Adolescent Psychiatry, Lafayette Clinic, Detroit, MI 1977-1979

Fornari, Victor MD (Child & Adolescent Psychiatry) - *Special Expertise: Eating Disorders;* **Admitting Hospital:** North Shore University Hospital at Manhasset; **Office Address:** 400 Community Drive, Manhasset, NY 11030; **Office Phone:** (516) 562-3051; **Board Certifications:** Psychiatry 1984, Child & Adolescent Psychiatry 1985; **Medical School:** SUNY Downstate 1979; **Residency:** Psychiatry, Hosp Univ PA, Philadelphia, PA 1980-1982; **Fellowship:** Child & Adolescent Psychiatry, LI Jewish Hosp, New Hyde Park, NY 1982-1984; **Faculty Appointment:** Assoc Prof Psychiatry, NYU Sch Med

Greenspan, Stanley MD (Child & Adolescent Psychiatry) - *Special Expertise: Autism; Infant/Toddler Psychiatry;* **Admitting Hospital:** George Washington University Hospital; **Office Address:** 7201 Glenbrook Rd Bethesda, MD 20814-1242; **Office Phone:** (301) 657-2348; **Board Certification:** Psychiatry 1972; **Medical School:** Yale Univ 1966; **Residency:** Psychiatry, Columbia-Presby Psych Inst, New York, NY 1967-1969; **Fellowship:** Child & Adolescent Psychiatry, Childrens Hosp-NMC, Washington, DC 1969-1971; **Faculty Appointment:** Clin Prof Psychiatry, Geo Wash Univ

Hertzig, Margaret MD (Child & Adolescent Psychiatry) - *Special Expertise: Developmental Disorders; ADD/ADHD;* **Admitting Hospital:** New York Weill Cornell Medical Center - NY Presbyterian Hospital (Page 72); **Office Address:** 525 E 68th St, Box 140 New York, NY 10021; **Office Phone:** (212) 746-5712; **Board Certifications:** Psychiatry 1968, Child & Adolescent Psychiatry 1975; **Medical School:** NYU Sch Med 1960; **Residencies:** Pediatrics, Jewish Hosp, Brooklyn, NY 1961-1962; Psychiatry, Bellevue Psych Hosp, New York, NY 1962-1964; **Fellowship:** Psychiatric Research, NYU Sch Med, New York, NY 1964-1966; **Faculty Appointment:** Prof Psychiatry, Cornell Univ-Weil Med Coll

Kestenbaum, Clarice J MD (Child & Adolescent Psychiatry) - *Special Expertise:* Anxiety *Disorders;* **Admitting Hospital:** New York Weill Cornell Medical Center - NY Presbyterian Hospital (Page 72); **Office Address:** MD 1051 Riverside Dr, Box 74 New York, NY 10032; **Office Phone:** (212) 543-5333; **Board Certifications:** Psychiatry 1971, Child & Adolescent Psychiatry 1975; **Medical School:** USC Sch Med 1960; **Residencies:** Psychiatry, Columbia Presby Med Ctr, New York, NY 1961-1963; Child & Adolescent Psychiatry, Columbia Presby Med Ctr, New York, NY 1963-1965; **Faculty Appointment:** Clin Prof Psychiatry, Columbia P&S

Koplewicz, Harold MD (Child & Adolescent Psychiatry) - *Special Expertise:* Anxiety *Disorders;* **Admitting Hospital:** NYU Medical Center (Page 70); **Office Address:** 550 1st Ave New York, NY 10021; **Office Phone:** (212) 879-4878; **Board Certifications:** Psychiatry 1983, Child & Adolescent Psychiatry 1984; **Medical School:** Albert Einstein Coll Med 1978; **Residencies:** Psychiatry, NY Hosp, White Plains, NY 1979-1981; Child & Adolescent Psychiatry, NYS Psyc Inst, New York, NY 1981-1983; **Fellowship:** Psychiatric Research, NYS Psyc Inst, NY 1983-1985; **Faculty Appointment:** Prof Psychiatry, NYU Sch Med

Pruitt, David B. MD (Child & Adolescent Psychiatry) - *Special Expertise:* Child & *Adolescent Psychiatry - General;* **Admitting Hospital:** University of Maryland Medical System; **Office Address:** U Maryland Sch Med, Div Child & Adol Psyc 701 W Pratt St, Fl 4th Baltimore, MD 21201; **Office Phone:** (410) 328-3522; **Board Certifications:** Psychiatry 1979, Child & Adolescent Psychiatry 1981; **Medical School:** Univ Tex, Houston 1974; **Residencies:** Psychiatry, Univ Penn, Philadelphia, PA 1975-1978; Child & Adolescent Psychiatry, Child Guidance Ctr, Philadelphia, PA 1977-1979; **Faculty Appointment:** Prof Child & Adolescent Psychiatry, Univ MD Sch Med

Rapoport, Judith MD (Child & Adolescent Psychiatry) - *Special Expertise:* Schizophrenia; *Obsessive Compulsive Disorder;* **Admitting Hospital:** National Institutes of Health - Clinical Center; **Office Address:** NIMH, Bldg 10 - rm 3N202 Bethesda, MD 20892-1600; **Office Phone:** (301) 496-6081; **Board Certifications:** Psychiatry 1969, Child & Adolescent Psychiatry 1969; **Medical School:** Harvard Med Sch 1959; **Residencies:** Psychiatry, Mass Mental Hlth Ctr, Boston, MA 1960-1961; Psychiatry, St Elizabeth Hosp, Washington, DC 1961-1962; **Fellowships:** Karolinska Inst, Stockholm, Sweden 1962-1964; Child & Adolescent Psychiatry, Chldns Hosp, Washington, DC 1964-1966

Riddle, Mark A. MD (Child & Adolescent Psychiatry) - *Special Expertise:* *Psychopharmacology;* **Admitting Hospital:** Johns Hopkins Hospital - Baltimore (Page 65); **Office Address:** Johns Hopkins Hosp, CMSC 346 600 N Wolfe St Baltimore, MD 21287-3325; **Office Phone:** (410) 955-2320; **Board Certifications:** Psychiatry 1982, Child & Adolescent Psychiatry 1986; **Medical School:** Indiana Univ 1977; **Residency:** Psychiatry, Yale-Schl Med, New Haven, CT 1978-1981; **Fellowship:** Child & Adolescent Psychiatry, Yale Child Study Ctr, New Haven, CT 1981-1983; **Faculty Appointment:** Assoc Prof Child & Adolescent Psychiatry, Johns Hopkins Univ

Ryan, Neal David MD (Child & Adolescent Psychiatry) - *Special Expertise:* Mood *Disorders; Depression;* **Admitting Hospital:** UPMC - Presbyterian University Hospital; **Office Address:** Western Psyc Inst & Clin 3811 O'Hara St Pittsburgh, PA 15213-2593; **Office Phone:** (416) 624-1241; **Board Certifications:** Psychiatry 1983, Child & Adolescent Psychiatry 1987; **Medical School:** Yale Univ 1978; **Residency:** Psychiatry, NY State Psych-Columbia Univ, New York, NY 1979-1982; **Fellowship:** Psychiatric Research, Columbia Univ, New York, NY 1981-1984; **Faculty Appointment:** Prof Psychiatry, Univ Pittsburgh

Walkup, John MD (Child & Adolescent Psychiatry) - *Special Expertise: Child & Adolescent Psychiatry - General;* **Admitting Hospital:** Johns Hopkins Hospital - Baltimore (Page 65); **Office Address:** Johns Hopkins Hosp, Dept Child Psyc 600 N Wolfe St, Bldg CMSC - rm 338 Baltimore, MD 21287; **Office Phone:** (410) 955-1925; **Board Certifications:** Psychiatry 1987, Child & Adolescent Psychiatry 1992; **Medical School:** Univ Minn 1982; **Residencies:** Psychiatry, Yale Univ Med Sch, New Haven, CT 1983-1985; Child & Adolescent Psychiatry, Yale Chld Study Ctr, New HAven, CT 1985-1988; **Faculty Appointment:** Asst Prof Psychiatry, Johns Hopkins Univ

Wiener, Jerry M MD (Child & Adolescent Psychiatry) - *Special Expertise: Psychiatry-Adolescent/College Age; Anxiety/Mood Disorders .;* **Admitting Hospital:** George Washington University Hospital; **Office Address:** George Washington Univ 2150 Pennsylvania Ave NW Washington, DC 20037-2396; **Office Phone:** (202) 994-8308; **Board Certifications:** Psychiatry 1963, Child & Adolescent Psychiatry 1965; **Medical School:** Baylor Coll Med 1956; **Residencies:** Psychiatry, Mayo Clinic 1957-1961; Child & Adolescent Psychiatry, Mayo Clinic 1960-1961; **Fellowship:** Child & Adolescent Psychiatry, Columbia-Presby Med Ctr 1961-1962; **Faculty Appointment:** Prof Emeritus Psychiatry, Geo Wash Univ

Southeast

Heston, Jerry D MD (Child & Adolescent Psychiatry) - *Special Expertise: Child & Adolescent Psychiatry - General;* **Admitting Hospital:** Le Bonheur Children's Medical Center; **Office Address:** Univ Tenn Hlth Sci Ctr, Dept Psyc 711 Jefferson Ave, Ste 137 Memphis, TN 38105; **Office Phone:** (901) 448-5944; **Board Certifications:** Psychiatry 1988, Pediatrics 1997; **Medical School:** Univ S Fla Coll Med 1981; **Residencies:** Pediatrics, LeBonheur Chldns Hosp, Memphis, TN 1982-1984; Psychiatry, Univ Tennessee, Memphis, TN 1984-1986; **Fellowship:** Child & Adolescent Psychiatry, Univ Tennessee, Memphis, TN 1986-1988; **Faculty Appointment:** Asst Prof Child & Adolescent Psychiatry, Univ Tenn Coll Med, Memphis

March, John MD (Child & Adolescent Psychiatry) - *Special Expertise: Anxiety Disorders; Obsessive-Compulsive Disorder;* **Admitting Hospital:** Duke University Medical Center (Page 60); **Office Address:** 2213 Elba St Durham, NC 27705; **Office Phone:** (919) 684-4950; **Board Certifications:** Psychiatry 1992, Child & Adolescent Psychiatry 1992; **Medical School:** UCLA 1978; **Residencies:** Family Practice, Santa Monica Hosp Med Ctr, Santa Monica, CA 1978-1981; Psychiatry, Univ of Wisconsin Hosp, Milwaukee, WI 1986-1988; **Fellowship:** Child & Adolescent Psychiatry, Univ of Wisconsin Hosp, Milwaukee, WI 1988-1990; **Faculty Appointment:** Prof Psychiatry, Duke Univ

Sexson, Sandra G B MD (Child & Adolescent Psychiatry) - *Special Expertise: Transplant Patients; Death & Dying;* **Admitting Hospital:** Emory University Hospital; **Office Address:** Emory West, Div Child & Adol Psyc 1256 Briarcliff Rd, Fl 313 S Atlanta, GA 30306; **Office Phone:** (404) 727-3963; **Board Certifications:** Psychiatry 1980, Child & Adolescent Psychiatry 1981; **Medical School:** Univ Miss 1971; **Residencies:** Psychiatry, Tex Hlth Sci Ctr, San Antonio, TX 1972-1974; Child & Adolescent Psychiatry, Washington Univ, St Louis, MO 1976-1978; **Fellowship:** Child & Adolescent Psychiatry, Washington Univ, St Louis, MO 1976-1978; **Faculty Appointment:** Assoc Prof Psychiatry, Emory Univ

Tanguay, Peter MD (Child & Adolescent Psychiatry) - *Special Expertise: Autism; Developmental Disorders;* **Admitting Hospital:** Kosair Children's Hospital; **Office Address:** Bingham Child Guidance Clinic 200 E Chestnut St Louisville, KY 40202; **Office Phone:** (502) 852-1045; **Board Certifications:** Psychiatry 1972, Child & Adolescent Psychiatry 1974; **Medical School:** Univ Ottawa 1960; **Residency:** Psychiatry, UCLA Med Ctr, Los Angeles, CA 1961-1964; **Fellowship:** Child & Adolescent Psychiatry, UCLA Med Ctr, Los Angeles, CA 1968-1970

CHILD & ADOLESCENT PSYCHIATRY   *Southeast*

Wright, Harry MD (Child & Adolescent Psychiatry) - *Special Expertise: Infant/Toddler Psychiatry; Autism & Developmental Disorders;* **Admitting Hospital:** William S Hall Psychiatric Institute; **Office Address:** 3555 Harden St Columbia, SC 29203; **Office Phone:** (803) 434-4250; **Board Certifications:** Psychiatry 1982, Child & Adolescent Psychiatry 1984; **Medical School:** Univ Penn 1976; **Residency:** Psychiatry, William S Hall Psyc Inst, Columbia, SC 1978-1979; **Fellowship:** Child & Adolescent Psychiatry, William S Hall Psyc Inst, Columbia, SC 1979-1981; **Faculty Appointment:** Prof Psychiatry, Univ SC Sch Med

Midwest

Alessi, Norman E MD (Child & Adolescent Psychiatry) - *Special Expertise: Mood Disorders; Aggressive Disorders;* **Admitting Hospital:** University of Michigan Health Center; **Office Address:** UMMC-Taubman Health Care Ctr, Dept Psyc 1500 E Medical Ctr Dr Ann Arbor, MI 48109-0390; **Office Phone:** (734) 763-2015; **Board Certifications:** Psychiatry 1982, Child & Adolescent Psychiatry 1985; **Medical School:** Emory Univ 1976; **Residencies:** Child & Adolescent Psychiatry, Univ Mich Med Ctr, Ann Arbor, MI 1980-1981; Psychiatry, Univ Mich Med Ctr, Ann Arbor, MI 1977-1980; **Fellowship:** Child & Adolescent Psychiatry, Univ Mich Med Ctr, Ann Arbor, MI 1981-1983; **Faculty Appointment:** Assoc Prof Psychiatry, Univ Mich Med Sch

Dulcan, Mina Karen MD (Child & Adolescent Psychiatry) - *Special Expertise: ADD/ADHD;* **Admitting Hospital:** Children's Memorial Hospital; **Office Address:** Chlns Meml Hosp-Dept Psyc 10 2300 Children Plaza, Box 10 Chicago, IL 60614; **Office Phone:** (773) 880-4811; **Board Certifications:** Psychiatry 1978, Child & Adolescent Psychiatry 1979; **Medical School:** Penn State Univ-Hershey Med Ctr 1974; **Residencies:** Child & Adolescent Psychiatry, Univ Pittsburgh, Pittsburgh, PA 1974-1978; Psychiatry, Univ Pittsburgh, Pittsburgh, PA 1974-1977; **Faculty Appointment:** Prof Psychiatry, Northwestern Univ

Luby, Joan Lida MD (Child & Adolescent Psychiatry) - *Special Expertise: Developmental Disorders;* **Admitting Hospital:** Barnes - Jewish Hospital; **Office Address:** Child & Adolescent Psychiatry Offices, Montclair Bldg 24 S Kingshighway St Louis, MO 63108; **Office Phone:** (314) 286-2730; **Board Certifications:** Psychiatry 1993, Child & Adolescent Psychiatry 1993; **Medical School:** Wayne State Univ 1985; **Residency:** Psychiatry, Stanford Univ Sch Med, Palo Alto, CA 1986-1988; **Fellowship:** Child & Adolescent Psychiatry, Stanford Univ Sch Med, Palo Alto, CA 1988-1990; **Faculty Appointment:** Asst Prof Psychiatry, Washington Univ, St Louis

Slomowitz, Marcia MD (Child & Adolescent Psychiatry) - *Special Expertise: Child & Adolescent Psychiatry - General;* **Admitting Hospital:** Northwestern Memorial Hospital; **Office Address:** 676 N St Clair, Ste 1760 Chicago, IL 60611; **Office Phone:** (312) 266-0757; **Board Certifications:** Psychiatry 1982, Child & Adolescent Psychiatry 1983; **Medical School:** Univ Wisc 1977; **Residency:** Psychiatry, Univ Cincinnati, Cincinnati, OH 1978-1980; **Fellowship:** Child & Adolescent Psychiatry, Univ Cincinnati, Cincinnati, OH 1980-1982; **Faculty Appointment:** Asst Prof Psychiatry, Northwestern Univ

Todd, Richard D MD/PhD (Child & Adolescent Psychiatry) - *Special Expertise: Autism;* **Admitting Hospital:** St Louis Children's Hospital; **Office Address:** 24 S Kings Hwy St. Louis, MO 36108; **Office Phone:** (314) 286-1740; **Board Certifications:** Psychiatry 1988, Child & Adolescent Psychiatry 1989; **Medical School:** Univ Tex, San Antonio 1981; **Residency:** Psychiatry, Stanford Med Sch, Palo Alto, CA 1982-1984; **Fellowship:** Child Psychiatry, Washington Univ Sch Med, St Louis, MO 1984-1986; **Faculty Appointment:** Prof Psychiatry

668

Great Plains and Mountains

Bleiberg, Efrain MD (Child & Adolescent Psychiatry) - *Special Expertise: Trauma Psychiatry; Personality Disorders;* **Admitting Hospital:** Menninger Clinic; **Office Address:** Menninger Hosp & Clinic 5800 SW 6th St, Box 829 Topeka, KS 66601-0829; **Office Phone:** (785) 350-5876; **Board Certifications:** Psychiatry 1985, Child & Adolescent Psychiatry 1986; **Medical School:** Mexico 1976; **Residency:** Psychiatry, Menninger Fdn, Topeka, KS 1977-1980; **Fellowship:** Child & Adolescent Psychiatry, Menninger Fdn, Topeka, KS 1979-1981; **Faculty Appointment:** Prof Psychiatry, Univ Kans

Sargent III, A John MD (Child & Adolescent Psychiatry) - *Special Expertise: Eating Disorders; Suicide; Family Therapy;* **Admitting Hospital:** Menninger Clinic; **Office Address:** Menninger Clinic Box 829 Topeka, KS 66601; **Office Phone:** (785) 350-5357; **Board Certifications:** Pediatrics 1979, Child & Adolescent Psychiatry 1989; **Medical School:** Univ Rochester 1973; **Residencies:** Pediatrics, Univ Wisconsin Hosp, Madison, WI 1973-1977; Psychiatry, Hosp Univ Penn, Philadelphia, PA 1984-1987; **Fellowships:** Pediatrics, Univ Wisconsin Hosp, Madison, WI 1975-1976; Child & Adolescent Psychiatry, Phila Child Guidance Ctr, Philadelphia, PA 1978-1980; **Faculty Appointment:** Prof Psychiatry, Karl Menninger Sch Psych

Sokol, Mae Sandra MD (Child & Adolescent Psychiatry) - *Special Expertise: Eating Disorders;* **Admitting Hospital:** Menninger Clinic; **Office Address:** Menninger Clinic 5800 SW 6th St, Bldg 12 Topeka, KS 66606; **Office Phone:** (785) 350-5000; **Board Certifications:** Psychiatry 1986, Child & Adolescent Psychiatry 1987; **Medical School:** Belgium 1980; **Residency:** Psychiatry, Bellevue Hosp-NYU, New York, NY 1981-1984; **Fellowship:** Child & Adolescent Psychiatry, Bellevue Hosp-NYU, New York, NY 1984-1986; **Faculty Appointment:** Asst Prof Psychiatry, Karl Menninger Sch Psych

Southwest

Drell, Martin J. MD (Child & Adolescent Psychiatry) - *Special Expertise: Infant/Toddler Psychiatry; Family Therapy;* **Admitting Hospital:** New Orleans Adolescent Hosp; **Office Address:** LSU Med Ctr, Child Psyc, 3rd Fl 1542 Tulane Ave New Orleans, LA 70112-2825; **Office Phone:** (504) 568-6350; **Board Certifications:** Psychiatry 1982, Child & Adolescent Psychiatry 1982; **Medical School:** Univ IL Coll Med 1974; **Residency:** Psychiatry, Cambridge Hospital, Cambridge, MA 1977-1979; **Fellowship:** Child & Adolescent Psychiatry, Boston Childrens Hospital JBGC, Boston, MA 1975-1977; **Faculty Appointment:** Prof Psychiatry, Louisiana State Univ

Zeanah Jr, Charles H MD (Child & Adolescent Psychiatry) - *Special Expertise: Attachment Disorders; Abuse/Neglect; International Adoption;* **Admitting Hospital:** Tulane University Medical Center Hospital & Clinic; **Office Address:** Tulane U Sch Med, Dept Psych & Neurology 1440 Canal St, Tidewater Bldg, TB52 New Orleans, LA 70112-2715; **Office Phone:** (504) 588-5401; **Board Certifications:** Psychiatry 1983, Child & Adolescent Psychiatry 1983; **Medical School:** Tulane Univ 1977; **Residencies:** Psychiatry, Duke Univ, Durham, NC 1978-1980; Child & Adolescent Psychiatry, Stanford Univ, Palo Alto, CA 1980-1982; **Fellowship:** Stanford Univ, Palo Alto, CA 1982-1984; **Faculty Appointment:** Prof Psychiatry, Tulane Univ

West Coast and Pacific

McCracken, James Thomas MD (Child & Adolescent Psychiatry) - *Special Expertise:* *Obsessive Compulsive Disorder; Tourette's Syndrome;* **Admitting Hospital:** UCLA Neuropsychiatric Hospital; **Office Address:** UCLA Neuropsychiatric Hospital 760 Westwood Plaza Los Angeles, CA 90024-1759; **Office Phone:** (310) 825-0470; **Board Certifications:** Psychiatry 1986, Child & Adolescent Psychiatry 1988; **Medical School:** Baylor Coll Med 1980; **Residency:** Psychiatry, Duke Univ Med Ctr, Durham, NC 1980-1984; **Fellowship:** Child & Adolescent Psychiatry, UCLA Neuropsych Inst, Los Angeles, CA 1984; **Faculty Appointment:** Prof Psychiatry, UCLA

Ponton, Lynn Elisabeth MD (Child & Adolescent Psychiatry) - *Special Expertise:* *Adolescent Risk-Taking; Eating Disorders;* **Admitting Hospital:** University of California - San Francisco Medical Center; **Office Address:** 206 Edgewood Ave San Francisco, CA 94117-3715; **Office Phone:** (415) 664-3039; **Board Certifications:** Psychiatry 1985, Child & Adolescent Psychiatry 1985; **Medical School:** Univ Wisc 1978; **Residencies:** Psychiatry, Univ Pennsylvania, Philadelphia, PA 1979-1980; Psychiatry, Univ Calif-San Francisco, San Francisco, CA 1980-1981; **Fellowship:** Child & Adolescent Psychiatry, Univ Calif-San Francisco, San Francisco, CA 1981-1983; **Faculty Appointment:** Prof Child & Adolescent Psychiatry, UCSF

Russak, Sidney MD (Child & Adolescent Psychiatry) - *Special Expertise: Family Therapy;* **Admitting Hospital:** LAC + USC Medical Center; **Office Address:** LAC-USC Med Ctr 1937 Hosp Place Los Angeles, CA 90033; **Office Phone:** (323) 226-5288; **Board Certifications:** Psychiatry 1974, Child & Adolescent Psychiatry 1975; **Medical School:** UC Irvine 1962; **Residencies:** Psychiatry, LAC-USC Med Ctr, Los Angeles, CA 1962-1965; Child & Adolescent Psychiatry, LAC-USC Med Ctr, Los Angeles, CA 1965-1967; **Faculty Appointment:** Asst Prof Psychiatry, USC Sch Med

Russell, Andrew Thomas MD (Child & Adolescent Psychiatry) - *Special Expertise:* *ADD/ADHD; Schizophrenia; Depression;* **Admitting Hospital:** UCLA Neuropsychiatric Hospital; **Office Address:** UCLA NPI 760 Westwood Plaza Los Angeles, CA 90024-8300; **Office Phone:** (310) 825-0389; **Board Certifications:** Psychiatry 1980, Child & Adolescent Psychiatry 1988; **Medical School:** Univ Colo 1970; **Residency:** Psychiatry, UCLA, Los Angeles, CA 1971-1973; **Fellowship:** Child & Adolescent Psychiatry, UCLA, Los Angeles, CA 1973-1977; **Faculty Appointment:** Prof Psychiatry, UCLA

Steiner, Hans MD (Child & Adolescent Psychiatry) - *Special Expertise: Aggressive* *Disorders; Eating Disorders;* **Admitting Hospital:** Stanford Medical Center; **Office Address:** 401 Quarry Rd Stanford U Sch Med, Div Chld Psy & Chld Devlp Stanford, CA 94305; **Office Phone:** (650) 723-5446; **Board Certifications:** Psychiatry 1979, Child & Adolescent Psychiatry 1981; **Medical School:** Austria 1972; **Residency:** Psychiatry, SUNY Syracuse Med Ctr, Syracuse, NY 1973-1976; **Fellowship:** Child & Adolescent Psychiatry, Univ Michigan, Ann Arbor, MI 1976-1978; **Faculty Appointment:** Prof Psychiatry, Stanford Univ

Terr, Lenore Cagen MD (Child & Adolescent Psychiatry) - *Special Expertise: Trauma* *Psychiatry;* **Admitting Hospital:** University of California - San Francisco Medical Center; **Office Address:** 450 Sutter St, Rm 2534 San Francisco, CA 94108; **Office Phone:** (415) 433-7800; **Board Certifications:** Psychiatry 1968, Child & Adolescent Psychiatry 1969; **Medical School:** Univ Mich Med Sch 1961; **Residency:** Psychiatry, Univ Michigan, Ann Arbor, MI 1962-1964; **Fellowship:** Child & Adolescent Psychiatry, Univ Mich, Ann Arbor, MI 1964-1966; **Faculty Appointment:** Clin Prof Psychiatry, UCSF

670

Yates, Alayne MD (Child & Adolescent Psychiatry) - *Special Expertise:* Eating Disorders;
Admitting Hospital: Kapiolani Medical Center for Women & Children; **Office Address:** Kapiolani
Med Ctr 1319 Punahou St, Fl 6th Honolulu, HI 96826-9931; **Office Phone:** (808) 945-1500; **Board
Certifications:** Psychiatry 1975, Child & Adolescent Psychiatry 1976; **Medical School:** Univ IL Coll
Med 1961; **Residencies:** Pediatrics, Michael Reese Hosp, Chicago, IL 1962-1964; Child &
Adolescent Psychiatry, UC Davis Affil Hosp, Sacramento, CA 1972-1973; **Faculty Appointment:**
Prof Psychiatry, Univ Hawaii JA Burns Sch Med

GERIATRIC PSYCHIATRY

Mid Atlantic

Butler, Robert MD (Geriatric Psychiatry) - *Special Expertise:* Geriatric Psychiatry - General; **Admitting Hospital:** Mount Sinai Hospital (Page 70); **Office Address:** International Longevity Center 60 E 86th St New York, NY 10028; **Office Phone:** (212) 517-1315; **Board Certification:** Psychiatry 1961; **Medical School:** Columbia P&S 1953; **Residencies:** Psychiatry, Langley Porter Psyc Inst, San Francisco, CA 1954-1955; Psychiatry, Chesnut Lodge Hosp, Rockville, ME 1958-1959; **Fellowship:** Psychiatry, Nat Inst Mental Hlth, Bethesda, MD 1959-1960; **Faculty Appointment:** Prof Medicine, Mount Sinai Sch Med

Greenwald, Blaine MD (Geriatric Psychiatry) - *Special Expertise:* Depression; Dementia; **Admitting Hospital:** Long Island Jewish Medical Center; **Office Address:** 75-59 263rd St Glen Oaks, NY 11004; **Office Phone:** (718) 470-8159; **Board Certifications:** Psychiatry 1983, Geriatric Psychiatry 1991; **Medical School:** NY Med Coll 1978; **Residency:** Psychiatry, Mount Sinai Hosp, New York, NY 1979-1982; **Fellowship:** Geriatric Psychiatry, Mount Sinai Hosp/Bronx VA, New York, NY 1982-1983; **Faculty Appointment:** Assoc Prof Psychiatry, Albert Einstein Coll Med

Katz, Ira Ralph MD (Geriatric Psychiatry) - *Special Expertise:* Geriatric Psychiatry - General; **Admitting Hospital:** Hospital of the University of Pennsylvania; **Office Address:** Univ Penn, Geriatric Psyc Sect 3600 Market St, rm 758 Philadelphia, PA 19104; **Office Phone:** (215) 349-8225; **Board Certifications:** Psychiatry 1989, Geriatric Psychiatry 2001; **Medical School:** Albert Einstein Coll Med 1973; **Residency:** Psychiatry, Bronx Muni Hosp Ctr, Bronx, NY 1975-1978; **Fellowship:** Psychopharmacology, Albert Einstein Coll Med, Bronx, NY 1978-1979; **Faculty Appointment:** Prof Psychiatry, Univ Penn

Kennedy, Gary MD (Geriatric Psychiatry) - *Special Expertise:* Geriatric Psychiatry - General; **Admitting Hospital:** Montefiore Medical Center; **Office Address:** Montefiore Med Ctr, Dept Psyc & Behavioral Sci 111 E 210th St Bronx, NY 10467-2490; **Office Phone:** (718) 920-4236; **Board Certifications:** Psychiatry 1980, Geriatric Psychiatry 1991; **Medical School:** Univ Tex, San Antonio 1975; **Residency:** Psychiatry, VA Hosp-Univ Texas, San Antonio, TX 1976-1979; **Fellowship:** Geriatric Psychiatry, Montefiore Hosp, Bronx, NY 1981-1984; **Faculty Appointment:** Prof Psychiatry, Albert Einstein Coll Med

Klement, Maria MD (Geriatric Psychiatry) - *Special Expertise:* Dementia; **Admitting Hospital:** Sheppard Pratt Healthsystem; **Office Address:** Sheppard Pratt Hlth System 6501 N Charles St Baltimore, MD 21204; **Office Phone:** (410) 938-3000; **Board Certification:** Psychiatry 1972; **Medical School:** Penn State Univ-Hershey Med Ctr 1959; **Residencies:** Psychiatry, Philadelphia Genl Hosp, Philadelphia, PA 1960-1962; Psychiatry, Sheppeard Pratt Hosp, Towson, MD 1962-1963

Lyketsos, Constantine G MD (Geriatric Psychiatry) - *Special Expertise:* Alzheimer's Disease; Neuro-Psychiatry; **Admitting Hospital:** Johns Hopkins Hospital - Baltimore (Page 65); **Office Address:** Johns Hopkins Hosp, Osler 320 600 N Wolfe St Baltimore, MD 21287; **Office Phone:** (410) 955-6158; **Board Certifications:** Geriatric Psychiatry 1995, Psychiatry 1994; **Medical School:** Washington Univ, St Louis 1988; **Residency:** Psychiatry, Johns Hopkins Hosp, Baltimore, MD 1989-1992; **Fellowship:** Psychiatry, Johns Hopkins Hosp, Baltimore, MD 1992-1994; **Faculty Appointment:** Assoc Prof Psychiatry, Johns Hopkins Univ

Rabins, Peter MD (Geriatric Psychiatry) - *Special Expertise:* Geriatric Psychiatry - General; **Admitting Hospital:** Johns Hopkins Hospital - Baltimore (Page 65); **Office Address:** Johns Hopkins Hospital 600 N Wolfe St, Meyer Bldg, rm 279 Baltimore, MD 21287; **Office Phone:** (410) 955-6736; **Board Certifications:** Psychiatry 1980, Geriatric Psychiatry 1991; **Medical School:** Tulane Univ 1973; **Residency:** Psychiatry, Univ Oregon Hlth Scis Ctr, Portland, OR 1974-1977; **Fellowship:** Neurology, Johns Hopkins Univ Sch Med, Baltimore, MD; **Faculty Appointment:** Prof Psychiatry, Johns Hopkins Univ

Reisberg, Barry MD (Geriatric Psychiatry) - *Special Expertise:* Alzheimer's Disease; *Dementia; Depression;* **Admitting Hospital:** NYU Medical Center (Page 70); **Office Address:** 550 1st Ave, Ste THN314 New York, NY 10016; **Office Phone:** (212) 263-8554; **Board Certifications:** Psychiatry 1976, Geriatric Psychiatry 1991; **Medical School:** NY Med Coll 1972; **Residency:** Psychiatry, NY Med-Metro Hosp, New York, NY 1972-1975; **Fellowship:** U London, London, England 1975; **Faculty Appointment:** Prof Psychiatry, NYU Sch Med

Sunderland, Trey MD (Geriatric Psychiatry) - *Special Expertise:* Geriatric Psychiatry - General; **Admitting Hospital:** National Institutes of Health - Clinical Center; **Office Address:** 10 Ctr Dr, Bldg 10 - rm 3N228, MC-1274 Bethesda, MD 20982-1274; **Office Phone:** (301) 496-0948; **Board Certifications:** Psychiatry 1983, Geriatric Psychiatry 1996; **Medical School:** Geo Wash Univ 1978; **Residency:** Psychiatry, McLean Hosp, Belmont, MA 1979-1982; **Fellowship:** Psychopharmacology, Natl Inst for Mental Hlth, Bethesda, MD 1982-1984

Southeast

Nemeroff, Charles Barnet MD (Geriatric Psychiatry) - *Special Expertise:* Geriatric Psychiatry - General; **Admitting Hospital:** Emory University Hospital; **Office Address:** Emory Univ Sch Med 1639 Pierce Atlanta, GA 30322; **Office Phone:** (404) 727-8382; **Board Certifications:** Psychiatry 1987, Geriatric Psychiatry 1991; **Medical School:** Univ NC Sch Med 1981; **Residencies:** NC Meml Hosp, Chapel Hill, NC 1982-1983; Duke Univ Med Ctr, Durham, NC 1983-1985; **Faculty Appointment:** Prof Psychiatry, Emory Univ

Stein, Elliott MD (Geriatric Psychiatry) - *Special Expertise:* Geriatric Psychiatry - General; **Admitting Hospital:** Mount Sinai Medical Center; **Office Address:** Mount Sinai Med Ctr 4300 Alton Rd, Warner Bldg, Ste 360 Miami Beach, FL 33140; **Office Phone:** (305) 534-3636; **Board Certifications:** Psychiatry 1979, Geriatric Psychiatry 1991; **Medical School:** Univ Miami Sch Med 1973; **Residency:** Psychiatry, Herrick Meml Hosp, Berkerley, CA 1973-1976; **Faculty Appointment:** Adjct Prof Psychiatry, Univ Miami Sch Med

Midwest

Goldman, Samuel MD (Geriatric Psychiatry) - *Special Expertise:* Depression; Anxiety *Disorders; Phobias;* **Admitting Hospital:** Advocate Lutheran General Hospital; **Office Address:** Advocate Hlth Care 401 S Milwaukee Ave, Ste 235 Wheeling, IL 60090; **Office Phone:** (312) 670-6444; **Board Certifications:** Psychiatry 1982, Geriatric Psychiatry 1996; **Medical School:** Univ Chicago-Pritzker Sch Med 1974; **Residency:** Psychiatry, Univ Chicago, Chicago, IL 1975-1978

Grossberg, George MD (Geriatric Psychiatry) - *Special Expertise:* Geriatric Psychiatry - General; **Admitting Hospital:** St Louis University Hospital; **Office Address:** St Louis Univ Sch Med, Dept Psyc 1221 S Grand Blvd St Louis, MO 63104; **Office Phone:** (314) 577-8721; **Board Certifications:** Psychiatry 1982, Geriatric Psychiatry 1992; **Medical School:** St Louis Univ 1975; **Residency:** Psychiatry, St Louis Univ Med Ctr, St Louis, MO 1976-1979; **Faculty Appointment:** Prof Psychiatry, St Louis Univ

GERIATRIC PSYCHIATRY *Midwest*

Isenberg, Keith Eugene MD (Geriatric Psychiatry) - *Special Expertise: Alzheimer's Disease; Anxiety Disorders;* **Admitting Hospital:** Barnes - Jewish Hospital; **Office Address:** Barnes Jewish Hosp 1 Barnes Plaza E Pavilion Ste 15500JJ, Fl 15 St. Louis, MO 63110; **Office Phone:** (314) 362-1819; **Board Certifications:** Geriatric Psychiatry 1994, Psychiatry 1984; **Medical School:** Indiana Univ 1978; **Residency:** Psychiatry, Wash Univ/Barnes Hosp, St Louis, MO 1978-1982; **Faculty Appointment:** Clin Inst Psychiatry, Washington Univ, St Louis

Lazarus, Lawrence W MD (Geriatric Psychiatry) - *Special Expertise: Obsessive-Compulsive Disorder; Anxiety Disorders;* **Admitting Hospital:** Rush/Presbyterian - St Luke's Medical Center - Chicago (Page 74); **Office Address:** 1725 W Harrison St Ste 960 Chicago, IL 60612; **Office Phone:** (312) 942-6018; **Board Certifications:** Geriatric Psychiatry 1991, Psychiatry 1991; **Medical School:** Hahnemann Univ 1967; **Residency:** Psychiatry, Michael Reese Hosp, Chicago, IL 1968-1971

Luchins, Daniel MD (Geriatric Psychiatry) - *Special Expertise: Psychiatry-Geriatric; Mental Retardation;* **Admitting Hospital:** University of Chicago Hospitals (Page 78); **Office Address:** 5841 S Maryland Ave, MC-3077 Chicago, IL 60637; **Office Phone:** (773) 702-9716; **Board Certifications:** Geriatric Psychiatry 1992, Psychiatry 1978; **Medical School:** Canada 1973; **Residencies:** Psychiatry, Douglas Hosp, Montreal, Canada 1975; Psychiatry, St Mary's Hosp, Montreal, Canada 1976; **Fellowship:** Psychiatry, Allan Meml Inst, Montreal, Canada 1976-1977; **Faculty Appointment:** Assoc Prof Unic Chicago - Pritzker Sch Med

Mellow, Alan M. MD/PhD (Geriatric Psychiatry) - *Special Expertise: Dementia; Depression;* **Admitting Hospital:** University of Michigan Health Center; **Office Address:** University of Michigan Department of Psychiatry 1500 E Medical Center Drive Ann Arbor, MI 48100-0704; **Office Phone:** (734) 930-5630; **Board Certifications:** Psychiatry 1988, Geriatric Psychiatry 1991; **Medical School:** Northwestern Univ 1981; **Residencies:** Internal Medicine, Univ Chicago Hosp, Chicago, IL 1981-1982; Psychiatry, McLean Hosp-Harvard, Belmont, MA 1982-1985; **Fellowship:** Psychiatry, Nat Inst Mental Health, Bethesda, MD 1985-1988; **Faculty Appointment:** Prof Psychiatry, Univ Mich Med Sch

West Coast and Pacific

Borson, Soo MD (Geriatric Psychiatry) - *Special Expertise: Alzheimer's Disease;* **Admitting Hospital:** University of Washington Medical Center; **Office Address:** 4245 Roosevelt Way NE, Box 354760 Seattle, WA 98105; **Office Phone:** (206) 598-8750; **Board Certifications:** Psychiatry 1985, Geriatric Psychiatry 1991; **Medical School:** Stanford Univ 1969; **Residency:** Psychiatry, Univ Wash, Seattle, WA 1977-1979; **Fellowship:** Geriatric Psychiatry, Univ Wash, Seattle, WA 1979-1981; **Faculty Appointment:** Prof Psychiatry, Univ Wash

Friedman, Barry MD (Geriatric Psychiatry) - *Special Expertise: Psychopharmacology;* **Admitting Hospital:** Cedars-Sinai Medical Center; **Office Address:** 435 N Bedford Dr, Ste 112 Beverly Hills, CA 90210-4330; **Office Phone:** (310) 274-4372; **Board Certifications:** Psychiatry 1974, Geriatric Psychiatry 1995; **Medical School:** UCSF 1965; **Residencies:** Neurology, UCLA, Los Angeles, CA 1968-1971; Psychiatry, UCLA, Los Angeles, CA 1968-1971; **Faculty Appointment:** Assoc Clin Prof Psychiatry, UCLA

Jeste, Dilip MD (Geriatric Psychiatry) - *Special Expertise: Psychotic Disorders; Dementia; Tardive Dyskinesia;* **Admitting Hospital:** University of California - San Diego Healthcare; **Office Address:** UCSD, Div Geriatric Psyc 9500 Gillman Dr, MC-0603V La Jolla, CA 92093-0603; **Office Phone:** (858) 534-4020; **Board Certifications:** Psychiatry 1979, Geriatric Psychiatry 1991; **Medical School:** India 1966; **Residencies:** Psychiatry, NY Hosp, White Plains, NY 1975-1977; Neurology, George Washington Univ Hosp, Washington, DC 1982-1984; **Faculty Appointment:** Prof Geriatric Psychiatry, UCSD

Kramer, Barry Alan MD (Geriatric Psychiatry) - *Special Expertise: Electroconvulsive Therapy (ECT); Depression;* **Admitting Hospital:** Cedars-Sinai Medical Center; **Office Address:** Cedars-Sinai Med Ctr, Dept Psyc 8730 Alden Drive, rm W-223 Los Angeles, CA 90048; **Office Phone:** (310) 423-4014; **Board Certifications:** Psychiatry 1978, Geriatric Psychiatry 1991; **Medical School:** Hahnemann Univ 1974; **Residency:** Psychiatry, Montefiore Hospital & Medical Ctr, Bronx, NY 1974-1978; **Fellowship:** Geriatric Psychiatry, UCLA-USC Long Term Gero Ctr, Los Angeles, CA 1985-1986

Leuchter, Andrew Francis MD (Geriatric Psychiatry) - *Special Expertise: Depression;* **Admitting Hospital:** UCLA Neuropsychiatric Hospital; **Office Address:** 760 Westwood Plaza, rm 37430 Los Angeles, CA 90024-8300; **Office Phone:** (310) 825-0207; **Board Certifications:** Psychiatry 1986, Geriatric Psychiatry 1991; **Medical School:** Baylor Coll Med 1980; **Residency:** Psychiatry, UCLA - NPI&H, Los Angeles, CA 1981-1984; **Fellowship:** Geriatric Psychiatry, UCLA, Los Angeles, CA 1984-1986; **Faculty Appointment:** Assoc Prof Psychiatry, UCLA

Schneider, Lon S MD (Geriatric Psychiatry) - *Special Expertise: Alzheimer's Disease; Depression; Psychopharmacology;* **Admitting Hospital:** USC University Hospital - Richard K. Eamer Medical Plaza; **Office Address:** USC Sch Med, Dept Psyc 1975 Zonal Ave, Bldg KAM-400 Los Angeles, CA 90033; **Office Phone:** (323) 442-3715; **Board Certifications:** Psychiatry 1984, Geriatric Psychiatry 1991; **Medical School:** Hahnemann Univ 1978; **Residency:** Psychiatry, USC Sch Med, Los Angeles, CA 1979-1982; **Fellowship:** Geriatric Psychiatry, USC Sch Med, Los Angeles, CA 1982-1983; **Faculty Appointment:** Prof Geriatric Psychiatry, USC Sch Med

Small, Gary William MD (Geriatric Psychiatry) - *Special Expertise: Dementia;* **Admitting Hospital:** UCLA Medical Center; **Office Address:** UCLA- Neuropsyc Inst 760 Westwood Plaza, Fl 88-201 Los Angeles, CA 90024-1759; **Office Phone:** (310) 825-0291; **Board Certifications:** Psychiatry 1983, Geriatric Psychiatry 1991; **Medical School:** USC Sch Med 1977; **Residency:** Psychiatry, Mass Genl Hosp, Boston, MA 1978-1981; **Fellowship:** Psychiatry, UCLA Med Ctr, Los Angeles, CA 1981-1983; **Faculty Appointment:** Prof Psychiatry, UCLA

Veith, Richard MD (Geriatric Psychiatry) - *Special Expertise: Depression in Cardiovascular Disease; Elderly Cardiovascular Affects;* **Admitting Hospital:** University of Washington Medical Center; **Office Address:** Univ Washington Medical Center 1959 NE Pacific St, Box 6560 Seattle, WA 98195; **Office Phone:** (206) 543-3926; **Board Certifications:** Psychiatry 1979, Geriatric Psychiatry 1991; **Medical School:** Univ Wash 1973; **Residency:** Psychiatry, Univ Washington, Seattle, WA 1974-1977; **Faculty Appointment:** Prof Psychiatry, Univ Wash

PSYCHIATRY

Baldessarini, Ross MD (Psychiatry) - *Special Expertise:* Bipolar/Mood Disorders; Schizophrenia; Psychotic Disorders; **Admitting Hospital:** McLean Hospital; **Office Address:** McLean Hosp, Mailman Rsch Ctr 115 Mill St Belmont, MA 02478; **Office Phone:** (617) 855-3203; **Board Certification:** Psychiatry 1972; **Medical School:** Johns Hopkins Univ 1963; **Residency:** Psychiatry, Johns Hopkins Hosp, Baltimore, MD 1966-1969; **Fellowship:** Natl Inst Mental Hlth 1964-1966; **Faculty Appointment:** Prof Psychiatry, Harvard Med Sch

Bowers Jr, Malcolm B MD (Psychiatry) - *Special Expertise:* Schizophrenia; **Admitting Hospital:** Yale - New Haven Hospital; **Office Address:** Yale Univ Hosp, Dept Psyc 25 Park St New Haven, CT 06519-1110; **Office Phone:** (203) 785-2121; **Board Certification:** Psychiatry 1970; **Medical School:** Washington Univ, St Louis 1958; **Residency:** Psychiatry, Yale-New Haven Hosp, New Haven, CT 1962-1965; **Fellowship:** Psychiatry, Yale-New Haven Hosp, New Haven, CT 1963-1964; **Faculty Appointment:** Prof Psychiatry, Yale Univ

Cohen, Bruce M MD (Psychiatry) - *Special Expertise:* Psychopharmacology; **Admitting Hospital:** McLean Hospital; **Office Address:** McLean Hospital 115 Mill St Belmont, MA 02478-1041; **Office Phone:** (617) 855-3227; **Board Certification:** Psychiatry 1979; **Medical School:** Case West Res Univ 1975; **Residency:** Psychiatry, McLean Hospital, Belmont, MA 1975-1978; **Faculty Appointment:** Prof Psychiatry, Harvard Med Sch

Herman, John Benjamin MD (Psychiatry) - *Special Expertise:* Psychiatry - General; **Admitting Hospital:** Massachusetts General Hospital; **Office Address:** Mass General Hospital 55 Fruit St, Bldg Bulfinch 351 Boston, MA 02114-3139; **Office Phone:** (617) 726-9921; **Board Certification:** Psychiatry 1987; **Medical School:** Univ Wisc 1980; **Residency:** Psychiatry, Mass Genl Hosp., Boston, MA 1981-1984; **Faculty Appointment:** Asst Prof Psychiatry, Harvard Med Sch

Hobson, John Allan MD (Psychiatry) - *Special Expertise:* Sleep Disorders/Apnea; **Admitting Hospital:** Massachusetts Mental Health Center; **Office Address:** Harvard Med Sch, Mass Mental Health Ctr 74 Fenwood Rd Boston, MA 02115; **Office Phone:** (617) 734-9645; **Board Certification:** Psychiatry 1968; **Medical School:** Harvard Med Sch 1959; **Residencies:** Psychiatry, Mass Mental Hlth Ctr, Boston, MA 1960-1961; Psychiatry, NIMH, Bethesda, MD 1961-1963; **Fellowship:** Clinical Neurophysiology, Univ Lyon, France 1963-1964; **Faculty Appointment:** Prof Psychiatry, Harvard Med Sch

Jenike, Michael Andrew MD (Psychiatry) - *Special Expertise:* Obsessive-Compulsive Disorder; Psychiatry-Geriatric; **Admitting Hospital:** Massachusetts General Hospital; **Office Address:** Mass Genl Hosp, Dept Psychiatry Bldg 149 - 13th St, Charlestown Navy Yard Fl 9 Charlestown, MA 02129; **Office Phone:** (617) 726-2998; **Board Certification:** Psychiatry 1984; **Medical School:** Univ Okla Coll Med 1978; **Residency:** Psychiatry, Mass Genl Hosp, Boston, MA 1979-1982; **Fellowships:** Psychiatry, Harvard Med Sch, Cambridge, MA 1982; Psychiatry, Mass Genl Hosp, Boston, MA 1983; **Faculty Appointment:** Prof Psychiatry, Harvard Med Sch

McGlashan, Thomas MD (Psychiatry) - *Special Expertise:* Schizophrenia; Personality Disorders-Borderline; **Admitting Hospital:** Yale - New Haven Hospital; **Office Address:** Yale Univ Sch Med, Dept Psyc 301 Cedar St, Fl 2 New Haven, CT 06519; **Office Phone:** (203) 785-7210; **Board Certification:** Psychiatry 1973; **Medical School:** Univ Penn 1967; **Residency:** Psychiatry, Mass Mental Hlth Ctr, Boston, MA 1968-1971; **Faculty Appointment:** Prof Psychiatry, Yale Univ

Nelson, J Craig MD (Psychiatry) - *Special Expertise:* Psychiatry-Geriatric; Psychopharmacology; Mood Disorders; **Admitting Hospital:** Yale - New Haven Hospital; **Office Address:** 20 York St New Haven, CT 06504; **Office Phone:** (203) 688-2157; **Board Certifications:** Psychiatry 1974, Geriatric Psychiatry 1992; **Medical School:** Univ Wisc 1968; **Residencies:** Psychiatry, Yale-New Hosp, New Haven, CT 1969-1970; Psychiatry, Yale-New Hosp, New Haven, CT 1973-1974; **Faculty Appointment:** Prof Psychiatry, Yale Univ

Pope Jr, Harrison G MD (Psychiatry) - *Special Expertise:* Addiction/Substance Abuse; Psychopharmacology; **Admitting Hospital:** McLean Hospital; **Office Address:** McLean Hosp, Dept Psyc 115 Mill St Belmont, MA 02478; **Office Phone:** (617) 855-2911; **Board Certification:** Psychiatry 1980; **Medical School:** Harvard Med Sch 1974; **Residency:** Psychiatry, McLean Hosp, Belmont, MA 1974-1977; **Faculty Appointment:** Prof Psychiatry, Harvard Med Sch

Rasmussen, Steven A MD (Psychiatry) - *Special Expertise:* Obsessive-Compulsive Disorder; **Admitting Hospital:** Butler Hospital; **Office Address:** Butler Hospital 345 Blackstone Blvd Providence, RI 02906-7010; **Office Phone:** (401) 455-6209; **Board Certification:** Psychiatry 1983; **Medical School:** Brown Univ 1977; **Residency:** Psychiatry, Yale U, New Haven, CT 1977-1981; **Faculty Appointment:** Assoc Prof Psychiatry, Brown Univ

Rosenbaum, Jerrold Frank MD (Psychiatry) - *Special Expertise:* Anxiety & Mood Disorders; **Admitting Hospital:** Massachusetts General Hospital; **Office Address:** Mass Genl Hosp 15 Parkman St, WAC 812 Boston, MA 02114; **Office Phone:** (617) 726-3482; **Board Certification:** Psychiatry 1978; **Medical School:** Yale Univ 1973; **Residency:** Psychiatry, Mass Genl Hosp, Boston, MA 1974-1977; **Faculty Appointment:** Prof Psychiatry, Harvard Med Sch

van der Kolk, Bessel MD (Psychiatry) - *Special Expertise:* Post Traumatic Stress Disorder; Child Abuse; **Admitting Hospital:** Boston Medical Center; **Office Address:** 16 Braddock Park Boston, MA 02116-5804; **Office Phone:** (617) 247-3918; **Board Certification:** Psychiatry 1976; **Medical School:** Univ Chicago-Pritzker Sch Med 1970; **Residency:** Psychiatry, Harvard Med Sch, Boston, MA 1971-1974; **Faculty Appointment:** Prof Psychiatry, Boston Univ

Yonkers, Kimberly A MD (Psychiatry) - *Special Expertise:* Anxiety & Mood Disorders; Premenstrual Dysphoric Disorder; **Admitting Hospital:** Yale - New Haven Hospital; **Office Address:** Yale Univ Sch Med, Dept Psyc 142 Temple St, Ste 301 New Haven, CT 06510; **Office Phone:** (203) 764-6621; **Board Certification:** Psychiatry 1991; **Medical School:** Columbia P&S 1986; **Residency:** Psychiatry, McLean Hosp- Harvard, Belmont, MA 1987-1990; **Fellowship:** Psychiatry, McLean Hosp-Harvard, Belmont, MA 1990-1992; **Faculty Appointment:** Assoc Prof Psychiatry, Yale Univ

Mid Atlantic

Alexopoulos, George MD (Psychiatry) - *Special Expertise:* Psychiatry-Geriatric; **Admitting Hospital:** New York Weill Cornell Medical Center - NY Presbyterian Hospital (Page 72); **Office Address:** 21 Bloomingdale Rd White Plains, NY 10605; **Office Phone:** (914) 997-5767; **Board Certifications:** Psychiatry 1978, Geriatric Psychiatry 1992; **Medical School:** Greece 1970; **Residencies:** Psychiatry, UMDNJ Univ Hosp, Newark, NJ 1974-1976; Psychiatry, NY Hosp-Cornell Univ, White Plains, NY 1976-1977; **Fellowship:** Biological Psychiatry, NY Hosp-Cornell Med Ctr, New York, NY 1977-1978; **Faculty Appointment:** Prof Psychiatry, Cornell Univ-Weil Med Coll

Boronow, John Joseph MD (Psychiatry) - *Special Expertise:* Psychotic Disorders; Schizophrenia; **Admitting Hospital:** Sheppard Pratt Healthsystem; **Office Address:** Sheppard & Enoch Pratt Hospital 6501 N Charles St Towson, MD 21204; **Office Phone:** (410) 938-4306; **Board Certification:** Psychiatry 1983; **Medical School:** Yale Univ 1977; **Residency:** Psychiatry, NY Hosp-Cornell Med Ctr, New York, NY 1978-1981; **Fellowship:** Psychopharmacology, Natl Inst Mntl Hlth, Bethesda, MD 1981-1983

PSYCHIATRY *Mid Atlantic*

Breitbart, William MD (Psychiatry) - *Special Expertise:* Pain-Cancer; AIDS/HIV; **Admitting Hospital:** Memorial Sloan Kettering Cancer Center; **Office Address:** Meml Sloan Kettering Cancer Ctr-Counseling Ctr 1246 2nd Ave New York, NY 10021; **Office Phone:** (212) 639-4770; **Board Certifications:** Internal Medicine 1982, Psychiatry 1986; **Medical School:** Albert Einstein Coll Med 1978; **Residencies:** Psychiatry, Bronx Muni Hosp Ctr, Bronx, NY 1979-1980; Psychiatry, Bronx Muni Hosp Ctr, Bronx, NY 1982-1984; **Fellowship:** Psychiatric Oncology, Meml Sloan Kettering Cancer Ctr, New York, NY 1984-1986; **Faculty Appointment:** Prof Psychiatry, Cornell Univ-Weil Med Coll

Cancro, Robert MD (Psychiatry) - *Special Expertise:* Schizophrenia; Depression; **Admitting Hospital:** NYU Medical Center (Page 70); **Office Address:** 550 1st Ave New York, NY 10016; **Office Phone:** (212) 263-6214; **Board Certification:** Psychiatry 1962; **Medical School:** SUNY Hlth Sci Ctr 1955; **Residency:** Psychiatry, Kings County Hosp, Brooklyn, NY 1956-1959; **Faculty Appointment:** Prof Psychiatry, NYU Sch Med

Carpenter Jr, William T MD (Psychiatry) - *Special Expertise:* Schizophrenia; **Admitting Hospital:** Maryland Psychiatric Research Center; **Office Address:** Maryland Psychiatric Rsch Ctr Univ MD Sch Med, Box 21247 Baltimore, MD 21228-0747; **Office Phone:** (410) 402-7101; **Board Certification:** Psychiatry 1972; **Medical School:** Wake Forest Univ Sch Med 1962; **Residency:** Psychiatry, Strong Meml Hosp-Univ Roch, Rochester, NY 1963-1966; **Faculty Appointment:** Prof Psychiatry, Univ MD Sch Med

Davis, Kenneth MD (Psychiatry) - *Special Expertise:* Alzheimer's Disease; Schizophrenia; **Admitting Hospital:** Mount Sinai Hospital (Page 70); **Office Address:** Mount Sinai Sch Med 1 Gustave Levy Pl New York, NY 10029-6504; **Office Phone:** (212) 824-7008; **Board Certification:** Psychiatry 1980; **Medical School:** Mount Sinai Sch Med 1973; **Residency:** Psychiatry, Stanford Med Ctr, Stanford, CA 1973-1976; **Faculty Appointment:** Prof Psychiatry, Mount Sinai Sch Med

DePaulo, Jr, J Raymond MD (Psychiatry) - *Special Expertise:* Mood Disorders; **Admitting Hospital:** Johns Hopkins Hospital - Baltimore (Page 65); **Office Address:** Johns Hopkins Hosp, Dept Psyc 601 N Wolfe St, Bldg Meyer 3-181 Baltimore, MD 21287-7381; **Office Phone:** (410) 955-3246; **Board Certification:** Psychiatry 1977; **Medical School:** Johns Hopkins Univ 1972; **Residency:** Psychiatry, Baltimore City Hospital, Baltimore, MD 1973-1977; **Faculty Appointment:** Prof Psychiatry, Johns Hopkins Univ

Eth, Spencer MD (Psychiatry) - *Special Expertise:* Forensic Psychiatry; Depression-Postpartum; **Admitting Hospital:** St Vincents Catholic Medical Center of New York; **Office Address:** 144 W 12th St, rm 174 New York, NY 10011-8202; **Office Phone:** (212) 604-8196; **Board Certifications:** Psychiatry 1980, Forensic Psychiatry 1994; **Medical School:** UCLA 1976; **Residency:** Psychiatry, NY Cornell Med CTr, New York, NY 1976-1979; **Fellowship:** Child & Adolescent Psychiatry, Cedars - Sinai Med Ctr, Los Angeles, CA 1979-1981; **Faculty Appointment:** Prof Psychiatry, NY Med Coll

Ganguli, Rohan MD (Psychiatry) - *Special Expertise:* Schizophrenia; **Admitting Hospital:** Western Psychiatric Institute & Clinic; **Office Address:** UPMC-Western Psyc Inst & Clin 3811 O'Hara St Pittsburgh, PA 15213; **Office Phone:** (412) 624-1103; **Board Certification:** Psychiatry 1980; **Medical School:** India 1973; **Residencies:** Psychiatry, Meml Univ, New Foundland, Canada 1975-1978; Psychiatry, Univ Pitts Med Ctr, Pittsburgh, PA 1978; **Faculty Appointment:** Prof Psychiatry, Univ Pittsburgh

Gorman, Jack Matthew MD (Psychiatry) - *Special Expertise:* Panic Disorder/Anxiety Disorders; Schizophrenia; **Admitting Hospital:** Columbia Presbyterian Medical Center (Page 72); **Office Address:** 15 W 81st St New York, NY 10024; **Office Phone:** (212) 543-5000; **Board Certification:** Psychiatry 1979; **Medical School:** Columbia P&S 1977; **Residency:** Psychiatry, Columbia-Presby Med Ctr, New York, NY 1978-1980; **Fellowship:** Psychopharmacology, Columbia-Presby Med Ctr, New York, NY 1980-1982; **Faculty Appointment:** Prof Psychiatry, Columbia P&S

Halmi, Katherine MD (Psychiatry) - *Special Expertise:* Eating Disorders; **Admitting Hospital:** New York Presbyterian - Westchester Division; **Office Address:** 21 Bloomingdale Rd White Plains, NY 10605; **Office Phone:** (914) 997-5875; **Board Certifications:** Pediatrics 1970, Psychiatry 1977; **Medical School:** Univ Iowa Coll Med 1965; **Residencies:** Pediatrics, Univ IA Hosp, Iowa City, IA 1967-1968; Psychiatry, Univ IA Hosp, Iowa City, IA 1969-1972; **Fellowship:** Child Development, Univ IA Hosp, Iowa City, IA 1969; **Faculty Appointment:** Prof Psychiatry, Cornell Univ-Weil Med Coll

Holland, Jimmie C B MD (Psychiatry) - *Special Expertise:* Psychiatry of Cancer; **Admitting Hospital:** Memorial Sloan Kettering Cancer Center; **Office Address:** Dept Psyc & Behav Sci 1242 Second Ave, Box 421 New York, NY 10021-6007; **Office Phone:** (212) 639-3904; **Board Certification:** Psychiatry 1967; **Medical School:** Baylor Coll Med 1952; **Residencies:** Psychiatry, Mass Genl Hosp, Boston, MA 1955; Psychiatry, EJ Meyer Meml Hosp, Buffalo, NY 1956-1957; **Faculty Appointment:** Prof Psychiatry, Cornell Univ-Weil Med Coll

Hollander, Eric MD (Psychiatry) - *Special Expertise:* Obsessive-Compulsive Disorder; Anxiety Disorders; **Admitting Hospital:** Mount Sinai Hospital (Page 70); **Office Address:** 300 Central Park West, Ste 1C New York, NY 10024-1513; **Office Phone:** (212) 698-4481; **Board Certification:** Psychiatry 1987; **Medical School:** SUNY Hlth Sci Ctr 1982; **Residencies:** Internal Medicine, Mount Sinai, New York, NY 1982-1983; Psychiatry, Mount Sinai, New York, NY 1983-1986; **Fellowship:** Psychiatry, Columbia-Presby, New York, NY 1986-1988; **Faculty Appointment:** Prof Psychiatry, Mount Sinai Sch Med

Klagsbrun, Samuel C MD (Psychiatry) - *Special Expertise:* Behavioral Problems; **Admitting Hospital:** Four Winds Hospital (Page 61); **Office Address:** Four Winds Hospital 800 Cross River Rd Katonah, NY 10536; **Office Phone:** (914) 763-8151; **Board Certification:** Psychiatry 1977; **Medical School:** Univ Hlth Sci/Chicago Med Sch 1962; **Residency:** Psychiatry, Yale-New Haven Hosp, New Haven, CT 1963-1966; **Faculty Appointment:** Prof Psychiatry, Albert Einstein Coll Med

Klein, Donald MD (Psychiatry) - *Special Expertise:* Psychopharmacology; Depression/Anxiety Disorders; **Admitting Hospital:** Columbia Presbyterian Medical Center (Page 72); **Office Address:** 182 E 79th St New York, NY 10021-0422; **Office Phone:** (212) 543-2366; **Board Certification:** Psychiatry 1959; **Medical School:** SUNY Hlth Sci Ctr 1952; **Residency:** Psychiatry, Creedmoor, Queens Village, NY 1953-1954; **Faculty Appointment:** Prof Psychiatry, Columbia P&S

Kupfer, David J. MD (Psychiatry) - *Special Expertise:* Bipolar/Mood Disorders; Sleep Disorders/Apnea; **Admitting Hospital:** UPMC - Presbyterian University Hospital; **Office Address:** Western Psychiatric Inst & Clin 3811 O'Hara St Pittsburgh, PA 15213; **Office Phone:** (412) 624-2353; **Board Certification:** Psychiatry 1978; **Medical School:** Yale Univ 1965; **Residencies:** Psychiatry, Yale-New Haven Hosp, New Haven, CT 1969-1970; Psychiatry, Natl Inst Mental Hlth, Bethesda, MD 1967-1969; **Fellowship:** Psychiatry, Yale-New Haven Hosp, New Haven, CT 1966-1967; **Faculty Appointment:** Prof Psychiatry, Univ Pittsburgh

PSYCHIATRY *Mid Atlantic*

Lederberg, Marguerite MD (Psychiatry) - *Special Expertise:* Psychiatry of Cancer; **Admitting Hospital:** Memorial Sloan Kettering Cancer Center; **Office Address:** Meml Sloan Kettering Cancer Ctr, Dept Psyc 1275 York Ave, Box 421 New York, NY 10021; **Office Phone:** (212) 639-3911; **Board Certifications:** Pediatrics 1970, Psychiatry 1980; **Medical School:** Yale Univ 1961; **Residencies:** Pediatrics, Stanford Med Ctr, Stanford, CA 1962-1964; Psychiatry, Stanford Med Ctr, Stanford, CA 1972-1977; **Fellowship:** Ambulatory Pediatrics, Stanford Med Ctr, Stanford, CA 1964-1968; **Faculty Appointment:** Clin Prof Psychiatry, Cornell Univ-Weil Med Coll

Liebowitz, Michael R MD (Psychiatry) - *Special Expertise:* Depression; Anxiety Disorders; **Admitting Hospital:** Columbia Presbyterian Medical Center (Page 72); **Office Address:** 10 E 90th St, Ste 1A New York, NY 10028; **Office Phone:** (212) 543-5366; **Board Certification:** Psychiatry 1978; **Medical School:** Yale Univ 1969; **Residencies:** Psychiatry, Med Ctr Hosp VT, Burlington, VT 1974-1975; Psychiatry, NY State Psyc Inst, New York, NY 1975-1977; **Fellowship:** Psychiatry, NY State Psyc Inst, New York, NY 1977-1979; **Faculty Appointment:** Prof Psychiatry, Columbia P&S

Loewenstein, Richard MD (Psychiatry) - *Special Expertise:* Trauma Psychiatry; Dissociative Disorders; **Admitting Hospital:** Sheppard Pratt Healthsystem; **Office Address:** Sheppard Pratt Hlth Sys 6501 N Charles St, Box 6815 Baltimore, MD 21285-6815; **Office Phone:** (410) 938-5070; **Board Certification:** Psychiatry 1980; **Medical School:** Yale Univ 1975; **Residency:** Psychiatry, Yale, New Haven, CT 1976-1979; **Fellowship:** NIH,NIMH-Biol Psych Br, Bethesda, MD 1980-1982; **Faculty Appointment:** Assoc Clin Prof Psychiatry, Univ MD Sch Med

Marin, Deborah B MD (Psychiatry) - *Special Expertise:* Alzheimer's Disease; **Admitting Hospital:** Mount Sinai Hospital (Page 70); **Office Address:** Mt Sinai Hosp, Dept Psyc 1 Gustave Levy Pl, Box 1230 New York, NY 10029; **Office Phone:** (212) 659-8840; **Board Certification:** Psychiatry 1990; **Medical School:** Mount Sinai Sch Med 1984; **Residency:** Psychiatry, Mount Sinai Hosp, New York, NY 1984-1988; **Fellowship:** Psychiatry, NY Hosp-Cornell Med Ctr, New York, NY 1988-1991; **Faculty Appointment:** Assoc Prof Psychiatry, Mount Sinai Sch Med

McCann, Merle Clements MD (Psychiatry) - *Special Expertise:* Psychiatry - General; **Admitting Hospital:** Sheppard Pratt Healthsystem; **Office Address:** Sheppard & Enoch Pratt Hosp 6501 N Charles St Towson, MD 21285; **Office Phone:** (410) 938-3000; **Board Certification:** Psychiatry 1986; **Medical School:** Med Coll VA 1981; **Residency:** Psychiatry, Geo Wash Univ Hosp, Washington, DC 1982-1985; **Faculty Appointment:** Asst Clin Prof Psychiatry, Univ MD Sch Med

McHugh, Paul MD (Psychiatry) - *Special Expertise:* Neuro-Psychiatry; Huntington's Disease; **Admitting Hospital:** Johns Hopkins Hospital - Baltimore (Page 65); **Office Address:** Johns Hopkins Hosp 600 N Wolfe St, Meyer Bldg, rm 4-113 Baltimore, MD 21287-7113; **Office Phone:** (410) 955-3130; **Board Certifications:** Neurology 1967, Psychiatry 1968; **Medical School:** Harvard Med Sch 1956; **Residencies:** Neurology, Mass Genl Hosp, Boston, MA 1957-1960; Psychiatry, Maudsley Hosp, London, England 1960-1961; **Faculty Appointment:** Prof Psychiatry, Johns Hopkins Univ

Pearlson, Godfrey D MD (Psychiatry) - *Special Expertise:* Schizophrenia; Psychiatric Neuro-Imaging; **Admitting Hospital:** Johns Hopkins Hospital - Baltimore (Page 65); **Office Address:** Johns Hopkins Hospital 600 N Wolfe St, Meyer Bldg, rm 3-166 Baltimore, MD 21287-7362; **Office Phone:** (410) 955-5135; **Board Certification:** Psychiatry 1980; **Medical School:** England 1974; **Residency:** Psychiatry, Johns Hopkins Hosp, Baltimore, MD 1975-1978; **Faculty Appointment:** Prof Psychiatry, Johns Hopkins Univ

Rosse, Richard B MD (Psychiatry) - *Special Expertise:* *Psychiatry - General;* **Admitting Hospital:** Veterans Affairs Medical Center - Washington; **Office Address:** Wash VA Med Ctr, Psyc Svc 50 Irving St NW, rm 3A154 , MC-116A Washington, DC 20422; **Office Phone:** (202) 745-8156; **Board Certification:** Psychiatry 1986; **Medical School:** Univ MD Sch Med 1980; **Residency:** Psychiatry, Georgetown Univ Med Ctr, Washington, DC 1981-1984; **Faculty Appointment:** Assoc Prof Psychiatry, Georgetown Univ

Sadock, Benjamin MD (Psychiatry) - *Special Expertise:* *Anxiety Disorders; Depression; Sexual Dysfunction;* **Admitting Hospital:** NYU Medical Center (Page 70); **Office Address:** 4 E 89th St, rm 1E New York, NY 10128-0656; **Office Phone:** (212) 263-6210; **Board Certification:** Psychiatry 1966; **Medical School:** NY Med Coll 1959; **Residency:** Psychiatry, Bellevue Psyc Hosp, New York, NY 1960-1963; **Faculty Appointment:** Prof Psychiatry, NYU Sch Med

Sadock, Virginia MD (Psychiatry) - *Special Expertise:* *Psychotherapy; Sexual Dysfunction;* **Admitting Hospital:** NYU Medical Center (Page 70); **Office Address:** 4 E 89th St New York, NY 10128; **Office Phone:** (212) 427-0885; **Board Certification:** Psychiatry 1975; **Medical School:** NY Med Coll 1970; **Residency:** Psychiatry, NY Metropolitan Hosp, New York, NY 1970-1973; **Faculty Appointment:** Clin Prof Psychiatry, NYU Sch Med

Shear, Mary Katherine MD (Psychiatry) - *Special Expertise:* *Panic Disorder & Agoraphobia; Anxiety Disorders; Bereavement/Traumatic Grief;* **Admitting Hospital:** UPMC - Presbyterian University Hospital; **Office Address:** Western Psych Inst & Clin 3811 O'Hara St Pittsburgh, PA 15213; **Office Phone:** (412) 624-1340; **Board Certifications:** Internal Medicine 1975, Psychiatry 1981; **Medical School:** Tufts Univ 1972; **Residencies:** Internal Medicine, Mt Sinai Hosp, New York, NY 1972-1976; Psychiatry, Payne Whitney Clin, New York, NY 1976-1979; **Fellowship:** Psychosomatic Medicine, Montefiore Hosp, Bronx, NY 1979-1980; **Faculty Appointment:** Prof Psychiatry, Univ Pittsburgh

Simon, Robert Isaac MD (Psychiatry) - *Special Expertise:* *Forensic Psychiatry;* **Admitting Hospital:** University of Maryland Medical System; **Office Address:** 7921D Glenbrook Rd Bethesda, MD 20814-2441; **Office Phone:** (410) 584-8181; **Board Certifications:** Psychiatry 1969, Forensic Psychiatry 1994; **Medical School:** Tufts Univ 1960; **Residency:** Psychiatry, Jackson Mem Hosp, Miami, FL 1963-1966; **Faculty Appointment:** Prof Psychiatry, Georgetown Univ

Stinnett, James MD (Psychiatry) - *Special Expertise:* *Psychiatry - General;* **Admitting Hospital:** Hospital of the University of Pennsylvania; **Office Address:** Hosp Univ Penn, Founders Bldg 3400 Spruce St, rm 10 Philadelphia, PA 19104; **Office Phone:** (215) 662-2815; **Board Certification:** Psychiatry 1972; **Medical School:** Univ Penn 1965; **Residency:** Psychiatry, Hosp Univ Penn, Philadelphia, PA 1965-1970; **Faculty Appointment:** Prof Psychiatry, Univ Penn

Sussman, Norman MD (Psychiatry) - *Special Expertise:* *Psychopharmacology; Anxiety Disorders;* **Admitting Hospital:** NYU Medical Center (Page 70); **Office Address:** 150 E 58th, Fl 27 New York, NY 10155; **Office Phone:** (212) 588-9722; **Board Certification:** Psychiatry 1980; **Medical School:** NY Med Coll 1975; **Residencies:** Psychiatry, Metropolitan Hosp Ctr, New York, NY 1975-1977; Psychiatry, Westchester Co Med Ctr, Westchester, NY 1977-1978; **Faculty Appointment:** Clin Prof Psychiatry, NYU Sch Med

Thase, Michael E MD (Psychiatry) - *Special Expertise:* *Anxiety & Mood Disorders; Psychopharmocology;* **Admitting Hospital:** UPMC - Presbyterian University Hospital; **Office Address:** Western Psyc Inst & Clin 3811 O'Hara St Pittsburgh, PA 15213; **Office Phone:** (412) 624-5070; **Board Certification:** Psychiatry 1984; **Medical School:** Ohio State Univ 1979; **Residency:** Psychiatry, Western Psych Inst Clin, Pittsburgh, PA 1980-1983; **Fellowship:** Research, Univ Pitts Sch Med, Pittsburgh, PA 1982-1984; **Faculty Appointment:** Prof Psychiatry, Univ Pittsburgh

PSYCHIATRY

Wait, Susan Braynard MD (Psychiatry) - *Special Expertise:* Post Traumatic Stress Disorder; Dissociative Disorders; **Admitting Hospital:** Sheppard Pratt Healthsystem; **Office Address:** Sheppard Pratt Hlth System 6501 N Charles St Baltimore, MD 21285-6815; **Office Phone:** (410) 938-5076; **Board Certification:** Psychiatry 1993; **Medical School:** Med Coll PA Hahnemann 1987; **Residency:** Psychiatry, Sheppard Pratt Hosp, Baltimore, MD 1987-1991; **Faculty Appointment:** Prof Psychiatry, Univ MD Sch Med

Walsh, B Timothy MD (Psychiatry) - *Special Expertise:* Eating Disorders; **Admitting Hospital:** New York State Psychiatric Institute; **Office Address:** NYS Psyc Inst-Unit 98 1051 Riverside Dr New York, NY 10032; **Office Phone:** (212) 543-5752; **Board Certification:** Psychiatry 1978; **Medical School:** Harvard Med Sch 1972; **Residency:** Psychiatry, Bronx Muni Hosp Ctr, Bronx, NY 1974-1977; **Faculty Appointment:** Prof Psychiatry, Columbia P&S

Southeast

Ballenger, James MD (Psychiatry) - *Special Expertise:* Anxiety & Mood Disorders; Forensic Psychiatry; **Admitting Hospital:** MUSC Medical Center; **Office Address:** Med Univ SC, Dept Psyc 67 President St, Box 250861 Charleston, SC 29425; **Office Phone:** (843) 792-0028; **Board Certifications:** Psychiatry 1977, Forensic Psychiatry 1999; **Medical School:** Duke Univ 1970; **Residency:** Psychiatry, Mass Genl Hosp-Harvard, Boston, MA 1971-1974; **Faculty Appointment:** Prof Psychiatry, Med Univ SC

Blazer II, Dan G MD/PhD (Psychiatry) - *Special Expertise:* Psychiatry-Geriatric; Mood Disorders; **Admitting Hospital:** Duke University Medical Center (Page 60); **Office Address:** Duke Med Ctr, Dept Psyc 3521 Hospital S, Box 3003 Durham, NC 27710-3003; **Office Phone:** (919) 684-4128; **Board Certifications:** Psychiatry 1977, Geriatric Psychiatry 1991; **Medical School:** Univ Tenn Coll Med, Memphis 1969; **Residency:** Psychiatry, Duke Univ Med Ctr, Durham, NC 1973-1975; **Fellowship:** Liason Psychiatry, Montefiore Hosp, Bronx, NY 1975-1976; **Faculty Appointment:** Prof Psychiatry, Duke Univ

Davidson, Jonathan MD (Psychiatry) - *Special Expertise:* Anxiety & Mood Disorders; **Admitting Hospital:** Duke University Medical Center (Page 60); **Office Address:** Duke Univ Med Ctr, Dept Psyc Hospital S, rm 40825, Box 3812 Durham, NC 27710; **Office Phone:** (919) 684-2880; **Board Certification:** Psychiatry 1979; **Medical School:** England 1967; **Residency:** Psychiatry, Royal Edinburgh Hosp, Edinburgh, Scotland 1969-1972; **Faculty Appointment:** Prof Psychiatry, Duke Univ

Eisdorfer, Carl MD/PhD (Psychiatry) - *Special Expertise:* Aging and Dementitia; Alzheimer's Disease; **Admitting Hospital:** University of Miami - Jackson Memorial Hospital; **Office Address:** Univ Miami Sch Med 1695 NW Ninth Ave, Ste 3100 Miami, FL 33136-1024; **Office Phone:** (305) 355-9105; **Board Certification:** Psychiatry 1974; **Medical School:** Duke Univ 1964; **Residency:** Psychiatry, Duke Univ Med Ctr, Durham, NC 1965-1967; **Faculty Appointment:** Prof Psychiatry, Univ Miami Sch Med

Kendler, Kenneth S MD (Psychiatry) - *Special Expertise:* Schizophrenia; Mood Disorders; **Admitting Hospital:** Medical College of Virginia Hospitals; **Office Address:** Med Coll VA, Dept Psyc Box 980126 Richmond, VA 23298; **Office Phone:** (804) 828-8590; **Board Certification:** Psychiatry 1981; **Medical School:** Stanford Univ 1976; **Residency:** Psychiatry, Yale-New Haven Hosp, New Haven, CT 1977-1980; **Faculty Appointment:** Prof Psychiatry, Med Coll VA

Powers, Pauline MD (Psychiatry) - *Special Expertise:* Eating Disorders; **Admitting Hospital:** Tampa General Hospital; **Office Address:** Univ S Fla, Dept Psych 3515 E Fletcher Ave Tampa, FL 33613-4706; **Office Phone:** (813) 974-2926; **Board Certification:** Psychiatry 1977; **Medical School:** Univ Iowa Coll Med 1971; **Residencies:** Psychiatry, Univ Iowa, Iowa City, IA 1972-1974; Psychiatry, Univ Calif-Davis, Santa Barbara, CA 1974-1975; **Faculty Appointment:** Prof Psychiatry, Univ S Fla Coll Med

Midwest

Andersen, Arnold MD (Psychiatry) - *Special Expertise:* Eating Disorders; **Admitting Hospital:** University of Iowa Hospitals and Clinics; **Office Address:** Univ Iowa Hosp & Clin, Dept Psyc 200 Hawkins Dr, rm 2880 Iowa City, IA 52242-1057; **Office Phone:** (319) 356-1354; **Board Certification:** Psychiatry 1980; **Medical School:** Cornell Univ-Weil Med Coll 1968; **Residencies:** Psychiatry, NY Hosp, New York, NY 1969-1970; Psychiatry, Johns Hopkins Hosp, Baltimore, MD 1975-1976; **Fellowship:** Psychiatry, Natl Inst Mental Hlth, Bethesda, MD 1974-1975; **Faculty Appointment:** Prof Psychiatry, Univ Iowa Coll Med

Cloninger, C Robert MD (Psychiatry) - *Special Expertise:* Personality Disorders; **Admitting Hospital:** Barnes - Jewish Hospital; **Office Address:** Wash Univ Sch Med 660 S Euclid Ave, Box 8134 St Louis, MO 63110; **Office Phone:** (314) 362-7005; **Board Certification:** Psychiatry 1975; **Medical School:** Washington Univ, St Louis 1970; **Residencies:** Psychiatry, Barnes Hosp, St Louis, MO 1970-1973; Psychiatry, Renard Hosp, St Louis, MO 1970-1973; **Faculty Appointment:** Prof Psychiatry, Washington Univ, St Louis

Fawcett, Jan A MD (Psychiatry) - *Special Expertise:* Depression; **Admitting Hospital:** Rush/Presbyterian - St Luke's Medical Center - Chicago (Page 74); **Office Address:** Rush Presbyterian, Dept Psyc 1725 W Harrison St, Ste 955 Chicago, IL 60612; **Office Phone:** (312) 942-5372; **Board Certification:** Psychiatry 1967; **Medical School:** Yale Univ 1960; **Residencies:** Psychiatry, Langley Porter Inst, San Francisco, CA 1961-1963; Psychiatry, Rochester Med Ctr, Rochester, NY 1963-1964

Greden, John MD (Psychiatry) - *Special Expertise:* Anxiety & Mood Disorders; Depression; **Admitting Hospital:** University of Michigan Health Center; **Office Address:** U Mich Med Ctr, Dept of Psyc 1500 E Med Ctr Dr Ann Arbor, MI 48109-0704; **Office Phone:** (734) 763-9629; **Board Certification:** Psychiatry 1975; **Medical School:** Univ Minn 1967; **Residencies:** Psychiatry, Univ Minn Med Ctr, Minneapolis, MN 1968-1969; Psychiatry, Walter Reed AMC, Washington, DC 1970-1972; **Faculty Appointment:** Prof Psychiatry, Univ Mich Med Sch

Greist, John MD (Psychiatry) - *Special Expertise:* Anxiety & Mood Disorders; Behavioral Problems; Psychopharmacology; **Admitting Hospital:** University of Wisconsin Hospital & Clinics; **Office Address:** Healthcare Technology Systems 7617 Mineral Point Rd, Ste 300 Madison, WI 53717; **Office Phone:** (608) 827-2440; **Board Certification:** Psychiatry 1974; **Medical School:** Indiana Univ 1965; **Residencies:** Internal Medicine, Univ Wisc Hosp & Clin, Madison, WI 1966-1967; Psychiatry, Univ Wisc Hosp & Clin, Madison, WI 1967-1970; **Fellowship:** Child & Adolescent Psychiatry, Univ Wisc Hosp & Clin, Madison, WI 1970-1971; **Faculty Appointment:** Clin Prof Psychiatry, Univ Wisc

Janicak, Philip G. MD (Psychiatry) - *Special Expertise:* Psychopharmacology; Mood Disorders; **Admitting Hospital:** University of Illinois at Chicago Medical Center; **Office Address:** Univ IL at Chicago, Dept Psyc 1601 W Taylor St Chicago, IL 60612; **Office Phone:** (312) 413-4507; **Board Certification:** Psychiatry 1978; **Medical School:** Loyola Univ-Stritch Sch Med 1973; **Residency:** Psychiatry, McGaw Hosp/Loyola Med Ctr, Maywood, IL 1973-1976; **Faculty Appointment:** Prof Psychiatry, Univ IL Coll Med

Levine, Stephen B MD (Psychiatry) - *Special Expertise:* Sexual Dysfuction; Relationship Problems; **Admitting Hospital:** University Hospital - Cleveland; **Office Address:** 23230 Chagrin Blvd, Ste 350 Beachwood, OH 44122-5402; **Office Phone:** (216) 831-2900; **Board Certification:** Psychiatry 1976; **Medical School:** Case West Res Univ 1967; **Residency:** Psychiatry, Univ Hosps, Cleveland, OH 1970-1973; **Faculty Appointment:** Clin Prof Psychiatry, Case West Res Univ

Uhde, Thomas W MD (Psychiatry) - *Special Expertise:* Anxiety & Mood Disorders; Depression; **Admitting Hospital:** Harper Hospital (Page 59); **Office Address:** Wayne State Univ 540 E Canfield Detroit, MI 48201; **Office Phone:** (313) 577-9553; **Board Certification:** Psychiatry 1984; **Medical School:** Univ Louisville Sch Med 1975; **Residency:** Psychiatry, Yale-New Haven Hosp, New Haven, CT 1976-1979; **Fellowship:** Psychiatry, Natl Inst Mental Hlth, Bethesda, MD 1979-1981; **Faculty Appointment:** Prof Psychiatry, Wayne State Univ

Zorumski, Charles F MD (Psychiatry) - *Special Expertise:* Neuro-Psychiatry; Psychopharmacology; **Admitting Hospital:** Barnes - Jewish Hospital; **Office Address:** Wash Univ Sch Med, Dept Psyc 660 S Euclid Ave St Louis, MO 63110; **Office Phone:** (314) 747-2680; **Board Certification:** Psychiatry 1984; **Medical School:** St Louis Univ 1978; **Residency:** Psychiatry, Barnes-Jewish Hosp, St Louis, MO 1978-1982; **Faculty Appointment:** Prof Psychiatry, Washington Univ, St Louis

Great Plains and Mountains

Davidson, Joyce Eileen MD (Psychiatry) - *Special Expertise:* Obsessive-Compulsive Disorder; Bipolar/Mood Disorders; Schizophrenia; **Admitting Hospital:** Menninger Clinic; **Office Address:** Menninger Clinic Box 829 Topeka, KS 66601-0829; **Office Phone:** (785) 350-5635; **Board Certification:** Psychiatry 1988; **Medical School:** Univ MO-Kansas City 1979; **Residency:** Psychiatry, Karl Menninger Sch Psyc, Topeka, KS 1980-1982; **Fellowship:** Child & Adolescent Psychiatry, Karl Menninger Sch Psyc, Topeka, KS 1982-1984; **Faculty Appointment:** Prof Psychiatry, Karl Menninger Sch Psych

Gabbard, Glen O. MD (Psychiatry) - *Special Expertise:* Personality Disorders-Borderline; Cognitive Psychiatry; **Admitting Hospital:** Menninger Clinic; **Office Address:** Menninger Clinic 5800 SW 6th St, Box 829 Topeka, KS 66601; **Office Phone:** (785) 350-4161; **Board Certification:** Psychiatry 1979; **Medical School:** Rush Med Coll 1975; **Residency:** Psychiatry, Menninger Sch Psyc, Topeka, KS 1975-1978; **Fellowship:** Psychoanalysis, Topeka Inst Psychoan, Topeka, KS 1977-1984; **Faculty Appointment:** Clin Prof Psychiatry, Univ Kans

Menninger, W Walter MD (Psychiatry) - *Special Expertise:* Post Traumatic Stress Disorder; Forensic Psychiatry; **Admitting Hospital:** Menninger Clinic; **Office Address:** 5800 SW 6th St Topeka, KS 66606; **Office Phone:** (785) 350-5830; **Board Certification:** Psychiatry 1963; **Medical School:** Columbia P&S 1957; **Residency:** Psychiatry, Topeka State Hosp, Topeka, KS 1958-1960; **Fellowship:** Psychiatry, Menninger Fdn, Topeka, KS 1960-1961; **Faculty Appointment:** Prof Psychiatry, Karl Menninger Sch Psych

Mitchell, James Edward MD (Psychiatry) - *Special Expertise:* Eating Disorders; **Admitting Hospital:** MeritCare Hospital; **Office Address:** NeuroPsychological Research Inst 700 1st Ave S, Box 1415 Fargo, ND 58107-1415; **Office Phone:** (701) 293-1335; **Board Certification:** Psychiatry 1979; **Medical School:** Northwestern Univ 1972; **Residency:** Psychiatry, Fairview-Univ Med Ctr, Minneapolis, MN 1973-1976; **Faculty Appointment:** Prof Psychiatry, Univ ND Sch Med

Munich, Richard MD (Psychiatry) - *Special Expertise:* Psychotic Disorders; Psychoanalysis; Hospice Care; **Admitting Hospital:** Menninger Clinic; **Office Address:** Menninger Clinic Box 829 Topeka, KS 66601; **Office Phone:** (785) 350-5530; **Board Certification:** Psychiatry 1982; **Medical School:** Univ KY Coll Med 1965; **Residencies:** Psychiatry, Yale New Haven Hosp, New Haven, CT 1966-1967; Psychiatry, Yale Psych Inst, New Haven, CT 1968-1970

Zerbe, Kathryn J MD (Psychiatry) - *Special Expertise:* Eating Disorders; Women's Health-Mental Health; Psychoanalysis; **Admitting Hospital:** Menninger Clinic; **Office Address:** Menninger Clinic 5800 SE 6th Ave, Box 829 Topeka, KS 66601; **Office Phone:** (785) 350-5391; **Board Certification:** Psychiatry 1984; **Medical School:** Temple Univ 1978; **Residency:** Psychiatry, Menninger Clin, Topeka, KS 1978-1982; **Faculty Appointment:** Prof Psychiatry, Karl Menninger Sch Psych

Southwest

Altshuler, Kenneth Z. MD (Psychiatry) - *Special Expertise:* Psychotherapy; **Admitting Hospital:** Zale Lipshy University Hospital; **Office Address:** 5323 Harry Hines Blvd Dallas, TX 75390-9070; **Office Phone:** (214) 648-5555; **Board Certification:** Psychiatry 1961; **Medical School:** SUNY Buffalo 1952; **Residencies:** Psychiatry, Kings Co. Hosp, New York, NY 1952-1953; Psychiatry, VA Hosp, Bronx, NY 1955-1956; **Fellowship:** Psychiatry, NY Psychatric Inst., New York, NY 1956-1958; **Faculty Appointment:** Prof Psychiatry, Univ Tex SW, Dallas

Bowden, Charles MD (Psychiatry) - *Special Expertise:* Bipolar/Mood Disorders; **Admitting Hospital:** University of Texas Health & Science Center; **Office Address:** Univ Tex Hlth Sci Ctr 7703 Floyd Curl Dr San Antonio, TX 78284-7792; **Office Phone:** (210) 567-5390; **Board Certification:** Psychiatry 1970; **Medical School:** Baylor Coll Med 1964; **Residency:** Psychiatry, NY State Psyc Inst/Columbia-Presby Med Ctr, New York, NY 1965-1968; **Faculty Appointment:** Prof Psychiatry, Univ Tex, San Antonio

Hirschfeld, Robert, M A MD (Psychiatry) - *Special Expertise:* Mood Disorders; **Admitting Hospital:** University of Texas Health & Science Center; **Office Address:** Univ Tex Med Branch, Dept Psyc & Behav Scis 301 University Blvd Galveston, TX 77555-0429; **Office Phone:** (409) 772-4956; **Board Certification:** Psychiatry 1975; **Medical School:** Univ Mich Med Sch 1968; **Residency:** Psychiatry, Stanford Med Ctr, Stanford, CA 1969-1972; **Faculty Appointment:** Prof Psychiatry, Univ Tex Med Br, Galveston

Mohl, Paul C. MD (Psychiatry) - *Special Expertise:* Psychopharmacology; Psychotherapy; **Admitting Hospital:** Zale Lipshy University Hospital; **Office Address:** Univ Tex SW Ctr, Dept Psyc 5323 Harry Hines Blvd Dallas, TX 75390-9070; **Office Phone:** (214) 648-7365; **Board Certification:** Psychiatry 1977; **Medical School:** Duke Univ 1971; **Residency:** Psychiatry, Duke Hospital, Durham, NC 1971-1974; **Faculty Appointment:** Prof Psychiatry, Univ Tex SW, Dallas

Moore, Constance A. MD (Psychiatry) - *Special Expertise:* Sleep Disorders/Apnea; **Admitting Hospital:** Baylor University Medical Center; **Office Address:** VA Affairs Med Ctr 2002 Holcomb Blvd, MS 6C344 Houston, TX 77030; **Office Phone:** (713) 942-9779; **Board Certification:** Psychiatry 1991; **Medical School:** Baylor Coll Med 1980; **Residency:** Psychiatry, Baylor Medical College, Houston, TX 1984; **Faculty Appointment:** Assoc Prof Psychiatry, Baylor Coll Med

Rush Jr, Augustus John MD (Psychiatry) - *Special Expertise:* Mood Disorders; **Admitting Hospital:** Zale Lipshy University Hospital; **Office Address:** Univ Tex-SW Med Ctr 5323 Harry Hines Blvd Dallas, TX 75390-9086; **Office Phone:** (214) 648-4600; **Board Certification:** Psychiatry 1976; **Medical School:** Columbia P&S 1968; **Residency:** Psychiatry, Univ Penn, Philadelphia, PA 1972-1975; **Faculty Appointment:** Prof Psychiatry, Univ Tex SW, Dallas

Weiner, Myron MD (Psychiatry) - *Special Expertise:* Psychiatry-Geriatric; Alzheimer's Disease; **Admitting Hospital:** Zale Lipshy University Hospital; **Office Address:** UT Southwestern Med Ctr 5323 Harry Hines Blvd, Bldg NC6.102 Dallas, TX 75235-7208; **Office Phone:** (214) 648-5591; **Board Certification:** Psychiatry 1966; **Medical School:** Tulane Univ 1957; **Residency:** Psychiatry, Parkland Hosp, Dallas, TX 1960-1963; **Fellowship:** Geriatric Psychiatry, Mt Sinai Med Ctr, New York, NY 1984-1985; **Faculty Appointment:** Prof Psychiatry, Univ Tex SW, Dallas

Yager, Joel MD (Psychiatry) - *Special Expertise:* Eating Disorders; **Admitting Hospital:** University of New Mexico Hospital; **Office Address:** Univ NM Sch Med, Dept Psyc 2400 Tucker NE Albuquerque, NM 87131-5326; **Office Phone:** (505) 272-5416; **Board Certification:** Psychiatry 1971; **Medical School:** Albert Einstein Coll Med 1965; **Residency:** Psychiatry, Bronx Muni Hosp Ctr, New York, NY 1966-1969; **Faculty Appointment:** Prof Psychiatry, Univ New Mexico

West Coast and Pacific

Burt, Vivien Kleinman MD/PhD (Psychiatry) - *Special Expertise:* Women's Health-Mental Health; Impulse-Control Disorders; **Admitting Hospital:** UCLA Neuropsychiatric Hospital; **Office Address:** UCLA Neuropsyc Inst 300 UCLA Med Plaza, Ste 2337 Los Angeles, CA 90095; **Office Phone:** (310) 206-5135; **Board Certification:** Psychiatry 1990; **Medical School:** McGill Univ 1984; **Residency:** Psychiatry, UCLA-Neurpsyc Inst, Los Angeles, CA 1985-1988; **Faculty Appointment:** Assoc Prof Psychiatry, UCLA

Bystritsky, Alexander MD (Psychiatry) - *Special Expertise:* Obsessive-Compulsive Disorder; Anxiety Disorders; **Admitting Hospital:** UCLA Neuropsychiatric Hospital; **Office Address:** Department of Psychiatry 300 UCLA Med Plaza, Ste 2200 Los Angeles, CA 90095-8346; **Office Phone:** (310) 206-5133; **Board Certification:** Psychiatry 1988; **Medical School:** Russia 1977; **Residency:** Psychiatry, NYU Med Ctr, New York, NY 1981-1985; **Fellowship:** RW Johnson/UCLA Sch Med, Los Angeles, CA 1985-1987; **Faculty Appointment:** Assoc Clin Prof Psychiatry, UCLA

Dunner, David Louis MD (Psychiatry) - *Special Expertise:* Anxiety & Mood Disorders; Bipolar/Mood Disorders; **Admitting Hospital:** University of Washington Medical Center; **Office Address:** Ctr for Anxiety & Depression 4225 Roosevelt Way, Ste 306 Seattle, WA 98105-6099; **Office Phone:** (206) 221-3925; **Board Certification:** Psychiatry 1971; **Medical School:** Washington Univ, St Louis 1965; **Residency:** Psychiatry, Barnes Hosp- Wash, Seattle, WA 1966-1969; **Faculty Appointment:** Prof Psychiatry, Univ Wash

Eisendrath, Stuart James MD (Psychiatry) - *Special Expertise:* Depression; Munchausen Syndrome; **Admitting Hospital:** University of California - San Francisco Medical Center; **Office Address:** UCSF Med Ctr 401 Parnassus Ave, MC-0984 San Francisco, CA 94143; **Office Phone:** (415) 476-7868; **Board Certification:** Psychiatry 1980; **Medical School:** Med Coll Wisc 1974; **Residency:** Psychiatry, Langley Porter NPI, San Francisco, CA 1975-1978; **Fellowship:** Liason Psychiatry, Langley Porter NPI, San Francisco, CA 1978-1979; **Faculty Appointment:** Prof Psychiatry, UCSF

Gitlin, Michael Jay MD (Psychiatry) - *Special Expertise:* Mood Disorders; **Admitting Hospital:** UCLA Neuropsychiatric Hospital; **Office Address:** 300 UCLA Med Plaza, Box 2200 Los Angeles, CA 90095; **Office Phone:** (310) 206-6546; **Board Certification:** Psychiatry 1981; **Medical School:** Univ Penn 1975; **Residency:** Psychiatry, UCLA Med Ctr, Los Angeles, CA 1976-1979; **Faculty Appointment:** Prof Psychiatry, UCLA

Guilleminault, Christian MD (Psychiatry) - *Special Expertise:* Sleep Disorders; Sleep Aprea; **Admitting Hospital:** Stanford Medical Center; **Office Address:** Sleep Disorder Clinic-Stanford Univ Hosp 401 Quarry Rd, Bldg Pysch - Fl 3 - Ste 3301- Palo Alto, CA 94304; **Office Phone:** (650) 723-6601; **Medical School:** France 1968; **Faculty Appointment:** Prof Psych, Stanford University

Liberman, Robert Paul MD (Psychiatry) - *Special Expertise:* Schizophrenia; Psychotic Disorders; Psychiatric Rehabilitation; **Admitting Hospital:** UCLA Neuropsychiatric Hospital; **Office Address:** UCLA 300 Med Plaza, Ste 2263 Los Angeles, CA 90095; **Office Phone:** (310) 478-3711; **Board Certification:** Psychiatry 1969; **Medical School:** Johns Hopkins Univ 1963; **Residency:** Psychiatry, Mass Mental Health Ctr, Boston, MA 1964-1967; **Fellowships:** Psychiatry, Harvard Med Sch, Boston, MA 1966-1968; Psychiatry, UCSF, San Francisco, CA 1960-1961; **Faculty Appointment:** Prof Emeritus Psychiatry, UCLA

Marder, Stephen Robert MD (Psychiatry) - *Special Expertise:* Schizophrenia; Psychopharmacology; **Admitting Hospital:** VA Medical Center - West Los Angeles; **Office Address:** West Los Angeles VA - Gr LA Hlth Svcs 11301 Wilshire Blvd, Bldg MIRECC 210A Los Angeles, CA 90073; **Office Phone:** (310) 268-3647; **Board Certification:** Psychiatry 1977; **Medical School:** SUNY Buffalo 1971; **Residency:** Psychiatry, LAC-USC Med Ctr, Los Angeles, CA 1972-1975; **Faculty Appointment:** Prof Psychiatry, UCLA

Neppe, Vernon Michael MD (Psychiatry) - *Special Expertise:* Forensic Psychiatry; Neuro-Psychiatry; **Admitting Hospital:** Northwest Hospital; **Office Address:** 10330 Meridian Ave N, Ste 380 Seattle, WA 98133-9463; **Office Phone:** (206) 527-6289; **Board Certifications:** Geriatric Psychiatry 1991, Forensic Psychiatry 1994; **Medical School:** South Africa 1973; **Residency:** Psychiatry, Johannesburgh, South Africa 1976-1980; **Fellowship:** Psychiatry, NY Cornell Med Ctr, New York, NY 1982-1983; **Faculty Appointment:** Adjct Prof Psychiatry, St Louis Univ

Norman, Kim Peter MD (Psychiatry) - *Special Expertise:* Eating Disorders-Obesity; Schizophrenia; Personality Disorders; **Admitting Hospital:** University of California - San Francisco Medical Center; **Office Address:** UCSF-Langely Porter Psyc Inst 505 Parnassus Avenue San Francisco, CA 94143-6401; **Office Phone:** (415) 476-7402; **Board Certification:** Psychiatry 1983; **Medical School:** Albert Einstein Coll Med 1977; **Residency:** Psychiatry, Langley Porter Psyc Inst, San Francisco, CA 1978-1981; **Faculty Appointment:** Asst Prof Psychiatry, UCSF

Pi, Edmond Hsin-Tung MD (Psychiatry) - *Special Expertise:* Psychiatry - General; **Admitting Hospital:** LAC - King/Drew Medical Center; **Office Address:** Charles R Drew Univ Med & Sci 1731 E 120 St Los Angeles, CA 90059; **Office Phone:** (310) 668-4803; **Board Certification:** Psychiatry 1980; **Medical School:** South Korea 1972; **Residencies:** Psychiatry, SUNY-Stony Brook, Stony Brook, NY 1975-1977; Psychiatry, Univ KY Hosp-Chandler Med Ctr, Lexington, KY 1977-1978; **Faculty Appointment:** Prof Psychiatry, Charles Drew Univ Med & Sci

Pomer, Sydney Lawrence MD (Psychiatry) - *Special Expertise:* Psychoanalysis; **Admitting Hospital:** Cedars-Sinai Medical Center; **Office Address:** 430 S Bundy Dr Los Angeles, CA 90049; **Office Phone:** (310) 472-1580; **Board Certification:** Psychiatry 1953; **Medical School:** Univ Toronto 1941; **Residency:** Psychiatry, VA Hosp, Palo Alto, CA 1946-1947; **Fellowship:** Psychiatry, MT. Zion Hosp, San Francisco, CA 1947-1948; **Faculty Appointment:** Asst Clin Prof Univ SC Sch Med

Reus, Victor Ivar MD (Psychiatry) - *Special Expertise:* Alzheimer's Disease; Bipolar/Mood Disorders; **Admitting Hospital:** University of California - San Francisco Medical Center; **Office Address:** UCSF, Langley Porter NPI 401 Parnassus Ave San Francisco, CA 94143; **Office Phone:** (415) 476-7478; **Board Certifications:** Psychiatry 1977, Geriatric Psychiatry 1991; **Medical School:** Univ MD Sch Med 1973; **Residency:** Psychiatry, Univ of WI, Madison, WI 1973-1976; **Fellowship:** Psychiatry, NIMH, Bethesda, MD 1976-1978; **Faculty Appointment:** Prof Psychiatry, UCSF

PSYCHIATRY

West Coast and Pacific

Roy-Byrne, Peter MD (Psychiatry) - *Special Expertise:* Anxiety & Mood Disorders; Panic Disorder; **Admitting Hospital:** University of Washington Medical Center; **Office Address:** Harborview Med Ctr, Dept Psyc & Behav Scis 325 9th Ave, Box 359911 Seattle, WA 98104; **Office Phone:** (206) 731-3404; **Board Certification:** Psychiatry 1983; **Medical School:** Tufts Univ 1978; **Residency:** Psychiatry, UCLA NPI, Los Angeles, CA 1979-1982; **Fellowship:** Biological Psychiatry, Natl Inst Hlth, Bethesda, MD 1982-1984; **Faculty Appointment:** Prof Psychiatry, Univ Wash

Schatzberg, Alan F MD (Psychiatry) - *Special Expertise:* Anxiety & Mood Disorders; Psychopharmacology; **Admitting Hospital:** Stanford Medical Center; **Office Address:** Stanford Univ Sch Med, Dept Psy & Behav Scis 401 Quarry Rd Stanford, CA 94305-5717; **Office Phone:** (650) 723-6811; **Board Certification:** Psychiatry 1975; **Medical School:** NYU Sch Med 1968; **Residency:** Psychiatry, Mass Mental Hlth Ctr, Boston, MA 1969-1972; **Fellowship:** Psychiatry, Mass Mental Hlth Ctr/Harvard, Boston, MA 1969-1972; **Faculty Appointment:** Prof Psychiatry, Stanford Univ

Simpson, George M MD (Psychiatry) - *Special Expertise:* Schizophrenia; Depression; **Admitting Hospital:** LAC + USC Medical Center; **Office Address:** LAC + USC Med Ctr, Psychiatric Outpatient Clinic 1937 Hospital Pl, Bldg Grad Hall - rm 240 Los Angeles, CA 90033; **Office Phone:** (323) 226-5363; **Board Certification:** Psychiatry 1962; **Medical School:** England 1955; **Residencies:** Psychiatry, Royal Victoria Hosp-McGill Univ, Montreal, Canada 1956-1957; Psychiatry, Rockland State Hosp, Orangeburg, NY 1957-1959; **Faculty Appointment:** Prof Psychiatry, USC Sch Med

Spiegel, David MD (Psychiatry) - *Special Expertise:* Hypnosis; Psychiatry of Cancer; **Admitting Hospital:** Stanford Medical Center; **Office Address:** Stanford Univ Sch Med, Dept Psyc-Behav Scis PBS C231, MC-5718 Stanford, CA 94305-5718; **Office Phone:** (650) 723-6421; **Board Certification:** Psychiatry 1976; **Medical School:** Harvard Med Sch 1971; **Residencies:** Psychiatry, Mass Mntl Hlth Ctr-Harvard Med Sch, Boston, MA 1971-1974; Psychiatry, Cambridge Hosp-Harvard Med Sch, Boston, MA 1972-1974; **Fellowship:** Community Psychiatry, Harvard Med Sch, Boston, MA 1973-1974; **Faculty Appointment:** Prof Emeritus Psychiatry, Stanford Univ

Stein, Murray Brent MD (Psychiatry) - *Special Expertise:* Anxiety Disorders; Panic Disorder; Post Traumatic Stress Disorder; **Admitting Hospital:** VA Medical Affairs - San Diego HealthCare Center; **Office Address:** UCSD Sch Med 9500 Gilman Dr, MC-0985 LA Jolla, CA 92093-0985; **Office Phone:** (858) 622-6112; **Board Certification:** Psychiatry 1989; **Medical School:** Univ Manitoba 1983; **Residencies:** Psychiatry, Univ Toronto, Toronto, Canada 1985-1986; Psychiatry, Natl Inst Mental Hlth-NIH, Bethesda, MD 1986-1987; **Fellowship:** Anxiety Disorder, Natl Inst Mental Hlth-NIH, Bethesda, MD 1987-1989; **Faculty Appointment:** Prof Psychiatry, UCSD

Zisook, Sidney MD (Psychiatry) - *Special Expertise:* Bereavement/Traumatic Grief; Depression; **Admitting Hospital:** University of California - San Diego Healthcare; **Office Address:** UCSD, Dept Psyc 9500 Gilman Dr, MS 0603-R La Jolla, CA 92093; **Office Phone:** (858) 534-4040; **Board Certification:** Psychiatry 1975; **Medical School:** Loyola Univ-Stritch Sch Med 1969; **Residency:** Psychiatry, Mass Genl Hosp, Boston, MA 1970-1973; **Fellowship:** Psychiatry, Harvard Med Sch, Boston, MA 1970-1973; **Faculty Appointment:** Prof Psychiatry, UCSD

PULMONOLOGY

(a subspecialty of INTERNAL MEDICINE)

An internist who treats diseases of the lungs and airways. The pulmonologist diagnoses and treats cancer, pneumonia, pleurisy, asthma, occupational diseases, bronchitis, sleep disorders, emphysema and other complex disorders of the lungs.

INTERNAL MEDICINE

An internist is a personal physician who provides long-term, comprehensive care in the office and the hospital, managing both common and complex illness of adolescents, adults and the elderly. Internists are trained in the diagnosis and treatment of cancer, infections and diseases affecting the heart, blood, kidneys, joints and digestive, respiratory and vascular systems. They are also trained in the essentials of primary care internal medicine which incorporates an understanding of disease prevention, wellness, substance abuse, mental health and effective treatment of common problems of the eyes, ears, skin, nervous system and reproductive organs.

Training required: Three years in internal medicine *plus* additional training and examination for certification in pulmonary disease

PHYSICIAN LISTINGS

Pulmonary Disease

New England

Braman, Sidney MD (Pulmonary Disease) - *Special Expertise:* Asthma; **Admitting Hospital:** Rhode Island Hospital; **Office Address:** Rhode Island Hosp, Div Pulm 593 Eddy St Providence, RI 02903; **Office Phone:** (401) 444-8410; **Board Certifications:** Internal Medicine 1971, Pulmonary Disease 1972; **Medical School:** Temple Univ 1967; **Residency:** Internal Medicine, Philadelphia Genl Hosp, Philadelphia, PA 1968-1969; **Fellowship:** Pulmonary Disease, Univ Penn Med Ctr, Philadelphia, PA 1969-1970; **Faculty Appointment:** Assoc Prof Medicine, Brown Univ

Celli, Bartolome MD (Pulmonary Disease) - *Special Expertise:* Chronic Lung Disease (COPD); Mechanical Ventilation; Respiratory Failure; **Admitting Hospital:** St Elizabeth's Medical Center; **Office Address:** St Elizabeth Med Ctr, Dept Pulm 736 Cambridge St Boston, MA 02135; **Office Phone:** (617) 789-2545; **Board Certifications:** Pulmonary Disease 1978, Critical Care Medicine 1987; **Medical School:** Venezuela 1971; **Residencies:** Internal Medicine, St Vincent Hosp, Worcester, MA 1972-1973; Internal Medicine, Boston City Hosp, Boston, MA 1973-1976; **Fellowship:** Pulmonary Disease, Boston Univ Med Ctr, Boston, MA 1974-1977; **Faculty Appointment:** Prof Medicine, Tufts Univ

Christiani, David MD (Pulmonary Disease) - *Special Expertise:* Occupational Lung Disease; **Admitting Hospital:** Massachusetts General Hospital; **Office Address:** 55 Fruit St, BUL-148 Boston, MA 02115; **Office Phone:** (617) 726-9274; **Board Certifications:** Occupational Medicine 1984, Pulmonary Disease 1988; **Medical School:** Tufts Univ 1976; **Residencies:** Internal Medicine, Boston City Hosp, Boston, MA 1976-1979; Occupational Medicine, Harvard Sch Pub Health, Boston, MA 1979-1981; **Fellowship:** Pulmonary Disease, Mass Genl Hosp, Boston, MA 1985-1987; **Faculty Appointment:** Prof Medicine, Harvard Med Sch

Fanta, Christopher MD (Pulmonary Disease) - *Special Expertise:* Asthma; **Admitting Hospital:** Brigham & Women's Hospital; **Office Address:** Brigham & Women's Hosp, Dept Pulm & Crit Care Med 75 Francis St Boston, MA 02115; **Office Phone:** (617) 732-7420; **Board Certifications:** Pulmonary Disease 1980, Critical Care Medicine 1991; **Medical School:** Harvard Med Sch 1975; **Residency:** Internal Medicine, Peter Bent Brigham Hosp, Boston, MA 1976-1978; **Fellowship:** Pulmonary Disease, Peter Bent Brigham Hosp, Boston, MA 1978-1980; **Faculty Appointment:** Assoc Prof Medicine, Harvard Med Sch

Friedman, Lloyd Neal MD (Pulmonary Disease) - *Special Expertise:* Tuberculosis; Critical Care; **Admitting Hospital:** Milford Hospital; **Office Address:** Milford Hospital 300 Seaside Ave Milford, CT 06460; **Office Phone:** (203) 876-4288; **Board Certifications:** Pulmonary Disease 1988, Critical Care Medicine 1999; **Medical School:** Yale Univ 1979; **Residencies:** Internal Medicine, Beth Israel Med Ctr, New York, NY 1979-1980; Internal Medicine, Oregon Hlth Scis Univ, Portland, OR 1981-1983; **Fellowship:** Pulmonary Intensive Care, Yale-New Haven Hosp, New Haven, CT 1985-1988; **Faculty Appointment:** Assoc Clin Prof Medicine, Yale Univ

Irwin, Richard Stephen MD (Pulmonary Disease) - *Special Expertise:* Chronic Cough; Cardiac Respiratory Problems; **Admitting Hospital:** UMASS Memorial Health Care - Worcester; **Office Address:** 55 Lake Ave N Worcester, MA 01655; **Office Phone:** (508) 856-3121; **Board Certifications:** Critical Care Medicine 1997, Pulmonary Disease 1974; **Medical School:** Tufts Univ 1968; **Residency:** Internal Medicine, Tufts-New England Med Ctr, Boston, MA 1969-1970; **Fellowship:** Cardiac Respiratory Physiology, Columbia-Presby Hosp, New York, NY 1970-1972; **Faculty Appointment:** Prof Medicine, Univ Mass Sch Med

Mahler, Donald A MD (Pulmonary Disease) - *Special Expertise:* Chronic Lung Disease *(COPD);* **Admitting Hospital:** Dartmouth - Hitchcock Medical Center; **Office Address:** Dartmouth-Hitchcock Med Ctr 1 Medical Ctr Dr Lebanon, NH 03756-0001; **Office Phone:** (603) 650-5533; **Board Certifications:** Internal Medicine 1978, Pulmonary Disease 1980; **Medical School:** Loyola Univ-Stritch Sch Med 1972; **Residency:** Internal Medicine, Dartmouth-Hitchcock Med Ctr, Lebanon, NH 1975-1977; **Fellowship:** Pulmonary Disease, Yale-New Haven Hosp, New Haven, CT 1977-1980

Matthay, Richard (Pulmonary Disease) - *Special Expertise:* Lung Cancer; **Admitting Hospital:** Yale - New Haven Hospital; **Office Address:** Yale Univ Sch Med, Dept Int Med, Sec Pulm 333 Cedar St, rm 1051c, Box 208057 New Haven, CT 06520; **Office Phone:** (203) 785-4196; **Board Certifications:** Internal Medicine 1973, Pulmonary Disease 1976; **Medical School:** Tufts Univ 1970; **Residency:** Internal Medicine, Univ Colo Med Ctr, Denver, CO 1971-1973; **Fellowship:** Pulmonary Disease, Univ Colo Med Ctr, Denver, CO 1973-1975; **Faculty Appointment:** Prof Medicine, Yale Univ

Metersky, Mark Lewis MD (Pulmonary Disease) - *Special Expertise:* Pulmonary Infections; Asthma; **Admitting Hospital:** University of Connecticut Health Center; **Office Address:** Univ Conn Hlth Ctr 263 Farmington Ave Farmington, CT 06030; **Office Phone:** (860) 679-3343; **Board Certifications:** Pulmonary Disease 1992, Critical Care Medicine 1993; **Medical School:** NYU Sch Med 1985; **Residency:** Internal Medicine, Boston City Hosp, Boston, MA 1985-1988; **Fellowship:** Pulmonary Critical Care Medicine, UCSD Med Ctr, San Diego, CA 1989-1992; **Faculty Appointment:** Assoc Prof Medicine, Univ Conn

Nardell, Edward MD (Pulmonary Disease) - *Special Expertise:* Tuberculosis; **Admitting Hospital:** Cambridge Hospital; **Office Address:** Cambridge Hosp. 1493 Cambridge Street Cambridge, MA 02139; **Office Phone:** (617) 665-1029; **Board Certifications:** Internal Medicine 1975, Pulmonary Disease 1982; **Medical School:** Hahnemann Univ 1972; **Residency:** Internal Medicine, Hahnemann U Hosp., Philadelphia, PA 1973-1975; **Fellowship:** Pulmonary Disease, Mass Genl Hosp., Boston, MA 1975-1977; **Faculty Appointment:** Assoc Prof Medicine, Harvard Med Sch

Parsons, Polly E. MD (Pulmonary Disease) - *Special Expertise:* Critical Care; **Admitting Hospital:** Fletcher Allen - Healthcare; **Office Address:** Fletcher Allen Health Care / Patrick 310 1111 Colchester Ave Burlington, VT 05495; **Office Phone:** (802) 847-6177; **Board Certifications:** Pulmonary Disease 1986, Critical Care Medicine 1989; **Medical School:** Univ Ariz Coll Med 1978; **Residency:** Internal Medicine, Univ Colo Hosp, Denver, CO 1978-1981; **Fellowship:** Pulmonary Disease, Univ Colo Hosp, Denver, CO 1982-1983; **Faculty Appointment:** Prof Pulmonary Disease, Univ VT Coll Med

Redlich, Carrie MD (Pulmonary Disease) - *Special Expertise:* Occupational Lung Disease; **Admitting Hospital:** Yale - New Haven Hospital; **Office Address:** Yale Occup & Env Med Prog 135 College Street 3rd Flr New Haven, CT 06511; **Office Phone:** (203) 737-2817; **Board Certifications:** Occupational Medicine 1990, Pulmonary Disease 1990; **Medical School:** Yale Univ 1982; **Residencies:** Internal Medicine, Yale-New Haven Hosp, New Haven, CT 1984-1986; Occupational Medicine, Yale-New Haven Hosp, New Haven, CT 1986-1987; **Fellowship:** Pulmonary Disease, Univ Seattle, Seattle, WA 1987-1989; **Faculty Appointment:** Asst Prof Medicine, Yale Univ

Reilly Jr, John Joseph MD (Pulmonary Disease) - *Special Expertise: Transplant Medicine-Lung; Emphysema;* **Admitting Hospital:** Brigham & Women's Hospital; **Office Address:** Brigham & Women's Hosp, Dept Pulm-Crit Care 75 Francis St, Fl tw4B Boston, MA 02115; **Office Phone:** (617) 732-7420; **Board Certifications:** Pulmonary Disease 1986, Critical Care Medicine 1987; **Medical School:** Harvard Med Sch 1981; **Residency:** Internal Medicine, Brigham & Women's Hosp, Boston, MA 1982-1984; **Fellowship:** Pulmonary Disease, Brigham & Women's Hosp, Boston, MA 1984-1987; **Faculty Appointment:** Assoc Prof Medicine, Harvard Med Sch

Rochester, Carolyn MD (Pulmonary Disease) - *Special Expertise: Chronic Lung Disease (COPD);* **Admitting Hospital:** Yale - New Haven Hospital; **Office Address:** Yale Univ Sch Med, Dept Pulm & Crit Care 333 Cedar St New Haven, CT 06520; **Office Phone:** (203) 785-3207; **Board Certifications:** Critical Care Medicine 1991, Internal Medicine 1986; **Medical School:** Columbia P&S 1983; **Residency:** Internal Medicine, Columbia Presby Med Ctr, New York, NY 1984-1986; **Fellowship:** Pulmonary Disease, Colombia Presby Med Ctr, New York, NY 1986-1988; **Faculty Appointment:** Asst Prof Pulmonary Disease, Yale Univ

White, David P MD (Pulmonary Disease) - *Special Expertise: Sleep Disorders/Apnea;* **Admitting Hospital:** Brigham & Women's Hospital; **Office Address:** Brigham & Women's Hosp-Sleep Disorders Prog 221 Longwood Ave Boston, MA 02115; **Office Phone:** (617) 732-5778; **Board Certifications:** Pulmonary Disease 1982, Critical Care Medicine 1997; **Medical School:** Emory Univ 1975; **Residency:** Internal Medicine, Univ Colo Med Ctr, Denver, CO 1976-1978; **Fellowship:** Pulmonary Disease, Univ Colo Med Ctr, Denver, CO 1979-1982; **Faculty Appointment:** Assoc Prof Medicine, Harvard Med Sch

Mid Atlantic

Greenberg, Harly MD (Pulmonary Disease) - *Special Expertise: Sleep Disorders/Apnea; Critical Care;* **Admitting Hospital:** Long Island Jewish Medical Center; **Office Address:** Long Island Jewish Med Ctr 270-05 76th Ave New Hyde Park, NY 11040; **Office Phone:** (718) 470-7058; **Board Certifications:** Pulmonary Disease 1988, Critical Care Medicine 1989; **Medical School:** NYU Sch Med 1982; **Residency:** Internal Medicine, N Shore Univ Hosp, Manhasset, NY 1982-1985; **Fellowship:** Pulmonary Disease, NYU-Bellevue Hosp Ctr, New York, NY 1985-1987; **Faculty Appointment:** Assoc Prof Medicine, Albert Einstein Coll Med

Hansen-Flaschen, John MD (Pulmonary Disease) - *Special Expertise: Lung Injury; Wegener's Granulomatosis;* **Admitting Hospital:** Hospital of the University of Pennsylvania; **Office Address:** Hosp Univ PA, Dept Pulm and CCM 3400 Spruce St, Bldg 3 Radvin - Ste F Philadelphia, PA 19104; **Office Phone:** (215) 662-6003; **Board Certifications:** Pulmonary Disease 1982, Critical Care Medicine 1988; **Medical School:** NYU Sch Med 1976; **Residency:** Internal Medicine, Hosp Univ PA, Philadelphia, PA 1977-1980; **Fellowships:** Pulmonary Disease, Hosp Univ PA, Philadelphia, PA 1980-1981; Critical Care Medicine, Hosp Univ PA, Philadelphia, PA 1981-1982; **Faculty Appointment:** Prof Medicine, Univ Penn

Haponik, Edward Francis MD (Pulmonary Disease) - *Special Expertise: Sleep Disorders/Apnea; Critical Care;* **Admitting Hospital:** Johns Hopkins Medical Center - Bayview; **Office Address:** Johns Hopkins Univ, Div Pulm & Crit Care 600 N Wolfe St Baltimore, MD 21287; **Office Phone:** (410) 550-5864; **Board Certifications:** Internal Medicine 1977, Pulmonary Disease 1980; **Medical School:** Wake Forest Univ Sch Med 1974; **Residency:** Internal Medicine, N Carolina Bapt Hosp-Bowman Gray, Winston Salem, NC 1975; **Fellowship:** Pulmonary Disease, Johns Hopkins Sch Med, Baltimore, MD 1978-1980; **Faculty Appointment:** Prof Medicine, Johns Hopkins Univ

Kamholz, Stephan MD (Pulmonary Disease) - *Special Expertise:* AIDS/HIV; **Admitting Hospital:** University Hospital - Brooklyn; **Office Address:** SUNY Downstate Med Ctr, Dept Med 450 Clarkson Ave, Bldg UHB - Fl 6 - rm B6518, Box 50 Brooklyn, NY 11203-2012; **Office Phone:** (718) 270-2030; **Board Certifications:** Internal Medicine 1975, Critical Care Medicine 1987; **Medical School:** NY Med Coll 1972; **Residency:** Internal Medicine, Montefiore Hosp Med Ctr, Bronx, NY 1972-1975; **Fellowship:** Pulmonary Disease, Montefiore Hosp Med Ctr, Bronx, NY 1975-1977; **Faculty Appointment:** Prof Medicine, SUNY Hlth Sci Ctr

Libby, Daniel MD (Pulmonary Disease) - *Special Expertise:* Asthma; **Admitting Hospital:** New York Weill Cornell Medical Center - NY Presbyterian Hospital (Page 72); **Office Address:** 407 E 70th St New York, NY 10021; **Office Phone:** (212) 628-6611; **Board Certifications:** Internal Medicine 1977, Pulmonary Disease 1987; **Medical School:** Baylor Coll Med 1974; **Residency:** Internal Medicine, NY Hosp-Cornell Med Ctr, New York, NY 1974-1977; **Fellowship:** Pulmonary Disease, NY Hosp-Cornell Med Ctr, New York, NY 1977-1979; **Faculty Appointment:** Assoc Clin Prof Medicine, Cornell Univ-Weil Med Coll

Niederman, Michael MD (Pulmonary Disease) - *Special Expertise:* Infectious Disease-Lung; *Emphysema; Respiratory Failure & Pneumonia;* **Admitting Hospital:** Winthrop - University Hospital; **Office Address:** Pulmonary Assoc Mineola 222 Station Plaza N, Ste 400 Mineola, NY 11501-3893; **Office Phone:** (516) 663-2834; **Board Certifications:** Pulmonary Disease 1983, Critical Care Medicine 1987; **Medical School:** Boston Univ 1977; **Residency:** Internal Medicine, Northwestern Univ Med Ctr, Chicago, IL 1977-1980; **Fellowship:** Pulmonary Disease, Yale-New Haven Hosp, New Haven, CT 1980-1983; **Faculty Appointment:** Prof Medicine, SUNY Stony Brook

Pack, Allan I MD/PhD (Pulmonary Disease) - *Special Expertise:* Sleep Disorders & Aging; *Sleep Disorders/Apnea;* **Admitting Hospital:** Hospital of the University of Pennsylvania; **Office Address:** Hosp Univ Penn, Dept Sleep & Respiratory Neurobiology 991 Maloney Bldg/ 3600 Spruce Street Philadelphia, PA 19104-4283; **Office Phone:** (215) 662-3302; **Medical School:** Scotland 1967; **Residency:** Internal Medicine, Univ Glasgow, Scotland; **Fellowship:** Pulmonary Disease, Univ Glasgow, Scotland; **Faculty Appointment:** Prof Medicine, Univ Penn

Reichman, Lee Brodersohn MD (Pulmonary Disease) - *Special Expertise:* Tuberculosis; *Mycobacterial Infections;* **Admitting Hospital:** UMDNJ-University Hospital-Newark; **Office Address:** NJ Med Sch, Natl Tuberculosis Ctr 65 Bergen St, Ste GB1 Newark, NJ 07107-3001; **Office Phone:** (973) 972-3270; **Board Certifications:** Internal Medicine 1972, Pulmonary Disease 1972; **Medical School:** NYU Sch Med 1964; **Residencies:** Internal Medicine, Bellevue Hosp, New York, NY 1967-1968; Pulmonary Disease, Harlem Hosp, New York, NY 1969-1970; **Faculty Appointment:** Prof Medicine, UMDNJ-NJ Med Sch, Newark

Rogers, Robert M MD (Pulmonary Disease) - *Special Expertise:* Pulmonary Alveolar *Proteinosis;* **Admitting Hospital:** UPMC - Presbyterian University Hospital; **Office Address:** UPMC, Dept Pulm Dis, Allergy, & Crit Care 3459 5th Ave NW, rm 628, Box MUH Pittsburgh, PA 15203; **Office Phone:** (412) 692-2210; **Board Certifications:** Pulmonary Disease 1969, Critical Care Medicine 1999; **Medical School:** Univ Penn 1960; **Residencies:** Internal Medicine, Univ Hosps Cleveland, Cleveland, OH 1961-1963; Pulmonary Disease, Case West Res, Cleveland, OH 1963-1964; **Fellowships:** Pulmonary Disease, Univ Penn, Philadephia, PA 1964-1965; Physiology, Univ Penn, Philadelphia, PA 1966-1968; **Faculty Appointment:** Prof Medicine, Univ Pittsburgh

Rosen, Mark J MD (Pulmonary Disease) - *Special Expertise:* AIDS/HIV; Chronic Lung Disease (COPD); **Admitting Hospital:** Beth Israel Medical Center - New York; **Office Address:** Beth Israel Med Ctr, Pul and CC Med 1st Ave & 16th St New York, NY 10003; **Office Phone:** (212) 420-2697; **Board Certifications:** Pulmonary Disease 1980, Critical Care Medicine 1987; **Medical School:** Brown Univ 1975; **Residency:** Internal Medicine, Mount Sinai Hosp, New York, NY 1975-1978; **Fellowships:** Pulmonary Disease, Mount Sinai Hosp, New York, NY 1978-1980; Critical Care Medicine, St Vincent's Hosp & Med Ctr, New York, NY 1980; **Faculty Appointment:** Prof Medicine, Albert Einstein Coll Med

Schluger, Neil MD (Pulmonary Disease) - *Special Expertise:* Tuberculosis; Pulmonary Infections; **Admitting Hospital:** Columbia Presbyterian Medical Center (Page 72); **Office Address:** Columbia Univ Coll Phys & Surgeons 630 W 168th St, Fl VC, Box 12-206 New York, NY 10032; **Office Phone:** (212) 305-9817; **Board Certifications:** Pulmonary Disease 1992, Critical Care Medicine 1993; **Medical School:** Univ Penn 1985; **Residency:** Internal Medicine, St Luke's Roosevelt Hosp Ctr, New York, NY 1985-1989; **Fellowship:** Pulmonary Critical Care Medicine, NY Hosp-Cornell Med Ctr, New York, NY 1989-1992; **Faculty Appointment:** Assoc Prof Medicine, Columbia P&S

Smith, James P MD (Pulmonary Disease) - *Special Expertise:* Emphysema; Lung Cancer; **Admitting Hospital:** New York Weill Cornell Medical Center - NY Presbyterian Hospital (Page 72); **Office Address:** 170 E 77th St New York, NY 10021; **Office Phone:** (212) 879-2180; **Board Certifications:** Internal Medicine 1967, Pulmonary Disease 1968; **Medical School:** Georgetown Univ 1960; **Residencies:** Internal Medicine, NY Hosp-Cornell Med Ctr, New York, NY 1960-1962; Internal Medicine, NY Hosp-Cornell Med Ctr, New York, NY 1964-1965; **Fellowship:** Pulmonary Disease, NY Hosp-Cornell Med Ctr, New York, NY 1964-1966; **Faculty Appointment:** Clin Prof Medicine, Cornell Univ-Weil Med Coll

Steiger, David MD (Pulmonary Disease) - *Special Expertise:* Critical Care; **Admitting Hospital:** Hospital for Joint Diseases; **Office Address:** 305 2nd Ave, Ste 16 New York, NY 10003; **Office Phone:** (212) 598-6091; **Board Certifications:** Pulmonary Disease 1992, Critical Care Medicine 1995; **Medical School:** England 1981; **Residency:** Internal Medicine, St Luke's Roosevelt Hosp Ctr, New York, NY 1984-1989; **Fellowship:** Pulmonary Disease, UCSF Med Ctr, San Francisco, CA 1989-1994; **Faculty Appointment:** Asst Prof Medicine, NYU Sch Med

Steinberg, Harry MD (Pulmonary Disease) - *Special Expertise:* Emphysema; Lung Cancer; **Admitting Hospital:** Long Island Jewish Medical Center; **Office Address:** Long Island Jewish Med Ctr, Dept Med 270-05 76th Ave New Hyde Park, NY 11040; **Office Phone:** (718) 470-7231; **Medical School:** Temple Univ 1966; **Residencies:** Temple Univ Hosp, Philadelphia, PA; Long Island Jewish, New Hyde Park, NY 1962; **Fellowships:** Critical Care Medicine, Long Island Jewish, New Hyde Park, NY 1967-1969; Hosp of U Penn, Philadelphia, PA 1972-1974; **Faculty Appointment:** Prof Medicine, Albert Einstein Coll Med

Stover-Pepe, Diane E MD (Pulmonary Disease) - *Special Expertise:* Lung Cancer; AIDS/HIV; Infectious Disease-Lung; **Admitting Hospital:** Memorial Sloan Kettering Cancer Center; **Office Address:** 1275 York Ave, Fl C678 New York, NY 10021; **Office Phone:** (212) 639-8380; **Board Certifications:** Internal Medicine 1975, Pulmonary Disease 1978; **Medical School:** Albert Einstein Coll Med 1970; **Residencies:** Internal Medicine, Harlem Hosp Ctr, New York, NY 1971-1972; Internal Medicine, NY Hosp-Cornell Med Ctr, New York, NY 1974-1975; **Fellowship:** Pulmonary Disease, Albert Einstein Med Ctr, Bronx, NY 1975; **Faculty Appointment:** Prof Medicine, Cornell Univ-Weil Med Coll

Teirstein, Alvin MD (Pulmonary Disease) - *Special Expertise: Sarcoidosis; Interstitial Lung Disease;* **Admitting Hospital:** Mount Sinai Hospital (Page 70); **Office Address:** 5 E 98th St, Fl 10 New York, NY 10029; **Office Phone:** (212) 241-5656; **Board Certifications:** Internal Medicine 1961, Pulmonary Disease 1969; **Medical School:** SUNY Downstate 1953; **Residency:** Internal Medicine, Mt Sinai Med Ctr, New York, NY 1955-1957; **Fellowships:** Pulmonary Disease, Mt Sinai Med Ctr, New York, NY 1953-1954; Pulmonary Disease, VA Med Ctr/nyu/bellevue, Bronx, NY 1954-1956; **Faculty Appointment:** Prof Medicine, Mount Sinai Sch Med

Terry, Peter Browne MD (Pulmonary Disease) - *Special Expertise: Pulmonary Disease - General;* **Admitting Hospital:** Johns Hopkins Hospital - Baltimore (Page 65); **Office Address:** Johns Hopkins Hosp 600 N Wolfe St Baltimore, MD; **Office Phone:** (410) 955-3467; **Board Certifications:** Internal Medicine 1973, Pulmonary Disease 1976; **Medical School:** St Louis Univ 1968; **Residencies:** Internal Medicine, Univ Conn Hlth Ctr, Farmington, CT 1969-1970; Internal Medicine, Johns Hopkins Hosp, Baltimore, MD 1972-1973; **Fellowships:** Pulmonary Disease, Johns Hopkins Hosp, Baltimore, MD 1973-1974; Pulmonary Disease, Mayo Clinic, Rochester, MN 1974-1975; **Faculty Appointment:** Prof Medicine, Johns Hopkins Univ

Thomashow, Byron MD (Pulmonary Disease) - *Special Expertise: Emphysema; Asthma;* **Admitting Hospital:** Columbia Presbyterian Medical Center (Page 72); **Office Address:** 161 Fort Washington Ave New York, NY 10032; **Office Phone:** (212) 305-5261; **Board Certifications:** Internal Medicine 1977, Pulmonary Disease 1980; **Medical School:** Columbia P&S 1974; **Residencies:** Internal Medicine, St Luke's-Roosevelt Hosp Ctr, New York, NY 1974-1977; Pulmonary Disease, St Luke's-Roosevelt Hosp Ctr, New York, NY 1977-1978; **Fellowship:** Pulmonary Disease, Harlem Hosp Ctr, New York, NY 1978-1979; **Faculty Appointment:** Assoc Clin Prof Medicine, Columbia P&S

Tino, Gregory MD (Pulmonary Disease) - *Special Expertise: Lung Volume Reduction; Chronic Lung Disease (COPD); Interstitial Lung Disease;* **Admitting Hospital:** Hospital of the University of Pennsylvania; **Office Address:** Univ Penn Med Ctr, Pulmonary & Critical Care Div 831 West Gates Bldg Philadelphia, PA 19104; **Office Phone:** (215) 349-5303; **Board Certifications:** Pulmonary Disease 1992, Critical Care Medicine 1995; **Medical School:** Mount Sinai Sch Med 1986; **Residency:** Internal Medicine, Hosp Univ Penn, Philadelphia, PA 1986-1989; **Fellowship:** Pulmonary Critical Care Medicine, Hosp Univ Penn, Philadelphia, PA 1989-1992; **Faculty Appointment:** Asst Prof Medicine, Univ Penn

White, Dorothy MD (Pulmonary Disease) - *Special Expertise: Lung Cancer; AIDS/HIV;* **Admitting Hospital:** Memorial Sloan Kettering Cancer Center; **Office Address:** 1275 York Ave, rm C671 New York, NY 10021; **Office Phone:** (212) 639-8022; **Board Certifications:** Pulmonary Disease 1984, Critical Care Medicine 1987; **Medical School:** SUNY Hlth Sci Ctr 1977; **Residency:** Pulmonary Disease, NY Hosp-Cornell Med Ctr, New York, NY 1977-1981; **Fellowship:** Pulmonary Disease, Yale-New Haven Hosp, New Haven, CT 1982-1984; **Faculty Appointment:** Assoc Prof Medicine, Cornell Univ-Weil Med Coll

Southeast

Bayly, Timothy C MD (Pulmonary Disease) - *Special Expertise: Pulmonary Disease - General;* **Admitting Hospital:** Fairfax Hospital; **Office Address:** Virginia Medical Alliance 5510 Alma Lane, Ste 300 Springfield, VA 22151; **Office Phone:** (703) 642-5990; **Board Certifications:** Internal Medicine 1975, Pulmonary Disease 1976; **Medical School:** Georgetown Univ 1972; **Residency:** Internal Medicine, Cornell Univ Med Coll, New York, NY 1974-1975; **Fellowship:** Pulmonary Disease, Georgetown Univ Hosp, Washington, DC 1975-1976; **Faculty Appointment:** Asst Clin Prof Medicine, Georgetown Univ

Brooks, Stuart M MD (Pulmonary Disease) - *Special Expertise: Occupational Lung Disease;* **Admitting Hospital:** Tampa General Hospital; **Office Address:** USF Coll Pub Hlth 13201 Bruce B Downs Blvd, Box 56 MDC Tampa, FL 33612-3805; **Office Phone:** (813) 974-6626; **Board Certifications:** Internal Medicine 1977, Pulmonary Disease 1969; **Medical School:** Univ Cincinnati 1962; **Residency:** Internal Medicine, Boston City Hosp, Boston, MA 1963-1967; **Fellowship:** Pulmonary Disease, Boston City Hosp, Boston, MA 1967-1969; **Faculty Appointment:** Prof Occupational Medicine, Univ S Fla Coll Med

Christman, Brian Wallace MD (Pulmonary Disease) - *Special Expertise: Pulmonary Hypertension; Lung Injury;* **Admitting Hospital:** Vanderbilt University Medical Center; **Office Address:** Vanderbilt Univ Med Ctr, Div Pulm Med 1161 21st Ave S, rm T1217 Nashville, TN 37232-2650; **Office Phone:** (615) 322-2386; **Board Certifications:** Internal Medicine 1984, Critical Care Medicine 1999; **Medical School:** Univ Okla Coll Med 1981; **Residency:** Internal Medicine, Vanderbilt Univ Med Ctr, Nashville, TN 1982-1984; **Fellowship:** Pulmonary Disease, Vanderbilt Univ Med Ctr, Nashville, TN 1984-1987; **Faculty Appointment:** Assoc Prof Medicine, Vanderbilt Univ

Cicale, Michael Jon MD (Pulmonary Disease) - *Special Expertise: Pulmonary Disease - General;* **Admitting Hospital:** Shands Healthcare at University Florida (Page 77); **Office Address:** Shands Healthcare at Univ FL 1600 SW Archer Rd, Box 100255 Gainesville, FL 32610-0225; **Office Phone:** (352) 392-2666; **Board Certifications:** Internal Medicine 1982, Pulmonary Disease 1984; **Medical School:** Georgetown Univ 1979; **Residency:** Internal Medicine, Univ FL Med Ctr, Gainesville, FL 1979-1982; **Fellowship:** Pulmonary Disease, Univ FL Med Ctr, Gainesville, FL 1982-1984; **Faculty Appointment:** Assoc Prof Medicine, Univ Fla Coll Med

Cooper, John Allen Dicks MD (Pulmonary Disease) - *Special Expertise: Drug Induced Lung Disease;* **Admitting Hospital:** University of Alabama Hospital at Birmingham; **Office Address:** 215 Pinsley Harrison Tower 1900 University Blvd Birmingham, AL 35233; **Office Phone:** (205) 934-7941; **Board Certifications:** Pulmonary Disease 1984, Critical Care Medicine 1999; **Medical School:** Duke Univ 1978; **Residency:** Internal Medicine, Univ VA, Charlottesville, VA 1979-1981; **Fellowship:** Pulmonary Disease, Yale Univ, New Haven, CT 1981-1985; **Faculty Appointment:** Prof Medicine, Univ Ala

Cooper, William MD (Pulmonary Disease) - *Special Expertise: Critical Care;* **Admitting Hospital:** Sentara Virginia Beach General Hospital; **Office Address:** Pulm Med VA Beach Inc 1008 First Colonial Rd, Ste 103 Virginia Beach, VA 23454; **Office Phone:** (757) 481-2515; **Board Certifications:** Internal Medicine 1972, Pulmonary Disease 1974; **Medical School:** Univ VA Sch Med 1969; **Residencies:** Internal Medicine, Univ VA Hosp, Richmond, VA 1971-1972; Pulmonary Disease, Univ VA Hosp, Richmond, VA 1972-1973; **Fellowship:** Pulmonary Disease, Mount Sinai Med Ctr, Miami Beach, FL 1973-1974

Donohue, James MD (Pulmonary Disease) - *Special Expertise: Asthma; Chronic Lung Disease; Sarcoidosis;* **Admitting Hospital:** University of North Carolina Hospitals; **Office Address:** Univ N. Carolina, Chapel Hill Sch Med, Div Pulm Dis & CCM 420 Burnett-Wolmack Bldg CB#7020, MC-CB#7020 Chapel Hill, NC 27599-7020; **Office Phone:** (919) 966-2531; **Board Certifications:** Internal Medicine 1975, Pulmonary Disease 1976; **Medical School:** UMDNJ-NJ Med Sch, Newark 1969; **Residencies:** UMDNJ, Newark, NJ 1970-1971; NC Meml Hosp, Chapel Hill, NC 1973-1974; **Fellowship:** Pulmonary Disease, Univ NC, Chapel Hill, NC 1974-1976; **Faculty Appointment:** Prof Medicine, Univ NC Sch Med

PULMONARY DISEASE

Southeast

Dunlap, Nancy Elizabeth MD/PhD (Pulmonary Disease) - *Special Expertise:* Tuberculosis; Critical Care; **Admitting Hospital:** University of Alabama Hospital at Birmingham; **Office Address:** 2000 6th Ave S, Fl 4 Birmingham, AL 35233; **Office Phone:** (205) 934-9876; **Board Certifications:** Pulmonary Disease 1988, Critical Care Medicine 1999; **Medical School:** Duke Univ 1981; **Residency:** Internal Medicine, Univ Ala, Birmingham, AL 1982-1984; **Fellowship:** Pulmonary Disease, Univ Ala, Birmingham, AL 1984-1987; **Faculty Appointment:** Prof Medicine, Univ Ala

Enelow, Richard Ian MD (Pulmonary Disease) - *Special Expertise:* Interstitial Lung Disease; Inflammatory Lung Disease; **Admitting Hospital:** University of Virginia Health Systems; **Office Address:** Univ VA Hlth Scis Ctr, Div Pulm & Crit Care Hosp Dr, Fl 6th - rm 6590 Charlottesville, VA 22908; **Office Phone:** (804) 924-5270; **Board Certifications:** Internal Medicine 1986, Pulmonary Disease 2002; **Medical School:** Boston Univ 1983; **Residency:** Internal Medicine, New Eng-Deaconess Med Ctr, Boston, MA 1984-1986; **Fellowship:** Pulmonary Disease, Univ VA Hlth Scis Ctr, Charlottesville, VA 1989-1992; **Faculty Appointment:** Assoc Prof Pulmonary Disease, Univ VA Sch Med

Fletcher, Eugene MD (Pulmonary Disease) - *Special Expertise:* Chronic Lung Disease (COPD); Pulmonary Disease; **Admitting Hospital:** University of Louisville Hospital; **Office Address:** Univ Louisville Sch Med 530 S Jackson St, A3L01 Louisville, KY 40292; **Office Phone:** (502) 852-5841; **Board Certifications:** Pulmonary Disease 1980, Critical Care Medicine 1987; **Medical School:** Temple Univ 1971; **Residencies:** Internal Medicine, Univ Colo Affil Hosp, Denver, CO 1972-1973; Internal Medicine, Fitzsimons Army Med Ctr, Denver, CO 1973-1974; **Fellowship:** Pulmonary Disease, Univ Okla Hlth Scis Ctr, Oklahoma City, OK; **Faculty Appointment:** Prof Medicine, Univ Louisville Sch Med

Fulkerson Jr, William J MD (Pulmonary Disease) - *Special Expertise:* Respiratory Failure-Acute; Thromboembolic Disorders; **Admitting Hospital:** Duke University Medical Center (Page 60); **Office Address:** Duke Univ Med Ctr Box 3121 Durham, NC 27710; **Office Phone:** (919) 684-8076; **Board Certifications:** Pulmonary Disease 1984, Critical Care Medicine 1996; **Medical School:** Univ NC Sch Med 1977; **Residency:** Internal Medicine, Vanderbilt Univ Hosp, Nashville, TN 1977-1980; **Fellowship:** Pulmonary Disease, Vanderbilt Univ Hosp, Nashville, TN 1981-1983; **Faculty Appointment:** Prof Medicine, Duke Univ

Goldman, Allan Larry MD (Pulmonary Disease) - *Special Expertise:* Occupational Lung Disease; Airway Disorders; **Admitting Hospital:** Tampa General Hospital; **Office Address:** USF Coll Med, Internal Med 12901 Bruce B Downs Blvd, Box MDC19 Tampa, FL 33612-4799; **Office Phone:** (813) 974-2271; **Board Certifications:** Pulmonary Disease 1972, Internal Medicine 1972; **Medical School:** Univ Minn 1968; **Residency:** Internal Medicine, Brooke Army Hosp, San Antonio, TX 1969-1970; **Fellowship:** Pulmonary Disease, Walter Reed Army Hosp, Washington, DC 1970-1972; **Faculty Appointment:** Prof Medicine, Univ S Fla Coll Med

Harman, Eloise M MD (Pulmonary Disease) - *Special Expertise:* Pulmonary Disease - General; **Admitting Hospital:** Shands Healthcare at University Florida (Page 77); **Office Address:** Shands Healthcare at Univ of FL 1600 SW Archer Rd, Box 100225 Gainesville, FL 32610-0225; **Office Phone:** (352) 392-2666; **Board Certifications:** Pulmonary Disease 1976, Critical Care Medicine 1997; **Medical School:** Johns Hopkins Univ 1970; **Residency:** Internal Medicine, Johns Hopkins Hosp, Baltimore, MD 1970-1972; **Fellowship:** Pulmonary Disease, NY Hosp-Cornell Med Ctr, New York, NY 1972-1974; **Faculty Appointment:** Prof Medicine, Univ Fla Coll Med

698

Haynes, Johnson MD (Pulmonary Disease) - *Special Expertise: Pulmonary Disease - General;* **Admitting Hospital:** University of South Alabama Medical Center; **Office Address:** Univ S AL Med Ctr 2451 Fillingim St Mobile, AL 36617; **Office Phone:** (334) 471-7888; **Board Certifications:** Internal Medicine 1983, Pulmonary Disease 1986; **Medical School:** Univ S Ala Coll Med 1980; **Residency:** Internal Medicine, Univ S AL Med Ctr, Mobile, AL 1981-1983; **Fellowship:** Pulmonary Disease, Univ S AL Med Ctr, Mobile, AL 1984-1986; **Faculty Appointment:** Prof Medicine, Univ S Ala Coll Med

Heffner, John E MD (Pulmonary Disease) - *Special Expertise: Critical Care;* **Admitting Hospital:** MUSC Medical Center; **Office Address:** Med Univ SC, Dept Pulm Med 96 Jonathan Lucas St, Fl 812, Box 250623 Charleston, SC 29425; **Office Phone:** (843) 792-2153; **Board Certifications:** Pulmonary Disease 1982, Critical Care Medicine 1987; **Medical School:** UCLA 1974; **Residency:** Internal Medicine, Univ Colo Med Ctr, Denver, CO 1973-1978; **Faculty Appointment:** Prof Medicine, Med Univ SC

Henke, David Carroll MD (Pulmonary Disease) - *Special Expertise: Asthma;* **Admitting Hospital:** University of North Carolina Hospitals; **Office Address:** Univ NC Med Sch-Chapel Hill, Dept Pulm Dis rm 420, Box 7020 Chapel Hill, NC 27599-7020; **Office Phone:** (919) 966-2531; **Board Certifications:** Pulmonary Disease 1988, Critical Care Medicine 1991; **Medical School:** Univ NC Sch Med 1977; **Residencies:** Internal Medicine, NC Memorial Hosp, Chapel Hill, NC 1978-1980; Dermatology, NC Meml NIEHS, Chapel Hill, NC 1982-1984; **Fellowship:** Pulmonary Disease, NC Memorial Hosp, Chapel Hill, NC 1984-1987; **Faculty Appointment:** Assoc Prof Medicine, Univ NC Sch Med

Johnson, Bruce Ellsworth (Pulmonary Disease) - *Special Expertise: Sleep Disorders/Apnea;* **Admitting Hospital:** Sentara Virginia Beach General Hospital; **Office Address:** 1008 First Colonial Rd Ste 103 Virginia Beach, VA; **Office Phone:** (757) 481-2515; **Board Certifications:** Pulmonary Disease 1986, Critical Care Medicine 1991; **Medical School:** Med Coll GA 1978; **Fellowship:** Pulmonary Disease, U Va, Charlottesville, VA 1981-1983

Koenig, Steven Michael MD (Pulmonary Disease) - *Special Expertise: Sleep Disorders/Apnea; Occupational Lung Disease;* **Admitting Hospital:** University of Virginia Health Systems; **Office Address:** Univ of VA Hlth Sci Ctr 100 Lee St W, Fl 6 - rm 6594, Box 800546 Charlottesville, VA 22908; **Office Phone:** (804) 924-2228; **Board Certifications:** Pulmonary Disease 1990, Critical Care Medicine 1991; **Medical School:** Univ Penn 1984; **Residency:** Internal Medicine, Univ Chicago, Chicago, IL 1984-1987; **Fellowship:** Pulmonary Critical Care Medicine, Univ Chicago, Chicago, IL 1987-1990; **Faculty Appointment:** Asst Prof Pulmonary Disease, Univ VA Sch Med

Light, Richard Wayne MD (Pulmonary Disease) - *Special Expertise: Pleural Disease;* **Admitting Hospital:** St Thomas Hospital - Nashville; **Office Address:** St Thomas Hosp 4220 Harding Rd Nashville, TN 37205; **Office Phone:** (615) 222-4445; **Board Certifications:** Internal Medicine 1972, Pulmonary Disease 1974; **Medical School:** Johns Hopkins Univ 1968; **Residency:** Internal Medicine, Johns Hopkins Hosp, Baltimore, MD 1969-1970; **Fellowship:** Pulmonary Disease, Johns Hopkins Hosp, Baltimore, MD 1970-1972; **Faculty Appointment:** Prof Medicine, Vanderbilt Univ

Lorusso, Thomas MD (Pulmonary Disease) - *Special Expertise: Critical Care;* **Admitting Hospital:** Fairfax Hospital; **Office Address:** 1800 Town Ctr Dr, Ste 419 Reston, VA 20190; **Office Phone:** (703) 620-3926; **Board Certifications:** Pulmonary Disease 1992, Critical Care Medicine 1993; **Medical School:** SUNY Syracuse 1987; **Residency:** Internal Medicine, Univ Hosp - SUNY, Stony Brook, NY 1988-1990; **Fellowship:** Pulmonary Disease, Cedars Sinai Med Ctr, Los Angeles, CA 1990-1993

PULMONARY DISEASE

Loyd, James Emory MD (Pulmonary Disease) - *Special Expertise:* Transplant Medicine-Lung; Interstitial Lung Disease; Pulmonary Fibrosis; **Admitting Hospital:** Vanderbilt University Medical Center; **Office Address:** Vanderbilt Univ Med Ctr, Div Pulm Med Med Ctr North, rm T-1217 Nashville, TN 37232; **Office Phone:** (615) 322-2386; **Board Certifications:** Pulmonary Disease 1984, Critical Care Medicine 1997; **Medical School:** W VA Univ 1973; **Residency:** Internal Medicine, Vanderbilt Univ Hosp, Nashville, TN; **Fellowship:** Pulmonary Disease, Vanderbilt Univ Hosp, Nashville, TN; **Faculty Appointment:** Prof Medicine, Vanderbilt Univ

MacIntyre, Neil Ross MD (Pulmonary Disease) - *Special Expertise:* Pulmonary Rehabilitation; Pulmonary Function Testing; **Admitting Hospital:** Duke University Medical Center (Page 60); **Office Address:** Duke Univ Med Ctr 400 Erwin Road Box 3911 Durham, NC 27710-0001; **Office Phone:** (919) 681-2720; **Board Certifications:** Internal Medicine 1975, Pulmonary Disease 1980; **Medical School:** Cornell Univ-Weil Med Coll 1972; **Residency:** Internal Medicine, NY Hosp-Cornell, New York, NY 1973-1975; **Fellowship:** Pulmonary Disease, UCSF Med Ctr, San Francisco, CA 1978-1981; **Faculty Appointment:** Prof Medicine, Duke Univ

O'Brien, Richard MD (Pulmonary Disease) - *Special Expertise:* Tuberculosis; **Admitting Hospital:** Grady Health System; **Office Address:** Chief of Rsch & Evaluation Br, TB Div CDC Ms E-10 1600 Clifton Rd NE Atlanta, GA 30333; **Office Phone:** (404) 639-8123; **Board Certifications:** Pulmonary Disease 1978, Public Health & General Preventive Medicine 1980; **Medical School:** Univ VA Sch Med 1969; **Residency:** Internal Medicine, Emory U-Grady Meml Hosp., Atlanta, GA 1972-1974; **Fellowship:** Pulmonary Disease, Emory U-Grady Meml Hosp., Atlanta, GA 1977-1978; **Faculty Appointment:** Asst Clin Prof Medicine, Emory Univ

Sahn, Steven A. MD (Pulmonary Disease) - *Special Expertise:* Pleural Disease; Asthma; **Admitting Hospital:** MUSC Medical Center; **Office Address:** MUSC, Dept Pulmonary Med 96 Jonathan Lucas St, Box 250623 Charleston, SC 19425; **Office Phone:** (843) 792-3167; **Board Certifications:** Pulmonary Disease 1974, Critical Care Medicine 1974; **Medical School:** Univ Louisville Sch Med 1968; **Residency:** Internal Medicine, Univ Iowa Hosp, Iowa City, IA 1968-1971; **Fellowship:** Pulmonary Disease, Univ Colorado Hlth Sci, Denver, CO 1971-1973; **Faculty Appointment:** Prof Medicine, Univ SC Sch Med

Schwartz, David A MD (Pulmonary Disease) - *Special Expertise:* Occupational Lung Disease; Pulmonary Fibrosis; Asthma; **Admitting Hospital:** Duke University Medical Center (Page 60); **Office Address:** Duke Univ Med Ctr PO Box 2629 Durham, NC 27710; **Office Phone:** (919) 668-0380; **Board Certifications:** Occupational Medicine 1987, Pulmonary Disease 1988; **Medical School:** UCSD 1979; **Residency:** Internal Medicine, Boston City Hosp, Boston, MA 1981-1984; **Fellowships:** Occupational Medicine, Harvard Sch Pub Hlth, Boston, MA 1984-1986; Pulmonary Disease, Univ of Seattle, Seattle, WA 1985-1988; **Faculty Appointment:** Asst Prof Medicine, Univ Iowa Coll Med

Shure, Deborah MD (Pulmonary Disease) - *Special Expertise:* Pulmonary Hypertension; Sarcoidosis; **Admitting Hospital:** University Hospital & Clinics- Mississippi; **Office Address:** Univ Miss Med Ctr, Dept Pulm 2500 N State St Jackson, MS 39216; **Office Phone:** (601) 984-5650; **Board Certifications:** Internal Medicine 1976, Pulmonary Disease 1980; **Medical School:** Albert Einstein Coll Med 1973; **Residencies:** Internal Medicine, Bellevue Hosp, New York, NY 1973-1976; Internal Medicine, Bellevue Hosp, New York, NY 1976-1977; **Fellowship:** Pulmonary Disease, UCSD Med Ctr, San Diego, CA 1977-1980; **Faculty Appointment:** Prof Medicine, Univ Miss

Sweet, Michael MD (Pulmonary Disease) - *Special Expertise:* Pulmonary Disease - General; **Admitting Hospital:** Martin Memorial Health System; **Office Address:** 1100 E Ocean Blvd Pulmonary Associates Stuart, FL 34996-2590; **Office Phone:** (561) 283-4428; **Board Certifications:** Internal Medicine 1977, Pulmonary Disease 1980; **Medical School:** Univ Miami Sch Med 1974; **Residency:** Internal Medicine, U South FL Hosp, Tampa, FL 1975-1977; **Fellowship:** Pulmonary Disease, U South Fl Hosp, Tampa, FL 1977-1979

Tapson, Victor MD/PhD (Pulmonary Disease) - *Special Expertise:* Pulmonary Vascular Disease; Thromboembolic Disorders; **Admitting Hospital:** Duke University Medical Center (Page 60); **Office Address:** Duke University Med Ctr, Dept PUL Critical Care Med Box 3822 Durham, NC 37715; **Office Phone:** (919) 684-6237; **Board Certifications:** Pulmonary Disease 1989, Internal Medicine 1986; **Medical School:** Hahnemann Univ 1982; **Residency:** Internal Medicine, Duke Univ Med Ctr, Durham, NC 1982-1986; **Fellowship:** Critical Care Obstetrics, Boston Univ, Boston, MA 1986-1989; **Faculty Appointment:** Assoc Clin Prof Medicine, Duke Univ

Vaughey, Ellen MD (Pulmonary Disease) - *Special Expertise:* Critical Care; **Admitting Hospital:** Inova Fairfax Hospital; **Office Address:** North Virginia Pulm-Critical Care Assoc 3289 Woodburn Rd, Ste 350 Annandale, VA 22003; **Office Phone:** (703) 641-8616; **Board Certifications:** Internal Medicine 1990, Pulmonary Disease 1992; **Medical School:** Georgetown Univ 1987; **Residency:** Internal Medicine, Thomas Jefferson Univ, Philadelphia, PA 1990; **Fellowship:** Pulmonary Disease, Roger Williams Hosp-Brown Univ, Prividence, RI 1993

Wanner, Adam MD (Pulmonary Disease) - *Special Expertise:* Asthma; **Admitting Hospital:** University of Miami - Jackson Memorial Hospital; **Office Address:** Univ Miami Sch Med, Div Pulm & Crit Care Box 016960 (R-47) Miami, FL 33140-2800; **Office Phone:** (305) 243-6387; **Board Certifications:** Internal Medicine 1973, Pulmonary Disease 1974; **Medical School:** Switzerland 1966; **Residency:** Internal Medicine, Kantonsspital Aarau, Switzerland 1968-1970; **Fellowship:** Pulmonary Disease, Mt Sinai Med Ctr, Miami Beach, FL 1970-1972; **Faculty Appointment:** Prof Medicine, Univ Miami Sch Med

Wunderink, Richard MD (Pulmonary Disease) - *Special Expertise:* Infectious Disease-Lung; **Admitting Hospital:** Methodist Health Care North - Memphis; **Office Address:** Univ Tenn Med Grp Heart Lung Ctr 930 Madison, Ste 850 Memphis, TN 38104; **Office Phone:** (901) 726-8078; **Board Certifications:** Pulmonary Disease 1986, Critical Care Medicine 1987; **Medical School:** Indiana Univ 1980; **Residency:** Internal Medicine, Butterworth Hosp, Grand Rapids, MI 1981-1983; **Fellowship:** Pulmonary Disease, Henry Ford Hosp, Detroit, MI 1983-1985; **Faculty Appointment:** Assoc Clin Prof Pulmonary Disease, Univ Tenn Coll Med, Memphis

Young, Keith Randall MD (Pulmonary Disease) - *Special Expertise:* Transplant Medicine-Lung; **Admitting Hospital:** University of Alabama Hospital at Birmingham; **Office Address:** Univ AL Sch Med, 215 Tinsley Harrison Tower 1900 University Blvd Birmingham, AL 35294; **Office Phone:** (205) 934-5400; **Board Certifications:** Pulmonary Disease 1986, Allergy & Immunology 1987; **Medical School:** Jefferson Med Coll 1978; **Residencies:** Internal Medicine, Yale-New Haven Hosp, New Haven, CT 1979-1982; Pulmonary Disease, Yale-New Haven Hosp, New Haven, CT 1982-1985; **Fellowship:** Allergy & Immunology, Nat Inst Hlth, Bethesda, MD 1985-1988; **Faculty Appointment:** Prof Medicine, Univ Ala

Midwest

Antony, Veena B. MD (Pulmonary Disease) - *Special Expertise:* Pleural Disease; **Admitting Hospital:** Indiana University Hospital & Medical Center - Indianapolis; **Office Address:** 926 W Michigan Street Indianapolis, IN 46202-5203; **Office Phone:** (317) 274-8660; **Board Certifications:** Internal Medicine 1979, Pulmonary Disease 1982; **Medical School:** India 1974; **Residencies:** Pulmonary Disease, Univ Co Hlth Sci Ctr; Pulmonary Disease, Natl Jewish Hosp-Asthma Ctr; **Fellowship:** Internal Medicine, Kingsbrook Jewish Med Ctr

Arroliga, Alejandro C MD (Pulmonary Disease) - *Special Expertise:* Pulmonary Hypertension; **Admitting Hospital:** Cleveland Clinic Foundation; **Office Address:** Cleveland Clinic Fdn, Dept Pulm & Crit Care 9500 Euclid Ave, Ste A-90 Cleveland, OH 44195; **Office Phone:** (216) 445-5765; **Board Certifications:** Pulmonary Disease 1992, Critical Care Medicine 1993; **Medical School:** Mexico 1984; **Residency:** Internal Medicine, Coney Island Hosp, Brooklyn, NY 1988-1990; **Fellowship:** Pulmonary Disease, Yale-New Haven Hosp, New Haven, CT 1990-1993

Balk, Robert MD (Pulmonary Disease) - *Special Expertise:* Asthma; Emphysema; **Admitting Hospital:** Rush/Presbyterian - St Luke's Medical Center - Chicago (Page 74); **Office Address:** 1725 W Harrison St, Bldg 3 - rm 054 Chicago, IL 60612; **Office Phone:** (312) 942-6744; **Board Certifications:** Pulmonary Disease 1986, Critical Care Medicine 1987; **Medical School:** Univ MO-Kansas City 1978; **Residency:** Internal Medicine, Univ MO-Kansas City Affil Hosps, Kansas City, MO 1978-1981; **Fellowship:** Pulmonary Intensive Care, Univ Arkansas, Little Rock, AR 1981-1983; **Faculty Appointment:** Prof Medicine, Rush Med Coll

Cromydas, George MD (Pulmonary Disease) - *Special Expertise:* Emphysema; Lung Disease; **Admitting Hospital:** Advocate Lutheran General Hospital; **Office Address:** North Shore Lung Specialists, SC 1614 W Central Rd, Ste 205 Arlington Heights, IL 60005; **Office Phone:** (847) 818-1184; **Board Certifications:** Pulmonary Disease 1984, Critical Care Medicine 1989; **Medical School:** Univ IL Coll Med 1977; **Residency:** Internal Medicine, Univ IL Hosp & Clin, Chicago, IL 1977-1980; **Fellowship:** Pulmonary Critical Care Medicine, Univ IL Hosp & Clin, Chicago, IL 1980-1982

Fahey, Patrick J MD (Pulmonary Disease) - *Special Expertise:* Lung Disease; **Admitting Hospital:** Loyola University Health System; **Office Address:** Loyola Univ Med Ctr 2160 S 1st Ave Maywood, IL 60153; **Office Phone:** (708) 216-3300; **Board Certifications:** Pulmonary Disease 1978, Critical Care Medicine 1989; **Medical School:** Univ Wisc 1973; **Residency:** Internal Medicine, St Elizabeth's Hosp, Boston, MA 1973-1976; **Fellowships:** Pulmonary Disease, St Elizabeth's Hosp, Boston, MA 1976-1977; Pulmonary Disease, Strong Meml, Rochester, NY 1977-1980; **Faculty Appointment:** Prof Medicine, Loyola Univ-Stritch Sch Med

Geppert, Eugene MD (Pulmonary Disease) - *Special Expertise:* Cystic Fibrosis; Asthma; **Admitting Hospital:** University of Chicago Hospitals (Page 78); **Office Address:** 5758 S Maryland Ave, Module 5D Chicago, IL 60637; **Office Phone:** (773) 702-9660; **Board Certifications:** Pulmonary Disease 1978, Critical Care Medicine 1987; **Medical School:** Yale Univ 1974; **Residency:** Internal Medicine, Univ Chicago Hosps, Chicago, IL 1975-1976; **Fellowship:** Pulmonary Disease, UCSF Med Ctr, San Francisco, CA 1976-1979; **Faculty Appointment:** Asst Prof Medicine, Univ Chicago-Pritzker Sch Med

Glassroth, Jeffrey MD (Pulmonary Disease) - *Special Expertise:* Pulmonary Fibrosis; AIDS/HIV & Tuberculosis; Infectious Disease-Lung; **Admitting Hospital:** University of Wisconsin Hospital & Clinics; **Office Address:** 600 Highland Ave Madison, WI 53792; **Office Phone:** (608) 631-1792; **Board Certifications:** Pulmonary Disease 1980, Critical Care Medicine 1989; **Medical School:** Univ Cincinnati 1973; **Residency:** Internal Medicine, Univ Cincinnati Med Ctr, Cincinnati, OH 1974-1978; **Fellowship:** Pulmonary Disease, Boston Univ Med Ctr, Boston, MA 1978-1981; **Faculty Appointment:** Prof Pulmonary Disease, Univ Wisc

Gracey, Douglas Robert MD (Pulmonary Disease) - *Special Expertise:* Respiratory Failure; Chronic Lung Disease (COPD); **Admitting Hospital:** Mayo Medical Center & Clinic - Rochester; **Office Address:** Mayo Clinic 200 1st St SW Rochester, MN 55905; **Office Phone:** (507) 284-2495; **Board Certifications:** Pulmonary Disease 1970, Internal Medicine 1969; **Medical School:** Northwestern Univ 1962; **Residency:** Internal Medicine, Mayo Grad Sch Med, Rochester, MN 1963-1966; **Fellowship:** Pulmonary Disease, Mayo Grad Sch Med, Rochester, MN 1968-1969; **Faculty Appointment:** Prof Medicine, Mayo Med Sch

Grum, Cyril M MD (Pulmonary Disease) - *Special Expertise:* Asthma; Cystic Fibrosis; **Admitting Hospital:** University of Michigan Health Center; **Office Address:** Univ Michigan Med Ctr - Taubman Hlth Care Ctr 1500 E Medical Center Dr, rm 3110-TC, Box 0368 Ann Arbor, MI 48109; **Office Phone:** (734) 936-5549; **Board Certifications:** Pulmonary Disease 1982, Internal Medicine 1980; **Medical School:** Med Coll Wisc 1977; **Residency:** Internal Medicine, Cleveland Clinic, Cleveland, OH; **Fellowship:** Pulmonary Disease, Univ Michigan Hosps, Ann Arbor, MI; **Faculty Appointment:** Prof Univ Mich Med Sch

Hall, Jesse MD (Pulmonary Disease) - *Special Expertise:* Respiratory Failure; Critical Care; **Admitting Hospital:** University of Chicago Hospitals (Page 78); **Office Address:** Ctr Advanced Medicine 5758 S Maryland Ave Chicago, IL 60637; **Office Phone:** (773) 702-6239; **Medical School:** Univ Chicago-Pritzker Sch Med 1977; **Residency:** Internal Medicine, Univ Chicago Hosps, Chicago, IL 1978-1982; **Faculty Appointment:** Prof Pulmonary Disease, Univ Chicago-Pritzker Sch Med

Hunninghake, Gary MD (Pulmonary Disease) - *Special Expertise:* Sarcoidosis; Interstitial Lung Disease; **Admitting Hospital:** University of Iowa Hospitals and Clinics; **Office Address:** Univ IA Hosps & Clinics, Dept of Pulm 200 Hawkins Dr, C33G-GH Iowa City, IA 52242; **Office Phone:** (319) 356-4187; **Board Certifications:** Critical Care Medicine 1989, Pulmonary Disease 1980; **Medical School:** Univ Kans 1972; **Residencies:** Internal Medicine, Univ of KS Med Sch, Kansas City, KS 1972-1974; Pulmonary Disease, Natl Inst Hlth, Bethesda, MD 1974-1976; **Faculty Appointment:** Prof Medicine, Univ Iowa Coll Med

Hyers, Thomas Morgan MD (Pulmonary Disease) - *Special Expertise:* Thromboembolic Disorders; **Admitting Hospital:** St Louis University Hospital; **Office Address:** 533 Couch Ave, Ste 140 St Louis, MO 63122; **Office Phone:** (314) 909-9779; **Board Certifications:** Pulmonary Disease 1980, Critical Care Medicine 1999; **Medical School:** Duke Univ 1968; **Residencies:** Internal Medicine, Univ Wash Med Ctr, Seattle, WA 1972-1975; Pulmonary Disease, Univ Hosp, Denver, CO 1975-1977; **Fellowship:** Pulmonary Disease, Natl Inst Hlth, Bethesda, MD 1969-1972; **Faculty Appointment:** Prof Medicine, St Louis Univ

Kaye, Mitchell MD (Pulmonary Disease) - *Special Expertise:* Chronic Lung Disease (COPD); Asthma; Sleep Disorders/Apnea; **Admitting Hospital:** Fairview-University Medical Center - University Campus; **Office Address:** 920 E 28th St, Ste 700 Minneapolis, MN 55407; **Office Phone:** (612) 863-3750; **Board Certifications:** Pulmonary Disease 1990, Critical Care Medicine 1991; **Medical School:** Univ Minn 1984; **Residency:** Internal Medicine, Univ IL Hosps & Clins, Chicago, IL 1984-1987; **Fellowship:** Pulmonary Disease, Northwestern Univ Med Sch, Chicago, IL 1987-1989

Kollef, Marin Hristo MD (Pulmonary Disease) - *Special Expertise:* Critical Care; Infectious Disease-Lung; **Admitting Hospital:** Barnes - Jewish Hospital; **Office Address:** 216 Kings Hwy St Louis, MO 63110; **Office Phone:** (314) 454-8764; **Board Certifications:** Pulmonary Disease 1988, Critical Care Medicine 1991; **Medical School:** Univ Rochester 1983; **Residency:** Internal Medicine, Madigan Army Med Ctr, Tacoma, WA 1984-1986; **Fellowship:** Pulmonary Disease, Madigan Army Med Ctr, Tacoma, WA 1986

Krowka, Michael Joseph MD (Pulmonary Disease) - *Special Expertise:* Hepatopulmonary Syndrome; **Admitting Hospital:** Mayo Medical Center & Clinic - Rochester; **Office Address:** Mayo Clinic 200 1st St SW Rochester, MN 55905; **Office Phone:** (507) 284-2921; **Board Certifications:** Internal Medicine 1983, Pulmonary Disease 1986; **Medical School:** Univ Nevada 1980; **Residency:** Internal Medicine, Evanston Hosp, Chicago, IL 1981-1983; **Fellowship:** Pulmonary Disease, Mayo Clinic, Rochester, MN 1983-1986; **Faculty Appointment:** Prof Pulmonary Disease, Mayo Med Sch

Lefrak, Stephen MD (Pulmonary Disease) - *Special Expertise:* Lung Volume Reduction; **Admitting Hospital:** Barnes - Jewish Hospital; **Office Address:** 4960 Children's Pl, Ste 4 St Louis, MO 63110; **Office Phone:** (314) 362-6044; **Board Certifications:** Pulmonary Disease 1972, Critical Care Medicine 1987; **Medical School:** SUNY Downstate 1965; **Residencies:** Internal Medicine, Boston Univ Hosp, Boston, MA 1967-1968; Pulmonary Disease, Kings Co Hosp Ctr, Brooklyn, NY 1968-1969; **Fellowship:** Cardiopulmonary Disease, Columbia-Presby Hosp, New York, NY 1969-1970

Lynch, Joseph P MD (Pulmonary Disease) - *Special Expertise:* Lung Transplant Care; Interstitial Lung Disease; Pulmonary Fibrosis; **Admitting Hospital:** University of Michigan Health Center; **Office Address:** Taubman Hlth Care Ctr 1500 E Medical Ctr Dr Ann Arbor, MI 48109-0360; **Office Phone:** (734) 647-9342; **Board Certifications:** Internal Medicine 1976, Pulmonary Disease 1980; **Medical School:** Harvard Med Sch 1973; **Residency:** Internal Medicine, Univ Mich Med Ctr, Ann Arbor, MI 1974-1976; **Fellowship:** Pulmonary Disease, Univ Mich Med Ctr, Ann Arbor, MI 1976-1978; **Faculty Appointment:** Prof Pulmonary Disease, Univ Mich Med Sch

Marini, John Joseph MD (Pulmonary Disease) - *Special Expertise:* Critical Care; **Admitting Hospital:** Regions Hospital - St Paul; **Office Address:** St Paul Ramsey Med Ctr 640 Jackson St St Paul, MN 55101-2502; **Office Phone:** (651) 221-3135; **Board Certifications:** Pulmonary Disease 1978, Critical Care Medicine 1987; **Medical School:** Johns Hopkins Univ 1973; **Residency:** Internal Medicine, Univ Wash Med Ctr, Seattle, WA 1974-1976; **Fellowship:** Pulmonary Disease, Univ Wash Med Ctr, Seattle, WA 1976-1978; **Faculty Appointment:** Prof Medicine, Univ Minn

Martinez, Fernando J MD (Pulmonary Disease) - *Special Expertise:* Pulmonary Disease; Critical Care; **Admitting Hospital:** University of Michigan Health Center; **Office Address:** 1500 E Med Ctr Dr 3916 Taubman Center Ann Arbor, MI 48109; **Office Phone:** (734) 936-5201; **Board Certifications:** Internal Medicine 1986, Critical Care Medicine 1999; **Medical School:** Univ Fla Coll Med 1983; **Residency:** Internal Medicine, Beth Israel Hosp, Boston, MA 1984-1986; **Fellowship:** Pulmonary Disease, Boston Univ, Boston, MA 1986-1989; **Faculty Appointment:** Prof Medicine, Univ Mich Med Sch

Maurer, Janet Rae MD (Pulmonary Disease) - *Special Expertise:* Transplant Medicine-Lung; **Admitting Hospital:** Cleveland Clinic Foundation; **Office Address:** Cleveland Clinic Foundation 9500 Euclid Ave Desk A90 Cleveland, OH 44195; **Office Phone:** (216) 444-6505; **Board Certifications:** Internal Medicine 1979, Pulmonary Disease 1982; **Medical School:** Univ Minn Residency: Internal Medicine, Emory Univ Hosp, Atlanta, GA 1977-1979; **Fellowship:** Pulmonary Disease, UCSD Med Ctr, San Diego, CA 1979-1981

Mehta, Atul Chandrakant MD (Pulmonary Disease) - *Special Expertise:* Transplant Medicine-Lung; Lung Volume Reduction; **Admitting Hospital:** Cleveland Clinic Foundation; **Office Address:** Cleveland Clinic Foundation 9500 Euclid Ave, Ste A-90 Cleveland, OH 44195; **Office Phone:** (216) 444-2911; **Board Certifications:** Pulmonary Disease 1984, Critical Care Medicine 1991; **Medical School:** India 1976; **Residencies:** Internal Medicine, St Francis Med Ctr, Trenton, NJ 1978-1980; Internal Medicine, Easton Hosp, Trenton, NJ 1980-1981; **Fellowship:** Pulmonary Disease, Cleveland Clin, Cleveland, OH 1981-1983; **Faculty Appointment:** Assoc Prof Medicine, Ohio State Univ

Popovich Jr, John MD (Pulmonary Disease) - *Special Expertise:* Lung Disease; Critical Care; **Admitting Hospital:** Henry Ford Health System (Page 62); **Office Address:** 2799 W Grand Blvd Detroit, MI 48202; **Office Phone:** (313) 916-1828; **Board Certifications:** Critical Care Medicine 1996, Pulmonary Disease 1980; **Medical School:** Univ Mich Med Sch 1975; **Residency:** Internal Medicine, Henry Ford Hosp, Detroit, MI 1975-1978; **Fellowship:** Pulmonary Disease, Henry Ford Hosp, Detroit, MI 1978-1980; **Faculty Appointment:** Asst Clin Prof Medicine, Univ Mich Med Sch

Prakash, Udaya MD (Pulmonary Disease) - *Special Expertise:* Bronchoscopy; **Admitting Hospital:** Mayo Medical Center & Clinic - Rochester; **Office Address:** Mayo Clinic 200 First St SW Rochester, MN 55905; **Office Phone:** (507) 284-4162; **Board Certifications:** Internal Medicine 1987, Pulmonary Disease 1976; **Medical School:** India 1969; **Residency:** Internal Medicine, Mayo Clin, Rochester, MN 1972-1973; **Fellowship:** Pulmonary Disease, Mayo Clin, Rochester, MN 1974-1976; **Faculty Appointment:** Prof Medicine, Mayo Med Sch

Silver, Michael MD (Pulmonary Disease) - *Special Expertise:* Chronic Lung Disease (COPD); **Admitting Hospital:** Rush/Presbyterian - St Luke's Medical Center - Chicago (Page 74); **Office Address:** Rush-Presby-St Luke's Med Ctr 1725 W Harrison St, Bldg 3 - rm 054 Chicago, IL 60612; **Office Phone:** (312) 942-6744; **Board Certifications:** Pulmonary Disease 1988, Critical Care Medicine 1999; **Medical School:** Albany Med Coll 1981; **Residency:** Internal Medicine, Rush-Presby-St Luke's Med Ctr, Chicago, IL 1981-1985; **Fellowship:** Pulmonary Critical Care Medicine, Rush-Presby-St Luke's Med Ctr, Chicago, IL 1985-1987; **Faculty Appointment:** Assoc Prof Medicine, Rush Med Coll

Stoller, James MD (Pulmonary Disease) - *Special Expertise:* Emphysema/Alpha-1 Antitrypsin Deficiency; **Admitting Hospital:** Cleveland Clinic Foundation; **Office Address:** 9500 Euclid Ave, rm A-90 Cleveland, OH 44195; **Office Phone:** (216) 444-1960; **Board Certifications:** Pulmonary Disease 1984, Internal Medicine 1982; **Medical School:** Yale Univ 1979; **Residency:** Internal Medicine, Peter Bent Brigham Hosp, Boston, MA 1980-1982; **Fellowship:** Pulmonary Disease, Brigham & Women's Hosp, Boston, MA 1982-1983

Tobin, Martin MD (Pulmonary Disease) - *Special Expertise:* Mechanical Ventilation; Chronic Lung Disease (COPD); **Admitting Hospital:** Loyola University Health System; **Office Address:** Loyola Univ Med Ctr, Dept Pulm & Critical Care 2160 S First Ave Maywood, IL 60153; **Office Phone:** (708) 202-2715; **Board Certifications:** Pulmonary Disease 1984, Critical Care Medicine 1987; **Medical School:** Ireland 1975; **Residencies:** Internal Medicine, Trinity Coll Hosps, Dublin, Ireland 1976-1979; Pulmonary Disease, Kings Coll Hosp, London, England 1979-1980; **Fellowships:** Pulmonary Critical Care Medicine, Mount Sinai Hosp, New York, NY 1980-1982; Pulmonary Critical Care Medicine, Univ Pittsburgh, Pittsburgh, PA 1982-1983; **Faculty Appointment:** Prof Medicine, Loyola Univ-Stritch Sch Med

Trulock, Elbert MD (Pulmonary Disease) - *Special Expertise: Transplant Medicine-Lung; Emphysema;* **Admitting Hospital:** Barnes - Jewish Hospital; **Office Address:** Wash Univ Sch Med, Dept Pulm 660 S Euclid Ave, Box 8052 St Louis, MO 63110; **Office Phone:** (314) 362-5409; **Board Certifications:** Internal Medicine 1981, Pulmonary Disease 1984; **Medical School:** Emory Univ 1978; **Residency:** Internal Medicine, Barnes Hosp, St Louis, MO 1978-1981; **Fellowship:** Pulmonary Disease, Wash Univ Med Ctr, St Louis, MO 1981-1983; **Faculty Appointment:** Assoc Prof Medicine, Washington Univ, St Louis

Wiedemann, Herbert P MD (Pulmonary Disease) - *Special Expertise: Interstitial Lung Disease; Critical Care;* **Admitting Hospital:** Cleveland Clinic Foundation; **Office Address:** Cleveland Clin Fdn 9500 Euclid Ave, Desk A90 Cleveland, OH 44195; **Office Phone:** (216) 444-8335; **Board Certifications:** Pulmonary Disease 1984, Critical Care Medicine 1987; **Medical School:** Cornell Univ-Weil Med Coll 1977; **Residencies:** Internal Medicine, Univ Wash Hosps, Seattle, WA 1977-1980; Internal Medicine, Harborview Hosp, Seattle, WA 1980-1981; **Fellowship:** Pulmonary Disease, Yale Univ Sch Med, New Haven, CT 1981-1984

Great Plains and Mountains

Brown, Kevin K MD (Pulmonary Disease) - *Special Expertise: Interstitial Lung Disease; Autoimmune Lung Disease;* **Admitting Hospital:** National Jewish Medical & Research Center; **Office Address:** Natl Jewish Med & Rsch Ctr 1400 Jackson St, rm F108 Denver, CO 80206; **Office Phone:** (303) 398-1621; **Board Certifications:** Internal Medicine 1989, Pulmonary Disease 1992; **Medical School:** Univ Minn 1984; **Residency:** Internal Medicine, Providence Med Ctr, Portland, OR 1986-1989; **Fellowships:** Pulmonary Disease, Maine Med Ctr, Portland, ME 1990-1992; Pulmonary Disease, Univ Colo Hlth Scis Ctr, Denver, CO 1992-1994; **Faculty Appointment:** Asst Prof Medicine, Univ Colo

Elliott, Charles Gregory MD (Pulmonary Disease) - *Special Expertise: Pulmonary Hypertension; Thromboembolic Disorders;* **Admitting Hospital:** LDS Hospital; **Office Address:** LDS Hosp, Dept Pulm 325 8th Ave Salt Lake City, UT 84143; **Office Phone:** (801) 408-1875; **Board Certifications:** Internal Medicine 1976, Pulmonary Disease 1978; **Medical School:** Univ MD Sch Med 1973; **Residency:** Internal Medicine, Univ Utah, Salt Lake City, UT 1976-1978; **Fellowship:** Pulmonary Disease, Univ MD Hosp, Baltimore, MD 1974-1976; **Faculty Appointment:** Prof Medicine, Univ Utah

Harmon, Gary MD (Pulmonary Disease) - *Special Expertise: Pulmonary Disease - General;* **Admitting Hospital:** Overland Park Regional Medical Center; **Office Address:** 10550 Quivira, Ste 480 Overland Park, KS 66215; **Office Phone:** (913) 599-3800; **Board Certifications:** Pulmonary Disease 1986, Critical Care Medicine 1989; **Medical School:** Univ Kans 1981; **Residencies:** Pulmonary Disease, Univ Kansas Med Ctr, Kansas City, KS; Internal Medicine, Univ Kansas Med Ctr, Kansas City, KS

Iseman, Michael MD (Pulmonary Disease) - *Special Expertise: Tuberculosis; Tuberculosis/Mycobacterial Infections;* **Admitting Hospital:** National Jewish Medical & Research Center; **Office Address:** Natl Jewish Med & Rsch Ctr 1400 Jackson St, rm J201 Denver, CO 80206; **Office Phone:** (303) 398-1667; **Board Certifications:** Internal Medicine 1972, Pulmonary Disease 1976; **Medical School:** Columbia P&S 1965 **Residencies:** Internal Medicine, Bellevue Hosp, New York, NY 1965-1967; Internal Medicine, Harlem Hosp, New York, NY 1968-1970; **Fellowship:** Pulmonary Disease, Harlem Hosp, New York, NY 1970-1972; **Faculty Appointment:** Prof Medicine, Univ Colo

Kaplan, James MD (Pulmonary Disease) - *Special Expertise:* *Pulmonary Disease - General;* **Admitting Hospital:** Overland Park Regional Medical Center; **Office Address:** 10550 Quivira , Ste 480 Overland Park, KS 66215; **Office Phone:** (913) 599-3800; **Board Certifications:** Pulmonary Disease 1990, Critical Care Medicine 1991; **Medical School:** Univ MO-Kansas City 1984; **Residency:** Internal Medicine, Barnes Hosp, St Louis, MO 1984-1987; **Fellowship:** Pulmonary Disease, Barnes Hosp-Wash Univ, St Louis, MO 1987-1989

Make, Barry J MD (Pulmonary Disease) - *Special Expertise:* *Chronic Lung Disease (COPD); Emphysema;* **Admitting Hospital:** National Jewish Medical & Research Center; **Office Address:** Natl Jewish Med & Research Ctr 1400 Jackson St, rm B107 Denver, CO 80206; **Office Phone:** (303) 398-1703; **Board Certifications:** Internal Medicine 1973, Critical Care Medicine 1997; **Medical School:** Jefferson Med Coll 1970; **Residency:** Internal Medicine, Univ Michigan, Ann Arbor, MI 1971-1973; **Fellowships:** Pulmonary Disease, West Virginia Med Ctr, Morgantown, WV 1973-1974; Pulmonary Disease, Boston Univ Med Ctr, Boston, MA 1975-1976; **Faculty Appointment:** Prof Medicine, Univ Colo

Martin, Richard Jay MD (Pulmonary Disease) - *Special Expertise:* *Asthma (Adult); Vocal Cord Disorders;* **Admitting Hospital:** National Jewish Medical & Research Center; **Office Address:** Natl Jewish Med & Res Ctr 1400 Jackson St, rm J-106 Denver, CO 80206-2761; **Office Phone:** (303) 398-1545; **Board Certifications:** Internal Medicine 1976, Pulmonary Disease 1978; **Medical School:** Univ Mich Med Sch 1971; **Residency:** Internal Medicine, Tulane, New Orleans, LA 1974-1976; **Fellowship:** Pulmonary Disease, University of Okla, Oklahoma City, OK 1976-1978; **Faculty Appointment:** Prof Pulmonary Disease, Univ Colo

Newman, Lee MD (Pulmonary Disease) - *Special Expertise:* *Occupational Lung Disease;* **Admitting Hospital:** National Jewish Medical & Research Center; **Office Address:** 1400 Jackson Street Denver, CO 80206; **Office Phone:** (303) 398-1725; **Board Certifications:** Internal Medicine 1983, Pulmonary Disease 1986; **Medical School:** Vanderbilt Univ 1980; **Residency:** Internal Medicine, Emory U Affil Prgm, Atlanta, GA 1982-1984; **Fellowship:** Pulmonary Disease, Univ of Colorado, Denver, CO 1984-1987; **Faculty Appointment:** Asst Prof Medicine, Univ Colorado

Petty, Thomas L MD (Pulmonary Disease) - *Special Expertise:* *Chronic Obstructive Lung Disease (COPD); Asthma; Respiratory Distress Syndrome(ARDS);* **Admitting Hospital:** Presbyterian - St Luke's Medical Center; **Office Address:** 1850 High St Denver, CO 80218-1235; **Office Phone:** (303) 839-6755; **Board Certifications:** Internal Medicine 1965, Pulmonary Disease 1966; **Medical School:** Univ Conn 1958; **Residencies:** Univ Mich Hosp, Ann Arbor, MI 1959-1960; Univ Colo Med Ctr, Denver, CO 1960-1962; **Fellowship:** Pulmonary Disease, Univ Colo Med Ctr, Denver, CO 1962-1963; **Faculty Appointment:** Prof Medicine, Univ Colo

Pingleton, Susan MD (Pulmonary Disease) - *Special Expertise:* *Critical Care;* **Admitting Hospital:** University of Kansas Medical Center; **Office Address:** 3901 Rainbow Blvd Kansas City, KS 66160; **Office Phone:** (913) 588-6044; **Board Certifications:** Pulmonary Disease 1978, Critical Care Medicine 1991; **Medical School:** Univ Kans 1972; **Residency:** Internal Medicine, Univ of Kansas Med Ctr, Kansas City, KS; **Faculty Appointment:** Prof Medicine, Univ Kans

Rodman, David MD (Pulmonary Disease) - *Special Expertise:* *Cystic Fibrosis; Emphysema;* **Admitting Hospital:** University of Colorado Health & Science Center; **Office Address:** Pulm Div, Sch Med 4200 E Ninth Ave, MS C272 Denver, CO 80220; **Office Phone:** (303) 315-7047; **Board Certifications:** Pulmonary Disease 1988, Critical Care Medicine 1991; **Medical School:** Univ Penn 1980; **Residencies:** Internal Medicine, Univ Colorado, Denver, CO 1980-1983; Pulmonary Disease, Univ Colorado, Denver, CO 1983-1984; **Fellowship:** Pulmonary Disease, Univ Colorado, Denver, CO 1985-1988; **Faculty Appointment:** Prof Medicine, Univ Colo

Rose, Cecile MD (Pulmonary Disease) - *Special Expertise: Occupational Lung Disease; Sarcoidosis;* **Admitting Hospital:** National Jewish Medical & Research Center; **Office Address:** 1400 Jackson Street Denver, CO 80206; **Office Phone:** (303) 398-1520; **Board Certifications:** Occupational Medicine 1987, Pulmonary Disease 1986; **Medical School:** Univ IL Coll Med 1980; **Residency:** Internal Medicine, Med Coll of VA, Richmond, VA 1981-1983; **Fellowship:** Pulmonary Disease, Med Coll of VA, Richmond, VA 1983-1985; **Faculty Appointment:** Assoc Prof Medicine, Univ Colo

Schwarz, Marvin Ira MD (Pulmonary Disease) - *Special Expertise: Interstitial Lung Disease; Pulmonary Vascular Disease; Lung Hemorrhage;* **Admitting Hospital:** University of Colorado Health & Science Center; **Office Address:** Univ Colo Hlth Scis Ctr, Div Pulm Sci & Crit Care 4200 Ninth Ave Denver, CO 80262; **Office Phone:** (303) 315-7047; **Board Certifications:** Internal Medicine 1970, Pulmonary Disease 1971; **Medical School:** Tulane Univ 1964; **Residency:** Internal Medicine, Charity Hosp, New Orleans, LA 1965-1967; **Fellowship:** Pulmonary Disease, Charity Hosp, New Orleans, LA 1967-1969; **Faculty Appointment:** Prof Medicine, Univ Colo

Voelkel, Norbert F MD (Pulmonary Disease) - *Special Expertise: Pulmonary Hypertension; Asthma; Emphysema;* **Admitting Hospital:** University of Colorado Health & Science Center; **Office Address:** Univ Colorado Hlth Sci Ctr 4200 E 9th Ave, rm 5525 Denver, CO 80262; **Office Phone:** (303) 315-4211; **Medical School:** Germany 1972; **Residency:** Internal Medicine, Univ Hamburg, Hamburg, Germany 1973-1977; **Fellowships:** Research, Univ Colorado, Denver, CO 1977-1978; Pulmonary Disease, Univ Colorado, Denver, CO 1978-1981; **Faculty Appointment:** Prof Medicine, Univ Colo

Wenzel, Sally E MD (Pulmonary Disease) - *Special Expertise: Asthma;* **Admitting Hospital:** National Jewish Medical & Research Center; **Office Address:** Natl Jewish Med & Research Ctr 1400 Jackson St, rm j114 Denver, CO 80206; **Office Phone:** (303) 398-1521; **Board Certifications:** Pulmonary Disease 1986, Internal Medicine 1984; **Medical School:** Univ Fla Coll Med 1981; **Residency:** Internal Medicine, NC Baptist Hosp, Winston Salem, NC 1981-1984; **Fellowship:** Pulmonary Disease, Med Coll VA, Richmond, VA 1984-1986; **Faculty Appointment:** Asst Prof Medicine, Univ Colo

Southwest

Campbell, G. Douglas MD (Pulmonary Disease) - *Special Expertise: Infectious Disease-Lung;* **Admitting Hospital:** Louisiana State University Hospital; **Office Address:** LSUMC-Shrvprt, Div Pulm & CritCare 1501 Kings Hwy Shreveport, LA 71103; **Office Phone:** (318) 675-5920; **Board Certifications:** Internal Medicine 1979, Pulmonary Disease 1986; **Medical School:** Univ Miss 1976; **Residency:** Internal Medicine, Univ Miss Hosp, Jackson, MS 1977-1979; **Fellowships:** Pulmonary Disease, Univ Tex Hlth Sci Ctr, San Antonio, TX 1981-1983; Infectious Disease, Univ Calgary HSC, Alberta, Canada 1983-1985; **Faculty Appointment:** Prof Medicine, Louisiana State Univ

Guidry, George Gary MD (Pulmonary Disease) - *Special Expertise: Chronic Lung Disease (COPD);* **Admitting Hospital:** Our Lady of Lourdes Regional Medical Center - Lafayette; **Office Address:** 155 Hosp Dr, Ste 206 Lafayette, LA 70503-2852; **Office Phone:** (337) 234-3204; **Board Certifications:** Internal Medicine 1988, Pulmonary Disease 1999; **Medical School:** Univ Louisville Sch Med 1985; **Residency:** Internal Medicine, LSU Med Ctr, Shreveport, LA 1985-1988; **Fellowship:** Pulmonary Disease, LSU Med Ctr, Shreveport, LA 1988

Jenkinson, Stephen George MD (Pulmonary Disease) - *Special Expertise:* Lung Cancer; Chronic Lung Disease (COPD); Asthma; **Admitting Hospital:** Audie L Murphy Memorial Veterans Hospital; **Office Address:** Audie Murphy VA Hosp, Dept Pulm 7400 Merton Minter Blvd San Antonio, TX 78284; **Office Phone:** (210) 617-5256; **Board Certifications:** Pulmonary Disease 1978, Critical Care Medicine 1987; **Medical School:** Louisiana State Univ 1973; **Residency:** Internal Medicine, LSU Med Ctr, Shreveport, LA 1973-1976; **Fellowship:** Pulmonary Disease, LSU Med Ctr, Shreveport, LA 1976-1978; **Faculty Appointment:** Prof Medicine, Univ Tex, San Antonio

Levin, David C MD (Pulmonary Disease) - *Special Expertise:* Critical Care; **Admitting Hospital:** University of Oklahoma Health Science Center; **Office Address:** Univ Okla Hlth Sci Ctr, Dept Med 921 NE 13th St, Ste 111E Oklahoma City, OK 73104; **Office Phone:** (405) 270-1573; **Board Certifications:** Pulmonary Disease 1976, Critical Care Medicine 1987; **Medical School:** Case West Res Univ 1970; **Residency:** Internal Medicine, Univ CO Hlth Sci Ctr, Denver, CO 1971-1974; **Fellowship:** Pulmonary Disease, Univ CO Hlth Sci Ctr, Denver, CO 1974-1975; **Faculty Appointment:** Prof Medicine, Univ Okla Coll Med

Perret, Phillip Samuel MD (Pulmonary Disease) - *Special Expertise:* Chronic Lung Disease (COPD); **Admitting Hospital:** Our Lady of Lourdes Regional Medical Center - Lafayette; **Office Address:** 614 W St Mary Blvd Lafayette, LA 70506; **Office Phone:** (337) 232-6435; **Board Certifications:** Pulmonary Disease 1980, Critical Care Medicine 2007; **Medical School:** Emory Univ 1974; **Residency:** Internal Medicine, Emory Univ Hosp, Atlanta, GA 1974-1977; **Fellowship:** Pulmonary Disease, Emory Univ Hosp, Atlanta, GA 1977-1979

Shellito, Judd Ernest MD (Pulmonary Disease) - *Special Expertise:* Pulmonary Infections; **Admitting Hospital:** Louisiana State University Hospital; **Office Address:** Louisiana State Univ Med Ctr 1901 Perdido, Ste 3205 New Orleans, LA 70112-2865; **Office Phone:** (504) 568-4634; **Board Certifications:** Pulmonary Disease 1980, Critical Care Medicine 1989; **Medical School:** Tulane Univ 1974; **Residency:** Internal Medicine, Evanston Hosp, Evanston, IL 1974-1978; **Fellowship:** Pulmonary Critical Care Medicine, Univ New Mexico Hosp, Albuquerque, NM 1978-1980; **Faculty Appointment:** Prof Medicine, Louisiana State Univ

Weissler, Jonathan C MD (Pulmonary Disease) - *Special Expertise:* Interstitial Lung Disease; **Admitting Hospital:** Zale Lipshy University Hospital; **Office Address:** 5323 Harry Hines Blvd Dallas, TX 75390-9034; **Office Phone:** (214) 648-2534; **Board Certifications:** Pulmonary Disease 1984, Critical Care Medicine 1997; **Medical School:** NYU Sch Med 1979; **Residency:** Internal Medicine, Univ Texas SW, Dallas, TX 1979-1982; **Fellowship:** Pulmonary Disease, Univ Texas SW, Dallas, TX 1982-1985; **Faculty Appointment:** Prof Medicine, Univ Tex SW, Dallas

West Coast and Pacific

Albertson, Timothy MD/PhD (Pulmonary Disease) - *Special Expertise:* Critical Care; **Admitting Hospital:** University of California - Davis Medical Center; **Office Address:** UC Davis, Div Pulm Crit Care 4150 V St, Fl 3400 Sacramento, CA 95817-9002; **Office Phone:** (916) 734-9564; **Board Certifications:** Pulmonary Disease 1984, Critical Care Medicine 1996; **Medical School:** UC Davis 1977; **Residencies:** Internal Medicine, Univ Arizona, Tuscon, AZ 1979-1980; Internal Medicine, UC Davis Med Ctr, Sacramento, CA 1980-1981; **Fellowship:** Pulmonary Critical Care Medicine, UC Davis Med Ctr, Sacramento, CA 1981-1983; **Faculty Appointment:** Prof Medicine, UC Davis

PULMONARY DISEASE

West Coast and Pacific

Balmes, John Randolph MD (Pulmonary Disease) - *Special Expertise: Occupational Lung Disease;* **Admitting Hospital:** San Francisco General Hospital; **Office Address:** 1001 Potrero Ave, Bldg 30 - Fl 5 San Francisco, CA 94110; **Office Phone:** (415) 206-4320; **Board Certifications:** Internal Medicine 1979, Pulmonary Disease 1984; **Medical School:** Mount Sinai Sch Med 1976; **Residency:** Internal Medicine, Mount Sinai Hosp, New York, NY 1977-1979; **Fellowship:** Pulmonary Disease, Yale-New Haven Hosp, New Haven, CT 1979-1981; **Faculty Appointment:** Prof Medicine, UCSF

Bellamy, Paul Eric MD (Pulmonary Disease) - *Special Expertise: Critical Care;* **Admitting Hospital:** UCLA Medical Center; **Office Address:** UCLA Med Sch, Dept Med 37-131 CHS, Box 951690 Los Angeles, CA 90095-1690; **Office Phone:** (310) 825-8061; **Board Certifications:** Pulmonary Disease 1980, Critical Care Medicine 1987; **Medical School:** SUNY Buffalo 1975; **Residency:** Internal Medicine, Univ Hosps, Cleveland, OH 1976-1978; **Fellowship:** Pulmonary Disease, UCLA Med Ctr, Los Angeles, CA 1978-1980; **Faculty Appointment:** Clin Prof Medicine, UCLA

Boushey Jr, Homer A MD (Pulmonary Disease) - *Special Expertise: Asthma; Bronchitis;* **Admitting Hospital:** University of California - San Francisco Medical Center; **Office Address:** UCSF Med Ctr, Dept Med 505 Parnassus Ave, Fl 12th - rm M1292, Box 0130 San Francisco, CA 94143-0130; **Office Phone:** (415) 476-8019; **Board Certifications:** Internal Medicine 1972, Pulmonary Disease 1974; **Medical School:** UCSF 1968; **Residencies:** Internal Medicine, UCSF Med Ctr, San Francisco, CA 1969-1970; Internal Medicine, Beth Israel Hosp, Boston, MA 1970-1971; **Fellowships:** Pulmonary Disease, Oxford Univ, Oxford, England 1971-1972; Pulmonary Disease, UCSF, San Francisco, CA 1972-1973; **Faculty Appointment:** Prof Medicine, UCSF

Catanzaro, Antonino MD (Pulmonary Disease) - *Special Expertise: Tuberculosis;* **Admitting Hospital:** University of California - San Diego Healthcare; **Office Address:** UCSD Med Ctr 200 W Arbor Dr, #8374 San Diego, CA 92103-8374; **Office Phone:** (619) 543-5550; **Board Certifications:** Internal Medicine 1972, Pulmonary Disease 1976; **Medical School:** SUNY Buffalo 1965; **Residency:** Internal Medicine, Georgetown Univ Hosp, Washington, DC 1968-1970; **Fellowships:** Pulmonary Critical Care Medicine, UCSD Med Ctr, San Diego, CA 1970-1972; Research, Scripps Clin Rsch Fdn, La Jolla, CA 1970-1972; **Faculty Appointment:** Prof Medicine, UCSD

Gong Jr, Henry MD (Pulmonary Disease) - *Special Expertise: Pulmonary Disease - General;* **Admitting Hospital:** LAC - Rancho Los Amigos Medical Center; **Office Address:** Rancho Los Amigos Med Ctr-Env Hlth Svc, Med Sci Bldg 7601 E Imperial Hwy, rm 145 Downey, CA 90242; **Office Phone:** (562) 401-3828; **Board Certifications:** Internal Medicine 1977, Pulmonary Disease 1980; **Medical School:** UC Davis 1973; **Residency:** Internal Medicine, Boston Hosp, Boston, MA 1974-1975; **Fellowship:** Pulmonary Disease, UCLA Med Ctr, Los Angeles, CA 1975-1977; **Faculty Appointment:** Prof Preventive Medicine, USC Sch Med

Hopewell, Philip MD (Pulmonary Disease) - *Special Expertise: AIDS/HIV; Tuberculosis; Infectious Disease-Lung;* **Admitting Hospital:** San Francisco General Hospital; **Office Address:** San Francisco Genl Hosp 1001 Potrero Ave Box 0841 San Francisco, CA 94110-1001; **Office Phone:** (415) 206-8313; **Board Certifications:** Internal Medicine 1973, Pulmonary Disease 1974; **Medical School:** W VA Univ 1965; **Residency:** Internal Medicine, U Calif San Fran Hospitals, San Francisco, CA 1968-1971; **Fellowship:** Pulmonary Disease, U Calif San Fran Hosps, San Francisco, CA 1971-1973; **Faculty Appointment:** Prof UCSF

Huang, Laurence MD (Pulmonary Disease) - *Special Expertise:* *AIDS/HIV;* **Admitting Hospital:** San Francisco General Hospital; **Office Address:** San Francisco Genl Hosp, AIDS Prog, Ward 84,Bldg #80 995 Potrero Ave San Francisco, CA 94110; **Office Phone:** (415) 476-4082; **Board Certifications:** Internal Medicine 1993, Pulmonary Disease 1996; **Medical School:** Columbia P&S 1989; **Residency:** Internal Medicine, Columbia-Presby Hosp, New York, NY 1990-1992; **Fellowship:** Pulmonary Critical Care Medicine, San Francisco General Hospital Medical Center, San Francisco, CA 1992-1995; **Faculty Appointment:** Asst Clin Prof Medicine, UCSF

Hudson, Leonard MD (Pulmonary Disease) - *Special Expertise:* *Critical Care;* **Admitting Hospital:** University of Washington Medical Center; **Office Address:** 325 9th Ave, Box 359762 Seattle, WA 98104; **Office Phone:** (206) 731-3533; **Board Certifications:** Internal Medicine 1973, Pulmonary Disease 1974; **Medical School:** Univ Wash 1964; **Residencies:** Internal Medicine, NY Hosp-Cornell Med Ctr, New York, NY 1965-1966; Internal Medicine, Univ Wash Hosps, Seattle, WA 1968-1969; **Fellowship:** Pulmonary Disease, Univ Colo Med Ctr, Denver, CO 1970-1971; **Faculty Appointment:** Prof Medicine, Univ Wash

King Jr, Talmadge Everett MD (Pulmonary Disease) - *Special Expertise:* *Interstitial Lung Disease; Bronchitis; Asthma;* **Admitting Hospital:** San Francisco General Hospital; **Office Address:** 1001 Potrero Ave, Bldg Rm 5H22 San Francisco, CA 94110; **Office Phone:** (415) 206-3465; **Board Certifications:** Internal Medicine 1977, Pulmonary Disease 1982; **Medical School:** Harvard Med Sch 1974; **Residency:** Internal Medicine, Emory Univ Hosp, Atlanta, GA 1975-1977; **Fellowship:** Pulmonary Disease, Univ Colorado Hlth Sci, Denver, CO 1977-1979; **Faculty Appointment:** Prof Medicine, UCSF

Matthay, Michael Anthony MD (Pulmonary Disease) - *Special Expertise:* *Critical Care;* **Admitting Hospital:** University of California - San Francisco Medical Center; **Office Address:** University of California Medical Center 505 Parnasas Ave San Francisco, CA 94143-0624; **Office Phone:** (415) 353-1206; **Board Certifications:** Critical Care Medicine 1987, Pulmonary Disease 1980; **Medical School:** Univ Penn 1973; **Residency:** Internal Medicine, U Colo Med Ctr, Denver, CO 1974-1976; **Fellowship:** Surgery, UCLA Med Ctr, Los Angeles, CA 1977-1979; **Faculty Appointment:** Prof Medicine, UCSF

Mohsenifar, Z MD (Pulmonary Disease) - *Special Expertise:* *Pulmonary Disease - General;* **Admitting Hospital:** Cedars-Sinai Medical Center; **Office Address:** Cedars-Sinai Med Ctr, Dept Pul 8700 Beverly Blvd Los Angeles, CA 90048-1804; **Office Phone:** (310) 423-4685; **Board Certifications:** Internal Medicine 1978, Pulmonary Disease 1980; **Medical School:** Iran 1973; **Residencies:** Internal Medicine, Thomas Jefferson Univ Hosp, Philadelphia, PA; Internal Medicine, UCLA Med Ctr, Los Angeles, CA; **Fellowship:** Pulmonary Disease, UCLA Med Ctr, Los Angeles, CA; **Faculty Appointment:** Prof Medicine, UCLA

Patterson, James R MD (Pulmonary Disease) - *Special Expertise:* *Pulmonary Disease - General;* **Admitting Hospital:** Providence Portland Medical Center; **Office Address:** 507 NE 47th Ave Portland, OR 97213; **Office Phone:** (503) 215-2300; **Board Certifications:** Internal Medicine 1972, Pulmonary Disease 1974; **Medical School:** Columbia P&S 1968; **Residency:** Internal Medicine, Columbia-Presby Med Ctr, New York, NY 1969-1970; **Fellowship:** Pulmonary Disease, Fitzsimons Army Med Ctr, Denver, CO 1971-1973; **Faculty Appointment:** Clin Prof Medicine, Oregon Hlth Scis Univ

Raffin, Thomas Alfred MD (Pulmonary Disease) - *Special Expertise: Pulmonary Disease - General;* **Admitting Hospital:** Stanford Medical Center; **Office Address:** Stanford Univ, Dept Pulm & Crit Care 300 Pasteur Dr Stanford, CA 94305-5236; **Office Phone:** (650) 723-6381; **Board Certifications:** Internal Medicine 1976, Pulmonary Disease 1978; **Medical School:** Stanford Univ 1973; **Residency:** Internal Medicine, Peter Bent Brigham Hosp, Boston, MA 1973-1975; **Fellowship:** Pulmonary Disease, Stanford Univ Med Ctr, Stanford, CA 1975-1978; **Faculty Appointment:** Prof Medicine, Stanford Univ

Raghu, Ganesh MD (Pulmonary Disease) - *Special Expertise: Interstitial Lung Disease; Pulmonary Fibrosis; Sarcoidosis;* **Admitting Hospital:** University of Washington Medical Center; **Office Address:** U of Wash-Pulmonary Medicine Campus Box 356522 Seattle, WA 98195; **Office Phone:** (206) 598-4615; **Board Certifications:** Pulmonary Disease 1990, Critical Care Medicine 1991; **Medical School:** India 1974; **Residencies:** Internal Medicine, SUNY Buffalo, Buffalo, NY 1978-1981; Internal Medicine, U Rochester 1977-1978; **Fellowship:** Critical Care Medicine, U Washington, Seattle, WA 1981-1984; **Faculty Appointment:** Prof Medicine, Univ Wash

Ries, Andrew MD (Pulmonary Disease) - *Special Expertise: Chronic Lung Disease (COPD);* **Admitting Hospital:** University of California - San Diego Healthcare; **Office Address:** UCSD Med Ctr 200 W Arbor Dr San Diego, CA 92103-8377; **Office Phone:** (619) 543-7350; **Board Certifications:** Pulmonary Disease 1980, Critical Care Medicine 1987; **Medical School:** Yale Univ 1974; **Residency:** Internal Medicine, Bellevue Hosp Ctr, New York, NY 1975-1977; **Fellowship:** Pulmonary Disease, UCSD Med Ctr, San Diego, CA 1977-1981; **Faculty Appointment:** Prof Medicine, UCSD

Rizk, Norman Wade MD (Pulmonary Disease) - *Special Expertise: Pulmonary & Critical Care; Asthma;* **Admitting Hospital:** Stanford Medical Center; **Office Address:** Stanford Univ Sch Med, Div Pulm & CritCare Med 300 Pasteur Dr, H3147 Stanford, CA 94305-5236; **Office Phone:** (650) 498-7746; **Board Certifications:** Internal Medicine 1979, Pulmonary Disease 1984; **Medical School:** Yale Univ 1976; **Residency:** Internal Medicine, San Fran Genl Hosp, San Francisco, CA 1977-1980; **Fellowship:** Pulmonary Disease, Moffitt Hosp-UCSF, San Francisco, CA 1981-1983; **Faculty Appointment:** Prof Medicine, Stanford Univ

Rubin, Lewis MD (Pulmonary Disease) - *Special Expertise: Pulmonary Hypertension; Pulmonary Vascular Disease;* **Admitting Hospital:** University of California - San Diego Healthcare; **Office Address:** UCSD Med Ctr 9300 Campus Pt Dr, Ste 7372 La Jolla, CA 92037; **Office Phone:** (858) 657-7105; **Board Certifications:** Pulmonary Disease 1980, Critical Care Medicine 1989; **Medical School:** Albert Einstein Coll Med 1975; **Residency:** Internal Medicine, Duke Univ Med Ctr, Durham, NC 1977-1978; **Fellowship:** Pulmonary Disease, Duke Univ Med Ctr, Durham, NC 1978-1979; **Faculty Appointment:** Prof Medicine, Univ SD Sch Med

Sharma, Om Prakash MD (Pulmonary Disease) - *Special Expertise: Sarcoidosis;* **Admitting Hospital:** LAC + USC Medical Center; **Office Address:** 1200 N State St, Bldg GNH 11900 Los Angeles, CA 90033; **Office Phone:** (323) 226-7923; **Board Certification:** Internal Medicine 1972; **Medical School:** India 1959; **Residencies:** Internal Medicine, Norwalk Hosp, Norwalk, CT 1962-1963; Internal Medicine, Einstein Med Coll Hosp, Bronx, NY 1963-1965; **Fellowships:** Pulmonary Disease, Einstein Med Coll Hosp, Bronx, NY 1965-1966; Research, Royal Coll of Phys, London, England 1966-1969; **Faculty Appointment:** Prof Medicine, USC Sch Med

Stansell, John Dee MD (Pulmonary Disease) - *Special Expertise: AIDS/HIV;* **Admitting Hospital:** University of California - San Francisco Medical Center; **Office Address:** San Francisco Genl Hosp Med Ctr, Dept Pulm & CCM 1001 Potrero Ave San Francisco, CA 94110; **Office Phone:** (415) 476-4082; **Board Certifications:** Internal Medicine 1989, Pulmonary Disease 1990; **Medical School:** Geo Wash Univ 1985; **Residency:** Internal Medicine, Stanford Univ Hosp, Stanford, CA 1985-1988; **Faculty Appointment:** Assoc Clin Prof Medicine, UCSF

Tashkin, Donald P MD (Pulmonary Disease) - *Special Expertise:* Asthma; Chronic Lung Disease (COPD); **Admitting Hospital:** UCLA Medical Center; **Office Address:** UCLA Med Ctr, Dept Med 200 UCLA Med Plaza, Ste 365B Los Angeles, CA 90095; **Office Phone:** (310) 825-8061; **Board Certifications:** Internal Medicine 1968, Pulmonary Disease 1972; **Medical School:** Univ Penn 1961; **Residency:** Internal Medicine, VA Hosp, Philadelphia, PA 1962-1965; **Fellowship:** Pulmonary Disease, UCLA Med Ctr, Los Angeles, CA 1967-1969; **Faculty Appointment:** Prof Medicine, UCLA

Tharratt, Robert S (Pulmonary Disease) - *Special Expertise:* Lung Cancer; **Admitting Hospital:** University of California - Davis Medical Center; **Office Address:** UC Davis Med Ctr, Div Pulm Crit Care 4150 V St, Ste 3400 Sacramento, CA 95817; **Office Phone:** (916) 734-3564; **Board Certifications:** Pulmonary Disease 1988, Medical Toxicology 1995; **Medical School:** UCLA 1983; **Residency:** Internal Medicine, UC Davis Med Ctr, Sacramento, CA 1984-1986; **Fellowship:** Pulmonary Critical Care Medicine, UC Davis Med Ctr, Sacramento, CA 1986-1989; **Faculty Appointment:** Prof Medicine, UC Davis

Theodore, James MD (Pulmonary Disease) - *Special Expertise:* Transplant Medicine-Heart & Lung; Pulmonary Fibrosis; Interstitial Lung Disease; **Admitting Hospital:** Stanford Medical Center; **Office Address:** Standford Univ Med Ctr, Dept Pulm Critical Care 300 Pasteur Dr, rm H3147 Stanford, CA 94305-5236; **Office Phone:** (650) 723-5200; **Board Certification:** Internal Medicine 1971; **Medical School:** Univ Pittsburgh 1962; **Residencies:** Internal Medicine, Univ Pitts Med Ctr, Pittsburgh, PA 1966-1967; Internal Medicine, Barnes Hosp, St Louis, MO 1967-1968; **Fellowship:** Pulmonary Disease, Univ Pitts Med Ctr, Pittsburgh, PA 1963-1966; **Faculty Appointment:** Prof Medicine, Stanford Univ

Wallace, Jeanne Marie MD (Pulmonary Disease) - *Special Expertise:* AIDS/HIV; **Admitting Hospital:** Olive View Medical Center; **Office Address:** Olive View UCLA Med Ctr 14445 Olive View Dr Sylmar, CA 91342-1437; **Office Phone:** (818) 364-3205; **Board Certifications:** Pulmonary Disease 1980, Critical Care Medicine 1991; **Medical School:** UCLA 1974; **Residency:** Internal Medicine, UCSF Med Ctr, San Francisco, CA 1975-1977; **Fellowship:** Pulmonary Disease, Univ Hosp, San Diego, CA 1978

Wilson, Archie MD/PhD (Pulmonary Disease) - *Special Expertise:* Pulmonary Disease - General; **Admitting Hospital:** University of California - Irvine Medical Center; **Office Address:** UC-Irvine Med Ctr, Dept Pulm 101 The City Dr, Bldg 53 - rm 119 Orange, CA 92868; **Office Phone:** (714) 456-5150; **Board Certifications:** Internal Medicine 1970, Pulmonary Disease 1971; **Medical School:** UCSF 1957; **Residencies:** Internal Medicine, San Fran VA Hosp, San Francisco, CA 1958-1959; Pulmonary Disease, UCSF Med Ctr, San Francisco, CA 1959-1960; **Fellowship:** Pulmonary Disease, UCLA Med Ctr, Los Angeles, CA 1966-1967; **Faculty Appointment:** Prof Medicine, UC Irvine

RADIATION ONCOLOGY

(a subspecialty of RADIOLOGY)

A subspecialist in radiation oncology deals with the therapeutic applications of radiant energy and its modifiers and the study and management of disease, especially malignant tumors.

RADIOLOGY

A radiologist utilizes radiologic methodologies to diagnose and treat disease. Physicians practicing in the field of radiology most often specialize in radiology, diagnostic radiology, radiation oncology or radiological physics.

Training required: Four years in radiology *plus* additional training and examination

PHYSICIAN LISTINGS

716

New England

Choi, Noah C MD (Radiation Oncology) - *Special Expertise:* Lung Cancer; Esophageal Cancer; **Admitting Hospital:** Massachusetts General Hospital; **Office Address:** Mass Genl Hosp, Dept Rad Onc 100 Blossom St, Bldg Cox - rm 307 Boston, MA 02114; **Office Phone:** (617) 726-8146; **Board Certification:** Therapeutic Radiology 1970; **Medical School:** South Korea 1963; **Residency:** Radiation Oncology, Princess Margaret Hosp, Toronto, Canada 1970

D'Amico, Anthony V MD/PhD (Radiation Oncology) - *Special Expertise:* Prostate Cancer; Brachytherapy Under MRI; **Admitting Hospital:** St Anne's Hospital; **Office Address:** Center for Radiation Oncology Therapy 480 Hawthorn St, Ste 102 North Dartmouth, MA 02747; **Office Phone:** (508) 979-5858; **Board Certification:** Radiation Oncology 1995; **Medical School:** Univ Penn 1990; **Residency:** Radiation Oncology, Penn U Hosp, Philadelphia, PA 1991-1994

Haffty, Bruce MD (Radiation Oncology) - *Special Expertise:* Breast Cancer; Lung Cancer; Head & Neck Cancer; **Admitting Hospital:** Yale - New Haven Hospital; **Office Address:** Yale U Sch Med HRT-133 333 Cedar St New Haven, CT 06520; **Office Phone:** (203) 785-2959; **Board Certification:** Radiation Oncology 1988; **Medical School:** Yale Univ 1984; **Residency:** Radiation Oncology, Yale Univ, New Haven, CT 1985-1988; **Faculty Appointment:** Assoc Prof Radiology, Yale Univ

Harris, Jay R MD (Radiation Oncology) - *Special Expertise:* Breast Cancer; **Admitting Hospital:** Brigham & Women's Hospital; **Office Address:** Dana Farber Cancer Inst 44 Binney St, rm 1622 Boston, MA 02115; **Office Phone:** (617) 632-2291; **Board Certifications:** Radiation Oncology 1999, Therapeutic Radiology 1976; **Medical School:** Stanford Univ 1970; **Residency:** Radiation Oncology, Joint Ctr Rad Ther, Boston, MA 1973-1976; **Fellowship:** Radium Therapy, Harvard Med Sch, Boston, MA 1976-1977; **Faculty Appointment:** Prof Radiation Oncology, Harvard Med Sch

Loeffler, Jay Steven MD (Radiation Oncology) - *Special Expertise:* Spinal Cord Tumors; Stereotactic Radiosurgery; Brain Tumors; **Admitting Hospital:** Massachusetts General Hospital; **Office Address:** Mass Genl Hosp, NE Proton Therapy Ctr 100 Blossom St Boston, MA 02114; **Office Phone:** (617) 724-1548; **Board Certification:** Therapeutic Radiology 1986; **Medical School:** Brown Univ 1982; **Residencies:** Radium Therapy, Harvard Joint Ctr, Boston, MA 1983-1986; Transplant Surgery, Harvard Joint Ctr, Boston, MA 1985-1986; **Fellowship:** Cancer Biology, Harvard Sch Pub Hlth, Boston, MA 1984-1985; **Faculty Appointment:** Prof Radiation Oncology, Harvard Med Sch

Recht, Abram MD (Radiation Oncology) - *Special Expertise:* Breast Cancer; **Admitting Hospital:** Beth Israel Deaconess Medical Center - Boston (Page 57); **Office Address:** Beth Israel Deaconess Med Ctr, Rad Onc 330 Brookline Ave Boston, MA 02215; **Office Phone:** (617) 667-2345; **Board Certification:** Therapeutic Radiology 1984; **Medical School:** Johns Hopkins Univ 1980; **Residency:** Radiology, Joint Ctr Radium Therapy, Boston, MA 1981-1984; **Faculty Appointment:** Assoc Prof Radiology, Harvard Med Sch

Shipley, William MD (Radiation Oncology) - *Special Expertise:* Bladder Cancer; Prostate Cancer; **Admitting Hospital:** Massachusetts General Hospital; **Office Address:** Mass Genl Hosp-Cox Bldg 55 Fruit St, Ste 302 Boston, MA 02114; **Office Phone:** (617) 726-8146; **Board Certification:** Therapeutic Radiology 1975; **Medical School:** Harvard Med Sch 1966; **Residencies:** Surgery, Mass Genl Hosp, Boston, MA 1967-1971; Radium Therapy, Mass Genl Hosp, Boston, MA 1971-1973; **Fellowship:** Radium Therapy, Royal Marsden Hosp, Sutton, England 1973-1974; **Faculty Appointment:** Prof Radiology, Harvard Med Sch

Suit, Herman MD (Radiation Oncology) - *Special Expertise:* Sarcoma; **Admitting Hospital:** Massachusetts General Hospital; **Office Address:** Mass Genl Hosp, Dept Rad Onc 100 Blossom St, Bldg Cox - rm 302 Boston, MA 02114; **Office Phone:** (617) 726-8150; **Board Certification:** Therapeutic Radiology 1958; **Medical School:** Baylor Coll Med 1952; **Residencies:** Radium Therapy, Jefferson Davis Hosp, Houston, TX 1953; Radium Therapy, Churchhill Hosp, Oxford, England 1954-1957; **Faculty Appointment:** Prof Radiation Oncology, Harvard Med Sch

Wazer, David E MD (Radiation Oncology) - *Special Expertise:* Breast Cancer; **Admitting Hospital:** New England Medical Center; **Office Address:** New England Med Ctr 750 Washington St, Ste 359 Boston, MA 02111; **Office Phone:** (617) 636-6161; **Board Certification:** Radiation Oncology 1988; **Medical School:** NYU Sch Med 1982; **Residency:** Radiation Oncology, Tufts New England Med Ctr, Boston, MA 1985-1988; **Fellowship:** Neurological Chemistry, NYU Med Ctr, New York, NY 1983-1984; **Faculty Appointment:** Prof Radiation Oncology, Tufts Univ

Willett, Chris MD (Radiation Oncology) - *Special Expertise:* Gastrointestinal Cancer; **Admitting Hospital:** Massachusetts General Hospital; **Office Address:** 100 Blossom St Boston, MA 02114; **Office Phone:** (617) 726-8650; **Board Certification:** Therapeutic Radiology 1986; **Medical School:** Tufts Univ 1981; **Residency:** Radiation Oncology, Mass Genl Hosp, Boston, MA 1982-1986; **Faculty Appointment:** Prof Radiation Oncology, Harvard Med Sch

Mid Atlantic

Berg, Christine Dorothy MD (Radiation Oncology) - *Special Expertise:* Breast Cancer; **Admitting Hospital:** Suburban Hospital Healthcare Systems; **Office Address:** 6410 Rockledge Dr Bethesda, MD 20817; **Office Phone:** (301) 896-3021; **Board Certifications:** Therapeutic Radiology 1986, Radiation Oncology 1999; **Medical School:** Northwestern Univ 1977; **Residencies:** Internal Medicine, Northwestern Meml Hosp, Chicago, IL 1978-1981; Radiation Oncology, Georgetown Univ Hosp, Washington, DC 1984-1986; **Fellowship:** Medical Oncology, Natl Cancer Inst-NIH, Bethesda, MD 1981-1984; **Faculty Appointment:** Assoc Prof Radiation Oncology, Georgetown Univ

Curran Jr, Walter J MD (Radiation Oncology) - *Special Expertise:* Lung Cancer; Brain Tumors; **Admitting Hospital:** Thomas Jefferson University Hospital; **Office Address:** Thomas Jefferson Univ Hosp, Dept Rad Onc 111 S 11TH St Philadelphia, PA 19107; **Office Phone:** (215) 955-6702; **Board Certification:** Therapeutic Radiology 1986; **Medical School:** Med Coll GA 1982; **Residency:** Radium Therapy, Hosp Univ Penn, Philadelphia, PA 1983-1986; **Faculty Appointment:** Prof Radiation Oncology, Jefferson Med Coll

Ennis, Ronald MD (Radiation Oncology) - *Special Expertise:* Stereotactic Radiosurgery; Brachytherapy; Prostate & Gynecologic Cancers; **Admitting Hospital:** NYU Medical Center (Page 70); **Office Address:** Columbia-Presby Med Ctr, Dept Rad Onc 622 W 168th St New York, NY; **Office Phone:** (212) 305-7997; **Board Certification:** Radiation Oncology 1995; **Medical School:** Yale Univ 1990; **Residency:** Therapeutic Radiology, Yale-New Haven Hosp, New Haven, CT 1991-1994; **Faculty Appointment:** Assoc Prof Radiation Oncology, Columbia P&S

Fountain, Karen MD (Radiation Oncology) - *Special Expertise:* Radiation Therapy-Cancer; **Admitting Hospital:** Columbia Presbyterian Medical Center (Page 72); **Office Address:** Columbia Presby Med Ctr, Dept Rad Onc 622 W 168th St New York, NY 10032-3702; **Office Phone:** (212) 305-5841; **Board Certification:** Radiology 1976; **Medical School:** Univ MD Sch Med 1972; **Residencies:** Therapeutic Radiology, Univ Maryland Hosp, Baltimore, MD 1973-1974; Therapeutic Radiology, Mayo Clinic, Rochester, MN 1974-1976; **Faculty Appointment:** Assoc Clin Prof Radiation Oncology, Columbia P&S

Fowble, Barbara MD (Radiation Oncology) - *Special Expertise: Breast Cancer;* **Admitting Hospital:** Fox Chase Cancer Center; **Office Address:** Fox Chase Cancer Ctr, Dept Rad Onc 7701 Burholme Ave Philadelphia, PA 19111; **Office Phone:** (215) 728-3053; **Board Certification:** Therapeutic Radiology 1976; **Medical School:** Jefferson Med Coll 1972; **Residencies:** Therapeutic Radiology, Bellevue Hosp Ctr-NYU, New York, NY 1973-1975; Therapeutic Radiology, Hahnemann, Philadelphia, PA 1975-1976; **Fellowship:** Radium Therapy, Jefferson Hosp, Philadelphia, PA 1976-1977; **Faculty Appointment:** Prof Radiation Oncology, Univ Penn

Glatstein, Eli MD (Radiation Oncology) - *Special Expertise: Lymphoma; Lung Cancer; Photodynamic Therapy;* **Admitting Hospital:** Hospital of the University of Pennsylvania; **Office Address:** HUP Dept of Radiation Oncology 3400 Spruce St. 2 Donner Philadelphia, PA 19104; **Office Phone:** (800) 789-7366; **Board Certification:** Therapeutic Radiology 1972; **Medical School:** Stanford Univ 1964; **Residency:** Radium Therapy, Stanford Med Ctr, Stanford, CA 1967-1970; **Fellowship:** Hammersmith Hosp, London, England 1970-1972; **Faculty Appointment:** Radiation Oncology, Univ Penn

Goodman, Robert L. MD (Radiation Oncology) - *Special Expertise: Breast Cancer; Lymphoma;* **Admitting Hospital:** St Barnabas Medical Center; **Office Address:** St Barnabus Med Ctr. , Radiation Oncology 94 Old Short Hills Rd Livingston, NJ 07039; **Office Phone:** (973) 322-5637; **Board Certifications:** Therapeutic Radiology 1974, Medical Oncology 1975; **Medical School:** Columbia P&S 1966; **Residencies:** Internal Medicine, Beth Israel Hosp, Boston, MA 1967-1968; Therapeutic Radiology, Harvard Joint Ctr, Boston, MA 1970-1972; **Fellowships:** Hematology, Presby Hosp, New York, NY 1968-1969; Radiation Oncology, Harvard Medical Center, Boston, MA 1970-1974; **Faculty Appointment:** Adjct Prof Radiation Oncology, Univ Penn

Harrison, Louis MD (Radiation Oncology) - *Special Expertise: Head & Neck Cancer;* **Admitting Hospital:** Beth Israel Medical Center - New York; **Office Address:** Beth Israel Med Ctr, Dept Rad Onc 10 Union Square East New York, NY 10003; **Office Phone:** (212) 844-8087; **Board Certification:** Radiation Oncology 1986; **Medical School:** SUNY Hlth Sci Ctr 1982; **Residencies:** Surgery, Mount Sinai Hosp, New York, NY 1982-1983; Radiation Oncology, Yale-New Haven Hosp, New Haven, CT 1983-1986; **Faculty Appointment:** Prof Radiation Oncology, Columbia P&S

Hilaris, Basil MD (Radiation Oncology) - *Special Expertise: Prostate Cancer;* **Admitting Hospital:** Our Lady of Mercy Medical Center; **Office Address:** 600 E 233rd St Radiation Oncology & Clinical Research Associates Bronx, NY 10466; **Office Phone:** (718) 920-9750; **Board Certification:** Radiation Oncology 1968; **Medical School:** Greece 1955; **Residency:** Radiology, Mem Sloan, New York, NY 1957-1959; **Fellowships:** Mem-Sloan, New York, NY 1959-1961; Mem-Sloan, New York, NY 1961-1963; **Faculty Appointment:** Prof Radiology, NY Med Coll

Isaacson, Steven MD (Radiation Oncology) - *Special Expertise: Brain Tumors;* **Admitting Hospital:** Columbia Presbyterian Medical Center (Page 72); **Office Address:** Columbia Presby Med Ctr, Dept Rad 622 W 168th St New York, NY 10032; **Office Phone:** (212) 305-2611; **Board Certifications:** Radiation Oncology 1988, Otolaryngology 1978; **Medical School:** Jefferson Med Coll 1973; **Residencies:** Otolaryngology, Hosp Univ Penn, Philadelphia, PA 1975-1978; Radiation Oncology, SUNY Hlth Sci Ctr, Brooklyn, NY 1985-1988; **Faculty Appointment:** Asst Prof Radiation Oncology, Columbia P&S

Leibel, Steven A MD (Radiation Oncology) - *Special Expertise: Prostate Cancer; Brain Tumors;* **Admitting Hospital:** Memorial Sloan Kettering Cancer Center; **Office Address:** Meml Sloan Kettering Canc Ctr 1275 York Ave New York, NY 10021-6007; **Office Phone:** (212) 639-6024; **Board Certifications:** Radiology 1976, Pulmonary Disease 1999; **Medical School:** UCSF 1972; **Residency:** Radiation Oncology, UCSF Med Ctr, San Francisco, CA 1973-1976

Lepanto, Philip Bliss MD (Radiation Oncology) - *Special Expertise:* Radiation Oncology - General; **Admitting Hospital:** St Mary's Hospital; **Office Address:** St Marys hosp Dept Rad Ther 2900 1St. Ave Huntington, WV 25702; **Office Phone:** (304) 526-1143; **Board Certification:** Therapeutic Radiology 1975; **Medical School:** Univ Louisville Sch Med 1970; **Residencies:** Hosp U Penn, Philadelphia, PA 1972-1975; Radiology, U Penn, Philadelphia, PA 1971-1972; **Faculty Appointment:** Clin Prof Radiology, Marshall Univ

Mandell, Lynda MD/PhD (Radiation Oncology) - *Special Expertise:* Radiation Oncology-Pediatric; Brain Tumors; **Admitting Hospital:** Mount Sinai Hospital (Page 70); **Office Address:** Radiation Oncology Assoc of Mt Sinai 1184 5th Ave New York, NY 10029-6574; **Office Phone:** (212) 241-7503; **Board Certification:** Therapeutic Radiology 1985; **Medical School:** Med Coll VA 1981; **Residency:** Radiation Oncology, Sloan-Kettering, New York, NY 1982-1985; **Faculty Appointment:** Prof Radiology, Mount Sinai Sch Med

McCormick, Beryl MD (Radiation Oncology) - *Special Expertise:* Breast Cancer; **Admitting Hospital:** Memorial Sloan Kettering Cancer Center; **Office Address:** 1275 York Ave New York, NY 10021-6007; **Office Phone:** (212) 639-6828; **Board Certification:** Therapeutic Radiology 1977; **Medical School:** UMDNJ-NJ Med Sch, Newark 1973; **Residency:** Therapeutic Radiology, Meml Sloan Kettering Canc Ctr, New York, NY 1974-1977; **Faculty Appointment:** Prof Radiation Oncology, Cornell Univ-Weil Med Coll

Minsky, Bruce MD (Radiation Oncology) - *Special Expertise:* Colon Cancer; **Admitting Hospital:** Memorial Sloan Kettering Cancer Center; **Office Address:** Meml Sloan Kettering Cancer Ctr, Dept Rad Therapy 1275 York Ave New York, NY 10021; **Office Phone:** (212) 639-6817; **Board Certification:** Radiation Oncology 1987; **Medical School:** Univ Mass Sch Med 1982; **Residency:** Radiation Oncology, Harvard Jt Ctr Rad Ther, Boston, MA 1983-1986

Nori, Dattatreyudu MD (Radiation Oncology) - *Special Expertise:* Prostate & Breast Cancer; Brachytherapy; **Admitting Hospital:** New York Weill Cornell Medical Center - NY Presbyterian Hospital (Page 72); **Office Address:** 525 E 68th St New York, NY 11355; **Office Phone:** (212) 746-3679; **Board Certification:** Radiation Oncology 1979; **Medical School:** India 1970; **Residency:** Radiation Oncology, Meml Sloan Kettering, New York, NY 1973-1975; **Fellowship:** Radiation Oncology, Meml Sloan Kettering, New York, NY 1976-1977; **Faculty Appointment:** Prof Radiation Oncology, Cornell Univ-Weil Med Coll

Pollack, Jed MD (Radiation Oncology) - *Special Expertise:* Brain Tumors; Prostate Cancer; **Admitting Hospital:** Long Island Jewish Medical Center; **Office Address:** Dept Rad Onc 27D-0 76th Ave New Hyde Park, NY 11040; **Office Phone:** (718) 470-7192; **Board Certification:** Therapeutic Radiology 1985; **Medical School:** Univ New Mexico 1981; **Residency:** Therapeutic Radiology, Mem Sloan-Kett Cancer Ctr, New York, NY 1985

Schiff, Peter B MD/PhD (Radiation Oncology) - *Special Expertise:* Prostate Cancer; **Admitting Hospital:** Columbia Presbyterian Medical Center (Page 72); **Office Address:** Columbia Presby Med Ctr, Dept Rad Onc 622 W 168th St New York, NY 10032-3702; **Office Phone:** (212) 305-2991; **Board Certification:** Radiation Oncology 1990; **Medical School:** Albert Einstein Coll Med 1984; **Residencies:** Internal Medicine, Meml Sloan Kettering Canc Ctr, New York, NY 1984-1985; Radiation Oncology, Meml Sloan Kettering Canc Ctr, New York, NY 1985-1988; **Faculty Appointment:** Prof Radiology, Columbia P&S

Solin, Lawrence MD (Radiation Oncology) - *Special Expertise: Breast Cancer;* **Admitting Hospital:** Hospital of the University of Pennsylvania; **Office Address:** Univ Penn Med Ctr, Dept Rad Onc 3400 Spruce St, 2 Donner Bldg Philadelphia, PA 19104; **Office Phone:** (215) 662-7267; **Board Certifications:** Therapeutic Radiology 1984, Radiation Oncology 1999; **Medical School:** Brown Univ 1978; **Residencies:** Surgery, Jefferson Univ Hosp, Philadelphia, PA 1979-1981; Radium Therapy, Jefferson Univ Hosp/Hosp Univ Penn, Philadelphia, PA 1981-1984; **Faculty Appointment:** Prof Therapeutic Radiology, Univ Penn

Stock, Richard MD (Radiation Oncology) - *Special Expertise: Radiation Oncology - General;* **Admitting Hospital:** Mount Sinai Hospital (Page 70); **Office Address:** 1184 5th Ave New York, NY 10029; **Office Phone:** (212) 241-7502; **Board Certification:** Radiation Oncology 1993; **Medical School:** Mount Sinai Sch Med 1988; **Residency:** Radiation Oncology, Meml Sloan Kettering Canc Ctr, New York, NY 1989-1992; **Faculty Appointment:** Assoc Prof Radiation Oncology, Mount Sinai Sch Med

Southeast

Anscher, Mitchell MD (Radiation Oncology) - *Special Expertise: Prostate Cancer; Brachytherapy;* **Admitting Hospital:** Duke University Medical Center (Page 60); **Office Address:** Duke Univ Med Ctr Box 3085 Durham, NC 27710; **Office Phone:** (919) 602-2113; **Board Certifications:** Internal Medicine 1984, Radiation Oncology 1987; **Medical School:** Med Coll VA 1981; **Residencies:** Internal Medicine, St Marys Hosp, Waterbury, CT 1982-1984; Radiation Oncology, Duke Univ Med Ctr, Durham, NC 1984-1987; **Faculty Appointment:** Prof Radiation Oncology, Duke Univ

Ferree, Carolyn Ruth Black MD (Radiation Oncology) - *Special Expertise: Breast Cancer; Hodgkin's Disease; Radiation Oncology-Pediatric;* **Admitting Hospital:** Wake Forest University Baptist Medical Center; **Office Address:** Wake Forest Univ Baptist Med Ctr Medical Center Blvd Winston Salem, NC 27157; **Office Phone:** (336) 716-4981; **Board Certification:** Therapeutic Radiology 1974; **Medical School:** Wake Forest Univ Sch Med 1970; **Residency:** Radiology, NC Baptist Hosp, Winston Salem, NC 1971-1974; **Faculty Appointment:** Prof Radiology, Wake Forest Univ Sch Med

Halle, Jan MD (Radiation Oncology) - *Special Expertise: Breast & Lung Cancer;* **Admitting Hospital:** University of North Carolina Hospitals; **Office Address:** Univ North Carolina Sch Med, Dept Rad Onc Chapel Hill, NC 27514; **Office Phone:** (919) 966-7700; **Board Certification:** Therapeutic Radiology 1982; **Medical School:** Tufts Univ 1975; **Residency:** Radiation Oncology, North Carolina Meml-UNC, Chapel Hill, NC 1975-1981

Lewin, Alan MD (Radiation Oncology) - *Special Expertise: Radiation Oncology - General;* **Admitting Hospital:** Baptist Hospital - Miami; **Office Address:** 8900 N Kendall Dr Lewin & Abitbol Miami, FL 33176-2118; **Office Phone:** (305) 596-6566; **Board Certifications:** Radiology 1982, Medical Oncology 1981; **Medical School:** Geo Wash Univ 1973; **Residency:** Internal Medicine, Mt Sinai Hosp, New york, NY 1974-1976; **Fellowships:** Radiation Oncology, Joint Ctr Rad Ther/ Harvard 1978-1980; Hematology and Oncology, Beth Israel Hosp/S. Far 1976-1978; **Faculty Appointment:** Prof Therapeutic Radiology, Univ Miami Sch Med

Marks, Lawrence MD (Radiation Oncology) - *Special Expertise: Breast Cancer; Lung Cancer; Radiation Therapy-Cancer;* **Admitting Hospital:** Duke University Medical Center (Page 60); **Office Address:** Duke University Medical Center Box 3085 Durham, NC 27710; **Office Phone:** (919) 660-2127; **Board Certification:** Radiation Oncology 1989; **Medical School:** Univ Rochester 1985; **Residency:** Radiation Oncology, Mass Genl Hosp, Boston, MA 1986-1989; **Faculty Appointment:** Prof Radiation Oncology, Duke Univ

Mendenhall, Nancy P MD (Radiation Oncology) - *Special Expertise: Breast Cancer; Lymphoma; Hodgkin's Disease;* **Admitting Hospital:** Shands Healthcare at University Florida (Page 77); **Office Address:** 2000 SW Archer Rd, Box 100385 Gainesville, FL 32610-0385; **Office Phone:** (352) 265-0287; **Board Certification:** Therapeutic Radiology 1985; **Medical School:** Univ Fla Coll Med 1980; **Residency:** Radiology, Shands-Univ of Florida, Gainesville, FL 1981-1984; **Faculty Appointment:** Prof Radiation Oncology, Univ Fla Coll Med

Mendenhall, William M MD (Radiation Oncology) - *Special Expertise: Head & Neck Cancer; Stereotactic Radiosurgery; Colon Cancer;* **Admitting Hospital:** Shands Healthcare at University Florida (Page 77); **Office Address:** 1600 SW Archer Rd, Box 100385 Gainesville, FL 32610-0385; **Office Phone:** (352) 395-0287; **Board Certification:** Radiology 1983; **Medical School:** Univ S Fla Coll Med 1978; **Residency:** Radiation Oncology, University of Florida, Gainesville, FL 1978-1983; **Faculty Appointment:** Prof Radiation Oncology, Univ Fla Coll Med

Prosnitz, Leonard MD (Radiation Oncology) - *Special Expertise: Lymphoma; Breast Cancer; Hyperthermia;* **Admitting Hospital:** Duke University Medical Center (Page 60); **Office Address:** Duke Univ Med Ctr, Dept Rad Onc Morris Bld, Box 3085 Durham, NC 27710; **Office Phone:** (919) 660-2110; **Board Certification:** Therapeutic Radiology 1970; **Medical School:** SUNY Downstate 1961; **Residencies:** Internal Medicine, Dartmouth Affil Hosps, New Haven, CT 1961-1963; Radiation Oncology, Yale-New Haven Hosp, New Haven, CT 1967-1969; **Fellowship:** Hematology and Oncology, Yale-New Haven Hosp, New Haven, CT 1965-1967; **Faculty Appointment:** Prof Radiation Oncology, Duke Univ

Rich, Tyvin Andrew MD (Radiation Oncology) - *Special Expertise: Colon Cancer; Gastrointestinal Cancer;* **Admitting Hospital:** University of Virginia Health Systems; **Office Address:** Univ Va Hlth Sci Ctr, Dept Rad Onc Box 800383 Charlottesville, VA 22908; **Office Phone:** (804) 924-5191; **Board Certification:** Radiation Oncology 1978; **Medical School:** Univ VA Sch Med 1973; **Residency:** Radiology, Mass Genl Hosp, Boston, MA 1975-1978; **Fellowship:** Mt Vernon Hosp/Gray Lab, England 1978; **Faculty Appointment:** Prof Radiation Oncology, Univ VA Sch Med

Rosenman, Julian MD (Radiation Oncology) - *Special Expertise: Lung Cancer; Breast Cancer; Prostate Cancer;* **Admitting Hospital:** University of North Carolina Hospitals; **Office Address:** NC Clinical Canc Ctr-Univ NC, Dept Rad Onc 101 Manning Dr, Campus Box 7512 Chapel Hill, NC 27514; **Office Phone:** (919) 966-1101; **Board Certification:** Therapeutic Radiology 1981; **Medical School:** Univ Tex SW, Dallas 1977; **Residency:** Therapeutic Radiology, Mass Genl Hosp, Boston, MA 1978-1981; **Faculty Appointment:** Prof Radiation Oncology, Univ NC Sch Med

Sailer, Scott MD (Radiation Oncology) - *Special Expertise: Head & Neck Tumors;* **Admitting Hospital:** University of North Carolina Hospitals; **Office Address:** Univ North Carolina Schl Med Dept Radiation Oncology CB 7512 Chapel Hill, NC 27599-7512; **Office Phone:** 919 9667700; **Board Certification:** Radiation Oncology 1988; **Medical School:** Harvard Med Sch 1984; **Residency:** Radium Therapy, Mass Genl Hosp, Boston, MA 1985-1988; **Faculty Appointment:** Assoc Clin Prof Univ NC Sch Med

Shaw, Edward Gus MD (Radiation Oncology) - *Special Expertise: Stereotactic Radiosurgery; Brain Tumors;* **Admitting Hospital:** Wake Forest University Baptist Medical Center; **Office Address:** Wake Forest Baptist Univ Med Ctr Medical Center Blvd Winston Salem, NC 27157-1029; **Office Phone:** (336) 716-4647; **Board Certification:** Radiation Oncology 1987; **Medical School:** Rush Med Coll 1983; **Residency:** Radiation Oncology, Mayo Grad Sch Med, Rochester, MN 1984-1987; **Faculty Appointment:** Prof Radiation Oncology, Wake Forest Univ Sch Med

Tepper, Joel MD (Radiation Oncology) - *Special Expertise:* *Gastrointestinal Cancer; Sarcoma; Colon Cancer;* **Admitting Hospital:** University of North Carolina Hospitals; **Office Address:** UNC Sch Med Dept Rad Onc - CB 7512 Chapel Hill, NC 27599-7512; **Office Phone:** (919) 966-0400; **Board Certification:** Therapeutic Radiology 1976; **Medical School:** Washington Univ, St Louis 1972; **Residencies:** Therapeutic Radiology, Mass General, Boston, MA 1973-1976; Therapeutic Radiology, Mass General, Boston, MA 1976-1977; **Faculty Appointment:** Prof Radiation Oncology, Univ NC Sch Med

Turrisi III, Andrew Thomas MD (Radiation Oncology) - *Special Expertise:* *Lung Cancer;* **Admitting Hospital:** MUSC Medical Center; **Office Address:** Med Univ SC, Dept Rad Onc 169 Ashley Ave, Box 250318 Charleston, SC 29425-0721; **Office Phone:** (843) 792-3273; **Board Certifications:** Medical Oncology 1981, Therapeutic Radiology 1984; **Medical School:** Georgetown Univ 1974; **Residencies:** Internal Medicine, Georgetown Univ Hosp, Washington, DC 1975-1977; Radiation Oncology, Univ Penn, Philadelphia, PA 1980-1982; **Fellowship:** Medical Oncology, Natl Cancer Inst-NIH, Bethesda, MD 1977-1980; **Faculty Appointment:** Prof Medicine, Med Univ SC

Midwest

Emami, Bahman MD (Radiation Oncology) - *Special Expertise:* *Head & Neck Cancer;* **Admitting Hospital:** Loyola University Health System; **Office Address:** Loyola Univ Med Ctr 2160 S First Ave, Ste 114B Maywood, IL 60153; **Office Phone:** (708) 202-2170; **Board Certification:** Therapeutic Radiology 1976; **Medical School:** Iran 1968; **Residency:** Radium Therapy, Tufts Univ-New Eng Med Ctr, Boston, MA 1973-1976; **Fellowship:** Radium Therapy, Tufts Univ-New England Med Ctr, Boston, MA 1976-1977; **Faculty Appointment:** Prof Radiation Oncology, Loyola Univ-Stritch Sch Med

Forman, Jeffrey D MD (Radiation Oncology) - *Special Expertise:* *Prostate Cancer; Genitourinary Cancer;* **Admitting Hospital:** Harper Hospital (Page 59); **Office Address:** Harper Hosp, Dept Rad Onc 3990 John R St Detroit, MI 48021; **Office Phone:** (313) 745-2593; **Board Certification:** Radiation Oncology 1986; **Medical School:** NY Med Coll 1982; **Residency:** Radiation Oncology, Johns Hopkins Hosp, Baltimore, MD 1983-1986; **Fellowship:** Therapeutic Radiology, Johns Hopkins Hosp, Baltimore, MD 1986-1987; **Faculty Appointment:** Prof Radiation Oncology, Wayne State Univ

Gunderson, Leonard MD (Radiation Oncology) - *Special Expertise:* *Colon Cancer;* **Admitting Hospital:** Mayo Medical Center & Clinic - Rochester; **Office Address:** Mayo Clinic, Dept Rad Onc 200 First St SW Rochester, MN 55905; **Office Phone:** (507) 284-3261; **Board Certification:** Therapeutic Radiology 1975; **Medical School:** Univ KY Coll Med 1969; **Residency:** Radiation Oncology, LDS Hosp, Salt Lake City, UT 1970-1974; **Faculty Appointment:** Prof Medical Oncology, Mayo Med Sch

Kinsella, Timothy James MD (Radiation Oncology) - *Special Expertise:* *Brain Tumors; Sarcoma;* **Admitting Hospital:** University Hospital - Cleveland; **Office Address:** U Hosp Cleveland-Dept. Rad Onc 1100 Euclid Ave, Bldg Bolwell B-200 Cleveland, OH; **Office Phone:** (216) 844-3100

Lichter, Allen MD (Radiation Oncology) - *Special Expertise:* *Lung Cancer; Breast Cancer; Prostate Cancer;* **Admitting Hospital:** University of Michigan Health Center; **Office Address:** U Mich Med Ctr UHB2 C490 Box0010 Ann Arbor, MI 48109-0010; **Office Phone:** (734) 936-8207; **Board Certification:** Therapeutic Radiology 1976; **Medical School:** Univ Mich Med Sch 1972; **Residency:** Radiation Oncology, U Calif, San Francisco, CA 1973-1976; **Faculty Appointment:** Prof Radiation Oncology, Univ Mich Med Sch

RADIATION ONCOLOGY

Myerson, Robert J MD (Radiation Oncology) - *Special Expertise:* Colon Cancer; **Admitting Hospital:** Barnes - Jewish Hospital; **Office Address:** Barnes Jewish Hospital 4939 Childrens Pl, Ste 5500 St. Louis, MO 63110; **Office Phone:** (314) 362-8510; **Board Certification:** Therapeutic Radiology 1985; **Medical School:** Univ Miami Sch Med 1980; **Residency:** Radium Therapy, Univ Penn, Philadelphia, PA 1981-1984; **Faculty Appointment:** Prof Therapeutic Radiology, Washington Univ, St Louis

Perez, Carlos A MD (Radiation Oncology) - *Special Expertise:* Breast Cancer; Lung *Radiation;* **Admitting Hospital:** Barnes - Jewish Hospital; **Office Address:** One Barnes Jewish Hosp Plaza Ground Floor- MIR St Louis, MO 63108; **Office Phone:** (314) 362-7030; **Board Certifications:** Radiation Oncology 1999, Radiology 1964; **Medical School:** Colombia 1960; **Residencies:** Radiology, Univ Del Valle Cali Hosp, Cali, Colombia 1959-1960; Radiology, Mallinckrodt Inst Rad, St Louis, MO 1960-1963; **Fellowship:** Radiation Oncology, MD Anderson Cancer Ctr, Houston, TX 1963-1964; **Faculty Appointment:** Prof Radiology, Washington Univ, St Louis

Pierce, Lori J MD (Radiation Oncology) - *Special Expertise:* Breast Cancer; **Admitting Hospital:** University of Michigan Health Center; **Office Address:** Univ Hosp, Dept Rad Onc 1500 E Med Ctr Dr, rm B2C440, Box 0010 Ann Arbor, MI 48109-0010; **Office Phone:** (734) 936-4319; **Board Certification:** Radiation Oncology 1989; **Medical School:** Duke Univ 1985; **Residency:** Radiation Oncology, Hosp Univ Penn, Philadelphia, PA 1986-1989; **Faculty Appointment:** Asst Prof Radiation Oncology, Univ Mich Med Sch

Taylor, Marie E MD (Radiation Oncology) - *Special Expertise:* Breast Cancer; **Admitting Hospital:** Barnes - Jewish Hospital; **Office Address:** 510 S KingsHighway Blvd St Louis, MO 63110; **Office Phone:** (314) 454-7000; **Board Certification:** Radiation Oncology 1987; **Medical School:** Univ Wash 1982; **Residency:** Radiation Oncology, Univ Wash, Seattle, WA 1983-1986

Vicini, Frank A MD (Radiation Oncology) - *Special Expertise:* Breast Cancer; Prostate *Cancer;* **Admitting Hospital:** William Beaumont Hospital; **Office Address:** William Beumont Hosp, Dept Rad Onc 3601 W 13 Mile Rd Royal Oak, MI 48073; **Office Phone:** (248) 551-1219; **Board Certification:** Radiation Oncology 1990; **Medical School:** Wayne State Univ 1985; **Residency:** Radiation Oncology, William Beaumont Hosp, Royal Oak, MI 1986-1989; **Fellowship:** Radiation Oncology, Harvard Med Sch, Boston, MA 1989-1990

Weichselbaum, Ralph R MD (Radiation Oncology) - *Special Expertise:* Gene-Targeted *Radiotherapy; Head & Neck Cancer; Chemoprevention of Cancer;* **Admitting Hospital:** University of Chicago Hospitals (Page 78); **Office Address:** Univ Chicago Hosps, Dept Rad Onc 5758 S Maryland Ave, MS 9006 Chicago, IL 60637; **Office Phone:** (773) 702-0817; **Board Certification:** Therapeutic Radiology 1975; **Medical School:** Univ IL Coll Med 1971; **Residency:** Therapeutic Radiology, Harvard Jt Ctr Rad Therapy, Cambridge, MA 1972-1975; **Fellowship:** Radiology, Harvard Med Sch, Cambridge, MA 1974-1976; **Faculty Appointment:** Prof Medical Oncology, Univ Chicago-Pritzker Sch Med

Wilson, J Frank MD (Radiation Oncology) - *Special Expertise:* Breast Cancer; Skin Cancer; **Admitting Hospital:** Froedtert Memorial Lutheran Hospital; **Office Address:** 8701 W Watertown Plank Rd Milwaukee, WI 53226-3548; **Office Phone:** (414) 805-4450; **Board Certification:** Therapeutic Radiology 1971; **Medical School:** Univ MO-Columbia Sch Med 1965; **Residency:** Radiation Oncology, Penrose Cancer Hosp, Colorado Springs, CO 1966-1969; **Fellowship:** Radium Therapy, NCI/NIH, Bethesda, MD 1969-1971; **Faculty Appointment:** Prof Radiation Oncology, Med Coll Wisc

Great Plains and Mountains

Smalley, Stephen R MD (Radiation Oncology) - *Special Expertise:* Colon Cancer; Gastrointestinal Cancer; **Admitting Hospital:** Olathe Medical Center; **Office Address:** Olathe Med Ctr 20375 W 151st St Olathe, KS 64131; **Office Phone:** (913) 768-7200; **Board Certifications:** Medical Oncology 1984; Radiation Oncology 1987; **Medical School:** Univ MO-Kansas City 1979; **Residencies:** Internal Medicine, Mayo Clinic, Rochester, MN 1979-1982; Radiation Oncology, Mayo Clinic, Rochester, MN 1984-1986; **Fellowship:** Medical Oncology, Mayo Clinic, Rochester, MN 1982-1984; **Faculty Appointment:** Prof Radiation Oncology, Univ Kans

Southwest

Ang, Kie-Kian MD/PhD (Radiation Oncology) - *Special Expertise:* Head & Neck Cancer; **Admitting Hospital:** University of Texas MD Anderson Cancer Center (Page 66); **Office Address:** UT MD Anderson Cancer Ctr 1515 Holcombe Blvd, Box 97 Houston, TX 77030; **Office Phone:** (713) 792-3409; **Board Certification:** Radiation Oncology 1987; **Medical School:** Belgium **Residency:** Radiation Oncology, Univ Hosp Louvian, Belgium 1976-1980; **Faculty Appointment:** Prof Radiology, Univ Tex, Houston

Cox, James D MD (Radiation Oncology) - *Special Expertise:* Lymphoma; Lung Cancer; **Admitting Hospital:** University of Texas MD Anderson Cancer Center (Page 66); **Office Address:** Univ Texas/MD Anderson Cancer Ctr 1515 Holcombe Blvd, Box 97 Houston, TX 77030; **Office Phone:** (713) 792-3411; **Board Certification:** Radiation Oncology 1999; **Medical School:** Univ Rochester 1965; **Residency:** Radiology, Penrose Cancer Hosp, Colorado Springs, CO 1966-1969; **Fellowship:** Radiology, Inst Gustave-Roussy, Villeuif, France 1969-1970; **Faculty Appointment:** Prof Radiation Oncology, Univ Tex, Houston

Herman, Terence Spencer MD (Radiation Oncology) - *Special Expertise:* Breast Cancer; Sarcoma; Brain Tumors; **Admitting Hospital:** University of Texas Health & Science Center; **Office Address:** Univ Texas Hlth Sci Ctr, Dept Radiation Onc 7703 Floyd Curl Dr, MC-7889 San Antonio, TX 78229-3900; **Office Phone:** (210) 616-5648; **Board Certifications:** Therapeutic Radiology 1985, Medical Oncology 1977; **Medical School:** Univ Conn 1972; **Residencies:** Internal Medicine, Univ Arizona, Tuscon, AZ 1973-1975; Radiation Oncology, Stanford Univ, Stanford, CA 1983-1985; **Fellowship:** Medical Oncology, Univ Arizona, Tucson, AZ 1975-1977; **Faculty Appointment:** Prof Radiation Oncology, Univ Tex, San Antonio

Komaki, Ritsuko MD (Radiation Oncology) - *Special Expertise:* Lung Cancer; Thymoma; **Admitting Hospital:** University of Texas MD Anderson Cancer Center (Page 66); **Office Address:** 1515 Holcombe Blvd, Box 0097 Houston, TX 77030-4095; **Office Phone:** (713) 792-3420; **Board Certification:** Therapeutic Radiology 1977; **Medical School:** Japan 1969; **Residency:** Radiation Oncology, Med Coll Wisc, Milwaukee, WI 1974-1978; **Faculty Appointment:** Prof Therapeutic Radiology, Univ Tex, Houston

McNeese, Marsha MD (Radiation Oncology) - *Special Expertise:* Breast Cancer; **Admitting Hospital:** University of Texas MD Anderson Cancer Center (Page 66); **Office Address:** Radiation Oncology 1515 Holcombe Blvd, Box 97 Houston, TX 77030-4009; **Office Phone:** (713) 792-3418; **Board Certification:** Therapeutic Radiology 1978; **Medical School:** Louisiana State Univ 1974; **Residency:** Radium Therapy, Univ Texas/MD Anderson Cancer Ctr, Houston, TX 1975-1977; **Fellowship:** Radiology, Univ Texas/MD Anderson Cancer Ctr, Houston, TX 1977; **Faculty Appointment:** Assoc Prof Radiation Oncology, Univ Tex, Houston

Pistenmaa, David A MD (Radiation Oncology) - *Special Expertise: Stereotactic Radiosurgery-CyberKnife;* **Admitting Hospital:** St Paul Medical Center; **Office Address:** Univ Texas SW Med Sch, Dept Rad Onc 5323 Harry Hines Blvd Dallas, TX 75390-9183; **Office Phone:** (214) 648-6765; **Board Certification:** Therapeutic Radiology 1974; **Medical School:** Stanford Univ 1970; **Fellowship:** Radium Therapy, Stanford Univ, Stanford, CA 1970-1973; **Faculty Appointment:** Prof Radiation Oncology, Univ Tex SW, Dallas

Senzer, Neil Nathan MD (Radiation Oncology) - *Special Expertise: Radiation Oncology - General;* **Admitting Hospital:** Baylor University Medical Center; **Office Address:** 3535 Worth St Dallas, TX 75246-2044; **Office Phone:** (214) 370-1400; **Board Certifications:** Pediatric Hematology-Oncology 1978, Therapeutic Radiology 1985; **Medical School:** SUNY Buffalo 1971; **Residencies:** Pediatrics, Johns Hopkins Hosp, Baltimore, MD 1971-1974; Radiation Oncology, St Barnabas Med Ctr, Livingston, NJ 1982-1985; **Fellowship:** Pediatric Hematology-Oncology, St Jude Chldns Rsch Hosp, Memphis, TN 1976-1978

Strom, Eric Alan MD (Radiation Oncology) - *Special Expertise: Breast Cancer;* **Admitting Hospital:** University of Texas MD Anderson Cancer Center (Page 66); **Office Address:** Dept Rad Onc 1515 Holcombe Blvd, Box 97 Houston, TX 77030; **Office Phone:** (713) 792-3437; **Board Certifications:** Internal Medicine 1985, Radiation Oncology 1990; **Medical School:** Northwestern Univ 1982; **Residencies:** Internal Medicine, Univ KY, Lexington, KY 1982-1985; Radiation Oncology, Univ TX-MD Anderson, Houston, TX 1986-1990; **Faculty Appointment:** Assoc Prof Radiation Oncology, Univ Tex, Houston

West Coast and Pacific

Blasko, John Charles MD (Radiation Oncology) - *Special Expertise: Radiation Therapy-Cancer; Prostate Cancer;* **Admitting Hospital:** University of Washington Medical Center; **Office Address:** Univ Wash Med Ctr, Dept Rad Onc 1959 NE Pacific St Seattle, WA 98195; **Office Phone:** (206) 548-7900; **Board Certification:** Therapeutic Radiology 1976; **Medical School:** Univ MD Sch Med 1969; **Residencies:** Diagnostic Radiology, Maine Med Ctr, Portland, ME 1973-1974; Radium Therapy, Univ Wash, St Louis, MO 1974-1976; **Faculty Appointment:** Prof Radiation Oncology, Univ Wash

Goffinet, Don R MD (Radiation Oncology) - *Special Expertise: Breast Cancer; Melanoma; Sarcoma;* **Admitting Hospital:** Stanford Medical Center; **Office Address:** Stanford Univ Hosp, Dept Rad Onc 300 Pasteur Dr Stanford, CA 94305; **Office Phone:** (650) 723-6195; **Board Certification:** Therapeutic Radiology 1973; **Medical School:** Stanford Univ 1964; **Residencies:** Surgery, Stanford Univ, Stanford, CA 1965-1966; Surgery, Stanford Univ, Stanford, CA 1968-1972; **Faculty Appointment:** Prof Therapeutic Radiology, Stanford Univ

Halberg, Francine Erna MD (Radiation Oncology) - *Special Expertise: Radiation Therapy-Cancer;* **Admitting Hospital:** Marin General Hospital; **Office Address:** Marin Cancer Inst-Dept of Rad.Oncology 1350 S Eliseo Greenbrae, CA 94904; **Office Phone:** (415) 925-7326; **Board Certifications:** Radiation Oncology 1984, Internal Medicine 1981; **Medical School:** Cornell Univ-Weil Med Coll 1978; **Residency:** Internal Medicine, USPHS Hosp, San Francisco, CA 1979-1981; **Fellowship:** Radiation Oncology, Stanford Med Ctr, Palo Alto, CA 1981-1984; **Faculty Appointment:** Assoc Clin Prof Radiation Oncology, UCSF

Juillard, Guy Jean-Felix MD (Radiation Oncology) - *Special Expertise: Head & Neck Cancer; Breast Cancer; Gynecologic Cancer;* **Admitting Hospital:** UCLA Medical Center; **Office Address:** 200 UCLA Med Plz, Ste B-265 Los Angeles, CA 90095; **Office Phone:** (310) 825-7145; **Board Certification:** Radiation Oncology 1991; **Medical School:** France 1963; **Residency:** Radium Therapy, Inst Gustave Roussy, Villejuif, France 1961-1963; **Faculty Appointment:** Prof Radiation Oncology, UCLA

Phillips, Theodore Locke MD (Radiation Oncology) - *Special Expertise:* *Radiation Therapy-Cancer;* **Admitting Hospital:** University of California - San Francisco Medical Center; **Office Address:** UCSF Med Ctr 505 Parnassus Ave, rm I-175 San Francisco, CA 94143-0226; **Office Phone:** (415) 353-8900; **Board Certification:** Therapeutic Radiology 1965; **Medical School:** Univ Penn 1959; **Residency:** Radium Therapy, UCSF Med Ctr, San Francisco, CA 1960-1963; **Faculty Appointment:** Prof Radiation Oncology, UCSF

Quivey, Jeanne Marie MD (Radiation Oncology) - *Special Expertise:* *Radium Therapy;* **Admitting Hospital:** St Francis Memorial Hospital; **Office Address:** UCSF, Dept Rad Onc 505 Parnassus Ave , rm L-08 San Francisco, CA 94143-0226; **Office Phone:** (415) 353-8900; **Board Certification:** Therapeutic Radiology 1974; **Medical School:** UCSF 1970; **Residency:** Radium Therapy, UC - San Francisco Med Ctr, San Francisco, CA 1971-1974; **Faculty Appointment:** Prof Radiation Oncology, UCSF

Rose, Christopher Marshall MD (Radiation Oncology) - *Special Expertise:* *Prostate Cancer;* **Admitting Hospital:** Providence Saint Joseph Medical Center; **Office Address:** St Joseph Med Ctr, Rad Ther 501 S Buena Vista St Burbank, CA 91505-4809; **Office Phone:** (818) 840-7925; **Board Certification:** Radiology 1979; **Medical School:** Harvard Med Sch 1974; **Residencies:** Internal Medicine, Beth Israel Deaconess, Boston, MA 1975-1976; Radium Therapy, Joint Ctr Rad Therapy, Boston, MA 1976-1979; **Fellowship:** Research, British Inst Cancer Rsch, London, England 1978-1979; **Faculty Appointment:** Assoc Clin Prof Radiology, UCLA

Seagren, Stephen L MD (Radiation Oncology) - *Special Expertise:* *Lung Cancer;* **Admitting Hospital:** University of California - San Diego Healthcare; **Office Address:** U California San Diego Med Ctr-Dept Rad Oncol 200 W Arbor Dr San Diego, CA 92103-8757; **Office Phone:** (619) 543-5303; **Board Certifications:** Therapeutic Radiology 1977, Internal Medicine 1972; **Medical School:** Northwestern Univ 1967; **Residencies:** Radiation Oncology, USCD, San Diego, CA 1976-1977; Internal Medicine, Univ Minn, Hennepin Co Genl Hosp, Minneapolis, MN 1968-1971; **Fellowships:** Medical Oncology, LA Co-USC Med Ctr, Los Angeles, CA 1974-1975; Harob Genl Hosp, Los Angeles, CA 1975-1976; **Faculty Appointment:** Prof Radiology, UCSD

Selch, Michael T MD (Radiation Oncology) - *Special Expertise:* *Brain Cancer; Lung Cancer; Cancer-Pediatric;* **Admitting Hospital:** UCLA Medical Center; **Office Address:** UCLA Med Ctr, Dept Rad Onc B-265 200 Med Plz Los Angeles, CA 90095-6591; **Office Phone:** (310) 825-4966; **Board Certification:** Radiology 1982; **Medical School:** UCLA 1977; **Residency:** Radiation Oncology, UCLA Med Ctr, Los Angeles, CA 1979-1982; **Faculty Appointment:** Clin Prof Radiation Oncology, UCLA

Shank, Brenda MD/PhD (Radiation Oncology) - *Special Expertise:* *Breast Cancer;* **Admitting Hospital:** Doctors Medical Center; **Office Address:** Doctors Medical Center 2000 Vale Rd San Pablo, CA 94806; **Office Phone:** (510) 970-5239; **Board Certification:** Therapeutic Radiology 1980; **Medical School:** UMDNJ-RW Johnson Med Sch 1976; **Residency:** Radium Therapy, Mem Sloan Kettering Cancer Ctr, New York, NY 1976-1979; **Fellowship:** Mem Sloan Kettering Cancer Ctr, New York, NY 1979-1980

Streeter Jr, Oscar E MD (Radiation Oncology) - *Special Expertise:* *Lung Cancer; Head & Neck Cancer;* **Admitting Hospital:** USC Norris Cancer Comprehensive Center; **Office Address:** Kenneth Norris Jr Cancer Hosp 1441 Eastlake Ave Los Angeles, CA 90033; **Office Phone:** (323) 865-3084; **Board Certification:** Radiation Oncology 1989; **Medical School:** Howard Univ 1982; **Residency:** Radiation Oncology, Howard Univ, Washington, DC 1983-1986; **Faculty Appointment:** Assoc Prof Radiation Oncology, USC Sch Med

RADIOLOGY

A radiologist utilizes radiologic methodologies to diagnose and treat disease. Physicians practicing in the field of radiology most often specialize in radiology, diagnostic radiology, radiation oncology or radiological physics.

DIAGNOSTIC RADIOLOGY
A radiologist who utilizes X-ray, radionuclides, ultrasound and electromagnetic radiation to diagnose and treat disease.

RADIATION ONCOLOGY
A radiologist who deals with the therapeutic applications of radiant energy and its modifiers and the study and management of disease, especially malignant tumors.

Training required: Four years

Certification in one of the following subspecialties requires additional training and examination.

Neuroradiology: A radiologist who diagnoses and treats diseases utilizing imaging procedures as they relate to the brain, spine and spinal cord, head, neck and organs of special sense in adults and children.

Pediatric Radiology: A radiologist who is proficient in all forms of diagnostic imaging as it pertains to the treatment of diseases in the newborn, infant, child and adolescent. This specialist has knowledge of both imaging and interventional procedures related to the care and manegemtn of diseases of children. A pediatric radiologist must be highly knowledgeable of all organ systems as they relate to growth and development, congenital malformations, diseases peculiar to infants and children and diseases that begin in childhood but cause substantial residual impairment in adulthood.

Vascular and Interventional Radiology: A radiologist who diagnoses and treats diseases by various radiologic imaging modalities. These include fluoroscopy, digital radiography, computed tomography, sonography and magnetic resonance imaging.

Physician Listings

New England

Kopans, Daniel B MD (Diagnostic Radiology) - *Special Expertise:* Breast Imaging; **Admitting Hospital:** Massachusetts General Hospital; **Office Address:** Mass Genl Hosp, WACC 15 Parkman St, Level 2, # 219 Boston, MA 02114; **Office Phone:** (617) 726-3093; **Board Certification:** Diagnostic Radiology 1977; **Medical School:** Harvard Med Sch 1973; **Residency:** Diagnostic Radiology, Mass Genl Hosp, Boston, MA 1974-1977; **Faculty Appointment:** Prof Radiology, Harvard Med Sch

McCarthy, Shirley MD/PhD (Diagnostic Radiology) - *Special Expertise:* Infertility; Gynecologic Cancer; **Admitting Hospital:** Yale - New Haven Hospital; **Office Address:** Yale Univ Med Sch, Dept Rad 333 Cedar St New Haven, CT 06520; **Office Phone:** (203) 785-5251; **Board Certification:** Diagnostic Radiology 1983; **Medical School:** Yale Univ 1979; **Residency:** Radiology, Yale-New Haven Hosp, New Haven, CT 1980-1983; **Fellowship:** Cross Sectional Imaging, UCSF Med Ctr, San Francisco, CA 1983-1984; **Faculty Appointment:** Prof Diagnostic Radiology, Yale Univ

Mid Atlantic

Austin, John MD (Diagnostic Radiology) - *Special Expertise:* Diagnostic Radiology - General; **Admitting Hospital:** Columbia Presbyterian Medical Center (Page 72); **Office Address:** Columbia Presby Med Ctr 622 W 168th St New York, NY 10032; **Office Phone:** (212) 305-2986; **Board Certification:** Radiology 1970; **Medical School:** Yale Univ 1965; **Residency:** Radiology, UC San Francisco Med Ctr, San Francisco, CA 1966-1970; **Faculty Appointment:** Prof Radiology

Dalinka, Murray MD (Diagnostic Radiology) - *Special Expertise:* Bone Disorders; Musculoskeletal Disorders; **Admitting Hospital:** Hospital of the University of Pennsylvania; **Office Address:** Hospital of Univ Pa, Dept of Radiology 3400 Spruce St Philadelphia, PA 19104; **Office Phone:** (215) 662-3019; **Board Certification:** Radiology 1969; **Medical School:** Univ Mich Med Sch 1964; **Residency:** Radiology, Montefiore Hosp, Bronx, NY 1965-1968; **Faculty Appointment:** Prof Radiology, Univ Penn

Edelstein, Barbara A MD (Diagnostic Radiology) - *Special Expertise:* Breast Cancer; Women's Radiology; **Admitting Hospital:** Lenox Hill Hospital; **Office Address:** Women's Radiology PC 1045 Park Ave New York, NY 10028; **Office Phone:** (212) 860-7700; **Board Certification:** Diagnostic Radiology 1983; **Medical School:** NY Med Coll 1977; **Residency:** Diagnostic Radiology, Montefiore Hosp, New York, NY 1979-1982

Fishman, Elliot MD (Diagnostic Radiology) - *Special Expertise:* Thoracic Imaging; Abdominal Imaging; **Admitting Hospital:** Johns Hopkins Hospital - Baltimore (Page 65); **Office Address:** Johns Hopkins Hosp, Dept Radiology 600 North Wolfe Street Baltimore, MD 21287; **Office Phone:** (410) 955-5173; **Board Certification:** Diagnostic Radiology 1981; **Medical School:** Univ MD Sch Med 1977; **Residency:** Diagnostic Radiology, Sinai Hospital, Baltimore, MD 1977-1980; **Fellowship:** Diagnostic Radiology, Johns Hopkins Hospital, Baltimore, MD 1980-1981; **Faculty Appointment:** Prof Radiology, Johns Hopkins Univ

Kurtz, Albert B MD (Diagnostic Radiology) - *Special Expertise:* Obstetrical Ultrasound; **Admitting Hospital:** Thomas Jefferson University Hospital; **Office Address:** Thomas Jefferson Univ Hosp, Dept Radiology 111 S 11th St, rm 3350AB Philadelphia, PA 19107; **Office Phone:** (215) 995-6343; **Board Certification:** Diagnostic Radiology 1977; **Medical School:** St Louis Univ 1972; **Residencies:** Internal Medicine, Montefiore Med Ctr, Bronx, NY 1973-1974; Diagnostic Radiology, Montefiore Med Ctr, Bronx, NY 1974-1977; **Fellowship:** Ultrasound, Thomas Jefferson Univ Hosp, Philadelphia, PA 1977-1978; **Faculty Appointment:** Prof Radiology, Jefferson Med Coll

Mitnick, Julie MD (Diagnostic Radiology) - *Special Expertise:* Mammography; Breast Cancer; **Admitting Hospital:** NYU Medical Center (Page 70); **Office Address:** 650 1st Ave New York, NY 10016; **Office Phone:** (212) 686-4440; **Board Certification:** Diagnostic Radiology 1977; **Medical School:** NYU Sch Med 1977; **Residency:** Diagnostic Radiology, NYU Med Ctr, New York, NY 1973-1977; **Fellowship:** Pediatric Radiology, NYU Med Ctr, New York, NY 1977-1978; **Faculty Appointment:** Diagnostic Radiology, NYU Sch Med

Panicek, David MD (Diagnostic Radiology) - *Special Expertise:* Bone/Soft Tissue Radiology; Cross Sectional Imaging; **Admitting Hospital:** Memorial Sloan Kettering Cancer Center; **Office Address:** Meml Sloan Kettering Cancer Ctr, Dept of Rad 1275 York Ave, rm C278 New York, NY 10021; **Office Phone:** (212) 639-5825; **Board Certification:** Diagnostic Radiology 1984; **Medical School:** Cornell Univ-Weil Med Coll 1980; **Residency:** Radiology, NY Hosp-Cornell, New York, NY 1981-1984; **Faculty Appointment:** Prof Radiology, Cornell Univ-Weill Med Coll

Sostman, H Dirk MD (Diagnostic Radiology) - *Special Expertise:* Diagnostic Radiology - General; **Admitting Hospital:** New York Weill Cornell Medical Center - NY Presbyterian Hospital (Page 72); **Office Address:** 525 E 68TH St, Starr Bldg, rm 8A37 New York, NY 10021; **Office Phone:** (212) 746-2520; **Board Certifications:** Diagnostic Radiology 1980, Nuclear Medicine 1996; **Medical School:** Yale Univ 1976; **Residencies:** Internal Medicine, Yale-New Haven Hosp, New Haven, CT 1976-1977; Diagnostic Radiology, Yale New Haven Hosp, New Haven, CT 1977-1979; **Fellowships:** Nuclear Medicine, Yale-New Haven Hosp, New Haven, CT 1979-1980; Pulmonary Disease, Yale-New Haven Hosp, New Haven, CT 1980-1981; **Faculty Appointment:** Prof Radiology, Cornell Univ-Weill Med Coll

Teal, James S MD (Diagnostic Radiology) - *Special Expertise:* Interventional Radiology; **Admitting Hospital:** Howard University Hospital; **Office Address:** Howard Univ Hosp, Dept Rad 2041 Georgia Ave NW Washington, DC 20060-0001; **Office Phone:** (202) 865-1571; **Board Certification:** Diagnostic Radiology 1970; **Medical School:** Univ Tex Med Br, Galveston 1965; **Residency:** Radiology, Mt Zion Hosp, San Francisco, CA 1965-1969; **Fellowship:** Neurology, LAC Univ of SCA, Los Angeles, CA 1969-1970; **Faculty Appointment:** Prof Radiology, Howard Univ

Templeton, Philip MD (Diagnostic Radiology) - *Special Expertise:* Lung Biopsy; **Admitting Hospital:** University of Maryland Medical System; **Office Address:** Univ of Maryland Hosp 22 South Greene Street Baltimore, MD 21201; **Office Phone:** (410) 328-3477; **Board Certification:** Diagnostic Radiology 1987; **Medical School:** Univ Rochester 1982; **Residency:** Radiology, Univ Maryland Hosp, Baltimore, MD 1983-1987; **Fellowship:** Thoracic Radiology, Mass Gnl Hosp, Boston, MA 1987-1988; **Faculty Appointment:** Prof Radiology, Univ MD Sch Med

White, Charles MD (Diagnostic Radiology) - *Special Expertise:* Thoracic Radiology; **Admitting Hospital:** University of Maryland Medical System; **Office Address:** Univ of MD Med Hosp 22 S Green St Baltimore, MD 21201; **Office Phone:** (410) 328-8667; **Board Certifications:** Internal Medicine 1987, Radiology 1991; **Medical School:** SUNY Buffalo 1984; **Residencies:** Internal Medicine, Columbia Presby, New York, NY 1984-1987; Diagnostic Radiology, Columbia Presby, New York, NY 1987-1991; **Faculty Appointment:** Assoc Prof Diagnostic Radiology, Univ MD Sch Med

Southeast

Hawkins Jr, Irvin MD (Diagnostic Radiology) - *Special Expertise: Interventional Radiology;* **Admitting Hospital:** Shands Healthcare at University Florida (Page 77); **Office Address:** Shands University of Florida Box 100374 Gainesville, FL 32610; **Office Phone:** (352) 395-0291; **Board Certification:** Diagnostic Radiology 1969; **Medical School:** Univ MD Sch Med 1962; **Residency:** Radiology, Ohio State Univ, Columbus, OH 1965-1968; **Fellowship:** Cardiology (Cardiovascular Disease), Shands Teaching Hosps, Gainesville, FL 1968-1970; **Faculty Appointment:** Prof Radiology, Univ Fla Coll Med

Mancuso, Anthony MD (Diagnostic Radiology) - *Special Expertise: Soft Tissue Tumors;* **Admitting Hospital:** Shands Healthcare at University Florida (Page 77); **Office Address:** Shands HealthCare at Univ Fla, Dept Rad 1600 SW Archer Rd Gainesville, FL 32601; **Office Phone:** (352) 395-0106; **Board Certifications:** Diagnostic Radiology 1978, Nuclear Radiology 1995; **Medical School:** Univ Miami Sch Med 1973; **Residencies:** Diagnostic Radiology, UCLA Med Ctr, Los Angeles, CA; Nuclear Medicine, UCLA Med Ctr, Los Angeles, CA; **Fellowship:** Radiology, UCLA Med Ctr, Los Angeles, CA; **Faculty Appointment:** Prof Radiology, Univ Fla Coll Med

Pisano, Etta Driscoll MD (Diagnostic Radiology) - *Special Expertise: Oncology; Breast Imaging;* **Admitting Hospital:** University of North Carolina Hospitals; **Office Address:** 101 Manning Dr, Box 7510 Chapel Hill, NC 27299-7510; **Office Phone:** (919) 966-6957; **Board Certification:** Diagnostic Radiology 1988; **Medical School:** Duke Univ 1983; **Residency:** Diagnostic Radiology, Beth Israel Deaconess Hosp, Boston, MA 1984-1988

Midwest

Cavallino, Robert MD (Diagnostic Radiology) - *Special Expertise: Musculoskeletal Radiology;* **Admitting Hospital:** Illinois Masonic Medical Center (Page 64); **Office Address:** IL Masonic Med Ctr, Dept of Radiology 836 W Wellington Ave Chicago, IL 60657-4421; **Office Phone:** (773) 296-7820; **Board Certification:** Diagnostic Radiology 1968; **Medical School:** Tufts Univ 1959; **Residency:** Radiology, New York Hosp, New York, NY 1964-1967; **Faculty Appointment:** Prof Radiology, Rush Med Coll

Sagel, Stuart Steven MD (Diagnostic Radiology) - *Special Expertise: Diagnostic Radiology - General;* **Admitting Hospital:** Barnes - Jewish Hospital; **Office Address:** Mallinckrodt Inst Rad-Barnes Hosp 510 S Kingshighway Blvd, Box 8131 St Louis, MO 63110-1016; **Office Phone:** (314) 362-2927; **Board Certification:** Diagnostic Radiology 1970; **Medical School:** Temple Univ 1965; **Residencies:** Diagnostic Radiology, Yale New Haven Hosp, New Haven, CT 1966-1968; Diagnostic Radiology, UCSF, San Francisco, CA 1968-1970; **Faculty Appointment:** Prof Radiology, Washington Univ, St Louis

Southwest

Dodd III, Gerald Dewey MD (Diagnostic Radiology) - *Special Expertise: Ultrasound;* **Admitting Hospital:** University of Texas Health & Science Center; **Office Address:** 7703 Floyd Curl Dr, MC-7800 San Antonio, TX 78229-3900; **Office Phone:** (210) 567-6470; **Board Certification:** Diagnostic Radiology 1987; **Medical School:** Univ Tex, Houston 1983; **Residencies:** Diagnostic Radiology, Univ Hosp, Cincinnati, OH 1984-1987; Diagnostic Radiology, Univ Hosp, Cincinnati, OH 1986-1987; **Fellowship:** Abdonimal Imaging & Angio-Interventional, Univ Hosp, Cincinnati, OH 1987-1988; **Faculty Appointment:** Prof Radiology, Univ Tex, San Antonio

Huynh, Phan Tuong MD (Diagnostic Radiology) - _Special Expertise:_ Mammography; **Admitting Hospital:** St Luke's Episcopal Hospital - Houston (Page 76); **Office Address:** Women's Center 6624 Fannin St, Fl 10 Houston, TX 77030; **Office Phone:** (713) 791-8120; **Board Certification:** Diagnostic Radiology 1994; **Medical School:** Univ VA Sch Med 1989; **Residency:** Radiology, Univ Virginia, Charlottesville, VA 1990-1994; **Fellowship:** Mammography, Iniv Virginia, Charlottesville, VA 1994

Otto, Pamela MD (Diagnostic Radiology) - _Special Expertise:_ Mammography; **Admitting Hospital:** University of Texas Health & Science Center; **Office Address:** UTHSCSA- Dept. of Radiology 7703 Floyd Curl Dr. San Antonio, TX 78229-3900; **Office Phone:** (210) 567-6488; **Board Certification:** Diagnostic Radiology 1993; **Medical School:** Univ MO-Columbia Sch Med 1988; **Residency:** Radiology, U of Tx Hlth Sci Ctr., San Antonio, TX 1990-1993; **Faculty Appointment:** Assoc Prof Radiology, Univ Tex, San Antonio

Rivera, Frank James MD (Diagnostic Radiology) - _Special Expertise:_ Interventional Radiology; **Admitting Hospital:** Parkland Memorial Hospital; **Office Address:** UT Southwestern Medical Center 5323 Harry Hines Blvd Dallas, TX 75390-8896; **Office Phone:** (214) 648-8011; **Board Certifications:** Diagnostic Radiology 1989, Vascular & Interventional Radiology 1998; **Medical School:** Univ Tex, San Antonio 1982; **Residency:** Diagnostic Radiology, SUNY, Syracuse, NY 1985-1989; **Fellowship:** Vascular & Interventional Radiology, SUNY, Syracuse, NY 1988-1989; **Faculty Appointment:** Asst Prof Radiology, Univ Tex, Houston

West Coast and Pacific

Gomes, Antoinette Susan MD (Diagnostic Radiology) - _Special Expertise:_ Cardiovascular Intervention Radiology; **Admitting Hospital:** UCLA Medical Center; **Office Address:** UCLA Med Ctr 10833 Le Conte Ave, Bldg CHS, Box 951721 Los Angeles, CA 90095-1721; **Office Phone:** (310) 206-8909; **Board Certifications:** Diagnostic Radiology 1975, Vascular & Interventional Radiology 1994; **Medical School:** Med Coll PA Hahnemann 1969; **Residencies:** Internal Medicine, LAC-USC MC, Los Angeles, CA 1970-1972; Diagnostic Radiology, Stanford Univ, CA 1972-1975; **Fellowship:** Univ Minn, MN 1976-1978; **Faculty Appointment:** Prof Radiology, UCLA

RADIOLOGY

New England

Benson, Carol MD (Radiology) - *Special Expertise: Obstetrical Ultrasound;* **Admitting Hospital:** Brigham & Women's Hospital; **Office Address:** Brigham & Womens Hosp 75 Francis St Boston, MA 02115-6110; **Office Phone:** (617) 732-6280; **Board Certification:** Diagnostic Radiology 1984; **Medical School:** Univ Penn 1980; **Residency:** Radiology, NY Hosp-Cornell Univ, New York, NY 1981-1984; **Fellowship:** Brigham Womens, Boston, MA 1984-1985; **Faculty Appointment:** Assoc Prof Harvard Med Sch

Mid Atlantic

Berdon, Walter MD (Radiology) - *Special Expertise: Radiology-Pediatric;* **Admitting Hospital:** Columbia Presbyterian Medical Center (Page 72); **Office Address:** Columbia Presby Med Ctr 3959 Broadway New York, NY 10032; **Office Phone:** (212) 305-9864; **Board Certifications:** Radiology 1962, Pediatric Radiology 1995; **Medical School:** SUNY Syracuse 1955; **Residencies:** Internal Medicine, Montefiore Hosp, New York, NY 1956-1957; Radiology, Montefiore Hosp, New York, NY 1959-1962; **Fellowship:** Pediatric Radiology, Coll P&S -Columbia Univ, New York, NY 1962-1964; **Faculty Appointment:** Prof Radiology, Columbia P&S

Berenstein, Alejandro MD (Radiology) - *Special Expertise: Neuro-Radiology;* **Admitting Hospital:** Beth Israel Medical Center - New York; **Office Address:** Hyman Newman Inst Neurolgy & Neuro Surg 170 E End Ave at 87th St, Fl 3 New York, NY 10128; **Office Phone:** (212) 870-9660; **Board Certifications:** Diagnostic Radiology 1976, Neuroradiology 1995; **Medical School:** Mexico 1970; **Residency:** Radiology, Mount Sinai Med Ctr, New York, NY 1973-1976; **Fellowship:** Neuroradiology, NYU Med Ctr, New York, NY 1976-1978; **Faculty Appointment:** Prof Radiology, Albert Einstein Coll Med

Coldwell, Douglas Michael MD (Radiology) - *Special Expertise: Vascular & Interventional Radiology; Chemoembolization;* **Admitting Hospital:** University of Maryland Medical System; **Office Address:** Univ of Maryland Med System, Dept Radiology 22 South Greene Street Baltimore, MD 21201; **Office Phone:** (410) 328-7490; **Board Certifications:** Diagnostic Radiology 1986, Vascular & Interventional Radiology 1995; **Medical School:** Univ Tex Med Br, Galveston 1980; **Residency:** Diagnostic Radiology, Hershey Med Ctr-Penn St U, Hershey, PA 1980-1983; **Fellowship:** Vascular & Interventional Radiology, MD Anderson Hosp-Tumor Inst, Houston, TX 1983-1984; **Faculty Appointment:** Prof Radiology, Univ MD Sch Med

Dershaw, D David MD (Radiology) - *Special Expertise: Breast Cancer; Radiology-Diagnostic;* **Admitting Hospital:** Memorial Sloan Kettering Cancer Center; **Office Address:** 1275 York Ave New York, NY 10021; **Office Phone:** (212) 639-7295; **Board Certification:** Diagnostic Radiology 1978; **Medical School:** Jefferson Med Coll 1974; **Residency:** Diagnostic Radiology, NY Hosp, New York, NY 1975-1978; **Fellowship:** Ultrasound, Thomas Jefferson Univ Hosp, Philadelphia, PA 1978-1979; **Faculty Appointment:** Prof Radiology, Cornell Univ-Weill Med Coll

Haskal, Ziv MD (Radiology) - *Special Expertise: Uterine Fibroid Embolization; Angiography; Vascular & Interventional Radiology;* **Admitting Hospital:** Columbia Presbyterian Medical Center (Page 72); **Office Address:** Vascular and Interventional Radiology 177 W Fort Washington Ave, Bldg MHB - Fl 4 - Ste 100 New York, NY 10032; **Office Phone:** (212) 305-8070; **Board Certifications:** Diagnostic Radiology 1991, Vascular & Interventional Radiology 1999; **Medical School:** Boston Univ 1986; **Residency:** Diagnostic Radiology, UCSF, San Francisco, CA 1987-1991; **Fellowship:** Vascular & Interventional Radiology, UCSF, San Francisco, CA 1991-1992; **Faculty Appointment:** Prof Radiology, Columbia P&S

Kandarpa, Krishna MD (Radiology) - *Special Expertise:* Vascular & Interventional Radiology; **Admitting Hospital:** New York Weill Cornell Medical Center - NY Presbyterian Hospital (Page 72); **Office Address:** NY Weill Cornell Med Ctr - NY Presby, Dept Rad 525 E 68th St, L-515 New York, NY 10021-4873; **Office Phone:** (212) 746-2604; **Board Certifications:** Diagnostic Radiology 1984, Vascular & Interventional Radiology 1996; **Medical School:** Univ Miami Sch Med 1980; **Residency:** Radiology, Brigham & Women's-Harvard, Boston, MA 1981-1984; **Fellowship:** Vascular & Interventional Radiology, Brigham & Women's-Harvard, Boston, MA 1984-1986; **Faculty Appointment:** Prof Radiology, Cornell Univ-Weil Med Coll

Leonidas, John MD (Radiology) - *Special Expertise:* Radiology-Pediatric; **Admitting Hospital:** Long Island Jewish Medical Center; **Office Address:** Pediatric Radiology 270-05 76th Ave New Hyde Park, NY 11040-1433; **Office Phone:** (718) 470-3404; **Board Certifications:** Pediatrics 1965, Radiology 1969; **Medical School:** Greece 1955; **Residency:** Pediatrics, Jewish Hosp, Brooklyn, NY 1961-1963; **Fellowship:** Diagnostic Radiology, Columbia-Presby Med Ctr, New York, NY 1966-1969; **Faculty Appointment:** Prof Radiology, Albert Einstein Coll Med

Norton, Karen MD (Radiology) - *Special Expertise:* Radiology-Pediatric; **Admitting Hospital:** Mount Sinai Hospital (Page 70); **Office Address:** 1 Gustave Levy Pl New York, NY 10029-6504; **Office Phone:** (212) 241-7418; **Board Certifications:** Radiology 1984, Pediatric Radiology 1995; **Medical School:** Mount Sinai Sch Med 1980; **Residencies:** Pediatrics, NYU Med Ctr, New York, NY 1980-1981; Radiology, Mount Sinai Hosp, New York, NY 1981-1984; **Fellowship:** Pediatric Pulmonology, Mount Sinai Hosp, New York, NY 1984-1985; **Faculty Appointment:** Asst Prof Pediatric Radiology, Mount Sinai Sch Med

Pile-Spellman, John MD (Radiology) - *Special Expertise:* Interventional Neuroradiology; **Admitting Hospital:** Columbia Presbyterian Medical Center (Page 72); **Office Address:** Interventional Neuroradiology 177 Fort Washington Ave, Bldg MHB 8SK New York, NY 10032; **Office Phone:** (212) 305-6384; **Board Certification:** Diagnostic Radiology 1984; **Medical School:** Tufts Univ 1978; **Residencies:** Neurological Surgery, New England Med Ctr, Boston, MA 1979-1981; Neurological Radiology, Mass Genl Hosp, Boston, MA 1984-1986; **Fellowship:** Interventional Neurological Radiology, NYU Med Ctr, New York, NY 1986; **Faculty Appointment:** Prof Radiology, Columbia P&S

Tenner, Michael MD (Radiology) - *Special Expertise:* Neuroradiology; **Admitting Hospital:** Westchester Medical Center; **Office Address:** NY Med Coll, Dept. Radiology Route 100 Munger Pavilion Valhalla, NY 10595; **Office Phone:** (914) 493-1927; **Board Certifications:** Radiology 1967, Neuroradiology 1995; **Medical School:** Univ MD Sch Med 1960; **Residencies:** Univ Maryland Hosp, Baltimore, MD 1961-1962; Univ Maryland Hosp, Baltimore, MD 1962-1964; **Fellowships:** Neuroradiology, Columbia-Presby, New York, NY 1966-1967; Neuro Inst 1966-1968; **Faculty Appointment:** Prof Neuroradiology, NY Med Coll

Yoon, Sydney MD (Radiology) - *Special Expertise:* Fibroid Embolization; Interventional Radiology; **Admitting Hospital:** St Francis Hospital (Page 75); **Office Address:** St Francis Hosp, Dept Radiology 100 Pt Washington Blvd Roslyn, NY 11576-1348; **Office Phone:** (516) 562-6517; **Board Certifications:** Diagnostic Radiology 1993, Neuroradiology 1995; **Medical School:** Univ Chicago-Pritzker Sch Med 1986; **Residencies:** Internal Medicine, Johns Hopkins Hosp, Baltimore, MD 1987-1989; Diagnostic Radiology, UCLA Med Ctr, Los Angeles, CA 1989-1993; **Fellowships:** Nuclear Radiology, Columbia Presby Med Ctr, New York, NY 1993-1995; Vascular & Interventional Radiology, UCLA Med Ctr, Los Angeles, CA 1996-1997

Southeast

Becker, Gary J. MD (Radiology) - *Special Expertise: Vascular & Interventional Radiology;* **Admitting Hospital:** Baptist Hospital - Miami; **Office Address:** Miami Cardiac&Vascular Institute 8900 N Kendall Drive Miami, FL 33176-2118; **Office Phone:** (305) 598-5990; **Board Certifications:** Vascular & Interventional Radiology 1994, Diagnostic Radiology 1981; **Medical School:** Indiana Univ 1977; **Residency:** Diagnostic Radiology, Ind Univ Med Ctr., Indianapolis, IN 1978-1981; **Faculty Appointment:** Clin Prof Radiology, Univ Miami Sch Med

Benenati, James Francis MD (Radiology) - *Special Expertise: Uterine Fibroid Embolization; Stentgraphs; Aneurysm-Abdominal Aortic;* **Admitting Hospital:** Baptist Hospital - Miami; **Office Address:** 8900 N Kendall Dr Miami, FL 33176-2118; **Office Phone:** (305) 598-5990; **Board Certifications:** Diagnostic Radiology 1988, Vascular & Interventional Radiology 1995; **Medical School:** Univ S Fla Coll Med 1984; **Residency:** Radiation Oncology, Indiana Univ Hosp, Indianapolis, IN 1984-1988; **Fellowship:** Cardiology (Cardiovascular Disease), Johns Hopkins Hosp, Baltimore, MD 1988-1989; **Faculty Appointment:** Prof Radiology, Univ Miami Sch Med

Katzen, Barry MD (Radiology) - *Special Expertise: Radiology - General;* **Admitting Hospital:** Baptist Hospital - Miami; **Office Address:** Miami Cardiac & Vascular Inst 8900 N Kendall Dr Miami, FL 33176-2118; **Office Phone:** (305) 598-5990; **Board Certifications:** Diagnostic Radiology 1974, Vascular & Interventional Radiology 1994; **Medical School:** Univ Miami Sch Med 1970; **Residency:** Radiology, NY Hosp Cornell Med Ctr, New York, NY 1971-1974

Midwest

Charboneau, J William MD (Radiology) - *Special Expertise: Ultrasound; Liver Cancer-Diagnosis & Ablation; Thyroid Cancer;* **Admitting Hospital:** Mayo Medical Center & Clinic - Rochester; **Office Address:** Mayo Clinic 200 First Street SW Rochester, MN 55905; **Office Phone:** (507) 284-2097; **Board Certification:** Diagnostic Radiology 1980; **Medical School:** Univ Wisc 1976; **Residency:** Radiology, Mayo Clinic, Rochester, MN 1976-1980; **Faculty Appointment:** Prof Radiology, Mayo Med Sch

Cross III, DeWitte T MD (Radiology) - *Special Expertise: Neuro-Radiology;* **Admitting Hospital:** Barnes - Jewish Hospital; **Office Address:** Wash Univ, Dept Rad 510 S Kingshighway Blvd St Louis, MO 63110-1016; **Office Phone:** (314) 362-5950; **Board Certifications:** Diagnostic Radiology 1985, Neuroradiology 1996; **Medical School:** Univ Ala 1980; **Residency:** Diagnostic Radiology, Naval Hosp, Bethesda, MD 1982-1985; **Fellowships:** Neuroradiology, NY Med Coll, Valhalla, NY 1987-1988; Neuroradiology, Columbia Univ, New York, NY 1988-1989; **Faculty Appointment:** Assoc Prof Radiology, Washington Univ, St Louis

Goodman, Lawrence R MD (Radiology) - *Special Expertise: Thoracic Radiology; Radiology-Diagnostic;* **Admitting Hospital:** Froedtert Memorial Lutheran Hospital; **Office Address:** Froedtert Meml Lutheran Hosp, Dept Radiology 9200 West Wisconsin Avenue Milwaukee, WI 53226; **Office Phone:** (414) 805-3700; **Board Certification:** Diagnostic Radiology 1973; **Medical School:** SUNY Downstate 1968; **Residency:** Radiology, Boston City Hosp, Boston, MA 1969-1972; **Fellowship:** Univ California Hosp, CA 1972-1973

Martenson Jr, James A MD (Radiology) - *Special Expertise: Mucositis; Espohagitis; Therapeutic Radiology;* **Admitting Hospital:** Mayo Medical Center & Clinic - Rochester; **Office Address:** Mayo Clinic, Dept Radiation Oncology 200 First St SW Rochester, MN 55905; **Office Phone:** (507) 284-4561; **Board Certification:** Therapeutic Radiology 1985; **Medical School:** Univ Wash 1981; **Residency:** Radiation Oncology, Mayo Grad Sch Med, Rochester, MN 1981-1985; **Faculty Appointment:** Assoc Prof Radiology, Mayo Med Sch

RADIOLOGY

Midwest

McAlister, Bill MD (Radiology) - *Special Expertise:* Radiology-Pediatric; **Admitting Hospital:** St Louis Children's Hospital; **Office Address:** 510 S Kingshighway Blvd Saint Louis, MO 63110; **Office Phone:** (314) 454-6229; **Board Certifications:** Pediatric Radiology 1994, Radiology 1961; **Medical School:** Wayne State Univ 1954; **Residency:** Radiology, Cincinnati Genl Hosp, Cincinnati, OH 1957-1960; **Faculty Appointment:** Prof Radiology, Washington Univ, St Louis

Modic, Michael MD (Radiology) - *Special Expertise:* Neuro-Radiology; MRI; **Admitting Hospital:** Cleveland Clinic Foundation; **Office Address:** Cleveland Clinic 9500 Euclid Ave Cleveland, OH 44195; **Office Phone:** (216) 444-9308; **Board Certifications:** Diagnostic Radiology 1979, Neuroradiology 1995; **Medical School:** Case West Res Univ 1975; **Residency:** Radiology, Cleveland Clin Fdn, Cleveland, OH; **Fellowship:** Radiology, Cleveland Clin Fdn, Cleveland, OH

Sivit, Carlos MD (Radiology) - *Special Expertise:* Radiology-Pediatric; Abdominal Imaging; Emergency Radiology; **Admitting Hospital:** Rainbow Babies & Children's Hospital; **Office Address:** Univ Hosps Cleveland, Dept Radiology 11100 Euclid Ave Cleveland, OH 44106; **Office Phone:** (216) 844-1172; **Board Certifications:** Radiology 1987, Pediatric Radiology 1995; **Medical School:** Univ VA Sch Med 1981; **Residencies:** Pediatrics, Vanderbilt Univ Hosp, Nashville, TN 1981-1984; Radiology, George Washington Univ Hosp, Washington, DC 1984-1987; **Fellowship:** Pediatric Radiology, Chldns Natl Med Ctr, Washington, DC 1987-1989; **Faculty Appointment:** Prof Radiology, Case West Res Univ

Great Plains and Mountains

Durham, Janette Denham MD (Radiology) - *Special Expertise:* Vascular & Interventional Radiology; **Admitting Hospital:** University of Colorado Health & Science Center; **Office Address:** Univ Colo Hlth Sci Ctr 4200 E Ninth Ave, Box A 030 Denver, CO 80262; **Office Phone:** (303) 372-6134; **Board Certifications:** Diagnostic Radiology 1987, Vascular & Interventional Radiology 1996; **Medical School:** Indiana Univ **Residency:** Ind Univ Hosp, Indianapolis, IN 1983-1987; **Fellowship:** Mass Genl Hosp, Boston, MA 1987-1988; **Faculty Appointment:** Assoc Prof Radiology, Univ Colo

Kumpe, David A MD (Radiology) - *Special Expertise:* Vascular & Interventional Radiology; Neurovascular Disease; **Admitting Hospital:** University of Colorado Health & Science Center; **Office Address:** Univ Hosp-Denver, Dept Radiology 4200 E 9th Ave, Box A030 Denver, CO 80626; **Office Phone:** (303) 372-6141; **Board Certifications:** Radiology 1972, Vascular & Interventional Radiology 1994; **Medical School:** Harvard Med Sch 1967; **Residency:** Radiology, Mass Genl Hosp, Boston, MA 1968-1971; **Fellowships:** Neurological Radiology, Zurich, Switzerland 1974-1975; Angiography, Zurich, Switzerland 1975-1976; **Faculty Appointment:** Prof Radiology, Univ Colo

Miller, Franklin MD (Radiology) - *Special Expertise:* Interventional Radiology; **Admitting Hospital:** University of Utah Hospital and Clinics; **Office Address:** Univ of Utah School of Medicine 50 N Medical Drive, rm 1A71 Salt Lake City, UT 84132-0002; **Office Phone:** (801) 581-8188; **Board Certifications:** Diagnostic Radiology 1973, Vascular & Interventional Radiology 1995; **Medical School:** Temple Univ 1966; **Residency:** Diagnostic Radiology, Johns Hopkins Hosp, Baltimore, MD 1969-1972; **Fellowship:** Vascular & Interventional Radiology, Johns Hopkins Hosp, Baltimore, MD 1972-1973; **Faculty Appointment:** Prof Radiology, Univ Utah

Southwest

Palmaz, Julio C. MD (Radiology) - *Special Expertise:* Interventional Radiology; Endovascular Therapy; Intravascular Stents; **Admitting Hospital:** University of Texas Health & Science Center; **Office Address:** 7703 Floyd Curl Dr. San Antonio, TX 78229-3900; **Office Phone:** (210) 567-5564; **Board Certifications:** Diagnostic Radiology 1981, Vascular & Interventional Radiology 1994; **Medical School:** Argentina 1971; **Residency:** Radiology, Rawson Hosp Bueno Aires, Argentina 1971-1974; **Fellowship:** Vascular & Interventional Radiology, UC Davis VA Med Ctr, Martinez, CA 1977-1980; **Faculty Appointment:** Prof Radiology, Univ Tex, San Antonio

Seibert, Joanna J MD (Radiology) - *Special Expertise:* Sickle Cell Screening; Radiology-Pediatric; **Admitting Hospital:** Arkansas Children's Hospital; **Office Address:** Arkansas Children's Hospital-Dept Rad 800 Marshall St Little Rock, AR 72202; **Office Phone:** (501) 320-1175; **Board Certifications:** Diagnostic Radiology 1974, Pediatric Radiology 1994; **Medical School:** Univ Tenn Coll Med, Memphis 1968; **Residencies:** Radiology, Univ Tenn Coll Med, Iowa City, IA 1972-1973; Radiology, Univ Tenn Coll Med, Memphis, TN 1970-1972; **Faculty Appointment:** Prof Radiology, Univ Ark

West Coast and Pacific

Atlas, Scott W MD (Radiology) - *Special Expertise:* Neuro-Radiology; Brain/Stroke-MRI; **Admitting Hospital:** Stanford Medical Center; **Office Address:** Stanford Univ Med Ctr 300 Pasteur, rm S047 Stanford, CA 94305-5105; **Office Phone:** (650) 723-7426; **Board Certifications:** Diagnostic Radiology 1985, Neuroradiology 1995; **Medical School:** Univ Chicago-Pritzker Sch Med 1981; **Residency:** Radiology, Northwestern Univ Med Ctr, Chicago, IL 1982-1985; **Fellowship:** Neuroradiology, Hosp of Univ Penn, Philadelphia, PA 1985-1987; **Faculty Appointment:** Prof Neuroradiology, Stanford Univ

Dake, Michael David MD (Radiology) - *Special Expertise:* Interventional Radiology; **Admitting Hospital:** Stanford Medical Center; **Office Address:** Stanford Univ Med Ctr 300 Pasteur Dr Stanford, CA 94305; **Office Phone:** (650) 725-5204; **Board Certifications:** Pulmonary Disease 1986, Vascular & Interventional Radiology 1994; **Medical School:** Baylor Coll Med 1978; **Residencies:** Internal Medicine, Baylor Hosp, Houston, TX 1978-1982; Radiology, UCSF, San Francisco, CA 1983-1986; **Fellowships:** Pulmonary Disease, UCSF, San Francisco, CA 1982-1983; Interventional Radiology, UCSF, San Francisco, CA 1986-1987; **Faculty Appointment:** Assoc Prof Radiology, Stanford Univ

Donaldson, Sarah S MD (Radiology) - *Special Expertise:* Radiology - General; **Admitting Hospital:** Stanford Medical Center; **Office Address:** 300 Pasteur Dr, Rm A083 Stanford U Med Ctr, Dept Rad/Onc Stanford, CA 94305; **Office Phone:** (650) 723-6195; **Board Certification:** Therapeutic Radiology 1974; **Medical School:** Harvard Med Sch 1968; **Residency:** Radiology, Stanford University, Stanford, CA 1969-1972; **Fellowships:** Medical Oncology, Inst Gustave-Roussy, France 1972-1973; Medical Oncology, MD Anderson, Houston, TX 1971; **Faculty Appointment:** Prof Radiation Oncology, Stanford Univ

Hasso, Anton N MD (Radiology) - *Special Expertise:* Neuro-Radiology; Epilepsy/Seizure Disorders; **Admitting Hospital:** University of California - Irvine Medical Center; **Office Address:** UC Irvine Med Ctr, Dept Rad 101 The City DR, Rt 140, ZC5005 S Orange, CA 92868-3298; **Office Phone:** (714) 456-6595; **Board Certifications:** Diagnostic Radiology 1972, Neuroradiology 1995; **Medical School:** Loma Linda Univ 1967; **Faculty Appointment:** Clin Prof Radiology, Loma Linda Univ

Keller, Frederick MD (Radiology) - *Special Expertise: Interventional Radiology;* **Admitting Hospital:** Oregon Health Science University Hospital and Clinics; **Office Address:** Dotter Interventional Inst 3181 SW Sam Jackson Park Rd, Ste L-605 Portland, OR 97201-3011; **Office Phone:** (503) 494-7660; **Board Certifications:** Diagnostic Radiology 1977, Vascular & Interventional Radiology 1994; **Medical School:** Univ Penn 1968; **Residency:** Diagnostic Radiology, Univ Oreg Hlth Scis Ctr, Portland, OR 1974-1977; **Faculty Appointment:** Prof Diagnostic Radiology, Oregon Hlth Scis Univ

Petrovich, Zbigniew MD (Radiology) - *Special Expertise: Stereotactic Radiology; Prostate Cancer;* **Admitting Hospital:** USC Norris Cancer Comprehensive Center; **Office Address:** USC, Dept Rad Onc 1441 Eastlake Ave, rm G-356 Los Angeles, CA 90033; **Office Phone:** (323) 865-3072; **Board Certification:** Radiology 1971; **Medical School:** Poland 1963; **Residency:** Radiology, St Boniface Genl Hosp, Winnipeg, Canada 1967-1968

Valji, Karim MD (Radiology) - *Special Expertise: Interventional Radiology;* **Admitting Hospital:** University of California - San Diego Healthcare; **Office Address:** UCSD Med Ctr 200 W Arbor Dr San Diego, CA 92103-8756; **Office Phone:** (619) 543-6607; **Board Certifications:** Diagnostic Radiology 1989, Vascular & Interventional Radiology 1998; **Medical School:** Harvard Med Sch 1982; **Residencies:** Internal Medicine, UCSF, San Francisco, CA 1982-1984; Diagnostic Radiology, UCSD, San Diego, CA 1985-1988; **Fellowship:** Angiography, UCSD, San Diego, CA 1988-1989; **Faculty Appointment:** Assoc Prof Radiology, Univ SD Sch Med

Vinuela, Fernando MD (Radiology) - *Special Expertise: Interventional Neuroradiology; Aneurysm;* **Admitting Hospital:** UCLA Medical Center; **Office Address:** UCLA Med Ctr- 10833 Le Conte Ave, rm BL-121 Los Angeles, CA 90095-1721; **Office Phone:** (310) 825-6576; **Board Certification:** Diagnostic Radiology 1979; **Medical School:** Uruguay 1970; **Residencies:** Radiology, Westminster Hosp, London, England 1974-1975; Radiology, Victoria Hosp, London, England 1975-1977; **Fellowship:** Neuroradiology, Univ Hosp, London, England 1977-1979; **Faculty Appointment:** Prof Radiology, UCLA

Wood, Beverly MD (Radiology) - *Special Expertise: Pediatric Radiology;* **Admitting Hospital:** LAC + USC Medical Center; **Office Address:** 4650 Sunset Blvd Los Angeles, CA 90033; **Office Phone:** (323) 442-2377; **Board Certifications:** Diagnostic Radiology 1972, Pediatric Radiology 1994; **Medical School:** Univ Rochester 1965; **Residency:** Radiology, Strong Meml Hosp, Rochester, NY 1968-1971; **Fellowship:** Pediatric Radiology, Strong Meml Hosp, Rochester, NY 1971-1972; **Faculty Appointment:** Prof Radiology, USC Sch Med

REPRODUCTIVE ENDOCRINOLOGY

(a subspecialty of OBSTETRICS AND GYNECOLOGY)

An obstetrician/gynecologist who is capable of managing complex problems relating to reproductive endocrinology and infertility.

OBSTETRICS AND GYNECOLOGY

An obstetrician/gynecologist possesses special knowledge, skills and professional capability in the medical and surgical care of the female reproductive system and associated disorders. This physician serves as a consultant to other physicians and as a primary physician for women.

Training required: Four years plus two years in clinical practice before certification in obstetrics and gynecology is complete *plus* additional training and examination in reproductive endocrinology

PHYSICIAN LISTINGS

Reproductive Endocrinology

New England

Barbieri, Robert MD (Reproductive Endocrinology) - *Special Expertise:* Fibroids; Infertility-Female; Endometriosis; **Admitting Hospital:** Brigham & Women's Hospital; **Office Address:** Brigham & Womens Hosp, Dept Ob/Gyn 75 Francis St Boston, MA 02482; **Office Phone:** (617) 732-4265; **Board Certifications:** Obstetrics & Gynecology 1997, Reproductive Endocrinology 1997; **Medical School:** Harvard Med Sch 1977; **Residencies:** Obstetrics & Gynecology, Peter Bent Brigham, Boston, MA 1980-1984; Internal Medicine, Peter Bent Brigham, Boston, MA 1977-1980; **Faculty Appointment:** Prof Obstetrics & Gynecology, Harvard Med Sch

Crowley, William MD (Reproductive Endocrinology) - *Special Expertise:* Gonadotropin Deficiency; Kallmann Syndrome; **Admitting Hospital:** Massachusetts General Hospital; **Office Address:** Mass Genl Hosp, Reproductive Sci Ctr Bartlett Hall, Exten 5, Bldg 2511 Boston, MA; **Office Phone:** (617) 726-5390; **Board Certifications:** Internal Medicine 1974, Endocrinology, Diabetes & Metabolism 1977; **Medical School:** Tufts Univ 1969; **Residencies:** Internal Medicine, Mass Genl Hosp, Boston, MA 1970-1971; Internal Medicine, Mass Genl Hosp, Boston, MA 1973-1974; **Fellowship:** Endocrinology, Diabetes & Metabolism, Mass Genl Hosp, Boston, MA 1974-1976; **Faculty Appointment:** Prof Medicine, Harvard Med Sch

Hill III, Joseph Albert MD (Reproductive Endocrinology) - *Special Expertise:* Miscarriage-Recurrent; Infertility-Female; **Admitting Hospital:** Brigham & Women's Hospital; **Office Address:** Brigham & Women's Hospital 75 Francis St. Dept. of OB/GYN Boston, MA 02118; **Office Phone:** (617) 732-4222; **Board Certifications:** Obstetrics & Gynecology 1989, Reproductive Endocrinology 1991; **Medical School:** Med Coll GA 1981; **Residency:** Obstetrics & Gynecology, Med Coll Ga, Augusta, GA 1982-1985; **Fellowship:** Reproductive Endocrinology, Brigham-Womens Hosp/Harvard, Boston, MA; **Faculty Appointment:** Prof Obstetrics & Gynecology, Harvard Med Sch

Isaacson, Keith B MD (Reproductive Endocrinology) - *Special Expertise:* Infertility; Endometriosis; **Admitting Hospital:** Massachusetts General Hospital; **Office Address:** Mass Genl Hosp 32 Fruit St, Bldg Vincent - rm 206 Boston, MA 02114; **Office Phone:** (617) 726-5523; **Board Certifications:** Reproductive Endocrinology 1991, Obstetrics & Gynecology 1990; **Medical School:** Med Coll GA 1983; **Residency:** Obstetrics & Gynecology, Ochsner Foundation Hosp., Houma, LA 1987; **Fellowship:** Reproductive Endocrinology, Univ Penn, Philadelphia, PA 1989; **Faculty Appointment:** Assoc Prof Obstetrics & Gynecology, Harvard Med Sch

Keefe, David Lawrence MD (Reproductive Endocrinology) - *Special Expertise:* Infertility; **Admitting Hospital:** Women & Infants Hospital - Rhode Island; **Office Address:** Women & Infants Hosp, Dept OB/GYN 101 Dudley St Providence, RI 02905; **Office Phone:** (401) 453-7500; **Board Certifications:** Obstetrics & Gynecology 1993, Reproductive Endocrinology 1995; **Medical School:** Georgetown Univ 1980; **Residencies:** Psychiatry, Harvard Psych Srv/Camb Hosp, Boston, MA 1981-1983; Psychiatry, Univ Chicago Hosp & Clins, Chicago, IL 1983-1985; **Fellowships:** Obstetrics & Gynecology, Yale New Haven Hosp, New Haven, CT 1985-1989; Reproductive Endocrinology, Yale New Haven Hosp, New Haven, CT 1989-1991; **Faculty Appointment:** Assoc Prof Obstetrics & Gynecology, Brown Univ

Luciano, Anthony Adolph MD (Reproductive Endocrinology) - *Special Expertise:* Infertility; Endometriosis; **Admitting Hospital:** New Britain General Hospital; **Office Address:** 100 Grand St, Ste N3 New Britain, CT 06050; **Office Phone:** (860) 224-5467; **Board Certifications:** Obstetrics & Gynecology 1980, Reproductive Endocrinology 1981; **Medical School:** Univ Conn 1973; **Residency:** Obstetrics & Gynecology, Hartford Hosp, Hartford, CT 1974-1977; **Fellowship:** Reproductive Endocrinology, Univ Conn Sch Med, Farmington, CT 1977-1979; **Faculty Appointment:** Prof Obstetrics & Gynecology, Univ Conn

REPRODUCTIVE ENDOCRINOLOGY *New England*

Schiff, Isaac MD (Reproductive Endocrinology) - *Special Expertise:* Menopause Problems; Infertility-Female; **Admitting Hospital:** Massachusetts General Hospital; **Office Address:** Mass Genl Hosp. 55 Fruit St., Bldg VBK - Ste 113 Boston, MA 02114; **Office Phone:** (617) 726-3001; **Board Certifications:** Obstetrics & Gynecology 1998, Reproductive Endocrinology 1979; **Medical School:** McGill Univ 1968; **Residencies:** Surgery, New England Med. Ctr, Boston, MA 1974; Obstetrics & Gynecology, Boston Hosp. Women, Boston, MA 1971-1973; **Fellowship:** Reproductive Endocrinology, Boston Hosp. Women, Boston, MA 1974-1976; **Faculty Appointment:** Prof Gynecologic Oncology, Harvard Med Sch

Mid Atlantic

Berga, Sarah Lee MD (Reproductive Endocrinology) - *Special Expertise:* Infertility-IVF; Hormonal Replacement; Menopause Problems; **Admitting Hospital:** Magee Women's Hospital; **Office Address:** Magee-Women's Hosp, Dept ObGyn 300 Halket St, Fl 4 - rm 4100 Pittsburgh, PA 15213-3181; **Office Phone:** (412) 641-1600; **Board Certifications:** Obstetrics & Gynecology 1998, Reproductive Endocrinology 1998; **Medical School:** Univ VA Sch Med 1980; **Residency:** Obstetrics & Gynecology, Harvard Med Sch/ Mass Genl Hosp, Boston, MA 1980-1984; **Fellowship:** Reproductive Endocrinology, UCSD, San Diego, CA 1984-1986; **Faculty Appointment:** Assoc Prof Obstetrics & Gynecology, Univ Pittsburgh

Grifo, James MD/PhD (Reproductive Endocrinology) - *Special Expertise:* Reproductive Endocrinology - General; **Admitting Hospital:** NYU Medical Center (Page 70); **Office Address:** 660 1st Ave, FL 5 New York, NY 10016; **Office Phone:** (212) 263-7978; **Board Certifications:** Obstetrics & Gynecology 1991, Reproductive Endocrinology 1994; **Medical School:** Case West Res Univ 1982; **Residency:** Obstetrics & Gynecology, NY Hosp-Columbia, New York, NY 1985-1988; **Fellowship:** Reproductive Endocrinology, Yale-New Haven Hosp, New Haven, CT 1988-1990; **Faculty Appointment:** Prof Reproductive Endocrinology, NYU Sch Med

Lobo, Rogerio MD (Reproductive Endocrinology) - *Special Expertise:* Menopause Problems; **Admitting Hospital:** Columbia Presbyterian Medical Center (Page 72); **Office Address:** Dept of Obstetrics & Gynecology 161 Ft Washington Ave, Ste 450 New York, NY 10032; **Office Phone:** (212) 305-3696; **Board Certifications:** Obstetrics & Gynecology 1981, Reproductive Endocrinology 1982; **Medical School:** Georgetown Univ 1974; **Residency:** Obstetrics & Gynecology, Univ Chicago, Chicago, IL 1975-1978; **Fellowship:** Reproductive Endocrinology, USC Med Ctr, Los Angeles, CA 1980; **Faculty Appointment:** Prof Obstetrics & Gynecology, Columbia P&S

McClamrock, Howard Dean MD (Reproductive Endocrinology) - *Special Expertise:* Infertility; Blastocyst Transfer; Infertility-IVF; **Admitting Hospital:** University of Maryland Medical System; **Office Address:** Univ Maryland, Dept OB/GYN 405 W Redwood St, Fl 3rd Baltimore, MD 21201; **Office Phone:** (800) 492-5538; **Board Certifications:** Reproductive Endocrinology 1998, Obstetrics & Gynecology 1998; **Medical School:** Univ NC Sch Med 1981; **Residency:** Obstetrics & Gynecology, Univ Maryland, Baltimore, MD 1982-1986; **Fellowship:** Reproductive Endocrinology, Univ Maryland, Baltimore, MD 1986-1988; **Faculty Appointment:** Assoc Prof Obstetrics & Gynecology, Univ MD Sch Med

Oktay, Kutluk MD (Reproductive Endocrinology) - *Special Expertise:* Transplant-Ovarian Tissue; Infertility-Female; **Admitting Hospital:** New York Weill Cornell Medical Center - NY Presbyterian Hospital (Page 72); **Office Address:** Ctr for Reproductive Med & Infertility 505 E 70TH St, Fl 3RD New York, NY 11215; **Office Phone:** (212) 746-1762; **Board Certifications:** Obstetrics & Gynecology 1997, Reproductive Endocrinology 1999; **Medical School:** Turkey 1986; **Residencies:** Internal Medicine, Cook Co Hosp, Chicago, IL 1986-1989; Obstetrics & Gynecology, Univ Conn Hlt, Farmington, CT 1989-1993; **Fellowships:** Reproductive Endocrinology, Univ Texas, San Antonio, TX 1993-1995; Reproductive Endocrinology, Univ Leeds, Leeds, England 1995-1996; **Faculty Appointment:** Asst Prof Obstetrics & Gynecology, Cornell Univ-Weil Med Coll

Rosenwaks, Zev MD (Reproductive Endocrinology) - *Special Expertise:* Infertility-IVF; Genetic Disorders; **Admitting Hospital:** New York Weill Cornell Medical Center - NY Presbyterian Hospital (Page 72); **Office Address:** Ctr for Reproductive Med and Infertility 505 E 70th St, Ste 320 New York, NY 10021; **Office Phone:** (212) 746-1743; **Board Certifications:** Obstetrics & Gynecology 1978, Reproductive Endocrinology 1981; **Medical School:** SUNY Downstate 1972; **Residency:** Obstetrics & Gynecology, LIJ Med Ctr, New Hyde Park, NY 1972-1976; **Fellowship:** Reproductive Endocrinology, Johns Hopkins Hosp, Baltimore, MD 1976-1978; **Faculty Appointment:** Prof Obstetrics & Gynecology, Cornell Univ-Weil Med Coll

Sauer, Mark MD (Reproductive Endocrinology) - *Special Expertise:* Reproductive Endocrinology - General; **Admitting Hospital:** Columbia Presbyterian Medical Center (Page 72); **Office Address:** Center for Women's Reproductive Care 161 Fort Washington Ave, rm 450 New York, NY 10032; **Office Phone:** (212) 305-4665; **Board Certifications:** Obstetrics & Gynecology 1987, Reproductive Endocrinology 1988; **Medical School:** Univ Hlth Sci/Chicago Med Sch 1980; **Residency:** Obstetrics & Gynecology, Univ IL Med Ctr, Chicago, IL 1980-1984; **Fellowship:** Reproductive Endocrinology, UCLA Med Ctr, Los Angeles, CA 1984-1986; **Faculty Appointment:** Prof Obstetrics & Gynecology, Columbia P&S

Wallach, Edward Eliot MD (Reproductive Endocrinology) - *Special Expertise:* Fibroids; Infertility-IVF; Myomectomy; **Admitting Hospital:** Johns Hopkins Hospital - Baltimore (Page 65); **Office Address:** Johns Hopkins Hosp 600 N Wolfe St Baltimore, MD 21287-0005; **Office Phone:** (410) 955-7800; **Board Certifications:** Reproductive Endocrinology 1975, Obstetrics & Gynecology 1979; **Medical School:** Cornell Univ-Weil Med Coll 1958; **Residency:** Obstetrics & Gynecology, Kings Co Hosp, New York, NY 1959-1963; **Fellowship:** Reproductive Endocrinology, Worcester Fdn Exptl Biol, Worcester, MA 1961-1962; **Faculty Appointment:** Prof Obstetrics & Gynecology, Johns Hopkins Univ

Zacur, Howard A. MD/PhD (Reproductive Endocrinology) - *Special Expertise:* Prolactin Disorders; Uterine Fibroids; **Admitting Hospital:** Johns Hopkins Hospital - Baltimore (Page 65); **Office Address:** Johns Hopkins Hosp 600 N Wolfe St, Phipps 247 Baltimore, MD 21205; **Office Phone:** (410) 583-2686; **Board Certifications:** Reproductive Endocrinology 1984, Obstetrics & Gynecology 1994; **Medical School:** Univ Miami Sch Med 1973; **Residency:** Obstetrics & Gynecology, Johns Hopkins Hosp, Baltimore, MD 1977-1980; **Fellowship:** Reproductive Endocrinology, Johns Hopkins Hosp, Baltimore, MD 1981-1982; **Faculty Appointment:** Prof Reproductive Endocrinology, Johns Hopkins Univ

REPRODUCTIVE ENDOCRINOLOGY *Southeast*

Southeast

Azziz, Ricardo MD (Reproductive Endocrinology) - *Special Expertise:* Infertility-IVF; Infertility-Female; **Admitting Hospital:** University of Alabama Hospital at Birmingham; **Office Address:** Old Hillman Bldg, Ste 549 618 S 20th St Birmingham, AL 35294; **Office Phone:** (205) 934-5708; **Board Certifications:** Obstetrics & Gynecology 1996, Reproductive Endocrinology 1996; **Medical School:** Penn State Univ-Hershey Med Ctr 1981; **Fellowship:** Reproductive Endocrinology, Johns Hopkins Hosp, Baltimore, MD 1985-1987; **Faculty Appointment:** Prof Obstetrics & Gynecology, Univ Ala

Blackwell, Richard MD (Reproductive Endocrinology) - *Special Expertise:* Infertility-Female; **Admitting Hospital:** University of Alabama Hospital at Birmingham; **Office Address:** 618 S 20th St Birmingham, AL 35294; **Office Phone:** (205) 934-6090; **Board Certifications:** Obstetrics & Gynecology 1982, Reproductive Endocrinology 1987; **Medical School:** Baylor Coll Med 1975; **Residency:** Obstetrics & Gynecology, Univ Alabama Hosp, Birmingham, AL 1975-1979; **Fellowship:** Reproductive Endocrinology, Univ Alabama Hosp, Birmingham, AL 1979-1981; **Faculty Appointment:** Prof Obstetrics & Gynecology, Univ Ala

DeVane, Gary Williams MD (Reproductive Endocrinology) - *Special Expertise:* Infertility; Miscarriage-Recurrent; **Admitting Hospital:** Florida Hospital; **Office Address:** 3435 Pinehurst Ave Orlando, FL 32804-4049; **Office Phone:** (407) 740-0909; **Board Certifications:** Obstetrics & Gynecology 1977, Reproductive Endocrinology 1982; **Medical School:** Baylor Coll Med 1971; **Residency:** Obstetrics & Gynecology, UCSD Hosp, San Diego, CA 1972-1975; **Fellowship:** Reproductive Endocrinology, Univ Texas SW Hosp, Dallas, TX 1978-1980

Fritz, Marc Anthony MD (Reproductive Endocrinology) - *Special Expertise:* Infertility; Menopause Problems; **Admitting Hospital:** University of North Carolina Hospitals; **Office Address:** Univ NC, Div Reproductive Endo & Fert CB 7570, 4001 Old Clinic Bldg Chapel Hill, NC 27599-7570; **Office Phone:** (919) 966-5283; **Board Certifications:** Reproductive Endocrinology 1996, Obstetrics & Gynecology 1996; **Medical School:** Tulane Univ 1977; **Residency:** Obstetrics & Gynecology, Wright State Univ, Dayton, OH 1978-1981; **Fellowship:** Reproductive Endocrinology, Oregon Hlth Sci Univ, Portland, OR 1981-1983; **Faculty Appointment:** Prof Obstetrics & Gynecology, Univ NC Sch Med

Goodman, Neil MD (Reproductive Endocrinology) - *Special Expertise:* Reproductive Endocrinology - General; **Admitting Hospital:** Baptist Hospital - Miami; **Office Address:** 9150 SW 87th Ave, Ste 210 Miami, FL 33176-2313; **Office Phone:** (305) 595-6855; **Board Certifications:** Internal Medicine 1973, Endocrinology, Diabetes & Metabolism 1975; **Medical School:** Columbia P&S 1970; **Residency:** Internal Medicine, Beth Israel Hosp, Boston, MA 1971-1972; **Fellowship:** Endocrinology, Diabetes & Metabolism, Mass Genl Hosp, Boston, MA 1972-1974; **Faculty Appointment:** Clin Prof Endocrinology, Diabetes & Metabolism, Univ Miami Sch Med

Hammond, Charles B MD (Reproductive Endocrinology) - *Special Expertise:* Menopause Problems; **Admitting Hospital:** Duke University Medical Center (Page 60); **Office Address:** Duke Univ Med Ctr Box 3853 Durham, NC 27710; **Office Phone:** (919) 684-3008; **Board Certifications:** Obstetrics & Gynecology 1972, Reproductive Endocrinology 1974; **Medical School:** Duke Univ 1961; **Residencies:** Obstetrics & Gynecology, Duke Med Ctr, Durham, NC 1966-1968; Obstetrics & Gynecology, Duke Med Ctr, Durham, NC 1962-1963; **Fellowship:** Gynecology, Duke Med Ctr, Durham, NC 1963-1964; **Faculty Appointment:** Prof Obstetrics & Gynecology, Duke Univ

746

Haney, Arthur MD (Reproductive Endocrinology) - *Special Expertise:* Infertility-Female; **Admitting Hospital:** Duke University Medical Center (Page 60); **Office Address:** Duke Univ Med Ctr Box 2971 Durham, NC 22715; **Office Phone:** (919) 684-2471; **Board Certifications:** Obstetrics & Gynecology 1989, Reproductive Endocrinology 1981; **Medical School:** Univ Ariz Coll Med 1972; **Residency:** Obstetrics & Gynecology, Duke Univ Med Ctr, Durham, NC 1972-1976; **Fellowship:** Reproductive Endocrinology, Duke Univ Med Ctr, Durham, NC 1976-1978; **Faculty Appointment:** Prof Obstetrics & Gynecology, Duke Univ

Murphy, Ana Alvarez MD (Reproductive Endocrinology) - *Special Expertise:* Infertility; Endometriosis; Pelvic Surgery; **Admitting Hospital:** Emory University Hospital; **Office Address:** Emory Univ 20 Linden Ave, Fl 4 Atlanta, GA 30308; **Office Phone:** (404) 686-1843; **Board Certifications:** Obstetrics & Gynecology 1987, Reproductive Endocrinology 1989; **Medical School:** Univ Mich Med Sch 1980; **Residency:** Obstetrics & Gynecology, Johns Hopkins Univ, Baltimore, MD 1980-1984; **Fellowship:** Reproductive Endocrinology, Johns Hopkins Univ, Baltimore, MD 1984-1986; **Faculty Appointment:** Prof Obstetrics & Gynecology, Emory Univ

Ory, Steven MD (Reproductive Endocrinology) - *Special Expertise:* Infertility; **Admitting Hospital:** Northwest Medical Center; **Office Address:** 2825 N State Road 7, Ste 302 Margate, FL 33063; **Office Phone:** (954) 247-6200; **Board Certifications:** Obstetrics & Gynecology 1983, Reproductive Endocrinology 1984; **Medical School:** Baylor Coll Med 1976; **Residency:** Obstetrics & Gynecology, Mayo Clinic, Rochester, MN 1976-1980; **Fellowship:** Reproductive Endocrinology, Duke Univ, Durham, NC 1980-1982; **Faculty Appointment:** Assoc Clin Prof Obstetrics & Gynecology, Univ Miami Sch Med

Rock, John A MD (Reproductive Endocrinology) - *Special Expertise:* Infertility-Female, Diagnostic; Endometriosis; Vaginal Abnormalities; **Admitting Hospital:** Emory University Hospital; **Office Address:** Emory Clinic 1365 Clifton Rd, Bldg A - Fl 4 Atlanta, GA 30322; **Office Phone:** (404) 727-8704; **Board Certifications:** Reproductive Endocrinology 1981, Obstetrics & Gynecology 1998; **Medical School:** Louisiana State Univ 1972; **Residency:** Obstetrics & Gynecology, Duke Med Ctr, Durham, NC 1973-1976; **Fellowship:** Reproductive Endocrinology, Johns Hopkins, Baltimore, MD 1976-1978; **Faculty Appointment:** Prof Obstetrics & Gynecology, Emory Univ

Steinkampf, Michael MD (Reproductive Endocrinology) - *Special Expertise:* Infertility; **Admitting Hospital:** University of Alabama Hospital at Birmingham; **Office Address:** 618 S 20th Birmingham, AL 35294-7333; **Office Phone:** (205) 934-1030; **Board Certifications:** Obstetrics & Gynecology 1997, Reproductive Endocrinology 1997; **Medical School:** Louisiana State Univ 1981; **Residency:** Obstetrics & Gynecology, Parkland Meml Hosp, Dallas, TX 1981-1985; **Fellowship:** Reproductive Endocrinology, Univ Texas SW Med Sch, Dallas, TX 1985-1987; **Faculty Appointment:** Prof Obstetrics & Gynecology, Univ Ala

Younger, J Benjamin MD (Reproductive Endocrinology) - *Special Expertise:* Infertility-Female; **Admitting Hospital:** University of Alabama Hospital at Birmingham; **Office Address:** American Soc Reproductive Med 1209 Montgomery Hwy Birmingham, AL 35216-2809; **Office Phone:** (205) 978-5000; **Board Certification:** Obstetrics & Gynecology 1989; **Medical School:** Tulane Univ 1962; **Residency:** Obstetrics & Gynecology, Duke Med Ctr, Durham, NC 1963-1965; **Fellowship:** Reproductive Endocrinology, Duke Med Ctr, Durham, NC 1965-1966

Midwest

Barnes, Randall B MD (Reproductive Endocrinology) - *Special Expertise:* Endometriosis; Infertility; **Admitting Hospital:** University of Chicago Hospitals (Page 78); **Office Address:** 5841 S Maryland Ave, MC-2050 Chicago, IL 60637; **Office Phone:** (773) 702-6642; **Board Certifications:** Obstetrics & Gynecology 1986, Reproductive Endocrinology 1987; **Medical School:** Johns Hopkins Univ 1979; **Residency:** Obstetrics & Gynecology, LAC-USC Med Ctr, Los Angeles, CA 1980-1983; **Fellowship:** Reproductive Endocrinology, LAC-USC Med Ctr, Los Angeles, CA 1983-1985; **Faculty Appointment:** Assoc Prof Obstetrics & Gynecology, Univ Chicago-Pritzker Sch Med

Bieber, Eric Joseph MD (Reproductive Endocrinology) - *Special Expertise:* Fibroids; Endometriosis; **Admitting Hospital:** University of Chicago Hospitals (Page 78); **Office Address:** 5841 S Maryland Ave, MS 2050 Chicago, IL 60637; **Office Phone:** (773) 702-6642; **Board Certifications:** Obstetrics & Gynecology 1994, Maternal & Fetal Medicine 1994; **Medical School:** Loyola Univ-Stritch Sch Med 1986; **Residency:** Obstetrics & Gynecology, Rush-Presby-St Lukes Med Ctr, Chicago, IL 1987-1990; **Fellowship:** Reproductive Endocrinology, Univ Chicago, Chicago, IL 1990-1993; **Faculty Appointment:** Assoc Prof Obstetrics & Gynecology, Univ Chicago-Pritzker Sch Med

Christman, Gregory MD (Reproductive Endocrinology) - *Special Expertise:* Infertility; **Admitting Hospital:** University of Michigan Health Center; **Office Address:** Univ Mich, Med Sci Bldg I 1301 Catherine St, rm 6428, Box 0617 Ann Arbor, MI 48109-0617; **Office Phone:** (734) 764-8142; **Board Certifications:** Obstetrics & Gynecology 1994, Reproductive Endocrinology 1996; **Medical School:** Univ Wisc 1983; **Residency:** Obstetrics & Gynecology, Univ Wisc Med Sch, Madison, WI 1983-1987; **Fellowship:** Reproductive Endocrinology, Univ NC, Chapel Hill, NC 1990-1992; **Faculty Appointment:** Asst Prof Obstetrics & Gynecology, Univ Mich Med Sch

Diamond, Michael MD (Reproductive Endocrinology) - *Special Expertise:* Infertility-IVF; Infertility-Female; Polycystic Ovary Disease; **Admitting Hospital:** Harper Hospital (Page 59); **Office Address:** Univ Ctr for Women's Med 28800 Ryan Rd, Fl 320 Warren, MI 48092; **Office Phone:** (810) 558-1100; **Board Certifications:** Obstetrics & Gynecology 1997, Reproductive Endocrinology 1997; **Medical School:** Vanderbilt Univ 1981; **Residencies:** Obstetrics & Gynecology, Vanderbilt Univ, Nashville, TN 1981-1985; Reproductive Endocrinology, Yale Univ, New Haven, CT 1985-1987; **Faculty Appointment:** Prof Obstetrics & Gynecology, Wayne State Univ

Dodds, William G MD (Reproductive Endocrinology) - *Special Expertise:* Infertility; Endometriosis; Infertility-IVF; **Admitting Hospital:** Spectrum Health East; **Office Address:** 630 Kenmore Ave SE Grand Rapids, MI 49546; **Office Phone:** (616) 988-2229; **Board Certifications:** Obstetrics & Gynecology 1999, Reproductive Endocrinology 2000; **Medical School:** Ohio State Univ 1982; **Residency:** Obstetrics & Gynecology, Ohio State Univ, Columbus, OH 1982-1986; **Fellowship:** Reproductive Endocrinology, Ohio State Univ, Columbus, OH 1986-1988; **Faculty Appointment:** Assoc Prof Obstetrics & Gynecology, Univ Mich Med Sch

Dumesic, Daniel Anthony MD (Reproductive Endocrinology) - *Special Expertise:* Infertility-Female/IVF; Hormonal Disorders; Endometriosis/Pelvic Pain; **Admitting Hospital:** Mayo Medical Center & Clinic - Rochester; **Office Address:** Mayo Clinic, Dept ObGyn-Div Repro Endo 200 1st St SW, Charlton Bldg Rochester, MN 55905; **Office Phone:** (507) 284-9792; **Board Certifications:** Obstetrics & Gynecology 1995, Reproductive Endocrinology 1999; **Medical School:** Univ Wisc 1978; **Residency:** Obstetrics & Gynecology, UCSF, San Francisco, CA 1980-1982; **Fellowship:** Reproductive Endocrinology, UCSF, San Francisco, CA 1985-1987; **Faculty Appointment:** Assoc Prof Reproductive Endocrinology, Mayo Med Sch

Falcone, Tommaso MD (Reproductive Endocrinology) - *Special Expertise:* Minimally Invasive Surgery; Infertility; Tubal Ligation Reversal-Microsurgery; **Admitting Hospital:** Cleveland Clinic Foundation; **Office Address:** Cleveland Clin, Dept Gyn 9500 Euclid Ave Cleveland, OH 44195-0001; **Office Phone:** (216) 444-1758; **Board Certifications:** Obstetrics & Gynecology 1998, Reproductive Endocrinology 1998; **Medical School:** McGill Univ 1981; **Residency:** Obstetrics & Gynecology, McGill Univ, Montreal, CN 1983-1986; **Fellowship:** Reproductive Endocrinology, McGill Univ, Montreal, CN 1987-1989

Jacobs, Laurence MD (Reproductive Endocrinology) - *Special Expertise:* Infertility-IVF; Polycystic Ovary Disease; Infertility; **Admitting Hospital:** Advocate Lutheran General Hospital; **Office Address:** 35 N Arlington Heights Rd, Ste 195 Buffalo Grove, IL 60089; **Office Phone:** (847) 215-8899; **Board Certification:** Obstetrics & Gynecology 1981; **Medical School:** Northwestern Univ 1975; **Residency:** Obstetrics & Gynecology, Northwestern, Chicago, IL 1975-1979; **Fellowship:** Reproductive Endocrinology, Mayo Clini, Rochester, MN 1986-1988; **Faculty Appointment:** Assoc Prof Obstetrics & Gynecology, Univ Chicago-Pritzker Sch Med

Kazer, Ralph MD (Reproductive Endocrinology) - *Special Expertise:* Endocrinology; Infertility; Infertility; **Admitting Hospital:** Northwestern Memorial Hospital; **Office Address:** 675 North St.Claire 314-200 Chicago, IL 60611; **Office Phone:** (312) 695-7269; **Board Certifications:** Obstetrics & Gynecology 1996, Reproductive Endocrinology 1996; **Medical School:** Tufts Univ 1979; **Residency:** Obstetrics & Gynecology, Tufts U, Boston, MA 1979-1983; **Fellowship:** Reproductive Endocrinology, UC San Die, San Diego, CA 1983-1986; **Faculty Appointment:** Assoc Prof Northwestern Univ

Milad, Magdy P MD (Reproductive Endocrinology) - *Special Expertise:* Reproductive Surgery; Tubal Reconstruction; **Admitting Hospital:** Northwestern Memorial Hospital; **Office Address:** Northwestern Med Fac Fdn 675 North St Clair Oak Park, IL 60611; **Office Phone:** (312) 695-7269; **Board Certifications:** Obstetrics & Gynecology 1994, Reproductive Endocrinology 1996; **Medical School:** Wayne State Univ 1987; **Fellowship:** Reproductive Endocrinology, Mayo Clinic, Rochester, NY 1991-1993; **Faculty Appointment:** Asst Prof Obstetrics & Gynecology, Northwestern Univ

Odem, Randall R MD (Reproductive Endocrinology) - *Special Expertise:* Reproductive Surgery; **Admitting Hospital:** Barnes - Jewish Hospital; **Office Address:** Washington Univ, Div Repro Endo Ste 3100 4444 Forest Park Ave St Louis, MO 63108; **Office Phone:** (314) 286-2400; **Board Certifications:** Obstetrics & Gynecology 1998, Reproductive Endocrinology 1998; **Medical School:** Univ Iowa Coll Med 1981; **Residency:** Obstetrics & Gynecology, U Ill Hosps, Chicago, IL 1981-1985; **Fellowship:** Reproductive Endocrinology, Wash U Sch Med, St Louis, MO 1985-1987; **Faculty Appointment:** Assoc Prof Obstetrics & Gynecology, Washington Univ, St Louis

Ratts, Valerie Sue MD (Reproductive Endocrinology) - *Special Expertise:* Polycystic Ovary Disease; Uterine Fibroids; **Admitting Hospital:** Barnes - Jewish Hospital; **Office Address:** Wash Univ Sch Med 4444 Forest Park Ave, Ste 3100 St Louis, MO 63108; **Office Phone:** (314) 286-2400; **Board Certifications:** Obstetrics & Gynecology 1995, Reproductive Endocrinology 1997; **Medical School:** Johns Hopkins Univ 1987; **Residency:** Obstetrics & Gynecology, Johns Hopkins Hosp, Baltimore, MD 1987-1991; **Fellowship:** Reproductive Endocrinology, Johns Hopkins Hosp, Baltimore, MD 1991-1993; **Faculty Appointment:** Asst Prof Obstetrics & Gynecology, Washington Univ, St Louis

Schreiber, James MD (Reproductive Endocrinology) - *Special Expertise:* Menstrual Disorders; Infertility; **Admitting Hospital:** Barnes - Jewish Hospital; **Office Address:** Obstetrics and Gynecology 4444 Forest Park Ave, Ste 3100 St Louis, MO 63110; **Office Phone:** (314) 362-7135; **Board Certifications:** Obstetrics & Gynecology 1981, Reproductive Endocrinology 1982; **Medical School:** Johns Hopkins Univ 1972; **Residencies:** Obstetrics & Gynecology, USC-LA County, Los Angeles, CA 1972-1974; Obstetrics & Gynecology, USC-LA County, Los Angeles, CA 1976-1978; **Fellowship:** Reproductive Endocrinology, Natl Inst of Hlth, Bethesda, MD 1974-1976; **Faculty Appointment:** Prof Obstetrics & Gynecology, Washington Univ, St Louis

Session, Donna Ruth MD (Reproductive Endocrinology) - *Special Expertise:* Ultrasound Guided Surgery; Sonohysterography; Infertility-Female; **Admitting Hospital:** Mayo Medical Center & Clinic - Rochester; **Office Address:** Mayo Clin, Dept Ob/Gyn 200 1st St SW, Bldg Charl - Fl 3A Rochester, MN 55905; **Office Phone:** (507) 284-3176; **Board Certifications:** Obstetrics & Gynecology 1994, Reproductive Endocrinology 1996; **Medical School:** Eastern VA Med Sch 1986; **Residency:** Obstetrics & Gynecology, Winthrop Hosp, Mineola, NY 1986-1990; **Fellowship:** Reproductive Endocrinology, Columbia Presby Med Ctr, New York, NY 1991-1993; **Faculty Appointment:** Asst Prof Obstetrics & Gynecology, Mayo Med Sch

Smith, Yolanda MD (Reproductive Endocrinology) - *Special Expertise:* Infertility; **Admitting Hospital:** University of Michigan Health Center; **Office Address:** Women's Hosp 1500 E Med Ctr Dr, Box 0276 Ann Arbor, MI 48109-0276; **Office Phone:** (734) 763-4323; **Board Certifications:** Obstetrics & Gynecology 1997, Reproductive Endocrinology 1999; **Medical School:** Wake Forest Univ Sch Med 1989; **Residency:** Obstetrics & Gynecology, Univ Mich Hosp, Ann Arbor, MI 1990-1993; **Fellowship:** Reproductive Endocrinology, Johns Hopkins Hosp, Baltimore, MD 1993-1995; **Faculty Appointment:** Asst Prof Obstetrics & Gynecology, Univ Mich Med Sch

Wood Molo, Mary MD (Reproductive Endocrinology) - *Special Expertise:* Infertility; Fibroids; Infertility-IVF; **Admitting Hospital:** Rush/Presbyterian - St Luke's Medical Center - Chicago (Page 74); **Office Address:** 1725 W Harrison St, Ste 408 East Chicago, IL 60612; **Office Phone:** (312) 997-2229; **Board Certifications:** Obstetrics & Gynecology 1991, Reproductive Endocrinology 1994; **Medical School:** Southern IL Univ 1982; **Residencies:** Obstetrics & Gynecology, SIU Affil, Springfield, IL 1983-1984; Obstetrics & Gynecology, Rush Presb, Chicago, IL 1984-1987; **Fellowship:** Reproductive Endocrinology, Rush Presb, Chicago, IL 1987-1989; **Faculty Appointment:** Asst Prof Obstetrics & Gynecology, Rush Med Coll

Zinaman, Michael MD (Reproductive Endocrinology) - *Special Expertise:* Endometriosis; Osteoporosis; **Admitting Hospital:** Loyola University Health System; **Office Address:** Loyola Univ Med Ctr, Dept ObGyn 2160 S First Ave Maywood, IL 60153; **Office Phone:** (708) 327-1000; **Board Certifications:** Obstetrics & Gynecology 1988, Reproductive Endocrinology 1996; **Medical School:** SUNY Downstate 1981; **Residency:** Obstetrics & Gynecology, Univ Chicago Hosps, Chicago, IL 1981-1985; **Fellowship:** Reproductive Endocrinology, Georgetown Univ, Washington, DC 1985-1987; **Faculty Appointment:** Assoc Prof Obstetrics & Gynecology, Loyola Univ-Stritch Sch Med

Great Plains and Mountains

Adashi, Eli Y MD (Reproductive Endocrinology) - *Special Expertise:* Infertility-Female; **Admitting Hospital:** University of Utah Hospital and Clinics; **Office Address:** Univ Utah Sch Med 50 N Medical Salt Lake City, UT 84132; **Office Phone:** (801) 581-5490; **Board Certifications:** Obstetrics & Gynecology 1991, Reproductive Endocrinology 1983; **Medical School:** Israel 1972; **Residency:** Obstetrics & Gynecology, Tufts Univ Sch Med, Boston, MA 1974-1977; **Fellowships:** Reproductive Endocrinology, Univ CA - San Diego, La Jolla, CA 1978-1981; Reproductive Endocrinology, Johns Hopkins Univ, Baltimore, MD 1977-1978; **Faculty Appointment:** Prof Obstetrics & Gynecology, Univ Utah

Schlaff, William D MD (Reproductive Endocrinology) - *Special Expertise:* Infertility/Uterine Fibroids; Endometriosis; **Admitting Hospital:** University of Colorado Health & Science Center; **Office Address:** Univ Colo Hlth Scis Ctr 4200 E 9th Ave, Box B198 Denver, CO 80262-0001; **Office Phone:** (303) 315-7128; **Board Certifications:** Obstetrics & Gynecology 1995, Reproductive Endocrinology 1997; **Medical School:** Univ Mich Med Sch 1977; **Residency:** Obstetrics & Gynecology, Univ Mich Hosps, Ann Arbor, MI 1978-1981; **Fellowship:** Reproductive Endocrinology, Johns Hopkins Med Ctr, Baltimore, MD 1983-1985; **Faculty Appointment:** Prof Obstetrics & Gynecology, Univ Colo

Surrey, Eric Shire MD (Reproductive Endocrinology) - *Special Expertise:* Reproductive Endocrinology - General; **Admitting Hospital:** University of Colorado Health Science Center, CO.; **Office Address:** 799 E Hamden Ave, Ste 430 Englewood, CO 80110; **Office Phone:** (303) 788-8300; **Board Certifications:** Obstetrics & Gynecology 1998, Reproductive Endocrinology 1998; **Medical School:** Univ Penn 1981; **Residency:** Obstetrics & Gynecology, UCLA Med. Ctr., Los Angeles, CA 1982-1986; **Fellowship:** Reproductive Endocrinology, UCLA Med.Ctr., Los Angeles, CA 1986-1988;

Southwest

Schenken, Robert S MD (Reproductive Endocrinology) - *Special Expertise:* Infertility-Female; Endometriosis; **Admitting Hospital:** University of Texas Health & Science Center; **Office Address:** Univ Tx Hlth Sci Ctr, Dept OB/GYN 7703 Floyd Curl, MC-7836 San Antonio, TX 78229-3900; **Office Phone:** (210) 567-4930; **Board Certifications:** Reproductive Endocrinology 1985, Obstetrics & Gynecology 1995; **Medical School:** Baylor Coll Med 1977; **Residency:** Obstetrics & Gynecology, Bexar Co Hosp, San Antonio, TX 1978-1981; **Fellowships:** Reproductive Endocrinology, Univ Tx Hlth Sci Ctr, San Antonio, TX 1982-1983; Reproductive Endocrinology, Natl Inst Hlth, Bethesda, MD 1981-1982; **Faculty Appointment:** Prof Obstetrics & Gynecology, Univ Tex, San Antonio

West Coast and Pacific

Burry, Kenneth Arnold MD (Reproductive Endocrinology) - *Special Expertise:* Infertility-IVF; Menopause Problems; **Admitting Hospital:** Oregon Health Science University Hospital and Clinics; **Office Address:** Sam Jackson Pkwy Oreg Hlth Scis Univ and Clinics, MC-L466 Portland, OR 97201-3098; **Office Phone:** (503) 418-3744; **Board Certifications:** Obstetrics & Gynecology 1977, Reproductive Endocrinology 1981; **Medical School:** UC Irvine 1968; **Residency:** Obstetrics & Gynecology, Oreg Hlth Sci Univ and Clinics, Portland, OR 1971-1974; **Fellowship:** Reproductive Endocrinology, Univ Wash Hosp, Seattle, WA 1974-1976; **Faculty Appointment:** Prof Obstetrics & Gynecology

Jaffe, Robert B MD (Reproductive Endocrinology) - *Special Expertise:* Hormonal Disorders; Menopause Problems; **Admitting Hospital:** University of California - San Francisco Medical Center; **Office Address:** UC San Francisco Med Ctr, Dept OB/GYN 505 Parnassus Ave, rm HSW1656 San Francisco, CA 94143-0566; **Office Phone:** (415) 476-2269; **Board Certifications:** Obstetrics & Gynecology 1967, Reproductive Endocrinology 1977; **Medical School:** Univ Mich Med Sch 1957; **Residency:** Obstetrics & Gynecology, Univ Colo Med Ctr, Denver, CO 1959-1963; **Fellowships:** Endocrinology, Diabetes & Metabolism, Univ Colo Med Ctr, Denver, CO 1958-1959; Reproductive Endocrinology, CtrKarolinska Sjuktuset, Stockholm, Sweden 1963-1964; **Faculty Appointment:** Prof Obstetrics & Gynecology, UCSF

Marrs, Richard P MD (Reproductive Endocrinology) - *Special Expertise: Infertility-Female; Endometriosis; Fibroids;* **Admitting Hospital:** Santa Monica - UCLA Medical Center; **Office Address:** 1245 16th St, Ste 220 Santa Monica, CA 90404-1240; **Office Phone:** (310) 828-4008; **Board Certifications:** Obstetrics & Gynecology 1980, Reproductive Endocrinology 1983; **Medical School:** Univ Tex Med Br, Galveston 1974; **Residency:** Obstetrics & Gynecology, Univ Tex Hosps, Galveston, TX 1974-1977; **Fellowship:** Reproductive Endocrinology, USC Med Ctr, Los Angeles, CA 1977-1979

Paulson, Richard John MD (Reproductive Endocrinology) - *Special Expertise: Infertility-IVF; Infertility-Egg Donation;* **Admitting Hospital:** LAC + USC Medical Center; **Office Address:** USC Med Ctr, Dept Repro Endo and Infertility 1245 Wilshire Blvd, - Ste 403 Los Angeles, CA 90017; **Office Phone:** (213) 975-9990; **Board Certifications:** Obstetrics & Gynecology 1997, Reproductive Endocrinology 1997; **Medical School:** UCLA 1980; **Residency:** Obstetrics & Gynecology, Harbor - UCLA Medical Center, Torrance, CA 1980-1984; **Fellowship:** Reproductive Endocrinology, LAC - USC Med Ctr, Los Angeles, CA 1984-1986; **Faculty Appointment:** Obstetrics & Gynecology, USC Sch Med

Polan, Mary Lake MD/PhD (Reproductive Endocrinology) - *Special Expertise: Menopause Problems;* **Admitting Hospital:** Stanford Medical Center; **Office Address:** Stanford Univ Med Ctr Dept Gyn/Ob, rm HH333 Stanford, CA 94305-5317; **Office Phone:** (650) 723-5533; **Board Certifications:** Obstetrics & Gynecology 1998, Reproductive Endocrinology 1999; **Medical School:** Yale Univ 1975; **Residency:** Obstetrics & Gynecology, Yale-New Haven Hosp, New Haven, CT 1975-1978; **Fellowship:** Reproductive Endocrinology, Yale New Haven Hosp, New Haven, CT 1979-1980; **Faculty Appointment:** Prof Obstetrics & Gynecology, Stanford Univ

Soules, Michael Roy MD (Reproductive Endocrinology) - *Special Expertise: Reproductive Medicine; Infertility-Female;* **Admitting Hospital:** University of Washington Medical Center; **Office Address:** Univ Wash, Dept OB/GYN 4225 Roosevelt Way NE, Ste 305 Seattle, WA 98105-6099; **Office Phone:** (206) 543-0670; **Board Certifications:** Obstetrics & Gynecology 1993, Reproductive Endocrinology 1981; **Medical School:** UCLA 1972; **Residency:** Obstetrics & Gynecology, Univ Colo Med Ctr, Denver, CO 1972-1976; **Fellowship:** Reproductive Endocrinology, Duke Univ Hosp, Durham, NC 1976-1978; **Faculty Appointment:** Prof Obstetrics & Gynecology, Univ Wash

Taylor, Robert N MD (Reproductive Endocrinology) - *Special Expertise: Endometriosis; Miscarriage-Recurrent;* **Admitting Hospital:** University of California - San Francisco Medical Center; **Office Address:** 350 Parnassus Ave, Ste 300 San Francisco, CA 94143-0310; **Office Phone:** (415) 476-2224; **Board Certifications:** Obstetrics & Gynecology 1997, Reproductive Endocrinology 1997; **Medical School:** Baylor Coll Med 1981; **Residency:** Obstetrics & Gynecology, UCSF Med Ctr, San Fransisco, CA 1981-1985; **Fellowship:** Reproductive Endocrinology, UCSF Med Ctr, San Fransisco, CA 1984-1986; **Faculty Appointment:** Assoc Prof Obstetrics & Gynecology, UCSF

Winer, Sharon Ann MD (Reproductive Endocrinology) - *Special Expertise: Hormonal Disorders; Infertility-Female;* **Admitting Hospital:** Cedars-Sinai Medical Center; **Office Address:** 9400 Brighton Way, Ste 206 Beverly Hills, CA 90210-4709; **Office Phone:** (310) 274-9100; **Board Certifications:** Obstetrics & Gynecology 1997, Reproductive Endocrinology 1997; **Medical School:** USC Sch Med 1978; **Residency:** Obstetrics & Gynecology, LAC-USC Med Ctr, Los Angeles, CA 1978-1979; **Fellowships:** Reproductive Endocrinology, USC Univ Hosp, Los Angeles, CA 1979-1982; Maternal & Fetal Medicine, Hammersmith, London, England 1982-1983; **Faculty Appointment:** Clin Prof Obstetrics & Gynecology, USC Sch Med

Yee, Billy MD (Reproductive Endocrinology) - *Special Expertise:* *Infertility;* **Admitting Hospital:** Long Beach Memorial Medical Center; **Office Address:** Reproductive Partners Med Grp 701 E 28th St, Ste 202 Long Beach, CA 90806; **Office Phone:** (562) 427-2229; **Board Certifications:** Obstetrics & Gynecology 1995, Reproductive Endocrinology 1989; **Medical School:** UC Davis 1978; **Residency:** Obstetrics & Gynecology, USC, Los Angeles, CA 1979-1982; **Fellowship:** Reproductive Endocrinology, USC, Los Angeles, CA 1983-1985; **Faculty Appointment:** Assoc Clin Prof Reproductive Endocrinology, UC Irvine

RHEUMATOLOGY

An internist who treats diseases of joints, muscle, bones and tendons. This specialist diagnoses and treats arthritis, back pain, muscle strains, common athletic injuries and "collagen" diseases.

INTERNAL MEDICINE

An internist is a personal physician who provides long-term, comprehensive care in the office and the hospital, managing both common and complex illness of adolescents, adults and the elderly. Internists are trained in the diagnosis and treatment of cancer, infections and diseases affecting the heart, blood, kidneys, joints and digestive, respiratory and vascular systems. They are also trained in the essentials of primary care internal medicine which incorporates an understanding of disease prevention, wellness, substance abuse, mental health and effective treatment of common problems of the eyes, ears, skin, nervous system and reproductive organs.

Training required: Three years in internal medicine *plus* additional training and examination for certification in rheumatology

Physician Listings

New England

Brenner, Michael B MD (Rheumatology) - *Special Expertise:* *Gout/Pseudogout; Rheumatoid Arthritis; Lupus/SLE;* **Admitting Hospital:** Brigham & Women's Hospital; **Office Address:** Brigham and Womens Hosp, Div Rheumatology 1 Jimmy Way, Bldg Smith 552 Boston, MA 02115; **Office Phone:** (617) 732-5325; **Board Certifications:** Internal Medicine 1978, Rheumatology 1982; **Medical School:** Vanderbilt Univ 1975; **Residency:** Internal Medicine, Vanderbilt Univ Hosp, Nashville, TN 1976-1979; **Fellowship:** Rheumatology, UCLA Med Ctr, Los Angeles, CA 1979-1981; **Faculty Appointment:** Prof Medicine, Harvard Med Sch

Polisson, Richard Paul MD (Rheumatology) - *Special Expertise:* *Rheumatoid Arthritis; Lupus/SLE;* **Admitting Hospital:** Massachusetts General Hospital; **Office Address:** The Arthritis Unit-Mass Genl Hosp Bldg Bulfinch - rm 165 Boston, MA 02114; **Office Phone:** (617) 726-1581; **Board Certifications:** Rheumatology 1984, Internal Medicine 1979; **Medical School:** Duke Univ 1976; **Residencies:** Natl Inst Hlth/NCI, Bethesda, MD 1978-1980; Internal Medicine, Duke U Med Ctr., Durham, NC 1977-1978; **Fellowship:** Rheumatology, Mass Genl Hosp., Boston, MA 1980-1982; **Faculty Appointment:** Assoc Prof Rheumatology, Harvard Med Sch

Schoen, Robert Taylor MD (Rheumatology) - *Special Expertise:* *Rheumatoid Arthritis; Lyme Disease;* **Admitting Hospital:** Yale - New Haven Hospital; **Office Address:** 60 Temple St, Ste 6A New Haven, CT 06510; **Office Phone:** (203) 789-2255; **Board Certifications:** Internal Medicine 1979, Rheumatology 1982; **Medical School:** Yale Univ 1976; **Residency:** Internal Medicine, Yale New haven Hosp, New Haven, CT 1977-1979; **Fellowship:** Rheumatology, Brigham & Womens Hosp, Boston, MA 1979-1981; **Faculty Appointment:** Clin Prof Medicine, Yale Univ

Shadick, Nancy A MD (Rheumatology) - *Special Expertise:* *Lyme Disease; Rheumatoid Arthritis;* **Admitting Hospital:** Brigham & Women's Hospital; **Office Address:** Brigham & Women's Hosp, Dept Rheum 45 Francis St Boston, MA 02115; **Office Phone:** (617) 732-5266; **Board Certifications:** Internal Medicine 1989, Rheumatology 1992; **Medical School:** NYU Sch Med 1986; **Residency:** Internal Medicine, Columbia Presby Hosp, New York, NY 1986-1989; **Fellowship:** Rheumatology, Brigham & Womens Hosp, Boston, MA 1989-1992; **Faculty Appointment:** Asst Prof Medicine, Harvard Med Sch

Weinblatt, Michael Eliot MD (Rheumatology) - *Special Expertise:* *Rheumatoid Arthritis;* **Admitting Hospital:** Brigham & Women's Hospital; **Office Address:** Brigham & Womens Hosp 75 Francis St Boston, MA 02115-6110; **Office Phone:** (617) 732-5331; **Board Certifications:** Internal Medicine 1978, Rheumatology 1980; **Medical School:** Univ MD Sch Med 1975; **Residency:** Internal Medicine, Univ Maryland Hosp, Baltimore, MD 1975-1978; **Fellowship:** Rheumatology, Peter Bent Brigham Hosp, Boston, MA 1978-1980; **Faculty Appointment:** Prof Medicine, Harvard Med Sch

Mid Atlantic

Abramson, Steven B MD (Rheumatology) - *Special Expertise:* *Arthritis;* **Admitting Hospital:** Hospital for Joint Diseases; **Office Address:** 301 E 17th St New York, NY 10003; **Office Phone:** (212) 598-6110; **Board Certifications:** Internal Medicine 1977, Rheumatology 1980; **Medical School:** Harvard Med Sch 1974; **Residency:** Internal Medicine, Bellevue Hosp/NYU, New York, NY 1974-1978; **Fellowships:** Rheumatology, Bellevue Hosp/NYU, New York, NY 1978-1980; Rheumatology, NYU Med Ctr, New York, NY 1980-1983; **Faculty Appointment:** Prof Medicine, NYU Sch Med

Argyros, Thomas MD (Rheumatology) - *Special Expertise:* Lyme Disease; Lupus/SLE; **Admitting Hospital:** Lenox Hill Hospital; **Office Address:** 122 E 76th St New York, NY 10021; **Office Phone:** (212) 988-7680; **Board Certification:** Internal Medicine 1961; **Medical School:** NYU Sch Med 1954; **Residency:** Internal Medicine, Lenox Hill Hosp, New York, NY 1957-1958; **Fellowship:** Rheumatology, New York Univ Med Ctr, New York, NY 1964-1965; **Faculty Appointment:** Clin Prof Medicine, NYU Sch Med

Blume, Ralph MD (Rheumatology) - *Special Expertise:* Rheumatology - General; **Admitting Hospital:** Columbia Presbyterian Medical Center (Page 72); **Office Address:** 161 Fort Washington Ave, Ste 537 New York, NY 10032-3713; **Office Phone:** (212) 305-5512; **Board Certifications:** Internal Medicine 1972, Rheumatology 1974; **Medical School:** Columbia P&S 1964; **Residencies:** Internal Medicine, Columbia Presby Hosp, New York, NY 1965-1966; Internal Medicine, Columbia Presby Hosp, New York, NY 1968-1969; **Fellowship:** Rheumatology, Columbia P&S, New York, NY 1968-1970; **Faculty Appointment:** Clin Prof Medicine, Columbia P&S

Bunning, Robert Daniel MD (Rheumatology) - *Special Expertise:* Exercise Therapy; Rheumatoid Arthritis; Musculoskeletal Disease; **Admitting Hospital:** National Rehabilitation Hospital; **Office Address:** Natl Rehab Hosp 102 Irving St NW, rm 2158 Washington, DC 20010-2921; **Office Phone:** (202) 877-1660; **Board Certifications:** Internal Medicine 1984, Rheumatology 1986; **Medical School:** Univ Cincinnati 1979; **Residencies:** Internal Medicine, Wash Hosp Ctr, Washington, DC 1979-1981; Internal Medicine, Wash Hosp Ctr, Washington, DC 1981-1984; **Fellowship:** Rheumatology, Wash Hosp Ctr, Washington, DC 1981-1983; **Faculty Appointment:** Asst Clin Prof Reproductive Endocrinology, Geo Wash Univ

Buyon, Jill MD (Rheumatology) - *Special Expertise:* Lupus/SLE-Pregnancy; Lupus/SLE-Menopause; **Admitting Hospital:** Hospital for Joint Diseases; **Office Address:** Rheumatology and Molecular Medicine 305 E 2nd Ave, Fl 16 New York, NY 10003; **Office Phone:** (212) 598-6516; **Board Certifications:** Rheumatology 1984, Internal Medicine 1981; **Medical School:** Albert Einstein Coll Med 1978; **Residency:** Internal Medicine, Albert Einstein, NY, NY 1978-1981; **Fellowship:** Rheumatology, NYU School of Medicine, New York, NY 1981-1983; **Faculty Appointment:** Prof Medicine, NYU Sch Med

Clauw, Daniel J MD (Rheumatology) - *Special Expertise:* Fibromyalgia; Chronic Fatigue Syndrome; **Admitting Hospital:** Georgetown University Hospital; **Office Address:** GUMC - Lower Level, Gorman Bldg 3800 Reservoir Rd NW Washington, DC 20007; **Office Phone:** (202) 687-8233; **Board Certifications:** Rheumatology 1990, Internal Medicine 1988; **Medical School:** Univ Mich Med Sch 1985; **Residencies:** Internal Medicine, Georgetown Univ Hosp, Washington, DC 1985-1988; Rheumatology, Georgetown Univ Hosp, Washington, DC 1988-1990; **Faculty Appointment:** Assoc Prof Medicine, Georgetown Univ

Cupps, Thomas R MD (Rheumatology) - *Special Expertise:* Vasculitis; Hepatitis B-Immune Response; **Admitting Hospital:** Georgetown University Hospital; **Office Address:** GUMC - Lower Level, Gorman Building 3800 Reservoir Rd NW Washington, DC 20007; **Office Phone:** (202) 687-8233; **Board Certifications:** Allergy & Immunology 1981, Internal Medicine 1978; **Medical School:** Stanford Univ 1975; **Residency:** Internal Medicine, Strong Meml Hosp, Rochester, NY 1975-1978; **Fellowship:** Allergy & Immunology, Natl Inst of All & Inf Dis, Bethesda, MD

Farber, Martin Stuart MD/PhD (Rheumatology) - *Special Expertise:* Rheumatology - General; **Admitting Hospital:** Sunnyview Hospital and Rehabilitation Center; **Office Address:** Sunnyview Hosp 1270 Belmont Ave Schenectady, NY 12308; **Office Phone:** (518) 386-3644; **Board Certifications:** Internal Medicine 1982, Rheumatology 1984; **Medical School:** Albert Einstein Coll Med 1979; **Residency:** Internal Medicine, City Hosp, Boston, MA 1980-1982; **Fellowship:** Rheumatology, Boston Univ Sch Med, Boston, MA 1982-1984; **Faculty Appointment:** Asst Clin Prof Medicine, Albany Med Coll

Ginzler, Ellen MD (Rheumatology) - *Special Expertise: Lupus/SLE;* **Admitting Hospital:** University Hospital - Brooklyn; **Office Address:** Dept Rheumatology 450 Clarkson Ave, Box 42 Brooklyn, NY 11203-0042; **Office Phone:** (718) 270-1662; **Board Certifications:** Internal Medicine 1972, Rheumatology 1974; **Medical School:** Case West Res Univ 1969; **Residencies:** Internal Medicine, Kings Co Hosp, Brooklyn, NY 1970-1971; Internal Medicine, Bellevue Hosp, New York, NY 1971-1972; **Fellowship:** Rheumatology, Univ Hosp, Brooklyn, NY 1972-1974; **Faculty Appointment:** Prof Medicine, SUNY Hlth Sci Ctr

Gourley, Mark MD (Rheumatology) - *Special Expertise: Rheumatology - General;* **Admitting Hospital:** Washington Hospital Center - DC (Page 79); **Office Address:** Washington Hosp Ctr, Dept Rheumatology 110 Irving St NW, rm 2A66 Washington, DC 20010; **Office Phone:** (202) 877-6274; **Board Certifications:** Rheumatology 1992, Internal Medicine 1988; **Medical School:** Tulane Univ 1985; **Residency:** Internal Medicine, Univ Wisconsin Hosps & Clins, Madison, WI 1985-1988; **Fellowship:** Rheumatology, Natl Inst Hlth, Bethesda, MD 1988-1996

Kagen, Lawrence MD (Rheumatology) - *Special Expertise: Musculoskeletal Disease;* **Admitting Hospital:** Hospital for Special Surgery (Page 63); **Office Address:** 535 E 70th St, Ste 71 W New York, NY 10021-4892; **Office Phone:** (212) 606-1449; **Board Certifications:** Internal Medicine 1967, Rheumatology 1974; **Medical School:** NYU Sch Med 1960; **Residency:** Internal Medicine, Presbyterian Hosp, New York, NY 1960-1965; **Fellowship:** Rheumatology, Columbia P&S, New York, NY 1965-1966

Katz, Paul MD (Rheumatology) - *Special Expertise: Vasculitis; Lupus/SLE; Immune Deficiency-Rheumatoid Arthritis;* **Admitting Hospital:** Georgetown University Hospital; **Office Address:** GUMC - Lower Level, Gorman Building 3800 Reservoir Rd NW Washington, DC 20007; **Office Phone:** (202) 687-8233; **Board Certifications:** Allergy & Immunology 1979, Rheumatology 1982; **Medical School:** Georgetown Univ 1973; **Residency:** Internal Medicine, Univ FL, Gainesville, FL 1974-1976; **Fellowship:** Immunology, Natl Inst Hlth, Bethesda, MD 1976-1980; **Faculty Appointment:** Prof Medicine, Georgetown Univ

Lahita, Robert MD (Rheumatology) - *Special Expertise: Lupus/SLE; Autoimmune Disease;* **Admitting Hospital:** St Vincents Catholic Medical Center of New York; **Office Address:** St Vincent's Hosp & Med Ctr, Dept Rheum 115 E 61st St, Fl 11 New York, NY 10021; **Office Phone:** (212) 556-6550; **Board Certifications:** Internal Medicine 1993, Rheumatology 1997; **Medical School:** Jefferson Med Coll 1973; **Residency:** Internal Medicine, NY Hosp-Cornell, New York, NY 1974-1976; **Fellowship:** Rheumatology, Rockefeller Hosp, New York, NY 1976-1978; **Faculty Appointment:** Prof Medicine, NY Med Coll

Lockshin, Michael Dan MD (Rheumatology) - *Special Expertise: Lupus/SLE;* **Admitting Hospital:** Hospital for Special Surgery (Page 63); **Office Address:** 535 E 70th St, FL 6 New York, NY 10021; **Office Phone:** (212) 606-1461; **Board Certifications:** Internal Medicine 1969, Rheumatology 1972; **Medical School:** Harvard Med Sch 1963; **Residency:** Internal Medicine, Bellevue Hosp, New York, NY 1966-1968; **Fellowship:** Rheumatology, Columbia-Presby Med Ctr, New York, NY 1968-1970; **Faculty Appointment:** Prof Rheumatology, Cornell Univ-Weil Med Coll

Medsger Jr, Thomas A MD (Rheumatology) - *Special Expertise: Scleroderma; Raynaud's Disease; Polymyositis & Dermatomyositis;* **Admitting Hospital:** UPMC - Presbyterian University Hospital; **Office Address:** Univ Arth Ctr - Liliane Kaufman Bldg, rm 900 3471 Fifth Ave Pittsburgh, PA 15213; **Office Phone:** (412) 648-6970; **Board Certifications:** Internal Medicine 1972, Rheumatology 1972; **Medical School:** Univ Penn 1962; **Residency:** Internal Medicine, Univ Pittsburgh, Pittsburgh, PA 1966-1968; **Fellowships:** Rheumatology, Univ Pittsburgh, Pittsburgh, PA 1965-1966; Rheumatology, Univ TN Coll Med, Memphis, TN 1968-1969; **Faculty Appointment:** Prof Medicine, Univ Pittsburgh

Mitnick, Hal J MD (Rheumatology) - *Special Expertise: Rheumatoid Arthritis; Psoriatic Arthritis;* **Admitting Hospital:** NYU Medical Center (Page 70); **Office Address:** 333 E 34th St, Ste 1C New York, NY 10016; **Office Phone:** (212) 889-7217; **Board Certifications:** Internal Medicine 1976, Rheumatology 1978; **Medical School:** NYU Sch Med 1972; **Residency:** Internal Medicine, Bellevue Hosp, New York, NY 1972-1976; **Fellowship:** Rheumatology, New York Univ Med Ctr, New York, NY 1976-1978; **Faculty Appointment:** Clin Prof Medicine, NYU Sch Med

Oddis, Chester MD (Rheumatology) - *Special Expertise: Myositis;* **Admitting Hospital:** UPMC - Presbyterian University Hospital; **Office Address:** University Of Pittsburgh-Dept Med Rheum 3471 Fifth Avenue #502 Kaufman Pittsburgh, PA 15213; **Office Phone:** (412) 383-8000; **Board Certifications:** Rheumatology 1986, Internal Medicine 1983; **Medical School:** Penn State Univ-Hershey Med Ctr 1980; **Residency:** Internal Medicine, Hershey Med Ctr-Penn Univ, Hershey, PA 1981-1983; **Fellowship:** Rheumatology, University of Pittsburgh, Pittsburgh, PA 1984-1986; **Faculty Appointment:** Assoc Prof Medicine, Univ Pittsburgh

Paget, Stephen MD (Rheumatology) - *Special Expertise: Rheumatoid Arthritis; Lupus/SLE;* **Admitting Hospital:** Hospital for Special Surgery (Page 63); **Office Address:** 535 E 70th St, Fl 7 New York, NY 10021; **Office Phone:** (212) 606-1845; **Board Certifications:** Internal Medicine 1974, Rheumatology 1976; **Medical School:** SUNY Downstate 1971; **Residency:** Internal Medicine, Johns Hopkins Hosp, Baltimore, MD 1972-1973; **Fellowship:** Rheumatology, Hosp Special Surg, New York, NY 1975; **Faculty Appointment:** Clin Prof Medicine, Cornell Univ-Weil Med Coll

Petri, Michelle Ann MD (Rheumatology) - *Special Expertise: Lupus/SLE;* **Admitting Hospital:** Johns Hopkins Hospital - Baltimore (Page 65); **Office Address:** 1830 E Monument St, Ste 7500 Baltimore, MD 21205; **Office Phone:** (410) 955-3052; **Board Certifications:** Internal Medicine 1983, Rheumatology 1986; **Medical School:** Harvard Med Sch 1980; **Residency:** Internal Medicine, Mass Genl Hosp, Boston, MA 1980-1983; **Fellowships:** Allergy & Immunology, UCSF, San Francisco, CA 1985; Rheumatology, UCSF, San Francisco, CA 1986; **Faculty Appointment:** Assoc Prof Medicine, Johns Hopkins Univ

Plotz, Paul MD (Rheumatology) - *Special Expertise: Rheumatology - General;* **Admitting Hospital:** National Institutes of Health - Clinical Center; **Office Address:** 9000 Rockville Pike Bethseda, MD; **Office Phone:** 301 4961474; **Board Certification:** Internal Medicine 1970; **Medical School:** Harvard Med Sch 1963; **Residency:** Beth Isrel Hosp, Boston, MA 1964-1965; **Fellowship:** Rheumatology, Clin Ctr- NIH, Bethesda, MD 1965-1968

Sigal, Leonard H MD (Rheumatology) - *Special Expertise: Lyme Disease; Lupus/SLE;* **Admitting Hospital:** Robert Wood Johnson University Hospital @ New Brunswick; **Office Address:** UMDNJ, Dept Medicine-Rheumatology 125 Paterson St New Brunswick, NJ 08901-1962; **Office Phone:** (732) 235-7210; **Board Certifications:** Internal Medicine 1979, Rheumatology 1984; **Medical School:** Stanford Univ 1976; **Residencies:** Internal Medicine, Mount Sinai, New York, NY 1976-1979; Rheumatology, Yale Univ Sch Med, New Haven, CT 1981-1984; **Faculty Appointment:** Prof Medicine, Robert W Johnson Med Sch

Solomon, Gary MD (Rheumatology) - *Special Expertise: Silicone Associated Disorders; Arthritis;* **Admitting Hospital:** Hospital for Joint Diseases; **Office Address:** Hosp Joint Dis, Dept Ortho 305 Second Ave, Ste 16 New York, NY 10003; **Office Phone:** (212) 598-6516; **Board Certifications:** Internal Medicine 1980, Rheumatology 1982; **Medical School:** Mount Sinai Sch Med 1977; **Residency:** Internal Medicine, Mount Sinai Med Ctr, New York, NY 1978-1980; **Fellowship:** Rheumatology, Albert Einstein Coll Med, Bronx, NY 1980-1982; **Faculty Appointment:** Assoc Clin Prof Medicine, NYU Sch Med

Spiera, Harry MD (Rheumatology) - *Special Expertise:* Temporal Arteritis; Connective Tissue Disorders; **Admitting Hospital:** Mount Sinai Hospital (Page 70); **Office Address:** 1088 Park Ave New York, NY 10128-1132; **Office Phone:** (212) 860-4000; **Board Certifications:** Internal Medicine 1965, Rheumatology 1972; **Medical School:** NYU Sch Med 1958; **Residencies:** Internal Medicine, VA Med Ctr, Brooklyn, NY 1959-1960; Internal Medicine, Mount Sinai Hosp, New York, NY 1960-1961; **Fellowship:** Rheumatology, Columbia-Presby Med Ctr, New York, NY 1961-1963; **Faculty Appointment:** Prof Medicine, Mount Sinai Sch Med

Weinstein, Arthur MD (Rheumatology) - *Special Expertise:* Lyme Disease; Lupus/SLE; **Admitting Hospital:** George Washington University Hospital; **Office Address:** 2150 Pennsylvania Ave NW, Ste 5-405 Washington, DC 20037; **Office Phone:** (202) 994-4624; **Board Certifications:** Rheumatology 1976, Diagnostic Lab Immunology 1986; **Medical School:** Univ Toronto 1967; **Residencies:** Internal Medicine, Toronto Genl Hosp, Toronto, Canada 1967-1968; Internal Medicine, Toronto Welleley Hosp, Toronto, Canada 1968-1969; **Fellowships:** Rheumatology, Hammersmith Hosp, London, England 1969-1971; Rheumatology, Toronto Wellesley Hosp, Toronto, Canada 1972-1973; **Faculty Appointment:** Prof Rheumatology, Geo Wash Univ

White, Barbara MD (Rheumatology) - *Special Expertise:* Scleroderma; **Admitting Hospital:** University of Maryland Medical System; **Office Address:** VA Med Ctr 10 N Greene St, MS 1515 Baltimore, MD 21201; **Office Phone:** (410) 328-8667; **Board Certifications:** Allergy & Immunology 1983, Rheumatology 1982; **Medical School:** Univ Penn 1975; **Residency:** Internal Medicine, Univ Iowa, Iowa City, IA 1976-1978; **Fellowships:** Allergy & Immunology, Univ Iowa, Iowa City, IA 1979-1981; Rheumatology, Univ Iowa, Iowa City, IA 1981-1982; **Faculty Appointment:** Prof Medicine, Univ MD Sch Med

Wigley, Frederick M MD (Rheumatology) - *Special Expertise:* Scleroderma; Raynaud's Disease; **Admitting Hospital:** Johns Hopkins Hospital - Baltimore (Page 65); **Office Address:** 1830 E Monument Street Suite 7500 Baltimore, MD 21205; **Office Phone:** (410) 955-3052; **Board Certifications:** Internal Medicine 1980, Rheumatology 1980; **Medical School:** Univ Fla Coll Med 1972; **Residency:** Internal Medicine, John Hopkins Hops, Baltimore, MD 1972-1975; **Fellowship:** Rheumatology, John Hopkins Hosp, Baltimore, MD 1977-1979; **Faculty Appointment:** Prof Medicine, Johns Hopkins Univ

Southeast

Allen, Nancy B MD (Rheumatology) - *Special Expertise:* Rheumatology - General; **Admitting Hospital:** Duke University Medical Center (Page 60); **Office Address:** Duke Univ Med Ctr Box 3440 Durham, NC 27710; **Office Phone:** (919) 684-2965; **Board Certifications:** Internal Medicine 1981, Rheumatology 1984; **Medical School:** Tufts Univ 1978; **Residency:** Internal Medicine, Duke U Med Ctr, Durham, NC 1979-1981; **Fellowship:** Rheumatology, Duke U Med Ctr, Durham, NC 1981-1983; **Faculty Appointment:** Assoc Clin Prof Medicine, Duke Univ

Chatham, Walter W MD (Rheumatology) - *Special Expertise:* Lupus/SLE; Fibromyalgia; Rheumatoid Arthritis; **Admitting Hospital:** University of Alabama Hospital at Birmingham; **Office Address:** Univ Alabama Birmingham Med Ctr 1530 3rd Ave S Birmingham, AL 35205-7005; **Office Phone:** (205) 934-4212; **Board Certifications:** Internal Medicine 1983, Rheumatology 1988; **Medical School:** Vanderbilt Univ 1980; **Residencies:** Internal Medicine, North Carolina Meml Hosp-UNC, Chapel Hill, NC 1980-1982; Internal Medicine, North Carolina Meml Hosp-UNC, Chapel Hill, NC 1982-1983; **Fellowship:** Rheumatology, Univ Alabama, Birmingham, AL 1986-1988; **Faculty Appointment:** Asst Prof Medicine, Univ Ala

Hadler, Nortin MD (Rheumatology) - *Special Expertise:* Occupational Musculosketeal Disorders; **Admitting Hospital:** University of North Carolina Hospitals; **Office Address:** University of NC, Dept Medicine 3330 Thurston Building, Box 7280 Chapel Hill, NC 27599-7280; **Office Phone:** (919) 966-0566; **Board Certifications:** Rheumatology 1974, Allergy & Immunology 1975; **Medical School:** Harvard Med Sch 1968; **Residency:** Internal Medicine, Mass Genl Hosp, Boston, MA 1969-1973; **Fellowships:** Rheumatology, Natl Inst Hlth, Bethesda, MD 1970-1972; Allergy & Immunology, Clin Res Ctr, London, England 1973-1974; **Faculty Appointment:** Prof Medicine, Univ NC Sch Med

Heck, Louis William MD (Rheumatology) - *Special Expertise:* Lupus/SLE; Rheumatoid Arthritis; **Admitting Hospital:** University of Alabama Hospital at Birmingham; **Office Address:** Univ of Alabama at Birmingham - Rheum Clinic 1530 3rd Ave S, Bldg SRC - rm 068 Birmingham, AL 35294; **Office Phone:** (205) 934-6485; **Board Certifications:** Internal Medicine 1974, Rheumatology 1988; **Medical School:** Indiana Univ 1970; **Residency:** Internal Medicine, Indiana Univ 1971-1972; **Fellowships:** Allergy & Immunology, Natl Inst of Allergy & Inf Dis, Bethesda, MD 1972-1975; Rheumatology, Robert Bronton Hosp, Boston, MA 1975-1979; **Faculty Appointment:** Assoc Prof Medicine, Univ Ala

Kaplan, Stanley MD (Rheumatology) - *Special Expertise:* Rheumatoid Arthritis; **Admitting Hospital:** Baptist Memorial Hospital Medical Center; **Office Address:** Univ Tenn Med Group 920 Madison Ave, Ste 434 Memphis, TN 38103; **Office Phone:** (901) 448-7260; **Board Certification:** Internal Medicine 1965; **Medical School:** Univ Tenn Coll Med, Memphis 1954; **Residencies:** Internal Medicine, Univ Tenn Hosps, Memphis, TN 1958-1960; Internal Medicine, Univ Tenn Hosps, Memphis, TN 1961-1962; **Fellowship:** Rheumatology, Univ Tenn Hosps, Memphis, TN 1960-1962; **Faculty Appointment:** Prof Medicine, Univ Tenn Coll Med, Memphis

Rahn, Daniel W MD (Rheumatology) - *Special Expertise:* Rheumatoid Arthritis; Lyme Disease; Lupus/SLE; **Admitting Hospital:** Medical College of Georgia Hospital; **Office Address:** MCG Health Inc 1120 15th St, rm BA3310 Augusta, GA 30912; **Office Phone:** (706) 721-7346; **Board Certifications:** Rheumatology 1982, Internal Medicine 1979; **Medical School:** Yale Univ 1976; **Residency:** Internal Medicine, Yale New Haven Hosp, New Haven, CT 1972-1976; **Fellowship:** Rheumatology, Yale Univ/Yale New Haven Hosp, New Haven, CT 1976-1978; **Faculty Appointment:** Prof Medicine, Med Coll GA

Sundy, John Sargent MD/PhD (Rheumatology) - *Special Expertise:* Rheumatoid Arthritis; Gout; Lupus/SLE; **Admitting Hospital:** Duke University Medical Center (Page 60); **Office Address:** Duke Univ Med Ctr Box 3278 Durham, NC 27710; **Office Phone:** (919) 684-3956; **Board Certifications:** Rheumatology 1998, Allergy & Immunology 1999; **Medical School:** Hahnemann Univ 1991; **Residency:** Internal Medicine, Duke Univ Med Ctr, Durham, NC 1992-1993; **Fellowships:** Rheumatology, Duke Univ Med Ctr, Durham, NC 1993-1996; Allergy & Immunology, Duke Univ Med Ctr, Durham, NC 1995-1998; **Faculty Appointment:** Assoc Prof Medicine, Duke Univ

Wise, Christopher Murray MD (Rheumatology) - *Special Expertise:* Lupus/SLE; Sjogren's Syndrome; **Admitting Hospital:** Medical College of Virginia Hospitals; **Office Address:** Med Coll Va Box 980647 Richmond, VA 23298; **Office Phone:** (804) 828-9341; **Board Certifications:** Internal Medicine 1980, Rheumatology 1982; **Medical School:** Univ NC Sch Med 1977; **Residency:** Internal Medicine, Med Coll VA, Richmond, VA 1978-1980; **Fellowship:** Rheumatology, Med Coll VA, Richmond, VA 1980; **Faculty Appointment:** Assoc Clin Prof Medicine, Va Commonwealth Univ

Midwest

Adams, Elaine MD (Rheumatology) - *Special Expertise: Rheumatoid Arthritis; Lupus/SLE;* **Admitting Hospital:** Loyola University Health System; **Office Address:** 2160 S First Ave Maywood, IL 60153; **Office Phone:** (708) 216-3313; **Board Certifications:** Internal Medicine 1981, Rheumatology 1984; **Medical School:** Loyola Univ-Stritch Sch Med 1978; **Residencies:** Internal Medicine, Loyola University, Maywood, IL 1978-1981; Rheumatology, University of Wisconsin, Madison, WI; **Fellowship:** Rheumatology, Univ Wisc, Madison 1981-1983; **Faculty Appointment:** Assoc Prof Medicine, Loyola Univ-Stritch Sch Med

Barr, Walter Gerard MD (Rheumatology) - *Special Expertise: Rheumatoid Arthritis; Vasculitis; Arthritis/Viscosupplementation;* **Admitting Hospital:** Northwestern Memorial Hospital; **Office Address:** 675 N Sinclair Ave, Ste 18250 Chicago, IL 60611; **Office Phone:** (312) 695-8628; **Board Certifications:** Internal Medicine 1978, Rheumatology 1982; **Medical School:** Loyola Univ-Stritch Sch Med **Residency:** Internal Medicine, Loyola Univ Med Ctr, Chicago, IL; **Fellowships:** Rheumatology, Loyola Univ Med Ctr, Chicago, IL; Rheumatology, Mayo Clinic and Hosp, Rochester, MN

Brasington, Richard MD (Rheumatology) - *Special Expertise: Rheumatology - General;* **Admitting Hospital:** Barnes - Jewish Hospital; **Office Address:** 4932 Forest Park St Louis, MO 63108; **Office Phone:** (314) 286-2635; **Board Certifications:** Internal Medicine 1985, Rheumatology 1986; **Medical School:** Duke Univ 1980; **Residencies:** Internal Medicine, Univ Iowa, Iowa City, IA 1981-1982; Internal Medicine, Univ Iowa, Iowa City, IA 1984-1985; **Fellowship:** Rheumatology, Univ Iowa, Iowa City, IA 1982-1986; **Faculty Appointment:** Assoc Prof Medicine, Washington Univ, St Louis

Chang, Rowland Waton MD (Rheumatology) - *Special Expertise: Rheumatoid Arthritis; Arthritis and Exercise;* **Admitting Hospital:** Northwestern Memorial Hospital; **Office Address:** 345 E Superior St, Fl 9 Chicago, IL 60611; **Office Phone:** (312) 238-1156; **Board Certifications:** Internal Medicine 1979, Rheumatology 1982; **Medical School:** Tufts Univ 1976; **Residency:** Internal Medicine, Mt Auburn Hosp, Cambridge, MA 1977-1979; **Fellowships:** Rheumatology, Hammersmith Hosp, London, England 1979-1980; Rheumatology, Brigham & Womens Hosp, Boston, MA 1980-1982; **Faculty Appointment:** Prof Medicine, Northwestern Univ

Chang-Miller, April MD (Rheumatology) - *Special Expertise: Connective Tissue Disorders; Spondyloarthropathies;* **Admitting Hospital:** Mayo Medical Center & Clinic - Rochester; **Office Address:** Mayo Clinic, Dept Rheumatology 200 1st St SW Rochester, MN 55905; **Office Phone:** (507) 284-2965; **Board Certifications:** Rheumatology 1992, Internal Medicine 1986; **Medical School:** Yale Univ 1983; **Residency:** Internal Medicine, Mayo Grad Sch Med, Rochester, MN 1983-1985; **Fellowships:** Rheumatology, Mayo Grad Sch Med, Rochester, MN 1986-1989; Biochemical and Molecular Biology, Mayo Grad Sch Med, Rochester, MN 1989-1990; **Faculty Appointment:** Asst Prof Medicine, Mayo Med Sch

Crofford, Leslie MD (Rheumatology) - *Special Expertise: Fibromyalgia;* **Admitting Hospital:** University of Michigan Health Center; **Office Address:** 5510 Medical Science Research Bldg I 1150 W MedCtr Ann Arbor, MI 48109-0680; **Office Phone:** (734) 647-5900; **Board Certifications:** Internal Medicine 1987, Rheumatology 1992; **Medical School:** Univ Tenn Coll Med, Memphis 1984; **Residency:** Internal Medicine, Barnes/Wash Univ, St. Louis, MO 1984-1987; **Fellowship:** Rheumatology, Natl Inst Hlth Clin Ctr, Bethesda, MD 1989-1992; **Faculty Appointment:** Assoc Prof Medicine, Univ Mich Med Sch

Curran, James Joseph MD (Rheumatology) - *Special Expertise:* Arthritis; Lupus/SLE; **Admitting Hospital:** University of Chicago Hospitals (Page 78); **Office Address:** 5841 S Maryland Ave, MS 0930 Chicago, IL 60637; **Office Phone:** (773) 702-1232; **Board Certifications:** Internal Medicine 1980, Rheumatology 1982; **Medical School:** Univ IL Coll Med 1976; **Residency:** Internal Medicine, Bethesda Naval Hosp, Bethesda, MD 1978-1980; **Fellowship:** Rheumatology, Univ Chicago Hosp, Chicago, IL 1980-1982; **Faculty Appointment:** Clin Prof Medicine, Univ Chicago-Pritzker Sch Med

Duffy, Joseph MD (Rheumatology) - *Special Expertise:* Eosinophilic Disorders; Spondyloarthropathies; Connective Tissue Disorders; **Admitting Hospital:** Mayo Medical Center & Clinic - Rochester; **Office Address:** Mayo Clinic 200 1st St SW Rochester, MN 55905; **Office Phone:** (507) 284-4550; **Board Certifications:** Internal Medicine 1973, Rheumatology 1974; **Medical School:** Univ Okla Coll Med **Residency:** Internal Medicine, Univ Cincinnati, Cincinnati, OH 1964-1965; **Fellowships:** Rheumatology, Boston Univ, Boston, MA 1967-1968; Rheumatology, Baylor Coll of Med, TX 1971-1972

Ellman, Michael H MD (Rheumatology) - *Special Expertise:* Scleroderma; **Admitting Hospital:** University of Chicago Hospitals (Page 78); **Office Address:** Univ Chicago-Pritzker Sch Med 5841 S Maryland Ave, MC-2050 Chicago, IL 60637-1463; **Office Phone:** (773) 702-1226; **Board Certifications:** Internal Medicine 1969, Rheumatology 1972; **Medical School:** Univ IL Coll Med 1964; **Residency:** Internal Medicine, Michael Reese Hosp, Chicago, IL 1968-1970; **Fellowship:** Rheumatology, Univ Chicago Hosps, Chicago, IL 1970-1972; **Faculty Appointment:** Prof Medicine, Univ Chicago-Pritzker Sch Med

Fischbein, Lewis Conrad MD (Rheumatology) - *Special Expertise:* Rheumatoid Arthritis; Lupus/SLE; **Admitting Hospital:** Barnes - Jewish Hospital; **Office Address:** One Barnes - Hospital Plz East Pavilion , Ste 16422 St. Louis, MO 63110; **Office Phone:** (314) 367-9595; **Board Certifications:** Internal Medicine 1977, Rheumatology 1980; **Medical School:** Washington Univ, St Louis 1974; **Residency:** Internal Medicine, Barnes Jewish Hosp, St. Louis, MO 1975-1977; **Fellowship:** Rheumatology, Barnes Jewish Hosp, St. Louis, MO 1977-1979; **Faculty Appointment:** Assoc Prof Medicine, Washington Univ, St Louis

Harrington, J Timothy MD (Rheumatology) - *Special Expertise:* Arthritis; **Admitting Hospital:** University of Wisconsin Hospital & Clinics; **Office Address:** Univ WI Hosp and Clinics, Dept Rheum 1 South Park St Madison, WI 53715; **Office Phone:** (608) 287-2800; **Board Certifications:** Internal Medicine 1972, Rheumatology 1972; **Medical School:** Univ Wisc 1965; **Residencies:** Internal Medicine, Mass Genl Hosp, Boston, MA 1966-1967; Internal Medicine, Parkland Meml Hosp, Dallas, TX 1969-1970; **Fellowship:** Rheumatology, Univ Texas SW, Dallas, TX 1970-1971; **Faculty Appointment:** Prof Medicine, Univ Wisc

Hoffman, Gary Stuart MD (Rheumatology) - *Special Expertise:* Vasculitis; **Admitting Hospital:** Cleveland Clinic Foundation; **Office Address:** 9500 Euclid Ave, MC-A50 Cleveland, OH 44195; **Office Phone:** (216) 445-6996; **Board Certifications:** Internal Medicine 1976, Rheumatology 1978; **Medical School:** Med Coll VA 1971; **Residency:** Internal Medicine, Dartmouth-Hitchcock Clin, Lebanon, NH 1972-1973; **Fellowship:** Rheumatology, Dartmouth Univ, Lebanon, NH 1973-1974; **Faculty Appointment:** Prof Medicine, Ohio State Univ

Houk, John L MD (Rheumatology) - *Special Expertise:* Rheumatology - General; **Admitting Hospital:** University Hospital - Cincinnati; **Office Address:** Cincinnati Arthritis Association 2123 Auburn Ave, Fl 630 Cincinnati, OH 45219; **Office Phone:** (513) 621-7070; **Board Certifications:** Internal Medicine 1972, Rheumatology 1994; **Medical School:** Univ Cincinnati 1965; **Residency:** Internal Medicine, University Hospital, Cincinnati, OH 1969-1971; **Fellowship:** Rheumatology, University Hospital, Cincinnati, OH 1971-1973; **Faculty Appointment:** Prof Medicine, Univ Cincinnati

Katz, Robert MD (Rheumatology) - *Special Expertise: Fibromyalgia; Lupus/SLE;* **Admitting Hospital:** Rush/Presbyterian - St Luke's Medical Center - Chicago (Page 74); **Office Address:** 1725 W Harrison St, Ste 1039 Chicago, IL 60612; **Office Phone:** (312) 942-2159; **Board Certifications:** Internal Medicine 1975, Rheumatology 1976; **Medical School:** Univ MD Sch Med 1970; **Residency:** Internal Medicine, Washington Univ Med Ctr, St Louis, MO 1970-1972; **Fellowship:** Rheumatology, Johns Hopkins, Baltimore, MD 1974-1976; **Faculty Appointment:** Assoc Prof Medicine, Rush Med Coll

Klearman, Micki MD (Rheumatology) - *Special Expertise: Scleroderma;* **Admitting Hospital:** Barnes - Jewish Hospital; **Office Address:** One Barnes-Jewish Hospital Plz East Pavilion, Ste 16422 St. Louis, MO 63110; **Office Phone:** (314) 367-9595; **Board Certifications:** Internal Medicine 1985, Rheumatology 1988; **Medical School:** Washington Univ, St Louis 1981; **Residency:** Internal Medicine, Jewish Hosp, St Louis, MO 1982-1985; **Fellowship:** Rheumatology, Wash University, St Louis, MO 1985-1987

Luggen, Michael MD (Rheumatology) - *Special Expertise: Rheumatology;* **Admitting Hospital:** University Hospital - Cincinnati; **Office Address:** Cincinnati Arthritis Association 2123 Auburn Ave, Ste 630 Cincinnati, OH 45219; **Office Phone:** (513) 621-7070; **Board Certifications:** Rheumatology 1982, Internal Medicine 1978; **Medical School:** Columbia P&S 1974; **Residency:** Internal Medicine, Cinn General Hosp, Cincinnati, OH 1975-1977; **Fellowship:** Rheumatology, University Cinn, Cincinnati, OH 1980-1982; **Faculty Appointment:** Assoc Prof Medicine, Univ Cincinnati

Luthra, Harvinder Singh MD (Rheumatology) - *Special Expertise: Rheumatoid Arthritis; Ankylosing Spondilitis; Relapsing Polychondritis;* **Admitting Hospital:** St Mary's Hospital; **Office Address:** Mayo Clinic 200 1st St SW Rochester, MN 55905; **Office Phone:** (507) 284-1227; **Board Certifications:** Internal Medicine 1973, Rheumatology 1974; **Medical School:** India 1967; **Residencies:** Ophthalmology, Christian Med Coll, India 1968; Internal Medicine, Mount Sinai Hosp Med Ctr, Chicago, IL 1970-1972; **Fellowship:** Rheumatology, Mayo Grad Sch, Rochester, MN 1972-1974; **Faculty Appointment:** Prof Medicine, Mayo Med Sch

Mayes, Maureen Davidica MD/PhD (Rheumatology) - *Special Expertise: Scleroderma;* **Admitting Hospital:** Harper Hospital (Page 59); **Office Address:** 4707 Saint Antoine St Detroit, MI 48201; **Office Phone:** (313) 577-1133; **Board Certifications:** Internal Medicine 1980, Rheumatology 1982; **Medical School:** Eastern VA Med Sch 1976; **Residency:** Internal Medicine, Cleveland Clinic Fnd, Cleveland, OH 1978-1979; **Fellowship:** Rheumatology, Cleveland Clinic Fnd, Cleveland, OH 1979-1981; **Faculty Appointment:** Prof Medicine, Wayne State Univ

McCune, W. Joseph MD (Rheumatology) - *Special Expertise: Lupus/SLE; Rheumatoid arthritis;* **Admitting Hospital:** University of Michigan Health Center; **Office Address:** A Alfred Taubman Hlth Care Ctr 1500 E Med Ctr Dr, rm 3918, Box 0356 Ann Arbor, MI 48109-0358; **Office Phone:** (734) 936-5561; **Board Certifications:** Rheumatology 1982, Internal Medicine 1978; **Medical School:** Univ Cincinnati 1975; **Residencies:** Rheumatology, Univ of Mich, Ann Arbor, MI 1975-1976; Internal Medicine, Brigham Womens Hosp, Boston, MA 1976-1978; **Fellowship:** Rheumatology, Brigham Womens Hosp, Boston, MA 1978-1981; **Faculty Appointment:** Assoc Prof Medicine, Univ Mich Med Sch

Michalska, Margaret MD (Rheumatology) - *Special Expertise: Rheumatoid Arthritis; Connective Tissue Disorders;* **Admitting Hospital:** Rush/Presbyterian - St Luke's Medical Center - Chicago (Page 74); **Office Address:** 1725 W Harriston St Bldg 1 - rm 1017 Chicago, IL 60612; **Office Phone:** (312) 942-6641; **Board Certifications:** Internal Medicine 1988, Rheumatology 1990; **Medical School:** Poland 1979; **Residency:** Internal Medicine, Hines VA Hosp, Chicago, IL 1985-1988; **Fellowships:** Biochemistry, Nortwestern Univ, Evanston, IL 1980-1985; Rheumatology, Rush - Presby St Lukes, Chicago, IL 1988-1990; **Faculty Appointment:** Asst Prof Medicine, Rush Med Coll

Moder, Kevin Gerard MD (Rheumatology) - *Special Expertise: Rheumatoid Arthritis;*
Admitting Hospital: Mayo Medical Center & Clinic - Rochester; **Office Address:** Mayo Clinic 200
1st St SW Rochester, MN 55905; **Office Phone:** (507) 284-4550; **Board Certifications:** Internal
Medicine 1990, Rheumatology 1994; **Medical School:** Univ MO-Columbia Sch Med 1987;
Residency: Internal Medicine, Mayo Med Clinic, Rochester, MN 1987-1990; **Fellowship:**
Rheumatology, Mayo Med Clinic, Rochester, MN 1990-1993; **Faculty Appointment:** Asst Prof
Medicine, Mayo Med Sch

Moskowitz, Roland MD (Rheumatology) - *Special Expertise: Connective Tissue Disorders;
Osteoarthritis;* **Admitting Hospital:** University Hospital - Cleveland; **Office Address:** University
Hospital of Cleveland Div Rheum Dis 11100 Euclid Avenue Cleveland, OH 44106; **Office Phone:**
(216) 844-8500; **Board Certifications:** Internal Medicine 1961, Rheumatology 1974; **Medical
School:** Temple Univ 1953; **Residency:** Internal Medicine, Mayo Clinic, Rochester, MN 1954-1955;
Fellowship: Internal Medicine, Mayo Clin, Rochetser, MN 1957-1960; **Faculty Appointment:** Prof
Medicine, Case West Res Univ

Nelson, Audrey May MD (Rheumatology) - *Special Expertise: Scleroderma; Rheumatoid
Arthritis-Juvenile;* **Admitting Hospital:** St Mary's Hospital; **Office Address:** Mayo Medical Center
200 1st St SW Rochester, MN 55905; **Office Phone:** (507) 284-4550; **Board Certifications:** Internal
Medicine 1971, Rheumatology 1972; **Medical School:** Univ Minn 1965; **Residency:** Internal
Medicine, Mayo Grad Sch, Rochester, MN 1966-1969; **Fellowship:** Rheumatology, Mayo Grad
Sch, Rochester, MN 1970-1971; **Faculty Appointment:** Prof Rheumatology, Mayo Med Sch

Pope, Richard M MD (Rheumatology) - *Special Expertise: Arthritis; Sjogren's Syndrome;*
Admitting Hospital: Northwestern Memorial Hospital; **Office Address:** 675 N St Claire St, Fl 18 - Ste
250 Chicago, IL 60611-3373; **Office Phone:** (312) 695-8628; **Board Certifications:** Internal
Medicine 1973, Rheumatology 1976; **Medical School:** Loyola Univ-Stritch Sch Med 1970;
Residency: Internal Medicine, Michael Reese Hosp, Chicago, IL 1971-1972; **Fellowship:**
Rheumatology, Univ WA Med Ctr, Seattle, WA 1972-1974; **Faculty Appointment:** Prof
Rheumatology, Northwestern Univ

Great Plains and Mountains

Arend, Wiiliam Phelps MD (Rheumatology) - *Special Expertise: Arthritis; Immune
Deficiency-Rheumatoid Arthritis;* **Admitting Hospital:** University of Colorado Health & Science
Center; **Office Address:** Univ CO Hlth Sci Ctr 4200 9th Ave Denver, CO 80220-3706; **Office Phone:**
(303) 315-6666; **Board Certifications:** Internal Medicine 1971, Rheumatology 1980; **Medical
School:** Columbia P&S 1964; **Residencies:** Internal Medicine, Univ Wash Hosp, Seattle, WA 1965-
1966; Internal Medicine, Univ Wash Hosp, Seattle, WA 1968-1969; **Fellowship:** Rheumatology,
Univ Wash Hosp, Seattle, WA 1969-1971; **Faculty Appointment:** Prof Rheumatology, Univ Colo

Kotzin, Brian Leslie MD (Rheumatology) - *Special Expertise: Lupus/SLE;* **Admitting Hospital:**
National Jewish Medical & Research Center; **Office Address:** Natl Jewish Med & Rsch Ctr 1400
Jackson St Denver, CO 80206; **Office Phone:** (303) 388-4461; **Board Certifications:** Internal
Medicine 1978, Rheumatology 1980; **Medical School:** Stanford Univ 1975; **Residency:** Internal
Medicine, Beth Israel Hosp, Boston, MA 1976-1977; **Fellowship:** Rheumatology, Stanford Med Ctr,
Palo Alto, CA 1978; **Faculty Appointment:** Prof Medicine, Univ Colo

West, Sterling MD (Rheumatology) - *Special Expertise: Lupus/SLE;* **Admitting Hospital:**
University of Colorado Health & Science Center; **Office Address:** Univ Colo Hlth Sci Ctr 4200 E
Ninth Ave, Box B 115 Denver, CO 80262; **Office Phone:** (303) 315-6665; **Board Certifications:**
Internal Medicine 1979, Rheumatology 1982; **Medical School:** Emory Univ 1976; **Residency:**
Internal Medicine, Fitzsimons Army Med Ctr, Aurora, CO 1976-1979; **Fellowship:** Rheumatology,
Fitzsimons Army Med Ctr, Aurora, CO 1979-1981; **Faculty Appointment:** Prof Medicine, Univ Colo

Williams, H James MD (Rheumatology) - *Special Expertise:* Arthritis; **Admitting Hospital:** University of Utah Hospital and Clinics; **Office Address:** Univ Utah Med Ctr, Med Div Rheum 50 N Med Dr, 4B 200 SOM Salt Lake City, UT 84132-0001; **Office Phone:** (801) 581-7724; **Board Certifications:** Internal Medicine 1972, Rheumatology 1978; **Medical School:** Univ Utah 1969; **Residencies:** Internal Medicine, Duke Med Ctr, Durham, NC 1970-1972; Internal Medicine, Univ Utah Med Ctr, Salt Lake City, UT 1972-1973; **Fellowship:** Rheumatology, Univ Utah Med Ctr, Salt Lake City, UT 1975-1977; **Faculty Appointment:** Prof Rheumatology, Univ Utah

Southwest

Arnett Jr, Frank Couchman MD (Rheumatology) - *Special Expertise:* Reiter's Syndrome; **Admitting Hospital:** University of Texas Health & Science Center; **Office Address:** Hermann Prof Bldg 6410 Fannin St, Ste 1100 Houston, TX 77030; **Office Phone:** (713) 704-6100; **Board Certifications:** Rheumatology 1976, Clinical & Laboratory Dematologic Immunology 1990; **Medical School:** Univ Cincinnati 1968; **Residency:** Internal Medicine, Johns Hopkins Hosp, Baltimore, MD 1969-1970; **Fellowship:** Rheumatology, Johns Hopkins Hosp, Baltimore, MD 1970-1972; **Faculty Appointment:** Prof Medicine, Univ Tex, Houston

Davis, William Eugene MD (Rheumatology) - *Special Expertise:* Lupus/SLE; Rheumatoid Arthritis; **Admitting Hospital:** Ochsner Foundation Hospital; **Office Address:** Ochsner Clinic, Rheum 1514 Jefferson Hwy, #7N New Orleans, LA 70121; **Office Phone:** (504) 842-3920; **Board Certifications:** Internal Medicine 1987, Rheumatology 1988; **Medical School:** Louisiana State Univ 1983; **Residency:** Internal Medicine, Ochsner Fdn Hosp, New Orleans, LA 1983-1986; **Fellowship:** Rheumatology, Univ Michigan, Ann Arbor, MI 1986-1988

Hurd, Eric MD (Rheumatology) - *Special Expertise:* Rheumatoid Arthritis; **Admitting Hospital:** Baylor University Medical Center; **Office Address:** 712 N Washington, Ste 200 Dallas, TX 75246; **Office Phone:** (214) 823-6503; **Board Certifications:** Internal Medicine, Rheumatology; **Medical School:** Univ Okla Coll Med 1962; **Residencies:** Internal Medicine, Parkland Meml, Dallas, TX; Internal Medicine, St Johns Med Ctr

Lindsey, Stephen M MD (Rheumatology) - *Special Expertise:* Osteoporosis; Lupus/SLE; **Admitting Hospital:** Ochsner Foundation Hospital; **Office Address:** 9001 Summa Ave Baton Rouge, LA 70809; **Office Phone:** (757) 460-5604; **Board Certifications:** Internal Medicine 1975, Rheumatology 1980; **Medical School:** Louisiana State Univ 1972; **Residency:** Letterman AMC, San Francisco, CA 1973-1975; **Fellowship:** Rheumatology, Walter Reed AMC, Washington, DC 1977-1979; **Faculty Appointment:** Asst Prof Medicine, Eastern VA Med Sch

Lipstate, James Mitchell MD (Rheumatology) - *Special Expertise:* Arthritis; Osteoporosis; **Admitting Hospital:** Our Lady of Lourdes Regional Medical Center - Lafayette; **Office Address:** 401B Audubon Blvd, Ste 102B Lafayette, LA 70503; **Office Phone:** (337) 237-7801; **Board Certifications:** Internal Medicine 1983, Rheumatology 1986; **Medical School:** Tulane Univ 1980; **Residency:** Internal Medicine, Univ AL Hosp, Birmingham, AL 1981-1983; **Fellowship:** Rheumatology, Univ AL Hosp, Birmingham, AL 1983-1986; **Faculty Appointment:** Asst Clin Prof Medicine, Louisiana State Univ

Malin, Jennifer MD (Rheumatology) - *Special Expertise:* Arthritis; **Admitting Hospital:** Our Lady of Lourdes Regional Medical Center - Lafayette; **Office Address:** 401 Audobon Blvd, Ste 102B Lafayette, LA 70503-2676; **Office Phone:** (337) 237-7801; **Board Certifications:** Internal Medicine 1991, Rheumatology 1996; **Medical School:** Tulane Univ 1987; **Residencies:** Obstetrics & Gynecology, Tulane Univ Sch Med, New Orleans, LA 1987-1988; Internal Medicine, Tulane Univ Sch Med, New Orleans, LA 1988-1991; **Fellowship:** Rheumatology, Tulane Univ Sch Med, New Orleans, LA 1991-1993

Sessoms, Sandra Lee MD (Rheumatology) - *Special Expertise:* Arthritis; Lupus/SLE; **Admitting Hospital:** Methodist Hospital - Houston (Page 69); **Office Address:** Methodist Hospital 6550 Fannin St, Smith Tower St, rm 2600 Houston, TX 77030; **Office Phone:** (713) 986-8190; **Board Certifications:** Internal Medicine 1981, Rheumatology 1984; **Medical School:** Baylor Coll Med 1978; **Residency:** Internal Medicine, Baylor Coll Med, Houston, TX 1978-1979; **Fellowship:** Rheumatology, Baylor Coll Med, Houston, TX 1981-1983; **Faculty Appointment:** Assoc Prof Medicine, Baylor Coll Med

West Coast and Pacific

Bobrove, Arthur M MD (Rheumatology) - *Special Expertise:* Inflammatory Muscle Disease; **Admitting Hospital:** Stanford Medical Center; **Office Address:** Palo Alto Med Fnd 795 El Camino Real Palo Alto, CA 94301; **Office Phone:** (650) 321-4121; **Board Certifications:** Internal Medicine 1972, Rheumatology 1976; **Medical School:** Temple Univ 1967; **Residencies:** Internal Medicine, Univ of MI Hosp, Ann Arbor, MI 1968-1969; Internal Medicine, Univ of MI Hosp, Ann Arbor, MI 1971-1972; **Fellowship:** Immunology, Stanford Univ, Stanford, CA 1972-1974; **Faculty Appointment:** Clin Prof Medicine, Stanford Univ

Clements, Philip Jordan MD (Rheumatology) - *Special Expertise:* Scleroderma; **Admitting Hospital:** UCLA Medical Center; **Office Address:** UCLA Sch Med, Rehab 32-59 1000 Veteran Ave Los Angeles, CA 90095-1670; **Office Phone:** (310) 825-5330; **Board Certifications:** Internal Medicine 1972, Rheumatology 1974; **Medical School:** Indiana Univ 1965; **Residency:** Internal Medicine, Cedars-Sinai Med Ctr, Los Angeles, CA 1969-1971; **Fellowship:** Rheumatology, UCLA, Los Angeles, CA 1971-1974; **Faculty Appointment:** Prof Medicine, UCLA

Ehresmann, Glenn Richard MD (Rheumatology) - *Special Expertise:* Rheumatology - General; **Admitting Hospital:** USC University Hospital - Richard K. Eamer Medical Plaza; **Office Address:** USC Univ Hosp Rehabilitation Center 1500 San Pablo St Los Angelas, CA 90033; **Office Phone:** (323) 342-5100; **Board Certifications:** Internal Medicine 1977, Rheumatology 1978; **Medical School:** UC Irvine 1973; **Residency:** Internal Medicine, Los Angeles Co-USC Med Ctr, Los Angeles, CA 1976-1978; **Fellowship:** Rheumatology, Los Angeles Co-USC Med Ctr, Los Angeles, CA 1976-1978

Gardner, Gregory MD (Rheumatology) - *Special Expertise:* Rheumatology - General; **Admitting Hospital:** University of Washington Medical Center; **Office Address:** UWMC-Arthritis Clinic 1959 NE Pacific St, Box 356166 Seattle, WA 98195; **Office Phone:** (206) 598-7600; **Board Certifications:** Internal Medicine 1987, Rheumatology 1990; **Medical School:** Baylor Coll Med 1984; **Residency:** Internal Medicine, Univ of NC Hosp, Charleston, NC 1984-1987; **Fellowship:** Rheumatology, Univ CA-San Diego Med Ctr, San Diego, CA 1987-1989

Gershwin, Merrill Eric MD (Rheumatology) - *Special Expertise:* Allergy; Immune Deficiency-Rheumatoid Arthritis; **Admitting Hospital:** University of California - Davis Medical Center; **Office Address:** UC Davis Med Ctr, Div Rheu Box PB192 Sacramento, CA 95616; **Office Phone:** (530) 752-2884; **Board Certifications:** Rheumatology 1976, Allergy & Immunology 1979; **Medical School:** Stanford Univ 1971; **Residency:** Internal Medicine, New England Med Ctr, Boston, MA 1972-1973; **Fellowship:** Rheumatology, Natl Inst Arth Met, Bethesda, MD 1973-1975; **Faculty Appointment:** Prof Medicine, UC Davis

Hahn, Bevra H MD (Rheumatology) - *Special Expertise:* Lupus/SLE; **Admitting Hospital:** UCLA Medical Center; **Office Address:** UCLA Medical 1000 Veteran Ave Los Angeles, CA 90095; **Office Phone:** (310) 825-2448; **Board Certifications:** Internal Medicine 1970, Rheumatology 1972; **Medical School:** Johns Hopkins Univ 1964; **Residency:** Internal Medicine, Washington Univ - Barnes Hosp, St. Louis, MO 1965-1966; **Fellowship:** Rheumatology, Johns Hopkins Hosp, Baltimore, MD 1966-1969; **Faculty Appointment:** Prof Medicine, UCLA

Harris Jr, Edward Day MD (Rheumatology) - *Special Expertise:* Rheumatology - General; **Admitting Hospital:** Stanford Medical Center; **Office Address:** Stanford Univ School of Med 1000 Welch Rd, Ste 203 Palo Alto, CA 94304; **Office Phone:** (415) 723-5455; **Board Certifications:** Internal Medicine 1968, Rheumatology 1976; **Medical School:** Harvard Med Sch 1962; **Residency:** Internal Medicine, Mass Genl Hosp, Boston, MA 1963-1967; **Fellowship:** Internal Medicine, Mass Genl Hosp, Boston, MA 1967-1969; **Faculty Appointment:** Prof Medicine, Stanford Univ

Kitridou, Rodanthi C MD (Rheumatology) - *Special Expertise:* Lupus/SLE; **Admitting Hospital:** USC University Hospital - Richard K. Eamer Medical Plaza; **Office Address:** 1200 N State St, Box 386 Los Angeles, CA 90033-1029; **Office Phone:** (323) 226-7873; **Board Certifications:** Internal Medicine 1972, Rheumatology 1972; **Medical School:** Greece 1962; **Residency:** Internal Medicine, Hahnemann Hosp, Philadelphia, PA 1964-1966; **Fellowships:** Rheumatology, Univ Penn Med Ctr, Philadelphia, PA 1967-1968; Rheumatology, VA Hosp, Philadephia, PA 1968-1969; **Faculty Appointment:** Prof Medicine, USC Sch Med

Quismorio Jr, Francisco P MD (Rheumatology) - *Special Expertise:* Lupus/SLE; Connective Tissue Disorders; **Admitting Hospital:** LAC + USC Medical Center; **Office Address:** USC Keck Sch Med 2011 Zonal Ave, MC-HMR-715 Los Angeles, CA 90033-1034; **Office Phone:** (323) 442-1946; **Board Certifications:** Internal Medicine 1975, Rheumatology 1976; **Medical School:** Philippines 1964; **Residencies:** Internal Medicine, Philippines General Hosp, Manila, Philippines 1964-1966; Internal Medicine, LAC USC Med Ctr, Los Angeles, CA 1970-1971; **Fellowships:** Rheumatology, Univ Penn Hosp, Philadelphia, PA 1966-1968; Rheumatology, LAC USC Med Ctr, Los Angeles, CA 1968-1970; **Faculty Appointment:** Prof Medicine, USC Sch Med

Sack, Kenneth Edward MD (Rheumatology) - *Special Expertise:* Rheumatology - General; **Admitting Hospital:** University of California - San Francisco Medical Center; **Office Address:** UCSF Sch Med 400 Parnassus Ave, rm A555 San Francisco, CA 94143; **Office Phone:** (415) 353-2497; **Board Certifications:** Internal Medicine 1973, Rheumatology 1978; **Medical School:** Tufts Univ 1968; **Residencies:** Internal Medicine, RI Hosp, Providence, RI 1969-1970; Internal Medicine, U Mich Hosp, Ann Arbor, MI 1972-1974; **Fellowship:** Rheumatology, Univ Ala Hosp, Birmingham, AL 1977-1978; **Faculty Appointment:** Clin Prof Medicine, UCSF

Stimmler, Mary McMillen MD (Rheumatology) - *Special Expertise:* Lupus/SLE; Vasculitis; **Admitting Hospital:** LAC + USC Medical Center; **Office Address:** 1200 N State St, rm 1110 Los Angeles, CA 90033; **Office Phone:** (323) 226-6738; **Board Certifications:** Internal Medicine 1983, Rheumatology 1986; **Medical School:** Mexico 1979; **Residency:** Internal Medicine, VA Hosp-UC Irvine, Long Beach, CA 1981-1983; **Fellowship:** Rheumatology, USC Sch Med, Los Angeles, CA 1984-1986; **Faculty Appointment:** Assoc Prof Medicine, USC Sch Med

Weiss, Arthur MD/PhD (Rheumatology) - *Special Expertise:* Rheumatology - General; **Admitting Hospital:** University of California - San Francisco Medical Center; **Office Address:** Arthritis Clin, UCSF Ambulatory Care Bldg 400 3rd and Parnassus Ave, Box 0795 San Francisco, CA 94143; **Office Phone:** (415) 476-1291; **Board Certifications:** Internal Medicine 1983, Rheumatology 1986; **Medical School:** Univ Chicago-Pritzker Sch Med 1979; **Residency:** Internal Medicine, UCSF, San Francisco, CA 1981-1983; **Fellowship:** Rheumatology, UCSF, San Francisco, CA 1983-1985; **Faculty Appointment:** Prof Medicine, UCSF

Wener, Mark MD (Rheumatology) - *Special Expertise:* Lupus/SLE; Vasculitis; **Admitting Hospital:** University of Washington Medical Center; **Office Address:** Univ Wash Med Ctr, Arthritis Clinic 1959 NE Pacific St, Box 356166 Seattle, WA 98195; **Office Phone:** (206) 598-7600; **Board Certifications:** Rheumatology 1980, Internal Medicine 1978; **Medical School:** Washington Univ, St Louis 1974; **Residency:** Internal Medicine, Univ Iowa Hosp, Iowa City, IA 1974-1978; **Fellowships:** Rheumatology, Univ Iowa Hosp, Iowa City, IA 1978-1980; Immunology, Univ Wash, Seattle, WA 1978-1983

Wofsy, David MD (Rheumatology) - *Special Expertise:* Lupus/SLE; **Admitting Hospital:** University of California - San Francisco Medical Center; **Office Address:** 533 Parnassus Ave, Box 0633 San Francisco, CA 94143; **Office Phone:** (415) 750-2104; **Board Certifications:** Internal Medicine 1977, Rheumatology 1980; **Medical School:** UCSD 1974; **Residency:** Internal Medicine, UCSF Hosps, San Francisco, CA 1975-1977; **Fellowship:** Rheumatology, UCSF, San Francisco, CA 1977-1979; **Faculty Appointment:** Prof Medicine, UCSF

SPORTS MEDICINE

(a subspecialty of INTERNAL MEDICINE)

An internist trained to be responsible for continuous care in the field of sports medicine, not only for the enhancement of health and fitness, but also for the prevention of injury and illness. A sports medicine physician must have knowledge and experience in the promotion of wellness and the prevention of injury. Knowledge about special areas of medicine such as exercise physiology, biomechanics, nutrition, psychology, physical rehabilitation, epidemiology, physical evaluation, injuries (treatment and prevention and referral practice) and the role of exercise in promoting a healthy life style are essential to the practice of sports medicine. The sports medicine physician requires special education to provide the knowledge to improve the healthcare of the individual engaged in physical exercise (sports) whether as an individual or in team participation.

INTERNAL MEDICINE

An internist is a personal physician who provides long-term, comprehensive care in the office and the hospital, managing both common and complex illness of adolescents, adults and the elderly. Internists are trained in the diagnosis and treatment of cancer, infections and diseases affecting the heart, blood, kidneys, joints and digestive, respiratory and vascular systems. They are also trained in the essentials of primary care internal medicine which incorporates an understanding of disease prevention, wellness, substance abuse, mental health and effective treatment of common problems of the eyes, ears, skin, nervous system and reproductive organs.

Training required: Three years in internal medicine *plus* additional training and examination for certification in sports medicine

PHYSICIAN LISTINGS

Mid Atlantic

Altchek, David MD (Sports Medicine) - *Special Expertise: Shoulder Surgery; Elbow Surgery; Knee Surgery;* **Admitting Hospital:** Hospital for Special Surgery (Page 63); **Office Address:** 525 E 71st St New York, NY 10021; **Office Phone:** (212) 606-1909; **Board Certification:** Orthopaedic Surgery 1990; **Medical School:** Cornell Univ-Weil Med Coll 1982; **Residency:** Orthopaedic Surgery, Hosp For Special Surgery, New York, NY 1983-1987; **Fellowship:** Sports Medicine, Hosp For Special Surgery, New York, NY 1987-1988; **Faculty Appointment:** Asst Prof Orthopaedic Surgery, Cornell Univ-Weil Med Coll

Kelly, Michael MD (Sports Medicine) - *Special Expertise: Knee Surgery;* **Admitting Hospital:** Beth Israel Medical Center - Herbert & Nell Singer Division (Page 58); **Office Address:** 170 East End Ave, Fl 4 New York, NY 10128; **Office Phone:** (212) 870-9747; **Board Certification:** Orthopaedic Surgery 1999; **Medical School:** Georgetown Univ 1979; **Residencies:** Surgery, St Vincent Hosp, New York, NY 1979-1981; Orthopaedic Surgery, Columbia-Presby Hosp, New York, NY 1981-1984; **Fellowship:** Knee Surgery, Hosp For Special Surgery, New York, NY 1984-1985; **Faculty Appointment:** Asst Prof Orthopaedic Surgery, Columbia P&S

Levine, William MD (Sports Medicine) - *Special Expertise: Arthroscopy; Sports Medicine; Shoulder & Knee Injuries;* **Admitting Hospital:** Columbia Presbyterian Medical Center (Page 72); **Office Address:** Herbert Irving Pavilion, Fl 2 161 Fort Washington Ave New York, NY 10032; **Office Phone:** (212) 305-0762; **Board Certification:** Orthopaedic Surgery 1999; **Medical School:** Case West Res Univ 1990; **Residencies:** Surgery, Beth Israel Hosp, Boston, MA 1990-1991; Orthopaedic Surgery, New Eng Med Ctr Hosps, Boston, MA 1991-1995; **Fellowships:** Shoulder Surgery, Columbia-Presby Med Ctr, New York, NY 1995-1996; Sports Medicine, Univ MD Med Ctr, Baltimore, MD 1997-1998; **Faculty Appointment:** Asst Prof Orthopaedic Surgery, Colombia

Maharam, Lewis MD (Sports Medicine) - *Special Expertise: Running Injuries;* **Admitting Hospital:** Hospital for Joint Diseases; **Office Address:** 800A Fifth Ave, Ste 302, MC-10021 New York, NY 10021; **Office Phone:** (212) 308-2348; **Board Certification:** Sports Medicine 1990; **Medical School:** Emory Univ 1985; **Residencies:** Internal Medicine, Danbury Hosp, Danbury, CT 1986-1987; Internal Medicine, NY Infirm/Beekman Downtown, New York, NY 1987-1989; **Fellowship:** Sports Medicine, Pascack Valley Hosp, Westwood, NJ 1989-1990

Nisonson, Barton MD (Sports Medicine) - *Special Expertise: Knee Injuries;* **Admitting Hospital:** Lenox Hill Hospital; **Office Address:** 130 E 77th St New York, NY 10021-1803; **Office Phone:** (212) 570-9120; **Board Certification:** Orthopaedic Surgery 1974; **Medical School:** Columbia P&S 1966; **Residency:** Surgery, Columbia-Presby Med Ctr, New York, NY 1967-1968; **Fellowship:** Orthopaedic Surgery, Columbia-Presby Med Ctr, New York, NY 1970-1973

Southeast

Andrews, James R MD (Sports Medicine) - *Special Expertise: Shoulder, Elbow, Knee Surgery;* **Admitting Hospital:** Healthsouth Medical Center - Birmingham; **Office Address:** Alabama Sports Medicine & Orthopaedic Center 1201 11th Ave, Fl 200 Birmingham, AL 35205-3410; **Office Phone:** (205) 930-0061; **Board Certification:** Orthopaedic Surgery 1974; **Medical School:** Louisiana State Univ 1967; **Residencies:** USPHS Hosp, San Francisco, CA 1968; Orthopaedic Surgery, Touro Infirm-Tulane, New Orleans, LA 1969-1970; **Fellowship:** Hand Surgery, VA Med Ctr, Charlottesville, VA 1972

Speer, Kevin MD (Sports Medicine) - *Special Expertise:* Irritated Cuff Repair; **Admitting Hospital:** Western Wake Medical Center; **Office Address:** Cary Ortho and Sport Med 101 SW Cary Pkwy, Ste 100 Cary, NC 27511; **Office Phone:** (919) 467-4992; **Board Certification:** Orthopaedic Surgery 1994; **Medical School:** Johns Hopkins Univ 1985; **Residency:** Orthopaedic Surgery, Duke Univ Med Ctr, Durham, NC 1987-1991; **Fellowship:** Sports Medicine, Hosp Special Surg, New York, NY 1991-1992; **Faculty Appointment:** Assoc Prof Orthopaedic Surgery, Duke Univ

Midwest

Noyes, Frank MD (Sports Medicine) - *Special Expertise:* Sports Medicine; Joint Surgery; **Admitting Hospital:** Deaconess Hospital; **Office Address:** 621 E Mehring Way , rm 415 One Lytle Place Cincinnati, OH 45202-3528; **Office Phone:** (513) 421-5100; **Board Certification:** Orthopaedic Surgery 1972; **Medical School:** Geo Wash Univ 1966; **Residencies:** University of Mich Med Ctr, Ann Arbor, MI 1967-1968; Orthopaedic Surgery, University of Mich Med Ctr, Ann Arbor, MI 1968-1971; **Faculty Appointment:** Clin Prof Orthopaedic Surgery, Univ Cincinnati

Paletta, George A MD (Sports Medicine) - *Special Expertise:* Ankle Surgery; Knee Surgery; **Admitting Hospital:** Barnes - Jewish Hospital; **Office Address:** Barnes Jewish Hospital, Dept Orthopaedic Surg, West Pavilion West Pavilion, Ste 11300 St Louis, MO 63110; **Office Phone:** (314) 747-2500; **Board Certification:** Orthopaedic Surgery 1998; **Medical School:** Johns Hopkins Univ 1988; **Residency:** Orthopaedic Surgery, Cornell Univ Med Ctr, New York, NY 1990-1994; **Fellowship:** Orthopaedic Surgery, Cleveland Clin Fnd, Cleveland, OH 1994-1995; **Faculty Appointment:** Asst Prof Orthopaedic Surgery, Washington Univ, St Louis

Schwenk, Thomas L MD (Sports Medicine) - *Special Expertise:* Sports Medicine - General; **Admitting Hospital:** University of Michigan Health Center; **Office Address:** 1500 S Medical Ctr, rm L2003 Ann Arbor, MI 48109; **Office Phone:** (734) 998-7390; **Board Certifications:** Family Practice 1996, Sports Medicine 1993; **Medical School:** Univ Mich Med Sch 1975; **Residency:** Family Practice, Univ Utah Affil Hosps, Salt Lake City, UT 1975-1978; **Fellowship:** Family Practice, Univ Utah Affil Hosps, Salt Lake City, UT 1980-1982; **Faculty Appointment:** Prof Family Practice, Univ Mich Med Sch

Shively, Robert A MD (Sports Medicine) - *Special Expertise:* Ankle & Knee surgery; Knee Replacement; **Admitting Hospital:** Barnes - Jewish Hospital; **Office Address:** Washington Univ 1 Barnes Plaza, Ste 11300 St Louis, MO 63110; **Office Phone:** (314) 362-4080; **Board Certification:** Orthopaedic Surgery 1981; **Medical School:** Univ IL Coll Med 1969; **Residencies:** Surgery, Carolinas Med Ctr Prgm, Charlotte, NC 1970-1971; Orthopaedic Surgery, St Louis Univ Sch Med, St Louis, MO 1975-1979; **Fellowship:** Sports Medicine, Univ Okla Hlth Scis Ctr-Presby Hosp, Oklahoma City, OK 1979-1980; **Faculty Appointment:** Asst Prof Orthopaedic Surgery, Washington Univ, St Louis

West Coast and Pacific

Jobe, Frank Wilson MD (Sports Medicine) - *Special Expertise:* Shoulder Surgery; Elbow Surgery; **Admitting Hospital:** Centinela Hospital Medical Center; **Office Address:** LA Co Genl Hosp 6801 Park Terr, Fl 500 Los Angeles, CA 90045; **Office Phone:** (310) 665-7200; **Board Certification:** Orthopaedic Surgery 1968; **Medical School:** Loma Linda Univ 1956; **Residency:** Orthopaedic Surgery, Los Angeles Co Genl Hosp, Los Angeles, CA 1960-1964; **Faculty Appointment:** Clin Prof Orthopaedic Surgery, USC Sch Med

Schechter, David Louis MD (Sports Medicine) - *Special Expertise:* Pain-Back; **Admitting Hospital:** California Hospital Medical Center; **Office Address:** 50 N La Cienega Blvd , Ste 100 Beverly Hills, CA 90211; **Office Phone:** (310) 659-7414; **Board Certifications:** Sports Medicine 1993, Family Practice 1994; **Medical School:** NYU Sch Med 1984; **Residency:** Family Practice, UCLA/Santa Monica Hosp, CA 1984-1987; **Faculty Appointment:** Assoc Clin Prof Family Practice, USC Sch Med

SURGERY

A surgeon manages a broad spectrum of surgical conditions affecting almost any area of the body. The surgeon establishes the diagnosis and provides the preoperative, operative and postoperative care to surgical patients and is usually responsible for the comprehensive management of the trauma victim and the critically ill surgical patient.

The surgeon uses a variety of diagnostic techniques, including endoscopy, for observing internal structures and may use specialized instruments during operative procedures. A general surgeon is expected to be familiar with the salient features of other surgical specialties in order to recognize problems in those areas and to know when to refer a patient to another specialist.

Training required: Five years

For a description of the subspecialty **Hand Surgery** *(see page 265)*, **Pediatric Surgery**, *(see page 545)* and **Vascular Surgery** *(see page 853)*

The University of Chicago Hospitals
Transplant Program

5841 S. Maryland Avenue
Chicago, Illinois 60637-1470
For help finding a physician: 1-888-UCH-0200

AT THE FOREFRONT OF TRANSPLANTATION

Clinical research, medical expertise, and superior patient care come together to make the University of Chicago Hospitals' transplant program one of the most innovative and active transplant programs in the United States. The program offers patients the finest treatment options and a comprehensive, multi-faceted approach to care.

Attending physicians in the transplantation program are faculty members who participate in medical education and research, as well as the treatment of patients. Collectively, these physicians have published or presented several thousand research papers. As a result, the University of Chicago Hospitals provide treatment alternatives not yet available anywhere else -- offering our patients truly state-of-the-art medical care.

INNOVATIONS IN TRANSPLANT CARE

The University of Chicago Hospitals have an international reputation in transplant research and patient care:

◎ Experts here performed the nation's first successful heart-liver-kidney transplant.

◎ The first successful liver transplant from a living donor was performed at the University of Chicago Hospitals.

◎ Our pediatric liver transplantation program is among the largest in the United States.

◎ This is the only facility in the region that can assist a failing liver with continuous support with human liver cells.

◎ Illinois' first pancreas transplant was performed here.

◎ The bone marrow transplant program at the University of Chicago Hospitals is an integral part of efforts here to provide every available treatment for cancer patients.

◎ We have the state's most active kidney transplant program.

**To Find a University of Chicago Specialist in
Transplant Services,
call 1-888-UCH-0200**
Visit our web site at www.uchospitals.edu

COORDINATED CARE FOR PATIENTS AND THEIR FAMILIES

With the goal of enhancing each patient's long-term well-being, our physicians and nurses work closely with patients and families before the transplant and long afterward to monitor progress. They also consult frequently with referring physicians, keeping them informed about the patient's status and working with them to provide appropriate follow-up care after the patient leaves.

PHYSICIAN LISTINGS

Surgery

New England

Auchincloss Jr, Hugh MD (Surgery) - *Special Expertise:* Transplant-Kidney & Pancreas; Vascular Access; **Admitting Hospital:** Massachusetts General Hospital; **Office Address:** Brigham & Women's Hosp, Dept Transplant Surg 75 Francis St Boston, MA 02115; **Office Phone:** (617) 732-6866; **Board Certification:** Surgery 1985; **Medical School:** Harvard Med Sch 1976; **Residency:** Surgery, Mass General Hosp, Boston, MA 1977-1985; **Fellowship:** Transplant Surgery, Mass General Hosp, Boston, MA 1985; **Faculty Appointment:** Assoc Prof Surgery, Harvard Med Sch

Blackburn, George L MD/PhD (Surgery) - *Special Expertise:* Obesity; Eating Disorders; **Admitting Hospital:** Beth Israel Deaconess Medical Center - Boston (Page 57); **Office Address:** 1 Autum St, Ste 1B Boston, MA 02215; **Office Phone:** (617) 632-8543; **Board Certification:** Surgery 1972; **Medical School:** Univ Kans 1965; **Residency:** Surgery, Boston City Hosp, Boston, MA 1965-1970; **Faculty Appointment:** Assoc Prof Surgery, Harvard Med Sch

Cady, Blake MD (Surgery) - *Special Expertise:* Breast Cancer; Thyroid Cancer; **Admitting Hospital:** Women & Infants Hospital - Rhode Island; **Office Address:** Women & Infants Hosp - Breast Hlth Ctr One Blackston Place Pl, Fl 2nd Providence, RI 02905; **Office Phone:** (401) 537-7540; **Board Certification:** Surgery 1966; **Medical School:** Cornell Univ-Weil Med Coll 1957; **Residencies:** Surgery, Boston City Hosp, Boston, MA 1961-1965; Surgery, NY Meml Cancer Hosp, New York, NY 1965-1967; **Faculty Appointment:** Prof Surgery, Brown Univ

Cioffi, William MD (Surgery) - *Special Expertise:* Trauma; **Admitting Hospital:** Rhode Island Hospital; **Office Address:** Rhode Island Hosp, Dept Surg 2 Dudley St, Ste 470 Providence, RI 02905; **Office Phone:** (401) 553-8348; **Board Certifications:** Surgery 1987, Surgical Critical Care 1988; **Medical School:** Univ VT Coll Med 1981; **Residency:** Surgery, Med Ctr Hosp VT, Burlington, VT 1981-1986; **Faculty Appointment:** Assoc Prof Surgery, Brown Univ

Dudrick, Stanley MD (Surgery) - *Special Expertise:* Critical Care; Total Parenteral Nutrition; Laparoscopic Surgery; **Admitting Hospital:** Bridgeport Hospital; **Office Address:** Bridgeport Hosp, Dept Surg 267 Grant St Bridgeport, CT 06610; **Office Phone:** (203) 384-3273; **Board Certification:** Surgery 1968; **Medical School:** Univ Penn 1961; **Residency:** Surgery, Hosp Univ Penn, Philadelphia, PA 1962-1967; **Fellowship:** Research, Hosp Univ Penn, Philadelphia, PA 1962-1967; **Faculty Appointment:** Prof Surgery, Yale Univ

Hebert, James C MD (Surgery) - *Special Expertise:* Biliary Surgery; **Admitting Hospital:** Fletcher Allen Health Care Medical Center - Campus; **Office Address:** Fletcher Allen Hlth Care 100 Colchester Ave, Fletcher 301 Burlington, VT 05401; **Office Phone:** (802) 656-5354; **Board Certification:** Surgery 1994; **Medical School:** Univ VT Coll Med 1977; **Residency:** Surgery, Med Ctr Hosp, Burlington, VT 1978-1982; **Faculty Appointment:** Prof Surgery, Univ VT Coll Med

Jenkins, Roger L MD (Surgery) - *Special Expertise:* Transplant-Liver; **Admitting Hospital:** Lahey Clinic; **Office Address:** Lahey Clinic 41 Mall Rd, Ste 4West Burlington, MA 01805; **Office Phone:** (781) 744-2500; **Board Certification:** Surgery 1993; **Medical School:** Univ VT Coll Med 1977; **Residency:** Surgery, New Eng Deaconess Hosp, Boston, MA 1977-1982; **Fellowship:** Transplant Surgery, Univ Pittsburgh Hosp, Pittsburgh, PA 1983; **Faculty Appointment:** Assoc Prof Surgery, Harvard Med Sch

Lipkowitz, George S. MD (Surgery) - *Special Expertise:* Transplant-Kidney; **Admitting Hospital:** Baystate Medical Center; **Office Address:** 208 Ashley Ave West Springfield, MA 01089; **Office Phone:** (413) 750-3440; **Board Certification:** Surgery 1986; **Medical School:** SUNY Downstate 1980; **Residency:** Surgery, SUNY Kings Co Hosp, Brooklyn, NY 1981-1985; **Fellowship:** Transplant Surgery, SUNY Hlth Scis Ctr, Brooklyn, NY 1985-1986; **Faculty Appointment:** Assoc Prof Surgery, Tufts Univ

Monaco, Anthony MD (Surgery) - *Special Expertise:* Transplant-Kidney; Transplant-Pancreas; **Admitting Hospital:** Beth Israel Deaconess Medical Center - Boston (Page 57); **Office Address:** Beth Israel Deaconess Med Ctr-The Transplant Center 1 Deaconess Rd Boston, MA 02214; **Office Phone:** (617) 632-8549; **Board Certifications:** Surgery 1963, Thoracic Surgery 1965; **Medical School:** Harvard Med Sch 1956; **Residency:** Surgery, Mass Genl Hosp, Boston, MA 1957-1963; **Fellowship:** Immunopathology, Harvard 1960; **Faculty Appointment:** Prof Surgery, Harvard Med Sch

Osteen, Robert T MD (Surgery) - *Special Expertise:* Breast Cancer; **Admitting Hospital:** Brigham & Women's Hospital; **Office Address:** Brigham & Women's Hosp- Dept Surgical Oncology 75 Francis St, Ste General Surgical Specialists Boston, MA 02115-6110; **Office Phone:** (617) 732-6718; **Board Certification:** Surgery 1995; **Medical School:** Duke Univ 1966; **Residencies:** Surgery, Duke University Med Ctr, Durham 1967-1968; Surgery, PB Brigham, Boston, MA 1970-1975; **Faculty Appointment:** Assoc Prof Surgery, Harvard Med Sch

Salem, Ronald MD (Surgery) - *Special Expertise:* Cancer Surgery; Transplant-Liver; **Admitting Hospital:** Yale - New Haven Hospital; **Office Address:** Yale Sch Med, Dept Surg 333 Cedar St, Box 3333 New Haven, CT 06510; **Office Phone:** (203) 785-3577; **Board Certification:** Surgery 1991; **Medical School:** Zimbabwe 1978; **Residencies:** Surgery, Hammersmith Hosp, London, England 1981-1985; Surgery, New Eng-Deaconess Hosp, Boston, MA 1987-1989; **Faculty Appointment:** Asst Prof Surgery, Yale Univ

Singer, Samuel MD (Surgery) - *Special Expertise:* Soft Tissue Sarcoma; Melanoma; **Admitting Hospital:** Brigham & Women's Hospital; **Office Address:** Brigham & Women's Hosp, Div Surg Onc 75 Francis St NE, Bldg Amb2 - Ste 3RD Boston, MA 02115-6195; **Office Phone:** (617) 732-6980; **Board Certification:** Surgery 1998; **Medical School:** Harvard Med Sch 1982; **Residency:** Surgery, Brigham & Women's Hosp, Boston, MA 1983-1988; **Fellowship:** Surgical Oncology, Dana Farber Cancer Inst, Boston, MA 1988-1990; **Faculty Appointment:** Asst Prof Surgery, Harvard Med Sch

Smego, Douglas MD (Surgery) - *Special Expertise:* Tumor Surgery; **Admitting Hospital:** Stamford Hospital (Page 72); **Office Address:** 1250 Summer St, Ste 303 Stamford, CT 06905-5300; **Office Phone:** (203) 327-6755; **Board Certification:** Surgery 1993; **Medical School:** UMDNJ-NJ Med Sch, Newark 1977; **Residency:** Surgery, NY Hosp-Cornell Med Ctr, New York, NY 1978-1982; **Fellowship:** U Louisville, Louisville, KY 1982-1983; **Faculty Appointment:** Surgery

Smith, Barbara Lynn MD (Surgery) - *Special Expertise:* Breast Cancer; **Admitting Hospital:** Massachusetts General Hospital; **Office Address:** Mass General Hosp-Gillette Center 100 Blossom St, Cox 120 Boston, MA 02114; **Office Phone:** (617) 724-4800; **Board Certification:** Surgery 1990; **Medical School:** Harvard Med Sch 1983; **Residency:** Surgery, Brigham & Women's Hosp, Boston, MA 1983-1989; **Faculty Appointment:** Asst Prof Surgery, Harvard Med Sch

Tilney, Nicholas MD (Surgery) - *Special Expertise:* Transplant-Kidney; **Admitting Hospital:** Brigham & Women's Hospital; **Office Address:** Brigham & Women's Hosp, Dept Transplant Surg 75 Francis St Boston, MA 02115; **Office Phone:** (617) 732-6817; **Board Certification:** Surgery 1972; **Medical School:** Cornell Univ-Weil Med Coll 1962; **Residency:** Surgery, Peter Bent Brigham Hosp, Boston, MA 1969-1971; **Fellowships:** Cellular Immunology, Sir William Dunn Sch Path, Oxford, England 1971-1972; Cellular Immunology, Western Infirm Univ, Glasgow, Scotland 1972-1973; **Faculty Appointment:** Prof Surgery, Harvard Med Sch

Ward, Barbara MD (Surgery) - *Special Expertise:* Breast Cancer; Tumor Surgery; **Admitting Hospital:** Greenwich Hospital; **Office Address:** 4 Deerfield Pl Greeenwich, CT 06831; **Office Phone:** (203) 869-0338; **Board Certification:** Surgery 1991; **Medical School:** Temple Univ 1983; **Residencies:** Surgery, Yale-New Haven Hosp, New Haven, CT 1984-1985; Surgery, Yale-New Haven Hosp, New Haven, CT 1987-1990; **Fellowship:** Surgical Oncology, Natl Cancer Inst, Bethesda, MD 1985-1987; **Faculty Appointment:** Assoc Prof Surgery, Yale Univ

Warshaw, Andrew L MD (Surgery) - *Special Expertise:* Pancreatic Cancer; Pancreatic Surgery; **Admitting Hospital:** Massachusetts General Hospital; **Office Address:** Mass Genl Hosp 55 Fruit St, Bldg WHT 506 Boston, MA 02114-3117; **Office Phone:** (617) 726-8254; **Board Certifications:** Surgery 1971, Surgical Critical Care 1986; **Medical School:** Harvard Med Sch 1963; **Residencies:** Surgery, Mass Genl Hosp, Boston, MA 1967-1971; Surgery, Mass Genl Hosp, Boston, MA 1964-1965; **Faculty Appointment:** Prof Surgery, Harvard Med Sch

Zinner, Michael MD (Surgery) - *Special Expertise:* Gastrointestinal Surgery; **Admitting Hospital:** Brigham & Women's Hospital; **Office Address:** Brigham & Women's Hosp, Dept Surg 75 Francis St Boston, MA 02115; **Office Phone:** (617) 732-8181; **Board Certification:** Surgery 1988; **Medical School:** Univ Fla Coll Med 1971; **Residencies:** Surgery, Johns Hopkins Hosp, Baltimore, MD 1973-1974; Surgery, Johns Hoskins Hosp, Baltimore, MD 1976-1979; **Faculty Appointment:** Prof Surgery, Harvard Med Sch

Mid Atlantic

Alfonso, Antonio MD (Surgery) - *Special Expertise:* Breast Cancer; Head & Neck Surgery; **Admitting Hospital:** Long Island College Hospital (Page 58); **Office Address:** 100 Amity St, FL 1 Brooklyn, NY 11201; **Office Phone:** (718) 875-3244; **Board Certification:** Surgery 1973; **Medical School:** Philippines 1968; **Residency:** Surgery, Temple U Hosp, Philadelphia, PA 1968-1972; **Fellowship:** Surgical Oncology, Meml Sloan Kettering Cancer Ctr, New York, NY 1972-1974; **Faculty Appointment:** Prof Surgery, SUNY Hlth Sci Ctr

Ashikari, Roy MD (Surgery) - *Special Expertise:* Breast Cancer; **Admitting Hospital:** St Agnes Hospital; **Office Address:** St Agnes Hosp 305 North St White Plains, NY 10605; **Office Phone:** (914) 681-9478; **Board Certification:** Surgery 1967; **Medical School:** Japan 1958; **Residencies:** Surgery, Mount Sinai Hosp, New York, NY 1961-1964; Surgery, Mem Sloan-Kettering Cancer Ctr, New York, NY 1966-1968; **Fellowship:** Surgery, Mount Sinai Hosp, New York, NY 1964-1965; **Faculty Appointment:** Prof Surgery, NY Med Coll

Axelrod, Deborah MD (Surgery) - *Special Expertise:* Breast Cancer; **Admitting Hospital:** St Vincents Catholic Medical Center of New York; **Office Address:** St Vincent's Hosp & Med Ctr, Breast Clinic 325 W 15th St New York, NY 10011; **Office Phone:** (212) 604-6004; **Board Certification:** Surgery 1989; **Medical School:** Israel 1982; **Residency:** Surgery, Beth Israel Med Ctr, New York, NY 1983-1988; **Fellowship:** Surgical Oncology, Meml Sloan Kettering Cancer Ctr, New York, NY 1985-1986; **Faculty Appointment:** Asst Prof Surgery, Albert Einstein Coll Med

Bartlett, Stephen Thomas MD (Surgery) - *Special Expertise:* Transplant-Pancreas; Transplant-Kidney; **Admitting Hospital:** University of Maryland Medical System; **Office Address:** 29 S Greene St, Ste 200 Baltimore, MD 21201; **Office Phone:** (410) 328-5408; **Board Certifications:** Surgery 1995, Vascular Surgery (General) 1996; **Medical School:** Univ Chicago-Pritzker Sch Med 1979; **Residency:** Surgery, Hosp Univ Penn, Philadelphia, PA 1980-1985; **Fellowship:** Vascular Surgery (General), Northwestern Univ, Chicago, IL 1985-1986; **Faculty Appointment:** Prof Surgery, Univ MD Sch Med

SURGERY

Bass, Barbara MD (Surgery) - *Special Expertise:* Surgery - General; **Admitting Hospital:** University of Maryland Medical System; **Office Address:** Univ MD Med Sys, Dept Genl Surg 22 S Greene St, rm S4B04 Baltimore, MD 21201; **Office Phone:** (410) 328-8346; **Board Certification:** Surgery 1996; **Medical School:** Univ VA Sch Med 1979; **Residencies:** Surgery, Geo Wash Univ, Washington, DC 1979-1982; Surgery, Geo Wash Univ, Washington, DC 1984-1986; **Fellowship:** Surgery, Walter Reed Inst, Washington, DC 1982-1984; **Faculty Appointment:** Prof Surgery, Univ MD Sch Med

Borgen, Patrick Ivan MD (Surgery) - *Special Expertise:* Breast Cancer; **Admitting Hospital:** Memorial Sloan Kettering Cancer Center; **Office Address:** 205 E 64th St New York, NY 10021; **Office Phone:** (212) 639-5248; **Board Certification:** Surgery 1991; **Medical School:** Louisiana State Univ 1984; **Residency:** Surgery, Ochsner Fdn Hosp, New Orleans, LA 1985-1989; **Fellowship:** Surgical Oncology, Meml Sloan Kettering Canc Ctr, New York, NY 1989-1990; **Faculty Appointment:** Prof Surgery, Cornell Univ-Weil Med Coll

Brennan, Murray MD (Surgery) - *Special Expertise:* Sarcoma; Tumor Surgery; **Admitting Hospital:** Memorial Sloan Kettering Cancer Center; **Office Address:** Meml Sloan-Kettering Cancer Ctr, rm C1265 1275 York Ave New York, NY 10021-6007; **Office Phone:** (212) 639-6586; **Board Certification:** Surgery 1975; **Medical School:** New Zealand 1964; **Residency:** Surgery, Univ Otago, Dunedin, New Zealand 1966-1969; **Fellowships:** Surgery, Harvard Med Sch, Boston, MA 1970-1972; Surgery, Peter Bent Brigham Hosp, Cambridge, MA 1973-1975; **Faculty Appointment:** Prof Surgery, Cornell Univ-Weil Med Coll

Burdick, James Frederick MD (Surgery) - *Special Expertise:* Transplant-Kidney; Vascular Surgery; **Admitting Hospital:** Johns Hopkins Hospital - Baltimore (Page 65); **Office Address:** 338 Dumbarton Rd Baltimore, MD 21212-1532; **Office Phone:** (410) 955-6875; **Board Certification:** Surgery 1997; **Medical School:** Harvard Med Sch 1968; **Residencies:** Surgery, Mass Genl Hosp, Boston, MA 1969-1970; Surgery, Mass Genl Hosp, Boston, MA 1973-1975; **Fellowship:** Research, Mass Genl Hosp, Boston, MA 1976-1977; **Faculty Appointment:** Prof Surgery, Johns Hopkins Univ

Cameron, John MD (Surgery) - *Special Expertise:* Pancreatic Cancer; **Admitting Hospital:** Johns Hopkins Hospital - Baltimore (Page 65); **Office Address:** Johns Hopkins Hosp, Dept Surg 720 Rutland Ave, Ross Bldg-rm 759 Baltimore, MD 21205; **Office Phone:** (410) 955-5166; **Board Certifications:** Surgery 1970, Thoracic Surgery 1971; **Medical School:** Johns Hopkins Univ 1962; **Residency:** Surgery, Johns Hopkins Hosp, Baltimore, MD 1965-1970; **Fellowship:** Thoracic Surgery, Johns Hopkins Hosp, Baltimore, MD 1970-1971; **Faculty Appointment:** Prof Surgery, Johns Hopkins Univ

Coit, Daniel G MD (Surgery) - *Special Expertise:* Melanoma; Pancreatic & Stomach Cancer; **Admitting Hospital:** Memorial Sloan Kettering Cancer Center; **Office Address:** Memorial Sloan-Kettering Cancer Ctr 1275 York Ave New York, NY 10021; **Office Phone:** (212) 639-8411; **Board Certification:** Surgery 1994; **Medical School:** Univ Cincinnati 1976; **Residencies:** Internal Medicine, New England Deaconess Hosp, Boston, MA 1977-1978; Surgery, New England Deaconess Hosp, Boston, MA 1978-1983; **Fellowship:** Surgery, NY Meml Hosp, New York, NY 1983-1985; **Faculty Appointment:** Assoc Prof Surgery, Cornell Univ-Weil Med Coll

Conti, David James MD (Surgery) - *Special Expertise:* Transplant-Kidney; **Admitting Hospital:** Albany Medical Center; **Office Address:** Albany Med Ctr 47 New Scotland Ave, MS AG1-GE61 Albany, NY 12208; **Office Phone:** (518) 262-5614; **Board Certification:** Surgery 1998; **Medical School:** Northwestern Univ 1981; **Residency:** Surgery, McGaw Med Ctr, Chicago, IL 1982-1987; **Fellowship:** Surgery, Mass Genl Hosp, Boston, MA 1987-1989; **Faculty Appointment:** Prof Surgery, Albany Med Coll

Deitch, Edwin MD (Surgery) - *Special Expertise: Trauma;* **Admitting Hospital:** UMDNJ-University Hospital-Newark; **Office Address:** UMDNJ-NJ Med Sch 185 S Orange Ave, Bldg MSB - Fl G - rm 506 Newark, NJ 07103; **Office Phone:** (973) 972-5045; **Board Certifications:** Surgery 1997, Surgical Critical Care 1995; **Medical School:** Univ MD Sch Med 1973; **Residencies:** Surgery, US Public Hlth Svc Hosp, Baltimore, MD 1974-1976; Surgery, US Public Hlth Svc Hosp, New Orleans, LA 1976-1978; **Faculty Appointment:** Prof Surgery, UMDNJ-NJ Med Sch, Newark

Dooley, William Chesnut MD (Surgery) - *Special Expertise: Breast Cancer; Metastatic Disease Mgmt; Tumors-Rare & Multiple;* **Admitting Hospital:** Johns Hopkins Hospital - Baltimore (Page 65); **Office Address:** 600 N Wolfe St Carnegie Rm 681 Baltimore, MD 21287-6681; **Office Phone:** (410) 955-2615; **Board Certification:** Surgery 1997; **Medical School:** Vanderbilt Univ 1982; **Residencies:** Surgery, Oxford Univ, Oxford, England 1986; Surgery, Johns Hopkins, Baltimore, MD 1982-1987; **Fellowship:** Medical Oncology, Johns Hopkins, Baltimore, MD 1987-1988; **Faculty Appointment:** Assoc Prof Surgery, Johns Hopkins Univ

Edge, Stephen B MD (Surgery) - *Special Expertise: Breast Cancer;* **Admitting Hospital:** Roswell Park Cancer Institute; **Office Address:** Rosewell Park Cancer Inst Elm & Carlton Streets Buffalo, NY 14263; **Office Phone:** (716) 845-5789; **Board Certification:** Surgery 1987; **Medical School:** Case West Res Univ 1979; **Residency:** Surgery, Univ Hosp Cleveland, Cleveland, OH 1979-1986; **Fellowship:** Surgical Oncology, Natl Cancer Inst, Bethesda, MD 1981-1984; **Faculty Appointment:** Assoc Prof Surgery, SUNY Buffalo

Emond, Jean Crawford MD (Surgery) - *Special Expertise: Transplant-Liver;* **Admitting Hospital:** Columbia Presbyterian Medical Center (Page 72); **Office Address:** 622 W 168th St, Ste PH14 Center for Liver Disease and Transplantation New York, NY 10032; **Office Phone:** (212) 305-0914; **Board Certification:** Surgery 1985; **Medical School:** Univ Chicago-Pritzker Sch Med 1979; **Residency:** Surgery, Univ Ill/Cook Cty Hosp, Chicago, IL 1980-1984; **Fellowships:** Surgery, Paris, France 1984-1985; Transplant Surgery, Univ Chicago Hosp, Chicago, IL 1985-1987; **Faculty Appointment:** Prof Surgery, Columbia P&S

Enker, Warren MD (Surgery) - *Special Expertise: Surgical Oncology;* **Admitting Hospital:** Beth Israel Medical Center - New York; **Office Address:** 350 E 17th St, Ste 1622 New York, NY 10003; **Office Phone:** (212) 420-3960; **Board Certification:** Surgery 1973; **Medical School:** SUNY Hlth Sci Ctr 1967; **Residency:** Surgery, Univ Chicago Hosps-Clinics, Chicago, IL 1968-1972; **Fellowships:** Immunopathology, Univ Chicago Hosps-Clinics, Chicago, IL 1972-1973; Immunopathology, Univ Minnesota, Minneapolis, MN 1973-1974; **Faculty Appointment:** Prof Medicine, Albert Einstein Coll Med

Estabrook, Alison MD (Surgery) - *Special Expertise: Breast Cancer;* **Admitting Hospital:** St Luke's - Roosevelt Hospital Center - Roosevelt Division (Page 58); **Office Address:** 425 W 59th St, Ste 7A New York, NY 10019; **Office Phone:** (212) 523-7500; **Board Certification:** Surgery 1985; **Medical School:** NYU Sch Med 1978; **Residency:** Surgery, Columbia Presby, New York, NY 1979-1984; **Fellowship:** Surgical Oncology, Columbia Presby, New York, NY 1981-1982; **Faculty Appointment:** Prof Surgery, Columbia P&S

Ferzli, George MD (Surgery) - *Special Expertise: Laparoscopic Surgery;* **Admitting Hospital:** Staten Island University Hospital - North; **Office Address:** 78 Cromwell Ave Staten Island, NY 10304-3945; **Office Phone:** (718) 667-8100; **Board Certifications:** Surgery 1993, Surgical Critical Care 1994; **Medical School:** Lebanon 1979; **Residency:** Surgery, Staten Is Univ Hosp, Staten Island, NY 1980-1985; **Faculty Appointment:** Assoc Clin Prof Surgery, SUNY Downstate

Fung, John J MD/PhD (Surgery) - *Special Expertise:* Transplant-Liver; Transplant-Kidney; **Admitting Hospital:** UPMC - Presbyterian University Hospital; **Office Address:** Falk Med Bldg 3601 Fifth Ave, Ste 4th Pittsburgh, PA 15213; **Office Phone:** (412) 648-3200; **Board Certification:** Surgery 1997; **Medical School:** Univ Chicago-Pritzker Sch Med 1982; **Residency:** Surgery, Strong Memorial Hosp, Rochester, NY 1983-1988; **Fellowship:** Transplant Surgery, Univ Pittsburgh, Pittsburgh, PA 1984-1986; **Faculty Appointment:** Assoc Prof Surgery, Univ Pittsburgh

Gagner, Michel MD (Surgery) - *Special Expertise:* Laparoscopic Surgery; Liver & Biliary Surgery; **Admitting Hospital:** Mount Sinai Hospital (Page 70); **Office Address:** 19 E 98th St, Ste 5A, Box 1103 New York, NY 10029; **Office Phone:** (212) 241-5339; **Board Certification:** Surgery 1990; **Medical School:** Canada 1982; **Residency:** Surgery, Royal Victoria Hosp/McGill, Montreal, Canada 1982-1988; **Fellowships:** Hepatobiliary Surgery, Hosp Paul-Brousse, Paris, France 1988-1989; Hepatobiliary Surgery, Lahey Clinic, Burlington, MA 1989-1990; **Faculty Appointment:** Assoc Prof Surgery, Mount Sinai Sch Med

Hardy, Mark MD (Surgery) - *Special Expertise:* Transplant-Kidney; Parathyroid Disease; **Admitting Hospital:** Columbia Presbyterian Medical Center (Page 72); **Office Address:** 161 Fort Washington Ave New York, NY 10032-3713; **Office Phone:** (212) 305-5502; **Board Certification:** Surgery 1972; **Medical School:** Albert Einstein Coll Med 1962; **Residencies:** Surgery, Strong Meml Hosp, Rochester, NY 1963-1964; Surgery, Albert Einstein Med Ctr, Bronx, NY 1966-1971; **Fellowship:** Transplant Surgery, Harvard Med Sch, Cambridge, MA 1968-1969; **Faculty Appointment:** Prof Surgery, Columbia P&S

Kinne, David W MD (Surgery) - *Special Expertise:* Breast Cancer; **Admitting Hospital:** Columbia Presbyterian Medical Center (Page 72); **Office Address:** 16 E 60th St, Ste 460 New York, NY 10022-1002; **Office Phone:** (212) 326-8550; **Board Certification:** Surgery 1971; **Medical School:** SUNY Hlth Sci Ctr 1964; **Residency:** Surgery, Columbia-Presby Med Ctr, New York, NY 1964-1970; **Fellowship:** Transplant Surgery, Univ MN Med Ctr, Minneapolis, MN 1970-1971; **Faculty Appointment:** Prof Surgery

Klein, Andrew S MD (Surgery) - *Special Expertise:* Surgery - General; **Admitting Hospital:** Johns Hopkins Hospital - Baltimore (Page 65); **Office Address:** Johns Hopkins Hosp 600 N Wolfe St, Harvey 611 Baltimore, MD 21287-8611; **Office Phone:** (410) 955-5662; **Board Certification:** Surgery 1996; **Medical School:** Jefferson Med Coll 1979; **Residencies:** Surgery, John Hopkins Hosp, Baltimore, MD 1980-1982; Surgery, John Hopkins Hosp, Baltimore, MD 1984-1986; **Fellowship:** Transplant Surgery, UCLA-CHS, Los Angeles, CA 1987-1988; **Faculty Appointment:** Assoc Prof Surgery, Johns Hopkins Univ

Leffall Jr, LaSalle D MD (Surgery) - *Special Expertise:* Breast Cancer; Head & Neck Surgery; **Admitting Hospital:** Howard University Hospital; **Office Address:** 2041 Georgia Ave NW Washington, DC 20060; **Office Phone:** (202) 865-6237; **Board Certification:** Surgery 1958; **Medical School:** Howard Univ 1952; **Residencies:** Surgery, Freedmens Hosp, Washington, DC 1953-1956; Surgery, DC Genl Hosp, Washington, DC 1954-1955; **Fellowship:** Surgery, New York Meml Ctr, New York, NY 1957-1959; **Faculty Appointment:** Prof Emeritus Surgery, Howard Univ

Lillemoe, Keith Douglas MD (Surgery) - *Special Expertise:* Surgery - General; **Admitting Hospital:** Johns Hopkins Hospital - Baltimore (Page 65); **Office Address:** Johns Hopkins Hosp Surg 600 N Wolfe St Baltimore, MD 21287-7495; **Office Phone:** (410) 955-7495; **Board Certification:** Surgery 1986; **Medical School:** Johns Hopkins Univ 1978; **Residency:** Surgery, Johns Hopkins Hosp, Baltimore, MD 1979-1985; **Faculty Appointment:** Prof Johns Hopkins Univ

Miller, Charles MD (Surgery) - *Special Expertise:* Transplant-Liver; Liver & Biliary Surgery; **Admitting Hospital:** Mount Sinai Hospital (Page 70); **Office Address:** Racanati/Miller Transplantation Inst 19 E 98 St, Fl 6 - rm 6F, Box 1104 New York, NY 10029; **Office Phone:** (212) 241-8035; **Board Certification:** Surgery 1994; **Medical School:** Mount Sinai Sch Med 1978; **Residencies:** Surgery, Mount Sinai Hosp, New York, NY 1978-1983; , , NY; **Fellowships:** Transplant Surgery, Mount Sinai Hosp, New York, NY 1980-1981; Vascular Surgery (General), Mount Sinai Hosp, New York, NY 1983-1984; **Faculty Appointment:** Prof Surgery, Mount Sinai Sch Med

Numann, Patricia MD (Surgery) - *Special Expertise:* Breast Cancer; Thyroid Surgery; **Admitting Hospital:** University Hospital - SUNY Upstate Medical University; **Office Address:** SUNY Hlth Sci Ctr, Dept Surg 750 E Adams Street Syracuse, NY 13210; **Office Phone:** (315) 464-4603; **Board Certification:** Surgery 1994; **Medical School:** SUNY Syracuse 1965; **Residency:** Surgery, SUNY Upstate Med Ctr, Albany, NY 1966-1970; **Faculty Appointment:** Prof Surgery, SUNY Syracuse

Pachter, H Leon MD (Surgery) - *Special Expertise:* Breast Cancer; **Admitting Hospital:** NYU Medical Center (Page 70); **Office Address:** 530 1st Ave, Ste 6C New York, NY 10016; **Office Phone:** (212) 263-7302; **Board Certification:** Surgery 1977; **Medical School:** NYU Sch Med 1971; **Residency:** Surgery, NYU Med Ctr, New York, NY 1972-1976; **Faculty Appointment:** Prof Surgery, NYU Sch Med

Peitzman, Andrew MD (Surgery) - *Special Expertise:* Trauma; **Admitting Hospital:** UPMC - Presbyterian University Hospital; **Office Address:** UPP-Trauma Surgery 3601 Fifth Ave, Bldg Falk - Ste 6B Pittsburgh, PA 15213; **Office Phone:** (412) 648-9863; **Board Certifications:** Surgery 1994, Surgical Critical Care 1997; **Medical School:** Univ Pittsburgh 1976; **Residencies:** Surgery, Univ Pittsburgh, Pittsburgh, PA 1977-1979; Surgery, Univ Pittsburgh, Pittsburgh, PA 1981-1984; **Fellowship:** Surgery, NY Hosp-Cornell Univ, New York, NY 1979-1981; **Faculty Appointment:** Prof Surgery, Univ Pittsburgh

Petrek, Jeanne MD (Surgery) - *Special Expertise:* Breast Cancer; **Admitting Hospital:** Memorial Sloan Kettering Cancer Center; **Office Address:** 205 E 64th St New York, NY 10021-6635; **Office Phone:** (212) 639-5246; **Board Certification:** Surgery 1978; **Medical School:** Case West Res Univ 1973; **Residency:** Surgery, Bringham and Woman's Hosp, Boston, MA 1974-1978; **Fellowship:** Surgery, Meml Sloan-Kettering, New York, NY 1978-1980

Pressman, Peter MD (Surgery) - *Special Expertise:* Surgery - General; **Admitting Hospital:** Beth Israel Medical Center - Herbert & Nell Singer Division (Page 58); **Office Address:** 425 E 61st St, Fl 8th New York, NY 10021-3513; **Office Phone:** (212) 249-8040; **Board Certification:** Surgery 1967; **Medical School:** Columbia P&S 1959; **Residencies:** Surgery, Columbia-Presby, New York, NY 1959-1961; Columbia-Presby, New York, NY 1961-1963; **Faculty Appointment:** Clin Prof Surgery, Albert Einstein Coll Med

Rosenberg, Steven MD (Surgery) - *Special Expertise:* Tumor Surgery; Melanoma; Kidney Cancer; **Admitting Hospital:** National Institutes of Health - Clinical Center; **Office Address:** 9000 Rockville Pike Bethesda, MD 22089; **Office Phone:** (301) 496-4164; **Board Certification:** Surgery 1975; **Medical School:** Jefferson Med Coll 1964; **Residency:** Surgery, Peter Bent Brigham Hosp, Boston, MA 1968-1974

Roses, Daniel F MD (Surgery) - *Special Expertise:* Melanoma; Breast Cancer; Thyroid & Parathyroid Surgery; **Admitting Hospital:** NYU Medical Center (Page 70); **Office Address:** M N Harris, D F Roses, MD's, - NYU Med Ctr 530 1st Ave, Ste 6E New York, NY 10016-6402; **Office Phone:** (212) 263-7330; **Board Certification:** Surgery 1975; **Medical School:** NYU Sch Med 1969; **Residency:** Surgery, NYU - Bellevue, New York, NY 1969-1974; **Fellowship:** Surgical Oncology, NYU - Bellevue, New York, NY 1976-1978; **Faculty Appointment:** Prof Surgery, NYU Sch Med

Salky, Barry A MD (Surgery) - *Special Expertise:* Laparoscopic Surgery; Laparoscopic Cholecystectomy; **Admitting Hospital:** Mount Sinai Hospital (Page 70); **Office Address:** 1010 5th Ave New York, NY 10028; **Office Phone:** (212) 987-0410; **Board Certification:** Surgery 1979; **Medical School:** Univ Tenn Coll Med, Memphis 1970; **Residencies:** Surgery, Mt Sinai Hosp, New York, NY 1972-1973; Surgery, Mt Sinai Hosp, New York, NY 1975-1978; **Faculty Appointment:** Prof Surgery, Mount Sinai Sch Med

Schnabel, Freya MD (Surgery) - *Special Expertise:* Breast Cancer; **Admitting Hospital:** Columbia Presbyterian Medical Center (Page 72); **Office Address:** 161 Fort Washington Ave, Ste 1011 New York, NY 10032; **Office Phone:** (212) 305-1534; **Board Certification:** Surgery 1988; **Medical School:** NYU Sch Med 1982; **Residency:** Surgery, NYU Med Ctr, New York, NY 1982-1987; **Fellowship:** Surgery, Univ Hosp, Brooklyn, NY 1987-1988; **Faculty Appointment:** Assoc Clin Prof Surgery, Columbia P&S

Schwab, Richard MD (Surgery) - *Special Expertise:* Lung Surgery; Sleep Disorders/Apnea; **Admitting Hospital:** Hospital of the University of Pennsylvania; **Office Address:** Univ of Penn Med Ctr, Dept Pulmonary and CCM 3400 Spruce St, Bldg Ravdin 3 - Ste F Philadelphia, PA 19104; **Office Phone:** (215) 662-3202; **Board Certifications:** Critical Care Medicine 1991, Pulmonary Disease 1990; **Medical School:** Univ Penn 1983; **Residency:** Internal Medicine, Jefferson Univ Hosp, Philadelphia, PA 1984-1986; **Fellowship:** Pulmonary Critical Care Medicine, Jefferson Univ Hosp, Philadelphia, PA 1988-1991; **Faculty Appointment:** Asst Prof Medicine, Univ Penn

Shah, Jatin P MD (Surgery) - *Special Expertise:* Head & Neck Surgery; Thyroid Surgery; **Admitting Hospital:** Memorial Sloan Kettering Cancer Center; **Office Address:** 1275 York Ave, Ste c979 New York, NY 10021-6007; **Office Phone:** (212) 639-7604; **Board Certification:** Surgery 1975; **Medical School:** India 1964; **Residencies:** Vascular Surgery (General), SSG Hosp, Baroda, India 1964-1967; Vascular Surgery (General), NY Infirm, New York, NY 1972-1974; **Fellowship:** Surgical Oncology, Meml Sloan-Kettering, New York, NY 1968-1972; **Faculty Appointment:** Prof Surgery, Cornell Univ-Weil Med Coll

Shaha, Ashok MD (Surgery) - *Special Expertise:* Head & Neck Cancer; **Admitting Hospital:** Memorial Sloan Kettering Cancer Center; **Office Address:** Meml Sloan Kettering Cancer Ctr, Dept HNS 1275 York Ave New York, NY; **Office Phone:** (212) 639-7649; **Board Certification:** Surgery 1992; **Medical School:** India 1970; **Residency:** Surgery, Downstate Med Ctr, Brooklyn, NY 1977-1981; **Fellowships:** Head and Neck Surgery, Meml Sloan Kettering Cancer Ctr, New York, NY 1981-1982; Surgical Oncology, Meml Sloan Kettering Cancer Ctr, New York, NY 1975-1976; **Faculty Appointment:** Prof Surgery, Cornell Univ-Weil Med Coll

Shapiro, Ron MD (Surgery) - *Special Expertise:* Transplant-Kidney; Transplant-Pancreas; **Admitting Hospital:** UPMC - Presbyterian University Hospital; **Office Address:** 3601 5th Ave, Fl 4 Pittsburgh, PA 15213; **Office Phone:** (412) 648-3921; **Board Certification:** Surgery; **Medical School:** Stanford Univ 1980; **Residency:** Surgery, Mt Sinai Hosp, New York, NY 1980-1986; **Faculty Appointment:** Assoc Prof Surgery, Univ Pittsburgh

Sugarbaker, Paul H MD (Surgery) - *Special Expertise:* Colon Cancer; **Admitting Hospital:** Washington Hospital Center - DC (Page 79); **Office Address:** Washington Cancer Inst 110 Irving St NW, rm CG 175 Washington, DC 20010; **Office Phone:** (202) 877-3908; **Board Certification:** Surgery 1973; **Medical School:** Cornell Univ-Weil Med Coll 1967; **Residency:** Surgery, Peter Bent Brigham Hosp, Boston, MA 1968-1973; **Fellowship:** Surgery, Mass Genl Hosp, Boston, MA 1973-1976

Teperman, Lewis William MD (Surgery) - *Special Expertise:* Transplant-Liver; Transplant-Kidney; **Admitting Hospital:** NYU Medical Center (Page 70); **Office Address:** NYU Med Ctr 403 E 34th St, Fl 3 New York, NY 10016; **Office Phone:** (212) 263-8134; **Board Certification:** Surgery 1997; **Medical School:** Mount Sinai Sch Med 1981; **Residencies:** Surgery, Columbia Presby Med Ctr, New York, NY 1981-1984; Surgery, LI Jewish Med Ctr, New Hyde Park, NY 1984-1986; **Fellowship:** Transplant Surgery, Univ Pittsburgh, Pittsburgh, PA 1986-1988; **Faculty Appointment:** Asst Prof Surgery, Univ Pittsburgh

Yurt, Roger MD (Surgery) - *Special Expertise:* Burns; Wound Healing/Care; **Admitting Hospital:** New York Weill Cornell Medical Center - NY Presbyterian Hospital (Page 72); **Office Address:** NY Hosp - Cornell Med Ctr 525 E 68th St, rm L706 New York, NY 10021; **Office Phone:** (212) 746-5410; **Board Certification:** Surgery 1980; **Medical School:** Univ Miami Sch Med 1972; **Residencies:** Surgery, Parkland Meml Hosp, Dallas, TX 1972-1974; Surgery, NY Hosp-Cornell Med Ctr, New York, NY 1978-1980; **Fellowship:** Internal Medicine, Brigham Hosp-Harvard, Cambridge, MA 1974-1978; **Faculty Appointment:** Prof Surgery, Cornell Univ-Weil Med Coll

Southeast

Albertson, David Allen MD (Surgery) - *Special Expertise:* Endocrinologic Surgery; **Admitting Hospital:** Wake Forest University Baptist Medical Center; **Office Address:** Wake Forest Univ Baptist Med Cntr Medical Center Blvd Winston Salem, NC 27157-1095; **Office Phone:** (336) 716-4442; **Board Certification:** Surgery 1998; **Medical School:** Univ VA Sch Med 1972; **Residency:** Surgery, NC Bapt Hosp, Winston Salem, NC 1973-1977; **Fellowship:** Endocrinology, Diabetes & Metabolism, Boston Univ, Boston, MA 1977-1978; **Faculty Appointment:** Assoc Prof Surgery, Wake Forest Univ Sch Med

Baker, Christopher MD (Surgery) - *Special Expertise:* Trauma; **Admitting Hospital:** University of North Carolina Hospitals; **Office Address:** Univ NC Bldg Burnett-Womack - rm 215, Box 7210 Chapel Hill, NC 27599; **Office Phone:** (919) 966-4389; **Board Certifications:** Surgery 1991, Surgical Critical Care 1996; **Medical School:** Harvard Med Sch 1970; **Residencies:** Surgery, UCSF, San Francisco, CA 1974-1975; Surgery, UCSF, San Francisco, CA 1975-1981; **Fellowship:** Surgery, Yale Univ, New Haven, CT 1982-1989; **Faculty Appointment:** Prof Surgery, Univ NC Sch Med

Balch, Charles MD (Surgery) - *Special Expertise:* Sentinel Node Surgery; Tumor Surgery; **Admitting Hospital:** Johns Hopkins Hospital - Baltimore (Page 65); **Office Address:** 1900 Duke St, Ste 200 Alexandria, VA 22314; **Office Phone:** (703) 299-1081; **Board Certification:** Surgery 1997; **Medical School:** Columbia P&S 1967; **Residencies:** Surgery, U Alabama Med Ctr, Birmingham, AL 1970-1971; Surgery, U Alabama Med Ctr, Birmingham, AL 1973-1975; **Fellowship:** Scripps Clin-Rsch Fdn, La Jolla, CA 1971-1973; **Faculty Appointment:** Prof Surgery, Johns Hopkins Univ

Beauchamp, Robert Daniel MD (Surgery) - *Special Expertise:* Breast Cancer; Colorectal Cancer; **Admitting Hospital:** Vanderbilt University Medical Center; **Office Address:** Vanderbilt Univ Med Ctr Med Ctr N, rm D-5230 Nashville, TN 37232-2729; **Office Phone:** (615) 322-2391; **Board Certifications:** Surgery 1997, Surgical Critical Care 1993; **Medical School:** Univ Tex Med Br, Galveston 1982; **Residency:** Surgery, Univ Tex Med Br, Galveston, TX 1982-1987; **Fellowship:** Cellular Molecular Biology, Vanderbilt Univ, Nashville, TN 1987-1989; **Faculty Appointment:** Prof Surgery, Vanderbilt Univ

Bland, Kirby MD (Surgery) - *Special Expertise:* Cancer Surgery; Breast Cancer; **Admitting Hospital:** University of Alabama Hospital at Birmingham; **Office Address:** Kirklin Clinic 2000 6th Ave South Birmingham, AL 35294; **Office Phone:** (205) 975-5000; **Board Certification:** Surgery 1991; **Medical School:** Univ Ala 1968; **Residencies:** Surgery, Univ Fla Hosp, Gainesville, FL 1969-1970; Surgery, Univ Fla Hosp, Gainesville, FL 1972-1976; **Fellowship:** Surgical Oncology, Univ Tex/Anderson Hosp, Houston, TX 1976-1977; **Faculty Appointment:** Prof Surgery, Univ Ala

Bollinger, R Randal MD/PhD (Surgery) - *Special Expertise:* Transplant-Kidney; Transplant-Pancreas; **Admitting Hospital:** Duke University Medical Center (Page 60); **Office Address:** Duke Univ Med Ctr Box 2910 Durham, NC 27710; **Office Phone:** (919) 684-5209; **Board Certification:** Surgery 1990; **Medical School:** Tulane Univ 1970; **Residencies:** Surgery, Duke Univ Med Ctr, Durham, NC 1970-1972; Surgery, Duke Univ Med Ctr, Durham, NC 1977-1980; **Fellowship:** Immunology, Duke Univ Med Ctr, Durham, NC 1974-1976; **Faculty Appointment:** Prof Surgery, Duke Univ

Britt, L D MD (Surgery) - *Special Expertise:* Surgery - General; **Admitting Hospital:** Sentara Norfolk General Hospital; **Office Address:** Eastern VA Med Sch, Dept Surg 825 Fairfax Ave, Ste 610 Norfolk, VA 23507; **Office Phone:** (757) 446-8950; **Board Certifications:** Surgery 1993, Surgical Critical Care 1997; **Medical School:** Harvard Med Sch 1977; **Residencies:** Surgery, Barnes Hosp-Wash Univ, St Louis, MO 1978-1979; Surgery, Univ IL, Chicago, IL 1981-1984; **Fellowship:** Trauma, Md Inst Emer Med Serv Sys, Baltimore, MD 1985-1986; **Faculty Appointment:** Prof Surgery, Eastern VA Med Sch

Cance, William George MD (Surgery) - *Special Expertise:* Tumor Surgery; **Admitting Hospital:** University of North Carolina Hospitals; **Office Address:** Univ NC - Chapel Hill, Dept of Surg 3010 Old Clinic Bldg, CB 7210 Chapel Hill, NC 27599; **Office Phone:** (919) 966-5221; **Board Certification:** Surgery 1998; **Medical School:** Duke Univ 1982; **Residency:** Surgery, Barnes Hosp-Wash Univ, St Louis, MO 1986-1988; **Fellowship:** Surgical Oncology, Meml Sloan Kettering Canc Ctr, New York, NY 1989-1990; **Faculty Appointment:** Assoc Prof Surgery, Univ NC Sch Med

Carey, Larry C MD (Surgery) - *Special Expertise:* Pancreatic Cancer; Bile Duct Cancer; **Admitting Hospital:** Tampa General Hospital; **Office Address:** Univ S FL Coll Med, Dept Surg 12901 Bruce B Downs Blvd, MDC Box 16 Tampa, FL 33606; **Office Phone:** (813) 259-0935; **Board Certifications:** Surgery 1965, Critical Care Medicine 1987; **Medical School:** Ohio State Univ 1959; **Residency:** Surgery, Milwaukee Co Genl Hosp, Milwaukee, WI 1960-1965; **Faculty Appointment:** Prof Surgery, Univ S Fla Coll Med

Copeland III, Edward M MD (Surgery) - *Special Expertise:* Breast Cancer; Colon Cancer; **Admitting Hospital:** Shands Healthcare at University Florida (Page 77); **Office Address:** Shands Hlthcare Univ FL 1600 Archer Rd SW, Box 100826 Gainesville, FL 32610; **Office Phone:** (352) 395-0622; **Board Certification:** Surgery 1971; **Medical School:** Cornell Univ-Weil Med Coll 1963; **Residencies:** Surgery, Univ Penn, Philadelphia, PA 1964-1969; Surgical Oncology, Univ TX MD Anderson Cancer Ctr, Houston, TX 1971-1972; **Fellowship:** Research, Univ Penn, Philadelphia, PA 1966-1967; **Faculty Appointment:** Prof Surgery, Univ Fla Coll Med

Cox, Charles E MD (Surgery) - *Special Expertise:* Surgery - General; **Admitting Hospital:** H Lee Moffitt Cancer Center & Research Institute; **Office Address:** Moffit Cancer Ctr 12902 Magnolia, Ste 3157 Tampa, FL 33612-9416; **Office Phone:** (813) 972-8410; **Board Certification:** Surgery 1994; **Medical School:** Univ Utah 1975; **Residency:** Surgery, Duke Univ Med Ctr, Durham, NC 1976-1983; **Faculty Appointment:** Prof Surgery, Univ S Fla Coll Med

Gadacz, Thomas R MD (Surgery) - *Special Expertise:* Laparoscopic Surgery; **Admitting Hospital:** Medical College of Georgia Hospital; **Office Address:** Med Coll GA, Dept Surg 1120 15th St Augusta, GA 30912-4000; **Office Phone:** (706) 721-4651; **Board Certification:** Surgery 1975; **Medical School:** St Louis Univ 1966; **Residencies:** Surgery, Univ Chicago Hosp, Chicago, IL 1967-1968; Surgery, Moffitt Hosp-UCSF, San Francisco, CA 1971-1974; **Fellowship:** Gastroenterology, Mayo Clinic, Rochester, MN 1974; **Faculty Appointment:** Prof Surgery, Med Coll GA

Hanks, John B MD (Surgery) - *Special Expertise:* Endocrinologic Surgery; Breast Surgery; Thyroid & Parathyroid Surgery; **Admitting Hospital:** University of Virginia Health Systems; **Office Address:** Univ Virginia Hlth Scis Ctr, Dept Surgery PO Box 800709 Charlottesville, VA 22908-0709; **Office Phone:** (804) 924-0376; **Board Certification:** Surgery 1991; **Medical School:** Univ Rochester 1973; **Residencies:** Surgery, Duke Univ Med Ctr, Durham, NC 1972-1975; Surgery, Duke Univ Med Ctr, Durham, NC 1977-1982; **Faculty Appointment:** Prof Surgery, Univ VA Sch Med

Howard, Richard J MD (Surgery) - *Special Expertise:* Transplant-Liver; Transplant-Kidney; Gastrointestinal Surgery; **Admitting Hospital:** Shands Healthcare at University Florida (Page 77); **Office Address:** Shands Healthcare at Univ FL 1600 SW Archer Rd, Ste 6142 Gainesville, FL 32610-0286; **Office Phone:** (352) 265-0606; **Board Certification:** Surgery 1976; **Medical School:** Yale Univ 1966; **Residency:** Surgery, Univ Minn Hosp, Minneapolis, MN 1969-1975; **Faculty Appointment:** Prof Surgery, Univ Fla Coll Med

Koruda, Mark Joseph MD (Surgery) - *Special Expertise:* Gastrointestinal Surgery; Laparoscopic Surgery; **Admitting Hospital:** University of North Carolina Hospitals; **Office Address:** Univ NC - Chapel Hill, Div Surg 405 Burnett Womack Bldg - CB 7210 Chapel Hill, NC 27599-0001; **Office Phone:** (919) 966-8436; **Board Certification:** Surgery 1999; **Medical School:** Yale Univ 1981; **Residency:** Surgery, Hosp Univ Penn, Philadelphia, PA 1981-1988; **Faculty Appointment:** Assoc Prof Surgery, Univ NC Sch Med

Luterman, Arnold MD (Surgery) - *Special Expertise:* Burns; **Admitting Hospital:** University of South Alabama Medical Center; **Office Address:** Univ S. Alabama Dept. of Surgery 2451 Fillingim St Mobile, AL 36617; **Office Phone:** (334) 471-7993; **Board Certifications:** Surgery 1996, Surgical Critical Care 1996; **Medical School:** McGill Univ 1970; **Residencies:** Surgery, Sinai Hospital, Baltimore, MD 1972; Surgery, Jewish Gen Hosp. McGill U, Montreal, Canada 1973-1976; **Fellowship:** Trauma, University Wash 1974-1976; **Faculty Appointment:** Prof Surgery, Univ Ala

Meyer, Anthony A MD (Surgery) - *Special Expertise:* Critical Care; **Admitting Hospital:** University of North Carolina Hospitals; **Office Address:** Univ NC - Chapel Hill, Sch Med, Dept Surg Burnett Womack Bldg, rm 164, Box 7210 Chapel Hill, NC 27599-7210; **Office Phone:** (919) 966-4321; **Board Certifications:** Surgery 1990, Surgical Critical Care 1994; **Medical School:** Univ Chicago-Pritzker Sch Med 1977; **Residency:** Surgery, UCSF Med Ctr, San Francisco, CA 1978-1982; **Faculty Appointment:** Prof Surgery, Univ NC Sch Med

Miller, Joshua MD (Surgery) - *Special Expertise:* Transplant-Kidney; Transplant-Pancreas; **Admitting Hospital:** University of Miami - Jackson Memorial Hospital; **Office Address:** 1801 NW 9th Ave, Ste 519 Miami, FL 33136; **Office Phone:** (305) 355-5100; **Board Certifications:** Thoracic Surgery 1971, Surgery 1970; **Medical School:** Albert Einstein Coll Med 1961; **Residencies:** Surgery, Yale-New Haven Hosp, New Haven, CT 1963-1966; Surgery, Yale-New Haven Hosp, New Haven, CT 1967-1968; **Fellowship:** Cardiothoracic Transplantation, Yale-US Public Hlth Svc, New Haven, CT 1964-1965; **Faculty Appointment:** Prof Surgery, Univ Miami Sch Med

Minervini, Donald MD (Surgery) - *Special Expertise:* Hernia; Laparoscopic Cholecystectomy; **Admitting Hospital:** Mount Sinai Medical Center; **Office Address:** 4302 Alton Rd, Ste 820 Miami Beach, FL 33140-2893; **Office Phone:** (305) 531-7409; **Board Certification:** Surgery 1970; **Medical School:** NY Med Coll 1964; **Residency:** Surgery, St Lukes Hosp, New York, NY 1965-1969

Pappas, Theodore N MD (Surgery) - *Special Expertise:* Laparoscopic Surgery; **Admitting Hospital:** Duke University Medical Center (Page 60); **Office Address:** Duke Univ Med Ctr Box 3479 Durham, NC 27710-0001; **Office Phone:** (919) 681-3442; **Board Certification:** Surgery 1989; **Medical School:** Ohio State Univ 1981; **Residency:** Surgery, Brigham & Womens Hosp, Boston, MA 1981-1988; **Fellowship:** Gastroenterology, Wadworth VA Med Ctr, Los Angeles, CA 1983-1985; **Faculty Appointment:** Prof Surgery, Duke Univ

Polk Jr, Hiram C MD (Surgery) - *Special Expertise:* Hiatal Hernia; Colon Cancer; **Admitting Hospital:** University of Louisville Hospital; **Office Address:** Univ Louisville, Dept Surgery Louisville, KY 40292; **Office Phone:** (502) 852-5442; **Board Certification:** Surgery 1966; **Medical School:** Harvard Med Sch 1960; **Residency:** Barnes Hosp, St. Louis, MO 1961-1965; **Faculty Appointment:** Prof Surgery, Univ Louisville Sch Med

Reintgen, Douglas Scott MD (Surgery) - *Special Expertise:* Melanoma-Sentinel Node; Breast Cancer-Sentinel Node; **Admitting Hospital:** H Lee Moffitt Cancer Center & Research Institute; **Office Address:** 12902 Magnolia Dr, Ste 3057A Tampa, FL 33612-9416; **Office Phone:** (813) 972-8482; **Board Certification:** Surgery 1997; **Medical School:** Duke Univ 1979; **Residency:** Surgery, Duke Univ Med Ctr, Durham, NC 1980-1987; **Faculty Appointment:** Prof Surgery, Univ S Fla Coll Med

Richardson, James David MD (Surgery) - *Special Expertise:* Surgery - General; **Admitting Hospital:** Norton Hospital; **Office Address:** Univ Louisville, Dept Surg 530 S Jackson St Louisville, KY 40202-1675; **Office Phone:** (502) 852-5453; **Board Certifications:** Surgery 1992, Thoracic Surgery 1999; **Medical School:** Univ KY Coll Med 1970; **Residencies:** Surgery, Univ Kentucky Med Ctr, Lexington, KY 1971-1972; Surgery, Univ Hosp-SW Texas Med Ctr, San Antonio, TX 1972-1976; **Faculty Appointment:** Prof Surgery, Univ Louisville Sch Med

Schirmer, Bruce David MD (Surgery) - *Special Expertise:* Laparoscopic Surgery; Gastrointestinal/Liver Surgery; Pancreatic Surgery; **Admitting Hospital:** University of Virginia Health Systems; **Office Address:** Univ VA Hlth Sci Ctr Box 800709 Charlottesville, VA 22908; **Office Phone:** (804) 924-2104; **Board Certification:** Surgery 1996; **Medical School:** Duke Univ 1978; **Residency:** Surgery, Duke Med Ctr, Durham, NC 1980-1985; **Faculty Appointment:** Prof Surgery, Univ VA Sch Med

Stratta, Robert MD (Surgery) - *Special Expertise:* Transplant-Pancreas; **Admitting Hospital:** University of Tennessee Bowld Hospital; **Office Address:** 956 Court Ave, Ste 202 Memphis, TN 38163-2116; **Office Phone:** (901) 448-5924; **Board Certifications:** Surgery 1996, Surgical Critical Care 1991; **Medical School:** Univ Chicago-Pritzker Sch Med 1980; **Residency:** Surgery, Univ Utah Med Ctr, Salt Lake City, UT 1980-1986; **Fellowship:** Transplant Surgery, Univ Wisc Hosps & Clins, Madison, WI 1986-1988; **Faculty Appointment:** Prof Surgery, Univ Tenn Coll Med, Memphis

Tzakis, Andreas MD (Surgery) - *Special Expertise:* Transplant-Liver; Transplant-Gastrointestinal; **Admitting Hospital:** University of Miami - Jackson Memorial Hospital; **Office Address:** 1801 NW 9th Ave, Fl 6 - Ste 511 Miami, FL 33136; **Office Phone:** (305) 355-5011; **Board Certification:** Surgery 1993; **Medical School:** Greece 1974; **Residencies:** Surgery, Mt Sinai Hosp, New York, NY 1977-1979; Surgery, SUNY Stony Brook, Stony Brook, NY 1979-1983; **Fellowship:** Transplant Surgery, Univ Pittsburgh Med Ctr, Pittsburgh, PA 1983-1985; **Faculty Appointment:** Prof Surgery, Univ Miami Sch Med

Urist, Marshall MD (Surgery) - *Special Expertise:* Cancer Surgery; Breast Cancer; Melanoma; **Admitting Hospital:** University of Alabama Hospital at Birmingham; **Office Address:** Univ Alabama Sch Med, Dept Surg 1922 7th Ave S, Bldg Kracke - Ste 321 Birmingham, AL 35294; **Office Phone:** (205) 934-3028; **Board Certification:** Surgery 2000; **Medical School:** Univ Chicago-Pritzker Sch Med 1971; **Residency:** Surgery, Johns Hopkins Hosp, Baltimore, MD 1971-1978; **Fellowship:** Surgical Oncology, Johns Hopkins Hosp, Baltimore, MD 1975-1976

Vogel, Stephen Burton MD (Surgery) - *Special Expertise:* Esophageal Cancer; Liver Cancer; **Admitting Hospital:** Shands at Vista; **Office Address:** Shands at Vista Pavillion Box 100286 Gainesville, FL 32610-0286; **Office Phone:** (352) 395-0604; **Board Certification:** Surgery 1976; **Medical School:** Univ Fla Coll Med 1967; **Residency:** Surgery, Univ Minn Hosp, Minneapolis, MN 1970-1975; **Faculty Appointment:** Prof Surgery, Univ Fla Coll Med

Willis, Irvin MD (Surgery) - *Special Expertise:* Pancreatic Surgery; **Admitting Hospital:** Mount Sinai Medical Center; **Office Address:** 4302 Alton Rd, Ste 630 Miami Beach, FL 33140-2876; **Office Phone:** (305) 534-6050; **Board Certification:** Surgery 1970; **Medical School:** Univ Cincinnati 1964; **Residency:** Surgery, Univ Miami-Jackson Meml, Miami, FL 1965-1969

Midwest

Aiken, John Judson MD (Surgery) - *Special Expertise:* Tumor Surgery-Pediatric; **Admitting Hospital:** Children's Hospital of Wisconsin; **Office Address:** Children's Hospital of WI 9000 W Wisconsin Ave Milwaukee, WI 53226; **Office Phone:** (414) 266-6550; **Board Certifications:** Surgery 1995, Pediatric Surgery; **Medical School:** Univ Cincinnati 1984; **Residency:** Mass Genl Hosp, Cambridge, MA 1985-1991; **Fellowship:** Pediatric Surgery, Chldns Hosp, Cincinnati, OH; **Faculty Appointment:** Asst Prof Surgery, Med Coll Wisc

Brems, John MD (Surgery) - *Special Expertise:* Transplant-Liver; Transplant-Liver; Obesity; **Admitting Hospital:** Loyola University Health System; **Office Address:** 2160 S 1st Ave, MC-EMS-3268 2160 S 1st Ave, MC-EMS 3268 Maywood, IL 60153; **Office Phone:** (708) 327-2774; **Board Certifications:** Surgery 1995, Critical Care Medicine 1991; **Medical School:** St Louis Univ 1981; **Residency:** Surgery, St Louis U, St. Louis, MO 1982-1986; **Fellowship:** Transplant Surgery, UCLA, Los Angeles, CA 1986-1987; **Faculty Appointment:** Assoc Prof Surgery, Loyola Univ-Stritch Sch Med

Crowe, Joseph MD (Surgery) - *Special Expertise:* Breast Cancer; Tumor Surgery; **Admitting Hospital:** Cleveland Clinic Foundation; **Office Address:** Cleveland Clinic, Dept Surg 9500 Euclid Ave, rm A80 Cleveland, OH 44195; **Office Phone:** (216) 444-3024; **Board Certification:** Surgery 1994; **Medical School:** Case West Res Univ 1978; **Residency:** Surgery, Univ Hosp Case-West Res, Cleveland, OH 1979-1983; **Fellowship:** Surgical Oncology, Sloan Kettering Ctr, New York, NY 1983-1985

Eberlein, Timothy J MD (Surgery) - *Special Expertise:* Breast Cancer; Tumor Surgery; **Admitting Hospital:** Barnes - Jewish Hospital; **Office Address:** 660 S Euclid Ave, Box 8109 St Louis, MO 63110; **Office Phone:** (314) 362-8021; **Board Certification:** Surgery 2007; **Medical School:** Univ Pittsburgh 1977; **Residencies:** Surgery, Peter Bent Brigham Hosp, Boston, MA 1978-1979; Surgery, Brigham-Womens Hosp, Boston, MA 1982-1985; **Fellowship:** Allergy & Immunology, Natl Inst Hlth, Bethesda, MD 1979-1982; **Faculty Appointment:** Prof Washington Univ, St Louis

Ellison, Edwin Christopher MD (Surgery) - *Special Expertise:* Transplant-Liver; Biliary Surgery; Pancreatic Cancer; **Admitting Hospital:** Ohio State University Medical Center; **Office Address:** OHSU, Div Surg - N729 Doan Hall 410 W 10th Ave Columbus, OH 43210-1236; **Office Phone:** (614) 293-4732; **Board Certification:** Surgery 1991; **Medical School:** Univ Wisc **Residency:** Surgery, Ohio State Univ, Columbus, OH; **Faculty Appointment:** Assoc Prof Surgery, Ohio State Univ

Ferguson, Ronald MD (Surgery) - *Special Expertise:* Transplant-Kidney; **Admitting Hospital:** Ohio State University Medical Center; **Office Address:** Ohio State Univ Hosp, Dept Surg 1654 Upham Dr, 327 Means Hall Columbus, OH 43210-1250; **Office Phone:** (614) 293-8701; **Board Certification:** Surgery 1981; **Medical School:** Washington Univ, St Louis 1971; **Residency:** Surgery, Univ Minn Hosp, Minneapolis, MN 1972-1979; **Fellowship:** Immunology, Univ Minn Hosp, Minneapolis, MN 1979-1980; **Faculty Appointment:** Prof Surgery, Ohio State Univ

Gamelli, Richard Louis MD (Surgery) - *Special Expertise:* Burns; Trauma/Critical Care; Obesity/Bariatric Surgery; **Admitting Hospital:** Loyola University Health System; **Office Address:** Loyola Univ, Stritch School of Medicine 2160 S First Ave, Bldg 110 - rm 3244 Maywood, IL 60153; **Office Phone:** (708) 327-2444; **Board Certification:** Surgery 1980; **Medical School:** Univ VT Coll Med 1974; **Residency:** Surgery, VT Med Ctr Hosp, Burlington, VT 1975-1979; **Faculty Appointment:** Prof Surgery, Loyola Univ-Stritch Sch Med

Kirby, Thomas MD (Surgery) - *Special Expertise:* Transplant-Lung; Thoracic Surgery; **Admitting Hospital:** University Hospital - Cleveland; **Office Address:** Univ Hosp 11100 Euclid Avenue Cleveland, OH 44106-5001; **Office Phone:** (216) 844-7267; **Board Certifications:** Surgery 1995, Surgical Critical Care 1991; **Medical School:** Univ Western Ontario 1978; **Residency:** Surgery, Univ Toronto, Toronto, Canada 1979-1984; **Faculty Appointment:** Prof Surgery, Case West Res Univ

Lewis Jr., Frank R. MD (Surgery) - *Special Expertise:* Trauma-Cardiac; Trauma-Pulmonary; Trauma-Complex; **Admitting Hospital:** Henry Ford Health System (Page 62); **Office Address:** Henry Ford Hosp.-Dept. Surgery 2799 W Grand Blvd Detroit, MI 48202; **Office Phone:** (313) 876-3152; **Board Certification:** Surgery 1973; **Medical School:** Univ MD Sch Med 1965; **Residency:** Surgery, UC San Francisco Med Ctr., San Francisco, CA 1967-1972; **Fellowship:** Surgery, Univ Calif Hosp., CA 1972-1973; **Faculty Appointment:** Prof Surgery, Case West Res Univ

Maker, Vijay MD (Surgery) - *Special Expertise:* Surgery - General; **Admitting Hospital:** Illinois Masonic Medical Center (Page 64); **Office Address:** 836 W Wellington Ave, Bldg 3516 Chicago, IL 60657-5147; **Office Phone:** (773) 883-2520; **Board Certification:** Surgery 1995; **Medical School:** India 1967; **Residency:** Surgery, Mount Sinai, Chicago, IL 1969-1973; **Faculty Appointment:** Assoc Prof Surgery, Rush Med Coll

Matas, Arthur J MD (Surgery) - *Special Expertise:* Transplant-Kidney; **Admitting Hospital:** Fairview-University Medical Center - University Campus; **Office Address:** Fairview Univ Medl Ctr 420 Delaware St SE, Box 328-Mail Bldg Minneapolis, MN 55455-0301; **Office Phone:** (612) 625-6460; **Board Certification:** Surgery 1989; **Medical School:** Univ Manitoba 1972; **Residency:** Surgery, Univ Minneapolis, Minneapolis, MN 1973-1979; **Fellowship:** Transplant Surgery, Univ Minneapolis, Minneapolis, MN 1979-1980; **Faculty Appointment:** Prof Surgery, Univ Minn

Melvin, W Scott MD (Surgery) - *Special Expertise:* Liver & Biliary Surgery; Pancreatic & Laparoscopic Surgery; **Admitting Hospital:** Ohio State University Medical Center; **Office Address:** Ohio State Univ Dept Surg Rm N-737 Doan Hall 410 W 10th Avenue Columbus, OH 43210-4030; **Office Phone:** (614) 293-4499

Millis, J. Michael MD (Surgery) - *Special Expertise:* Transplant-Liver; Transplant-Pancreas; **Admitting Hospital:** University of Chicago Hospitals (Page 78); **Office Address:** Univ Chicago, Dept Surg 5841 S Maryland Ave Chiciago, IL 60637; **Office Phone:** (773) 834-3537; **Board Certifications:** Surgery 1993, Surgical Critical Care 1993; **Medical School:** Univ Tenn Coll Med, Memphis 1985; **Residency:** Surgery, UCLA Med Ctr, Los Angeles, CA 1986-1992; **Fellowship:** Transplant Surgery, UCLA Med Ctr, Los Angeles, CA 1992-1994; **Faculty Appointment:** Assoc Prof Surgery, Univ Chicago-Pritzker Sch Med

Morrow, Monica MD (Surgery) - *Special Expertise:* Breast Cancer; **Admitting Hospital:** Northwestern Memorial Hospital; **Office Address:** Northwestern Memorial Hospital 675 N. St. Clair Street 13th Fl Rm13-174 Chicago, IL 60611; **Office Phone:** (312) 926-9039; **Board Certification:** Surgery 1992; **Medical School:** Jefferson Med Coll 1976; **Residency:** Surgery, Med Ctr Hosp of Vermont, Burlington, Ct 1976-1981; **Fellowship:** Surgical Oncology, Meml Sloan Kettering Cancer Ctr 1981-1983; **Faculty Appointment:** Prof Surgery, Northwestern Univ

Najarian, John S MD (Surgery) - *Special Expertise:* Transplant-Kidney; Transplant-Pediatric; **Admitting Hospital:** Fairview-University Medical Center - University Campus; **Office Address:** Univ Minn, Dept Surg 420 Delaware St SE, Mayo Bldg, Box 195 Minneapolis, MN 55455; **Office Phone:** (612) 625-8444; **Board Certification:** Surgery 1961; **Medical School:** UCSF 1952; **Residency:** Surgery, Moffitt Hosp-UCSF, San Francisco, CA 1955-1960; **Fellowship:** Pathology, Univ Pitts Med Ctr, Pittsburgh, PA 1960-1961; **Faculty Appointment:** Prof Emeritus Surgery, Univ Minn

Newell, Kenneth MD/PhD (Surgery) - *Special Expertise: Transplant-Small Bowel; Transplant-Kidney; Transplant-Pancreas/Liver;* **Admitting Hospital:** University of Chicago Hospitals (Page 78); **Office Address:** 5841 South Maryland Avenue Chicago, IL 60637; **Office Phone:** (773) 702-4315; **Board Certification:** Surgery 1999; **Medical School:** Univ Mich Med Sch 1984; **Residency:** Surgery, Loyola University Med Ctr, Maywood 1984-1989; **Fellowship:** Transplant Surgery, University of Chicago 1989

Prinz, Richard MD (Surgery) - *Special Expertise: Endocrinologic Surgery;* **Admitting Hospital:** Rush/Presbyterian - St Luke's Medical Center - Chicago (Page 74); **Office Address:** Affiliated Clinical Surgeons 1725 W Harrison St, Ste 834 Chicago, IL 60612; **Office Phone:** (312) 942-6511; **Board Certification:** Surgery 1995; **Medical School:** Loyola Univ-Stritch Sch Med 1972; **Residencies:** Surgery, Barnes Hosp, St Louis, MO 1972-1974; Surgery, Loyola, Chicago, IL 1974-1977; **Fellowship:** Endocrinology, Diabetes & Metabolism, Hammersmit, London, England 1979-1980; **Faculty Appointment:** Prof Surgery, Rush Med Coll

Rikkers, Layton F MD (Surgery) - *Special Expertise: Liver & Biliary Surgery;* **Admitting Hospital:** University of Wisconsin Hospital & Clinics; **Office Address:** Univ Wisc, Dept Surg 600 Highland Ave, Clinic Sci Ctr, rm H4 710 Madison, WI 53792; **Office Phone:** (608) 265-8854; **Board Certification:** Surgery 1996; **Medical School:** Stanford Univ 1970; **Residencies:** Surgery, Univ Utah Hosp, Salt Lake City, UT 1971-1973; Surgery, Univ Utah Hosp, Salt Lake City, UT 1974-1976; **Fellowship:** Hepatology, Royal Free Hosp, LondonEngland 1973-1974; **Faculty Appointment:** Prof Surgery, Univ Wisc

Rosen, Charles Burke MD (Surgery) - *Special Expertise: Transplant-Liver; Transplant-Liver;* **Admitting Hospital:** Mayo Medical Center & Clinic - Rochester; **Office Address:** Mayo Clinic, Liver Transplant Pgrm,Charlton 10A 200 First St SW Rochester, MN 55905; **Office Phone:** (507) 266-6640; **Board Certification:** Surgery 1990; **Medical School:** Mayo Med Sch 1984; **Residency:** Surgery, Mayo Clinic, Rochester, MN 1984-1989; **Fellowship:** Transplant Surgery, Mayo Clinic, Rochester, MN 1989-1991

Saha, Sukamal MD (Surgery) - *Special Expertise: Sentinel Node Surgery; Colon Cancer;* **Admitting Hospital:** Tulane University Medical Center Hospital & Clinic; **Office Address:** 3500 Calkins Rd Flint, MI 48532; **Office Phone:** (810) 230-9600; **Board Certification:** Surgery 1989; **Medical School:** India 1977; **Residencies:** Surgery, Hahnemann Univ Hosp, Philadelphia, PA 1984-1985; Surgery, Easton Hosp, Easton, PA 1985-1987; **Fellowship:** Surgical Oncology, Tulane Univ Med Ctr, New Orleans, LA 1987-1989

Shuck, Jerry M MD (Surgery) - *Special Expertise: Thyroid Surgery;* **Admitting Hospital:** University Hospital - Cleveland; **Office Address:** 11100 Euclid Ave, Box LKS 5047 Cleveland, OH 44106-2602; **Office Phone:** (216) 844-3871; **Board Certifications:** Surgery 1967, Thoracic Surgery 1967; **Medical School:** Univ Cincinnati 1959; **Residency:** Surgery, Cincinnati Genl Hosp, Cincinnati, OH 1960-1966; **Faculty Appointment:** Prof Surgery, Case West Res Univ

Sollinger, Hans W MD (Surgery) - *Special Expertise: Transplant-Kidney; Transplant-Pancreas;* **Admitting Hospital:** University of Wisconsin Hospital & Clinics; **Office Address:** Univ Wisc Hosp, Dept Surg 600 Highland Ave Madison, WI 53792; **Office Phone:** (608) 263-9903; **Board Certification:** Surgery 1996; **Medical School:** Germany 1974; **Residency:** Surgery, Univ Wisc Hosp, Madison, WI 1976-1980; **Fellowship:** Immunological BIology, Univ Wisc Hosp, Madison, WI 1975-1977; **Faculty Appointment:** Prof Surgery, Univ Wisc

Soper, Nathaniel MD (Surgery) - *Special Expertise:* Laparoscopic Surgery; Nissen Fundoplication; **Admitting Hospital:** Barnes - Jewish Hospital; **Office Address:** Barnes Jewish Hosp, Dept Surg One Barnes Hosp Plaza, Ste 6108, Box 8109 St Louis, MO 63110-1036; **Office Phone:** (314) 454-8877; **Board Certification:** Surgery 1996; **Medical School:** Univ Iowa Coll Med 1980; **Residency:** Surgery, Univ Utah Hosps, Salt Lake City, UT 1980-1986; **Fellowship:** Digestive Dis, Mayo Clinic, Rochester, MN 1986-1988; **Faculty Appointment:** Prof Surgery, Washington Univ, St Louis

Steele, Glenn D MD/PhD (Surgery) - *Special Expertise:* Rectal Cancer; Colon Cancer; **Admitting Hospital:** University of Chicago Hospitals (Page 78); **Office Address:** Univ Chicago 5841 S Maryland, MC-1000 Chicago, IL 60637-1470; **Office Phone:** (773) 702-3004; **Board Certification:** Surgery 1993; **Medical School:** NYU Sch Med 1970; **Residency:** Surgery, Colorado Med Ctr, Denver, CO 1971-1976; **Faculty Appointment:** Prof Surgery, Univ Chicago-Pritzker Sch Med

Sutherland, David MD (Surgery) - *Special Expertise:* Transplant-Pancreas; **Admitting Hospital:** Fairview-University Medical Center - University Campus; **Office Address:** 427 Harvard St SE Minneapolis, MN 55455; **Office Phone:** (612) 625-7600; **Board Certification:** Surgery 1978; **Medical School:** Univ Minn 1966; **Residency:** Surgery, West Virginia Univ Hosp, Morgantown, VA 1966-1968; **Fellowship:** Transplant Surgery, Univ Minn Hosps, Minneapolis, MN 1970-1975; **Faculty Appointment:** Prof Surgery, Univ Minn

Thistlethwaite, J Richard MD (Surgery) - *Special Expertise:* Transplant-Kidney; Transplant-Pancreas/Liver; Transplant-Pediatric; **Admitting Hospital:** University of Chicago Hospitals (Page 78); **Office Address:** Center for Advanced Medicine 5758 S Maryland Ave Chicago, IL 60637; **Office Phone:** (773) 702-6104; **Board Certification:** Surgery 1996; **Medical School:** Duke Univ 1977; **Residency:** Surgery, Mass Genl Hosp, Boston, MA 1983; **Faculty Appointment:** Prof Transplant Surgery, Univ Chicago-Pritzker Sch Med

Great Plains and Mountains

Karrer, Frederick Merrill MD (Surgery) - *Special Expertise:* Liver Surgery-Complex; Transplant-Liver; Critical Care; **Admitting Hospital:** The Children's Hospital - Denver; **Office Address:** Children's Hospital 1950 Oden St Denver, CO 80218-1022; **Office Phone:** (303) 861-6571; **Board Certifications:** Surgery 1987, Pediatric Surgery 1990; **Medical School:** Univ Nebr Coll Med 1979; **Residencies:** Surgery, Univ Ariz, Tucson, AZ 1979-1984; Pediatric Surgery, Children's Meml Hosp, Chicago, IL 1986-1988; **Fellowship:** Transplant Surgery, Univ Pittsburgh, Pittsburgh, PA 1985-1986; **Faculty Appointment:** Assoc Prof Surgery, Univ Colo

Saffle, Jeffrey MD (Surgery) - *Special Expertise:* Burns; Wound Healing/Care; **Admitting Hospital:** University of Utah Hospital and Clinics; **Office Address:** Univ Utah Hlth Sci Ctr, Dept Surg 50 N Medical Dr Salt Lake City, UT 84132; **Office Phone:** (801) 581-2700; **Board Certifications:** Surgery 1983, Surgical Critical Care 1998; **Medical School:** Univ Chicago-Pritzker Sch Med 1976; **Residency:** Surgery, Univ Utah Med Ctr, Salt Lake City, UT 1977-1982; **Fellowship:** Burn Surgery, Univ Utah Med Ctr, Salt Lake City, UT 1979-1980; **Faculty Appointment:** Prof Surgery, Univ Utah

Shaw Jr, Byers Wendell MD (Surgery) - *Special Expertise:* Transplant-Liver; **Admitting Hospital:** University of Nebraska Medical Center; **Office Address:** Nebraska Med Ctr, Transplant Ctr Box 983280 Omaha, NE 68198-3285; **Office Phone:** (402) 559-4076; **Board Certifications:** Surgery 1992, Surgical Critical Care 1996; **Medical School:** Case West Res Univ 1976; **Residency:** Surgery, Univ Utah, Salt Lake City, UT 1977-1981; **Fellowship:** Transplant Surgery, Univ Pittsburgh, Piitsburgh, PA 1981-1983; **Faculty Appointment:** Prof Surgery, Univ Nebr Coll Med

Southwest

Curley, Steven Alan MD (Surgery) - *Special Expertise:* Colorectal Cancer; Liver Cancer; **Admitting Hospital:** University of Texas MD Anderson Cancer Center (Page 66); **Office Address:** Univ TX MD Anderson Cancer Ctr, Dept Surg Onc 1515 Holcombe Blvd, Box 106 Houston, TX 77030; **Office Phone:** (713) 794-4957; **Board Certification:** Surgery 1997; **Medical School:** Univ Tex, Houston 1982; **Residency:** Surgery, Univ NM, Albuquerque, NM 1982-1988; **Fellowship:** Surgical Oncology, Univ TX - MD Anderson Cancer Ctr, Houston, TX 1988-1990

Evans, Douglas Brian MD (Surgery) - *Special Expertise:* Pancreatic Cancer; Thyroid Cancer; Endocrinologic Cancers; **Admitting Hospital:** University of Texas MD Anderson Cancer Center (Page 66); **Office Address:** UT MD Anderson Cancer Ctr 1515 Holcombe Blvd, Box 106 Houston, TX 77030-4095; **Office Phone:** (713) 794-4324; **Board Certification:** Surgery 1996; **Medical School:** Boston Univ 1983; **Residency:** Surgery, Dartmouth, Hanover 1984-1988; **Fellowship:** Surgical Oncology, MD Anderson Cancer Inst, Houston, TX 1988-1990; **Faculty Appointment:** Assoc Prof Univ Tex, Houston

Griswold, John A MD (Surgery) - *Special Expertise:* Burns; **Admitting Hospital:** University Medical Center; **Office Address:** Texas Tech Univ Hlth Scis Ctr, Dept Surgery 3601 4th St Lubbock, TX 79430; **Office Phone:** (806) 743-1615; **Board Certifications:** Surgery 1999, Surgical Critical Care 1991; **Medical School:** Creighton Univ 1981; **Residency:** Surgery, Texas Tech Univ Hlth Scis Ctr, Lubbock, TX 1982-1986; **Fellowship:** Burn Surgery, Univ Washington, Seattle, WA 1986-1988

Halff, Glenn Alexander MD (Surgery) - *Special Expertise:* Transplant-Liver; Liver Surgery; **Admitting Hospital:** University Health System; **Office Address:** Univ TX Hlth Sci Ctr San Antonio, Dept of Surg 7703 Floyd Curl, MC-7858 San Antonio, TX 78229-3900; **Office Phone:** (210) 567-5777; **Board Certifications:** Surgical Critical Care 1990, Surgery 1998; **Medical School:** Univ Tex, Houston **Residency:** Surgery, NYU Med Ctr, New York, NY 1983-1987; **Fellowship:** Transplant Surgery, Univ of Pittsburgh, Pittsburgh, PA 1988-1989; **Faculty Appointment:** Assoc Prof Surgery, Univ Tex, San Antonio

Jackson, Gilchrist MD (Surgery) - *Special Expertise:* Laparoscopic Surgery-Gastrointestinal; Tumor Surgery; **Admitting Hospital:** St Luke's Episcopal Hospital - Houston (Page 76); **Office Address:** 6624 Fannin St, Ste 1700 Houston, TX 77030-2329; **Office Phone:** (713) 442-1132; **Board Certification:** Surgery 1980; **Medical School:** Univ KY Coll Med 1974; **Residency:** Parkland SW Hosps, Dallas, TX 1975-1979; **Fellowship:** Surgical Oncology, MD Anderson Hosp, Houston, TX 1979-1980; **Faculty Appointment:** Assoc Clin Prof Baylor Coll Med

Kahan, Barry MD (Surgery) - *Special Expertise:* Transplant-Kidney; **Admitting Hospital:** Memorial Hermann Healthcare System; **Office Address:** 6431 Fannin St, rm 6-240 Houston, TX 77030-1501; **Office Phone:** (713) 500-7400; **Board Certification:** Surgery 1973; **Medical School:** Univ Chicago-Pritzker Sch Med 1965; **Residency:** Surgery, Mass Genl Hosp, Boston, MA 1968-1972; **Faculty Appointment:** Prof Surgery, Univ Tex, Houston

Kelly, Keith A MD (Surgery) - *Special Expertise:* Colon Cancer; **Admitting Hospital:** Mayo Medical Center & Clinic - Scottsdale; **Office Address:** Mayo Clinic, Dept Genl Surg 13400 E Shea Blvd Scottsdale, AZ 85259; **Office Phone:** (480) 301-8000; **Board Certifications:** Surgery 1989, Thoracic Surgery 1967; **Medical School:** Univ Chicago-Pritzker Sch Med 1956; **Residencies:** Surgery, Univ Wash Med Ctr, Seattle, WA 1957-1958; Surgery, Univ Wash Med Ctr, Seattle, WA 1961-1966; **Fellowship:** Thoracic Surgery, Mayo Grad Sch Med, Rochester, MN 1966-1968; **Faculty Appointment:** Prof Surgery, Mayo Med Sch

Klimberg, V Suzanne MD (Surgery) - *Special Expertise:* Breast Cancer; **Admitting Hospital:** University of Arkansas for Medical Sciences; **Office Address:** University of Arkansas Medical Sciences 4301 W Markham, MC-725 Little Rock, AR 72205; **Office Phone:** (501) 686-6504; **Board Certification:** Surgery 1991; **Medical School:** Univ Fla Coll Med 1984; **Residency:** Surgery, Univ Fla, Gainesville, FL 1985-1990; **Fellowships:** Clinical Oncology, Univ Fla, Gainnsville, FL 1990-1991; Clinical Oncology, Univ Arkansas, AR 1990-1991; **Faculty Appointment:** Assoc Prof Surgery, Univ Ark

Lee, Jeffrey Edwin MD (Surgery) - *Special Expertise:* Melanoma; Pancreatic Cancer; Adrenal Tumors; **Admitting Hospital:** University of Texas MD Anderson Cancer Center (Page 66); **Office Address:** UT MD Anderson Cancer Ctr 1515 Holcombe Blvd, Box 106 Houston, TX 77030; **Office Phone:** (713) 792-7218; **Board Certification:** Surgery 2012; **Medical School:** Stanford Univ 1984; **Residencies:** Surgery, Stanford Univ Hosp, Palo Alto, CA 1985-1987; Surgery, Stanford Univ Hosp, Palo Alto, CA 1989-1991; **Fellowships:** Allergy & Immunology, Stanford Univ Sch Med, Palo Alto, CA 1987-1989; Surgical Oncology, Univ Tex-MD Anderson Cancer Ctr, Houston, TX 1991-1993; **Faculty Appointment:** Assoc Prof Surgery, Univ Tex, Houston

MacFadyen, Bruce MD (Surgery) - *Special Expertise:* Laparoscopic Surgery; Gastrointestinal Surgery; Endoscopy; **Admitting Hospital:** Memorial Hermann Healthcare System; **Office Address:** 6410 Fannin Street Suite 1400 Houston, TX 77030-1501; **Office Phone:** (713) 704-6025; **Board Certification:** Surgery 1975; **Medical School:** Hahnemann Univ 1968; **Residencies:** Surgery, Hosp Univ Penn, Philadelphia, PA 1969-1972; Surgery, Hermann Hosp, Houston, TX 1972-1974; **Faculty Appointment:** Prof Surgery, Univ Tex, Houston

Ross, Merrick I MD (Surgery) - *Special Expertise:* Sentinel Node Surgery; Breast Cancer; Melanoma; **Admitting Hospital:** University of Texas MD Anderson Cancer Center (Page 66); **Office Address:** Univ TX MD Anderson Cancer Ctr 1515 Holcombe Blvd, Box 106 Houston, TX 77030; **Office Phone:** (713) 792-7217; **Board Certification:** Surgery 1997; **Medical School:** Univ IL Coll Med 1980; **Residencies:** Surgery, Univ IL Hosp & Clin, Chicago, IL 1980-1982; Surgery, Univ IL Hosp & Clin, Chicago, IL 1984-1987; **Fellowships:** Research, Scripps Clin & Rsch, La Jolla, CA 1982-1984; Surgical Oncology, Univ TX-MD Anderson Cancer Ctr, Houston, TX 1987-1989; **Faculty Appointment:** Prof Surgery, Univ Tex, Houston

Singletary, S Eva MD (Surgery) - *Special Expertise:* Breast Cancer; Breast Cancer; Breast Reconstruction; **Admitting Hospital:** University of Texas MD Anderson Cancer Center (Page 66); **Office Address:** Univ Tex MD Anderson Canc Ctr 1515 Holcombe Blvd, Box 106 Houston, TX 77030-4009; **Office Phone:** (713) 792-6937; **Board Certification:** Surgery 1994; **Medical School:** Med Univ SC 1977; **Residency:** Surgery, Shands Hosp-Univ FL, Gainesville, FL 1977-1983; **Fellowship:** Surgery, MD Anderson Hosp, Houston, TX 1983-1985; **Faculty Appointment:** Prof Surgery, Univ Tex, Houston

Snyder III, William Henry MD (Surgery) - *Special Expertise:* Endocrinologic Surgery; **Admitting Hospital:** Parkland Memorial Hospital; **Office Address:** Univ Texas SW Med Ctr, Dept Surg 5323 Harry Hines Blvd, MC-9156 Dallas, TX 75235; **Office Phone:** (214) 648-3510; **Board Certifications:** Thoracic Surgery 1972, Surgery 1971; **Medical School:** Baylor Coll Med 1962; **Residency:** Thoracic Surgery, Univ Cincinnati Affil Hosps, Cincinnati, OH 1965-1971; **Faculty Appointment:** Prof Surgery, Univ Tex SW, Dallas

Stewart, Ronald Mack MD (Surgery) - *Special Expertise: Trauma;* **Admitting Hospital:** University of Texas Health & Science Center; **Office Address:** Univ Texas Hlth Sci Ctr, Dept Surgery 7703 Floyd Curl Dr, MC-7740 San Antonio, TX 78229-3900; **Office Phone:** (210) 567-3623; **Board Certifications:** Surgery 1992, Surgical Critical Care 1994; **Medical School:** Univ Tex, San Antonio 1985; **Residency:** Surgery, Univ Tex Hlth Sci Ctr, San Antonio, TX 1985-1991; **Fellowship:** Trauma, Univ Tenn Coll Med, Memphis, TN 1991-1993; **Faculty Appointment:** Assoc Prof Surgery, Univ Tex, San Antonio

Wood, R Patrick MD (Surgery) - *Special Expertise: Transplant-Liver; Liver Disease; Liver Cancer;* **Admitting Hospital:** St Luke's Episcopal Hospital - Houston (Page 76); **Office Address:** U Tx Med Sch/ Dept Surg 6431 Fannin St, Ste 6246 Houston, TX 77030; **Office Phone:** (713) 704-6801; **Board Certifications:** Surgery 1995, Surgical Critical Care 1992; **Medical School:** Univ Rochester 1979; **Residency:** Surgery, NYU Med-Bellevue, New York, NY 1980-1984; **Fellowship:** Transplant Surgery, U Pittsburgh, Pittsburgh, PA 1984-1985

West Coast and Pacific

Ascher, Nancy L MD (Surgery) - *Special Expertise: Transplant-Liver; Transplant-Kidney;* **Admitting Hospital:** University of California - San Francisco Medical Center; **Office Address:** 513 Parnassus Ave San Francisco, CA 94143-0780; **Office Phone:** (415) 353-2318; **Board Certification:** Surgery 1991; **Medical School:** Univ Mich Med Sch 1974; **Residency:** Surgery, Univ Minn Hosp, Minneapolis, MN 1975-1981; **Fellowship:** Transplant Surgery, Univ Minn Hosp, Minneapolis, MN 1981-1982; **Faculty Appointment:** Prof Surgery, UCSF

Bilchik, Anton Joel MD (Surgery) - *Special Expertise: Surgery - General;* **Admitting Hospital:** St John's Health Center; **Office Address:** John Wayne Cancer Institute 2200 Santa Monica Blvd Santa Monica, CA 90404; **Office Phone:** (310) 449-5206; **Board Certification:** Surgery 1997; **Medical School:** South Africa 1985; **Residency:** Surgery, UCLA, Los Angeles, CA 1991-1996; **Fellowship:** John Wayne Cancer Inst., Santa Monica, CA 1996-1998; **Faculty Appointment:** Asst Clin Prof Surgery, UCLA

Busuttil, Ronald Wilfred MD/PhD (Surgery) - *Special Expertise: Transplant-Liver;* **Admitting Hospital:** UCLA Medical Center; **Office Address:** UCLA Med Ctr - Dumont, UCLA Transpl Ctr 10833 Le Conte Av, rm 77-120 Los Angeles, CA 90095-7054; **Office Phone:** (310) 825-5318; **Board Certification:** Surgery 1997; **Medical School:** Tulane Univ 1971; **Residency:** Surgery, UCLA, Los Angeles, CA 1972-1976; **Fellowship:** Surgery, UCLA, Los Angeles, CA 1973-1975; **Faculty Appointment:** Prof Surgery, UCLA

Byrd, David MD (Surgery) - *Special Expertise: Tumor Surgery; Breast Cancer;* **Admitting Hospital:** University of Washington Medical Center; **Office Address:** Univ Wash Med Ctr, Dept Surg 1959 NE Pacific St Seattle, WA 98195-6165; **Office Phone:** (206) 598-4477; **Board Certification:** Surgery 1998; **Medical School:** Tulane Univ 1982; **Residency:** Surgery, Univ Wash Med Ctr, Seattle, WA 1983-1987; **Fellowship:** Surgery, Univ Tex-Anderson Canc Ctr, Houston, TX 1989-1992; **Faculty Appointment:** Assoc Prof Surgery, Univ Wash

Clark, Orlo H MD (Surgery) - *Special Expertise: Thyroid Cancer; Pancreatic Cancer; Hyperparathyroidism;* **Admitting Hospital:** UCSF - Mount Zion Medical Center; **Office Address:** UCSF/Mt Zion Med Ctr, Dept Surg 1600 Divisadero St, rm C347 San Francisco, CA 94115; **Office Phone:** (415) 883-7616; **Board Certification:** Surgery 1974; **Medical School:** Cornell Univ-Weil Med Coll 1967; **Residencies:** Surgery, UCSF, San Francisco, CA 1967-1970; Surgery, UCSF, San Francisco, CA 1971-1973; **Fellowship:** Surgery, Royal Med Sch London, London 1970-1971; **Faculty Appointment:** Prof Surgery, UCSF

Eilber, Frederick Richard MD (Surgery) - *Special Expertise:* Tumor Surgery; Sarcoma; **Admitting Hospital:** UCLA Medical Center; **Office Address:** Ctr for Hlth Scis 10833 Le Conte Ave, rm 54-14 Los Angeles, CA 90095-3075; **Office Phone:** (310) 825-7086; **Board Certification:** Surgery 1973; **Medical School:** Univ Mich Med Sch 1965; **Residency:** Surgery, Univ MD Hosp, Baltimore, MD 1966-1972; **Fellowship:** Surgery, Univ TX MD Anderson Hosp, Houston, TX 1972-1973; **Faculty Appointment:** Prof Surgery, UCLA

Esquivel, Carlos Orlando MD (Surgery) - *Special Expertise:* Transplant-Liver; **Admitting Hospital:** Stanford Medical Center; **Office Address:** Stanford Hosps & Clin.-Surg. Spec. Clin. 300 Pasteur Drive, A-160 Stanford, CA 94305-5731; **Office Phone:** (650) 498-5689; **Board Certifications:** Surgery 1994, Surgical Critical Care 1989; **Medical School:** Costa Rica 1975; **Residency:** Surgery, UC- Davis Med Ctr, Sacramento, CA 1977-1984; **Fellowship:** Surgical Critical Care, Univ Hlth Ctr Pittsburgh, Pittsburgh, PA 1984-1985; **Faculty Appointment:** Prof Surgery, Stanford Univ

Essner, Richard MD (Surgery) - *Special Expertise:* Sentinel Node Surgery; Melanoma; **Admitting Hospital:** St John's Health Center; **Office Address:** John Wayne Cancer Inst 2200 Santa Monica Blvd Santa Monica, CA 90404; **Office Phone:** (310) 998-3906; **Board Certification:** Surgery 1994; **Medical School:** Emory Univ 1985; **Residency:** Surgery, Univ NC Sch Med, Chapel Hill, NC 1985-1992; **Faculty Appointment:** Asst Clin Prof Surgery, USC Sch Med

Giuliano, Armando E MD (Surgery) - *Special Expertise:* Sentinel Node Surgery; Breast Cancer; **Admitting Hospital:** St John Hospital and Medical Center; **Office Address:** John Wayne Cancer Inst 1328 22nd St Santa Monica, CA 90404; **Office Phone:** (310) 829-8089; **Board Certification:** Surgery 1999; **Medical School:** Univ Chicago-Pritzker Sch Med 1973; **Residency:** Surgery, UCSF Med Ctr, San Francisco, CA 1974-1980; **Fellowship:** Surgical Oncology, UCLA Med Ctr, Los Angeles, CA 1976-1980; **Faculty Appointment:** Prof Surgery, UCLA

Hansen, Nora Marie MD (Surgery) - *Special Expertise:* Sentinel Node Surgery; Breast Cancer; **Admitting Hospital:** St John's Health Center; **Office Address:** St John's Hlth Ctr - John Wayne Canc Inst 1328 22nd St, Fl 4, West Wing Santa Monica, CA 90404; **Office Phone:** (310) 829-8089; **Board Certification:** Surgery 1996; **Medical School:** NY Med Coll 1988; **Residencies:** Univ Chicago, Chicago, IL 1989-1990; Univ Chicago, Chicago, IL 1992-1995; **Fellowships:** Surgical Oncology, Univ Chicago, Chicago, IL 1990-1992; Surgical Oncology, Univ Chicago, Chicago, IL 1995-1996

Hoyt, David MD (Surgery) - *Special Expertise:* Trauma; Burns; **Admitting Hospital:** University of California - San Diego Healthcare; **Office Address:** 200 W Arbor Dr San Diego, CA 92103-8896; **Office Phone:** (619) 294-6400; **Board Certifications:** Surgery 1994, Surgical Critical Care 1997; **Medical School:** Case West Res Univ 1976; **Residencies:** Surgery, UC - San Diego Med Ctr, San Diego, CA 1977-1979; Surgery, UC - Sand Diego Med Ctr, San Diego, CA 1982-1984; **Fellowships:** Research, UC - San Diego Med Ctr, San Diego, CA 1979-1980; Immunopathology, Scripps Clin, La Jolla, CA 1980-1982; **Faculty Appointment:** Prof Surgery, UCSD

Knudson, Mary Margaret MD (Surgery) - *Special Expertise:* Breast Cancer; Trauma; **Admitting Hospital:** University of California - San Francisco Medical Center; **Office Address:** UCSF 400 Parnassus Avenue-Rm.655 San Fransisco, CA 94143; **Office Phone:** (415) 353-2161; **Board Certifications:** Surgery 1992, Surgical Critical Care 1998; **Medical School:** Univ Mich Med Sch 1976; **Residencies:** Surgery, Beth Israel Hosp, Boston, MA 1977-1979; Surgery, Univ Mich Med Ctr, Ann Arbor, MI 1979-1982; **Fellowship:** Pediatric Surgery, Stanford Univ Hosps, Stanford, CA 1982; **Faculty Appointment:** Assoc Prof Surgery, UCSF

Pellegrini, Carlos MD (Surgery) - *Special Expertise:* Esophageal Surgery; Barrett's Esophagus; Laparoscopic Surgery; **Admitting Hospital:** University of Washington Medical Center; **Office Address:** Univ Washington Med Ctr, Dept Surg 1959 NE Pacific St, Box 356410 Seattle, WA 98195; **Office Phone:** (206) 543-3106; **Board Certification:** Surgery 1998; **Medical School:** Argentina 1971; **Residencies:** Surgery, Granadero Hosp, Argentina 1971-1975; Surgery, Chicago Hosps, Chicago, IL 1975-1979; **Faculty Appointment:** Prof Surgery, Univ Wash

Peters, Jeffrey Harold MD (Surgery) - *Special Expertise:* Esophageal Surgery; **Admitting Hospital:** USC University Hospital - Richard K. Eamer Medical Plaza; **Office Address:** USC Hlthcare Consultation Ctr 1510 San Pablo St, Bldg 514 Los Angeles, CA 90033-4612; **Office Phone:** (323) 442-5926; **Board Certifications:** Surgical Critical Care 1994, Surgery 1998; **Medical School:** Ohio State Univ 1981; **Residency:** Surgery, Johns Hopkins Hosp, Baltimore, MD 1985-1988; **Fellowships:** Allergy & Immunology, John Hopkins Hosp, Baltimore, MD 1983-1985; Esophagy, Creighton Univ, Omaha, OK 1990; **Faculty Appointment:** Prof Surgery, USC Sch Med

Rassman, William Richard MD (Surgery) - *Special Expertise:* Hair Restoration/Tranplant; **Office Address:** New Hair Inst 9911 W Pico Blvd, Bldg 301 Los Angeles, CA 90035-2709; **Office Phone:** (310) 553-9113; **Board Certification:** Surgery 1975; **Medical School:** Med Coll VA 1966; **Residencies:** Surgery, Cornell Med Ctr, New York, NY 1967-1969; Surgery, Dartmouth Med Ctr, Lebannon, NH 1971-1973

Silverstein, Melvin J MD (Surgery) - *Special Expertise:* Breast Cancer; **Admitting Hospital:** USC Norris Cancer Comprehensive Center; **Office Address:** USC Norris Cancer Center 1441 Eastlake Ave, rm 7415, MC-74 Los Angeles, CA 90033; **Office Phone:** (323) 865-3535; **Board Certification:** Surgery 1971; **Medical School:** Albany Med Coll 1965; **Residency:** Surgery, Boston City Hosp-Tufts Univ, Boston, MA 1966-1970; **Fellowship:** Surgical Oncology, UCLA, Los Angeles, CA 1972-1975; **Faculty Appointment:** Prof Surgery, USC Sch Med

THORACIC SURGERY

A thoracic surgeon provides the operative, perioperative care and critical care of patients with pathologic conditions within the chest. Included is the surgical care of coronary artery disease, cancers of the lung, esophagus and chest wall, abnormalities of the trachea, abnormalities of the great vessels and heart valves, congenital anomalies, tumors of the mediastinum and diseases of the diaphragm. The management of the airway and injuries of the chest is within the scope of the specialty.

Thoracic surgeons have the knowledge, experience and technical skills to accurately diagnose, operate upon safely and effectively manage patients with thoracic diseases of the chest. This requires substantial knowledge of cardiorespiratory physiology and oncology, as well as capability in the use of heart assist devices, management of abnormal heart rhythms and drainage of the chest cavity, respiratory support systems, endoscopy and invasive and noninvasive diagnostic techniques.

Training required: Seven to eight years

PHYSICIAN LISTINGS

Thoracic Surgery

New England

Akins, Cary W MD (Thoracic Surgery) - *Special Expertise: Heart Valve Surgery; Coronary Artery Surgery; Aneurysm;* **Admitting Hospital:** Massachusetts General Hospital; **Office Address:** Mass Genl Hosp- Surg WHT 503 55 Fruit St Boston, MA 02114; **Office Phone:** (617) 726-8218; **Board Certifications:** Thoracic Surgery 1997, Surgery 1976; **Medical School:** Harvard Med Sch 1970; **Residency:** Surgery, Mass Genl Hosp, Boston, MA 1971-1975; **Faculty Appointment:** Clin Prof Surgery, Harvard Med Sch

Austen, W. Gerald MD (Thoracic Surgery) - *Special Expertise: Thoracic Surgery - General;* **Admitting Hospital:** Massachusetts General Hospital; **Office Address:** Mass Genl Hosp- Surg 55 Fruit St Boston, MA 02114; **Office Phone:** (617) 726-2050; **Board Certifications:** Surgery 1962, Thoracic Surgery 1964; **Medical School:** Harvard Med Sch 1955; **Residency:** Surgery, Mass General Hospital, Boston, MA 1956-1961; **Faculty Appointment:** Prof Surgery, Harvard Med Sch

Bredenberg, Carl Eric MD (Thoracic Surgery) - *Special Expertise: Esophageal Surgery;* **Admitting Hospital:** Maine Medical Center; **Office Address:** Maine Heart Surgical Assoc 887 Congress St, Ste 300 Portland, ME 04102; **Office Phone:** (207) 773-8161; **Board Certifications:** Thoracic Surgery 1974, Vascular Surgery (General) 1993; **Medical School:** Johns Hopkins Univ 1964; **Residency:** Surgery, Johns Hopkins Hosp, Baltimore, MD 1967-1972; **Fellowship:** Research, Walter Reed Army Inst Rsch, Washington, DC 1965-1967; **Faculty Appointment:** Prof Surgery, Univ VT Coll Med

Cohn, Lawrence H MD (Thoracic Surgery) - *Special Expertise: Heart Valve Surgery; Heart Disease-Congenital;* **Admitting Hospital:** Brigham & Women's Hospital; **Office Address:** Brigham & Women's Hosp 75 Francis Street Boston, MA 02115-6110; **Office Phone:** (617) 732-7678; **Board Certifications:** Surgery 1970, Thoracic Surgery 1971; **Medical School:** Stanford Univ 1962; **Residencies:** Surgery, UCSF Med Ctr, San Francisco, CA 1966-1969; Cardiothoracic Surgery, Stanford Univ, Stanford, CA 1969-1971; **Fellowship:** Surgery, Boston City Hosp, Boston, MA 1962-1964; **Faculty Appointment:** Prof Surgery, Harvard Med Sch

Elefteriades, John MD (Thoracic Surgery) - *Special Expertise: Transplant-Heart; Aneurysm-Abdominal Aortic;* **Admitting Hospital:** Yale - New Haven Hospital; **Office Address:** Yale University School of Medicine 333 Cedar St-121FMB New Haven, CT 06520; **Office Phone:** (203) 785-2705; **Board Certification:** Thoracic Surgery 1994; **Medical School:** Yale Univ 1976; **Residencies:** Surgery, Yale-New H, New Haven, CT 1977-1981; Thoracic Surgery, Yale-New H, New Haven, CT 1981-1983; **Fellowship:** Thoracic Surgery, Yale-New H, New Haven, CT 1981-1983; **Faculty Appointment:** Prof Surgery, Yale Univ

Jonas, Richard A MD (Thoracic Surgery) - *Special Expertise: Cardiac Surgery-Pediatric;* **Admitting Hospital:** Children's Hospital; **Office Address:** Children's Hospital- Cardiac Surgery 300 Longwood Ave Boston, MA 02115; **Office Phone:** (617) 355-7930; **Medical School:** Australia 1974; **Residencies:** Surgery, Royal Childrens Hosp, Australia; Pediatric Surgery, Green Lane Hosp, New Zealand; **Fellowship:** Thoracic Surgery, Brigham & Women's Hosp, Boston, MA 1982-1984; **Faculty Appointment:** Prof Surgery, Harvard Med Sch

Kopf, Gary MD (Thoracic Surgery) - *Special Expertise: Cardiac Surgery-Adult & Pediatric;* **Admitting Hospital:** Yale - New Haven Hospital; **Office Address:** 330 Orchard St, Ste 107 New Haven, CT 06511; **Office Phone:** (203) 785-2702; **Board Certification:** Thoracic Surgery 1982; **Medical School:** Harvard Med Sch 1970; **Residencies:** Surgery, Peter Bent Brigham Hosp, Boston, MA 1973-1977; Thoracic Surgery, Chldns Hosp Med Ctr, Boston, MA 1977-1980; **Fellowship:** Surgery, Harvard/Brigham Hosp, Boston, MA 1973-1980; **Faculty Appointment:** Prof Surgery, Yale Univ

Mathisen, Douglas MD (Thoracic Surgery) - *Special Expertise: Tracheal Surgery; Lung Cancer; Esophageal Cancer;* **Admitting Hospital:** Massachusetts General Hospital; **Office Address:** Mass Genl Hosp 55 Fruit St, Bldg Blake 1570 Boston, MA 02114; **Office Phone:** (617) 726-6826; **Board Certifications:** Surgery 1982, Thoracic Surgery 1984; **Medical School:** Univ IL Coll Med 1974; **Residencies:** Surgery, Mass Genl Hosp, Boston, MA 1974-1981; Thoracic Surgery, Mass Genl Hosp, Boston, MA 1981-1982; **Fellowship:** Surgical Oncology, Natl Cancer Inst, Bethesda, MD 1977-1979; **Faculty Appointment:** Prof Surgery, Harvard Med Sch

Moncure, Ashby MD (Thoracic Surgery) - *Special Expertise: Esophageal Cancer;* **Admitting Hospital:** Massachusetts General Hospital; **Office Address:** MGH-WANG ACC 15 Parkman St Boston, MA 02114; **Office Phone:** (617) 726-2819; **Board Certifications:** Thoracic Surgery 1971, Vascular Surgery (General) 1989; **Medical School:** Univ VA Sch Med 1960; **Residencies:** Surgery, Mass Genl Hosp, Boston, MA 1961-1962; Thoracic Surgery, Frenchy Hosp, Bristol England 1967; **Faculty Appointment:** Assoc Prof Surgery, Harvard Med Sch

Shahian, David MD (Thoracic Surgery) - *Special Expertise: Lung Cancer;* **Admitting Hospital:** Lahey Clinic; **Office Address:** Lahey Clinic, Dept Thor and CV Surg 41 Mall Rd Burlington, MA 01805; **Office Phone:** (781) 744-8575; **Board Certification:** Thoracic Surgery 1990; **Medical School:** Harvard Med Sch 1973; **Residency:** Surgery, Mass Genl Hosp, Boston, MA 1974-1978; **Fellowship:** Thoracic Surgery, Rush Presby-St Lukes Hosp, Chicago, IL 1978-1980; **Faculty Appointment:** Assoc Clin Prof Surgery, Harvard Med Sch

Sugarbaker, David John MD (Thoracic Surgery) - *Special Expertise: Mesothelioma;* **Admitting Hospital:** Brigham & Women's Hospital; **Office Address:** Brigham & Women's Hosp, Dept Thor Surg 75 Francis St Boston, MA 02115-6110; **Office Phone:** (617) 732-5004; **Board Certifications:** Surgery 1987, Thoracic Surgery 1999; **Medical School:** Cornell Univ-Weil Med Coll 1979; **Residencies:** Surgery, Brigham & Women's Hosp, Boston, MA 1980-1982; Surgery, Brigham & Women's Hosp, Boston, MA 1984-1986; **Fellowship:** Thoracic Surgery, Toronto Genl Hosp, Toronto, CN 1986-1988; **Faculty Appointment:** Assoc Prof Surgery, Harvard Med Sch

Vander Salm, Thomas MD (Thoracic Surgery) - *Special Expertise: Mitral Valve Surgery; Cardiovascular Surgery;* **Admitting Hospital:** UMASS Memorial Health Care - Worcester; **Office Address:** 55 Lake Ave N Worcester, MA 01655; **Office Phone:** (508) 856-2216; **Board Certifications:** Surgery 1974, Thoracic Surgery 1994; **Medical School:** Johns Hopkins Univ 1966; **Residencies:** Surgery, Mass Genl Hosp, Boston, MA 1967-1968; Surgery, Johns Hopkins Hosp, Baltimore, MD 1968; **Faculty Appointment:** Prof Surgery, Univ Mass Sch Med

Wain, John MD (Thoracic Surgery) - *Special Expertise: Transplant-Lung; Emphysema;* **Admitting Hospital:** Massachusetts General Hospital; **Office Address:** Mass Genl Hosp 55 Fruit St, Blake 1570 Boston, MA 02114; **Office Phone:** (617) 726-5200; **Board Certifications:** Surgery 1986, Thoracic Surgery 1990; **Medical School:** Jefferson Med Coll 1980; **Residencies:** Surgery, Mass Genl Hosp, Boston, MA 1980-1985; Medical Oncology, City Hope Med Ctr, Duarte, CA 1985-1986; **Fellowship:** Cardiothoracic Surgery, Mass Genl Hosp, Bostn, MA 1986-1988; **Faculty Appointment:** Asst Prof Thoracic Surgery, Harvard Med Sch

Wright, Cameron MD (Thoracic Surgery) - *Special Expertise: Lung Cancer; Thoracic Cancers;* **Admitting Hospital:** Massachusetts General Hospital; **Office Address:** Mass Genl Hosp 55 Fruit St, Blake 1570 Boston, MA 02114; **Office Phone:** (617) 726-5801; **Board Certifications:** Surgery 1995, Thoracic Surgery 1997; **Medical School:** Univ Mich Med Sch 1980; **Residencies:** Surgery, Mass Genl Hosp, Boston, MA 1980-1986; Thoracic Surgery, Mass Genl Hosp, Boston, MA 1986-1988

Mid Atlantic

Acinapura, Anthony MD (Thoracic Surgery) - *Special Expertise:* Cardiothoracic Surgery; Vascular Surgery; **Admitting Hospital:** Maimonides Medical Center (Page 67); **Office Address:** Lutheran Med Ctr 150 55th St, Ste 3524 Brooklyn, NY 11220; **Office Phone:** (718) 630-7351; **Board Certifications:** Surgery 1971, Thoracic Surgery 1972; **Medical School:** Georgetown Univ 1969; **Residencies:** Surgery, Bellevue Hosp, New York, NY 1966-1969; Thoracic Surgery, Bellevue Hosp, New York, NY 1969-1971; **Fellowship:** Surgery, Duke Univ Med Ctr 1965-1966; **Faculty Appointment:** Prof Surgery, NY Med Coll

Acker, Michael Andrew MD (Thoracic Surgery) - *Special Expertise:* Transplant-Heart; Heart Assistance Devices; **Admitting Hospital:** University of Pennsylvania - Presbyterian Medical Center; **Office Address:** Univ PA - Presby Med Ctr 39th and Market Streets Philadelphia, PA 19104; **Office Phone:** (215) 349-8305; **Board Certifications:** Thoracic Surgery 1992, Surgery 2000; **Medical School:** Brown Univ 1981; **Residencies:** Surgery, Hosp Univ Pennsylvania Hlth Sys, Philadelphia, PA 1982-1988; Thoracic Surgery, Johns Hopkins Hosp, Baltimore, MD 1988-1991; **Faculty Appointment:** Assoc Prof Surgery, Univ Penn

Bains, Manjit MD (Thoracic Surgery) - *Special Expertise:* Cardiothoracic Surgery; Esophageal Cancer; **Admitting Hospital:** Memorial Sloan Kettering Cancer Center; **Office Address:** 1275 York Ave New York, NY 10021; **Office Phone:** (212) 639-7450; **Board Certification:** Thoracic Surgery 1972; **Medical School:** India 1963; **Residency:** Rochester, Rochester, NY 1966-1970; **Fellowships:** Thoracic Surgery, Sloan Kett, New York, NY; Cornel Uni, New York, NY 1970-1972; **Faculty Appointment:** Thoracic Surgery, Cornell Univ-Weil Med Coll

Baumgartner, William MD (Thoracic Surgery) - *Special Expertise:* Thoracic Surgery - General; **Admitting Hospital:** Johns Hopkins Hospital - Baltimore (Page 65); **Office Address:** Johns Hopkins Hospital 600 N Wolfe St, Bldg Blalock 618 Baltimore, MD 21287; **Office Phone:** (410) 955-5248; **Board Certifications:** Surgery 1990, Thoracic Surgery 1991; **Medical School:** Univ KY Coll Med 1973; **Residencies:** Surgery, Stanford U Med Ctr, Stanford, CA 1974-1975; Thoracic Surgery, Stanford U Med Ctr, Stanford, CA 1975-1976; **Faculty Appointment:** Prof Surgery, Johns Hopkins Univ

Bavaria, Joseph MD (Thoracic Surgery) - *Special Expertise:* Aortic Surgery-Thoracic; Transplant-Lung; Heart Valve Surgery; **Admitting Hospital:** Hospital of the University of Pennsylvania; **Office Address:** Hosp of Univ Pennsylvania 3400 Spruce St Philadelphia, PA 19104; **Office Phone:** (215) 662-2017; **Board Certifications:** Surgery 1992, Thoracic Surgery 1993; **Medical School:** Tulane Univ 1983; **Residencies:** Thoracic Surgery, U Penn, Philadelphia, PA 1990-1992; Thoracic Surgery, Children's Hosp Philadelphia, Philadelphia, PA 1991-1992; **Fellowship:** U Penn, Philadelphia, PA 1986-1988; **Faculty Appointment:** Assoc Prof Surgery, Univ Penn

Boyd, Arthur D MD (Thoracic Surgery) - *Special Expertise:* Thoracic Surgery - General; **Admitting Hospital:** NYU Medical Center (Page 70); **Office Address:** 530 1st Ave, Ste 6D New York, NY 10016; **Office Phone:** (212) 263-7287; **Board Certifications:** Surgery 1966, Thoracic Surgery 1967; **Medical School:** Univ Pittsburgh 1957; **Residencies:** Surgery, Johns Hopkins, Baltimore, MD 1958-1960; Surgery, Cincinnati Genl Hosp, Cincinnati, OH 1960-1965; **Fellowships:** Surgery, Johns Hopkins, Baltimore, MD 1958-1959; Cincinnati Genl Hosp, Cincinnati, OH 1962-1963; **Faculty Appointment:** Prof Surgery, NYU Sch Med

THORACIC SURGERY   *Mid Atlantic*

Brodman, Richard Ferris MD (Thoracic Surgery) - *Special Expertise:* Thoracic Surgery - General; **Admitting Hospital:** New York Weill Cornell Medical Center - NY Presbyterian Hospital (Page 72); **Office Address:** NY Presby Hosp, Cardiothoracic Surgery 525 E 68th St, MS F2103 New York, NY 10021; **Office Phone:** (212) 746-1100; **Board Certifications:** Thoracic Surgery 1978, Surgery 1976; **Medical School:** Univ Fla Coll Med 1972; **Residencies:** Surgery, Montefiore Hosp Med Ctr, Bronx, NY 1972-1976; Thoracic Surgery, Montefiore Hosp Med Ctr, Bronx, NY 1976-1978; **Fellowship:** Univ Florida Sch Med, Gainesville, FL 1969-1970; **Faculty Appointment:** Prof Thoracic Surgery, Albert Einstein Coll Med

Conte Jr, John V MD (Thoracic Surgery) - *Special Expertise:* Transplant-Heart; Transplant-Lung; **Admitting Hospital:** Johns Hopkins Hospital - Baltimore (Page 65); **Office Address:** Johns Hopkins Hosp 600 N Wolfe St, Bldg Blalock - rm 618 Baltimore, MD 21287-4618; **Office Phone:** (410) 955-1753; **Board Certifications:** Surgery 1993, Thoracic Surgery 1997; **Medical School:** Georgetown Univ 1986; **Residencies:** Thoracic Surgery, Standford Univ, Palo Alto, CA 1992-1995; Surgery, Georgetown Univ, Washington, DC 1987-1992

Furukawa, Satoshi MD (Thoracic Surgery) - *Special Expertise:* Transplant-Heart; Transplant-Lung; Cardiac Surgery-High Risk; **Admitting Hospital:** Temple University Hospital; **Office Address:** Temple Univ Hosp 3401 N Broad St, Ste 300 Philadelphia, PA 19140; **Office Phone:** (215) 707-3601; **Board Certifications:** Surgery 1993, Thoracic Surgery 1996; **Medical School:** Univ Penn 1984; **Residencies:** Surgery, Univ of PA Hlth Sys, PA 1984-1991; Thoracic Surgery, Univ of PA Hlth Sys, PA 1991-1993; **Faculty Appointment:** Assoc Prof Thoracic Surgery, Temple Univ

Gardner, Timothy Joseph MD (Thoracic Surgery) - *Special Expertise:* Heart Failure; Bypass Surgery-High Risk; Heart Disease-Congenital; **Admitting Hospital:** University of Pennsylvania - Presbyterian Medical Center; **Office Address:** Hosp Univ Penn, Dept Cardiothoracic Surgery 3400 Spruce St , Bldg Silverstein - Fl 4 Philadelphia, PA 19104-4283; **Office Phone:** (215) 662-2022; **Board Certifications:** Surgery 1975, Thoracic Surgery 1996; **Medical School:** Georgetown Univ 1966; **Residencies:** Surgery, Johns Hopkins Hosp, Baltimore, MD 1967-1968; Surgery, Johns Hopkins Hosp, Baltimore, MD 1971-1976; **Fellowship:** Research, John Hopkins Hosp, Baltimore, MD 1970-1971; **Faculty Appointment:** Prof Surgery, Univ Penn

Graver, L. Michael MD (Thoracic Surgery) - *Special Expertise:* Cardiac Surgery; Heart Valve Surgery; **Admitting Hospital:** Long Island Jewish Medical Center; **Office Address:** Long Island Jewish Medical Center 270-05 76th Ave, Ste 2123 New Hyde Park, NY 11040; **Office Phone:** (718) 470-7464; **Board Certifications:** Surgery 1993, Thoracic Surgery 1995; **Medical School:** Albany Med Coll 1977; **Residencies:** Surgery, Roosevelt Hosp, New York, NY 1977-1982; Deaconess Hosp, Boston, MA 1983-1985; **Fellowship:** Cardiology (Cardiovascular Disease), NY Hosp-Cornell Med Ctr, New York, NY 1982-1983; **Faculty Appointment:** Assoc Prof Surgery, Albert Einstein Coll Med

Griepp, Randall MD (Thoracic Surgery) - *Special Expertise:* Aneurysm-Abdominal Aortic; **Admitting Hospital:** Mount Sinai Hospital (Page 70); **Office Address:** Mount Sinai Med Ctr, Dept Thoracic Surgery ANBG Bldg, Fl 7 - rm 54, Box 1028 New York, NY 10029; **Office Phone:** (212) 241-8181; **Board Certifications:** Thoracic Surgery 1997, Surgery 1977; **Medical School:** Stanford Univ 1967; **Residencies:** Thoracic Surgery, Stanford Univ Hosp, Stanford, CA 1968-1973; Internal Medicine, Bellevue Hosp Ctr, New York, NY 1967-1968; **Fellowship:** Thoracic Surgery, Stanford Univ Hosp, Stanford, CA 1971-1972

Griffith, Bartley MD (Thoracic Surgery) - *Special Expertise:* Transplant-Heart; **Admitting Hospital:** UPMC - Presbyterian University Hospital; **Office Address:** UPMC - Presbyterian Univ Hosp - CTS 20 Lothrop St, Ste C700 Pittsburgh, PA 15213-2582; **Office Phone:** (412) 648-9254; **Board Certifications:** Thoracic Surgery 1992, Surgery 1982; **Medical School:** Jefferson Med Coll 1974; **Residencies:** Surgery, Univ Hlth Ctr Hosp, Pittsburgh, PA 1978-1979; Thoracic Surgery, Univ Hlth Ctr Hosp, Pittsburgh, PA 1978-1979; **Fellowship:** Research, Univ Hlth Ctr Hosp, Pittsburgh, PA 1977-1978; **Faculty Appointment:** Prof Surgery, Univ Pittsburgh

Heitmiller, Richard F MD (Thoracic Surgery) - *Special Expertise:* Esophageal Surgery; Esophageal Cancer; Lung Cancer; **Admitting Hospital:** Johns Hopkins Hospital - Baltimore (Page 65); **Office Address:** Johns Hopkins Hosp- Dept. Surgery 600 N Wolfe St, rm Osler 624 Baltimore, MD; **Office Phone:** (410) 955-4408; **Board Certifications:** Surgery 1997, Thoracic Surgery 1999; **Medical School:** Johns Hopkins Univ 1979; **Residency:** Surgery, Mass Genl Hosp., Boston, MA 1980-1985; **Fellowship:** Thoracic Surgery, Mass Genl Hosp., Boston, MA 1985-1987; **Faculty Appointment:** Assoc Prof Surgery

Isom, O Wayne MD (Thoracic Surgery) - *Special Expertise:* Cardiac Surgery; **Admitting Hospital:** New York Weill Cornell Medical Center - NY Presbyterian Hospital (Page 72); **Office Address:** 525 E 68th St New York, NY 10021-4873; **Office Phone:** (212) 746-5151; **Board Certifications:** Surgery 1971, Thoracic Surgery 1972; **Medical School:** Univ Tex, Houston 1965; **Residency:** Surgery, Parkland Meml Hosp, Dallas, TX 1965-1970; **Fellowship:** Thoracic Surgery, NYU Med Ctr, New York, NY 1970-1972

Kaiser, Larry Robert MD (Thoracic Surgery) - *Special Expertise:* Lung Cancer; Emphysema; **Admitting Hospital:** Hospital of the University of Pennsylvania; **Office Address:** Hosp Univ Penn #4 Silverstien 3400 Spruce St Philadelphia, PA 19104-4219; **Office Phone:** (215) 662-7538; **Board Certification:** Thoracic Surgery 1996; **Medical School:** Tulane Univ 1977; **Residencies:** Surgery, UCLA Med Ctr, Los Angeles, CA 1978-1983; Thoracic Surgery, Univ Toronto, Canada 1983-1985; **Fellowship:** Surgical Oncology, UCLA Med Ctr, Los Angeles, CA 1979-1981; **Faculty Appointment:** Prof Surgery, Univ Penn

Kanda, Louis T MD (Thoracic Surgery) - *Special Expertise:* Heart Valve Surgery; **Admitting Hospital:** Washington Hospital Center - DC (Page 79); **Office Address:** Cardio & Thor Surg Assocs 106 Irving St NW, Bldg POB N. Tower - Fl 4300-N Washington, DC 20010; **Office Phone:** (202) 829-5602; **Board Certification:** Thoracic Surgery 1991; **Medical School:** Geo Wash Univ 1970; **Residency:** Surgery, Washington Hosp Ctr, Washington, DC 1971-1975; **Fellowship:** Thoracic Surgery, Cleveland Clin Fdn, Cleveland, OH 1978-1980; **Faculty Appointment:** Asst Prof Surgery, Howard Univ

Katz, Nevin M MD (Thoracic Surgery) - *Special Expertise:* Coronary Artery Surgery; Heart Valve Surgery; **Admitting Hospital:** Georgetown University Hospital; **Office Address:** Georgetown Univ, Dept Surg 3800 Reservoir Rd NW Washington, DC 20007; **Office Phone:** (202) 687-8725; **Board Certification:** Thoracic Surgery 1990; **Medical School:** Case West Res Univ 1971; **Residencies:** Cardiovascular Surgery, Boston Chldns Hosp, Birmingham, AL 1976; Thoracic Surgery, Univ Alabama, Birmingham, AL 1978-1980; **Fellowship:** Cardiovascular Surgery, Univ Alabama, Birmingham, AL 1977-1978; **Faculty Appointment:** Prof Surgery, Georgetown Univ

Keenan, Robert MD (Thoracic Surgery) - *Special Expertise:* Transplant-Lung; Lung Surgery; **Admitting Hospital:** UPMC - Presbyterian University Hospital; **Office Address:** University of Pittsburgh Medical Center Pittsburgh, PA; **Board Certification:** Surgery 1990; **Medical School:** Canada 1984; **Residency:** Surgery, Univ Toronto, Toronto Canada 1985-1989; **Fellowship:** Thoracic Surgery, Univ Pittsburgh Med Ctr, Pittsburgh, PA 1989

THORACIC SURGERY

Kormos, Robert MD (Thoracic Surgery) - *Special Expertise: Transplant-Heart; Heart-Artificial;* **Admitting Hospital:** UPMC - Presbyterian University Hospital; **Office Address:** UPMC Presbyterian 200 Lothrop St, Ste c700 Pittsburgh, PA 15213; **Office Phone:** (412) 648-8107; **Medical School:** Canada 1976; **Residency:** Surgery, Toronto Western Hosp, Toronto, Canada; **Fellowships:** Cardiothoracic Surgery, Toronto Genl Hosp, Toronto, Canada; Transplant Surgery, Univ Pitts Med Ctr, Pittsburgh, PA 1985-1987; **Faculty Appointment:** Assoc Prof Surgery, Univ Pittsburgh

Krellenstein, Daniel MD (Thoracic Surgery) - *Special Expertise: Thoracic Surgery - General;* **Admitting Hospital:** Mount Sinai Hospital (Page 70); **Office Address:** 16 E 98th St, Ste 1F New York, NY 10029-6545; **Office Phone:** (212) 423-9311; **Board Certifications:** Thoracic Surgery 1977, Surgery 1974; **Medical School:** SUNY Buffalo 1964; **Residency:** Surgery, SUNY Downstate, Brooklyn, NY 1965-1972; **Faculty Appointment:** Assoc Clin Prof Thoracic Surgery, Mount Sinai Sch Med

Landreneau, Rodney MD (Thoracic Surgery) - *Special Expertise: Thoracoscopy;* **Admitting Hospital:** Allegheny General Hospital; **Office Address:** Allegheny Genl Hosp, Dept Thor Surg 320 E North Ave Pittsburgh, PA 15212-4772; **Office Phone:** (412) 359-6412; **Board Certifications:** Surgery 1984, Thoracic Surgery 1994; **Medical School:** Louisiana State Univ 1965; **Residency:** Surgery, Parkland Meml Hosp, Dallas, TX 1978-1983; **Fellowship:** Cardiothoracic Surgery, Univ Mich Med Ctr, Ann Arbor, MI 1983-1985; **Faculty Appointment:** Prof Surgery, Hahnemann Univ

Lang, Samuel MD (Thoracic Surgery) - *Special Expertise: Coronary Artery Surgery; Heart Valve Surgery;* **Admitting Hospital:** St Vincents Catholic Medical Center of New York; **Office Address:** 170 W 12th St New York, NY 10011; **Office Phone:** (212) 604-2488; **Board Certification:** Thoracic Surgery 1996; **Medical School:** Univ Ala 1978; **Residencies:** Surgery, Center for Health Sci, Los Angeles, CA 1978-1982; Thoracic Surgery, NYU Medical, New York, NY 1982-1983; **Faculty Appointment:** Prof Surgery, Cornell Univ-Weil Med Coll

Mindich, Bruce MD (Thoracic Surgery) - *Special Expertise: Cardiac Surgery;* **Admitting Hospital:** The Valley Hospital (Page 72); **Office Address:** Valley Hosp-Ridgewood, Dept Cardiothoracic Surgery 223 N Van Dien Ave Ridgewood, NJ 07450-2736; **Office Phone:** (201) 447-8377; **Board Certification:** Thoracic Surgery 1979; **Medical School:** SUNY Downstate 1972; **Residencies:** Surgery, Jewish Hosp Med Ctr, Brooklyn, NY 1972-1975; Thoracic Surgery, Mt Sinai Hosp, New York, NY 1975-1977; **Fellowships:** Surgery, Cleveland Clinic, Cleveland, OH 1977-1978; Cardiology (Cardiovascular Disease), Univ Alabama Med Ctr, Birmingham, AL 1978

Oz, Mehmet Cengiz MD (Thoracic Surgery) - *Special Expertise: Transplant Medicine-Heart; Coronary Artery Surgery;* **Admitting Hospital:** Columbia Presbyterian Medical Center (Page 72); **Office Address:** New York Presbyterian Hospital, Dept of Surgery 177 Ft. Washington Ave, Bldg MHB - Fl 7GN - Ste 435 New York, NY 10032; **Office Phone:** (212) 305-4434; **Board Certifications:** Surgery 1992, Thoracic Surgery 1994; **Medical School:** Univ Penn 1986; **Residency:** Surgery, Columbia Presby Med Ctr, New York, NY 1987-1991; **Fellowship:** Thoracic Surgery, Columbia Presby Med Ctr, New York, NY 1991-1993; **Faculty Appointment:** Asst Prof Surgery, Columbia P&S

Rose, Eric A MD (Thoracic Surgery) - *Special Expertise: Transplant-Heart; Cardiothoracic Surgery;* **Admitting Hospital:** Columbia Presbyterian Medical Center (Page 72); **Office Address:** 177 Ft Washington Ave, Ste 7-435 New York, NY 10032; **Office Phone:** (212) 305-6380; **Board Certifications:** Thoracic Surgery 1992, Surgery 1975; **Medical School:** Columbia P&S 1975; **Residencies:** Surgery, Columbia Presby Med Ctr, New York, NY 1976-1979; Thoracic Surgery, Columbia Presby Med Ctr, New York, NY 1980-1981; **Faculty Appointment:** Prof Thoracic Surgery, Columbia P&S

Rusch, Valerie MD (Thoracic Surgery) - *Special Expertise:* Mesothelioma; **Admitting Hospital:** Memorial Sloan Kettering Cancer Center; **Office Address:** Meml Sloan Kettering Canc Ctr 1275 York Ave, Ste 867 New York, NY 10021; **Office Phone:** (212) 639-5873; **Board Certifications:** Surgery 1981, Thoracic Surgery 1983; **Medical School:** Columbia P&S 1975; **Residencies:** Surgery, Univ WA Med Ctr, Seattle, WA 1975-1980; Cardiothoracic Surgery, Univ WA Med Ctr, Seattle, WA 1980-1982; **Faculty Appointment:** Prof Surgery, Cornell Univ-Weil Med Coll

Samuels, Louis MD (Thoracic Surgery) - *Special Expertise:* Transplant-Heart; Artificial Heart; **Admitting Hospital:** Hahnemann University Hospital; **Office Address:** Hahnemann Univ Hosp, Dept Cardiothor Surg Broad & Vine St Philadelphia, PA 19102; **Office Phone:** (215) 762-7802; **Board Certifications:** Surgery 1994, Thoracic Surgery 1996; **Medical School:** Hahnemann Univ 1987; **Residencies:** Surgery, Hahnemann Hosp, Philadelphia, PA 1987-1992; Thoracic Surgery, Hahnemann Hosp, Philadelphia, PA 1992-1995; **Faculty Appointment:** Asst Prof Thoracic Surgery, Hahnemann Univ

Shennib, Hani MD (Thoracic Surgery) - *Special Expertise:* Coronary Artery Surgery; Robotics in Surgery; **Admitting Hospital:** Beth Israel Medical Center - New York; **Office Address:** 1090 Amsterdam Ave, Fl 7 - Ste 7A New York, NY 10025; **Office Phone:** (212) 523-2798; **Board Certifications:** Surgery 1987, Thoracic Surgery 1998; **Medical School:** Egypt 1975; **Residencies:** Surgery, C Middlesex Hosp/London Univ, London, England 1978-1979; Surgery, McGill Univ, Montreal, Canada 1980-1985; **Fellowship:** Thoracic Surgery, Univ Toronto, Toronto, Canada 1987-1988

Smith, Craig R MD (Thoracic Surgery) - *Special Expertise:* Coronary Artery Surgery; Transplant-Heart; **Admitting Hospital:** Columbia Presbyterian Medical Center (Page 72); **Office Address:** 177 Fort Washington Ave, Fl 7th - rm 435 New York, NY 10032; **Office Phone:** (212) 305-8312; **Board Certification:** Thoracic Surgery 1986; **Medical School:** Case West Res Univ 1977; **Residency:** Surgery, Strong Meml Hosp, Rochester, NY 1978-1982; **Fellowship:** Cardiothoracic Surgery, Columbia Presby Med Ctr, New York, NY 1982-1984

Strong III, Michael D MD (Thoracic Surgery) - *Special Expertise:* Coronary Artery Surgery-Off Pump; Heart Valve Surgery; **Admitting Hospital:** Hahnemann University Hospital; **Office Address:** Hahnemann Univ Hosp, Dept Cardiothor Surg Broad & Vine Sts, N Tower Bldg, Ste 744, MS 111 Philadelphia, PA 19102; **Office Phone:** (215) 762-7802; **Board Certifications:** Surgery 1974, Thoracic Surgery 1996; **Medical School:** Jefferson Med Coll 1966; **Residencies:** Surgery, Jefferson Hosp, Philadelphia, PA 1969-1973; Thoracic Surgery, Temple Univ Hosp, Philadelphia, PA 1973-1975; **Faculty Appointment:** Assoc Prof Thoracic Surgery, Hahnemann Univ

Stuart, Richard Scott MD (Thoracic Surgery) - *Special Expertise:* Cardiac Surgery; **Admitting Hospital:** Johns Hopkins Hospital - Baltimore (Page 65); **Office Address:** 600 N Wolfe St, Blalock 618 Baltimore, MD 21287; **Office Phone:** (410) 955-9780; **Board Certifications:** Thoracic Surgery 1990, Surgical Critical Care 1993; **Medical School:** Johns Hopkins Univ 1981; **Residency:** Surgery, Johns Hopkins Hosp, Baltimore, MD 1982-1986; **Fellowship:** Thoracic Surgery, Johns Hopkins Hosp, Baltimore, MD 1988-1989; **Faculty Appointment:** Assoc Prof Surgery, Johns Hopkins Univ

Tranbaugh, Robert MD (Thoracic Surgery) - *Special Expertise:* Thoracic Surgery - General; **Admitting Hospital:** Beth Israel Medical Center - Herbert & Nell Singer Division (Page 58); **Office Address:** Beth Israel Med Ctr 1st Ave at 16th St New York, NY 10003; **Office Phone:** (212) 420-2584; **Board Certifications:** Thoracic Surgery 1986, Surgery 1984; **Medical School:** Univ Penn 1976; **Residencies:** Surgery, UCSF, San Francisco, CA 1976-1983; Thoracic Surgery, UCSF, San Francisco, CA 1983-1985; **Faculty Appointment:** Asst Prof Thoracic Surgery, Albert Einstein Coll Med

Southeast

Alexander, James A MD (Thoracic Surgery) - *Special Expertise:* Transplant-Lung; Transplant-Heart; Cardiac Surgery-Adult & Pediatric; **Admitting Hospital:** Shands Healthcare at University Florida (Page 77); **Office Address:** Shands Healthcare at Univ of FL 1600 SW Archer Rd Gainesville, FL 32610-0286; **Office Phone:** (352) 846-0364; **Board Certifications:** Thoracic Surgery 1976, Surgical Critical Care 1993; **Medical School:** Duke Univ 1966; **Residency:** Thoracic Surgery, Duke Univ, Durham, NC 1967-1974; **Fellowship:** Thoracic Surgery, Duke Univ, Durham, NC; **Faculty Appointment:** Prof Thoracic Surgery, Univ Fla Coll Med

Craver, Joseph MD (Thoracic Surgery) - *Special Expertise:* Heart Bypass(off pump); **Admitting Hospital:** Emory University Hospital; **Office Address:** Emory Clinic 1365 Clifton Rd NE Atlanta, GA 30322; **Office Phone:** (404) 778-3480; **Board Certifications:** Surgery 1973, Thoracic Surgery 1975; **Medical School:** Univ NC Sch Med 1967; **Residencies:** Surgery, Mass Genl Hosp, Boston, MA 1968-1972; Thoracic Surgery, Univ of Virginia Hosp, Charlottesville, VA 1973-1974; **Fellowship:** Cardiology (Cardiovascular Disease), Mass Genl Hosp, Boston, MA 1972; **Faculty Appointment:** Prof Surgery, Emory Univ

Daniel, Thomas M MD (Thoracic Surgery) - *Special Expertise:* Esophageal Surgery; Thoracoscopy; Laparoscopic Surgery; **Admitting Hospital:** University of Virginia Health Systems; **Office Address:** Univ Virginia Hlth Scis Ctr, Dept of Surgery Box 800679 Charlottesville, VA 22908; **Office Phone:** (804) 924-5052; **Board Certifications:** Thoracic Surgery 1975, Vascular Surgery (General) 2006; **Medical School:** Univ VA Sch Med 1964; **Residencies:** Internal Medicine, Grady Meml Hosp-Emory Univ, Atlanta, GA 1965-1966; Surgery, Duke Med Ctr, Durham, NC 1968-1975; **Faculty Appointment:** Prof Surgery, Univ VA Sch Med

Egan, Thomas MD (Thoracic Surgery) - *Special Expertise:* Transplant-Lung; Thoracic Cancers; **Admitting Hospital:** University of North Carolina Hospitals; **Office Address:** Univ NC Hosp 108 Burnett Womack Bldg, CB 7065 Chapel Hill, NC 27599; **Office Phone:** (919) 966-3381; **Board Certification:** Thoracic Surgery 1999; **Medical School:** Univ Toronto 1984; **Residencies:** Surgery, Univ Toronto, Toronto, Canada 1980-1982; Thoracic Surgery, Univ Toronto, Toronto, Canada 1984-1988; **Fellowships:** Thoracic Surgery, Univ Toronto, Toronto, Canada 1982-1984; Thoracic Surgery, Washington Univ, St. Louis, MO 1988-1989; **Faculty Appointment:** Prof Surgery, Univ NC Sch Med

Glassford Jr, David M MD (Thoracic Surgery) - *Special Expertise:* Cardiac Surgery; **Admitting Hospital:** St Thomas Hospital - Nashville; **Office Address:** St Thomas Heart Inst-Cardio Surg Assocs PC 4230 Harding Rd, Ste 501 Nashville, TN 37205; **Office Phone:** (615) 385-4781; **Board Certifications:** Surgery 1988, Thoracic Surgery 1997; **Medical School:** Univ Tex Med Br, Galveston 1970; **Residencies:** Surgery, Unix Texas Med Br, Galveston, TX 1971-1975; Thoracic Surgery, Ochsner Clinic, New Orleans, LA 1975-1977; **Faculty Appointment:** Asst Clin Prof Thoracic Surgery, Vanderbilt Univ

Gray, Laman MD (Thoracic Surgery) - *Special Expertise:* Thoracic Surgery - General; **Admitting Hospital:** Jewish Hospital & Medical Center - Louisville; **Office Address:** 201 Abraham Flexner Way, Ste 1200 Louisville, KY 40202-3841; **Office Phone:** (502) 583-8383; **Board Certifications:** Thoracic Surgery 1975, Surgery 1973; **Medical School:** Johns Hopkins Univ 1967; **Residency:** Surgery, Univ Hosp, Ann Arbor, MI 1968-1972; **Faculty Appointment:** Prof Surgery, Univ Louisville Sch Med

Guyton, Robert A MD (Thoracic Surgery) - *Special Expertise:* Cardiac Surgery-Adult; **Admitting Hospital:** Emory University Hospital; **Office Address:** Emory Clinic 1365 Clifton Rd, Ste 2223 Atlanta, GA 30322; **Office Phone:** (404) 778-3836; **Board Certifications:** Thoracic Surgery 1990, Surgery 1989; **Medical School:** Harvard Med Sch 1971; **Residencies:** Mass Genl Hosp, Boston, MA 1973-1975; Mass Genl Hosp, Boston, MA 1979; **Fellowship:** Natl Heart Lung Inst 1973-1975

Hammon Jr, John W MD (Thoracic Surgery) - *Special Expertise:* Cardiac Surgery; **Admitting Hospital:** Wake Forest University Baptist Medical Center; **Office Address:** Wake Forest Univ Sch Med Medical Center Blvd Winston Salem, NC 27157-1096; **Office Phone:** (336) 716-6002; **Board Certifications:** Thoracic Surgery 1997, Surgery 1978; **Medical School:** Tulane Univ 1968; **Residency:** Duke Univ Med Ctr, Durham, NC 1969-1978; **Faculty Appointment:** Prof Thoracic Surgery, Wake Forest Univ Sch Med

Jones, Ellis MD (Thoracic Surgery) - *Special Expertise:* Coronary Artery Surgery; **Admitting Hospital:** Emory University Hospital; **Office Address:** Emory Univ Sch Med 1365 Clifton Rd Atlanta, GA; **Office Phone:** (404) 778-3484; **Board Certifications:** Surgery 1972, Thoracic Surgery 1972; **Medical School:** Emory Univ 1963; **Residency:** Surgery, Johns Hopkins Hosp, Baltimore, MD 1964-1965; **Fellowship:** Thoracic Surgery, Johns Hopkins Hosp, Baltimore, MD 1967-1972; **Faculty Appointment:** Prof Thoracic Surgery, Emory Univ

Kiernan, Paul Chapman MD (Thoracic Surgery) - *Special Expertise:* Vascular Surgery; **Admitting Hospital:** Fairfax Hospital; **Office Address:** Cardiovascular&Thoracic Surgery Assocs 3301 Woodburn Road, Ste 301 Annandale, VA 22003-1229; **Office Phone:** (703) 280-5858; **Board Certification:** Thoracic Surgery 1992; **Medical School:** Georgetown Univ 1974; **Residencies:** Surgery, Mayo Clin, Rochester 1975-1979; Thoracic Surgery, Mayo Clin, Rochester 1979-1981; **Fellowship:** Vascular Surgery (General), Mayo Clin, Rochester 1981-1982; **Faculty Appointment:** Assoc Clin Prof Surgery, Georgetown Univ

Kirklin, James MD (Thoracic Surgery) - *Special Expertise:* Transplant-Heart-Pediatric; Cardiac Surgery-Adult & Pediatric; **Admitting Hospital:** University of Alabama Hospital at Birmingham; **Office Address:** Univ AL Med Ctr, Dept Thoracic Surg 1530 3rd Ave S, Bldg Zeigler - rm 739 Birmingham, AL 35294; **Office Phone:** (205) 934-5167; **Board Certifications:** Surgery 1990, Thoracic Surgery 1981; **Medical School:** Harvard Med Sch 1973; **Residencies:** Surgery, Mass Genl Hosp, Boston, MA 1973-1974; Mass genl Hosp, Boston, MA 1978; **Fellowship:** Cardiothoracic Surgery, Chldns Hosp Ctr, Boston, MA 1979; **Faculty Appointment:** Prof Surgery, Univ Ala

Kron, Irving L MD (Thoracic Surgery) - *Special Expertise:* Coronary Artery Surgery; Transplant-Lung; **Admitting Hospital:** University of Virginia Health Systems; **Office Address:** Univ of Virginia Hlth Scis Ctr, Dept of Thoracic Surgery Box 800679 Charlottesville, VA 22908; **Office Phone:** (804) 924-2158; **Board Certifications:** Thoracic Surgery 1991, Surgical Critical Care 1996; **Medical School:** Med Coll Wisc 1975; **Residencies:** Surgery, Maine Med Ctr, Portland, ME 1975-1980; Thoracic Surgery, Univ Virginia Med Ctr, Charlottesville, NC 1980-1982; **Fellowship:** Thoracic Surgery, Univ Virginia Med Ctr, Charlottesville, NC 1980-1982; **Faculty Appointment:** Prof Thoracic Surgery, Univ VA Sch Med

Merrill, Walter H MD (Thoracic Surgery) - *Special Expertise:* Cardiothoracic Surgery; Cardiac Surgery-Adult & Pediatric; **Admitting Hospital:** Vanderbilt University Medical Center; **Office Address:** Vanderbilt Cardiac and Thoracic Surg Clin 1301 S 22ND Ave, rm 2986T Nashville, TN 37232-0001; **Office Phone:** (615) 322-0064; **Board Certifications:** Thoracic Surgery 1991, Surgical Critical Care 1999; **Medical School:** Johns Hopkins Univ 1974; **Residencies:** Thoracic Surgery, Natl Inst Hlth, Bethesda, MD 1976-1978; Thoracic Surgery, Johns Hopkins Hosp, Baltimore, MD 1980-1982; **Fellowship:** Pediatric Surgery, Hosp Sick Children, London England 1982-1983; **Faculty Appointment:** Prof Surgery, Vanderbilt Univ

Pacifico, Albert D MD (Thoracic Surgery) - *Special Expertise:* Cardiac Surgery; Heart Disease-Congenital; **Admitting Hospital:** University of Alabama Hospital at Birmingham; **Office Address:** Univ AL Hosp Birmingham 1900 University Blvd, Ste 760 Birmingham, AL 35294-0016; **Office Phone:** (205) 934-2344; **Board Certifications:** Surgery 1971, Thoracic Surgery 1971; **Medical School:** UMDNJ-NJ Med Sch, Newark 1964; **Residencies:** Surgery, Mayo Grad Sch Med, Rochester, MN 1965-1966; Thoracic Surgery, Univ AL Hosp, Birmingham, AL 1970-1972; **Fellowship:** Surgery, Univ AL Hosp, Birmingham, AL 1967-1968; **Faculty Appointment:** Prof Thoracic Surgery, Univ Ala

Perryman, Richard A MD (Thoracic Surgery) - *Special Expertise:* Cardiac Surgery-Adult & Pediatric; Cardiac Surgery-Adult; **Admitting Hospital:** Memorial Regional Hospital- Hollywood; **Office Address:** Memorial Heart Ctr 1150 N 35th Ave, Ste 440 Hollywood, FL 33021; **Office Phone:** (954) 962-5400; **Board Certification:** Thoracic Surgery 1994; **Medical School:** England 1967; **Residencies:** Thoracic Surgery, Duke Univ Med Ctr, Durham, NC 1969-1977; Thoracic Surgery, Univ Florida Med Coll, Gainesville, FL 1980-1981; **Fellowship:** Cardiology (Cardiovascular Disease), Duke Univ Med Ctr, Durham, NC 1970-1971; **Faculty Appointment:** Prof Thoracic Surgery, Univ Miami Sch Med

Pierson III, Richard Norris MD (Thoracic Surgery) - *Special Expertise:* Thoracic Surgery - General; **Admitting Hospital:** Vanderbilt University Medical Center; **Office Address:** The Vanderbilt Clinic Dept of Cardiac and Thor Surg Nashville, TN 37232; **Office Phone:** (615) 322-0069; **Board Certifications:** Surgery 1991, Therapeutic Radiology 1994; **Medical School:** Columbia P&S 1983; **Residency:** Surgery, Univ Mich, Ann Arbor, MI 1983-1990; **Fellowship:** Thoracic Surgery, Mass General Hosp, Boston, MA 1990-1992; **Faculty Appointment:** Asst Prof Thoracic Surgery, Vanderbilt Univ

Quintessenza, James MD (Thoracic Surgery) - *Special Expertise:* Transplant Medicine-Heart; Coronary Artery Surgery; Cardiovascular Surgery; **Admitting Hospital:** All Children's Hospital; **Office Address:** 603 7th St S, Ste 450 St Petersburg, FL 33701-4734; **Office Phone:** (727) 822-6666; **Board Certifications:** Thoracic Surgery 1989, Surgery 1987; **Medical School:** Univ Fla Coll Med 1981; **Residency:** Surgery, Univ FL, Gainesville, FL 1982-1986; **Fellowship:** Thoracic Surgery, UCSD, San Diego, CA 1986-1988

Smith, Peter Kent MD (Thoracic Surgery) - *Special Expertise:* Coronary Artery Surgery; Heart Valve Surgery; **Admitting Hospital:** Duke University Medical Center (Page 60); **Office Address:** Duke Univ Med Ctr Box 3442 Durham, NC 27710; **Office Phone:** (919) 684-2890; **Board Certifications:** Surgery 1995, Thoracic Surgery 1998; **Medical School:** Duke Univ 1977; **Residencies:** Surgery, Duke Univ, Durham, NC 1977-1987; Thoracic Surgery, Duke Univ, Durham, NC 1984-1987; **Faculty Appointment:** Prof Surgery, Duke Univ

Staples, Edward D MD (Thoracic Surgery) - *Special Expertise:* Transplant-Heart & Lung; Ventricular Assist Devices; **Admitting Hospital:** Shands Healthcare at University Florida (Page 77); **Office Address:** Shands Hlthcare at Univ FL, Dept CardioThoracic Surg 1600 SW Archer Rd, Box 100286 Gainesville, FL 32610-0268; **Office Phone:** (352) 846-0362; **Board Certifications:** Thoracic Surgery 1997, Surgical Critical Care 1993; **Medical School:** Univ S Fla Coll Med 1977; **Residencies:** Med Coll Virginia, Richmond, VA 1978-1979; Surgery, Univ Hosp, Jacksonville, FL 1979-1982; **Fellowship:** Cardiothoracic Surgery, Univ Florida, Gainesville, FL 1982-1984; **Faculty Appointment:** Assoc Prof Surgery, Univ Fla Coll Med

Tedder, Mark MD (Thoracic Surgery) - *Special Expertise: Transplant Medicine-Heart; Cardiac Surgery;* **Admitting Hospital:** St Thomas Hospital - Nashville; **Office Address:** St Thomas Heart Inst-Cardio Surg Assocs PC 4230 Harding Rd, Ste 501 Nashville, TN 37205; **Office Phone:** (615) 385-4781; **Board Certifications:** Surgery 1996, Thoracic Surgery 1998; **Medical School:** Duke Univ 1988; **Residencies:** Surgery, Duke Univ Med Ctr, Durham, NC 1988-1990; Thoracic Surgery, Duke Univ Med Ctr, Durham, NC 1995-1996; **Fellowship:** Surgery, Duke Univ Med Ctr, Durham, NC 1990-1992

Ungerleider, Ross M MD (Thoracic Surgery) - *Special Expertise: Heart Disease-Congenital; Cardiac Surgery-Adult & Pediatric;* **Admitting Hospital:** Duke University Medical Center (Page 60); **Office Address:** Duke Univ Med Ctr Box 3178 Durham, NC 27710; **Office Phone:** (919) 681-2343; **Board Certification:** Thoracic Surgery 1997; **Medical School:** Rush Med Coll 1977; **Residencies:** Surgery, Duke Univ Med Ctr, Durham, NC 1978-1979; Thoracic Surgery, Duke Univ Med Ctr, Durham, NC 1981-1987; **Fellowship:** Thoracic Surgery, Duke Univ Med Ctr, Durham, NC 1979-1981; **Faculty Appointment:** Prof Surgery, Duke Univ

Wilcox, Benson MD (Thoracic Surgery) - *Special Expertise: Cardiothoracic Surgery;* **Admitting Hospital:** University of North Carolina Hospitals; **Office Address:** Univ NC Hosp 108 Burnett-Womack, Box 7065 Chapel Hill, NC 27599-7065; **Office Phone:** (919) 966-3381; **Board Certifications:** Surgery 1965, Thoracic Surgery 1966; **Medical School:** Univ NC Sch Med 1957; **Residencies:** Surgery, Barnes Jewish Hosp, St Louis, MO 1958-1959; Surgery, NC Meml Hosp, Chapel Hill, NC 1959-1964; **Fellowship:** Thoracic Surgery, Natl Inst Hlth, Bethesda, MD 1960-1962; **Faculty Appointment:** Prof Surgery, Univ NC Sch Med

Williams, Donald B MD (Thoracic Surgery) - *Special Expertise: Cardiac Surgery;* **Admitting Hospital:** Mount Sinai Medical Center; **Office Address:** 4300 Alton Rd, Ste 211 Miami Beach, FL 33140-2800; **Office Phone:** (305) 674-2780; **Board Certifications:** Anatomic Pathology 1988, Thoracic Surgery 1990; **Medical School:** Jefferson Med Coll 1974; **Residency:** Surgery, Dartmouth-Hitchcock Med Ctr, Lebanon, NH 1975-1979; **Fellowship:** Thoracic Surgery, Mayo Clinic, Rochester, MN 1979-1981

Zorn, George L. MD (Thoracic Surgery) - *Special Expertise: Transplant-Lung; Lung Cancer;* **Admitting Hospital:** University of Alabama Hospital at Birmingham; **Office Address:** Univ Ala at Birm - Bldg 720THT 1900 Univ Blvd Birmingham, AL 35294; **Office Phone:** (205) 934-2536; **Board Certifications:** Thoracic Surgery 1987, Surgery 1974; **Medical School:** Emory Univ 1968; **Residencies:** Surgery, Columbia - Presby Hosp, New York, NY 1969-1973; Thoracic Surgery, Univ Alabama, Birmingham, IL 1975-1977; **Faculty Appointment:** Assoc Prof Surgery, Univ Ala

Midwest

Bassett, Joseph MD (Thoracic Surgery) - *Special Expertise: Heart Valve Surgery; Coronary Artery Surgery;* **Admitting Hospital:** William Beaumont Hospital; **Office Address:** 1663 W Big Beaver Rd Troy, MI 48084; **Office Phone:** (248) 643-8633; **Board Certifications:** Surgery 1967, Transplant Surgery 1969; **Medical School:** Wayne State Univ 1961; **Residencies:** Surgery, Wayne State Univ Affil Hosp, Detroit, MI 1962-1966; Thoracic Surgery, Wayne State Univ Affil Hosp, Detroit, MI 1966-1968; **Faculty Appointment:** Assoc Clin Prof Surgery, Wayne State Univ

Behrendt, Douglas M. MD (Thoracic Surgery) - *Special Expertise: Cardiothoracic Surgery;* **Admitting Hospital:** University of Iowa Hospitals and Clinics; **Office Address:** U Iowa Hosps & Clinics-Dept Surg-Div CTS 200 Hawkins Iowa City, IA 52242; **Office Phone:** (319) 356-2761; **Board Certifications:** Surgery 1972, Thoracic Surgery 1972; **Medical School:** Harvard Med Sch 1963; **Residencies:** Surgery, Mass Genl Hosp, Boston, MA 1964-1971; NIH, Bethesda, MD 1967-1968; **Fellowship:** Pediatric Cardiology, Hosp Sick Chldns, London England 1969-1970; **Faculty Appointment:** Prof Thoracic Surgery, Univ Iowa Coll Med

Bolman III, Ralph Morton MD (Thoracic Surgery) - *Special Expertise:* Transplant-Heart; Cardiothoracic Surgery; **Admitting Hospital:** Fairview-University Medical Center - University Campus; **Office Address:** Fairview Univ Med Ctr, Dept CV & Thor Surg 420 Deleware St SE, Box 207 Minneapolis, MN 55455; **Office Phone:** (612) 625-3902; **Board Certifications:** Surgery 1991, Thoracic Surgery 1993; **Medical School:** St Louis Univ 1973; **Residency:** Surgery, Duke Univ Med Ctr, Durham, NC 1974-1980; **Fellowship:** Thoracic Surgery, Univ Minn Hosp, Minneapolis, MN 1980-1982

Brown, John W MD (Thoracic Surgery) - *Special Expertise:* Cardiac Surgery-Adult & Pediatric; **Admitting Hospital:** Riley Hospital for Children; **Office Address:** 545 Barnhill Dr, Emerson Hall 215 Indianapolis, IN 46202-5112; **Office Phone:** (317) 274-7150; **Board Certifications:** Surgery 1977, Thoracic Surgery 1998; **Medical School:** Indiana Univ 1970; **Residencies:** Surgery, Univ Mich Med Ctr, Ann Arbor, MI 1974-1976; Cardiothoracic Surgery, Univ Mich Med Ctr, Ann Arbor, MI 1976-1978; **Fellowship:** Natl Heart Lung-Blood Inst 1972-1974; **Faculty Appointment:** Prof Surgery, Indiana Univ

Cooper, Joel David MD (Thoracic Surgery) - *Special Expertise:* Transplant-Lung; Lung Volume Reduction; **Admitting Hospital:** Barnes - Jewish Hospital; **Office Address:** Barnes-Jewish Hosp, Queeny Tower 1 Barnes-Jewish Hosp Plaza, Fl 3108 St Louis, MO 63110-1013; **Office Phone:** (314) 362-6021; **Board Certifications:** Surgery 1971, Thoracic Surgery 1972; **Medical School:** Harvard Med Sch 1964; **Residencies:** Surgery, Mass Genl Hosp, Boston, MA 1965-1968; Frenchay Hosp, Bristol England 1968; **Fellowship:** Hammersmith Hosp, London England 1969; **Faculty Appointment:** Prof Surgery, Washington Univ, St Louis

Cosgrove III, Delos M MD (Thoracic Surgery) - *Special Expertise:* Heart Valve Surgery; Minimally Invasive Surgery; **Admitting Hospital:** Cleveland Clinic Foundation; **Office Address:** Cleveland Clinic Fdn, Dept Thor & CV Surg 9500 Euclid Ave, MS F25 Cleveland, OH 44195; **Office Phone:** (216) 444-6733; **Board Certifications:** Surgery 1975, Thoracic Surgery 1996; **Medical School:** Univ VA Sch Med 1966; **Residencies:** Surgery, Strong Meml Hosp, Rochester, NY 1967-1968; Surgery, Mass Genl Hosp, Boston, MA 1970-1972

Danielson, Gordon MD (Thoracic Surgery) - *Special Expertise:* Heart Disease-Congenital; Ebstein's Anomaly; Hypertrophic Obstructive Cardiomyopathy; **Admitting Hospital:** Mayo Medical Center & Clinic - Rochester; **Office Address:** Mayo Med Ctr 200 1st St SW Rochester, MN 55905-0001; **Office Phone:** (507) 255-7062; **Board Certifications:** Surgery 1963, Thoracic Surgery 1963; **Medical School:** Univ Penn 1956; **Residencies:** Surgery, Univ Hosp - Univ MI, Ann Arbor, MI 1956-1957; Thoracic Surgery, Hosp Univ Penn, Philadelphia, PA 1957-1961; **Fellowships:** Thoracic Surgery, Univ Hosp - Univ Penn, Philadelphia, PA 1962-1963; Cardiothoracic Surgery, Karolinska Sjukhuset, Stokholm, Sweden 1963-1964; **Faculty Appointment:** Prof Surgery, Mayo Med Sch

DeCamp Jr, Malcolm M MD (Thoracic Surgery) - *Special Expertise:* Cardiac Surgery; **Admitting Hospital:** Cleveland Clinic Foundation; **Office Address:** Cleveland Clinic Foundation 9500 Euclid Ave, Desk A-25 Cleveland, OH 44195; **Office Phone:** (216) 444-2200; **Board Certifications:** Thoracic Surgery 2004, Surgery 2002; **Medical School:** Univ Louisville Sch Med 1983; **Residencies:** Surgery, Brighams & Womens Hosp, Boston, MA 1984-1986; Surgery, Brighams & Womens Hosp, Boston, MA 1988-1993; **Faculty Appointment:** Asst Prof Surgery, Harvard Med Sch

Deschamps, Claude MD (Thoracic Surgery) - *Special Expertise:* Gastroesophageal Reflux; Achalasia; Esophageal/Lung Cancer; **Admitting Hospital:** St Mary's Hospital; **Office Address:** Mayo Clinic 200 First St SW Rochester, MN 55905; **Office Phone:** (507) 284-2644; **Board Certification:** Surgery 1994; **Medical School:** Univ Montreal 1979; **Residencies:** Surgery, Univ Montreal Hosps, Canada 1980-1984; Thoracic Surgery, Univ Montreal Hosp, Montreal, Canada 1984-1985; **Fellowship:** Thoracic Surgery, Mayo Clinic, Rochester, MN 1985-1987

Faber, L Penfield MD (Thoracic Surgery) - *Special Expertise:* Lung Cancer; Thoracic Cancers; **Admitting Hospital:** Rush/Presbyterian - St Luke's Medical Center - Chicago (Page 74); **Office Address:** 1725 W Harrison St, Ste 218 Chicago, IL 60612; **Office Phone:** (312) 738-3732; **Board Certifications:** Surgery 1962, Thoracic Surgery 1963; **Medical School:** Northwestern Univ 1956; **Residencies:** Surgery, Presbyterian-St Lukes Hosp, Chicago, IL 1957-1961; Thoracic Surgery, Hines VA Hosp 1961-1963; **Faculty Appointment:** Prof Surgery, Rush Med Coll

Ferguson, Mark MD (Thoracic Surgery) - *Special Expertise:* Barrett's Esophagus; Esophageal Cancer; **Admitting Hospital:** University of Chicago Hospitals (Page 78); **Office Address:** Univ Chicago Hosp 5841 S Maryland Ave # Mc5035 Chicago, IL 60637-1463; **Office Phone:** (773) 702-3551; **Board Certifications:** Surgery 1993, Thoracic Surgery 1985; **Medical School:** Univ Chicago-Pritzker Sch Med 1977; **Residency:** Surgery, Univ Chicago Hosps, Chicago, IL 1978-1982; **Fellowship:** Cardiothoracic Surgery, Univ Chicago Hosps, Chicago, IL 1982-1984; **Faculty Appointment:** Prof Thoracic Surgery, Univ Chicago-Pritzker Sch Med

Frederiksen, James W MD (Thoracic Surgery) - *Special Expertise:* Cardiothoracic Surgery; **Admitting Hospital:** Northwestern Memorial Hospital; **Office Address:** Northwestern Univ Med Sch 251 E Chicago Ave, Ste 628 Chicago, IL 60611-2643; **Office Phone:** (312) 908-3121; **Board Certifications:** Surgery 1980, Thoracic Surgery 1982; **Medical School:** Harvard Med Sch 1972; **Residencies:** Surgery, Peter Bent Brigham Hosp, Boston, MA 1973-1978; Cardiothoracic Surgery, Northwestern Meml Hosp, Chicago, IL 1978-1980; **Fellowship:** Cardiothoracic Surgery, Johns Hopkins Hosp, Baltimore, MD 1974-1976; **Faculty Appointment:** Assoc Prof Surgery, Northwestern Univ

Iannettoni, Mark D. MD (Thoracic Surgery) - *Special Expertise:* Transplant-Lung; **Admitting Hospital:** University of Michigan Health Center; **Office Address:** Univ of Michigan Taubman Hlth Care Ctr 1500 E Med Ctr Dr, RM 2120, Box 0344 Ann Arbor, MI 48109-0344; **Office Phone:** (734) 763-7418; **Board Certifications:** Thoracic Surgery 1994, Surgery 1993; **Medical School:** SUNY Syracuse 1985; **Residencies:** Thoracic Surgery, Univ Mich Med Sch, Ann Arbor, MI 1991-1993; Thoracic Surgery, SUNY Upstate, New York, NY 1986-1991; **Fellowship:** Thoracic Surgery, Univ Mich Med Sch, Ann Arbor, MI 1993-1994; **Faculty Appointment:** Assoc Prof Thoracic Surgery, Univ Mich Med Sch

Karp, Robert Bruce MD (Thoracic Surgery) - *Special Expertise:* Transplant-Heart; Aortic Surgery-Thoracic; Heart Valve Surgery; **Admitting Hospital:** University of Chicago Hospitals (Page 78); **Office Address:** 5841 S Maryland Ave, Box MC 5040 Chicago, IL 60637-1463; **Office Phone:** (773) 702-2500; **Board Certifications:** Thoracic Surgery 1970, Surgery 1967; **Medical School:** UCSF 1958; **Residencies:** Univ Alabama, Birmingham, AL 1967-1969; UCSF, San Francisco, CA 1962-1967; **Faculty Appointment:** Prof Thoracic Surgery, Univ Chicago-Pritzker Sch Med

Lytle, Bruce Whitney MD (Thoracic Surgery) - *Special Expertise:* Heart Valve Surgery-Mitral; Coronary Artery Surgery; **Admitting Hospital:** Cleveland Clinic Foundation; **Office Address:** Cleveland Clinic Fdn 9500 Euclid Ave, MS F25 Cleveland, OH 44195; **Office Phone:** (216) 444-6962; **Board Certification:** Thoracic Surgery 1998; **Medical School:** Harvard Med Sch 1971; **Residencies:** Surgery, Mass Genl Hsop, Boston, MA 1971-1975; Shotley Bridge Hosp, England 1975-1976; **Fellowship:** Thoracic Surgery, Mass Genl Hosp, Boston, MA 1977

McCarthy, Patrick McGuane MD (Thoracic Surgery) - *Special Expertise:* Transplant-Heart; *Maze Procedure;* **Admitting Hospital:** Cleveland Clinic Foundation; **Office Address:** Cleveland Clinic Foundation 9500 Euclid Ave, MS F25 Cleveland, OH 44195-0001; **Office Phone:** (216) 444-0648; **Board Certification:** Thoracic Surgery 1998; **Medical School:** Loyola Univ-Stritch Sch Med 1980; **Residencies:** Thoracic Surgery, Mayo Clinic, Rochester, MN 1985-1988; Surgery, Mayo Clinic, Rochester, MN 1980-1985; **Fellowship:** Cardiothoracic Surgery, Stanford Univ, Palo Alto, CA 1988-1989

McGregor, Christopher MD (Thoracic Surgery) - *Special Expertise:* Transplant-Heart & Lung; Cardiac Surgery; **Admitting Hospital:** Mayo Medical Center & Clinic - Rochester; **Office Address:** Mayo Clinic - St Mary's Hospital 2-716 Mary Brigh D Bldg Rochester, MN 55905; **Office Phone:** (507) 255-6038; **Medical School:** Scotland 1972; **Residencies:** Surgery, Edinburgh Royal Infirm, Scotland 1973-1978; Surgery, Glasgow Royal Infirm, Scotland 1979-1981; **Fellowship:** Cardiothoracic Transplantation, Stanford Univ Hosp, Stanford, CA 1983-1984; **Faculty Appointment:** Prof Surgery, Mayo Med Sch

Meyers, Bryan MD (Thoracic Surgery) - *Special Expertise:* Lung Cancer; Esophageal Cancer; **Admitting Hospital:** Barnes - Jewish Hospital; **Office Address:** 3108 Queeny Tower 1 Barnes Hospital Plaza St Louis, MO 63110; **Office Phone:** (314) 362-8598; **Board Certifications:** Surgery 1998, Thoracic Surgery 1999; **Medical School:** Univ Chicago-Pritzker Sch Med 1986; **Residency:** Surgery, Mass Genl Hosp, Boston, MA 1990-1996; **Fellowship:** Cardiothoracic Surgery, Barnes Hosp-Wash Univ, St Louis, MO 1996-1998; **Faculty Appointment:** Asst Prof Surgery, Washington Univ, St Louis

Michler, Robert MD (Thoracic Surgery) - *Special Expertise:* Transplant-Heart; Coronary Artery Surgery; **Admitting Hospital:** Ohio State University Medical Center; **Office Address:** Ohio State Univ Med Ctr 410 W 10th Ave Doan Bldg N847 Columbus, OH 43210; **Office Phone:** (614) 935-5502; **Board Certifications:** Surgery 1990, Thoracic Surgery 1988; **Medical School:** Dartmouth Med Sch 1981; **Residencies:** Surgery, Columbia Presby Med Ctr, New York, NY 1981-1987; Transplant Surgery, Columbia Presby Med Ctr, New York, NY 1984-1985; **Fellowships:** Thoracic Surgery, Columbia Presby Med Ctr, New York, NY 1987-1989; Pediatric Surgery, Harvard Med Sch, Cambridge, MA 1989-1990; **Faculty Appointment:** Prof Surgery, Ohio State Univ

Orringer, Mark B MD (Thoracic Surgery) - *Special Expertise:* Esophageal Cancer; Esophageal Disease, Benign; Cardiothoracic Surgery; **Admitting Hospital:** University of Michigan Health Center; **Office Address:** 1500 E Medical Ctr. Dr., rm 2120, Box 0344 Taubman Health Care Ctr. Ann Arbor, MI 48109-0344; **Office Phone:** (734) 936-5800; **Board Certifications:** Thoracic Surgery 1974, Surgery 1973; **Medical School:** Univ Pittsburgh 1967; **Residencies:** Surgery, Frenchay Hosp., Bristol 1970; Johns Hopkins Hosp., Baltimore, MD 1968-1973; **Faculty Appointment:** Prof Surgery, Univ Mich Med Sch

Pagani, Francis Domenic MD (Thoracic Surgery) - *Special Expertise:* Transplant-Heart; **Admitting Hospital:** University of Michigan Health Center; **Office Address:** 1500 E Medical Center Drive Ann Arbor, MI 48109; **Office Phone:** (734) 647-2894; **Board Certifications:** Surgery 1994, Thoracic Surgery 1996; **Medical School:** Georgetown Univ 1986; **Residencies:** Surgery, Georgetown Univ Med Ctr, Washinton, DC 1986-1993; Thoracic Surgery, Univ Michigan Hosp, Ann Arbor, MI 1993-1995; **Faculty Appointment:** Asst Prof Thoracic Surgery, Univ Mich Med Sch

Pairolero, Peter MD (Thoracic Surgery) - *Special Expertise:* Chest Wall Tumors; **Admitting Hospital:** Mayo Medical Center & Clinic - Rochester; **Office Address:** Mayo Clinic 200 1st St SW Rochester, MN 55905-4317; **Office Phone:** (507) 284-2511; **Board Certifications:** Thoracic Surgery 1974, Surgery 1972; **Medical School:** Univ Mich Med Sch 1963; **Residencies:** Surgery, Mayo Grad Sch Med, Rochester, MN 1966-1971; Thoracic Surgery, Mayo Grad Sch Med, Rochetser, MN 1971-1973; **Fellowship:** Cerebrovascular Disease, Mayo Grad Sch Med, Rochester, MN 1968-1969

Pass, Harvey MD (Thoracic Surgery) - *Special Expertise:* Cardiothoracic Surgery; **Admitting Hospital:** Harper Hospital (Page 59); **Office Address:** Harper Hosp - Wayne State Univ 3990 John R St, Ste 2102 Detroit, MI 48201; **Office Phone:** (313) 745-1413; **Board Certifications:** Surgery 1981, Thoracic Surgery 1992; **Medical School:** Duke Univ 1973; **Residencies:** Surgery, Duke Univ Med Ctr, Durham, NC 1973-1975; Surgery, Univ Miss Med Ctr, Jackson, MI 1977-1980; **Fellowship:** Cardiothoracic Surgery, MUSC Med Ctr, Charleston, SC 1980-1982; **Faculty Appointment:** Prof Surgery, Wayne State Univ

Patterson, George Alexander MD (Thoracic Surgery) - *Special Expertise:* Transplant-Lung; **Admitting Hospital:** Barnes - Jewish Hospital; **Office Address:** One Barnes Jewish Hospital Plaza Queens Tower, Ste 3108 St Louis, MO 63110; **Office Phone:** (314) 362-6025; **Board Certifications:** Surgery 1978, Thoracic Surgery 1981; **Medical School:** Canada 1974; **Residencies:** Surgery, Queens Univ, Kingston 1975-1978; Vascular Surgery (General), Unniv of Toronto 1978-1979; **Fellowships:** Research, Toronto Genl Hosp, Toronto Canada 1980-1981; Research, John Hopkins Univ, Baltimore, MD 1981-1982; **Faculty Appointment:** Prof Surgery, Washington Univ, St Louis

Piccione, William MD (Thoracic Surgery) - *Special Expertise:* Transplant Medicine-Heart; **Admitting Hospital:** Rush/Presbyterian - St Luke's Medical Center - Chicago (Page 74); **Office Address:** 1725 W Harrison St, Ste 425 Chicago, IL 60612; **Office Phone:** (312) 563-2235; **Board Certifications:** Surgery 1997, Thoracic Surgery 1999; **Medical School:** Univ Rochester 1980; **Residency:** Surgery, Harvard Surg Svc-New England Deaconess Hosp, Boston, MA 1981-1986; **Fellowships:** Cardiothoracic Surgery, Rush Presbyterian-St Lukes Med Ctr, Chicago, IL 1986-1988; Thoracic Surgery, Meml Sloan Kettering 1988; **Faculty Appointment:** Prof Medicine, Rush Med Coll

Schaff, Hartzell MD (Thoracic Surgery) - *Special Expertise:* Heart Valve Surgery; Heart Disease-Congenital; **Admitting Hospital:** St Mary's Hospital; **Office Address:** Mayo Clin, Dept Cardiovasc Surg 200 First St SW Rochester, MN 55905; **Office Phone:** (507) 255-7068; **Board Certifications:** Surgery 1980, Thoracic Surgery 1992; **Medical School:** Univ Okla Coll Med 1973; **Residencies:** Surgery, Johns Hopkins Hosp, Baltimore, MD 1974-1978; Thoracic Surgery, Johns Hopkins Hosp, Baltimore, MD 1978-1980; **Fellowship:** Surgery, Johns Hopkins Hosp, Baltimore, MD 1975-1975; **Faculty Appointment:** Prof Surgery, Mayo Med Sch

Silverman, Norman A MD (Thoracic Surgery) - *Special Expertise:* Heart Valve Surgery; Aneurysm-Abdominal Aortic; **Admitting Hospital:** Henry Ford Health System (Page 62); **Office Address:** Henry Ford Hosp, Div Cardiothor Surg 2799 W Grand Blvd Detroit, MI 48202; **Office Phone:** (313) 876-2692; **Board Certifications:** Surgery 1989, Thoracic Surgery 1990; **Medical School:** Boston Univ 1971; **Residencies:** Surgery, Duke Univ Med Ctr, Durham, NC 1972-1973; Thoracic Surgery, Duke Univ Med Ctr, Durham, NC 1975-1980

Smedira, Nicholas MD (Thoracic Surgery) - *Special Expertise:* Transplant-Heart; Transplant-Lung; **Admitting Hospital:** Cleveland Clinic Foundation; **Office Address:** Cleveland Clinic Foundation 9500 Euclid Ave, Ste F25, MS Desk F25 Cleveland, OH 44195; **Office Phone:** (216) 445-7052; **Board Certifications:** Surgery 1992, Thoracic Surgery 1995; **Medical School:** Univ Rochester 1995; **Residencies:** Surgery, UCSF Med Ctr, San Francisco, CA 1984-1991; Thoracic Surgery, UCSF Med Ctr, San Francisco, CA 1992-1994

Sundt III, Thoralf Mauritz MD (Thoracic Surgery) - *Special Expertise: Transplant-Heart & Lung; Aneurysm; Cardiothoracic Surgery;* **Admitting Hospital:** Barnes - Jewish Hospital; **Office Address:** 1 Barnes-Jewish Hosp Plaza Queeny Tower, Ste 4105 St Louis, MO 63110; **Office Phone:** (314) 362-8008; **Board Certifications:** Surgery 1987, Thoracic Surgery 1993; **Medical School:** Johns Hopkins Univ 1984; **Residencies:** Surgery, Mass Genl Hosp, Boston, MA 1985-1991; Cardiothoracic Surgery, Wash Univ Sch Med, St Louis, MO 1991-1993; **Fellowship:** Cardiothoracic Surgery, Harefield Hosp, London, England 1993-1994; **Faculty Appointment:** Asst Prof Surgery, Washington Univ, St Louis

Turrentine, Mark W MD (Thoracic Surgery) - *Special Expertise: Cardiac Surgery-Pediatric; Transplant-Heart & Lung;* **Admitting Hospital:** Riley Hospital for Children; **Office Address:** 545 Barnhill Dr, Emerson Hall, Ste 215 Indianapolis, IN 46202; **Office Phone:** (317) 274-1121; **Board Certifications:** Surgery 1989, Thoracic Surgery 1992; **Medical School:** Univ Kans 1983; **Residencies:** Surgery, Univ Kansas, Wichita, KS 1984-1988; Cardiothoracic Surgery, Indiana Univ Med Ctr, Indianapolis, IN 1989-1991; **Fellowships:** Cardiothoracic Surgery, Texas Heart Inst, Houston, TX 1986; Transplant Surgery, Indiana Univ Med Ctr, Indianapolis, IN 1988-1989; **Faculty Appointment:** Assoc Prof Surgery, Indiana Univ

Great Plains and Mountains

Doty, Donald B. MD (Thoracic Surgery) - *Special Expertise: Cardiac Surgery-Adult;* **Admitting Hospital:** LDS Hospital; **Office Address:** 324 10th Ave, Ste 160 Salt Lake City, UT 84103; **Office Phone:** (801) 322-0563; **Board Certifications:** Thoracic Surgery 1971, Surgery 1968; **Medical School:** Stanford Univ 1962; **Residency:** Los Angeles Co Hosp, Los Angeles, CA 1963-1967; **Fellowship:** Thoracic Surgery, Univ Ala Med Ctr, Birmingham, AL 1969-1971; **Faculty Appointment:** Clin Prof Thoracic Surgery, Univ Utah

Karwande, Shreekanth V MD (Thoracic Surgery) - *Special Expertise: Thoracic Surgery - General;* **Admitting Hospital:** University of Utah Hospital and Clinics; **Office Address:** Univ Utah Med Ctr, Cardio Thors 50 N Med Dr Salt Lake City, UT 84132-0001; **Office Phone:** (801) 581-5311; **Board Certifications:** Surgical Critical Care 1989, Thoracic Surgery 1993; **Medical School:** India 1973; **Residencies:** Surgery, Erie Co Med Ctr, Buffalo, NY 1976-1981; Surgery, NY Hosp-Cornell Med Ctr, New York, NY 1982-1985; **Faculty Appointment:** Assoc Prof Surgery, Univ Utah

Pomerantz, Marvin MD (Thoracic Surgery) - *Special Expertise: Tuberculosis;* **Admitting Hospital:** University of Colorado Health & Science Center; **Office Address:** 4200 E Ninth Ave Denver, CO; **Office Phone:** 303 3153035; **Board Certifications:** Surgery 1968, Thoracic Surgery 1968; **Medical School:** Univ Rochester 1959; **Residencies:** Surgery, Duke Univ Med Ctr, Durham, NC 1959-1963; Thoracic Surgery, Duke Univ Med Ctr, Durham, NC 1963-1967; **Faculty Appointment:** Prof Surgery, Univ Colo

Southwest

Antakli, Tamim MD (Thoracic Surgery) - *Special Expertise: Thoracic Surgery - General;* **Admitting Hospital:** University of Arkansas for Medical Sciences; **Office Address:** Univ Hosp of AR Med Scis Dept of Thor Surg Slot 713, MC-713 Little Rock, AR 72205; **Office Phone:** (501) 686-7884; **Board Certifications:** Surgery 1994, Thoracic Surgery 1997; **Medical School:** Syria 1983; **Residencies:** Surgery, Meth Hosp, Brooklyn, NY 1988-1993; Thoracic Surgery, Univ Arkansas Med Ctr, Little Rock, AR 1993-1996; **Faculty Appointment:** Asst Prof Surgery, Univ Ark

Cooley, Denton A MD (Thoracic Surgery) - *Special Expertise:* Heart Valve Surgery; Aneurysm-Abdominal Aortic; **Admitting Hospital:** St Luke's Episcopal Hospital - Houston (Page 76); **Office Address:** Surg Assocs of Tex PA, Tex Heart Inst 1101 Bates Ave, Fl P-514 Houston, TX 77030-2607; **Office Phone:** (713) 791-4900; **Board Certifications:** Surgery 1951, Thoracic Surgery 1952; **Medical School:** Johns Hopkins Univ 1944; **Residency:** Surgery, Johns Hopkins Hosp, Baltimore, MD 1945-1950; **Fellowship:** Thoracic Surgery, Brompton Hosp Chest Dis, London England 1950-1951; **Faculty Appointment:** Clin Prof Surgery, Univ Tex, Houston

Copeland III, Jack G MD (Thoracic Surgery) - *Special Expertise:* Transplant-Heart; Artificial Heart; **Admitting Hospital:** University Medical Center; **Office Address:** Univ Ariz Hlth Sci Ctr 1501 N Campbell Rd, rm 4402 Tucson, AZ 85724-5071; **Office Phone:** (520) 626-6339; **Board Certifications:** Surgery 1988, Thoracic Surgery 1997; **Medical School:** Stanford Univ 1969; **Residencies:** Surgery, UC-San DiegoNatl Inst Hlth, San Diego, CA 1970-1971; Cardiology (Cardiovascular Disease), Natl Inst Hlth, Bethesda, MD 1971-1973; **Fellowship:** Cardiothoracic Surgery, Stanford Univ, Stanford, CA 1973-1977; **Faculty Appointment:** Prof Thoracic Surgery, Univ Ariz Coll Med

Coselli, Joseph Stapleton MD (Thoracic Surgery) - *Special Expertise:* Aneurysm-Abdominal Aortic; Marfan's Syndrome; Vascular Surgery; **Admitting Hospital:** Methodist Hospital - Houston (Page 69); **Office Address:** Methodist Hosp 6560 Fannin St, Fl 11 - Ste 1100 Houston, TX 77030; **Office Phone:** (713) 790-4313; **Board Certifications:** Surgery 1992, Thoracic Surgery 1993; **Medical School:** Univ Tex Med Br, Galveston 1977; **Residencies:** Surgery, Baylor Coll Med, Houston, TX 1977-1982; Thoracic Surgery, Baylor Coll Med, Houston, TX 1982-1984; **Faculty Appointment:** Assoc Prof Surgery, Baylor Coll Med

Frazier, Oscar Howard MD (Thoracic Surgery) - *Special Expertise:* Transplant-Heart; Lung Surgery; **Admitting Hospital:** St Luke's Episcopal Hospital - Houston (Page 76); **Office Address:** Texas Heart Inst 1101 Bates, MC-3-147 Houston, TX 77030; **Office Phone:** (713) 791-4900; **Board Certifications:** Surgery 1975, Thoracic Surgery 1997; **Medical School:** Baylor Coll Med 1967; **Residencies:** Surgery, Baylor Affil Hosp, Houston, TX 1970-1974; Thoracic Surgery, Texas Heart Inst, Houston, TX 1974-1976; **Faculty Appointment:** Prof Surgery, Univ Tex, Houston

Harrell Jr, James E MD (Thoracic Surgery) - *Special Expertise:* Transplant-Heart; **Admitting Hospital:** Arkansas Children's Hospital; **Office Address:** Chldrn's Hosp, Dept Cardiac Surg 800 Marshall St, Slot 835, Ste S-341 Little Rock, AR 72202; **Office Phone:** (501) 320-1809; **Board Certifications:** Surgery 1995, Thoracic Surgery 1996; **Medical School:** Baylor Coll Med 1978; **Residencies:** Surgery, Univ Texas hlth Science Ctr, Houston, TX 1982-1984; Thoracic Surgery, Baylor Coll Med, Houston, TX 1984-1986; **Fellowship:** Thoracic Surgery, Hosp Sick Chldrn, London England 1986-1987; **Faculty Appointment:** Assoc Prof Surgery, Univ Ark

Harrison, Lynn MD (Thoracic Surgery) - *Special Expertise:* Coronary Revascularization; **Admitting Hospital:** West Jefferson Medical Center; **Office Address:** Louisiana St Univ Med Ctr Clins 1111 Medical Center Blvd, Ste N504 Marrero, LA 70072; **Office Phone:** (504) 349-6606; **Board Certifications:** Thoracic Surgery 1989, Surgery 1980; **Medical School:** Univ Okla Coll Med 1970; **Residencies:** Thoracic Surgery, Duke Univ Hosp, Durham, NC 1971-1972; Thoracic Surgery, Duke Univ Hosp, Durham, NC 1974-1979; **Fellowship:** Cardiothoracic Surgery, Duke Univ, Durham, NC 1978-1979

THORACIC SURGERY

Livesay, James J MD (Thoracic Surgery) - *Special Expertise:* Coronary Artery Surgery; Heart Valve Surgery; **Admitting Hospital:** St Luke's Episcopal Hospital - Houston (Page 76); **Office Address:** Surg Assocs of Texas Ste 20345 Houston, TX 77225-0345; **Office Phone:** (713) 791-4976; **Board Certifications:** Thoracic Surgery 1993, Surgery 1999; **Medical School:** Baylor Coll Med 1973; **Residencies:** Surgery, UCLA, Los Angeles, CA 1973-1979; Thoracic Surgery, Tex Heart Inst, Houston, TX 1979-1981; **Fellowship:** Research, UCLA, Los Angeles, CA 1975-1976; **Faculty Appointment:** Assoc Prof Surgery, Univ Tex, Houston

Noon, George P MD (Thoracic Surgery) - *Special Expertise:* Transplant-Heart; Transplant-Lung; Thoracic Vascular Surgery; **Admitting Hospital:** Methodist Hospital - Houston (Page 69); **Office Address:** Methodist Hosp, Dept Surg One Baylor Plaza Houston, TX 77030-3411; **Office Phone:** (713) 790-3155; **Board Certifications:** Thoracic Surgery 1966, Surgery 1966; **Medical School:** Baylor Coll Med 1960; **Residencies:** Surgery, Baylor Coll Med, Houston, TX 1961-1966; Surgery, Ben Taub Genl Hosp, Houston, TX 1965-1966; **Faculty Appointment:** Prof Surgery, Baylor Coll Med

Ott, David A MD (Thoracic Surgery) - *Special Expertise:* Thoracic Surgery - General; **Admitting Hospital:** St Luke's Episcopal Hospital - Houston (Page 76); **Office Address:** 1101 Bates Ave, Ste P-514 Houston, TX 77030-2607; **Office Phone:** (713) 791-4900; **Board Certification:** Thoracic Surgery 1997; **Medical School:** Baylor Coll Med 1972; **Residencies:** Surgery, Baylor Coll Med, Houston, TX 1972-1976; Vascular Surgery (General), Tex Heart Inst, Houston, TX 1976-1978; **Faculty Appointment:** Clin Prof Surgery, Baylor Coll Med

Putnam Jr, Joe B MD (Thoracic Surgery) - *Special Expertise:* Lung Cancer; Esophageal Cancer; Sarcoma-Soft Tissue; **Admitting Hospital:** University of Texas MD Anderson Cancer Center (Page 66); **Office Address:** UT MD Anderson Cancer Ctr 1515 Holcombe Blvd, Box 109 Houston, TX 77030; **Office Phone:** (713) 792-6934; **Board Certifications:** Thoracic Surgery 1997, Surgery 1987; **Medical School:** Univ NC Sch Med 1979; **Residencies:** Thoracic Surgery, U Mich., Ann Arbor, MI 1986-1988; Surgery, U Rochester, Rochester, NY 1984-1986; **Fellowship:** Medical Oncology, NCI/NIH-Surg. Branch, Bethesda, MD 1981-1984; **Faculty Appointment:** Assoc Prof Surgery, Univ Tex, Houston

Reul, George J MD (Thoracic Surgery) - *Special Expertise:* Coronary Artery Surgery; Aneurysm; Heart Valve Surgery; **Admitting Hospital:** St Luke's Episcopal Hospital - Houston (Page 76); **Office Address:** Surg Assocs-Tex Heart Inst 1101 Bates Ave Houston, TX 77030-2607; **Office Phone:** (713) 791-4900; **Board Certifications:** Surgery 1971, Thoracic Surgery 1971; **Medical School:** Med Coll Wisc 1962; **Residencies:** Surgery, Marquette Sch Med, Milwaukee, WI 1969; Thoracic Surgery, Baylor Coll Med, Houston, TX 1971; **Faculty Appointment:** Clin Prof Surgery, Univ Tex, Houston

Trastek, Victor MD (Thoracic Surgery) - *Special Expertise:* Lung Cancer; Esophageal Cancer; **Admitting Hospital:** Mayo Medical Center & Clinic - Scottsdale; **Office Address:** Mayo Clinic 13400 E Shea Blvd Scottsdale, AZ 85259; **Office Phone:** (480) 301-4608; **Board Certifications:** Thoracic Surgery 1994, Surgery 1982; **Medical School:** Univ Wisc 1976; **Residencies:** Surgery, Mayo Clinic, Rochester, MN 1977-1981; Thoracic Surgery, Mayo Clinic, Rochester, MN 1981-1984; **Fellowship:** Thoracic Surgery, Toronto Genl Hosp, Toronto, Canada 1985

Turner, William F MD (Thoracic Surgery) - *Special Expertise:* Coronary Artery Surgery; Cardiac Surgery; **Admitting Hospital:** East Texas Medical Center; **Office Address:** Cardiovascular Surgery Box 150 Tyler, TX 75710; **Office Phone:** (903) 595-6680; **Board Certifications:** Surgery 1997, Thoracic Surgery 1998; **Medical School:** Baylor Coll Med 1981; **Residencies:** Surgery, Baylor Coll Med, Houston, TX 1983-1987; Thoracic Surgery, Baylor Coll Med, Houston, TX 1987-1989

Urschel Jr, Harold C MD (Thoracic Surgery) - *Special Expertise:* *Thoracic Outlet Syndrome;* **Admitting Hospital:** Baylor University Medical Center; **Office Address:** 3600 Gaston Ave, Ste 1201 Dallas, TX 75246-1800; **Office Phone:** (214) 824-2503; **Board Certifications:** Thoracic Surgery 1963, Surgery 1963; **Medical School:** Harvard Med Sch 1955; **Residencies:** Thoracic Surgery, Mass Genl Hosp, Boston, MA 1959-1961; Vascular Surgery (General), Mass Genl Hosp, Boston, MA 1956-1957; **Faculty Appointment:** Prof Thoracic Surgery, Univ Tex SW, Dallas

West Coast and Pacific

Bailey, Leonard Lee MD (Thoracic Surgery) - *Special Expertise:* *Transplant-Heart-Infant;* *Heart Disease-Congenital;* **Admitting Hospital:** Loma Linda University Medical Center; **Office Address:** Loma Linda U Med Ctr- Surg 11175 Campus St, Ste 21120 Loma Linda, CA 92354; **Office Phone:** (909) 824-4200; **Board Certifications:** Thoracic Surgery 1988, Surgery 1975; **Medical School:** Loma Linda Univ 1969; **Residencies:** Surgery, Loma Linda Univ Med Ctr, Loma Linda, CA 1970-1973; Thoracic Surgery, Loma Linda Univ Med Ctr, Loma Linda, CA 1973-1974; **Fellowship:** Cardiology (Cardiovascular Disease), Hosp Sick Chldn, Toronto, Canada 1974-1975; **Faculty Appointment:** Prof Surgery, Loma Linda Univ

De Meester, Tom R MD (Thoracic Surgery) - *Special Expertise:* *Gastric Diseases; Esophageal Surgery;* **Admitting Hospital:** USC University Hospital - Richard K. Eamer Medical Plaza; **Office Address:** USC Sch Med 1510 San Pablo St, Ste 514 Los Angeles, CA 90033-4612; **Office Phone:** (323) 442-5925; **Board Certifications:** Surgery 1971, Thoracic Surgery 1971; **Medical School:** Univ Mich Med Sch 1963; **Residencies:** Surgery, Univ Mich Hosp, Ann Arbor, MI 1964-1965; Surgery, Johns Hopkins Hosp, Baltimore, MD 1965-1966; **Fellowship:** Surgery, Johns Hopkins Hosp, Baltimore, MD 1967-1968; **Faculty Appointment:** Prof Surgery, USC Sch Med

Flachsbart, Keith D MD (Thoracic Surgery) - *Special Expertise:* *Thoracic Surgery - General;* **Admitting Hospital:** KFH San Francisco Medical Center; **Office Address:** Permanente Medical Group 2350 Geary Blvd San Francisco, CA 94115; **Office Phone:** (415) 202-3800; **Board Certification:** Thoracic Surgery 1990; **Medical School:** Univ Nebr Coll Med 1971; **Residencies:** Surgery, Rush-Presby St Lukes, Chicago, IL 1974-1978; Thoracic Surgery, Hosp Good Samaritan, Los Angeles, CA 1978-1980

Fontana, Gregory MD (Thoracic Surgery) - *Special Expertise:* *Minimally Invasive Surgery;* *Cardiac Surgery-Pediatric;* **Admitting Hospital:** Cedars-Sinai Medical Center; **Office Address:** Cedars-Sinai Med Ctr, Dept Cardithor Surg 8700 Beverly Blvd, Ste 6215 Los Angeles, CA 90048; **Office Phone:** (310) 423-3851; **Board Certifications:** Surgery 1993, Thoracic Surgery 1994; **Medical School:** UCLA 1984; **Residencies:** Surgery, Duke Univ Med Ctr, Durham, NC 1985-1986; Thoracic Surgery, Duke Univ Med Ctr, Durham, NC 1988-1991; **Fellowships:** Cardiac Electrophysiology, Duke Univ Med Ctr, Durham, NC 1986-1988; Pediatric Cardiac Surgery, UCLA, Los Angeles, CA 1993; **Faculty Appointment:** Asst Clin Prof Surgery, UCLA

Gundry, Steven MD (Thoracic Surgery) - *Special Expertise:* *Cardiac Surgery-Adult & Pediatric;* **Admitting Hospital:** Loma Linda University Medical Center; **Office Address:** Loma Linda Univ Med Ctr, Div Cardiothoracic Surg 11175 Campus St, Ste 21121 Loma Linda, CA 92354; **Office Phone:** (909) 824-4354; **Board Certifications:** Surgery 1993, Thoracic Surgery 1995; **Medical School:** Med Coll GA 1977; **Residencies:** Surgery, Univ Michigan Hosps, Ann Arbor, MI 1980-1983; Thoracic Surgery, Univ Michigan Hosps, Ann Arbor, MI 1983-1985; **Fellowship:** Pediatric Cardiac Surgery, Hosp-Sick Chldn, London, England 1985-1986; **Faculty Appointment:** Prof Surgery, Loma Linda Univ

THORACIC SURGERY

Hanley, Frank Louis MD (Thoracic Surgery) - *Special Expertise:* Thoracic Surgery-Pediatric; **Admitting Hospital:** University of California - San Francisco Medical Center; **Office Address:** 505 Parnassus Ave, Bldg S543 San Francisco, CA 94143; **Office Phone:** (415) 476-3501; **Board Certifications:** Thoracic Surgery 1990, Surgery 1987; **Medical School:** Tufts Univ 1978; **Residencies:** Surgery, UCSF Med Ctr, San Francisco, CA 1978-1981; Cardiothoracic Surgery, UCSF Med Ctr, San Francisco, CA 1986-1988; **Fellowship:** Research, UCSF Sch Med, San Francisco, CA 1981-1984; **Faculty Appointment:** Prof Surgery, UCSF

Holmes, E Carmack MD (Thoracic Surgery) - *Special Expertise:* Lung Cancer; **Admitting Hospital:** UCLA Medical Center; **Office Address:** UCLA Med Ctr, Dept of Surgery 10833 Le Conte Ave Los Angeles, CA 90095-1749; **Office Phone:** (310) 825-7017; **Board Certifications:** Thoracic Surgery 1974, Surgery 1973; **Medical School:** Univ NC Sch Med 1964; **Residencies:** Surgery, John Hopkins Hosp, Baltimore, MD 1965-1973; Surgery, Natl Cancer Inst 1966-1969; **Faculty Appointment:** Prof Surgery, UCLA

Kay, Jerome Harold MD (Thoracic Surgery) - *Special Expertise:* Cardiac Surgery; Lung Surgery; **Admitting Hospital:** Good Samaritan Hospital - Los Angeles; **Office Address:** 1127 Wilshire Blvd, Fl 600 Los Angeles, CA 90017-3907; **Office Phone:** (213) 250-5711; **Board Certifications:** Surgery 1955, Thoracic Surgery 1957; **Medical School:** UCSF **Residencies:** Surgery, McKinney VA Hosp 1946-1950; Surgery, Johns Hopkins Hosp, Baltimore, MD 1950-1954; **Fellowship:** Thoracic Surgery, Johns Hopkins Hosp, BAltimore, MD 1950-1952

Laks, Hillel MD (Thoracic Surgery) - *Special Expertise:* Heart Disease-Congenital; Transplant-Heart; **Admitting Hospital:** UCLA Medical Center; **Office Address:** UCLA Med Ctr, Div Cardiothoracic Surg 10833 Le Conte Ave, rm 62-182 A Los Angeles, CA 90095-1741; **Office Phone:** (310) 206-8232; **Board Certifications:** Surgery 1975, Thoracic Surgery 1996; **Medical School:** Africa 1965; **Residencies:** Surgery, Peter Bent Brigham Hosp, Boston, MA 1967-1969; Thoracic Surgery, Peter Bent Brigham Hosp, Boston, MA 1969-1973; **Faculty Appointment:** Prof Surgery, UCLA

Little, Alex G MD (Thoracic Surgery) - *Special Expertise:* Thoracic Surgery - General; **Admitting Hospital:** University Medical Center - Fresno; **Office Address:** Univ Nevada Sch Med 2040 W Charleston Blvd, Ste 601 Las Vegas, NV 89102-2245; **Office Phone:** (702) 385-1980; **Board Certifications:** Surgery 1998, Thoracic Surgery 1990; **Medical School:** Johns Hopkins Univ 1974; **Residencies:** Thoracic Surgery, Univ Chicago Hosp, Chicago, IL 1979-1981; Surgery, Univ Chicago Hosp, Chicago, IL 1977-1979; **Faculty Appointment:** Prof Thoracic Surgery, Univ Nevada

McKenna Jr, Robert J MD (Thoracic Surgery) - *Special Expertise:* Lung Cancer; **Admitting Hospital:** Cedars-Sinai Medical Center; **Office Address:** 8635 W 3rd St, Ste 975W Los Angeles, CA 90048-6101; **Office Phone:** (310) 652-0530; **Board Certifications:** Thoracic Surgery 1997, Surgery 1983; **Medical School:** USC Sch Med 1977; **Residencies:** Surgery, Stanford University Hosp 1978-1982; Surgery, Hosp Good Samaritan, Los Angeles, CA 1985-1987; **Fellowship:** Thoracic Surgery, MD Anderson Hosp-Tumor Inst 1982-1983; **Faculty Appointment:** Clin Prof Thoracic Surgery, UCLA

Miller, David Craig MD (Thoracic Surgery) - *Special Expertise:* Thoracic Surgery - General; **Admitting Hospital:** Stanford Medical Center; **Office Address:** Stanford Univ Sch Med, Dept Cardiothoracic Surg, Falk Res Ctr 300 Pasteur Dr Stanford, CA 94305-5247; **Office Phone:** (650) 725-3826; **Board Certifications:** Thoracic Surgery 1988, Vascular Surgery (General) 1993; **Medical School:** Stanford Univ 1972; **Residency:** Thoracic Surgery, Standford Univ Med Ctr, Standford, CA 1973-1978; **Faculty Appointment:** Prof Thoracic Surgery, Stanford Univ

Morton, Donald Lee MD (Thoracic Surgery) - *Special Expertise:* Melanoma; Sentinel Node Surgery; Cancer Resch & Prevention; **Admitting Hospital:** St John's Health Center; **Office Address:** John Wayne Cancer Inst 2200 Santa Monica Blvd Santa Monica, CA 90404; **Office Phone:** (310) 829-8363; **Board Certifications:** Thoracic Surgery 1969, Surgery 1967; **Medical School:** UCSF 1958; **Residencies:** Surgery, Natnl Cancer Inst-NIH, Bethesda, MD 1960-1962; Thoracic Surgery, UC- San Francisco, San Francisco, CA 1962-1966; **Fellowship:** Surgery, Cancer Rsch Inst- UCSF, San Francisco, CA 1962-1966; **Faculty Appointment:** Prof Emeritus Surgery, UCLA

Reitz, Bruce Arnold MD (Thoracic Surgery) - *Special Expertise:* Transplant-Heart; Heart Valve Surgery; **Admitting Hospital:** Stanford Medical Center; **Office Address:** Stanford Hosp, Dept Cardiothoracic Falk CVRB ULN, 300 Pasteur Drive Stanford, CA 94305-5407; **Office Phone:** (650) 725-4497; **Board Certifications:** Thoracic Surgery 1991, Surgery 1980; **Medical School:** Yale Univ 1970; **Residencies:** Thoracic Surgery, Stanford Univ Hosp, Palo Alto, CA 1971-1972; Thoracic Surgery, Natl Heart Inst-NIH, Bethesda, MD 1972-1974; **Faculty Appointment:** Prof Thoracic Surgery, Stanford Univ

Robbins, Robert Clayton MD (Thoracic Surgery) - *Special Expertise:* Thoracic Surgery - General; **Admitting Hospital:** Stanford Medical Center; **Office Address:** Stanford Univ Falk CVRB Dept Cardiothoracic Surgery Stanford, CA 94305; **Office Phone:** (650) 723-4000; **Board Certifications:** Thoracic Surgery 1994, Surgery 1990; **Medical School:** Univ Miss 1983; **Residency:** Surgery, Univ Miss Med Ctr, Jackson, MS 1984-1988; **Fellowship:** Thoracic Surgery, Stanford Univ, Stanford, CA 1989-1991; **Faculty Appointment:** Asst Prof Thoracic Surgery, Stanford Univ

Shumway, Norman Edward MD (Thoracic Surgery) - *Special Expertise:* Transplant-Heart; Transplant-Lung; **Admitting Hospital:** Stanford Medical Center; **Office Address:** 300 Pasteur Dr Stanford, CA 94305; **Office Phone:** (650) 725-3816; **Board Certifications:** Surgery 1957, Thoracic Surgery 1957; **Medical School:** Vanderbilt Univ 1949; **Residency:** Surgery, Univ Minn Hosp, Minneapolis, MN 1950-1957; **Fellowship:** Surgery, Univ Minn Hosp, Minneapolis, MN 1954-1956

Starnes, Vaughn Alden MD (Thoracic Surgery) - *Special Expertise:* Transplant-Heart-Pediatric; Cardiac Surgery-Adult & Pediatric; **Admitting Hospital:** USC University Hospital - Richard K. Eamer Medical Plaza; **Office Address:** USC Cardiothoracic Surg 1510 San Pablo Rd, HCC 415 Los Angeles, CA 90033; **Office Phone:** (323) 442-5849; **Board Certifications:** Surgery 1985, Thoracic Surgery 1998; **Medical School:** Univ NC Sch Med 1977; **Residencies:** Surgery, Vanderbilt Univ Hosp, Nashville, TN 1977-1984; Cardiovascular Surgery, Stanford Unv Hosp, Stanford, CA 1984-1986; **Fellowships:** Cardiothoracic Transplantation, Stanford Unv Hosp, Stanford, CA 1986-1987; Pediatric Cardiac Surgery, Univ NC Hosp, Chapel Hill, NC 1987; **Faculty Appointment:** Prof Surgery, USC Sch Med

Trento, Alfredo MD (Thoracic Surgery) - *Special Expertise:* Transplant-Heart; Cardiac Surgery-Adult & Pediatric; **Admitting Hospital:** Cedars-Sinai Medical Center; **Office Address:** Cedars-Sinai Med Ctr, Dept Cardiothor Surg 8700 Beverly Blvd, North Tower - rm 6215 Los Angeles, CA 90048; **Office Phone:** (310) 423-3851; **Board Certifications:** Surgery 1984, Thoracic Surgery 1995; **Medical School:** Italy 1975; **Residencies:** Surgery, Univ Mass Med Ctr, Worcester, MA 1977-1982; Thoracic Surgery, Univ Pittsburgh, Pittsburgh, PA 1983-1985; **Fellowship:** Cardiothoracic Surgery, Univ Mass-Coord Surg Prog, Worcester, MA 1982; **Faculty Appointment:** Prof Surgery, UCLA

Verrier, Edward MD (Thoracic Surgery) - *Special Expertise:* Coronary Artery Surgery; Heart Valve Surgery; **Admitting Hospital:** University of Washington Medical Center; **Office Address:** Univ Wash Med Ctr, Div Cardiothor Surg 1959 NE Pacific St, Bldg HSC - Fl 1st - Ste AA115 Seattle, WA 98195-6310; **Office Phone:** (206) 685-3370; **Board Certifications:** Surgery 1992, Thoracic Surgery 1993; **Medical School:** Tufts Univ 1974; **Residencies:** Surgery, UCSF Med Ctr, San Francisco, CA 1980-1982; Thoracic Surgery, UCSF Med Ctr, San Francisco, CA 1982-1984; **Fellowship:** Thoracic Surgery, UCSF Med Ctr, San Francisco, CA 1977-1980; **Faculty Appointment:** Prof Thoracic Surgery, Univ Wash

Whyte, Richard MD (Thoracic Surgery) - *Special Expertise:* Lung Cancer; Esophageal Cancer; **Admitting Hospital:** Stanford Medical Center; **Office Address:** Stanford Univ Sch Med, Div Thor Surg 300 Pasteur Dr, Bldg CVRB - rm 205 Stanford, CA 94305; **Office Phone:** (650) 723-6649; **Board Certifications:** Surgery 1991, Thoracic Surgery 1993; **Medical School:** Univ Pittsburgh 1983; **Residencies:** Surgery, Mass Genl Hosp, Boston, MA 1983-1990; Thoracic Surgery, Univ Michigan Hosp, Ann Arbor, MI 1991-1992; **Faculty Appointment:** Assoc Prof Thoracic Surgery, Stanford Univ

Wood, Douglas MD (Thoracic Surgery) - *Special Expertise:* Tracheal Surgery; Lung Cancer; Esophageal Cancer; **Admitting Hospital:** University of Washington Medical Center; **Office Address:** Univ Wash, Dept CardioThoracic Surgery 1959 NE Pacific, Box 356310 Seattle, WA 98195-6310; **Office Phone:** (206) 685-3228; **Board Certifications:** Thoracic Surgery 1993, Surgery 1999; **Medical School:** Harvard Med Sch 1983; **Residency:** Surgery, Mass Genl Hosp, Boston, MA 1983-1989; **Fellowship:** Thoracic Surgery, Mass Genl Hosp, Boston, MA 1989-1991; **Faculty Appointment:** Assoc Prof Surgery, Univ Wash

UROLOGY

A urologist manages benign and malignant medical and surgical disorders of the genitourinary system and the adrenal gland. This specialist has comprehensive knowledge of, and skills in, endoscopic, percutaneous and open surgery of congenital and acquired conditions of the urinary and reproductive systems and their contiguous structures.

Training required: Five years

PHYSICIAN LISTINGS

Urology

New England

Dretler, Stephen P. MD (Urology) - *Special Expertise:* Kidney Stones; **Admitting Hospital:** Massachusetts General Hospital; **Office Address:** Mass Genl Hosp 15 Parkman St, Fl 4 - Ste 486 Boston, MA 02114-3139; **Office Phone:** (617) 726-3512; **Board Certification:** Urology 1975; **Medical School:** Tufts Univ 1964; **Residencies:** Surgery, Mass Genl Hosp, Boston, MA 1965; Urology, Mass Genl Hosp, Boston, MA 1971; **Fellowship:** Nephrology, Mass Genl Hosp, Boston, MA 1968; **Faculty Appointment:** Clin Prof Surgery, Harvard Med Sch

Goldstein, Irwin MD (Urology) - *Special Expertise:* Erectile Dysfunction; **Admitting Hospital:** Boston University Medical Center-East Newton Street Campus; **Office Address:** 720 Harrison Ave, Ste 606 Boston, MA 02118-2334; **Office Phone:** (617) 638-8485; **Board Certification:** Urology 1982; **Medical School:** McGill Univ 1975; **Residencies:** Urology, Boston Univ Med Ctr, Boston, MA 1977-1980; Surgery, Boston Univ Med Ctr, Boston, MA 1977; **Fellowship:** Urology, Boston Univ Med Ctr, Boston, MA 1981; **Faculty Appointment:** Assoc Prof Urology, Boston Univ

Gomery, Pablo MD (Urology) - *Special Expertise:* Neuro-Urology; Erectile Dysfunction; **Admitting Hospital:** Massachusetts General Hospital; **Office Address:** Genl Med Assoc - Mass Genl Hosp 275 Cambridge St, Bldg Prof Office Boston, MA 02116; **Office Phone:** (617) 724-6208; **Board Certification:** Urology 1990; **Medical School:** Albert Einstein Coll Med 1974; **Residencies:** Urology, Mass Genl Hosp, Boston, MA 1977-1980; Surgery, New England Deaconess, Boston, MA 1975-1977; **Faculty Appointment:** Clin Inst Surgery, Harvard Med Sch

Heney, Niall M MD (Urology) - *Special Expertise:* Urologic Cancer; **Admitting Hospital:** Massachusetts General Hospital; **Office Address:** Mass General Hosp, Dept Urology 15 Parkman St Boston, MA 02114; **Office Phone:** (617) 726-3011; **Board Certification:** Urology 1977; **Medical School:** Ireland 1965; **Residencies:** Urology, Reg Hosp, Galway, Ireland 1968-1972; Urology, Mass Genl Hosp, Boston, MA; **Faculty Appointment:** Prof Medicine, Harvard Med Sch

Libertino, John A. MD (Urology) - *Special Expertise:* Kidney Reconstruction; **Admitting Hospital:** Lahey Clinic; **Office Address:** 41 Mall Rd Lahey Medical Clinic Burlington, MA 01803; **Office Phone:** (781) 744-8420; **Board Certification:** Urology 1973; **Medical School:** Georgetown Univ 1965; **Residencies:** Urology, Yale-New Haven Hosp., New Haven, CT 1967-1970; Urology, U Rochester-Strong Meml Hosp., Rochester, NY 1967; **Fellowship:** Surgery, Yale-New Haven Hosp., New Haven, CT 1968; **Faculty Appointment:** Assoc Clin Prof Surgery, Harvard Med Sch

McDougal, William Scott MD (Urology) - *Special Expertise:* Urinary Reconstruction; **Admitting Hospital:** Massachusetts General Hospital; **Office Address:** Mass Genl Hosp 55 Fruit St, Bldg GRB - rm 1102 Boston, MA 02114; **Office Phone:** (617) 726-3010; **Board Certifications:** Urology 1992, Surgery 1975; **Medical School:** Cornell Univ-Weil Med Coll 1968; **Residency:** Surgery, Univ Hosps, Cleveland, OH 1969-1975; **Fellowship:** Physiology, Yale Med Sch, New Haven, CT 1971-1972; **Faculty Appointment:** Prof Urology, Harvard Med Sch

McGovern, Francis MD (Urology) - *Special Expertise:* Prostate Cancer; **Admitting Hospital:** Massachusetts General Hospital; **Office Address:** 1 Hawthorne Pl, Ste 109 Boston, MA 02114; **Office Phone:** (617) 523-5250; **Board Certification:** Urology 1999; **Medical School:** Case West Res Univ 1983; **Residency:** Urology, Mass Genl Hosp., Boston, MA 1984-1989; **Faculty Appointment:** Clin Inst Surgery, Harvard Med Sch

Oates, Robert Davis MD (Urology) - *Special Expertise: Infertility-Male; Vasectomy Reversal;* **Admitting Hospital:** Boston Medical Center; **Office Address:** Boston Univ Med Ctr, Dept Urology 720 Harrison Ave, Fl 606 Boston, MA 02118-2334; **Office Phone:** (617) 638-8485; **Board Certification:** Urology 1990; **Medical School:** Boston Univ 1982; **Residencies:** Urology, Boston Univ Hosp, Boston, MA 1984-1987; Surgery, Boston Univ Hosp, Boston, MA 1983-1984; **Fellowship:** Reproductive Medicine, Baylor Coll Med, Houston, TX 1987-1988; **Faculty Appointment:** Assoc Prof Urology, Boston Univ

Retik, Alan MD (Urology) - *Special Expertise: Urinary Reconstruction-Pediatric;* **Admitting Hospital:** Children's Hospital; **Office Address:** Chldn's Hosp, Hunnewell Bldg, Dept Urology 300 Longwood Ave, rm 390 Boston, MA 02115-5724; **Office Phone:** (617) 731-6220; **Board Certification:** Urology 1969; **Medical School:** Cornell Univ-Weil Med Coll 1957; **Residencies:** Surgery, Strong Meml Hosp, Rochester, MN 1958-1961; Urology, Peter Bent Brigham Hosp, Boston, MA 1962-1965; **Fellowship:** Pediatric Urology, Hosp Sich Chldn, London, England 1966-1967; **Faculty Appointment:** Prof Urology, Harvard Med Sch

Richie, Jerome MD (Urology) - *Special Expertise: Prostate Cancer; Testicular Cancer; Kidney Cancer;* **Admitting Hospital:** Brigham & Women's Hospital; **Office Address:** Brigham & Women's Hosp 75 Francis St Boston, MA 02115; **Office Phone:** (617) 732-6325; **Board Certification:** Urology 1977; **Medical School:** Univ Tex Med Br, Galveston 1969; **Residencies:** Surgery, UCLA, Los Angeles, CA 1969-1971; Urology, UCLA, Los Angeles, CA 1971-1975; **Faculty Appointment:** Prof Urology, Harvard Med Sch

Sigman, Mark MD (Urology) - *Special Expertise: Infertility-Male;* **Admitting Hospital:** Rhode Island Hospital; **Office Address:** Univ Urological Assoc 2 Dudley St, Ste 175 Providence, RI 02905-3247; **Office Phone:** (401) 421-0710; **Board Certification:** Urology 2000; **Medical School:** Univ Conn 1981; **Residencies:** Urology, Univ VA, Charlottesville, VA 1983-1987; Surgery, Univ VA, Charlottesville, VA 1982-1983; **Fellowship:** Male Reproduction, Baylor Coll Med, Houston, TX 1987-1989; **Faculty Appointment:** Assoc Prof Urology, Brown Univ

Weiss, Robert M MD (Urology) - *Special Expertise: Urology-Pediatric;* **Admitting Hospital:** Yale - New Haven Hospital; **Office Address:** Yale Univ Sch Med, Dept of Urol 800 Howard Ave New Haven, CT 06520; **Office Phone:** (203) 785-2815; **Board Certification:** Urology 1970; **Medical School:** SUNY Downstate 1960; **Residencies:** Surgery, Beth Israel Hosp, New York, NY 1963-1967; Urology, Columbia Presby, New York, NY 1963-1967; **Fellowship:** Pharmacology, Columbia Presby, New York, NY 1964-1965; **Faculty Appointment:** Prof Urology, Yale Univ

Mid Atlantic

Alexander, Richard B MD (Urology) - *Special Expertise: Prostate Disease; Prostate Disease;* **Admitting Hospital:** University of Maryland Medical System; **Office Address:** Maryland Prostate Center 419 W Redwood St, Ste 320 Baltimore, MD 21201; **Office Phone:** (410) 328-5544; **Board Certification:** Urology 1999; **Medical School:** Johns Hopkins Univ 1981; **Residencies:** Urology, Johns Hopkins, Baltimore, MD 1983-1988; Surgery, Vanderbilt Univ Affl Hosps, Nashville, TN 1981-1983; **Faculty Appointment:** Assoc Prof Urology, Univ MD Sch Med

Bander, Neil MD (Urology) - *Special Expertise: Prostate Cancer;* **Admitting Hospital:** New York Weill Cornell Medical Center - NY Presbyterian Hospital (Page 72); **Office Address:** 428 E 72nd St, Ste 400 New York, NY 10021; **Office Phone:** (212) 746-5460; **Board Certification:** Urology 1983; **Medical School:** Univ Conn 1974; **Residencies:** Urology, Bellevue Hosp, New York, NY 1975-1977; Urology, U Conn, Farmington, CT 1977-1980; **Fellowship:** Urologic Oncology, Meml Sloan Kettering Cancer Ctr, New York, NY 1980-1983; **Faculty Appointment:** Prof Urology, Cornell Univ-Weil Med Coll

Belman, A Barry MD (Urology) - *Special Expertise:* Urology-Pediatric; **Admitting Hospital:** Children's National Medical Center - DC; **Office Address:** Chldns Natl Med Ctr 111 Michigan Ave NW Washington, DC 20010; **Office Phone:** (202) 884-5042; **Board Certification:** Urology 1973; **Medical School:** Northwestern Univ 1964; **Residency:** Urology, Northwestern Univ Med Ctr, Chicago, IL 1964-1970; **Faculty Appointment:** Prof Urology, Geo Wash Univ

Benson, Mitchell C MD (Urology) - *Special Expertise:* Prostate Cancer; Incontinence; **Admitting Hospital:** Columbia Presbyterian Medical Center (Page 72); **Office Address:** 161 Ft Washington Ave New York, NY 10032-3713; **Office Phone:** (212) 305-5201; **Board Certification:** Urology 1984; **Medical School:** Columbia P&S 1977; **Residencies:** Surgery, Mount Sinai Med Ctr, New York, NY 1977-1979; Urology, Columbia-Presby, New York, NY 1979-1982; **Fellowship:** Medical Oncology, Johns Hopkins Hosp, Baltimore, MD 1982-1984; **Faculty Appointment:** Prof Urology, Columbia P&S

Blaivas, Jerry G MD (Urology) - *Special Expertise:* Uro-Gynecology; Bladder/Prostate Problems; Urology-Female; **Admitting Hospital:** New York Weill Cornell Medical Center - NY Presbyterian Hospital (Page 72); **Office Address:** 400 E 56th St New York, NY 10022; **Office Phone:** (212) 308-6565; **Board Certification:** Urology 1978; **Medical School:** Tufts Univ 1964; **Residencies:** Surgery, Boston Med Ctr, Boston, MA 1969-1971; Urology, New England Med Ctr, Boston, MA 1973-1976; **Faculty Appointment:** Clin Prof Urology, Cornell Univ-Weil Med Coll

Burnett II, Arthur L MD (Urology) - *Special Expertise:* Prostate Cancer; Erectile Dysfunction; **Admitting Hospital:** Johns Hopkins Hospital - Baltimore (Page 65); **Office Address:** Johns Hopkins Bayview Med Ctr 4940 Eastern Ave Baltimore, MD 21224; **Office Phone:** (410) 550-3506; **Board Certification:** Urology 1998; **Medical School:** Johns Hopkins Univ 1988; **Residencies:** Urology, Johns Hopkins Hosp, Baltimore, MD 1990-1994; Surgery, Johns Hopkins Hosp, Baltimore, MD 1989-1990; **Faculty Appointment:** Prof Urology, Johns Hopkins Univ

Droller, Michael J MD (Urology) - *Special Expertise:* Urologic Cancer; Bladder/Prostate Cancer; **Admitting Hospital:** Mount Sinai Hospital (Page 70); **Office Address:** Mt Sinai Urological Assoc 5 E 98th St, 6th Fl, Box 1272 New York, NY 10029; **Office Phone:** (212) 241-3868; **Board Certification:** Urology 1979; **Medical School:** Harvard Med Sch 1968; **Residencies:** Peter Bent Brigham Hosp, Boston, MA 1969-1970; Stanford Univ Med Ctr, Palo Alto, CA 1972-1976; **Fellowship:** Allergy & Immunology, Univ Stockholm, Sweden 1976-1977; **Faculty Appointment:** Prof Urology, Mount Sinai Sch Med

Eid, Jean Francois MD (Urology) - *Special Expertise:* Erectile Dysfunction; **Admitting Hospital:** New York Weill Cornell Medical Center - NY Presbyterian Hospital (Page 72); **Office Address:** 428 E 72nd Street, Ste 400 New York, NY 10021; **Office Phone:** (212) 746-5473; **Board Certification:** Urology 1999; **Medical School:** Cornell Univ-Weil Med Coll 1982; **Residencies:** Surgery, NY Hosp-Cornell, New York, NY 1983-1984; Urology, NY Hosp-Cornell, New York, NY 1984-1988; **Faculty Appointment:** Asst Prof Urology, Cornell Univ-Weil Med Coll

Fisch, Harry MD (Urology) - *Special Expertise:* Infertility-Male; **Admitting Hospital:** Columbia Presbyterian Medical Center (Page 72); **Office Address:** 944 Park Ave, Ste 1C New York, NY 10028-0319; **Office Phone:** (212) 879-0800; **Board Certification:** Urology 1991; **Medical School:** Mount Sinai Sch Med 1983; **Residencies:** Surgery, Montefiore Hosp Med Ctr, Bronx, NY 1983-1985; Urology, Montefiore Hosp Med Ctr, Bronx, NY 1985-1989; **Faculty Appointment:** Asst Prof Urology, Columbia P&S

Goldstein, Marc MD (Urology) - *Special Expertise: Infertility-Male; Vasectomy Reversal; Vasectomy-Scalpelless;* **Admitting Hospital:** New York Weill Cornell Medical Center - NY Presbyterian Hospital (Page 72); **Office Address:** Cornell Inst for Repro Med 525 E 68th St, rm F900, Box 580 New York, NY 10021; **Office Phone:** (212) 746-5470; **Board Certification:** Urology 1982; **Medical School:** SUNY Downstate 1972; **Residencies:** Surgery, Columb-Presby Med Ctr, New York, NY 1972-1974; Urology, SUNY Hlth Science Ctr, Brooklyn, NY 1977-1980; **Fellowship:** Reproductive Endocrinology, Rockefeller Univ, New York, NY 1980-1982; **Faculty Appointment:** Prof Urology, Cornell Univ-Weil Med Coll

Gribetz, Michael MD (Urology) - *Special Expertise: Prostate Disease;* **Admitting Hospital:** Mount Sinai Hospital (Page 70); **Office Address:** 1155 Park Ave New York, NY 10128-1209; **Office Phone:** (212) 831-1300; **Board Certification:** Urology 1980; **Medical School:** Albert Einstein Coll Med 1973; **Residencies:** Surgery, Montefiore Hosp Med Ctr, Bronx, NY 1973-1975; Urology, Mount Sinai, New York, NY 1975-1978; **Faculty Appointment:** Assoc Prof Urology, Mount Sinai Sch Med

Hensle, Terry MD (Urology) - *Special Expertise: Urology-Pediatric;* **Admitting Hospital:** Columbia Presbyterian Medical Center (Page 72); **Office Address:** 3959 Broadway, Ste 219N New York, NY 10032-1537; **Office Phone:** (212) 305-8510; **Board Certification:** Urology 1978; **Medical School:** Cornell Univ-Weil Med Coll 1968; **Residencies:** Surgery, Boston City Hosp, Boston, MA 1969-1973; Urology, Mass Genl Hosp, Boston, MA 1973-1976; **Fellowship:** Pediatrics, Mass Genl Hosp, Boston, MA 1976-1977; **Faculty Appointment:** Prof Urology, Columbia P&S

Herr, Harry Wallace MD (Urology) - *Special Expertise: Bladder Cancer; Urologic Tumors; Laparoscopic Surgery;* **Admitting Hospital:** Memorial Sloan Kettering Cancer Center; **Office Address:** Meml Sloan Kettering Canc Ctr, Dept Urology 1275 York Ave New York, NY 10021; **Office Phone:** (212) 639-8264; **Board Certification:** Urology 1976; **Medical School:** UCSF 1969; **Residency:** Urology, UC Irvine, Orange, CA 1970-1974; **Fellowship:** Urology, Meml Sloan Kettering Canc Ctr, New York, NY 1974-1976; **Faculty Appointment:** Surgery, Cornell Univ-Weil Med Coll

Huben, Robert P MD (Urology) - *Special Expertise: Prostate Cancer; Urologic Cancer;* **Admitting Hospital:** Roswell Park Cancer Institute; **Office Address:** Roswell Park Cancer Inst, Urology Clin Elm & Carlton Sts Buffalo, NY 14263-0001; **Office Phone:** (716) 845-3159; **Board Certification:** Urology 1983; **Medical School:** Cornell Univ-Weil Med Coll 1976; **Residency:** Urology, East Virginia Med Ctr, Norfolk, VA 1977-1981; **Fellowship:** Medical Oncology, Roswell Park Meml Inst, Buffalo, NY 1981-1982

Irwin, Robert MD (Urology) - *Special Expertise: Urology - General;* **Admitting Hospital:** UMDNJ-University Hospital-Newark; **Office Address:** 185 S Orange Ave, rm G536 Newark, NJ 07103; **Office Phone:** (973) 972-4488; **Board Certification:** Urology 1976; **Medical School:** Harvard Med Sch 1967; **Residency:** Urology, Mass Genl Hosp, Boston, MA 1971-1974; **Fellowship:** Chemical Pathology, Guys Hosp Med Sch, London England 1964-1965; **Faculty Appointment:** Prof UMDNJ-NJ Med Sch, Newark

Jacobs, Stephen C MD (Urology) - *Special Expertise: Laparoscopic Nephrectomy; Prostate Cancer; Kidney Cancer;* **Admitting Hospital:** University of Maryland Medical System; **Office Address:** Maryland Prostate Ctr 22 S Greene St, Rm S8D18 Baltimore, MD 21201; **Office Phone:** (410) 328-5544; **Board Certification:** Urology 1979; **Medical School:** Case West Res Univ 1971; **Residencies:** Urology, Peter Bent Brigham Hosp, Boston, MA 1975-1977; Surgery, UC San Diego, San Diego, CA 1972-1975; **Faculty Appointment:** Prof Urology, Univ MD Sch Med

Jarow, Jonathan MD (Urology) - *Special Expertise:* Infertility-Male; Prostate Cancer; Erectile Dysfunction; **Admitting Hospital:** Johns Hopkins Hospital - Baltimore (Page 65); **Office Address:** 601 N Caroline St Baltimore, MD 21287; **Office Phone:** (410) 955-3617; **Board Certification:** Urology 1999; **Medical School:** Northwestern Univ 1980; **Residencies:** Urology, Johns Hopkins, Baltimore, MD 1982-1986; Surgery, Johns Hopkins, Baltimore, MD 1981-1982; **Fellowship:** Baylor U., Houston, TX 1987; **Faculty Appointment:** Asst Prof Urology, Wake Forest Univ Sch Med

Kavoussi, Louis Rapheal MD (Urology) - *Special Expertise:* Laparoscopic Surgery; Endourology; Kidney Stones; **Admitting Hospital:** Johns Hopkins Hospital - Baltimore (Page 65); **Office Address:** Johns Hopkins Hospital 601 N Wolfe St Baltimore, MD 21287; **Office Phone:** (410) 955-6101; **Board Certification:** Urology 1999; **Medical School:** SUNY Buffalo 1983; **Residencies:** Surgery, Barnes Hosp/Wash Univ Sch Med, St Louis, MO 1983-1985; Urologic Surgery, Barnes Hosp/Wash Univ Sch Med, St Louis, MO 1985-1989; **Faculty Appointment:** Prof Urology, Johns Hopkins Univ

Kirschenbaum, Alexander Michael MD (Urology) - *Special Expertise:* Prostate Cancer; Bladder Surgery; **Admitting Hospital:** Mount Sinai Hospital (Page 70); **Office Address:** 5 E 98th St New York, NY 10029; **Office Phone:** (212) 241-8711; **Board Certification:** Urology 1997; **Medical School:** Mount Sinai Sch Med 1980; **Residencies:** Surgery, Mount Sinai, New York, NY 1980-1982; Urology, Mount Sinai, New York, NY 1982-1985; **Fellowship:** Urologic Oncology, Mount Sinai, New York, NY 1985-1987; **Faculty Appointment:** Assoc Prof Urology, Mount Sinai Sch Med

Lepor, Herbert MD (Urology) - *Special Expertise:* Prostate Cancer; Kidney Cancer; **Admitting Hospital:** NYU Medical Center (Page 70); **Office Address:** New York Sch of Med 550 1st Ave, Ste 10R New York, NY 10016; **Office Phone:** (212) 263-6420; **Board Certification:** Urology 1987; **Medical School:** Johns Hopkins Univ 1975; **Residency:** Urology, John Hopkins Hosp, Baltimore, MD 1981-1986; **Faculty Appointment:** Prof Urology, NYU Sch Med

Levitt, Selwyn MD (Urology) - *Special Expertise:* Urology-Pediatric; Voiding Dysfunction; **Admitting Hospital:** Long Island Jewish Medical Center; **Office Address:** Ped Urol Assoc 833 Northern Blvd, Ste 270 Great Neck, NY 11021; **Office Phone:** (516) 466-6953; **Board Certification:** Urology 1972; **Medical School:** South Africa 1961; **Residency:** Urology, Bronx Muni Hosp, Bronx, NY 1963-1967; **Fellowships:** Pediatric Urology, Babies Hosp, New York, NY 1967-1968; Pediatric Urology, Hosp for Sick Chldrn, London, England 1968-1969; **Faculty Appointment:** Clin Prof Urology, NY Med Coll

Lowe, Franklin MD (Urology) - *Special Expertise:* Prostate Disease; Prostate Disease-Alternative Medicine; **Admitting Hospital:** St Luke's - Roosevelt Hospital Center - Roosevelt Division (Page 58); **Office Address:** 425 W 59th St, Ste 3A New York, NY 10019; **Office Phone:** (212) 523-7790; **Board Certification:** Urology 1995; **Medical School:** Columbia P&S 1979; **Residencies:** Surgery, Johns Hopkins, Baltimore, MD 1979-1981; Urology, Johns Hopkins, Baltimore, MD 1981-1984; **Faculty Appointment:** Assoc Clin Prof Urology, Columbia P&S

Macchia, Richard MD (Urology) - *Special Expertise:* Incontinence-Fecal; Prostate Disease; **Admitting Hospital:** University Hospital - Brooklyn; **Office Address:** 445 Lenox Rd Brooklyn, NY 11203-0079; **Office Phone:** (718) 270-2554; **Board Certification:** Urology 1977; **Medical School:** NY Med Coll 1969; **Residencies:** Surgery, St Vincent's Hosp & Med Ctr, Brooklyn, NY 1970; Urology, Univ Hosp, Brooklyn, NY 1971-1974; **Fellowship:** Urologic Oncology, Meml Sloan Kettering Cancer Ctr, New York, NY 1975-1976; **Faculty Appointment:** Prof Urology, SUNY Hlth Sci Ctr

Malkowicz, Bruce MD (Urology) - *Special Expertise:* Urologic Cancer; **Admitting Hospital:** Hospital of the University of Pennsylvania; **Office Address:** 3400 Spruce St. Philadelphia, PA 19104; **Office Phone:** (215) 662-2891; **Board Certification:** Urology 2000; **Medical School:** Univ Penn 1981; **Residencies:** Surgery, Hosp Univ Penn, Philadelphia, PA 1982-1983; Urology, Hosp Univ Penn, Philadelphia, PA 1983-1987; **Fellowships:** Urologic Oncology, USC Med Ctr, Los Angeles, CA 1987-1998; Urologic Oncology, Hosp Univ Penn/Wistar Inst, Philadelphia, PA 1988-1990; **Faculty Appointment:** Assoc Prof Urology, Univ Penn

Melman, Arnold MD (Urology) - *Special Expertise:* Erectile Dysfunction; Incontinence; **Admitting Hospital:** Montefiore Medical Center; **Office Address:** 969 Park Ave, Ste 1G New York, NY 10028; **Office Phone:** (212) 639-1561; **Board Certification:** Urology 1976; **Medical School:** Univ Rochester 1966; **Residencies:** Urology, Strong Meml Hosp, Rochester, NY 1966-1968; Urology, UCLA Med Ctr, Los Angeles, CA 1970-1974; **Fellowship:** Nephrology, Cedars-Sinai Med Ctr, Los Angeles, CA 1971-1972; **Faculty Appointment:** Prof Urology, Albert Einstein Coll Med

Mostwin, Jacek Lech MD/PhD (Urology) - *Special Expertise:* Prostate Cancer; **Admitting Hospital:** Johns Hopkins Hospital - Baltimore (Page 65); **Office Address:** 600 N Wolfe St, Bldg Marburg - Ste 401C John Hopkins Hosp. Baltimore, MD 21287-2411; **Office Phone:** (410) 955-4461; **Board Certification:** Urology 1997; **Medical School:** Univ MD Sch Med 1975; **Residencies:** Urology, Johns Hopkins Hosp., Baltimore, MD 1979-1983; Surgery, U Mich., Ann Arbor, MI 1976-1978; **Faculty Appointment:** Prof Urology, Johns Hopkins Univ

Nagler, Harris M MD (Urology) - *Special Expertise:* Urology - General; **Admitting Hospital:** Beth Israel Medical Center - New York; **Office Address:** 10 Union Square E, Ste 3A New York, NY 10003; **Office Phone:** (212) 844-8900; **Board Certification:** Urology 1982; **Medical School:** Temple Univ 1975; **Residency:** Urology, Columbia Presby, New York, NY 1976-1980; **Fellowship:** Reproductive Medicine, Columbia Presby, New York, NY 1980-1981; **Faculty Appointment:** Prof Urology, Albert Einstein Coll Med

Naslund, Michael MD (Urology) - *Special Expertise:* Prostate Cancer; Prostate Disease; **Admitting Hospital:** University of Maryland Medical System; **Office Address:** Maryland Prostate Ctr 419 W Redwood St, Fl 320 Baltimore, MD 21201; **Office Phone:** (410) 328-0800; **Board Certification:** Urology 2000; **Medical School:** Johns Hopkins Univ 1981; **Residencies:** Urology, Johns Hopkins Hosp, Baltimore, MD 1983-1987; Surgery, Johns Hopkins Hosp, Baltimore, MD 1982-1983; **Faculty Appointment:** Assoc Prof Surgery, Univ MD Sch Med

Nelson, Joel Byron MD (Urology) - *Special Expertise:* Prostate Cancer; **Admitting Hospital:** UPMC - Presbyterian University Hospital; **Office Address:** UPMC Shadyside Med Ctr 5200 Centre Ave, Ste 209 Pittsburgh, PA 15232; **Office Phone:** (412) 605-3013; **Board Certification:** Urology 1998; **Medical School:** Northwestern Univ 1988; **Residency:** Urology, Northwestern Mem Hosp, Chicago, IL 1988-1994; **Fellowship:** Urology, Johns Hopkins Hosp, Baltimore, MD; **Faculty Appointment:** Prof Urology, Univ Pittsburgh

Nitti, Victor MD (Urology) - *Special Expertise:* Voiding Dysfunction; Urology-Female; **Admitting Hospital:** NYU Medical Center (Page 70); **Office Address:** NYU Med Ctr 540 First Ave New York, NY 10016-6402; **Office Phone:** (212) 263-1086; **Board Certification:** Urology 1994; **Medical School:** UMDNJ-NJ Med Sch, Newark 1985; **Residencies:** Surgery, Univ Hosp- SUNY Hlth Sci Ctr, Brooklyn, NY 1985-1987; Urology, Univ Hosp-SUNY Hlth Sci Ctr, Brooklyn, NY 1987-1991; **Fellowship:** Urology, UCLA, Los Angeles, CA 1991-1992; **Faculty Appointment:** Assoc Prof Urology, NYU Sch Med

Olsson, Carl MD (Urology) - *Special Expertise:* Urology - General; **Admitting Hospital:** Columbia Presbyterian Medical Center (Page 72); **Office Address:** 161 Ft Washington Ave Bldg DAP - Fl 11 - rm 1102 New York, NY 10032; **Office Phone:** (212) 305-0100; **Board Certification:** Urology 1972; **Medical School:** Boston Univ 1963; **Residency:** Urology, Boston VA, Boston, MA 1966-1969; **Fellowship:** Urology, Cleveland Clinic Fdn, Cleveland, OH 1967-1968; **Faculty Appointment:** Prof Urology, Columbia P&S

Scardino, Peter MD (Urology) - *Special Expertise:* Bladder Cancer; Prostate Cancer; **Admitting Hospital:** Memorial Sloan Kettering Cancer Center; **Office Address:** Memorial Sloan-Kettering Cancer Ctr 1275 York Ave, Bldg Rm C1061 New York, NY 10021; **Office Phone:** (212) 639-8193; **Board Certification:** Urology 1981; **Medical School:** Duke Univ 1971; **Residencies:** Internal Medicine, Mass Genl, Boston, MA 1972-1973; Urology, UCLA, Los Angeles, CA 1976-1979; **Fellowship:** Urology, Natl Cancer Inst, Bethesda, MD 1973-1976; **Faculty Appointment:** Prof Urology, Baylor Coll Med

Schlegel, Peter MD (Urology) - *Special Expertise:* Prostate Cancer; Infertility-Male; **Admitting Hospital:** New York Weill Cornell Medical Center - NY Presbyterian Hospital (Page 72); **Office Address:** Brady Urological Assocs 525 E 68th St, Fl F907A New York, NY 10021-4873; **Office Phone:** (212) 746-5491; **Board Certification:** Urology 1993; **Medical School:** Univ Mass Sch Med 1983; **Residencies:** Surgery, Johns Hopkins Hosp, Baltimore, MD 1983-1985; Urology, Johns Hopkins Hosp, Baltimore, MD 1985-1989; **Fellowships:** Medical Oncology, Johns Hopkins Hosp, Baltimore, MD 1986-1987; Male Reproduction, NY Hosp-Cornell Med Ctr, New York, NY 1989-1991; **Faculty Appointment:** Assoc Prof Urology, Cornell Univ-Weil Med Coll

Smith, Arthur D MD (Urology) - *Special Expertise:* Kidney Stones; Laparoscopic Surgery; **Admitting Hospital:** Long Island Jewish Medical Center; **Office Address:** Long Island Jewish Med Ctr 270-05 76th Ave, Fl 4th New Hyde Park, NY 11040; **Office Phone:** (718) 470-7221; **Board Certification:** Urology 1980; **Medical School:** South Africa 1962; **Residencies:** Surgery, Baragwanannath Hosp, Johannesburg, So Africa 1966; Genl Hosp, Johannesburg, So Africa; **Fellowship:** Urology, Johannesburg Hosp, Johannesburg, So Africa; **Faculty Appointment:** Prof Urology, Albert Einstein Coll Med

Snyder III, Howard M MD (Urology) - *Special Expertise:* Urology-Pediatric; **Admitting Hospital:** The Children's Hospital of Philadelphia; **Office Address:** Chldrns Hosp, Dept Ped Urology 34th St & Civic Ctr Blvd, Wood Bldg, Fl 3 Philadelphia, PA 19104; **Office Phone:** (215) 590-2754; **Board Certifications:** Urology 1982, Pediatric Surgery 1995; **Medical School:** Harvard Med Sch 1969; **Residencies:** Surgery, Peter Bent Brigham Hosp, Boston, MA 1970-1973; Pediatric Surgery, Boston Chldns Hosp Med Ctr, Boston, MA 1973-1974; **Faculty Appointment:** Prof Urology, Univ Penn

Sosa, R Ernest MD (Urology) - *Special Expertise:* Kidney Stones; Laparoscopic Surgery; **Admitting Hospital:** New York Weill Cornell Medical Center - NY Presbyterian Hospital (Page 72); **Office Address:** Brady Urol Assocs 525 E 68th St, Fl 9 - rm F940 New York, NY 10021-0005; **Office Phone:** (212) 746-5362; **Board Certification:** Urology 1996; **Medical School:** Cornell Univ-Weil Med Coll 1978; **Residencies:** Surgery, NY Hosp-Cornell Med Ctr, New York, NY 1979-1980; Urology, NY Hosp-Cornell Med Ctr, New York, NY 1980-1984; **Fellowship:** Renal Physiology, NY Hosp-Cornell Med Ctr, New York, NY 1984-1986; **Faculty Appointment:** Assoc Prof Urology, Cornell Univ-Weil Med Coll

Vapnek, Jonathan M MD (Urology) - *Special Expertise:* Incontinence; **Admitting Hospital:** Mount Sinai Hospital (Page 70); **Office Address:** Mount Sinai Hosp 5 E 98th St, Fl 6 New York, NY 10029; **Office Phone:** (212) 241-4812; **Board Certification:** Urology 1995; **Medical School:** UCSD 1986; **Residencies:** Surgery, UCSD, San Diego, CA 1987-1988; Urology, UCSF, San Francisco, CA 1988-1992; **Fellowship:** Urology, UC Davis, Sacramento, CA 1992-1993; **Faculty Appointment:** Asst Prof Urology, Mount Sinai Sch Med

Vaughan, Edwin D MD (Urology) - *Special Expertise:* Urology - General; **Admitting Hospital:** New York Weill Cornell Medical Center - NY Presbyterian Hospital (Page 72); **Office Address:** New York Presby Hosp, Dept Urology 525 E 68th St, Ste F901, Box 94 New York, NY 10021; **Office Phone:** (212) 746-5480; **Board Certification:** Urology 1986; **Medical School:** Univ VA Sch Med 1965; **Residencies:** Surgery, Vanderbilt Univ, Nashville, TN 1966-1967; Urology, Univ VA Hlth Sci Ctr, Charlottesville, VA 1969-1971; **Faculty Appointment:** Prof Urology, Cornell Univ-Weil Med Coll

Waldbaum, Robert MD (Urology) - *Special Expertise:* Urology - General; **Admitting Hospital:** North Shore University Hospital at Manhasset; **Office Address:** Urology Associates 535 Plandome Rd, Ste 3 Manhasset, NY 11030-1961; **Office Phone:** (516) 627-6188; **Board Certification:** Urology 1973; **Medical School:** Columbia P&S 1962; **Residencies:** Surgery, Columbia Presby, New York, NY 1965-1966; Urology, NY Hosp, New York, NY 1966-1970; **Faculty Appointment:** Clin Prof Urology, Cornell Univ-Weil Med Coll

Walsh, Patrick MD (Urology) - *Special Expertise:* Prostate Cancer; Urologic Cancer; **Admitting Hospital:** Johns Hopkins Hospital - Baltimore (Page 65); **Office Address:** Johns Hopkins Hosp-Brady Urological Inst 600 N Wolfe St, Bldg Marbu - Fl rg - rm 134 Baltimore, MD 21287-2101; **Office Phone:** (410) 614-3377; **Board Certification:** Urology 1975; **Medical School:** Case West Res Univ 1964; **Residencies:** Urology, UCLA Med Ctr, Los Angeles, CA 1967-1971; Pediatric Surgery, Boston Chldn's Hosp, Boston, MA 1966-1967; **Fellowship:** Endocrinology, Diabetes & Metabolism, Harbor Genl Hospital, Torrance, CA 1968-1970; **Faculty Appointment:** Prof Urology, Johns Hopkins Univ

Wein, Alan J MD (Urology) - *Special Expertise:* Neuro-Urology; Prostate Cancer; Incontinence; **Admitting Hospital:** Hospital of the University of Pennsylvania; **Office Address:** Hosp Univ Penn, 1 Rhoads Pavilion 3400 Spruce St, Bldg Rhoad - Ste 1 Philadelphia, PA 19104-4204; **Office Phone:** (215) 662-2891; **Board Certification:** Urology 1995; **Medical School:** Univ Penn 1966; **Residencies:** Surgery, Hosp Univ Penn, Philadelphia, PA 1969-1972; Urology, Hosp Univ Penn, Philadelphia, PA 1967-1968; **Fellowship:** Urology, Hosp Univ Penn, Philadelphia, PA 1968-1969; **Faculty Appointment:** Prof Urology, Univ Penn

Southeast

Abramson, Edward G MD (Urology) - *Special Expertise:* Urology - General; **Admitting Hospital:** Inova Alexandria Hospital; **Office Address:** 1707 Osage St, Ste 301 Alexandria, VA 22302; **Office Phone:** (703) 836-8010; **Board Certification:** Urology 1969; **Medical School:** Univ VA Sch Med 1967; **Residencies:** Surgery, George Washington Univ Hosp, Washington, DC 1968-1969; Urology, George Washington Univ Hosp, Washington, DC 1969-1972; **Faculty Appointment:** Asst Clin Prof Urology, Geo Wash Univ

Assimos, Dean George MD (Urology) - *Special Expertise:* Kidney & Ureteral Stones; Reconstructive Renal Surgery; **Admitting Hospital:** Wake Forest University Baptist Medical Center; **Office Address:** Wake Forest Univ Baptist Med Ctr Medical Center Blvd Winston-Salem, NC 27157; **Office Phone:** (336) 716-4131; **Board Certification:** Urology 1995; **Medical School:** Loyola Univ-Stritch Sch Med 1977; **Residencies:** Surgery, Northwestern Univ Hosp, Chicago, IL 1978-1979; Urology, Northwestern Univ Hosp, Chicago, IL 1979-1983; **Fellowship:** Urology, Bowman Gray Sch Med, Winston-Salem, NC 1983-1984; **Faculty Appointment:** Prof Surgery, Wake Forest Univ Sch Med

Beall, Michael E MD (Urology) - *Special Expertise:* Urology - General; **Admitting Hospital:** Fairfax Hospital; **Office Address:** 3299 Woodburn Rd, Ste 200 Annandale, VA 22003-7316; **Office Phone:** (703) 876-1791; **Board Certification:** Urology 1979; **Medical School:** Geo Wash Univ 1972; **Residencies:** Surgery, Geo Wash Univ Hosp, Washington, DC 1972-1974; Urology, Geo Wash Univ Hosp, Washington, DC 1974-1977; **Faculty Appointment:** Assoc Clin Prof Urology, Geo Wash Univ

Belker, Arnold MD (Urology) - *Special Expertise:* *Infertility-Male; Vasectomy Reversal;* **Admitting Hospital:** Jewish Hospital & Medical Center - Louisville; **Office Address:** Urology Surgical Assoc PSC 250 E Liberty St, Ste 602 Louisville, KY 40202; **Office Phone:** (502) 584-0651; **Board Certification:** Urology 1969; **Medical School:** Univ Louisville Sch Med 1958; **Residencies:** Urology, Univ Iowa Hosps, Iowa City, IA 1962-1965; Surgery, Louisville Genl Hosp, Louisville, KY 1961-1962; **Fellowship:** Nephrology, Louisville Genl Hosp, Louisville, KY 1965-1966; **Faculty Appointment:** Clin Prof Surgery, Univ Louisville Sch Med

Broderick, Gregory MD (Urology) - *Special Expertise:* *Erectile Dysfunction; Voiding Dysfunction;* **Admitting Hospital:** Mayo/St Luke's Hospital; **Office Address:** Mayo Clinic, Dept Urol 4500 San Pablo Rd Jacksonville, FL 32224; **Office Phone:** (904) 953-7330; **Board Certification:** Urology 1992; **Medical School:** UCSF 1983; **Residencies:** Surgery, UCSF Med Ctr, San Francisco, CA 1983-1985; Urology, UCSF Med Ctr, San Francisco, CA 1985-1988; **Fellowship:** Neurourology, UC Davis, Sacramento, CA 1989-1990; **Faculty Appointment:** Prof Urology, Mayo Med Sch

Carson, Culley MD (Urology) - *Special Expertise:* *Erectile Dysfunction; Kidney Stones;* **Admitting Hospital:** University of North Carolina Hospitals; **Office Address:** Univ North Carolina, Dept Urol 427 Burnett-Womack Bldg, rm 427 Chapel Hill, NC 27599-7235; **Office Phone:** (919) 966-2571; **Board Certification:** Urology 1980; **Medical School:** Geo Wash Univ 1971; **Residency:** Surgery, Dartmouth Hitchcock Med Ctr, Hanover, NH 1972-1973; **Fellowship:** Urology, Mayo Clinic, Rochester, MN 1975-1978; **Faculty Appointment:** Prof Urology, Univ NC Sch Med

Harty, James MD (Urology) - *Special Expertise:* *Urologic Cancer;* **Admitting Hospital:** University of Louisville Hospital; **Office Address:** Univ Surgical Assocs 210 E Gray St, Ste 1000 Louisville, KY 40202; **Office Phone:** (502) 629-5904; **Board Certification:** Urology 1979; **Medical School:** Ireland 1969; **Residencies:** Surgery, Johns Hopkins Hosp, Baltimore, MD 1972-1973; Urology, Johns Hopkins Hosp, Baltimore, MD 1973-1977; **Faculty Appointment:** Prof Surgery, Univ Louisville Sch Med

Howards, Stuart S MD (Urology) - *Special Expertise:* *Infertility-Male; Urology-Pediatric;* **Admitting Hospital:** University of Virginia Health Systems; **Office Address:** Univ VA Hlth Sci Ctr, Dept Urol Jefferson Park Ave, Ste 2, Box 800422 Charlottesville, VA 22098; **Office Phone:** (804) 924-9559; **Board Certification:** Urology 1975; **Medical School:** Columbia P&S 1963; **Residencies:** Surgery, Peter Bent Brigham-Chldns Hosp, Boston, MA 1963-1965; Urology, Peter Bent Brigham Hosp, Boston, MA 1968-1971; **Fellowship:** Renal Physiology, Natl Inst Hlth, Bethesda, MD 1965-1968; **Faculty Appointment:** Prof Urology, Univ VA Sch Med

Irby III, Pierce B MD (Urology) - *Special Expertise:* *Kidney Stones;* **Admitting Hospital:** Carolinas Medical Center; **Office Address:** 1416 E Moorehead St, Ste 101 Charlotte, NC 28204; **Office Phone:** (704) 355-8686; **Board Certification:** Urology 1994; **Medical School:** Uniformed Srvs Univ, Bethesda 1983; **Residency:** Urology, Letterman Army Med Ctr, San Francisco, CA 1986-1990; **Fellowship:** Endourology, UCSF Med Ctr, San Francisco, CA 1991-1992

Jordan, Gerald MD (Urology) - *Special Expertise:* *Incontinence; Urethral Reconstruction;* **Admitting Hospital:** Sentara Norfolk General Hospital; **Office Address:** 400 W Brambleton Ave, Ste 100 Norfolk, VA 23510-1196; **Office Phone:** (757) 668-4131; **Board Certification:** Urology 1984; **Medical School:** Univ Tex, San Antonio 1977; **Residency:** Urology, Naval Reg Med Ctr., Portsmouth, VA 1977-1978; **Fellowship:** Reconstructive Surgery, Eastern Va Med Sch., Norfolk, VA 1982-1984; **Faculty Appointment:** Prof Urology, Eastern VA Med Sch

UROLOGY

Southeast

Kennelly, Michael Joseph MD (Urology) - *Special Expertise:* Incontinence; Voiding Dysfunction; Pelvic Reconstruction; **Admitting Hospital:** Carolinas Medical Center; **Office Address:** McKay Urology 1416 E Morehead St, Ste 101 Charlotte, NC 28204; **Office Phone:** (704) 355-8686; **Board Certification:** Urology 1997; **Medical School:** Univ Cincinnati 1989; **Residency:** Urology, Univ Mich Med Ctr, Ann Arbor, MI 1991-1994; **Fellowship:** Neurology, Univ Tex Hlth Sci Ctr, Houston, TX 1994-1995; **Faculty Appointment:** Clin Prof Urology, Univ NC Sch Med

Lewis, Ronald W MD (Urology) - *Special Expertise:* Erectile Dysfunction; **Admitting Hospital:** Medical College of Georgia Hospital; **Office Address:** Med Coll GA, Dept Urol 1120 15th St, rm BA-8412 Augusta, GA 30912-4050; **Office Phone:** (706) 721-2546; **Board Certification:** Urology 1976; **Medical School:** Tulane Univ 1968; **Residency:** Urology, Naval Reg Med Ctr, Oakland, CA 1970-1974; **Fellowship:** Research, Tulane Univ-Delta Reg, Covington, LA 1976-1977; **Faculty Appointment:** Prof Urology, Med Coll GA

Lloyd Jr, Lewis K MD (Urology) - *Special Expertise:* Interstitial Cystitis; **Admitting Hospital:** University of Alabama Hospital at Birmingham; **Office Address:** Univ Ala Med Ctr, Div Urol 1530 3rd Ave S Birmingham, AL 35294-0001; **Office Phone:** (205) 934-1459; **Board Certification:** Urology 1976; **Medical School:** Tulane Univ 1966; **Residency:** Urology, Tulane Univ Hosp, New Orleans, LA 1970-1974; **Faculty Appointment:** Prof Surgery, Univ Ala

Lockhart, Jorge L MD (Urology) - *Special Expertise:* Kidney Stones; **Admitting Hospital:** Tampa General Hospital; **Office Address:** Harborside Med Tower, Dept Surg 4 Columbia Dr, Ste 650 Tampa, FL 33606-3589; **Office Phone:** (813) 259-0862; **Board Certification:** Urology 1980; **Medical School:** Uruguay 1973; **Residency:** Urology, Duke Univ Med Ctr, Durham, NC 1974-1977; **Fellowship:** Urodynamics, Duke Univ Med Ctr, Durham, NC 1977-1978; **Faculty Appointment:** Prof Surgery, Univ S Fla Coll Med

Marshall, Fray F MD (Urology) - *Special Expertise:* Urologic Cancer; Prostate Cancer; **Admitting Hospital:** Emory University Hospital; **Office Address:** Emory Clin, Dept Urology 1365 Clifton Rd, Fl A3225 Atlanta, GA 30322; **Office Phone:** (404) 778-5951; **Board Certification:** Urology 1977; **Medical School:** Univ VA Sch Med 1969; **Residencies:** Urology, Mass Genl Hosp, Boston, MA 1972-1975; Surgery, Univ Mich Hosp, Ann Arbor, MI 1970-1972; **Faculty Appointment:** Prof Urology, Emory Univ

McCullough, David L MD (Urology) - *Special Expertise:* Genitourinary Cancer; Kidney Stones; **Admitting Hospital:** Wake Forest University Baptist Medical Center; **Office Address:** Wake Forest Univ Baptist Med Ctr - Dept Urology Med Ctr Blvd Winston Salem, NC 27157; **Office Phone:** (336) 716-4131; **Board Certification:** Urology 1995; **Medical School:** Wake Forest Univ Sch Med 1964; **Residencies:** Urology, Mass Genl Hosp, Boston, MA 1969-1972; Surgery, Univ Hosp-Case Western Res Univ, Cleveland, OH 1965-1966; **Faculty Appointment:** Prof Urology, Wake Forest Univ Sch Med

Milam, Douglas F MD (Urology) - *Special Expertise:* Urodynamics; Voiding Dysfunction; **Admitting Hospital:** Vanderbilt University Medical Center; **Office Address:** Vanderbilt Univ Med Ctr North Dept Urol, rm A-1302 Nashville, TN 37232-2765; **Office Phone:** (615) 322-2142; **Board Certification:** Urology 1994; **Medical School:** W VA Univ 1986; **Residencies:** Urology, Univ Utah, Salt Lake City, UT 1988-1991; Surgery, Univ Utah, Salt Lake City, UT 1987-1988; **Faculty Appointment:** Asst Prof Urology, Vanderbilt Univ

838

Noseworthy, John MD (Urology) - *Special Expertise: Multiple Sclerosis; Urologic Surgery-Pediatric;* **Admitting Hospital:** Mayo Medical Center & Clinic - Rochester; **Office Address:** 807 Nira Street Jacksonville, FL 32207; **Office Phone:** (904) 390-3740; **Board Certifications:** Urology 1981, Pediatric Surgery 1991; **Medical School:** Harvard Med Sch 1970; **Residencies:** Surgery, Univ Hosps-Case West Res, Cleveland, OH 1971-1978; Urology, Univ Hosps-Case West Res, Cleveland, OH 1974-1978; **Fellowship:** Pediatric Surgery, Chldns Hosp Med Ctr, Boston, MA 1978-1980; **Faculty Appointment:** Assoc Prof Surgery, Mayo Med Sch

Paulson, David F MD (Urology) - *Special Expertise: Urologic Cancer;* **Admitting Hospital:** Duke University Medical Center (Page 60); **Office Address:** Duke Univ Med Ctr Box 2977 Durham, NC 27710; **Office Phone:** (919) 684-5057; **Board Certification:** Urology 1974; **Medical School:** Duke Univ 1964; **Residencies:** Surgery, Duke Univ Med Ctr, Durham, NC 1965-1966; Urology, Duke Univ Med Ctr, Durham, NC 1969-1972; **Fellowship:** Surgery, Natl Cancer Inst, Bethesda, MD 1966-1969; **Faculty Appointment:** Prof Urology, Duke Univ

Sanders, William Holt MD (Urology) - *Special Expertise: Prostate Cancer; Kidney Stones;* **Admitting Hospital:** Emory University Hospital; **Office Address:** Emory Clinic 5669 Peachtree Dunwoody Rd, Ste 350 Atlanta, GA 30342; **Office Phone:** (404) 255-3822; **Board Certification:** Urology 1996; **Medical School:** Emory Univ 1988; **Residency:** Urology, Yale Sch of Med, New Haven, CT 1991-1993

Schellhammer, Paul MD (Urology) - *Special Expertise: Urologic Cancer;* **Admitting Hospital:** Sentara Norfolk General Hospital; **Office Address:** 600 Gresham Dr Norfolk, VA 23507; **Office Phone:** (757) 668-3000; **Board Certification:** Urology 1999; **Medical School:** Cornell Univ-Weil Med Coll 1966; **Residencies:** Surgery, U Hosps, Cleveland, OH 1967-1968; Urology, Med Coll Va, Richmond, VA 1970-1973; **Fellowship:** Urology, Meml Hosp-Am Canc Soc, New York, NY 1973-1974; **Faculty Appointment:** Prof Neurology, Eastern VA Med Sch

Shaban, Stephen F MD (Urology) - *Special Expertise: Infertility-Male;* **Admitting Hospital:** University of North Carolina Hospitals; **Office Address:** Univ NC - Chapel Hill 427 Burnett-Womack - CB 7235 Chapel Hill, NC 27599-7235; **Office Phone:** (919) 966-8217; **Board Certification:** Urology 1993; **Medical School:** Mount Sinai Sch Med 1982; **Residency:** Urology, Univ S Fla, Tampa, FL 1983-1987; **Fellowship:** Male Reproduction, Baylor Coll Med, Houston, TX 1987-1988; **Faculty Appointment:** Assoc Prof Surgery, Univ NC Sch Med

Smith, Joseph MD (Urology) - *Special Expertise: Urologic Cancer; Prostate Cancer; Bladder Cancer;* **Admitting Hospital:** Vanderbilt University Medical Center; **Office Address:** Vanderbilt Univ Med Ctr, Dept Urol Surgery A-1302 MCN Nashville, TN 37232-2765; **Office Phone:** (615) 343-0234; **Board Certification:** Urology 1981; **Medical School:** Univ Tenn Coll Med, Memphis 1974; **Residencies:** Urology, Univ Utah, Salt Lake City, UT 1976-1979; Surgery, Parkland Meml Hosp., Dallas, TX 1975-1976; **Fellowship:** Urology, Meml Sloan Kettering, New York, NY 1979-1980; **Faculty Appointment:** Prof Urology, Vanderbilt Univ

Soloway, Mark MD (Urology) - *Special Expertise: Urologic Cancer; Kidney Cancer; Bladder Cancer;* **Admitting Hospital:** University of Miami - Jackson Memorial Hospital; **Office Address:** Univ Miami, Dept Urol 1150 NW 14th St, Ste 309 Miami, FL 33136; **Office Phone:** (305) 243-6596; **Board Certification:** Urology 1977; **Medical School:** Case West Res Univ 1968; **Residencies:** Surgery, Univ Hosps, Cleveland, OH 1969-1970; Urology, Univ Hosps, Cleveland, OH 1972-1975; **Fellowship:** Surgery, Natl Cancer Inst, Bethesda, MD 1970-1972; **Faculty Appointment:** Prof Urology, Univ Miami Sch Med

UROLOGY

Steers, William D MD (Urology) - *Special Expertise:* Incontinence; Impotence; **Admitting Hospital:** University of Virginia Health Systems; **Office Address:** Univ Va Hlth Scis Ctr, Dept Urol Hospital Dr, Box 800422 Charlotteville, VA 22908; **Office Phone:** (804) 924-9107; **Board Certification:** Urology 1999; **Medical School:** Ohio Univ, Coll Osteo Med 1980; **Residency:** Urology, Univ Tex Hlth Sci Ctr, Houston, TX 1981-1986; **Fellowship:** Neurology, Univ Pitts Med Ctr, Pittsburgh, PA 1986-1988; **Faculty Appointment:** Prof Urology, Univ VA Sch Med

Teigland, Chris Michael MD (Urology) - *Special Expertise:* Urologic Cancer; **Admitting Hospital:** Carolinas Medical Center; **Office Address:** Mckay Urology 1461 E Morehead St, Ste 101 Charlotte, NC 28204; **Office Phone:** (704) 355-8686; **Board Certification:** Urology 1999; **Medical School:** Duke Univ 1980; **Residencies:** Surgery, Univ Utah Affil Hosps, UT 1981-1982; Urology, Univ Texas SW Med Ctr, TX 1983-1987; **Faculty Appointment:** Assoc Clin Prof Surgery, Univ NC Sch Med

Wajsman, Zew Lew MD (Urology) - *Special Expertise:* Urologic Cancer; **Admitting Hospital:** Shands Healthcare at University Florida (Page 77); **Office Address:** Shands Hlthcare at Univ Florida 1600 SW Archer Rd, Box 100247 Gainesville, FL 32610-0247; **Office Phone:** (352) 392-2501; **Board Certification:** Urology 1979; **Medical School:** Israel 1965; **Residencies:** Surgery, Central Emek Hosp, Afula, Israel 1969-1970; Urology, Central Emek Hosp, Afula, Israel 1970-1973; **Fellowship:** Urology, Rosewell Park Meml Inst, Buffalo, NY 1973-1975; **Faculty Appointment:** Prof Urology, Univ Fla Coll Med

Walker III, R Dixon MD (Urology) - *Special Expertise:* Urology-Pediatric; Genitourinary Congenital Abnormality; **Admitting Hospital:** Shands Healthcare at University Florida (Page 77); **Office Address:** Shands Hlthcare at Univ FL 1600 SW Archer Rd, Box 100247 Gainesville, FL 32610-0247; **Office Phone:** (352) 392-2501; **Board Certification:** Urology 1972; **Medical School:** Univ Miami Sch Med 1963; **Residency:** Surgery, Shands Hosp-Univ Fla, Gainesville, FL 1964-1968; **Faculty Appointment:** Prof Surgery, Univ Fla Coll Med

Webster, George David MD (Urology) - *Special Expertise:* Reconstructive Urology; Urology-Female; Urodynamics; **Admitting Hospital:** Duke University Medical Center (Page 60); **Office Address:** Duke Univ Med Ctr, Dept Urol Box 3146 Durham, NC 27710; **Office Phone:** (919) 684-2516; **Board Certification:** Urology 1981; **Medical School:** England 1968; **Residencies:** Urology, Inst Urol, London UK 1973-1974; Harare Hosp, Salisbury, UK 1970-1972; **Fellowship:** Urology, Duke Univ Med Ctr, Durham, NC 1975-1978; **Faculty Appointment:** Prof Urology, Duke Univ

Midwest

Albala, David Mois MD (Urology) - *Special Expertise:* Laparoscopic Surgery; Kidney Stones; **Admitting Hospital:** Loyola University Health System; **Office Address:** 2160 S 1st Ave Maywood, IL 60153-3304; **Office Phone:** (708) 216-4076; **Board Certification:** Urology 1994; **Medical School:** Mich State Univ Coll Osteo Med 1983; **Residencies:** Surgery, Dartmouth, Lebanon, NH 1984-1985; Urology, Dartmouth, Lebanon, NH 1986-1990; **Fellowship:** Endocrinology, Diabetes & Metabolism, Wash Univ Med Ctr, St Louis, MO 1990-1991; **Faculty Appointment:** Prof Urology, Loyola Univ-Stritch Sch Med

Bahnson, Robert MD (Urology) - *Special Expertise:* Urology - General; **Admitting Hospital:** Ohio State University Medical Center; **Office Address:** 456 West 10th Avenue Div of Urology4960 UHC Columbus, OH 43210-1228; **Office Phone:** (614) 293-3648; **Board Certification:** Urology 1987; **Medical School:** Tufts Univ 1979; **Residencies:** Surgery, Northwestern U, Chicago, IL 1980-1981; Urology, Northwestern U, Chicago, IL 1981-1983; **Fellowship:** Northwestern U, Chicago, IL 1983-1984; **Faculty Appointment:** Prof Urology, Ohio State Univ

Bloom, David A MD (Urology) - *Special Expertise:* Urology-Pediatric; Voiding Dysfunction; **Admitting Hospital:** University of Michigan Health Center; **Office Address:** Taubman Health Care Center- Urology Dept 1500 E Medical Ctr Dr Ann Arbor, MI 48109-0330; **Office Phone:** (734) 936-7030; **Board Certifications:** Urology 1982, Surgery 1977; **Medical School:** SUNY Buffalo 1971; **Residencies:** Urology, UCLA Med Ctr, Los Angeles, CA 1976-1980; Surgery, UCLA Med Ctr, Los Angeles, CA 1972-1976; **Fellowship:** Pediatrics, Inst Urol-St Peters Hosp, London, England 1977-1978; **Faculty Appointment:** Prof Urology, Univ Mich Med Sch

Brendler, Charles B MD (Urology) - *Special Expertise:* Prostate Cancer; **Admitting Hospital:** University of Chicago Hospitals (Page 78); **Office Address:** 5841 S Maryland Ave, MC-6038 Chicago, IL 60637; **Office Phone:** (773) 702-1860; **Board Certification:** Urology 1981; **Medical School:** Univ VA Sch Med 1974; **Residencies:** Surgery, Duke U Med, Durham, NC 1975-1976; Urology, Duke U Med, Durham, NC 1976-1979; **Fellowship:** Johns Hopkins, Baltimore, MD 1980-1981; **Faculty Appointment:** Prof Urology, Univ Chicago-Pritzker Sch Med

Bruskewitz, Reginald C MD (Urology) - *Special Expertise:* Urologic Cancer; Prostate Disease; **Admitting Hospital:** University of Wisconsin Hospital & Clinics; **Office Address:** 600 Highland Avenue, rm G5343 Madison, WI 53792-0001; **Office Phone:** (608) 263-4757; **Board Certification:** Urology 1981; **Medical School:** Univ Wisc 1973; **Residency:** Urology, Univ Wisc, Madsion, WI 1974-1978; **Fellowship:** Urology, UCLA, Los Angeles, CA 1978-1979; **Faculty Appointment:** Assoc Prof Surgery, Univ Wisc

Bushman, Wade MD (Urology) - *Special Expertise:* Incontinence; Urodynamics; **Admitting Hospital:** Northwestern Memorial Hospital; **Office Address:** Northwestern Univ Med Sch, Dept Urol 303 E Chicago Ave, Bldg Tarry 11-715 Chicago, IL 60611-3008; **Office Phone:** (312) 695-8146; **Board Certification:** Urology 1997; **Medical School:** Univ Chicago-Pritzker Sch Med 1986; **Residency:** Urology, Univ VA Med Ctr, Charlottesville, VA 1988-1992; **Faculty Appointment:** Asst Prof Urology, Northwestern Univ

Catalona, William J MD (Urology) - *Special Expertise:* Urologic Cancer; Prostate Cancer; **Admitting Hospital:** Barnes - Jewish Hospital; **Office Address:** Washington Univ Med Ctr, Dept Urology 4960 Chldns Pl St Louis, MO 63110-1002; **Office Phone:** (314) 362-8200; **Board Certification:** Urology 1978; **Medical School:** Yale Univ 1968; **Residencies:** Urology, UC San Francisco, San Francisco, CA 1969-1970; Urology, Johns Hopkins Hosp, Baltimore, MD 1972-1976; **Fellowship:** Urologic Oncology, Natl Cancer Inst, Bethesda, MD 1970-1972; **Faculty Appointment:** Prof Urology, Washington Univ, St Louis

Chodak, Gerald MD (Urology) - *Special Expertise:* Prostate Cancer; Prostate Cancer; **Admitting Hospital:** Louis A Weiss Memorial Hospital; **Office Address:** 4646 N Marine Rd Chicago, IL 60640; **Office Phone:** (773) 564-5006; **Board Certification:** Urology 1984; **Medical School:** SUNY Buffalo 1975; **Residencies:** Surgery, UCLA Med Ctr, California, CA 1976-1977; Urology, Brigham Hosp, Boston, MA 1977-1979; **Fellowship:** Research, Harvard Chldns Hosp, Boston, MA 1981-1982; **Faculty Appointment:** Prof Surgery

Clayman, Ralph V MD (Urology) - *Special Expertise:* Kidney Stones; Endourology; **Admitting Hospital:** Barnes - Jewish Hospital; **Office Address:** 4960 Children's Pl St Louis, MO 63110; **Office Phone:** (314) 362-8200; **Board Certification:** Urology 1981; **Medical School:** UCSD 1973; **Residency:** Urology, Univ Minn, Minneapolis, MN 1974-1979; **Faculty Appointment:** Prof Urology, Washington Univ, St Louis

Flanigan, Robert MD (Urology) - *Special Expertise:* Prostate CAncer; Bladder Cancer; Transplant-Kidney; **Admitting Hospital:** Loyola University Health System; **Office Address:** Loyola Univ Med-Fahey Bldg 54 2160 S First Ave, rm 245 Maywood, IL 60153; **Office Phone:** (708) 216-5100; **Board Certifications:** Urology 1980, Surgery 1988; **Medical School:** Case West Res Univ 1972; **Residencies:** Surgery, Case West U, Cleveland, OH 1973-1978; Urology; **Faculty Appointment:** Prof Urology, Loyola Univ-Stritch Sch Med

Gluckman, Gordon MD (Urology) - *Special Expertise:* Urinary Tract Infections; Erectile Dysfunction; **Admitting Hospital:** Lutheran Medical Center; **Office Address:** Parkside Center 1875 Dempster St, Ste 506 Park Ridge, IL 60068; **Office Phone:** (847) 823-4700; **Board Certification:** Urology 1997; **Medical School:** Northwestern Univ 1989; **Residencies:** Surgery, UCSF, San Francisco, CA 1990-1991; Urology, UCSF, San Francisco, CA 1991-1995

Klein, Eric A MD (Urology) - *Special Expertise:* Prostate Cancer; Bladder Cancer; Urologic Cancer; **Admitting Hospital:** Cleveland Clinic Foundation; **Office Address:** Cleveland Clinic Fdn, Dept Urol, Sect Urol-Onc 9500 Euclid Ave, Fl A100 Cleveland, OH 44195-0001; **Office Phone:** (216) 444-5591; **Board Certification:** Urology 1999; **Medical School:** Univ Pittsburgh 1981; **Residency:** Urology, Cleveland Clinic Fdn, Cleveland, OH 1981-1986; **Fellowship:** Urologic Oncology, Meml Sloan Kettering Canc Ctr, New York, NY 1986-1989; **Faculty Appointment:** Assoc Prof Surgery, Ohio State Univ

Kozlowski, James Michael MD (Urology) - *Special Expertise:* Prostate Cancer; Continent Urinary Diversions; Laparoscopic Surgery; **Admitting Hospital:** Northwestern Memorial Hospital; **Office Address:** 675 N St Clair Galter 20-150 Chicago, IL 60611; **Office Phone:** (312) 695-8146; **Board Certifications:** Urology 1983, Surgery 1993; **Medical School:** Northwestern Univ 1975; **Residencies:** Surgery, Northwestern Univ-McGraw, Chicago, IL 1977-1979; Urology, Northwestern Univ-McGraw, Chicago, IL 1979-1981; **Fellowship:** Research, Natl Cancer Inst-Frederick Canc Rsch, Chicago, IL 1982-1984; **Faculty Appointment:** Assoc Prof Urology, Northwestern Univ

Levine, Laurence Adan MD (Urology) - *Special Expertise:* Erectile Dysfunction; Infertility-Male; Impotence-Peyronies Disease; **Admitting Hospital:** Rush/Presbyterian - St Luke's Medical Center - Chicago (Page 74); **Office Address:** 1725 W Harrison St, Bldg 917 Chicago, IL 60612; **Office Phone:** (312) 829-1820; **Board Certification:** Urology 1999; **Medical School:** Univ Colo 1980; **Residencies:** Surgery, Tufts-New England Med Ctr, Boston, MA 1980-1982; Urology, Harvard/Brigham-Womens, Boston, MA 1983-1987; **Faculty Appointment:** Prof Urology, Rush Med Coll

Mc Vary, Kevin MD (Urology) - *Special Expertise:* Prostate Cancer; Erectile Dysfunction; **Admitting Hospital:** Northwestern Memorial Hospital; **Office Address:** 675 N St. Clair Galter Pavillion Court 20th FL Suite 150 Chicago, IL 60611-4813; **Office Phone:** (312) 695-8146; **Board Certification:** Urology 1991; **Medical School:** Northwestern Univ 1983; **Residencies:** Surgery, Northwestern Meml Hosp, Chicago, IL 1984-1985; Urology, Northwestern Meml Hosp, Chicago, IL 1985-1988; **Fellowship:** Urology, Northwestern Meml Hosp, Chicago, IL; **Faculty Appointment:** Assoc Prof Urology, Northwestern Univ

Menon, Mani MD (Urology) - *Special Expertise:* Prostate Cancer; Transplant-Kidney; **Admitting Hospital:** Henry Ford Health System (Page 62); **Office Address:** Henry Ford Hlth Sys, Dept Urol 1 Ford Pl, Ste 2F Detroit, MI 48202-2689; **Office Phone:** (313) 874-4754; **Board Certification:** Urology 1982; **Medical School:** India 1969; **Residencies:** Urology, Bryn Mawr Hosp, Bryn Mawr, PA 1973-1974; Urology, John Hopkins Hosp, Baltimore, MD 1974-1980; **Fellowship:** Transplant Surgery, John Hopkins Univ, Baltimore, MD 1976-1977; **Faculty Appointment:** Prof Surgery, Univ Mass Sch Med

Montague, Drogo K. MD (Urology) - *Special Expertise: Erectile Dysfunction; Incontinence;* **Admitting Hospital:** Cleveland Clinic Foundation; **Office Address:** Cleveland Clinic Foundation-Urological Inst 9500 Euclid Ave Cleveland, OH 44195-5041; **Office Phone:** (216) 444-5590; **Board Certification:** Urology 1975; **Medical School:** Univ Mich Med Sch 1968; **Residencies:** Urology, Cleveland Clinic, Cleveland, OH 1970-1973; Surgery, Cleveland Clinic, Cleveland, OH 1969-1970; **Faculty Appointment:** Prof Urology, Ohio State Univ

Montie, James MD (Urology) - *Special Expertise: Bladder Cancer; Prostate Cancer;* **Admitting Hospital:** University of Michigan Health Center; **Office Address:** 1500 E Medical Ctr Dr A. Alfred Taubman Hlth Care Ctr-Sec Urol, rm 2918, Box 0330 Ann Arbor, MI 48109; **Office Phone:** (734) 647-8903; **Board Certification:** Urology 1978; **Medical School:** Univ Mich Med Sch 1971; **Residency:** Urology, Cleveland Clinic Foundation 1973-1976; **Fellowship:** Urology, Memorial Sloan-Kettering, NY, NY 1978-1979; **Faculty Appointment:** Prof Surgery, Univ Mich Med Sch

Mulcahy, John J. MD (Urology) - *Special Expertise: Erectile Dysfunction; Incontinence; Penile Prostheses;* **Admitting Hospital:** Indiana University Hospital & Medical Center - Indianapolis; **Office Address:** 535 Barnhill, Ste 420 Indianapolis, IN 46202-2859; **Office Phone:** (317) 278-7560; **Board Certification:** Urology 1976; **Medical School:** Georgetown Univ 1966; **Residencies:** Urology, Mayo Clinic, Rochester, MN 1972-1974; Urology, Mayo Clinic, Rochester, MN 1967-1969; **Fellowship:** Physiology, Univ Mich, Ann Arbor, MI 1969-1972; **Faculty Appointment:** Prof Urology, Indiana Univ

Novick, Andrew MD (Urology) - *Special Expertise: Transplant-Kidney; Adrenal Disorders; Urologic Cancer;* **Admitting Hospital:** Cleveland Clinic Foundation; **Office Address:** Chairman, Urological Institute, Cleveland Clinic 9500 Euclid Ave, rm A-100 Cleveland, OH 44195; **Office Phone:** (216) 444-5584; **Board Certification:** Urology 1979; **Medical School:** McGill Univ 1972; **Residencies:** Cleveland Clinic, Cleveland, OH 1974-1977; Royal Victoria Hosp, Montreal, CN 1973-1974

Ohl, Dana Alan MD (Urology) - *Special Expertise: Infertility-Male; Kidney Stones;* **Admitting Hospital:** University of Michigan Health Center; **Office Address:** Univ Mich Med Ctr, Dept Urology 1500 E Med Ctr Ann Arbor, MI 48109-0330; **Office Phone:** (734) 936-7030; **Board Certification:** Urology 1999; **Medical School:** Univ Mich Med Sch 1982; **Residency:** Urology, Univ Mich Hosps, Ann Arbor, MI 1983-1987; **Faculty Appointment:** Assoc Prof Urology, Univ Mich Med Sch

Pryor, Jon L. MD (Urology) - *Special Expertise: Infertility-Male; Erectile Dysfunction;* **Admitting Hospital:** Fairview-University Medical Center - University Campus; **Office Address:** Fairview University Medical Center 420 Delaware St SE, Box 394 Minneapolis, MN 55455-0374; **Office Phone:** (612) 625-0662; **Board Certification:** Urology 1994; **Medical School:** Univ Minn 1983; **Residency:** U Va., Charlottesville, VA 1985-1989; **Fellowship:** Urology, U Minn., Minneapolis, MN 1989-1991

Resnick, Martin MD (Urology) - *Special Expertise: Prostate Cancer;* **Admitting Hospital:** University Hospital - Cleveland; **Office Address:** Univ Hosp - Case Western Reserve 11100 Euclid Ave Cleveland, OH 44106-5046; **Office Phone:** (216) 844-3011; **Board Certification:** Urology 1977; **Medical School:** Wake Forest Univ Sch Med 1969; **Residencies:** Surgery, Univ Hosps, Cleveland, OH 1970-1971; Urology, Northwestern Med Ctr, Cleveland, OH 1971-1975; **Faculty Appointment:** Prof Urology, Case West Res Univ

Rink, Richard C (Urology) - *Special Expertise:* Urology-Pediatric; **Admitting Hospital:** Riley Hospital for Children; **Office Address:** Indiana Univ Med Ctr 702 Barhill Ave, Ste 1739 Indianapolis, IN 46202; **Office Phone:** (317) 274-5000; **Board Certification:** Urology 1996; **Medical School:** Indiana Univ 1978; **Residencies:** Surgery, Emory Univ Med Ctr, Atlanta, GA 1979-1980; Urology, Indiana Univ Med Ctr, Indianapolis, IN 1980-1984; **Fellowship:** Pediatrics, Chldns Hosp-Harvard, Boston, MA 1984-1985; **Faculty Appointment:** Prof Pediatrics, Indiana Univ

Ross, Lawrence S MD (Urology) - *Special Expertise:* Infertility-Male; **Admitting Hospital:** Michael Reese Hospital & Medical Center; **Office Address:** 900 N Michigan Ave, Ste 1420 Chicago, IL 60611; **Office Phone:** (312) 440-5128; **Board Certification:** Urology 1974; **Medical School:** Univ Chicago-Pritzker Sch Med 1965; **Residency:** Urology, Michael Reese Hosp, Chicago, IL 1966-1970; **Faculty Appointment:** Prof Urology, Univ IL Coll Med

Schaeffer, Anthony MD (Urology) - *Special Expertise:* Interstitial Cystitis; Incontinence; **Admitting Hospital:** Northwestern Memorial Hospital; **Office Address:** 675 N St. Clair, Ste 20 Chicago, IL 60611; **Office Phone:** (312) 908-8146; **Board Certification:** Urology 1978; **Medical School:** Northwestern Univ 1968; **Residencies:** Surgery, Northwestern, Chicago, IL 1969-1970; Urology, Stanford Med Ctr, Stanford, CA 1972-1976; **Faculty Appointment:** Prof Urology, Northwestern Univ

Seftel, Allen D MD (Urology) - *Special Expertise:* Erectile Dysfunction; Infertility-Male; **Admitting Hospital:** MacDonald Womens Hospital; **Office Address:** Urology of Cleveland Inc 11100 Euclid Ave, MS 5046 Cleveland, OH 44106-5046; **Office Phone:** (216) 844-7632; **Board Certification:** Urology 1995; **Medical School:** SUNY Downstate 1984; **Residencies:** Urology, SUNY Downstate Med Ctr, Brooklyn, NY 1986-1987; Urology, Univ Hosps-Case West Res, Cleveland, OH 1987-1990; **Fellowship:** Urology, Boston Univ Med Ctr, Boston, MA 1990-1992; **Faculty Appointment:** Assoc Prof Urology, Case West Res Univ

Thomas, Anthony J. MD (Urology) - *Special Expertise:* Erectile Dysfunction; Vasectomy Reversal; **Admitting Hospital:** Cleveland Clinic Foundation; **Office Address:** Cleveland Clinic, Dept Urology 9500 Euclid Ave, rm A-100 Cleveland, OH 44195; **Office Phone:** (216) 444-5600; **Board Certification:** Urology 1978; **Medical School:** Univ Cincinnati 1969; **Residency:** Urology, Wayne St Univ Affil Hosp, Detroit, MI 1973-1976

Totonchi, Emil MD (Urology) - *Special Expertise:* Urology - General; **Admitting Hospital:** Illinois Masonic Medical Center (Page 64); **Office Address:** 860 N Clark St Chicago, IL 60610-3218; **Office Phone:** (312) 944-2848; **Board Certification:** Urology 1984; **Medical School:** Iraq 1968; **Residencies:** Surgery, United Kingdom 1972-1977; Urology, Cook County Hosp, Chicago, IL 1978-1982; **Fellowship:** Otolaryngology, Univ Illinois, Chicago, IL 1977-1978

Uehling, David T MD (Urology) - *Special Expertise:* Urology-Pediatric; **Admitting Hospital:** University of Wisconsin Hospital & Clinics; **Office Address:** 600 Highland Ave, G5-339 Madison, WI 53792-3236; **Office Phone:** (608) 263-4757; **Board Certification:** Urology 1967; **Medical School:** Northwestern Univ 1959; **Residency:** Urology, Northwestern Univ, Chicago, IL 1960-1964; **Fellowship:** Pediatric Urology, Chldns Meml Hosp, Chicago, IL 1964; **Faculty Appointment:** Prof Surgery, Univ Wisc

Williams, Richard D MD (Urology) - *Special Expertise:* Kidney Cancer; Bladder Cancer; Prostate Cancer; **Admitting Hospital:** University of Iowa Hospitals and Clinics; **Office Address:** Univ Iowa, Dept Urol 200 Hawkins Dr Iowa City, IA 52242-1089; **Office Phone:** (319) 356-0760; **Board Certification:** Urology 1979; **Medical School:** Univ Kans 1970; **Residencies:** Surgery, Univ Minn Hosps & Clins, Minneapolis, MN 1971-1972; Urology, Univ Minn Hosps & Clins, Minneapolis, MN 1972-1976; **Fellowship:** Urologic Oncology, Univ Minn Hosps & Clins, Minneapolis, MN 1976-1979; **Faculty Appointment:** Prof Urology, Univ Iowa Coll Med

Great Plains and Mountains

Cartwright, Patrick MD (Urology) - *Special Expertise: Urology-Pediatric;* **Admitting Hospital:** Primary Children's Medical Center; **Office Address:** Primary Chldns Hosp 100 N Medical Dr, Ste 2200 Salt Lake City, UT 84113-1100; **Office Phone:** (801) 588-3300; **Board Certification:** Urology 1992; **Medical School:** Univ Tex SW, Dallas 1984; **Residency:** Urology, Univ Utah Affil Hosp, Salt Lake City, UT 1984-1989; **Fellowship:** Pediatric Urology, Chldns Hosp, Philadelphia, PA 1989-1990; **Faculty Appointment:** Asst Prof Surgery, Univ Utah

Koyle, Martin Allan MD (Urology) - *Special Expertise: Genitourinary Reconstruction-Complex; Transplant-Kidney-Pediatric; Urologic Surgery-Pediatric;* **Admitting Hospital:** The Children's Hospital - Denver; **Office Address:** Chldrn's Hosp 1056 E 19th Ave, rm B-463 Denver, CO 80218-1007; **Office Phone:** (303) 837-2680; **Board Certification:** Urology 1986; **Medical School:** Canada 1976; **Residencies:** Surgery, Hlth Scis Ctr, Winnipeg, Canada 1977-1978; Urology, Brigham-Womens Hosp, Boston, MA 1980-1984; **Fellowship:** Transplant Surgery, Pacific Med Ctr, San Francisco, CA 1981-1982; **Faculty Appointment:** Prof Surgery, Univ Colo

Middleton, Richard MD (Urology) - *Special Expertise: Urology - General;* **Admitting Hospital:** University of Utah Hospital and Clinics; **Office Address:** University of Utah Med Ctr 50 N Med Dr. Salt Lake City, UT 84132-1001; **Office Phone:** (801) 581-4703; **Board Certification:** Urology 1970; **Medical School:** Cornell Univ-Weil Med Coll 1958; **Residencies:** Surgery, NY Hosp-Cornell Med Ctr, New York, NY 1963-1967; Urology, NY Hosp-Cornell Med Ctr, New York, NY 1963-1967; **Faculty Appointment:** Prof Urology, Univ Utah

Southwest

Bardot, Stephen F MD (Urology) - *Special Expertise: Urologic Cancer; Prostate Cancer;* **Admitting Hospital:** Ochsner Foundation Hospital; **Office Address:** Ochsner Clinic 1514 Jefferson Hwy New Orleans, LA 70121; **Office Phone:** (504) 842-4083; **Board Certification:** Urology 1993; **Medical School:** Univ Kans 1985; **Residencies:** Surgery, St Luke's Hosp, Kansas City, MO 1985-1987; Urology, Kansas City Univ Med Ctr, Kansas City, KS 1987-1990; **Fellowship:** Urologic Oncology, Cleveland Clinic, Cleveland, OH 1990-1991

Basler, Joseph W MD (Urology) - *Special Expertise: Prostate Cancer; Urologic Cancer;* **Admitting Hospital:** Audie L Murphy Memorial Veterans Hospital; **Office Address:** 7703 Floyd Curl Dr, MC-7845 San Antonio, TX 78229-3900; **Office Phone:** (210) 567-5640; **Board Certification:** Urology 1992; **Medical School:** Univ MO-Columbia Sch Med 1984; **Residency:** Urology, Barnes-Jewish Hosp, St.Louis, MO 1986-1990; **Faculty Appointment:** Assoc Prof Surgery, Univ Tex, San Antonio

Boone, Timothy Bolton MD/PhD (Urology) - *Special Expertise: Neuro-Urology; Urinary Reconstruction; Urinary Reconstruction;* **Admitting Hospital:** Methodist Hospital - Houston (Page 69); **Office Address:** Scurlock Tower 6560 Fannin, Ste 2100 Houston, TX 77030; **Office Phone:** (713) 798-4001; **Board Certification:** Urology 1995; **Medical School:** Univ Tex, Houston 1985; **Residencies:** Urology, U Tex Southwestern, Dallas, TX 1987-1991; Surgery, U Tex Southwestern, Dallas, TX 1986-1987; **Faculty Appointment:** Assoc Prof Urology, Baylor Coll Med

Buch, Jeffrey Phillip MD (Urology) - *Special Expertise: Infertility-Male;* **Admitting Hospital:** Baylor-Richardson Medical Center; **Office Address:** North Dallas Urol & Male Infertility Ctr 1600 Coit, Ste 304 Plano, TX 75075; **Office Phone:** (972) 612-8037; **Board Certification:** Urology 1997; **Medical School:** Univ Mich Med Sch 1980; **Residencies:** Surgery, Albany Med Ctr, Albany, NY 1981-1982; Urology, Albany Med Ctr, Albany, NY 1982-1985; **Fellowship:** Urology, Baylor Coll Med, Houston, TX 1985-1987

Culkin, Daniel J MD (Urology) - *Special Expertise:* Urology-Pediatric; **Admitting Hospital:** Veterans Affairs Medical Center - Oklahoma City; **Office Address:** OUHSC, Div Urol 920 S L Young Blvd Oklahoma City, OK 73104-5020; **Office Phone:** (405) 271-6900; **Board Certification:** Urology 1987; **Medical School:** Creighton Univ 1979; **Residencies:** Surgery, Loyola Univ Med Ctr, Maywood, IL 1980-1981; Urology, Loyola Univ Med Ctr, Maywood, IL 1981-1983; **Fellowship:** Endourology, Loyola Univ Med Ctr, Maywood, IL 1983-1984; **Faculty Appointment:** Prof Urology, Univ Okla Coll Med

Fuselier Jr, Harold A MD (Urology) - *Special Expertise:* Kidney Stones; Prostate Disease; Erectile Dysfunction; **Admitting Hospital:** Ochsner Foundation Hospital; **Office Address:** Ochsner Clinic 1514 Jefferson Hwy, Bldg LT - Fl 10N New Orleans, LA 70121-2483; **Office Phone:** (504) 842-4083; **Board Certification:** Urology 1974; **Medical School:** Louisiana State Univ 1967; **Residency:** Urology, Alton Ochsner Med Fdn, New Orleans, LA 1970-1974; **Faculty Appointment:** Clin Prof Urology, Louisiana State Univ

Greene, Graham MD (Urology) - *Special Expertise:* Urologic Cancer; **Admitting Hospital:** University of Arkansas for Medical Sciences; **Office Address:** Univ Hosp of AR for Med Sci 4301 W Markham Slot 774 Little Rock, AR 72205-7199; **Office Phone:** (501) 296-1545; **Board Certifications:** Urology 1999, Surgery 2000; **Medical School:** Dalhousie Univ 1994; **Residency:** Urology, Victoria Genl, Halifax 1990-1994; **Fellowship:** Medical Oncology, M.D. Anderson Cancer Ctr, Houston, TX 1994-1997; **Faculty Appointment:** Asst Prof Urology, Univ Ark

Lipshultz, Larry MD (Urology) - *Special Expertise:* Infertility-Male; Microsurgery; Erectile Dysfunction; **Admitting Hospital:** St Luke's Episcopal Hospital - Houston (Page 76); **Office Address:** Baylor College of Med, Scott Dept Urology 6560 Fannin, Ste 2100 Houston, TX 77030-2706; **Office Phone:** (713) 798-4001; **Board Certification:** Urology 1977; **Medical School:** Univ Penn 1968; **Residency:** U Penn Hosp., Philadelphia, PA 1969-1971; **Fellowship:** U Tex., Houston, TX; **Faculty Appointment:** Prof Urology, Baylor Coll Med

McConnell, John Dowling MD (Urology) - *Special Expertise:* Prostate Cancer; **Admitting Hospital:** Zale Lipshy University Hospital; **Office Address:** Univ Texas SW Med Ctr, Dept Urology 5323 Harry Hines Blvd Dallas, TX 75235; **Office Phone:** (214) 648-5630; **Board Certification:** Urology 1996; **Medical School:** Loyola Univ-Stritch Sch Med 1978; **Residencies:** Urology, Univ Tex Hlth Sci-Parkland, Dallas, TX 1980-1984; Surgery, Univ Tex Hlth Sci-Parkland, Dallas, TX 1979-1980; **Faculty Appointment:** Prof Urology, Univ Tex SW, Dallas

Miles, Brian J MD (Urology) - *Special Expertise:* Prostate Cancer; Incontinence; Bladder Cancer; **Admitting Hospital:** Methodist Hospital - Houston (Page 69); **Office Address:** Scurlock Tower 6560 Fannin St, Ste 2100 Houston, TX 77030; **Office Phone:** (713) 798-4001; **Board Certification:** Urology 1984; **Medical School:** Univ Mich Med Sch 1974; **Residency:** Urology, Walter Reed Army Med Ctr, Washington, DC 1978-1982; **Faculty Appointment:** Prof Urology, Baylor Coll Med

Sagalowsky, Arthur I MD (Urology) - *Special Expertise:* Urologic Cancer; Transplant-Kidney; **Admitting Hospital:** Zale Lipshy University Hospital; **Office Address:** Univ Tex SW Med Ctr, Dept Urol 5323 Harry Hines Blvd Dallas, TX 75390-9110; **Office Phone:** (214) 648-3976; **Board Certification:** Urology 1980; **Medical School:** Indiana Univ 1973; **Residencies:** Surgery, Indiana Univ Hosps, Indianapolis, IN 1973-1975; Urology, Indiana Univ Hosps, Indianapolis, IN 1975-1978; **Fellowship:** Clinical Pharmacology, Univ Tex SW Med Ctr, Dallas, TX 1978-1980; **Faculty Appointment:** Prof Urology, Univ Tex SW, Dallas

Strand, William MD (Urology) - *Special Expertise:* Urology-Pediatric; Laparoscopic Nephrectomy; **Admitting Hospital:** Children's Medical Center of Dallas; **Office Address:** Children's Med Ctr, Dept Urol 6300 Harry Hines Blvd, Ste 1401 Dallas, TX 75235; **Office Phone:** (214) 456-2444; **Board Certification:** Urology 1991; **Medical School:** Mayo Med Sch 1983; **Residencies:** Surgery, Naval Med Ctr, San Diego, CA 1983-1984; National Naval Med Ctr, Bethesda, MD 1984-1988; **Faculty Appointment:** Assoc Prof Urology, Univ Tex SW, Dallas

Swanson, David A MD (Urology) - *Special Expertise:* Genitourinary Cancer; Organ-Conserving Surgery; **Admitting Hospital:** University of Texas MD Anderson Cancer Center (Page 66); **Office Address:** Univ Tex MD Anderson Cancer Ctr, Div Urol 1515 Holcombe Blvd, Box 110 Houston, TX 77030-4095; **Office Phone:** (713) 792-3250; **Board Certification:** Urology 1977; **Medical School:** Univ Penn 1967; **Residencies:** Surgery, Harbor Genl Hosp, Torrance, CA 1968-1969; Urology, UC Davis, Sacramento, CA 1972-1975; **Fellowship:** Urologic Oncology, Univ Tex-MD Anderson Hosp, Houston, TX 1976-1978; **Faculty Appointment:** Prof Urology, Univ Tex, Houston

Thompson Jr, Ian M MD (Urology) - *Special Expertise:* Prostate Cancer; Prostate Surgery; **Admitting Hospital:** University of Texas Health & Science Center; **Office Address:** Univ Tex Hlth Scis Ctr, Dept Surg 7703 Floyd Curl Dr San Antonio, TX 78284-3900; **Office Phone:** (210) 567-5643; **Board Certification:** Urology 1997; **Medical School:** Tulane Univ 1980; **Residency:** Urology, Brooke Army Med Ctr, San Antonio, TX 1981-1985; **Fellowship:** Medical Oncology, Meml Sloan-Kettering Canc Ctr, New York, NY 1987-1988; **Faculty Appointment:** Prof Urology, Univ Tex, San Antonio

Von Eschenbach, Andrew C MD (Urology) - *Special Expertise:* Prostate Cancer; **Admitting Hospital:** University of Texas MD Anderson Cancer Center (Page 66); **Office Address:** Univ Tex - MD Anderson Cancer Ctr 1515 Holcombe Blvd, Box 328 Houston, TX 77030-4009; **Office Phone:** (713) 792-2570; **Board Certification:** Urology 1978; **Medical School:** Georgetown Univ 1967; **Residencies:** Surgery, Penn Hosp, Philadelphia, PA 1971-1972; Transplant Surgery, Penn Hosp, Philadelphia, PA 1972-1975; **Fellowship:** Urologic Oncology, Univ Texas-MD Anderson Hosp, Houston, TX 1976-1977; **Faculty Appointment:** Prof Urology, Univ Tex, Houston

Winters, Jack Christian MD (Urology) - *Special Expertise:* Voiding Dysfunction; Urology-Female; Urinary Reconstruction; **Admitting Hospital:** Ochsner Foundation Hospital; **Office Address:** 1514 Jefferson Hwy Dr New Orleans, LA 70121; **Office Phone:** (504) 842-4083; **Board Certification:** Urology 1997; **Medical School:** Louisiana State Univ 1988; **Residencies:** Surgery, Ochner Fdn Hosp, New Orleans, LA 1988-1990; Urology, Ochner Fdn Hosp, New Orleans, LA 1990-1994; **Fellowship:** Female Urology, Cleveland Clinic Fdn, Cleveland, OH 1994-1995

West Coast and Pacific

Berger, Richard E MD (Urology) - *Special Expertise:* Infertility-Male; Infectious Disease; Urologic Surgery; **Admitting Hospital:** University of Washington Medical Center; **Office Address:** Univ Wash Med Ctr 1959 NE Pacific St, Box 356510 Seattle, WA 98195; **Office Phone:** (206) 598-4203; **Board Certification:** Urology 1981; **Medical School:** Univ Chicago-Pritzker Sch Med 1973; **Residencies:** Surgery, Univ Colo Hlth Sci Ctr, Denver, CO 1974-1975; Urology, Univ Wash Med Ctr, Seattle, WA 1975-1979; **Fellowship:** Infectious Disease, Univ Wash Med Ctr, Seattle, WA 1976-1977; **Faculty Appointment:** Prof Urology, Univ Wash

Boyd, Stuart D MD (Urology) - *Special Expertise:* Incontinence; Impotence; Urologic Cancer; **Admitting Hospital:** USC Norris Cancer Comprehensive Center; **Office Address:** USC Dept Urol 1441 Eastlake, Ste 7414 Los Angeles, CA 90033-4525; **Office Phone:** (323) 865-3704; **Board Certification:** Urology 1984; **Medical School:** UCLA 1975; **Residency:** Urology, UCLA, Los Angeles, CA 1978-1982; **Faculty Appointment:** Prof Urology, USC Sch Med

Carroll, Peter Robert MD (Urology) - *Special Expertise:* Urology - General; **Admitting Hospital:** University of California - San Francisco Medical Center; **Office Address:** 400 Parnassus Ave, Ste 610 San Francisco, CA 94143-0330; **Office Phone:** (415) 476-1611; **Board Certification:** Urology 1998; **Medical School:** Georgetown Univ 1979; **Residency:** Surgery, UC San Francisco Med Ctr, San Francisco, CA 1980-1984; **Fellowship:** Urology, Mem Sloan Kettering Cancer Ctr, New York, NY 1984-1986; **Faculty Appointment:** Prof Urology, UCSF

Danoff, Dudley S MD (Urology) - *Special Expertise:* Prostate Cancer; Bladder Cancer; Kidney Cancer; **Admitting Hospital:** Cedars-Sinai Medical Center; **Office Address:** Cedars-Sinai Med Office Tower 8631 W 3rd St, Ste 915E Los Angeles, CA 90048-5912; **Office Phone:** (310) 854-9898; **Board Certification:** Urology 1974; **Medical School:** Yale Univ 1963; **Residencies:** Urology, Yale Med Ctr, New Haven, CT 1964-1965; Urology, Columbia P&S, New York, NY 1965-1969

de Kernion, Jean Bayhi MD (Urology) - *Special Expertise:* Urologic Cancer; Kidney Cancer; **Admitting Hospital:** UCLA Medical Center; **Office Address:** UCLA Med Ctr, Dept Urol 10833 Le Conte Ave, Box 951738 Los Angeles, CA 90095-1738; **Office Phone:** (310) 206-6453; **Board Certifications:** Surgery 1973, Urology 1975; **Medical School:** Louisiana State Univ 1965; **Residencies:** Surgery, Univ Hosps-Case West Res, Cleveland, OH 1966-1967; Urology, Univ Hosps-Case West Res, Cleveland, OH 1969-1973; **Fellowship:** Urologic Oncology, Natl Cancer Inst, Bethesda, MD 1967-1969; **Faculty Appointment:** Prof Urology, UCLA

Fuchs, Eugene F MD (Urology) - *Special Expertise:* Infertility-Male; Kidney Stones; Vasectomy Reversal; **Admitting Hospital:** Oregon Health Science University Hospital and Clinics; **Office Address:** 1750 SW Harbor Way, Ste 230 Portland, OR 97201-5164; **Office Phone:** (503) 525-0071; **Board Certification:** Urology 1977; **Medical School:** Univ VT Coll Med 1970; **Residency:** Urology, U Oregon, Portland, OR 1971-1975; **Faculty Appointment:** Prof Urology, Oregon Hlth Scis Univ

Gill, Harcharan Singh MD (Urology) - *Special Expertise:* Urologic Cancer; **Admitting Hospital:** Stanford Medical Center; **Office Address:** Stanford Hlth Svcs, Dept Urol 300 Pasteur Dr Stanford, CA 94305; **Office Phone:** (650) 723-6024; **Board Certification:** Urology 1995; **Medical School:** Kenya 1977; **Residencies:** Urology, Inst of Urol, London, England; Urology, Univ Penn, Philidelphia, PA 1986-1991; **Fellowship:** Urology, Univ Penn, Philidelphia, PA 1985-1986; **Faculty Appointment:** Prof Urology, Stanford Univ

Holden, Stuart MD (Urology) - *Special Expertise:* Kidney Cancer; **Admitting Hospital:** Cedars-Sinai Medical Center; **Office Address:** 8631 W 3rd St, Ste 915-E Los Angeles, CA 90048; **Office Phone:** (310) 854-9898; **Board Certification:** Urology 1977; **Medical School:** Cornell Univ-Weil Med Coll 1968; **Residencies:** Surgery, NY Hosp-Cornell, New York, NY 1969-1970; Urology, Emory Univ Hosp, Atlanta, GA 1972-1975; **Fellowship:** Urology, Sloan Kettering Cancer Ctr, New York, NY 1976-1978

Huffman, Jeffry Lee MD (Urology) - *Special Expertise:* Kidney Stones; Kidney Cancer; Bladder/Prostate Cancer; **Admitting Hospital:** USC University Hospital - Richard K. Eamer Medical Plaza; **Office Address:** USC Care Med Grp 1510 San Pablo St, Ste 649 Los Angeles, CA 90033; **Office Phone:** (323) 442-5955; **Board Certification:** Urology 1995; **Medical School:** Loyola Univ-Stritch Sch Med 1978; **Residency:** Medical Oncology, Memorial Sloan Kettering Cancer Ctr, New York, NY 1983-1985; **Fellowship:** Urologic Oncology, Memorial Sloan Kettering Cancer Ctr, New York, NY 1983-1985; **Faculty Appointment:** Prof Urology, USC Sch Med

Lieskovsky, Gary MD (Urology) - *Special Expertise:* Prostate Cancer; **Admitting Hospital:** USC Norris Cancer Comprehensive Center; **Office Address:** 1441 Eastlake Ave, Ste 7416 Los Angeles, CA 90089; **Office Phone:** (323) 865-3702; **Board Certification:** Urology 1980; **Medical School:** Canada 1973; **Residency:** Urology, Univ Alberta Hosp, Edmonton,Canada 1974-1978; **Fellowship:** Urology, UCLA Med Ctr, Los Angeles, CA 1979-1980; **Faculty Appointment:** Prof Urology, USC Sch Med

Lue, Tom F MD (Urology) - *Special Expertise:* Impotence; Peyronie's disease; **Admitting Hospital:** University of California - San Francisco Medical Center; **Office Address:** 2330 Post St, Ste 600 San Francisco, CA 94115; **Office Phone:** (415) 353-7344; **Board Certification:** Urology 1983; **Medical School:** Taiwan 1972; **Residencies:** Surgery, Brookdale Hosp, Brooklyn, NY 1976-1978; Urology, SUNY Downstate Med Ctr, Brooklyn, NY 1978-1981; **Fellowship:** Urology, UCSF, San Francisco, CA 1981-1982; **Faculty Appointment:** Prof Urology, UCSF

McAninch, Jack MD (Urology) - *Special Expertise:* Trauma; **Admitting Hospital:** San Francisco General Hospital; **Office Address:** 100 1 Potrero U California - San Francisco Gen Hosp Urol, Ste 3A20 San Francisco, CA 94110-3518; **Office Phone:** (415) 476-3372; **Board Certification:** Urology 1972; **Medical School:** Univ Tex Med Br, Galveston 1964; **Residencies:** Darnall Army Hosp, Fort Hood, TX; Letterman AMC, San Francisco, CA 1966-1969; **Faculty Appointment:** Prof Urology, UCSF

Padma-Nathan, Harin MD (Urology) - *Special Expertise:* Erectile Dysfunction; **Admitting Hospital:** USC Norris Cancer Comprehensive Center; **Office Address:** 9100 Wilshire Blvd East Wilshire Tower, Ste 360E Beverly Hills, CA 90212; **Office Phone:** (310) 858-4455; **Medical School:** Dalhousie Univ 1980; **Residency:** Urology, Dalhoise Univ, Halifax, Canada 1981-1985; **Fellowship:** Urology, Boston Univ Med Ctr, Boston, MA 1985-1988; **Faculty Appointment:** Clin Prof Urology, USC Sch Med

Payne, Christopher K MD (Urology) - *Special Expertise:* Neurogenic Bladder-Female; Bladder Prolapse; Incontinence-Female; **Admitting Hospital:** Stanford Medical Center; **Office Address:** Stanford Med Ctr MC-5314 300 Pasteur Dr, Ste 287 Stanford, CA 94305; **Office Phone:** (650) 723-6024; **Board Certification:** Urology 1995; **Medical School:** Vanderbilt Univ 1986; **Residency:** Urology, Univ Penn, Philadelphia, PA 1987-1992; **Fellowship:** Urology, UCLA, Los Angeles, CA 1992-1993; **Faculty Appointment:** Asst Prof Urology, Stanford Univ

Rajfer, Jacob MD (Urology) - *Special Expertise:* Erectile Dysfunction; **Admitting Hospital:** LAC - Harbor - UCLA Medical Center; **Office Address:** 1000 W Carson St, Box 5 Torrance, CA 90509; **Office Phone:** (310) 222-2727; **Board Certification:** Urology 1980; **Medical School:** Northwestern Univ 1972; **Residencies:** Surgery, St Josephs Hosp, Denver, CO 1973-1974; Urology, Johns Hopkins Hosp, Baltimore, MD 1976-1978; **Fellowship:** Research, Johns Hopkins Hosp, Baltimore, MD 1975-1976; **Faculty Appointment:** Prof Urology, UCLA

Raz, Shlomo MD (Urology) - *Special Expertise:* Incontinence-Female; Urology-Female; **Admitting Hospital:** UCLA Medical Center; **Office Address:** 924 Westwood Blvd, Ste 520 Los Angeles, CA 90024-2926; **Office Phone:** (310) 794-0206; **Board Certification:** Urology 1979; **Medical School:** Uruguay 1938; **Residency:** Surgery, Hadassah Univ Hosp, Jerusalem, Israel 1967-1973; **Fellowship:** Urology, UCLA Med Ctr, Los Angeles, CA 1974-1975; **Faculty Appointment:** Assoc Prof Urology, UCLA

Salvatierra, Oscar MD (Urology) - *Special Expertise:* Transplant-Kidney; **Admitting Hospital:** Stanford Medical Center; **Office Address:** Stanford Univ Med Ctr 703 Welch Rd, Ste H2 Palo Alto, CA 94304; **Office Phone:** (650) 498-5481; **Board Certification:** Urology 1970; **Medical School:** USC Sch Med 1961; **Residency:** Urology, LAC-USC Med Ctr, Los Angeles, CA 1962-1966; **Fellowship:** Transplant Surgery, UCSF, San Francisco, CA 1972-1973; **Faculty Appointment:** Prof Urology, Stanford Univ

Schmidt, Joseph MD (Urology) - *Special Expertise:* Prostate Cancer; **Admitting Hospital:** University of California - San Diego Healthcare; **Office Address:** UCSD Med Ctr, Div Urol 200 W Arbor Dr San Diego, CA 92103-8897; **Office Phone:** (619) 543-5904; **Board Certification:** Urology 1971; **Medical School:** Univ IL Coll Med 1961; **Residencies:** Surgery, Rush-Presby-St Lukes Hosp, Chicago, IL 1962-1963; Urology, Johns Hopkins Hosp, Baltimore, MD 1963-1967; **Faculty Appointment:** Prof Urology, UCSD

Sharlip, Ira Dorian MD (Urology) - *Special Expertise:* Erectile Dysfunction; **Admitting Hospital:** California Pacific Medical Center; **Office Address:** Pan Pacific Urol 2100 Webster St, Ste 222 San Francisco, CA 94115-2376; **Office Phone:** (415) 202-0250; **Board Certifications:** Urology 1977, Internal Medicine 1972; **Medical School:** Univ Penn 1965; **Residencies:** Internal Medicine, Hosp U Penn, Philadelphia, PA 1966-1967; Urology, UC San Francisco, San Francisco, CA 1972-1975; **Fellowship:** Urology, Middlesex Hosp, Waltham, MA 1975-1976; **Faculty Appointment:** Asst Clin Prof Urology, UCSF

Shortliffe, Linda MD (Urology) - *Special Expertise:* Urology-Pediatric; **Admitting Hospital:** Stanford Medical Center; **Office Address:** Stanford U Med Ctr, Dept. Urol, S-287 300 Pasteur Dr Stanford, CA 94305-5118; **Office Phone:** (650) 725-5530; **Board Certification:** Urology 1983; **Medical School:** Stanford Univ 1975; **Residencies:** Surgery, Tufts Med Ctr, Boston, MA 1976-1977; Urology, Stanford U Med Ctr, Stanford, CA 1977-1981; **Faculty Appointment:** Prof Urology, Stanford Univ

Skinner, Donald George MD (Urology) - *Special Expertise:* Bladder Cancer; Urologic Cancer; **Admitting Hospital:** USC University Hospital - Richard K. Eamer Medical Plaza; **Office Address:** 2025 Zonal Ave, rm #NO-5900 Los Angeles, CA 90033; **Office Phone:** (323) 865-3707; **Board Certification:** Urology 1974; **Medical School:** Yale Univ 1964; **Residencies:** Urology, Mass Genl Hosp, Boston, MA 1964-1966; Surgery, Mass Genl Hosp, Boston, MA 1968-1971; **Faculty Appointment:** Prof Urology, USC Sch Med

Skinner, Eila C MD (Urology) - *Special Expertise:* Urologic Cancer; Urinary Reconstruction; Urology-Female; **Admitting Hospital:** LAC + USC Medical Center; **Office Address:** USC-Keck Sch Med, Dept Urol NOR 7416 Bldg, MC-9178 Los Angeles, CA 90033-1034; **Office Phone:** (323) 865-3705; **Board Certification:** Urology 1992; **Medical School:** USC Sch Med 1983; **Residency:** Urology, LAC-USC Med Ctr, Los Angeles, CA 1984-1988; **Fellowship:** Urologic Oncology, LAC-USC Med Ctr, Los Angeles, CA 1988-1990; **Faculty Appointment:** Assoc Clin Prof Urology, USC Sch Med

Smith, Robert B MD (Urology) - *Special Expertise:* Urologic Cancer; **Admitting Hospital:** UCLA Medical Center; **Office Address:** UCLA Sch Med, Div Urology 760 Westwood Plaza Los Angeles, CA 90024; **Office Phone:** (310) 825-9273; **Board Certification:** Urology 1972; **Medical School:** UCLA 1963; **Residencies:** Surgery, UCLA, Los Angeles, CA 1964-1965; Urology, UCLA, Los Angeles, CA 1965-1969; **Faculty Appointment:** Prof Surgery, UCLA

Stoller, Marshall Leedy MD (Urology) - *Special Expertise:* Kidney Stones; Laparoscopic Surgery; **Admitting Hospital:** University of California - San Francisco Medical Center; **Office Address:** UCSF, Dept Urology 400 Parnassus Ave, Fl A-61 San Francisco, CA 94143-0738; **Office Phone:** (415) 353-2200; **Board Certification:** Urology 1999; **Medical School:** Baylor Coll Med 1981; **Residencies:** Urology, UCSF, San Francisco, CA 1983-1987; Surgery, UCSF, San Francisco, CA 1981-1983; **Fellowship:** Urology, Prince Henry Hosptial, Sydney, Australia 1985-1986; **Faculty Appointment:** Prof Urology, UCSF

Stone, Anthony MD (Urology) - *Special Expertise:* Urology-Female; Voiding Dysfunction; **Admitting Hospital:** University of California - Davis Medical Center; **Office Address:** 4860 1st St, Ste 3500 Sacramento, CA 95817-2214; **Office Phone:** (916) 734-8135; **Board Certification:** Urology 1997; **Medical School:** Scotland 1972; **Residencies:** Urological Renal Transplant, Western Genl Hosp, Glasgow, Scotland 1978-1980; Urology, Cardiff Royal Infirm, Cardiff, Wales 1980-1983; **Fellowship:** Urodynamics, Duke Univ Med Ctr, Durham, NC 1983-1986; **Faculty Appointment:** Prof Urology, UC Davis

Winfield, Howard Neil MD (Urology) - *Special Expertise:* Minimally Invasive Surgery; **Admitting Hospital:** Stanford Medical Center; **Office Address:** Stanford Hlth Svcs, Dept Urol 300 Pasteur Dr, S287 Stanford, CA 94305; **Office Phone:** (650) 858-3916; **Board Certification:** Urology 1999; **Medical School:** McGill Univ 1978; **Residency:** Urology, McGill Univ Tchg Hosp, Montreal, Canada 1981-1984; **Fellowships:** Endourology, Wash Univ, St Louis, MO 1984-1985; Endourology, UCLA, Los Angeles, CA 1985-1986; **Faculty Appointment:** Assoc Prof Urology, Stanford Univ

VASCULAR SURGERY (GENERAL)

(a subspecialty of SURGERY)

A surgeon with expertise in the management of surgical disorders of the blood vessels, excluding the intercranial vessels or the heart.

SURGERY

A surgeon manages a broad spectrum of surgical conditions affecting almost any area of the body. The surgeon establishes the diagnosis and provides the preoperative, operative and postoperative care to surgical patients and is usually responsible for the comprehensive management of the trauma victim and the critically ill surgical patient.

The surgeon uses a variety of diagnostic techniques, including endoscopy, for observing internal structures and may use specialized instruments during operative procedures. A general surgeon is expected to be familiar with the salient features of other surgical specialties in order to recognize problems in those areas and to know when to refer a patient to another specialist.

Training required: Five years in surgery *plus* additional training and examination

THE VASCULAR INSTITUTE
MAIMONIDES MEDICAL CENTER

4802 Tenth Avenue   Brooklyn, NY 11219

Tel. 718.283.7957   Fax. 718.283.8599   www.maimonidesmed.org

The Vascular Institute at Maimonides Medical Center has helped thousands of patients prevent the most serious circulatory complications of hypertension, diabetes, arteriosclerosis and other diseases. A nationally recognized Center of Excellence established in 1992 by Enrico Ascher MD, the Institute is setting the standard for medical quality in stroke prevention, chronic wound treatment, limb salvage surgery, varicose vein treatment, balloon angioplasties and stents, as well as diagnosis and treatment of circulatory blockages.

The Vascular Institute consists of the following divisions and services:

THE VASCULAR DIAGNOSTIC LABORATORY

This is the largest noninvasive lab in New York State and employs the most advanced technology to assess all patients. Thanks to dedicated physicians and a multimillion-dollar investment in sophisticated equipment, patients receive full and speedy evaluations—and most can do so without undergoing invasive angiograms.

THE WOUND TREATMENT CENTER

The first in Brooklyn and Staten Island to focus on the needs of patients with chronic non-healing wounds of the extremities, the Center has had a remarkable number of patients reporting dramatic improvements in their condition.

THE DIVISION OF VASCULAR SURGERY

Stroke prevention: Through balloon angioplasty and stents as well as a simplified technique for carotid endarterectomy, Dr. Ascher and his colleagues have pioneered innovative and less invasive approaches to stroke prevention.

The Vein Center: Several effective and safe procedures are used to remove unwanted varicose veins.

The Endovascular Center: One of the busiest of its kind, the center uses minimally invasive techniques to repair aneurysms and blocked arteries.

THE VASCULAR INSTITUTE

Enrico Ascher MD, founder of The Vascular Institute, is known as the best option to save a dying limb. By following an aggressive treatment program, he views amputation as a rare last resort. As a result, The Vascular Institute saves almost two-thirds of limbs that had been deemed unreconstructable.

Vascular Surgery
A Kinder, Gentler Approach to Aneurysm Repair

Only ten years ago, a patient with an aortic aneurysm would have undergone an extensive operation to repair this life-threatening swelling in the body's most important artery. Today, **The Mount Sinai Hospital** and **NYU Hospitals Center** are among a select group of institutions worldwide that offer minimally invasive surgical solutions to complex aortic problems.

The new, minimally invasive procedure used at both hospitals involves making small incisions in the groin and inserting a stent graft, which the surgeon guides to the exact position in the artery needed to ease pressure and prevent rupture. Usually, patients require no blood transfusion and are able to leave the hospital just one to two days after surgery.

As the site of early FDA testing of one of the newest devices used in endovascular surgery, **NYU Hospitals Center** is leading the way in both clinical and scientific research in the burgeoning field of vascular surgery. It also is a major training center, where vascular surgeons learn and perfect the latest minimally invasive techniques. NYU's outstanding specialists continue to achieve high rates of success with the new stent graft procedure, even in patients over 75 years of age. Judging from the pace of research at NYU, it is extremely likely that the new techniques will be used to treat other types of conditions in the very near future.

The Mount Sinai Hospital's endovascular aneurysm program is among the busiest in the United States. As a first line of defense against aortic disease, the hospital's vascular surgeons promote prevention through early diagnosis. They have pioneered and perfected a number of minimally invasive techniques, including the stent-graft procedure described above. In active partnership with cardiologists, radiologists, and other specialists throughout the institution, Mount Sinai's vascular surgeons are saving and extending lives in greater numbers than ever before.

At Mount Sinai NYU Health, we pride ourselves on delivering the highest-quality care in a patient-centered environment. Our emphasis on the newest surgical technologies is not an end in itself, but a way to ease pain and decrease recovery time, as well as achieve the best possible outcomes. In conventional aneurysm repair, the surgeon performs an open-chest procedure, involving blood transfusions, intensive care, and lengthy hospital stays. With the new devices and minimally invasive techniques, our patients not only get well—they return to normal activity and improved quality of life as soon as a week after surgery.

800-MD-YOURS
(800-639-6877)
www.msnyuhealth.org

MOUNT SINAI NYU
HEALTH

PHYSICIAN LISTINGS

New England

Abbott, William Martin MD (Vascular Surgery (General)) - *Special Expertise:* *Vascular Surgery (General) - General;* **Admitting Hospital:** Massachusetts General Hospital; **Office Address:** Mass Genl Hosp, Dept Surg 15 Parkman St Boston, MA 02114; **Office Phone:** (617) 726-8250; **Board Certifications:** Surgery 1971, Vascular Surgery (General) 1992; **Medical School:** Stanford Univ 1961; **Residencies:** Surgery, Mass Genl Hosp, Boston, MA 1962-1965; Surgery, Mass Genl Hosp, Boston, MA 1969-1971; **Fellowship:** Surgery, Mass Genl Hosp, Boston, MA 1965-1966; **Faculty Appointment:** Prof Surgery, Harvard Med Sch

Belkin, Michael MD (Vascular Surgery (General)) - *Special Expertise:* *Aneurysm; Arterial Bypass Surgery; Carotid Artery Disease;* **Admitting Hospital:** Brigham & Women's Hospital; **Office Address:** Brigham & Women's Hosp 75 Francis St Boston, MA 02115; **Office Phone:** (617) 732-6816; **Board Certifications:** Vascular Surgery (General) 2010, Surgical Critical Care 2003; **Medical School:** Univ Conn 1982; **Residency:** Surgery, Hartford Hosp, Hartford, CT 1982-1987; **Fellowship:** Vascular Surgery (General), Boston Univ/Brigham-Womens Hosp, Boston, MA 1987-1989; **Faculty Appointment:** Assoc Prof Surgery, Harvard Med Sch

Brewster, David Charles MD (Vascular Surgery (General)) - *Special Expertise:* *Aneurysm-Abdominal Aortic; Endovascular Surgery;* **Admitting Hospital:** Massachusetts General Hospital; **Office Address:** Mass Genl Hosp One Hawthorne Pl Boston, MA 02114-2333; **Office Phone:** (617) 523-4293; **Board Certifications:** Surgery 1975, Vascular Surgery (General) 1991; **Medical School:** Columbia P&S 1967; **Residency:** Surgery, Mass Genl Hosp, Boston, MA 1968-1975; **Fellowship:** Vascular Surgery (General), Mass Genl Hosp, Boston, MA 1975-1976; **Faculty Appointment:** Clin Prof Surgery, Harvard Med Sch

Cambria, Richard P MD (Vascular Surgery (General)) - *Special Expertise:* *Aneurysm-Abdominal Aortic; Cerebrovascular Surgery; Renovascular Disease;* **Admitting Hospital:** Massachusetts General Hospital; **Office Address:** Mass Genl Hosp, Surgery 15 Parkman St, MS WAC 458 Boston, MA 02114-3117; **Office Phone:** (617) 726-8278; **Board Certifications:** Surgery 1994, Vascular Surgery (General) 1994; **Medical School:** Columbia P&S 1977; **Residency:** Surgery, Mass Genl Hosp, Boston, MA 1977-1978; **Fellowship:** Vascular Surgery (General), Mass Genl Hosp, Boston, MA 1983-1984; **Faculty Appointment:** Prof Surgery, Harvard Med Sch

Cronenwett, Jack MD (Vascular Surgery (General)) - *Special Expertise:* *Peripheral Vascular Surgery; Aneurysm-Abdominal Aortic;* **Admitting Hospital:** Dartmouth - Hitchcock Medical Center; **Office Address:** Dartmouth Hitchcock Med Ctr, Sect Vasc Surg One Med Ctr Lebanon, NH 03756; **Office Phone:** (603) 650-8670; **Board Certifications:** Vascular Surgery (General) 1991, Surgery 1989; **Medical School:** Stanford Univ 1973; **Residency:** Surgery, Univ Mich Hosp, Ann Arbor, MI 1974-1979; **Fellowship:** Vascular Surgery (General), Univ Tenn Hosp, Memphis, TN 1979-1980; **Faculty Appointment:** Prof Surgery, Dartmouth Med Sch

Gertler, Jonathan P MD (Vascular Surgery (General)) - *Special Expertise:* *Aneurysm; Thoracic Outlet Syndrome;* **Admitting Hospital:** Massachusetts General Hospital; **Office Address:** Mass Genl Hosp 15 Parkman St, Ste 464 Boston, MA 02114-3117; **Office Phone:** (617) 724-0785; **Board Certifications:** Surgery 1997, Vascular Surgery (General) 1997; **Medical School:** Columbia P&S 1981; **Residency:** Surgery, Yale-New Haven Hosp, New Haven, CT 1981-1986; **Fellowship:** Vascular Surgery (General), Mass Genl Hosp, Boston, MA 1987-1988; **Faculty Appointment:** Assoc Prof Vascular Surgery (General), Harvard Med Sch

VASCULAR SURGERY (GENERAL) New England

Gibbons, Gary William MD (Vascular Surgery (General)) - *Special Expertise:* Diabetic Leg/Foot; **Admitting Hospital:** Boston Medical Center; **Office Address:** 930 Commonwealth Ave Boston, MA 02215; **Office Phone:** (617) 414-6843; **Board Certifications:** Vascular Surgery (General) 1992, Surgery 1988; **Medical School:** Univ Cincinnati 1971; **Residency:** Surgery, New Eng Deaconess Hosp, Boston, MA 1972-1976; **Faculty Appointment:** Assoc Clin Prof Surgery, Harvard Med Sch

Lo Gerfo, Frank W MD (Vascular Surgery (General)) - *Special Expertise:* Arterial Bypass Surgery-Leg; Diabetic Leg/Foot; **Admitting Hospital:** Beth Israel Deaconess Medical Center - Boston (Page 57); **Office Address:** Beth Israel Deaconess Med Ctr - Vasc Surg 110 Francis St, Ste 5B Boston, MA 02215; **Office Phone:** (617) 632-9955; **Board Certifications:** Surgery 1972, Vascular Surgery (General) 2004; **Medical School:** Univ Rochester 1966; **Residency:** Surgery, Boston Univ Hosp, Boston, MA 1967-1971; **Faculty Appointment:** Prof Surgery, Harvard Med Sch

Mackey, William C. MD (Vascular Surgery (General)) - *Special Expertise:* Carotid Artery Disease; Aneurysm-Abdominal Aortic; **Admitting Hospital:** New England Medical Center; **Office Address:** 750 Washington St, Ste 1035 Boston, MA 02111-1526; **Office Phone:** (617) 636-5927; **Board Certifications:** Vascular Surgery (General) 1995, Surgical Critical Care 1997; **Medical School:** Duke Univ 1977; **Residency:** Surgery, NY Hosp-Cornell Med Ctr, New York, NY 1978-1982; **Fellowship:** Vascular Surgery (General), Tufts Univ-New Eng Med Ctr, Boston, MA 1982-1984; **Faculty Appointment:** Prof Surgery, Tufts Univ

Whittemore, Anthony D MD (Vascular Surgery (General)) - *Special Expertise:* Carotid Artery Surgery; Aortic Surgery; Aneurysm-Abdominal Aortic; **Admitting Hospital:** Brigham & Women's Hospital; **Office Address:** Brigham & Women's Hosp 75 Francis St Boston, MA 02115; **Office Phone:** (617) 732-8515; **Board Certifications:** Surgery 1987, Vascular Surgery (General) 1992; **Medical School:** Columbia P&S 1970; **Residency:** Surgery, Columbia-Presby Med Ctr, New York, NY 1970-1976; **Fellowship:** Vascular Surgery (General), Peter Bent Brigham Hosp, Boston, MA 1976-1977; **Faculty Appointment:** Prof Surgery, Harvard Med Sch

Mid Atlantic

Adelman, Mark MD (Vascular Surgery (General)) - *Special Expertise:* Carotid Artery Surgery; Aneurysm-Abdominal Aortic; Varicose Veins; **Admitting Hospital:** NYU Medical Center (Page 70); **Office Address:** Vascular Surgery 530 1st Ave, Bldg 6F New York, NY 10016; **Office Phone:** (212) 263-7311; **Board Certifications:** Surgery 1991, Vascular Surgery (General) 1993; **Medical School:** NYU Sch Med 1985; **Residency:** Surgery, New York Univ, New York, NY 1986-1990; **Fellowship:** Vascular Surgery (General), New York Univ, New York, NY 1990-1991; **Faculty Appointment:** Assoc Prof Vascular Surgery (General), NYU Sch Med

Ascher, Enrico MD (Vascular Surgery (General)) - *Special Expertise:* Carotid Artery Surgery; **Admitting Hospital:** Maimonides Medical Center (Page 67); **Office Address:** Maimonedes Med Ctr-Admin Bldg 4802 10th Ave, Fl 4 - rm O Brooklyn, NY 11219; **Office Phone:** (718) 283-7957; **Board Certifications:** Surgery 1984, Vascular Surgery (General) 1995; **Medical School:** Brazil 1974; **Residency:** Surgery, NY Med Coll, Valhalla, NY 1976-1981; **Fellowship:** Vascular Surgery (General), Montefiore Hosp Med Ctr, Bronx, NY 1981-1982; **Faculty Appointment:** Prof Surgery, SUNY Downstate

Atnip, Robert MD (Vascular Surgery (General)) - *Special Expertise: Aneurysm-Abdominal Aortic; Aneurysm-Peripheral;* **Admitting Hospital:** Penn State University Hospital - Milton S.Hershey Medical Center; **Office Address:** Hershey Med Ctr, Po Box 850- Rm C4628, Hershey, PA 17033; **Office Phone:** (717) 318-8888; **Board Certifications:** Surgery 1985, Surgical Critical Care 1990; **Medical School:** Univ Ala 1978; **Residency:** Surgery, Mass Genl Hospital, Boston, MA 1979-1984; **Fellowship:** Vascular Surgery (General), Mass Genl Hospital, Boston, MA 1984-1985; **Faculty Appointment:** Assoc Prof Surgery, Penn State Univ-Hershey Med Ctr

Benvenisty, Alan I MD (Vascular Surgery (General)) - *Special Expertise: Cardiovascular Surgery; Peripheral Vascular Surgery;* **Admitting Hospital:** Columbia Presbyterian Medical Center (Page 72); **Office Address:** 161 Fort Washington Ave, rm 638 New York, NY 10032; **Office Phone:** (212) 305-8055; **Board Certifications:** Surgery 1999, Vascular Surgery (General) 1999; **Medical School:** Columbia P&S 1978; **Residency:** Surgery, Columbia-Presby Hosp, New York, NY 1979-1983; **Fellowship:** Vascular Surgery (General), Columbia-Presby Hosp, New York, NY 1983-1984; **Faculty Appointment:** Assoc Prof Surgery, Columbia P&S

Brener, Bruce MD (Vascular Surgery (General)) - *Special Expertise: Peripheral Vascular Surgery; Minimally Invasive Surgery;* **Admitting Hospital:** Newark Beth Israel Medical Center; **Office Address:** Millburn Surgical Assoc 225 Millburn Ave, Ste 104B Millburn, NJ 07041; **Office Phone:** (973) 379-5888; **Board Certifications:** Surgery 1972, Vascular Surgery (General) 1993; **Medical School:** Harvard Med Sch 1966; **Residencies:** Surgery, Chldns Hosp, Boston, MA 1967-1968; Surgery, Peter Bent Hosp, Boston, MA 1968-1972; **Fellowship:** Surgery, Mass Genl Hosp, Boston, MA 1972-1973; **Faculty Appointment:** Clin Prof Surgery, UMDNJ-NJ Med Sch, Newark

Calligaro, Keith Don MD (Vascular Surgery (General)) - *Special Expertise: Aneurysm-Abdominal Aortic;* **Admitting Hospital:** Pennsylvania Hospital; **Office Address:** 700 Spruce St Philadelphia, PA 19106; **Office Phone:** (215) 829-5000; **Board Certifications:** Surgery 1997, Vascular Surgery (General) 1990; **Medical School:** Rutgers Univ 1982; **Residencies:** Surgery, U Hlth Scis/Chicago Med. Sch, Chicago, IL 1984-1987; Surgery, St. Barnabas Med. Ctr., Livingston, NJ 1982-1984; **Faculty Appointment:** Assoc Clin Prof Surgery, Univ Penn

Cohen, Jon MD (Vascular Surgery (General)) - *Special Expertise: Aneurysm-Abdominal Aortic; Carotid Artery Surgery;* **Admitting Hospital:** Long Island Jewish Medical Center; **Office Address:** Long Island Jewish Med Ctr 270-05 76th Ave New Hyde Park, NY 11040-1433; **Office Phone:** (718) 470-7377; **Board Certifications:** Surgery 1985, Vascular Surgery (General) 1987; **Medical School:** Univ Miami Sch Med 1979; **Residencies:** Surgery, Cornell Med Ctr, New York, NY 1980-1984; Vascular Surgery (General), Brigham & Women's, Boston, MA 1984-1985; **Fellowship:** Vascular Surgery (General), Brigham & Women's, Boston, MA 1984-1985; **Faculty Appointment:** Prof Surgery, Albert Einstein Coll Med

Comerota, Anthony J MD (Vascular Surgery (General)) - *Special Expertise: Endovascular Surgery;* **Admitting Hospital:** Temple University Hospital; **Office Address:** Temple Univ Hosp, Dept Surg Broad & Ontario Sts, Parkinsons Pavilion- FL 14 Philadelphia, PA 19140; **Office Phone:** (215) 707-3622; **Board Certifications:** Surgery 1987, Vascular Surgery (General) 1994; **Medical School:** Temple Univ 1974; **Residency:** Surgery, Temple Univ Hosp, Philadelphia, PA 1974-1978; **Fellowship:** Vascular Surgery (General), Good Samaritan Hosp, Cincinnati, OH 1979-1981; **Faculty Appointment:** Prof Surgery, Temple Univ

Dardik, Herbert MD (Vascular Surgery (General)) - *Special Expertise: Limb Salvage; Stroke;* **Admitting Hospital:** Englewood Hospital & Medical Center; **Office Address:** Englewood Surg Assoc, PA 375 Engle St Englewood, NJ 07631; **Office Phone:** (201) 894-0400; **Board Certifications:** Surgery 1966, Vascular Surgery (General) 1983; **Medical School:** NYU Sch Med 1960; **Residency:** Surgery, Montefiore Hosp Med Ctr, Bronx, NY 1960-1965; **Faculty Appointment:** Clin Prof Surgery, Mount Sinai Sch Med

Darling, Ralph Clement MD (Vascular Surgery (General)) - *Special Expertise:* Aneurysm-Abdominal Aortic; Carotid Artery Surgery; **Admitting Hospital:** Albany Medical Center; **Office Address:** Albany Med Coll MC-157 47 New Scotland Ave Albany, NY 12208; **Office Phone:** (518) 262-5640; **Board Certifications:** Vascular Surgery (General) 1995, Surgical Critical Care 1995; **Medical School:** Univ Cincinnati 1984; **Residency:** Vascular Surgery (General), Havard-Deaconess, Boston, MA 1984-1989; **Fellowship:** Vascular Surgery (General), Albany Med Ctr Hosp, Albany, NY 1990-1991; **Faculty Appointment:** Prof Surgery, Albany Med Coll

Giangola, Gary MD (Vascular Surgery (General)) - *Special Expertise:* Vascular Surgery (General) - General; **Admitting Hospital:** St Luke's - Roosevelt Hospital Center - Roosevelt Division (Page 58); **Office Address:** St Luke's-Roosevelt Hosp Ctr 425 W 59th St, Ste 7B New York, NY 10019; **Office Phone:** (212) 523-8700; **Board Certifications:** Surgery 1986, Vascular Surgery (General) 1988; **Medical School:** NYU Sch Med 1980; **Residencies:** Internal Medicine, New York Univ Med Ctr, New York, NY 1980-1981; Surgery, New York Univ Med Ctr, New York, NY 1981-1985; **Fellowship:** Vascular Surgery (General), New York Univ Med Ctr, New York, NY 1985-1986; **Faculty Appointment:** Asst Prof Surgery, NYU Sch Med

Green, Richard MD (Vascular Surgery (General)) - *Special Expertise:* Aneurysm-Abdominal Aortic; Carotid Artery Surgery; **Admitting Hospital:** Strong Memorial Hospital - Medical Center; **Office Address:** Univ Rochester, Dept Surg 601 Elmwood Ave Rochester, NY 14642; **Office Phone:** (716) 275-6772; **Board Certifications:** Surgery 1993, Vascular Surgery (General) 1993; **Medical School:** Univ Rochester 1970; **Residency:** Surgery, Strong Meml Hosp, Rochester, NY 1971-1976; **Faculty Appointment:** Prof Surgery, Univ Rochester

Harrington, Elizabeth MD (Vascular Surgery (General)) - *Special Expertise:* Carotid Artery Surgery; **Admitting Hospital:** Mount Sinai Hospital (Page 70); **Office Address:** 1225 Park Ave, Ste 1D New York, NY 10128; **Office Phone:** (212) 876-7400; **Board Certifications:** Surgery 1981, Vascular Surgery (General) 1989; **Medical School:** NY Med Coll 1975; **Residency:** Surgery, Mount Sinai, New York, NY 1975-1980; **Fellowship:** Vascular Surgery (General), Mount Sinai, New York, NY 1980-1981; **Faculty Appointment:** Assoc Prof Vascular Surgery (General), Mount Sinai Sch Med

Hobson II, Robert Wayne MD (Vascular Surgery (General)) - *Special Expertise:* Vascular Surgery (General) - General; **Admitting Hospital:** St Michael's Medical Center; **Office Address:** UMDNJ Medical School, Medical Science Bldg, G532 185 S Orange Ave Newark, NJ 07103; **Office Phone:** (973) 972-6633; **Board Certifications:** Surgery 1972, Vascular Surgery (General) 1992; **Medical School:** Geo Wash Univ 1963; **Residency:** Surgery, Walter Reed AMC, Washington, DC 1967-1971; **Fellowship:** Vascular Surgery (General), Walter Reed AMC, Washington, DC 1972-1973; **Faculty Appointment:** Prof Surgery, UMDNJ-NJ Med Sch, Newark

Hollier, Larry Harold MD (Vascular Surgery (General)) - *Special Expertise:* Aortic Surgery; Carotid Artery Surgery; **Admitting Hospital:** Mount Sinai Hospital (Page 70); **Office Address:** Professor and Chairman, Dept Surg 5 E 98th St, Fl 14th, Box 1263 New York, NY 10029; **Office Phone:** (212) 241-7646; **Board Certifications:** Surgery 1976, Vascular Surgery (General) 1983; **Medical School:** Louisiana State Univ 1968; **Residency:** Surgery, Charity Hosp, New Orleans, LA 1968-1973; **Fellowship:** Vascular Surgery (General), Baylor Med Ctr, Dallas, TX 1973-1974; **Faculty Appointment:** Prof Surgery, Mount Sinai Sch Med

Kent, K Craig MD (Vascular Surgery (General)) - *Special Expertise: Vascular Surgery (General) - General;* **Admitting Hospital:** New York Weill Cornell Medical Center - NY Presbyterian Hospital (Page 72); **Office Address:** NY Hosp Cornell Med Ctr 530 E 70th St, rm M014 New York, NY 10021; **Office Phone:** (212) 746-5192; **Board Certifications:** Surgery 1988, Vascular Surgery (General) 1990; **Medical School:** UCSF 1981; **Residency:** Surgery, UCSF, San Francisco, CA 1981-1986; **Fellowship:** Vascular Surgery (General), Brigham & Women's Hosp, Boston, MA 1986-1988; **Faculty Appointment:** Prof Vascular Surgery (General), Cornell Univ-Weil Med Coll

Makaroun, Michel MD (Vascular Surgery (General)) - *Special Expertise: Vascular Surgery (General) - General;* **Admitting Hospital:** UPMC - Presbyterian University Hospital; **Office Address:** Presby-Univ Hosp. A-1011 Pittsburgh, PA 15213; **Office Phone:** (412) 648-2060; **Board Certifications:** Surgery 1993, Vascular Surgery (General) 1998; **Medical School:** Lebanon 1978; **Residencies:** Surgery, Anerican U Hosp., Lebanon 1978-1980; Surgery, U Pittsburgh, Pittsburgh, PA 1980-1985; **Faculty Appointment:** Assoc Prof Surgery, Univ Pittsburgh

Perler, Bruce Alan MD (Vascular Surgery (General)) - *Special Expertise: Carotid Artery Disease; Aneurysm; Stroke;* **Admitting Hospital:** Johns Hopkins Hospital - Baltimore (Page 65); **Office Address:** Johns Hopkins Hosp-Surg 600 N Wolfe St, Bldg Harvey - Ste 611 Baltimore, MD 21287-8611; **Office Phone:** (410) 955-2618; **Board Certifications:** Vascular Surgery (General) 1997, Surgery 1982; **Medical School:** Duke Univ 1976; **Residency:** Surgery, Mass Genl Hosp, Boston, MA 1976-1981; **Fellowship:** Vascular Surgery (General), Mass Genl Hosp, Boston, MA 1981-1982; **Faculty Appointment:** Prof Surgery, Johns Hopkins Univ

Ricotta, John MD (Vascular Surgery (General)) - *Special Expertise: Aneurysm; Carotid Artery Surgery;* **Admitting Hospital:** University Hospital & Medical Center at Stony Brook; **Office Address:** SUNY at Stony Brook, Dept Surgery HSC, Fl 19 - rm 020 Stony Brook, NY 11794-8191; **Office Phone:** (631) 444-7875; **Board Certification:** Vascular Surgery (General) 1980; **Medical School:** Johns Hopkins Univ 1973; **Residencies:** Surgery, Johns Hopkins, Baltimore, MD 1973-1976; Surgery, Johns Hopkins, Baltimore, MD 1976-1977; **Fellowship:** Surgery, Johns Hopkins, Baltimore, MD 1977-1979; **Faculty Appointment:** Prof Surgery, SUNY Stony Brook

Riles, Thomas MD (Vascular Surgery (General)) - *Special Expertise: Aneurysm-Abdominal Aortic; Carotid Artery Surgery;* **Admitting Hospital:** NYU Medical Center (Page 70); **Office Address:** NYU Med Ctr, Univ Vascular Assoc 530 1st Ave, Fl 6F New York, NY 10016; **Office Phone:** (212) 263-7311; **Board Certifications:** Vascular Surgery (General) 1992, Surgery 1990; **Medical School:** Baylor Coll Med 1969; **Residency:** Surgery, NYU Med Ctr, New York, NY 1970-1976; **Fellowship:** Vascular Surgery (General), NYU Med Ctr, New York, NY 1976-1977; **Faculty Appointment:** Prof Surgery, NYU Sch Med

Shah, Dhiraj MD (Vascular Surgery (General)) - *Special Expertise: Carotid Artery Surgery;* **Admitting Hospital:** Albany Medical Center; **Office Address:** Albany Med Coll-Dept Surg 47 New Scotland Ave MC 157 Albany, NY 12208-3412; **Office Phone:** (518) 262-5640; **Board Certifications:** Vascular Surgery (General) 1983, Surgery 1977; **Medical School:** Bangladesh 1965; **Residency:** Surgery, St Peters Hosp, Albany, NY 1971-1975; **Fellowship:** Research, Albany Med Ctr, Albany, NY 1975-1976; **Faculty Appointment:** Prof Surgery, Albany Med Coll

Sobel, Michael MD (Vascular Surgery (General)) - *Special Expertise: Carotid Artery Disease; Vein Disease;* **Admitting Hospital:** Upstate University Medical Hospital; **Office Address:** Upstate Med Univ, Dept Surg 750 E Adam St Syracuse, NY 13210; **Office Phone:** (315) 464-5829; **Board Certifications:** Vascular Surgery (General) 1996, Surgery 1992; **Medical School:** Albert Einstein Coll Med 1975; **Residency:** Surgery, Beth Israel Hosp/Harvard, Boston, MA 1976-1982; **Fellowship:** Vascular Surgery (General), NYU Med Ctr, New York, NY 1982-1983; **Faculty Appointment:** Prof Vascular Surgery (General), SUNY Syracuse

Steed, David Luther MD (Vascular Surgery (General)) - *Special Expertise:* Wound Healing/Care; **Admitting Hospital:** UPMC - Presbyterian University Hospital; **Office Address:** UPMC-Presby Hosp 200 Lothrop St, rm a1011 Pittsburgh, PA 15213; **Office Phone:** (412) 648-9910; **Board Certifications:** Surgical Critical Care 1995, Vascular Surgery (General) 1997; **Medical School:** Univ Pittsburgh 1973; **Residencies:** Surgery, Univ Pitts Med Ctr, Pittsburgh, PA 1974-1976; Surgery, Univ Pitts Med Ctr, Pittsburgh, PA 1977-1980; **Fellowship:** Thoracic Surgery, UCLA Med Ctr, Los Angeles, CA 1976-1977; **Faculty Appointment:** Prof Surgery, Univ Pittsburgh

Todd, George MD (Vascular Surgery (General)) - *Special Expertise:* Carotid Artery Surgery; Aneurysm; **Admitting Hospital:** St Luke's - Roosevelt Hospital Center - Roosevelt Division (Page 58); **Office Address:** Surgery 1000 10th Ave, Fl 5 - rm RG77 New York, NY 10019; **Office Phone:** (212) 305-5505; **Board Certifications:** Surgery 1980, Vascular Surgery (General) 1986; **Medical School:** Penn State Univ-Hershey Med Ctr 1974; **Residency:** Vascular Surgery (General), Columbia-Presby, New York, NY 1974-1979; **Fellowship:** Vascular Surgery (General), Columbia-Presby, New York, NY 1979-1980; **Faculty Appointment:** Prof Surgery, Columbia P&S

Turner, James MD (Vascular Surgery (General)) - *Special Expertise:* Esophageal Surgery; Laparoscopic Abdominal Surgery; **Admitting Hospital:** New York Hospital Medical Center of Queens; **Office Address:** CRT Surgical Assoc-NYHQ 56-45 Main St Flushing, NY 11355; **Office Phone:** (718) 445-0220; **Board Certifications:** Surgery 1995, Surgical Critical Care 1995; **Medical School:** Eastern VA Med Sch 1970; **Residency:** Surgery, NYU Med Ctr, New York, NY 1970-1975; **Faculty Appointment:** Assoc Clin Prof Surgery, Cornell Univ-Weil Med Coll

Veith, Frank James MD (Vascular Surgery (General)) - *Special Expertise:* Limb Salvage; Aneurysm; Endovascular Surgery; **Admitting Hospital:** Montefiore Medical Center; **Office Address:** Montefiore Med Ctr-Vascular 111 E 210th St Bronx, NY 10467-2490; **Office Phone:** (718) 920-4757; **Board Certifications:** Surgery 1961, Vascular Surgery (General) 1991; **Medical School:** Cornell Univ-Weil Med Coll 1955; **Residency:** Surgery, Peter Bent Brigham Hosp, Boston, MA 1955-1960; **Fellowship:** Vascular Surgery (General), Harvard Med, Cambridge, MA 1962-1963; **Faculty Appointment:** Prof Surgery, Albert Einstein Coll Med

Webster Jr., Marshall W. MD (Vascular Surgery (General)) - *Special Expertise:* Thoracic Vascular Surgery; **Admitting Hospital:** UPMC - Presbyterian University Hospital; **Office Address:** Univ Pittsburgh Med Ctr 200 Lothrop St, Ste A1011 Pittsburgh, PA 15213; **Office Phone:** (412) 648-9867; **Board Certifications:** Surgery 1971, Vascular Surgery (General) 1971; **Medical School:** Johns Hopkins Univ 1964; **Residency:** Surgery, U Pittsburgh, Pittsburgh, PA 1965-1970; **Faculty Appointment:** Prof Surgery, Univ Pittsburgh

Williams, G. Melville MD (Vascular Surgery (General)) - *Special Expertise:* Peripheral Vascular Surgery; Aneurysm-Abdominal Aortic; **Admitting Hospital:** Johns Hopkins Hospital - Baltimore (Page 65); **Office Address:** 600 N Wolfe St, Bldg Harvey - Ste 611 Baltimore, MD 21287; **Office Phone:** (410) 955-5165; **Board Certifications:** Vascular Surgery (General) 1994, Surgery 1966; **Medical School:** Harvard Med Sch 1957; **Residencies:** Surgery, Mass Genl Hosp, Boston, MA 1962-1964; Surgery, Mass Genl Hosp, Boston, MA 1958-1960; **Faculty Appointment:** Prof Surgery, Johns Hopkins Univ

Southeast

Bandyk, Dennis MD (Vascular Surgery (General)) - *Special Expertise: Vascular Graft Infection; Infrainguinal Bypass;* **Admitting Hospital:** Tampa General Hospital; **Office Address:** Univ So Fla Coll Med, Harborside Med Tower 4 Columbia Dr, Ste 650 Tampa, FL 33606-3589; **Office Phone:** (813) 259-0921; **Board Certifications:** Surgery 1988, Vascular Surgery (General) 1991; **Medical School:** Univ Mich Med Sch 1975; **Residency:** Surgery, Univ Wash Hosp, Seattle, WA 1976-1980; **Fellowship:** Vascular Surgery (General), Univ Wash Hosp, Seattle, WA 1980-1981; **Faculty Appointment:** Prof Surgery, Univ S Fla Coll Med

Dean, Richard H MD (Vascular Surgery (General)) - *Special Expertise: Hypertension-Renovascular;* **Admitting Hospital:** Wake Forest University Baptist Medical Center; **Office Address:** Wake Forest Univ Sch Med Med Ctr Blvd Winston Salem, NC 27157; **Office Phone:** (336) 716-4424; **Board Certifications:** Surgery 1975, Vascular Surgery (General) 1983; **Medical School:** Med Coll VA 1968; **Residency:** Surgery, Vanderbilt Univ Hosp, Nashville, TN 1969-1974; **Fellowship:** Vascular Surgery (General), Northwestern Univ Hosp, Chicago, IL 1974-1975; **Faculty Appointment:** Prof Surgery, Wake Forest Univ Sch Med

Flynn, Timothy Carlyle MD (Vascular Surgery (General)) - *Special Expertise: Aneurysm; Carotid Artery Disease;* **Admitting Hospital:** Shands Healthcare at University Florida (Page 77); **Office Address:** Shands Hlthcare Univ FL, Dept Surg 1600 SW Archer Rd, Box 100286 Gainesville, FL 32610-0286; **Office Phone:** (352) 374-6013; **Board Certifications:** Vascular Surgery (General) 1994, Surgical Critical Care 1998; **Medical School:** Baylor Coll Med 1974; **Residency:** Surgery, Univ Texas, Houston, TX 1977-1980; **Faculty Appointment:** Prof Surgery, Univ Fla Coll Med

Hansen, Kimberley J MD (Vascular Surgery (General)) - *Special Expertise: Aortic & Visceral Artery Reconstruction; Renovascular Disease; Carotid Artery Surgery;* **Admitting Hospital:** Wake Forest University Baptist Medical Center; **Office Address:** Wake Forest Univ Sch Med, Dept Genl Surg Medical Center Blvd Winston-Salem, NC 27157-1095; **Office Phone:** (336) 716-4151; **Board Certifications:** Vascular Surgery (General) 1998, Surgical Critical Care 1992; **Medical School:** Univ Ala 1980

Keagy, Blair Allen MD (Vascular Surgery (General)) - *Special Expertise: Mesenteric Occlusive Disease;* **Admitting Hospital:** University of North Carolina Hospitals; **Office Address:** Univ North Carolina Hosp Bldg Burnett-Womack - rm 210 Chapel Hill, NC 27599; **Office Phone:** (919) 966-3391; **Board Certifications:** Vascular Surgery (General) 1998, Surgery 1989; **Medical School:** Univ Pittsburgh 1970; **Residency:** Surgery, Univ North Carolina, Chapel Hill, NC 1971-1977; **Fellowship:** Vascular Surgery (General), Univ North Carolina, Chapel Hill, NC 1978; **Faculty Appointment:** Prof Thoracic Surgery, Univ NC Sch Med

Lumsden, Alan Boyd MD (Vascular Surgery (General)) - *Special Expertise: Aortic Stent Grafts; Minimally Invasive Surgery;* **Admitting Hospital:** Emory University Hospital; **Office Address:** Emory Univ Hosp 1364 Clifton Rd NE, Box M-11 Atlanta, GA 30322; **Office Phone:** (404) 727-7246; **Board Certifications:** Surgery 1990, Vascular Surgery (General) 1993; **Medical School:** Scotland 1981; **Residency:** Surgery, Emory Univ Hosp, Atlanta, GA 1983-1989; **Fellowship:** Vascular Surgery (General), Emory Univ Hosp, Atlanta, GA 1990; **Faculty Appointment:** Prof Vascular Surgery (General), Emory Univ

McCann, Richard L MD (Vascular Surgery (General)) - *Special Expertise: Vascular Surgery (General) - General;* **Admitting Hospital:** Duke University Medical Center (Page 60); **Office Address:** Duke Univ Med Ctr Box 2990 Durham, NC 27710; **Office Phone:** (919) 684-2620; **Board Certifications:** Surgery 1992, Vascular Surgery (General) 1996; **Medical School:** Cornell Univ-Weil Med Coll 1974; **Residency:** Surgery, Duke Univ Med Ctr, Durham, NC 1975-1983; **Faculty Appointment:** Prof Surgery, Duke Univ

Rosenthal, David MD (Vascular Surgery (General)) - *Special Expertise: Stroke; Aneurysm;* **Admitting Hospital:** Atlanta Medical Center; **Office Address:** 315 Blvd NE, Ste 412 Atlanta, GA 30312-1264; **Office Phone:** (404) 524-0095; **Board Certifications:** Vascular Surgery (General) 1991, Surgery 1979; **Medical School:** SUNY Downstate 1973; **Residency:** Surgery, Tufts-New Eng Med Ctr, Boston, MA 1973-1977; **Fellowship:** Vascular Surgery (General), Tufts-New Eng Med Ctr, Boston, MA 1977-1978; **Faculty Appointment:** Clin Prof Surgery, Med Coll GA

Seeger, James M MD (Vascular Surgery (General)) - *Special Expertise: Lower Extremity Arterial Disease; Aneurysm-Aortic;* **Admitting Hospital:** Shands Healthcare at University Florida (Page 77); **Office Address:** Univ FL, Dept Vasc Surg 1600 SW Archer Rd, Bldg JHMHC - rm 6165, Box 100286 Gainesville, FL 32610-0286; **Office Phone:** (352) 395-0605; **Board Certifications:** Surgery 1990, Vascular Surgery (General) 1992; **Medical School:** Med Coll GA 1973; **Residency:** Surgery, Univ UT Med Ctr, Salt Lake City, UT; **Fellowship:** Vascular Surgery (General), Eastern VA Med Sch, Norfolk, VA; **Faculty Appointment:** Prof Surgery, Univ Fla Coll Med

Sivina, Manuel MD (Vascular Surgery (General)) - *Special Expertise: Vascular Surgery (General) - General;* **Admitting Hospital:** Mount Sinai Medical Center; **Office Address:** Mt Sinai Med Ctr 4300 Alton Rd, Greenspan Bldg, Ste 212A Miami Beach, FL 33140-2800; **Office Phone:** (305) 674-2760; **Board Certification:** Surgery 1987; **Medical School:** Peru 1969; **Residency:** Surgery, Mt Sinai Med Ctr, Miami Beach, FL 1970-1975; **Fellowship:** Vascular Surgery (General), Mt Sinai Med Ctr, Miami Beach, FL 1975-1976

Midwest

Baker, William MD (Vascular Surgery (General)) - *Special Expertise: Carotid Artery Disease; Aneurysm-Abdominal Aortic;* **Admitting Hospital:** Loyola University Health System; **Office Address:** Loyola Univ Med Ctr 2160 S 1st Ave, Fl 3 Maywood, IL 60153-5590; **Office Phone:** (708) 327-2685; **Board Certifications:** Surgery 1970, Vascular Surgery (General) 1991; **Medical School:** Univ Chicago-Pritzker Sch Med 1962; **Residencies:** Surgery, Univ Iowa Hosp, Iowa City, IA 1963-1964; Surgery, Univ Chicago Hosp, Chicago, IL 1966-1969; **Fellowship:** Vascular Surgery (General), UCSF, San Francisco, CA 1969-1970; **Faculty Appointment:** Prof Vascular Surgery (General), Loyola Univ-Stritch Sch Med

Beebe, Hugh Grenville MD (Vascular Surgery (General)) - *Special Expertise: Endovascular Surgery;* **Admitting Hospital:** Toledo Hospital; **Office Address:** Jobst Vasc Ctr 2109 Hughes Drive, Ste 400 Toledo, OH 43606; **Office Phone:** (419) 471-2088; **Board Certifications:** Surgery 1971, Vascular Surgery (General) 1995; **Medical School:** Univ Rochester 1964; **Residency:** Surgery, Strong Meml Hosp, Rochester, NY 1965-1969; **Faculty Appointment:** Clin Prof Surgery, Univ Mich Med Sch

Berguer, Ramon MD (Vascular Surgery (General)) - *Special Expertise: Cerebrovascular Surgery; Aortic Branch Surgery;* **Admitting Hospital:** Harper Hospital - Detroit; **Office Address:** DMC-WSU Harper Hosp. Dept. Vascular Surgery 3990 John R Detroit, MI 48201; **Office Phone:** (313) 745-8637; **Board Certifications:** Vascular Surgery (General) 1983, Surgery 1970; **Medical School:** Spain 1963; **Residency:** Surgery, Henry Ford Hospital

Cherry Jr., Kenneth J. MD (Vascular Surgery (General)) - *Special Expertise: Vascular Reconstruction; Aortic Graft Infection;* **Admitting Hospital:** St Mary's Hospital; **Office Address:** St Mary's Hospital 1216 2nd St SW Rochester, MN 55905; **Office Phone:** (507) 284-2644; **Board Certifications:** Surgery 1981, Vascular Surgery (General) 1993; **Medical School:** Univ VA Sch Med 1974; **Residencies:** Surgery, Univ VA, Charlottesville, VA 1975-1980; Vascular Surgery (General), Univ Calif, San Francisco, CA 1980-1981; **Faculty Appointment:** Prof Surgery, Mayo Med Sch

Corson, John MD (Vascular Surgery (General)) - *Special Expertise:* Cerebrovascular Surgery; Vascular Disease in the Elderly; **Admitting Hospital:** University of Iowa Hospitals and Clinics; **Office Address:** Univ Iowa Hosps, Div Vas Surg 200 Hawkins Drive Iowa City, IA 52242-1009; **Office Phone:** (319) 356-1639; **Board Certifications:** Surgery 1991, Vascular Surgery (General) 1992; **Medical School:** Scotland 1968; **Residencies:** Surgery, Boston Univ Med Ctr, Boston, MA 1977-1980; Vascular Surgery (General), Harvard Univ, Boston, MA 1980-1981; **Faculty Appointment:** Prof Surgery, Univ Iowa Coll Med

Gewertz, Bruce MD (Vascular Surgery (General)) - *Special Expertise:* Carotid Artery Disease; Peripheral Vascular Surgery; Arterial Disease; **Admitting Hospital:** University of Chicago Hospitals (Page 78); **Office Address:** Univ Chicago, Dept Vascular Surgery 5841 S Maryland Ave, Bldg SBRI - rm J557, MC-5028 Chicago, IL 60637-1463; **Office Phone:** (773) 702-6128; **Board Certifications:** Vascular Surgery (General) 1993, Surgery 1989; **Medical School:** Jefferson Med Coll 1972; **Residency:** Surgery, Univ Mich Hosp, Ann Arbor, MI 1972-1977; **Faculty Appointment:** Prof Surgery, Univ Chicago-Pritzker Sch Med

Gloviczki, Peter MD (Vascular Surgery (General)) - *Special Expertise:* Aneurysm-Abdominal Aortic; Ischemia-Critical Limb; Vein Disease; **Admitting Hospital:** St Mary's Hospital; **Office Address:** Mayo Clin, Div Vasc Surg, West 6B 200 First Street SW Rochester, MN 55905-0001; **Office Phone:** (507) 284-4652; **Board Certifications:** Surgery 1988, Vascular Surgery (General) 1989; **Medical School:** Hungary 1972; **Residencies:** Vascular Surgery (General), Semmelweis Med Sch, Budapest,Hungary 1977-1980; Surgery, Mayo Clin, Rochester, MN 1984-1987; **Fellowship:** Vascular Surgery (General), Mayo Clin, Rochester, MN 1983; **Faculty Appointment:** Prof Surgery, Mayo Med Sch

Greenfield, Lazar MD (Vascular Surgery (General)) - *Special Expertise:* Pulmonary Embolism; Deep Venous Thrombosis; Carotid Artery Disease; **Admitting Hospital:** University of Michigan Health Center; **Office Address:** Univ Michigan - Taubman Hlth Care Ctr, Dept Surgery 1500 E Medical Center Dr Ann Arbor, MI 48109-0346; **Office Phone:** (734) 936-5850; **Board Certifications:** Thoracic Surgery 1967, Surgery 1980; **Medical School:** Baylor Coll Med 1958; **Residency:** Johns Hopkins Hosp, Baltimore, MD 1961-1966; **Fellowship:** Natl Heart Inst, Washington, DC 1959-1961; **Faculty Appointment:** Prof Surgery

Hallett Jr, John MD (Vascular Surgery (General)) - *Special Expertise:* Aneurysm-Abdominal Aortic; **Admitting Hospital:** Mayo Medical Center & Clinic - Rochester; **Office Address:** Mayo Clinic, Dept Vascular Surg 200 1st St SW Rochester, MN 55905; **Office Phone:** (507) 284-4751; **Board Certifications:** Vascular Surgery (General) 1993, Surgery 1999; **Medical School:** Duke Univ 1973; **Residency:** Surgery, Wilford Hall USAF Med Ctr, San Antonio, TX 1974-1978; **Fellowship:** Vascular Surgery (General), Mass Genl Hosp-Harvard Med Sch, Boston, MA 1979; **Faculty Appointment:** Prof Surgery, Mayo Med Sch

Hertzer, Norman Ray MD (Vascular Surgery (General)) - *Special Expertise:* Carotid Artery Disease; Aneurysm-Abdominal Aortic; **Admitting Hospital:** Cleveland Clinic Foundation; **Office Address:** Cleveland Clinic Foundation 9500 Euclid Ave, Ste S-61 Cleveland, OH 44195-0001; **Office Phone:** (216) 444-5705; **Board Certifications:** Vascular Surgery (General) 1993, Surgery 1973; **Medical School:** Indiana Univ 1967; **Residencies:** Vascular Surgery (General), Cleveland Clin Hosp, Cleveland, OH 1974-1975; Surgery, Cleveland Clin Hosp, Cleveland, OH 1968-1972

Hodgson, Kim John MD (Vascular Surgery (General)) - *Special Expertise:* Aneurysm; Carotid Angioplasty; Endovascular Surgery; **Admitting Hospital:** St John Hospital and Medical Center; **Office Address:** S Ill Univ Sch Med 800 N Rutledge, rm D346 Springfield, IL 62702; **Office Phone:** (217) 782-8856; **Board Certifications:** Vascular Surgery (General) 1995, Surgery 1995; **Medical School:** Univ Penn 1981; **Residency:** Surgery, Albany Med Ctr, Albany, NY 1982-1986; **Fellowship:** Vascular Surgery (General), Southern Ill Univ, Springfield, IL 1986-1987; **Faculty Appointment:** Prof Vascular Surgery (General), Southern IL Univ

Merrick III, Hollis W. MD (Vascular Surgery (General)) - *Special Expertise:* Vascular Surgery (General) - General; **Admitting Hospital:** Medical College of Ohio Hospitals; **Office Address:** Medical College Hospital-Dept. Surgery 3065 Arlington Ave Toledo, OH 43614-2570; **Office Phone:** (419) 383-4421; **Board Certification:** Surgery 1988; **Medical School:** McGill Univ 1964; **Residency:** Surgery, Royal Victoria Hospital, Montreal, CN 1967-1972; **Faculty Appointment:** Prof Surgery

Ouriel, Kenneth MD (Vascular Surgery (General)) - *Special Expertise:* Thrombolytic Therapy; **Admitting Hospital:** Cleveland Clinic Foundation; **Office Address:** Cleveland Clinic Desk S61 9500 Euclid Ave Cleveland, OH 44195; **Office Phone:** (216) 445-3464; **Board Certifications:** Vascular Surgery (General) 1995, Surgery 1995; **Medical School:** Univ Chicago-Pritzker Sch Med 1981; **Residency:** Vascular Surgery (General), Strong Meml Hosp-Univ Roch, Rochester, MN 1982-1986; **Fellowship:** Vascular Surgery (General), Strong Meml Hosp-Univ Roch, Rochester, MN 1986-1987

Pearce, William MD (Vascular Surgery (General)) - *Special Expertise:* Aneurysm-Abdominal Aortic; Carotid Artery Disease; Claudication; **Admitting Hospital:** Northwestern Memorial Hospital; **Office Address:** Northwestern Meml Hosp - Galter Pavlin 675 N St Clair St, Ste 19-100 Chicago, IL 60611-2647; **Office Phone:** (312) 695-2714; **Board Certifications:** Surgical Critical Care 1999, Vascular Surgery (General) 1992; **Medical School:** Univ Colo 1975; **Residencies:** Internal Medicine, Mayo Grad Sch Med/Mayo Fdn, Rochester, MN 1975-1976; Surgery, Univ Co Hlth Sci Ctr, Denver, CO 1976-1980; **Fellowship:** Cardiology (Cardiovascular Disease), Northwestern Meml Hosp, Chicago, IL 1981-1982; **Faculty Appointment:** Prof Surgery, Northwestern Univ

Reddy, Daniel MD (Vascular Surgery (General)) - *Special Expertise:* Aneurysm-Abdominal Aortic; Carotid Artery Surgery; **Admitting Hospital:** Henry Ford Health System (Page 62); **Office Address:** Henry Ford Hosp, Dept of Vascular Surgery 2799 W Grand Blvd Detroit, MI 48202-2608; **Office Phone:** (313) 916-3156; **Board Certifications:** Surgery 1998, Vascular Surgery (General) 1991; **Medical School:** Univ Mich Med Sch 1973; **Residency:** Vascular Surgery (General), Wayne State Univ, Detroit, MI 1974-1978; **Fellowship:** Vascular Surgery (General), Wayne State Univ, Detroit, MI 1978-1979

Shepard, Alexander D MD (Vascular Surgery (General)) - *Special Expertise:* Arterial Bypass Surgery-Leg; **Admitting Hospital:** Henry Ford Health System (Page 62); **Office Address:** 2799 West Grand Blvd Detroit, MI 48202; **Office Phone:** (313) 916-3155; **Board Certifications:** Surgery 1992, Vascular Surgery (General) 1994; **Medical School:** Johns Hopkins Univ 1976; **Residency:** Surgery, Johns Hopkins Hosp, Baltimore, MD 1976-1982; **Fellowship:** Vascular Surgery (General), New England Med Ctr, Boston, MA 1983-1985; **Faculty Appointment:** Asst Prof Surgery, Johns Hopkins Univ

Sicard, Gregorio Arquel MD (Vascular Surgery (General)) - *Special Expertise:* *Aneurysm-Abdominal Aortic;* **Admitting Hospital:** Barnes - Jewish Hospital; **Office Address:** Washington Univ Barnes Jewish Hosp One Barnes Jewish Hospital Plaza, Ste 5103 St Louis, MO 63110; **Office Phone:** (314) 362-7841; **Board Certifications:** Vascular Surgery (General) 1992, Surgery 1996; **Medical School:** Univ Puerto Rico 1972; **Residency:** Surgery, Barnes Hosp, St Louis, MO 1973-1977; **Fellowship:** Transplant Surgery, Wash Univ Hosp, St Louis, MO 1977-1978; **Faculty Appointment:** Prof Surgery, Washington Univ, St Louis

Stanley, James MD (Vascular Surgery (General)) - *Special Expertise:* Peripheral Vascular Surgery; Renovascular Disease; **Admitting Hospital:** University of Michigan Health Center; **Office Address:** Univ Hosp, Dept Vasc Surg 1500 E Med Ctr Ann Arbor, MI 48109-0329; **Office Phone:** (734) 936-5786; **Board Certifications:** Surgery 1973, Vascular Surgery (General) 1991; **Medical School:** Univ Mich Med Sch 1964; **Residency:** Surgery, Univ Mich Med Ctr, Ann Arbor, MI 1967-1972; **Faculty Appointment:** Prof Surgery, Univ Mich Med Sch

Towne, Jonathan MD (Vascular Surgery (General)) - *Special Expertise:* Peripheral Vascular Surgery; Thoracic Outlet Syndrome; **Admitting Hospital:** Froedtert Memorial Lutheran Hospital; **Office Address:** Med Coll Wisconsin 9200 W Wisconsin Ave Milwaukee, WI 53226; **Office Phone:** (414) 456-6970; **Board Certifications:** Surgery 1973, Vascular Surgery (General) 1991; **Medical School:** Univ Rochester 1967; **Residencies:** Surgery, Univ Mich Med Ctr, Michigan, MI 1968-1969; Surgery, Univ Nebraska Coll Med, Nebraska, WI 1969-1972; **Fellowship:** Vascular Surgery (General), Baylor Coll Med, Houston, TX 1974-1975; **Faculty Appointment:** Prof Vascular Surgery (General), Med Coll Wisc

Yao, James MD (Vascular Surgery (General)) - *Special Expertise:* Vascular Surgery (General) - General; **Admitting Hospital:** Northwestern Memorial Hospital; **Office Address:** Northwestern Meml Hosp 675 St Clare, Ste 19-100 Chicago, IL 60611-2647; **Office Phone:** (312) 695-2714; **Board Certifications:** Surgery 1967, Vascular Surgery (General) 1983; **Medical School:** Taiwan 1961; **Residency:** Surgery, Cook Co Hosp, Chicago, IL 1962-1967; **Fellowship:** Vascular Surgery (General), St Mary's, London, England 1967-1968; **Faculty Appointment:** Prof Surgery, Northwestern Univ

Zelenock, Gerald MD (Vascular Surgery (General)) - *Special Expertise:* Vascular Surgery (General) - General; **Admitting Hospital:** William Beaumont Hospital; **Office Address:** WM Beaumont Hosp Med Admin 3601 W 13 Mile Rd Royal Oak, MI 48073; **Office Phone:** (248) 551-4165; **Board Certifications:** Surgery 1979, Vascular Surgery (General) 1983; **Medical School:** Univ Mich Med Sch 1973; **Residency:** Surgery, Univ Mich Hosps, MI 1974-1978; **Faculty Appointment:** Prof Surgery, Univ Mich Med Sch

Southwest

Clagett, George Patrick MD (Vascular Surgery (General)) - *Special Expertise:* *Aneurysm-Abdominal Aortic;* **Admitting Hospital:** Parkland Memorial Hospital; **Office Address:** Univ Tex SW Med Ctr 5323 Harry Hines Blvd Dallas, TX 75390; **Office Phone:** (214) 648-3516; **Board Certifications:** Surgery 1987, Vascular Surgery (General) 1991; **Medical School:** Univ VA Sch Med **Residency:** Surgery, Univ Mich, Ann Harbor, MI 1974-1976; **Fellowships:** Vascular Surgery (General), Walter Reed Army Med Ctr, Washington, DC 1978-1979; Research, Harvard Med Sch, Boston, MA 1972-1974; **Faculty Appointment:** Prof Surgery, Univ Tex SW, Dallas

Eidt, John MD (Vascular Surgery (General)) - *Special Expertise:* Arterial Bypass Surgery; Critical Care; **Admitting Hospital:** University of Arkansas for Medical Sciences; **Office Address:** 4301 W Markham St, MS 520-2 Llittle Rock, AR 72205-7101; **Office Phone:** (501) 686-6176; **Board Certifications:** Surgical Critical Care 1990, Vascular Surgery (General) 1996; **Medical School:** Univ Tex SW, Dallas 1981; **Residency:** Surgery, Brigham-Womens Hosp, Boston, MA 1981-1986; **Fellowship:** Vascular Surgery (General), Univ Tex SW Med Ctr, Dallas, TX 1987; **Faculty Appointment:** Assoc Prof Surgery, Univ Ark

Money, Samuel MD (Vascular Surgery (General)) - *Special Expertise:* Aneurysm-Abdominal Aortic; Arterial Bypass Surgery-Leg; **Admitting Hospital:** Ochsner Foundation Hospital; **Office Address:** Department of Surgery 1514 Jefferson Hwy New Orleans, LA 70121; **Office Phone:** (504) 842-4070; **Board Certifications:** Surgery 1991, Vascular Surgery (General) 1995; **Medical School:** SUNY Downstate 1983; **Residency:** Surgery, Kings Co Med Ctr, Brooklyn, NY 1983-1990; **Fellowship:** Vascular Surgery (General), Ochsner Clinic, New Orleans, LA 1991-1993; **Faculty Appointment:** Asst Clin Prof Surgery, Tulane Univ

Safi, Hazim Jawad MD (Vascular Surgery (General)) - *Special Expertise:* Aneurysm-Abdominal Aortic; **Admitting Hospital:** Memorial Hermann Healthcare System; **Office Address:** 6410 Fannin St, Ste 450 Houston, TX 77030; **Office Phone:** (713) 500-5304; **Board Certifications:** Thoracic Surgery 1989, Vascular Surgery (General) 1984; **Medical School:** Iraq 1970; **Residencies:** Surgery, Baylor Coll Of Med, Houston, TX 1977-1980; Radiation Oncology, Baylor Coll Of Med, Houston, TX 1980-1981; **Fellowship:** Thoracic Surgery, Baylor Coll Of Med, Houston, TX 1981-1983; **Faculty Appointment:** Assoc Prof Surgery, Univ Tex, Houston

West Coast and Pacific

Ahn, Samuel S MD (Vascular Surgery (General)) - *Special Expertise:* Thoracic Outlet Syndrome; **Admitting Hospital:** UCLA Medical Center; **Office Address:** UCLA Med Ctr 200 UCLA Medical Plaza, Ste 526 Los Angeles, CA 90095; **Office Phone:** (310) 206-3885; **Board Certifications:** Surgery 1994, Vascular Surgery (General) 1997; **Medical School:** Univ Tex SW, Dallas 1978; **Residency:** Surgery, UCLA Med Ctr, Los Angeles, CA 1979-1984; **Fellowship:** Vascular Surgery (General), UCLA Med Ctr, Los Angeles, CA 1984-1986; **Faculty Appointment:** Prof Surgery, UCLA

Andros, George MD (Vascular Surgery (General)) - *Special Expertise:* Aneurysm-Aortic; Carotid Artery Surgery; **Admitting Hospital:** Providence Saint Joseph Medical Center; **Office Address:** 16500 Ventura Blvd, Ste 360 Encino, CA 91436; **Office Phone:** (818) 845-7242; **Board Certifications:** Surgery 1970, Vascular Surgery (General) 1983; **Medical School:** Univ Chicago-Pritzker Sch Med 1960; **Residency:** Surgery, Mass Genl Hosp, Boston, MA 1965-1969

Bergan, John Jerome MD (Vascular Surgery (General)) - *Special Expertise:* Vein Disease; Vein Disease/Leg Ulcers; **Admitting Hospital:** Scripps Hospital - La Jolla; **Office Address:** 9850 Genesee Ave, Ste 410 La Jolla, CA 92037-1229; **Office Phone:** (858) 550-0330; **Board Certifications:** Vascular Surgery (General) 1991, Surgery 1960; **Medical School:** Indiana Univ 1954; **Residency:** Surgery, Northwestern Meml Hosp, Chicago, IL 1955-1959; **Faculty Appointment:** Clin Prof Surgery, UCSD

Flanigan, Preston D. MD (Vascular Surgery (General)) - *Special Expertise:* Aneurysm-Abdominal Aortic; **Admitting Hospital:** St Joseph's Hospital - Orange; **Office Address:** 1310 W Stewart Dr, Ste 407 Orange, CA 92868-3855; **Office Phone:** (714) 997-4961; **Board Certifications:** Surgery 1978, Vascular Surgery (General) 1983; **Medical School:** Jefferson Med Coll 1972; **Residency:** Surgery, St Joseph-Mercy Hosp, Ann Arbor, MI 1974-1977; **Fellowship:** Vascular Surgery (General), Northwest Med Ctr 1977-1978; **Faculty Appointment:** Clin Prof Surgery, UC Irvine

Grey, Douglas P MD (Vascular Surgery (General)) - *Special Expertise:* *Vascular Surgery (General) - General;* **Admitting Hospital:** KFH San Francisco Medical Center; **Office Address:** 2238 Geary Blvd San Francisco, CA 94115-3394; **Office Phone:** (415) 333-3385; **Board Certifications:** Thoracic Surgery 1993, Vascular Surgery (General) 1993; **Medical School:** UC Irvine 1975; **Residencies:** Surgery, Peter Bent Brigham Hosp, Boston, MA 1976-1980; Thoracic Surgery, Texas Heart Inst, Houston, TX 1980-1982; **Faculty Appointment:** Clin Prof Surgery, UCSF

Johansen, Kaj MD/PhD (Vascular Surgery (General)) - *Special Expertise:* *Portal Hypertension; Trauma; Vascular Access;* **Admitting Hospital:** Swedish Medical Center Providence Campus; **Office Address:** Providence Seattle Med Ctr 1600 E Jefferson St, rm 110 Seattle, WA 98124-1008; **Office Phone:** (206) 616-1130; **Board Certifications:** Surgery 1979, Vascular Surgery (General) 1983; **Medical School:** Univ Wash 1970; **Residencies:** Surgery, UCSD, San Diego, CA 1975-1978; Surgery, UCSD, San Diego, CA 1971-1972; **Fellowship:** Vascular Surgery (General), UCSD, San Diego, CA 1972-1977; **Faculty Appointment:** Prof Surgery, Univ Wash

Moore, Wesley Sanford MD (Vascular Surgery (General)) - *Special Expertise:* *Aneurysm-Abdominal Aortic; Carotid Artery Surgery; Arterial Reconstruction;* **Admitting Hospital:** UCLA Medical Center; **Office Address:** UCLA Ctr Hlth Sciences- Dept Surgery Box 956904 Los Angeles, CA 90095-6904; **Office Phone:** (310) 825-9641; **Board Certifications:** Surgery 1966, Vascular & Interventional Radiology 1983; **Medical School:** UCSF 1959; **Residency:** Surgery, UCSF Med Ctr, San Francisco, CA 1960-1964; **Fellowship:** Research, VA Hosp-NIH, San Francisco, CA 1966-1967; **Faculty Appointment:** Prof Surgery, UCLA

Porter, John M. MD (Vascular Surgery (General)) - *Special Expertise:* *Raynaud's Disease; Thoracic Outlet Syndrome; Carotid Artery Surgery;* **Admitting Hospital:** Oregon Health Science University Hospital and Clinics; **Office Address:** OHSU, Div Vasc Surg 3181 SW Sam Jackson Park Rd Portland, OR 97201-3011; **Office Phone:** (503) 494-7593; **Board Certifications:** Vascular Surgery (General) 1991, Thoracic Surgery 1971; **Medical School:** Duke Univ 1963; **Residency:** Surgery, Duke Univ, Durham, NC 1964-1971; **Fellowship:** Vascular Surgery (General), Duke Univ, Durham, NC 1965-1966; **Faculty Appointment:** Prof Surgery, Oregon Hlth Scis Univ

Taylor, Lloyd M MD (Vascular Surgery (General)) - *Special Expertise:* *Vascular Surgery (General) - General;* **Admitting Hospital:** Oregon Health Science University Hospital and Clinics; **Office Address:** OHSU Hosp & Clinics 3181 SW Sam Jackson Park Rd, MC-OP11 Portland, OR 97201-3011; **Office Phone:** (503) 494-7593; **Board Certifications:** Surgery 1983, Vascular Surgery (General) 1987; **Medical School:** Duke Univ 1973; **Residencies:** Surgery, U Oreg Hlth Sci Ctr, Portland, OR 1977-1981; Surgery, U Oreg Hlth Sci Ctr, Portland, OR 1981-1982; **Fellowship:** Vascular Surgery (General), Oreg Hlth Sci U, Portland, OR 1982-1983; **Faculty Appointment:** Prof Surgery, Oregon Hlth Scis Univ

White, Rodney Allen MD (Vascular Surgery (General)) - *Special Expertise:* *Vascular Surgery (General) - General;* **Admitting Hospital:** LAC - Harbor - UCLA Medical Center; **Office Address:** Harbor-UCLA Med Ctr 1000 W Carson St, Box 11 Torrance, CA 90509-9823; **Office Phone:** (310) 222-2704; **Board Certifications:** Surgery 1988, Vascular Surgery (General) 1994; **Medical School:** SUNY Syracuse 1974; **Residency:** Surgery, LA Co Harbor-UCLA, Torrance, CA 1975-1979; **Fellowship:** Vascular Surgery (General), LA Co Harbor-UCLA, Torrance, CA 1979-1980; **Faculty Appointment:** Prof Surgery, UCLA

VASCULAR SURGERY (GENERAL)

Yellin, Albert E MD (Vascular Surgery (General)) - *Special Expertise:* *Vascular Surgery (General) - General;* **Admitting Hospital:** LAC + USC Medical Center; **Office Address:** LAC & USC Med Ctr 1200 N Date St, rm 9610 Los Angeles, CA 90033; **Office Phone:** (323) 226-7737; **Board Certifications:** Surgery 1970, Vascular Surgery (General) 1991; **Medical School:** USC Sch Med 1962; **Residency:** Surgery, LAC-USC Med Ctr, Los Angeles, CA 1965-1969; **Fellowship:** Vascular Surgery (General), LAC-USC Med Ctr, Los Angeles, CA 1969-1970; **Faculty Appointment:** Prof Surgery, USC Sch Med

Zarins, Christopher Kristaps MD (Vascular Surgery (General)) - *Special Expertise:* *Carotid Artery Surgery; Aneurysm-Abdominal Aortic;* **Admitting Hospital:** Stanford Medical Center; **Office Address:** Standford Univ, Dept Surg 300 Pasteur Ave, Ste H3630 Stanford, CA 94305-5642; **Office Phone:** (650) 725-5227; **Board Certifications:** Surgery 1975, Vascular Surgery (General) 1991; **Medical School:** Johns Hopkins Univ 1968; **Residency:** Surgery, Univ Michigan Hosp, Ann Arbor, MI 1969-1974; **Fellowship:** Surgery, Johns Hopkins Hosp, Baltimore, MD 1971-1972; **Faculty Appointment:** Prof Surgery, Stanford Univ

APPENDICES

APPENDICES

APPENDIX A

ADDITIONAL MEDICAL SPECIALTIES AND
SUBSPECIALTIES RECOGNIZED BY THE
ABMS

All specialties in this section are in capital letters and boldface type (e.g., **INTERNAL MEDICINE**). All subspecialties in this section are in initial capitals and boldface type (e.g., Critical Care Medicine).

Some specialties have a page number following the name of the specialty. This page number indicates where you will find a description of that specialty in this Guide.

Subspecialties require board certification in the specialty plus additional training and examination in the subspecialty.

ALLERGY-IMMUNOLOGY *(see page 93)*

Clinical & Laboratory Immunology: A subspecialist who utilizes various laboratory procedures to diagnose and treat disorders characterized by defective responses of the body's immune system. These results are used for patient management.

ANESTHESIOLOGY
An anesthesiologist is trained to provide pain relief and maintenance, or restoration, of a stable condition during and immediately following an operation, an obstetric or diagnostic procedure. The anesthesiologist assesses the risk of the patient undergoing surgery and optimizes the patient's condition prior to, during, and after surgery. In addition to these management responsibilities, the anesthesiologist provides medical management and consultation in pain management and critical care medicine. Anesthesiologists diagnose and treat acute, long-standing and cancer pain problems; diagnose and treat patients with critical illnesses or severe injuries; direct resuscitation in the care of patients with cardiac or respiratory emergencies, including the need for artificial ventilation; and supervise post anesthesia recovery.

Training required: Four years

Critical Care Medicine: An anesthesiologist who specializes in critical care medicine diagnoses, treats and supports patients with multiple organ dysfunction. This specialist may have administrative responsibilities for intensive care units and may also facilitate and coordinate patient care among the primary physician, the critical care staff, and other specialists.

APPENDIX A

DERMATOLOGY (*see page 179*)

Clinical and Laboratory Dermatological Immunology: A dermatologist who utilizes various specialized laboratory procedures to diagnose disorders characterized by defective responses of the body's immune system. *Immunodermatologists* also may provide consultation in the management of these disorders and administer specialized forms of therapy for these diseases.

EMERGENCY MEDICINE

An emergency physician focuses on the immediate decision making and action necessary to prevent death or any further disability both in the pre-hospital setting by directing emergency medical technicians and in the emergency department. The emergency physician provides immediate recognition, evaluation, care, stabilization and disposition of a generally diversified population of adult and pediatric patients in response to acute illness and injury.

Training required: Three years

Certification in one of the following subspecialties requires additional training and examination.

Medical Toxicology: An emergency physician who has special knowledge about the evaluation and management of patients with accidental or purposeful poisoning through exposure to prescription and nonprescription medications, drugs of abuse, household or industrial toxins and environmental toxins. Areas of medical toxicology include acute pediatric and adult drug ingestion; drug abuse, addiction and withdrawal; chemical poisoning exposure and toxicity; hazardous materials exposure and toxicity and occupational toxicology.

Pediatric Emergency Medicine: An emergency physician who has special qualifications to manage emergencies in infants and children.

Sports Medicine: An emergency physician with special knowledge in sports medicine is responsible for continuous care in the field of sports medicine, not only for the enhancement of health and fitness, but also for the prevention and management of injury and illness. A sports medicine physician has knowledge and experience in the promotion of wellness and the role of exercise in promoting a healthy lifestyle. Knowledge of exercise physiology, biomechanics, nutrition, psychology, physical rehabilitation and epidemiology is essential to the practice of sports medicine.

874

FAMILY PRACTICE

A family physician is concerned with the total healthcare of the individual and the family, and is trained to diagnose and treat a wide variety of ailments in patients of all ages. The family physician receives a broad range of training that includes internal medicine, pediatrics, obstetrics and gynecology, psychiatry and geriatrics. Special emphasis is placed on prevention and the primary care of entire families, utilizing consultations and community resources when appropriate.

Training required: Three years

Certification in one of the following subspecialties requires additional training and examination.

Geriatric Medicine: A family physician with special knowledge of the aging process and special skills in the diagnostic, therapeutic, preventive and rehabilitative aspects of illness in the elderly. This specialist cares for geriatric patients in the patient's home, the office, long-term care settings such as nursing homes and the hospital.

Sports Medicine: A family practice physician who is trained to be responsible for continuous care in the field of sports medicine, not only for the enhancement of health and fitness, but also for the prevention of injury and illness. A sports medicine physician must have knowledge and experience in the promotion of wellness and the prevention of injury. Knowledge about special areas of medicine such as exercise physiology, biomechanics, nutrition, psychology, physical rehabilitation, epidemiology, physical evaluation, injuries (treatment and prevention and referral practice) and the role of exercise in promoting a healthy life style are essential to the practice of sports medicine. The sports medicine physician requires special education to provide the knowledge to improve the healthcare of the individual engaged in physical exercise (sports) whether as an individual or in team participation.

INTERNAL MEDICINE (*see page 331*)

Clinical and Laboratory Immunology: An internist who uses laboratory tests and complex procedures to diagnose and treat disorders characterized by defective responses of the body's immune system.

Critical Care Medicine: An internist who diagnoses, treats and supports patients with multiple organ dysfunction. This specialist may have administrative responsibilities for intensive care units and may also facilitate and coordinate patient care among the primary physician, the critical care staff and other specialists.

APPENDIX A

MEDICAL GENETICS *(see Clinical Genetics page 157)*

The Board issues multiple general certificates in the following areas of genetics:

Clinical Biochemical Genetics: A clinical biochemical geneticist demonstrates competence in performing and interpreting biochemical analyses relevant to the diagnosis and management of human genetic diseases, and is a consultant regarding laboratory diagnosis of a broad range of inherited disorders.

Clinical Cytogenetics: A clinical cytogeneticist demonstrates competence in providing laboratory diagnostic and clinical interpretive services dealing with cellular components, particularly chromosomes, associated with heredity.

Ph.D. Medical Genetics: A medical geneticist works in association with a medical specialist, is affiliated with a clinical genetics program, and serves as a consultant to medical and dental specialists.

Molecular Genetic Pathology: A molecular genetic pathologist is expert in the principles, theory, and technologies of molecular biology and molecular genetics. This expertise is used to make or confirm diagnoses of Mendelian genetic disorders, of human development, infectious diseases and malignancies, and to assess the natural history of those disorders. A molecular genetic pathologist provides information about gene structure, function, and alteration and applies laboratory techniques for diagnosis, treatment, and prognosis for individuals with related disorders.

NEUROLOGY *(see page 391)*

Clinical Neurophysiology: A neurologist who specializes in the diagnosis and management of central, peripheral and autonomic nervous system disorders using a combination of clinical evaluation and electrophysiologic testing such as electroencephalography (EEG), electromyography (EMG) and nerve conduction studies (NCS), among others.

Neurodevelopmental Disabilities: A pediatrician or neurologist who specializes in the diagnosis and management of chronic conditions that affect the developing and mature nervous system such as cerebral palsy, mental retardation and chronic behavioral syndromes, or neurologic conditions.

OBSTETRICS AND GYNECOLOGY *(see page 429)*

Critical Care Medicine: An obstetrician-gynecologist who specializes in critical care medicine diagnoses, treats and supports female patients with multiple organ dysfunc-

876

tion. This specialist may have administrative responsibilities for intensive care units and may also facilitate and coordinate patient care among the primary physician, the critical care staff, and other specialists.

OTOLARYNGOLOGY *(see page 499)*

Plastic Surgery within the Head and Neck: An otolaryngologist with additional training in plastic and reconstructive procedures within the head, face, neck and associated structures, including cutaneous head and neck oncology and reconstruction, management of maxillofacial trauma, soft tissue repair and neural surgery. The field is diverse and involves a wide age range of patients, from the newborn to the aged. While both cosmetic and reconstructive surgery are practiced, there are many additional procedures which interface with them.

Otology/Neurotology: An otolaryngologist who treats diseases of the ear and temporal bone, including disorders of hearing and balance. The additional training in otology and neurotology emphasizes the study of embryology, anatomy, physiology, epidemiology, pathophysiology, pathology, genetics, immunology, microbiology and the etiology of diseases of the ear and temporal bone.

PATHOLOGY *(see page 533)*

Blood Banking/Transfusion Medicine: A physician who specializes in blood banking/transfusion medicine is responsible for the maintenance of an adequate blood supply, blood donor and patient-recipient safety and appropriate blood utilization. Pretransfusion compatibility testing and antibody testing assure that blood transfusions, when indicated, are as safe as possible. This physician directs the preparation and safe use of specially prepared blood components, including red blood cells, white blood cells, platelets and plasma constituents.

Chemical Pathology: A chemical pathologist has expertise in the biochemistry of the human body as it applies to the understanding of the cause and progress of disease. This physician functions as a clinical consultant in the diagnosis and treatment of human disease. Chemical pathology entails the application of biochemical data to the detection, confirmation or monitoring of disease.

Cytopathology: A cytopathologist is an anatomic pathologist trained in the diagnosis of human disease by means of the study of cells obtained from body secretions and fluids, by scraping, washing or sponging the surface of a lesion, or by the aspiration of a tumor mass or body organ with a fine needle. A major aspect of a cytopathologist's practice is the interpretation of Papanicolaou-stained smears of cells from the female reproductive systems, the "Pap" test. However, the cytopathologist's expertise is applied to the diagnosis of cells from all systems and areas of the body. He/she is a consultant to all medical specialists.

APPENDIX A

Forensic Pathology: A forensic pathologist is expert in investigating and evaluating cases of sudden, unexpected, suspicious and violent death as well as other specific classes of death defined by law. The forensic pathologist serves the public as coroner or medical examiner, or by performing medicolegal autopsies for such officials.

Hematology: A physician who is expert in diseases that affect blood cells, blood clotting mechanisms, bone marrow and lymph nodes. He/she has the knowledge and technical skills essential for the laboratory diagnosis of anemias, leukemias, lymphomas, bleeding disorders and blood clotting disorders.

Medical Microbiology: A physician who is expert in the isolation and identification of microbial agents that cause infectious disease. Viruses, bacteria and fungi, as well as parasites are identified and, where possible, tested for susceptibility to appropriate antimicrobial agents.

Molecular Genetic Pathology: A molecular genetic pathologist is expert in the principles, theory and technologies of molecular biology and molecular genetics. This expertise is used to make or confirm diagnoses of Mendelian genetic disorders, disorders of human development, infectious diseases and malignancies, and to assess the natural history of those disorders. A molecular genetic pathologist provides information about gene structure, function and alteration and applies laboratory techniques for diagnosis, treatment and prognosis for individuals with related disorders.

Neuropathology: A neuropathologist is expert in the diagnosis of diseases of the nervous system and skeletal muscles and functions as a consultant primarily to neurologists and neurosurgeons. The neuropathologist is knowledgeable in the infirmities of humans as they affect the nervous and neuromuscular systems, be they degenerative, infectious, metabolic, immunologic, neoplastic, vascular or physical in nature.

Pediatric Pathology: A pediatric pathologist is expert in the laboratory diagnosis of diseases that occur during fetal growth, infancy and child development. The practice requires a strong foundation in general pathology and substantial understanding of normal growth and development, along with extensive knowledge of pediatric medicine.

PEDIATRICS *(see page 545)*

Clinical & Laboratory Immunology: A pediatrician who utilizes laboratory tests and complex procedures to diagnose and treat disorders characterized by defective responses of the body's immune system.

Medical Toxicology: A pediatrician who focuses on the evaluation and management of patients with accidental or intentional poisoning through exposure to prescription and non-prescription medications, drugs of abuse, household or industrial toxins and environmental toxins. Important areas of medical toxicology include acute pediatric and adult drug ingestion; drug abuse, addiction and withdrawal; chemical poisoning exposure and toxicity; hazardous materials exposure and toxicity and occupational toxicology.

Neurodevelopmental Disabilities: A pediatrician who treats children having developmental delays or learning disorders, including those associated with visual and hearing impairment, mental retardation, cerebral palsy, spina bifida, autism and other chronic neurologic conditions. This specialist provides medical consultation and education and assumes leadership in the interdisciplinary management of children with neurodevelopmental disorders. They may also focus on the early identification and diagnosis of neurodevelopmental disabilities in infants and young children as well as on changes that occur as the child with developmental disabilities grows.

Pediatric Critical Care Medicine: A pediatrician expert in advanced life support for children from the term or near-term neonate to the adolescent. This competence extends to the critical care management of life-threatening organ system failure from any cause in both medical and surgical patients, and to the support of vital physiological functions. This specialist may have administrative responsibilities for intensive care units and also facilitate patient care among other specialists.

Pediatric Emergency Medicine: A pediatrician who has special qualifications to manage emergencies in infants and children.

Sports Medicine: A pediatrician who is responsible for continuous care in the field of sports medicine, not only for the enhancement of health and fitness, but also for the prevention of injury and illness. A sports medicine physician must have knowledge and experience in the promotion of wellness and the prevention of injury. Knowledge about special areas of medicine such as exercise physiology, biomechanics, nutrition, psychology, physical rehabilitation, epidemiology, physical evaluation, injuries (treatment and prevention and referral practice) and the role of exercise in promoting a healthy life style are essential to the practice of sports medicine. The sports medicine physician requires special education to provide the knowledge to improve the healthcare of the individual engaged in physical exercise (sports) whether as an individual or in team participation.

PHYSICAL MEDICINE & REHABILITATION *(see page 621)*

Pain Management: A physician who provides a high level of care, either as a primary physician or consultant, for patients experiencing problems with acute, chronic or cancer pain in both hospital and ambulatory settings.

Pediatric Rehabilitation Medicine: A physiatrist who utilizes an interdisciplinary approach and addresses the prevention, diagnosis, treatment, and management of congenital and childhood onset physical impairments including related or secondary medical, physical, functional, psychosocial, and vocational limitations or conditions, with an understanding of the life course of disability.

PREVENTIVE MEDICINE
A preventive medicine specialist focuses on the health of individuals and defined populations in order to protect, promote and maintain health and well being, and to prevent disease, disability and premature death. The distinctive components of preventive medicine include:
 1. Biostatistics and the application of biostatistical principles and methodology;
 2. Epidemiology and its application to population-based medicine and research;
 3. Health services management and administration including: developing, assessing and assuring health policies; planning, implementing, directing, budgeting and evaluating population health and disease management programs; and utilizing legislative and regulatory processes to enhance health;
 4. Control of environmental factors that may adversely affect health;
 5. Control and prevention of occupational factors that may adversely affect health safety;
 6. Clinical preventive medicine activities, including measures to promote health and prevent the occurrence, progression and disabling effects of disease and injury; and
 7. Assessment of social, cultural and behavioral influences on health.

A preventive medicine physician may be a specialist in general preventive medicine, public health, occupational medicine, or aerospace medicine. This specialist works with large population groups as well as with individual patients to promote health and understand the risks of disease, injury, disability and death, seeking to modify and eliminate these risks.

Training required: Three years

Certification in one of the following subspecialties requires additional training and examination.

Medical Toxicology: A specialist who is expert in the evaluation and management of patients with accidental or intentional poisoning through exposure to prescription and nonprescription medications, drugs of abuse, household or industrial toxins and environmental toxins. Important areas of medical toxicology include acute pediatric and adult drug ingestion; drug abuse, addiction and withdrawal; chemical poisoning exposure and toxicity; hazardous materials exposure and toxicity and occupational toxicology.

ADDITIONAL ABMS SPECIALTIES AND SUBSPECIALTIES

Undersea and Hyperbaric Medicine: A specialist who treats decompression illness and diving accident cases and uses hyperbaric oxygen therapy to treat such conditions as carbon monoxide poisoning, gas gangrene, non-healing wounds, tissue damage from radiation and burns and bone infections. This specialist also serves as consultant to other physicians in all aspects of hyperbaric chamber operations, and assesses risks and applies appropriate standards to prevent disease and disability in divers and other persons working in altered atmospheric conditions.

PSYCHIATRY *(see page 657)*

Clinical Neurophysiology: A psychiatrist with expertise in the diagnosis and management of central, peripheral, and autonomic nervous system disorders using a combination of clinical evaluation and electrophysiologic testing such as electroencephalography (EEG), electromyography (EMG), and nerve conduction studies (NCS).

Forensic Psychiatry: A psychiatrist who focuses on the interrelationships between psychiatry and civil, criminal and administrative law. This specialist evaluates individuals involved with the legal system and provides specialized treatment to those incarcerated in jails, prisons and forensic psychiatry hospitals.

Pain Management: A psychiatrist who provides a high level of care, either as a primary physician or consultant, for patients experiencing problems with acute, chronic or cancer pain in both hospital and ambulatory settings.

RADIOLOGY *(see page 729)*

Radiological Physics: A radiological physicist deals with the diagnostic and therapeutic applications of roentgen rays, gamma rays from sealed sources, ultrasonic radiation and radio-frequency radiation, as well as the equipment associated with their production and use, including radiation safety.

Nuclear Radiology: A radiologist who is involved in the analysis and imaging of radionuclides and radiolabeled substances in vitro and in vivo for diagnosis, and the administration of radionuclides and radiolabeled substances for the treatment of disease.

SURGERY *(see page 777)*

Surgical Critical Care: A surgeon with expertise in the management of the critically ill and postoperative patient, particularly the trauma victim, who specializes in critical care medicine diagnoses, treats and supports patients with multiple organ dysfunction. This specialist may have administrative responsibilities for intensive care units and may also facilitate and coordinate patient care among the primary physician, the critical care staff and other specialists.

APPENDIX B

PURPOSE OF THE AMERICAN BOARD OF MEDICAL SPECIALTIES

THE STATEMENT OF PURPOSE INCLUDED IN THE ARTICLES OF INCORPORATION IS:

- *To improve the standards of medical care.*

- *To act as spokesman for all approved specialty boards, as a group.*

- *To resolve problems encountered among and between specialty boards.*

- *To deal with the applications for approval of proposed new specialty boards, new types of certification, modification of existing types of certification, and related matters.*

- *To endeavor to avoid duplication of effort by specialty boards.*

- *To establish and maintain standards of organization and operation of specialty boards.*

Following is a list of the addresses of the various medical specialty boards approved by the ABMS. Note that there are 24 board organizations for 25 medical specialties. Psychiatry and Neurology share the same board.

To find out if a physician is certified, consumers can call the individual boards which will provide information for a fee, or they can call the ABMS at (800) 776-2378 (no fee).

BOARD SPECIALTIES

■ **American Board of Allergy and Immunology**
510 Walnut Street, Suite 1701
Philadelphia, PA 19106-3699
(215) 592-9466
General Certification in Allergy and Immunology; with Added Qualification in Diagnostic Laboratory Immunology. Certifications awarded since 1989 are valid for 10 years. For those certified prior to 1989 there is no recertification requirement.

■ **American Board of Anesthesiology**
4101 Lake Boone Trail
Suite 510
Raleigh, NC 27607-7506
(919) 881-2570
General Certification in Anesthesiology; with Special and Added Qualifications in Critical Care Medicine and Pain Management. Certifications awarded since 2000 are valid for 10 years.

■ **American Board of Colon and Rectal Surgery**
20600 Eureka Road, Suite 713
Taylor, MI 48180
(734) 282-9400
General Certification is in Colon and Rectal Surgery. Certifications awarded since 1991 are valid for 8 years.

■ **American Board of Dermatology**
Henry Ford Hospital
One Ford Place
Detroit, MI 48202
(313) 874-1088
General Certification in Dermatology; with Special Qualifications in Dermatopathology, Dermatological Immunology/Diagnostic and Laboratory Immunology. Certifications awarded since 1991 are valid for 10 years. For those certified prior to 1991, there is no recertification requirement.

■ **American Board of Emergency Medicine**
3000 Coolidge Road
East Lansing, MI 48823
(517) 332-4800
General Certification in Emergency Medicine; with Special and Added Qualifications in Pediatric Emergency Medicine and Sports Medicine. Certifications are valid for a 10-year period.

American Board of Family Practice
2228 Young Drive
Lexington, KY 40505
(606) 269-5626
General Certification in Family Practice; with Added Qualifications in Geriatric Medicine and Sports Medicine. Certifications are valid for a 7-year period.

American Board of Internal Medicine
510 Walnut Street, Suite 1700
Philadelphia, PA 19106-3699
(215) 446-3500, (800) 441-ABIM
General Certification in Internal Medicine; with Special Qualifications in Cardiovascular Disease, Critical Care Medicine, Endocrinology, Diabetes and Metabolism, Gastroenterology, Hematology, Infectious Disease, Medical Oncology, Nephrology, Pulmonary Disease, and Rheumatology; and Added Qualifications in Adolescent Medicine, Cardiac Electrophysiology, Diagnostic Laboratory Immunology, Geriatric Medicine and Sports Medicine. Certifications awarded since 1990 are valid for 10 years. For those certified prior to 1990 there is no recertification requirement.

American Board of Medical Genetics
9650 Rockville Pike
Bethesda, MD 20814
(301) 571-1825
General Certification in Clinical Genetics, Medical Genetics, Clinical Biochemical Genetics, Clinical Cytogenetics, Clinical Biochemical/Molecular Genetics and Clinical Molecular Genetics. Certifications are valid for a 10-year period.

American Board of Neurological Surgery
6550 Fannin Street
Suite 2139
Houston, TX 77030-2701
(713) 790-6015
General Certification in Neurological Surgery. Certifications awarded since 1999 are valid for 10 years.

American Board of Nuclear Medicine
900 Veteran Avenue, Room 12-200
Los Angeles, CA 90024-1786
(310) 825-6787
General Certification in Nuclear Medicine. Certifications awarded since 1992 are valid for 10 years. For those certified prior to 1992, there is no recertification requirement.

APPENDIX B

■ **American Board of Obstetrics and Gynecology**
2915 Vine Street
Dallas, TX 75204
(214) 871-1619
General Certification in Obstetrics and Gynecology; with Special Qualifications in Gynecologic Oncology, Maternal and Fetal Medicine, Reproductive Endocrinology and Added Qualification in Critical Care. Certifications awarded since 1986 are valid for 10 years. For those certified prior to 1986, there is no recertification requirement.

■ **American Board of Ophthalmology**
111 Presidential Boulevard, Suite 241
Bala Cynwyd, PA 19004
(610) 664-1175
Certifications awarded since 1992 are valid for 10 years. For those certified prior to 1992, there is no recertification requirement.

■ **American Board of Orthopaedic Surgery**
400 Silver Cedar Court
Chapel Hill, NC 27514
(919) 929-7103
General Certification in Orthopaedic Surgery; with Added Qualification in Hand Surgery. Certifications awarded since 1986 are valid for 10 years. For those certified prior to 1986, there is no recertification requirement.

■ **American Board of Otolaryngology**
2211 Norfolk, Suite 800
Houston, TX 77098-4044
(713) 528-6200
General Certification in Otolaryngology; with Added Qualification in Otology/Neurotology and Pediatric Otolaryngology. Presently, there is no recertification requirement.

■ **American Board of Pathology**
P.O. Box 25915
Tampa, FL 33622-5915
(813) 286-2444
General Certification in Anatomic and Clinical Pathology, Anatomic Pathology and Clinical Pathology; with Special Qualifications in Blood Banking/Transfusion Medicine, Chemical Pathology, Dermatopathology, Forensic Pathology, Hematology, Immunopathology, Medical Microbiology, Neuropathology and Pediatric Pathology and Added Qualification in Cytopathology. Certifications awarded since 1997 are valid for 10 years.

American Board of Pediatrics
111 Silver Cedar Court
Chapel Hill, NC 27514-1651
(919) 929-0461
General Certification in Pediatrics; with Special Qualifications in Adolescent Medicine, Allergy & Immunology, Pediatric Cardiology, Pediatric Critical Care Medicine, Pediatric Emergency Medicine, Pediatric Endocrinology, Pediatric Gastroenterology, Pediatric Hematology-Oncology, Pediatric Infectious Diseases, Pediatric Nephrology, Pediatric Pulmonology, Neonatal-Perinatal Medicine and Pediatric Rheumatology. Added Qualifications in Diagnostic Laboratory Immunology, Medical Toxicology and Sports Medicine. Certifications valid for 7 years.

American Board of Physical Medicine and Rehabilitation
Norwest Center, Suite 674
21 First Street, S.W.
Rochester, MN 55902
(507) 282-1776
General Certification in Physical Medicine and Rehabilitation; with Special Qualifications in Spinal Cord Injury Medicine. Certifications awarded since 1993 are valid for 10 years.

American Board of Plastic Surgery
Seven Penn Center, Suite 400
1635 Market Street
Philadelphia, PA 19103-2204
(215) 587-9322
General Certification in Plastic Surgery; with Added Qualification in Hand Surgery. Certifications are valid for a 10-year period.

American Board of Preventive Medicine
9950 W. Lawrence Avenue, Suite 106
Schiller Park, IL 60176
(847) 671-1750
General Certification in Aerospace Medicine, Occupational Medicine and Public Health and General Preventive Medicine; with Added Qualification in Underseas Medicine and Medical Toxicology. In the subspecialty of Underseas Medicine and Medical Toxicology certifications are valid for a 10-year period.

American Board of Psychiatry & Neurology
500 Lake Cook Road, Suite 335
Deerfield, IL 60015
(847) 945-7900
General Certification in Psychiatry, Neurology and Neurology with Special Qualification in Child Neurology; with Special Qualification in Child and Adolescent Psychiatry and Added Qualification in Addiction Psychiatry, Clinical Neurophysiology, Forensic Psychiatry and Geriatric Psychiatry. Certifications are valid for a 10-year period.

APPENDIX B

■ **American Board of Radiology**
5255 E. Williams Circle, Suite 3200
Tucson, AZ 85711
(520) 790-2900
General Certification in Diagnostic Radiology or Radiation Oncology; with Special Competency in Nuclear Radiology and Added Qualifications in Neuroradiology, Pediatric Radiology and Vascular and Interventional Radiology. Radiation Physics is a non-clinical certification. Certificates are valid for a 10-year period.

■ **American Board of Surgery**
1617 John F. Kennedy Boulevard, Suite 860
Philadelphia, PA 19103-1847
(215) 568-4000
General Certification in Surgery; with Special Qualifications in Pediatric Surgery and General Vascular Surgery and Added Qualifications in Surgery of the Hand, Surgical Critical Care and General Vascular Surgery. Certifications are valid for a 10-year period.

■ **American Board of Thoracic Surgery**
One Rotary Center, Suite 803
Evanston, IL 60201
(847) 475-1520
General Certification in Thoracic Surgery. Certifications awarded since 1976 are valid for 10 years. For those certified prior to 1976, there is no recertification requirement.

■ **American Board of Urology**
2216 Ivy Road, Suite 210
Charlottesville, VA 22903
(248) 646-9720
General Certification in Urology. Certifications awarded as of 1985 are valid for 10 years. For those certified prior to 1985, there is no recertification requirement.

APPENDIX C

OSTEOPATHIC BOARDS

American Osteopathic Association
142 E Ontario Street
Chicago, IL 60611
(800) 621-1773

GENERAL CERTIFICATION

◼ **American Osteopathic Board of Anesthesiology**
Anesthesiology
- No time-limited certificates

◼ **American Osteopathic Board of Dermatology**
Dermatology
- No time-limited certificates

◼ **American Osteopathic Board of Emergency Medicine**
Emergency Medicine
- Beginning 1/1/94, 10-year certificates

◼ **American Osteopathic Board of Family Physicians**
Family Practice
- Beginning 3/1/97, 8-year certificates

◼ **American Osteopathic Board of Internal Medicine**
Internal Medicine
- Beginning 1/1/93, 10-year certificates

◼ **American Osteopathic Board of Neurology and Psychiatry**
Neurology
Psychiatry
- Beginning 1/1/96, 10-year certificates

◼ **American Osteopathic Board of Obstetrics and Gynecology**
Obstetrics and Gynecology
- No time-limited certificates

APPENDIX C

■ **American Osteopathic Board of Ophthalmology and Otorhinolaryngology**
Ophthalmology
• Beginning 1/1/00, 10-year certificates
Otorhinolaryngology
Facial Plastic Surgery
Otorhinolaryngology and Facial Plastic Surgery
• Beginning 1/1/02, 10-year certificates

■ **American Osteopathic Board of Orthopaedic Surgery**
Orthopaedic Surgery
• Beginning 1/1/94, 10-year certificates

■ **American Osteopathic Board of Pathology**
Laboratory Medicine
Anatomic Pathology
Anatomic Pathology and Laboratory Medicine
• Beginning 1/1/95, 10-year certificates

■ **American Osteopathic Board of Pediatrics**
Pediatrics
• Beginning 1/1/95, 7-year certificates

■ **American Osteopathic Board of Preventive Medicine**
Preventive Medicine/Aerospace Medicine
Preventive Medicine/Occupational-Environmental Medicine
Preventive Medicine/Public Health
• Beginning 1/1/94, 10-year certificates

■ **American Osteopathic Board of Proctology**
Proctology
• No time-limited certificates

■ **American Osteopathic Board of Radiology**
Diagnostic Radiology
Radiation Oncology
• No time-limited certificates

■ **American Osteopathic Board of Rehabilitation Medicine**
Rehabilitation Medicine
• No time-limited certificates

■ **American Osteopathic Board of Special Proficiency in Osteopathic Manipulative Medicine**
   Special Proficiency in Osteopathic Manipulative Medicine
   • Beginning 1/1/95, 10-year certificates

■ **American Osteopathic Board of Surgery**
   Surgery (general)
   Plastic and Reconstructive Surgery
   Thoracic Cardiovascular Surgery
   Urological Surgery
   General Vascular Surgery
   • Beginning 1/1/97, 10-year certificates

Consumers may call the American Osteopathic Association at (800) 621-1773 for general certification information.

APPENDIX D

SELF-DESIGNATED MEDICAL SPECIALTIES

This list of self-designated medical specialty groups was obtained from the American Board of Medical Specialties. However, it is important to point out that these groups are not recognized by the ABMS, the governing board for the recognized twenty-four medical specialty boards (listed in Appendix B).

The organizations listed below range from highly organized groups that are attempting to formalize training and certification in their field to informal groups interested in a particular aspect of medicine.

If you wish to obtain information from any of these groups you will have to do some detective work. Because so many are informal, the location, phone and mailing addresses change frequently, depending upon the person who is functioning as secretary or administrator.

The best way to track down one of these groups is to consult the doctor listings to find a doctor who has expressed a special interest in that field, and call his or her office. You might also call a nearby academic health center in the area to see if they have a faculty or staff member known to be involved in that particular medical interest. If that fails, take the same approach with your community hospital.

APPENDIX D

A

Abdominal Surgeons
Acupuncture Medicine
Addiction Medicine
Addictionology
Adolescent Psychiatry
Aesthetic Plastic Surgery
Alcoholism and Other Drug
    Dependencies (AMSAODD)
Algology (Chronic Pain)
Alternative Medicine
Ambulatory Anesthesia
Ambulatory Foot Surgery
Anesthesia
Arthroscopic Surgery
Arthroscopy (Board of North America)

B

Bariatric Medicine
Bionic Psychology
Bloodless Medicine & Surgery

C

Chelation Therapy
Chemical Dependence
Clinical Chemistry
Clinical Ecology
Clinical Medicine and Surgery
Clinical Neurology
Clinical Neurophysiology
Clinical Neurosurgery
Clinical Nutrition
Clinical Orthopaedic Surgery
Clinical Pharmacology
Clinical Polysomnography
Clinical Psychiatry
Clinical Psychology
Clinical Toxicology
Cosmetic Plastic Surgery
Cosmetic Surgery
Council of Non-Board Certified Physicians
Critical Care in Medicine & Surgery

D

Dermalogy
Disability Analysis
Disability Evaluating Physicians

E

Electrodiagnostic Medicine
Electroencephalography
Electromyography & Electrodiagnosis
Environmental Medicine
Epidemiology (College)
Eye Surgery

F

Facial Cosmetic Surgery
Facial Plastic & Reconstructive Surgery
Family Practice, Certification
Forensic Examiners
Forensic Psychiatry
Forensic Toxicology

H

Hand Surgery
Head, Facial & Neck Pain & TMJ Orthopaedics
Health Physics
Homeopathic Physicians
Homeotherapeutics
Hypnotic Anesthesiology, National Board for

I

Independent Medical Examiners
Industrial Medicine & Surgery
Insurance Medicine
International Cosmetic & Plastic
    Facial Reconstructive Standards
Interventional Radiology

L

Laser Surgery
Law in Medicine
Longevity Medicine/Surgery

M

Malpractice Physicians
Maxillofacial Surgeons
Medical Accreditation (American Federation for)
Medical Hypnosis
Medical Laboratory Immunology
Medical-Legal Analysis of Medicine & Surgery
Medical Legal & Workers
    Comp. Medicine & Surgery
Medical-Legal Consultants
Medical Management
Medical Microbiology
Medical Preventics (Academy)
Medical Psychotherapists
Medical Toxicology
Microbiology (Medical Microbiology)
Military Medicine
Mohs Micrographic Surgery &
    Cutaneous Oncology

N

Neuroimaging
Neurologic & Orthopaedic Dental
    Medicine and Surgery
Neurological & Orthopaedic Medicine
Neurological & Orthopaedic Surgery
Neurological Microsurgery
Neurology
Neuromuscular Thermography
Neuro-Orthopaedic Dental Medicine & Surgery
Neuro-Orthopaedic Electrodiagnosis
Neuro-Orthopaedic Laser Surgery
Neuro-Orthopaedic Psychiatry
Neuro-Orthopaedic Thoracic Medicine/Surgery
Neurorehabilitation
Nutrition

O

Orthopaedic Medicine
Orthopaedic Microneurosurgery
Otorhinolaryngology

P

Pain Management (American Academy of)

Pain Management Specialties
Pain Medicine
Palliative Medicine
Percutaneous Diskectomy
Plastic Esthetic Surgeons
Prison Medicine
Professional Disability Consultants
Psychiatric Medicine
Psychiatry (American National Board of)
Psychoanalysis (American Examining
    Board in)
Psychological Medicine (International)

Q

Quality Assurance & Utilization Review

R

Radiology & Medical Imaging
Rheumatologic Surgery
Rheumatological & Reconstructive Medicine
Ringside Medicine & Surgery

S

Skin Specialists
Sleep Medicine (Polysomnography)
Spinal Cord Injury
Spinal Surgery
Sports Medicine
Sports Medicine/Surgery

T

Toxicology
Trauma Surgery
Traumatologic Medicine & Surgery
Tropical Medicine

U

Ultrasound Technology
Urologic Allied Health Professionals
Urological Surgery

W

Weight Reduction Medicine

APPENDIX E

HOSPITAL LISTINGS

Following is an alphabetical listing of hospitals noted in doctors' entries. Due to the many mergers taking place in the hospital industry these days, the names on this list periodically may change.

Abbott - Northwestern Hospital
Abbott - Northwestern Hosp
800 E 28th St
Minneapolis, MN 55407
Midwest
(612) 863-4000

Advocate Lutheran General Hospital
Advocate Lutheran Gen Hosp
1775 Dempster St
Park Ridge, IL 60068
Midwest
(847) 723-2210

Albany Medical Center
Albany Medical Center
43 New Scotland Ave
Albany, NY 12208
Mid Atlantic
(518) 262-3125

Albert Einstein Medical Center
Albert Einstein Med Ctr
5501 Old York Road
Philadelphia, PA 19141
Mid Atlantic
(215) 456-7890

Alfred I Dupont Hospital for Children
Alfred I Dupont Hosp for Children
1600 Rockland Rd
Wilmington, DE 19803
Mid Atlantic
(302) 651-6600

All Children's Hospital
All Children's Hosp
801 Sixth Street South
St. Petersburg, FL 33701
Southeast
(727) 898-7451

Allegheny General Hospital
Allegheny General Hosp
320 E. North Avenue
Pittsburgh, PA 15212
Mid Atlantic
(412) 359-3131

Alta Bates Summit Medical Center
Alta Bates Summit Med Ctr
2450 Ashby Avenue
Berkeley, CA 94705
West Coast and Pacific
(510) 204-4444

APPENDIX E

Anne Bates Leach Eye Hosp
Anne B Leach Eye Hosp
900 NW 17th St PO Box 16680
Miami, FL 33136
Southeast
(305) 326-6000

Arkansas Children's Hospital
Arkansas Chldns Hosp
800 Marshall St
Little Rock, AR 72202
Southwest
(501) 320-1100

Arlington Hospital
Arlington Hosp
1701 N George Mason Dr
Arlington, VA 22205-3698
Southeast
(703) 558-5000

Armed Forces Institute of Pathology
Armed Forces Inst of Path
6825 16th St NW
Washington, DC 20306-6000
Mid Atlantic
(202) 782-2100

Arthur G. James Cancer Hospital & Research
Institute
A G James Cancer Hosp & Research Inst
300 West 10th Avenue
Columbus, OH 43210
Midwest
(614) 293-5485

Atlanta Medical Center
Atlanta Medical Center
303 Parkway Dr. NE
Atlanta, GA 3031
Southeast
(404) 265-4000

Audie L Murphy Memorial Veterans Hospital
Audie L Murphy Memorial Veterans Hosp
7400 Merton Minter Boulevard
San Antonio, TX 78284
Southwest
(210) 617-5300

Baptist Hospital
Baptist Hosp
2000 Church St
Nashville, TN 37236
Southeast
(615) 284-5555

Baptist Hospital - Miami
Baptist Hosp - Miami
8900 N Kendall Dr
Miami, FL 33176
Southeast
(305) 596-1960

Baptist Medical Center
Baptist Med Ctr
111 Dallas St
San Antonio, TX 78205
Southwest
(210) 297-7000

Baptist Memorial Hospital Medical Center
Baptist Mem Hosp Med Ctr
899 Madison Ave
Memphis, TN 38146
Southeast
(901) 227-2727

Barbara Ann Karmanos Cancer Institute
Barbara Ann Karmanos Cancer Inst
110 East Warren Ave
Detroit, MI 48201
Midwest
(800) 527-6266

Barnes - Jewish Hospital
Barnes - Jewish Hosp
One Barnes-Jewish Hospital Plaza
St. Louis, MO 63110
Midwest
(314) 286-2000

Baylor University Medical Center
Baylor Univ Medical Ctr
3500 Gaston Avenue
Dallas, TX 75246
Southwest
(214) 820-0111

Baylor-Richardson Medical Center
Baylor-Richardson Med Ctr
401 West Campbell Road
Richardson, TX 75080
Southwest
(972) 498-4000

Baystate Medical Center
Baystate Med Ctr
759 Chestnut Street
Springfield, MA 01199
New England
(413) 794-0000

Bellevue Hospital Center
Bellevue Hosp Ctr
462 First Avenue
New York, NY 10016
Mid Atlantic
(212) 562-4141

Bergen Regional Medical Center
Bergen Regional Med Ctr
230 East Ridgewood Avenue
Paramus, NJ 07652
Mid Atlantic
(201) 967-4000

Beth Israel Deaconess Medical Center - Boston
Affiliate, CareGroup
Beth Israel Deaconess Med Ctr - Boston
330 Brookline Ave
Boston, MA 02215
New England
(617) 667-7000

Beth Israel Medical Center
Beth Israel Med Ctr
First Avenue @ 16th Street
New York, NY 10003
Mid Atlantic
(212) 420-2000

Beth Israel Medical Center - Herbert & Nell Singer Division
Affiliate, Continuum Health Partners
Beth Israel Med Ctr - Singer Div
170 East End Avenue @ 87th Street
New York, NY 10128
Mid Atlantic
(212) 870-9000

Boca Raton Community Hosp
Boca Raton Comm Hosp
800 Meadows Road
Boca Raton, FL 33486
Southeast
(561) 395-7100

Boston Medical Center
Boston Medical Ctr
1 Boston Medical Center Place
Boston, MA 02118
New England
(617) 638-8000

APPENDIX E

Boston University Medical Center-East Newton
Street Campus
BUMC - E Newton St Cam
88 East Newton Street
Boston, MA 02118
New England
(617) 638-8000

Bridgeport Hospital
Bridgport Hosp
267 Grant St
Bridgeport, CT 06610
New England
(203) 384-3000

Brigham & Women's Hospital
Brigham & Women's Hospital
75 Francis Street
Boston, MA 02115
New England
(617) 732-5500

Brooklyn Hospital Center-Downtown
Brooklyn Hosp Ctr-Downtown
121 DeKalb Avenue
Brooklyn, NY 11201
Mid Atlantic
(718) 250-8000

Broward General Medical Center
Broward General Med Ctr
1600 S Andrews Ave
Fort Lauderdale, FL 33316
Southeast
(954) 355-4400

Buffalo General Hospital
Buffalo General Hosp
100 High Street
Buffalo, NY 14203
Mid Atlantic
(716) 859-5600

Burke Rehabilitation Hospital
Burke Rehabilitation Hosp
785 Mamaroneck Avenue
White Plains, NY 10605
Mid Atlantic
(914) 597-2500

Butler Hospital
Butler Hosp
345 Blackstone Blvd
Providence, RI 02906
New England
(401) 455-6200

Cabrini Medical Center
Cabrini Med Ctr
227 East 19th Street
New York, NY 10003
Mid Atlantic
(212) 995-6000

California Hospital Medical Center
California Hosp Med Ctr
1401 S. Grand Avenue
Los Angeles, CA 90015
West Coast and Pacific
(213) 748-2411

California Pacific Medical Center
California Pacific Med Ctr
2333 Buchanan Street
San Francisco, CA 94120
West Coast and Pacific
(415) 600-6000

Cambridge Hospital
Cambridge Hospital
1493 Cambridge Street
Cambridge, MA 02139
New England
(617) 665-1000

Campbell Clinic
Campbell Clinic
1400 Germantown Road
Germantown, TN 38138
Southeast
(901) 759-3100

Cancer Institute of New Jersey, The
Cancer Inst of NJ, The
195 Little Albany St
New Brunswick, NJ 08901
Mid Atlantic
(732) 235-2465

Carolinas Medical Center
Carolinas Med Ctr
1000 Blythe Blvd0
Charlotte, NC 28203-5871
Southeast
(704) 355-2000

Cedars Medical Center - Miami
Cedars Med Ctr - Miami
1400 NW 12 Ave
Miami, FL 33136
Southeast
(305) 325-5511

Cedars-Sinai Medical Center
Cedars-Sinai Med Ctr
8700 Beverly Boulevard
Los Angeles, CA 90048
West Coast and Pacific
(310) 423-5000

Centennial Medical Center
Centennial Medical Ctr
2300 Patterson Street
Nashville, TN 37203
Southeast
(615) 342-1000

Centinela Hospital Medical Center
Centinela Hosp Med Ctr
555 East Hardy Street
Inglewood, CA 90301
West Coast and Pacific
(310) 673-4660

Century City Hospital
Century City Hosp
2070 Century Park East
Los Angeles, CA 90067
West Coast and Pacific
(310) 553-6211

Children's Healthcare of Atlanta
Children's Healthcare of Atlanta
1405 Clifton Road
Atlanta, GA 30322
Southeast
(404) 250-5437

Children's Healthcare of Atlanta at Scottish Rite
Children's Hlthcre of Atl at Scottish Rite
1001 Johnson Ferry Road
Atlanta, GA 30342
Southeast
(404) 256-5252

Children's Hospital
Children's Hospital
1600 7th Ave South
Birmingham, AL 35233
Southeast
(205) 939-9100

Children's Hospital
Chldn's Hosp
700 Children's Drive
Columbus, OH 43205
Midwest
(614) 722-2000

APPENDIX E

Children's Hospital
Children's Hospital
300 Longwood Avenue
Boston, MA 02115
New England
(617) 355-6000

Children's Hospital Medical Center
Children's Hosp and Med Ctr-Cincinnati
3333 Burnet Ave
Cincinnati, OH 45229
Midwest
(800) 344-2462

Children's Hospital - Los Angeles
Children's Hosp - Los Angeles
4650 Sunset Boulevard
Los Angeles, CA 90027
West Coast and Pacific
(323) 660-2450

Children's Hospital - New Orleans
Children's Hospital - New Orleans
200 Henry Clay Ave
New Orleans, LA 70118
Southwest
(504) 899-9511

Children's Hospital and Clinics
Children's Hosp and Clins - Minneapolis
2525 Chicago Ave S
Minneapolis, MN 55404
Midwest
(612) 813-6111

Children's Hospital and Health Center
Children's Hosp and Hlth Ctr - San Diego
3020 Childrens Way
San Diego, CA 92123
West Coast and Pacific
(858) 576-1700

Children's Hospital and Regional Medical Center - Seattle
Children's Hospital and Reg Med Ctr - Seattle
4800 Sand Point Way NE
Seattle, WA 98105
West Coast and Pacific
(206) 526-2000

Children's Hospital of Michigan
Chldn's Hosp of Michigan
3901 Beaubian Blvd
Detroit, MI 48201
Midwest
(313) 745-5437

Children's Hospital of Oklahoma
Chldn's Hosp of Oklahoma
940 NE13th Street
Oklahoma City, OK 73104
Southwest
(405) 271-5437

Children's Hospital of Pittsburgh
Chldn's Hosp of Pittsbrgh
3705 Fifth Avenue
Pittsburgh, PA 15213
Mid Atlantic
(412) 692-5325

Children's Hospital of Wisconsin
Children's Hospital - Wisconsin
9000 West Wisconsin Avenue
Milwaukee, WI 53201
Midwest
(414) 266-2000

Children's Medical Center - Oakland
Children's Hosp Med Ctr - Oakland
747 52nd Street
Oakland, CA 94609
West Coast and Pacific
(800) 400-7337

Children's Medical Center of Dallas
Children's Medical Center of Dallas
1935 Motor Street
Dallas, TX 75235
Southwest
(214) 456-7000

Children's Memorial Hospital
Children's Mem Hosp
2300 Children's Plaza
Chicago, IL 60614
Midwest
(773) 880-4000

Children's Mercy Hospital & Clinics
Children's Mercy Hosp & Clinics
1401 Gilham Road
Kansas City, MO 64108
Midwest
(816) 234-3000

Children's National Medical Center - DC
Children's National Med Ctr - DC
111 Michigan Avenue NorthWest
Washington, DC 20010
Mid Atlantic
(202) 884-5000

Christ Hospital, The
Christ Hospital
2139 Auburn Ave
Cincinnati, OH 45219
Midwest
(513) 585-2000

Christus St Joseph's Hospital
Christus St Joseph's Hosp
1919 La Branch Street
Houston, TX 77002
Southwest
(713) 757-1000

City of Hope National Medical Center
City of Hope National Med Ctr
1500 East Duarte Road
Duarte, CA 91010
West Coast and Pacific
(626) 359-8111

Cleveland Clinic Florida
Cleveland Clinic FL
3000 W Cypress Creek Rd
Fort Lauderdale, FL 33309
Southeast
(954) 978-5000

Cleveland Clinic Foundation
Cleveland Clinic Foundation
9500 Euclid Avenue
Cleveland, OH 44195
Midwest
(800) 223-2273

**Columbia Presbyterian Medical Center
Affiliate, NewYork-Presbyterian Health
System**
Columbia Presby Med Ctr
622 West 168th Street
New York, NY 10032
Mid Atlantic
(212) 305-2500

Columbus Hospital
Columbus Hosp
495 N 13th Street
Newark, NJ 07107
Mid Atlantic
(973) 268-1400

Cook Children's Medical Center
Cook Children's Med Ctr
801 7th Ave
Fort Worth, TX 76104-2796
Southwest
(817) 885-4000

APPENDIX E

Craig Hospital
Craig hospital
3425 S Clarkson
Englewood, CO 80110-2899
Great Plains and Mountains
(303) 789-8000

Crouse Hospital
Crouse Hosp
736 Irving Ave
Syracuse, NY 13210-1607
Mid Atlantic
(315) 470-7111

Dana Farber Cancer Institute
Dana Farber cancer Inst
44 Binney Street
Boston, MA 02115
New England
(617) 632-3000

Dartmouth - Hitchcock Medical Center
Dartmouth - Hitchcock Med Ctr
1 Medical Center Dr
Lebanon, NH 03756-0002
New England
(603) 650-5000

Davies Medical Center
Davies Med Ctr
3700 California Street
San Francisco, CA 94114
West Coast and Pacific
(415) 565-6000

Deaconess Hospital
Deaconess Hosp
600 Mary Street
Evansville, IN 47747-0002
Midwest
(812) 426-3000

Denver Health Medical Center
Denver Health Med Ctr
777 Bannock St
Denver, CO 80204
Great Plains and Mountains
(303) 436-6000

Doctors Medical Center
Doctors Med Ctr
2000 Vale Road
San Pablo, CA 94806
West Coast and Pacific
(510) 970-5000

Duke University Medical Center
Duke Univ Med Ctr
Box 3708
Durham, NC 27710
Southeast
(919) 684-8026

East Jefferson General Hospital
E Jefferson Gen Hosp
4200 Houma Blvd
Metairie, LA 70006-2973
Southwest
(504) 454-4000

East Texas Medical Center
E TX Med Ctr
1000 South Beckham Ave.
Tyler, TX 75711
Southwest
(903) 597-0351

Eastmoreland Hospital
Eastmoreland Hosp
2900 SE Steele St
Portland, OR 97202-4590
West Coast and Pacific
(503) 234-0411

904

Eden Medical Center
Eden Med Ctr
20103 Lake Chabot Road
Castro Valley, CA 94546
West Coast and Pacific
(510) 537-1234

Emory - Adventist Hospital
Emory - Adventist Hosp
3949 South Cobb Drive
Smyrna, GA 30080
Southeast
(770) 434-0710

Emory University Hospital
Emory Univ Hosp
1364 Clifton Road NorthEast
Atlanta, GA 30322
Southeast
(404) 712-7021

Englewood Hospital & Medical Center
Englewood Hosp & Med Ctr
350 Engle Street
Englewood, NJ 07631
Mid Atlantic
(201) 894-3000

Evanston Hospital
Evanston Hosp
2650 Ridge Ave
Evanston, IL 60201
Midwest
(847) 570-2000

Fairfax Hospital
Fairfax Hospital
3300 Gallows Road
Falls Church, VA 22042
Southeast
(703) 698-1110

Fairview Southdale Hospital
Fairview Southdale Hosp
6401 France Ave. S
Edina, MN 55435-2199
Midwest
(952) 924-5000

Fairview-University Medical Center - University Campus
Fairview-Univ Med Ctr - Univ Campus
2450 Riverside Avenue
Minneapolis, MN 55454
Midwest
(612) 273-3000

Fletcher Allen - Healthcare
Fletcher Allen - Healthcare
1 South Prospect St
Burlington, VT 05401
New England
(802) 656-2345

Fletcher Allen Health Care Medical Center - Campus
Fletcher Allen Hlth Care Med Ctr - Campus
111 Colchester Avenue (Burgess 1)
Burlington, VT 05011
New England
(802) 656-2345

Florida Hospital
Florida Hosp
400 Celebration Place
Celebration, FL 34742
Southeast
(407) 896-6611

Florida Hospital
FL Hosp
601 East Rollins Street
Orlando, FL 32803
Southeast
(407) 896-6611

Foster G McGaw Hospital/Loyola Univ Med Ctr
Foster G McGaw Hosp/Loyola Univ Med Ctr
2160 S 1st Ave
Maywood, IL 60153
Midwest
(708) 216-9000

Four Winds Hospital
Four Winds Hosp
800 Cross River Road
Katonah, NY 11580
Mid Atlantic
(914) 763-8151

Fox Chase Cancer Center
Fox Chase Cancer Ctr
7701 Burholme Avenue
Philadelphia, PA 19111
Mid Atlantic
(215) 728-6900

Froedtert Memorial Lutheran Hospital
Froedtert Mem Lutheran Hosp
9200 West Wisconsin Avenue
Milwaukee, WI 53226
Midwest
(414) 805-2606

George Washington University Hospital
G Washington Univ Hosp
901 23rd Street NW
Washington, DC 20037
Mid Atlantic
(202) 715-4000

Georgetown University Hospital
Georgetown Univ Hosp
3800 Reservoir Road NorthWest
Washington, DC 20007
Mid Atlantic
(202) 784-3000

Gillette Children's Specialty Healthcare
Gillette Chldn's Specialty Hlthcre
200 University Ave E
St Paul , MN 55101
Midwest
(651) 291-2848

Goleta Valley Cottage Hospital
Goleta Valley Cottage Hosp
351 S Patterson Ave
Santa Barbara, CA 93111
West Coast and Pacific
(805) 967-3411

Good Samaritan Hosp - Cincinnati
Good Samaritan Hosp - Cincinnati
375 Dixmyth Avenue
Cincinnati, OH 45220
Midwest
(513) 872-1400

Good Samaritan Hospital - Los Angeles
Good Samaritan Hosp - Los Angeles
1225 Wilshire Boulevard
Los Angeles, CA 90017
West Coast and Pacific
(213) 977-2121

Good Samaritan Regional Medical Center - Phoenix
Good Samaritan Regionl - Phoenix
1111 E. McDowell Road
Phoenix, AZ 85062
Southwest
(602) 239-2000

Grady Health System
Grady Hlth Sys
80 Butler Street SouthEast
Atlanta, GA 30335
Southeast
(404) 616-4307

Greater Baltimore Medical Center
Greater Baltimore Med Ctr
6701 N. Charles Street
Baltimore, MD 21204
Mid Atlantic
(410) 828-2000

Greenwich Hospital
Greenwich Hosp
Five Perryridge Road
Greenwich, CT 06830
New England
(203) 863-3000

H Lee Moffitt Cancer Center & Research Institute
H Lee Moffitt Cancer Ctr & Research Inst
12902 Magnolia Drive
Tampa, FL 33612
Southeast
(813) 972-4673

Hackensack University Medical Center
Hackensack Univ Med Ctr
30 Prospect Avenue
Hackensack, NJ 07601
Mid Atlantic
(201) 996-2000

Hahnemann University Hospital
Hahnemann Univ Hosp
Broad & Vine Street
Philadelphia, PA 19102
Mid Atlantic
(215) 762-7000

Hamot Medical Center
Hamot Med Ctr
201 State Street
Erie, PA 16550-0001
Mid Atlantic
(814) 877-6000

Harbor Hospital
Harbor Hosp
3001 S. Hanover
Baltimore, MD 21225
Mid Atlantic
(410) 350-3200

Harlem Hospital Center
Harlem Hosp Ctr
506 Lenox Avenue
New York, NY 10037
Mid Atlantic
(212) 939-1000

Harper Hospital
Harper Hospital
3990 John R St
Detroit, MI 48201-2097
Midwest
(313) 745-8040

Hartford Hospital
Hartford Hosp
80 Seymour Street, P.O. Box 5037
Hartford, CT 06102
New England
(860) 545-5000

Healthsouth Doctor's Hospital
Healthsouth Doctor's Hosp
5000 University Drive
Coral Gables, FL 33146
Southeast
(305) 669-3401

Healthsouth Medical Center - Birmingham
Healthsouth Med Ctr - Birmingham
1201 11th Ave S
Birmingham, AL 35205-5299
Southeast
(205) 930-7000

Hebrew Rehabilitation Center for the Aged
Hebrew Rehab Center
1200 Centre St
Boston, MA 02131
New England
(617) 325-8000

Helen Ellis Memorial Hospital
Helen Ellis Memorial Hosp
1395 S Pinellas Avenue
Tarpon Springs, FL 34689
Southeast
(813) 947-5000

Hennepin County Medical Center
Hennepin Coutny Med Ctr
701 Park Avenue South
Minneapolis, MN 55415
Midwest
(612) 347-2121

Henry Ford Health System
Henry Ford Hlth Sys
One Ford Place
Detroit, MI 48202-2600
Midwest
(313) 876-2600

Hoag Memorial Hospital Presbyterian
Hoag Mem Hosp Presby
One Hoag Drive
Newport Beach, CA 92663
West Coast and Pacific
(949) 645-8600

Hospital for Joint Diseases
Hosp For Joint Diseases
301 East 17th Street
New York, NY 10003
Mid Atlantic
(212) 598-6000

Hospital for Special Surgery
Affiliate, NewYork-Presbyterian Health
System
Hosp For Special Surgery
535 East 70th Street
New York, NY 10021
Mid Atlantic
(212) 606-1000

Hospital of the University of Pennsylvania
Hosp Univ Penn
3400 Spruce Street
Philadelphia, PA 19104
Mid Atlantic
(215) 898-5181

Howard University Hospital
Howard Univ Hosp
2041 Georgia Avenue NorthWest
Washington, DC 20060
Mid Atlantic
(202) 865-6660

Hutzel Hospital - Detroit
Hutzel Hosp - Detroit
4707 St Antoint Blvd
Detroit, MI 48201-1498
Midwest
(313) 745-7552

Illinois Masonic Medical Center
IL Masonic Med Ctr
836 W Wellington Ave
Chicago, IL 60657-5147
Midwest
(773) 975-1600

Indian River Memorial Hosp
Indian River Mem Hosp
1000 36th St
Vero Beach, FL 32960 |
Southeast
(561) 567-4311

Indiana University Hospital & Medical Center -
Indianapolis
IN Univ Hosp & Med Ctr - Indianapolis
550 N University Blvd
Indianapolis, IN 46202
Midwest
(317) 274-4862

Inova Alexandria Hospital
Inova Alexandria Hosp
4320 Seminary Rd
Alexandria, VA 22304
Southeast
(703) 504-3000

Inova Fairfax Hospital
Inova Fairfax Hosp
3300 Gallows Rd
Falls Church, VA 22042-3300
Southeast
(703) 289-2068

Intergris Baptist Medical Center - Oklahoma
Integris Baptist Med Ctr - OK
3300 NW Expressway
Oklahoma City, OK 73112-9028
Southwest
(405) 949-3011

Jewish Hospital & Medical Center - Louisville
Jewish Hosp & Med Ctr - Louisvile
217 E. Chestnut Street
Louisville, KY 40202
Southeast
(502) 587-4011

John Dempsey Hospital - University Connecticut
Health Center
John Dempsey Hosp - Univ Conn Hlth Ctr
263 Farmington Ave
Farmington, CT 06030
New England
(860) 679-2000

Johns Hopkins Hospital - Baltimore
Johns Hopkins Hosp - Baltimore
550 North Broadway
Baltimore, MD 21205
Mid Atlantic
(410) 955-0620

Johns Hopkins Medical Center - Bayview
Johns Hopkins Bayview Med Ctr |
4940 Eastern Avenue
Baltimore, MD 21224
Mid Atlantic
(410) 550-0516

Kaiser Permanente Medical Center
Kaiser Permanente Med Ctr
1200 El Camino Real
South San Francisco, CA 94080
West Coast and Pacific
(650) 742-2000

Kapiolani Medical Center for Women & Children
Kapiolani Med Ctr for Women & Children
1319 Punahou Street
Honolulu, HI 96826
West Coast and Pacific
(808) 983-6000

Kessler Institute for Rehabilitation - East Orange
Kessler Inst For Rehab - East Orange
240 Central Avenue
East Orange, NJ 07018
Mid Atlantic
(973) 414-4700

APPENDIX E

KFH San Francisco Medical Center
KFH San Francisco Med Ctr
2425 Geary Boulevard
San Francisco, CA 94115
West Coast and Pacific
(415) 202-2000

Kosair Children's Hospital
Kosair Chldn's Hosp
31 E Chestnut St
Louisville, KY 40202
Southeast
(502) 629-6000

KPH Panorama City Medical Center
KPH Panorama City Med Ctr
13652 Cantara Street
Panorama City, CA 91402
West Coast and Pacific
(818) 375-2000

LAC + USC Medical Center
LAC + USC Med Ctr
1200 N State Street
Los Angeles, CA 90033-4525
West Coast and Pacific
(323) 226-2622

LAC - Harbor - UCLA Medical Center
LAC - Harbor - UCLA Med Ctr
1000 W Carson St
Torrance, CA 90509-2059
West Coast and Pacific
(310) 222-2345

LAC - King/Drew Medical Center
LAC - King/Drew Med Ctr
12021 South Wilmington Avenue
Los Angeles, CA 90059
West Coast and Pacific
(310) 668-4321

LAC - Rancho Los Amigos Medical Center
LAC - Rancho Los Amigos Med Ctr
7601 East Imperial Highway
Downey, CA 90242
West Coast and Pacific
(562) 401-7111

Lahey Clinic
Lahey Cli.
41 Mall Road
Burlington, MA 01805
New England
(781) 744-5100

LDS Hospital
LDSHospital
8th Ave & C Street
Salt Lake City, UT 84143
Great Plains and Mountains
(801) 408-1100

Le Bonheur Children's Medical Center
LeBonheur Chldn Med Ctr
50 N Dunlap
Memphis, TN 38103-2893
Southeast
(901) 572-3000

Legacy Good Samaritan Hospital and Medical Center
Legacy Good Samaritan Hosp and Med Ctr
1015 NW 22nd Ave
Portland, OR 97210-3025
West Coast and Pacific
(503) 413-7711

Lenox Hill Hospital
Lenox Hill Hosp
100 East 77th Street
New York, NY 10021
Mid Atlantic
(212) 434-2000

Loma Linda University Behavioral Medical Center - Redlands
Loma Linda Univ Behav Med Ctr - Redlands
1710 Barton Road
Redlands, CA 92373
West Coast and Pacific
(909) 793-9333

Loma Linda University Medical Center
Loma Linda University Med Ctr
11234 Anderson St
Loma Linda, CA 92354
West Coast and Pacific
(909) 824-0800

Long Beach Memorial Medical Center
Long Beach Memorial Med Ctr
2801 Atlantic Avenue
Long Beach, CA 90801
West Coast and Pacific
(562) 933-2000

Long Island College Hospital
Affiliate, Continuum Health Partners
Long Island Coll Hosp
339 Hicks Street
Brooklyn, NY 11201
Mid Atlantic
(718) 780-1000

Long Island Jewish Medical Center
Long Island Jewish Med Ctr
270-05 76th Avenue
New Hyde Park, NY 11040
Mid Atlantic
(516) 470-7000

Los Alamitos Medical Center
Los Alamitos Med Ctr
3751 Katella Avenue
Los Alamitos, CA 90720
West Coast and Pacific
(562) 598-1311

Louis A Weiss Memorial Hospital
Louis A Weiss Mem Hosp
4646 N Marine Dr
Chicago, IL 60640
Midwest
(773) 878-8700

Louisiana State University Hospital
Louisiana State Univ Hosp
1501 Kings Highway P.O. Box 33932
Shreveport, LA 71130
Southwest
(318) 675-4239

Loyola University Health System
Loyola Univ Hlth Sys
2160 S 1st Ave
Maywood, IL 60153
Midwest
(708) 216-9000

Lutheran Medical Center
Lutheran Med Ctr
1730 W 25th St
Cleveland, OH 44113
Midwest
(216) 696-4300

MacDonald Womens Hospital
MacDonald Women's Hosp
11100 Euclid Ave
Cleveland, OH 44106
Midwest
(216) 844-7565

Magee Rehabilitation Hospital
Magee Rehab Hosp
Six Franklin Plaza
Philadelphia, PA 19102-1177
Mid Atlantic
(215) 587-3000

Magee Women's Hospital
Mage Women's Hosp
300 Halket Street
Pittsburgh, PA 15213
Mid Atlantic
(412) 641-1000

Maimonides Medical Center
Maimonides Med Ctr
4802 Tenth Avenue
Brooklyn, NY 11219
Mid Atlantic
(718) 283-6000

Maine Medical Center
Maine Med Ctr
22 Bramhall Street
Portland, ME 04102
New England
(207) 871-0111

Manhattan Eye, Ear & Throat Hospital
Manhattan Eye, Ear & Throat Hosp
210 East 64th Street
New York, NY 10021
Mid Atlantic
(212) 838-9200

Marin General Hospital
Marin General Hosp
250 Bon Air Road
Greenbrae, CA 94904
West Coast and Pacific
(415) 925-7000

Martin Memorial Health System
Martin Memorial Health System
300 Hospital Drive
Stuart, FL 34994
Southeast
(561) 287-5200

Mary Shiels Hospital
Mary Shiels Hosp
3515 Howell Street
Dallas, TX 75204
Southwest
(214) 443-3000

Maryland General Hospital
Maryland General Hosp
827 Linden Ave
Baltimore, MD 21201
Mid Atlantic
(410) 225-8000

Maryland Psychiatric Research Center
Maryland Psyc Research Ctr
Maple & Locust, PO Box 21247
Baltimore, MD 21228
Mid Atlantic
(410) 402-7666

Massachusetts Eye & Ear Infirmary
Mass Eye & Ear Infirmary
243 Charles Street
Boston, MA 02114
New England
(617) 573-5520

Massachusetts General Hospital
Mass Gen Hosp
55 Fruit Street
Boston, MA 02114
New England
(617) 726-2000

Massachusetts Mental Health Center
Mass Mental Hlth Ctr
74 Fenwood Road
Boston, MA 02115
New England
(617) 626-9300

Mayo Medical Center & Clinic - Rochester
Mayo - Rochester
200 First Street SW
Rochester, MN 55905
Midwest
(507) 284-2511

Mayo Medical Center & Clinic - Scottsdale
Mayo - Scottsdale
13400 E Shea Boulevard
Scottsdale, AZ 85259
Southwest
(480) 301-8000

Mayo/St Luke's Hospital
Mayo/St Luke's Hosp
4201 Belfort Road
Jacksonville, FL 32216
Southeast
(904) 296-3700

McLaren Regional Medical Center
McLaren Reg Med Ctr
401 S. Ballenger Highway
Flint, MI 48532
Midwest
(810) 342-2000

McLean Hospital
McLean Hosp
115 Mill Street
Belmont, MA 02478
New England
(617) 855-2000

Medical Center of Central Georgia
Med Ctr of Central GA
777 Hemlock Street
Macon, GA 31201
Southeast
(912) 633-1000

Medical College of Georgia Hospital
Med Coll of GA Hosp
1120 15th Street
Augusta, GA 30912
Southeast
(706) 721-0211

Medical College of Ohio Hospitals
Med Coll of Ohio Hosp
3000 Arlington Ave
Toledo, OH 43614
Midwest
(419) 383-4000

Medical College of Virginia Hospitals
Med Coll of VA Hosp
P.O. Box 980510
Richmond, VA 23298-0570
Southeast
(804) 828-9000

Memorial Hermann Healthcare System
Meml Hermann Hlthcare Sys
7737 SW Freeway
Houston, TX 77074
Southwest
(713) 776-5484

Memorial Medical Center - Baptist Campus
Memorial Med Ctr - Baptist Campus
2700 Napoleon Ave
New Orleans, LA 70115
Southwest
(504) 899-9311

Memorial Medical Center - Savannah
Memorial Med Ctr - Savannah
4700 Waters Avenue
Savannah, GA 31404
Southeast
(912) 350-8000

APPENDIX E

Memorial Regional Hospital- Hollywood
Mem Reg Hosp - Hollywood
3501 Johnson Street
Hollywood, FL 33021
Southeast
(954) 987-2000

Memorial Sloan Kettering Cancer Center
Mem Sloan Kettering Cancer Ctr
1275 York Avenue
New York, NY 10021
Mid Atlantic
(212) 639-2000

Menninger Clinic
Menninger Clinic
5800 SW 6th Ave or PO Box 829
Topeka, KS 66601-0829
Great Plains and Mountains
(785) 350-5000

Mercy Health Center - Oklahoma City
Mercy Hlth Ctr - Oklahoma City
4300 W Memorial Road
Oklahoma City, OK 73120
Southwest
(405) 755-1515

Mercy Hospital & Medical Center - San Diego
Mercy Hosp & Med Ctr - San Diego
4077 5th Ave
San Diego, CA 92103
West Coast and Pacific
(619) 294-8111

Mercy Hospital - Coon Rapids
Mercy Hosp - Coon Rapids
4050 Coon Rapids Blvd
Coon Rapids, MN 55433-2522
Midwest
(763) 421-8888

Mercy Hospital - Miami
Mercy Hosp- Miami
3663 S Miami Ave
Miami, FL 33133
Southeast
(305) 854-4400

MeritCare Hospital
MeritCare Hosp
720 Fourth Street North
Fargo, ND 58122
Great Plains and Mountains
(701) 234-6000

Methodist Health Care North - Memphis
Meth Hlth Care N - Memphis
4960 Covington Pike
Memphis, TN 38128
Southeast
(901) 384-5200

Methodist Healthcare Central - Memphis Hospital
Meth Healthcare Central - Memphis Hosp
1265 Union Ave
Memphis, TN 38104
Southeast
(901) 726-7000

Methodist Hospital - Houston
Methodist Hosp - Houston
6565 Fannin Street
Houston, TX 77030
Southwest
(713) 790-3311

Methodist Hospital - Indianapolis
Methodist Hosp - Indianapolis
1701 N Senate Boulevard, Box 1367
Indianapolis, IN 46206
Midwest
(317) 929-2000

914

Miami Children's Hospital
Miami Children's Hosp
3100 SW 62nd Ave
Miami, FL 33155
Southeast
(305) 666-6511

Miami Heart Institute - North Campus
Miami Heart Inst - North Campus
4701 Meridian Ave
Miami Beach, FL 33140
Southeast
(305) 672-1111

Michael Reese Hospital & Medical Center
Michael Reese Hosp & Med Ctr
2929 S Ellis Ave
Chicago, IL 60616
Midwest
(312) 791-2000

Millard Fillmore Hospitals
Millard Fillmore Hosp
Three Gates Hospital
Buffalo, NY 14209
Mid Atlantic
(716) 887-4600

Mills - Peninsula Health Center Hospital
Mills - Peninsula Hlth Ctr Hosp
1783 El Camino Real
Burlingame, CA 94010
West Coast and Pacific
(650) 696-5400

Montclair - Baptist Medical Center
Montclair - Baptist Med Ctr
800 Montclair Rd
Birmingham, AL 35213-1984
Southeast
(205) 592-1000

Montefiore Medical Center
Montefiore Med Ctr
111 East 210 Street
Bronx, NY 10467
Mid Atlantic
(718) 920-4321

Montefiore Medical Center - Weiler/Einstein Division
Montefiore Med Ctr - Weiler/Einstein Div
1825 Eastchester Road
Bronx, NY 10461
Mid Atlantic
(718) 904-2000

Moss Rehab Hospital
Moss Rehab Hosp
1200 W Tabor Rd
Philadelphia, PA 19141
Mid Atlantic
(215) 456-9900

Motts Children's Hospital
Motts Chldns Hosp
1500 E Medical Center Drive
Ann Arbor, MI 48109
Midwest
(734) 936-4000

Mount Auburn Hospital
Mount Auburn Hosp
330 Mount Auburn Street
Cambridge, MA 02238
New England
(617) 492-3500

Mount Sinai Hospital
Affiliate, Mount Sinai NYU Health System
Mount Sinai Hosp
One Gustave L. Levy Place, Box 1037
New York, NY 10029
Mid Atlantic
(212) 241-6500

Mount Sinai Medical Center
Mount Sinai Med Ctr
4300 Alton Rd
Miami Beach, FL 33140
Southeast
(305) 674-2121

Muhlenberg Regional Medical Center
Muhlenberg Regional Med Ctr
Park Avenue and Randolph Road
Plainfield, NJ 07061
Mid Atlantic
(908) 668-2000

MUSC Medical Center
Med Univ of SC
169 Ashley Ave
Charleston, SC 29425
Southeast
(843) 792-2300

National Institutes of Health - Clinical Center
Natl Inst of Hlth - Clin Ctr
9000 Rockville Pike, Building 10, Room 2C146
Bethesda, MD 20892
Mid Atlantic
(301) 496-2563

National Jewish Medical & Research Center
Natl Jewish Med & Rsrch Ctr
1400 Jackson Street
Denver, CO 80206-2762
Great Plains and Mountains
(303) 388-4461

National Rehabilitation Hospital
Natl Rehab Hosp
102 Irving Street NorthWest
Washington, DC 20010
Mid Atlantic
(202) 877-1000

Nebraska Health System - Clarkson
Nebraska Hlth Sys - Clarkson
4350 Dewey Ave
Omaha, NE 68105-1018
Great Plains and Mountains
(402) 552-2000

Nebraska Methodist Hospital
Nebraska Meth Hosp
8303 Dodge St
Omaha, NE 68114
Great Plains and Mountains
(402) 354-4000

New Britain General Hospital
New Britain Gen Hosp
100 Grand Street
New Britain, CT 06050
New England
(860) 224-5666

**New England Baptist Hospital
Affiliate, CareGroup**
New England Baptist
125 Parker Hill Avenue
Boston, MA 02120
New England
(617) 754-5800

New England Medical Center
New England Med Ctr - Boston
750 Washington Street
Boston, MA 02111
New England
(617) 636-5000

New Orleans Adolescent Hosp
New Orleans Adol Hosp
210 State St
New Orleans, LA 70118-5735
Southwest
(504) 897-3400

New York Eye & Ear Infirmary
Affiliate, Continuum Health Partners
New York Eye & Ear Infirm
310 East 14th Street
New York, NY 10003
Mid Atlantic
(212) 979-4000

New York Hospital Medical Center of Queens
NY Hosp Med Ctr of Queens
56-45 Main Street
Flushing, NY 11355
Mid Atlantic
(718) 670-1231

New York Methodist Hospital
Affiliate, NewYork-Presbyterian Health System
New York Methodist Hosp
506 Sixth Street
Brooklyn, NY 11215
Mid Atlantic
(718) 780-3000

New York Presbyterian - Westchester Division
NY Presby - Westchester Div
21 Bloomingdale Rd
White Plains, NY 10605
Mid Atlantic
(914) 682-9100

New York State Psychiatric Institute
NYS Psychiatric Institute
1051 Riverside Drive
New York, NY 10032
Mid Atlantic
(212) 543-5000

New York Weill Cornell Medical Center - NY
Presbyterian Hospital
Affiliate, NewYork-Presbyterian Health
System
NY Weill Cornell Med Ctr - NY Presby Hosp
525 East 68th Street
New York, NY 10021
Mid Atlantic
(212) 821-0560

Newark Beth Israel Medical Center
Newark Beth Israel Med Ctr
201 Lyons Avenue
Newark, NJ 07112
Mid Atlantic
(973) 926-7000

Newton - Wellesley Hospital
Newton - Wellesley Hosp
2014 Washington Street
Newton, MA 02462
New England
(617) 243-6000

North Central Baptist Hospital
N Central Baptist Hosp
520 Madison Oak
San Antonio, TX 78258
Southwest
(210) 297-4000

North Oaks Medical Center
North Oaks Med Ctr
15790 Medical Center Dr
Hammond, LA 70403
Southwest
(504) 230-6601

North Shore University Hospital at Manhasset
N Shore Univ Hosp at Manhasset
300 Community Drive
Manhasset, NY 11030
Mid Atlantic
(516) 562-0100

APPENDIX E

Northern Westchester Hospital Center
Northern Westchester Hosp Ctr
400 East Main Street
Mount Kisco, NY 10549
Mid Atlantic
(914) 666-1200

Northwest Hospital
NW Hosp
1550 N 115th St
Seattle, WA 98133-0806
West Coast and Pacific
(206) 364-0500

Northwest Medical Center
Northwest Med Ctr
2801 N State Rd 7
Margate, FL 33063
Southeast
(954) 974-0400

Northwestern Memorial Hospital
Northwestern Mem Hosp
251 E Huron Street
Chicago, IL 60611
Midwest
(312) 926-2000

Norton Hospital
Norton Hospital
200 E Chestnut St
Louisville, KY 40202
Southeast
(502) 629-8000

NYU Downtown Hospital
NYU Downtown Hosp
170 William Street
New York, NY 10038
Mid Atlantic
(212) 312-5000

NYU Medical Center
Affiliate, Mount Sinai NYU Health System
NYU Med Ctr
540 First Avenue
New York, NY 10016
Mid Atlantic
(212) 263-7300

Ochsner Foundation Hospital
Ochsner Found Hosp
1516 Jefferson Hwy
New Orleans, LA 70121-2484
Southwest
(504) 842-3000

Ohio State University Medical Center
Ohio St Univ Med Ctr
410 W 10th Avenue
Columbus, OH 43210
Midwest
(614) 293-8000

Olathe Medical Center
Olathe Med Ctr
20333 W 151st St
Olathe, KS 66061-5352
Great Plains and Mountains
(913) 791-4200

Olive View Medical Center
Olive View Med Ctr
14445 Olive View Dr
Sylmar, CA 91342
West Coast and Pacific
(818) 364-1555

Oregon Health Science University Hospital and Clinics
OR Hlth Sci Univ Hosp and Clinics
3181 SW Sam Jackson Park Rd
Portland, OR 97201-3098
West Coast and Pacific
(503) 494-8311

Orlando Regional Medical Center
Orlando Reg Med Ctr
1414 Kuhl Avenue
Orlando, FL 32806
Southeast
(407) 841-5111

Orthopaedic Hospital
Orthopaedic Hosp
2400 South Flower Street
Los Angeles, CA 90007
West Coast and Pacific
(213) 742-1000

Orthopedic Specialty Hospital, The
TOSH - The Ortho Spec Hosp
5848 S 300 East
Salt Lake City, UT 84107
Great Plains and Mountains
(801) 269-4000

Our Lady of Lourdes Regional Medical Center -
Lafayette
Our Lady of Lordes Reg Med Ctr - Lafayette
611 ST Landry St
Lafayette, LA 70506-4697
Southwest
(337) 289-2000

Our Lady of Mercy Medical Center
Our Lady of Mercy Med Ctr
600 East 233rd Street
Bronx, NY 10466
Mid Atlantic
(718) 920-9000

Overlake Hospital Medical Center
Ovelake Hosp Med Ctr
1035 116th Ave
Bellevue, WA 98004-4687
West Coast and Pacific
(425) 688-5000

Overland Park Regional Medical Center
Overland Park Reg Med Ctr
10500 Quivira Rd
Overland Park, KS 66215
Great Plains and Mountains
(913) 541-5000

Parkland Memorial Hospital
Parkland Mem Hosp
5201 Harry Hines Boulevard
Dallas, TX 75235
Southwest
(214) 590-8000

Penn State University Hospital - Milton S.Hershey
Medical Center
Penn State Univ Hosp - Milton S Hershey Med Ctr
500 University Drive, P.O. Box 850
Hershey, PA 17033
Mid Atlantic
(717) 531-8803

Pennsylvania Hospital
Pennsylvania Hosp
800 Spruce Street
Philadelphia, PA 19107
Mid Atlantic
(215) 829-3000

Phillips Eye Institute
Phillips Eye Inst
2215 Park Ave S
Minneapolis, MN 55404
Midwest
(612) 336-6000

Piedmont Hospital
Piedmont Hosp
1968 Peachtree Road NorthWest
Atlanta, GA 30309
Southeast
(404) 605-5000

Presbyterian - St Luke's Medical Center
Presby - St Luke's Med Ctr
1719 E 19th Ave
Denver, CO 80218
Great Plains and Mountains
(303) 839-6000

Presbyterian Hospital - Albuquerque
Presbyterian Hospital - Albuquerque
1100 Central Ave SE
Albuquerque, NM 87106
Southwest
(505) 841-1234

Presbyterian Hospital of Dallas
Presby Hosp - Dallas
8200 Walnut Hill Lane
Dallas, TX 75231
Southwest
(214) 345-8400

Primary Children's Medical Center
Primary Children's Med Ctr
100 N Medical Drive
Salt Lake City, UT 84113-1100
Great Plains and Mountains
(801) 588-2000

Providence Hospital - Southfield
Providence Hosp - Southfield
16001 Nine Mile Road
Southfield, MI 48075
Midwest
(248) 424-3000

Providence Portland Medical Center
Providence Portland Med Ctr
4805 NE Glisan
Portland, OR 97213-2967
West Coast and Pacific
(503) 215-1111

Providence Saint Joseph Medical Center
Providence St Joseph Med Ctr
501 South Buena Vista St.
Burbank, CA 91505
West Coast and Pacific
(818) 843-5111

Queen's Medical Center - Honolulu
Queen's Med Ctr - Honolulu
1301 Punchbowl Street
Honolulu, HI 96813
West Coast and Pacific
(808) 547-4688

Rainbow Babies & Children's Hospital
Rainbow Babies & Chldns Hosp
11100 Euclid Ave
Cleveland, OH 44106
Midwest
(216) 844-1000

Regions Hospital - St Paul
Regions Hosp - St Paul
640 Jackson Street
St Paul, MN 55101
Midwest
(651) 221-3456

Rehabilitation Institute - Chicago
Rehab Inst - Chicago
345 E. Superior Street
Chicago, IL 60611
Midwest
(312) 238-1000

Rhode Island Hospital
Rhode Island Hosp
593 Eddy Street
Providence, RI 02903
New England
(401) 444-4000

Riley Hospital for Children
Riley Hosp for Children
702 Barnhill Drive
Indianapolis, IN 46202
Midwest
(317) 274-5000

Robert Wood Johnson University Hospital
R W Johnson Univ Hosp
One Robert Wood Johnson Place
New Brunswick, NJ 08901
Mid Atlantic
(732) 828-3000

Robert Wood Johnson University Hospital @ New Brunswick
RWJ Univ Hosp @ New Brnsw
One Robert Wood Johnson Place
New Brunswick, NJ 08903
Mid Atlantic
(732) 828-3000

Rochester General Hospital
Rochester Gen Hosp
1425 Portland Avenue
Rochester, NY 14621
Mid Atlantic
(716) 338-4000

Roswell Park Cancer Institute
Roswell Park Cancer Inst
Elm and Carlton Streets
Buffalo, NY 14263
Mid Atlantic
(716) 845-5772

Rush/Presbyterian - St Luke's Medical Center - Chicago
Affiliate, Rush/Presbyterian - St Luke's Medical Center
Rush/Presby - St Luke's Med Ctr - Chicago
1653 W Congress Parkway
Chicago, IL 60612-3833
Midwest
(312) 942-5000

Sacred Heart Hospital
Sacred Heart Hosp
3240 W Franklin Blvd
Chicago, IL 60624
Midwest
(773) 722-3020

San Francisco General Hospital
San Francisco Gen Hosp
1001 Potrero Avenue
San Francisco, CA 94110
West Coast and Pacific
(415) 206-8000

Santa Clara Valley Medical Center
Santa Clara Valley Med Ctr
751 S Bascom Avenue
San Jose, CA 95128
West Coast and Pacific
(408) 885-5000

Santa Monica - UCLA Medical Center
Santa Monica - UCLA Med Ctr
1250 16th Street
Santa Monica, CA 90404
West Coast and Pacific
(310) 319-4000

Sarasota Memorial Hospital
Sarasota Mem Hosp
1700 S Tamiami Trail
Sarasota, FL 34239
Southeast
(941) 917-9000

APPENDIX E

Schneider Children's Hospital
Schneider Children's Hosp
269-01 76th Avenue
New Hyde Park, NY 11040
Mid Atlantic
(718) 470-3000

Scripps Hospital - La Jolla
Scripps Hosp - La Jolla
9888 Genese Ave
La Jolla, CA 92037
West Coast and Pacific
(858) 626-4123

Self Memorial Hospital
Self Mem Hosp
1325 Spring St
Greenwood, SC 29646
Southeast
(864) 227-4111

Sentara Norfolk General Hospital
Sentara Norfolk Gen Hosp
600 Gresham Drive
Norfolk, VA 23507
Southeast
(757) 668-3000

Sentara Virginia Beach General Hospital
Sentara Virginia Beach Gen Hosp
1060 First Colonial Rd
Virginia Beach, VA 23454
Southeast
(757) 395-8000

Shands at Jacksonville
Shands at Jacksonville
655 W 8th St
Jacksonville, FL 32209
Southeast
(904) 244-0411

Shands at Vista
Shands at Vista
8900 NW 39th Ave
Gainesville, FL 32606
Southeast
(352) 338-0097

Shands Healthcare at University Florida
Shands at Univ FL
1600 SW Archer Road
Gainesville, FL 32610
Southeast
(352) 395-0111

Shands Jacksonville Medical Center
Shands Jacksonville Med Ctr
655 West 8th Street
Jacksonville, FL 32209
Southeast
(904) 549-5000

Sharp Memorial Hospital
Sharp Mem Hosp
7901 Frost Street
San Diego, CA 92103
West Coast and Pacific
(858) 541-3400

Sheppard Pratt Healthsystem
Sheppard Pratt Hlth Sys
6501 N Charles St
Baltimore, MD 21285-6815
Mid Atlantic
(410) 938-3000

Sinai Hospital - Baltimore
Sinai Hosp - Baltimore
2401 West Belvedere Avenue
Baltimore, MD 21215
Mid Atlantic
(410) 601-5134

Sinai-Grace Hospital - Detroit
Sinai-Grace Hosp - Detroit
6071 W. Outer Drive
Detroit, MI 48235
Midwest
(313) 966-3300

South Shore Hospital - Miami Beach
South Shore Hosp - Miami Bch
630 ALton Rd
Miami Beach, FL 33139
Southeast
(305) 672-2100

Southern New Hampshire Medical Center
Southern NH Med Ctr
8 Prospect St
Nashua, NH 03060
New England
(603) 577-2000

Southwest Texas Methodist Hospital
SW Texas Methodist Hosp
7700 Floyd Curl Drive
San Antonio, TX
Southwest

Spectrum Health East
Spectrum Health East
1840 Wealthy St SE
Grand Rapids, MI 49506
Midwest
(616) 774-7444

St. Agnes Hospital
St Agnes Hosp
305 North Street
White Plains, NY 10605
Mid Atlantic
(914) 681-4500

St. Alphonsus Regional Medical Center
St Alphonsus Reg Med Ctr
1055 N Curtis Rd
Boise, ID 83706-1370
Great Plains and Mountains
(208) 367-2121

St. Anne's Hospital
St Anne's Hosp
795 Middle Street
Fall River, MA 02721
New England
(508) 674-5741

St. Barnabas Medical Center
St Barnabas Med Ctr
94 Old Short Hills Road
Livingston, NJ 07039-5672
Mid Atlantic
(973) 533-5000

St. Christopher's Hospital for Children
St Christopher's Hosp for Children
Erie Avenue at Front Street
Philadelphia, PA 19134
Mid Atlantic
(215) 427-5337

St. Elizabeth's Medical Center
St Elizabeth's Med Ctr
736 Cambridge Street
Brighton, MA 02135
New England
(617) 789-3000

St. Francis Hospital
St Francis Hosp
100 Port Washington Boulevard
Roslyn, NY 11576
Mid Atlantic
(516) 562-6000

APPENDIX E

St. Francis Hospital & Medical Center
St Francis Hosp & Med Ctr
114 Woodland Street
Hartford, CT 06105
New England
(860) 714-4000

St. Francis Medical Center of Santa Barbara
St Francis Med Ctr of Santa Barbara
601 E. Micheltorena St
Santa Barbara, CA 93103
West Coast and Pacific
(805) 962-7661

St. Francis Memorial Hospital
St Francis Memorial Hosp
900 Hyde Street
San Francisco, CA 94109
West Coast and Pacific
(415) 353-6000

St. John Hospital and Medical Center
St John Hosp and Med Ctr
22101 Moross Road
Detroit, MI 48236-2172
Midwest
(313) 343-4000

St. John's Health Center
St John's Hlth Ctr
1328 22nd St
Santa Monica, CA 90404
West Coast and Pacific
(310) 829-5511

St. John's Mercy Medical Center - St Louis
St John's Mercy Med Ctr - St Louis
615 South New Ballas Road
St Louis, MO 63141
Midwest
(314) 569-6908

St. John's Regional Medical Center
St John's Regional Med Ctr
1600 N Rose Ave
Oxnard, CA 93030
West Coast and Pacific
(805) 988-2500

St. Joseph's Hospital & Medical Center - Phoenix
St Joseph's Hosp & Med Ctr - Phoenix
350 West Thomas Road
Phoenix, AZ 85013-4496
Southwest
(602) 406-3000

St. Joseph's Hospital - Atlanta
St Joseph's Hosp - Atlanta
5665 Peachtree Dunwoody Road NorthEast
Atlanta, GA 30342
Southeast
(404) 851-7001

St. Joseph's Hospital - Chicago
St Joseph's Hosp - Chicago
2900 N Lake Shore Dr
Chicago, IL 60657
Midwest
(773) 665-3000

St. Joseph's Hospital - Orange
St Joseph's Hosp - Orange
1100 West Stewart Drive
Orange, CA 92868
West Coast and Pacific
(714) 633-9111

St. Joseph's Hospital - Tampa
St Joseph's Hosp - Tampa
3001 W Martin Luther King Jr Blvd
Tampa, FL 33607
Southeast
(813) 870-4000

St. Joseph's Mercy - Oakland
St Joseph Mercy - Oakland
Oakland, MI
Midwest

St. Jude Children's Research Hospital
St Jude Children's Research Hosp
332 N Lauderdale St
Memphis, TN 38105
Southeast
(901) 495-3300

St. Louis Children's Hospital
St Louis Children's Hospital
One Children's Place
St Louis, MO 63110
Midwest
(314) 454-6000

St. Louis University Hospital
St Louis Univ Hospital
3635 Vista at Grand Blvd
St. Louis, MO 63110
Midwest
(314) 577-8000

**St Luke's - Roosevelt Hospital Center -
Roosevelt Division
Affiliate, Continuum Health Partners
St Luke's - Roosevelt Hosp Ctr - Roosevelt Div
1000 Tenth Avenue
New York, NY 10019
Mid Atlantic
(212) 523-4000**

**St Luke's Episcopal Hospital - Houston
St Luke's Episcopal Hosp - Houston
6720 Bertner Avenue
Houston, TX 77030
Southwest
(713) 791-3006**

St Luke's Hospital
St Luke's Hosp
4401 Wornhall Road
Kansas City, MO 64111
Midwest
(816) 932-2000

St. Lukes Hospital
St Lukes Hosp
232 S Woods Mill Rd
Chesterfield, MO 63017
Midwest
(314) 434-1500

St. Mary's Health Center - St Louis
St Mary's Hlth Ctr - St Louis
6420 Clayton Road
St. Louis, MO 63117
Midwest
(314) 768-8000

St. Mary's Hospital
St Mary's Hosp
2900 1st Ave
Huntington, WV 25702-1272
Mid Atlantic
(304) 526-1234

St. Mary's Hospital
St Mary's Hosp
1216 Second Street, S.W.
Rochester, MN 55902
Midwest
(507) 255-4400

St. Mary's Medical Center
St Mary's Med Ctr
1050 Linden Avenue
Long Beach, CA 90813
West Coast and Pacific
(562) 491-9000

St. Mary's Medical Center - Duluth
St Mary's Med Ctr - Duluth
407 E 3rd St
Duluth, MN 55805-1984
Midwest
(218) 726-4000

St. Mary's Medical Center - West Palm Beach
St Mary's Med Ctr - W Palm Bch
901 45th St
West Palm Beach, FL 33407
Southeast
(561) 844-6300

St. Mary's Mercy Medical Center
St. Mary's Mercy Med Ctr
200 Jefferson Ave,S.E.
Grand Rapids, MI 49503
Midwest
(616) 752-6090

St. Michael's Medical Center
St Michael's Med Ctr
268 Dr. Martin Luther King, Jr. Boulevard
Newark, NJ 07102
Mid Atlantic
(973) 877-5000

St. Paul Medical Center
St Paul Medical Ctr
5909 Harry Hines Boulevard
Dallas, TX 75235
Southwest
(214) 879-1000

St. Thomas Hospital - Nashville
St Thomas Hosp - Nashville
4220 Harding Road
Nashville, TN 37205
Southeast
(615) 222-2111

St. Vincent's Hospital - Carmel
St Vincent's Hosp - Carmel
13500 N Meridian Street
Carmel, IN 46032-1496
Midwest
(317) 573-7000

St. Vincent's Hospital and Health Center - Indianapolis
St Vincent's Hosp and Hlth Ctr - Indianapolis
2001 West 86th Street
Indianapolis, IN 46260-1991
Midwest
(317) 338-7000

St. Vincent's Medical Center - Jacksonville
St Vincent's Med Ctr - Jacksonville
1800 Barrs Street
Jacksonville, FL 32214
Southeast
(904) 308-7300

St. Vincent's Medical Center - Los Angeles
St Vincent's Med Ctr - Los Angeles
2131 West Third Street
Los Angeles, CA 90057
West Coast and Pacific
(213) 484-7111

Saint Vincents Catholic Medical Center of New York
St Vincents Cath Med Ctr of New York
170 West 12th Street
New York, NY 10011
Mid Atlantic
(212) 604-7000

Saint Vincents Hospital & Med Center of N.Y.- Westchester Branch
St Vincents Hosp & Med Ctr of N.Y.-Westchester
275 North Street
Harrison, NY 10528
Mid Atlantic
(914) 967-6500

Stamford Hospital
Affiliate, NewYork-Presbyterian Health System
Stamford Hosp
Shelburn Road @ W Broad St
Stamford, CT 06902
New England
(203) 325-7000

Stanford Medical Center
Stanford Med Ctr
300 Pasteur Drive
Stanford, CA 94305
West Coast and Pacific
(650) 723-4000

Staten Island University Hospital - North
Staten Island Univ Hosp-North
475 Seaview Avenue
Staten Island, NY 10305
Mid Atlantic
(718) 226-9000

Staten Island University Hospital - South
Staten Island Univ Hosp - South
375 Seguine Avenue
Staten Island, NY 10309
Mid Atlantic
(718) 226-2000

Strong Memorial Hospital - Medical Center
Strong Memorial Hosp - URMC
601 Elmwood Avenue
Rochester, NY 14642
Mid Atlantic
(716) 275-7685

Suburban Hospital Healthcare Systems
Suburban Hosp - Bethesda
8600 Old Georgetown Road
Bethesda, MD 20814
Mid Atlantic
(301) 896-3100

Sunnyview Hospital and Rehabilitation Center
Sunnyview Hosp
1270 Belmont Ave
Schenectady, NY 12308-2198
Mid Atlantic
(518) 382-4500

Sunrise Hospital & Medical Center
Sunrise Hosp & Med Ctr
3186 Maryland Pkwy
Las Vegas, NV 89109-2306
West Coast and Pacific
(702) 731-8000

Swedish Covenant Hospital
Swedish Covenant Hosp
5145 N California Ave
Chicago, IL 60625
Midwest
(773) 878-8200

Swedish Medical Center
Swedish Med Ctr
747 Broadway
Seattle, WA 98122
West Coast and Pacific
(206) 386-6000

Swedish Medical Center - Englewood
Swedish Med Ctr - Englewood
501 E Hampden Ave
Englewood, CO 80110-2795
Great Plains and Mountains
(303) 788-5000

Swedish Medical Center Providence Campus
Swedish Med Ctr Providence Campus
500 17th Ave
Seattle, WA 98122
West Coast and Pacific
(206) 320-2000

APPENDIX E

Tampa General Hospital
Tampa Genl Hosp
PO BOX 1289
Tampa, FL 33601
Southeast
(813) 251-7000

Temple University Hospital
Temple Univ Hosp
3401 N Broad St
Philadelphia, PA 19140-5189
Mid Atlantic
(215) 707-2000

Texas Children's Hospital - Houston
TX Chldns Hosp - Houston
6621 Fannin
Houston, TX 77030
Southwest
(832) 824-1000

Texas Scottish Rite Hospital for Children - Dallas
Texas Scottish Rite Hosp for Children - Dallas
2222 Welborn
Dallas, TX 75219
Southwest
(214) 521-3168

The Children's Hospital - Denver
The Chldn's Hosp - Denver
1056 east 19th Ave
Denver, CO 80218
Great Plains and Mountains
(303) 861-8888

The Children's Hospital of Buffalo
The Chldn's Hosp of Buffalo
219 Bryant St.
Buffalo, NY 14222
Mid Atlantic
(716) 878-7000

The Children's Hospital of Philadelphia
The Chldn's Hosp of Philadelphia
34th and Civic Center Boulevard
Philadelphia, PA 19104
Mid Atlantic
(215) 590-1000

The Parkinson's Institute/Movement Disorders
Treament Center
Parkinson's Inst/Movement Disorders Treatmt Ctr
1170 Morse Ave
Sunnyvale, CA 94089-1605
West Coast and Pacific
(408) 734-2800

The Valley Hospital
Affiliate, NewYork-Presbyterian Health System
The Valley Hosp
223 North Van Dien Avenue
Ridgewood, NJ 07450
Mid Atlantic
(201) 447-8000

The Woman's Hospital of Texas
The Woman's Hosp TX
7600 Fannin St
Houston, TX 77054
Southwest
(713) 790-1234

Thomas Jefferson University Hospital
Thomas Jefferson Univ Hosp
111 S 11th St
Philadelphia, PA 19107
Mid Atlantic
(215) 955-6000

TIRR LifeBridge Hospital
TIRR Lifebridge
1333 Moursund 3rd FL Clinic Bldg
Houston, TX 77030
Southwest
(713) 799-6969

Toledo Hospital
Toledo Hosp
2142 North Cove Boulevard
Toledo, OH 43606
Midwest
(419) 471-4000

Touro Infirmary
Tourp Infirmary
1401 Foucher Street
New Orleans, LA 70115
Southwest
(504) 897-8246

Truman Medical Center
Truman Med Ctr
2301 Holmes Street
Kansas City, MO 64108
Midwest
(816) 556-3153

Tulane University Medical Center Hospital & Clinic
Tulane Univ MEd Ctr Hosp & Clinic
1415 Tulane Avenue
New Orleans, LA 70112
Southwest
(504) 588-5263

UCLA Medical Center
UCLA Med Ctr
10833 Le Conte Avenue
Los Angeles, CA 90095
West Coast and Pacific
(310) 825-9111

UCLA Neuropsychiatric Hospital
UCLA Neuropsychiatric Hosp
760 Westwood Plaza
Los Angeles, CA 90024
West Coast and Pacific
(310) 825-9989

UCLA-Sepulveda VA Greater LA Health Care System
UCLA-Sepulveda VA Grtr LA Hlth Care Sys
16111 Plummer St
North Hills, CA 91343
West Coast and Pacific
(818) 891-7711

UCSF - Mount Zion Medical Center
UCSF - Mount Zion Med Ctr
1600 Divisadero Street
San Francisco, CA 94115
West Coast and Pacific
(415) 567-6600

UMASS Memorial Health Care - Worcester
UMASS Memorial Hlth Care - Worcester
55 Lake Avenue North
Worcester, MA 01655-0002
New England
(508) 856-0011

UMDNJ-University Hospital-Newark
UMDNJ-Univ Hosp-Newark
150 Bergen Street
Newark, NJ 07103-2406
Mid Atlantic
(973) 972-6273

Union Memorial Hospital - Baltimore
Union Memorial Hosp - Baltimore
201 E University Pkwy
Baltimore, MD 21218
Mid Atlantic
(410) 554-2000

University Community Hospital
University Comm Hosp
3100 E Fletcher Avenue
Tampa, FL 33613
Southeast
(813) 971-6000

APPENDIX E

University Community Hospital of Carrollwood
University Comm Hosp of Carrollwood
7171 N Dale Mabry
Tampa, FL 33614
Southeast
(813) 932-2222

University Health System
Univ Hlth Sys - San Antonio
4502 Medical Drive
San Antonio, TX 78229
Southwest
(210) 358-4000

University Hospital
Univesity Hosp - OK
1200 Everett Drive
Oklahoma City, OK 73104
Southwest
(405) 271-5911

University Hospital
Univ Hosp-San Antonio
4502 Medical Drive
San Antonio, TX 78229
Southwest
(210) 358-4000

University Hospital & Clinics- Mississippi
Univ Hosps & Clins - Mississippi
2500 North State Street
Jackson, MS 39216
Southeast
(601) 984-1000

University Hospital & Medical Center at Stony Brook
Univ Hosp & Med Ctr @ Stony Brook
Nicolls Road
Stony Brook, NY 11794
Mid Atlantic
(631) 689-8333

University Hospital - Brooklyn
Univ Hosp - Brklyn
450 Clarkson Ave
Brooklyn, NY 11203
Mid Atlantic
(718) 270-1000

University Hospital - Charlotte
Unv Hosp- Charlotte, NC
8800 N Tryon St
Charlotte, NC 28262-8415
Southeast
(704) 548-6000

University Hospital - Cincinnati
Univ Hosp - Cincinnati
234 Goodman Street
Cincinnati, OH 45219
Midwest
(513) 584-1000

University Hospital - Cleveland
Univ Hosp of Cleveland
11100 Euclid Ave
Cleveland, OH 44106
Midwest
(216) 844-1000

University Hospital - SUNY Upstate Medical University
Univ. Hosp.- SUNY Upstate Med. Univ.
750 E Adams Street
Syracuse, NY 13210
Mid Atlantic
(315) 464-5540

University Hospital, Hahnemann
Univ Hosp, Hahnemann
Broad and Vine Streets-MS #300
Philadelphia, PA 19102
Mid Atlantic
(215) 762-7000

University Medical Center
Univ Med Ctr
1501 N. Campbell Ave
Tucson, AZ 85724-5018
Southwest
(520) 694-0111

University Medical Center
Univ Med Ctr-Las Vegas
1800 W Charleston Blvd
Las Vegas, NV 89102
West Coast and Pacific
(702) 383-2000

University Medical Center
Univ Med Ctr
602 Indiana Ave, Box 5980
Lubbock, TX 79410
Southwest
(806) 743-3111

University Medical Center - Fresno
Univ Med Ctr - Fresno
445 South Cedar Avenue
Fresno, CA 93702
West Coast and Pacific
(559) 459-4000

University of Alabama Hospital at Birmingham
Univ of Ala Hosp at Birmingham
619 South 19th Street
Birmingham, AL 35249-6544
Southeast
(205) 934-4011

University of Arkansas for Medical Sciences
UAMS
4301 W Markham St
Little Rock, AR 72205
Southwest
(501) 686-7000

University of California - Davis Medical Center
Univ CA - Davis Med Ctr
2315 Stockton Boulevard
Sacramento, CA 95817
West Coast and Pacific
(916) 734-3096

University of California - Irvine Medical Center
UCI Med Ctr
101 The City Drive
Orange, CA 92868
West Coast and Pacific
(714) 456-6011

University of California - San Diego Healthcare
UCSD Healthcare
200 West Arbor Drive
San Diego, CA 92103
West Coast and Pacific
(619) 543-6222

University of California - San Francisco Medical Center
UCSF Med Ctr
505 Parnassus Avenue
San Francisco, CA 94143
West Coast and Pacific
(415) 476-1000

**University of Chicago Hospitals
Affiliate, University of Chicago Hospitals and
Health System**
Univ Chicago Hospitals
**5841 S Maryland Avenue
Chicago, IL 60637
Midwest
(773) 702-1000**

University of Colorado Health & Science Center
Univ Colo HSC - Denver
4200 E. 9th Avenue
Denver, CO 80262
Great Plains and Mountains
(303) 499-5900

APPENDIX E

University of Connecticut Health Center
Univ Conn Hlth Ctr
263 Farmington Ave
Farmington, CT 06030
New England
(860) 679-2100

University of Illinois at Chicago Eye and Ear Infirmary
Univ of IL at Chicago Eye and Ear Infi
1855 W Taylor St
Chicago, IL 60612
Midwest
(312) 996-6500

University of Illinois at Chicago Medical Center
Univ of IL at Chicago Med Ctr
1740 W Taylor St.
Chicago, IL 60612
Midwest
(312) 996-7000

University of Iowa Hospitals and Clinics
Univ of IA Hosp and Clinics
200 Hawkins Drive
Iowa City , IA 52242
Midwest
(319) 356-3155

University of Kansas Medical Center
Univ Kansas Med Ctr
3901 Rainbow Boulevard
Kansas City, KS 66160
Great Plains and Mountains
(913) 588-5000

University of Kentucky Medical Center
Univ Kentucky Med Ctr
800 Rose Street
Lexington, KY 40536
Southeast
(859) 323-5000

University of Louisville Hospital
Univ Louisville Hosp
530 S. Jackson Street
Louisville, KY 40202
Southeast
(502) 562-3000

University of Maryland Medical System
University of MD Med Sys
22 S Greene St
Baltimore, MD 21201
Mid Atlantic
(410) 328-8667

University of Miami - Jackson Memorial Hospital
Univ of Miami - Jackson Meml Hosp
1611 NW 12th Ave
Miami, FL 33136
Southeast
(305) 585-1111

University of Miami Hosp & Clinics/Sylvestor Comp Cancer Cntr
Univ of Miami & Clinics/Sylvestor Comp Cancer Ctr
1475 NW 12th Ave
Miami, FL 33136
Southeast
(305) 243-6418

University of Michigan Health Center
Univ of MI Hlth Ctr
1500 E. Medical Center Drive
Ann Arbor, MI 48109
Midwest
(734) 936-4000

University of Missouri Hospitals & Clinics
Univ of Missouri Hosp & Clinics
One Hospital Drive
Columbia, MO 65212
Midwest
(573) 882-4141

University of Nebraska Medical Center
University of NE Med Ctr
980159 Univ of Nebraska Med Ctr
Omaha, NE 68106-0159
Great Plains and Mountains
(402) 559-4000

University of New Mexico Hospital
Univ NM Hosp
2211 Lomas Boulevard, N.E.
Albuquerque, NM 87106
Southwest
(505) 272-2111

University of North Carolina Hospitals
Univ of NC Hosp
101 Manning Drive, Box 7600
Chapel Hill, NC 27514-4335
Southeast
(919) 966-4131

University of Oklahoma Health Science Center
Univ OK Hlth Sci Ctr
1100 N Lindsay
Oklahoma City, OK 73104
Southwest
(405) 271-4000

University of Pennsylvania - Presbyterian Medical Center
Univ Penn - Presby Med Ctr
51 N 39th St
Philadelphia, PA 19104
Mid Atlantic
(215) 662-8000

University of South Alabama Medical Center
Univ of S Ala Med Ctr
2451 Fillingim Street
Mobile, AL 36617
Southeast
(334) 471-7000

University of Tennessee Bowld Hospital
Univ of Tenn Bowld Hosp
951 Court Ave
Memphis, TN 38103
Southeast
(901) 448-4000

University of Texas Health & Science Center
Univ of Texas Hlth & Sci Ctr
7703 Floyd Curl Drive
San Antonio, TX 78229
Southwest
(210) 567-7000

University of Texas MD Anderson Cancer Center
Univ of TX MD Anderson Cancer Ctr
1515 Holcombe Boulevard
Houston, TX 77030
Southwest
(713) 792-2121

University of Texas Medical Branch Hospitals at Galveston
Univ of TX Med Brch Hosps at Galveston
301 University Boulevard
Galveston, TX 77555
Southwest
(409) 772-1011

University of Utah Hospital and Clinics
Univ Utah Hosp and Clin
50 N Medical Dr
Salt Lake City, UT 84132-0001
Great Plains and Mountains
(801) 581-2121

University of Virginia Health Systems
Univ VA Hlth Sci Ctr
1215 Lee Street
Charlottesville, VA 22908-0001
Southeast
(804) 924-0211

University of Washington Medical Center
Univ WA Med Ctr
1959 NE Pacific Street, RC-35
Seattle, WA 98195
West Coast and Pacific
(206) 598-3300

University of Wisconsin Hospital & Clinics
Univ WI Hosp & Clins
600 Highland Avenue
Madison, WI 53792
Midwest
(608) 263-6400

UPMC - Presbyterian University Hospital
UPMC - Presbyterian Univ Hosp
200 Lothrop Street
Pittsburgh, PA 15213
Mid Atlantic
(412) 647-7808

Upstate University Medical Hospital
Upstate Univ Med Hosp
750 E Adams St
Syracuse, NY 13210-2306
Mid Atlantic
(315) 464-5540

USC Norris Cancer Comprehensive Center
USC Norris Cancer Comp Ctr
1441 Eastlake Avenue
Los Angeles, CA 90033
West Coast and Pacific
(323) 865-3000

USC University Hospital - Richard K. Eamer Medical Plaza
USC Univ Hosp - R K Eamer Med Plz
1500 San Pablo
Los Angeles, CA 90033
West Coast and Pacific
(323) 442-8444

VA Medical Affairs - San Diego HealthCare Center
VA Med Aff - San Diego HlthCare Ctr
3350 La Jolla Village Drive
San Diego, CA 92161
West Coast and Pacific
(858) 552-8585

VA Medical Center - Dallas
VA Med Ctr - Dallas
4500 South Lancaster Road
Dallas, TX 75216
Southwest
(214) 742-8387

VA Medical Center - Palo Alto
VA Med Ctr - Palo Alto
3801 Miranda Avenue
Palo Alto, CA 94304
West Coast and Pacific
(650) 493-5000

VA Medical Center - San Francisco
VA Med Ctr - San Francisco
4150 Clement Street
San Francisco, CA 94121
West Coast and Pacific
(415) 750-2041

VA Medical Center - West Los Angeles
VA Med Ctr - West LA
11301 Wilshire Boulevard
Los Angeles, CA 90073
West Coast and Pacific
(310) 478-3711

VA Pittsburgh Health Care System
VA Pittsburgh Hlth Care Sys
University Drive
Pittsburgh, PA 15240
Mid Atlantic
(412) 784-3900

Valley Children's Hospital
Valley Chldns Hosp
9300 Valley Children's Pl
Madera, CA 93638
West Coast and Pacific
(559) 353-3000

Vanderbilt University Medical Center
Vanderbilt Univ Med Ctr
University Hospital 1161 21st Ave. South
Nashville, TN 37232
Southeast
(615) 322-5000

Ventura County Medical Center
Ventura County Med Ctr
3291 Loma Vista Road
Ventura, CA 93003
West Coast and Pacific
(805) 652-6000

Veterans Affairs Medical Center - Indianapolis
VA Med Ctr - Indianapolis
1481 W 10th St
Indianapolis, IN 46202
Midwest
(317) 554-0000

Veterans Affairs Medical Center - Oklahoma City
VA Med Ctr - Oklahoma City
921 NE 13th St
Oklahoma City, OK 73104
Southwest
(405) 270-5133

Veterans Affairs Medical Center - Washington
VA Medical Center - Washington
50 Irving Street, N.W.
Washington, DC 20422
Mid Atlantic
(202) 745-8100

Via Health System-Genesee Hospital
Via Hlth Sys-Genesee Hosp
224 Alexander Street
Rochester, NY 14607
Mid Atlantic
(716) 922-6000

Virginia Beach General Hospital
Virginia Beach Gen Hosp
1060 First Colonial Rd
Virginia Beach, VA 23454
Southeast
(757) 395-8000

Virginia Mason Medical Center
Virginia Mason Med Ctr
925 Seneca Street/PO Box 900
Seattle, WA 98111
West Coast and Pacific
(206) 223-6600

Wake Forest University Baptist Medical Center
Wake Forest Univ Baptist Med Ctr
Medical Center Blvd
Winston-Salem, NC 27157-0001
Southeast
(336) 716-2011

WakeMed New Bern Avenue Campus
WakeMed New Bern
3000 New Bern Ave
Raleigh, NC 27610
Southeast
(919) 350-8000

Washington Hospital
Washington Hosp
155 Wilson Avenue
Washington, PA 15301
Mid Atlantic
(724) 225-7000

Washington Hospital Center - DC
Washington Hosp Ctr - DC
110 Irving Street NorthWest
Washington, DC 20010
Mid Atlantic
(202) 877-7000

Wesley Woods Geriatric Hospital
Wesley Woods Ger Hosp
1821 Clifton Road
Atlanta, GA 30329
Southeast
(404) 728-6200

West Hills Medical Center
West Hills Med Ctr
7300 Medical Center drive
West Hills, CA 91307
West Coast and Pacific
(818) 676-4100

West Jefferson Medical Center
West Jefferson Med Ctr
1101 Medical Ctr Blvd
Marrero, LA 70072
Southwest
(504) 347-5511

West Virginia University Hospital - Ruby Memorial
WV Univ Hosp - Ruby Memorial
1 Medical Center Drive
Morgantown, WV 26506
Mid Atlantic
(304) 598-4200

Westchester Medical Center
Westchester Med Ctr
95 Grasslands Road
Valhalla, NY 10595
Mid Atlantic
(914) 493-7000

Western Psychiatric Institute & Clinic
Western Psy Inst & Clin
3811 O'Hara St
Pittsburgh, PA 15213-2593
Mid Atlantic
(412) 624-2100

Western Wake Medical Center
Western Wake Med Ctr
1900 Kildaire Farm Rd
Cary , NC 27511-6616
Southeast
(919) 233-2300

Wilford Hall Medical Center
Wilford Hall Medical Ctr
2200 Bergquist
Lackland AFB, TX 78236
Southwest
(210) 292-7412

William Beaumont Hospital
William Beaumont Hosp
3601 West 13 Mile Road
Royal Oak, MI 48073
Midwest
(248) 551-5000

William S Hall Psychiatric Institute
William S Hall Psyc Inst
1800 Colonial Drive, PO Box 202
Columbia, SC 29202-6827
Southeast
(803) 898-1693

Wills Eye Hospital
Wills Eye Hosp
900 Walnut Street
Philadelphia, PA 19107-5598
Mid Atlantic
(215) 928-3000

Winter Park Memorial Hospital
Winter Park Memorial Hosp
200 North Lakemont Avenue
Winter Park, FL 32792
Southeast
(407) 646-7000

Winthrop - University Hospital
Winthrop - Univ Hosp
259 First Street
Mineola, NY 11501
Mid Atlantic
(516) 663-0333

Wolfson Children's Hospital @ Baptist Medical
Center
Wolfson Children's Hosp @ Baptist Med Cen
800 Prudential Drive
Jacksonville, FL 32207
Southeast
(904) 393-2000

Women & Infants Hospital - Rhode Island
Women & Infants Hosp - Rhode Island
101 Dudley Street
Providence, RI 02905
New England
(401) 274-1100

Yale - New Haven Hospital
Yale - New Haven Hosp
20 York Street
New Haven, CT 06512
New England
(203) 688-4242

Zale Lipshy University Hospital
Zale Lipshy Univ Hosp
5151 Harry Hines Boulevard
Dallas, TX 75235
Southwest
(214) 590-3101

APPENDIX F

PATIENT RIGHTS

YOUR RIGHTS IN THE HOSPITAL

The following bill of rights is one that has been adopted by the American Hospital Association (AHA) and is in use in many hospitals throughout the nation.

The patient has the right to:

■ *Considerate and respectful care.*

■ *Complete information about his/her treatment and condition in terms the patient can reasonably understand.*

■ *Know the identity of physicians, nurses, and others involved in their care, as well as when those involved are students, residents, or other trainees.*

■ *Information necessary to give informed consent prior to the start of any procedure or treatment.*

■ *Refuse treatment and be informed of the consequences.*

■ *Have an advance directive (such as a living will, health care proxy, or durable power of attorney) for health care.*

■ *Privacy concerning his/her treatment.*

■ *Have all records and communications regarding medical treatment kept confidential.*

■ *Expect the hospital, within the limits of its capabilities, to respond to a request for services.*

■ *Obtain information regarding the relationship of the hospital to any other health care institutions.*

■ *Be advised if the hospital proposes human experimentation which affects his/her care.*

APPENDIX F

- *Reasonable continuity of care.*

- *An explanation of the bill, regardless of payment source.*

- *Know what hospital rules and regulations apply to patient contact.*

(Source: American Hospital Association, Chicago, IL)

According to the American Hospital Association, this was last edited in 1992, so this version should be up-to-date. However, the AHA now has a "Fax on Demand" service at (312) 422-2020 through which consumers can obtain an up-to-date copy, free of charge, by sending their name, fax# and specifying document # 471124.

APPENDIX G

RESOURCES

American Ambulance Association (AAA)
1255 Twenty-Third Street, NW, Suite 200
Washington, DC 20037-1174
202-452-8888
fax 202-452-0005
http://www.the-aaa.org/
The American Ambulance Association represents emergency and non-emergency medical transportation providers, advocating high quality pre-hospital care and keeping these providers aware of legislation and news that may affect them.

American Association of Health Plans (AAHP)
1129 20th Street, NW, Suite 600
Washington, DC 20036-3421
202-778-3200
http://www.aahp.org/
The American Association of Health Plans is the national trade association that speaks on behalf of over 1,000 health plans regarding regulatory and legislative issues.

American Board of Medical Specialties (ABMS)
1007 Church Street, Suite 404
Evanston, Illinois 60201-5913
847-481-9091
fax 847-328-3596
http://www.abms.org
The ABMS is the authoritative body for the recognition of medical specialties, coordinating 24 medical specialty boards (including 25 medical specialties) and providing information on the board certification of doctors.

American Hospital Association (AHA)
800-424-4301
http://www.aha.org/
A national health advocacy organization, the AHA represents hospitals and health-care networks in legislative and regulatory matters. In 1973 the AHA adopted the Patient Bill of Rights to help patients understand their rights and responsibilities.

American Medical Association (AMA)
515 North State Street
Chicago, IL 60610
312-464-5000
http://www.ama-assn.org/
The AMA is an association that maintains information on physicians practicing throughout the nation. Healthcare consumers can use their database to check the location, licensing, education and specialty of many doctors in the United States.

Center for Medical Consumers
130 Macdougal Street
New York, NY 10012
212-674-7105
fax 212-674-7100
http://medicalconsumers.org
Provides volume and outcome data on certain medical procedures performed in New York state.

Centers for Disease Control and Prevention (CDC)
1-800-311-3435
http://www.cdc.gov/netinfo.htm
Part of the Department of Health and Human Services, the CDC's mission is to prevent and manage diseases and illnesses. Its Web site contains information on a range of illnesses and the research being pursued to manage them.

The CenterWatch Clinical Trials Listing Service
22 Thomson Place, 36T1
Boston, MA 02210-1212
617-856-5900
fax 617-856-5901
http://www.centerwatch.com
Profiles centers conducting clinical research by therapeutic area and geographic region, including more than 41,000 international industry and government-sponsored clinical trials and new FDA approved drug therapies, as well as 5,200 clinical trials that are actively recruiting patients.

Health Care Choices
P.O. Box 21039
Columbus Circle Station
New York, NY 10023
http://www.healthcarechoices.org
Provides information on volume and outcomes of certain medical procedures performed in hospitals in various states throughout the country.

Medline
One Medline Place
Mundelein, Illinois 60060
1-800-MEDLINE
fax 1-800-351-1512
http://www.medline.com
A medical database including millions of medical references and abstracts from thousands of scientific and medical journals.

The National Cancer Institute (NCI)
Clinical Studies Support Center (CSSC)
6116 Executive Boulevard
Bethesda, MD 20892-8329
800-4-CANCER (800-422-6237)
http://www.nci.nih.gov
Part of the NIH, the NCI sponsors cancer clinical trials at more than 100 sites in the United States. Trials are carried out in major medical research centers, such as teaching hospitals, as well as in community hospitals, specialized medical clinics and even in doctors' offices.

The National Institutes of Health (NIH)
Patient Recruitment Referral Center
10 Cloister Court
Bethesda, MD 20892-4754
800-411-1222
http://www.nih.gov
http://www.clinicaltrials.gov
An organization operated by the U.S. government, the NIH operates its own hospital at which the care provided is usually related to clinical studies its researchers are undertaking. Information about the Warren G. Magnuson Clinical Center is also available.

APPENDIX G

The Patient Advocate Foundation
753 Thimble Shoals Boulevard, Suite B
Newport News, VA 23606
800-532-5274
http://www.patientadvocate.org/
A national non-profit organization that provides consultation, referrals and case management to patients to ensure that they are not denied access to healthcare, insurance coverage, employment and public assistance programs during an illness. In particular, the organization maintains comprehensive information on cancer treatment options that are available to consumers through a separate Web site: http://www.oncology.com.

People's Medical Society
462 Walnut Street
Allentown, PA 18102
610-770-1670
fax:610-770-0607
http://www.peoplesmed.org/index.html
The People's Medical Society, a nonprofit organization, is focused on educating the healthcare consumer about healthcare issues and medical rights. Their Web site provides information on useful books and publications as well as the latest healthcare developments.

Persons United Limiting Substandards and Errors in Healthcare (P.U.L.S.E.)
PO Box 353
Wanatgh NY 11793 - 0353
www.PULSEofNY.com
A support group for the survivors of medical malpractice and substandard healthcare, this nonprofit group also advocates patient education and patient-doctor communication.

Physicians Who Care
10615 Perrin Beitel, Suite 201
San Antonio, Texas 78217
http://www.pwc.org/
Physicians Who Care is a non-profit organization devoted to the doctor-patient relationship and maintaining high standards in healthcare.

Public Citizen's Health and Research Group

1600 20th Street NW
Washington, D.C. 20009
202-588-1000
http://www.citizen.org/hrg/
A non-profit organization, the Public Citizen's Group acts as a watchdog agency by
advocating accountability and the open use of doctors' disciplinary backgrounds.

Veritas Medicine
238 Main Street Suite 501
Cambridge, Massachusetts 02142
617-234-1500
fax 617-234-1555
www.veritasmedicine.com
An organization that allows individuals to perform confidential, personalized searches
of their clinical trials database and to access information on new treatment and drug
options. The text is submitted by Harvard-affiliated doctors.

INDICES

SUBJECT INDEX

SPECIAL EXPERTISE INDEX

Interchangeable Terms and Cross References
The following are terms that you may find helpful. These are medical synonyms or cross references that often are used interchangeably. While this list is not all-inclusive, it is offered to assist you both in understanding your medical records and in discussions you may have with your doctors.

If you are unable to find the term you are seeking in the **Special Expertise Index** that follows, we suggest looking under the synonym or cross reference for the term since it is likely that you will find what you need there.

Since this list contains only those terms that relate to the special expertise of doctors in this Guide, you may wish to consult a medical dictionary either in print format or online for other terms.

ACOUSTIC NEUROMA . . . . ACOUSTIC NERVE TUMORS
AMYOTROPHIC LATERAL SCLEROSIS (ALS) . . LOU GEHRIG'S DISEASE
ANXIETY DISORDERS . . . . MOOD DISORDERS, DEPRESSION
AORTIC VALVE DISEASE . . . . HEART VALVE DISEASE
CARDIAC . . . . HEART
CIRRHOSIS . . . . LIVER DISEASE
CROHN'S DISEASE . . . . INFLAMMATORY BOWEL DISEASE
DIPLOPIA . . . . DOUBLE VISION
EPILEPSY . . . . SEIZURE DISORDERS
ERECTILE DYSFUNCTION . . . . IMPOTENCE
HEMATOLOGY . . . . BLOOD DISORDERS
HEPATIC DISEASE . . . . LIVER DISEASE
HEPATIC . . . . LIVER
KNEE/SHOULDER SURGERY . . . . SHOULDER/KNEE SURGERY
MITRAL VALVE DISEASE . . . . HEART VALVE DISEASE
MOHS' SURGERY . . . . MELANOMA / SKIN CANCER
NEPHROLOGY . . . . KIDNEY
OCULAR . . . . EYE
ONCOLOGY . . . . SOLIID TUMORS
OPHTHALMIC . . . . EYE
PARKINSON'S DISEASE . . . . MOVEMENT DISORDERS
PEPTIC . . . . GASTRIC
PULMONARY . . . . LUNG
REFLEX SYMPATHETIC DYSTROPHY (RSD) . . . SHOULDER-HANDSYNDROME
RENAL . . . . KIDNEY
STRABISMUS . . . . SQUINT, LAZY EYE

SPECIAL EXPERTISE INDEX

Some Common Medical Abbreviations and Acronyms

Following is a list of some commonly used medical abbreviations or acronyms that healthcare professionals frequently use as a "shorthand" way to record information. These sometimes make a medical record difficult for a non-professional to understand. Therefore, we are providing their complete meaning.

Abbreviation . . Medical Term
Acronym

Abbreviation/Acronym	Medical Term
ACL	Anterior Cruciate Ligament
ADD	Attention Deficit Disorder
ADHD	Attention Deficit Hyperactivity Disorder
AIDS	Acquired ImmunoDeficiency Syndrome
ALS	Amyotrophic lateral sclerosis (Lou Gehrig's Disease)
ARDS	Adult respiratory distress syndrome
BPH	Benign prostatic hypertrophy
CABG	Coronary artery bypass graft
CAD	Coronary artery disease
CBC	Complete blood count
CNS	Central nervous system
COPD	Chronic obstructive pulmonary disease
CSF	Cerebrospinal fluid
CT	Computerized tomography
ECG	Electrocardiogram
EEG	Electroencephalogram
EKG	Electrocardiogram
ERCP	Biliary/Pancreatic Endoscopy
GERD	Gastroesophageal reflux disease
HDL	High density lipoprotein
HTN	Hypertension
IBD	Inflammatory Bowel Disease
IBS	Irritable bowel syndrome
IVP	Intravenous pyelogram
LDL	Low density lipoprotein
MRI	Magnetic resonance imaging
MS	Multiple sclerosis
OCD	Obsessive compulsive disorder
PID	Pelvic inflammatory disease
PKU	Phenylketonuria
PTSD	Post traumatic stress disorder

RSD ....Reflex sympathetic dystrophy (Pain)
SIDS ....Sudden infant death syndrome
SLE ....Systemic lupus erythematosus (Lupus)
STD ....Sexually transmitted disease
TB ....Tuberculosis
TCIC ....Trans abdominal cervical cerclage
TIA ....Transient ischemic attack
TMJ ....Temperomandibular joint

Special Expertise	Specialty	Doctor's Name	Page
A			
Abdominal Imaging	Diagnostic Radiology	Fishman, Elliot (MD)	731
Abdominal Imaging	Radiology	Sivit, Carlos (MD)	738
Abdominal Pain-Recurrent	Pediatric Gastroenterology	Kirschner, Barbara S (MD)	580
Abdominal Plasty	Plastic Surgery	Eriksson, Elof (MD)	635
Abuse/Neglect	Child & Adolescent Psychiatry	Zeanah Jr, Charles H (MD)	669
Achalasia	Gastroenterology	Ravich, William Jay (MD)	225
Achalasia	Thoracic Surgery	Deschamps, Claude (MD)	817
Acid-Base Disorders	Nephrology	Aronson, Peter Samuel (MD)	359
Acid-Base Disorders	Nephrology	Weiner, Irving David (MD)	364
Acne	Dermatology	Gordon, Marsha (MD)	184
Acne	Dermatology	Granstein, Richard (MD)	184
Acne	Dermatology	Leyden, James (MD)	184
Acne	Dermatology	Paller, Amy Susan (MD)	190
Acne	Dermatology	Shalita, Alan (MD)	186
Acne	Pediatric Endocrinology	Rosenfield, Robert (MD)	576
Acoustic Nerve Tumors	Neurological Surgery	Eisenberg, Howard M (MD)	375
Acoustic Nerve Tumors	Neurological Surgery	Jacobson , Jeff (MD)	376
Acoustic Nerve Tumors	Neurological Surgery	Long, Donlin M (MD/PhD)	377
Acoustic Nerve Tumors	Neurological Surgery	Ojemann, Robert G. (MD)	373
Acoustic Nerve Tumors	Neurological Surgery	Pitts, Lawrence H (MD)	389
Acoustic Nerve Tumors	Neurological Surgery	Post, Kalmon (MD)	378
Acoustic Nerve Tumors	Neurological Surgery	Rhoton Jr, Albert L (MD)	381
Acoustic Nerve Tumors	Neurological Surgery	Stieg, Philip E (MD/PhD)	379
Acoustic Nerve Tumors	Otolaryngology	Cohen, Noel L (MD)	503
Acoustic Nerve Tumors	Otolaryngology	De la Cruz, Antonio (MD)	521
Acoustic Nerve Tumors	Otolaryngology	Jenkins, Herman A. (MD)	519
Acoustic Nerve Tumors	Otolaryngology	Miyamoto, Richard (MD)	515
Acoustic Nerve Tumors	Otolaryngology	Wackym, Phillip (MD)	517
Acoustic Nerve Tumors	Otolaryngology	Wazen, Jack (MD)	506
Acromegaly	Endocrinology, Diabetes & Metabolism	Biller, Beverly M K (MD)	197
Acromegaly	Endocrinology, Diabetes & Metabolism	Melmed, Shlomo (MD)	212
Acupuncture	Pain Management	Ngeow, Jeffrey (MD)	528
ADD/ADHD	Child & Adolescent Psychiatry	Abright, Arthur Reese (MD)	664
ADD/ADHD	Child & Adolescent Psychiatry	Biederman, Joseph (MD)	663
ADD/ADHD	Child & Adolescent Psychiatry	Bogrov, Michael (MD)	665
ADD/ADHD	Child & Adolescent Psychiatry	Dulcan, Mina Karen (MD)	668
ADD/ADHD	Child & Adolescent Psychiatry	Hertzig, Margaret (MD)	665
ADD/ADHD	Child & Adolescent Psychiatry	Russell, Andrew Thomas (MD)	670
ADD/ADHD	Child & Adolescent Psychiatry	Spencer, Thomas (MD)	664
ADD/ADHD	Child & Adolescent Psychiatry	Wilens, Timothy (MD)	664
Addiction	Addiction Psychiatry	Gorelick, David Alan (MD)	661

SPECIAL EXPERTISE INDEX

Special Expertise	Specialty	Doctor's Name	Page
Addiction	Internal Medicine	Eustace, John C (MD)	335
Addiction	Internal Medicine	Selwyn, Peter (MD)	334
Addiction/Substance Abuse	Psychiatry	Pope Jr, Harrison G (MD)	677
ADHD/Headaches	Neurology	Finkel, Michael (MD)	407
Adolescent Chronic Illness	Adolescent Medicine	Schwarz, Donald F. (MD)	89
Adolescent Medicine	Pediatrics	Zeltzer, Lonnie Kaye (MD)	619
Adolescent Mothers	Adolescent Medicine	Schwarz, Donald F. (MD)	89
Adolescent Risk-Taking	Child & Adolescent Psychiatry	Ponton, Lynn Elisabeth (MD)	670
Adoption	Child & Adolescent Psychiatry	Nickman, Steven L (MD)	664
Adrenal & Gonadal Disorders	Endocrinology, Diabetes & Metabolism	Veldhuis, Johannes D (MD)	205
Adrenal Disorders	Endocrinology, Diabetes & Metabolism	Fleischer, Norman (MD)	200
Adrenal Disorders	Endocrinology, Diabetes & Metabolism	Jacobs, Thomas (MD)	200
Adrenal Disorders	Endocrinology, Diabetes & Metabolism	Ontjes, David A (MD)	204
Adrenal Disorders	Pediatric Endocrinology	Levy, Richard Alshuler (MD)	575
Adrenal Disorders	Pediatric Endocrinology	New, Maria Iandolo (MD)	573
Adrenal Disorders	Pediatric Endocrinology	Oberfield, Sharon (MD)	573
Adrenal Disorders	Urology	Novick, Andrew (MD)	843
Adrenal Tumors	Internal Medicine	Vance, Mary Lee (MD)	335
Adrenal Tumors	Surgery	Lee, Jeffrey Edwin (MD)	798
Advanced Maternal Age	Obstetrics & Gynecology	Toig, Randall (MD)	437
Aggressive Disorders	Child & Adolescent Psychiatry	Alessi, Norman E (MD)	668
Aggressive Disorders	Child & Adolescent Psychiatry	Steiner, Hans (MD)	670
Aging	Geriatric Medicine	Gambert, Steven (MD)	244
Aging	Geriatric Medicine	Minaker, Kenneth (MD)	243
Aging	Geriatric Medicine	Reuben, David (MD)	251
Aging and Dementitia	Psychiatry	Eisdorfer, Carl (MD/PhD)	682
Aging Skin	Dermatology	Fenske, Neil (MD)	187
Aging Skin	Dermatology	Voorhees, John (MD)	190
AIDS/HIV	Allergy & Immunology	Beall, Gildon N (MD)	103
AIDS/HIV	Child Neurology	Epstein, Leon G (MD)	153
AIDS/HIV	Gastroenterology	Brandt, Lawrence (MD)	222
AIDS/HIV	Gastroenterology	Dieterich, Douglas (MD)	223
AIDS/HIV	Geriatric Medicine	McCormick, Wayne (MD)	251
AIDS/HIV	Gynecologic Oncology	Goodman, Annekathryn (MD)	255
AIDS/HIV	Infectious Disease	Ballon-Landa, Gonzalo (MD)	328
AIDS/HIV	Infectious Disease	Bartlett, John A (MD)	322
AIDS/HIV	Infectious Disease	Bartlett, John Gill (MD)	318
AIDS/HIV	Infectious Disease	Campbell, J William (MD)	325
AIDS/HIV	Infectious Disease	Cancio, Margarita (MD)	322
AIDS/HIV	Infectious Disease	Chaisson, Richard Ernest (MD)	318
AIDS/HIV	Infectious Disease	Chan, Joseph (MD)	323
AIDS/HIV	Infectious Disease	Cohn, David (MD)	326
AIDS/HIV	Infectious Disease	Craven, Donald Edward (MD)	317
AIDS/HIV	Infectious Disease	Droller, David G (MD)	323
AIDS/HIV	Infectious Disease	Ellner, Jerrold Jay (MD)	318
AIDS/HIV	Infectious Disease	Fauci, Anthony Stephen (MD)	319
AIDS/HIV	Infectious Disease	Frank, Ian (MD)	319
AIDS/HIV	Infectious Disease	Friedman, Harvey Michael (MD)	319
AIDS/HIV	Infectious Disease	Hammer, Glenn (MD)	319
AIDS/HIV	Infectious Disease	Hirsch, Martin Stanley (MD)	317
AIDS/HIV	Infectious Disease	Hollander, Harry (MD)	328
AIDS/HIV	Infectious Disease	Holmes, King K (MD)	328
AIDS/HIV	Infectious Disease	Kaplan, Mark H (MD)	320
AIDS/HIV	Infectious Disease	Katner, Harold (MD)	323
AIDS/HIV	Infectious Disease	Kazanjian Jr, Powel H (MD)	325
AIDS/HIV	Infectious Disease	Keiser, Philip (MD)	327
AIDS/HIV	Infectious Disease	Masur, Henry (MD)	320
AIDS/HIV	Infectious Disease	Mildvan, Donna (MD)	320
AIDS/HIV	Infectious Disease	Patterson, Thomas F. (MD)	327
AIDS/HIV	Infectious Disease	Paya, Carlos Vicente (MD)	326
AIDS/HIV	Infectious Disease	Pegram Jr., Paul Samuel (MD)	324
AIDS/HIV	Infectious Disease	Perlman, David (MD)	320

Special Expertise	Specialty	Doctor's Name	Page
AIDS/HIV	Infectious Disease	Polsky, Bruce (MD)	321
AIDS/HIV	Infectious Disease	Powderly, William (MD)	326
AIDS/HIV	Infectious Disease	Ratzan, Kenneth (MD)	324
AIDS/HIV	Infectious Disease	Richman, Douglas (MD)	329
AIDS/HIV	Infectious Disease	Saag, Michael S (MD)	324
AIDS/HIV	Infectious Disease	Sepkowitz, Kent (MD)	321
AIDS/HIV	Infectious Disease	Smith, Leon G (MD)	321
AIDS/HIV	Infectious Disease	Van Der Horst, Charles (MD)	325
AIDS/HIV	Infectious Disease	Wallace Jr, Richard James (MD)	328
AIDS/HIV	Infectious Disease	Wiviott, Lory David (MD)	329
AIDS/HIV	Infectious Disease	Wormser, Gary (MD)	322
AIDS/HIV	Infectious Disease	Yancovitz, Stanley (MD)	322
AIDS/HIV	Internal Medicine	Schooley, Robert Turner (MD)	336
AIDS/HIV	Internal Medicine	Selwyn, Peter (MD)	334
AIDS/HIV	Medical Oncology	Abrams, Donald Ira (MD)	312
AIDS/HIV	Medical Oncology	Volberding, Paul Arthur (MD)	314
AIDS/HIV	Neurology	Berger, Joseph (MD)	407
AIDS/HIV	Pediatric Allergy & Immunology	Church, Joseph August (MD)	558
AIDS/HIV	Pediatric Allergy & Immunology	Shearer, William T (MD)	558
AIDS/HIV	Pediatric Allergy & Immunology	Stiehm, E Richard (MD)	559
AIDS/HIV	Pediatric Allergy & Immunology	Wara, Diane Wickizer (MD)	560
AIDS/HIV	Pediatric Infectious Disease	Andiman, Warren A. (MD)	590
AIDS/HIV	Pediatric Infectious Disease	Borkowsky, William (MD)	590
AIDS/HIV	Pediatric Infectious Disease	Bryson, Yvonne Joyce (MD)	594
AIDS/HIV	Pediatric Infectious Disease	Givner, Laurence Bruce (MD)	592
AIDS/HIV	Pediatric Infectious Disease	Gorensek, Margaret (MD)	592
AIDS/HIV	Pediatric Infectious Disease	Kline, Mark (MD)	594
AIDS/HIV	Pediatric Infectious Disease	Mitchell, Charles (MD)	592
AIDS/HIV	Pediatric Infectious Disease	Scott, Gwendolyn (MD)	592
AIDS/HIV	Pediatrics	Pizzo, Philip Anthony (MD)	617
AIDS/HIV	Psychiatry	Breitbart, William (MD)	678
AIDS/HIV	Pulmonary Disease	Hopewell, Philip (MD)	710
AIDS/HIV	Pulmonary Disease	Huang, Laurence (MD)	711
AIDS/HIV	Pulmonary Disease	Kamholz, Stephan (MD)	694
AIDS/HIV	Pulmonary Disease	Rosen, Mark J (MD)	695
AIDS/HIV	Pulmonary Disease	Stansell, John Dee (MD)	712
AIDS/HIV	Pulmonary Disease	Stover-Pepe, Diane E (MD)	695
AIDS/HIV	Pulmonary Disease	Wallace, Jeanne Marie (MD)	713
AIDS/HIV	Pulmonary Disease	White, Dorothy (MD)	696
AIDS/HIV & Tuberculosis	Pulmonary Disease	Glassroth, Jeffrey (MD)	703
AIDS/HIV in Pregnancy	Maternal & Fetal Medicine	Bardeguez-Brown, Arlene D (MD)	341
AIDS/HIV in Pregnancy	Obstetrics & Gynecology	Ledger, William (MD)	432
AIDS/HIV in Pregnancy	Obstetrics & Gynecology	Minkoff, Howard L (MD)	432
AIDS/HIV-Gastro Comp	Gastroenterology	Forsmark, Christopher (MD)	228
AIDS/HIV-Kaposi's Sarcoma	Dermatology	Conant, Marcus A (MD)	192
AIDS/HIV-Nutrition	Gastroenterology	Kotler, Donald P (MD)	224
Airway Disorders	Otolaryngology	Bower, Charles (MD)	518
Airway Disorders	Otolaryngology	Zalzal, George (MD)	507
Airway Disorders	Pediatric Otolaryngology	Crockett, Dennis M (MD)	603
Airway Disorders	Pediatric Otolaryngology	Holinger, Lauren (MD)	602
Airway Disorders	Pediatric Otolaryngology	Inglis, Andrew (MD)	603
Airway Disorders	Pediatric Otolaryngology	Miller, Robert (MD)	602
Airway Disorders	Pediatric Otolaryngology	Milmoe, Gregory J (MD)	601
Airway Disorders	Pulmonary Disease	Goldman, Allan Larry (MD)	698
Alcoholism	Addiction Psychiatry	Galanter, Marc (MD)	661
Alcoholism	Addiction Psychiatry	Kosten, Thomas (MD)	661
Alcoholism	Addiction Psychiatry	Schuckit, Marc A (MD)	662
Allergies-Pediatric	Allergy & Immunology	Nelson, Harold (MD)	102
Allergy	Allergy & Immunology	Korenblat, Phillip Erwin (MD)	101
Allergy	Allergy & Immunology	Levinson, Arnold (MD)	96
Allergy	Allergy & Immunology	MacLean, James Andrew (MD)	95
Allergy	Allergy & Immunology	Sanders, Georgiana (MD)	101

SPECIAL EXPERTISE INDEX

Special Expertise	Specialty	Doctor's Name	Page
Anal Sphincter Repair	Colon & Rectal Surgery	Lowry, Ann (MD)	174
Anaphylaxis	Allergy & Immunology	Greenberger, Paul A (MD)	101
Anaphylaxis	Allergy & Immunology	Wasserman, Stephen (MD)	103
Andrology	Endocrinology, Diabetes & Metabolism	Swerdloff, Ronald Sherwin (MD)	213
Anemia	Hematology	Blinder, Morey (MD)	288
Anemia	Hematology	Zalusky, Ralph (MD)	286
Anemias & Red Cell Disorders	Hematology	Benz, Edward (MD)	285
Aneurysm	Neurology	Rothrock, John (MD)	409
Aneurysm	Radiology	Vinuela, Fernando (MD)	740
Aneurysm	Thoracic Surgery	Akins, Cary W (MD)	805
Aneurysm	Thoracic Surgery	Reul, George J (MD)	822
Aneurysm	Thoracic Surgery	Sundt III, Thoralf Mauritz (MD)	820
Aneurysm	Vascular Surgery (General)	Belkin, Michael (MD)	857
Aneurysm	Vascular Surgery (General)	Flynn, Timothy Carlyle (MD)	863
Aneurysm	Vascular Surgery (General)	Gertler, Jonathan P (MD)	857
Aneurysm	Vascular Surgery (General)	Hodgson, Kim John (MD)	866
Aneurysm	Vascular Surgery (General)	Perler, Bruce Alan (MD)	861
Aneurysm	Vascular Surgery (General)	Ricotta, John (MD)	861
Aneurysm	Vascular Surgery (General)	Rosenthal, David (MD)	864
Aneurysm	Vascular Surgery (General)	Todd, George (MD)	862
Aneurysm	Vascular Surgery (General)	Veith, Frank James (MD)	862
Aneurysm-Abdominal Aortic	Radiology	Benenati, James Francis (MD)	737
Aneurysm-Abdominal Aortic	Thoracic Surgery	Cooley, Denton A (MD)	821
Aneurysm-Abdominal Aortic	Thoracic Surgery	Coselli, Joseph Stapleton (MD)	821
Aneurysm-Abdominal Aortic	Thoracic Surgery	Elefteriades, John (MD)	805
Aneurysm-Abdominal Aortic	Thoracic Surgery	Griepp, Randall (MD)	808
Aneurysm-Abdominal Aortic	Thoracic Surgery	Silverman, Norman A (MD)	819
Aneurysm-Abdominal Aortic	Vascular Surgery (General)	Adelman, Mark (MD)	858
Aneurysm-Abdominal Aortic	Vascular Surgery (General)	Atnip, Robert (MD)	859
Aneurysm-Abdominal Aortic	Vascular Surgery (General)	Baker, William (MD)	864
Aneurysm-Abdominal Aortic	Vascular Surgery (General)	Brewster, David Charles (MD)	857
Aneurysm-Abdominal Aortic	Vascular Surgery (General)	Calligaro, Keith Don (MD)	859
Aneurysm-Abdominal Aortic	Vascular Surgery (General)	Cambria, Richard P (MD)	857
Aneurysm-Abdominal Aortic	Vascular Surgery (General)	Clagett, George Patrick (MD)	867
Aneurysm-Abdominal Aortic	Vascular Surgery (General)	Cohen, Jon (MD)	859
Aneurysm-Abdominal Aortic	Vascular Surgery (General)	Cronenwett, Jack (MD)	857
Aneurysm-Abdominal Aortic	Vascular Surgery (General)	Darling, Ralph Clement (MD)	860
Aneurysm-Abdominal Aortic	Vascular Surgery (General)	Flanigan, Preston D. (MD)	868
Aneurysm-Abdominal Aortic	Vascular Surgery (General)	Gloviczki, Peter (MD)	865
Aneurysm-Abdominal Aortic	Vascular Surgery (General)	Green, Richard (MD)	860
Aneurysm-Abdominal Aortic	Vascular Surgery (General)	Hallett Jr, John (MD)	865
Aneurysm-Abdominal Aortic	Vascular Surgery (General)	Hertzer, Norman Ray (MD)	865
Aneurysm-Abdominal Aortic	Vascular Surgery (General)	Mackey, William C. (MD)	858
Aneurysm-Abdominal Aortic	Vascular Surgery (General)	Money, Samuel (MD)	868
Aneurysm-Abdominal Aortic	Vascular Surgery (General)	Moore, Wesley Sanford (MD)	869
Aneurysm-Abdominal Aortic	Vascular Surgery (General)	Pearce, William (MD)	866
Aneurysm-Abdominal Aortic	Vascular Surgery (General)	Reddy, Daniel (MD)	866
Aneurysm-Abdominal Aortic	Vascular Surgery (General)	Riles, Thomas (MD)	861
Aneurysm-Abdominal Aortic	Vascular Surgery (General)	Safi, Hazim Jawad (MD)	868
Aneurysm-Abdominal Aortic	Vascular Surgery (General)	Sicard, Gregorio Arquel (MD)	867
Aneurysm-Abdominal Aortic	Vascular Surgery (General)	Whittemore, Anthony D (MD)	858
Aneurysm-Abdominal Aortic	Vascular Surgery (General)	Williams, G. Melville (MD)	862
Aneurysm-Abdominal Aortic	Vascular Surgery (General)	Zarins, Christopher Kristaps (MD)	870
Aneurysm-Aortic	Vascular Surgery (General)	Andros, George (MD)	868
Aneurysm-Aortic	Vascular Surgery (General)	Seeger, James M (MD)	864
Aneurysm-Cerebral	Neurological Surgery	Batjer, H. Hunt (MD)	382
Aneurysm-Cerebral	Neurological Surgery	Dacey Jr., Ralph Gerald (MD)	383
Aneurysm-Cerebral	Neurological Surgery	Giannotta, Steven L (MD)	389
Aneurysm-Cerebral	Neurological Surgery	Sekhar, Laligam N (MD)	381
Aneurysm-Cerebral	Neurological Surgery	Steinberg, Gary K (MD)	390

SPECIAL EXPERTISE INDEX

Special Expertise	Specialty	Doctor's Name	Page
Aneurysm-Peripheral	Vascular Surgery (General)	Atnip, Robert (MD)	859
Angelman Syndrome	Clinical Genetics	Driscoll, Daniel J (MD)	161
Angina	Cardiology (Cardiovascular Disease)	Achuff, Stephen Charles (MD)	123
Angina-Unstable	Cardiology (Cardiovascular Disease)	Borzak, Steven (MD)	133
Angioedema	Allergy & Immunology	Frigas, Evangelo (MD)	100
Angiography	Radiology	Haskal, Ziv (MD)	735
Angiography-Coronary	Cardiology (Cardiovascular Disease)	Abittan, Meyer H (MD)	123
Angiography-Coronary	Cardiology (Cardiovascular Disease)	Douglas Jr, John Simonton (MD)	131
Angiography-Coronary	Cardiology (Cardiovascular Disease)	Moses, Jeffrey W (MD)	127
Angiography-Coronary	Cardiology (Cardiovascular Disease)	Ramee, Stephen Robert (MD)	140
Angiography-Coronary	Cardiology (Cardiovascular Disease)	Sacchi, Terrence J (MD)	127
Angioplasty	Cardiology (Cardiovascular Disease)	Behar, Victor Samuel (MD)	129
Angioplasty	Cardiology (Cardiovascular Disease)	Conti, Charles Richard (MD)	130
Angioplasty	Cardiology (Cardiovascular Disease)	Isner, Jeffrey Michael (MD)	121
Angioplasty	Cardiology (Cardiovascular Disease)	Klapholz, Marc (MD)	126
Angioplasty	Cardiology (Cardiovascular Disease)	Phillips III, Harry Rissler (MD)	132
Angioplasty	Cardiology (Cardiovascular Disease)	Shani, Jacob (MD)	128
Angioplasty	Interventional Cardiology	Applegate, Robert Joseph (MD)	144
Angioplasty	Interventional Cardiology	Diver, Daniel Joseph (MD)	144
Angioplasty	Interventional Cardiology	Kleiman, Neal Stephen (MD)	147
Angioplasty	Interventional Cardiology	Matar, Fadi (MD)	145
Angioplasty	Interventional Cardiology	Pichard, Augusto (MD)	144
Angioplasty	Pediatric Cardiology	Cutilletta , Anthony F (MD)	564
Angioplasty	Pediatric Cardiology	Kan, Jean (MD)	562
Angioplasty-Pulmonary Artery	Pediatric Cardiology	Lock, James E (MD)	561
Ankle & Knee surgery	Sports Medicine	Shively, Robert A (MD)	774
Ankle Joint Replacement	Hand Surgery	Nunley, James (MD)	270
Ankle Surgery	Orthopaedic Surgery	Waller, John F (MD)	484
Ankle Surgery	Sports Medicine	Paletta , George A (MD)	774
Ankylosing Spondilitis	Rheumatology	Luthra, Harvinder Singh (MD)	765
Anorectal Disorders	Colon & Rectal Surgery	Abcarian, Herand (MD)	173
Anorectal Disorders	Colon & Rectal Surgery	Nivatvongs, Santhat (MD)	174
Anorectal Disorders	Colon & Rectal Surgery	Shellito, Paul C (MD)	170
Antiemetic Therapy	Medical Oncology	Kris, Mark (MD)	297
Anxiety & Mood Disorders	Child & Adolescent Psychiatry	Biederman, Joseph (MD)	663
Anxiety & Mood Disorders	Psychiatry	Ballenger, James (MD)	682
Anxiety & Mood Disorders	Psychiatry	Davidson, Jonathan (MD)	682
Anxiety & Mood Disorders	Psychiatry	Dunner, David Louis (MD)	686
Anxiety & Mood Disorders	Psychiatry	Greden, John (MD)	683
Anxiety & Mood Disorders	Psychiatry	Greist, John (MD)	683
Anxiety & Mood Disorders	Psychiatry	Rosenbaum, Jerrold Frank (MD)	677
Anxiety & Mood Disorders	Psychiatry	Roy-Byrne, Peter (MD)	688
Anxiety & Mood Disorders	Psychiatry	Schatzberg, Alan F (MD)	688
Anxiety & Mood Disorders	Psychiatry	Thase, Michael E (MD)	681
Anxiety & Mood Disorders	Psychiatry	Uhde, Thomas W (MD)	684
Anxiety & Mood Disorders	Psychiatry	Yonkers, Kimberly A (MD)	677
Anxiety Disorders	Child & Adolescent Psychiatry	Kestenbaum, Clarice J (MD)	666
Anxiety Disorders	Child & Adolescent Psychiatry	Koplewicz, Harold (MD)	666
Anxiety Disorders	Child & Adolescent Psychiatry	March, John (MD)	667
Anxiety Disorders	Geriatric Psychiatry	Goldman, Samuel (MD)	673
Anxiety Disorders	Geriatric Psychiatry	Isenberg, Keith Eugene (MD)	674
Anxiety Disorders	Geriatric Psychiatry	Lazarus, Lawrence W (MD)	674
Anxiety Disorders	Psychiatry	Bystritsky, Alexander (MD)	686
Anxiety Disorders	Psychiatry	Hollander, Eric (MD)	679
Anxiety Disorders	Psychiatry	Liebowitz, Michael R (MD)	680
Anxiety Disorders	Psychiatry	Sadock, Benjamin (MD)	681
Anxiety Disorders	Psychiatry	Shear, Mary Katherine (MD)	681
Anxiety Disorders	Psychiatry	Stein, Murray Brent (MD)	688
Anxiety Disorders	Psychiatry	Sussman, Norman (MD)	681
Anxiety/Mood Disorders .	Child & Adolescent Psychiatry	Wiener, Jerry M (MD)	667

958

Special Expertise	Specialty	Doctor's Name	Page
Aortic & Visceral Artery Reconstruction	Vascular Surgery (General)	Hansen, Kimberley J (MD)	863
Aortic Branch Surgery	Vascular Surgery (General)	Berguer, Ramon (MD)	864
Aortic Diseases & Dissection	Cardiology (Cardiovascular Disease)	Braverman, Alan Charles (MD)	133
Aortic Dissection	Cardiology (Cardiovascular Disease)	Eagle, Kim A (MD)	135
Aortic Graft Infection	Vascular Surgery (General)	Cherry Jr., Kenneth J. (MD)	864
Aortic Stent Grafts	Vascular Surgery (General)	Lumsden, Alan Boyd (MD)	863
Aortic Surgery	Vascular Surgery (General)	Hollier, Larry Harold (MD)	860
Aortic Surgery	Vascular Surgery (General)	Whittemore, Anthony D (MD)	858
Aortic Surgery-Thoracic	Thoracic Surgery	Bavaria, Joseph (MD)	807
Aortic Surgery-Thoracic	Thoracic Surgery	Karp, Robert Bruce (MD)	817
Aphasia	Neurology	Kirshner, Howard S (MD)	408
Aphasia	Neurology	Mohr, Jay Preston (MD)	404
Aplastic Anemia	Hematology	Silverstein, Roy (MD)	286
Arrhythmias	Cardiac Electrophysiology	Cain, Michael Edwin (MD)	117
Arrhythmias	Cardiac Electrophysiology	DiMarco, John Philip (MD/PhD)	116
Arrhythmias	Cardiac Electrophysiology	Ellenbogen, Kenneth A. (MD)	116
Arrhythmias	Cardiac Electrophysiology	Epstein, Andrew Ernest (MD)	117
Arrhythmias	Cardiac Electrophysiology	Gomes, J Anthony (MD)	115
Arrhythmias	Cardiac Electrophysiology	Levine, Joseph H (MD)	115
Arrhythmias	Cardiac Electrophysiology	Marchlinski, Francis Edward (MD)	116
Arrhythmias	Cardiac Electrophysiology	Morady, Fred (MD)	117
Arrhythmias	Cardiac Electrophysiology	Prystowsky, Eric Neal (MD)	118
Arrhythmias	Cardiac Electrophysiology	Rothman, Steven Alan (MD)	116
Arrhythmias	Cardiac Electrophysiology	Stevenson, William G. (MD)	115
Arrhythmias	Cardiac Electrophysiology	Swerdlow, Charles Dennis (MD)	119
Arrhythmias	Cardiology (Cardiovascular Disease)	Josephson, Mark Eric (MD)	121
Arrhythmias	Cardiology (Cardiovascular Disease)	Sacchi, Terrence J (MD)	127
Arrhythmias	Cardiology (Cardiovascular Disease)	Zipes, Douglas P (MD)	139
Arrhythmias	Pediatric Cardiology	Gillette, Paul Crawford (MD)	566
Arrhythmias	Pediatric Cardiology	Porter, Co-burn Joseph (MD)	565
Arrhythmias	Pediatric Cardiology	Sodt, Peter (MD)	566
Arrhythmias	Pediatric Cardiology	Walsh, Edward Patrick (MD)	561
Arrhythmias	Pediatric Cardiology	Wolff, Grace Susan (MD)	563
Arrhythmias	Pediatric Cardiology	Young, Ming-Lon (MD)	564
Arrhythmias-Atrial	Cardiac Electrophysiology	Morady, Fred (MD)	117
Arrhythmias-Atrial	Cardiac Electrophysiology	Waldo, Albert (MD)	118
Arrhythmias-Atrial	Cardiology (Cardiovascular Disease)	Manning, Warren (MD)	122
Arrhythmias-Defibrillators/Pacemakers	Cardiology (Cardiovascular Disease)	Myerburg, Robert (MD)	131
Arrhythmias-Fetal	Pediatric Cardiology	Porter, Co-burn Joseph (MD)	565
Arterial Bypass Surgery	Vascular Surgery (General)	Belkin, Michael (MD)	857
Arterial Bypass Surgery	Vascular Surgery (General)	Eidt, John (MD)	868
Arterial Bypass Surgery-Leg	Vascular Surgery (General)	Lo Gerfo, Frank W (MD)	858
Arterial Bypass Surgery-Leg	Vascular Surgery (General)	Money, Samuel (MD)	868
Arterial Bypass Surgery-Leg	Vascular Surgery (General)	Shepard, Alexander D (MD)	866
Arterial Disease	Vascular Surgery (General)	Gewertz, Bruce (MD)	865
Arterial Reconstruction	Vascular Surgery (General)	Moore, Wesley Sanford (MD)	869
Arterial Switch	Pediatric Surgery	Quaegebeur, Jan Modest (MD)	612
Arteriovenous Malformations	Neurological Surgery	Batjer, H. Hunt (MD)	382
Arteriovenous Malformations	Neurological Surgery	Grubb, Robert (MD)	383
Arteriovenous Malformations	Neurological Surgery	Sekhar, Laligam N (MD)	381
Arteriovenous Malformations	Neurological Surgery	Steinberg, Gary K (MD)	390
Arteriovenous Malformations	Neurological Surgery	Winn, H Richard (MD)	390
Arthritis	Internal Medicine	Robinson, Dwight R. (MD)	333
Arthritis	Orthopaedic Surgery	Goldberg, Victor M (MD)	490
Arthritis	Orthopaedic Surgery	Stulberg, Samuel David (MD)	493
Arthritis	Orthopaedic Surgery	Thornhill, Thomas S (MD)	477
Arthritis	Orthopaedic Surgery	Vail, Thomas Parker (MD)	488
Arthritis	Pediatric Rheumatology	Lehman, Thomas (MD)	608
Arthritis	Pediatric Rheumatology	McCarthy, Paul L (MD)	608
Arthritis	Rheumatology	Abramson, Steven B (MD)	757

SPECIAL EXPERTISE INDEX

Special Expertise	Specialty	Doctor's Name	Page
Arthritis	Rheumatology	Arend, William Phelps (MD)	766
Arthritis	Rheumatology	Curran, James Joseph (MD)	764
Arthritis	Rheumatology	Harrington, J Timothy (MD)	764
Arthritis	Rheumatology	Lipstate, James Mitchell (MD)	768
Arthritis	Rheumatology	Malin, Jennifer (MD)	768
Arthritis	Rheumatology	Pope, Richard M (MD)	766
Arthritis	Rheumatology	Sessoms, Sandra Lee (MD)	768
Arthritis	Rheumatology	Solomon, Gary (MD)	761
Arthritis	Rheumatology	Williams, H James (MD)	767
Arthritis and Exercise	Rheumatology	Chang, Rowland Waton (MD)	763
Arthritis Hand Surgery	Hand Surgery	Beasley, Robert (MD)	267
Arthritis Hand Surgery	Hand Surgery	Mass, Daniel (MD)	273
Arthritis Hand Surgery	Hand Surgery	McCormack Jr, Richard R (MD)	268
Arthritis Hand Surgery	Hand Surgery	Melone Jr, Charles P (MD)	268
Arthritis Hand Surgery	Hand Surgery	Nunley, James (MD)	270
Arthritis Hand Surgery	Hand Surgery	Taleisnik, Julio (MD)	276
Arthritis-Juvenile	Pediatric Rheumatology	Wagner-Weiner, Linda (MD)	609
Arthritis-Septic	Infectious Disease	Bayer, Arnold Sander (MD)	328
Arthritis/Viscosupplementation	Rheumatology	Barr, Walter Gerard (MD)	763
Arthrogryposis-Limb Deficiency	Physical Medicine & Rehabilitation	Jaffe, Kenneth M (MD)	630
Arthroscopic Surgery	Orthopaedic Surgery	Goitz, Henry (MD)	490
Arthroscopic Surgery	Orthopaedic Surgery	Nuber, Gordon (MD)	492
Arthroscopic Surgery	Orthopaedic Surgery	Sherman, Orrin (MD)	484
Arthroscopic Surgery	Orthopaedic Surgery	Spindler, Kurt Paul (MD)	488
Arthroscopic Surgery	Orthopaedic Surgery	Zarins, Bertram (MD)	477
Arthroscopy	Sports Medicine	Levine, William (MD)	773
Artificial Bowel Sphincter	Colon & Rectal Surgery	Thorson, Alan (MD)	175
Artificial Heart	Thoracic Surgery	Copeland III, Jack G (MD)	821
Artificial Heart	Thoracic Surgery	Samuels, Louis (MD)	811
Artificial Sphincter-Anal	Colon & Rectal Surgery	Wong, Westley Douglas (MD)	171
Asperger's Syndrome	Child & Adolescent Psychiatry	Volkmar, Fred R (MD)	664
Aspiration	Pediatric Otolaryngology	Holinger, Lauren (MD)	602
Assisted Breathing	Pediatric Pulmonology	Warren, Robert Hughes (MD)	606
Asthma	Allergy & Immunology	Aaronson, Donald W (MD)	99
Asthma	Allergy & Immunology	Adkinson, Franklin (MD)	95
Asthma	Allergy & Immunology	Atkins, Paul Charles (MD)	95
Asthma	Allergy & Immunology	Benenati, Susan (MD)	98
Asthma	Allergy & Immunology	Buchbinder, Ellen (MD)	95
Asthma	Allergy & Immunology	Busse, William (MD)	100
Asthma	Allergy & Immunology	Chandler, Michael (MD)	96
Asthma	Allergy & Immunology	Friedman, Stuart (MD)	98
Asthma	Allergy & Immunology	Grammer, Leslie C (MD)	100
Asthma	Allergy & Immunology	Grant, Evalyn N (MD)	100
Asthma	Allergy & Immunology	Greenberger, Paul A (MD)	101
Asthma	Allergy & Immunology	Korenblat, Phillip Erwin (MD)	101
Asthma	Allergy & Immunology	Ledford, Dennis (MD)	99
Asthma	Allergy & Immunology	MacLean, James Andrew (MD)	95
Asthma	Allergy & Immunology	Macris, Nicholas T (MD)	96
Asthma	Allergy & Immunology	Nelson, Harold (MD)	102
Asthma	Allergy & Immunology	Neustrom, Mark Ray (DO)	102
Asthma	Allergy & Immunology	Rosenwasser, Lanny Jeffrey (MD)	102
Asthma	Allergy & Immunology	Sanders, Georgiana (MD)	101
Asthma	Allergy & Immunology	Slankard, Marjorie (MD)	97
Asthma	Allergy & Immunology	Slavin, Raymond (MD)	101
Asthma	Allergy & Immunology	Ten, Rosa Maria (MD/PhD)	101
Asthma	Allergy & Immunology	Togias, Alkis George (MD)	97
Asthma	Allergy & Immunology	Wald, Jeffrey A (MD)	102
Asthma	Allergy & Immunology	Wong, Johnson T (MD)	95
Asthma	Allergy & Immunology	Wood, John (MD)	102
Asthma	Geriatric Medicine	Williamson, Wayne (MD)	249

SPECIAL EXPERTISE INDEX

Special Expertise	Specialty	Doctor's Name	Page
Asthma	Pediatric Allergy & Immunology	Bahna, Sami Labib (MD)	556
Asthma	Pediatric Allergy & Immunology	Blum, Paul (MD)	556
Asthma	Pediatric Allergy & Immunology	Epstein, Stuart Zane (MD)	559
Asthma	Pediatric Allergy & Immunology	Evans III, Richard (MD)	557
Asthma	Pediatric Allergy & Immunology	Gelfand, Erwin (MD)	558
Asthma	Pediatric Allergy & Immunology	Lemanske Jr, Robert F (MD)	557
Asthma	Pediatric Allergy & Immunology	Pongracic, Jacqueline (MD)	557
Asthma	Pediatric Allergy & Immunology	Skoner, David Peter (MD)	555
Asthma	Pediatric Allergy & Immunology	Sly, Ridge Michael (MD)	555
Asthma	Pediatric Allergy & Immunology	Strunk, Robert (MD)	557
Asthma	Pediatric Allergy & Immunology	Umetsu, Dale T (MD/PhD)	559
Asthma	Pediatric Allergy & Immunology	Wolf, Raoul (MD)	557
Asthma	Pediatric Allergy & Immunology	Wood, Robert Alan (MD)	556
Asthma	Pediatric Pulmonology	Kim, Young-Jee (MD)	605
Asthma	Pediatric Pulmonology	Kurachek, Stephen Charles (MD)	605
Asthma	Pediatric Pulmonology	Lapey, Allen (MD)	604
Asthma	Pediatric Pulmonology	Loughlin, Gerald M (MD)	604
Asthma	Pediatric Pulmonology	Mellins, Robert (MD)	604
Asthma	Pediatric Pulmonology	Redding , Gregory (MD)	607
Asthma	Pulmonary Disease	Balk, Robert (MD)	702
Asthma	Pulmonary Disease	Boushey Jr, Homer A (MD)	710
Asthma	Pulmonary Disease	Braman, Sidney (MD)	691
Asthma	Pulmonary Disease	Donohue, James (MD)	697
Asthma	Pulmonary Disease	Fanta, Christopher (MD)	691
Asthma	Pulmonary Disease	Geppert, Eugene (MD)	702
Asthma	Pulmonary Disease	Grum, Cyril M (MD)	703
Asthma	Pulmonary Disease	Henke, David Carroll (MD)	699
Asthma	Pulmonary Disease	Jenkinson, Stephen George (MD)	709
Asthma	Pulmonary Disease	Kaye, Mitchell (MD)	703
Asthma	Pulmonary Disease	King Jr, Talmadge Everett (MD)	711
Asthma	Pulmonary Disease	Libby, Daniel (MD)	694
Asthma	Pulmonary Disease	Metersky, Mark Lewis (MD)	692
Asthma	Pulmonary Disease	Nash, Thomas (MD)	334
Asthma	Pulmonary Disease	Petty, Thomas L (MD)	707
Asthma	Pulmonary Disease	Rizk, Norman Wade (MD)	712
Asthma	Pulmonary Disease	Sahn, Steven A. (MD)	700
Asthma	Pulmonary Disease	Schwartz, David A (MD)	700
Asthma	Pulmonary Disease	Tashkin, Donald P (MD)	713
Asthma	Pulmonary Disease	Thomashow, Byron (MD)	696
Asthma	Pulmonary Disease	Voelkel, Norbert F (MD)	708
Asthma	Pulmonary Disease	Wanner, Adam (MD)	701
Asthma	Pulmonary Disease	Wenzel, Sally E (MD)	708
Asthma & Allergy	Pediatric Allergy & Immunology	Berger, Melvin (MD/PhD)	556
Asthma & Allergy	Pediatric Allergy & Immunology	Fanous, Yvonne F (MD)	559
Asthma & Allergy	Pediatric Allergy & Immunology	Ostrom, Nancy Kay (MD)	559
Asthma & Allergy	Pediatric Allergy & Immunology	Shapiro, Gail Greenberg (MD)	559
Asthma (Adult)	Pulmonary Disease	Martin, Richard Jay (MD)	707
Asthma and Sinusitis	Allergy & Immunology	Baraniuk, James N (MD)	95
Asthma in Pregnancy	Allergy & Immunology	Gluck, Joan (MD)	98
Asthma-Adult & Pediatric	Allergy & Immunology	Mazza, David S (MD)	96
Asthma/Allergies-Pediatric	Allergy & Immunology	Gluck, Joan (MD)	98
Ataxia	Child Neurology	Stumpf, David A (MD)	154
Ataxia	Neurology	Burns , R Stanley (MD)	412
Ataxia	Neurology	Gilman, Sid (MD)	413
Atherosclerosis	Cardiology (Cardiovascular Disease)	Fuster, Valentin (MD)	125
Atherosclerosis	Cardiology (Cardiovascular Disease)	Libby, Peter (MD)	122
Atopic Dermatitis	Dermatology	Gurevitch, Arnold William (MD)	193
Atopic Dermatitis	Pediatric Allergy & Immunology	Leung, Donald (MD/PhD)	558
Attachment Disorders	Child & Adolescent Psychiatry	Zeanah Jr, Charles H (MD)	669
Autism	Child & Adolescent Psychiatry	Cohen, Donald (MD)	663

SPECIAL EXPERTISE INDEX

Special Expertise	Specialty	Doctor's Name	Page
Autism	Child & Adolescent Psychiatry	Greenspan, Stanley (MD)	665
Autism	Child & Adolescent Psychiatry	Tanguay, Peter (MD)	667
Autism	Child & Adolescent Psychiatry	Todd, Richard D (MD/PhD)	668
Autism	Child & Adolescent Psychiatry	Volkmar, Fred R (MD)	664
Autism	Child Neurology	Trauner, Doris Ann (MD)	156
Autism & Developmental Disorders	Child & Adolescent Psychiatry	Wright, Harry (MD)	668
Autoimmune Disease	Allergy & Immunology	Busse, William (MD)	100
Autoimmune Disease	Allergy & Immunology	Levinson, Arnold (MD)	96
Autoimmune Disease	Neurology	Weiner, Howard (MD)	399
Autoimmune Disease	Rheumatology	Lahita, Robert (MD)	759
Autoimmune Lung Disease	Pulmonary Disease	Brown, Kevin K (MD)	706
Autonomic Disorders	Cardiology (Cardiovascular Disease)	Grubb, Blair Paul (MD)	135
Autonomic Disorders	Cardiology (Cardiovascular Disease)	Robertson, Rose Marie (MD)	132

B

Balance Disorders	Otolaryngology	Daspit, C Phillip (MD)	518
Balance Disorders	Otolaryngology	Farmer, Joseph (MD)	508
Barrett's Esophagus	Gastroenterology	Aronchick, Craig Alan (MD)	222
Barrett's Esophagus	Gastroenterology	Boyce Jr, H Worth (MD)	226
Barrett's Esophagus	Gastroenterology	Brazer, Scott Robert (MD)	226
Barrett's Esophagus	Gastroenterology	Fleischer, David (MD)	223
Barrett's Esophagus	Gastroenterology	Lightdale, Charles (MD)	224
Barrett's Esophagus	Surgery	Pellegrini, Carlos (MD)	801
Barrett's Esophagus	Thoracic Surgery	Ferguson, Mark (MD)	817
Behavioral Neurology	Neurology	Heilman, Kenneth (MD)	408
Behavioral Problems	Psychiatry	Greist, John (MD)	683
Behavioral Problems	Psychiatry	Klagsbrun, Samuel C (MD)	679
Bereavement/Traumatic Grief	Psychiatry	Shear, Mary Katherine (MD)	681
Bereavement/Traumatic Grief	Psychiatry	Zisook, Sidney (MD)	688
Bile Duct Cancer	Surgery	Carey, Larry C (MD)	790
Biliary Disease	Gastroenterology	Cotton, Peter (MD)	227
Biliary Disease	Gastroenterology	Edmundowicz, Steven (MD)	231
Biliary Disease	Gastroenterology	Elta, Grace Helen (MD)	231
Biliary Surgery	Surgery	Ellison, Edwin Christopher (MD)	793
Biliary Surgery	Surgery	Hebert, James C (MD)	781
Biochemical Genetics	Clinical Genetics	Charrow, Joel (MD)	162
Biochemical Genetics	Clinical Genetics	Craigen, William (MD)	163
Biochemical Genetics	Clinical Genetics	Jonas, Adam Jonathan (MD)	165
Biochemical Genetics	Clinical Genetics	Northrup, Hope (MD)	163
Biomechanics-Arms	Hand Surgery	Trumble, Thomas (MD)	276
Biotechnology	Medical Oncology	Garnick, Marc Bennett (MD)	292
Bipolar/Mood Disorders	Psychiatry	Baldessarini, Ross (MD)	676
Bipolar/Mood Disorders	Psychiatry	Bowden, Charles (MD)	685
Bipolar/Mood Disorders	Psychiatry	Davidson, Joyce Eileen (MD)	684
Bipolar/Mood Disorders	Psychiatry	Dunner, David Louis (MD)	686
Bipolar/Mood Disorders	Psychiatry	Kupfer, David J. (MD)	679
Bipolar/Mood Disorders	Psychiatry	Reus, Victor Ivar (MD)	687
Birth Defects	Clinical Genetics	Carey, John (MD)	163
Birth Defects	Clinical Genetics	Cunniff, Christopher (MD)	163
Birth Defects	Clinical Genetics	Desposito, Franklin (MD)	160
Birth Defects	Clinical Genetics	Holmes, Lewis B (MD)	159
Birth Defects	Clinical Genetics	Rimoin, David L (MD/PhD)	165
Birth Defects	Clinical Genetics	Saul, Robert (MD)	161
Birth Defects	Clinical Genetics	Stevenson, Roger E (MD)	161
Birth Defects	Clinical Genetics	Willner, Judith P (MD)	160
Birth Defects-Cardiac	Pediatric Cardiology	Sodt, Peter (MD)	566
Birthmarks	Dermatology	Treadwell, Patricia (MD)	190
Bladder Cancer	Medical Oncology	Roth, Bruce Joseph (MD)	303
Bladder Cancer	Medical Oncology	Scher, Howard (MD)	299

Special Expertise	Specialty	Doctor's Name	Page
Bladder Cancer	Pathology	Cote, Richard (MD)	542
Bladder Cancer	Radiation Oncology	Shipley, William (MD)	717
Bladder Cancer	Urology	Danoff, Dudley S (MD)	848
Bladder Cancer	Urology	Flanigan, Robert (MD)	842
Bladder Cancer	Urology	Herr, Harry Wallace (MD)	832
Bladder Cancer	Urology	Klein, Eric A (MD)	842
Bladder Cancer	Urology	Miles, Brian J (MD)	846
Bladder Cancer	Urology	Montie, James (MD)	843
Bladder Cancer	Urology	Scardino, Peter (MD)	835
Bladder Cancer	Urology	Skinner, Donald George (MD)	850
Bladder Cancer	Urology	Smith, Joseph (MD)	839
Bladder Cancer	Urology	Soloway, Mark (MD)	839
Bladder Cancer	Urology	Williams, Richard D (MD)	844
Bladder Prolapse	Urology	Payne, Christopher K (MD)	849
Bladder Surgery	Urology	Kirschenbaum, Alexander M (MD)	833
Bladder/Prostate Cancer	Urology	Droller, Michael J (MD)	831
Bladder/Prostate Cancer	Urology	Huffman, Jeffry Lee (MD)	848
Bladder/Prostate Problems	Urology	Blaivas, Jerry G (MD)	831
Blastocyst Transfer	Reproductive Endocrinology	McClamrock, Howard Dean (MD)	744
Bleeding-Gastrointestinal	Gastroenterology	Cunningham, John (MD)	227
Bleeding/Coagulation Disorders	Hematology	Baron, Joseph M (MD)	288
Bleeding/Coagulation Disorders	Hematology	Blinder, Morey (MD)	288
Bleeding/Coagulation Disorders	Hematology	Bockenstedt, Paula (MD)	288
Bleeding/Coagulation Disorders	Hematology	Cobos, Everardo (MD)	290
Bleeding/Coagulation Disorders	Hematology	Coller, Barry (MD)	285
Bleeding/Coagulation Disorders	Hematology	Diuguid, David Lincoln (MD)	285
Bleeding/Coagulation Disorders	Hematology	Feinstein, Donald Ivan (MD)	291
Bleeding/Coagulation Disorders	Hematology	Green, David (MD)	289
Bleeding/Coagulation Disorders	Pathology	Kao, Kuo-Jang (MD/PhD)	539
Bleeding/Coagulation Disorders	Pediatric Hematology-Oncology	Bussel, James (MD)	583
Bleeding/Coagulation Disorders	Pediatric Hematology-Oncology	Castle, Valerie (MD)	586
Bleeding/Coagulation Disorders	Pediatric Hematology-Oncology	Pegelow Jr, Charles Henry (MD)	586
Bleeding/Coagulation Disorders	Pediatric Hematology-Oncology	Valentino, Leonard A (MD)	587
Blistering Diseases	Dermatology	Anhalt, Grant James (MD)	182
Blistering Diseases	Dermatology	Bystryn, Jean-Claude (MD)	183
Blistering Diseases	Dermatology	Fivenson, David (MD)	189
Blistering Diseases	Dermatology	Sobel, Stuart (MD)	188
Blistering Diseases	Dermatology	Stanley, John R (MD)	186
Bone Densitometry	Obstetrics & Gynecology	Scialli, Anthony R (MD)	433
Bone Disorders	Diagnostic Radiology	Dalinka, Murray (MD)	731
Bone Disorders-Metabolic	Endocrinology, Diabetes & Metabolism	Bockman, Richard (MD/PhD)	199
Bone Disorders-Metabolic	Endocrinology, Diabetes & Metabolism	Dalkin, Alan Craig (MD)	203
Bone Disorders-Metabolic	Endocrinology, Diabetes & Metabolism	Khosla, Sundeep (MD)	208
Bone Disorders-Metabolic	Endocrinology, Diabetes & Metabolism	Licata, Angelo A (MD)	208
Bone Disorders-Metabolic	Endocrinology, Diabetes & Metabolism	Mundy, Gregory Robert (MD)	210
Bone Disorders-Metabolic	Endocrinology, Diabetes & Metabolism	Sizemore, Glenn (MD)	209
Bone Disorders-Metabolic	Endocrinology, Diabetes & Metabolism	Watts, Nelson B (MD)	205
Bone Disorders-Metabolic	Geriatric Medicine	Lyles, Kenneth W (MD)	246
Bone Disorders-Metabolic	Orthopaedic Surgery	Rosier, Randy (MD/PhD)	483
Bone Disorders-Metabolic	Pediatric Endocrinology	Friedman, Nancy Eisenberg (MD)	574
Bone Marrow & Stem Cell Transplant	Medical Oncology	Ball, Edward David (MD)	313
Bone Marrow Pathology	Pathology	Schiller, Alan (MD)	538
Bone Marrow Transplant	Allergy & Immunology	Good, Robert (MD/PhD)	98
Bone Marrow Transplant	Hematology	Barlogie, Bartholomew (MD/PhD)	290
Bone Marrow Transplant	Hematology	Benz, Edward (MD)	285
Bone Marrow Transplant	Hematology	Bitran, Jacob (MD)	288
Bone Marrow Transplant	Hematology	Cobos, Everardo (MD)	290
Bone Marrow Transplant	Hematology	Litzow, Mark Robert (MD)	289
Bone Marrow Transplant	Hematology	Miller, Kenneth B. (MD)	285
Bone Marrow Transplant	Hematology	Schuster, Michael (MD)	286

SPECIAL EXPERTISE INDEX

Special Expertise	Specialty	Doctor's Name	Page
Bone Marrow Transplant	Hematology	Solberg, Lawrence (MD)	287
Bone Marrow Transplant	Hematology	Stiff, Patrick J (MD)	290
Bone Marrow Transplant	Hematology	Winter, Jane N. (MD)	290
Bone Marrow Transplant	Medical Oncology	Antin, Joseph Harry (MD)	292
Bone Marrow Transplant	Medical Oncology	Armitage, James (MD)	310
Bone Marrow Transplant	Medical Oncology	Davidson, Nancy E (MD)	295
Bone Marrow Transplant	Medical Oncology	Di Persio, John (MD/PhD)	306
Bone Marrow Transplant	Medical Oncology	Jillella, Anand (MD)	301
Bone Marrow Transplant	Medical Oncology	Livingston, Robert B (MD)	314
Bone Marrow Transplant	Medical Oncology	Press, Oliver William (MD/PhD)	314
Bone Marrow Transplant	Medical Oncology	Shea, Thomas (MD)	303
Bone Marrow Transplant	Medical Oncology	Wingard, John R (MD)	305
Bone Marrow Transplant	Pediatric Hematology-Oncology	Abella, Esteban (MD)	586
Bone Marrow Transplant	Pediatric Hematology-Oncology	Cairo, Mitchell (MD)	583
Bone Marrow Transplant	Pediatric Hematology-Oncology	Ferrara, James (MD)	587
Bone Marrow Transplant	Pediatric Hematology-Oncology	Kushner, Brian (MD)	584
Bone Marrow Transplant	Pediatric Hematology-Oncology	O'Reilly, Richard (MD)	584
Bone Marrow Transplant	Pediatric Hematology-Oncology	Weinstein, Howard (MD)	583
Bone Tumor Pathology	Pathology	Dorfman, Howard (MD)	536
Bone Tumor Pathology	Pathology	Unni, K Krishnan (MD)	540
Bone Tumors	Orthopaedic Surgery	Eckardt, Jeffrey J (MD)	497
Bone Tumors	Orthopaedic Surgery	Friedlaender, Gary (MD)	475
Bone Tumors	Orthopaedic Surgery	Gebhardt, Mark (MD)	475
Bone Tumors	Orthopaedic Surgery	Healey, John (MD)	481
Bone Tumors	Orthopaedic Surgery	Scarborough, Mark (MD)	487
Bone Tumors	Orthopaedic Surgery	Simon, Michael (MD)	492
Bone Tumors	Orthopaedic Surgery	Springfield, Dempsey (MD)	484
Bone Tumors	Pediatric Hematology-Oncology	Meyers, Paul (MD)	584
Bone-Calcium Problems	Endocrinology, Diabetes & Metabolism	Jacobs, Thomas (MD)	200
Bone/Bone Marrow Pathology	Pathology	Huvos, Andrew (MD)	536
Bone/Bone Marrow Pathology	Pathology	Knowles, Daniel (MD)	537
Bone/Joint Infections	Infectious Disease	Brause, Barry (MD)	318
Bone/Soft Tissue Disorders	Diagnostic Radiology	Panicek, David (MD)	732
Botox Therapy	Neurology	Sethi, Kapil (MD)	410
Botox Therapy	Neurology	Stern, Matthew (MD)	406
Botulinum Toxin Injections	Physical Medicine & Rehabilitation	Robinson, Lawrence (MD)	631
Brachial Plexus	Hand Surgery	Waters, Peter Michael (MD)	267
Brachial Plexus-Pediatric	Plastic Surgery	Nath, Rahul Kamur (MD)	650
Brachytherapy	Radiation Oncology	Anscher, Mitchell (MD)	721
Brachytherapy	Radiation Oncology	Ennis, Ronald (MD)	718
Brachytherapy	Radiation Oncology	Nori, Dattatreyudu (MD)	720
Brachytherapy Under MRI	Radiation Oncology	D'Amico, Anthony V (MD/PhD)	717
Brain & Spinal Cord Tumors	Neurological Surgery	Black, Peter (MD)	373
Brain & Spinal Cord Tumors	Neurological Surgery	Carson, Benjamin S (MD)	375
Brain & Spinal Cord Tumors	Neurological Surgery	Kobrine, Arthur (MD/PhD)	377
Brain & Spinal Cord Tumors	Neurological Surgery	Piepmeier, Joseph (MD)	374
Brain & Spinal Cord Tumors	Pediatric Hematology-Oncology	Bleyer, W Archie (MD)	588
Brain & Spinal Cord Tumors-Pediatric	Neurological Surgery	O'Brien, Mark S. (MD)	381
Brain & Spinal Surgery	Neurological Surgery	Dennis, Gary Creed (MD)	375
Brain & Spinal Surgery	Neurological Surgery	Hoff, Julian T (MD)	383
Brain Cancer	Nuclear Medicine	Alavi, Abass (MD)	425
Brain Cancer	Radiation Oncology	Selch, Michael T (MD)	727
Brain Hemorrage	Neurological Surgery	Atkinson, John (MD)	382
Brain Infections	Pathology	Bollen, Andrew W (MD)	542
Brain Infections	Pediatric Infectious Disease	Bradley, John S (MD)	594
Brain Injury	Neurological Surgery	Carson, Benjamin S (MD)	375
Brain Injury	Neurology	Cilo, Mark P (MD)	416
Brain Injury Rehabilitation	Physical Medicine & Rehabilitation	Ivanhoe, Cindy (MD)	629
Brain Injury Rehabilitation	Physical Medicine & Rehabilitation	Matthews, Dennis Jerome (MD)	628
Brain Injury Rehabilitation	Physical Medicine & Rehabilitation	Zafonte, Ross (DO)	625

Special Expertise	Specialty	Doctor's Name	Page
Brain Stem Tumors-Pediatric	Neurological Surgery	Epstein, Fred Jacob (MD)	376
Brain Tumors	Child Neurology	Packer, Roger (MD)	153
Brain Tumors	Neurological Surgery	Albright, Leland (MD)	374
Brain Tumors	Neurological Surgery	Barnett, Gene H (MD)	382
Brain Tumors	Neurological Surgery	Bauer, Jerry (MD)	382
Brain Tumors	Neurological Surgery	Chandler, William F (MD)	382
Brain Tumors	Neurological Surgery	Cosgrove, G. Rees (MD)	373
Brain Tumors	Neurological Surgery	Ferraz, Francisco M (MD)	379
Brain Tumors	Neurological Surgery	Friedman, William A (MD)	380
Brain Tumors	Neurological Surgery	Germano, Isabelle M (MD)	376
Brain Tumors	Neurological Surgery	Grubb, Robert (MD)	383
Brain Tumors	Neurological Surgery	Gutierrez, Francisco A (MD)	383
Brain Tumors	Neurological Surgery	Hankinson, Hal L. (MD)	386
Brain Tumors	Neurological Surgery	Hekmatpanah, Javad (MD)	383
Brain Tumors	Neurological Surgery	Kelly, Patrick J. (MD)	377
Brain Tumors	Neurological Surgery	Kranzler, Leonard I (MD)	383
Brain Tumors	Neurological Surgery	Levy, Robert M (MD)	384
Brain Tumors	Neurological Surgery	Mangiardi, John (MD)	377
Brain Tumors	Neurological Surgery	Marion, Donald W (MD)	378
Brain Tumors	Neurological Surgery	Ojemann, Robert G. (MD)	373
Brain Tumors	Neurological Surgery	Pollack, Ian (MD)	378
Brain Tumors	Neurological Surgery	Rosenblum, Mark (MD)	385
Brain Tumors	Neurological Surgery	Ruge, John (MD)	385
Brain Tumors	Neurological Surgery	Scott, R. Michael (MD)	374
Brain Tumors	Neurological Surgery	Walker, Marion L. (MD)	386
Brain Tumors	Neurological Surgery	Weiss, Martin Harvey (MD)	390
Brain Tumors	Neurological Surgery	Wilson, Charles B (MD)	390
Brain Tumors	Neurology	Greenberg, Harry S. (MD)	413
Brain Tumors	Neurology	Hochberg, Fred (MD)	398
Brain Tumors	Neurology	Levin, Victor Alan (MD)	418
Brain Tumors	Neurology	Posner, Jerome (MD)	405
Brain Tumors	Neurology	Schold Jr., S. Clifford (MD)	405
Brain Tumors	Pathology	Bollen, Andrew W (MD)	542
Brain Tumors	Pathology	Burger, Peter (MD)	536
Brain Tumors	Pathology	Davis, Richard L (MD)	542
Brain Tumors	Pathology	Scheithauer, Bernd (MD)	540
Brain Tumors	Pediatric Hematology-Oncology	Puccetti, Diane (MD)	587
Brain Tumors	Pediatric Hematology-Oncology	Siegel, Stuart E (MD)	589
Brain Tumors	Radiation Oncology	Curran Jr, Walter J (MD)	718
Brain Tumors	Radiation Oncology	Herman, Terence Spencer (MD)	725
Brain Tumors	Radiation Oncology	Isaacson, Steven (MD)	719
Brain Tumors	Radiation Oncology	Kinsella, Timothy James (MD)	723
Brain Tumors	Radiation Oncology	Leibel, Steven A (MD)	719
Brain Tumors	Radiation Oncology	Loeffler, Jay Steven (MD)	717
Brain Tumors	Radiation Oncology	Mandell, Lynda (MD/PhD)	720
Brain Tumors	Radiation Oncology	Pollack, Jed (MD)	720
Brain Tumors	Radiation Oncology	Shaw, Edward Gus (MD)	722
Brain Tumors & Hemifacial Spasms	Neurological Surgery	Harper, Richard L (MD)	387
Brain Tumors-Adult & Pedatric	Neurological Surgery	Berger, Mitchel Stuart (MD)	388
Brain Tumors-Pediatric	Neurological Surgery	Carmel, Peter (MD)	375
Brain/Skull Base Tumors	Neurological Surgery	Sekhar, Laligam N (MD)	381
Brain/Spinal Cord Injury	Physical Medicine & Rehabilitation	Jaffe, Kenneth M (MD)	630
Brain/Stroke-MRI	Radiology	Atlas, Scott W (MD)	739
Breast & Esophageal Cancer	Medical Oncology	Mortimer, Joanne (MD)	307
Breast & Lung Cancer	Radiation Oncology	Halle, Jan (MD)	721
Breast Augmentation	Plastic Surgery	Horowitz, Jed H (MD)	652
Breast Augmentation	Plastic Surgery	Meltzer, Toby R (MD)	653
Breast Augmentation	Plastic Surgery	Tebbetts, John B (MD)	650
Breast Augmentation	Plastic Surgery	Young, Vernon Leroy (MD)	647
Breast Cancer	Diagnostic Radiology	Edelstein, Barbara A (MD)	731

SPECIAL EXPERTISE INDEX

Special Expertise	Specialty	Doctor's Name	Page
Breast Cancer	Diagnostic Radiology	Mitnick, Julie (MD)	732
Breast Cancer	Gynecologic Oncology	Fiorica, James Vincent (MD)	258
Breast Cancer	Hematology	Bitran, Jacob (MD)	288
Breast Cancer	Medical Oncology	Abeloff, Martin (MD)	294
Breast Cancer	Medical Oncology	Albain, Kathy (MD)	305
Breast Cancer	Medical Oncology	Anderson, Joseph (MD)	305
Breast Cancer	Medical Oncology	Antman, Karen (MD)	294
Breast Cancer	Medical Oncology	Baker, Laurence H (DO)	305
Breast Cancer	Medical Oncology	Balducci, Lodovico (MD)	300
Breast Cancer	Medical Oncology	Canellos, George Peter (MD)	292
Breast Cancer	Medical Oncology	Carlson, Robert Wells (MD)	313
Breast Cancer	Medical Oncology	Chlebowski, Rowan Thomas (MD)	313
Breast Cancer	Medical Oncology	Cohen, Seymour (MD)	295
Breast Cancer	Medical Oncology	Come, Steven Eliot (MD)	292
Breast Cancer	Medical Oncology	Davidson, Nancy E (MD)	295
Breast Cancer	Medical Oncology	Fabian, Carol J (MD)	310
Breast Cancer	Medical Oncology	Ganz, Patricia Anne (MD)	313
Breast Cancer	Medical Oncology	Garber, Judy E (MD)	292
Breast Cancer	Medical Oncology	Glick, John H (MD)	296
Breast Cancer	Medical Oncology	Goldstein, Lori J (MD)	296
Breast Cancer	Medical Oncology	Graham, Mark (MD)	300
Breast Cancer	Medical Oncology	Hait, William (MD/PhD)	296
Breast Cancer	Medical Oncology	Hande, Kenneth (MD)	301
Breast Cancer	Medical Oncology	Hayes, Daniel Fleming (MD)	297
Breast Cancer	Medical Oncology	Holland, James F (MD)	297
Breast Cancer	Medical Oncology	Horton, John (MD)	301
Breast Cancer	Medical Oncology	Hutchins, Laura (MD)	311
Breast Cancer	Medical Oncology	Ingle, James N (MD)	306
Breast Cancer	Medical Oncology	Jones, Stephen E (MD)	311
Breast Cancer	Medical Oncology	Kosova, Leonard (MD)	307
Breast Cancer	Medical Oncology	Legha, Sewa Singh (MD)	312
Breast Cancer	Medical Oncology	Levine, Ellis (MD)	298
Breast Cancer	Medical Oncology	Lippman, Marc E (MD)	307
Breast Cancer	Medical Oncology	Livingston, Philip (MD)	298
Breast Cancer	Medical Oncology	Livingston, Robert B (MD)	314
Breast Cancer	Medical Oncology	Moore, Anne (MD)	298
Breast Cancer	Medical Oncology	Muss, Hyman (MD)	293
Breast Cancer	Medical Oncology	Nissenblatt, Michael (MD)	299
Breast Cancer	Medical Oncology	Norton, Larry (MD)	299
Breast Cancer	Medical Oncology	Olopade, Olufunmilayo I F (MD)	307
Breast Cancer	Medical Oncology	Osborne, Charles Kent (MD)	312
Breast Cancer	Medical Oncology	Oster, Martin (MD)	299
Breast Cancer	Medical Oncology	Peters, William P (MD/PhD)	308
Breast Cancer	Medical Oncology	Robert, Nicholas J (MD)	303
Breast Cancer	Medical Oncology	Rosen, Steven T (MD)	308
Breast Cancer	Medical Oncology	Salem, Philip Adeeb (MD)	312
Breast Cancer	Medical Oncology	Schwartz, Burton (MD)	309
Breast Cancer	Medical Oncology	Shapiro, Charles L (MD)	309
Breast Cancer	Medical Oncology	Sledge Jr, George W (MD)	309
Breast Cancer	Medical Oncology	Smith, Thomas Joseph (MD)	304
Breast Cancer	Medical Oncology	Speyer, James (MD)	299
Breast Cancer	Medical Oncology	Stone, Joel (MD)	304
Breast Cancer	Medical Oncology	Valero, Vicente (MD)	312
Breast Cancer	Medical Oncology	Weber, Barbara L (MD)	300
Breast Cancer	Medical Oncology	Wicha, Max S (MD)	310
Breast Cancer	Medical Oncology	Winer, Eric P (MD)	293
Breast Cancer	Nuclear Medicine	Podoloff, Donald (MD)	427
Breast Cancer	Pathology	Carter, Darryl (MD)	535
Breast Cancer	Pathology	Page, David L (MD)	540
Breast Cancer	Pathology	Sanchez, Miguel (MD)	538

SPECIAL EXPERTISE INDEX

Special Expertise	Specialty	Doctor's Name	Page
Breast Cancer	Pathology	Turner, Roderick Randolph (MD)	543
Breast Cancer	Pathology	Woodruff, James M. (MD)	538
Breast Cancer	Radiation Oncology	Berg, Christine Dorothy (MD)	718
Breast Cancer	Radiation Oncology	Ferree, Carolyn Ruth Black (MD)	721
Breast Cancer	Radiation Oncology	Fowble, Barbara (MD)	719
Breast Cancer	Radiation Oncology	Goffinet, Don R (MD)	726
Breast Cancer	Radiation Oncology	Goodman, Robert L (MD)	719
Breast Cancer	Radiation Oncology	Haffty, Bruce (MD)	717
Breast Cancer	Radiation Oncology	Harris, Jay R (MD)	717
Breast Cancer	Radiation Oncology	Herman, Terence Spencer (MD)	725
Breast Cancer	Radiation Oncology	Juillard, Guy Jean-Felix (MD)	726
Breast Cancer	Radiation Oncology	Lichter, Allen (MD)	723
Breast Cancer	Radiation Oncology	Marks, Lawrence (MD)	721
Breast Cancer	Radiation Oncology	McCormick, Beryl (MD)	720
Breast Cancer	Radiation Oncology	McNeese, Marsha (MD)	725
Breast Cancer	Radiation Oncology	Mendenhall, Nancy P (MD)	722
Breast Cancer	Radiation Oncology	Perez, Carlos A (MD)	724
Breast Cancer	Radiation Oncology	Pierce, Lori J (MD)	724
Breast Cancer	Radiation Oncology	Prosnitz, Leonard (MD)	722
Breast Cancer	Radiation Oncology	Recht, Abram (MD)	717
Breast Cancer	Radiation Oncology	Rosenman, Julian (MD)	722
Breast Cancer	Radiation Oncology	Shank, Brenda (MD/PhD)	727
Breast Cancer	Radiation Oncology	Solin, Lawrence (MD)	721
Breast Cancer	Radiation Oncology	Strom, Eric Alan (MD)	726
Breast Cancer	Radiation Oncology	Taylor, Marie E (MD)	724
Breast Cancer	Radiation Oncology	Vicini, Frank A (MD)	724
Breast Cancer	Radiation Oncology	Wazer, David E (MD)	718
Breast Cancer	Radiation Oncology	Wilson, J Frank (MD)	724
Breast Cancer	Radiology	Dershaw, D David (MD)	735
Breast Cancer	Surgery	Alfonso, Antonio (MD)	783
Breast Cancer	Surgery	Ashikari, Roy (MD)	783
Breast Cancer	Surgery	Axelrod, Deborah (MD)	783
Breast Cancer	Surgery	Beauchamp, Robert Daniel (MD)	789
Breast Cancer	Surgery	Bland, Kirby (MD)	789
Breast Cancer	Surgery	Borgen, Patrick Ivan (MD)	784
Breast Cancer	Surgery	Byrd, David (MD)	799
Breast Cancer	Surgery	Cady, Blake (MD)	781
Breast Cancer	Surgery	Copeland lll, Edward M (MD)	790
Breast Cancer	Surgery	Crowe, Joseph (MD)	793
Breast Cancer	Surgery	Dooley, William Chesnut (MD)	785
Breast Cancer	Surgery	Eberlein, Timothy J (MD)	793
Breast Cancer	Surgery	Edge, Stephen B (MD)	785
Breast Cancer	Surgery	Estabrook, Alison (MD)	785
Breast Cancer	Surgery	Giuliano, Armando E (MD)	800
Breast Cancer	Surgery	Hansen, Nora Marie (MD)	800
Breast Cancer	Surgery	Kinne, David W (MD)	786
Breast Cancer	Surgery	Klimberg, V Suzanne (MD)	798
Breast Cancer	Surgery	Knudson, Mary Margaret (MD)	800
Breast Cancer	Surgery	Leffall Jr, LaSalle D (MD)	786
Breast Cancer	Surgery	Morrow, Monica (MD)	794
Breast Cancer	Surgery	Numann, Patricia (MD)	787
Breast Cancer	Surgery	Osteen, Robert T (MD)	782
Breast Cancer	Surgery	Pachter, H Leon (MD)	787
Breast Cancer	Surgery	Petrek, Jeanne (MD)	787
Breast Cancer	Surgery	Roses, Daniel F (MD)	787
Breast Cancer	Surgery	Ross, Merrick I (MD)	798
Breast Cancer	Surgery	Schnabel, Freya (MD)	788
Breast Cancer	Surgery	Silverstein, Melvin J (MD)	801
Breast Cancer	Surgery	Singletary, S Eva (MD)	798
Breast Cancer	Surgery	Smith, Barbara Lynn (MD)	782

SPECIAL EXPERTISE INDEX

Special Expertise	Specialty	Doctor's Name	Page
Breast Cancer	Surgery	Urist, Marshall (MD)	792
Breast Cancer	Surgery	Ward, Barbara (MD)	783
Breast Cancer-Sentinel Node	Surgery	Reintgen, Douglas Scott (MD)	792
Breast Cosmetic Surgery	Plastic Surgery	Mustoe, Thomas (MD)	646
Breast Imaging	Diagnostic Radiology	Kopans, Daniel B (MD)	731
Breast Imaging	Diagnostic Radiology	Pisano, Etta Driscoll (MD)	733
Breast Imaging	Nuclear Medicine	Scheff, Alice M (MD)	427
Breast Pathology	Pathology	Connolly, James Leo (MD)	535
Breast Pathology	Pathology	Kempson, Richard (MD)	543
Breast Pathology	Pathology	Mills, Stacey E (MD)	539
Breast Pathology	Pathology	Rosen, Paul Peter (MD)	538
Breast Pathology	Pathology	Schnitt, Stuart (MD)	536
Breast Pathology	Pathology	Young, Robert Henry (MD)	536
Breast Reconstruction	Plastic Surgery	Bostwick III, John J (MD)	641
Breast Reconstruction	Plastic Surgery	Bucky, Louis P (MD)	637
Breast Reconstruction	Plastic Surgery	Fisher, Jack (MD)	642
Breast Reconstruction	Plastic Surgery	Fix, R Jobe (MD)	642
Breast Reconstruction	Plastic Surgery	Georgiade, Gregory (MD)	642
Breast Reconstruction	Plastic Surgery	Hidalgo, David (MD)	637
Breast Reconstruction	Plastic Surgery	Hoffman, Lloyd (MD)	638
Breast Reconstruction	Plastic Surgery	Kroll, Stephen S (MD)	649
Breast Reconstruction	Plastic Surgery	Mathes, Stephen (MD)	653
Breast Reconstruction	Plastic Surgery	Maxwell, G Patrick (MD)	644
Breast Reconstruction	Plastic Surgery	May Jr, James W (MD)	635
Breast Reconstruction	Plastic Surgery	Mullin, Walter (MD)	644
Breast Reconstruction	Plastic Surgery	Schusterman, Mark A (MD)	650
Breast Reconstruction	Plastic Surgery	Sherman, Randolph (MD)	655
Breast Reconstruction	Plastic Surgery	Spear, Scott L (MD)	639
Breast Reconstruction	Plastic Surgery	Sultan, Mark (MD)	640
Breast Reconstruction	Plastic Surgery	Vasconez, Luis O (MD)	645
Breast Reconstruction	Plastic Surgery	Walton, Robert Lee (MD)	647
Breast Reconstruction	Surgery	Singletary, S Eva (MD)	798
Breast Reconstruction & Augmentation	Plastic Surgery	Eriksson, Elof (MD)	635
Breast Surgery	Plastic Surgery	Baker Jr, Thomas J (MD)	641
Breast Surgery	Plastic Surgery	Beasley, Michael (MD)	641
Breast Surgery	Plastic Surgery	Hammond, Dennis (MD)	646
Breast Surgery	Plastic Surgery	Kelly, John Michael (MD)	649
Breast Surgery	Plastic Surgery	Mladick, Richard (MD)	644
Breast Surgery	Plastic Surgery	Puckett, Charles Linwood (MD)	647
Breast Surgery	Plastic Surgery	Rand, Richard Pierce (MD)	654
Breast Surgery	Plastic Surgery	Shaw, William Wei-Lien (MD)	655
Breast Surgery	Plastic Surgery	Stuzin, James M (MD)	645
Breast Surgery	Plastic Surgery	Wells, James H (MD)	655
Breast Surgery	Plastic Surgery	Zarem, Harvey Alan (MD)	655
Breast Surgery	Surgery	Hanks, John B (MD)	791
Breathing Disorders	Neonatal-Perinatal Medicine	Lawson, Edward Earle (MD)	352
Breech Birth	Maternal & Fetal Medicine	Collea, Joseph Vincent (MD)	342
Bronchitis	Pulmonary Disease	Boushey Jr, Homer A (MD)	710
Bronchitis	Pulmonary Disease	King Jr, Talmadge Everett (MD)	711
Bronchopulmonary Dysplasia	Pediatric Pulmonology	Kim, Young-Jee (MD)	605
Bronchopulmonary Dysplasia	Pediatric Pulmonology	Murphy, Thomas M (MD)	604
Bronchoscopy	Pulmonary Disease	Prakash, Udaya (MD)	705
Burkett's Lymphoma	Pediatric Hematology-Oncology	Steinherz, Peter G (MD)	585
Burns	Physical Medicine & Rehabilitation	Sisung, Charles (MD)	628
Burns	Plastic Surgery	Cruse, C Wayne (MD)	642
Burns	Plastic Surgery	Hoffman, Lloyd (MD)	638
Burns	Plastic Surgery	Jewell, Mark L (MD)	652
Burns	Plastic Surgery	Krizek, Thomas (MD)	643
Burns	Plastic Surgery	Molnar, Joseph (MD)	644
Burns	Surgery	Gamelli, Richard Louis (MD)	793

Special Expertise	Specialty	Doctor's Name	Page
Burns	Surgery	Griswold, John A (MD)	797
Burns	Surgery	Hoyt, David (MD)	800
Burns	Surgery	Luterman, Arnold (MD)	791
Burns	Surgery	Saffle, Jeffrey (MD)	796
Burns	Surgery	Yurt, Roger (MD)	789
Bypass Surgery-High Risk	Thoracic Surgery	Gardner, Timothy Joseph (MD)	808

C

Special Expertise	Specialty	Doctor's Name	Page
Calcium Disorders	Endocrinology, Diabetes & Metabolism	Mandel, Susan (MD)	201
Calcium Disorders	Pediatric Endocrinology	Friedman, Nancy Eisenberg (MD)	574
Cancer & General Surgery	Pediatric Surgery	Ziegler, Moritz M (MD)	611
Cancer & Infections	Pediatric Hematology-Oncology	Siegel, Stuart E (MD)	589
Cancer Detection & Staging	Nuclear Medicine	Siegel, Barry (MD)	427
Cancer Prevention	Medical Oncology	Ganz, Patricia Anne (MD)	313
Cancer Reconstruction	Plastic Surgery	Coleman, John (MD)	646
Cancer Reconstruction	Plastic Surgery	Kroll, Stephen S (MD)	649
Cancer Resch & Prevention	Thoracic Surgery	Morton, Donald Lee (MD)	825
Cancer Surgery	Pediatric Surgery	Grosfeld, Jay L (MD)	615
Cancer Surgery	Pediatric Surgery	LaQuaglia, Michael (MD)	612
Cancer Surgery	Pediatric Surgery	Wiener, Eugene (MD)	613
Cancer Surgery	Surgery	Bland, Kirby (MD)	789
Cancer Surgery	Surgery	Salem, Ronald (MD)	782
Cancer Surgery	Surgery	Urist, Marshall (MD)	792
Cancer Survivors	Pediatric Hematology-Oncology	Rosoff, Phillip Martin (MD)	586
Cancer-Hormonal Influences	Endocrinology, Diabetes & Metabolism	Earp III, Henry Shelton (MD)	203
Cancer-Pediatric	Radiation Oncology	Selch, Michael T (MD)	727
Carcinoid Tumors	Medical Oncology	Grosh, William W (MD)	301
Cardiac Catheter Ablation	Cardiac Electrophysiology	Wilber, David James (MD)	118
Cardiac Catheterization	Cardiology (Cardiovascular Disease)	Ambrose, John (MD)	123
Cardiac Catheterization	Cardiology (Cardiovascular Disease)	Behar, Victor Samuel (MD)	129
Cardiac Catheterization	Cardiology (Cardiovascular Disease)	Clements, Stephen (MD)	130
Cardiac Catheterization	Cardiology (Cardiovascular Disease)	Coppola, John (MD)	125
Cardiac Catheterization	Cardiology (Cardiovascular Disease)	Criley, John Michael (MD)	141
Cardiac Catheterization	Cardiology (Cardiovascular Disease)	Garcia-Gonzalez, Efrain (MD)	139
Cardiac Catheterization	Cardiology (Cardiovascular Disease)	Gulotta, Stephen J (MD)	126
Cardiac Catheterization	Cardiology (Cardiovascular Disease)	Isner, Jeffrey Michael (MD)	121
Cardiac Catheterization	Cardiology (Cardiovascular Disease)	Margolis, James (MD)	131
Cardiac Catheterization	Cardiology (Cardiovascular Disease)	Phillips III, Harry Rissler (MD)	132
Cardiac Catheterization	Cardiology (Cardiovascular Disease)	Sacchi, Terrence J (MD)	127
Cardiac Catheterization	Cardiology (Cardiovascular Disease)	Schwartz, Allan (MD)	128
Cardiac Catheterization	Cardiology (Cardiovascular Disease)	Shani, Jacob (MD)	128
Cardiac Catheterization	Interventional Cardiology	Applegate, Robert Joseph (MD)	144
Cardiac Catheterization	Interventional Cardiology	Braden, Gregory Alan (MD)	145
Cardiac Catheterization	Interventional Cardiology	Clark, Vivian (MD)	145
Cardiac Catheterization	Interventional Cardiology	Jacobs, Alice K (MD)	144
Cardiac Catheterization	Pediatric Cardiology	Boucek, Mark M. (MD)	566
Cardiac Catheterization	Pediatric Cardiology	O'Laughlin, Martin P (MD)	563
Cardiac Catheterization	Pediatric Cardiology	Takahashi, Masato (MD)	567
Cardiac Catheterization/Angioplasty	Cardiology (Cardiovascular Disease)	Kirshenbaum, James M (MD)	121
Cardiac Disease	Pediatric Cardiology	Teitel, David F (MD)	568
Cardiac Electrophysiology	Cardiology (Cardiovascular Disease)	Batsford, William P (MD)	120
Cardiac Electrophysiology	Cardiology (Cardiovascular Disease)	Grubb, Blair Paul (MD)	135
Cardiac Electrophysiology	Cardiology (Cardiovascular Disease)	Josephson, Mark Eric (MD)	121
Cardiac Electrophysiology	Cardiology (Cardiovascular Disease)	Myerburg, Robert (MD)	131
Cardiac Electrophysiology	Cardiology (Cardiovascular Disease)	Naccarelli, Gerald V (MD)	127
Cardiac Electrophysiology	Pediatric Cardiology	Walsh, Edward Patrick (MD)	561
Cardiac Electrophysiology	Pediatric Cardiology	Wolff, Grace Susan (MD)	563
Cardiac Electrophysiology	Pediatric Cardiology	Young, Ming-Lon (MD)	564
Cardiac Imaging	Cardiology (Cardiovascular Disease)	Cerqueira, Manuel (MD)	124

SPECIAL EXPERTISE INDEX

Special Expertise	Specialty	Doctor's Name	Page
Cardiac Imaging	Nuclear Medicine	Sandler, Martin P (MD)	427
Cardiac Pathology	Pathology	Mark, Eugene J. (MD)	535
Cardiac Pathology	Pathology	Roberts, William (MD)	541
Cardiac Rehabilitation	Cardiology (Cardiovascular Disease)	Vander Laan, Ronald Lee (MD)	138
Cardiac Respiratory Problems	Pulmonary Disease	Irwin, Richard Stephen (MD)	691
Cardiac Surgery	Pediatric Surgery	Mayer, John (MD)	611
Cardiac Surgery	Pediatric Surgery	Quaegebeur, Jan Modest (MD)	612
Cardiac Surgery	Pediatric Surgery	Spray, Thomas L (MD)	612
Cardiac Surgery	Thoracic Surgery	DeCamp Jr, Malcolm M (MD)	816
Cardiac Surgery	Thoracic Surgery	Glassford Jr, David M (MD)	812
Cardiac Surgery	Thoracic Surgery	Hammon Jr, John W (MD)	813
Cardiac Surgery	Thoracic Surgery	Isom, O Wayne (MD)	809
Cardiac Surgery	Thoracic Surgery	Kay, Jerome Harold (MD)	824
Cardiac Surgery	Thoracic Surgery	McGregor, Christopher (MD)	818
Cardiac Surgery	Thoracic Surgery	Mindich, Bruce (MD)	810
Cardiac Surgery	Thoracic Surgery	Pacifico, Albert D (MD)	814
Cardiac Surgery	Thoracic Surgery	Stuart, Richard Scott (MD)	811
Cardiac Surgery	Thoracic Surgery	Tedder, Mark (MD)	815
Cardiac Surgery	Thoracic Surgery	Turner, William F (MD)	822
Cardiac Surgery	Thoracic Surgery	Williams, Donald B (MD)	815
Cardiac Surgery-Adult	Thoracic Surgery	Doty, Donald B. (MD)	820
Cardiac Surgery-Adult	Thoracic Surgery	Guyton, Robert A (MD)	813
Cardiac Surgery-Adult	Thoracic Surgery	Perryman, Richard A (MD)	814
Cardiac Surgery-Adult & Pediatric	Thoracic Surgery	Alexander, James A (MD)	812
Cardiac Surgery-Adult & Pediatric	Thoracic Surgery	Brown, John W (MD)	816
Cardiac Surgery-Adult & Pediatric	Thoracic Surgery	Gundry, Steven (MD)	823
Cardiac Surgery-Adult & Pediatric	Thoracic Surgery	Kirklin, James (MD)	813
Cardiac Surgery-Adult & Pediatric	Thoracic Surgery	Kopf, Gary (MD)	805
Cardiac Surgery-Adult & Pediatric	Thoracic Surgery	Merrill, Walter H (MD)	813
Cardiac Surgery-Adult & Pediatric	Thoracic Surgery	Perryman, Richard A (MD)	814
Cardiac Surgery-Adult & Pediatric	Thoracic Surgery	Starnes, Vaughn Alden (MD)	825
Cardiac Surgery-Adult & Pediatric	Thoracic Surgery	Trento, Alfredo (MD)	825
Cardiac Surgery-Adult & Pediatric	Thoracic Surgery	Ungerleider, Ross M (MD)	815
Cardiac Surgery-High Risk	Thoracic Surgery	Furukawa, Satoshi (MD)	808
Cardiac Surgery-Pediatric	Thoracic Surgery	Fontana, Gregory (MD)	823
Cardiac Surgery-Pediatric	Thoracic Surgery	Jonas, Richard A (MD)	805
Cardiac Surgery-Pediatric	Thoracic Surgery	Turrentine, Mark W (MD)	820
Cardiology	Nuclear Medicine	Schelbert, Heinrich R (MD/PhD)	428
Cardiology Research	Cardiology (Cardiovascular Disease)	Braunwald, Eugene (MD)	120
Cardiology-Geriatric	Cardiology (Cardiovascular Disease)	Herling, Irving M (MD)	126
Cardiology-Pediatric	Cardiology (Cardiovascular Disease)	Seward, James Bernard (MD)	137
Cardiomyopathy	Cardiology (Cardiovascular Disease)	Baughman, Kenneth (MD)	124
Cardiomyopathy	Pediatric Cardiology	Bernstein, Daniel (MD)	567
Cardiomyopathy	Pediatric Cardiology	Boucek, Robert (MD)	562
Cardiomyopathy	Pediatric Cardiology	Cutilletta , Anthony F (MD)	564
Cardiomyopathy	Pediatric Cardiology	Driscoll, David J (MD)	564
Cardiothoracic Surgery	Pediatric Surgery	Bove, Edward (MD)	614
Cardiothoracic Surgery	Pediatric Surgery	Oldham, Keith T (MD)	615
Cardiothoracic Surgery	Thoracic Surgery	Acinapura, Anthony (MD)	807
Cardiothoracic Surgery	Thoracic Surgery	Bains, Manjit (MD)	807
Cardiothoracic Surgery	Thoracic Surgery	Behrendt, Douglas M. (MD)	815
Cardiothoracic Surgery	Thoracic Surgery	Bolman III, Ralph Morton (MD)	816
Cardiothoracic Surgery	Thoracic Surgery	Frederiksen, James W (MD)	817
Cardiothoracic Surgery	Thoracic Surgery	Merrill, Walter H (MD)	813
Cardiothoracic Surgery	Thoracic Surgery	Orringer, Mark B (MD)	818
Cardiothoracic Surgery	Thoracic Surgery	Pass, Harvey (MD)	819
Cardiothoracic Surgery	Thoracic Surgery	Rose, Eric A (MD)	810
Cardiothoracic Surgery	Thoracic Surgery	Sundt III, Thoralf Mauritz (MD)	820
Cardiothoracic Surgery	Thoracic Surgery	Wilcox, Benson (MD)	815
Cardiovascular Disease	Geriatric Medicine	Minaker, Kenneth (MD)	243

Special Expertise	Specialty	Doctor's Name	Page
Cardiovascular Disease-Pregnancy	Maternal & Fetal Medicine	Hibbard, Judith (MD)	345
Cardiovascular Imaging-Non-Invasive	Cardiology (Cardiovascular Disease)	Schnittger, Ingela (MD)	143
Cardiovascular Intervention Radiology	Diagnostic Radiology	Gomes, Antoinette Susan (MD)	734
Cardiovascular Surgery	Thoracic Surgery	Quintessenza, James (MD)	814
Cardiovascular Surgery	Thoracic Surgery	Vander Salm, Thomas (MD)	806
Cardiovascular Surgery	Vascular Surgery (General)	Benvenisty, Alan I (MD)	859
Carotid Angioplasty	Vascular Surgery (General)	Hodgson, Kim John (MD)	866
Carotid Artery Disease	Neurological Surgery	Day, Arthur L (MD)	379
Carotid Artery Disease	Neurological Surgery	Diaz, Fernando G (MD)	383
Carotid Artery Disease	Neurological Surgery	Stieg, Philip E (MD/PhD)	379
Carotid Artery Disease	Neurology	Goldstein, Larry Bruce (MD)	408
Carotid Artery Surgery	Vascular Surgery (General)	Adelman, Mark (MD)	858
Carotid Artery Surgery	Vascular Surgery (General)	Andros, George (MD)	868
Carotid Artery Surgery	Vascular Surgery (General)	Ascher, Enrico (MD)	858
Carotid Artery Surgery	Vascular Surgery (General)	Baker, William (MD)	864
Carotid Artery Surgery	Vascular Surgery (General)	Belkin, Michael (MD)	857
Carotid Artery Surgery	Vascular Surgery (General)	Cohen, Jon (MD)	859
Carotid Artery Surgery	Vascular Surgery (General)	Darling, Ralph Clement (MD)	860
Carotid Artery Surgery	Vascular Surgery (General)	Flynn, Timothy Carlyle (MD)	863
Carotid Artery Surgery	Vascular Surgery (General)	Gewertz, Bruce (MD)	865
Carotid Artery Surgery	Vascular Surgery (General)	Green, Richard (MD)	860
Carotid Artery Surgery	Vascular Surgery (General)	Greenfield, Lazar (MD)	865
Carotid Artery Surgery	Vascular Surgery (General)	Hansen, Kimberley J (MD)	863
Carotid Artery Surgery	Vascular Surgery (General)	Harrington, Elizabeth (MD)	860
Carotid Artery Surgery	Vascular Surgery (General)	Hertzer, Norman Ray (MD)	865
Carotid Artery Surgery	Vascular Surgery (General)	Hollier, Larry Harold (MD)	860
Carotid Artery Surgery	Vascular Surgery (General)	Mackey, William C. (MD)	858
Carotid Artery Surgery	Vascular Surgery (General)	Moore, Wesley Sanford (MD)	869
Carotid Artery Surgery	Vascular Surgery (General)	Pearce, William (MD)	866
Carotid Artery Surgery	Vascular Surgery (General)	Perler, Bruce Alan (MD)	861
Carotid Artery Surgery	Vascular Surgery (General)	Porter, John M. (MD)	869
Carotid Artery Surgery	Vascular Surgery (General)	Reddy, Daniel (MD)	866
Carotid Artery Surgery	Vascular Surgery (General)	Ricotta, John (MD)	861
Carotid Artery Surgery	Vascular Surgery (General)	Riles, Thomas (MD)	861
Carotid Artery Surgery	Vascular Surgery (General)	Shah, Dhiraj (MD)	861
Carotid Artery Surgery	Vascular Surgery (General)	Sobel, Michael (MD)	861
Carotid Artery Surgery	Vascular Surgery (General)	Todd, George (MD)	862
Carotid Artery Surgery	Vascular Surgery (General)	Whittemore, Anthony D (MD)	858
Carotid Artery Surgery	Vascular Surgery (General)	Zarins, Christopher Kristaps (MD)	870
Carotid Artery,Gamma Knife Surgery	Neurological Surgery	Loftus, Christopher M. (MD)	387
Carpal Tunnel Syndrome	Hand Surgery	Carroll, Charles (MD)	271
Carpal Tunnel Syndrome	Hand Surgery	Derman, Gordon Harris (MD)	272
Carpal Tunnel Syndrome	Hand Surgery	Koman, L Andrew (MD)	270
Carpal Tunnel Syndrome	Hand Surgery	Schenck, Robert Roy (MD)	274
Carpal Tunnel Syndrome	Hand Surgery	Weiss, Arnold Peter (MD)	267
Carpal Tunnel Syndrome	Orthopaedic Surgery	Rosenwasser, Melvin (MD)	483
Cartilage Problems	Orthopaedic Surgery	Nuber, Gordon (MD)	492
Cataract Surgery	Ophthalmology	Crandall, Alan Slade (MD)	461
Cataract Surgery	Ophthalmology	Farrell, Thomas A. (MD)	457
Cataract Surgery	Ophthalmology	Feder, Robert S (MD)	457
Cataract Surgery	Ophthalmology	Forster, Richard K (MD)	453
Cataract Surgery	Ophthalmology	Foster, Charles Stephen (MD)	443
Cataract Surgery	Ophthalmology	Hersh, Peter (MD)	447
Cataract Surgery	Ophthalmology	Holladay, Jack T. (MD)	461
Cataract Surgery	Ophthalmology	Holland, Edward J. (MD)	457
Cataract Surgery	Ophthalmology	Koch, Douglas D (MD)	462
Cataract Surgery	Ophthalmology	Lichter, Paul R. (MD)	458
Cataract Surgery	Ophthalmology	Lindstrom, Richard Lyndon (MD)	458
Cataract Surgery	Ophthalmology	Mackool, Richard (MD)	448
Cataract Surgery	Ophthalmology	Magramm, Irene (MD)	448

SPECIAL EXPERTISE INDEX

Special Expertise	Specialty	Doctor's Name	Page
Chemoembolization	Radiology	Coldwell, Douglas Michael (MD)	735
Chemoprevention of Cancer	Medical Oncology	Hong, Waun Ki (MD)	311
Chemoprevention of Cancer	Radiation Oncology	Weichselbaum, Ralph R (MD)	724
Chest Wall Deformities	Pediatric Surgery	Paidas, Charles Nicholas (MD)	612
Chest Wall Reconstruction	Plastic Surgery	Seyfer, Alan (MD)	654
Chest Wall Tumors	Thoracic Surgery	Pairolero, Peter (MD)	818
Chiari's Deformity	Neurological Surgery	Batzdorf, Ulrich (MD)	388
Chiari's Deformity	Neurological Surgery	Ellenbogen, Richard (MD)	389
Chiari's Deformity	Neurological Surgery	Luken, Martin (MD)	384
Chiari's Deformity	Neurological Surgery	Milhorat, Thomas H (MD)	378
Chiari's Deformity	Neurological Surgery	Oakes, W Jerry (MD)	381
Child Abuse	Psychiatry	van der Kolk, Bessel (MD)	677
Child Abuse & Neglect	Pediatrics	Ludwig, Stephen (MD)	617
Child Development	Pediatrics	Levine, Melvin David (MD)	618
Cholesterol/Lipid Disorders	Cardiology (Cardiovascular Disease)	Herling, Irving M (MD)	126
Cholesterol/Lipid Disorders	Endocrinology, Diabetes & Metabolism	Barrett, Eugene Joseph (MD)	203
Cholesterol/Lipid Disorders	Endocrinology, Diabetes & Metabolism	Semenkovich, Clay F (MD)	209
Cholesterol/Lipid Disorders	Pediatric Cardiology	Liebman, Jerome (MD)	565
Cholesterol/Lipid Disorders	Pediatric Cardiology	Moodie, Douglas (MD)	565
Cholesterol/Lipid Disorders	Pediatric Cardiology	Newburger, Jane (MD)	561
Chronic Cough	Pulmonary Disease	Irwin, Richard Stephen (MD)	691
Chronic Disease	Adolescent Medicine	Slap, Gail (MD)	89
Chronic Disease	Pediatrics	Lantos, John (MD)	618
Chronic Fatigue Syndrome	Allergy & Immunology	Jones, James F (MD)	102
Chronic Fatigue Syndrome	Infectious Disease	Straus, Stephen (MD)	321
Chronic Fatigue Syndrome	Pediatric Infectious Disease	Gorensek, Margaret (MD)	592
Chronic Fatigue Syndrome	Pediatrics	Pasquariello Jr, Patrick S (MD)	617
Chronic Fatigue Syndrome	Rheumatology	Clauw, Daniel J (MD)	758
Chronic Lung Disease (COPD)	Pulmonary Disease	Celli, Bartolome (MD)	691
Chronic Lung Disease (COPD)	Pulmonary Disease	Donohue, James (MD)	697
Chronic Lung Disease (COPD)	Pulmonary Disease	Fletcher, Eugene (MD)	698
Chronic Lung Disease (COPD)	Pulmonary Disease	Gracey, Douglas Robert (MD)	703
Chronic Lung Disease (COPD)	Pulmonary Disease	Guidry, George Gary (MD)	708
Chronic Lung Disease (COPD)	Pulmonary Disease	Jenkinson, Stephen George (MD)	709
Chronic Lung Disease (COPD)	Pulmonary Disease	Kaye, Mitchell (MD)	703
Chronic Lung Disease (COPD)	Pulmonary Disease	Mahler, Donald A (MD)	692
Chronic Lung Disease (COPD)	Pulmonary Disease	Make, Barry J (MD)	707
Chronic Lung Disease (COPD)	Pulmonary Disease	Perret, Phillip Samuel (MD)	709
Chronic Lung Disease (COPD)	Pulmonary Disease	Petty, Thomas L (MD)	707
Chronic Lung Disease (COPD)	Pulmonary Disease	Ries, Andrew (MD)	712
Chronic Lung Disease (COPD)	Pulmonary Disease	Rochester, Carolyn (MD)	693
Chronic Lung Disease (COPD)	Pulmonary Disease	Rosen, Mark J (MD)	695
Chronic Lung Disease (COPD)	Pulmonary Disease	Silver, Michael (MD)	705
Chronic Lung Disease (COPD)	Pulmonary Disease	Tashkin, Donald P (MD)	713
Chronic Lung Disease (COPD)	Pulmonary Disease	Tino, Gregory (MD)	696
Chronic Lung Disease (COPD)	Pulmonary Disease	Tobin, Martin (MD)	705
Claudication	Vascular Surgery (General)	Pearce, William (MD)	866
Cleft Palate/Lip	Clinical Genetics	Saal, Howard (MD)	162
Cleft Palate/Lip	Plastic Surgery	Bauer, Bruce (MD)	645
Cleft Palate/Lip	Plastic Surgery	Cutting, Court (MD)	637
Cleft Palate/Lip	Plastic Surgery	Georgiade, Gregory (MD)	642
Cleft Palate/Lip	Plastic Surgery	Ketch, Lawrence Levant (MD)	648
Cleft Palate/Lip	Plastic Surgery	Marsh, Jeffrey L (MD)	646
Cleft Palate/Lip	Plastic Surgery	Mulliken, John B. (MD)	635
Cleft Palate/Lip	Plastic Surgery	Reinisch, John F (MD)	654
Cleft Palate/Lip	Plastic Surgery	Seyfer, Alan (MD)	654
Cleft Palate/Lip	Plastic Surgery	Vander Kolk, Craig Alan (MD)	640
Cleft Palate/Lip	Plastic Surgery	Wells, James H (MD)	655
Clinical Genetics-Birth Defects	Pediatrics	Hall, Bryan Davis (MD)	161
Clinical Genetics-Dysmorphology	Pediatrics	Jones, Kenneth L (MD)	165

SPECIAL EXPERTISE INDEX

Special Expertise	Specialty	Doctor's Name	Page
Clinical Trials	Gynecologic Oncology	De Geest, Koen (MD)	259
Clostridium Difficile Disease	Gastroenterology	Surawicz, Christina (MD)	238
Clubfoot	Orthopaedic Surgery	Aronson, James (MD)	494
Cocaine Addiction	Addiction Psychiatry	Kosten, Thomas (MD)	661
Coccidioidomycosis	Infectious Disease	Bayer, Arnold Sander (MD)	328
Cochlear Implant Surgery	Otolaryngology	Wackym, Phillip (MD)	517
Cochlear Implants	Otolaryngology	Cohen, Noel L (MD)	503
Cochlear Implants	Otolaryngology	Parisier, Simon (MD)	505
Cochlear Implants	Otolaryngology	Pillsbury, Harold Crockett (MD)	510
Cochlear Implants	Otolaryngology	Poe, Dennis (MD)	501
Cochlear Implants	Otolaryngology	Schindler, Robert Allen (MD)	523
Cochlear Implants	Otolaryngology	Telian, Steven Allen (MD)	517
Cochlear Implants	Pediatric Otolaryngology	Belenky, Walter (MD)	602
Cochlear Implants	Pediatric Otolaryngology	Lusk, Rodney (MD)	602
Cognitive Psychiatry	Psychiatry	Gabbard, Glen O. (MD)	684
Collagen Vascular Disease	Neurology	Nadeau, Stephen E (MD)	409
Colon & Rectal Cancer	Colon & Rectal Surgery	Beart Jr, Robert W (MD)	176
Colon & Rectal Cancer	Colon & Rectal Surgery	Fazio, Victor (MD)	173
Colon & Rectal Cancer	Colon & Rectal Surgery	Galandiuk, Susan (MD)	172
Colon & Rectal Cancer	Colon & Rectal Surgery	Golub, Richard (MD)	170
Colon & Rectal Cancer	Colon & Rectal Surgery	Kodner, Ira Joe (MD)	174
Colon & Rectal Cancer	Colon & Rectal Surgery	Nelson, Heidi (MD)	174
Colon & Rectal Cancer	Colon & Rectal Surgery	Nivatvongs, Santhat (MD)	174
Colon & Rectal Cancer	Colon & Rectal Surgery	Rothenberger, David (MD)	175
Colon & Rectal Cancer	Colon & Rectal Surgery	Schoetz, David (MD)	169
Colon & Rectal Cancer	Colon & Rectal Surgery	Senagore, Anthony (MD)	175
Colon & Rectal Cancer	Colon & Rectal Surgery	Shellito, Paul C (MD)	170
Colon & Rectal Cancer	Colon & Rectal Surgery	Steinhagen, Randolph (MD)	171
Colon & Rectal Cancer	Colon & Rectal Surgery	Wolff, Bruce (MD)	175
Colon & Rectal Cancer	Gastroenterology	Levin, Bernard (MD)	236
Colon & Rectal Cancer	Medical Oncology	Haller, Daniel (MD)	296
Colon & Rectal Cancer	Medical Oncology	Rothenberg, Mace (MD)	303
Colon & Rectal Cancer	Surgery	Beauchamp, Robert Daniel (MD)	789
Colon & Rectal Cancer	Surgery	Curley, Steven Alan (MD)	797
Colon & Rectal Surgery	Colon & Rectal Surgery	Fleshman, James (MD)	173
Colon & Rectal Surgery	Colon & Rectal Surgery	Foley, Eugene F (MD)	172
Colon & Rectal Surgery	Colon & Rectal Surgery	Milsom, Jeffrey (MD)	171
Colon & Rectal Surgery	Colon & Rectal Surgery	Opelka, Frank (MD)	176
Colon Cancer	Colon & Rectal Surgery	Beck, David (MD)	176
Colon Cancer	Colon & Rectal Surgery	Becker, James (MD)	169
Colon Cancer	Colon & Rectal Surgery	Bleday, Ronald (MD)	169
Colon Cancer	Colon & Rectal Surgery	Coller, John (MD)	169
Colon Cancer	Colon & Rectal Surgery	Larach, Sergio (MD)	173
Colon Cancer	Colon & Rectal Surgery	Opelka, Frank (MD)	176
Colon Cancer	Colon & Rectal Surgery	Roberts, Patricia L (MD)	169
Colon Cancer	Colon & Rectal Surgery	Smith, Lee (MD)	171
Colon Cancer	Colon & Rectal Surgery	Stryker, Steven J (MD)	175
Colon Cancer	Colon & Rectal Surgery	Whelan, Richard (MD)	171
Colon Cancer	Gastroenterology	Lipshutz, William H. (MD)	224
Colon Cancer	Gastroenterology	Waye, Jerome (MD)	226
Colon Cancer	Gastroenterology	Winawer, Sidney J (MD)	226
Colon Cancer	Medical Oncology	Ahlgren, James David (MD)	294
Colon Cancer	Medical Oncology	Benson, Al B (MD)	305
Colon Cancer	Medical Oncology	Donehower, Ross Carl (MD)	295
Colon Cancer	Medical Oncology	Kemeny, Nancy (MD)	297
Colon Cancer	Medical Oncology	MacDonald, John (MD)	298
Colon Cancer	Radiation Oncology	Gunderson, Leonard (MD)	723
Colon Cancer	Radiation Oncology	Mendenhall, William M (MD)	722
Colon Cancer	Radiation Oncology	Minsky, Bruce (MD)	720
Colon Cancer	Radiation Oncology	Myerson, Robert J (MD)	724

Special Expertise	Specialty	Doctor's Name	Page
Colon Cancer	Radiation Oncology	Rich, Tyvin Andrew (MD)	722
Colon Cancer	Radiation Oncology	Smalley, Stephen R (MD)	725
Colon Cancer	Radiation Oncology	Tepper, Joel (MD)	723
Colon Cancer	Surgery	Copeland lll, Edward M (MD)	790
Colon Cancer	Surgery	Kelly, Keith A (MD)	797
Colon Cancer	Surgery	Polk Jr, Hiram C (MD)	792
Colon Cancer	Surgery	Saha, Sukamal (MD)	795
Colon Cancer	Surgery	Steele, Glenn D (MD/PhD)	796
Colon Cancer	Surgery	Sugarbaker, Paul H (MD)	788
Colonoscopy	Colon & Rectal Surgery	Christie, John (MD)	172
Colonoscopy	Gastroenterology	Ostroff, James Warren (MD)	238
Colonoscopy	Internal Medicine	Yaffe, Bruce (MD)	334
Colonoscopy/Polypectomy	Colon & Rectal Surgery	Forde, Kenneth (MD)	170
Colonoscopy/Polypectomy	Gastroenterology	Winawer, Sidney J (MD)	226
Colorectal Cancer-Liver Metastasis	Colon & Rectal Surgery	Cohen, Alfred M (MD)	172
Colorectal Surgery	Pediatric Surgery	Fonkalsrud, Eric W (MD)	616
Colostomy Avoidance	Colon & Rectal Surgery	Gingold, Bruce (MD)	170
Coma	Neurology	Plum, Fred (MD)	405
Congenital Abnormalities	Maternal & Fetal Medicine	Mennuti, Michael (MD)	343
Congenital Abnormalities	Maternal & Fetal Medicine	Wilkins, Isabelle (MD)	347
Congenital Abnormalities-Limb	Clinical Genetics	Hudgins, Louanne (MD)	164
Congenital Birth Defects	Plastic Surgery	Bauer, Bruce (MD)	645
Congenital Defect Repair	Pediatric Surgery	Sato, Thomas Tad (MD)	615
Congenital Malformations & Syndromes	Orthopaedic Surgery	Goldberg, Michael Jay (MD)	476
Congestive Heart Failure	Cardiology (Cardiovascular Disease)	Baughman, Kenneth (MD)	124
Congestive Heart Failure	Cardiology (Cardiovascular Disease)	Brozena, Susan Celia (MD)	124
Congestive Heart Failure	Cardiology (Cardiovascular Disease)	Chatterjee, Kanu (MD)	141
Congestive Heart Failure	Cardiology (Cardiovascular Disease)	Cody Jr., Robert James (MD)	134
Congestive Heart Failure	Cardiology (Cardiovascular Disease)	Costanzo, Maria Rosa (MD)	134
Congestive Heart Failure	Cardiology (Cardiovascular Disease)	Douglas Jr, John Simonton (MD)	131
Congestive Heart Failure	Cardiology (Cardiovascular Disease)	Eisen, Howard J (MD)	125
Congestive Heart Failure	Cardiology (Cardiovascular Disease)	Elkayam, Uri (MD)	141
Congestive Heart Failure	Cardiology (Cardiovascular Disease)	Fishbein, Daniel P (MD)	141
Congestive Heart Failure	Cardiology (Cardiovascular Disease)	Johnson, Maryl R (MD)	136
Congestive Heart Failure	Cardiology (Cardiovascular Disease)	Klapholz, Marc (MD)	126
Congestive Heart Failure	Cardiology (Cardiovascular Disease)	Konstam, Marvin Amnon (MD)	121
Congestive Heart Failure	Cardiology (Cardiovascular Disease)	Lindenfeld, JoAnn (MD)	139
Congestive Heart Failure	Cardiology (Cardiovascular Disease)	Massin, Edward Krauss (MD)	140
Congestive Heart Failure	Cardiology (Cardiovascular Disease)	Packer, Milton (MD)	127
Congestive Heart Failure	Cardiology (Cardiovascular Disease)	Plehn, Jonathan (MD)	127
Congestive Heart Failure	Cardiology (Cardiovascular Disease)	Rahko, Peter (MD)	137
Congestive Heart Failure	Cardiology (Cardiovascular Disease)	Rich, Stuart (MD)	137
Congestive Heart Failure	Cardiology (Cardiovascular Disease)	Rogers, Joseph (MD)	137
Congestive Heart Failure	Cardiology (Cardiovascular Disease)	Schroeder, John S (MD)	143
Congestive Heart Failure	Cardiology (Cardiovascular Disease)	Stevenson, Lynne W (MD)	122
Congestive Heart Failure	Cardiology (Cardiovascular Disease)	Thames, Marc (MD)	129
Congestive Heart Failure	Cardiology (Cardiovascular Disease)	Vander Ark, Condon R (MD)	138
Congestive Heart Failure	Cardiology (Cardiovascular Disease)	Young, James B (MD)	138
Congestive Heart Failure	Geriatric Medicine	Supiano, Mark A. (MD)	249
Congestive Heart Failure	Internal Medicine	Messer, Joseph V (MD)	336
Connective Tissue Disorders	Clinical Genetics	Cassidy, Suzanne (MD)	162
Connective Tissue Disorders	Pediatric Rheumatology	Kredich, Deborah Welt (MD)	608
Connective Tissue Disorders	Rheumatology	Chang-Miller, April (MD)	763
Connective Tissue Disorders	Rheumatology	Duffy, Joseph (MD)	764
Connective Tissue Disorders	Rheumatology	Michalska, Margaret (MD)	766
Connective Tissue Disorders	Rheumatology	Moskowitz, Roland (MD)	766
Connective Tissue Disorders	Rheumatology	Quismorio Jr, Francisco P (MD)	769
Connective Tissue Disorders	Rheumatology	Spiera, Harry (MD)	761
Constipation	Gastroenterology	Rao, Satish S C (MD)	233
Constipation	Gastroenterology	Wald, Arnold (MD)	225

SPECIAL EXPERTISE INDEX

Special Expertise	Specialty	Doctor's Name	Page
Contact Dermatitis	Dermatology	DeLeo, Vincent A. (MD)	183
Continent Urinary Diversions	Urology	Kozlowski, James Michael (MD)	842
Cornea Plastic Surgery	Ophthalmology	Katowitz, James A (MD)	447
Cornea Transplant	Ophthalmology	Boniuk, Milton (MD)	461
Cornea Transplant	Ophthalmology	Driebe Jr, William T (MD)	452
Cornea Transplant	Ophthalmology	Forster, Richard K (MD)	453
Cornea Transplant	Ophthalmology	Steinert, Roger F (MD)	444
Cornea Transplant	Ophthalmology	Waring III, George Oral (MD)	455
Cornea Transplant	Ophthalmology	Wilhelmus, Kirk R (MD)	463
Cornea Transplant	Ophthalmology	Zaidman, Gerald (MD)	451
Corneal & External Eye Disease	Ophthalmology	Alfonso, Eduardo (MD)	451
Corneal & External Eye Disease	Ophthalmology	Irvine, John Alexander (MD)	465
Corneal & External Eye Disease	Ophthalmology	McCulley, James P (MD)	462
Corneal & External Eye Disease	Ophthalmology	Mondino, Bartly John (MD)	466
Corneal & External Eye Disease	Ophthalmology	Pepose, Jay (MD)	459
Corneal & External Eye Disease	Ophthalmology	Wilhelmus, Kirk R (MD)	463
Corneal Disease	Ophthalmology	Culbertson, William (MD)	452
Corneal Disease	Ophthalmology	Durrie, Daniel (MD)	461
Corneal Disease	Ophthalmology	Feder, Robert S (MD)	457
Corneal Disease	Ophthalmology	Foster, Charles Stephen (MD)	443
Corneal Disease	Ophthalmology	Hersh, Peter (MD)	447
Corneal Disease	Ophthalmology	Holland, Edward J. (MD)	457
Corneal Disease	Ophthalmology	Holliday, James N (MD/PhD)	454
Corneal Disease	Ophthalmology	Koch, Douglas D (MD)	462
Corneal Disease	Ophthalmology	Krachmer, Jay H. (MD)	457
Corneal Disease	Ophthalmology	Kramer, Steven G (MD)	465
Corneal Disease	Ophthalmology	Krueger, Ronald (MD)	457
Corneal Disease	Ophthalmology	Laibson, Peter R (MD)	447
Corneal Disease	Ophthalmology	Lindstrom, Richard Lyndon (MD)	458
Corneal Disease	Ophthalmology	Manche, Edward Emanuel (MD)	466
Corneal Disease	Ophthalmology	Nesburn, Anthony B (MD)	467
Corneal Disease & Transplant	Ophthalmology	Stark, Walter J (MD)	450
Corneal Disease & Transplant	Ophthalmology	Stulting, R. Doyle (MD)	455
Corneal Disease-Pediatric	Ophthalmology	Medow, Norman (MD)	448
Coronal Canthopexy	Plastic Surgery	Flowers, Robert (MD)	651
Coronary Angioplasty	Cardiology (Cardiovascular Disease)	Konstam, Marvin Amnon (MD)	121
Coronary Artery Disease	Cardiology (Cardiovascular Disease)	Beller, George Allan (MD)	129
Coronary Artery Disease	Cardiology (Cardiovascular Disease)	Chatterjee, Kanu (MD)	141
Coronary Artery Disease	Cardiology (Cardiovascular Disease)	Moran, John (MD)	136
Coronary Artery Disease	Cardiology (Cardiovascular Disease)	O'Gara, Patrick Thomas (MD)	122
Coronary Artery Disease	Cardiology (Cardiovascular Disease)	Parmley, William Watts (MD)	142
Coronary Artery Disease	Cardiology (Cardiovascular Disease)	Reiss, Craig (MD)	137
Coronary Artery Disease	Cardiology (Cardiovascular Disease)	Schroeder, John S (MD)	143
Coronary Artery Disease	Cardiology (Cardiovascular Disease)	Thames, Marc (MD)	129
Coronary Artery Disease	Cardiology (Cardiovascular Disease)	Topol, Eric Jeffrey (MD)	138
Coronary Artery Disease	Cardiology (Cardiovascular Disease)	Zaret, Barry L. (MD)	123
Coronary Artery Disease	Internal Medicine	Messer, Joseph V (MD)	336
Coronary Artery Disease	Interventional Cardiology	Diver, Daniel Joseph (MD)	144
Coronary Artery Surgery	Thoracic Surgery	Akins, Cary W (MD)	805
Coronary Artery Surgery	Thoracic Surgery	Bassett, Joseph (MD)	815
Coronary Artery Surgery	Thoracic Surgery	Jones, Ellis (MD)	813
Coronary Artery Surgery	Thoracic Surgery	Katz, Nevin M (MD)	809
Coronary Artery Surgery	Thoracic Surgery	Kron, Irving L (MD)	813
Coronary Artery Surgery	Thoracic Surgery	Lang, Samuel (MD)	810
Coronary Artery Surgery	Thoracic Surgery	Livesay, James J (MD)	822
Coronary Artery Surgery	Thoracic Surgery	Lytle, Bruce Whitney (MD)	817
Coronary Artery Surgery	Thoracic Surgery	Michler, Robert (MD)	818
Coronary Artery Surgery	Thoracic Surgery	Oz, Mehmet Cengiz (MD)	810
Coronary Artery Surgery	Thoracic Surgery	Quintessenza, James (MD)	814
Coronary Artery Surgery	Thoracic Surgery	Reul, George J (MD)	822

Special Expertise	Specialty	Doctor's Name	Page
Coronary Artery Surgery	Thoracic Surgery	Shennib, Hani (MD)	811
Coronary Artery Surgery	Thoracic Surgery	Smith, Craig R (MD)	811
Coronary Artery Surgery	Thoracic Surgery	Smith, Peter Kent (MD)	814
Coronary Artery Surgery	Thoracic Surgery	Strong III, Michael D (MD)	811
Coronary Artery Surgery	Thoracic Surgery	Turner, William F (MD)	822
Coronary Artery Surgery	Thoracic Surgery	Verrier, Edward (MD)	826
Coronary Disease-Complex	Interventional Cardiology	Klein, Lloyd (MD)	146
Coronary Revascularization	Thoracic Surgery	Harrison, Lynn (MD)	821
Cosmetic & Reconstructive Surgery	Plastic Surgery	Puckett, Charles Linwood (MD)	647
Cosmetic Dematology	Dermatology	Cohen, Bernard Hershel (MD)	187
Cosmetic Dematology	Dermatology	Kane, Bryna (MD)	193
Cosmetic Dematology	Dermatology	Safai , Bijan (MD)	185
Cosmetic Dematology	Dermatology	Wheeland, Ronald (MD)	192
Cosmetic Dermatology	Dermatology	Arndt, Kenneth (MD)	181
Cosmetic Dermatology	Dermatology	Glogau, Richard Gordon (MD)	193
Cosmetic Dermatology	Dermatology	Lask, Gary P (MD)	193
Cosmetic Dermatology	Dermatology	Safai , Bijan (MD)	185
Cosmetic Surgery	Hand Surgery	Chiu, David (MD)	267
Cosmetic Surgery	Plastic Surgery	Baker Jr, Thomas J (MD)	641
Cosmetic Surgery	Plastic Surgery	Berner, Carl Frederick (MD)	651
Cosmetic Surgery	Plastic Surgery	Brink, Robert Ross (MD)	651
Cosmetic Surgery	Plastic Surgery	Burns, Alton Jay (MD)	649
Cosmetic Surgery	Plastic Surgery	Colon, Gustavo (MD)	649
Cosmetic Surgery	Plastic Surgery	Fodor, Peter Bela (MD)	651
Cosmetic Surgery	Plastic Surgery	Gold, Alan (MD)	637
Cosmetic Surgery	Plastic Surgery	Grossman, John A (MD)	652
Cosmetic Surgery	Plastic Surgery	Grotting, James (MD)	643
Cosmetic Surgery	Plastic Surgery	Kawamoto Jr, Henry K (MD)	652
Cosmetic Surgery	Plastic Surgery	Markowitz, Bernard Lloyd (MD)	653
Cosmetic Surgery	Plastic Surgery	Marten, Timothy James (MD)	653
Cosmetic Surgery	Plastic Surgery	May Jr, James W (MD)	635
Cosmetic Surgery	Plastic Surgery	Nahai, Foad (MD)	645
Cosmetic Surgery	Plastic Surgery	Rand, Richard Pierce (MD)	654
Cosmetic Surgery	Plastic Surgery	Stevenson, Thomas Ray (MD)	655
Cosmetic Surgery	Plastic Surgery	Sultan, Mark (MD)	640
Cosmetic Surgery	Plastic Surgery	Vogt, Peter (MD)	647
Cosmetic Surgery-Body	Plastic Surgery	Jelks, Glenn (MD)	638
Cosmetic Surgery-Body	Plastic Surgery	Klatsky, Stanley A (MD)	638
Cosmetic Surgery-Body	Plastic Surgery	Lockwood, Ted (MD)	648
Cosmetic Surgery-Body	Plastic Surgery	Stuzin, James M (MD)	645
Cosmetic Surgery-Eyelid	Ophthalmology	Della Rocca, Robert (MD)	445
Cosmetic Surgery-Face	Dermatology	Johnson, Timothy M (MD)	189
Cosmetic Surgery-Face	Otolaryngology	Baker, Shan Ray (MD)	512
Cosmetic Surgery-Face	Otolaryngology	Cheney, Mack Lowell (MD)	501
Cosmetic Surgery-Face	Otolaryngology	Cook, Ted (MD)	521
Cosmetic Surgery-Face	Otolaryngology	Denenberg, Steven M (MD)	518
Cosmetic Surgery-Face	Otolaryngology	Donovan, Donald Thomas (MD)	519
Cosmetic Surgery-Face	Otolaryngology	Farrior, Edward (MD)	508
Cosmetic Surgery-Face	Otolaryngology	Glasgold, Alvin (MD)	503
Cosmetic Surgery-Face	Otolaryngology	Hansen, Lori Eldean (MD)	519
Cosmetic Surgery-Face	Otolaryngology	Haughey, Bruce (MD)	514
Cosmetic Surgery-Face	Otolaryngology	Hilger, Peter A. (MD)	514
Cosmetic Surgery-Face	Otolaryngology	Johnson Jr, Calvin M (MD)	520
Cosmetic Surgery-Face	Otolaryngology	Kamer, Frank M (MD)	522
Cosmetic Surgery-Face	Otolaryngology	Keller, Gregory Steele (MD)	522
Cosmetic Surgery-Face	Otolaryngology	Larrabee Jr., Wayne F. (MD)	522
Cosmetic Surgery-Face	Otolaryngology	Mangat, Devinder Singh (MD)	515
Cosmetic Surgery-Face	Otolaryngology	Papel, Ira David (MD)	505
Cosmetic Surgery-Face	Otolaryngology	Quatela, Vito Charles (MD)	506
Cosmetic Surgery-Face	Otolaryngology	Romo III, Thomas (MD)	506

SPECIAL EXPERTISE INDEX

Special Expertise	Specialty	Doctor's Name	Page
Cosmetic Surgery-Face	Otolaryngology	Szachowicz II, Edward H (MD)	516
Cosmetic Surgery-Face	Otolaryngology	Toriumi, Dean (MD)	517
Cosmetic Surgery-Face	Otolaryngology	Wolf, Gregory (MD)	517
Cosmetic Surgery-Face	Plastic Surgery	Arnold, Phillip (MD)	645
Cosmetic Surgery-Face	Plastic Surgery	Aston, Sherrell (MD)	636
Cosmetic Surgery-Face	Plastic Surgery	Baker, Daniel (MD)	636
Cosmetic Surgery-Face	Plastic Surgery	Barton Jr, Fritz (MD)	648
Cosmetic Surgery-Face	Plastic Surgery	Becker, Ferdinand Francis (MD)	641
Cosmetic Surgery-Face	Plastic Surgery	Biggs Jr, Thomas M (MD)	648
Cosmetic Surgery-Face	Plastic Surgery	Bostwick III, John J (MD)	641
Cosmetic Surgery-Face	Plastic Surgery	Burget, Gary C (MD)	645
Cosmetic Surgery-Face	Plastic Surgery	Byrd, Henry S (MD)	649
Cosmetic Surgery-Face	Plastic Surgery	Carraway, James Howard (MD)	642
Cosmetic Surgery-Face	Plastic Surgery	Daniel, Rollin K (MD)	651
Cosmetic Surgery-Face	Plastic Surgery	Feldman, Joel (MD)	635
Cosmetic Surgery-Face	Plastic Surgery	Gregory, Richard (MD)	643
Cosmetic Surgery-Face	Plastic Surgery	Hamra, Sameer T (MD)	649
Cosmetic Surgery-Face	Plastic Surgery	Hester Jr, Thomas R (MD)	643
Cosmetic Surgery-Face	Plastic Surgery	Hoefflin, Steven M (MD)	652
Cosmetic Surgery-Face	Plastic Surgery	Horowitz, Jed H (MD)	652
Cosmetic Surgery-Face	Plastic Surgery	Jelks, Glenn (MD)	638
Cosmetic Surgery-Face	Plastic Surgery	Kelly, John Michael (MD)	649
Cosmetic Surgery-Face	Plastic Surgery	Ketch, Lawrence Levant (MD)	648
Cosmetic Surgery-Face	Plastic Surgery	Klatsky, Stanley A (MD)	638
Cosmetic Surgery-Face	Plastic Surgery	Knize, David Maurice (MD)	648
Cosmetic Surgery-Face	Plastic Surgery	Koplin, Lawrence Mark (MD)	653
Cosmetic Surgery-Face	Plastic Surgery	Krizek, Thomas (MD)	643
Cosmetic Surgery-Face	Plastic Surgery	Leipziger, Lyle S (MD)	638
Cosmetic Surgery-Face	Plastic Surgery	Little, John W (MD)	638
Cosmetic Surgery-Face	Plastic Surgery	Marten, Timothy James (MD)	653
Cosmetic Surgery-Face	Plastic Surgery	McCarthy, Joseph (MD)	639
Cosmetic Surgery-Face	Plastic Surgery	Mustoe, Thomas (MD)	646
Cosmetic Surgery-Face	Plastic Surgery	Nahai, Foad (MD)	645
Cosmetic Surgery-Face	Plastic Surgery	Paul, Malcolm D (MD)	654
Cosmetic Surgery-Face	Plastic Surgery	Pitman, Gerald (MD)	639
Cosmetic Surgery-Face	Plastic Surgery	Posnick, Jeffrey Craig (MD/DMD)	639
Cosmetic Surgery-Face	Plastic Surgery	Ristow, Brunno (MD)	654
Cosmetic Surgery-Face	Plastic Surgery	Schusterman, Mark A (MD)	650
Cosmetic Surgery-Face	Plastic Surgery	Shaw, William Wei-Lien (MD)	655
Cosmetic Surgery-Face	Plastic Surgery	Spear, Scott L (MD)	639
Cosmetic Surgery-Face	Plastic Surgery	Thorne, Charles (MD)	640
Cosmetic Surgery-Face	Plastic Surgery	Vasconez, Luis O (MD)	645
Cosmetic Surgery-Face	Plastic Surgery	Walton, Robert Lee (MD)	647
Cosmetic Surgery-Face	Plastic Surgery	Whitaker, Linton A (MD)	640
Cosmetic Surgery-Face	Plastic Surgery	Zarem, Harvey Alan (MD)	655
Cosmetic Surgery-Face	Plastic Surgery	Zins, James (MD)	648
Cosmetic Surgery-Face & Body	Plastic Surgery	Hunstad, Joseph P. (MD)	643
Cosmetic Surgery-Face & Breast	Plastic Surgery	Hidalgo, David (MD)	637
Cosmetic Surgery-Face & Breast	Plastic Surgery	Rohrich, Rodney James (MD)	650
Cosmetic Surgery-Liposuction	Plastic Surgery	Mladick, Richard (MD)	644
Cosmetic Surgery-Liposuction	Plastic Surgery	Nahai, Foad (MD)	645
Cosmetic Surgery-Liposuction	Plastic Surgery	Pitman, Gerald (MD)	639
Cosmetic Surgery-Liposuction	Plastic Surgery	Rohrich, Rodney James (MD)	650
Cosmetic Surgery-Liposuction	Plastic Surgery	Tebbetts, John B (MD)	650
Cranial Plastic Surgery	Plastic Surgery	Thorne, Charles (MD)	640
Cranial/Orbital Tumors	Neurological Surgery	Day, Arthur L (MD)	379
Craniocervical Abnormalities	Neurological Surgery	Menezes, Arnold (MD)	384
Craniofacial Disorders	Clinical Genetics	Graham Jr, John M (MD)	164
Craniofacial Disorders	Clinical Genetics	Jones, Marilyn (MD)	165
Craniofacial Disorders	Clinical Genetics	Saal, Howard (MD)	162

Special Expertise	Specialty	Doctor's Name	Page
Craniofacial Surgery	Neurological Surgery	Morrison, Glenn (MD)	381
Craniofacial Surgery	Neurological Surgery	Pollack, Ian (MD)	378
Craniofacial Surgery/Reconstruction	Plastic Surgery	Bartlett, Scott P (MD)	636
Craniofacial Surgery/Reconstruction	Plastic Surgery	Cutting, Court (MD)	637
Craniofacial Surgery/Reconstruction	Plastic Surgery	Kawamoto Jr, Henry K (MD)	652
Craniofacial Surgery/Reconstruction	Plastic Surgery	Markowitz, Bernard Lloyd (MD)	653
Craniofacial Surgery/Reconstruction	Plastic Surgery	Marsh, Jeffrey L (MD)	646
Craniofacial Surgery/Reconstruction	Plastic Surgery	Matthews, David (MD)	644
Craniofacial Surgery/Reconstruction	Plastic Surgery	McCarthy, Joseph (MD)	639
Craniofacial Surgery/Reconstruction	Plastic Surgery	Newman, M Haskell (MD)	647
Craniofacial Surgery/Reconstruction	Plastic Surgery	Posnick, Jeffrey Craig (MD/DMD)	639
Craniofacial Surgery/Reconstruction	Plastic Surgery	Reinisch, John F (MD)	654
Craniofacial Surgery/Reconstruction	Plastic Surgery	Spinelli, Henry M (MD)	640
Craniofacial Surgery/Reconstruction	Plastic Surgery	Sullivan, Patrick Kevin (MD)	636
Craniofacial Surgery/Reconstruction	Plastic Surgery	Vander Kolk, Craig Alan (MD)	640
Craniofacial Surgery/Reconstruction	Plastic Surgery	Whitaker, Linton A (MD)	640
Craniofacial Surgery/Reconstruction	Plastic Surgery	Wolfe, S Anthony (MD)	645
Craniosynostosis	Clinical Genetics	Zackai, Elaine (MD)	160
Craniosynostosis	Neurological Surgery	Winston, Ken R. (MD)	386
Critical Care	Infectious Disease	Masur, Henry (MD)	320
Critical Care	Neonatal-Perinatal Medicine	Ehrenkranz, Richard (MD)	351
Critical Care	Neurology	Gress, Daryl Ray (MD)	421
Critical Care	Pain Management	Abram, Stephen Edward (MD)	530
Critical Care	Pain Management	Berde, Charles Benjamin (MD)	527
Critical Care	Pediatric Critical Care Medicine	Anand, Kanwaljeet Singh (MD/PhD)	571
Critical Care	Pediatric Critical Care Medicine	Sarnaik, Ashok P (MD)	570
Critical Care	Pediatric Critical Care Medicine	Thompson, Ann Ellen (MD)	570
Critical Care	Pediatric Pulmonology	Kurachek, Stephen Charles (MD)	605
Critical Care	Pediatric Surgery	Reynolds, Marleta (MD)	615
Critical Care	Pediatric Surgery	Tapper, David (MD)	616
Critical Care	Pulmonary Disease	Albertson, Timothy (MD/PhD)	709
Critical Care	Pulmonary Disease	Bellamy, Paul Eric (MD)	710
Critical Care	Pulmonary Disease	Cooper, William (MD)	697
Critical Care	Pulmonary Disease	Dunlap, Nancy Elizabeth (MD/PhD)	698
Critical Care	Pulmonary Disease	Friedman, Lloyd Neal (MD)	691
Critical Care	Pulmonary Disease	Greenberg, Harly (MD)	693
Critical Care	Pulmonary Disease	Hall, Jesse (MD)	703
Critical Care	Pulmonary Disease	Haponik, Edward Francis (MD)	693
Critical Care	Pulmonary Disease	Heffner, John E (MD)	699
Critical Care	Pulmonary Disease	Hudson, Leonard (MD)	711
Critical Care	Pulmonary Disease	Kollef, Marin Hristo (MD)	704
Critical Care	Pulmonary Disease	Levin, David C (MD)	709
Critical Care	Pulmonary Disease	Lorusso, Thomas (MD)	699
Critical Care	Pulmonary Disease	Marini, John Joseph (MD)	704
Critical Care	Pulmonary Disease	Martinez, Fernando J (MD)	704
Critical Care	Pulmonary Disease	Matthay, Michael Anthony (MD)	711
Critical Care	Pulmonary Disease	Parsons, Polly E. (MD)	692
Critical Care	Pulmonary Disease	Pingleton, Susan (MD)	707
Critical Care	Pulmonary Disease	Popovich Jr, John (MD)	705
Critical Care	Pulmonary Disease	Steiger, David (MD)	695
Critical Care	Pulmonary Disease	Vaughey, Ellen (MD)	701
Critical Care	Pulmonary Disease	Wiedemann, Herbert P (MD)	706
Critical Care	Surgery	Dudrick, Stanley (MD)	781
Critical Care	Surgery	Karrer, Frederick Merrill (MD)	796
Critical Care	Surgery	Meyer, Anthony A (MD)	791
Critical Care	Vascular Surgery (General)	Eidt, John (MD)	868
Critically Ill Infants	Neonatal-Perinatal Medicine	Perlman, Jeffrey (MD)	354
Cross Sectional Imaging	Diagnostic Radiology	Panicek, David (MD)	732
Cushing's Syndrome	Endocrinology, Diabetes & Metabolism	Biller, Beverly M K (MD)	197
Cushing's Syndrome	Pediatric Endocrinology	Levitsky, Lynne Lipton (MD)	572

SPECIAL EXPERTISE INDEX

Special Expertise	Specialty	Doctor's Name	Page
Cutaneous T-Cell Lymphoma	Dermatology	Duvic, Madeleine (MD)	191
Cystic Fibrosis	Pediatric Allergy & Immunology	Fanous, Yvonne F (MD)	559
Cystic Fibrosis	Pediatric Pulmonology	Accurso, Frank J (MD)	605
Cystic Fibrosis	Pediatric Pulmonology	Lapey, Allen (MD)	604
Cystic Fibrosis	Pediatric Pulmonology	Morgan, Wayne J. (MD)	606
Cystic Fibrosis	Pediatric Pulmonology	Murphy, Thomas M (MD)	604
Cystic Fibrosis	Pediatric Pulmonology	Quittell, Lynne (MD)	604
Cystic Fibrosis	Pediatric Pulmonology	Ramsey, Bonnie W (MD)	606
Cystic Fibrosis	Pediatric Pulmonology	Sherman, James (MD)	605
Cystic Fibrosis	Pediatric Pulmonology	Stern, Robert C (MD)	605
Cystic Fibrosis	Pediatric Pulmonology	Zeitlin, Pamela Leslie (MD)	604
Cystic Fibrosis	Pulmonary Disease	Geppert, Eugene (MD)	702
Cystic Fibrosis	Pulmonary Disease	Grum, Cyril M (MD)	703
Cystic Fibrosis	Pulmonary Disease	Rodman, David (MD)	707
Cystic Fibrosis Infection	Pediatric Infectious Disease	Saiman, Lisa (MD)	591
Cysticercosis	Child Neurology	Mitchell, Wendy Gayle (MD)	156
Cytogenetic Disorders	Clinical Genetics	Hoyme, Harold Eugene (MD)	164
Cytogenetic Disorders	Clinical Genetics	Zackai, Elaine (MD)	160
Cytomegalovirus PTLD	Infectious Disease	Paya, Carlos Vicente (MD)	326

D

Dance/Ballet Injuries	Orthopaedic Surgery	Micheli, Lyle J (MD)	476
Deafness & Ear Disorders	Otolaryngology	Balkany, Thomas Jay (MD)	507
Death & Dying	Child & Adolescent Psychiatry	Sexson, Sandra G B (MD)	667
Deep Venous Thrombosis	Vascular Surgery (General)	Greenfield, Lazar (MD)	865
Defibrillators	Cardiac Electrophysiology	DiMarco, John Philip (MD/PhD)	116
Defibrillators	Cardiac Electrophysiology	Epstein, Andrew Ernest (MD)	117
Defibrillators	Cardiac Electrophysiology	Swerdlow, Charles Dennis (MD)	119
Defibrillators	Cardiac Electrophysiology	Wilber, David James (MD)	118
Dementia	Geriatric Medicine	Blass, John (MD/PhD)	244
Dementia	Geriatric Medicine	Bloom, Harrison (MD)	244
Dementia	Geriatric Medicine	Bloom, Patricia (MD)	244
Dementia	Geriatric Medicine	Liem, Pham (MD)	250
Dementia	Geriatric Medicine	McCormick, Wayne (MD)	251
Dementia	Geriatric Medicine	Snustad, Diane Gail (MD)	246
Dementia	Geriatric Medicine	Von Sternberg, Thomas (MD)	249
Dementia	Geriatric Psychiatry	Greenwald, Blaine (MD)	672
Dementia	Geriatric Psychiatry	Jeste, Dilip (MD)	674
Dementia	Geriatric Psychiatry	Klement, Maria (MD)	672
Dementia	Geriatric Psychiatry	Mellow, Alan M. (MD/PhD)	674
Dementia	Geriatric Psychiatry	Reisberg, Barry (MD)	673
Dementia	Geriatric Psychiatry	Small, Gary William (MD)	675
Dementia	Neurology	Fox, Jacob H (MD)	412
Dementia	Neurology	Gendelman, Seymour (MD)	402
Dementia	Neurology	Levine, David (MD)	403
Dementia	Neurology	Mesulam, Marek Marsel (MD)	414
Dementia	Neurology	Nadeau, Stephen E (MD)	409
Dementia	Neurology	Reder, Anthony T (MD)	414
Dementia & Depression	Geriatric Medicine	Gorbien, Martin (MD)	248
Dementia/Alzheimer's	Neurology	Chui, Helena Chang (MD)	419
Depression	Child & Adolescent Psychiatry	Russell, Andrew Thomas (MD)	670
Depression	Child & Adolescent Psychiatry	Ryan, Neal David (MD)	666
Depression	Geriatric Psychiatry	Goldman, Samuel (MD)	673
Depression	Geriatric Psychiatry	Greenwald, Blaine (MD)	672
Depression	Geriatric Psychiatry	Kramer, Barry Alan (MD)	675
Depression	Geriatric Psychiatry	Leuchter, Andrew Francis (MD)	675
Depression	Geriatric Psychiatry	Mellow, Alan M. (MD/PhD)	674
Depression	Geriatric Psychiatry	Reisberg, Barry (MD)	673
Depression	Geriatric Psychiatry	Schneider, Lon S (MD)	675

Special Expertise	Specialty	Doctor's Name	Page
Diabetes	Endocrinology, Diabetes & Metabolism	Kamdar, Vikram V (MD)	212
Diabetes	Endocrinology, Diabetes & Metabolism	Korytkowski, Mary T (MD)	200
Diabetes	Endocrinology, Diabetes & Metabolism	Kreisberg, Robert Alan (MD)	204
Diabetes	Endocrinology, Diabetes & Metabolism	Lavis, Victor Ralph (MD)	210
Diabetes	Endocrinology, Diabetes & Metabolism	Levy, Philip (MD)	210
Diabetes	Endocrinology, Diabetes & Metabolism	Mersey, James Harris (MD)	201
Diabetes	Endocrinology, Diabetes & Metabolism	Moses, Alan Charles (MD)	198
Diabetes	Endocrinology, Diabetes & Metabolism	Ovalle, Fernando (MD)	204
Diabetes	Endocrinology, Diabetes & Metabolism	Polonsky, Kenneth S (MD)	208
Diabetes	Endocrinology, Diabetes & Metabolism	Powers, Alvin C (MD)	205
Diabetes	Endocrinology, Diabetes & Metabolism	Raskin, Philip (MD)	210
Diabetes	Endocrinology, Diabetes & Metabolism	Ratner, Robert (MD)	201
Diabetes	Endocrinology, Diabetes & Metabolism	Rudnick, Paul Arthur (MD)	212
Diabetes	Endocrinology, Diabetes & Metabolism	Saudek, Christopher D (MD)	202
Diabetes	Endocrinology, Diabetes & Metabolism	Schwartz, Stanley (MD)	202
Diabetes	Endocrinology, Diabetes & Metabolism	Semenkovich, Clay F (MD)	209
Diabetes	Endocrinology, Diabetes & Metabolism	Sherwin, Robert (MD)	198
Diabetes	Endocrinology, Diabetes & Metabolism	Shuldiner, Alan Rodney (MD)	202
Diabetes	Endocrinology, Diabetes & Metabolism	Skyler, Jay S (MD)	205
Diabetes	Endocrinology, Diabetes & Metabolism	Weissman, Peter (MD)	205
Diabetes	Endocrinology, Diabetes & Metabolism	Werner, Phillip Ladd (MD)	209
Diabetes	Geriatric Medicine	Schwartz, Robert S (MD)	249
Diabetes	Internal Medicine	Beaser, Richard Seth (MD)	333
Diabetes	Internal Medicine	Braunstein, Seth N (MD/PhD)	333
Diabetes	Internal Medicine	Corbett Jr, Eugene Charles (MD)	335
Diabetes	Internal Medicine	De Fronzo, Ralph Anthony (MD)	337
Diabetes	Pediatric Endocrinology	Allen, David Bruce (MD)	575
Diabetes	Pediatric Endocrinology	Becker, Dorothy Joan (MD)	572
Diabetes	Pediatric Endocrinology	Dahms, William (MD)	575
Diabetes	Pediatric Endocrinology	Foster, Carol M (MD)	575
Diabetes	Pediatric Endocrinology	Freemark, Michael Scott (MD)	574
Diabetes	Pediatric Endocrinology	Kaufman, Francine R (MD)	577
Diabetes	Pediatric Endocrinology	Klingensmith, Georgeanna (MD)	577
Diabetes	Pediatric Endocrinology	Levitsky, Lynne Lipton (MD)	572
Diabetes	Pediatric Endocrinology	Mahoney, Charles Patrick (MD)	577
Diabetes	Pediatric Endocrinology	New, Maria Iandolo (MD)	573
Diabetes	Pediatric Endocrinology	Plotnick, Leslie Parker (MD)	573
Diabetes	Pediatric Endocrinology	Rogers, Douglas G (MD)	576
Diabetes	Pediatric Endocrinology	Silverstein, Janet H (MD)	575
Diabetes	Pediatric Endocrinology	Sperling, Mark Alexander (MD)	573
Diabetes	Pediatric Endocrinology	Tamborlane, William V (MD)	572
Diabetes in Pregnancy	Endocrinology, Diabetes & Metabolism	Ratner, Robert (MD)	201
Diabetes in Pregnancy	Obstetrics & Gynecology	Socol, Michael (MD)	437
Diabetes Insipidus	Endocrinology, Diabetes & Metabolism	Robertson, Gary Lee (MD)	209
Diabetes-Amputation	Orthopaedic Surgery	Chambers, Richard Byron (MD)	496
Diabetes-Gastrointestinal Complications	Gastroenterology	Sninsky, Charles (MD)	229
Diabetes-Gestational	Maternal & Fetal Medicine	Gabbe, Steven G (MD)	347
Diabetes-Insulin Pump Therapy	Endocrinology, Diabetes & Metabolism	Bell, David S H (MD)	203
Diabetes-Insulin-dependent	Endocrinology, Diabetes & Metabolism	Bell, David S H (MD)	203
Diabetes-Lipid Disorders	Endocrinology, Diabetes & Metabolism	Rizza, Robert Alan (MD)	208
Diabetic Eye Disease	Ophthalmology	Gentile, Ronald (MD)	446
Diabetic Eye Disease/Retinopathy	Ophthalmology	Aiello, Lloyd (MD)	443
Diabetic Eye Disease/Retinopathy	Ophthalmology	Flynn, Harry W (MD)	453
Diabetic Eye Disease/Retinopathy	Ophthalmology	Fuchs, Wayne (MD)	446
Diabetic Eye Disease/Retinopathy	Ophthalmology	Goldberg, Morton (MD)	446
Diabetic Eye Disease/Retinopathy	Ophthalmology	Guyer, David (MD)	446
Diabetic Eye Disease/Retinopathy	Ophthalmology	Lambert, H. Michael (MD)	462
Diabetic Eye Disease/Retinopathy	Ophthalmology	Nussbaum, Julian (MD)	459
Diabetic Eye Disease/Retinopathy	Ophthalmology	Rosen, Richard (MD)	450
Diabetic Kidney Disease	Nephrology	Brenner, Barry M (MD)	359

Special Expertise	Specialty	Doctor's Name	Page
Diabetic Kidney Disease	Nephrology	Friedman, Eli A (MD)	361
Diabetic Kidney Disease	Nephrology	Lewis, Edmund J (MD)	365
Diabetic Kidney Disease	Nephrology	Seifter, Julian L (MD)	360
Diabetic Leg Reconstruction	Plastic Surgery	Attinger, Chris (MD)	636
Diabetic Leg/Foot	Vascular Surgery (General)	Gibbons, Gary William (MD)	858
Diabetic Leg/Foot	Vascular Surgery (General)	Lo Gerfo, Frank W (MD)	858
Diagnostic Problems	Internal Medicine	Sarosi, George (MD)	336
Dialysis Care	Nephrology	Swartz, Richard D (MD)	366
Dialysis-Peritoneal	Pediatric Nephrology	Bergstein, Jerry (MD)	597
Diarrhea	Gastroenterology	Fordtran, John (MD)	236
Diarrhea	Gastroenterology	Holt, Peter R (MD)	223
Diarrhea	Gastroenterology	Roche, James Kenneth (MD/PhD)	229
Diarrhea	Infectious Disease	Bartlett, John Gill (MD)	318
Diarrhea	Infectious Disease	DuPont, Herbert Lancashire (MD)	327
Digestion	Gastroenterology	Owyang, Chung (MD)	233
Digestion-Motility Disorders	Gastroenterology	Drossman, Douglas Arnold (MD)	228
Diplopia	Ophthalmology	Hall, Lisabeth (MD)	446
Disc Disease	Neurological Surgery	Branch Jr, Charles L (MD)	379
Disc Disease	Neurological Surgery	Kelly Jr, David L (MD)	380
Disc Disease-Lumbar	Neurological Surgery	Hoff, Julian T (MD)	383
Dissociative Disorders	Psychiatry	Loewenstein, Richard (MD)	680
Dissociative Disorders	Psychiatry	Wait, Susan Braynard (MD)	682
Diverticulitis	Colon & Rectal Surgery	Goldberg, Stanley (MD)	174
Diverticulitis	Colon & Rectal Surgery	Roberts, Patricia L (MD)	169
Diverticulitis	Colon & Rectal Surgery	Steinhagen, Randolph (MD)	171
Dizziness	Neurology	Troost, Bradley Todd (MD)	410
Dizziness	Otolaryngology	Brookler, Kenneth (MD)	502
Dizziness	Otolaryngology	Goebel, Joel Alan (MD)	514
Down Syndrome	Child Neurology	Lott, Ira T (MD)	156
Down Syndrome	Pediatric Hematology-Oncology	Rosoff, Phillip Martin (MD)	586
Drug Abuse	Addiction Psychiatry	Galanter, Marc (MD)	661
Drug Hepatotoxicity	Gastroenterology	Raiford, David S (MD)	229
Drug Induced Lung Disease	Pulmonary Disease	Cooper, John Allen Dicks (MD)	697
Drug Sensitivity	Allergy & Immunology	Adkinson, Franklin (MD)	95
Drug Toxicity-Kidneys	Nephrology	Bennett, William M (MD)	368
Dupuytren's Contracture	Hand Surgery	McCormack Jr, Richard R (MD)	268
Dyslexia	Child Neurology	Shaywitz, Bennett (MD)	151
Dyslexia	Pediatrics	Shaywitz, Sally Epstein (MD)	617
Dysmorphology	Clinical Genetics	Graham Jr, John M (MD)	164
Dysmorphology	Clinical Genetics	Hoyme, Harold Eugene (MD)	164
Dysmorphology	Clinical Genetics	Jones, Marilyn (MD)	165
Dysmorphology	Clinical Genetics	Martin, Rick A (MD)	162
Dysmorphology	Clinical Genetics	Willner, Judith P (MD)	160
Dysmorphology	Pediatrics	Hall, Bryan Davis (MD)	161
Dysphagia	Gastroenterology	Brazer, Scott Robert (MD)	226
Dysphagia	Gastroenterology	Ravich, William Jay (MD)	225

E

Ear & Nasal Disorders/Surgery	Otolaryngology	Johnson Jr, Calvin M (MD)	520
Ear Disorders/Surgery	Otolaryngology	Antonelli, Patrick (MD)	507
Ear Disorders/Surgery	Otolaryngology	Farmer, Joseph (MD)	508
Ear Disorders/Surgery	Otolaryngology	Farrior, Joseph Brown (MD)	508
Ear Disorders/Surgery	Otolaryngology	Gantz, Bruce (MD)	513
Ear Disorders/Surgery	Otolaryngology	Jenkins, Herman A. (MD)	519
Ear Disorders/Surgery	Otolaryngology	Kartush, Jack (MD)	514
Ear Disorders/Surgery	Otolaryngology	Nadol, Joseph (MD)	501
Ear Disorders/Surgery	Otolaryngology	Niparko, John (MD)	505
Ear Disorders/Surgery	Otolaryngology	Roland, Peter S (MD)	520
Ear Disorders/Surgery	Otolaryngology	Silverstein, Herbert (MD)	511

SPECIAL EXPERTISE INDEX

SPECIAL EXPERTISE INDEX

Special Expertise	Specialty	Doctor's Name	Page
Epilepsy/Seizure Disorders	Neurology	French, Jacqueline (MD)	402
Epilepsy/Seizure Disorders	Neurology	Krumholz, Allan (MD)	403
Epilepsy/Seizure Disorders	Neurology	Pedley, Timothy A. (MD)	404
Epilepsy/Seizure Disorders	Neurology	Spencer, Susan S (MD)	399
Epilepsy/Seizure Disorders	Radiology	Hasso, Anton N (MD)	739
Epstein-Barr Virus	Pediatric Infectious Disease	Jenson, Hal B (MD)	593
Erectile Dysfunction	Urology	Broderick, Gregory (MD)	837
Erectile Dysfunction	Urology	Burnett II, Arthur L (MD)	831
Erectile Dysfunction	Urology	Carson, Culley (MD)	837
Erectile Dysfunction	Urology	Eid, Jean Francois (MD)	831
Erectile Dysfunction	Urology	Fuselier Jr, Harold A (MD)	846
Erectile Dysfunction	Urology	Gluckman, Gordon (MD)	842
Erectile Dysfunction	Urology	Goldstein, Irwin (MD)	829
Erectile Dysfunction	Urology	Gomery, Pablo (MD)	829
Erectile Dysfunction	Urology	Jarow, Jonathan (MD)	833
Erectile Dysfunction	Urology	Levine, Laurence Adan (MD)	842
Erectile Dysfunction	Urology	Lewis, Ronald W (MD)	838
Erectile Dysfunction	Urology	Lipshultz, Larry (MD)	846
Erectile Dysfunction	Urology	Mc Vary, Kevin (MD)	842
Erectile Dysfunction	Urology	Melman, Arnold (MD)	834
Erectile Dysfunction	Urology	Montague, Drogo K. (MD)	843
Erectile Dysfunction	Urology	Mulcahy, John J. (MD)	843
Erectile Dysfunction	Urology	Padma-Nathan, Harin (MD)	849
Erectile Dysfunction	Urology	Pryor, Jon L. (MD)	843
Erectile Dysfunction	Urology	Rajfer, Jacob (MD)	849
Erectile Dysfunction	Urology	Seftel, Allen D (MD)	844
Erectile Dysfunction	Urology	Sharlip, Ira Dorian (MD)	850
Erectile Dysfunction	Urology	Thomas, Anthony J. (MD)	844
Esophageal & Swallowing Disorders	Gastroenterology	Winans, Charles (MD)	235
Esophageal Cancer	Gastroenterology	Brazer, Scott Robert (MD)	226
Esophageal Cancer	Gastroenterology	Fleischer, David (MD)	223
Esophageal Cancer	Medical Oncology	Leichman, Lawrence Peter (MD)	298
Esophageal Cancer	Medical Oncology	Masters, Gregory (MD)	307
Esophageal Cancer	Radiation Oncology	Choi, Noah C (MD)	717
Esophageal Cancer	Surgery	Vogel, Stephen Burton (MD)	792
Esophageal Cancer	Thoracic Surgery	Bains, Manjit (MD)	807
Esophageal Cancer	Thoracic Surgery	Ferguson, Mark (MD)	817
Esophageal Cancer	Thoracic Surgery	Heitmiller, Richard F (MD)	809
Esophageal Cancer	Thoracic Surgery	Mathisen, Douglas (MD)	806
Esophageal Cancer	Thoracic Surgery	Meyers, Bryan (MD)	818
Esophageal Cancer	Thoracic Surgery	Moncure, Ashby (MD)	806
Esophageal Cancer	Thoracic Surgery	Orringer, Mark B (MD)	818
Esophageal Cancer	Thoracic Surgery	Putnam Jr, Joe B (MD)	822
Esophageal Cancer	Thoracic Surgery	Trastek, Victor (MD)	822
Esophageal Cancer	Thoracic Surgery	Whyte, Richard (MD)	826
Esophageal Cancer	Thoracic Surgery	Wood, Douglas (MD)	826
Esophageal Disease, Benign	Thoracic Surgery	Orringer, Mark B (MD)	818
Esophageal Disorders	Gastroenterology	Achkar, Edgar (MD)	230
Esophageal Disorders	Gastroenterology	Benjamin, Stanley (MD)	222
Esophageal Disorders	Gastroenterology	Brady III, Charles Elmer (MD)	235
Esophageal Disorders	Gastroenterology	Clouse, Ray Eugene (MD)	231
Esophageal Disorders	Gastroenterology	Kahrilas, Peter (MD)	232
Esophageal Disorders	Gastroenterology	Kotler, Donald P (MD)	224
Esophageal Disorders	Gastroenterology	Lipshutz, William H. (MD)	224
Esophageal Disorders	Gastroenterology	Richter, Joel (MD)	234
Esophageal Disorders	Pediatric Gastroenterology	Wyllie, Robert (MD)	581
Esophageal Surgery	Pediatric Surgery	Othersen, H Biemann (MD)	614
Esophageal Surgery	Surgery	Pellegrini, Carlos (MD)	801
Esophageal Surgery	Surgery	Peters, Jeffrey Harold (MD)	801
Esophageal Surgery	Thoracic Surgery	Bredenberg, Carl Eric (MD)	805

SPECIAL EXPERTISE INDEX

Special Expertise	Specialty	Doctor's Name	Page
Family Therapy	Child & Adolescent Psychiatry	Russak, Sidney (MD)	670
Family Therapy	Child & Adolescent Psychiatry	Sargent III, A John (MD)	669
Febrile Infants	Pediatrics	Pantell, Robert Howard (MD)	619
Feeding & Nutrition	Pediatric Gastroenterology	Berman, James (MD)	580
Fetal Alcohol Syndrome	Clinical Genetics	Hoyme, Harold Eugene (MD)	164
Fetal Alcohol Syndrome	Clinical Genetics	Seaver, Laurie Heron (MD)	161
Fetal Anomaly	Maternal & Fetal Medicine	Dooley, Sharon L (MD)	345
Fetal Assessment	Obstetrics & Gynecology	Johnson, Timothy R.B. (MD)	436
Fetal Cardiology	Pediatric Cardiology	Sanders, Stephen Pruett (MD)	563
Fetal Diagnosis	Maternal & Fetal Medicine	Koos, Brian John (MD)	348
Fetal Echogram	Pediatric Cardiology	Colvin, Edward V (MD)	563
Fetal Macrosomia	Maternal & Fetal Medicine	Benedetti, Thomas J (MD)	347
Fetal Pathology	Clinical Genetics	Seaver, Laurie Heron (MD)	161
Fetal Stress	Maternal & Fetal Medicine	Hobel, Calvin John (MD)	348
Fetal Surgery	Maternal & Fetal Medicine	Chescheir, Nancy Custer (MD)	344
Fetal Surgery	Pediatric Surgery	Adzick, Nick Scott (MD)	611
Fetal Surgery	Pediatric Surgery	Harrison, Michael R (MD)	616
Fetal Therapy	Maternal & Fetal Medicine	Goldberg, James David (MD)	348
Fetal Transfusion	Maternal & Fetal Medicine	Strassner, Howard T (MD)	346
Fevers-Unknown Origin	Pediatric Infectious Disease	Givner, Laurence Bruce (MD)	592
Fibroid Embolization	Radiology	Yoon, Sydney (MD)	736
Fibroids	Reproductive Endocrinology	Barbieri, Robert (MD)	743
Fibroids	Reproductive Endocrinology	Bieber, Eric Joseph (MD)	748
Fibroids	Reproductive Endocrinology	Marrs, Richard P (MD)	752
Fibroids	Reproductive Endocrinology	Wallach, Edward Eliot (MD)	745
Fibroids	Reproductive Endocrinology	Wood Molo, Mary (MD)	750
Fibromyalgia	Pediatric Rheumatology	Schanberg, Laura Eve (MD)	609
Fibromyalgia	Rheumatology	Chatham, Walter W (MD)	762
Fibromyalgia	Rheumatology	Clauw, Daniel J (MD)	758
Fibromyalgia	Rheumatology	Crofford, Leslie (MD)	764
Fibromyalgia	Rheumatology	Katz, Robert (MD)	765
Fistula	Colon & Rectal Surgery	Bailey, Harold Randolph (MD)	176
Flexor Tendon Surgery	Hand Surgery	Gelberman, Richard (MD)	272
Fluid/Electrolyte Balance	Internal Medicine	Coe, Fredric (MD)	364
Fluid/Electrolyte Balance	Nephrology	Berl, Tomas (MD)	366
Fluid/Electrolyte Balance	Nephrology	Olivero, Juan Jose (MD)	367
Food Allergy	Allergy & Immunology	Metcalfe, Dean D (MD)	97
Food Allergy	Pediatric Allergy & Immunology	Bahna, Sami Labib (MD)	556
Food Allergy	Pediatric Allergy & Immunology	Wood, Robert Alan (MD)	556
Food Allergy	Pediatric Pulmonology	Lapey, Allen (MD)	604
Foot & Ankle Surgery	Orthopaedic Surgery	Bauman, Phillip (MD)	478
Foot & Ankle Surgery	Orthopaedic Surgery	Brage, Michael (MD)	496
Foot & Ankle Surgery	Orthopaedic Surgery	Coughlin, Michael (MD)	493
Foot & Ankle Surgery	Orthopaedic Surgery	Deland, Jonathan T (MD)	480
Foot & Ankle Surgery	Orthopaedic Surgery	Hansen Jr., Sigvard (MD)	497
Foot & Ankle Surgery	Orthopaedic Surgery	Myerson, Mark (MD)	482
Foot & Ankle Surgery	Orthopaedic Surgery	Saltzman, Charles Louis (MD)	492
Foot & Ankle Surgery	Orthopaedic Surgery	Webb, Lawrence (MD)	488
Foot Surgery	Orthopaedic Surgery	Brodsky, James White (MD)	494
Foot Surgery	Orthopaedic Surgery	Manoli II, Arthur (MD)	491
Foot Surgery	Orthopaedic Surgery	Waller, John F (MD)	484
Foot Surgery	Orthopaedic Surgery	Wapner, Keith Leslie (MD)	485
Forehead Lift-Endoscpic	Otolaryngology	Quatela, Vito Charles (MD)	506
Forensic Psychiatry	Psychiatry	Ballenger, James (MD)	682
Forensic Psychiatry	Psychiatry	Eth, Spencer (MD)	678
Forensic Psychiatry	Psychiatry	Menninger, W Walter (MD)	684
Forensic Psychiatry	Psychiatry	Neppe, Vernon Michael (MD)	687
Forensic Psychiatry	Psychiatry	Simon, Robert Isaac (MD)	681
Fott & Ankle Surgery	Orthopaedic Surgery	Sangeorzan, Bruce J. (MD)	498
Fractures-Complex	Orthopaedic Surgery	Browner, Bruce D (MD)	475

SPECIAL EXPERTISE INDEX

Special Expertise	Specialty	Doctor's Name	Page
Fractures-Complex	Orthopaedic Surgery	Helfet, David L (MD)	481
Fractures-Non Union	Orthopaedic Surgery	Swiontkowski, Marc F (MD)	493
Frail Elderly	Geriatric Medicine	Hanson, Laura Catherine ()	246
Frailty	Physical Medicine & Rehabilitation	De Lateur, Barbara J (MD)	623
Fungal Infection	Pediatric Infectious Disease	Saiman, Lisa (MD)	591
Fungal Infections	Infectious Disease	Dismukes, William Ernest (MD)	323
Fungal Infections	Infectious Disease	Edwards Jr., John Ellis (MD)	328
Fungal Infections	Infectious Disease	Van Der Horst, Charles (MD)	325
Fungal Infections	Internal Medicine	Graybill, John Richard (MD)	337
Fungal Lung Disease	Internal Medicine	Sarosi, George (MD)	336

G

Special Expertise	Specialty	Doctor's Name	Page
Gallbladder & Swallowing Disorders	Gastroenterology	Craig, Robert M (MD)	231
Gastric Diseases	Gastroenterology	Schulze, Konrad S (MD)	234
Gastric Diseases	Thoracic Surgery	De Meester, Tom R (MD)	823
Gastroenterology	Pediatric Gastroenterology	Christie, Dennis (MD)	581
Gastroenterology	Pediatric Gastroenterology	Levy, Joseph (MD)	578
Gastroesophageal Reflux	Gastroenterology	Clouse, Ray Eugene (MD)	231
Gastroesophageal Reflux	Gastroenterology	Diamond, Jeffrey (MD)	227
Gastroesophageal Reflux	Gastroenterology	Kodsi, Baroukh (MD)	223
Gastroesophageal Reflux	Gastroenterology	Richter, Joel (MD)	234
Gastroesophageal Reflux	Gastroenterology	Schulze, Konrad S (MD)	234
Gastroesophageal Reflux	Gastroenterology	Winans, Charles (MD)	235
Gastroesophageal Reflux	Internal Medicine	Roth, Bennett E (MD)	337
Gastroesophageal Reflux	Pediatric Gastroenterology	Hillemeier, A Craig (MD)	580
Gastroesophageal Reflux	Pediatric Gastroenterology	Schwarz, Steven M (MD)	579
Gastroesophageal Reflux	Pediatric Surgery	Fonkalsrud, Eric W (MD)	616
Gastroesophageal Reflux	Thoracic Surgery	Deschamps, Claude (MD)	817
Gastrointestinal Cancer	Gastroenterology	Barkin, Jamie (MD)	226
Gastrointestinal Cancer	Gastroenterology	Bresalier, Robert (MD)	230
Gastrointestinal Cancer	Gastroenterology	Chuttani, Ram (MD)	221
Gastrointestinal Cancer	Gastroenterology	Forsmark, Christopher (MD)	228
Gastrointestinal Cancer	Gastroenterology	Levin, Bernard (MD)	236
Gastrointestinal Cancer	Gastroenterology	Liddle, Rodger Alan (MD)	228
Gastrointestinal Cancer	Medical Oncology	Abbruzzese, James L (MD)	310
Gastrointestinal Cancer	Medical Oncology	Grossbard, Michael Laurence (MD)	296
Gastrointestinal Cancer	Medical Oncology	Haller, Daniel (MD)	296
Gastrointestinal Cancer	Medical Oncology	Horton, John (MD)	301
Gastrointestinal Cancer	Medical Oncology	Leichman, Lawrence Peter (MD)	298
Gastrointestinal Cancer	Medical Oncology	Todd III, Robert F (MD/PhD)	309
Gastrointestinal Cancer	Medical Oncology	Vogelzang, Nicholas (MD)	309
Gastrointestinal Cancer	Medical Oncology	Weiner, Louis M (MD)	300
Gastrointestinal Cancer	Radiation Oncology	Rich, Tyvin Andrew (MD)	722
Gastrointestinal Cancer	Radiation Oncology	Smalley, Stephen R (MD)	725
Gastrointestinal Cancer	Radiation Oncology	Tepper, Joel (MD)	723
Gastrointestinal Cancer	Radiation Oncology	Willett, Chris (MD)	718
Gastrointestinal Motility Disorders	Gastroenterology	Wald, Arnold (MD)	225
Gastrointestinal Motility Disorders	Pediatric Gastroenterology	Boyle, John T (MD)	580
Gastrointestinal Pathology	Pathology	Appelman, Henry (MD)	540
Gastrointestinal Pathology	Pathology	Bostwick, David (MD)	539
Gastrointestinal Pathology	Pathology	Chandrasoma, Parakrama T (MD)	542
Gastrointestinal Pathology	Pathology	Lewin, Klaus J (MD)	543
Gastrointestinal Surgery	Surgery	Howard, Richard J (MD)	791
Gastrointestinal Surgery	Surgery	Koruda, Mark Joseph (MD)	791
Gastrointestinal Surgery	Surgery	MacFadyen, Bruce (MD)	798
Gastrointestinal Surgery	Surgery	Zinner, Michael (MD)	783
Gastrointestinal/Liver Surgery	Surgery	Schirmer, Bruce David (MD)	792
Gastroparesis	Gastroenterology	Schulze, Konrad S (MD)	234
Gastroscopy	Gastroenterology	Gostout, Christopher John (MD)	232

SPECIAL EXPERTISE INDEX

Special Expertise	Specialty	Doctor's Name	Page
Gastroscopy	Internal Medicine	Yaffe, Bruce (MD)	334
Gene-Targeted Radiotherapy	Radiation Oncology	Weichselbaum, Ralph R (MD)	724
Genetic Disorders	Child Neurology	Menkes, John H (MD)	156
Genetic Disorders	Clinical Genetics	Desposito, Franklin (MD)	160
Genetic Disorders	Clinical Genetics	Grody, Wayne W (MD)	164
Genetic Disorders	Clinical Genetics	Huff, Robert Whitley (MD)	438
Genetic Disorders	Clinical Genetics	Nussbaum, Robert (MD)	159
Genetic Disorders	Clinical Genetics	Weaver, David Dawson (MD)	162
Genetic Disorders	Maternal & Fetal Medicine	Landy, Helain Jody (MD)	342
Genetic Disorders	Reproductive Endocrinology	Rosenwaks, Zev (MD)	745
Genetic Kidney Disease	Pediatric Nephrology	Kashtan, Clifford (MD)	598
Genitourinary Cancer	Medical Oncology	Balducci, Lodovico (MD)	300
Genitourinary Cancer	Medical Oncology	Hudes, Gary Robert (MD)	297
Genitourinary Cancer	Medical Oncology	Scher, Howard (MD)	299
Genitourinary Cancer	Radiation Oncology	Forman, Jeffrey D (MD)	723
Genitourinary Cancer	Urology	McCullough, David L (MD)	838
Genitourinary Cancer	Urology	Swanson, David A (MD)	847
Genitourinary Congenital Abnormality	Urology	Walker lll, R Dixon (MD)	840
Genitourinary Reconstruction-Complex	Urology	Koyle, Martin Allan (MD)	845
Genitourinary-Congenital Anomaly	Pediatrics	Zilleruelo, Gaston E (MD)	618
Geriatric Endocrinology	Endocrinology, Diabetes & Metabolism	Axelrod, Lloyd (MD)	197
Geriatric Endocrinology	Geriatric Medicine	Carter, William Jerry (MD)	250
Geriatric Infectious Disease	Infectious Disease	Yoshikawa, Thomas T (MD)	329
Geriatric Medicine	Allergy & Immunology	de Shazo, Richard Denson (MD)	98
Geriatric Medicine	Internal Medicine	Esch, Peter (MD)	335
Geriatric Medicine	Neurology	Ferrendelli, James A (MD)	416
GI Surgery	Colon & Rectal Surgery	Huber, Philip (MD)	176
Glanzmann's Thrombasthenia	Hematology	Coller, Barry (MD)	285
Glaucoma	Ophthalmology	Alward, Wallace (MD)	456
Glaucoma	Ophthalmology	Burde, Ronald (MD)	444
Glaucoma	Ophthalmology	Caprioli, Joseph (MD)	464
Glaucoma	Ophthalmology	Crandall, Alan Slade (MD)	461
Glaucoma	Ophthalmology	Kass, Michael A (MD)	457
Glaucoma	Ophthalmology	Lee, Paul P (MD)	454
Glaucoma	Ophthalmology	Lichter, Paul R. (MD)	458
Glaucoma	Ophthalmology	Liebmann, Jeffrey (MD)	447
Glaucoma	Ophthalmology	Medow, Norman (MD)	448
Glaucoma	Ophthalmology	Minckler, Donald Saier (MD)	466
Glaucoma	Ophthalmology	Palmberg, Paul (MD/PhD)	454
Glaucoma	Ophthalmology	Parrish, Richard K (MD)	454
Glaucoma	Ophthalmology	Pepose, Jay (MD)	459
Glaucoma	Ophthalmology	Podos, Steven M (MD)	449
Glaucoma	Ophthalmology	Quigley, Harry Alan (MD)	449
Glaucoma	Ophthalmology	Raab, Edward (MD)	449
Glaucoma	Ophthalmology	Ritch, Robert (MD)	450
Glaucoma	Ophthalmology	Samuelson, Thomas ()	460
Glaucoma & Strabismus-Pediatric	Ophthalmology	Jaafar, Mohamad S (MD)	447
Glaucoma-Congenital/Pediatric	Ophthalmology	Freedman, Sharon (MD)	453
Glaucoma-Pediatric	Ophthalmology	Traboulsi, Elias Iskan (MD)	460
Glaucoma-Pediatric	Ophthalmology	Walton, David S (MD)	444
Gonadotropin Deficiency	Reproductive Endocrinology	Crowley, William (MD)	743
Gout	Rheumatology	Sundy, John Sargent (MD/PhD)	762
Gout/Pseudogout	Rheumatology	Brenner, Michael B (MD)	757
Graft vs Host Disease	Pediatric Hematology-Oncology	Ferrara, James (MD)	587
Graft vs. Host Disease	Dermatology	Horn, Thomas (MD)	191
Graves' Disease	Endocrinology, Diabetes & Metabolism	Bahn, Rebecca Sue (MD)	206
Graves' Disease	Endocrinology, Diabetes & Metabolism	De Groot, Leslie (MD)	206
Graves' Disease	Endocrinology, Diabetes & Metabolism	Hurley, James (MD)	200
Growth/Development Disorders	Pediatric Endocrinology	Casella, Samuel Joseph (MD)	572
Growth/Development Disorders	Pediatric Endocrinology	Dahms, William (MD)	575

SPECIAL EXPERTISE INDEX

Special Expertise	Specialty	Doctor's Name	Page
Growth/Development Disorders	Pediatric Endocrinology	Foster, Carol M (MD)	575
Growth/Development Disorders	Pediatric Endocrinology	Freemark, Michael Scott (MD)	574
Growth/Development Disorders	Pediatric Endocrinology	Friedman, Nancy Eisenberg (MD)	574
Growth/Development Disorders	Pediatric Endocrinology	Geffner, Mitchell Eugene (MD)	577
Growth/Development Disorders	Pediatric Endocrinology	Kappy, Michael Steven (MD/PhD)	576
Growth/Development Disorders	Pediatric Endocrinology	Kaufman, Francine R (MD)	577
Growth/Development Disorders	Pediatric Endocrinology	Levitsky, Lynne Lipton (MD)	572
Growth/Development Disorders	Pediatric Endocrinology	Mahoney, Charles Patrick (MD)	577
Growth/Development Disorders	Pediatric Endocrinology	Maurer, William (MD)	576
Growth/Development Disorders	Pediatric Endocrinology	Moshang Jr., Thomas (MD)	573
Growth/Development Disorders	Pediatric Endocrinology	New, Maria Iandolo (MD)	573
Growth/Development Disorders	Pediatric Endocrinology	Rogers, Douglas G (MD)	576
Growth/Development Disorders	Pediatric Endocrinology	Silverstein, Janet H (MD)	575
Growth/Development Disorders	Pediatric Endocrinology	Zimmerman, Donald (MD)	576
Growth/Development Disorders	Pediatrics	Underwood, Louis (MD)	618
Guillain-Barre Syndrome	Neurology	Arnason, Barry G W (MD)	411
Guillain-Barre Syndrome	Neurology	Asbury, Arthur K (MD)	399
Guillain-Barre Syndrome	Neurology	Ropper, Allan (MD)	398
Gynecologic Cancer	Diagnostic Radiology	McCarthy, Shirley (MD/PhD)	731
Gynecologic Cancer	Gynecologic Oncology	Carlson, John (MD)	256
Gynecologic Cancer	Gynecologic Oncology	Chalas, Eva (MD)	256
Gynecologic Cancer	Gynecologic Oncology	Fiorica, James Vincent (MD)	258
Gynecologic Cancer	Gynecologic Oncology	Johnston, Carolyn Marie (MD)	260
Gynecologic Cancer	Gynecologic Oncology	Roberts, James A (MD)	264
Gynecologic Cancer	Gynecologic Oncology	Taylor Jr., Peyton T. (MD)	259
Gynecologic Cancer	Gynecologic Oncology	Teng, Nelson NH (MD/PhD)	264
Gynecologic Cancer	Gynecologic Oncology	Yordan, Edgardo (MD)	262
Gynecologic Cancer	Obstetrics & Gynecology	Berman, Michael Leonard (MD)	438
Gynecologic Cancer	Obstetrics & Gynecology	Boyce, John G (MD)	432
Gynecologic Cancer	Obstetrics & Gynecology	Morgan, Linda S (MD)	434
Gynecologic Cancer	Radiation Oncology	Juillard, Guy Jean-Felix (MD)	726
Gynecologic Pathology	Pathology	Hart, William (MD)	540
Gynecologic Pathology	Pathology	Hendrickson, Michael (MD)	543
Gynecologic Pathology	Pathology	Kempson, Richard (MD)	543
Gynecologic Pathology	Pathology	Kurman, Robert J (MD)	537
Gynecologic Surgery	Gynecologic Oncology	Massad, L Stewart (MD)	260
Gynecologic Surgery	Obstetrics & Gynecology	Eschenbach, David Arthur (MD)	438
Gynecologic Surgery	Obstetrics & Gynecology	Merrick, Frank W (MD)	436
Gynecologic Surgery	Obstetrics & Gynecology	Reilly, Raymond J (MD)	431
Gynecologic Surgery	Obstetrics & Gynecology	Sciarra, John J (MD)	437
Gynecologic Surgery-Benign	Obstetrics & Gynecology	Steege, John Francis (MD)	434
Gynecologic Surgery-Complex	Gynecologic Oncology	Clarke-Pearson, Daniel L (MD)	258
Gynecologic Surgery-Complex	Gynecologic Oncology	Johnston, Carolyn Marie (MD)	260
Gynecologic Surgery-Complex	Gynecologic Oncology	Taylor Jr., Peyton T. (MD)	259
Gynecology	Obstetrics & Gynecology	Gluck, Paul (MD)	434
Gynecology-Adolescent	Obstetrics & Gynecology	Merritt, Diane (MD)	436
Gynecology-Adolescent	Obstetrics & Gynecology	Wylen, Michele (MD)	433

H

Hair Loss & Restoration Surgery	Dermatology	Cohen, Bernard Hershel (MD)	187
Hair Problems	Dermatology	Nigra, Thomas P (MD)	185
Hair Removal	Dermatology	Grossman, Melanie (MD)	184
Hair Restoration/Transplant	Dermatology	Bernstein, Robert M (MD)	183
Hair Restoration/Transplant	Surgery	Rassman, William Richard (MD)	801
Hair Transplantation & Laser Surgery	Dermatology	Fitzpatrick, Richard (MD)	192
Hand & Microvascular Surgery	Hand Surgery	Chiu, David (MD)	267
Hand & Microvascular Surgery	Hand Surgery	Chung, Kevin (MD)	271
Hand & Microvascular Surgery	Hand Surgery	Greene, Thomas (MD)	270
Hand & Wrist Fractures	Hand Surgery	McCormack Jr, Richard R (MD)	268

SPECIAL EXPERTISE INDEX

Special Expertise	Specialty	Doctor's Name	Page
Head & Neck Cancer	Otolaryngology	Kern, Robert (MD)	514
Head & Neck Cancer	Otolaryngology	Levine, Paul (MD)	509
Head & Neck Cancer	Otolaryngology	McGuirt, W Fredrick (MD)	509
Head & Neck Cancer	Otolaryngology	Medina, Jesus (MD)	520
Head & Neck Cancer	Otolaryngology	Myers, Eugene (MD)	505
Head & Neck Cancer	Otolaryngology	Otto, Randal A (MD)	520
Head & Neck Cancer	Otolaryngology	Pelzer, Harold J (MD/DDS)	515
Head & Neck Cancer	Otolaryngology	Persky, Mark (MD)	505
Head & Neck Cancer	Otolaryngology	Peters, Glenn Eidson (MD)	510
Head & Neck Cancer	Otolaryngology	Rice, Dale (MD)	523
Head & Neck Cancer	Otolaryngology	Sasaki, Clarence T (MD)	501
Head & Neck Cancer	Otolaryngology	Schuller, David (MD)	516
Head & Neck Cancer	Otolaryngology	Siegel, Gordon J (MD)	516
Head & Neck Cancer	Otolaryngology	Sinha, Uttam Kumar (MD)	523
Head & Neck Cancer	Otolaryngology	Stringer, Scott Pearson (MD)	511
Head & Neck Cancer	Otolaryngology	Suen, James (MD)	520
Head & Neck Cancer	Otolaryngology	Valentino, Joseph (MD)	511
Head & Neck Cancer	Otolaryngology	Weinstein, Gregory (MD)	507
Head & Neck Cancer	Otolaryngology	Weissler, Mark Christian (MD)	512
Head & Neck Cancer	Otolaryngology	Weymuller, Ernest (MD)	523
Head & Neck Cancer	Radiation Oncology	Ang, Kie-Kian (MD/PhD)	725
Head & Neck Cancer	Radiation Oncology	Emami, Bahman (MD)	723
Head & Neck Cancer	Radiation Oncology	Haffty, Bruce (MD)	717
Head & Neck Cancer	Radiation Oncology	Harrison, Louis (MD)	719
Head & Neck Cancer	Radiation Oncology	Juillard, Guy Jean-Felix (MD)	726
Head & Neck Cancer	Radiation Oncology	Mendenhall, William M (MD)	722
Head & Neck Cancer	Radiation Oncology	Sailer, Scott (MD)	722
Head & Neck Cancer	Radiation Oncology	Streeter Jr, Oscar E (MD)	727
Head & Neck Cancer	Radiation Oncology	Weichselbaum, Ralph R (MD)	724
Head & Neck Cancer	Surgery	Shaha, Ashok (MD)	788
Head & Neck Reconstruction	Otolaryngology	Levine, Paul (MD)	509
Head & Neck Reconstruction	Otolaryngology	Picken, Catherine A (MD)	505
Head & Neck Reconstruction	Plastic Surgery	Ketch, Lawrence Levant (MD)	648
Head & Neck Surgery	Otolaryngology	Abramson, Allan (MD)	502
Head & Neck Surgery	Otolaryngology	Bailey, Byron J (MD)	518
Head & Neck Surgery	Otolaryngology	Baim, Howard (MD)	512
Head & Neck Surgery	Otolaryngology	Berke, Gerald Spencer (MD)	521
Head & Neck Surgery	Otolaryngology	Cummings, Charles (MD)	503
Head & Neck Surgery	Otolaryngology	De la Cruz, Antonio (MD)	521
Head & Neck Surgery	Otolaryngology	Gluckman, Jack L (MD)	513
Head & Neck Surgery	Otolaryngology	Goepfert, Helmuth (MD)	519
Head & Neck Surgery	Otolaryngology	Hayden, Richard Earle (MD)	504
Head & Neck Surgery	Otolaryngology	Johnson, Jonas Talmadge (MD)	504
Head & Neck Surgery	Otolaryngology	Myers, Eugene (MD)	505
Head & Neck Surgery	Otolaryngology	Netterville, James (MD)	510
Head & Neck Surgery	Otolaryngology	Pearson, Bruce (MD)	510
Head & Neck Surgery	Otolaryngology	Robbins, Thomas (MD)	511
Head & Neck Surgery	Otolaryngology	Schaefer, Steven (MD)	506
Head & Neck Surgery	Otolaryngology	Schuller, David (MD)	516
Head & Neck Surgery	Otolaryngology	Urken, Mark (MD)	506
Head & Neck Surgery	Otolaryngology	Wackym, Phillip (MD)	517
Head & Neck Surgery	Otolaryngology	Zeitels, Steven (MD)	502
Head & Neck Surgery	Pediatric Otolaryngology	Cotton, Robin (MD)	602
Head & Neck Surgery	Pediatric Otolaryngology	Drake, Amelia (MD)	601
Head & Neck Surgery	Pediatric Otolaryngology	Duncan III, Newton Oran (MD)	603
Head & Neck Surgery	Pediatric Otolaryngology	Rosenfeld, Richard M (MD)	601
Head & Neck Surgery	Pediatric Otolaryngology	Tunkel, David Eric (MD)	601
Head & Neck Surgery	Plastic Surgery	Ariyan, Stephan (MD)	635
Head & Neck Surgery	Surgery	Alfonso, Antonio (MD)	783
Head & Neck Surgery	Surgery	Leffall Jr, LaSalle D (MD)	786

Special Expertise	Specialty	Doctor's Name	Page
Head & Neck Surgery	Surgery	Shah, Jatin P (MD)	788
Head & Neck Trauma	Otolaryngology	Funk, Gerry Franklin (MD)	513
Head & Spinal Cord Injury	Neurological Surgery	Eisenberg, Howard M (MD)	375
Head Injury	Neurological Surgery	Clifton, Guy (MD)	386
Head Injury	Neurology	Bernad, Peter (MD)	400
Head Injury	Pediatric Critical Care Medicine	Kochanek, Patrick (MD)	569
Headache	Child Neurology	Prensky, Arthur (MD)	154
Headache	Child Neurology	Turk, William (MD)	153
Headache	Neurology	Lopez, Raul (MD)	409
Headache	Neurology	Petito, Frank (MD)	404
Headache	Neurology	Rothrock, John (MD)	409
Headache	Neurology	Troost, Bradley Todd (MD)	410
Headache	Neurology	Weinberg, Harold (MD)	406
Headache-Migraine	Neurology	Bernad, Peter (MD)	400
Hearing Disorders	Otolaryngology	Antonelli, Patrick (MD)	507
Hearing Disorders	Otolaryngology	Daspit, C Phillip (MD)	518
Hearing Disorders	Otolaryngology	Farmer, Joseph (MD)	508
Hearing Disorders	Otolaryngology	Goebel, Joel Alan (MD)	514
Hearing Disorders	Otolaryngology	Nadol, Joseph (MD)	501
Hearing Disorders	Pediatric Otolaryngology	Potsic, William Paul (MD)	601
Hearing Loss/Tinnitus	Otolaryngology	Brookler, Kenneth (MD)	502
Heart Assistance Devices	Thoracic Surgery	Acker, Michael Andrew (MD)	807
Heart Attack/ Sudden Death	Cardiac Electrophysiology	Gomes, J Anthony (MD)	115
Heart Bypass(off pump)	Thoracic Surgery	Craver, Joseph (MD)	812
Heart Disease	Cardiology (Cardiovascular Disease)	Segal, Bernard L (MD)	128
Heart Disease	Cardiology (Cardiovascular Disease)	Shlofmitz, Richard A (MD)	128
Heart Disease Imaging-Congenital	Pediatric Cardiology	Moodie, Douglas (MD)	565
Heart Disease in Pregnancy	Cardiology (Cardiovascular Disease)	Wilansky, Susan (MD)	140
Heart Disease in the Elderly	Cardiology (Cardiovascular Disease)	Wenger, Nanette Kass (MD)	133
Heart Disease in Women	Cardiology (Cardiovascular Disease)	Wenger, Nanette Kass (MD)	133
Heart Disease in Women	Cardiology (Cardiovascular Disease)	Wilansky, Susan (MD)	140
Heart Disease-Congenital	Cardiology (Cardiovascular Disease)	Byrd III, Benjamin F (MD)	130
Heart Disease-Congenital	Cardiology (Cardiovascular Disease)	Fuster, Valentin (MD)	125
Heart Disease-Congenital	Cardiology (Cardiovascular Disease)	Perloff, Joseph Kayle (MD)	142
Heart Disease-Congenital	Pediatric Cardiology	Boucek, Robert (MD)	562
Heart Disease-Congenital	Pediatric Cardiology	Brenner, Joel I (MD)	561
Heart Disease-Congenital	Pediatric Cardiology	Colvin, Edward V (MD)	563
Heart Disease-Congenital	Pediatric Cardiology	Dreyer, William Jeffrey (MD)	566
Heart Disease-Congenital	Pediatric Cardiology	Epstein, Michael (MD)	564
Heart Disease-Congenital	Pediatric Cardiology	Gersony, Welton Mark (MD)	562
Heart Disease-Congenital	Pediatric Cardiology	Hijazi, Ziyad M (MD)	565
Heart Disease-Congenital	Pediatric Cardiology	Liebman, Jerome (MD)	565
Heart Disease-Congenital	Pediatric Cardiology	Mahony, Lynn (MD)	566
Heart Disease-Congenital	Pediatric Cardiology	Mullins, Charles (MD)	567
Heart Disease-Congenital	Pediatric Cardiology	Newburger, Jane (MD)	561
Heart Disease-Congenital	Pediatric Cardiology	Rocchini, Albert P (MD)	565
Heart Disease-Congenital	Pediatric Cardiology	Rogers Jr, James Henry (MD)	567
Heart Disease-Congenital	Pediatric Cardiology	Rosenthal, Amnon (MD)	565
Heart Disease-Congenital	Pediatric Critical Care Medicine	Latson, Larry Allen (MD)	570
Heart Disease-Congenital	Thoracic Surgery	Bailey, Leonard Lee (MD)	823
Heart Disease-Congenital	Thoracic Surgery	Cohn, Lawrence H (MD)	805
Heart Disease-Congenital	Thoracic Surgery	Danielson, Gordon (MD)	816
Heart Disease-Congenital	Thoracic Surgery	Gardner, Timothy Joseph (MD)	808
Heart Disease-Congenital	Thoracic Surgery	Laks, Hillel (MD)	824
Heart Disease-Congenital	Thoracic Surgery	Pacifico, Albert D (MD)	814
Heart Disease-Congenital	Thoracic Surgery	Schaff, Hartzell (MD)	819
Heart Disease-Congenital	Thoracic Surgery	Ungerleider, Ross M (MD)	815
Heart Disease-Ischemic	Cardiology (Cardiovascular Disease)	Pepine, Carl J (MD)	131
Heart Disease-Ischemic	Cardiology (Cardiovascular Disease)	Reiss, Craig (MD)	137
Heart Disease-Ischemic	Cardiology (Cardiovascular Disease)	Williams, Kim A (MD)	138

SPECIAL EXPERTISE INDEX

Special Expertise	Specialty	Doctor's Name	Page
Heart Failure	Cardiology (Cardiovascular Disease)	Califf, Robert M (MD)	130
Heart Failure	Cardiology (Cardiovascular Disease)	Parmley, William Watts (MD)	142
Heart Failure	Cardiology (Cardiovascular Disease)	Zaret, Barry L. (MD)	123
Heart Failure	Pediatric Cardiology	Bayron, Harry (MD)	562
Heart Failure	Thoracic Surgery	Gardner, Timothy Joseph (MD)	808
Heart Murmurs	Pediatric Cardiology	Bayron, Harry (MD)	562
Heart Valve Disease	Cardiology (Cardiovascular Disease)	Achuff, Stephen Charles (MD)	123
Heart Valve Disease	Cardiology (Cardiovascular Disease)	Bashore, Thomas (MD)	129
Heart Valve Disease	Cardiology (Cardiovascular Disease)	Blumenthal, David S (MD)	124
Heart Valve Disease	Cardiology (Cardiovascular Disease)	Borer, Jeffrey (MD)	124
Heart Valve Disease	Cardiology (Cardiovascular Disease)	Gliklich, Jerry (MD)	125
Heart Valve Disease	Cardiology (Cardiovascular Disease)	Harrison, John Kevin (MD)	131
Heart Valve Disease	Cardiology (Cardiovascular Disease)	O'Gara, Patrick Thomas (MD)	122
Heart Valve Disease	Cardiology (Cardiovascular Disease)	Powers, Eric Randall (MD)	132
Heart Valve Disease	Cardiology (Cardiovascular Disease)	Rahko, Peter (MD)	137
Heart Valve Disease	Cardiology (Cardiovascular Disease)	Stewart, William (MD)	138
Heart Valve Surgery	Pediatric Surgery	Quaegebeur, Jan Modest (MD)	612
Heart Valve Surgery	Thoracic Surgery	Akins, Cary W (MD)	805
Heart Valve Surgery	Thoracic Surgery	Bassett, Joseph (MD)	815
Heart Valve Surgery	Thoracic Surgery	Bavaria, Joseph (MD)	807
Heart Valve Surgery	Thoracic Surgery	Cohn, Lawrence H (MD)	805
Heart Valve Surgery	Thoracic Surgery	Cooley, Denton A (MD)	821
Heart Valve Surgery	Thoracic Surgery	Cosgrove III, Delos M (MD)	816
Heart Valve Surgery	Thoracic Surgery	Kanda, Louis T (MD)	809
Heart Valve Surgery	Thoracic Surgery	Karp, Robert Bruce (MD)	817
Heart Valve Surgery	Thoracic Surgery	Katz, Nevin M (MD)	809
Heart Valve Surgery	Thoracic Surgery	Lang, Samuel (MD)	810
Heart Valve Surgery	Thoracic Surgery	Livesay, James J (MD)	822
Heart Valve Surgery	Thoracic Surgery	Reitz, Bruce Arnold (MD)	825
Heart Valve Surgery	Thoracic Surgery	Reul, George J (MD)	822
Heart Valve Surgery	Thoracic Surgery	Schaff, Hartzell (MD)	819
Heart Valve Surgery	Thoracic Surgery	Silverman, Norman A (MD)	819
Heart Valve Surgery	Thoracic Surgery	Smith, Peter Kent (MD)	814
Heart Valve Surgery	Thoracic Surgery	Strong III, Michael D (MD)	811
Heart Valve Surgery	Thoracic Surgery	Verrier, Edward (MD)	826
Heart Valve Surgery-Aortic & Mitral	Cardiology (Cardiovascular Disease)	Stewart, William (MD)	138
Heart Valve Surgery-Mitral	Thoracic Surgery	Lytle, Bruce Whitney (MD)	817
Heart Valve Surgery-Mitral	Thoracic Surgery	Vander Salm, Thomas (MD)	806
Heart-Artificial	Thoracic Surgery	Kormos, Robert (MD)	810
Helicobacter Pylori	Infectious Disease	Blaser, Martin Jack (MD)	318
Hemangioma	Dermatology	Burton III, Claude Shreve (MD)	186
Hemangioma	Dermatology	Orlow, Seth (MD)	185
Hemangioma	Otolaryngology	Waner, Milton (MD)	520
Hematology	Medical Oncology	Di Persio, John (MD/PhD)	306
Hematology	Medical Oncology	Robert, Nicholas J (MD)	303
Hematology	Pediatric Hematology-Oncology	Falletta, John (MD)	585
Hematology	Pediatric Hematology-Oncology	Suarez, Carlos (MD)	587
Hematology	Pediatric Hematology-Oncology	Valentino, Leonard A (MD)	587
Hematology/Oncology	Pediatric Hematology-Oncology	Matthay, Katherine Kurshan (MD)	589
Hematopathology	Pathology	Banks, Peter (MD)	539
Hematopathology	Pathology	Frizzera, Glauco (MD)	536
Hematopathology	Pathology	Harris, Nancy L (MD)	535
Hematopathology	Pathology	Weisenburger, Dennis ()	541
Hematuria	Pediatric Nephrology	Richard, George (MD)	596
Hemolytic Anemia	Hematology	Telen, Marilyn J (MD)	287
Hemolytic Uremic Syndrome	Pediatric Nephrology	Kaplan, Bernard S (MD)	595
Hemolytic Uremic Syndrome	Pediatric Nephrology	Watkins, Sandra (MD)	599
Hemophilia-Adult	Hematology	Lutcher, Charles (MD)	287
Hemophilia/Bleeding Disorders	Internal Medicine	Seremetis, Stephanie (MD)	334
Hemophilla Related Disease	Orthopaedic Surgery	Luck Jr, James Vernon (MD)	497

Special Expertise	Specialty	Doctor's Name	Page
Hepatic Iron Metabolism	Gastroenterology	Bacon, Bruce (MD)	230
Hepatitis	Gastroenterology	Bacon, Bruce (MD)	230
Hepatitis	Gastroenterology	Davis, Gary L (MD)	227
Hepatitis	Gastroenterology	Dienstag, Jules Leonard (MD)	221
Hepatitis	Gastroenterology	Dieterich, Douglas (MD)	223
Hepatitis	Gastroenterology	Hunter, Ellen B (MD)	228
Hepatitis	Gastroenterology	Schiff, Eugene (MD)	229
Hepatitis	Gastroenterology	Sorrell, Michael (MD)	235
Hepatitis	Gastroenterology	Van Thiel, David (MD)	235
Hepatitis B	Pediatric Gastroenterology	Schwarz, Kathleen (MD)	578
Hepatitis B-Immune Response	Rheumatology	Cupps, Thomas R (MD)	758
Hepatitis C	Gastroenterology	Blei, Andres T (MD)	230
Hepatitis C	Gastroenterology	Pimstone, Neville R (MD)	238
Hepatitis C	Infectious Disease	Craven, Donald Edward (MD)	317
Hepatitis C	Pediatric Gastroenterology	Schwarz, Kathleen (MD)	578
Hepatitis C & B	Gastroenterology	Maddrey, Willis Crocker (MD)	236
Hepatitis-Antiviral Therapy	Gastroenterology	Glombicki, Alan Paul (MD)	236
Hepatitis-Antiviral Therapy	Gastroenterology	Keeffe, Emmet B (MD)	237
Hepatoma	Medical Oncology	Grosh, William W (MD)	301
Hepatopulmonary Syndrome	Pulmonary Disease	Krowka, Michael Joseph (MD)	704
Hereditary Metabolic Diseases	Child Neurology	Patterson, Marc (MD)	154
Hernia	Pediatric Surgery	Toufanian, Ahmad (MD)	614
Hernia	Surgery	Minervini, Donald (MD)	791
Herpes	Ophthalmology	Nesburn, Anthony B (MD)	467
Herpes	Pediatric Infectious Disease	Gershon, Anne (MD)	590
Herpes Simplex	Infectious Disease	Friedman, Harvey Michael (MD)	319
Herpetic Neuralgia	Pain Management	Rowbotham, Michael Charles (MD)	532
Hiatal Hernia	Surgery	Polk Jr, Hiram C (MD)	792
Hip & Knee Replacement	Orthopaedic Surgery	Blaha, J David (MD)	478
Hip & Knee Replacement	Orthopaedic Surgery	Brick, Gregory (MD)	475
Hip & Knee Replacement	Orthopaedic Surgery	Callaghan, John J (MD)	490
Hip & Knee Replacement	Orthopaedic Surgery	Cuckler, John (MD)	486
Hip & Knee Replacement	Orthopaedic Surgery	Dorr, Lawrence Douglas (MD)	497
Hip & Knee Replacement	Orthopaedic Surgery	Finerman, Gerald (MD)	497
Hip & Knee Replacement	Orthopaedic Surgery	Galante, Jorge O (MD)	490
Hip & Knee Replacement	Orthopaedic Surgery	Goldberg, Victor M (MD)	490
Hip & Knee Replacement	Orthopaedic Surgery	Grant, Richard E (MD)	481
Hip & Knee Replacement	Orthopaedic Surgery	Grelsamer, Ronald (MD)	481
Hip & Knee Replacement	Orthopaedic Surgery	Luck Jr, James Vernon (MD)	497
Hip & Knee Replacement	Orthopaedic Surgery	Mallory, Thomas (MD)	491
Hip & Knee Replacement	Orthopaedic Surgery	Martell, John Mark (MD)	491
Hip & Knee Replacement	Orthopaedic Surgery	Nelson, Carl (MD)	495
Hip & Knee Replacement	Orthopaedic Surgery	Perry, James (MD)	487
Hip & Knee Replacement	Orthopaedic Surgery	Reilly, Donald T. (MD)	477
Hip & Knee Replacement	Orthopaedic Surgery	Rothman, Richard (MD)	483
Hip & Knee Replacement	Orthopaedic Surgery	Salvati, Eduardo Augustin (MD)	483
Hip & Knee Replacement	Orthopaedic Surgery	Sculco, Thomas Peter (MD)	484
Hip & Knee Replacement	Orthopaedic Surgery	Stulberg, Samuel David (MD)	493
Hip & Knee Replacement	Orthopaedic Surgery	Thornhill, Thomas S (MD)	477
Hip & Knee Replacement	Orthopaedic Surgery	Trick, Lorence Wain (MD)	495
Hip & Knee Replacement	Orthopaedic Surgery	Vail, Thomas Parker (MD)	488
Hip & Knee Replacement	Orthopaedic Surgery	Wixson, Richard L (MD)	493
Hip & Knee Replacement	Orthopaedic Surgery	Zuckerman, Joseph (MD)	485
Hip Disorders	Orthopaedic Surgery	Aronson, James (MD)	494
Hip Replacement	Orthopaedic Surgery	Bierbaum, Benjamin (MD)	475
Hip Replacement	Orthopaedic Surgery	Goldstein, Wayne (MD)	490
Hip Replacement	Orthopaedic Surgery	Schmalzried, Thomas P (MD)	498
Hip Replacement	Orthopaedic Surgery	Tischler, Henry (MD)	484
Hip Surgery	Orthopaedic Surgery	Dunn, Harold Kenneth (MD)	493
Hip Surgery	Orthopaedic Surgery	Nelson, Carl (MD)	495

SPECIAL EXPERTISE INDEX

Special Expertise	Specialty	Doctor's Name	Page
Hip Surgery	Orthopaedic Surgery	Ranawat, Chitranjan (MD)	483
Hip Surgery	Orthopaedic Surgery	Salvati, Eduardo Augustin (MD)	483
Hip Surgery Rehabilitation	Physical Medicine & Rehabilitation	Munin, Michael Craig (MD)	625
Hirschsprung's Disease	Pediatric Surgery	Coran, Arnold G (MD)	615
Hirschsprung's Disease	Pediatric Surgery	Georgeson, Keith E (MD)	613
Hodgkin's Disease	Hematology	Winter, Jane N. (MD)	290
Hodgkin's Disease	Medical Oncology	Come, Steven Eliot (MD)	292
Hodgkin's Disease	Medical Oncology	De Vita Jr, Vincent T (MD)	292
Hodgkin's Disease	Medical Oncology	Fisher, Richard I (MD)	306
Hodgkin's Disease	Medical Oncology	Glick, John H (MD)	296
Hodgkin's Disease	Medical Oncology	Gordon, Leo I (MD)	306
Hodgkin's Disease	Pediatric Hematology-Oncology	Schwartz, Cindy Lee (MD)	585
Hodgkin's Disease	Radiation Oncology	Ferree, Carolyn Ruth Black (MD)	721
Hodgkin's Disease	Radiation Oncology	Mendenhall, Nancy P (MD)	722
Hormonal Disorders	Endocrinology, Diabetes & Metabolism	Collins, Francis M (MD)	206
Hormonal Disorders	Endocrinology, Diabetes & Metabolism	Dobs, Adrian Sandra (MD)	199
Hormonal Disorders	Geriatric Medicine	Tenover, Joyce Sander (MD/PhD)	246
Hormonal Disorders	Reproductive Endocrinology	Dumesic, Daniel Anthony (MD)	748
Hormonal Disorders	Reproductive Endocrinology	Jaffe, Robert B (MD)	751
Hormonal Disorders	Reproductive Endocrinology	Winer, Sharon Ann (MD)	752
Hormonal Replacement	Reproductive Endocrinology	Berga , Sarah Lee (MD)	744
Hospice Care	Hematology	Bricker, Leslie J (MD)	288
Hospice Care	Psychiatry	Munich, Richard (MD)	685
Hospital Epidemiology	Pediatric Infectious Disease	Saiman, Lisa (MD)	591
Hospital Infection Control	Infectious Disease	Patterson, Jan E Evans (MD)	327
Huntington's Disease	Neurology	Beal, Myron Flint (MD)	400
Huntington's Disease	Neurology	Koroshetz, Walter J. (MD)	398
Huntington's Disease	Neurology	Shoulson, Ira (MD)	405
Huntington's Disease	Neurology	Weiner, William J. (MD)	411
Huntington's Disease	Neurology	Young, Anne (MD)	399
Huntington's Disease	Psychiatry	McHugh, Paul (MD)	680
Hydrocephalus	Neurological Surgery	Canady, Alexa I (MD)	382
Hydrocephalus	Neurological Surgery	Milhorat, Thomas H (MD)	378
Hydrocephalus	Neurological Surgery	Morrison, Glenn (MD)	381
Hydrocephalus	Neurological Surgery	Walker, Marion L. (MD)	386
Hydrocephalus-Pediatric	Neurological Surgery	O'Brien, Mark S. (MD)	381
Hyperparathyroidism	Surgery	Clark, Orlo H (MD)	799
Hypertension	Cardiology (Cardiovascular Disease)	Kostis, John B (MD)	126
Hypertension	Cardiology (Cardiovascular Disease)	Shlofmitz, Richard A (MD)	128
Hypertension	Endocrinology, Diabetes & Metabolism	Hsueh, Willa Ann (MD)	211
Hypertension	Endocrinology, Diabetes & Metabolism	Williams, Gordon H (MD)	198
Hypertension	Geriatric Medicine	Applegate, William (MD)	245
Hypertension	Geriatric Medicine	Supiano, Mark A. (MD)	249
Hypertension	Geriatric Medicine	Williamson, Wayne (MD)	249
Hypertension	Internal Medicine	Schwartz, Gary Lee (MD)	336
Hypertension	Internal Medicine	Weder, Alan B (MD)	336
Hypertension	Nephrology	Ahmad, Suhail (MD)	368
Hypertension	Nephrology	Black, Henry R (MD)	364
Hypertension	Nephrology	Bourgoignie, Jacques (MD)	362
Hypertension	Nephrology	Brenner, Barry M (MD)	359
Hypertension	Nephrology	Buckalew Jr., Vardaman Moore (MD)	362
Hypertension	Nephrology	Coffman, Thomas Myron (MD)	363
Hypertension	Nephrology	Coggins, Cecil (MD)	359
Hypertension	Nephrology	Gluck, Stephen (MD)	363
Hypertension	Nephrology	Harris, Raymond C (MD)	363
Hypertension	Nephrology	Johnston, James (MD)	361
Hypertension	Nephrology	Massry, Shaul Gourgi (MD)	369
Hypertension	Nephrology	Myers, Bryan David (MD)	369
Hypertension	Nephrology	Perrone, Ronald (MD)	360
Hypertension	Nephrology	Pohl, Marc (MD)	365

Special Expertise	Specialty	Doctor's Name	Page
Hypertension	Nephrology	Schrier, Robert William (MD)	367
Hypertension	Nephrology	Tolkoff-Rubin, Nina (MD)	360
Hypertension	Nephrology	Umans, Jason (MD/PhD)	362
Hypertension	Pediatric Cardiology	Hohn, Arno R (MD)	567
Hypertension	Pediatric Nephrology	Bergstein, Jerry (MD)	597
Hypertension	Pediatric Nephrology	Richard, George (MD)	596
Hypertension-Drug Resistent	Nephrology	Wilcox, Christopher S (MD)	362
Hypertension-Renovascular	Vascular Surgery (General)	Dean, Richard H (MD)	863
Hypertension-Renovascular/Adrenal	Nephrology	Wilcox, Christopher S (MD)	362
Hyperthermia	Radiation Oncology	Prosnitz, Leonard (MD)	722
Hyperthyroidism	Pediatric Endocrinology	Zimmerman, Donald (MD)	576
Hypertrophic Obstructive Cardio	Thoracic Surgery	Danielson, Gordon (MD)	816
Hypnosis	Psychiatry	Spiegel, David (MD)	688
Hypoglycemia	Endocrinology, Diabetes & Metabolism	Ovalle, Fernando (MD)	204
Hypoglycemia	Endocrinology, Diabetes & Metabolism	Rizza, Robert Alan (MD)	208
Hypogonadism-Male	Endocrinology, Diabetes & Metabolism	Griffin, James Emmet (MD)	209
Hypoplastic Left Heart Syndrome	Pediatric Surgery	Bove, Edward (MD)	614
Hypotension	Internal Medicine	Schwartz, Gary Lee (MD)	336
Hypothalamic Dysfunction	Endocrinology, Diabetes & Metabolism	Lechan, Ronald (MD/PhD)	198
Hypothalamic Dysfunction	Endocrinology, Diabetes & Metabolism	Marshall, John Crook (MD/PhD)	204
Hysteroscopic Surgery	Obstetrics & Gynecology	Sanz, Luis E (MD)	433

I

Ilizarov Procedure	Orthopaedic Surgery	Aronson, James (MD)	494
Ilizarov Procedure	Orthopaedic Surgery	Lowenberg, David W (MD)	497
Immune Deficiency	Allergy & Immunology	Baraniuk, James N (MD)	95
Immune Deficiency	Allergy & Immunology	Beall, Gildon N (MD)	103
Immune Deficiency	Allergy & Immunology	Cunningham-Rundles, C (MD/PhD)	96
Immune Deficiency	Allergy & Immunology	Good, Robert (MD/PhD)	98
Immune Deficiency	Allergy & Immunology	Levinson, Arnold (MD)	96
Immune Deficiency	Allergy & Immunology	Lockey, Richard (MD)	99
Immune Deficiency	Allergy & Immunology	Stein, Mark R (MD)	99
Immune Deficiency	Allergy & Immunology	Strober, Warren (MD)	97
Immune Deficiency	Allergy & Immunology	Ten, Rosa Maria (MD/PhD)	101
Immune Deficiency	Gynecologic Oncology	Freedman, Ralph (MD)	262
Immune Deficiency	Pediatric Allergy & Immunology	Barrett, Douglas John (MD)	556
Immune Deficiency	Pediatric Allergy & Immunology	Berger, Melvin (MD/PhD)	556
Immune Deficiency	Pediatric Allergy & Immunology	Buckley, Rebecca Hatcher (MD)	556
Immune Deficiency	Pediatric Allergy & Immunology	Church, Joseph August (MD)	558
Immune Deficiency	Pediatric Allergy & Immunology	Fanous, Yvonne F (MD)	559
Immune Deficiency	Pediatric Allergy & Immunology	Gelfand, Erwin (MD)	558
Immune Deficiency	Pediatric Allergy & Immunology	Shearer, William T (MD)	558
Immune Deficiency	Pediatric Allergy & Immunology	Stiehm, E Richard (MD)	559
Immune Deficiency	Pediatric Allergy & Immunology	Umetsu, Dale T (MD/PhD)	559
Immune Deficiency	Pediatric Allergy & Immunology	Winkelstein, Jerry Allen (MD)	555
Immune Deficiency	Pediatric Hematology-Oncology	Bussel, James (MD)	583
Immune Deficiency-Lung	Allergy & Immunology	Slavin, Raymond (MD)	101
Immune Deficiency-Skin	Dermatology	Granstein, Richard (MD)	184
Immune Deficiency-Skin	Dermatology	Katz, Stephen ()	184
Immune Deficiency-Thyroid	Allergy & Immunology	Baker Jr., James Russell (MD)	100
Immunogenetics	Nephrology	Carpenter, Charles B (MD)	359
Immunology	Medical Oncology	Chapman, Paul (MD)	295
Immunopathology	Pathology	Bhan, Atul Kumar (MD)	535
Immunopathology	Pathology	Grogan, Thomas (MD)	541
Immunosuppression-Kidney Transplant	Nephrology	Neylan, John Francis (MD)	363
Immunotherapy	Medical Oncology	Weiner, Louis M (MD)	300
Impotence	Urology	Boyd, Stuart D (MD)	847
Impotence	Urology	Lue, Tom F (MD)	849
Impotence	Urology	Steers, William D (MD)	840

SPECIAL EXPERTISE INDEX

Special Expertise	Specialty	Doctor's Name	Page
Impotence-Peyronies Disease	Urology	Levine, Laurence Adan (MD)	842
Impulse-Control Disorders	Psychiatry	Burt, Vivien Kleinman (MD/PhD)	686
Inborn Errors of Metabolism	Clinical Genetics	Cederbaum, Stephen D (MD)	164
Inborn Errors of Metabolism	Clinical Genetics	Wilcox, William (MD)	166
Incontinence	Geriatric Medicine	Ouslander, Joseph (MD)	246
Incontinence	Urology	Benson, Mitchell C (MD)	831
Incontinence	Urology	Boyd, Stuart D (MD)	847
Incontinence	Urology	Bushman, Wade (MD)	841
Incontinence	Urology	Jordan, Gerald (MD)	837
Incontinence	Urology	Kennelly, Michael Joseph (MD)	838
Incontinence	Urology	Melman, Arnold (MD)	834
Incontinence	Urology	Miles, Brian J (MD)	846
Incontinence	Urology	Montague, Drogo K. (MD)	843
Incontinence	Urology	Mulcahy, John J. (MD)	843
Incontinence	Urology	Schaeffer, Anthony (MD)	844
Incontinence	Urology	Steers, William D (MD)	840
Incontinence	Urology	Vapnek, Jonathan M (MD)	835
Incontinence	Urology	Wein, Alan J (MD)	836
Incontinence-Fecal	Colon & Rectal Surgery	Fleshman, James (MD)	173
Incontinence-Fecal	Colon & Rectal Surgery	Saclarides, Theodore John (MD)	175
Incontinence-Fecal	Colon & Rectal Surgery	Thorson, Alan (MD)	175
Incontinence-Fecal	Colon & Rectal Surgery	Wong, Westley Douglas (MD)	171
Incontinence-Fecal	Gastroenterology	Rao, Satish S C (MD)	233
Incontinence-Fecal	Urology	Macchia, Richard (MD)	833
Incontinence-Female	Urology	Payne, Christopher K (MD)	849
Incontinence-Female	Urology	Raz, Shlomo (MD)	849
Infant/Toddler Psychiatry	Child & Adolescent Psychiatry	Drell, Martin J. (MD)	669
Infant/Toddler Psychiatry	Child & Adolescent Psychiatry	Greenspan, Stanley (MD)	665
Infant/Toddler Psychiatry	Child & Adolescent Psychiatry	Wright, Harry (MD)	668
Infection in Newborns	Pediatrics	Regan, Joan (MD)	352
Infection-B Strep	Pediatric Infectious Disease	Baker, Carol (MD)	593
Infection-Respiratory	Internal Medicine	Sarosi, George (MD)	336
Infection-Respiratory	Pediatric Infectious Disease	Wald, Ellen (MD)	591
Infection-Respiratory	Pediatric Pulmonology	Redding , Gregory (MD)	607
Infections	Maternal & Fetal Medicine	Ismail, Mahmoud (MD)	345
Infections In Cancer Patients	Infectious Disease	Sepkowitz, Kent (MD)	321
Infections in Immune Deficient	Infectious Disease	Brennan, Patrick J (MD)	318
Infections in Immune Deficient	Infectious Disease	Edwards Jr., John Ellis (MD)	328
Infections in Immune Deficient	Pediatric Infectious Disease	Emmanuel, Patricia (MD)	591
Infections in Immune Deficient	Pediatric Infectious Disease	McKinney Jr, Ross E (MD)	592
Infections-Cancer Patients	Pediatrics	Pizzo, Philip Anthony (MD)	617
Infections-Hospital Acquired	Infectious Disease	Hopkins, Cyrus Clark (MD)	317
Infections-Hospital Acquired	Infectious Disease	McGowan Jr, John E (MD)	324
Infections-Transplant	Infectious Disease	Houston, Sally (MD)	323
Infectious & Demyelinating Diseases	Neurology	Berger, Joseph (MD)	407
Infectious & Demyelinating Diseases	Neurology	Cook, Stuart (MD)	400
Infectious Diarrhea	Infectious Disease	Guerrant, Richard (MD)	323
Infectious Disease	Dermatology	Gurevitch, Arnold William (MD)	193
Infectious Disease	Dermatology	Leyden, James (MD)	184
Infectious Disease	Internal Medicine	Graybill, John Richard (MD)	337
Infectious Disease	Obstetrics & Gynecology	Amstey, Marvin S. (MD)	431
Infectious Disease	Obstetrics & Gynecology	Duff, W Patrick (MD)	433
Infectious Disease	Obstetrics & Gynecology	Eschenbach, David Arthur (MD)	438
Infectious Disease	Obstetrics & Gynecology	Faro, Sebastian (MD)	437
Infectious Disease	Obstetrics & Gynecology	Galask, Rudolph P. (MD)	435
Infectious Disease	Obstetrics & Gynecology	Hager, William David (MD)	434
Infectious Disease	Obstetrics & Gynecology	Ledger, William (MD)	432
Infectious Disease	Obstetrics & Gynecology	Linn, Edward S (MD)	436
Infectious Disease	Pathology	Walker, David H (MD)	541
Infectious Disease	Pediatric Infectious Disease	Gorensek, Margaret (MD)	592

SPECIAL EXPERTISE INDEX

Special Expertise	Specialty	Doctor's Name	Page
Infertility-IVF	Reproductive Endocrinology	Azziz, Ricardo (MD)	746
Infertility-IVF	Reproductive Endocrinology	Berga , Sarah Lee (MD)	744
Infertility-IVF	Reproductive Endocrinology	Burry, Kenneth Arnold (MD)	751
Infertility-IVF	Reproductive Endocrinology	Diamond, Michael (MD)	748
Infertility-IVF	Reproductive Endocrinology	Dodds, William G (MD)	748
Infertility-IVF	Reproductive Endocrinology	Jacobs, Laurence (MD)	749
Infertility-IVF	Reproductive Endocrinology	McClamrock, Howard Dean (MD)	744
Infertility-IVF	Reproductive Endocrinology	Paulson, Richard John (MD)	752
Infertility-IVF	Reproductive Endocrinology	Rosenwaks, Zev (MD)	745
Infertility-IVF	Reproductive Endocrinology	Wallach, Edward Eliot (MD)	745
Infertility-IVF	Reproductive Endocrinology	Wood Molo, Mary (MD)	750
Infertility-Male	Urology	Belker, Arnold (MD)	837
Infertility-Male	Urology	Berger, Richard E (MD)	847
Infertility-Male	Urology	Buch, Jeffrey Phillip (MD)	845
Infertility-Male	Urology	Fisch, Harry (MD)	831
Infertility-Male	Urology	Fuchs, Eugene F (MD)	848
Infertility-Male	Urology	Goldstein, Marc (MD)	832
Infertility-Male	Urology	Howards, Stuart S (MD)	837
Infertility-Male	Urology	Jarow, Jonathan (MD)	833
Infertility-Male	Urology	Levine, Laurence Adan (MD)	842
Infertility-Male	Urology	Lipshultz, Larry (MD)	846
Infertility-Male	Urology	Oates, Robert Davis (MD)	830
Infertility-Male	Urology	Ohl, Dana Alan (MD)	843
Infertility-Male	Urology	Pryor, Jon L. (MD)	843
Infertility-Male	Urology	Ross, Lawrence S (MD)	844
Infertility-Male	Urology	Schlegel, Peter (MD)	835
Infertility-Male	Urology	Seftel, Allen D (MD)	844
Infertility-Male	Urology	Shaban, Stephen F (MD)	839
Infertility-Male	Urology	Sigman, Mark (MD)	830
Infertility/Uterine Fibroids	Reproductive Endocrinology	Schlaff, William D (MD)	751
Inflammatory Bowel Disease/Crohn's	Allergy & Immunology	Strober, Warren (MD)	97
Inflammatory Bowel Disease/Crohn's	Colon & Rectal Surgery	Abcarian, Herand (MD)	173
Inflammatory Bowel Disease/Crohn's	Colon & Rectal Surgery	Beart Jr, Robert W (MD)	176
Inflammatory Bowel Disease/Crohn's	Colon & Rectal Surgery	Becker, James (MD)	169
Inflammatory Bowel Disease/Crohn's	Colon & Rectal Surgery	Dozois, Roger R (MD)	173
Inflammatory Bowel Disease/Crohn's	Colon & Rectal Surgery	Fazio, Victor (MD)	173
Inflammatory Bowel Disease/Crohn's	Colon & Rectal Surgery	Fry, Robert Dean (MD)	170
Inflammatory Bowel Disease/Crohn's	Colon & Rectal Surgery	Galandiuk, Susan (MD)	172
Inflammatory Bowel Disease/Crohn's	Colon & Rectal Surgery	Gingold, Bruce (MD)	170
Inflammatory Bowel Disease/Crohn's	Colon & Rectal Surgery	Kodner, Ira Joe (MD)	174
Inflammatory Bowel Disease/Crohn's	Colon & Rectal Surgery	Larach, Sergio (MD)	173
Inflammatory Bowel Disease/Crohn's	Colon & Rectal Surgery	Medich, David (MD)	171
Inflammatory Bowel Disease/Crohn's	Colon & Rectal Surgery	Pemberton, John (MD)	174
Inflammatory Bowel Disease/Crohn's	Colon & Rectal Surgery	Schoetz, David (MD)	169
Inflammatory Bowel Disease/Crohn's	Colon & Rectal Surgery	Steinhagen, Randolph (MD)	171
Inflammatory Bowel Disease/Crohn's	Colon & Rectal Surgery	Stryker, Steven J (MD)	175
Inflammatory Bowel Disease/Crohn's	Colon & Rectal Surgery	Wexner, Steven (MD)	173
Inflammatory Bowel Disease/Crohn's	Colon & Rectal Surgery	Wolff, Bruce (MD)	175
Inflammatory Bowel Disease/Crohn's	Gastroenterology	Banks, Peter Alan (MD)	221
Inflammatory Bowel Disease/Crohn's	Gastroenterology	Bayless, Theodore (MD)	222
Inflammatory Bowel Disease/Crohn's	Gastroenterology	Cominelli, Fabio (MD/PhD)	227
Inflammatory Bowel Disease/Crohn's	Gastroenterology	Craig, Robert M (MD)	231
Inflammatory Bowel Disease/Crohn's	Gastroenterology	Deren, Julius Jay (MD)	222
Inflammatory Bowel Disease/Crohn's	Gastroenterology	Diamond, Jeffrey (MD)	227
Inflammatory Bowel Disease/Crohn's	Gastroenterology	Elliott, David (MD)	231
Inflammatory Bowel Disease/Crohn's	Gastroenterology	Elta, Grace Helen (MD)	231
Inflammatory Bowel Disease/Crohn's	Gastroenterology	Farmer, Richard G (MD)	223
Inflammatory Bowel Disease/Crohn's	Gastroenterology	Hanauer, Stephen (MD)	232
Inflammatory Bowel Disease/Crohn's	Gastroenterology	Hodges, David S (MD)	236
Inflammatory Bowel Disease/Crohn's	Gastroenterology	Holt, Peter R (MD)	223

Special Expertise	Specialty	Doctor's Name	Page
Inflammatory Bowel Disease/Crohn's	Gastroenterology	Korelitz, Burton I (MD)	224
Inflammatory Bowel Disease/Crohn's	Gastroenterology	Mayer, Lloyd (MD)	224
Inflammatory Bowel Disease/Crohn's	Gastroenterology	Peppercorn, Mark (MD)	222
Inflammatory Bowel Disease/Crohn's	Gastroenterology	Present, Daniel (MD)	225
Inflammatory Bowel Disease/Crohn's	Gastroenterology	Roche, James Kenneth (MD/PhD)	229
Inflammatory Bowel Disease/Crohn's	Gastroenterology	Rogers, Arvey (MD)	229
Inflammatory Bowel Disease/Crohn's	Gastroenterology	Sachar, David (MD)	225
Inflammatory Bowel Disease/Crohn's	Gastroenterology	Sandborn, William Jeffery (MD)	234
Inflammatory Bowel Disease/Crohn's	Gastroenterology	Targan, Stephan Raoul (MD)	238
Inflammatory Bowel Disease/Crohn's	Gastroenterology	Tremaine, William John (MD)	234
Inflammatory Bowel Disease/Crohn's	Internal Medicine	Roth, Bennett E (MD)	337
Inflammatory Bowel Disease/Crohn's	Pediatric Gastroenterology	Berman, James (MD)	580
Inflammatory Bowel Disease/Crohn's	Pediatric Gastroenterology	Heyman, Melvin Bernard (MD)	581
Inflammatory Bowel Disease/Crohn's	Pediatric Gastroenterology	Hillemeier, A Craig (MD)	580
Inflammatory Bowel Disease/Crohn's	Pediatric Gastroenterology	Kirschner, Barbara S (MD)	580
Inflammatory Bowel Disease/Crohn's	Pediatric Gastroenterology	Oliva-Hemker, Maria M (MD)	578
Inflammatory Bowel Disease/Crohn's	Pediatric Gastroenterology	Rothbaum, Robert Jay (MD)	581
Inflammatory Bowel Disease/Crohn's	Pediatric Gastroenterology	Schwarz, Steven M (MD)	579
Inflammatory Bowel Disease/Crohn's	Pediatric Gastroenterology	Thompson, John (MD)	579
Inflammatory Bowel Disease/Crohn's	Pediatric Gastroenterology	Treem, William R (MD)	579
Inflammatory Bowel Disease/Crohn's	Pediatric Gastroenterology	Wyllie, Robert (MD)	581
Inflammatory Bowel Disease/Crohn's	Pediatric Surgery	Neblett, Wallace W (MD)	613
Inflammatory Diseases of Skin	Dermatology	Ackerman, A Bernard (MD)	182
Inflammatory Muscle Disease	Rheumatology	Bobrove, Arthur M (MD)	768
Infrainguinal Bypass	Vascular Surgery (General)	Bandyk, Dennis (MD)	863
Inhalant Addiction	Addiction Psychiatry	Crowley, Thomas J. (MD)	662
Inherited Bone Disorders	Clinical Genetics	Weaver, David Dawson (MD)	162
Inherited Diseases	Clinical Genetics	Holmes, Lewis B (MD)	159
Inherited Diseases	Clinical Genetics	Jonas, Adam Jonathan (MD)	165
Inherited Diseases	Clinical Genetics	Korf, Bruce (MD/PhD)	159
Inherited Diseases	Clinical Genetics	Morris, Colleen A. (MD)	165
Inherited Metabolic Disorders	Clinical Genetics	Desnick, Robert J (MD/PhD)	160
Inherited Metabolic Disorders	Clinical Genetics	Seashore, Margretta (MD)	159
Insect Allergies	Allergy & Immunology	Freeman, Theodore (MD)	103
Insect Allergies	Allergy & Immunology	Pacin, Michael (MD)	99
Insect Allergy	Allergy & Immunology	de Shazo, Richard Denson (MD)	98
Insect Sting Allergy	Allergy & Immunology	Reisman, Robert E (MD)	97
Internal Medicine	Nephrology	Riordan, John William (MD)	369
International Adoption	Child & Adolescent Psychiatry	Zeanah Jr, Charles H (MD)	669
Interstitial Cystitis	Urology	Lloyd Jr, Lewis K (MD)	838
Interstitial Cystitis	Urology	Schaeffer, Anthony (MD)	844
Interstitial Lung Disease	Pathology	Katzenstein, Anna-Luise A. (MD)	537
Interstitial Lung Disease	Pediatric Pulmonology	Fan, Leland Lane (MD)	606
Interstitial Lung Disease	Pulmonary Disease	Brown, Kevin K (MD)	706
Interstitial Lung Disease	Pulmonary Disease	Enelow, Richard Ian (MD)	698
Interstitial Lung Disease	Pulmonary Disease	Hunninghake, Gary (MD)	703
Interstitial Lung Disease	Pulmonary Disease	King Jr, Talmadge Everett (MD)	711
Interstitial Lung Disease	Pulmonary Disease	Loyd, James Emory (MD)	700
Interstitial Lung Disease	Pulmonary Disease	Lynch, Joseph P (MD)	704
Interstitial Lung Disease	Pulmonary Disease	Raghu, Ganesh (MD)	712
Interstitial Lung Disease	Pulmonary Disease	Schwarz, Marvin Ira (MD)	708
Interstitial Lung Disease	Pulmonary Disease	Teirstein, Alvin (MD)	696
Interstitial Lung Disease	Pulmonary Disease	Theodore, James (MD)	713
Interstitial Lung Disease	Pulmonary Disease	Tino, Gregory (MD)	696
Interstitial Lung Disease	Pulmonary Disease	Weissler, Jonathan C (MD)	709
Interstitial Lung Disease	Pulmonary Disease	Wiedemann, Herbert P (MD)	706
Interventional Cardiology	Cardiac Electrophysiology	Cohen, Martin (MD)	115
Interventional Cardiology	Cardiology (Cardiovascular Disease)	Califf, Robert M (MD)	130
Interventional Cardiology	Cardiology (Cardiovascular Disease)	Cohen, Howard Arthur (MD)	124
Interventional Cardiology	Cardiology (Cardiovascular Disease)	Faxon, David P (MD)	135

SPECIAL EXPERTISE INDEX

Special Expertise	Specialty	Doctor's Name	Page
Interventional Cardiology	Cardiology (Cardiovascular Disease)	Freeman, Gregory Lane (MD)	139
Interventional Cardiology	Cardiology (Cardiovascular Disease)	Harrison, John Kevin (MD)	131
Interventional Cardiology	Cardiology (Cardiovascular Disease)	Kereiakes, Dean J (MD)	136
Interventional Cardiology	Cardiology (Cardiovascular Disease)	O'Neill, William (MD)	136
Interventional Cardiology	Cardiology (Cardiovascular Disease)	Palacios, Igor F (MD)	122
Interventional Cardiology	Cardiology (Cardiovascular Disease)	Powers, Eric Randall (MD)	132
Interventional Cardiology	Cardiology (Cardiovascular Disease)	Safian, Robert D (MD)	137
Interventional Cardiology	Cardiology (Cardiovascular Disease)	Schwartz, Allan (MD)	128
Interventional Cardiology	Cardiology (Cardiovascular Disease)	Shani, Jacob (MD)	128
Interventional Cardiology	Cardiology (Cardiovascular Disease)	Topol, Eric Jeffrey (MD)	138
Interventional Cardiology	Cardiology (Cardiovascular Disease)	Vetrovec, George (MD)	132
Interventional Cardiology	Cardiology (Cardiovascular Disease)	Vignola, Paul (MD)	133
Interventional Cardiology	Cardiology (Cardiovascular Disease)	Williams, David (MD)	123
Interventional Cardiology	Interventional Cardiology	Holmes Jr., David Richard (MD)	146
Interventional Cardiology	Interventional Cardiology	Morris, Douglas (MD)	145
Interventional Cardiology	Pediatric Cardiology	Hellenbrand, William E (MD)	562
Interventional Cardiology	Pediatric Cardiology	Hijazi, Ziyad M (MD)	565
Interventional Cardiology	Pediatric Cardiology	Lock, James E (MD)	561
Interventional Cardiology	Pediatric Cardiology	Perry, Stanton Bruce (MD)	561
Interventional Cardiology	Pediatric Cardiology	Pitlick, Paul T (MD)	567
Interventional Cardiology	Pediatric Cardiology	Rocchini, Albert P (MD)	565
Interventional Cardiology	Pediatric Critical Care Medicine	Latson, Larry Allen (MD)	570
Interventional Neuroradiology	Radiology	Pile-Spellman, John (MD)	736
Interventional Neuroradiology	Radiology	Vinuela, Fernando (MD)	740
Interventional Radiology	Diagnostic Radiology	Hawkins Jr, Irvin (MD)	733
Interventional Radiology	Diagnostic Radiology	Rivera, Frank James (MD)	734
Interventional Radiology	Diagnostic Radiology	Teal, James S (MD)	732
Interventional Radiology	Radiology	Dake, Michael David (MD)	739
Interventional Radiology	Radiology	Keller, Frederick (MD)	740
Interventional Radiology	Radiology	Miller, Franklin (MD)	738
Interventional Radiology	Radiology	Palmaz, Julio C. (MD)	739
Interventional Radiology	Radiology	Valji, Karim (MD)	740
Interventional Radiology	Radiology	Yoon, Sydney (MD)	736
Intestinal Disease	Pediatric Gastroenterology	Ulshen, Martin H (MD)	579
Intestinal Parasites	Gastroenterology	Elliott, David (MD)	231
Intra Operative MRI Surgery	Neurological Surgery	Black, Peter (MD)	373
Intratumoral Chemotherapy	Neurological Surgery	Hassenbusch, Samuel J (MD/PhD)	387
Intravascular Stents	Radiology	Palmaz, Julio C. (MD)	739
Invasive Cardiology	Cardiology (Cardiovascular Disease)	Margolis, James (MD)	131
Irregular Heartbeat	Cardiology (Cardiovascular Disease)	Del Negro, Albert Anthony (MD)	130
Irritable Bowel Syndrome	Gastroenterology	Shenk, Ian (MD)	229
Irritable Bowel Syndrome	Gastroenterology	Sninsky, Charles (MD)	229
Irritable Bowel Syndrome	Gastroenterology	Wald, Arnold (MD)	225
Irritable Bowel Syndrome	Internal Medicine	Roth, Bennett E (MD)	337
Irritated Cuff Repair	Sports Medicine	Speer, Kevin (MD)	774
Ischemia-Critical Limb	Vascular Surgery (General)	Gloviczki, Peter (MD)	865
Ischemic Bowel Disease	Gastroenterology	Brandt, Lawrence (MD)	222
Ischemic/Optic/Neuropathy	Ophthalmology	Burde, Ronald (MD)	444
IVIG Infusion	Pediatric Allergy & Immunology	Barrett, Douglas John (MD)	556

J

Joint Pathology	Pathology	Dorfman, Howard (MD)	536
Joint Revision	Orthopaedic Surgery	Trick, Lorence Wain (MD)	495
Joint Surgery	Sports Medicine	Noyes, Frank (MD)	774
Juvenile Arthritis	Pediatric Rheumatology	Sills, Edward M (MD)	608
Juvenile Dermatomyositis, Sclerdoma	Pediatric Rheumatology	Myones, Barry Lee (MD)	609

Special Expertise	Specialty	Doctor's Name	Page
K			
Kallmann Syndrome	Reproductive Endocrinology	Crowley, William (MD)	743
Kawasaki Disease	Pediatric Allergy & Immunology	Leung, Donald (MD/PhD)	558
Kawasaki Disease	Pediatric Cardiology	Newburger, Jane (MD)	561
Kawasaki Disease	Pediatric Cardiology	Takahashi, Masato (MD)	567
Kawasaki Disease	Pediatric Cardiology	Tamer, Dolores (MD)	563
Kawasaki Disease	Pediatric Infectious Disease	Mason, Wilbert Henry (MD)	594
Kawasaki Disease	Pediatric Rheumatology	Lehman, Thomas (MD)	608
Kawasaki Disease	Pediatric Rheumatology	Myones, Barry Lee (MD)	609
Kidney & Ureteral Stones	Urology	Assimos, Dean George (MD)	836
Kidney Cancer	Medical Oncology	Motzer, Robert J (MD)	298
Kidney Cancer	Surgery	Rosenberg, Steven (MD)	787
Kidney Cancer	Urology	Danoff, Dudley S (MD)	848
Kidney Cancer	Urology	de Kernion, Jean Bayhi (MD)	848
Kidney Cancer	Urology	Holden, Stuart (MD)	848
Kidney Cancer	Urology	Huffman, Jeffry Lee (MD)	848
Kidney Cancer	Urology	Jacobs, Stephen C (MD)	832
Kidney Cancer	Urology	Lepor, Herbert (MD)	833
Kidney Cancer	Urology	Richie, Jerome (MD)	830
Kidney Cancer	Urology	Soloway, Mark (MD)	839
Kidney Cancer	Urology	Williams, Richard D (MD)	844
Kidney Cancer-Renal Cell	Hematology	Bukowski, Ronald Mathew (MD)	288
Kidney Development	Pediatric Nephrology	Davis, Ira D (MD)	597
Kidney Disease	Nephrology	Bolton, Warren Kline (MD)	362
Kidney Disease	Nephrology	Brazy, Peter C (MD)	364
Kidney Disease	Nephrology	Buckalew Jr., Vardaman Moore (MD)	362
Kidney Disease	Nephrology	Coggins, Cecil (MD)	359
Kidney Disease	Nephrology	Delmez, James Albert (MD)	365
Kidney Disease	Nephrology	Harris, Raymond C (MD)	363
Kidney Disease	Nephrology	Hruska, Keith Anthony (MD)	365
Kidney Disease	Nephrology	Kliger, Alan (MD)	359
Kidney Disease	Nephrology	Myers, Bryan David (MD)	369
Kidney Disease	Nephrology	Roguska-Kyts, Jadwiga (MD)	366
Kidney Disease	Nephrology	Sapir, Daniel Gustave (MD)	361
Kidney Disease	Nephrology	Umans, Jason (MD/PhD)	362
Kidney Disease	Nephrology	Weiner, Irving David (MD)	364
Kidney Disease	Pediatric Nephrology	Andreoli, Sharon (MD)	596
Kidney Disease	Pediatric Nephrology	Bergstein, Jerry (MD)	597
Kidney Disease	Pediatric Nephrology	Dabbagh, Shermine (MD)	597
Kidney Disease	Pediatric Nephrology	Richard, George (MD)	596
Kidney Disease-Diabetic	Nephrology	Johnston, James (MD)	361
Kidney Disease-Geriatric	Nephrology	Kasiske, Bertram (MD)	365
Kidney Disease-Glomerular	Nephrology	Appel, Gerald (MD)	360
Kidney Disease-Glomerular	Nephrology	Bolton, Warren Kline (MD)	362
Kidney Disease-Glomerular	Nephrology	Couser, William (MD)	368
Kidney Disease-Glomerular	Nephrology	Falk, Ronald J (MD)	363
Kidney Disease-Glomerular	Nephrology	Gluck, Stephen (MD)	363
Kidney Disease-Glomerular	Nephrology	Rakowski, Thomas A (MD)	361
Kidney Disease-Glomerular	Nephrology	Salant, David (MD)	360
Kidney Disease-Immunologic	Nephrology	Salant, David (MD)	360
Kidney Disease-Metabolic	Nephrology	Brazy, Peter C (MD)	364
Kidney Disease-Metabolic	Nephrology	Kaysen, George Alan (MD/PhD)	368
Kidney Disease-Metabolic	Nephrology	Kliger, Alan (MD)	359
Kidney Disease-Metabolic	Nephrology	Massry, Shaul Gourgi (MD)	369
Kidney Disease-Nutrition	Nephrology	Kopple, Joel David (MD)	369
Kidney Failure	Nephrology	Olivero, Juan Jose (MD)	367
Kidney Failure	Nephrology	Owen, William F. (MD)	359
Kidney Failure	Nephrology	Scheel Jr, Paul Joseph (MD)	361
Kidney Failure	Nephrology	Schwab, Steve Joseph (MD)	364

SPECIAL EXPERTISE INDEX

Special Expertise	Specialty	Doctor's Name	Page
Kidney Failure	Nephrology	Swartz, Richard D (MD)	366
Kidney Failure	Pediatric Nephrology	Alexander, Steven R (MD)	598
Kidney Failure-Acute	Nephrology	Brenner, Barry M (MD)	359
Kidney Failure-Acute	Nephrology	Tolkoff-Rubin, Nina (MD)	360
Kidney Failure-Chronic	Nephrology	Ahmad, Suhail (MD)	368
Kidney Failure-Chronic	Nephrology	Bourgoignie, Jacques (MD)	362
Kidney Failure-Chronic	Nephrology	Brennan, Thomas Stephen (MD)	367
Kidney Failure-Chronic	Nephrology	Fang, Leslie (MD)	359
Kidney Failure-Chronic	Nephrology	Kaysen, George Alan (MD/PhD)	368
Kidney Failure-Chronic	Nephrology	Okusa, Mark D (MD)	363
Kidney Failure-Chronic	Nephrology	Paganini, Emil (MD)	365
Kidney Failure-Chronic	Nephrology	Roth, David (MD)	364
Kidney Failure-Chronic	Nephrology	Seifter, Julian L (MD)	360
Kidney Failure-Chronic	Nephrology	Williams, Gail S (MD)	362
Kidney Failure-Chronic	Nephrology	Zimmerman, Stephen W (MD)	366
Kidney Failure-Chronic	Pediatric Nephrology	Dabbagh, Shermine (MD)	597
Kidney Failure-Chronic	Pediatric Nephrology	Davis, Ira D (MD)	597
Kidney Failure-Chronic	Pediatric Nephrology	Fennell III, Robert Samuel (MD)	596
Kidney Failure-Chronic	Pediatric Nephrology	Nevins, Thomas E (MD)	598
Kidney Failure-Chronic	Pediatric Nephrology	Watkins, Sandra (MD)	599
Kidney Reconstruction	Urology	Libertino, John A. (MD)	829
Kidney Stones	Internal Medicine	Coe, Fredric (MD)	364
Kidney Stones	Nephrology	Ahmad, Suhail (MD)	368
Kidney Stones	Nephrology	Brennan, Thomas Stephen (MD)	367
Kidney Stones	Nephrology	Hoffman, David (MD)	363
Kidney Stones	Nephrology	Saleh, Saleh (MD)	369
Kidney Stones	Nephrology	Seifter, Julian L (MD)	360
Kidney Stones	Nephrology	Weiner, Irving David (MD)	364
Kidney Stones	Pediatric Nephrology	Langman, Craig (MD)	598
Kidney Stones	Pediatric Nephrology	Stapleton, F Bruder (MD)	599
Kidney Stones	Urology	Albala, David Mois (MD)	840
Kidney Stones	Urology	Carson, Culley (MD)	837
Kidney Stones	Urology	Clayman, Ralph V (MD)	841
Kidney Stones	Urology	Dretler, Stephen P. (MD)	829
Kidney Stones	Urology	Fuchs, Eugene F (MD)	848
Kidney Stones	Urology	Fuselier Jr, Harold A (MD)	846
Kidney Stones	Urology	Huffman, Jeffry Lee (MD)	848
Kidney Stones	Urology	Irby III, Pierce B (MD)	837
Kidney Stones	Urology	Kavoussi, Louis Rapheal (MD)	833
Kidney Stones	Urology	Lockhart, Jorge L (MD)	838
Kidney Stones	Urology	McCullough, David L (MD)	838
Kidney Stones	Urology	Ohl, Dana Alan (MD)	843
Kidney Stones	Urology	Sanders, William Holt (MD)	839
Kidney Stones	Urology	Smith, Arthur D (MD)	835
Kidney Stones	Urology	Sosa, R Ernest (MD)	835
Kidney Stones	Urology	Stoller, Marshall Leedy (MD)	851
Klippel-Trenaunay Syndrome	Pediatric Cardiology	Driscoll, David J (MD)	564
Knee & Hip Surgery	Orthopaedic Surgery	Galante, Jorge O (MD)	490
Knee Injuries	Orthopaedic Surgery	Johnson, Darren Lee (MD)	486
Knee Injuries	Orthopaedic Surgery	Scott, W Norman (MD)	483
Knee Injuries	Orthopaedic Surgery	Zarins, Bertram (MD)	477
Knee Injuries	Sports Medicine	Nisonson, Barton (MD)	773
Knee Injuries-Women	Orthopaedic Surgery	Anderson, Lesley J (MD)	496
Knee Injuries/Ligament Surgery	Orthopaedic Surgery	Sherman, Orrin (MD)	484
Knee Replacement	Orthopaedic Surgery	Booth, Robert (MD)	479
Knee Replacement	Orthopaedic Surgery	Goldstein, Wayne (MD)	490
Knee Replacement	Orthopaedic Surgery	Scott, W Norman (MD)	483
Knee Replacement	Sports Medicine	Shively, Robert A (MD)	774
Knee Surgery	Orthopaedic Surgery	Bach Jr, Bernard R (MD)	489
Knee Surgery	Orthopaedic Surgery	Bauman, Phillip (MD)	478

Special Expertise	Specialty	Doctor's Name	Page
Knee Surgery	Orthopaedic Surgery	Bierbaum, Benjamin (MD)	475
Knee Surgery	Orthopaedic Surgery	Boland Jr., Arthur L (MD)	475
Knee Surgery	Orthopaedic Surgery	Cannon Jr, W Dilworth (MD)	496
Knee Surgery	Orthopaedic Surgery	Johnson, Carl A (MD)	482
Knee Surgery	Orthopaedic Surgery	Jokl, Peter (MD)	476
Knee Surgery	Orthopaedic Surgery	Mabrey, Jay D (MD)	495
Knee Surgery	Orthopaedic Surgery	Martell, John Mark (MD)	491
Knee Surgery	Orthopaedic Surgery	Ranawat, Chitranjan (MD)	483
Knee Surgery	Orthopaedic Surgery	Rosenberg, Thomas D (MD)	494
Knee Surgery	Orthopaedic Surgery	Shelbourne, K Donald (MD)	492
Knee Surgery	Orthopaedic Surgery	Warren, Russell (MD)	485
Knee Surgery	Sports Medicine	Altchek, David (MD)	773
Knee Surgery	Sports Medicine	Kelly, Michael (MD)	773
Knee Surgery	Sports Medicine	Paletta , George A (MD)	774

L

Special Expertise	Specialty	Doctor's Name	Page
Labor-Abnormal	Maternal & Fetal Medicine	Hayashi, Robert H. (MD)	345
Lacrimal Gland Disorders	Ophthalmology	Fein, William (MD)	464
Lacrimal Gland Disorders	Ophthalmology	Hornblass, Albert (MD)	447
Lacrimal Gland Disorders	Ophthalmology	Robb, Richard M (MD)	443
Lacrimal Gland Disorders	Ophthalmology	Tse, David (MD)	455
Laparoscopic Abdominal Surgery	Vascular Surgery (General)	Turner, James (MD)	862
Laparoscopic Cholecystectomy	Surgery	Minervini, Donald (MD)	791
Laparoscopic Cholecystectomy	Surgery	Salky, Barry A (MD)	788
Laparoscopic Nephrectomy	Urology	Jacobs, Stephen C (MD)	832
Laparoscopic Nephrectomy	Urology	Strand, William (MD)	847
Laparoscopic Surgery	Colon & Rectal Surgery	Bailey, Harold Randolph (MD)	176
Laparoscopic Surgery	Colon & Rectal Surgery	Forde, Kenneth (MD)	170
Laparoscopic Surgery	Colon & Rectal Surgery	Senagore, Anthony (MD)	175
Laparoscopic Surgery	Colon & Rectal Surgery	Whelan, Richard (MD)	171
Laparoscopic Surgery	Gynecologic Oncology	Barter, James (MD)	255
Laparoscopic Surgery	Gynecologic Oncology	Curtin, John P (MD)	256
Laparoscopic Surgery	Obstetrics & Gynecology	Sanz, Luis E (MD)	433
Laparoscopic Surgery	Pediatric Surgery	Cohen, Roger David (MD)	614
Laparoscopic Surgery	Pediatric Surgery	Georgeson, Keith E (MD)	613
Laparoscopic Surgery	Surgery	Dudrick, Stanley (MD)	781
Laparoscopic Surgery	Surgery	Ferzli, George (MD)	785
Laparoscopic Surgery	Surgery	Gadacz, Thomas R (MD)	790
Laparoscopic Surgery	Surgery	Gagner, Michel (MD)	786
Laparoscopic Surgery	Surgery	Koruda, Mark Joseph (MD)	791
Laparoscopic Surgery	Surgery	MacFadyen, Bruce (MD)	798
Laparoscopic Surgery	Surgery	Pappas, Theodore N (MD)	791
Laparoscopic Surgery	Surgery	Pellegrini, Carlos (MD)	801
Laparoscopic Surgery	Surgery	Salky, Barry A (MD)	788
Laparoscopic Surgery	Surgery	Schirmer, Bruce David (MD)	792
Laparoscopic Surgery	Surgery	Soper, Nathaniel (MD)	796
Laparoscopic Surgery	Thoracic Surgery	Daniel, Thomas M (MD)	812
Laparoscopic Surgery	Urology	Albala, David Mois (MD)	840
Laparoscopic Surgery	Urology	Herr, Harry Wallace (MD)	832
Laparoscopic Surgery	Urology	Kavoussi, Louis Rapheal (MD)	833
Laparoscopic Surgery	Urology	Kozlowski, James Michael (MD)	842
Laparoscopic Surgery	Urology	Smith, Arthur D (MD)	835
Laparoscopic Surgery	Urology	Sosa, R Ernest (MD)	835
Laparoscopic Surgery	Urology	Stoller, Marshall Leedy (MD)	851
Laparoscopic Surgery (Advanced)	Obstetrics & Gynecology	Steege, John Francis (MD)	434
Laparoscopic Surgery-Gastrointestinal	Surgery	Jackson, Gilchrist (MD)	797
Laparoscopy & Thoracostomy	Pediatric Surgery	Sato, Thomas Tad (MD)	615
Laryngeal & Tracheal Disorders	Otolaryngology	Zalzal, George (MD)	507
Laryngeal Cancer	Otolaryngology	Pearson, Bruce (MD)	510

SPECIAL EXPERTISE INDEX

Special Expertise	Specialty	Doctor's Name	Page
Laryngeal Cancer	Otolaryngology	Wolf, Gregory (MD)	517
Laryngeal Disorders	Otolaryngology	Courey, Mark Sam (MD)	508
Laryngeal Disorders	Otolaryngology	Cummings, Charles (MD)	503
Laryngeal Disorders	Otolaryngology	Koufman, James Alan (MD)	509
Laryngeal Disorders	Otolaryngology	McGuirt, W Fredrick (MD)	509
Laryngeal Disorders	Otolaryngology	Sataloff, Robert (MD)	506
Laryngeal Disorders	Otolaryngology	Suen, James (MD)	520
Laryngeal Disorders	Otolaryngology	Woo, Peak (MD)	507
Laryngeal Disorders	Otolaryngology	Zeitels, Steven (MD)	502
Larynx & Vocal Cord Surgery	Otolaryngology	Caldarelli, David D (MD)	512
Laser Surgery	Obstetrics & Gynecology	Tan, Merita R.C. (MD)	437
Laser Surgery	Otolaryngology	Chernoff, William Gregory (MD)	512
Laser Surgery-Larynx	Otolaryngology	Davis, Roy Kim (MD)	517
Laser Vision Surgery	Ophthalmology	Zaidman, Gerald (MD)	451
Latex Allergy	Allergy & Immunology	Benenati, Susan (MD)	98
Latex Allergy	Pediatric Allergy & Immunology	Pongracic, Jacqueline (MD)	557
Learning Disorders	Child Neurology	Lell, Mary-Elizabeth (MD)	152
Learning Disorders	Child Neurology	Shaywitz, Bennett (MD)	151
Learning Disorders	Pediatrics	Levine, Melvin David (MD)	618
Learning Disorders	Pediatrics	Shaywitz, Sally Epstein (MD)	617
LEEP Procedure	Gynecologic Oncology	Lurain, John R (MD)	260
Leg Ulcers	Dermatology	Burton III, Claude Shreve (MD)	186
Legionnaire's Disease	Infectious Disease	Yu, Victor (MD)	322
Lens Implant Complications	Ophthalmology	Driebe Jr, William T (MD)	452
Lens Implants	Ophthalmology	Serafano, Donald Natale (MD)	467
Leukemia	Hematology	Adler, Solomon Stanley (MD)	287
Leukemia	Hematology	Gregory, Stephanie (MD/PhD)	289
Leukemia	Hematology	Kantarjian, Hagop M (MD)	290
Leukemia	Hematology	Kempin, Sanford Jay (MD)	286
Leukemia	Hematology	Miller, Kenneth B. (MD)	285
Leukemia	Hematology	Zuckerman, Kenneth (MD)	287
Leukemia	Medical Oncology	Canellos, George Peter (MD)	292
Leukemia	Medical Oncology	Gabrilove, Janice (MD)	296
Leukemia	Medical Oncology	Gockerman, Jon Paul (MD)	300
Leukemia	Medical Oncology	Mitchell, Beverly (MD)	302
Leukemia	Medical Oncology	Powell, Bayard Lowery (MD)	303
Leukemia	Medical Oncology	Scheinberg, David (MD/PhD)	299
Leukemia	Medical Oncology	Schiffer, Charles Alan (MD)	308
Leukemia	Medical Oncology	Williams, Michael (MD)	304
Leukemia	Medical Oncology	Wingard, John R (MD)	305
Leukemia	Pediatric Hematology-Oncology	Bleyer, W Archie (MD)	588
Leukemia	Pediatric Hematology-Oncology	Cairo, Mitchell (MD)	583
Leukemia	Pediatric Hematology-Oncology	Nachman, James (MD)	587
Leukemia	Pediatric Hematology-Oncology	Odom , Lorrie Furman (MD)	588
Leukemia	Pediatric Hematology-Oncology	Reaman, Gregory (MD)	585
Leukemia	Pediatric Hematology-Oncology	Rosoff, Phillip Martin (MD)	586
Leukemia	Pediatric Hematology-Oncology	Steinherz, Peter G (MD)	585
Leukemia	Pediatric Hematology-Oncology	Weinstein, Howard (MD)	583
Leukemia-Acute Lymphcytic	Pediatric Hematology-Oncology	Crist, William (MD)	586
Leukemia-Adult	Hematology	Stone, Richard Maury (MD)	285
Leukemia-Pathology	Pathology	Braylan, Raul (MD)	539
Leukemia/Hematopoietic Malignancy	Hematology	Bockenstedt, Paula (MD)	288
Leukemia/Hematopoietic Malignancy	Hematology	Levine, Alexandra Mary (MD)	291
Leukemia/Hematopoietic Malignancy	Medical Oncology	Gordon, Leo I (MD)	306
Leukemia/Hematopoietic Malignancy	Medical Oncology	Mitchell, Beverly (MD)	302
Leukemia/Lymphoma	Medical Oncology	Ball, Edward David (MD)	313
Ligament Injuries	Orthopaedic Surgery	Taft, Timothy (MD)	488
Limb Salvage	Vascular Surgery (General)	Dardik, Herbert (MD)	859
Limb Salvage	Vascular Surgery (General)	Veith, Frank James (MD)	862
Limb Surgery	Orthopaedic Surgery	Aamoth, Gordon (MD)	489

Special Expertise	Specialty	Doctor's Name	Page
Limb Surgery/Reconstruction	Plastic Surgery	Sherman, Randolph (MD)	655
Liquid Ventilation	Pediatric Critical Care Medicine	Fuhrman, Bradley P (MD)	569
Liver & Biliary Disease	Gastroenterology	Hoffman, Brenda (MD)	228
Liver & Biliary Disease	Gastroenterology	La Russo, Nicholas Francis (MD)	232
Liver & Biliary Surgery	Surgery	Gagner, Michel (MD)	786
Liver & Biliary Surgery	Surgery	Melvin, W Scott (MD)	794
Liver & Biliary Surgery	Surgery	Miller, Charles (MD)	787
Liver & Biliary Surgery	Surgery	Rikkers, Layton F (MD)	795
Liver Cancer	Surgery	Curley, Steven Alan (MD)	797
Liver Cancer	Surgery	Vogel, Stephen Burton (MD)	792
Liver Cancer	Surgery	Wood, R Patrick (MD)	799
Liver Cancer-Diagnosis & Ablation	Radiology	Charboneau, J William (MD)	737
Liver Disease	Gastroenterology	Blei, Andres T (MD)	230
Liver Disease	Gastroenterology	Bloomer, Joseph (MD)	226
Liver Disease	Gastroenterology	Bonkovsky, Herbert (MD)	221
Liver Disease	Gastroenterology	Brown, Kimberly A (MD)	230
Liver Disease	Gastroenterology	Davis, Gary L (MD)	227
Liver Disease	Gastroenterology	Dienstag, Jules Leonard (MD)	221
Liver Disease	Gastroenterology	Friedman, Lawrence S. (MD)	221
Liver Disease	Gastroenterology	Galati, Joseph Steven (MD)	236
Liver Disease	Gastroenterology	Jacobson, Ira (MD)	223
Liver Disease	Gastroenterology	Keeffe, Emmet B (MD)	237
Liver Disease	Gastroenterology	Martin, Paul (MD)	238
Liver Disease	Gastroenterology	Raiford, David S (MD)	229
Liver Disease	Gastroenterology	Schiff, Eugene (MD)	229
Liver Disease	Gastroenterology	Schmidt, Warren Norman (MD)	234
Liver Disease	Gastroenterology	Silverman, William Bruce (MD)	234
Liver Disease	Gastroenterology	Vierling, John Moore (MD)	238
Liver Disease	Pathology	Bhan, Atul Kumar (MD)	535
Liver Disease	Pathology	Kanel, Gary Craig (MD)	543
Liver Disease	Pathology	Lewin, Klaus J (MD)	543
Liver Disease	Pediatric Gastroenterology	Boyle, John T (MD)	580
Liver Disease	Pediatric Gastroenterology	El-Youssef, Mounif (MD)	580
Liver Disease	Pediatric Gastroenterology	Novak, Donald A (MD)	579
Liver Disease	Pediatric Gastroenterology	Treem, William R (MD)	579
Liver Disease	Pediatric Gastroenterology	Ulshen, Martin H (MD)	579
Liver Disease	Pediatric Gastroenterology	Whitington, Peter (MD)	581
Liver Disease-Drug Induced	Gastroenterology	Maddrey, Willis Crocker (MD)	236
Liver Disease/Biliary Cirrhosis	Gastroenterology	Lindor, Keith Douglas (MD)	233
Liver Metabolic Disorders	Pathology	Norenberg, Michael D (MD)	539
Liver Pathology	Pathology	Govindarajan, Sugantha (MD)	543
Liver Pathology	Pathology	Ishak, Kamal G. (MD)	537
Liver Surgery	Surgery	Halff, Glenn Alexander (MD)	797
Liver Surgery	Surgery	Wood, R Patrick (MD)	799
Liver Surgery-Complex	Surgery	Karrer, Frederick Merrill (MD)	796
Liver Tumors	Gastroenterology	Raiford, David S (MD)	229
Liver Tumors	Pediatric Surgery	LaQuaglia, Michael (MD)	612
Liver/Pancreas Diseases	Gastroenterology	Dienstag, Jules Leonard (MD)	221
Lower Extremities Reconstruction	Plastic Surgery	Attinger, Chris (MD)	636
Lower Extremity Arterial Disease	Vascular Surgery (General)	Seeger, James M (MD)	864
Lung Biopsy	Diagnostic Radiology	Templeton, Philip (MD)	732
Lung Cancer	Medical Oncology	Aisner, Joseph (MD)	294
Lung Cancer	Medical Oncology	Albain, Kathy (MD)	305
Lung Cancer	Medical Oncology	Belani, Chandra (MD)	294
Lung Cancer	Medical Oncology	Bonomi, Philip (MD)	305
Lung Cancer	Medical Oncology	Bunn Jr, Paul (MD)	310
Lung Cancer	Medical Oncology	Cohen, Seymour (MD)	295
Lung Cancer	Medical Oncology	Comis, Robert L (MD)	295
Lung Cancer	Medical Oncology	Crawford, Jeffrey (MD)	300
Lung Cancer	Medical Oncology	Einhorn, Lawrence (MD)	306

SPECIAL EXPERTISE INDEX

Special Expertise	Specialty	Doctor's Name	Page
Lung Cancer	Medical Oncology	Ettinger, David Seymour (MD)	295
Lung Cancer	Medical Oncology	Fossella, Frank V (MD)	311
Lung Cancer	Medical Oncology	Gandara, David R (MD)	313
Lung Cancer	Medical Oncology	Glisson, Bonnie S (MD)	311
Lung Cancer	Medical Oncology	Greco, F Anthony (MD)	301
Lung Cancer	Medical Oncology	Green, Mark (MD)	301
Lung Cancer	Medical Oncology	Hait, William (MD/PhD)	296
Lung Cancer	Medical Oncology	Hong, Waun Ki (MD)	311
Lung Cancer	Medical Oncology	Johnson, Bruce Evan (MD)	293
Lung Cancer	Medical Oncology	Johnson, David (MD)	301
Lung Cancer	Medical Oncology	Karp, Daniel David (MD)	293
Lung Cancer	Medical Oncology	Kris, Mark (MD)	297
Lung Cancer	Medical Oncology	Langer, Corey Jay (MD)	297
Lung Cancer	Medical Oncology	Lee, Jin Soo (MD)	311
Lung Cancer	Medical Oncology	Livingston, Robert B (MD)	314
Lung Cancer	Medical Oncology	Lynch, Thomas (MD)	293
Lung Cancer	Medical Oncology	Masters, Gregory (MD)	307
Lung Cancer	Medical Oncology	McCarley, Dean L (MD)	302
Lung Cancer	Medical Oncology	Natale, Ronald B (MD)	314
Lung Cancer	Medical Oncology	Nissenblatt, Michael (MD)	299
Lung Cancer	Medical Oncology	Oster, Martin (MD)	299
Lung Cancer	Medical Oncology	Perry, Michael (MD)	307
Lung Cancer	Medical Oncology	Pisters, Katherine M W (MD)	312
Lung Cancer	Medical Oncology	Ruckdeschel, John C (MD)	303
Lung Cancer	Medical Oncology	Schiller, Joan H ()	309
Lung Cancer	Medical Oncology	Socinski, Mark A (MD)	304
Lung Cancer	Medical Oncology	Stone, Joel (MD)	304
Lung Cancer	Medical Oncology	Todd III, Robert F (MD/PhD)	309
Lung Cancer	Medical Oncology	Treat, Joseph (MD)	300
Lung Cancer	Medical Oncology	Vokes, Everett Emmett (MD)	309
Lung Cancer	Pulmonary Disease	Jenkinson, Stephen George (MD)	709
Lung Cancer	Pulmonary Disease	Matthay, Richard ()	692
Lung Cancer	Pulmonary Disease	Smith, James P (MD)	695
Lung Cancer	Pulmonary Disease	Steinberg, Harry (MD)	695
Lung Cancer	Pulmonary Disease	Stover-Pepe, Diane E (MD)	695
Lung Cancer	Pulmonary Disease	Tharratt, Robert S ()	713
Lung Cancer	Pulmonary Disease	White, Dorothy (MD)	696
Lung Cancer	Radiation Oncology	Choi, Noah C (MD)	717
Lung Cancer	Radiation Oncology	Cox, James D (MD)	725
Lung Cancer	Radiation Oncology	Curran Jr, Walter J (MD)	718
Lung Cancer	Radiation Oncology	Glatstein, Eli (MD)	719
Lung Cancer	Radiation Oncology	Haffty, Bruce (MD)	717
Lung Cancer	Radiation Oncology	Komaki, Ritsuko (MD)	725
Lung Cancer	Radiation Oncology	Lichter, Allen (MD)	723
Lung Cancer	Radiation Oncology	Marks, Lawrence (MD)	721
Lung Cancer	Radiation Oncology	Perez, Carlos A (MD)	724
Lung Cancer	Radiation Oncology	Rosenman, Julian (MD)	722
Lung Cancer	Radiation Oncology	Seagren, Stephen L (MD)	727
Lung Cancer	Radiation Oncology	Selch, Michael T (MD)	727
Lung Cancer	Radiation Oncology	Streeter Jr, Oscar E (MD)	727
Lung Cancer	Radiation Oncology	Turrisi III, Andrew Thomas (MD)	723
Lung Cancer	Thoracic Surgery	Faber, L Penfield (MD)	817
Lung Cancer	Thoracic Surgery	Heitmiller, Richard F (MD)	809
Lung Cancer	Thoracic Surgery	Holmes, E Carmack (MD)	824
Lung Cancer	Thoracic Surgery	Kaiser, Larry Robert (MD)	809
Lung Cancer	Thoracic Surgery	Mathisen, Douglas (MD)	806
Lung Cancer	Thoracic Surgery	McKenna Jr, Robert J (MD)	824
Lung Cancer	Thoracic Surgery	Meyers, Bryan (MD)	818
Lung Cancer	Thoracic Surgery	Putnam Jr, Joe B (MD)	822
Lung Cancer	Thoracic Surgery	Shahian, David (MD)	806

Special Expertise	Specialty	Doctor's Name	Page
Lung Cancer	Thoracic Surgery	Trastek, Victor (MD)	822
Lung Cancer	Thoracic Surgery	Whyte, Richard (MD)	826
Lung Cancer	Thoracic Surgery	Wood, Douglas (MD)	826
Lung Cancer	Thoracic Surgery	Wright, Cameron (MD)	806
Lung Cancer	Thoracic Surgery	Zorn, George L. (MD)	815
Lung Disease	Pathology	Cole, Solon R (MD)	535
Lung Disease	Pathology	Mark, Eugene J. (MD)	535
Lung Disease	Pathology	Yousem, Samuel A. (MD)	539
Lung Disease	Pediatric Pulmonology	Larsen, Gary (MD)	606
Lung Disease	Pediatric Pulmonology	Stern, Robert C (MD)	605
Lung Disease	Pulmonary Disease	Cromydas, George (MD)	702
Lung Disease	Pulmonary Disease	Enelow, Richard Ian (MD)	698
Lung Disease	Pulmonary Disease	Fahey, Patrick J (MD)	702
Lung Disease	Pulmonary Disease	Popovich Jr, John (MD)	705
Lung Disease-Newborn	Neonatal-Perinatal Medicine	Adams, James M (MD)	354
Lung Disease-Newborn	Neonatal-Perinatal Medicine	Garcia-Prats, Joseph (MD)	354
Lung Disease-Pediatric	Allergy & Immunology	Sanders, Georgiana (MD)	101
Lung Hemorrhage	Pulmonary Disease	Schwarz, Marvin Ira (MD)	708
Lung Injury	Pediatric Critical Care Medicine	Zimmerman, Jerry John (MD)	571
Lung Injury	Pulmonary Disease	Christman, Brian Wallace (MD)	697
Lung Injury	Pulmonary Disease	Hansen-Flaschen, John (MD)	693
Lung Surgery	Pediatric Surgery	Othersen, H Biemann (MD)	614
Lung Surgery	Surgery	Schwab, Richard (MD)	788
Lung Surgery	Thoracic Surgery	Frazier, Oscar Howard (MD)	821
Lung Surgery	Thoracic Surgery	Kay, Jerome Harold (MD)	824
Lung Surgery	Thoracic Surgery	Keenan, Robert (MD)	809
Lung Transplant Care	Pulmonary Disease	Lynch, Joseph P (MD)	704
Lung Volume Reduction	Pulmonary Disease	Lefrak, Stephen (MD)	704
Lung Volume Reduction	Pulmonary Disease	Mehta, Atul Chandrakant (MD)	705
Lung Volume Reduction	Pulmonary Disease	Tino, Gregory (MD)	696
Lung Volume Reduction	Thoracic Surgery	Cooper, Joel David (MD)	816
Lupus Dermatomysitis Vasculitis	Dermatology	Callen, Jeffrey P (MD)	187
Lupus Nephritis	Nephrology	Appel, Gerald (MD)	360
Lupus Nephritis	Nephrology	Falk, Ronald J (MD)	363
Lupus Nephritis	Nephrology	Lewis, Edmund J (MD)	365
Lupus Nephritis	Pediatric Nephrology	Bunchman, Timothy E (MD)	596
Lupus/SLE	Dermatology	Fivenson, David (MD)	189
Lupus/SLE	Dermatology	Sontheimer, Richard (MD)	190
Lupus/SLE	Pediatric Rheumatology	Lehman, Thomas (MD)	608
Lupus/SLE	Pediatric Rheumatology	Sills, Edward M (MD)	608
Lupus/SLE	Pediatric Rheumatology	Wagner-Weiner, Linda (MD)	609
Lupus/SLE	Rheumatology	Adams, Elaine (MD)	763
Lupus/SLE	Rheumatology	Argyros, Thomas (MD)	758
Lupus/SLE	Rheumatology	Brenner, Michael B (MD)	757
Lupus/SLE	Rheumatology	Chatham, Walter W (MD)	762
Lupus/SLE	Rheumatology	Curran, James Joseph (MD)	764
Lupus/SLE	Rheumatology	Davis, William Eugene (MD)	767
Lupus/SLE	Rheumatology	Fischbein, Lewis Conrad (MD)	764
Lupus/SLE	Rheumatology	Ginzler, Ellen (MD)	759
Lupus/SLE	Rheumatology	Hahn, Bevra H (MD)	769
Lupus/SLE	Rheumatology	Heck, Louis William (MD)	762
Lupus/SLE	Rheumatology	Katz, Paul (MD)	759
Lupus/SLE	Rheumatology	Katz, Robert (MD)	765
Lupus/SLE	Rheumatology	Kitridou, Rodanthi C (MD)	769
Lupus/SLE	Rheumatology	Kotzin, Brian Leslie (MD)	767
Lupus/SLE	Rheumatology	Lahita, Robert (MD)	759
Lupus/SLE	Rheumatology	Lindsey, Stephen M (MD)	767
Lupus/SLE	Rheumatology	Lockshin, Michael Dan (MD)	759
Lupus/SLE	Rheumatology	McCune, W. Joseph (MD)	765
Lupus/SLE	Rheumatology	Paget, Stephen (MD)	760

SPECIAL EXPERTISE INDEX

Special Expertise	Specialty	Doctor's Name	Page
Lupus/SLE	Rheumatology	Petri, Michelle Ann (MD)	760
Lupus/SLE	Rheumatology	Polisson, Richard Paul (MD)	757
Lupus/SLE	Rheumatology	Quismorio Jr, Francisco P (MD)	769
Lupus/SLE	Rheumatology	Rahn, Daniel W (MD)	762
Lupus/SLE	Rheumatology	Sessoms, Sandra Lee (MD)	768
Lupus/SLE	Rheumatology	Sigal, Leonard H (MD)	760
Lupus/SLE	Rheumatology	Stimmler, Mary McMillen (MD)	770
Lupus/SLE	Rheumatology	Sundy, John Sargent (MD/PhD)	762
Lupus/SLE	Rheumatology	Weinstein, Arthur (MD)	761
Lupus/SLE	Rheumatology	Wener, Mark (MD)	770
Lupus/SLE	Rheumatology	West, Sterling (MD)	767
Lupus/SLE	Rheumatology	Wise, Christopher Murray (MD)	763
Lupus/SLE	Rheumatology	Wofsy, David (MD)	770
Lupus/SLE-Menopause	Rheumatology	Buyon, Jill (MD)	758
Lupus/SLE-Neonatal	Dermatology	Weston, William Lee (MD)	191
Lupus/SLE-Pregnancy	Maternal & Fetal Medicine	Hibbard, Judith (MD)	345
Lupus/SLE-Pregnancy	Rheumatology	Buyon, Jill (MD)	758
Lyme Disease	Allergy & Immunology	Dattwyler, Raymond (MD)	96
Lyme Disease	Infectious Disease	Brause, Barry (MD)	318
Lyme Disease	Infectious Disease	Welch, Peter (MD)	321
Lyme Disease	Infectious Disease	Wormser, Gary (MD)	322
Lyme Disease	Infectious Disease	Yancovitz, Stanley (MD)	322
Lyme Disease	Internal Medicine	Fisher, Laura (MD)	334
Lyme Disease	Neurology	Coyle, Patricia K (MD)	401
Lyme Disease	Neurology	Finkel, Michael (MD)	407
Lyme Disease	Neurology	Logigian, Eric L (MD)	403
Lyme Disease	Neurology	Petito, Frank (MD)	404
Lyme Disease	Pediatric Infectious Disease	Shapiro, Eugene D (MD)	590
Lyme Disease	Pediatric Rheumatology	Ilowite, Norman T (MD)	608
Lyme Disease	Rheumatology	Argyros, Thomas (MD)	758
Lyme Disease	Rheumatology	Rahn, Daniel W (MD)	762
Lyme Disease	Rheumatology	Schoen, Robert Taylor (MD)	757
Lyme Disease	Rheumatology	Shadick, Nancy A (MD)	757
Lyme Disease	Rheumatology	Sigal, Leonard H (MD)	760
Lyme Disease	Rheumatology	Weinstein, Arthur (MD)	761
Lymph Node Pathology	Pathology	Knowles, Daniel (MD)	537
Lymphedema	Physical Medicine & Rehabilitation	Francis, Kathleen (MD)	624
Lymphoma	Hematology	Adler, Solomon Stanley (MD)	287
Lymphoma	Hematology	Baron, Joseph M (MD)	288
Lymphoma	Hematology	Gaynor, Ellen (MD)	288
Lymphoma	Hematology	Gregory, Stephanie (MD/PhD)	289
Lymphoma	Hematology	Kempin, Sanford Jay (MD)	286
Lymphoma	Hematology	Preisler, Harvey D (MD)	290
Lymphoma	Hematology	Wisch, Nathaniel (MD)	286
Lymphoma	Medical Oncology	Armitage, James (MD)	310
Lymphoma	Medical Oncology	Bunn Jr, Paul (MD)	310
Lymphoma	Medical Oncology	Canellos, George Peter (MD)	292
Lymphoma	Medical Oncology	De Vita Jr, Vincent T (MD)	292
Lymphoma	Medical Oncology	Fisher, Richard I (MD)	306
Lymphoma	Medical Oncology	Gockerman, Jon Paul (MD)	300
Lymphoma	Medical Oncology	Grossbard, Michael Laurence (MD)	296
Lymphoma	Medical Oncology	Kosova, Leonard (MD)	307
Lymphoma	Medical Oncology	Mitchell, Beverly (MD)	302
Lymphoma	Medical Oncology	Nadler, Lee Marshall (MD)	293
Lymphoma	Medical Oncology	Nissenblatt, Michael (MD)	299
Lymphoma	Medical Oncology	Olopade, Olufunmilayo I F (MD)	307
Lymphoma	Medical Oncology	Press, Oliver William (MD/PhD)	314
Lymphoma	Medical Oncology	Rosen, Peter J (MD)	314
Lymphoma	Medical Oncology	Salem, Philip Adeeb (MD)	312
Lymphoma	Medical Oncology	Schiffer, Charles Alan (MD)	308

Special Expertise	Specialty	Doctor's Name	Page
Lymphoma	Medical Oncology	Schwartz, Burton (MD)	309
Lymphoma	Medical Oncology	Williams, Michael (MD)	304
Lymphoma	Pathology	Banks, Peter (MD)	539
Lymphoma	Pathology	Braylan, Raul (MD)	539
Lymphoma	Pathology	Grogan, Thomas (MD)	541
Lymphoma	Pathology	Harris, Nancy L (MD)	535
Lymphoma	Pathology	Jaffe, Elaine Sarkin (MD)	537
Lymphoma	Pathology	Nathwani, Bharat N (MD)	543
Lymphoma	Pathology	Swerdlow, Steven Howard (MD)	538
Lymphoma	Pathology	Warnke, Roger Allen (MD)	544
Lymphoma	Pathology	Weisenburger, Dennis ()	541
Lymphoma	Pathology	Weiss, Lawrence M (MD)	544
Lymphoma	Pediatric Hematology-Oncology	Weinstein, Howard (MD)	583
Lymphoma	Radiation Oncology	Cox, James D (MD)	725
Lymphoma	Radiation Oncology	Glatstein, Eli (MD)	719
Lymphoma	Radiation Oncology	Goodman, Robert L (MD)	719
Lymphoma	Radiation Oncology	Mendenhall, Nancy P (MD)	722
Lymphoma	Radiation Oncology	Prosnitz, Leonard (MD)	722

M

Special Expertise	Specialty	Doctor's Name	Page
Macular Degeneration	Ophthalmology	Gentile, Ronald (MD)	446
Macular Degeneration	Ophthalmology	Nussbaum, Julian (MD)	459
Macular Disease/Degeneration	Ophthalmology	Fuchs, Wayne (MD)	446
Macular Disease/Degeneration	Ophthalmology	Goldberg, Morton (MD)	446
Macular Disease/Degeneration	Ophthalmology	Guyer, David (MD)	446
Macular Disease/Degeneration	Ophthalmology	Lambert, H. Michael (MD)	462
Macular Disease/Degeneration	Ophthalmology	Muldoon, Thomas O (MD)	448
Macular Disease/Degeneration	Ophthalmology	Rosen, Richard (MD)	450
Macular Disease/Degeneration	Ophthalmology	Sternberg Jr, Paul (MD)	455
Macular Disease/Degeneration	Ophthalmology	Yannuzzi, Lawrence (MD)	451
Malabsorption	Gastroenterology	Fordtran, John (MD)	236
Malabsorption	Gastroenterology	Toskes, Phillip (MD)	230
Mammography	Diagnostic Radiology	Huynh, Phan Tuong (MD)	734
Mammography	Diagnostic Radiology	Mitnick, Julie (MD)	732
Mammography	Diagnostic Radiology	Otto, Pamela (MD)	734
Maple Syrup Urine Disease	Clinical Genetics	Elsas II, Louis Jacob (MD)	161
Marcus Gunn Syndrome	Ophthalmology	Jaafar, Mohamad S (MD)	447
Marfan's Syndrome	Cardiology (Cardiovascular Disease)	Braverman, Alan Charles (MD)	133
Marfan's Syndrome	Clinical Genetics	Davis, Jessica S (MD)	160
Marfan's Syndrome	Clinical Genetics	Rimoin, David L (MD/PhD)	165
Marfan's Syndrome	Thoracic Surgery	Coselli, Joseph Stapleton (MD)	821
Mast Cell Diseases	Allergy & Immunology	Metcalfe, Dean D (MD)	97
Maternal & Fetal Medicine	Obstetrics & Gynecology	Divon, Michael Y (MD)	432
Maternal & Fetal Medicine	Obstetrics & Gynecology	Gonik, Bernard (MD)	435
Maternal & Fetal Medicine	Obstetrics & Gynecology	Platt, Lawrence David (MD)	439
Maxillofacial & Craniofacial Surgery	Plastic Surgery	Gruss, Joseph (MD)	652
Maxillofacial Surgery	Otolaryngology	Powell, Nelson Bert (MD/DDS)	522
Maxillofacial Surgery	Otolaryngology	Stringer, Scott Pearson (MD)	511
Maxillofacial Surgery	Plastic Surgery	Kawamoto Jr, Henry K (MD)	652
Maxillofacial Surgery	Plastic Surgery	Manson, Paul (MD)	638
Maxillofacial Surgery	Plastic Surgery	Posnick, Jeffrey Craig (MD/DMD)	639
Maxillofacial Surgery	Plastic Surgery	Wolfe, S Anthony (MD)	645
Maze Procedure	Thoracic Surgery	McCarthy, Patrick McGuane (MD)	818
Mechanical Ventilation	Pediatric Critical Care Medicine	Nichols, David Gregory (MD)	570
Mechanical Ventilation	Pediatric Critical Care Medicine	Thompson, Ann Ellen (MD)	570
Mechanical Ventilation	Pulmonary Disease	Celli, Bartolome (MD)	691
Mechanical Ventilation	Pulmonary Disease	Tobin, Martin (MD)	705
Mediastinal Tumors	Medical Oncology	Kris, Mark (MD)	297
Melanoma	Dermatology	Ackerman, A Bernard (MD)	182

SPECIAL EXPERTISE INDEX

Special Expertise	Specialty	Doctor's Name	Page
Mesothelioma	Medical Oncology	Bonomi, Philip (MD)	305
Mesothelioma	Medical Oncology	Vogelzang, Nicholas (MD)	309
Mesothelioma	Thoracic Surgery	Rusch, Valerie (MD)	811
Mesothelioma	Thoracic Surgery	Sugarbaker, David John (MD)	806
Metabolic Disorders	Endocrinology, Diabetes & Metabolism	Mazzone, Theodore (MD)	208
Metabolic Disorders	Endocrinology, Diabetes & Metabolism	Moses, Alan Charles (MD)	198
Metabolic Genetic Disorders	Clinical Genetics	Willner, Judith P (MD)	160
Metastatic Disease Mgmt	Surgery	Dooley, William Chesnut (MD)	785
Microsurgery	Hand Surgery	Culp, Randall (MD)	268
Microsurgery	Hand Surgery	Lubahn, John D (MD)	268
Microsurgery	Hand Surgery	Mih, Alexander (MD)	273
Microsurgery	Hand Surgery	Rayan, Ghazi M. (MD)	275
Microsurgery	Hand Surgery	Stern, Peter (MD)	274
Microsurgery	Hand Surgery	Tsai, Tsu-Min (MD)	271
Microsurgery	Plastic Surgery	Buncke Jr, Harry J (MD)	651
Microsurgery	Plastic Surgery	Pribaz, Julian (MD)	636
Microsurgery	Plastic Surgery	Shaw, William Wei-Lien (MD)	655
Microsurgery	Plastic Surgery	Shenaq, Saleh (MD)	650
Microsurgery	Urology	Lipshultz, Larry (MD)	846
Microtia Reconstruction	Pediatric Otolaryngology	Eavey, Roland Douglas (MD)	600
Microvascular Reconstruction	Otolaryngology	Urken, Mark (MD)	506
Middle Ear Disorders	Otolaryngology	Miyamoto, Richard (MD)	515
Middle Ear Disorders	Otolaryngology	Tucci, Debara Lyn (MD)	511
Migraine	Child Neurology	Maytal, Joseph (MD)	152
Minimally Invasive Surgery	Pediatric Surgery	Krummel, Thomas M. (MD)	616
Minimally Invasive Surgery	Pediatric Surgery	Nakayama, Don Ken (MD)	613
Minimally Invasive Surgery	Reproductive Endocrinology	Falcone, Tommaso (MD)	749
Minimally Invasive Surgery	Thoracic Surgery	Cosgrove III, Delos M (MD)	816
Minimally Invasive Surgery	Thoracic Surgery	Fontana, Gregory (MD)	823
Minimally Invasive Surgery	Urology	Winfield, Howard Neil (MD)	851
Minimally Invasive Surgery	Vascular Surgery (General)	Brener, Bruce (MD)	859
Minimally Invasive Surgery	Vascular Surgery (General)	Lumsden, Alan Boyd (MD)	863
Miscarriage-Recurrent	Maternal & Fetal Medicine	Landy, Helain Jody (MD)	342
Miscarriage-Recurrent	Obstetrics & Gynecology	Baxi, Laxmi V (MD)	431
Miscarriage-Recurrent	Reproductive Endocrinology	DeVane, Gary Williams (MD)	746
Miscarriage-Recurrent	Reproductive Endocrinology	Hill III, Joseph Albert (MD)	743
Miscarriage-Recurrent	Reproductive Endocrinology	Taylor, Robert N (MD)	752
Mitochondrial Dis/Maternal Inheritance	Clinical Genetics	Boles, Richard Gregory (MD)	163
Mitochondrial Disorders	Child Neurology	Haas, Richard H (MD)	155
Mitochondrial Disorders	Clinical Genetics	Boles, Richard Gregory (MD)	163
Mitral Valve Disease	Cardiology (Cardiovascular Disease)	Russell Jr, Richard (MD)	132
Mobility Evaluation & Treatment	Physical Medicine & Rehabilitation	Esquenazi, Alberto (MD)	624
Mohs' Surgery	Dermatology	Amonette, Rex A (MD)	186
Mohs' Surgery	Dermatology	Bailin, Philip Lawrence (MD)	188
Mohs' Surgery	Dermatology	Dzubow, Leonard (MD)	183
Mohs' Surgery	Dermatology	Flowers, Franklin P (MD)	187
Mohs' Surgery	Dermatology	Geronemus, Roy (MD)	183
Mohs' Surgery	Dermatology	Glogau, Richard Gordon (MD)	193
Mohs' Surgery	Dermatology	Green, Howard (MD)	187
Mohs' Surgery	Dermatology	Hruza, George J (MD)	189
Mohs' Surgery	Dermatology	Leshin, Barry (MD)	188
Mohs' Surgery	Dermatology	Maloney, Mary (MD)	182
Mohs' Surgery	Dermatology	Neuberg, Marcy (MD)	190
Mohs' Surgery	Dermatology	Robins, Perry (MD)	185
Mohs' Surgery	Dermatology	Taylor, R Stan (MD)	192
Mohs' Surgery	Dermatology	Wheeland, Ronald (MD)	192
Mohs' Surgery	Dermatology	Zitelli, John (MD)	186
Mood Disorders	Child & Adolescent Psychiatry	Alessi, Norman E (MD)	668
Mood Disorders	Child & Adolescent Psychiatry	Bogrov, Michael (MD)	665
Mood Disorders	Child & Adolescent Psychiatry	Foley, Carmel (MD)	665

SPECIAL EXPERTISE INDEX

Special Expertise	Specialty	Doctor's Name	Page
Multiple Gestation	Maternal & Fetal Medicine	D'Alton, Mary Elizabeth (MD)	342
Multiple Gestation	Maternal & Fetal Medicine	Dooley, Sharon L (MD)	345
Multiple Gestation	Maternal & Fetal Medicine	Greene, Michael F. (MD)	341
Multiple Gestation	Maternal & Fetal Medicine	Thorp Jr, John Mercer (MD)	344
Multiple Gestation	Maternal & Fetal Medicine	Wilkins, Isabelle (MD)	347
Multiple Gestation	Maternal & Fetal Medicine	Winn, Hung (MD)	346
Multiple Gestation	Obstetrics & Gynecology	Baxi, Laxmi V (MD)	431
Multiple Gestation	Obstetrics & Gynecology	Socol, Michael (MD)	437
Multiple Gestation	Obstetrics & Gynecology	Witter, Frank Robert (MD)	433
Multiple Myeloma	Hematology	Greipp, Philip R (MD)	289
Multiple Myeloma	Medical Oncology	Rosen, Steven T (MD)	308
Multiple Myeloma	Medical Oncology	Williams, Michael (MD)	304
Multiple Myeloma	Medical Oncology	Wingard, John R (MD)	305
Multiple Sclerosis	Neurology	Apatoff, Brian R (MD/PhD)	399
Multiple Sclerosis	Neurology	Arnason, Barry G W (MD)	411
Multiple Sclerosis	Neurology	Berger, Joseph (MD)	407
Multiple Sclerosis	Neurology	Bourdette, Dennis (MD)	419
Multiple Sclerosis	Neurology	Brooks, Benjamin (MD)	411
Multiple Sclerosis	Neurology	Cohen, Jeffrey Alan (MD)	412
Multiple Sclerosis	Neurology	Corbett, James (MD)	407
Multiple Sclerosis	Neurology	Coyle, Patricia K (MD)	401
Multiple Sclerosis	Neurology	Elias, Stanton B (MD)	412
Multiple Sclerosis	Neurology	Goodin, Douglas (MD)	420
Multiple Sclerosis	Neurology	Hafler, David A. (MD)	397
Multiple Sclerosis	Neurology	Hauser, Stephen Lawrence (MD)	421
Multiple Sclerosis	Neurology	Hurwitz, Barrie (MD)	408
Multiple Sclerosis	Neurology	Johnson, Kenneth P (MD)	403
Multiple Sclerosis	Neurology	Lisak, Robert Philip (MD)	413
Multiple Sclerosis	Neurology	Lublin, Fred (MD)	404
Multiple Sclerosis	Neurology	Petito, Frank (MD)	404
Multiple Sclerosis	Neurology	Reder, Anthony T (MD)	414
Multiple Sclerosis	Neurology	Reed, Robert L (MD)	415
Multiple Sclerosis	Neurology	Richert, John R (MD)	405
Multiple Sclerosis	Neurology	Roos, Raymond (MD)	415
Multiple Sclerosis	Neurology	Rubin, Susan (MD)	415
Multiple Sclerosis	Neurology	Schapiro, Randall (MD)	415
Multiple Sclerosis	Neurology	Vollmer, Timothy Lee (MD)	399
Multiple Sclerosis	Neurology	Waxman, Stephen G. (MD/PhD)	399
Multiple Sclerosis	Neurology	Weiner, Howard (MD)	399
Multiple Sclerosis	Neurology	Weiner, Leslie P (MD)	422
Multiple Sclerosis	Neurology	Whitaker, John N (MD)	411
Multiple Sclerosis	Neurology	Wolinsky, Jerry (MD)	418
Multiple Sclerosis	Physical Medicine & Rehabilitation	Kraft, George Howard (MD)	631
Multiple Sclerosis	Physical Medicine & Rehabilitation	Sliwa, James (DO)	628
Multiple Sclerosis (Incontinence)	Urology	Noseworthy, John (MD)	839
Munchausen Syndrome	Psychiatry	Eisendrath, Stuart James (MD)	686
Muscular Disorders-Metabolic	Pediatric Endocrinology	Slonim, Alfred (MD)	573
Muscular Dystrophy	Child Neurology	Crawford, Thomas Owen (MD)	152
Muscular Dystrophy	Neurology	Drachman, Daniel Bruce (MD)	401
Muscular Dystrophy	Neurology	Garcia, Carlos (MD)	417
Muscular Dystrophy	Neurology	Porth, Karen (MD)	414
Muscular Dystrophy	Neurology	Siddique, Teepu (MD)	415
Muscular Dystrophy	Neurology	Weinberg, Harold (MD)	406
Muscular Dystrophy	Pediatric Pulmonology	Warren, Robert Hughes (MD)	606
Muscular Dystrophy	Physical Medicine & Rehabilitation	Jaffe, Kenneth M (MD)	630
Musculoskeletal Disorders	Diagnostic Radiology	Cavallino, Robert (MD)	733
Musculoskeletal Disorders	Diagnostic Radiology	Dalinka, Murray (MD)	731
Musculoskeletal Disorders	Physical Medicine & Rehabilitation	Ma, Dong M (MD)	625
Musculoskeletal Disorders	Physical Medicine & Rehabilitation	Matthews, Dennis Jerome (MD)	628
Musculoskeletal Disorders	Rheumatology	Bunning, Robert Daniel (MD)	758

SPECIAL EXPERTISE INDEX

Special Expertise	Specialty	Doctor's Name	Page
Musculoskeletal Disorders	Rheumatology	Kagen, Lawrence (MD)	759
Musculoskeletal Infections	Infectious Disease	Wilson, Walter Ray (MD)	326
Musculoskeletal Injuries	Physical Medicine & Rehabilitation	Press, Joel (MD)	627
Musculoskeletal Tumors	Orthopaedic Surgery	Benevenia, Joseph (MD)	478
Musculoskeletal Tumors	Orthopaedic Surgery	Gebhardt, Mark (MD)	475
Musculoskeletal Tumors	Orthopaedic Surgery	Luck Jr, James Vernon (MD)	497
Musculoskeletal Tumors	Orthopaedic Surgery	Neff, James R (MD)	494
Myasthenia Gravis	Neurology	Arnason, Barry G W (MD)	411
Myasthenia Gravis	Neurology	Elias, Stanton B (MD)	412
Myasthenia Gravis	Neurology	Garcia, Carlos (MD)	417
Myasthenia Gravis	Neurology	Lisak, Robert Philip (MD)	413
Myasthenia Gravis	Neurology	Reder, Anthony T (MD)	414
Myasthenia Gravis	Neurology	Seybold, Marjorie (MD)	421
Myasthenia Gravis	Neurology	Swerdlow, Michael (MD)	406
Myasthenia Gravis	Neurology	Wright, Robert B (MD)	415
Mycobacterial Infections	Pulmonary Disease	Iseman, Michael (MD)	706
Mycobacterial Infections	Pulmonary Disease	Reichman, Lee Brodersohn (MD)	694
Myelodysplastic Syndromes	Hematology	Adler, Solomon Stanley (MD)	287
Myelodysplastic Syndromes	Medical Oncology	Gabrilove, Janice (MD)	296
Myelodysplastic Syndromes	Medical Oncology	Powell, Bayard Lowery (MD)	303
Myeloproliferative Disorders	Hematology	Baron, Joseph M (MD)	288
Myeloproliferative Disorders	Hematology	Spivak, Jerry L. (MD)	286
Myeloproliferative Disorders	Hematology	Zuckerman, Kenneth (MD)	287
Myocardial Infarction	Cardiology (Cardiovascular Disease)	Borzak, Steven (MD)	133
Myocardial Infarction	Cardiology (Cardiovascular Disease)	Conti, Charles Richard (MD)	130
Myocardial Infarction	Interventional Cardiology	Holmes Jr., David Richard (MD)	146
Myomectomy	Reproductive Endocrinology	Wallach, Edward Eliot (MD)	745
Myositis	Rheumatology	Oddis, Chester (MD)	760

N

Nail Diseases	Dermatology	Scher, Richard K (MD)	185
Nasal & Sinus Disorders	Otolaryngology	Benninger, Michael S (MD)	512
Nasal & Sinus Disorders	Otolaryngology	Josephson, Jordan S (MD)	504
Nasal & Sinus Disorders	Otolaryngology	Kuhn, Frederick (MD)	509
Nasal & Sinus Disorders	Otolaryngology	Siegel, Gordon J (MD)	516
Nasal & Sinus Disorders	Otolaryngology	Sillers, Michael (MD)	511
Nasal & Sinus Disorders	Otolaryngology	Stringer, Scott Pearson (MD)	511
Nasal Allergy	Otolaryngology	Hurst, Michael K (MD)	504
Nasal Disorders	Otolaryngology	Corey, Jacquelynne P (MD)	513
Nasal Injuries	Otolaryngology	Donovan, Donald Thomas (MD)	519
Nasal Reconstruction	Plastic Surgery	Burget, Gary C (MD)	645
Nasal Reconstruction	Plastic Surgery	Constantian, Mark B (MD)	635
Nasal Reconstruction	Plastic Surgery	Walton, Robert Lee (MD)	647
Nasal Surgery	Plastic Surgery	Rohrich, Rodney James (MD)	650
Neck & Carotid Reconstruction	Neurological Surgery	Diaz, Fernando G (MD)	383
Neonatal Cardiology	Neonatal-Perinatal Medicine	Bucciarelli, Richard L (MD)	352
Neonatal Genetics	Pediatrics	McCabe, Edward (MD)	619
Neonatal Infections	Pediatric Infectious Disease	Baker, Carol (MD)	593
Neonatal Neurology	Child Neurology	Lell, Mary-Elizabeth (MD)	152
Neonatal Neurology	Child Neurology	Volpe, Joseph J. (MD)	151
Neonatal Nutrition	Neonatal-Perinatal Medicine	Neu, Josef (MD)	353
Neonatal Respiratory Disease	Neonatal-Perinatal Medicine	Martin, Richard (MD)	353
Neonatal Sepsis	Neonatal-Perinatal Medicine	Polin, Richard (MD)	352
Neonatal Surgery	Pediatric Surgery	Ginsburg, Howard (MD)	611
Neonatal Surgery	Pediatric Surgery	Nakayama, Don Ken (MD)	613
Neonatal Surgery	Pediatric Surgery	Oldham, Keith T (MD)	615
Neonatal Surgery	Pediatric Surgery	Sato, Thomas Tad (MD)	615
Neonatal Surgery-Gastrointestinal	Pediatric Surgery	Adkins, John Crawford (MD)	611
Neonatal-Perinatal Medicine	Pediatrics	Regan, Joan (MD)	352

Special Expertise	Specialty	Doctor's Name	Page
Neonatology	Neonatal-Perinatal Medicine	Bancalari, Eduardo (MD)	352
Neonatology	Neonatal-Perinatal Medicine	Boyle, Robert John (MD)	352
Neonatology	Neonatal-Perinatal Medicine	Cloherty, John ()	351
Neonatology	Neonatal-Perinatal Medicine	Denson, Susan Ellen (MD)	354
Neonatology	Neonatal-Perinatal Medicine	Ehrenkranz, Richard (MD)	351
Neonatology	Neonatal-Perinatal Medicine	Hurt, Hallam (MD)	351
Neonatology	Neonatal-Perinatal Medicine	Lemons, James A (MD)	353
Neonatology	Neonatal-Perinatal Medicine	Martin, Richard (MD)	353
Neonatology	Neonatal-Perinatal Medicine	Odom, Michael W (MD)	354
Neonatology	Neonatal-Perinatal Medicine	Stevenson, David K (MD)	355
Neonatology	Neonatal-Perinatal Medicine	Stiles, Alan (MD)	353
Neonatology	Neonatal-Perinatal Medicine	Tyson, Jon Edward (MD)	355
Nephrology	Internal Medicine	Coe, Fredric (MD)	364
Nephrotic Syndrome	Nephrology	Black, Henry R (MD)	364
Nephrotic Syndrome	Nephrology	Couser, William (MD)	368
Nephrotic Syndrome	Nephrology	Okusa, Mark D (MD)	363
Nephrotic Syndrome	Pediatrics	Zilleruelo, Gaston E (MD)	618
Nerve Regeneration	Hand Surgery	Trumble, Thomas (MD)	276
Nerve Transplantation	Plastic Surgery	Mackinnon, Susan (MD)	646
Nervous System Tumors	Neurological Surgery	Apuzzo, Michael L J (MD)	388
Neural Regulation of Mucosal Secretion	Allergy & Immunology	Baraniuk, James N (MD)	95
Neuro-Behavioral Disorder	Neurology	Jackson, John Kevin (MD)	417
Neuro-Endocrinology	Child Neurology	Ferriero, Donna Marie (MD)	155
Neuro-Endocrinology	Endocrinology, Diabetes & Metabolism	Marshall, John Crook (MD/PhD)	204
Neuro-Endocrinology	Obstetrics & Gynecology	Naftolin, Frederick (MD)	431
Neuro-Genetics	Clinical Genetics	Korf, Bruce (MD/PhD)	159
Neuro-Genetics	Clinical Genetics	Northrup, Hope (MD)	163
Neuro-Immunology	Neurology	Apatoff, Brian R (MD/PhD)	399
Neuro-Immunology	Neurology	Cohen, Jeffrey Alan (MD)	412
Neuro-Immunology	Neurology	Coyle, Patricia K (MD)	401
Neuro-Immunology	Neurology	Richert, John R (MD)	405
Neuro-Oncology	Neurological Surgery	Al-Mefty, Ossama (MD)	386
Neuro-Oncology	Neurological Surgery	Piepmeier, Joseph (MD)	374
Neuro-Oncology	Neurology	Cloughesy, Timothy Francis (MD)	419
Neuro-Oncology	Neurology	De Angelis, Lisa (MD)	401
Neuro-Oncology	Neurology	Greenberg, Harry S. (MD)	413
Neuro-Oncology	Neurology	Hiesiger, Emile (MD)	403
Neuro-Oncology	Neurology	Posner, Jerome (MD)	405
Neuro-Oncology	Neurology	Rogers, Lisa R (DO)	415
Neuro-Oncology	Neurology	Shapiro, William R. (MD)	418
Neuro-Oncology	Neurology	Spence, Alexander Morton (MD)	422
Neuro-Oncology	Pediatric Hematology-Oncology	Puccetti, Diane (MD)	587
Neuro-Onocology	Medical Oncology	Lyckholm, Laurel Jean (MD)	302
Neuro-Ophthalmology	Neurology	Carter, John E (MD)	416
Neuro-Ophthalmology	Neurology	Corbett, James (MD)	407
Neuro-Ophthalmology	Neurology	Galetta, Steven (MD)	402
Neuro-Ophthalmology	Neurology	Newman, Nancy Jean (MD)	409
Neuro-Ophthalmology	Neurology	Schatz, Norman Joseph (MD)	410
Neuro-Ophthalmology	Neurology	Seybold, Marjorie (MD)	421
Neuro-Ophthalmology	Neurology	Troost, Bradley Todd (MD)	410
Neuro-Ophthalmology	Ophthalmology	Arnold, Anthony C (MD)	463
Neuro-Ophthalmology	Ophthalmology	Behrens, Myles (MD)	444
Neuro-Ophthalmology	Ophthalmology	Capo, Hilda (MD)	452
Neuro-Ophthalmology	Ophthalmology	Feldon, Steven E (MD)	464
Neuro-Ophthalmology	Ophthalmology	Glaser, Joel (MD)	453
Neuro-Ophthalmology	Ophthalmology	Hoyt, William Fletcher (MD)	465
Neuro-Ophthalmology	Ophthalmology	Kupersmith, Mark (MD)	447
Neuro-Ophthalmology	Ophthalmology	Miller, Neil (MD)	448
Neuro-Ophthalmology	Ophthalmology	Pollock, Stephen (MD)	455
Neuro-Ophthalmology	Ophthalmology	Rosenberg, Michael A (MD)	459

SPECIAL EXPERTISE INDEX

Special Expertise	Specialty	Doctor's Name	Page
Neuro-Ophthalmology	Ophthalmology	Savino, Peter (MD)	450
Neuro-Ophthalmology	Ophthalmology	Sergott, Robert C (MD)	450
Neuro-Ophthalmology	Ophthalmology	Walton, David S (MD)	444
Neuro-Ophthalmology	Ophthalmology	Younge, Brian R (MD)	460
Neuro-Otolaryngology	Otolaryngology	Arriaga, Moises Alberto (MD)	502
Neuro-Otolaryngology	Otolaryngology	Poe, Dennis (MD)	501
Neuro-Otolaryngology	Otolaryngology	Roland, Peter S (MD)	520
Neuro-Otology	Otolaryngology	Balkany, Thomas Jay (MD)	507
Neuro-Otology	Otolaryngology	Brackmann, Derald E (MD)	521
Neuro-Otology	Otolaryngology	Gantz, Bruce (MD)	513
Neuro-Otology	Otolaryngology	Jackler, Robert K (MD)	522
Neuro-Otology	Otolaryngology	Jenkins, Herman A. (MD)	519
Neuro-Otology	Otolaryngology	Lambert, Paul R (MD)	509
Neuro-Otology	Otolaryngology	Mattox, Douglas (MD)	509
Neuro-Otology	Otolaryngology	Miyamoto, Richard (MD)	515
Neuro-Otology	Otolaryngology	Niparko, John (MD)	505
Neuro-Otology	Otolaryngology	Perkins, Rodney (MD)	522
Neuro-Pathology	Pathology	Chandrasoma, Parakrama T (MD)	542
Neuro-Pathology	Pathology	Davis, Richard L (MD)	542
Neuro-Pathology	Pathology	Petito, Carol (MD)	540
Neuro-Pathology	Pathology	Scheithauer, Bernd (MD)	540
Neuro-Pathology	Pathology	Schlaepfer, William W (MD)	538
Neuro-Pharmacology	Neurology	Hubble, Jean Pintar (MD)	413
Neuro-Psychiatry	Child & Adolescent Psychiatry	Leonard, Henrietta (MD)	663
Neuro-Psychiatry	Geriatric Psychiatry	Lyketsos, Constantine G (MD)	672
Neuro-Psychiatry	Neurology	Cummings, Jeffrey Lee (MD)	419
Neuro-Psychiatry	Neurology	Jackson, John Kevin (MD)	417
Neuro-Psychiatry	Psychiatry	McHugh, Paul (MD)	680
Neuro-Psychiatry	Psychiatry	Neppe, Vernon Michael (MD)	687
Neuro-Psychiatry	Psychiatry	Zorumski, Charles F (MD)	684
Neuro-Radiology	Radiology	Atlas, Scott W (MD)	739
Neuro-Radiology	Radiology	Berenstein, Alejandro (MD)	735
Neuro-Radiology	Radiology	Cross III, DeWitte T (MD)	737
Neuro-Radiology	Radiology	Hasso, Anton N (MD)	739
Neuro-Radiology	Radiology	Modic, Michael (MD)	738
Neuro-Radiology	Radiology	Tenner, Michael (MD)	736
Neuro-Rehabilitation	Orthopaedic Surgery	Riew, K Daniel (MD)	492
Neuro-Rehabilitation	Physical Medicine & Rehabilitation	Roth, Elliot (MD)	628
Neuro-Urology	Urology	Boone, Timothy Bolton (MD/PhD)	845
Neuro-Urology	Urology	Gomery, Pablo (MD)	829
Neuro-Urology	Urology	Wein, Alan J (MD)	836
Neurobiology	Neurology	Selkoe, Dennis (MD)	398
Neuroblastoma	Pediatric Hematology-Oncology	Brodeur, Garrett (MD)	583
Neuroblastoma	Pediatric Hematology-Oncology	Castle, Valerie (MD)	586
Neuroblastoma	Pediatric Hematology-Oncology	Kushner, Brian (MD)	584
Neuroblastoma	Pediatric Surgery	LaQuaglia, Michael (MD)	612
Neuroblastoma/Solid Tumors	Pediatric Hematology-Oncology	Matthay, Katherine Kurshan (MD)	589
Neurocutaneous Disorders	Clinical Genetics	Cassidy, Suzanne (MD)	162
Neurodegenerative Disease	Neurology	Beal, Myron Flint (MD)	400
Neurodegenerative Disease	Neurology	Burns , R Stanley (MD)	412
Neurodegenerative Disease	Physical Medicine & Rehabilitation	Francis, Kathleen (MD)	624
Neuroendocrine Disease	Geriatric Medicine	Minaker, Kenneth (MD)	243
Neuroendocrine Tumors	Gastroenterology	Metz, David C. (MD)	224
Neurofibromatosis	Child Neurology	Aron, Alan (MD)	151
Neurofibromatosis	Clinical Genetics	Carey, John (MD)	163
Neurofibromatosis	Clinical Genetics	Saal, Howard (MD)	162
Neurofibromatosis	Neurological Surgery	Hoff, Julian T (MD)	383
Neurofilament Metabolism	Pathology	Schlaepfer, William W (MD)	538
Neurogenic Bladder-Female	Urology	Payne, Christopher K (MD)	849
Neurologic Disorders	Child Neurology	Holmes, Gregory Lawrence (MD)	151

SPECIAL EXPERTISE INDEX

Special Expertise	Specialty	Doctor's Name	Page
Oculoplastic Surgery	Ophthalmology	McCord, Clinton (MD)	454
Oculoplastic Surgery	Ophthalmology	Putterman, Allen M. (MD)	459
Oculoplastic Surgery	Ophthalmology	Shorr, Norman (MD)	467
Oculoplastic Surgery	Plastic Surgery	Carraway, James Howard (MD)	642
Olfactory Disorders	Otolaryngology	Leopold, Donald Arthur (MD)	518
Oncology	Diagnostic Radiology	Pisano, Etta Driscoll (MD)	733
Oncology	Geriatric Medicine	Cohen, Harvey (MD)	245
Oncology	Medical Oncology	Comis, Robert L (MD)	295
Oncology	Medical Oncology	Schiller, Joan H ()	309
Oncology	Pediatric Hematology-Oncology	Barbosa, Jerry L (MD)	585
Oncology	Pediatric Hematology-Oncology	Reaman, Gregory (MD)	585
Ophthalmic Pathology	Ophthalmology	Albert, Daniel M. (MD)	456
Ophthalmologic Pathology	Pathology	McCormick, Steven (MD)	537
Ophthalmologic Plastic Surgery	Ophthalmology	Boxrud, Cynthia Ann (MD)	463
Ophthalmologic Plastic Surgery	Ophthalmology	Piest, Kenneth L (MD)	462
Ophthalmology-Genetics	Ophthalmology	Mets, Marilyn (MD)	458
Ophthalmology-Pediatric	Ophthalmology	Archer, Steven M (MD)	456
Ophthalmology-Pediatric	Ophthalmology	Aronian, Dianne D (MD)	444
Ophthalmology-Pediatric	Ophthalmology	Baker, John D (MD)	456
Ophthalmology-Pediatric	Ophthalmology	Bateman, Jane Bronwyn (MD)	461
Ophthalmology-Pediatric	Ophthalmology	Biglan, Albert William (MD)	444
Ophthalmology-Pediatric	Ophthalmology	Borchert, Mark S (MD)	463
Ophthalmology-Pediatric	Ophthalmology	Burke, Miles Joseph (MD)	456
Ophthalmology-Pediatric	Ophthalmology	Capo, Hilda (MD)	452
Ophthalmology-Pediatric	Ophthalmology	Caputo, Anthony R (MD)	445
Ophthalmology-Pediatric	Ophthalmology	Cibis, Gerhard W (MD)	456
Ophthalmology-Pediatric	Ophthalmology	Day, Susan H (MD)	464
Ophthalmology-Pediatric	Ophthalmology	Del Monte, Monte A (MD)	456
Ophthalmology-Pediatric	Ophthalmology	Demer, Joseph L (MD/PhD)	464
Ophthalmology-Pediatric	Ophthalmology	Eggers, Howard M (MD)	445
Ophthalmology-Pediatric	Ophthalmology	Ellis Jr, George S (MD)	461
Ophthalmology-Pediatric	Ophthalmology	Eustis, Horatio Sprague (MD)	461
Ophthalmology-Pediatric	Ophthalmology	France, Thomas D (MD)	457
Ophthalmology-Pediatric	Ophthalmology	Freedman, Sharon (MD)	453
Ophthalmology-Pediatric	Ophthalmology	Granet, David Bruce (MD)	465
Ophthalmology-Pediatric	Ophthalmology	Hall, Lisabeth (MD)	446
Ophthalmology-Pediatric	Ophthalmology	Hess, J Bruce (MD)	453
Ophthalmology-Pediatric	Ophthalmology	Isenberg, Sherwin Jay (MD)	465
Ophthalmology-Pediatric	Ophthalmology	Katowitz, James A (MD)	447
Ophthalmology-Pediatric	Ophthalmology	Kushner, Burton J (MD)	458
Ophthalmology-Pediatric	Ophthalmology	Lambert, Scott (MD)	454
Ophthalmology-Pediatric	Ophthalmology	Magramm, Irene (MD)	448
Ophthalmology-Pediatric	Ophthalmology	Mahon, Kathleen MK (MD)	465
Ophthalmology-Pediatric	Ophthalmology	Mets, Marilyn (MD)	458
Ophthalmology-Pediatric	Ophthalmology	Metz, Henry (MD)	448
Ophthalmology-Pediatric	Ophthalmology	Miller, Marilyn T (MD)	459
Ophthalmology-Pediatric	Ophthalmology	Mims III, James Luther (MD)	462
Ophthalmology-Pediatric	Ophthalmology	Mitchell, Paul Ralph (MD)	443
Ophthalmology-Pediatric	Ophthalmology	Murphree, A. Linn (MD)	466
Ophthalmology-Pediatric	Ophthalmology	Olitsky, Scott Eric (MD)	449
Ophthalmology-Pediatric	Ophthalmology	Palmer, Earl A. (MD)	467
Ophthalmology-Pediatric	Ophthalmology	Paul, Theodore Otis (MD)	467
Ophthalmology-Pediatric	Ophthalmology	Petersen, Robert Allen (MD)	443
Ophthalmology-Pediatric	Ophthalmology	Pollard, Zane F (MD)	454
Ophthalmology-Pediatric	Ophthalmology	Price, Ronald (MD)	459
Ophthalmology-Pediatric	Ophthalmology	Quinn, Graham Earl (MD)	449
Ophthalmology-Pediatric	Ophthalmology	Raab, Edward (MD)	449
Ophthalmology-Pediatric	Ophthalmology	Reynolds, James D. (MD)	449
Ophthalmology-Pediatric	Ophthalmology	Richard, James Marshall (MD)	463
Ophthalmology-Pediatric	Ophthalmology	Scott, William (MD)	460

SPECIAL EXPERTISE INDEX

Special Expertise	Specialty	Doctor's Name	Page
Ovarian Cancer	Gynecologic Oncology	Berek, Jonathan S (MD)	263
Ovarian Cancer	Gynecologic Oncology	Caputo, Thomas A (MD)	256
Ovarian Cancer	Gynecologic Oncology	Cohen, Carmel (MD)	256
Ovarian Cancer	Gynecologic Oncology	Copeland, Larry James (MD)	259
Ovarian Cancer	Gynecologic Oncology	Curtin, John P (MD)	256
Ovarian Cancer	Gynecologic Oncology	De Geest, Koen (MD)	259
Ovarian Cancer	Gynecologic Oncology	Freedman, Ralph (MD)	262
Ovarian Cancer	Gynecologic Oncology	Fuller, Arlan F. (MD)	255
Ovarian Cancer	Gynecologic Oncology	Gershenson, David Marc (MD)	263
Ovarian Cancer	Gynecologic Oncology	Herbst, Arthur (MD)	259
Ovarian Cancer	Gynecologic Oncology	Kim, Woo Shin (MD)	260
Ovarian Cancer	Gynecologic Oncology	Kwon, Tae (MD)	257
Ovarian Cancer	Gynecologic Oncology	Lagasse, Leo D (MD)	264
Ovarian Cancer	Gynecologic Oncology	Look, Katherine (MD)	260
Ovarian Cancer	Gynecologic Oncology	Moore, David H (MD)	260
Ovarian Cancer	Gynecologic Oncology	Partridge, Edward E (MD)	258
Ovarian Cancer	Gynecologic Oncology	Potkul, Ronald (MD)	261
Ovarian Cancer	Gynecologic Oncology	Smith, Donna Marie (MD)	262
Ovarian Cancer	Gynecologic Oncology	Van Nagell Jr., John R. (MD)	259
Ovarian Cancer	Gynecologic Oncology	Waggoner, Steven (MD)	262
Ovarian Cancer	Gynecologic Oncology	Webb, Maurice James (MD)	262
Ovarian Cancer	Medical Oncology	Markman, Maurie (MD)	307
Ovarian Cancer	Medical Oncology	Ozols, Robert Felix (MD/PhD)	299
Ovarian Cancer	Medical Oncology	Speyer, James (MD)	299
Ovarian Cancer-Hereditary	Gynecologic Oncology	Berchuck, Andrew ()	257
Ovarian Failure-Recurrent	Obstetrics & Gynecology	Simpson, Joe Leigh (MD)	438

P

Pacemakers	Cardiac Electrophysiology	Curtis, Anne B (MD)	116
Pacemakers	Cardiac Electrophysiology	DiMarco, John Philip (MD/PhD)	116
Pacemakers	Cardiac Electrophysiology	Hammill, Stephen Charles (MD)	117
Pacemakers	Cardiac Electrophysiology	Levine, Joseph H (MD)	115
Pacemakers	Cardiac Electrophysiology	Marchlinski, Francis Edward (MD)	116
Pacemakers	Cardiac Electrophysiology	Sorrentino, Robert A. (MD)	117
Pacemakers	Cardiology (Cardiovascular Disease)	Naccarelli, Gerald V (MD)	127
Pain Management	Neurological Surgery	Burchiel, Kim James (MD)	388
Pain Management	Neurological Surgery	Dennis, Gary Creed (MD)	375
Pain Management	Neurological Surgery	Hassenbusch, Samuel J (MD/PhD)	387
Pain Management	Neurological Surgery	Loeser, John D (MD)	389
Pain Management	Neurological Surgery	Rosomoff, Hubert L (MD)	381
Pain Management	Neurology	Hiesiger, Emile (MD)	403
Pain Management	Neurology	Max, Mitchell Bruce (MD)	404
Pain Management	Pain Management	Ashburn, Michael (MD)	530
Pain Management	Pain Management	Du Pen, Stuart L (MD)	531
Pain Management	Pain Management	Green, Carmen R (MD)	529
Pain Management	Pain Management	Lema, Mark J (MD)	527
Pain Management	Pain Management	Mullin, Vildan (MD)	530
Pain Management	Pain Management	Portenoy, Russell (MD)	528
Pain Management	Pain Management	Racz, Gabor (MD)	531
Pain Management	Pediatric Critical Care Medicine	Anand, Kanwaljeet Singh (MD/PhD)	571
Pain Management	Pediatrics	Zeltzer, Lonnie Kaye (MD)	619
Pain Management	Physical Medicine & Rehabilitation	Clairmont, Albert (MD)	626
Pain Management	Physical Medicine & Rehabilitation	Walsh, Nicolas Eugene (MD)	630
Pain Management-Back & Headache	Pain Management	Harden, Norman (MD)	529
Pain Management-Cancer	Pain Management	Ready, L Brian (MD)	531
Pain Management-Pediatric	Pain Management	Berde, Charles Benjamin (MD)	527
Pain Management-Pediatric	Pain Management	Weisman, Steven Jay (MD)	530
Pain Management-Pre Operative	Pain Management	Fitzgibbon, Dermot Richard (MD)	531
Pain-Acute	Pain Management	Rogers, James N (MD)	531

SPECIAL EXPERTISE INDEX

Special Expertise	Specialty	Doctor's Name	Page
Pain-Back	Orthopaedic Surgery	Riew, K Daniel (MD)	492
Pain-Back	Pain Management	Benzon, Honorio T (MD)	529
Pain-Back	Pain Management	Kreitzer, Joel (MD)	527
Pain-Back	Pain Management	Ramamurthy, Somayaji (MD)	531
Pain-Back	Pain Management	Smith, Joanne (MD)	530
Pain-Back	Pain Management	Weinberger, Michael (MD)	529
Pain-Back	Physical Medicine & Rehabilitation	Lipkin, David L (MD)	626
Pain-Back	Physical Medicine & Rehabilitation	Press, Joel (MD)	627
Pain-Back	Physical Medicine & Rehabilitation	Sliwa, James (DO)	628
Pain-Back	Sports Medicine	Schechter, David Louis (MD)	775
Pain-Back & Neck	Neurological Surgery	Bauer, Jerry (MD)	382
Pain-Back & Neck	Physical Medicine & Rehabilitation	Haig, Andrew (MD)	627
Pain-Cancer	Pain Management	Fitzgibbon, Dermot Richard (MD)	531
Pain-Cancer	Pain Management	Jain, Subhash (MD)	527
Pain-Cancer	Pain Management	Kreitzer, Joel (MD)	527
Pain-Cancer	Pain Management	Staats, Peter (MD)	528
Pain-Cancer	Pain Management	Weinberger, Michael (MD)	529
Pain-Cancer	Psychiatry	Breitbart, William (MD)	678
Pain-Chronic	Neurological Surgery	Brown, Frederick (MD)	382
Pain-Chronic	Neurological Surgery	Levy, Robert M (MD)	384
Pain-Chronic	Neurological Surgery	Rezai, Ali R (MD)	385
Pain-Chronic	Pain Management	Ramamurthy, Somayaji (MD)	531
Pain-Chronic	Pain Management	Rogers, James N (MD)	531
Pain-Facial	Neurological Surgery	Ruge, John (MD)	385
Pain-Musculoskeletal	Pain Management	Ngeow, Jeffrey (MD)	528
Pain-Musculoskeletal	Pain Management	Smith, Joanne (MD)	530
Pain-Orofacial	Otolaryngology	Blitzer, Andrew (MD)	502
Pain-Shoulder/Hand Syndrome(RSD)	Pain Management	Rowbotham, Michael Charles (MD)	532
Pain-Soft Tissue	Physical Medicine & Rehabilitation	Aseff, John Namer (MD)	623
Pain-Sympathetic	Pain Management	Raja, Srinivasa (MD)	528
Pain/Seizures	Neurological Surgery	Dogali, Michael (MD)	389
Palliative Care	Geriatric Medicine	Hanson, Laura Catherine ()	246
Palliative Care	Hematology	Bricker, Leslie J (MD)	288
Palliative Care	Internal Medicine	Selwyn, Peter (MD)	334
Palliative Care	Medical Oncology	Anderson, Joseph (MD)	305
Palliative Care	Medical Oncology	Smith, Thomas Joseph (MD)	304
Palliative Care	Pain Management	Payne, Richard (MD)	528
Palliative Care	Pain Management	Portenoy, Russell (MD)	528
Palliative Care-Pediatric	Pain Management	Weisman, Steven Jay (MD)	530
Pancreatc Disease	Gastroenterology	Cotton, Peter (MD)	227
Pancreatic & Biliary Disease	Gastroenterology	Barkin, Jamie (MD)	226
Pancreatic & Biliary Disease	Gastroenterology	Carr-Locke, David L (MD)	221
Pancreatic & Laparoscopic Surgery	Surgery	Melvin, W Scott (MD)	794
Pancreatic & Stomach Cancer	Surgery	Coit, Daniel G (MD)	784
Pancreatic Cancer	Gastroenterology	Forsmark, Christopher (MD)	228
Pancreatic Cancer	Medical Oncology	Abbruzzese, James L (MD)	310
Pancreatic Cancer	Medical Oncology	Donehower, Ross Carl (MD)	295
Pancreatic Cancer	Medical Oncology	Rothenberg, Mace (MD)	303
Pancreatic Cancer	Surgery	Cameron, John (MD)	784
Pancreatic Cancer	Surgery	Carey, Larry C (MD)	790
Pancreatic Cancer	Surgery	Clark, Orlo H (MD)	799
Pancreatic Cancer	Surgery	Ellison, Edwin Christopher (MD)	793
Pancreatic Cancer	Surgery	Evans, Douglas Brian (MD)	797
Pancreatic Cancer	Surgery	Lee, Jeffrey Edwin (MD)	798
Pancreatic Cancer	Surgery	Warshaw, Andrew L (MD)	783
Pancreatic Disease	Gastroenterology	Di Magno, Eugene (MD)	231
Pancreatic Disease	Gastroenterology	Jacobson, Ira (MD)	223
Pancreatic Disease	Pediatric Surgery	Neblett, Wallace W (MD)	613
Pancreatic Surgery	Surgery	Schirmer, Bruce David (MD)	792
Pancreatic Surgery	Surgery	Warshaw, Andrew L (MD)	783

Special Expertise	Specialty	Doctor's Name	Page
Pancreatic Surgery	Surgery	Willis, Irvin (MD)	793
Pancreatic/Biliary Dis Endoscopy (ERCP)	Gastroenterology	Carr-Locke, David L (MD)	221
Pancreatic/Biliary Dis Endoscopy (ERCP)	Gastroenterology	Kimmey, Michael Bryant (MD)	237
Pancreatic/Biliary Dis Endoscopy(ERCP)	Gastroenterology	Aronchick, Craig Alan (MD)	222
Pancreatic/Biliary Dis Endoscopy(ERCP)	Gastroenterology	Benjamin, Stanley (MD)	222
Pancreatic/Biliary Dis Endoscopy(ERCP)	Gastroenterology	Chuttani, Ram (MD)	221
Pancreatic/Biliary Dis Endoscopy(ERCP)	Gastroenterology	Ostroff, James Warren (MD)	238
Pancreatic/Biliary Dis Endoscopy(ERCP)	Gastroenterology	Siegel, Jerome (MD)	225
Pancreatic/Biliary Dis Endoscopy(ERCP)	Gastroenterology	Silverman, William Bruce (MD)	234
Pancreatitis	Gastroenterology	Cunningham, John (MD)	227
Pancreatitis	Gastroenterology	Lambiase, Louis (MD)	228
Pancreatitis	Gastroenterology	Toskes, Phillip (MD)	230
Panic Disorder	Psychiatry	Roy-Byrne, Peter (MD)	688
Panic Disorder	Psychiatry	Stein, Murray Brent (MD)	688
Panic Disorder & Agoraphobia	Psychiatry	Shear, Mary Katherine (MD)	681
Panic Disorder/Anxiety Disorders	Psychiatry	Gorman, Jack Matthew (MD)	679
Paralytic Disorders	Hand Surgery	Beasley, Robert (MD)	267
Parasitic Infections	Infectious Disease	Johnson, Warren (MD)	320
Parasitic Infections	Infectious Disease	Maguire, James (MD)	317
Parathyroid Disease	Endocrinology, Diabetes & Metabolism	Blum, Manfred (MD)	198
Parathyroid Disease	Geriatric Medicine	Lyles, Kenneth W (MD)	246
Parathyroid Disease	Nephrology	Massry, Shaul Gourgi (MD)	369
Parathyroid Surgery	Surgery	Hardy, Mark (MD)	786
Parkinson's Disease	Neurological Surgery	Baltuch, Gordon (MD/PhD)	374
Parkinson's Disease	Neurological Surgery	Dogali, Michael (MD)	389
Parkinson's Disease	Neurological Surgery	Freeman, Thomas B (MD)	380
Parkinson's Disease	Neurological Surgery	Friedman, William A (MD)	380
Parkinson's Disease	Neurological Surgery	Nazzaro, Jules M. (MD)	373
Parkinson's Disease	Neurological Surgery	Rezai, Ali R (MD)	385
Parkinson's Disease	Neurology	Ahlskog, J. Eric (MD)	411
Parkinson's Disease	Neurology	Cummings, Jeffrey Lee (MD)	419
Parkinson's Disease	Neurology	De Long, Mahlon R. (MD)	407
Parkinson's Disease	Neurology	Fahn, Stanley (MD)	402
Parkinson's Disease	Neurology	Feldman, Robert G (MD)	397
Parkinson's Disease	Neurology	Fink, J. Stephen (MD)	397
Parkinson's Disease	Neurology	Gendelman, Seymour (MD)	402
Parkinson's Disease	Neurology	Goetz, Christopher (MD)	413
Parkinson's Disease	Neurology	Goodgold, Albert (MD)	402
Parkinson's Disease	Neurology	Hubble, Jean Pintar (MD)	413
Parkinson's Disease	Neurology	Hurtig, Howard (MD)	403
Parkinson's Disease	Neurology	Jankovic, Joseph (MD)	417
Parkinson's Disease	Neurology	Koller, William C (MD)	408
Parkinson's Disease	Neurology	Langston, J William (MD)	421
Parkinson's Disease	Neurology	Nutt Jr, John G. (MD)	421
Parkinson's Disease	Neurology	Olanow, C Warren (MD)	404
Parkinson's Disease	Neurology	Perlmutter, Joel S (MD)	414
Parkinson's Disease	Neurology	Rubin, Susan (MD)	415
Parkinson's Disease	Neurology	Sethi, Kapil (MD)	410
Parkinson's Disease	Neurology	Shoulson, Ira (MD)	405
Parkinson's Disease	Neurology	Shults, Clifford Walter (MD)	422
Parkinson's Disease	Neurology	Stern, Matthew (MD)	406
Parkinson's Disease	Neurology	Tanner, Caroline M (MD/PhD)	422
Parkinson's Disease	Neurology	Tetrud, James W (MD)	422
Parkinson's Disease	Neurology	Watts, Ray Lannon (MD)	410
Parkinson's Disease	Neurology	Weiner, William J. (MD)	411
Parkinson's Disease	Neurology	Wooten, George Frederick (MD)	411
Parkinson's Disease	Neurology	Young, Anne (MD)	399
Parkinson's Disease	Pathology	Norenberg, Michael D (MD)	539
Parotid Gland Tumors	Otolaryngology	Burkey, Brian (MD)	507
Patella Problems	Orthopaedic Surgery	Grelsamer, Ronald (MD)	481

SPECIAL EXPERTISE INDEX

Special Expertise	Specialty	Doctor's Name	Page
Paternity Testing	Pathology	Kao, Kuo-Jang (MD/PhD)	539
Pediatric & Adolscent Gynecology	Adolescent Medicine	Emans, Sarah Jean Herriot (MD)	89
Pediatric Surgery	Pediatric Otolaryngology	Drake, Amelia (MD)	601
Pelvic Cancer	Gynecologic Oncology	FInan, Michael A (MD)	262
Pelvic Prolapse Repair	Obstetrics & Gynecology	McLeod, Allan G W (MD)	434
Pelvic Reconstruction	Gynecologic Oncology	Clarke-Pearson, Daniel L (MD)	258
Pelvic Reconstruction	Gynecologic Oncology	Mutch, David (MD)	261
Pelvic Reconstruction	Gynecologic Oncology	Podratz, Karl C (MD/PhD)	261
Pelvic Reconstruction	Gynecologic Oncology	Webb, Maurice James (MD)	262
Pelvic Reconstruction	Obstetrics & Gynecology	Cundiff, Geoffrey Williams (DO)	432
Pelvic Reconstruction	Obstetrics & Gynecology	Hunt, Robert Bridger (MD)	431
Pelvic Reconstruction	Obstetrics & Gynecology	McLeod, Allan G W (MD)	434
Pelvic Reconstruction	Urology	Kennelly, Michael Joseph (MD)	838
Pelvic Surgery	Gynecologic Oncology	Copeland, Larry James (MD)	259
Pelvic Surgery	Reproductive Endocrinology	Murphy, Ana Alvarez (MD)	747
Pelvic Tumors	Gynecologic Oncology	Barnes, Willard (MD)	255
Pemphigus	Dermatology	Anhalt, Grant James (MD)	182
Pemphigus	Dermatology	Bystryn, Jean-Claude (MD)	183
Pemphigus	Dermatology	Stanley, John R (MD)	186
Penile Inversion Technique	Plastic Surgery	Meltzer, Toby R (MD)	653
Penile Prostheses	Urology	Mulcahy, John J. (MD)	843
Peptic Acid Disorders	Gastroenterology	Bresalier, Robert (MD)	230
Peptic Acid Disorders	Gastroenterology	Feldman, Mark (MD)	236
Peptic Acid Disorders	Gastroenterology	Metz, David C. (MD)	224
Perinatal Medicine	Maternal & Fetal Medicine	Gianopoulos, John (MD)	345
Perinatal Medicine	Maternal & Fetal Medicine	Hussey, Michael J (MD)	345
Perinatal Medicine	Maternal & Fetal Medicine	Ismail, Mahmoud (MD)	345
Perinatal Medicine	Maternal & Fetal Medicine	Pielet, Bruce (MD)	346
Perinatal Medicine	Maternal & Fetal Medicine	Wapner, Ronald (MD)	343
Perinatal Medicine	Neonatal-Perinatal Medicine	Lemons, James A (MD)	353
Perinatal Medicine	Pediatric Critical Care Medicine	Sarnaik, Ashok P (MD)	570
Peripheral Nerve Surgery	Hand Surgery	Gelberman, Richard (MD)	272
Peripheral Nerve Surgery	Hand Surgery	Szabo, Robert (MD)	276
Peripheral Nerve Surgery	Hand Surgery	Urbaniak, James R (MD)	271
Peripheral Nerve Surgery	Plastic Surgery	Mackinnon, Susan (MD)	646
Peripheral Neuropathy	Neurology	Asbury, Arthur K (MD)	399
Peripheral Neuropathy	Neurology	Cornblath, David R. (MD)	401
Peripheral Neuropathy	Neurology	Olney, Richard Koch (MD)	421
Peripheral Vascular Disease	Cardiology (Cardiovascular Disease)	Halperin, Jonathan (MD)	126
Peripheral Vascular Intervention	Cardiology (Cardiovascular Disease)	Burket, Mark W. (MD)	134
Peripheral Vascular Surgery	Vascular Surgery (General)	Benvenisty, Alan I (MD)	859
Peripheral Vascular Surgery	Vascular Surgery (General)	Brener, Bruce (MD)	859
Peripheral Vascular Surgery	Vascular Surgery (General)	Cronenwett, Jack (MD)	857
Peripheral Vascular Surgery	Vascular Surgery (General)	Gewertz, Bruce (MD)	865
Peripheral Vascular Surgery	Vascular Surgery (General)	Stanley, James (MD)	867
Peripheral Vascular Surgery	Vascular Surgery (General)	Towne, Jonathan (MD)	867
Peripheral Vascular Surgery	Vascular Surgery (General)	Williams, G. Melville (MD)	862
Peritoneal Dialysis	Pediatric Nephrology	Warady, Bradley (MD)	598
Personality Disorders	Child & Adolescent Psychiatry	Bleiberg, Efrain (MD)	669
Personality Disorders	Psychiatry	Cloninger, C Robert (MD)	683
Personality Disorders	Psychiatry	Norman, Kim Peter (MD)	687
Personality Disorders-Borderline	Psychiatry	Gabbard, Glen O. (MD)	684
Personality Disorders-Borderline	Psychiatry	McGlashan, Thomas (MD)	676
PET Imaging	Cardiology (Cardiovascular Disease)	Gould, K Lance (MD)	139
PET Imaging	Nuclear Medicine	Coleman, Ralph Edward (MD)	426
PET Imaging	Nuclear Medicine	Larson, Steven (MD)	425
PET Imaging	Nuclear Medicine	Siegel, Barry (MD)	427
PET Imaging	Nuclear Medicine	Wahl, Richard (MD)	427
PET Scans	Neurology	Fox, Peter Thornton (MD)	416
Peyronie's disease	Urology	Lue, Tom F (MD)	849

SPECIAL EXPERTISE INDEX

Special Expertise	Specialty	Doctor's Name	Page
Phen/Fen Heart Valve Pathology	Pathology	Roberts, William (MD)	541
Phobias	Geriatric Psychiatry	Goldman, Samuel (MD)	673
Phosphate Homeostasis	Nephrology	Brazy, Peter C (MD)	364
Photoaging	Dermatology	DeLeo, Vincent A. (MD)	183
Photoaging	Dermatology	Fitzpatrick, Richard (MD)	192
Photoaging	Dermatology	Gilchrest, Barbara ()	181
Photoaging	Dermatology	Gordon, Marsha (MD)	184
Photoaging	Dermatology	Voorhees, John (MD)	190
Photodynamic Therapy	Gastroenterology	Lightdale, Charles (MD)	224
Photodynamic Therapy	Radiation Oncology	Glatstein, Eli (MD)	719
Photomedicine	Dermatology	Dover, Jeffrey (MD)	181
Pigment Disorders	Dermatology	Grimes, Pearl E (MD)	193
Pigmented Lesions	Dermatology	Neuberg, Marcy (MD)	190
Pituitary Disorders	Endocrinology, Diabetes & Metabolism	Biller, Beverly M K (MD)	197
Pituitary Disorders	Endocrinology, Diabetes & Metabolism	Hoffman, Andrew R (MD)	211
Pituitary Disorders	Endocrinology, Diabetes & Metabolism	Jacobs, Thomas (MD)	200
Pituitary Disorders	Endocrinology, Diabetes & Metabolism	Klibanski, Anne (MD)	197
Pituitary Disorders	Endocrinology, Diabetes & Metabolism	Lechan, Ronald (MD/PhD)	198
Pituitary Disorders	Endocrinology, Diabetes & Metabolism	Veldhuis, Johannes D (MD)	205
Pituitary Disorders	Endocrinology, Diabetes & Metabolism	Williams, Gordon H (MD)	198
Pituitary Disorders	Internal Medicine	Vance, Mary Lee (MD)	335
Pituitary Disorders	Pathology	Scheithauer, Bernd (MD)	540
Pituitary Disorders	Pediatric Endocrinology	Levy, Richard Alshuler (MD)	575
Pituitary Surgery	Neurological Surgery	Atkinson, John (MD)	382
Pituitary Surgery	Neurological Surgery	Chandler, William F (MD)	382
Pituitary Surgery	Neurological Surgery	Laws Jr., Edward R (MD)	380
Pituitary Surgery	Neurological Surgery	Mayberg, Marc (MD)	384
Pituitary Surgery	Neurological Surgery	Post, Kalmon (MD)	378
Pituitary Surgery	Neurological Surgery	Rhoton Jr, Albert L (MD)	381
Pituitary Surgery	Neurological Surgery	Selman, Warren R (MD)	385
Pituitary Surgery	Neurological Surgery	Shucart, William A (MD)	374
Pituitary Surgery	Neurological Surgery	Wilson, Charles B (MD)	390
Pituitary Tumors	Endocrinology, Diabetes & Metabolism	Melmed, Shlomo (MD)	212
Pituitary Tumors	Endocrinology, Diabetes & Metabolism	Snyder, Peter Joseph (MD)	202
Pituitary Tumors	Endocrinology, Diabetes & Metabolism	Swerdloff, Ronald Sherwin (MD)	213
Pituitary/Hypothalamic Disease	Endocrinology, Diabetes & Metabolism	Robertson, Gary Lee (MD)	209
Plasma Cell Disorders	Hematology	Barlogie, Bartholomew (MD/PhD)	290
Plastic Surgery	Pediatric Surgery	Stylianos, Steven (MD)	613
Plastic Surgery of Hand	Hand Surgery	Beasley, Robert (MD)	267
Plastic Surgery of Hand	Hand Surgery	Freshwater, M Felix (MD)	270
Plastic Surgery-Pediatric	Plastic Surgery	Boyajian, Michael (MD)	637
Plastic Surgery-Pediatric	Plastic Surgery	Mulliken, John B. (MD)	635
Platelet Disorders	Pediatric Hematology-Oncology	Bussel, James (MD)	583
Pleural Disease	Pulmonary Disease	Antony, Veena B. (MD)	702
Pleural Disease	Pulmonary Disease	Light, Richard Wayne (MD)	699
Pleural Disease	Pulmonary Disease	Sahn, Steven A. (MD)	700
Pneumonia	Infectious Disease	Bartlett, John Gill (MD)	318
Pneumonia	Infectious Disease	Craven, Donald Edward (MD)	317
Pneumonia-Chronic	Pediatric Pulmonology	Murphy, Thomas M (MD)	604
Polio Rehabilitation	Physical Medicine & Rehabilitation	Esquenazi, Alberto (MD)	624
Polycystic Kidney Disease	Nephrology	Bennett, William M (MD)	368
Polycystic Kidney Disease	Nephrology	Rakowski, Thomas A (MD)	361
Polycystic Kidney Disease	Nephrology	Schwab, Steve Joseph (MD)	364
Polycystic Kidney Disease	Nephrology	Torres, Vincente Esbarranch (MD)	366
Polycystic Kidney Disease	Pediatric Nephrology	Avner, Ellis D (MD)	597
Polycystic Kidney Disease	Pediatric Nephrology	Kaplan, Bernard S (MD)	595
Polycystic Ovary Disease	Endocrinology, Diabetes & Metabolism	Ehrmann, David Alan (MD)	207
Polycystic Ovary Disease	Endocrinology, Diabetes & Metabolism	Korytkowski, Mary T (MD)	200
Polycystic Ovary Disease	Reproductive Endocrinology	Diamond, Michael (MD)	748
Polycystic Ovary Disease	Reproductive Endocrinology	Jacobs, Laurence (MD)	749

SPECIAL EXPERTISE INDEX

Special Expertise	Specialty	Doctor's Name	Page
Polycystic Ovary Disease	Reproductive Endocrinology	Ratts, Valerie Sue (MD)	749
Polycythemia Vera	Hematology	Spivak, Jerry L. (MD)	286
Polymyositis & Dermatomyositis	Rheumatology	Medsger Jr, Thomas A (MD)	760
Polyposis Syndromes	Colon & Rectal Surgery	Dozois, Roger R (MD)	173
Porphyria	Clinical Genetics	Desnick, Robert J (MD/PhD)	160
Porphyria	Gastroenterology	Anderson, Karl (MD)	235
Porphyria	Gastroenterology	Bloomer, Joseph (MD)	226
Porphyria	Gastroenterology	Bonkovsky, Herbert (MD)	221
Porphyria	Gastroenterology	Brenner, David Allen (MD)	227
Porphyria	Gastroenterology	Pimstone, Neville R (MD)	238
Porphyria	Hematology	White, Peter (MD)	290
Porphyria	Internal Medicine	Bissell Jr, Dwight Montgomery (MD)	337
Porphyria	Internal Medicine	Pierach, Claus (MD)	336
Portal Hypertension	Vascular Surgery (General)	Johansen, Kaj (MD/PhD)	869
Post Traumatic Stress Disorder	Psychiatry	Menninger, W Walter (MD)	684
Post Traumatic Stress Disorder	Psychiatry	Stein, Murray Brent (MD)	688
Post Traumatic Stress Disorder	Psychiatry	van der Kolk, Bessel (MD)	677
Post Traumatic Stress Disorder	Psychiatry	Wait, Susan Braynard (MD)	682
Prader-Willi Syndrome	Clinical Genetics	Cassidy, Suzanne (MD)	162
Prader-Willi Syndrome	Clinical Genetics	Driscoll, Daniel J (MD)	161
Pregnancy-High Risk	Maternal & Fetal Medicine	Acker, David B. (MD)	341
Pregnancy-High Risk	Maternal & Fetal Medicine	Bartelsmeyer, James (MD)	344
Pregnancy-High Risk	Maternal & Fetal Medicine	Boehm, Frank Henry (MD)	343
Pregnancy-High Risk	Maternal & Fetal Medicine	Chervenak, Francis Anthony (MD)	342
Pregnancy-High Risk	Maternal & Fetal Medicine	D'Alton, Mary Elizabeth (MD)	342
Pregnancy-High Risk	Maternal & Fetal Medicine	Dooley, Sharon L (MD)	345
Pregnancy-High Risk	Maternal & Fetal Medicine	Ferguson II, James E (MD)	344
Pregnancy-High Risk	Maternal & Fetal Medicine	Fox, Harold E (MD/PhD)	342
Pregnancy-High Risk	Maternal & Fetal Medicine	Gabbe, Steven G (MD)	347
Pregnancy-High Risk	Maternal & Fetal Medicine	Greene, Michael F. (MD)	341
Pregnancy-High Risk	Maternal & Fetal Medicine	Hayashi, Robert H. (MD)	345
Pregnancy-High Risk	Maternal & Fetal Medicine	Heffner, Linda (MD/PhD)	341
Pregnancy-High Risk	Maternal & Fetal Medicine	Ismail, Mahmoud (MD)	345
Pregnancy-High Risk	Maternal & Fetal Medicine	Koos, Brian John (MD)	348
Pregnancy-High Risk	Maternal & Fetal Medicine	Lockwood, Charles (MD)	343
Pregnancy-High Risk	Maternal & Fetal Medicine	McLaren, Rodney A (MD)	344
Pregnancy-High Risk	Maternal & Fetal Medicine	Mennuti, Michael (MD)	343
Pregnancy-High Risk	Maternal & Fetal Medicine	O'Sullivan, Mary Jo (MD)	344
Pregnancy-High Risk	Maternal & Fetal Medicine	Philipson, Elliot (MD)	346
Pregnancy-High Risk	Maternal & Fetal Medicine	Tomich, Paul (MD)	346
Pregnancy-High Risk	Maternal & Fetal Medicine	Treadwell, Marjorie Clarke (MD)	346
Pregnancy-High Risk	Maternal & Fetal Medicine	Winn, Hung (MD)	346
Pregnancy-High Risk	Neonatal-Perinatal Medicine	Lawson, Edward Earle (MD)	352
Pregnancy-High Risk	Obstetrics & Gynecology	Baxi, Laxmi V (MD)	431
Pregnancy-High Risk	Obstetrics & Gynecology	Divon, Michael Y (MD)	432
Pregnancy-High Risk	Obstetrics & Gynecology	Duff, W Patrick (MD)	433
Pregnancy-High Risk	Obstetrics & Gynecology	Moawad, Atef H (MD)	436
Pregnancy-High Risk	Obstetrics & Gynecology	Witter, Frank Robert (MD)	433
Premature Labor	Maternal & Fetal Medicine	Hayashi, Robert H. (MD)	345
Premature Labor	Maternal & Fetal Medicine	Thorp Jr, John Mercer (MD)	344
Premature Labor	Obstetrics & Gynecology	Moawad, Atef H (MD)	436
Premature Labor	Obstetrics & Gynecology	Socol, Michael (MD)	437
Prematurity Prevention	Maternal & Fetal Medicine	Benedetti, Thomas J (MD)	347
Prematurity Prevention	Maternal & Fetal Medicine	Hobel, Calvin John (MD)	348
Prematurity/Low Birth Weight Infants	Neonatal-Perinatal Medicine	Perlman, Jeffrey (MD)	354
Premenstrual Dysphoric Disorder	Psychiatry	Yonkers, Kimberly A (MD)	677
Prenatal Diagnosis	Clinical Genetics	Gray, Diana Lee (MD)	162
Prenatal Diagnosis	Clinical Genetics	Weaver, David Dawson (MD)	162
Prenatal Diagnosis	Maternal & Fetal Medicine	Goldberg, James David (MD)	348
Prenatal Diagnosis	Maternal & Fetal Medicine	McLaren, Rodney A (MD)	344

Special Expertise	Specialty	Doctor's Name	Page
Prenatal Diagnosis	Obstetrics & Gynecology	Elias, Sherman (MD)	435
Prenatal Diagnosis	Obstetrics & Gynecology	Johnson, Timothy R.B. (MD)	436
Prenatal Diagnosis	Obstetrics & Gynecology	Simpson, Joe Leigh (MD)	438
Prenatal Genetic Diagnosis	Clinical Genetics	Anyane-Yeboa, Kwame (MD)	159
Prenatal Ultrasound	Maternal & Fetal Medicine	Wilkins, Isabelle (MD)	347
Preventive Cardiology	Cardiology (Cardiovascular Disease)	Balady, Gary (MD)	120
Preventive Cardiology	Cardiology (Cardiovascular Disease)	Gould, K Lance (MD)	139
Preventive Cardiology	Pediatric Cardiology	Bricker, John Timothy (MD)	566
Preventive Cardiology	Pediatric Cardiology	Hohn, Arno R (MD)	567
Preventive Medicine	Geriatric Medicine	Barnhart, William (MD)	247
Prolactin Disorders	Endocrinology, Diabetes & Metabolism	Klibanski, Anne (MD)	197
Prolactin Disorders	Reproductive Endocrinology	Zacur, Howard A. (MD/PhD)	745
Prostate & Breast Cancer	Radiation Oncology	Nori, Dattatreyudu (MD)	720
Prostate & Gynecologic Cancers	Radiation Oncology	Ennis, Ronald (MD)	718
Prostate Cancer	Medical Oncology	Donehower, Ross Carl (MD)	295
Prostate Cancer	Medical Oncology	Garnick, Marc Bennett (MD)	292
Prostate Cancer	Medical Oncology	Hudes, Gary Robert (MD)	297
Prostate Cancer	Medical Oncology	Myers, Charles E (MD)	302
Prostate Cancer	Medical Oncology	Oster, Martin (MD)	299
Prostate Cancer	Medical Oncology	Richards, Jon (MD/PhD)	308
Prostate Cancer	Medical Oncology	Roth, Bruce Joseph (MD)	303
Prostate Cancer	Medical Oncology	Scher, Howard (MD)	299
Prostate Cancer	Medical Oncology	Torti, Frank M (MD)	304
Prostate Cancer	Medical Oncology	Vogelzang, Nicholas (MD)	309
Prostate Cancer	Nuclear Medicine	Podoloff, Donald (MD)	427
Prostate Cancer	Radiation Oncology	Anscher, Mitchell (MD)	721
Prostate Cancer	Radiation Oncology	Blasko, John Charles (MD)	726
Prostate Cancer	Radiation Oncology	D'Amico, Anthony V (MD/PhD)	717
Prostate Cancer	Radiation Oncology	Forman, Jeffrey D (MD)	723
Prostate Cancer	Radiation Oncology	Hilaris, Basil (MD)	719
Prostate Cancer	Radiation Oncology	Leibel, Steven A (MD)	719
Prostate Cancer	Radiation Oncology	Lichter, Allen (MD)	723
Prostate Cancer	Radiation Oncology	Pollack, Jed (MD)	720
Prostate Cancer	Radiation Oncology	Rose, Christopher Marshall (MD)	727
Prostate Cancer	Radiation Oncology	Rosenman, Julian (MD)	722
Prostate Cancer	Radiation Oncology	Schiff, Peter B (MD/PhD)	720
Prostate Cancer	Radiation Oncology	Shipley, William (MD)	717
Prostate Cancer	Radiation Oncology	Vicini, Frank A (MD)	724
Prostate Cancer	Radiology	Petrovich, Zbigniew (MD)	740
Prostate Cancer	Urology	Bander, Neil (MD)	830
Prostate Cancer	Urology	Bardot, Stephen F (MD)	845
Prostate Cancer	Urology	Basler, Joseph W (MD)	845
Prostate Cancer	Urology	Benson, Mitchell C (MD)	831
Prostate Cancer	Urology	Brendler, Charles B (MD)	841
Prostate Cancer	Urology	Burnett II, Arthur L (MD)	831
Prostate Cancer	Urology	Catalona, William J (MD)	841
Prostate Cancer	Urology	Chodak, Gerald (MD)	841
Prostate Cancer	Urology	Danoff, Dudley S (MD)	848
Prostate CAncer	Urology	Flanigan, Robert (MD)	842
Prostate Cancer	Urology	Huben, Robert P (MD)	832
Prostate Cancer	Urology	Jacobs, Stephen C (MD)	832
Prostate Cancer	Urology	Jarow, Jonathan (MD)	833
Prostate Cancer	Urology	Kirschenbaum, Alexander M (MD)	833
Prostate Cancer	Urology	Klein, Eric A (MD)	842
Prostate Cancer	Urology	Kozlowski, James Michael (MD)	842
Prostate Cancer	Urology	Lepor, Herbert (MD)	833
Prostate Cancer	Urology	Lieskovsky, Gary (MD)	849
Prostate Cancer	Urology	Marshall, Fray F (MD)	838
Prostate Cancer	Urology	Mc Vary, Kevin (MD)	842
Prostate Cancer	Urology	McConnell, John Dowling (MD)	846

SPECIAL EXPERTISE INDEX

Special Expertise	Specialty	Doctor's Name	Page
Prostate Cancer	Urology	McGovern, Francis (MD)	829
Prostate Cancer	Urology	Menon, Mani (MD)	842
Prostate Cancer	Urology	Miles, Brian J (MD)	846
Prostate Cancer	Urology	Montie, James (MD)	843
Prostate Cancer	Urology	Mostwin, Jacek Lech (MD/PhD)	834
Prostate Cancer	Urology	Naslund, Michael (MD)	834
Prostate Cancer	Urology	Nelson, Joel Byron (MD)	834
Prostate Cancer	Urology	Resnick, Martin (MD)	843
Prostate Cancer	Urology	Richie, Jerome (MD)	830
Prostate Cancer	Urology	Sanders, William Holt (MD)	839
Prostate Cancer	Urology	Scardino, Peter (MD)	835
Prostate Cancer	Urology	Schlegel, Peter (MD)	835
Prostate Cancer	Urology	Schmidt, Joseph (MD)	850
Prostate Cancer	Urology	Smith, Joseph (MD)	839
Prostate Cancer	Urology	Thompson Jr, Ian M (MD)	847
Prostate Cancer	Urology	Von Eschenbach, Andrew C (MD)	847
Prostate Cancer	Urology	Walsh, Patrick (MD)	836
Prostate Cancer	Urology	Wein, Alan J (MD)	836
Prostate Cancer	Urology	Williams, Richard D (MD)	844
Prostate Disease	Urology	Alexander, Richard B (MD)	830
Prostate Disease	Urology	Bruskewitz, Reginald C (MD)	841
Prostate Disease	Urology	Fuselier Jr, Harold A (MD)	846
Prostate Disease	Urology	Gribetz, Michael (MD)	832
Prostate Disease	Urology	Lowe, Franklin (MD)	833
Prostate Disease	Urology	Macchia, Richard (MD)	833
Prostate Disease	Urology	Naslund, Michael (MD)	834
Prostate Disease-Alternative Medicine	Urology	Lowe, Franklin (MD)	833
Prostate Surgery	Urology	Thompson Jr, Ian M (MD)	847
Prosthetic Nose	Plastic Surgery	Tabbal, Nicolas (MD)	640
Pseudotumor Cerebri	Ophthalmology	Burde, Ronald (MD)	444
Psoriasis	Dermatology	Fenske, Neil (MD)	187
Psoriasis	Dermatology	Freedberg, Irwin M (MD)	183
Psoriasis	Dermatology	Krueger, Gerald (MD)	191
Psoriasis	Dermatology	Lebwohl, Mark (MD)	184
Psoriasis	Dermatology	Lowe, Nicholas J (MD)	194
Psoriasis	Dermatology	Menter, M Alan (MD)	192
Psoriasis	Dermatology	Nigra, Thomas P (MD)	185
Psoriasis	Dermatology	Voorhees, John (MD)	190
Psoriasis/Lupus	Dermatology	Braverman, Irwin (MD)	181
Psoriatic Arthritis	Rheumatology	Mitnick, Hal J (MD)	760
Psychiatric Neuro-Imaging	Psychiatry	Pearlson, Godfrey D (MD)	680
Psychiatric Rehabilitation	Psychiatry	Liberman, Robert Paul (MD)	687
Psychiatry of Cancer	Psychiatry	Holland, Jimmie C B (MD)	679
Psychiatry of Cancer	Psychiatry	Lederberg, Marguerite (MD)	680
Psychiatry of Cancer	Psychiatry	Spiegel, David (MD)	688
Psychiatry-Adolescent/College Age	Child & Adolescent Psychiatry	Wiener, Jerry M (MD)	667
Psychiatry-Geriatric	Geriatric Psychiatry	Luchins, Daniel (MD)	674
Psychiatry-Geriatric	Psychiatry	Alexopoulos, George (MD)	677
Psychiatry-Geriatric	Psychiatry	Blazer II, Dan G (MD/PhD)	682
Psychiatry-Geriatric	Psychiatry	Jenike, Michael Andrew (MD)	676
Psychiatry-Geriatric	Psychiatry	Nelson, J Craig (MD)	677
Psychiatry-Geriatric	Psychiatry	Weiner, Myron (MD)	686
Psychoanalysis	Psychiatry	Munich, Richard (MD)	685
Psychoanalysis	Psychiatry	Pomer, Sydney Lawrence (MD)	687
Psychoanalysis	Psychiatry	Zerbe, Kathryn J (MD)	685
Psychopharmacology	Addiction Psychiatry	Schuckit, Marc A (MD)	662
Psychopharmacology	Child & Adolescent Psychiatry	Riddle, Mark A (MD)	666
Psychopharmacology	Geriatric Psychiatry	Friedman, Barry (MD)	674
Psychopharmacology	Geriatric Psychiatry	Schneider, Lon S (MD)	675
Psychopharmacology	Psychiatry	Cohen, Bruce M (MD)	676

Special Expertise	Specialty	Doctor's Name	Page
Psychopharmacology	Psychiatry	Greist, John (MD)	683
Psychopharmacology	Psychiatry	Janicak, Philip G. (MD)	683
Psychopharmacology	Psychiatry	Klein, Donald (MD)	679
Psychopharmacology	Psychiatry	Marder, Stephen Robert (MD)	687
Psychopharmacology	Psychiatry	Mohl, Paul C. (MD)	685
Psychopharmacology	Psychiatry	Nelson, J Craig (MD)	677
Psychopharmacology	Psychiatry	Pope Jr, Harrison G (MD)	677
Psychopharmacology	Psychiatry	Schatzberg, Alan F (MD)	688
Psychopharmacology	Psychiatry	Sussman, Norman (MD)	681
Psychopharmacology	Psychiatry	Zorumski, Charles F (MD)	684
Psychopharmocology	Child & Adolescent Psychiatry	Egan, James Harold (MD)	665
Psychopharmocology	Psychiatry	Thase, Michael E (MD)	681
Psychotherapy	Child & Adolescent Psychiatry	Egan, James Harold (MD)	665
Psychotherapy	Psychiatry	Altshuler, Kenneth Z. (MD)	685
Psychotherapy	Psychiatry	Mohl, Paul C. (MD)	685
Psychotherapy	Psychiatry	Sadock, Virginia (MD)	681
Psychotic Disorders	Geriatric Psychiatry	Jeste, Dilip (MD)	674
Psychotic Disorders	Psychiatry	Baldessarini, Ross (MD)	676
Psychotic Disorders	Psychiatry	Boronow, John Joseph (MD)	677
Psychotic Disorders	Psychiatry	Liberman, Robert Paul (MD)	687
Psychotic Disorders	Psychiatry	Munich, Richard (MD)	685
Pubertal Disorders	Pediatric Endocrinology	Foster, Carol M (MD)	575
Pubertal Disorders	Pediatric Endocrinology	Geffner, Mitchell Eugene (MD)	577
Pubertal Disorders	Pediatric Endocrinology	Kappy, Michael Steven (MD/PhD)	576
Pubertal Disorders	Pediatric Endocrinology	Rosenfield, Robert (MD)	576
Pulmonary & Critical Care	Pulmonary Disease	Rizk, Norman Wade (MD)	712
Pulmonary Alveolar Proteinosis	Pulmonary Disease	Rogers, Robert M (MD)	694
Pulmonary Disease	Internal Medicine	Shore, Bernard L (MD)	336
Pulmonary Disease	Pulmonary Disease	Fletcher, Eugene (MD)	698
Pulmonary Disease	Pulmonary Disease	Martinez, Fernando J (MD)	704
Pulmonary Embolism	Vascular Surgery (General)	Greenfield, Lazar (MD)	865
Pulmonary Fibrosis	Pulmonary Disease	Glassroth, Jeffrey (MD)	703
Pulmonary Fibrosis	Pulmonary Disease	Loyd, James Emory (MD)	700
Pulmonary Fibrosis	Pulmonary Disease	Lynch, Joseph P (MD)	704
Pulmonary Fibrosis	Pulmonary Disease	Raghu, Ganesh (MD)	712
Pulmonary Fibrosis	Pulmonary Disease	Schwartz, David A (MD)	700
Pulmonary Fibrosis	Pulmonary Disease	Theodore, James (MD)	713
Pulmonary Function Testing	Pulmonary Disease	MacIntyre, Neil Ross (MD)	700
Pulmonary Hypertension	Cardiology (Cardiovascular Disease)	Rich, Stuart (MD)	137
Pulmonary Hypertension	Neonatal-Perinatal Medicine	Steinhorn, Robin (MD)	353
Pulmonary Hypertension	Pulmonary Disease	Arroliga, Alejandro C (MD)	702
Pulmonary Hypertension	Pulmonary Disease	Christman, Brian Wallace (MD)	697
Pulmonary Hypertension	Pulmonary Disease	Elliott, Charles Gregory (MD)	706
Pulmonary Hypertension	Pulmonary Disease	Rubin, Lewis (MD)	712
Pulmonary Hypertension	Pulmonary Disease	Shure, Deborah (MD)	700
Pulmonary Hypertension	Pulmonary Disease	Voelkel, Norbert F (MD)	708
Pulmonary Imaging	Nuclear Medicine	Alavi, Abass (MD)	425
Pulmonary Infections	Pulmonary Disease	Metersky, Mark Lewis (MD)	692
Pulmonary Infections	Pulmonary Disease	Schluger, Neil (MD)	695
Pulmonary Infections	Pulmonary Disease	Shellito, Judd Ernest (MD)	709
Pulmonary Pathology	Pathology	Colby, Thomas V (MD)	541
Pulmonary Pathology	Pathology	Katzenstein, Anna-Luise A. (MD)	537
Pulmonary Rehabilitation	Physical Medicine & Rehabilitation	Bach, John (MD)	623
Pulmonary Rehabilitation	Pulmonary Disease	MacIntyre, Neil Ross (MD)	700
Pulmonary Vascular Disease	Pulmonary Disease	Rubin, Lewis (MD)	712
Pulmonary Vascular Disease	Pulmonary Disease	Schwarz, Marvin Ira (MD)	708
Pulmonary Vascular Disease	Pulmonary Disease	Tapson, Victor (MD/PhD)	701

SPECIAL EXPERTISE INDEX

Special Expertise	Specialty	Doctor's Name	Page
R			
Radial Artery Catherization	Cardiology (Cardiovascular Disease)	Cooper, Christopher (MD)	134
Radiation Oncology-Pediatric	Radiation Oncology	Ferree, Carolyn Ruth Black (MD)	721
Radiation Oncology-Pediatric	Radiation Oncology	Mandell, Lynda (MD/PhD)	720
Radiation Therapy-Cancer	Radiation Oncology	Blasko, John Charles (MD)	726
Radiation Therapy-Cancer	Radiation Oncology	Fountain, Karen (MD)	718
Radiation Therapy-Cancer	Radiation Oncology	Halberg, Francine Erna (MD)	726
Radiation Therapy-Cancer	Radiation Oncology	Marks, Lawrence (MD)	721
Radiation Therapy-Cancer	Radiation Oncology	Phillips, Theodore Locke (MD)	727
Radioimmunotherapy of Cancer	Nuclear Medicine	Wahl, Richard (MD)	427
Radiology-Diagnostic	Radiology	Dershaw, D David (MD)	735
Radiology-Diagnostic	Radiology	Goodman, Lawrence R (MD)	737
Radiology-Pediatric	Radiology	Berdon, Walter (MD)	735
Radiology-Pediatric	Radiology	Leonidas, John (MD)	736
Radiology-Pediatric	Radiology	McAlister, Bill (MD)	738
Radiology-Pediatric	Radiology	Norton, Karen (MD)	736
Radiology-Pediatric	Radiology	Seibert, Joanna J (MD)	739
Radiology-Pediatric	Radiology	Sivit, Carlos (MD)	738
Radiology-Pediatric	Radiology	Wood, Beverly (MD)	740
Radium Therapy	Radiation Oncology	Quivey, Jeanne Marie (MD)	727
Raynaud's Disease	Rheumatology	Medsger Jr, Thomas A (MD)	760
Raynaud's Disease	Rheumatology	Wigley, Frederick M (MD)	761
Raynaud's Disease	Vascular Surgery (General)	Porter, John M. (MD)	869
Reconstructive Microsurgery	Plastic Surgery	Hidalgo, David (MD)	637
Reconstructive Microvascular Surgery	Hand Surgery	Hanel, Douglas (MD)	275
Reconstructive Microvascular Surgery	Plastic Surgery	Levin, L Scott (MD)	643
Reconstructive Microvascular Surgery	Plastic Surgery	Markowitz, Bernard Lloyd (MD)	653
Reconstructive Microvascular Surgery	Plastic Surgery	Molnar, Joseph (MD)	644
Reconstructive Plastic Surgery	Plastic Surgery	Argenta, Louis Charles (MD)	641
Reconstructive Plastic Surgery Face	Plastic Surgery	Baker, Daniel (MD)	636
Reconstructive Renal Surgery	Urology	Assimos, Dean George (MD)	836
Reconstructive Surgery	Otolaryngology	Denenberg, Steven M (MD)	518
Reconstructive Surgery	Plastic Surgery	Ariyan, Stephan (MD)	635
Reconstructive Surgery	Plastic Surgery	Burget, Gary C (MD)	645
Reconstructive Surgery	Plastic Surgery	Feldman, Joel (MD)	635
Reconstructive Surgery	Plastic Surgery	Gold, Alan (MD)	637
Reconstructive Surgery	Plastic Surgery	Hagan, Kevin Francis (MD)	643
Reconstructive Surgery	Plastic Surgery	Hoefflin, Steven M (MD)	652
Reconstructive Surgery	Plastic Surgery	Hurwitz, Dennis (MD)	638
Reconstructive Surgery	Plastic Surgery	Lesavoy, Malcolm A (MD)	653
Reconstructive Surgery	Plastic Surgery	Luce, Edward (MD)	646
Reconstructive Surgery	Plastic Surgery	Sanger, James (MD)	647
Reconstructive Surgery	Plastic Surgery	Singer, Robert (MD)	655
Reconstructive Surgery	Plastic Surgery	Stevenson, Thomas Ray (MD)	655
Reconstructive Surgery-Hip/Knee	Orthopaedic Surgery	Poss, Robert (MD)	477
Reconstructive Urology	Urology	Webster, George David (MD)	840
Rectal Cancer	Colon & Rectal Surgery	Fry, Robert Dean (MD)	170
Rectal Cancer	Colon & Rectal Surgery	MacKeigan, John (MD)	174
Rectal Cancer	Colon & Rectal Surgery	Medich, David (MD)	171
Rectal Cancer	Colon & Rectal Surgery	Wexner, Steven (MD)	173
Rectal Cancer	Colon & Rectal Surgery	Wong, Westley Douglas (MD)	171
Rectal Cancer	Medical Oncology	Ahlgren, James David (MD)	294
Rectal Cancer	Medical Oncology	Benson, Al B (MD)	305
Rectal Cancer	Medical Oncology	Kemeny, Nancy (MD)	297
Rectal Cancer	Surgery	Steele, Glenn D (MD/PhD)	796
Rectal Cancer-Sphincter Preservation	Colon & Rectal Surgery	Saclarides, Theodore John (MD)	175
Rectal Cancer/Sphincter Preservation	Colon & Rectal Surgery	Abcarian, Herand (MD)	173
Rectal Surgery	Colon & Rectal Surgery	Pemberton, John (MD)	174
Rectovaginal Fistula	Colon & Rectal Surgery	Lowry, Ann (MD)	174

Special Expertise	Specialty	Doctor's Name	Page
Reflex Sympathetic Dystrophy(RSD)	Pain Management	Harden, Norman (MD)	529
Reflex Sympathetic Dystrophy(RSD)	Pain Management	Rosner, Howard L (MD)	528
Reflex Sympathetic Dystrophy(RSD)	Pain Management	Rowbotham, Michael Charles (MD)	532
Reflex Sympathetic Dystrophy(RSD)	Pediatric Rheumatology	Sherry, David (MD)	610
Refractive Surgery	Ophthalmology	Binder, Perry Scott (MD)	463
Refractive Surgery	Ophthalmology	Holland, Edward J. (MD)	457
Refractive Surgery	Ophthalmology	Koch, Douglas D (MD)	462
Refractive Surgery	Ophthalmology	Krueger, Ronald (MD)	457
Refractive Surgery	Ophthalmology	Lindstrom, Richard Lyndon (MD)	458
Refractive Surgery	Ophthalmology	Maloney, Robert Keller (MD)	466
Refractive Surgery	Ophthalmology	Manche, Edward Emanuel (MD)	466
Refractive Surgery	Ophthalmology	McDonald, Marguerite B. (MD)	462
Refractive Surgery	Ophthalmology	Rosenberg, Michael A (MD)	459
Refractive Surgery	Ophthalmology	Stark, Walter J (MD)	450
Refractive Surgery	Ophthalmology	Teplick, Stanley (MD)	468
Refractive Surgery	Ophthalmology	Turner, Stephen Gordon (MD)	468
Refractive Surgery-Laser	Ophthalmology	McCulley, James P (MD)	462
Refractive Surgery-Laser	Ophthalmology	Nesburn, Anthony B (MD)	467
Refractive Surgery-Laser	Ophthalmology	Stulting, R. Doyle (MD)	455
Refractive Surgery-LASIK	Ophthalmology	Culbertson, William (MD)	452
Refractive Surgery-LASIK	Ophthalmology	Durrie, Daniel (MD)	461
Refractive Surgery-LASIK	Ophthalmology	Feder, Robert S (MD)	457
Refractive Surgery-LASIK	Ophthalmology	Hersh, Peter (MD)	447
Refractive Surgery-LASIK	Ophthalmology	Holladay, Jack T. (MD)	461
Refractive Surgery-LASIK	Ophthalmology	Mackool, Richard (MD)	448
Refractive Surgery-LASIK	Ophthalmology	Maloney, Robert Keller (MD)	466
Refractive Surgery-LASIK	Ophthalmology	Pepose, Jay (MD)	459
Refractive Surgery-LASIK	Ophthalmology	Serafano, Donald Natale (MD)	467
Refractive Surgery-LASIK	Ophthalmology	Waring III, George Oral (MD)	455
Refractive, Cataract Surgery	Ophthalmology	Steinert, Roger F (MD)	444
Rehabilitation-Pediatric	Physical Medicine & Rehabilitation	Nelson, Maureen R (MD)	630
Reheumatic Diseases of Childhood	Pediatric Rheumatology	Bernstein, Bram Henry (MD)	610
Reiter's Syndrome	Rheumatology	Arnett Jr, Frank Couchman (MD)	767
Relapsing Polychondritis	Rheumatology	Luthra, Harvinder Singh (MD)	765
Relationship Problems	Psychiatry	Levine, Stephen B (MD)	684
Renal Nuclear Medicine	Nuclear Medicine	Dubovsky, Eva V (MD/PhD)	426
Renal Research	Nephrology	Hoffman, David (MD)	363
Renovascular Disease	Vascular Surgery (General)	Cambria, Richard P (MD)	857
Renovascular Disease	Vascular Surgery (General)	Hansen, Kimberley J (MD)	863
Renovascular Disease	Vascular Surgery (General)	Stanley, James (MD)	867
Reperfusion Injury	Vascular Surgery (General)	Zelenock, Gerald (MD)	867
Repetitive Motion Injuries	Hand Surgery	Derman, Gordon Harris (MD)	272
Reproductive Endocrinology	Endocrinology, Diabetes & Metabolism	Marshall, John Crook (MD/PhD)	204
Reproductive Endocrinology	Endocrinology, Diabetes & Metabolism	Veldhuis, Johannes D (MD)	205
Reproductive Endocrinology	Obstetrics & Gynecology	DeCherney, Alan Hersh (MD)	438
Reproductive Endocrinology	Obstetrics & Gynecology	Naftolin, Frederick (MD)	431
Reproductive Endocrinology	Obstetrics & Gynecology	Nahmias, Jaime Pablo (MD)	434
Reproductive Endocrinology	Obstetrics & Gynecology	Novy, Miles (MD)	438
Reproductive Endocrinology-Male	Endocrinology, Diabetes & Metabolism	Snyder, Peter Joseph (MD)	202
Reproductive Genetics	Obstetrics & Gynecology	Evans, Mark Ira (MD)	435
Reproductive Immunology	Obstetrics & Gynecology	Beer, Alan Earl (MD)	435
Reproductive Infectious Disease	Maternal & Fetal Medicine	Landers, Daniel V. (MD)	342
Reproductive Medicine	Reproductive Endocrinology	Soules, Michael Roy (MD)	752
Reproductive Surgery	Reproductive Endocrinology	Milad, Magdy P (MD)	749
Reproductive Surgery	Reproductive Endocrinology	Odem, Randall R (MD)	749
Reproductive Toxicology	Obstetrics & Gynecology	Scialli, Anthony R (MD)	433
Respiratory Distress Syndrome(ARDS)	Pulmonary Disease	Petty, Thomas L (MD)	707
Respiratory Failure	Pediatric Critical Care Medicine	Nichols, David Gregory (MD)	570
Respiratory Failure	Pediatric Critical Care Medicine	Perez Fontan, J Julio (MD)	570
Respiratory Failure	Pediatric Critical Care Medicine	Thompson, Ann Ellen (MD)	570

SPECIAL EXPERTISE INDEX

SPECIAL EXPERTISE INDEX

Special Expertise	Specialty	Doctor's Name	Page
Rheumatoid Arthritis-Reconstruction	Orthopaedic Surgery	Deland, Jonathan T (MD)	480
Rheumatologic & Immunologic Derm	Dermatology	Jorizzo, Joseph L. (MD)	188
Rheumatological Surgery	Orthopaedic Surgery	Patzakis, Michael J (MD)	498
Rheumatology	Allergy & Immunology	de Shazo, Richard Denson (MD)	98
Rheumatology	Rheumatology	Luggen, Michael (MD)	765
Rhinitis	Allergy & Immunology	Neustrom, Mark Ray (DO)	102
Rhinitis	Allergy & Immunology	Slankard, Marjorie (MD)	97
Rhinitis	Allergy & Immunology	Togias, Alkis George (MD)	97
Rhinitis	Allergy & Immunology	Wald, Jeffrey A (MD)	102
Rhinitis	Allergy & Immunology	Wong, Johnson T (MD)	95
Rhinitis	Otolaryngology	Lanza, Donald (MD)	515
Rhinitis	Pediatric Allergy & Immunology	Skoner, David Peter (MD)	555
Rhinoplasty	Otolaryngology	Kamer, Frank M (MD)	522
Rhinoplasty	Otolaryngology	Quatela, Vito Charles (MD)	506
Rhinoplasty	Otolaryngology	Szachowicz II, Edward H (MD)	516
Rhinoplasty	Otolaryngology	Toriumi, Dean (MD)	517
Rhinoplasty	Plastic Surgery	Aston, Sherrell (MD)	636
Rhinoplasty	Plastic Surgery	Gunter, Jack (MD)	649
Rhinoplasty	Plastic Surgery	Hamra, Sameer T (MD)	649
Rhinoplasty	Plastic Surgery	Matarasso, Alan (MD)	639
Rhinoplasty	Plastic Surgery	Sheen, Jack (MD)	655
Rhinoplasty	Plastic Surgery	Tabbal, Nicolas (MD)	640
Rhinoplasty	Plastic Surgery	Tebbetts, John B (MD)	650
Rhinoplasty-Secondary Surgery	Plastic Surgery	Gunter, Jack (MD)	649
Rhinosinusitis	Otolaryngology	Stankiewicz, James (MD)	516
Robotics in Surgery	Thoracic Surgery	Shennib, Hani (MD)	811
Rocky Mountain Spotted Fever	Infectious Disease	Sexton, Daniel John (MD)	325
Rosacea	Dermatology	Paller, Amy Susan (MD)	190
Rosacea	Dermatology	Shalita, Alan (MD)	186
Ross Procedure	Pediatric Surgery	Spray, Thomas L (MD)	612
Rrheumatic Diseases of Childhood	Pediatric Rheumatology	Schanberg, Laura Eve (MD)	609
Running Injuries	Sports Medicine	Maharam, Lewis (MD)	773

S

Salivary Gland Surgery	Otolaryngology	Clayman, Gary Lee (MD)	518
Salivary Gland Tumors	Otolaryngology	Eisele, David (MD)	503
Salpingitis	Obstetrics & Gynecology	Hager, William David (MD)	434
Sarcoidosis	Pulmonary Disease	Donohue, James (MD)	697
Sarcoidosis	Pulmonary Disease	Hunninghake, Gary (MD)	703
Sarcoidosis	Pulmonary Disease	Raghu, Ganesh (MD)	712
Sarcoidosis	Pulmonary Disease	Rose, Cecile (MD)	708
Sarcoidosis	Pulmonary Disease	Sharma, Om Prakash (MD)	712
Sarcoidosis	Pulmonary Disease	Shure, Deborah (MD)	700
Sarcoidosis	Pulmonary Disease	Teirstein, Alvin (MD)	696
Sarcoma	Medical Oncology	Antman, Karen (MD)	294
Sarcoma	Orthopaedic Surgery	Scarborough, Mark (MD)	487
Sarcoma	Orthopaedic Surgery	Simon, Michael (MD)	492
Sarcoma	Radiation Oncology	Goffinet, Don R (MD)	726
Sarcoma	Radiation Oncology	Herman, Terence Spencer (MD)	725
Sarcoma	Radiation Oncology	Kinsella, Timothy James (MD)	723
Sarcoma	Radiation Oncology	Suit, Herman (MD)	718
Sarcoma	Radiation Oncology	Tepper, Joel (MD)	723
Sarcoma	Surgery	Brennan, Murray (MD)	784
Sarcoma	Surgery	Eilber, Frederick Richard (MD)	800
Sarcoma-Bone	Medical Oncology	Benjamin, Robert S (MD)	311
Sarcoma-Soft Tissue	Medical Oncology	Benjamin, Robert S (MD)	311
Sarcoma-Soft Tissue	Thoracic Surgery	Putnam Jr, Joe B (MD)	822
Sarcoma-Soft Tissue & Bone	Medical Oncology	Baker, Laurence H (DO)	305
Schizophrenia	Child & Adolescent Psychiatry	Rapoport, Judith (MD)	666

SPECIAL EXPERTISE INDEX

Special Expertise	Specialty	Doctor's Name	Page
Schizophrenia	Child & Adolescent Psychiatry	Russell, Andrew Thomas (MD)	670
Schizophrenia	Psychiatry	Baldessarini, Ross (MD)	676
Schizophrenia	Psychiatry	Boronow, John Joseph (MD)	677
Schizophrenia	Psychiatry	Bowers Jr, Malcolm B (MD)	676
Schizophrenia	Psychiatry	Cancro, Robert (MD)	678
Schizophrenia	Psychiatry	Carpenter Jr, William T (MD)	678
Schizophrenia	Psychiatry	Davidson, Joyce Eileen (MD)	684
Schizophrenia	Psychiatry	Davis, Kenneth (MD)	678
Schizophrenia	Psychiatry	Ganguli, Rohan (MD)	678
Schizophrenia	Psychiatry	Gorman, Jack Matthew (MD)	679
Schizophrenia	Psychiatry	Kendler, Kenneth S (MD)	682
Schizophrenia	Psychiatry	Liberman, Robert Paul (MD)	687
Schizophrenia	Psychiatry	Marder, Stephen Robert (MD)	687
Schizophrenia	Psychiatry	McGlashan, Thomas (MD)	676
Schizophrenia	Psychiatry	Norman, Kim Peter (MD)	687
Schizophrenia	Psychiatry	Pearlson, Godfrey D (MD)	680
Schizophrenia	Psychiatry	Simpson, George M (MD)	688
Scleroderma	Rheumatology	Clements, Philip Jordan (MD)	768
Scleroderma	Rheumatology	Ellman, Michael H (MD)	764
Scleroderma	Rheumatology	Klearman, Micki (MD)	765
Scleroderma	Rheumatology	Mayes, Maureen Davidica (MD/PhD)	765
Scleroderma	Rheumatology	Medsger Jr, Thomas A (MD)	760
Scleroderma	Rheumatology	Nelson, Audrey May (MD)	766
Scleroderma	Rheumatology	White, Barbara (MD)	761
Scleroderma	Rheumatology	Wigley, Frederick M (MD)	761
Sclerosing Cholangitis	Gastroenterology	Lindor, Keith Douglas (MD)	233
Scoliosis	Orthopaedic Surgery	Balderston, Richard (MD)	477
Scoliosis	Orthopaedic Surgery	Boachie, Oheneba (MD)	479
Scoliosis	Orthopaedic Surgery	Bridwell, Keith (MD)	489
Scoliosis	Orthopaedic Surgery	Roye, David (MD)	483
Scoliosis	Orthopaedic Surgery	Sponseller, Paul D (MD)	484
Scoliosis	Orthopaedic Surgery	Weinstein, Stuart L (MD)	493
Scoliosis & Kyphosis	Orthopaedic Surgery	Green, Neil Edward (MD)	486
Scoliosis/Spine Deformities	Orthopaedic Surgery	Bradford, David S (MD)	496
Seizure Disorders	Child Neurology	Aron, Alan (MD)	151
Seizure Disorders	Neurology	Cloughesy, Timothy Francis (MD)	419
Seizure Disorders	Neurology	Kase, Carlos S. (MD)	398
Seizure Disorders	Neurology	Rubin, Susan (MD)	415
Seizure Disorders-Pregnancy	Maternal & Fetal Medicine	Greene, Michael F. (MD)	341
Seizure Surgery	Neurological Surgery	Black, Peter (MD)	373
Sentinel Node Assessment	Medical Oncology	Kirkwood, John Munn (MD)	297
Sentinel Node Pathology	Pathology	Cote, Richard (MD)	542
Sentinel Node Pathology	Pathology	Turner, Roderick Randolph (MD)	543
Sentinel Node Surgery	Surgery	Balch, Charles (MD)	789
Sentinel Node Surgery	Surgery	Essner, Richard (MD)	800
Sentinel Node Surgery	Surgery	Giuliano, Armando E (MD)	800
Sentinel Node Surgery	Surgery	Hansen, Nora Marie (MD)	800
Sentinel Node Surgery	Surgery	Ross, Merrick I (MD)	798
Sentinel Node Surgery	Surgery	Saha, Sukamal (MD)	795
Sentinel Node Surgery	Thoracic Surgery	Morton, Donald Lee (MD)	825
Sepsis & Septic Shock	Pediatric Critical Care Medicine	Zimmerman, Jerry John (MD)	571
Septic Shock	Infectious Disease	Garvey, Glenda Josephine (MD)	319
Sexual Development	Pediatric Endocrinology	Levine, Lenore (MD)	572
Sexual Dysfunction	Psychiatry	Levine, Stephen B (MD)	684
Sexual Dysfunction	Psychiatry	Sadock, Benjamin (MD)	681
Sexual Dysfunction	Psychiatry	Sadock, Virginia (MD)	681
Sexually Transmitted Diseases	Infectious Disease	Holmes, King K (MD)	328
Sexually Transmitted Diseases	Infectious Disease	Sobel, Jack (MD)	326
Sexually Transmitted Diseases	Infectious Disease	Sparling, Philip Frederick (MD)	325
Sexually Transmitted Diseases	Obstetrics & Gynecology	Sweet, Richard Lance (MD)	433

Special Expertise	Specialty	Doctor's Name	Page
Short Bowel Syndrome	Pediatric Gastroenterology	Heyman, Melvin Bernard (MD)	581
Short Bowel Syndrome	Pediatric Gastroenterology	Thompson, John (MD)	579
Shoulder & Elbow Surgery	Orthopaedic Surgery	Uribe, John (MD)	488
Shoulder & Knee Injuries	Sports Medicine	Levine, William (MD)	773
Shoulder & Knee Reconstruction	Orthopaedic Surgery	Garrett, William (MD)	486
Shoulder & Knee Surgery	Orthopaedic Surgery	Garrett, William (MD)	486
Shoulder & Knee Surgery	Orthopaedic Surgery	Paulos, Leon (MD)	494
Shoulder & Knee Surgery	Orthopaedic Surgery	Pettrone, Frank A (MD)	487
Shoulder Impingement Syndrome	Orthopaedic Surgery	Taft, Timothy (MD)	488
Shoulder Reconstruction	Orthopaedic Surgery	Warren, Russell (MD)	485
Shoulder Surgery	Orthopaedic Surgery	Bigliani, Louis (MD)	478
Shoulder Surgery	Orthopaedic Surgery	Cofield, Robert H (MD)	490
Shoulder Surgery	Orthopaedic Surgery	Crossett, Lawrence (MD)	479
Shoulder Surgery	Orthopaedic Surgery	Dines, David Michael (MD)	480
Shoulder Surgery	Orthopaedic Surgery	Flatow, Evan (MD)	480
Shoulder Surgery	Orthopaedic Surgery	Iannotti, Joseph (MD)	491
Shoulder Surgery	Orthopaedic Surgery	Rockwood Jr, Charles A (MD)	495
Shoulder Surgery	Orthopaedic Surgery	Sherman, Orrin (MD)	484
Shoulder Surgery	Orthopaedic Surgery	Wickiewicz, Thomas (MD)	485
Shoulder Surgery	Orthopaedic Surgery	Wirth, Michael A (MD)	495
Shoulder Surgery	Orthopaedic Surgery	Zuckerman, Joseph (MD)	485
Shoulder Surgery	Sports Medicine	Altchek, David (MD)	773
Shoulder Surgery	Sports Medicine	Jobe, Frank Wilson (MD)	774
Shoulder, Elbow, Knee Surgery	Sports Medicine	Andrews, James R (MD)	773
Sickle Cell Disease	Pediatric Hematology-Oncology	Dover, George Joseph (MD)	583
Sickle Cell Disease	Pediatric Hematology-Oncology	Pegelow Jr, Charles Henry (MD)	586
Sickle Cell Disease	Pediatrics	Berman, Brian (MD)	618
Sickle Cell Screening	Radiology	Seibert, Joanna J (MD)	739
Sigmoidoscopy	Geriatric Medicine	Garb, Leslie Julian (MD)	250
Silicone Associated Disorders	Rheumatology	Solomon, Gary (MD)	761
Sinus & Skull Base Surgery	Otolaryngology	Har-El, Gady (MD)	504
Sinus Disorders	Allergy & Immunology	Aaronson, Donald W (MD)	99
Sinus Disorders	Allergy & Immunology	Atkins, Paul Charles (MD)	95
Sinus Disorders	Allergy & Immunology	Benenati, Susan (MD)	98
Sinus Disorders	Allergy & Immunology	Friedman, Stuart (MD)	98
Sinus Disorders	Allergy & Immunology	Mazza, David S (MD)	96
Sinus Disorders	Allergy & Immunology	Slavin, Raymond (MD)	101
Sinus Disorders	Allergy & Immunology	Wasserman, Stephen (MD)	103
Sinus Disorders	Allergy & Immunology	Wong, Johnson T (MD)	95
Sinus Disorders/Surgery	Otolaryngology	Bower, Charles (MD)	518
Sinus Disorders/Surgery	Otolaryngology	Calcaterra, Thomas Charles (MD)	521
Sinus Disorders/Surgery	Otolaryngology	Close, Lanny Garth (MD)	503
Sinus Disorders/Surgery	Otolaryngology	Friedman, Michael (MD)	513
Sinus Disorders/Surgery	Otolaryngology	Kuhn, Frederick (MD)	509
Sinus Disorders/Surgery	Otolaryngology	Kveton, John (MD)	501
Sinus Disorders/Surgery	Otolaryngology	Lanza, Donald (MD)	515
Sinus Disorders/Surgery	Otolaryngology	Lawson, William (MD)	504
Sinus Disorders/Surgery	Otolaryngology	Leopold, Donald Arthur (MD)	518
Sinus Disorders/Surgery	Otolaryngology	Piccirillo, Jay (MD)	516
Sinus Disorders/Surgery	Otolaryngology	Picken, Catherine A (MD)	505
Sinus Disorders/Surgery	Otolaryngology	Rice, Dale (MD)	523
Sinus Disorders/Surgery	Otolaryngology	Schaefer, Steven (MD)	506
Sinus Disorders/Surgery	Otolaryngology	Sillers, Michael (MD)	511
Sinus Disorders/Surgery	Otolaryngology	Vining, Eugenia (MD)	501
Sinus Disorders/Surgery	Otolaryngology	Ward, Robert (MD)	506
Sinus Disorders/Surgery	Otolaryngology	Weymuller, Ernest (MD)	523
Sinus Disorders/Surgery	Pediatric Otolaryngology	Gross, Charles (MD)	602
Sinus Disorders/Surgery	Pediatric Otolaryngology	Katz, Robert L (MD)	602
Sinus Disorders/Surgery	Pediatric Otolaryngology	Lusk, Rodney (MD)	602
Sinus Disorders/Surgery	Pediatric Otolaryngology	Milmoe, Gregory J (MD)	601

SPECIAL EXPERTISE INDEX

Special Expertise	Specialty	Doctor's Name	Page
Sinus Disorders/Surgery	Pediatric Otolaryngology	Rosenfeld, Richard M (MD)	601
Sjogren's Syndrome	Rheumatology	Pope, Richard M (MD)	766
Sjogren's Syndrome	Rheumatology	Wise, Christopher Murray (MD)	763
Skeletal Dysplasias	Clinical Genetics	Rimoin, David L (MD/PhD)	165
Skeletal Dysplasias	Clinical Genetics	Wilcox, William (MD)	166
Skeletal Dysplasias	Orthopaedic Surgery	Tolo, Vernon Thorpe (MD)	498
Skin & Collagen Disorders	Dermatology	Pinnell, Sheldon (MD)	188
Skin Cancer	Dermatology	Amonette, Rex A (MD)	186
Skin Cancer	Dermatology	Anderson, Richard Rox (MD)	181
Skin Cancer	Dermatology	Berg, Daniel (MD)	192
Skin Cancer	Dermatology	Butler, David F (MD)	191
Skin Cancer	Dermatology	Cohen, Bernard Hershel (MD)	187
Skin Cancer	Dermatology	Duvic, Madeleine (MD)	191
Skin Cancer	Dermatology	Edelson, Richard (MD)	181
Skin Cancer	Dermatology	Eichler, Craig (MD)	187
Skin Cancer	Dermatology	Fenske, Neil (MD)	187
Skin Cancer	Dermatology	Hanke, C William (MD)	189
Skin Cancer	Dermatology	Horn, Thomas (MD)	191
Skin Cancer	Dermatology	Johr, Robert (MD)	187
Skin Cancer	Dermatology	Lebwohl, Mark (MD)	184
Skin Cancer	Dermatology	McDonald, Charles J (MD)	182
Skin Cancer	Dermatology	Miller, Stanley (MD)	185
Skin Cancer	Dermatology	Neuberg, Marcy (MD)	190
Skin Cancer	Dermatology	Sobel, Stuart (MD)	188
Skin Cancer	Dermatology	Spielvogel, Richard Lee (MD)	186
Skin Cancer	Dermatology	Tabak, Brian (MD)	194
Skin Cancer	Dermatology	Taylor, R Stan (MD)	192
Skin Cancer	Dermatology	Zitelli, John (MD)	186
Skin Cancer	Pathology	Page, David L (MD)	540
Skin Cancer	Radiation Oncology	Wilson, J Frank (MD)	724
Skin Cancer-Melanoma	Dermatology	Kopf, Alfred (MD)	184
Skin Cancer-Melanoma	Dermatology	Robins, Perry (MD)	185
Skin Diseases	Dermatology	Braverman, Irwin (MD)	181
Skin Diseases	Dermatology	Shupack, Jerome L (MD)	186
Skin Diseases-Immunologic	Dermatology	Edelson, Richard (MD)	181
Skin Laser Surgery	Dermatology	Anderson, Richard Rox (MD)	181
Skin Laser Surgery	Dermatology	Arndt, Kenneth (MD)	181
Skin Laser Surgery	Dermatology	Bailin, Philip Lawrence (MD)	188
Skin Laser Surgery	Dermatology	Berg, Daniel (MD)	192
Skin Laser Surgery	Dermatology	Dzubow, Leonard (MD)	183
Skin Laser Surgery	Dermatology	Garden, Jerome (MD)	189
Skin Laser Surgery	Dermatology	Geronemus, Roy (MD)	183
Skin Laser Surgery	Dermatology	Grossman, Melanie (MD)	184
Skin Laser Surgery	Dermatology	Hruza, George J (MD)	189
Skin Laser Surgery	Dermatology	Kilmer, Suzanne L (MD)	193
Skin Laser Surgery	Dermatology	Maloney, Mary (MD)	182
Skin Laser Surgery	Dermatology	Wheeland, Ronald (MD)	192
Skin Laser Surgery	Dermatology	Zelickson, Brian D (MD)	190
Skin Laser Surgery	Plastic Surgery	Baker Jr, Thomas J (MD)	641
Skin Laser Surgery	Plastic Surgery	Burns, Alton Jay (MD)	649
Skin Laser Surgery	Plastic Surgery	Eriksson, Elof (MD)	635
Skin Laser Surgery	Plastic Surgery	Gregory, Richard (MD)	643
Skin Laser Surgery-Birthmarks	Dermatology	Shwayder, Tor A (MD)	190
Skin Laser Surgery-Resurfacing	Dermatology	Alster, Tina (MD)	182
Skin Laser Surgery-Resurfacing	Dermatology	Dover, Jeffrey (MD)	181
Skin Laser Surgery-Resurfacing	Dermatology	Garden, Jerome (MD)	189
Skin Laser Surgery-Resurfacing	Dermatology	Lask, Gary P (MD)	193
Skin Laser Surgery-Resurfacing	Plastic Surgery	Young, Vernon Leroy (MD)	647
Skin Pathology	Pathology	McNutt, N Scott (MD)	538
Skull Base Surgery	Neurological Surgery	Al-Mefty, Ossama (MD)	386

Special Expertise	Specialty	Doctor's Name	Page
Skull Base Surgery	Neurological Surgery	Benjamin, Vallo (MD)	374
Skull Base Surgery	Neurological Surgery	Carmel, Peter (MD)	375
Skull Base Surgery	Neurological Surgery	Khan, Agha S (MD)	377
Skull Base Surgery	Neurological Surgery	Pitts, Lawrence H (MD)	389
Skull Base Surgery	Neuroloegical Surgery	Stieg, Philip E (MD/PhD)	379
Skull Base Surgery	Otolaryngology	Carrau, Ricardo L. (MD)	503
Skull Base Surgery	Otolaryngology	Close, Lanny Garth (MD)	503
Skull Base Surgery	Otolaryngology	Daspit, C Phillip (MD)	518
Skull Base Surgery	Otolaryngology	Donald, Paul (MD)	521
Skull Base Surgery	Otolaryngology	Goodwin, Jerry (MD)	508
Skull Base Surgery	Otolaryngology	Hanna, Ehab (MD)	519
Skull Base Surgery	Otolaryngology	Jackler, Robert K (MD)	522
Skull Base Surgery	Otolaryngology	Leonetti, John (MD)	515
Skull Base Surgery	Otolaryngology	Peters, Glenn Eidson (MD)	510
Skull Base Surgery	Otolaryngology	Poe, Dennis (MD)	501
Skull Base Surgery	Otolaryngology	Roland, Peter S (MD)	520
Skull Base Surgery	Otolaryngology	Tucci, Debara Lyn (MD)	511
Skull Base Surgery	Otolaryngology	Wazen, Jack (MD)	506
Skull Base Tumors	Neurological Surgery	Giannotta, Steven L (MD)	389
Skull Base Tumors	Neurological Surgery	Long, Donlin M (MD/PhD)	377
Skull Base Tumors	Neurological Surgery	Mayberg, Marc (MD)	384
Skull Base Tumors	Otolaryngology	Lanza, Donald (MD)	515
Skull Base Tumors	Otolaryngology	Pensak, Myles (MD)	516
Skull Base Tumors	Otolaryngology	Weber, Randal Scott (MD)	507
Sleep & Breathing Disorders	Pediatric Pulmonology	Loughlin, Gerald M (MD)	604
Sleep Apnea	Psychiatry	Guilleminault, Christian (MD)	686
Sleep Disorders	Psychiatry	Guilleminault, Christian (MD)	686
Sleep Disorders & Aging	Pulmonary Disease	Pack, Allan I (MD/PhD)	694
Sleep Disorders/Apnea	Geriatric Medicine	Groene, Linda A (MD)	246
Sleep Disorders/Apnea	Neurology	Adornato, Bruce T. (MD)	418
Sleep Disorders/Apnea	Neurology	Logigian, Eric L (MD)	403
Sleep Disorders/Apnea	Neurology	Mahowald, Mark W (MD)	414
Sleep Disorders/Apnea	Neurology	Nolan, Bruce A (MD)	409
Sleep Disorders/Apnea	Otolaryngology	Friedman, Michael (MD)	513
Sleep Disorders/Apnea	Otolaryngology	Piccirillo, Jay (MD)	516
Sleep Disorders/Apnea	Otolaryngology	Powell, Nelson Bert (MD/DDS)	522
Sleep Disorders/Apnea	Otolaryngology	Strome, Marshall (MD)	516
Sleep Disorders/Apnea	Pediatric Otolaryngology	Lusk, Rodney (MD)	602
Sleep Disorders/Apnea	Pediatric Pulmonology	Kim, Young-Jee (MD)	605
Sleep Disorders/Apnea	Psychiatry	Hobson, John Allan (MD)	676
Sleep Disorders/Apnea	Psychiatry	Kupfer, David J. (MD)	679
Sleep Disorders/Apnea	Psychiatry	Moore, Constance A. (MD)	685
Sleep Disorders/Apnea	Pulmonary Disease	Greenberg, Harly (MD)	693
Sleep Disorders/Apnea	Pulmonary Disease	Haponik, Edward Francis (MD)	693
Sleep Disorders/Apnea	Pulmonary Disease	Johnson, Bruce Ellsworth ()	699
Sleep Disorders/Apnea	Pulmonary Disease	Kaye, Mitchell (MD)	703
Sleep Disorders/Apnea	Pulmonary Disease	Koenig, Steven Michael (MD)	699
Sleep Disorders/Apnea	Pulmonary Disease	Pack, Allan I (MD/PhD)	694
Sleep Disorders/Apnea	Pulmonary Disease	White, David P (MD)	693
Sleep Disorders/Apnea	Surgery	Schwab, Richard (MD)	788
Smell/Taste Disorders	Otolaryngology	Kern, Robert (MD)	514
Snoring-Surgery	Otolaryngology	Friedman, Michael (MD)	513
Soft Tissue Pathology	Pathology	Weiss, Sharon (MD)	540
Soft Tissue Sarcoma	Surgery	Singer, Samuel (MD)	782
Soft Tissue Tumors	Diagnostic Radiology	Mancuso, Anthony (MD)	733
Soft Tissue Tumors	Orthopaedic Surgery	Simon, Michael (MD)	492
Soft Tissue Tumors	Pathology	Dorfman, Howard (MD)	536
Soft-Tissue Tumors/Sarcomas	Pathology	Fletcher, Christopher (MD)	535
Solid Tumors	Medical Oncology	McCarley, Dean L (MD)	302
Solid Tumors	Medical Oncology	Ratain, Mark J (MD)	308

SPECIAL EXPERTISE INDEX

Special Expertise	Specialty	Doctor's Name	Page
Solid Tumors	Pediatric Hematology-Oncology	Meyers, Paul (MD)	584
Solid Tumors	Pediatric Hematology-Oncology	Odom , Lorrie Furman (MD)	588
Sonohysterography	Reproductive Endocrinology	Session, Donna Ruth (MD)	750
Spasticity & Movement Disorders	Neurological Surgery	Albright, Leland (MD)	374
Spasticity Management	Physical Medicine & Rehabilitation	Ballard, Pamela H (MD)	623
Spasticity Management	Physical Medicine & Rehabilitation	Mayer, Nathaniel (MD)	625
Spasticity Management	Physical Medicine & Rehabilitation	Munin, Michael Craig (MD)	625
Speech Disorders	Child Neurology	Trauner, Doris Ann (MD)	156
Sphincter of Oddi Dysfunction	Gastroenterology	Cunningham, John (MD)	227
Spinal Cord Injury	Neurology	Dobkin, Bruce H (MD)	420
Spinal Cord Injury	Neurology	Waxman, Stephen G. (MD/PhD)	399
Spinal Cord Injury	Orthopaedic Surgery	Alander, Dirk Huntley (MD)	489
Spinal Cord Injury	Physical Medicine & Rehabilitation	Ahn, Jung Hwan (MD)	623
Spinal Cord Injury	Physical Medicine & Rehabilitation	Bach, John (MD)	623
Spinal Cord Injury	Physical Medicine & Rehabilitation	Barber, Douglas Byron (MD)	629
Spinal Cord Injury	Physical Medicine & Rehabilitation	Cardenas, Diana (MD)	630
Spinal Cord Injury	Physical Medicine & Rehabilitation	Chen, David (MD)	626
Spinal Cord Injury	Physical Medicine & Rehabilitation	Colachis III, Samuel C (MD)	627
Spinal Cord Injury	Physical Medicine & Rehabilitation	Creamer, Michael (DO)	626
Spinal Cord Injury	Physical Medicine & Rehabilitation	Ditunno, John Francis (MD)	624
Spinal Cord Injury	Physical Medicine & Rehabilitation	Donovan, William Henry (MD)	629
Spinal Cord Injury	Physical Medicine & Rehabilitation	Gittler, Michelle (MD)	627
Spinal Cord Injury	Physical Medicine & Rehabilitation	Jackson, Amie Brown (MD)	626
Spinal Cord Injury	Physical Medicine & Rehabilitation	Kirshblum, Steven C (MD)	624
Spinal Cord Injury	Physical Medicine & Rehabilitation	Kraft, George Howard (MD)	631
Spinal Cord Injury	Physical Medicine & Rehabilitation	Lammertse, Daniel (MD)	628
Spinal Cord Injury	Physical Medicine & Rehabilitation	Nobunaga , Austin (MD)	627
Spinal Cord Injury	Physical Medicine & Rehabilitation	Parsons, Kenneth C. (MD)	630
Spinal Cord Injury	Physical Medicine & Rehabilitation	Ragnarsson, Kristjan (MD)	625
Spinal Cord Injury	Physical Medicine & Rehabilitation	Staas Jr, William E (MD)	625
Spinal Cord Injury	Physical Medicine & Rehabilitation	Volshteyn, Oksana (MD)	628
Spinal Cord Injury	Physical Medicine & Rehabilitation	Zafonte, Ross (DO)	625
Spinal Cord Injury-Pediatric	Physical Medicine & Rehabilitation	Massagli, Teresa Luisa (MD)	631
Spinal Cord Surgery	Neurological Surgery	Clifton, Guy (MD)	386
Spinal Cord Surgery	Neurological Surgery	Hadley, Mark (MD)	380
Spinal Cord Surgery	Neurological Surgery	Kobrine, Arthur (MD/PhD)	377
Spinal Cord Tumors	Neurological Surgery	Batzdorf, Ulrich (MD)	388
Spinal Cord Tumors	Neurological Surgery	Flamm, Eugene (MD)	376
Spinal Cord Tumors	Neurological Surgery	Ojemann, Robert G. (MD)	373
Spinal Cord Tumors	Neurological Surgery	Weiss, Martin Harvey (MD)	390
Spinal Cord Tumors	Neurological Surgery	Wilson, Charles B (MD)	390
Spinal Cord Tumors	Radiation Oncology	Loeffler, Jay Steven (MD)	717
Spinal Cord Tumors-Pediatric	Neurological Surgery	Epstein, Fred Jacob (MD)	376
Spinal Deformities-Adult & Pediatric	Orthopaedic Surgery	Lauerman, William (MD)	482
Spinal Deformity-Pediatric	Orthopaedic Surgery	Tolo, Vernon Thorpe (MD)	498
Spinal Diseases	Neurological Surgery	Long, Donlin M (MD/PhD)	377
Spinal Stenosis	Neurological Surgery	Hekmatpanah, Javad (MD)	383
Spinal Surgery	Neurological Surgery	Benjamin, Vallo (MD)	374
Spinal Surgery	Neurological Surgery	Borges, Lawrence F. (MD)	373
Spinal Surgery	Neurological Surgery	Branch Jr, Charles L (MD)	379
Spinal Surgery	Neurological Surgery	Brown, Frederick (MD)	382
Spinal Surgery	Neurological Surgery	Camins, Martin B (MD)	375
Spinal Surgery	Neurological Surgery	Caputy, Anthony J. (MD)	375
Spinal Surgery	Neurological Surgery	Ferraz, Francisco M (MD)	379
Spinal Surgery	Neurological Surgery	Green, Barth (MD)	380
Spinal Surgery	Neurological Surgery	Harper, Richard L (MD)	387
Spinal Surgery	Neurological Surgery	Khan, Agha S (MD)	377
Spinal Surgery	Neurological Surgery	Lavyne, Michael H (MD)	377
Spinal Surgery	Neurological Surgery	Mangiardi, John (MD)	377
Spinal Surgery	Neurological Surgery	Marion, Donald W (MD)	378

Special Expertise	Specialty	Doctor's Name	Page
Spinal Surgery	Neurological Surgery	Papadopoulos, Stephen M. (MD)	385
Spinal Surgery	Neurological Surgery	Pitts, Lawrence H (MD)	389
Spinal Surgery	Neurological Surgery	Rockswold, Gaylan (MD)	385
Spinal Surgery	Neurological Surgery	Rosenblum, Mark (MD)	385
Spinal Surgery	Neurological Surgery	Shaffrey, Christopher I (MD)	390
Spinal Surgery	Neurological Surgery	Sonntag, Volker (MD)	387
Spinal Surgery	Orthopaedic Surgery	Alander, Dirk Huntley (MD)	489
Spinal Surgery	Orthopaedic Surgery	Boachie, Oheneba (MD)	479
Spinal Surgery	Orthopaedic Surgery	Bohlman, Henry H (MD)	489
Spinal Surgery	Orthopaedic Surgery	Bradford, David S (MD)	496
Spinal Surgery	Orthopaedic Surgery	Brick, Gregory (MD)	475
Spinal Surgery	Orthopaedic Surgery	Bridwell, Keith (MD)	489
Spinal Surgery	Orthopaedic Surgery	Donaldson III, William F (MD)	480
Spinal Surgery	Orthopaedic Surgery	Dunn, Harold Kenneth (MD)	493
Spinal Surgery	Orthopaedic Surgery	Eismont, Frank (MD)	486
Spinal Surgery	Orthopaedic Surgery	Farcy, Jean-Pierre (MD)	480
Spinal Surgery	Orthopaedic Surgery	Lauerman, William (MD)	482
Spinal Surgery	Orthopaedic Surgery	Lipson, Stephen Jay (MD)	476
Spinal Surgery	Orthopaedic Surgery	O'Leary, Patrick (MD)	482
Spinal Surgery	Orthopaedic Surgery	Rechtine, Glenn (MD)	487
Spinal Surgery	Orthopaedic Surgery	Schafer, Michael F (MD)	492
Spinal Surgery	Orthopaedic Surgery	Spengler, Dan M (MD)	487
Spinal Surgery	Orthopaedic Surgery	Watkins, Robert Green (MD)	498
Spinal Surgery	Orthopaedic Surgery	Wiesel, Sam W (MD)	485
Spinal Surgery	Orthopaedic Surgery	Zdeblick, Thomas (MD)	493
Spinal Surgery-Low Back	Orthopaedic Surgery	Grant, Richard E (MD)	481
Spinal Surgery-Pediatric	Orthopaedic Surgery	Hensinger, Robert (MD)	491
Spine & Nerve Injuries	Physical Medicine & Rehabilitation	Feinberg, Joseph Hunt (MD)	624
Spine Surgery-Degenerative	Neurological Surgery	Kelly Jr, David L (MD)	380
Spondyloarthropathies	Rheumatology	Chang-Miller, April (MD)	763
Spondyloarthropathies	Rheumatology	Duffy, Joseph (MD)	764
Spontaneous Abortion	Obstetrics & Gynecology	Simpson, Joe Leigh (MD)	438
Sports Medicine	Orthopaedic Surgery	Anderson, Lesley J (MD)	496
Sports Medicine	Orthopaedic Surgery	Bach Jr, Bernard R (MD)	489
Sports Medicine	Orthopaedic Surgery	Bartolozzi, Arthur R. (MD)	478
Sports Medicine	Orthopaedic Surgery	Bergfeld, John (MD)	489
Sports Medicine	Orthopaedic Surgery	Bigliani, Louis (MD)	478
Sports Medicine	Orthopaedic Surgery	Boland Jr., Arthur L (MD)	475
Sports Medicine	Orthopaedic Surgery	Bradley, James P. (MD)	479
Sports Medicine	Orthopaedic Surgery	Callaghan, John J (MD)	490
Sports Medicine	Orthopaedic Surgery	Cannon Jr, W Dilworth (MD)	496
Sports Medicine	Orthopaedic Surgery	Curl, Walton Wright (MD)	486
Sports Medicine	Orthopaedic Surgery	Deland, Jonathan T (MD)	480
Sports Medicine	Orthopaedic Surgery	Finerman, Gerald (MD)	497
Sports Medicine	Orthopaedic Surgery	Fu, Freddie (MD)	480
Sports Medicine	Orthopaedic Surgery	Garrett, William (MD)	486
Sports Medicine	Orthopaedic Surgery	Goitz, Henry (MD)	490
Sports Medicine	Orthopaedic Surgery	Graf, Ben K (MD)	491
Sports Medicine	Orthopaedic Surgery	Grelsamer, Ronald (MD)	481
Sports Medicine	Orthopaedic Surgery	Johnson, Darren Lee (MD)	486
Sports Medicine	Orthopaedic Surgery	Lock, Terrence Ralph (MD)	491
Sports Medicine	Orthopaedic Surgery	Micheli, Lyle J (MD)	476
Sports Medicine	Orthopaedic Surgery	Minkoff, Jeffrey (MD)	487
Sports Medicine	Orthopaedic Surgery	Paulos, Leon (MD)	494
Sports Medicine	Orthopaedic Surgery	Pettrone, Frank A (MD)	487
Sports Medicine	Orthopaedic Surgery	Rosenberg, Thomas D (MD)	494
Sports Medicine	Orthopaedic Surgery	Schafer, Michael F (MD)	492
Sports Medicine	Orthopaedic Surgery	Scheller, Arnold (MD)	477
Sports Medicine	Orthopaedic Surgery	Shelbourne, K Donald (MD)	492
Sports Medicine	Orthopaedic Surgery	Spindler, Kurt Paul (MD)	488

SPECIAL EXPERTISE INDEX

Special Expertise	Specialty	Doctor's Name	Page
Sports Medicine	Orthopaedic Surgery	Taft, Timothy (MD)	488
Sports Medicine	Orthopaedic Surgery	Wickiewicz, Thomas (MD)	485
Sports Medicine	Orthopaedic Surgery	Zarins, Bertram (MD)	477
Sports Medicine	Physical Medicine & Rehabilitation	Haig, Andrew (MD)	627
Sports Medicine	Physical Medicine & Rehabilitation	Lipkin, David L (MD)	626
Sports Medicine	Physical Medicine & Rehabilitation	Press, Joel (MD)	627
Sports Medicine	Sports Medicine	Levine, William (MD)	773
Sports Medicine	Sports Medicine	Noyes, Frank (MD)	774
Sports Medicine-Women	Orthopaedic Surgery	Hannafin, Jo (MD/PhD)	481
Sports Vision	Ophthalmology	Granet, David Bruce (MD)	465
Sports-Orthopedic Related Injuries	Physical Medicine & Rehabilitation	Feinberg, Joseph Hunt (MD)	624
Sports/Dance Medicine	Orthopaedic Surgery	Bauman, Phillip (MD)	478
Staphylococcal Infections	Infectious Disease	Archer, Gordon Lee (MD)	322
Staphylococcal Infections	Internal Medicine	Schaberg, Dennis Ray (MD)	335
Stealth Guided Surgery	Neurological Surgery	Papadopoulos, Stephen M. (MD)	385
Stem Cell Transplantation	Medical Oncology	Jillella, Anand (MD)	301
Stentgraphs	Radiology	Benenati, James Francis (MD)	737
Stereotactic Radiology	Radiology	Petrovich, Zbigniew (MD)	740
Stereotactic Radiosurgery	Neurological Surgery	Adler Jr, John R (MD)	388
Stereotactic Radiosurgery	Neurological Surgery	Barnett, Gene H (MD)	382
Stereotactic Radiosurgery	Neurological Surgery	Branch Jr, Charles L (MD)	379
Stereotactic Radiosurgery	Neurological Surgery	Burchiel, Kim James (MD)	388
Stereotactic Radiosurgery	Neurological Surgery	Chapman, Paul H. (MD)	373
Stereotactic Radiosurgery	Neurological Surgery	Freeman, Thomas B (MD)	380
Stereotactic Radiosurgery	Neurological Surgery	Friedman, William A (MD)	380
Stereotactic Radiosurgery	Neurological Surgery	Hassenbusch, Samuel J (MD/PhD)	387
Stereotactic Radiosurgery	Neurological Surgery	Heilbrun, M Peter (MD)	386
Stereotactic Radiosurgery	Neurological Surgery	Kelly, Patrick J. (MD)	377
Stereotactic Radiosurgery	Neurological Surgery	Levy, Robert M (MD)	384
Stereotactic Radiosurgery	Neurological Surgery	Lunsford, L Dade (MD)	377
Stereotactic Radiosurgery	Neurological Surgery	Nazzaro, Jules M. (MD)	373
Stereotactic Radiosurgery	Neurological Surgery	Papadopoulos, Stephen M. (MD)	385
Stereotactic Radiosurgery	Radiation Oncology	Ennis, Ronald (MD)	718
Stereotactic Radiosurgery	Radiation Oncology	Loeffler, Jay Steven (MD)	717
Stereotactic Radiosurgery	Radiation Oncology	Mendenhall, William M (MD)	722
Stereotactic Radiosurgery	Radiation Oncology	Pistenmaa, David A (MD)	726
Stereotactic Radiosurgery	Radiation Oncology	Shaw, Edward Gus (MD)	722
Strabismus	Ophthalmology	Buckley, Edward G (MD)	452
Strabismus	Ophthalmology	Capo, Hilda (MD)	452
Strabismus	Ophthalmology	Caputo, Anthony R (MD)	445
Strabismus	Ophthalmology	Cibis, Gerhard W (MD)	456
Strabismus	Ophthalmology	Diamond, Gary Richard (MD)	445
Strabismus	Ophthalmology	Eggers, Howard M (MD)	445
Strabismus	Ophthalmology	Feldon, Steven E (MD)	464
Strabismus	Ophthalmology	France, Thomas D (MD)	457
Strabismus	Ophthalmology	Guyton, David Lee (MD)	446
Strabismus	Ophthalmology	Hall, Lisabeth (MD)	446
Strabismus	Ophthalmology	Hess, J Bruce (MD)	453
Strabismus	Ophthalmology	Isenberg, Sherwin Jay (MD)	465
Strabismus	Ophthalmology	Magramm, Irene (MD)	448
Strabismus	Ophthalmology	Mims III, James Luther (MD)	462
Strabismus	Ophthalmology	Olitsky, Scott Eric (MD)	449
Strabismus	Ophthalmology	Paul, Theodore Otis (MD)	467
Strabismus	Ophthalmology	Pollard, Zane F (MD)	454
Strabismus	Ophthalmology	Raab, Edward (MD)	449
Strabismus	Ophthalmology	Reynolds, James D. (MD)	449
Strabismus	Ophthalmology	Robb, Richard M (MD)	443
Strabismus	Ophthalmology	Simon, John W (MD)	450
Strabismus	Ophthalmology	Stern, Kathleen (MD)	451
Strabismus (Adult & Pediatric)	Ophthalmology	Rogers, Gary L (MD)	459

Special Expertise	Specialty	Doctor's Name	Page
Strabismus (Eye Muscle Disorders)	Ophthalmology	Burke, Miles Joseph (MD)	456
Strabismus (Eye Muscle Disorders)	Ophthalmology	Price, Ronald (MD)	459
Strabismus and Amblyopia	Ophthalmology	Weiss, Avery (MD)	468
Stress Disorders	Pediatric Endocrinology	Chrousos, George (MD)	572
Stroke	Cardiology (Cardiovascular Disease)	Segal, Bernard L (MD)	128
Stroke	Interventional Cardiology	Smalling, Richard W (MD/PhD)	147
Stroke	Neurological Surgery	Awad, Issam A (MD)	373
Stroke	Neurological Surgery	Grady, M Sean (MD)	376
Stroke	Neurology	Adams Jr., Harold Pomeroy (MD)	411
Stroke	Neurology	Adams, Robert Joseph (MD)	407
Stroke	Neurology	Adornato, Bruce T. (MD)	418
Stroke	Neurology	Albers, Gregory William (MD)	418
Stroke	Neurology	Bernad, Peter (MD)	400
Stroke	Neurology	Brust, John C (MD)	400
Stroke	Neurology	Caplan, Louis Robert (MD)	397
Stroke	Neurology	Caronna, John J (MD)	400
Stroke	Neurology	Chui, Helena Chang (MD)	419
Stroke	Neurology	Coull, Bruce (MD)	416
Stroke	Neurology	Dobkin, Bruce H (MD)	420
Stroke	Neurology	Easton, J Donald (MD)	397
Stroke	Neurology	Feldmann, Edward (MD)	397
Stroke	Neurology	Furlan, Anthony J (MD)	413
Stroke	Neurology	Goldstein, Larry Bruce (MD)	408
Stroke	Neurology	Gress, Daryl Ray (MD)	421
Stroke	Neurology	Grotta, James (MD)	417
Stroke	Neurology	Haley Jr, Elliott Clarke (MD)	408
Stroke	Neurology	Hart, Robert G. (MD)	417
Stroke	Neurology	Hess, David Charles (MD)	408
Stroke	Neurology	Kase, Carlos S. (MD)	398
Stroke	Neurology	Kirshner, Howard S (MD)	408
Stroke	Neurology	Kistler, John Philip (MD)	398
Stroke	Neurology	Koroshetz, Walter J. (MD)	398
Stroke	Neurology	Levine, David (MD)	403
Stroke	Neurology	Levine, Steven R (MD)	413
Stroke	Neurology	Mohr, Jay Preston (MD)	404
Stroke	Neurology	Plum, Fred (MD)	405
Stroke	Neurology	Reed, Robert L (MD)	415
Stroke	Neurology	Sherman, David (MD)	418
Stroke	Neurology	Smith, Wade S (MD/PhD)	422
Stroke	Neurology	Vas, George A (MD)	406
Stroke	Neurology	Wechsler, Lawrence Richard (MD)	406
Stroke	Neurology	Weisberg, Leon (MD)	418
Stroke	Vascular Surgery (General)	Dardik, Herbert (MD)	859
Stroke	Vascular Surgery (General)	Perler, Bruce Alan (MD)	861
Stroke	Vascular Surgery (General)	Rosenthal, David (MD)	864
Stroke Rehabilitation	Physical Medicine & Rehabilitation	Ahn, Jung Hwan (MD)	623
Stroke Rehabilitation	Physical Medicine & Rehabilitation	Kevorkian, Charles George (MD)	629
Stroke Rehabilitation	Physical Medicine & Rehabilitation	King, John Chandler (MD)	630
Stroke Rehabilitation	Physical Medicine & Rehabilitation	Mason, Kristin Denise (MD)	627
Stroke Rehabilitation	Physical Medicine & Rehabilitation	Roth, Elliot (MD)	628
Stroke-Microsurgery	Neurological Surgery	Selman, Warren R (MD)	385
Stroke/Cerebrovascular Disease	Neurological Surgery	Mayberg, Marc (MD)	384
Subarachnoid Hemorrhage	Neurological Surgery	Dennis, Gary Creed (MD)	375
Sudden Cardiac Death	Cardiology (Cardiovascular Disease)	Myerburg, Robert (MD)	131
Suicide	Child & Adolescent Psychiatry	Sargent III, A John (MD)	669
Surfactant Biology	Neonatal-Perinatal Medicine	Jobe, Alan Hall (MD/PhD)	353
Surgical Oncology	Surgery	Enker, Warren (MD)	785
Surgical Pathology	Pathology	Colby, Thomas V (MD)	541
Surgical Pathology	Pathology	Fletcher, Christopher (MD)	535
Surgical Pathology	Pathology	Katzenstein, Anna-Luise A. (MD)	537

SPECIAL EXPERTISE INDEX

SPECIAL EXPERTISE INDEX

Special Expertise	Specialty	Doctor's Name	Page
Thyroid & Parathyroid Surgery	Otolaryngology	Davis, Roy Kim (MD)	517
Thyroid & Parathyroid Surgery	Otolaryngology	Weber, Randal Scott (MD)	507
Thyroid & Parathyroid Surgery	Surgery	Hanks, John B (MD)	791
Thyroid & Parathyroid Surgery	Surgery	Roses, Daniel F (MD)	787
Thyroid & Pituitary Disorders	Endocrinology, Diabetes & Metabolism	Ontjes, David A (MD)	204
Thyroid Cancer	Endocrinology, Diabetes & Metabolism	De Groot, Leslie (MD)	206
Thyroid Cancer	Endocrinology, Diabetes & Metabolism	Wartofsky, Leonard (MD)	202
Thyroid Cancer	Nuclear Medicine	Larson, Steven (MD)	425
Thyroid Cancer	Pediatric Endocrinology	Zimmerman, Donald (MD)	576
Thyroid Cancer	Radiology	Charboneau, J William (MD)	737
Thyroid Cancer	Surgery	Cady, Blake (MD)	781
Thyroid Cancer	Surgery	Clark, Orlo H (MD)	799
Thyroid Cancer	Surgery	Evans, Douglas Brian (MD)	797
Thyroid Disease	Nuclear Medicine	Dubovsky, Eva V (MD/PhD)	426
Thyroid Disorders	Endocrinology, Diabetes & Metabolism	Bahn, Rebecca Sue (MD)	206
Thyroid Disorders	Endocrinology, Diabetes & Metabolism	Berkson, Richard Alan (MD)	210
Thyroid Disorders	Endocrinology, Diabetes & Metabolism	Blum, Manfred (MD)	198
Thyroid Disorders	Endocrinology, Diabetes & Metabolism	Brennan, Michael Desmond (MD)	206
Thyroid Disorders	Endocrinology, Diabetes & Metabolism	Burke, Susan F (MD)	206
Thyroid Disorders	Endocrinology, Diabetes & Metabolism	Cooper, David Stephen (MD)	199
Thyroid Disorders	Endocrinology, Diabetes & Metabolism	Daniels, Gilbert (MD)	197
Thyroid Disorders	Endocrinology, Diabetes & Metabolism	Davies, Terry (MD)	199
Thyroid Disorders	Endocrinology, Diabetes & Metabolism	Fleischer, Norman (MD)	200
Thyroid Disorders	Endocrinology, Diabetes & Metabolism	Gorman, Colum (MD)	207
Thyroid Disorders	Endocrinology, Diabetes & Metabolism	Graber, Alan (MD)	204
Thyroid Disorders	Endocrinology, Diabetes & Metabolism	Griffin, James Emmet (MD)	209
Thyroid Disorders	Endocrinology, Diabetes & Metabolism	Hurley, James (MD)	200
Thyroid Disorders	Endocrinology, Diabetes & Metabolism	Ladenson, Paul William (MD)	200
Thyroid Disorders	Endocrinology, Diabetes & Metabolism	Levy, Philip (MD)	210
Thyroid Disorders	Endocrinology, Diabetes & Metabolism	Mahler, Richard J (MD)	201
Thyroid Disorders	Endocrinology, Diabetes & Metabolism	Mandel, Susan (MD)	201
Thyroid Disorders	Endocrinology, Diabetes & Metabolism	Marcus, Robert A (MD)	212
Thyroid Disorders	Endocrinology, Diabetes & Metabolism	McConnell, Robert John (MD)	201
Thyroid Disorders	Endocrinology, Diabetes & Metabolism	Reasner, Charles A (MD)	210
Thyroid Disorders	Endocrinology, Diabetes & Metabolism	Singer, Peter Albert (MD)	212
Thyroid Disorders	Endocrinology, Diabetes & Metabolism	Surks, Martin (MD)	202
Thyroid Disorders	Endocrinology, Diabetes & Metabolism	Woeber, Kenneth Alois (MD)	213
Thyroid Disorders	Endocrinology, Diabetes & Metabolism	Young, Iven (MD)	203
Thyroid Disorders	Internal Medicine	Wood, Lawrence Crane (MD)	333
Thyroid Disorders	Otolaryngology	Davidson, Bruce J (MD)	503
Thyroid Disorders	Otolaryngology	Picken, Catherine A (MD)	505
Thyroid Disorders	Otolaryngology	Weber, Randal Scott (MD)	507
Thyroid Disorders	Pathology	Wheeler, Thomas M (MD)	542
Thyroid Disorders	Pediatric Endocrinology	Casella, Samuel Joseph (MD)	572
Thyroid Disorders	Pediatric Endocrinology	Freemark, Michael Scott (MD)	574
Thyroid Disorders	Pediatric Endocrinology	Kappy, Michael Steven (MD/PhD)	576
Thyroid Disorders	Pediatric Endocrinology	Levy, Richard Alshuler (MD)	575
Thyroid Disorders	Pediatric Endocrinology	Maurer, William (MD)	576
Thyroid Disorders	Pediatric Endocrinology	Oberfield, Sharon (MD)	573
Thyroid Disorders	Pediatric Endocrinology	Rogers, Douglas G (MD)	576
Thyroid Disorders & Diabetes	Endocrinology, Diabetes & Metabolism	Gonzalez, Martha (MD/PhD)	211
Thyroid Eye Disease	Ophthalmology	Char, Devron H (MD)	464
Thyroid Imaging	Nuclear Medicine	Scheff, Alice M (MD)	427
Thyroid Surgery	Otolaryngology	Alford, Bobby R (MD)	518
Thyroid Surgery	Otolaryngology	Clayman, Gary Lee (MD)	518
Thyroid Surgery	Pediatric Surgery	Neblett, Wallace W (MD)	613
Thyroid Surgery	Surgery	Numann, Patricia (MD)	787
Thyroid Surgery	Surgery	Shah, Jatin P (MD)	788
Thyroid Surgery	Surgery	Shuck, Jerry M (MD)	795
Thyroid/Lipid Disorders	Endocrinology, Diabetes & Metabolism	Ratner, Robert (MD)	201

SPECIAL EXPERTISE INDEX

Special Expertise	Specialty	Doctor's Name	Page
Tick-borne Diseases	Infectious Disease	Auwaerter, Paul (MD)	317
Tick-borne Diseases	Infectious Disease	Bakken, Johan Septimus (MD)	325
Tick-borne Diseases	Infectious Disease	Mann, John (MD)	320
Tobacco Abuse	Geriatric Medicine	Dale, Lowell C (MD)	247
Total Parenteral Nutrition	Surgery	Dudrick, Stanley (MD)	781
Tourette's Syndrome	Child & Adolescent Psychiatry	Cohen, Donald (MD)	663
Tourette's Syndrome	Child & Adolescent Psychiatry	McCracken, James Thomas (MD)	670
Tourette's Syndrome	Child Neurology	Eviatar, Lydia (MD)	152
Tourette's Syndrome	Neurology	Jankovic, Joseph (MD)	417
Tourette's Syndrome	Neurology	Mesulam, Marek Marsel (MD)	414
Toxoplasmosis, Amebiasis	Infectious Disease	Johnson, Warren (MD)	320
Tracheal Reconstruction	Pediatric Otolaryngology	Cotton, Robin (MD)	602
Tracheal Surgery	Pediatric Surgery	Othersen, H Biemann (MD)	614
Tracheal Surgery	Thoracic Surgery	Mathisen, Douglas (MD)	806
Tracheal Surgery	Thoracic Surgery	Wood, Douglas (MD)	826
Transabdominal Cervical Cerclage (TCIC)	Obstetrics & Gynecology	Novy, Miles (MD)	438
Transcranial Doppler	Neurology	Wechsler, Lawrence Richard (MD)	406
Transfusion Medicine	Hematology	Telen, Marilyn J (MD)	287
Transfusion Medicine	Pathology	Kao, Kuo-Jang (MD/PhD)	539
Transgender Surgery	Plastic Surgery	Meltzer, Toby R (MD)	653
Transplant Immunology	Pediatric Gastroenterology	McDiarmid, Suzanne V (MD)	582
Transplant Medicine-Heart	Cardiology (Cardiovascular Disease)	Bourge, Robert Charles (MD)	130
Transplant Medicine-Heart	Cardiology (Cardiovascular Disease)	Brozena, Susan Celia (MD)	124
Transplant Medicine-Heart	Cardiology (Cardiovascular Disease)	Cody Jr., Robert James (MD)	134
Transplant Medicine-Heart	Cardiology (Cardiovascular Disease)	Costanzo, Maria Rosa (MD)	134
Transplant Medicine-Heart	Cardiology (Cardiovascular Disease)	Eisen, Howard J (MD)	125
Transplant Medicine-Heart	Cardiology (Cardiovascular Disease)	Fishbein, Daniel P (MD)	141
Transplant Medicine-Heart	Cardiology (Cardiovascular Disease)	Hunt, Sharon Ann (MD)	142
Transplant Medicine-Heart	Cardiology (Cardiovascular Disease)	Johnson, Maryl R (MD)	136
Transplant Medicine-Heart	Cardiology (Cardiovascular Disease)	Kobashigawa, Jon Akira (MD)	142
Transplant Medicine-Heart	Cardiology (Cardiovascular Disease)	Konstam, Marvin Amnon (MD)	121
Transplant Medicine-Heart	Cardiology (Cardiovascular Disease)	Lindenfeld, JoAnn (MD)	139
Transplant Medicine-Heart	Cardiology (Cardiovascular Disease)	Massin, Edward Krauss (MD)	140
Transplant Medicine-Heart	Cardiology (Cardiovascular Disease)	Rogers, Joseph (MD)	137
Transplant Medicine-Heart	Pediatric Cardiology	Beerman, Lee (MD)	561
Transplant Medicine-Heart	Pediatric Cardiology	Bernstein, Daniel (MD)	567
Transplant Medicine-Heart	Pediatric Cardiology	Boucek, Mark M. (MD)	566
Transplant Medicine-Heart	Pediatric Cardiology	Boucek, Robert (MD)	562
Transplant Medicine-Heart	Pediatric Cardiology	Bricker, John Timothy (MD)	566
Transplant Medicine-Heart	Pediatric Cardiology	Caldwell, Randall (MD)	564
Transplant Medicine-Heart	Pediatric Cardiology	Colvin, Edward V (MD)	563
Transplant Medicine-Heart	Pediatric Cardiology	Fricker, Frederick Jay (MD)	563
Transplant Medicine-Heart	Pediatric Cardiology	Porter, Co-burn Joseph (MD)	565
Transplant Medicine-Heart	Thoracic Surgery	Oz, Mehmet Cengiz (MD)	810
Transplant Medicine-Heart	Thoracic Surgery	Piccione, William (MD)	819
Transplant Medicine-Heart	Thoracic Surgery	Quintessenza, James (MD)	814
Transplant Medicine-Heart	Thoracic Surgery	Tedder, Mark (MD)	815
Transplant Medicine-Heart & Lung	Pulmonary Disease	Theodore, James (MD)	713
Transplant Medicine-Intestine	Pediatric Gastroenterology	McDiarmid, Suzanne V (MD)	582
Transplant Medicine-Kidney	Nephrology	Amend Jr, William JC (MD)	368
Transplant Medicine-Kidney	Nephrology	Barcenas, Camilo Gustavo (MD)	367
Transplant Medicine-Kidney	Nephrology	Bennett, William M (MD)	368
Transplant Medicine-Kidney	Nephrology	Carpenter, Charles B (MD)	359
Transplant Medicine-Kidney	Nephrology	Coffman, Thomas Myron (MD)	363
Transplant Medicine-Kidney	Nephrology	Cohen, David (MD)	360
Transplant Medicine-Kidney	Nephrology	Dosa, Stefan (MD)	361
Transplant Medicine-Kidney	Nephrology	Friedman, Eli A (MD)	361
Transplant Medicine-Kidney	Nephrology	Gluck, Stephen (MD)	363
Transplant Medicine-Kidney	Nephrology	Josephson, Michelle Ann (MD)	365
Transplant Medicine-Kidney	Nephrology	Kasiske, Bertram (MD)	365

SPECIAL EXPERTISE INDEX

Special Expertise	Specialty	Doctor's Name	Page
Transplant Medicine-Lung	Pulmonary Disease	Young, Keith Randall (MD)	701
Transplant Patients	Child & Adolescent Psychiatry	Sexson, Sandra G B (MD)	667
Transplant-Gastrointestinal	Surgery	Tzakis, Andreas (MD)	792
Transplant-Heart	Thoracic Surgery	Acker, Michael Andrew (MD)	807
Transplant-Heart	Thoracic Surgery	Alexander, James A (MD)	812
Transplant-Heart	Thoracic Surgery	Bolman III, Ralph Morton (MD)	816
Transplant-Heart	Thoracic Surgery	Conte Jr, John V (MD)	808
Transplant-Heart	Thoracic Surgery	Copeland III, Jack G (MD)	821
Transplant-Heart	Thoracic Surgery	Elefteriades, John (MD)	805
Transplant-Heart	Thoracic Surgery	Frazier, Oscar Howard (MD)	821
Transplant-Heart	Thoracic Surgery	Furukawa, Satoshi (MD)	808
Transplant-Heart	Thoracic Surgery	Griffith, Bartley (MD)	809
Transplant-Heart	Thoracic Surgery	Harrell Jr, James E (MD)	821
Transplant-Heart	Thoracic Surgery	Karp, Robert Bruce (MD)	817
Transplant-Heart	Thoracic Surgery	Kormos, Robert (MD)	810
Transplant-Heart	Thoracic Surgery	Laks, Hillel (MD)	824
Transplant-Heart	Thoracic Surgery	McCarthy, Patrick McGuane (MD)	818
Transplant-Heart	Thoracic Surgery	Michler, Robert (MD)	818
Transplant-Heart	Thoracic Surgery	Noon, George P (MD)	822
Transplant-Heart	Thoracic Surgery	Pagani, Francis Domenic (MD)	818
Transplant-Heart	Thoracic Surgery	Reitz, Bruce Arnold (MD)	825
Transplant-Heart	Thoracic Surgery	Rose, Eric A (MD)	810
Transplant-Heart	Thoracic Surgery	Samuels, Louis (MD)	811
Transplant-Heart	Thoracic Surgery	Shumway, Norman Edward (MD)	825
Transplant-Heart	Thoracic Surgery	Smedira, Nicholas (MD)	819
Transplant-Heart	Thoracic Surgery	Smith, Craig R (MD)	811
Transplant-Heart	Thoracic Surgery	Trento, Alfredo (MD)	825
Transplant-Heart & Lung	Pediatric Surgery	Spray, Thomas L (MD)	612
Transplant-Heart & Lung	Thoracic Surgery	McGregor, Christopher (MD)	818
Transplant-Heart & Lung	Thoracic Surgery	Staples, Edward D (MD)	814
Transplant-Heart & Lung	Thoracic Surgery	Sundt III, Thoralf Mauritz (MD)	820
Transplant-Heart & Lung	Thoracic Surgery	Turrentine, Mark W (MD)	820
Transplant-Heart-Infant	Thoracic Surgery	Bailey, Leonard Lee (MD)	823
Transplant-Heart-Pediatric	Thoracic Surgery	Kirklin, James (MD)	813
Transplant-Heart-Pediatric	Thoracic Surgery	Starnes, Vaughn Alden (MD)	825
Transplant-Kidney & Pancreas	Surgery	Auchincloss Jr, Hugh (MD)	781
Transplant-Kidney-Pediatric	Urology	Koyle, Martin Allan (MD)	845
Transplant-Liver	Surgery	Ascher, Nancy L (MD)	799
Transplant-Liver	Surgery	Brems, John (MD)	793
Transplant-Liver	Surgery	Busuttil, Ronald Wilfred (MD/PhD)	799
Transplant-Liver	Surgery	Ellison, Edwin Christopher (MD)	793
Transplant-Liver	Surgery	Emond, Jean Crawford (MD)	785
Transplant-Liver	Surgery	Esquivel, Carlos Orlando (MD)	800
Transplant-Liver	Surgery	Fung, John J (MD/PhD)	786
Transplant-Liver	Surgery	Halff, Glenn Alexander (MD)	797
Transplant-Liver	Surgery	Howard, Richard J (MD)	791
Transplant-Liver	Surgery	Jenkins, Roger L (MD)	781
Transplant-Liver	Surgery	Karrer, Frederick Merrill (MD)	796
Transplant-Liver	Surgery	Miller, Charles (MD)	787
Transplant-Liver	Surgery	Millis, J. Michael (MD)	794
Transplant-Liver	Surgery	Rosen, Charles Burke (MD)	795
Transplant-Liver	Surgery	Salem, Ronald (MD)	782
Transplant-Liver	Surgery	Shaw Jr, Byers Wendell (MD)	796
Transplant-Liver	Surgery	Teperman, Lewis William (MD)	789
Transplant-Liver	Surgery	Tzakis, Andreas (MD)	792
Transplant-Liver	Surgery	Wood, R Patrick (MD)	799
Transplant-Lung	Surgery	Kirby, Thomas (MD)	794
Transplant-Lung	Thoracic Surgery	Alexander, James A (MD)	812
Transplant-Lung	Thoracic Surgery	Bavaria, Joseph (MD)	807
Transplant-Lung	Thoracic Surgery	Conte Jr, John V (MD)	808

Special Expertise	Specialty	Doctor's Name	Page
Transplant-Lung	Thoracic Surgery	Cooper, Joel David (MD)	816
Transplant-Lung	Thoracic Surgery	Egan, Thomas (MD)	812
Transplant-Lung	Thoracic Surgery	Furukawa, Satoshi (MD)	808
Transplant-Lung	Thoracic Surgery	Iannettoni, Mark D. (MD)	817
Transplant-Lung	Thoracic Surgery	Keenan, Robert (MD)	809
Transplant-Lung	Thoracic Surgery	Kron, Irving L (MD)	813
Transplant-Lung	Thoracic Surgery	Noon, George P (MD)	822
Transplant-Lung	Thoracic Surgery	Patterson, George Alexander (MD)	819
Transplant-Lung	Thoracic Surgery	Shumway, Norman Edward (MD)	825
Transplant-Lung	Thoracic Surgery	Smedira, Nicholas (MD)	819
Transplant-Lung	Thoracic Surgery	Wain, John (MD)	806
Transplant-Lung	Thoracic Surgery	Zorn, George L. (MD)	815
Transplant-Ovarian Tissue	Reproductive Endocrinology	Oktay, Kutluk (MD)	745
Transplant-Pancreas	Surgery	Bartlett, Stephen Thomas (MD)	783
Transplant-Pancreas	Surgery	Bollinger, R Randal (MD/PhD)	790
Transplant-Pancreas	Surgery	Miller, Joshua (MD)	791
Transplant-Pancreas	Surgery	Millis, J. Michael (MD)	794
Transplant-Pancreas	Surgery	Monaco, Anthony (MD)	782
Transplant-Pancreas	Surgery	Shapiro, Ron (MD)	788
Transplant-Pancreas	Surgery	Sollinger, Hans W (MD)	795
Transplant-Pancreas	Surgery	Stratta, Robert (MD)	792
Transplant-Pancreas	Surgery	Sutherland, David (MD)	796
Transplant-Pancreas/Liver	Surgery	Newell, Kenneth (MD/PhD)	795
Transplant-Pancreas/Liver	Surgery	Thistlethwaite, J Richard (MD)	796
Transplant-Pediatric	Surgery	Najarian, John S (MD)	794
Transplant-Pediatric	Surgery	Thistlethwaite, J Richard (MD)	796
Transplant-Small Bowel	Surgery	Newell, Kenneth (MD/PhD)	795
Transplant-Toe to Hand	Plastic Surgery	Levin, L Scott (MD)	643
Trauma	Orthopaedic Surgery	Beaty, James Harold (MD)	485
Trauma	Orthopaedic Surgery	Bucholz, Robert (MD)	494
Trauma	Orthopaedic Surgery	Burgess, Andrew (MD)	479
Trauma	Orthopaedic Surgery	Delahay, John Norris (MD)	479
Trauma	Orthopaedic Surgery	Helfet, David L (MD)	481
Trauma	Orthopaedic Surgery	Swiontkowski, Marc F (MD)	493
Trauma	Orthopaedic Surgery	Webb, Lawrence (MD)	488
Trauma	Pediatric Critical Care Medicine	Fleisher, Gary Robert (MD)	569
Trauma	Pediatric Surgery	Reynolds, Marleta (MD)	615
Trauma	Pediatric Surgery	Stylianos, Steven (MD)	613
Trauma	Physical Medicine & Rehabilitation	Sisung, Charles (MD)	628
Trauma	Surgery	Baker, Christopher (MD)	789
Trauma	Surgery	Cioffi, William (MD)	781
Trauma	Surgery	Deitch, Edwin (MD)	785
Trauma	Surgery	Hoyt, David (MD)	800
Trauma	Surgery	Knudson, Mary Margaret (MD)	800
Trauma	Surgery	Peitzman, Andrew (MD)	787
Trauma	Surgery	Stewart, Ronald Mack (MD)	799
Trauma	Urology	McAninch, Jack (MD)	849
Trauma	Vascular Surgery (General)	Johansen, Kaj (MD/PhD)	869
Trauma Neurology	Neurology	Ropper, Allan (MD)	398
Trauma Psychiatry	Child & Adolescent Psychiatry	Bleiberg, Efrain (MD)	669
Trauma Psychiatry	Child & Adolescent Psychiatry	Terr, Lenore Cagen (MD)	670
Trauma Psychiatry	Psychiatry	Loewenstein, Richard (MD)	680
Trauma-Brain Injury	Neurological Surgery	Marion, Donald W (MD)	378
Trauma-Cardiac	Surgery	Lewis Jr., Frank R. (MD)	794
Trauma-Complex	Surgery	Lewis Jr., Frank R. (MD)	794
Trauma-Pulmonary	Surgery	Lewis Jr., Frank R. (MD)	794
Trauma/Critical Care	Surgery	Gamelli, Richard Louis (MD)	793
Travel Medicine	Infectious Disease	Corey, G Ralph (MD)	323
Travel Medicine	Infectious Disease	Guerrant, Richard (MD)	323
Travel Medicine	Infectious Disease	Johnson, Warren (MD)	320

SPECIAL EXPERTISE INDEX

SPECIAL EXPERTISE INDEX

Special Expertise	Specialty	Doctor's Name	Page
Vascular & Interventional Radiology	Radiology	Kandarpa, Krishna (MD)	736
Vascular & Interventional Radiology	Radiology	Kumpe, David A (MD)	738
Vascular Access	Surgery	Auchincloss Jr, Hugh (MD)	781
Vascular Access	Vascular Surgery (General)	Johansen, Kaj (MD/PhD)	869
Vascular Birthmarks	Dermatology	Mihm Jr., Martin C. (MD)	182
Vascular Disease in the Elderly	Vascular Surgery (General)	Corson, John (MD)	865
Vascular Graft Infection	Vascular Surgery (General)	Bandyk, Dennis (MD)	863
Vascular Lesions-Head & Neck	Otolaryngology	Suen, James (MD)	520
Vascular Malformations	Dermatology	Levy, Moise (MD)	192
Vascular Malformations	Otolaryngology	Waner, Milton (MD)	520
Vascular Malformations	Plastic Surgery	Bauer, Bruce (MD)	645
Vascular Malformations	Plastic Surgery	Mulliken, John B. (MD)	635
Vascular Medicine	Cardiology (Cardiovascular Disease)	Dzau, Victor J (MD)	121
Vascular Medicine	Cardiology (Cardiovascular Disease)	Moses, Jeffrey W (MD)	127
Vascular Medicine	Internal Medicine	Weder, Alan B (MD)	336
Vascular Neurosurgery	Neurological Surgery	Dacey Jr., Ralph Gerald (MD)	383
Vascular Neurosurgery	Neurological Surgery	Hodge Jr., Charles J. (MD)	376
Vascular Neurosurgery	Neurological Surgery	Malik, Ghaus (MD)	384
Vascular Neurosurgery	Neurological Surgery	Piepgras, David (MD)	385
Vascular Neurosurgery	Neurological Surgery	Samson, Duke (MD)	387
Vascular Neurosurgery	Neurological Surgery	Spetzler, Robert (MD)	387
Vascular Reconstruction	Vascular Surgery (General)	Cherry Jr., Kenneth J. (MD)	864
Vascular Surgery	Surgery	Burdick, James Frederick (MD)	784
Vascular Surgery	Thoracic Surgery	Acinapura, Anthony (MD)	807
Vascular Surgery	Thoracic Surgery	Coselli, Joseph Stapleton (MD)	821
Vascular Surgery	Thoracic Surgery	Kiernan, Paul Chapman (MD)	813
Vasculitis	Nephrology	Falk, Ronald J (MD)	363
Vasculitis	Pediatric Rheumatology	Myones, Barry Lee (MD)	609
Vasculitis	Rheumatology	Barr, Walter Gerard (MD)	763
Vasculitis	Rheumatology	Cupps, Thomas R (MD)	758
Vasculitis	Rheumatology	Hoffman, Gary Stuart (MD)	764
Vasculitis	Rheumatology	Katz, Paul (MD)	759
Vasculitis	Rheumatology	Stimmler, Mary McMillen (MD)	770
Vasculitis	Rheumatology	Wener, Mark (MD)	770
Vasectomy Reversal	Urology	Belker, Arnold (MD)	837
Vasectomy Reversal	Urology	Fuchs, Eugene F (MD)	848
Vasectomy Reversal	Urology	Goldstein, Marc (MD)	832
Vasectomy Reversal	Urology	Oates, Robert Davis (MD)	830
Vasectomy Reversal	Urology	Thomas, Anthony J. (MD)	844
Vasectomy-Scalpelless	Urology	Goldstein, Marc (MD)	832
Vein Disease	Vascular Surgery (General)	Bergan, John Jerome (MD)	868
Vein Disease	Vascular Surgery (General)	Gloviczki, Peter (MD)	865
Vein Disease	Vascular Surgery (General)	Sobel, Michael (MD)	861
Vein Disease/Leg Ulcers	Vascular Surgery (General)	Bergan, John Jerome (MD)	868
Ventilator Dependent Children	Pediatric Pulmonology	Redding , Gregory (MD)	607
Ventricular Assist Devices	Thoracic Surgery	Staples, Edward D (MD)	814
Ventricular Tachycardia	Cardiac Electrophysiology	Wilber, David James (MD)	118
Vertigo	Otolaryngology	Pensak, Myles (MD)	516
Viral Infections	Infectious Disease	Luby, James P (MD)	327
Viral Infections	Infectious Disease	Van Der Horst, Charles (MD)	325
Viral Infections	Pediatric Infectious Disease	Mitchell, Charles (MD)	592
Vision Development	Ophthalmology	France, Thomas D (MD)	457
Vision-Unexplained Loss	Ophthalmology	Borchert, Mark S (MD)	463
Vitamin B-12 Metabolism	Geriatric Medicine	Groene, Linda A (MD)	246
Vitiligo	Dermatology	Bystryn, Jean-Claude (MD)	183
Vitiligo	Dermatology	Nigra, Thomas P (MD)	185
Vocal Cord Disorders	Otolaryngology	Benninger, Michael S (MD)	512
Vocal Cord Disorders	Pulmonary Disease	Martin, Richard Jay (MD)	707
Voice Disorders	Otolaryngology	Aviv, Jonathan (MD)	502
Voice Disorders	Otolaryngology	Berke, Gerald Spencer (MD)	521

SPECIAL EXPERTISE INDEX

Special Expertise	Specialty	Doctor's Name	Page
Voice Disorders	Otolaryngology	Cassisi, Nicholas J (MD)	508
Voice Disorders	Otolaryngology	Ford, Charles N (MD)	513
Voice Disorders	Otolaryngology	Koufman, James Alan (MD)	509
Voice Disorders	Otolaryngology	Postma, Gregory N (MD)	510
Voice Disorders	Otolaryngology	Sinha, Uttam Kumar (MD)	523
Voice Disorders	Otolaryngology	Weissler, Mark Christian (MD)	512
Voice Disorders	Otolaryngology	Woo, Peak (MD)	507
Voice Disorders	Otolaryngology	Woodson, Gayle Ellen (MD)	512
Voice Disorders	Otolaryngology	Zeitels, Steven (MD)	502
Voice Disorders	Pediatric Otolaryngology	Inglis, Andrew (MD)	603
Voice Disorders	Pediatric Otolaryngology	Katz, Robert L (MD)	602
Voice/Swallowing Disorders	Otolaryngology	Sasaki, Clarence T (MD)	501
Voiding Dysfunction	Geriatric Medicine	Resnick, Neil M. (MD)	243
Voiding Dysfunction	Urology	Bloom, David A (MD)	841
Voiding Dysfunction	Urology	Broderick, Gregory (MD)	837
Voiding Dysfunction	Urology	Kennelly, Michael Joseph (MD)	838
Voiding Dysfunction	Urology	Levitt, Selwyn (MD)	833
Voiding Dysfunction	Urology	Milam, Douglas F (MD)	838
Voiding Dysfunction	Urology	Nitti, Victor (MD)	834
Voiding Dysfunction	Urology	Stone, Anthony (MD)	851
Voiding Dysfunction	Urology	Winters, Jack Christian (MD)	847
Von Willebrand's Disease	Hematology	Bockenstedt, Paula (MD)	288
Vulva Disease/Neoplasia	Gynecologic Oncology	Fowler Jr, Wesley C (MD)	258
Vulva Disease/Neoplasia	Obstetrics & Gynecology	Amstey, Marvin S. (MD)	431
Vulva Disease/Neoplasia	Obstetrics & Gynecology	Galask, Rudolph P. (MD)	435

W

Wegener's Granulomatosis	Pulmonary Disease	Hansen-Flaschen, John (MD)	693
West Nile Virus	Infectious Disease	Rahal, James (MD)	321
White Cell Defects(Agranulocytosis)	Infectious Disease	Mandell, Gerald (MD)	324
Williams Syndrome	Clinical Genetics	Morris, Colleen A. (MD)	165
Women's Health	Internal Medicine	Seremetis, Stephanie (MD)	334
Women's Health	Medical Oncology	Chlebowski, Rowan T (MD/PhD)	313
Women's Health-Mental Health	Psychiatry	Burt, Vivien Kleinman (MD/PhD)	686
Women's Health-Mental Health	Psychiatry	Zerbe, Kathryn J (MD)	685
Women's Medicine	Pain Management	Smith, Joanne (MD)	530
Women's Radiology	Diagnostic Radiology	Edelstein, Barbara A (MD)	731
Wound Healing/Care	Dermatology	Burton III, Claude Shreve (MD)	186
Wound Healing/Care	Dermatology	Eaglstein, William (MD)	187
Wound Healing/Care	Dermatology	Fivenson, David (MD)	189
Wound Healing/Care	Plastic Surgery	Mustoe, Thomas (MD)	646
Wound Healing/Care	Surgery	Saffle, Jeffrey (MD)	796
Wound Healing/Care	Surgery	Yurt, Roger (MD)	789
Wound Healing/Care	Vascular Surgery (General)	Steed, David Luther (MD)	862
WPW Syndrome	Cardiac Electrophysiology	Morady, Fred (MD)	117
Wrist Arthroscopy	Orthopaedic Surgery	Osterman Jr, Arthur Lee (MD)	482
Wrist Surgery	Hand Surgery	Hunt III, Thomas (MD)	272
Wrist Surgery	Hand Surgery	Melone Jr, Charles P (MD)	268
Wrist/Hand Injuries	Hand Surgery	Cooney, William (MD)	271
Wrist/Hand Injuries	Hand Surgery	Koman, L Andrew (MD)	270
Wrist/Hand Injuries	Hand Surgery	Taleisnik, Julio (MD)	276
Wrist/Hand Injuries	Hand Surgery	Weiland, Andrew J (MD)	269

Y

Yeast Infection-Chronic	Obstetrics & Gynecology	Hager, William David (MD)	434

ALPHABETICAL LISTING OF DOCTORS

Name	Specialty	Page
A		
Aaberg Sr, Thomas Marshall (MD)	Ophthalmology	451
Aamoth, Gordon (MD)	Orthopaedic Surgery	489
Aaronson, Donald W (MD)	Allergy & Immunology	99
Abbott, William Martin (MD)	Vascular Surgery (General)	857
Abbruzzese, James L (MD)	Medical Oncology	310
Abcarian, Herand (MD)	Colon & Rectal Surgery	173
Abella, Esteban (MD)	Pediatric Hematology-Oncology	586
Abeloff, Martin (MD)	Medical Oncology	294
Abittan, Meyer H (MD)	Cardiology (Cardiovascular Disease)	123
Abram, Stephen Edward (MD)	Pain Management	530
Abrams, Donald Ira (MD)	Medical Oncology	312
Abrams, Gary W (MD)	Ophthalmology	455
Abramson, Allan (MD)	Otolaryngology	502
Abramson, David Harold (MD)	Ophthalmology	444
Abramson, Edward G (MD)	Urology	836
Abramson, Steven B (MD)	Rheumatology	757
Abrass, Itamar (MD)	Geriatric Medicine	250
Abright, Arthur Reese (MD)	Child & Adolescent Psychiatry	664
Accurso, Frank J (MD)	Pediatric Pulmonology	605
Achkar, Edgar (MD)	Gastroenterology	230
Achuff, Stephen Charles (MD)	Cardiology (Cardiovascular Disease)	123
Acinapura, Anthony (MD)	Thoracic Surgery	807
Acker, David B. (MD)	Maternal & Fetal Medicine	341
Acker, Michael Andrew (MD)	Thoracic Surgery	807
Ackerman, A Bernard (MD)	Dermatology	182
Adams Jr., Harlold Pomeroy (MD)	Neurology	411
Adams, Elaine (MD)	Rheumatology	763
Adams, James M (MD)	Neonatal-Perinatal Medicine	354
Adams, Robert Joseph (MD)	Neurology	407
Adashi, Eli Y (MD)	Reproductive Endocrinology	750
Adelman, Mark (MD)	Vascular Surgery (General)	858
Adkins, John Crawford (MD)	Pediatric Surgery	611
Adkinson, Franklin (MD)	Allergy & Immunology	95
Adler Jr, John R (MD)	Neurological Surgery	388
Adler, Solomon Stanley (MD)	Hematology	287
Adornato, Bruce T. (MD)	Neurology	418
Adzick, Nick Scott (MD)	Pediatric Surgery	611
Agarwala, Brojendra (MD)	Pediatric Cardiology	564
Ahlgren, James David (MD)	Medical Oncology	294
Ahlskog, J. Eric (MD)	Neurology	411
Ahmad, Suhail (MD)	Nephrology	368
Ahn, Jung Hwan (MD)	Physical Medicine & Rehabilitation	623
Ahn, Samuel S (MD)	Vascular Surgery (General)	868
Aiello, Lloyd (MD)	Ophthalmology	443
Aiken, John Judson (MD)	Surgery	793

ALPHABETICAL LISTING OF DOCTORS

Name	Specialty	Page
Aisner, Joseph (MD)	Medical Oncology	294
Akins, Cary W (MD)	Thoracic Surgery	805
Al-Mefty, Ossama (MD)	Neurological Surgery	386
Alander, Dirk Huntley (MD)	Orthopaedic Surgery	489
Alavi, Abass (MD)	Nuclear Medicine	425
Alazraki, Naomi Parver (MD)	Nuclear Medicine	426
Albain, Kathy (MD)	Medical Oncology	305
Albala, David Mois (MD)	Urology	840
Albers, Gregory William (MD)	Neurology	418
Albert, Daniel M. (MD)	Ophthalmology	456
Albertson, David Allen (MD)	Surgery	789
Albertson, Timothy (MD/PhD)	Pulmonary Disease	709
Albright, Leland (MD)	Neurological Surgery	374
Alessi, Norman E (MD)	Child & Adolescent Psychiatry	668
Alexander, James A (MD)	Thoracic Surgery	812
Alexander, Richard B (MD)	Urology	830
Alexander, Steven R (MD)	Pediatric Nephrology	598
Alexopoulos, George (MD)	Psychiatry	677
Alfonso, Antonio (MD)	Surgery	783
Alfonso, Eduardo (MD)	Ophthalmology	451
Alford, Bobby R (MD)	Otolaryngology	518
Allen, David Bruce (MD)	Pediatric Endocrinology	575
Allen, Nancy B (MD)	Rheumatology	761
Alleyn, James (MD)	Gynecologic Oncology	257
Alpern, Robert (MD)	Nephrology	367
Alster, Tina (MD)	Dermatology	182
Altchek, David (MD)	Sports Medicine	773
Altshuler, Kenneth Z. (MD)	Psychiatry	685
Alward, Wallace (MD)	Ophthalmology	456
Ambrose, John (MD)	Cardiology (Cardiovascular Disease)	123
Amend Jr, William JC (MD)	Nephrology	368
Aminoff, Michael J (MD)	Neurology	419
Amonette, Rex A (MD)	Dermatology	186
Amstey, Marvin S. (MD)	Obstetrics & Gynecology	431
Anand, Kanwaljeet Singh (MD/PhD)	Pediatric Critical Care Medicine	571
Andersen, Arnold (MD)	Psychiatry	683
Anderson, Douglas R (MD)	Ophthalmology	452
Anderson, Joseph (MD)	Medical Oncology	305
Anderson, Karl (MD)	Gastroenterology	235
Anderson, Kathryn D (MD)	Pediatric Surgery	615
Anderson, Lesley J (MD)	Orthopaedic Surgery	496
Anderson, Mark (MD)	Cardiac Electrophysiology	116
Anderson, Martin Mathew (MD)	Adolescent Medicine	90
Anderson, Richard Rox (MD)	Dermatology	181
Andiman, Warren A. (MD)	Pediatric Infectious Disease	590
Andreoli, Sharon (MD)	Pediatric Nephrology	596
Andrews, James R (MD)	Sports Medicine	773
Andros, George (MD)	Vascular Surgery (General)	868
Ang, Kie-Kian (MD/PhD)	Radiation Oncology	725
Anhalt, Grant James (MD)	Dermatology	182
Anscher, Mitchell (MD)	Radiation Oncology	721
Antakli, Tamim (MD)	Thoracic Surgery	820

Name	Specialty	Page
Antin, Joseph Harry (MD)	Medical Oncology	292
Antman, Karen (MD)	Medical Oncology	294
Antonelli, Patrick (MD)	Otolaryngology	507
Antony, Veena B. (MD)	Pulmonary Disease	702
Anyane-Yeboa, Kwame (MD)	Clinical Genetics	159
Apatoff, Brian R (MD/PhD)	Neurology	399
Appel, Gerald (MD)	Nephrology	360
Appelman, Henry (MD)	Pathology	540
Applegate, Robert Joseph (MD)	Interventional Cardiology	144
Applegate, William (MD)	Geriatric Medicine	245
Apuzzo, Michael L J (MD)	Neurological Surgery	388
Archer, Gordon Lee (MD)	Infectious Disease	322
Archer, Steven M (MD)	Ophthalmology	456
Arend, Wiiliam Phelps (MD)	Rheumatology	766
Argenta, Louis Charles (MD)	Plastic Surgery	641
Argyros, Thomas (MD)	Rheumatology	758
Ariyan, Stephan (MD)	Plastic Surgery	635
Armitage, James (MD)	Medical Oncology	310
Armon, Carmel (MD)	Neurology	419
Armstrong, William F (MD)	Cardiology (Cardiovascular Disease)	133
Arnason, Barry G W (MD)	Neurology	411
Arndt, Kenneth (MD)	Dermatology	181
Arnett Jr, Frank Couchman (MD)	Rheumatology	767
Arnold, Anthony C (MD)	Ophthalmology	463
Arnold, Phillip (MD)	Plastic Surgery	645
Aron, Alan (MD)	Child Neurology	151
Aronchick, Craig Alan (MD)	Gastroenterology	222
Aronian, Dianne D (MD)	Ophthalmology	444
Aronson, James (MD)	Orthopaedic Surgery	494
Aronson, Peter Samuel (MD)	Nephrology	359
Arriaga, Moises Alberto (MD)	Otolaryngology	502
Arroliga, Alejandro C (MD)	Pulmonary Disease	702
Asbury, Arthur K (MD)	Neurology	399
Ascher, Enrico (MD)	Vascular Surgery (General)	858
Ascher, Nancy L (MD)	Surgery	799
Aseff, John Namer (MD)	Physical Medicine & Rehabilitation	623
Ashburn, Michael (MD)	Pain Management	530
Ashikari, Roy (MD)	Surgery	783
Ashwal, Stephen (MD)	Child Neurology	155
Assimos, Dean George (MD)	Urology	836
Aston, Sherrell (MD)	Plastic Surgery	636
Atkins, Paul Charles (MD)	Allergy & Immunology	95
Atkinson, James B (MD)	Pediatric Surgery	616
Atkinson, John (MD)	Neurological Surgery	382
Atlas, Scott W (MD)	Radiology	739
Atnip, Robert (MD)	Vascular Surgery (General)	859
Attinger, Chris (MD)	Plastic Surgery	636
Auchincloss Jr, Hugh (MD)	Surgery	781
Austen, W. Gerald (MD)	Thoracic Surgery	805
Austin, John (MD)	Diagnostic Radiology	731
Auwaerter, Paul (MD)	Infectious Disease	317
Aviv, Jonathan (MD)	Otolaryngology	502

ALPHABETICAL LISTING OF DOCTORS

Name	Specialty	Page
Avner, Ellis D (MD)	Pediatric Nephrology	597
Awad, Issam A (MD)	Neurological Surgery	373
Axelrod, Deborah (MD)	Surgery	783
Axelrod, Lloyd (MD)	Endocrinology, Diabetes & Metabolism	197
Azziz, Ricardo (MD)	Reproductive Endocrinology	746

B

Name	Specialty	Page
Bach Jr, Bernard R (MD)	Orthopaedic Surgery	489
Bach, John (MD)	Physical Medicine & Rehabilitation	623
Bacon, Bruce (MD)	Gastroenterology	230
Bahn, Rebecca Sue (MD)	Endocrinology, Diabetes & Metabolism	206
Bahna, Sami Labib (MD)	Pediatric Allergy & Immunology	556
Bahnson, Robert (MD)	Urology	840
Bailey, Byron J (MD)	Otolaryngology	518
Bailey, Harold Randolph (MD)	Colon & Rectal Surgery	176
Bailey, Leonard Lee (MD)	Thoracic Surgery	823
Bailey, Steven Roderick (MD)	Interventional Cardiology	147
Bailin, Philip Lawrence (MD)	Dermatology	188
Baim, Howard (MD)	Otolaryngology	512
Bains, Manjit (MD)	Thoracic Surgery	807
Baker Jr, James L (MD)	Plastic Surgery	641
Baker Jr, Thomas J (MD)	Plastic Surgery	641
Baker Jr., James Russell (MD)	Allergy & Immunology	100
Baker, Carol (MD)	Pediatric Infectious Disease	593
Baker, Christopher (MD)	Surgery	789
Baker, Daniel (MD)	Plastic Surgery	636
Baker, John D (MD)	Ophthalmology	456
Baker, Laurence H (DO)	Medical Oncology	305
Baker, Shan Ray (MD)	Otolaryngology	512
Baker, William (MD)	Vascular Surgery (General)	864
Bakken, Johan Septimus (MD)	Infectious Disease	325
Balady, Gary (MD)	Cardiology (Cardiovascular Disease)	120
Balch, Charles (MD)	Surgery	789
Balderston, Richard (MD)	Orthopaedic Surgery	477
Baldessarini, Ross (MD)	Psychiatry	676
Balducci, Lodovico (MD)	Medical Oncology	300
Bale Jr, James (MD)	Child Neurology	154
Balk, Robert (MD)	Pulmonary Disease	702
Balkany, Thomas Jay (MD)	Otolaryngology	507
Ball, Edward David (MD)	Medical Oncology	313
Ballard, Pamela H (MD)	Physical Medicine & Rehabilitation	623
Ballenger, James (MD)	Psychiatry	682
Ballon-Landa, Gonzalo (MD)	Infectious Disease	328
Balmes, John Randolph (MD)	Pulmonary Disease	710
Baltuch, Gordon (MD/PhD)	Neurological Surgery	374
Bancalari, Eduardo (MD)	Neonatal-Perinatal Medicine	352
Bander, Neil (MD)	Urology	830
Bandyk, Dennis (MD)	Vascular Surgery (General)	863
Banks, Peter (MD)	Pathology	539
Banks, Peter Alan (MD)	Gastroenterology	221
Baraniuk, James N (MD)	Allergy & Immunology	95
Baratz, Mark E (MD)	Orthopaedic Surgery	478

Name	Specialty	Page
Barber, Douglas Byron (MD)	Physical Medicine & Rehabilitation	629
Barbieri, Robert (MD)	Reproductive Endocrinology	743
Barbosa, Jerry L (MD)	Pediatric Hematology-Oncology	585
Barcenas, Camilo Gustavo (MD)	Nephrology	367
Bardeguez-Brown, Arlene D (MD)	Maternal & Fetal Medicine	341
Bardot, Stephen F (MD)	Urology	845
Barkin, Jamie (MD)	Gastroenterology	226
Barlogie, Bartholomew (MD/PhD)	Hematology	290
Barnes, Randall B (MD)	Reproductive Endocrinology	748
Barnes, Willard (MD)	Gynecologic Oncology	255
Barnett, Gene H (MD)	Neurological Surgery	382
Barnhart, William (MD)	Geriatric Medicine	247
Baron, Joseph M (MD)	Hematology	288
Barr, Mark Lee (MD)	Cardiology (Cardiovascular Disease)	140
Barr, Walter Gerard (MD)	Rheumatology	763
Barrett, Douglas John (MD)	Pediatric Allergy & Immunology	556
Barrett, Eugene Joseph (MD)	Endocrinology, Diabetes & Metabolism	203
Barry, Michele (MD)	Internal Medicine	333
Bartelsmeyer, James (MD)	Maternal & Fetal Medicine	344
Barter, James (MD)	Gynecologic Oncology	255
Bartlett, John A (MD)	Infectious Disease	322
Bartlett, John Gill (MD)	Infectious Disease	318
Bartlett, Scott P (MD)	Plastic Surgery	636
Bartlett, Stephen Thomas (MD)	Surgery	783
Bartolozzi, Arthur R. (MD)	Orthopaedic Surgery	478
Barton Jr, Fritz (MD)	Plastic Surgery	648
Bashore, Thomas (MD)	Cardiology (Cardiovascular Disease)	129
Basler, Joseph W (MD)	Urology	845
Bass, Barbara (MD)	Surgery	784
Bass, Theodore Adam (MD)	Cardiology (Cardiovascular Disease)	129
Bassett, Joseph (MD)	Thoracic Surgery	815
Bateman, Jane Bronwyn (MD)	Ophthalmology	461
Batjer, H. Hunt (MD)	Neurological Surgery	382
Batsford, William P (MD)	Cardiology (Cardiovascular Disease)	120
Batzdorf, Ulrich (MD)	Neurological Surgery	388
Bauer, Bruce (MD)	Plastic Surgery	645
Bauer, Jerry (MD)	Neurological Surgery	382
Baughman, Kenneth (MD)	Cardiology (Cardiovascular Disease)	124
Bauman, Phillip (MD)	Orthopaedic Surgery	478
Baumgartner, William (MD)	Thoracic Surgery	807
Bavaria, Joseph (MD)	Thoracic Surgery	807
Baxi, Laxmi V (MD)	Obstetrics & Gynecology	431
Bayer, Arnold Sander (MD)	Infectious Disease	328
Bayless, Theodore (MD)	Gastroenterology	222
Baylis, Henry I (MD)	Ophthalmology	463
Bayly, Timothy C (MD)	Pulmonary Disease	696
Bayron, Harry (MD)	Pediatric Cardiology	562
Beal, Myron Flint (MD)	Neurology	400
Beall, Gildon N (MD)	Allergy & Immunology	103
Beall, Michael E (MD)	Urology	836
Beart Jr, Robert W (MD)	Colon & Rectal Surgery	176
Beaser, Richard Seth (MD)	Internal Medicine	333

ALPHABETICAL LISTING OF DOCTORS

Name	Specialty	Page
Beasley, Michael (MD)	Plastic Surgery	641
Beasley, Robert (MD)	Hand Surgery	267
Beaty, James Harold (MD)	Orthopaedic Surgery	485
Beauchamp, Robert Daniel (MD)	Surgery	789
Beck, David (MD)	Colon & Rectal Surgery	176
Becker, Dorothy Joan (MD)	Pediatric Endocrinology	572
Becker, Ferdinand Francis (MD)	Plastic Surgery	641
Becker, Gary J. (MD)	Radiology	737
Becker, James (MD)	Colon & Rectal Surgery	169
Beebe, Hugh Grenville (MD)	Vascular Surgery (General)	864
Beer, Alan Earl (MD)	Obstetrics & Gynecology	435
Beerman, Lee (MD)	Pediatric Cardiology	561
Behar, Victor Samuel (MD)	Cardiology (Cardiovascular Disease)	129
Behrendt, Douglas M. (MD)	Thoracic Surgery	815
Behrens, Myles (MD)	Ophthalmology	444
Belani, Chandra (MD)	Medical Oncology	294
Belenky, Walter (MD)	Pediatric Otolaryngology	602
Belinson, Jerome Leslie (MD)	Gynecologic Oncology	259
Belker, Arnold (MD)	Urology	837
Belkin, Michael (MD)	Vascular Surgery (General)	857
Bell, David S H (MD)	Endocrinology, Diabetes & Metabolism	203
Bellamy, Paul Eric (MD)	Pulmonary Disease	710
Beller, George Allan (MD)	Cardiology (Cardiovascular Disease)	129
Belman, A Barry (MD)	Urology	831
Belsky, Mark R (MD)	Hand Surgery	267
Benedetti, Thomas J (MD)	Maternal & Fetal Medicine	347
Benenati, James Francis (MD)	Radiology	737
Benenati, Susan (MD)	Allergy & Immunology	98
Benevenia, Joseph (MD)	Orthopaedic Surgery	478
Benjamin, Robert S (MD)	Medical Oncology	311
Benjamin, Stanley (MD)	Gastroenterology	222
Benjamin, Vallo (MD)	Neurological Surgery	374
Bennett, Richard Gordan (MD)	Geriatric Medicine	243
Bennett, William M (MD)	Nephrology	368
Benninger, Michael S (MD)	Otolaryngology	512
Benson, Al B (MD)	Medical Oncology	305
Benson, Carol (MD)	Radiology	735
Benson, Mitchell C (MD)	Urology	831
Bentley, David Warren (MD)	Geriatric Medicine	247
Benvenisty, Alan I (MD)	Vascular Surgery (General)	859
Benz, Edward (MD)	Hematology	285
Benzon, Honorio T (MD)	Pain Management	529
Berchuck, Andrew ()	Gynecologic Oncology	257
Berde, Charles Benjamin (MD)	Pain Management	527
Berdon, Walter (MD)	Radiology	735
Berek, Jonathan S (MD)	Gynecologic Oncology	263
Berenstein, Alejandro (MD)	Radiology	735
Berg, Christine Dorothy (MD)	Radiation Oncology	718
Berg, Daniel (MD)	Dermatology	192
Berg, Stacy (MD)	Pediatric Hematology-Oncology	588
Berga , Sarah Lee (MD)	Reproductive Endocrinology	744
Bergan, John Jerome (MD)	Vascular Surgery (General)	868

Name	Specialty	Page
Berger, Jerry (MD)	Pain Management	529
Berger, Joseph (MD)	Neurology	407
Berger, Melvin (MD/PhD)	Pediatric Allergy & Immunology	556
Berger, Mitchel Stuart (MD)	Neurological Surgery	388
Berger, Richard E (MD)	Urology	847
Bergfeld, John (MD)	Orthopaedic Surgery	489
Bergstein, Jerry (MD)	Pediatric Nephrology	597
Berguer, Ramon (MD)	Vascular Surgery (General)	864
Berke, Gerald Spencer (MD)	Otolaryngology	521
Berkowitz, Leonard B (MD)	Infectious Disease	318
Berkowitz, Richard (MD)	Obstetrics & Gynecology	432
Berkson, Richard Alan (MD)	Endocrinology, Diabetes & Metabolism	210
Berl, Tomas (MD)	Nephrology	366
Berman, Brian (MD)	Pediatrics	618
Berman, James (MD)	Pediatric Gastroenterology	580
Berman, Michael Leonard (MD)	Obstetrics & Gynecology	438
Bernad, Peter (MD)	Neurology	400
Berner, Carl Frederick (MD)	Plastic Surgery	651
Bernstein, Bram Henry (MD)	Pediatric Rheumatology	610
Bernstein, Daniel (MD)	Pediatric Cardiology	567
Bernstein, Robert M (MD)	Dermatology	183
Bhan, Atul Kumar (MD)	Pathology	535
Bieber, Eric Joseph (MD)	Reproductive Endocrinology	748
Biederman, Joseph (MD)	Child & Adolescent Psychiatry	663
Bierbaum, Benjamin (MD)	Orthopaedic Surgery	475
Biesecker, Leslie Glenn (MD)	Clinical Genetics	159
Biggs Jr, Thomas M (MD)	Plastic Surgery	648
Biglan, Albert William (MD)	Ophthalmology	444
Bigliani, Louis (MD)	Orthopaedic Surgery	478
Bilchik, Anton Joel (MD)	Surgery	799
Biller, Beverly M K (MD)	Endocrinology, Diabetes & Metabolism	197
Binder, Perry Scott (MD)	Ophthalmology	463
Bird, Hector (MD)	Child & Adolescent Psychiatry	664
Bishop, Allen Thorp (MD)	Hand Surgery	271
Bissell Jr, Dwight Montgomery (MD)	Internal Medicine	337
Bitran, Jacob (MD)	Hematology	288
Black, Henry R (MD)	Nephrology	364
Black, Keith Lanier (MD)	Neurological Surgery	388
Black, Peter (MD)	Neurological Surgery	373
Blackburn, George L (MD/PhD)	Surgery	781
Blackwell, Richard (MD)	Reproductive Endocrinology	746
Blaha, J David (MD)	Orthopaedic Surgery	478
Blaivas, Jerry G (MD)	Urology	831
Bland, Kirby (MD)	Surgery	789
Blaser, Martin Jack (MD)	Infectious Disease	318
Blasko, John Charles (MD)	Radiation Oncology	726
Blass, John (MD/PhD)	Geriatric Medicine	244
Blazer II, Dan G (MD/PhD)	Psychiatry	682
Bleday, Ronald (MD)	Colon & Rectal Surgery	169
Blei, Andres T (MD)	Gastroenterology	230
Bleiberg, Efrain (MD)	Child & Adolescent Psychiatry	669
Bleifer, Selvyn Burton (MD)	Cardiology (Cardiovascular Disease)	140

ALPHABETICAL LISTING OF DOCTORS

Name	Specialty	Page
Bleyer, W Archie (MD)	Pediatric Hematology-Oncology	588
Blinder, Morey (MD)	Hematology	288
Blitzer, Andrew (MD)	Otolaryngology	502
Bloom, David A (MD)	Urology	841
Bloom, Harrison (MD)	Geriatric Medicine	244
Bloom, Patricia (MD)	Geriatric Medicine	244
Bloomer, Joseph (MD)	Gastroenterology	226
Bluestone, Charles D (MD)	Pediatric Otolaryngology	600
Blum, Manfred (MD)	Endocrinology, Diabetes & Metabolism	198
Blum, Paul (MD)	Pediatric Allergy & Immunology	556
Blum, Robert W (MD/PhD)	Adolescent Medicine	89
Blume, Ralph (MD)	Rheumatology	758
Blumenthal, David S (MD)	Cardiology (Cardiovascular Disease)	124
Boachie, Oheneba (MD)	Orthopaedic Surgery	479
Bobrove, Arthur M (MD)	Rheumatology	768
Bockenstedt, Paula (MD)	Hematology	288
Bockman, Richard (MD/PhD)	Endocrinology, Diabetes & Metabolism	199
Boehm, Frank Henry (MD)	Maternal & Fetal Medicine	343
Bogrov, Michael (MD)	Child & Adolescent Psychiatry	665
Bohlman, Henry H (MD)	Orthopaedic Surgery	489
Boland Jr., Arthur L (MD)	Orthopaedic Surgery	475
Boles, Richard Gregory (MD)	Clinical Genetics	163
Bollen, Andrew W (MD)	Pathology	542
Bollinger, R Randal (MD/PhD)	Surgery	790
Bolman III, Ralph Morton (MD)	Thoracic Surgery	816
Bolton, Warren Kline (MD)	Nephrology	362
Boniuk, Milton (MD)	Ophthalmology	461
Bonkovsky, Herbert (MD)	Gastroenterology	221
Bonomi, Philip (MD)	Medical Oncology	305
Bonow, Robert O (MD)	Cardiology (Cardiovascular Disease)	133
Boone, Timothy Bolton (MD/PhD)	Urology	845
Booth, Robert (MD)	Orthopaedic Surgery	479
Borchert, Mark S (MD)	Ophthalmology	463
Borer, Jeffrey (MD)	Cardiology (Cardiovascular Disease)	124
Borgen, Patrick Ivan (MD)	Surgery	784
Borges, Lawrence F. (MD)	Neurological Surgery	373
Borkowsky, William (MD)	Pediatric Infectious Disease	590
Boronow, John Joseph (MD)	Psychiatry	677
Borson, Soo (MD)	Geriatric Psychiatry	674
Borzak, Steven (MD)	Cardiology (Cardiovascular Disease)	133
Bosl, George (MD)	Medical Oncology	294
Bostwick III, John J (MD)	Plastic Surgery	641
Bostwick, David (MD)	Pathology	539
Boucek, Mark M. (MD)	Pediatric Cardiology	566
Boucek, Robert (MD)	Pediatric Cardiology	562
Bourdette, Dennis (MD)	Neurology	419
Bourge, Robert Charles (MD)	Cardiology (Cardiovascular Disease)	130
Bourgoignie, Jacques (MD)	Nephrology	362
Boushey Jr, Homer A (MD)	Pulmonary Disease	710
Bove, Edward (MD)	Pediatric Surgery	614
Bowden, Charles (MD)	Psychiatry	685
Bowen, James (MD)	Neurology	419

Name	Specialty	Page
Bower, Charles (MD)	Otolaryngology	518
Bowers Jr, Malcolm B (MD)	Psychiatry	676
Boxrud, Cynthia Ann (MD)	Ophthalmology	463
Boyajian, Michael (MD)	Plastic Surgery	637
Boyce Jr, H Worth (MD)	Gastroenterology	226
Boyce, John G (MD)	Obstetrics & Gynecology	432
Boyd, Arthur D (MD)	Thoracic Surgery	807
Boyd, Robert (MD)	Pediatrics	619
Boyd, Stuart D (MD)	Urology	847
Boyle, John T (MD)	Pediatric Gastroenterology	580
Boyle, Robert John (MD)	Neonatal-Perinatal Medicine	352
Brackmann, Derald E (MD)	Otolaryngology	521
Braden, Gregory Alan (MD)	Interventional Cardiology	145
Bradford, David S (MD)	Orthopaedic Surgery	496
Bradley, James P. (MD)	Orthopaedic Surgery	479
Bradley, John S (MD)	Pediatric Infectious Disease	594
Brady III, Charles Elmer (MD)	Gastroenterology	235
Brage, Michael (MD)	Orthopaedic Surgery	496
Braman, Sidney (MD)	Pulmonary Disease	691
Branch Jr, Charles L (MD)	Neurological Surgery	379
Brandt, Lawrence (MD)	Gastroenterology	222
Brasington, Richard (MD)	Rheumatology	763
Braunstein, Seth N (MD/PhD)	Internal Medicine	333
Braunwald, Eugene (MD)	Cardiology (Cardiovascular Disease)	120
Brause, Barry (MD)	Infectious Disease	318
Braverman, Alan Charles (MD)	Cardiology (Cardiovascular Disease)	133
Braverman, Irwin (MD)	Dermatology	181
Braylan, Raul (MD)	Pathology	539
Brazer, Scott Robert (MD)	Gastroenterology	226
Brazy, Peter C (MD)	Nephrology	364
Bredenberg, Carl Eric (MD)	Thoracic Surgery	805
Breitbart, William (MD)	Psychiatry	678
Brems, John (MD)	Surgery	793
Brendler, Charles B (MD)	Urology	841
Brener, Bruce (MD)	Vascular Surgery (General)	859
Brennan, Michael Desmond (MD)	Endocrinology, Diabetes & Metabolism	206
Brennan, Murray (MD)	Surgery	784
Brennan, Patrick J (MD)	Infectious Disease	318
Brennan, Thomas Stephen (MD)	Nephrology	367
Brenner, Barry M (MD)	Nephrology	359
Brenner, David Allen (MD)	Gastroenterology	227
Brenner, Joel I (MD)	Pediatric Cardiology	561
Brenner, Michael B (MD)	Rheumatology	757
Bresalier, Robert (MD)	Gastroenterology	230
Brewster, David Charles (MD)	Vascular Surgery (General)	857
Brick, Gregory (MD)	Orthopaedic Surgery	475
Bricker, John Timothy (MD)	Pediatric Cardiology	566
Bricker, Leslie J (MD)	Hematology	288
Bridwell, Keith (MD)	Orthopaedic Surgery	489
Brill, Judith Eileen (MD)	Pediatric Critical Care Medicine	571
Brindis, Ralph Gerard (MD)	Cardiology (Cardiovascular Disease)	141
Brink, Robert Ross (MD)	Plastic Surgery	651

ALPHABETICAL LISTING OF DOCTORS

Name	Specialty	Page
Britt, L D (MD)	Surgery	790
Broderick, Gregory (MD)	Urology	837
Brodeur, Garrett (MD)	Pediatric Hematology-Oncology	583
Brodman, Richard Ferris (MD)	Thoracic Surgery	808
Brodsky, James White (MD)	Orthopaedic Surgery	494
Brody, Garry S (MD)	Plastic Surgery	651
Brookler, Kenneth (MD)	Otolaryngology	502
Brooks, Benjamin (MD)	Neurology	411
Brooks, Stuart M (MD)	Pulmonary Disease	697
Brown, Frederick (MD)	Neurological Surgery	382
Brown, John W (MD)	Thoracic Surgery	816
Brown, Kevin K (MD)	Pulmonary Disease	706
Brown, Kimberly A (MD)	Gastroenterology	230
Browner, Bruce D (MD)	Orthopaedic Surgery	475
Brozena, Susan Celia (MD)	Cardiology (Cardiovascular Disease)	124
Brushart, Thomas M (MD)	Orthopaedic Surgery	479
Bruskewitz, Reginald C (MD)	Urology	841
Brust, John C (MD)	Neurology	400
Bryson, Yvonne Joyce (MD)	Pediatric Infectious Disease	594
Bucciarelli, Richard L (MD)	Neonatal-Perinatal Medicine	352
Buch, Jeffrey Phillip (MD)	Urology	845
Buchbinder, Ellen (MD)	Allergy & Immunology	95
Bucholz, Robert (MD)	Orthopaedic Surgery	494
Buckalew Jr., Vardaman Moore (MD)	Nephrology	362
Buckley, Edward G (MD)	Ophthalmology	452
Buckley, Rebecca Hatcher (MD)	Pediatric Allergy & Immunology	556
Bucky, Louis P (MD)	Plastic Surgery	637
Bukowski, Ronald Mathew (MD)	Hematology	288
Bunchman, Timothy E (MD)	Pediatric Nephrology	596
Buncke Jr, Harry J (MD)	Plastic Surgery	651
Bunn Jr, Paul (MD)	Medical Oncology	310
Bunning, Robert Daniel (MD)	Rheumatology	758
Burchiel, Kim James (MD)	Neurological Surgery	388
Burde, Ronald (MD)	Ophthalmology	444
Burdick, James Frederick (MD)	Surgery	784
Burger, Peter (MD)	Pathology	536
Burgess, Andrew (MD)	Orthopaedic Surgery	479
Burget, Gary C (MD)	Plastic Surgery	645
Burke, Allan M (MD)	Neurology	412
Burke, Miles Joseph (MD)	Ophthalmology	456
Burke, Susan F (MD)	Endocrinology, Diabetes & Metabolism	206
Burket, Mark W. (MD)	Cardiology (Cardiovascular Disease)	134
Burkey, Brian (MD)	Otolaryngology	507
Burnett II, Arthur L (MD)	Urology	831
Burns , R Stanley (MD)	Neurology	412
Burns, Alton Jay (MD)	Plastic Surgery	649
Burry, Kenneth Arnold (MD)	Reproductive Endocrinology	751
Burt, Vivien Kleinman (MD/PhD)	Psychiatry	686
Burton III, Claude Shreve (MD)	Dermatology	186
Burton, John Russell (MD)	Geriatric Medicine	244
Bush, Robert (MD)	Allergy & Immunology	100
Bushman, Wade (MD)	Urology	841

ALPHABETICAL LISTING OF DOCTORS

Name	Specialty	Page
Carneiro, Ronaldo Dos Santos (MD)	Hand Surgery	269
Caronna, John J (MD)	Neurology	400
Carpenter Jr, William T (MD)	Psychiatry	678
Carpenter, Charles B (MD)	Nephrology	359
Carr, Bruce (MD)	Obstetrics & Gynecology	437
Carr, David Brian (MD)	Geriatric Medicine	247
Carr-Locke, David L (MD)	Gastroenterology	221
Carrasquillo, Jorge Amilcar (MD)	Nuclear Medicine	425
Carrau, Ricardo L. (MD)	Otolaryngology	503
Carraway, James Howard (MD)	Plastic Surgery	642
Carroll, Charles (MD)	Hand Surgery	271
Carroll, Peter Robert (MD)	Urology	848
Carroll, William L (MD)	Pediatric Hematology-Oncology	588
Carson, Benjamin S (MD)	Neurological Surgery	375
Carson, Culley (MD)	Urology	837
Carter, Darryl (MD)	Pathology	535
Carter, John E (MD)	Neurology	416
Carter, William Jerry (MD)	Geriatric Medicine	250
Cartwright, Patrick (MD)	Urology	845
Casella, Samuel Joseph (MD)	Pediatric Endocrinology	572
Cassel, Christine (MD)	Geriatric Medicine	244
Cassidy, Suzanne (MD)	Clinical Genetics	162
Cassisi, Nicholas J (MD)	Otolaryngology	508
Castle, Valerie (MD)	Pediatric Hematology-Oncology	586
Catalona, William J (MD)	Urology	841
Catanzaro, Antonino (MD)	Pulmonary Disease	710
Cavallino, Robert (MD)	Diagnostic Radiology	733
Cederbaum, Stephen D (MD)	Clinical Genetics	164
Cefalo, Robert Charles (MD)	Maternal & Fetal Medicine	343
Celli, Bartolome (MD)	Pulmonary Disease	691
Cello, John Patrick (MD)	Gastroenterology	237
Cerqueira, Manuel (MD)	Cardiology (Cardiovascular Disease)	124
Chaisson, Richard Ernest (MD)	Infectious Disease	318
Chaitman, Bernard R. (MD)	Cardiology (Cardiovascular Disease)	134
Chalas, Eva (MD)	Gynecologic Oncology	256
Chambers, Richard Byron (MD)	Orthopaedic Surgery	496
Chan, Joseph (MD)	Infectious Disease	323
Chandar, Jayanthi (MD)	Pediatric Nephrology	596
Chandler, Michael (MD)	Allergy & Immunology	96
Chandler, William F (MD)	Neurological Surgery	382
Chandrasoma, Parakrama T (MD)	Pathology	542
Chang, Rowland Waton (MD)	Rheumatology	763
Chang, Stanley (MD)	Ophthalmology	445
Chang-Miller, April (MD)	Rheumatology	763
Chapman, Paul (MD)	Medical Oncology	295
Chapman, Paul H. (MD)	Neurological Surgery	373
Char, Devron H (MD)	Ophthalmology	464
Charboneau, J William (MD)	Radiology	737
Charney, Jonathan (MD)	Neurology	400
Charrow, Joel (MD)	Clinical Genetics	162
Chatham, Walter W (MD)	Rheumatology	762
Chatterjee, Kanu (MD)	Cardiology (Cardiovascular Disease)	141

Name	Specialty	Page
Chen, David (MD)	Physical Medicine & Rehabilitation	626
Cheney, Mack Lowell (MD)	Otolaryngology	501
Chernoff, William Gregory (MD)	Otolaryngology	512
Cherry Jr., Kenneth J. (MD)	Vascular Surgery (General)	864
Cherry, James Donald (MD)	Pediatric Infectious Disease	594
Chervenak, Francis Anthony (MD)	Maternal & Fetal Medicine	342
Chescheir, Nancy Custer (MD)	Maternal & Fetal Medicine	344
Chiu, David (MD)	Hand Surgery	267
Chlebowski, Rowan Thomas (MD/PhD)	Medical Oncology	313
Chodak, Gerald (MD)	Urology	841
Choe, Soo-Sang (MD)	Cardiology (Cardiovascular Disease)	141
Choi, Dennis W (MD)	Neurology	412
Choi, Noah C (MD)	Radiation Oncology	717
Chopra, Inder Jit (MD)	Endocrinology, Diabetes & Metabolism	211
Choy, Andrew Eng (MD)	Ophthalmology	464
Christiani, David (MD)	Pulmonary Disease	691
Christiansen, Thomas (MD)	Otolaryngology	513
Christie, Dennis (MD)	Pediatric Gastroenterology	581
Christie, John (MD)	Colon & Rectal Surgery	172
Christman, Brian Wallace (MD)	Pulmonary Disease	697
Christman, Gregory (MD)	Reproductive Endocrinology	748
Chrousos, George (MD)	Pediatric Endocrinology	572
Chui, Helena Chang (MD)	Neurology	419
Chung, Kevin (MD)	Hand Surgery	271
Church, Joseph August (MD)	Pediatric Allergy & Immunology	558
Chutorian, Abraham (MD)	Child Neurology	151
Chuttani, Ram (MD)	Gastroenterology	221
Cibis, Gerhard W (MD)	Ophthalmology	456
Cicale, Michael Jon (MD)	Pulmonary Disease	697
Cilo, Mark P (MD)	Neurology	416
Ciocon, Jerry (MD)	Geriatric Medicine	245
Cioffi, William (MD)	Surgery	781
Cirigliano, Michael (MD)	Internal Medicine	334
Civin, Curt Ingraham (MD)	Pediatric Hematology-Oncology	583
Clagett, George Patrick (MD)	Vascular Surgery (General)	867
Clairmont, Albert (MD)	Physical Medicine & Rehabilitation	626
Clark, Orlo H (MD)	Surgery	799
Clark, Vivian (MD)	Interventional Cardiology	145
Clarke-Pearson, Daniel L (MD)	Gynecologic Oncology	258
Clauw, Daniel J (MD)	Rheumatology	758
Clayman, Gary Lee (MD)	Otolaryngology	518
Clayman, Ralph V (MD)	Urology	841
Clements III, Dennis Alfred (MD/PhD)	Pediatric Infectious Disease	591
Clements, Philip Jordan (MD)	Rheumatology	768
Clements, Stephen (MD)	Cardiology (Cardiovascular Disease)	130
Cleveland, William (MD)	Pediatric Endocrinology	574
Clifton, Guy (MD)	Neurological Surgery	386
Cloherty, John ()	Neonatal-Perinatal Medicine	351
Cloninger, C Robert (MD)	Psychiatry	683
Close, Lanny Garth (MD)	Otolaryngology	503
Cloughesy, Timothy Francis (MD)	Neurology	419
Clouse, Ray Eugene (MD)	Gastroenterology	231

ALPHABETICAL LISTING OF DOCTORS

Name	Specialty	Page
Cobos, Everardo (MD)	Hematology	290
Cochran, Alistair J (MD)	Pathology	542
Cockerell, Clay J (MD)	Dermatology	191
Cody Jr., Robert James (MD)	Cardiology (Cardiovascular Disease)	134
Coe, Fredric (MD)	Internal Medicine	364
Coffman, Thomas Myron (MD)	Nephrology	363
Cofield, Robert H (MD)	Orthopaedic Surgery	490
Coggins, Cecil (MD)	Nephrology	359
Cohen, Alfred M (MD)	Colon & Rectal Surgery	172
Cohen, Bernard Hershel (MD)	Dermatology	187
Cohen, Bruce M (MD)	Psychiatry	676
Cohen, Carmel (MD)	Gynecologic Oncology	256
Cohen, David (MD)	Nephrology	360
Cohen, Donald (MD)	Child & Adolescent Psychiatry	663
Cohen, Harvey (MD)	Geriatric Medicine	245
Cohen, Herbert J (MD)	Pediatrics	617
Cohen, Howard Arthur (MD)	Cardiology (Cardiovascular Disease)	124
Cohen, Jeffrey Alan (MD)	Neurology	412
Cohen, Jon (MD)	Vascular Surgery (General)	859
Cohen, Jonathan (MD)	Gastroenterology	222
Cohen, Lawrence Sorel (MD)	Cardiology (Cardiovascular Disease)	120
Cohen, Martin (MD)	Cardiac Electrophysiology	115
Cohen, Noel L (MD)	Otolaryngology	503
Cohen, Roger David (MD)	Pediatric Surgery	614
Cohen, Seymour (MD)	Medical Oncology	295
Cohn, David (MD)	Infectious Disease	326
Cohn, Lawrence H (MD)	Thoracic Surgery	805
Cohn, Richard (MD)	Pediatric Nephrology	597
Coit, Daniel G (MD)	Surgery	784
Colachis III, Samuel C (MD)	Physical Medicine & Rehabilitation	627
Colby, Thomas V (MD)	Pathology	541
Coldwell, Douglas Michael (MD)	Radiology	735
Cole, Andrew J. (MD)	Neurology	397
Cole, Barbara R (MD)	Pediatric Nephrology	597
Cole, Norman M (MD)	Plastic Surgery	642
Cole, Solon R (MD)	Pathology	535
Coleman, John (MD)	Plastic Surgery	646
Coleman, Morton (MD)	Medical Oncology	295
Coleman, Ralph Edward (MD)	Nuclear Medicine	426
Collea, Joseph Vincent (MD)	Maternal & Fetal Medicine	342
Coller, Barry (MD)	Hematology	285
Coller, John (MD)	Colon & Rectal Surgery	169
Collins, Francis M (MD)	Endocrinology, Diabetes & Metabolism	206
Colombani, Paul M (MD)	Pediatric Surgery	611
Colon, Gustavo (MD)	Plastic Surgery	649
Colvin, Edward V (MD)	Pediatric Cardiology	563
Come, Steven Eliot (MD)	Medical Oncology	292
Comerota, Anthony J (MD)	Vascular Surgery (General)	859
Cominelli, Fabio (MD/PhD)	Gastroenterology	227
Comis, Robert L (MD)	Medical Oncology	295
Compton III, Wilson M (MD)	Addiction Psychiatry	661
Conant, Marcus A (MD)	Dermatology	192

Name	Specialty	Page
Connolly, James Leo (MD)	Pathology	535
Constantian, Mark B (MD)	Plastic Surgery	635
Conte Jr, John V (MD)	Thoracic Surgery	808
Conti, Charles Richard (MD)	Cardiology (Cardiovascular Disease)	130
Conti, David James (MD)	Surgery	784
Cook, Stuart (MD)	Neurology	400
Cook, Ted (MD)	Otolaryngology	521
Cooley, Denton A (MD)	Thoracic Surgery	821
Cooney, Leo (MD)	Geriatric Medicine	243
Cooney, William (MD)	Hand Surgery	271
Cooper, Christopher (MD)	Cardiology (Cardiovascular Disease)	134
Cooper, David Stephen (MD)	Endocrinology, Diabetes & Metabolism	199
Cooper, Joel David (MD)	Thoracic Surgery	816
Cooper, John Allen Dicks (MD)	Pulmonary Disease	697
Cooper, William (MD)	Pulmonary Disease	697
Copel, Joshua (MD)	Maternal & Fetal Medicine	341
Copeland III, Jack G (MD)	Thoracic Surgery	821
Copeland lll, Edward M (MD)	Surgery	790
Copeland, Larry James (MD)	Gynecologic Oncology	259
Coppola, John (MD)	Cardiology (Cardiovascular Disease)	125
Coran, Arnold G (MD)	Pediatric Surgery	615
Corbett Jr, Eugene Charles (MD)	Internal Medicine	335
Corbett, James (MD)	Neurology	407
Corey, G Ralph (MD)	Infectious Disease	323
Corey, Jacquelynne P (MD)	Otolaryngology	513
Cornblath, David R. (MD)	Neurology	401
Cornelius, Lynne A (MD)	Dermatology	189
Corson, John (MD)	Vascular Surgery (General)	865
Coselli, Joseph Stapleton (MD)	Thoracic Surgery	821
Cosgrove III, Delos M (MD)	Thoracic Surgery	816
Cosgrove, G. Rees (MD)	Neurological Surgery	373
Costanzo, Maria Rosa (MD)	Cardiology (Cardiovascular Disease)	134
Cote, Richard (MD)	Pathology	542
Cotton, Peter (MD)	Gastroenterology	227
Cotton, Robin (MD)	Pediatric Otolaryngology	602
Couch, Nancy (MD)	Geriatric Medicine	247
Coughlin, Michael (MD)	Orthopaedic Surgery	493
Coull, Bruce (MD)	Neurology	416
Courey, Mark Sam (MD)	Otolaryngology	508
Couser, William (MD)	Nephrology	368
Coutsoftides, Theodore (MD)	Colon & Rectal Surgery	176
Cox, Charles E (MD)	Surgery	790
Cox, James D (MD)	Radiation Oncology	725
Coyle, Joseph (MD)	Child & Adolescent Psychiatry	663
Coyle, Patricia K (MD)	Neurology	401
Craig, Robert M (MD)	Gastroenterology	231
Craigen, William (MD)	Clinical Genetics	163
Crandall, Alan Slade (MD)	Ophthalmology	461
Craven, Donald Edward (MD)	Infectious Disease	317
Craver, Joseph (MD)	Thoracic Surgery	812
Crawford, Jeffrey (MD)	Medical Oncology	300
Crawford, Thomas Owen (MD)	Child Neurology	152

ALPHABETICAL LISTING OF DOCTORS

Name	Specialty	Page
Creamer, Michael (DO)	Physical Medicine & Rehabilitation	626
Criley, John Michael (MD)	Cardiology (Cardiovascular Disease)	141
Crist, William (MD)	Pediatric Hematology-Oncology	586
Crockett, Dennis M (MD)	Pediatric Otolaryngology	603
Crofford, Leslie (MD)	Rheumatology	764
Cromydas, George (MD)	Pulmonary Disease	702
Cronenwett, Jack (MD)	Vascular Surgery (General)	857
Cross III, DeWitte T (MD)	Radiology	737
Crossett, Lawrence (MD)	Orthopaedic Surgery	479
Crowe, Joseph (MD)	Surgery	793
Crowley, Thomas J. (MD)	Addiction Psychiatry	662
Crowley, William (MD)	Reproductive Endocrinology	743
Cruse, C Wayne (MD)	Plastic Surgery	642
Cryer, Philip E (MD)	Endocrinology, Diabetes & Metabolism	206
Cuckler, John (MD)	Orthopaedic Surgery	486
Culbertson, William (MD)	Ophthalmology	452
Culkin, Daniel J (MD)	Urology	846
Culp, Randall (MD)	Hand Surgery	268
Cummings, Charles (MD)	Otolaryngology	503
Cummings, Jeffrey Lee (MD)	Neurology	419
Cundiff, Geoffrey Williams (DO)	Obstetrics & Gynecology	432
Cunniff, Christopher (MD)	Clinical Genetics	163
Cunningham, John (MD)	Gastroenterology	227
Cunningham-Rundles, Charlotte (MD/PhD)	Allergy & Immunology	96
Cupps, Thomas R (MD)	Rheumatology	758
Curl, Walton Wright (MD)	Orthopaedic Surgery	486
Curley, Steven Alan (MD)	Surgery	797
Curran Jr, Walter J (MD)	Radiation Oncology	718
Curran, James Joseph (MD)	Rheumatology	764
Curry, Cynthia J (MD)	Clinical Genetics	164
Curtin, John P (MD)	Gynecologic Oncology	256
Curtis, Anne B (MD)	Cardiac Electrophysiology	116
Cutilletta , Anthony F (MD)	Pediatric Cardiology	564
Cutting, Court (MD)	Plastic Surgery	637

D

Name	Specialty	Page
D'Alton, Mary Elizabeth (MD)	Maternal & Fetal Medicine	342
D'Amico, Anthony V (MD/PhD)	Radiation Oncology	717
Dabbagh, Shermine (MD)	Pediatric Nephrology	597
Dabezies, Eugene (MD)	Orthopaedic Surgery	495
Dacey Jr., Ralph Gerald (MD)	Neurological Surgery	383
Dahms, William (MD)	Pediatric Endocrinology	575
Dake, Michael David (MD)	Radiology	739
Dale, Lowell C (MD)	Geriatric Medicine	247
Dalinka, Murray (MD)	Diagnostic Radiology	731
Dalkin, Alan Craig (MD)	Endocrinology, Diabetes & Metabolism	203
Daniel, Rollin K (MD)	Plastic Surgery	651
Daniel, Thomas M (MD)	Thoracic Surgery	812
Daniels, Gilbert (MD)	Endocrinology, Diabetes & Metabolism	197
Danielson, Gordon (MD)	Thoracic Surgery	816
Danoff, Dudley S (MD)	Urology	848
Dardik, Herbert (MD)	Vascular Surgery (General)	859

Name	Specialty	Page
Darling, Ralph Clement (MD)	Vascular Surgery (General)	860
Darras, Basil Theodore (MD)	Child Neurology	151
Daspit, C Phillip (MD)	Otolaryngology	518
Dattwyler, Raymond (MD)	Allergy & Immunology	96
Davidson, Bruce J (MD)	Otolaryngology	503
Davidson, Jonathan (MD)	Psychiatry	682
Davidson, Joyce Eileen (MD)	Psychiatry	684
Davidson, Nancy E (MD)	Medical Oncology	295
Davies, Terry (MD)	Endocrinology, Diabetes & Metabolism	199
Davis Jr, James William (MD)	Geriatric Medicine	251
Davis, Gary L (MD)	Gastroenterology	227
Davis, Ira D (MD)	Pediatric Nephrology	597
Davis, Jessica S (MD)	Clinical Genetics	160
Davis, Kenneth (MD)	Psychiatry	678
Davis, Richard L (MD)	Pathology	542
Davis, Roy Kim (MD)	Otolaryngology	517
Davis, William Eugene (MD)	Rheumatology	767
Day, Arthur L (MD)	Neurological Surgery	379
Day, Susan H (MD)	Ophthalmology	464
De Angelis, Lisa (MD)	Neurology	401
De Franco, Anthony (MD)	Cardiology (Cardiovascular Disease)	134
De Fronzo, Ralph Anthony (MD)	Internal Medicine	337
De Geest, Koen (MD)	Gynecologic Oncology	259
De Groot, Leslie (MD)	Endocrinology, Diabetes & Metabolism	206
De Juan Jr, Eugene (MD)	Ophthalmology	445
de Kernion, Jean Bayhi (MD)	Urology	848
De la Cruz, Antonio (MD)	Otolaryngology	521
De Lateur, Barbara J (MD)	Physical Medicine & Rehabilitation	623
De Long, Mahlon R. (MD)	Neurology	407
De Meester, Tom R (MD)	Thoracic Surgery	823
De Sanctis, Roman (MD)	Cardiology (Cardiovascular Disease)	120
de Shazo, Richard Denson (MD)	Allergy & Immunology	98
De Simone, Philip A (MD)	Hematology	287
De Vita Jr, Vincent T (MD)	Medical Oncology	292
De Vivo, Darryl C (MD)	Child Neurology	152
Dean, Richard H (MD)	Vascular Surgery (General)	863
DeCamp Jr, Malcolm M (MD)	Thoracic Surgery	816
DeCherney, Alan Hersh (MD)	Obstetrics & Gynecology	438
Deitch, Edwin (MD)	Surgery	785
DeKosky, Steven T. (MD)	Neurology	401
Del Monte, Monte A (MD)	Ophthalmology	456
Del Negro, Albert Anthony (MD)	Cardiology (Cardiovascular Disease)	130
Delahay, John Norris (MD)	Orthopaedic Surgery	479
Deland, Jonathan T (MD)	Orthopaedic Surgery	480
DeLeo, Vincent A. (MD)	Dermatology	183
Della Rocca, Robert (MD)	Ophthalmology	445
Delmez, James Albert (MD)	Nephrology	365
Demer, Joseph L (MD/PhD)	Ophthalmology	464
Denenberg, Steven M (MD)	Otolaryngology	518
Dennis, Gary Creed (MD)	Neurological Surgery	375
Denson, Susan Ellen (MD)	Neonatal-Perinatal Medicine	354
DePaulo, Jr, J Raymond (MD)	Psychiatry	678

ALPHABETICAL LISTING OF DOCTORS

Name	Specialty	Page
Deren, Julius Jay (MD)	Gastroenterology	222
Derman, Gordon Harris (MD)	Hand Surgery	272
Dershaw, D David (MD)	Radiology	735
Deschamps, Claude (MD)	Thoracic Surgery	817
Desnick, Robert J (MD/PhD)	Clinical Genetics	160
Desposito, Franklin (MD)	Clinical Genetics	160
DeVane, Gary Williams (MD)	Reproductive Endocrinology	746
Dewberry, Robert Gerard (MD)	Neurology	401
Di Magno, Eugene (MD)	Gastroenterology	231
Di Persio, John (MD/PhD)	Medical Oncology	306
Di Spaltro, Franklin (MD)	Plastic Surgery	637
Diamond, Frank (MD)	Pediatric Endocrinology	574
Diamond, Gary Richard (MD)	Ophthalmology	445
Diamond, Jeffrey (MD)	Gastroenterology	227
Diamond, Michael (MD)	Reproductive Endocrinology	748
Diao, Edward (MD)	Hand Surgery	275
Diaz, Angela (MD)	Adolescent Medicine	89
Diaz, Fernando G (MD)	Neurological Surgery	383
Dichter, Marc Allen (MD)	Neurology	401
Dienstag, Jules Leonard (MD)	Gastroenterology	221
Dieterich, Douglas (MD)	Gastroenterology	223
Dillingham, Michael Francis (MD)	Orthopaedic Surgery	496
Dillingham, Timothy R (MD)	Physical Medicine & Rehabilitation	623
DiMarco, John Philip (MD/PhD)	Cardiac Electrophysiology	116
Dines, David Michael (MD)	Orthopaedic Surgery	480
Dismukes, William Ernest (MD)	Infectious Disease	323
Ditunno, John Francis (MD)	Physical Medicine & Rehabilitation	624
Diuguid, David Lincoln (MD)	Hematology	285
Diver, Daniel Joseph (MD)	Interventional Cardiology	144
Divon, Michael Y (MD)	Obstetrics & Gynecology	432
Dobkin, Bruce H (MD)	Neurology	420
Dobs, Adrian Sandra (MD)	Endocrinology, Diabetes & Metabolism	199
Dodd III, Gerald Dewey (MD)	Diagnostic Radiology	733
Dodds, William G (MD)	Reproductive Endocrinology	748
Dodick, Jack M (MD)	Ophthalmology	445
Dogali, Michael (MD)	Neurological Surgery	389
Dokson, Joel (MD)	Neurology	407
Donald, Paul (MD)	Otolaryngology	521
Donaldson III, William F (MD)	Orthopaedic Surgery	480
Donaldson, Sarah S (MD)	Radiology	739
Donehower, Ross Carl (MD)	Medical Oncology	295
Donohue, James (MD)	Pulmonary Disease	697
Donovan, Donald Thomas (MD)	Otolaryngology	519
Donovan, William Henry (MD)	Physical Medicine & Rehabilitation	629
Dooley, Sharon L (MD)	Maternal & Fetal Medicine	345
Dooley, William Chesnut (MD)	Surgery	785
Dorfman, Howard (MD)	Pathology	536
Dorr, Lawrence Douglas (MD)	Orthopaedic Surgery	497
Dosa, Stefan (MD)	Nephrology	361
Doty, Donald B. (MD)	Thoracic Surgery	820
Douglas Jr, John Simonton (MD)	Cardiology (Cardiovascular Disease)	131
Dover, George Joseph (MD)	Pediatric Hematology-Oncology	583

ALPHABETICAL LISTING OF DOCTORS

Name	Specialty	Page
Edmundowicz, Steven (MD)	Gastroenterology	231
Edwards Jr., John Ellis (MD)	Infectious Disease	328
Egan, James Harold (MD)	Child & Adolescent Psychiatry	665
Egan, Thomas (MD)	Thoracic Surgery	812
Eggers, Howard M (MD)	Ophthalmology	445
Eggleston, Peyton Archer (MD)	Pediatric Allergy & Immunology	555
Ehrenkranz, Richard (MD)	Neonatal-Perinatal Medicine	351
Ehresmann, Glenn Richard (MD)	Rheumatology	768
Ehrmann, David Alan (MD)	Endocrinology, Diabetes & Metabolism	207
Eichler, Craig (MD)	Dermatology	187
Eid, Jean Francois (MD)	Urology	831
Eidt, John (MD)	Vascular Surgery (General)	868
Eilber, Frederick Richard (MD)	Surgery	800
Einhorn, Lawrence (MD)	Medical Oncology	306
Eisdorfer, Carl (MD/PhD)	Psychiatry	682
Eisele, David (MD)	Otolaryngology	503
Eisen, Howard J (MD)	Cardiology (Cardiovascular Disease)	125
Eisenberg, Howard M (MD)	Neurological Surgery	375
Eisendrath, Stuart James (MD)	Psychiatry	686
Eismont, Frank (MD)	Orthopaedic Surgery	486
El-Youssef, Mounif (MD)	Pediatric Gastroenterology	580
Elefteriades, John (MD)	Thoracic Surgery	805
Elias, Sherman (MD)	Obstetrics & Gynecology	435
Elias, Stanton B (MD)	Neurology	412
Elkayam, Uri (MD)	Cardiology (Cardiovascular Disease)	141
Ellenbogen, Kenneth A. (MD)	Cardiac Electrophysiology	116
Ellenbogen, Richard (MD)	Neurological Surgery	389
Elliott, Charles Gregory (MD)	Pulmonary Disease	706
Elliott, David (MD)	Gastroenterology	231
Ellis III, George John (MD)	Endocrinology, Diabetes & Metabolism	203
Ellis Jr, George S (MD)	Ophthalmology	461
Ellis, Jonathan C (MD)	Gastroenterology	237
Ellis, Stephen Geoffrey (MD)	Interventional Cardiology	145
Ellison, Edwin Christopher (MD)	Surgery	793
Ellman, Michael H (MD)	Rheumatology	764
Ellner, Jerrold Jay (MD)	Infectious Disease	318
Elsas II, Louis Jacob (MD)	Clinical Genetics	161
Elta, Grace Helen (MD)	Gastroenterology	231
Emami, Bahman (MD)	Radiation Oncology	723
Emans, Sarah Jean Herriot (MD)	Adolescent Medicine	89
Emanuele, Mary Ann (MD)	Endocrinology, Diabetes & Metabolism	207
Emanuele, Nicholas Victor (MD)	Endocrinology, Diabetes & Metabolism	207
Emery, Helen Margaret (MD)	Pediatric Rheumatology	610
Emmanuel, Patricia (MD)	Pediatric Infectious Disease	591
Emond, Jean Crawford (MD)	Surgery	785
Enelow, Richard Ian (MD)	Pulmonary Disease	698
Engel, William King (MD)	Neurology	420
Engstrom, John Walter (MD)	Neurology	420
Enker, Warren (MD)	Surgery	785
Ennis, Ronald (MD)	Radiation Oncology	718
Epstein, Andrew Ernest (MD)	Cardiac Electrophysiology	117
Epstein, Fred Jacob (MD)	Neurological Surgery	376

Name	Specialty	Page
Epstein, Jonathan (MD)	Pathology	536
Epstein, Leon G (MD)	Child Neurology	153
Epstein, Michael (MD)	Pediatric Cardiology	564
Epstein, Stuart Zane (MD)	Pediatric Allergy & Immunology	559
Eriksson, Elof (MD)	Plastic Surgery	635
Esch, Peter (MD)	Internal Medicine	335
Eschenbach, David Arthur (MD)	Obstetrics & Gynecology	438
Escobedo, Marilyn Barnard (MD)	Neonatal-Perinatal Medicine	354
Esquenazi, Alberto (MD)	Physical Medicine & Rehabilitation	624
Esquivel, Carlos Orlando (MD)	Surgery	800
Essner, Richard (MD)	Surgery	800
Estabrook, Alison (MD)	Surgery	785
Eth, Spencer (MD)	Psychiatry	678
Ettenger, Robert Bruce (MD)	Pediatric Nephrology	598
Ettinger, David Seymour (MD)	Medical Oncology	295
Eustace, John C (MD)	Internal Medicine	335
Eustis, Horatio Sprague (MD)	Ophthalmology	461
Evans III, Richard (MD)	Pediatric Allergy & Immunology	557
Evans, Douglas Brian (MD)	Surgery	797
Evans, Mark Ira (MD)	Obstetrics & Gynecology	435
Eviatar, Lydia (MD)	Child Neurology	152
Ezaki, Marybeth (MD)	Hand Surgery	274

F

Name	Specialty	Page
Faber, L Penfield (MD)	Thoracic Surgery	817
Fabian, Carol J (MD)	Medical Oncology	310
Fabian, Richard (MD)	Otolaryngology	501
Fagien, Steven (MD)	Ophthalmology	452
Fahey, Patrick J (MD)	Pulmonary Disease	702
Fahn, Stanley (MD)	Neurology	402
Failla, Joseph M (MD)	Hand Surgery	272
Faillace, Walter (MD)	Neurological Surgery	379
Falcone, Tommaso (MD)	Reproductive Endocrinology	749
Falk, Rena Ellen (MD)	Clinical Genetics	164
Falk, Ronald J (MD)	Nephrology	363
Falletta, John (MD)	Pediatric Hematology-Oncology	585
Fan, Leland Lane (MD)	Pediatric Pulmonology	606
Fang, Leslie (MD)	Nephrology	359
Fanous, Yvonne F (MD)	Pediatric Allergy & Immunology	559
Fanta, Christopher (MD)	Pulmonary Disease	691
Farber, Martin Stuart (MD/PhD)	Rheumatology	759
Farcy, Jean-Pierre (MD)	Orthopaedic Surgery	480
Farmer, Joseph (MD)	Otolaryngology	508
Farmer, Richard G (MD)	Gastroenterology	223
Faro, Sebastian (MD)	Obstetrics & Gynecology	437
Farrell, Thomas A. (MD)	Ophthalmology	457
Farrior, Edward (MD)	Otolaryngology	508
Farrior, Joseph Brown (MD)	Otolaryngology	508
Fauci, Anthony Stephen (MD)	Infectious Disease	319
Fawcett, Jan A (MD)	Psychiatry	683
Faxon, David P (MD)	Cardiology (Cardiovascular Disease)	135
Fazio, Victor (MD)	Colon & Rectal Surgery	173

ALPHABETICAL LISTING OF DOCTORS

Name	Specialty	Page
Feder, Robert S (MD)	Ophthalmology	457
Fee Jr, Willard E (MD)	Otolaryngology	521
Feig, Stephen A (MD)	Pediatric Hematology-Oncology	588
Fein, William (MD)	Ophthalmology	464
Feinberg, Joseph Hunt (MD)	Physical Medicine & Rehabilitation	624
Feinglos, Mark (MD)	Endocrinology, Diabetes & Metabolism	204
Feinstein, Donald Ivan (MD)	Hematology	291
Feldman, Eva L. (MD/PhD)	Neurology	412
Feldman, Joel (MD)	Plastic Surgery	635
Feldman, Mark (MD)	Gastroenterology	236
Feldman, Robert G (MD)	Neurology	397
Feldman, Ted (MD)	Interventional Cardiology	146
Feldmann, Edward (MD)	Neurology	397
Feldon, Steven E (MD)	Ophthalmology	464
Felig, Philip (MD)	Endocrinology, Diabetes & Metabolism	199
Fenichel, Gerald M (MD)	Child Neurology	153
Fennell III, Robert Samuel (MD)	Pediatric Nephrology	596
Fenske, Neil (MD)	Dermatology	187
Ferguson II, James E (MD)	Maternal & Fetal Medicine	344
Ferguson, Mark (MD)	Thoracic Surgery	817
Ferguson, Ronald (MD)	Surgery	793
Ferlic, Donald C. (MD)	Hand Surgery	274
Ferrante, F Michael (MD)	Pain Management	527
Ferrara, James (MD)	Pediatric Hematology-Oncology	587
Ferraz, Francisco M (MD)	Neurological Surgery	379
Ferree, Carolyn Ruth Black (MD)	Radiation Oncology	721
Ferrell, Linda (MD)	Pathology	542
Ferrendelli, James A (MD)	Neurology	416
Ferriero, Donna Marie (MD)	Child Neurology	155
Ferzli, George (MD)	Surgery	785
Filip, Stanley John (MD)	Obstetrics & Gynecology	434
FInan, Michael A (MD)	Gynecologic Oncology	262
Finerman, Gerald (MD)	Orthopaedic Surgery	497
Fink, J. Stephen (MD)	Neurology	397
Finkel, Michael (MD)	Neurology	407
Fiorica, James Vincent (MD)	Gynecologic Oncology	258
Fisch, Harry (MD)	Urology	831
Fischbein, Lewis Conrad (MD)	Rheumatology	764
Fischer, Thomas James (MD)	Hand Surgery	272
Fishbein, Daniel P (MD)	Cardiology (Cardiovascular Disease)	141
Fisher, Jack (MD)	Plastic Surgery	642
Fisher, Laura (MD)	Internal Medicine	334
Fisher, Mark (MD)	Neurology	420
Fisher, Michael (MD)	Dermatology	183
Fisher, Richard I (MD)	Medical Oncology	306
Fisher, Robert (MD)	Neurology	420
Fishman, Elliot (MD)	Diagnostic Radiology	731
Fishman, Marvin Allen (MD)	Child Neurology	155
Fitz, John Gregory (MD)	Gastroenterology	235
Fitzgerald, Paul Anthony (MD)	Endocrinology, Diabetes & Metabolism	211
Fitzgibbon, Dermot Richard (MD)	Pain Management	531
Fitzpatrick, Richard (MD)	Dermatology	192

ALPHABETICAL LISTING OF DOCTORS

Name	Specialty	Page
Fivenson, David (MD)	Dermatology	189
Fivush, Barbara A (MD)	Pediatric Nephrology	595
Fix, R Jobe (MD)	Plastic Surgery	642
Flachsbart, Keith D (MD)	Thoracic Surgery	823
Flamm, Eugene (MD)	Neurological Surgery	376
Flanigan, Preston D. (MD)	Vascular Surgery (General)	868
Flanigan, Robert (MD)	Urology	842
Flatow, Evan (MD)	Orthopaedic Surgery	480
Fleischer, David (MD)	Gastroenterology	223
Fleischer, Norman (MD)	Endocrinology, Diabetes & Metabolism	200
Fleisher, Gary Robert (MD)	Pediatric Critical Care Medicine	569
Fleshman, James (MD)	Colon & Rectal Surgery	173
Fletcher, Christopher (MD)	Pathology	535
Fletcher, Eugene (MD)	Pulmonary Disease	698
Flowers, Franklin P (MD)	Dermatology	187
Flowers, Robert (MD)	Plastic Surgery	651
Flynn, Harry W (MD)	Ophthalmology	453
Flynn, Patrick (MD)	Medical Oncology	306
Flynn, Timothy Carlyle (MD)	Vascular Surgery (General)	863
Fodor, Peter Bela (MD)	Plastic Surgery	651
Foley, Carmel (MD)	Child & Adolescent Psychiatry	665
Foley, Eugene F (MD)	Colon & Rectal Surgery	172
Foley, Kathleen M (MD)	Pain Management	527
Follansbee, William (MD)	Cardiology (Cardiovascular Disease)	125
Fonkalsrud, Eric W (MD)	Pediatric Surgery	616
Fontana, Gregory (MD)	Thoracic Surgery	823
Ford, Carol Ann (MD)	Adolescent Medicine	89
Ford, Charles N (MD)	Otolaryngology	513
Forde, Kenneth (MD)	Colon & Rectal Surgery	170
Fordtran, John (MD)	Gastroenterology	236
Forman, Jeffrey D (MD)	Radiation Oncology	723
Fornari, Victor (MD)	Child & Adolescent Psychiatry	665
Forsmark, Christopher (MD)	Gastroenterology	228
Forster, Richard K (MD)	Ophthalmology	453
Fossella, Frank V (MD)	Medical Oncology	311
Foster, Carol M (MD)	Pediatric Endocrinology	575
Foster, Charles Stephen (MD)	Ophthalmology	443
Fountain, Karen (MD)	Radiation Oncology	718
Fowble, Barbara (MD)	Radiation Oncology	719
Fowler Jr, Wesley C (MD)	Gynecologic Oncology	258
Fox, Harold E (MD/PhD)	Maternal & Fetal Medicine	342
Fox, Jacob H (MD)	Neurology	412
Fox, Peter Thornton (MD)	Neurology	416
Fox, Roger W (MD)	Allergy & Immunology	98
France, Thomas D (MD)	Ophthalmology	457
Francis, Kathleen (MD)	Physical Medicine & Rehabilitation	624
Francisco, Gerard E (MD)	Physical Medicine & Rehabilitation	629
Frank, Ian (MD)	Infectious Disease	319
Frankel, Jeffrey (MD)	Neurology	402
Frassica, Frank John (MD)	Orthopaedic Surgery	480
Frazier, Oscar Howard (MD)	Thoracic Surgery	821
Frederiksen, James W (MD)	Thoracic Surgery	817

ALPHABETICAL LISTING OF DOCTORS

Name	Specialty	Page
Freedberg, Irwin M (MD)	Dermatology	183
Freedman, Michael L (MD)	Geriatric Medicine	244
Freedman, Ralph (MD)	Gynecologic Oncology	262
Freedman, Sharon (MD)	Ophthalmology	453
Freeland, Alan Edward (MD)	Hand Surgery	269
Freeman, Gregory Lane (MD)	Cardiology (Cardiovascular Disease)	139
Freeman, John M (MD)	Child Neurology	152
Freeman, Theodore (MD)	Allergy & Immunology	103
Freeman, Thomas B (MD)	Neurological Surgery	380
Freemark, Michael Scott (MD)	Pediatric Endocrinology	574
French, Jacqueline (MD)	Neurology	402
Freshwater, M Felix (MD)	Hand Surgery	270
Fricker, Frederick Jay (MD)	Pediatric Cardiology	563
Frieden, Ilona J (MD)	Dermatology	193
Friedlaender, Gary (MD)	Orthopaedic Surgery	475
Friedman, Aaron (MD)	Pediatric Nephrology	597
Friedman, Barry (MD)	Geriatric Psychiatry	674
Friedman, Eli A (MD)	Nephrology	361
Friedman, Ellen (MD)	Otolaryngology	519
Friedman, Harvey Michael (MD)	Infectious Disease	319
Friedman, Lawrence S. (MD)	Gastroenterology	221
Friedman, Lloyd Neal (MD)	Pulmonary Disease	691
Friedman, Michael (MD)	Otolaryngology	513
Friedman, Nancy Eisenberg (MD)	Pediatric Endocrinology	574
Friedman, Stuart (MD)	Allergy & Immunology	98
Friedman, William A (MD)	Neurological Surgery	380
Frigas, Evangelo (MD)	Allergy & Immunology	100
Frigoletto Jr., Fredric D. (MD)	Maternal & Fetal Medicine	341
Fritz, Marc Anthony (MD)	Reproductive Endocrinology	746
Frizzera, Glauco (MD)	Pathology	536
Fromm, Geri Lynn (MD)	Gynecologic Oncology	263
Fry, Robert Dean (MD)	Colon & Rectal Surgery	170
Fu, Freddie (MD)	Orthopaedic Surgery	480
Fuchs, Eugene F (MD)	Urology	848
Fuchs, Wayne (MD)	Ophthalmology	446
Fuhrman, Bradley P (MD)	Pediatric Critical Care Medicine	569
Fulkerson Jr, William J (MD)	Pulmonary Disease	698
Fuller, Arlan F. (MD)	Gynecologic Oncology	255
Fung, John J (MD/PhD)	Surgery	786
Funk, Gerry Franklin (MD)	Otolaryngology	513
Furlan, Anthony J (MD)	Neurology	413
Furukawa, Satoshi (MD)	Thoracic Surgery	808
Fuselier Jr, Harold A (MD)	Urology	846
Fuster, Carlos Daniel (MD)	Adolescent Medicine	90
Fuster, Valentin (MD)	Cardiology (Cardiovascular Disease)	125

G

Name	Specialty	Page
Gabbard, Glen O. (MD)	Psychiatry	684
Gabbe, Steven G (MD)	Maternal & Fetal Medicine	347
Gabrilove, Janice (MD)	Medical Oncology	296
Gadacz, Thomas R (MD)	Surgery	790
Gage, James ()	Orthopaedic Surgery	490

ALPHABETICAL LISTING OF DOCTORS

Name	Specialty	Page
Gagner, Michel (MD)	Surgery	786
Galandiuk, Susan (MD)	Colon & Rectal Surgery	172
Galante, Jorge O (MD)	Orthopaedic Surgery	490
Galanter, Marc (MD)	Addiction Psychiatry	661
Galask, Rudolph P. (MD)	Obstetrics & Gynecology	435
Galati, Joseph Steven (MD)	Gastroenterology	236
Galetta, Steven (MD)	Neurology	402
Gallico, G Gregory (MD)	Plastic Surgery	635
Gambert, Steven (MD)	Geriatric Medicine	244
Gamelli, Richard Louis (MD)	Surgery	793
Gandara, David R (MD)	Medical Oncology	313
Gang, Eli Shimshon (MD)	Cardiac Electrophysiology	119
Ganguli, Rohan (MD)	Psychiatry	678
Gantz, Bruce (MD)	Otolaryngology	513
Ganz, Patricia Anne (MD)	Medical Oncology	313
Garb, Leslie Julian (MD)	Geriatric Medicine	250
Garber, Judy E (MD)	Medical Oncology	292
Garcia, Carlos (MD)	Neurology	417
Garcia-Gonzalez, Efrain (MD)	Cardiology (Cardiovascular Disease)	139
Garcia-Prats, Joseph (MD)	Neonatal-Perinatal Medicine	354
Garden, Jerome (MD)	Dermatology	189
Gardin, Julius Markus (MD)	Cardiology (Cardiovascular Disease)	135
Gardner, Gregory (MD)	Rheumatology	769
Gardner, Timothy Joseph (MD)	Thoracic Surgery	808
Garin, Eduardo Humberto (MD)	Pediatric Nephrology	596
Garnick, Marc Bennett (MD)	Medical Oncology	292
Garrett, William (MD)	Orthopaedic Surgery	486
Garvey, Glenda Josephine (MD)	Infectious Disease	319
Garvin, James (MD/PhD)	Pediatric Hematology-Oncology	584
Gass, James Donald (MD)	Ophthalmology	453
Gaynor, Ellen (MD)	Hematology	288
Gebhardt, Mark (MD)	Orthopaedic Surgery	475
Geffner, Mitchell Eugene (MD)	Pediatric Endocrinology	577
Gelberman, Richard (MD)	Hand Surgery	272
Gelfand, Erwin (MD)	Pediatric Allergy & Immunology	558
Geller, Kenneth Allen (MD)	Otolaryngology	522
Gendelman, Seymour (MD)	Neurology	402
Gentile, Ronald (MD)	Ophthalmology	446
Georgeson, Keith E (MD)	Pediatric Surgery	613
Georgiade, Gregory (MD)	Plastic Surgery	642
Geppert, Eugene (MD)	Pulmonary Disease	702
Germano, Isabelle M (MD)	Neurological Surgery	376
Geronemus, Roy (MD)	Dermatology	183
Gershengorn, Kent N (MD)	Cardiology (Cardiovascular Disease)	142
Gershenson, David Marc (MD)	Gynecologic Oncology	263
Gershon, Anne (MD)	Pediatric Infectious Disease	590
Gershwin, Merrill Eric (MD)	Rheumatology	769
Gersony, Welton Mark (MD)	Pediatric Cardiology	562
Gertler, Jonathan P (MD)	Vascular Surgery (General)	857
Gewertz, Bruce (MD)	Vascular Surgery (General)	865
Gewitz, Michael (MD)	Pediatric Cardiology	562
Gewurz, Anita (MD)	Pediatric Allergy & Immunology	557

ALPHABETICAL LISTING OF DOCTORS

Name	Specialty	Page
Giangola, Gary (MD)	Vascular Surgery (General)	860
Giannotta, Steven L (MD)	Neurological Surgery	389
Gianoli, Gerard (MD)	Otolaryngology	519
Gianopoulos, John (MD)	Maternal & Fetal Medicine	345
Gibbons, Gary William (MD)	Vascular Surgery (General)	858
Gibbons, Raymond John (MD)	Cardiology (Cardiovascular Disease)	135
Gibbs, Ronald Steven (MD)	Maternal & Fetal Medicine	347
Gilchrest, Barbara ()	Dermatology	181
Gill, Harcharan Singh (MD)	Urology	848
Gillette, Paul Crawford (MD)	Pediatric Cardiology	566
Gills Jr, James P (MD)	Ophthalmology	453
Gilman, Sid (MD)	Neurology	413
Gingold, Bruce (MD)	Colon & Rectal Surgery	170
Ginsburg, Howard (MD)	Pediatric Surgery	611
Ginzler, Ellen (MD)	Rheumatology	759
Gitlin, Michael Jay (MD)	Psychiatry	686
Gitlow, Stanley (MD)	Internal Medicine	334
Gittler, Michelle (MD)	Physical Medicine & Rehabilitation	627
Giuliano, Armando E (MD)	Surgery	800
Givner, Laurence Bruce (MD)	Pediatric Infectious Disease	592
Glader, Bertil E (MD)	Pediatric Hematology-Oncology	589
Glaser, Joel (MD)	Ophthalmology	453
Glasgold, Alvin (MD)	Otolaryngology	503
Glass, Jonathan (MD)	Neurology	407
Glassford Jr, David M (MD)	Thoracic Surgery	812
Glassroth, Jeffrey (MD)	Pulmonary Disease	703
Glatstein, Eli (MD)	Radiation Oncology	719
Glick, John H (MD)	Medical Oncology	296
Glickel, Steven (MD)	Hand Surgery	268
Gliklich, Jerry (MD)	Cardiology (Cardiovascular Disease)	125
Glisson, Bonnie S (MD)	Medical Oncology	311
Glogau, Richard Gordon (MD)	Dermatology	193
Glombicki, Alan Paul (MD)	Gastroenterology	236
Gloviczki, Peter (MD)	Vascular Surgery (General)	865
Gluck, Joan (MD)	Allergy & Immunology	98
Gluck, Paul (MD)	Obstetrics & Gynecology	434
Gluck, Stephen (MD)	Nephrology	363
Gluckman, Gordon (MD)	Urology	842
Gluckman, Jack L (MD)	Otolaryngology	513
Gockerman, Jon Paul (MD)	Medical Oncology	300
Godine, John Elliott (MD/PhD)	Endocrinology, Diabetes & Metabolism	197
Godwin, John (MD)	Hematology	289
Godzik, Cathleen (MD)	Hand Surgery	275
Goebel, Joel Alan (MD)	Otolaryngology	514
Goepfert, Helmuth (MD)	Otolaryngology	519
Goetz, Christopher (MD)	Neurology	413
Goffinet, Don R (MD)	Radiation Oncology	726
Goitz, Henry (MD)	Orthopaedic Surgery	490
Gold, Alan (MD)	Plastic Surgery	637
Goldberg, James David (MD)	Maternal & Fetal Medicine	348
Goldberg, Michael Jay (MD)	Orthopaedic Surgery	476
Goldberg, Morton (MD)	Ophthalmology	446

Name	Specialty	Page
Goldberg, Stanley (MD)	Colon & Rectal Surgery	174
Goldberg, Victor M (MD)	Orthopaedic Surgery	490
Goldman, Allan Larry (MD)	Pulmonary Disease	698
Goldman, Samuel (MD)	Geriatric Psychiatry	673
Goldner, Richard (MD)	Orthopaedic Surgery	486
Goldsmith, Ari (MD)	Pediatric Otolaryngology	600
Goldsmith, Stanley J (MD)	Nuclear Medicine	425
Goldstein, Irwin (MD)	Urology	829
Goldstein, Larry Bruce (MD)	Neurology	408
Goldstein, Lori J (MD)	Medical Oncology	296
Goldstein, Marc (MD)	Urology	832
Goldstein, Wayne (MD)	Orthopaedic Surgery	490
Golub, Richard (MD)	Colon & Rectal Surgery	170
Gomery, Pablo (MD)	Urology	829
Gomes, Antoinette Susan (MD)	Diagnostic Radiology	734
Gomes, J Anthony (MD)	Cardiac Electrophysiology	115
Gong Jr, Henry (MD)	Pulmonary Disease	710
Gonik, Bernard (MD)	Obstetrics & Gynecology	435
Gonzalez, Martha (MD/PhD)	Endocrinology, Diabetes & Metabolism	211
Gonzalez-Loya, Juan (MD)	Obstetrics & Gynecology	435
Good, Robert (MD/PhD)	Allergy & Immunology	98
Goodgold, Albert (MD)	Neurology	402
Goodin, Douglas (MD)	Neurology	420
Goodman, Annekathryn (MD)	Gynecologic Oncology	255
Goodman, Lawrence R (MD)	Radiology	737
Goodman, Neil (MD)	Reproductive Endocrinology	746
Goodman, Robert L (MD)	Radiation Oncology	719
Goodman, Stuart Barry (MD/PhD)	Orthopaedic Surgery	497
Goodwin, Jerry (MD)	Otolaryngology	508
Goodwin, W Jarrard (MD)	Otolaryngology	508
Gorbien, Martin (MD)	Geriatric Medicine	248
Gorchesky, Mark (MD)	Pain Management	529
Gordon, Leo I (MD)	Medical Oncology	306
Gordon, Marsha (MD)	Dermatology	184
Gorelick, David Alan (MD)	Addiction Psychiatry	661
Gorensek, Margaret (MD)	Pediatric Infectious Disease	592
Gorfine, Stephen (MD)	Colon & Rectal Surgery	170
Gorman, Colum (MD)	Endocrinology, Diabetes & Metabolism	207
Gorman, Jack Matthew (MD)	Psychiatry	679
Gostout, Christopher John (MD)	Gastroenterology	232
Gottdiener, John (MD)	Cardiology (Cardiovascular Disease)	125
Gould, K Lance (MD)	Cardiology (Cardiovascular Disease)	139
Gourley, Mark (MD)	Rheumatology	759
Govindarajan, Sugantha (MD)	Pathology	543
Graber, Alan (MD)	Endocrinology, Diabetes & Metabolism	204
Gracey, Douglas Robert (MD)	Pulmonary Disease	703
Grady, M Sean (MD)	Neurological Surgery	376
Graf, Ben K (MD)	Orthopaedic Surgery	491
Graham Jr, John M (MD)	Clinical Genetics	164
Graham, Mark (MD)	Medical Oncology	300
Graham-Pole, John R (MD)	Pediatric Hematology-Oncology	586
Grammer, Leslie C (MD)	Allergy & Immunology	100

ALPHABETICAL LISTING OF DOCTORS

Name	Specialty	Page
Granet, David Bruce (MD)	Ophthalmology	465
Granstein, Richard (MD)	Dermatology	184
Grant, Evalyn N (MD)	Allergy & Immunology	100
Grant, Richard E (MD)	Orthopaedic Surgery	481
Graves, Michael Clark (MD)	Neurology	420
Gravett, Michael Glen (MD)	Maternal & Fetal Medicine	348
Gray, Diana Lee (MD)	Clinical Genetics	162
Gray, Laman (MD)	Thoracic Surgery	812
Graybill, John Richard (MD)	Internal Medicine	337
Greco, F Anthony (MD)	Medical Oncology	301
Greden, John (MD)	Psychiatry	683
Green, Barth (MD)	Neurological Surgery	380
Green, Carmen R (MD)	Pain Management	529
Green, David (MD)	Hematology	289
Green, Howard (MD)	Dermatology	187
Green, Mark (MD)	Medical Oncology	301
Green, Neil Edward (MD)	Orthopaedic Surgery	486
Green, Richard (MD)	Vascular Surgery (General)	860
Greenberg, Harly (MD)	Pulmonary Disease	693
Greenberg, Harry S. (MD)	Neurology	413
Greenberger, Paul A (MD)	Allergy & Immunology	101
Greene Jr, Clarence S (MD)	Neurological Surgery	389
Greene, Graham (MD)	Urology	846
Greene, Loren Wissner (MD)	Endocrinology, Diabetes & Metabolism	200
Greene, Michael F. (MD)	Maternal & Fetal Medicine	341
Greene, Thomas (MD)	Hand Surgery	270
Greenfield, Lazar (MD)	Vascular Surgery (General)	865
Greenspan, Francis S (MD)	Endocrinology, Diabetes & Metabolism	211
Greenspan, Stanley (MD)	Child & Adolescent Psychiatry	665
Greenwald, Blaine (MD)	Geriatric Psychiatry	672
Greenwood, Robert Samuel (MD)	Child Neurology	153
Greer, Benjamin (MD)	Gynecologic Oncology	263
Greganti, Mac Andrew (MD)	Geriatric Medicine	246
Gregory, Richard (MD)	Plastic Surgery	643
Gregory, Stephanie (MD/PhD)	Hematology	289
Greipp, Philip R (MD)	Hematology	289
Greist, John (MD)	Psychiatry	683
Grelsamer, Ronald (MD)	Orthopaedic Surgery	481
Gress, Daryl Ray (MD)	Neurology	421
Grey, Douglas P (MD)	Vascular Surgery (General)	869
Gribetz, Michael (MD)	Urology	832
Griepp, Randall (MD)	Thoracic Surgery	808
Griffin, James Emmet (MD)	Endocrinology, Diabetes & Metabolism	209
Griffin, John Wesley (MD)	Neurology	402
Griffith, Bartley (MD)	Thoracic Surgery	809
Grifo, James (MD/PhD)	Reproductive Endocrinology	744
Grimes, Pearl E (MD)	Dermatology	193
Griswold, John A (MD)	Surgery	797
Grobman, Lawrence R (MD)	Otolaryngology	509
Grody, Wayne W (MD)	Clinical Genetics	164
Groene, Linda A (MD)	Geriatric Medicine	246
Grogan, Thomas (MD)	Pathology	541

Name	Specialty	Page
Grosfeld, Jay L (MD)	Pediatric Surgery	615
Grosh, William W (MD)	Medical Oncology	301
Gross, Charles (MD)	Pediatric Otolaryngology	602
Gross, Ian (MD)	Neonatal-Perinatal Medicine	351
Grossbard, Michael Laurence (MD)	Medical Oncology	296
Grossberg, George (MD)	Geriatric Psychiatry	673
Grossman, John A (MD)	Plastic Surgery	652
Grossman, Melanie (MD)	Dermatology	184
Grotta, James (MD)	Neurology	417
Grotting, James (MD)	Plastic Surgery	643
Grubb, Blair Paul (MD)	Cardiology (Cardiovascular Disease)	135
Grubb, Robert (MD)	Neurological Surgery	383
Grum, Cyril M (MD)	Pulmonary Disease	703
Grundfast, Kenneth (MD)	Pediatric Otolaryngology	600
Gruss, Joseph (MD)	Plastic Surgery	652
Guerrant, Richard (MD)	Infectious Disease	323
Guidry, George Gary (MD)	Pulmonary Disease	708
Guilleminault, Christian (MD)	Psychiatry	686
Gulotta, Stephen J (MD)	Cardiology (Cardiovascular Disease)	126
Gunasekaran, T S (MD)	Pediatric Gastroenterology	580
Gunderson, Leonard (MD)	Radiation Oncology	723
Gundry, Steven (MD)	Thoracic Surgery	823
Gunter, Jack (MD)	Plastic Surgery	649
Gurevitch, Arnold William (MD)	Dermatology	193
Gutai, James (MD)	Pediatric Endocrinology	575
Gutierrez, Francisco A (MD)	Neurological Surgery	383
Guyer, David (MD)	Ophthalmology	446
Guyton, David Lee (MD)	Ophthalmology	446
Guyton, Robert A (MD)	Thoracic Surgery	813

H

Name	Specialty	Page
Haas, Richard H (MD)	Child Neurology	155
Hadler, Nortin (MD)	Rheumatology	762
Hadley, Mark (MD)	Neurological Surgery	380
Haffty, Bruce (MD)	Radiation Oncology	717
Hafler, David A. (MD)	Neurology	397
Hagan, Kevin Francis (MD)	Plastic Surgery	643
Hager, William David (MD)	Obstetrics & Gynecology	434
Hahn, Bevra H (MD)	Rheumatology	769
Haig, Andrew (MD)	Physical Medicine & Rehabilitation	627
Haik, Barrett (MD)	Ophthalmology	453
Haines, Kathleen (MD)	Pediatric Rheumatology	608
Hait, William (MD/PhD)	Medical Oncology	296
Halberg, Francine Erna (MD)	Radiation Oncology	726
Haley Jr, Elliott Clarke (MD)	Neurology	408
Halff, Glenn Alexander (MD)	Surgery	797
Hall, Bryan Davis (MD)	Pediatrics	161
Hall, Jesse (MD)	Pulmonary Disease	703
Hall, Lisabeth (MD)	Ophthalmology	446
Halle, Jan (MD)	Radiation Oncology	721
Haller, Daniel (MD)	Medical Oncology	296
Hallett Jr, John (MD)	Vascular Surgery (General)	865

ALPHABETICAL LISTING OF DOCTORS

Name	Specialty	Page
Halmi, Katherine (MD)	Psychiatry	679
Halperin, Jonathan (MD)	Cardiology (Cardiovascular Disease)	126
Halter, Jeffrey Brian (MD)	Geriatric Medicine	248
Hamaker, Ronald (MD)	Otolaryngology	514
Hammer, Glenn (MD)	Infectious Disease	319
Hammill, Stephen Charles (MD)	Cardiac Electrophysiology	117
Hammon Jr, John W (MD)	Thoracic Surgery	813
Hammond, Charles B (MD)	Reproductive Endocrinology	746
Hammond, Dennis (MD)	Plastic Surgery	646
Hamra, Sameer T (MD)	Plastic Surgery	649
Hanauer, Stephen (MD)	Gastroenterology	232
Hande, Kenneth (MD)	Medical Oncology	301
Hanel, Douglas (MD)	Hand Surgery	275
Haney, Arthur (MD)	Reproductive Endocrinology	747
Hanke, C William (MD)	Dermatology	189
Hankinson, Hal L. (MD)	Neurological Surgery	386
Hanks, John B (MD)	Surgery	791
Hanley, Frank Louis (MD)	Thoracic Surgery	824
Hanna, Ehab (MD)	Otolaryngology	519
Hannafin, Jo (MD/PhD)	Orthopaedic Surgery	481
Hansen Jr., Sigvard (MD)	Orthopaedic Surgery	497
Hansen, Kimberley J (MD)	Vascular Surgery (General)	863
Hansen, Lori Eldean (MD)	Otolaryngology	519
Hansen, Nora Marie (MD)	Surgery	800
Hansen, Ronald (MD)	Dermatology	191
Hansen-Flaschen, John (MD)	Pulmonary Disease	693
Hanson, Laura Catherine ()	Geriatric Medicine	246
Haponik, Edward Francis (MD)	Pulmonary Disease	693
Har-El, Gady (MD)	Otolaryngology	504
Harden, Norman (MD)	Pain Management	529
Hardesty, Robert (MD)	Plastic Surgery	652
Hardy, Mark (MD)	Surgery	786
Hare, John W (MD)	Endocrinology, Diabetes & Metabolism	197
Harman, Eloise M (MD)	Pulmonary Disease	698
Harmon, Gary (MD)	Pulmonary Disease	706
Harmon, William E (MD)	Pediatric Nephrology	595
Harper, Richard L (MD)	Neurological Surgery	387
Harrell Jr, James E (MD)	Thoracic Surgery	821
Harrington, Elizabeth (MD)	Vascular Surgery (General)	860
Harrington, J Timothy (MD)	Rheumatology	764
Harris Jr, Edward Day (MD)	Rheumatology	769
Harris, Jay R (MD)	Radiation Oncology	717
Harris, Nancy L (MD)	Pathology	535
Harris, Raymond C (MD)	Nephrology	363
Harrison, John Kevin (MD)	Cardiology (Cardiovascular Disease)	131
Harrison, Louis (MD)	Radiation Oncology	719
Harrison, Lynn (MD)	Thoracic Surgery	821
Harrison, Michael R (MD)	Pediatric Surgery	616
Hart, Robert G. (MD)	Neurology	417
Hart, William (MD)	Pathology	540
Hartman, Barry Jay (MD)	Infectious Disease	319
Hartmann, Rene (MD)	Colon & Rectal Surgery	172

ALPHABETICAL LISTING OF DOCTORS

Name	Specialty	Page
Harty, James (MD)	Urology	837
Haskal, Ziv (MD)	Radiology	735
Hassenbusch, Samuel J (MD/PhD)	Neurological Surgery	387
Hasso, Anton N (MD)	Radiology	739
Hastings II, Hill (MD)	Hand Surgery	272
Haughey, Bruce (MD)	Otolaryngology	514
Hauser, Stephen Lawrence (MD)	Neurology	421
Hawkins Jr, Irvin (MD)	Diagnostic Radiology	733
Hayashi, Robert H. (MD)	Maternal & Fetal Medicine	345
Hayden, Richard Earle (MD)	Otolaryngology	504
Hayes, Daniel Fleming (MD)	Medical Oncology	297
Haynes, Johnson (MD)	Pulmonary Disease	699
Healey, John (MD)	Orthopaedic Surgery	481
Healy, Gerald (MD)	Pediatric Otolaryngology	600
Hebert, James C (MD)	Surgery	781
Heck, Louis William (MD)	Rheumatology	762
Heffner, John E (MD)	Pulmonary Disease	699
Heffner, Linda (MD/PhD)	Maternal & Fetal Medicine	341
Heger, Joel William (MD)	Cardiology (Cardiovascular Disease)	142
Heilbrun, M Peter (MD)	Neurological Surgery	386
Heilman, Kenneth (MD)	Neurology	408
Heitmiller, Richard F (MD)	Thoracic Surgery	809
Hekmatpanah, Javad (MD)	Neurological Surgery	383
Helfet, David L (MD)	Orthopaedic Surgery	481
Hellenbrand, William E (MD)	Pediatric Cardiology	562
Hendrickson, Michael (MD)	Pathology	543
Heney, Niall M (MD)	Urology	829
Henke, David Carroll (MD)	Pulmonary Disease	699
Hensinger, Robert (MD)	Orthopaedic Surgery	491
Hensle, Terry (MD)	Urology	832
Hentz, Vincent R (MD)	Hand Surgery	275
Herbst, Arthur (MD)	Gynecologic Oncology	259
Herling, Irving M (MD)	Cardiology (Cardiovascular Disease)	126
Herman, John Benjamin (MD)	Psychiatry	676
Herman, Terence Spencer (MD)	Radiation Oncology	725
Herman, William H (MD)	Endocrinology, Diabetes & Metabolism	207
Heros, Roberto (MD)	Neurological Surgery	380
Herr, Harry Wallace (MD)	Urology	832
Hersh, Peter (MD)	Ophthalmology	447
Hertzer, Norman Ray (MD)	Vascular Surgery (General)	865
Hertzig, Margaret (MD)	Child & Adolescent Psychiatry	665
Herzog, David B (MD)	Child & Adolescent Psychiatry	663
Hess, David Charles (MD)	Neurology	408
Hess, J Bruce (MD)	Ophthalmology	453
Hester Jr, Thomas R (MD)	Plastic Surgery	643
Heston, Jerry D (MD)	Child & Adolescent Psychiatry	667
Heyman, Melvin Bernard (MD)	Pediatric Gastroenterology	581
Hibbard, Judith (MD)	Maternal & Fetal Medicine	345
Hidalgo, David (MD)	Plastic Surgery	637
Hiesiger, Emile (MD)	Neurology	403
Hijazi, Ziyad M (MD)	Pediatric Cardiology	565
Hilaris, Basil (MD)	Radiation Oncology	719

ALPHABETICAL LISTING OF DOCTORS

Name	Specialty	Page
Hilger, Peter A. (MD)	Otolaryngology	514
Hill III, Joseph Albert (MD)	Reproductive Endocrinology	743
Hillemeier, A Craig (MD)	Pediatric Gastroenterology	580
Hirsch, Martin Stanley (MD)	Infectious Disease	317
Hirschfeld, Robert, M A (MD)	Psychiatry	685
Hobel, Calvin John (MD)	Maternal & Fetal Medicine	348
Hobson II, Robert Wayne (MD)	Vascular Surgery (General)	860
Hobson, John Allan (MD)	Psychiatry	676
Hochberg, Fred (MD)	Neurology	398
Hodge Jr., Charles J. (MD)	Neurological Surgery	376
Hodges, David S (MD)	Gastroenterology	236
Hodgson, Kim John (MD)	Vascular Surgery (General)	866
Hoefflin, Steven M (MD)	Plastic Surgery	652
Hoff, Julian T (MD)	Neurological Surgery	383
Hoffman, Andrew R (MD)	Endocrinology, Diabetes & Metabolism	211
Hoffman, Brenda (MD)	Gastroenterology	228
Hoffman, David (MD)	Nephrology	363
Hoffman, Gary Stuart (MD)	Rheumatology	764
Hoffman, Lloyd (MD)	Plastic Surgery	638
Hofkosh, Dena (MD)	Pediatrics	617
Hohn, Arno R (MD)	Pediatric Cardiology	567
Holbrook, Peter (MD)	Pediatric Critical Care Medicine	569
Holden, Stuart (MD)	Urology	848
Holinger, Lauren (MD)	Pediatric Otolaryngology	602
Holladay, Jack T. (MD)	Ophthalmology	461
Holland, Edward J. (MD)	Ophthalmology	457
Holland, James F (MD)	Medical Oncology	297
Holland, Jimmie C B (MD)	Psychiatry	679
Hollander, Eric (MD)	Psychiatry	679
Hollander, Harry (MD)	Infectious Disease	328
Holliday, James N (MD/PhD)	Ophthalmology	454
Hollier, Larry Harold (MD)	Vascular Surgery (General)	860
Holmes Jr., David Richard (MD)	Interventional Cardiology	146
Holmes, E Carmack (MD)	Thoracic Surgery	824
Holmes, Gregory Lawrence (MD)	Child Neurology	151
Holmes, King K (MD)	Infectious Disease	328
Holmes, Lewis B (MD)	Clinical Genetics	159
Holt, Peter R (MD)	Gastroenterology	223
Hong, Waun Ki (MD)	Medical Oncology	311
Hopewell, Philip (MD)	Pulmonary Disease	710
Hopkins, Cyrus Clark (MD)	Infectious Disease	317
Hopkins, Leo Nelson (MD)	Neurological Surgery	376
Horbar, Jeffrey David (MD)	Neonatal-Perinatal Medicine	351
Horn, Thomas (MD)	Dermatology	191
Hornblass, Albert (MD)	Ophthalmology	447
Horowitz, Jed H (MD)	Plastic Surgery	652
Horton, John (MD)	Medical Oncology	301
Horwitz, Ralph (MD)	Internal Medicine	333
Hoskins, William (MD)	Gynecologic Oncology	256
Hotchkiss, Robert (MD)	Orthopaedic Surgery	481
Houk, John L (MD)	Rheumatology	765
Houston, Sally (MD)	Infectious Disease	323

ALPHABETICAL LISTING OF DOCTORS

Name	Specialty	Page
Howard, Richard J (MD)	Surgery	791
Howards, Stuart S (MD)	Urology	837
Hoyme, Harold Eugene (MD)	Clinical Genetics	164
Hoyt, Creig S (MD)	Ophthalmology	465
Hoyt, David (MD)	Surgery	800
Hoyt, William Fletcher (MD)	Ophthalmology	465
Hruska, Keith Anthony (MD)	Nephrology	365
Hruza, George J (MD)	Dermatology	189
Hsueh, Willa Ann (MD)	Endocrinology, Diabetes & Metabolism	211
Huang, Laurence (MD)	Pulmonary Disease	711
Hubble, Jean Pintar (MD)	Neurology	413
Huben, Robert P (MD)	Urology	832
Huber, Philip (MD)	Colon & Rectal Surgery	176
Hudes, Gary Robert (MD)	Medical Oncology	297
Hudgins, Louanne (MD)	Clinical Genetics	164
Hudson, Leonard (MD)	Pulmonary Disease	711
Huff, Robert Whitley (MD)	Clinical Genetics	438
Huffman, Jeffry Lee (MD)	Urology	848
Hunninghake, Gary (MD)	Pulmonary Disease	703
Hunstad, Joseph P. (MD)	Plastic Surgery	643
Hunt III, Thomas (MD)	Hand Surgery	272
Hunt, Robert Bridger (MD)	Obstetrics & Gynecology	431
Hunt, Sharon Ann (MD)	Cardiology (Cardiovascular Disease)	142
Hunter, Ellen B (MD)	Gastroenterology	228
Hurd, Eric (MD)	Rheumatology	767
Hurley, James (MD)	Endocrinology, Diabetes & Metabolism	200
Hurst, Michael K (MD)	Otolaryngology	504
Hurt, Hallam (MD)	Neonatal-Perinatal Medicine	351
Hurtig, Howard (MD)	Neurology	403
Hurwitz, Barrie (MD)	Neurology	408
Hurwitz, Dennis (MD)	Plastic Surgery	638
Hussey, Michael J (MD)	Maternal & Fetal Medicine	345
Hutchins, Laura (MD)	Medical Oncology	311
Hutter Jr, Adolph M (MD)	Cardiology (Cardiovascular Disease)	121
Huvos, Andrew (MD)	Pathology	536
Huynh, Phan Tuong (MD)	Diagnostic Radiology	734
Hyers, Thomas Morgan (MD)	Pulmonary Disease	703

I

Name	Specialty	Page
Iannaccone, Susan (MD)	Child Neurology	155
Iannettoni, Mark D. (MD)	Thoracic Surgery	817
Iannotti, Joseph (MD)	Orthopaedic Surgery	491
Idler, Richard S. (MD)	Hand Surgery	273
Ilowite, Norman T (MD)	Pediatric Rheumatology	608
Infante, Ernesto (MD)	Neurology	417
Ingle, James N (MD)	Medical Oncology	306
Inglis, Andrew (MD)	Pediatric Otolaryngology	603
Ingram, David (MD)	Pediatric Infectious Disease	592
Interian Jr, Alberto (MD)	Cardiac Electrophysiology	117
Ipp, Eli (MD)	Endocrinology, Diabetes & Metabolism	212
Irby III, Pierce B (MD)	Urology	837
Irvine, John Alexander (MD)	Ophthalmology	465

ALPHABETICAL LISTING OF DOCTORS

Name	Specialty	Page
Irwin Jr, Charles Edwin (MD)	Adolescent Medicine	90
Irwin, Richard Stephen (MD)	Pulmonary Disease	691
Irwin, Robert (MD)	Urology	832
Isaacson, Keith B (MD)	Reproductive Endocrinology	743
Isaacson, Steven (MD)	Radiation Oncology	719
Iseman, Michael (MD)	Pulmonary Disease	706
Isenberg, Keith Eugene (MD)	Geriatric Psychiatry	674
Isenberg, Sherwin Jay (MD)	Ophthalmology	465
Ishak, Kamal G. (MD)	Pathology	537
Ismail, Mahmoud (MD)	Maternal & Fetal Medicine	345
Isner, Jeffrey Michael (MD)	Cardiology (Cardiovascular Disease)	121
Isom, O Wayne (MD)	Thoracic Surgery	809
Ivanhoe, Cindy (MD)	Physical Medicine & Rehabilitation	629

J

Name	Specialty	Page
Jaafar, Mohamad S (MD)	Ophthalmology	447
Jackler, Robert K (MD)	Otolaryngology	522
Jackman, Warren (MD)	Cardiac Electrophysiology	118
Jackson, Amie Brown (MD)	Physical Medicine & Rehabilitation	626
Jackson, Gilchrist (MD)	Surgery	797
Jackson, John Kevin (MD)	Neurology	417
Jackson, Neil (MD)	Obstetrics & Gynecology	431
Jacob, Molly (MD)	Pediatrics	618
Jacobs, Alice K (MD)	Interventional Cardiology	144
Jacobs, Charlotte DeCroes (MD)	Medical Oncology	313
Jacobs, Laurence (MD)	Reproductive Endocrinology	749
Jacobs, Richard (MD)	Pediatric Infectious Disease	593
Jacobs, Stephen C (MD)	Urology	832
Jacobs, Thomas (MD)	Endocrinology, Diabetes & Metabolism	200
Jacobson , Jeff (MD)	Neurological Surgery	376
Jacobson, Ira (MD)	Gastroenterology	223
Jaffe, Allan S. (MD)	Cardiology (Cardiovascular Disease)	135
Jaffe, Elaine Sarkin (MD)	Pathology	537
Jaffe, Kenneth M (MD)	Physical Medicine & Rehabilitation	630
Jaffe, Robert B (MD)	Reproductive Endocrinology	751
Jain, Subhash (MD)	Pain Management	527
Jakobiec, Frederick A. (MD)	Ophthalmology	443
Janicak, Philip G. (MD)	Psychiatry	683
Jankovic, Joseph (MD)	Neurology	417
Jarow, Jonathan (MD)	Urology	833
Jelks, Glenn (MD)	Plastic Surgery	638
Jenike, Michael Andrew (MD)	Psychiatry	676
Jenkins, Herman A. (MD)	Otolaryngology	519
Jenkins, Roger L (MD)	Surgery	781
Jenkinson, Stephen George (MD)	Pulmonary Disease	709
Jensen, Michael D. (MD)	Endocrinology, Diabetes & Metabolism	207
Jenson, Hal B (MD)	Pediatric Infectious Disease	593
Jeste, Dilip (MD)	Geriatric Psychiatry	674
Jewell, Mark L (MD)	Plastic Surgery	652
Jillella, Anand (MD)	Medical Oncology	301
Jobe, Alan Hall (MD/PhD)	Neonatal-Perinatal Medicine	353
Jobe, Frank Wilson (MD)	Sports Medicine	774

Name	Specialty	Page
Johansen, Kaj (MD/PhD)	Vascular Surgery (General)	869
Johnson Jr, Calvin M (MD)	Otolaryngology	520
Johnson, Bruce Ellsworth ()	Pulmonary Disease	699
Johnson, Bruce Evan (MD)	Medical Oncology	293
Johnson, Carl A (MD)	Orthopaedic Surgery	482
Johnson, Darren Lee (MD)	Orthopaedic Surgery	486
Johnson, David (MD)	Medical Oncology	301
Johnson, Jonas Talmadge (MD)	Otolaryngology	504
Johnson, Kenneth P (MD)	Neurology	403
Johnson, Maryl R (MD)	Cardiology (Cardiovascular Disease)	136
Johnson, Timothy M (MD)	Dermatology	189
Johnson, Timothy R.B. (MD)	Obstetrics & Gynecology	436
Johnson, Warren (MD)	Infectious Disease	320
Johnston, Carolyn Marie (MD)	Gynecologic Oncology	260
Johnston, James (MD)	Nephrology	361
Johr, Robert (MD)	Dermatology	187
Jokl, Peter (MD)	Orthopaedic Surgery	476
Jonas, Adam Jonathan (MD)	Clinical Genetics	165
Jonas, Richard A (MD)	Thoracic Surgery	805
Jones III, Howard Wilbur (MD)	Gynecologic Oncology	258
Jones, Ellis (MD)	Thoracic Surgery	813
Jones, Jacqueline (MD)	Pediatric Otolaryngology	600
Jones, James F (MD)	Allergy & Immunology	102
Jones, Kenneth L (MD)	Pediatrics	165
Jones, Marilyn (MD)	Clinical Genetics	165
Jones, Neil (MD)	Hand Surgery	275
Jones, Paul John (MD)	Otolaryngology	514
Jones, Stephen E (MD)	Medical Oncology	311
Jordan, Gerald (MD)	Urology	837
Jorizzo, Joseph L. (MD)	Dermatology	188
Josephson, Jordan S (MD)	Otolaryngology	504
Josephson, Mark Eric (MD)	Cardiology (Cardiovascular Disease)	121
Josephson, Michelle Ann (MD)	Nephrology	365
Juillard, Guy Jean-Felix (MD)	Radiation Oncology	726
Jupiter, Jesse B (MD)	Orthopaedic Surgery	476

K

Name	Specialty	Page
Kagen, Lawrence (MD)	Rheumatology	759
Kahan, Barry (MD)	Surgery	797
Kahrilas, Peter (MD)	Gastroenterology	232
Kaiser, Harold (MD)	Allergy & Immunology	101
Kaiser, Larry Robert (MD)	Thoracic Surgery	809
Kalloo, Anthony Nicholas (MD)	Gastroenterology	223
Kamdar, Vikram V (MD)	Endocrinology, Diabetes & Metabolism	212
Kamer, Frank M (MD)	Otolaryngology	522
Kamholz, Stephan (MD)	Pulmonary Disease	694
Kan, Jean (MD)	Pediatric Cardiology	562
Kanda, Louis T (MD)	Thoracic Surgery	809
Kandarpa, Krishna (MD)	Radiology	736
Kane, Bryna (MD)	Dermatology	193
Kanel, Gary Craig (MD)	Pathology	543
Kantarjian, Hagop M (MD)	Hematology	290

ALPHABETICAL LISTING OF DOCTORS

Name	Specialty	Page
Kao, Kuo-Jang (MD/PhD)	Pathology	539
Kaplan, Allen (MD)	Allergy & Immunology	99
Kaplan, Bernard S (MD)	Pediatric Nephrology	595
Kaplan, David William (MD)	Adolescent Medicine	90
Kaplan, James (MD)	Pulmonary Disease	707
Kaplan, Mark H (MD)	Infectious Disease	320
Kaplan, Sheldon (MD)	Pediatric Infectious Disease	593
Kaplan, Stanley (MD)	Rheumatology	762
Kappy, Michael Steven (MD/PhD)	Pediatric Endocrinology	576
Karchmer, Adolph W (MD)	Infectious Disease	317
Karp, Daniel David (MD)	Medical Oncology	293
Karp, Robert Bruce (MD)	Thoracic Surgery	817
Karrer, Frederick Merrill (MD)	Surgery	796
Kartush, Jack (MD)	Otolaryngology	514
Karwande, Shreekanth V (MD)	Thoracic Surgery	820
Kase, Carlos S. (MD)	Neurology	398
Kashtan, Clifford (MD)	Pediatric Nephrology	598
Kasinath, Balakuntalam S (MD)	Nephrology	367
Kasiske, Bertram (MD)	Nephrology	365
Kass, Michael A (MD)	Ophthalmology	457
Kasser, James (MD)	Orthopaedic Surgery	476
Katner, Harold (MD)	Infectious Disease	323
Katowitz, James A (MD)	Ophthalmology	447
Katz, Ira Ralph (MD)	Geriatric Psychiatry	672
Katz, Nevin M (MD)	Thoracic Surgery	809
Katz, Paul (MD)	Rheumatology	759
Katz, Robert (MD)	Rheumatology	765
Katz, Robert L (MD)	Pediatric Otolaryngology	602
Katz, Stephen ()	Dermatology	184
Katzen, Barry (MD)	Radiology	737
Katzenstein, Anna-Luise A. (MD)	Pathology	537
Kaufman, Francine R (MD)	Pediatric Endocrinology	577
Kaushansky, Kenneth (MD)	Hematology	291
Kavoussi, Louis Rapheal (MD)	Urology	833
Kawamoto Jr, Henry K (MD)	Plastic Surgery	652
Kay, Jerome Harold (MD)	Thoracic Surgery	824
Kaye, Mitchell (MD)	Pulmonary Disease	703
Kaysen, George Alan (MD/PhD)	Nephrology	368
Kazanjian Jr, Powel H (MD)	Infectious Disease	325
Kazer, Ralph (MD)	Reproductive Endocrinology	749
Keagy, Blair Allen (MD)	Vascular Surgery (General)	863
Keefe, David Lawrence (MD)	Reproductive Endocrinology	743
Keeffe, Emmet B (MD)	Gastroenterology	237
Keenan, Robert (MD)	Thoracic Surgery	809
Keiser, Philip (MD)	Infectious Disease	327
Keller Jr, Frank G (MD)	Pediatric Hematology-Oncology	584
Keller, Frederick (MD)	Radiology	740
Keller, Gregory Steele (MD)	Otolaryngology	522
Kelly Jr, David L (MD)	Neurological Surgery	380
Kelly, John Michael (MD)	Plastic Surgery	649
Kelly, Keith A (MD)	Surgery	797
Kelly, Michael (MD)	Sports Medicine	773

ALPHABETICAL LISTING OF DOCTORS

Name	Specialty	Page
Kelly, Patrick J. (MD)	Neurological Surgery	377
Kemeny, Nancy (MD)	Medical Oncology	297
Kempin, Sanford Jay (MD)	Hematology	286
Kempson, Richard (MD)	Pathology	543
Kendler, Kenneth S (MD)	Psychiatry	682
Kennedy, David (MD)	Otolaryngology	504
Kennedy, Gary (MD)	Geriatric Psychiatry	672
Kennelly, Michael Joseph (MD)	Urology	838
Kent, K Craig (MD)	Vascular Surgery (General)	861
Kereiakes, Dean J (MD)	Cardiology (Cardiovascular Disease)	136
Kern, Robert (MD)	Otolaryngology	514
Kestenbaum, Clarice J (MD)	Child & Adolescent Psychiatry	666
Ketch, Lawrence Levant (MD)	Plastic Surgery	648
Kevorkian, Charles George (MD)	Physical Medicine & Rehabilitation	629
Khan, Agha S (MD)	Neurological Surgery	377
Khosla, Sundeep (MD)	Endocrinology, Diabetes & Metabolism	208
Kiernan, Paul Chapman (MD)	Thoracic Surgery	813
Killip, Thomas (MD)	Cardiology (Cardiovascular Disease)	126
Kilmer, Suzanne L (MD)	Dermatology	193
Kim, Woo Shin (MD)	Gynecologic Oncology	260
Kim, Young-Jee (MD)	Pediatric Pulmonology	605
Kimbrough, Robert (MD)	Infectious Disease	327
Kimmey, Michael Bryant (MD)	Gastroenterology	237
King III, Spencer (MD)	Interventional Cardiology	145
King Jr, Talmadge Everett (MD)	Pulmonary Disease	711
King, Bryan Harry (MD)	Child & Adolescent Psychiatry	663
King, John Chandler (MD)	Physical Medicine & Rehabilitation	630
Kinne, David W (MD)	Surgery	786
Kinsella, Timothy James (MD)	Radiation Oncology	723
Kirby, Thomas (MD)	Surgery	794
Kirkland III, John Lindsey (MD)	Pediatric Endocrinology	577
Kirklin, James (MD)	Thoracic Surgery	813
Kirkwood, John Munn (MD)	Medical Oncology	297
Kirschenbaum, Alexander Michael (MD)	Urology	833
Kirschner, Barbara S (MD)	Pediatric Gastroenterology	580
Kirshblum, Steven C (MD)	Physical Medicine & Rehabilitation	624
Kirshenbaum, James M (MD)	Cardiology (Cardiovascular Disease)	121
Kirshner, Howard S (MD)	Neurology	408
Kistler, John Philip (MD)	Neurology	398
Kitridou, Rodanthi C (MD)	Rheumatology	769
Kitterman, Joseph A (MD)	Neonatal-Perinatal Medicine	355
Klagsbrun, Samuel C (MD)	Psychiatry	679
Klamut, Michael (MD)	Gastroenterology	232
Klapholz, Marc (MD)	Cardiology (Cardiovascular Disease)	126
Klatsky, Stanley A (MD)	Plastic Surgery	638
Klearman, Micki (MD)	Rheumatology	765
Kleber, Herbert (MD)	Addiction Psychiatry	661
Kleiman, Martin (MD)	Pediatric Infectious Disease	593
Kleiman, Neal Stephen (MD)	Interventional Cardiology	147
Klein, Andrew S (MD)	Surgery	786
Klein, Donald (MD)	Psychiatry	679
Klein, Eric A (MD)	Urology	842

ALPHABETICAL LISTING OF DOCTORS

Name	Specialty	Page
Klein, Lloyd (MD)	Interventional Cardiology	146
Kleinman, Ronald Ellis (MD)	Pediatric Gastroenterology	578
Klement, Maria (MD)	Geriatric Psychiatry	672
Klibanski, Anne (MD)	Endocrinology, Diabetes & Metabolism	197
Kliger, Alan (MD)	Nephrology	359
Klimberg, V Suzanne (MD)	Surgery	798
Kline, Mark (MD)	Pediatric Infectious Disease	594
Klingensmith, Georgeanna (MD)	Pediatric Endocrinology	577
Klish, William John (MD)	Pediatric Gastroenterology	581
Knize, David Maurice (MD)	Plastic Surgery	648
Knoefel, Janice E (MD)	Neurology	417
Knowles, Daniel (MD)	Pathology	537
Knudson, Mary Margaret (MD)	Surgery	800
Kobashigawa, Jon Akira (MD)	Cardiology (Cardiovascular Disease)	142
Kobrine, Arthur (MD/PhD)	Neurological Surgery	377
Koch, Douglas D (MD)	Ophthalmology	462
Kochanek, Patrick (MD)	Pediatric Critical Care Medicine	569
Kodner, Ira Joe (MD)	Colon & Rectal Surgery	174
Kodsi, Baroukh (MD)	Gastroenterology	223
Koenig, Steven Michael (MD)	Pulmonary Disease	699
Kollef, Marin Hristo (MD)	Pulmonary Disease	704
Koller, William C (MD)	Neurology	408
Kolodny, Edwin H (MD)	Neurology	403
Komaki, Ritsuko (MD)	Radiation Oncology	725
Koman, L Andrew (MD)	Hand Surgery	270
Konicek, Frank (MD)	Gastroenterology	232
Konstam, Marvin Amnon (MD)	Cardiology (Cardiovascular Disease)	121
Koos, Brian John (MD)	Maternal & Fetal Medicine	348
Kopans, Daniel B (MD)	Diagnostic Radiology	731
Kopf, Alfred (MD)	Dermatology	184
Kopf, Gary (MD)	Thoracic Surgery	805
Koplewicz, Harold (MD)	Child & Adolescent Psychiatry	666
Koplin, Lawrence Mark (MD)	Plastic Surgery	653
Kopple, Joel David (MD)	Nephrology	369
Korelitz, Burton I (MD)	Gastroenterology	224
Korenblat, Phillip Erwin (MD)	Allergy & Immunology	101
Korf, Bruce (MD/PhD)	Clinical Genetics	159
Kormos, Robert (MD)	Thoracic Surgery	810
Koroshetz, Walter J. (MD)	Neurology	398
Koruda, Mark Joseph (MD)	Surgery	791
Korytkowski, Mary T (MD)	Endocrinology, Diabetes & Metabolism	200
Kosova, Leonard (MD)	Medical Oncology	307
Kosten, Thomas (MD)	Addiction Psychiatry	661
Kostis, John B (MD)	Cardiology (Cardiovascular Disease)	126
Kotler, Donald P (MD)	Gastroenterology	224
Kotzin, Brian Leslie (MD)	Rheumatology	767
Koufman, James Alan (MD)	Otolaryngology	509
Koyle, Martin Allan (MD)	Urology	845
Kozarek, Richard (MD)	Gastroenterology	237
Kozlowski, James Michael (MD)	Urology	842
Krachmer, Jay H. (MD)	Ophthalmology	457
Kraft, George Howard (MD)	Physical Medicine & Rehabilitation	631

ALPHABETICAL LISTING OF DOCTORS

Name	Specialty	Page
Kramer, Barry Alan (MD)	Geriatric Psychiatry	675
Kramer, Steven G (MD)	Ophthalmology	465
Kranzler, Leonard I (MD)	Neurological Surgery	383
Kredich, Deborah Welt (MD)	Pediatric Rheumatology	608
Kreisberg, Robert Alan (MD)	Endocrinology, Diabetes & Metabolism	204
Kreitzer, Joel (MD)	Pain Management	527
Krellenstein, Daniel (MD)	Thoracic Surgery	810
Kris, Mark (MD)	Medical Oncology	297
Krizek, Thomas (MD)	Plastic Surgery	643
Kroll, Stephen S (MD)	Plastic Surgery	649
Kron, Irving L (MD)	Thoracic Surgery	813
Krowka, Michael Joseph (MD)	Pulmonary Disease	704
Krueger, Gerald (MD)	Dermatology	191
Krueger, Ronald (MD)	Ophthalmology	457
Krumholz, Allan (MD)	Neurology	403
Krummel, Thomas M. (MD)	Pediatric Surgery	616
Kuhn, Frederick (MD)	Otolaryngology	509
Kumpe, David A (MD)	Radiology	738
Kupersmith, Mark (MD)	Ophthalmology	447
Kupfer, David J. (MD)	Psychiatry	679
Kurachek, Stephen Charles (MD)	Pediatric Pulmonology	605
Kurman, Robert J (MD)	Pathology	537
Kurtz, Albert B (MD)	Diagnostic Radiology	731
Kurtzke, Robert (MD)	Neurology	409
Kushner, Brian (MD)	Pediatric Hematology-Oncology	584
Kushner, Burton J (MD)	Ophthalmology	458
Kveton, John (MD)	Otolaryngology	501
Kwon, Tae (MD)	Gynecologic Oncology	257

L

Name	Specialty	Page
La Russo, Nicholas Francis (MD)	Gastroenterology	232
Ladenson, Paul William (MD)	Endocrinology, Diabetes & Metabolism	200
Lagasse, Leo D (MD)	Gynecologic Oncology	264
Lahita, Robert (MD)	Rheumatology	759
Laibson, Peter R (MD)	Ophthalmology	447
Laks, Hillel (MD)	Thoracic Surgery	824
Lambert, H. Michael (MD)	Ophthalmology	462
Lambert, Paul R (MD)	Otolaryngology	509
Lambert, Scott (MD)	Ophthalmology	454
Lambiase, Louis (MD)	Gastroenterology	228
Lammertse, Daniel (MD)	Physical Medicine & Rehabilitation	628
Landefeld, Charles Seth (MD)	Geriatric Medicine	251
Landers, Daniel V. (MD)	Maternal & Fetal Medicine	342
Landreneau, Rodney (MD)	Thoracic Surgery	810
Landy, Helain Jody (MD)	Maternal & Fetal Medicine	342
Lang, Samuel (MD)	Thoracic Surgery	810
Langer, Corey Jay (MD)	Medical Oncology	297
Langman, Craig (MD)	Pediatric Nephrology	598
Langston, J William (MD)	Neurology	421
Lantos, John (MD)	Pediatrics	618
Lanza, Donald (MD)	Otolaryngology	515
Lapey, Allen (MD)	Pediatric Pulmonology	604

ALPHABETICAL LISTING OF DOCTORS

Name	Specialty	Page
LaQuaglia, Michael (MD)	Pediatric Surgery	612
Larach, Sergio (MD)	Colon & Rectal Surgery	173
Larrabee Jr., Wayne F. (MD)	Otolaryngology	522
Larsen, Gary (MD)	Pediatric Pulmonology	606
Larson, Steven (MD)	Nuclear Medicine	425
Lask, Gary P (MD)	Dermatology	193
Latson, Larry Allen (MD)	Pediatric Critical Care Medicine	570
Lauerman, William (MD)	Orthopaedic Surgery	482
Lavis, Victor Ralph (MD)	Endocrinology, Diabetes & Metabolism	210
Lavyne, Michael H (MD)	Neurological Surgery	377
Laws Jr., Edward R (MD)	Neurological Surgery	380
Lawson, Edward Earle (MD)	Neonatal-Perinatal Medicine	352
Lawson, William (MD)	Otolaryngology	504
Lazarus, Lawrence W (MD)	Geriatric Psychiatry	674
Leaf, Norman (MD)	Plastic Surgery	653
Lebwohl, Mark (MD)	Dermatology	184
Lechan, Ronald (MD/PhD)	Endocrinology, Diabetes & Metabolism	198
Lederberg, Marguerite (MD)	Psychiatry	680
Ledford, Dennis (MD)	Allergy & Immunology	99
Ledger, William (MD)	Obstetrics & Gynecology	432
Lee, Jeffrey Edwin (MD)	Surgery	798
Lee, Jin Soo (MD)	Medical Oncology	311
Lee, Paul P (MD)	Ophthalmology	454
Leffall Jr, LaSalle D (MD)	Surgery	786
Leffert, Robert D. (MD)	Orthopaedic Surgery	476
Lefrak, Stephen (MD)	Pulmonary Disease	704
Legha, Sewa Singh (MD)	Medical Oncology	312
Lehman, Thomas (MD)	Pediatric Rheumatology	608
Lehman, Wallace B (MD)	Pediatric Surgery	612
Leibel, Steven A (MD)	Radiation Oncology	719
Leichman, Lawrence Peter (MD)	Medical Oncology	298
Leipziger, Lyle S (MD)	Plastic Surgery	638
Lell, Mary-Elizabeth (MD)	Child Neurology	152
Lema, Mark J (MD)	Pain Management	527
Lemanske Jr, Robert F (MD)	Pediatric Allergy & Immunology	557
Lemons, James A (MD)	Neonatal-Perinatal Medicine	353
Leon, Martin (MD)	Interventional Cardiology	144
Leonard Jr., James A. (MD)	Physical Medicine & Rehabilitation	627
Leonard, Henrietta (MD)	Child & Adolescent Psychiatry	663
Leonetti, John (MD)	Otolaryngology	515
Leonidas, John (MD)	Radiology	736
Leopold, Donald Arthur (MD)	Otolaryngology	518
Lepanto, Philip Bliss (MD)	Radiation Oncology	720
Lepor, Herbert (MD)	Urology	833
Lerman, Bruce (MD)	Cardiac Electrophysiology	115
Lesavoy, Malcolm A (MD)	Plastic Surgery	653
Leshin, Barry (MD)	Dermatology	188
Leuchter, Andrew Francis (MD)	Geriatric Psychiatry	675
Leung, Donald (MD/PhD)	Pediatric Allergy & Immunology	558
Leung, Lawrence L (MD)	Hematology	291
Levin, Bernard (MD)	Gastroenterology	236
Levin, David C (MD)	Pulmonary Disease	709

Name	Specialty	Page
Levin, L Scott (MD)	Plastic Surgery	643
Levin, Victor Alan (MD)	Neurology	418
Levine, Alexandra Mary (MD)	Hematology	291
Levine, David (MD)	Neurology	403
Levine, Elliot Mark (MD)	Obstetrics & Gynecology	436
Levine, Ellis (MD)	Medical Oncology	298
Levine, Joseph H (MD)	Cardiac Electrophysiology	115
Levine, Laurence Adan (MD)	Urology	842
Levine, Lenore (MD)	Pediatric Endocrinology	572
Levine, Melvin David (MD)	Pediatrics	618
Levine, Paul (MD)	Otolaryngology	509
Levine, Stephen B (MD)	Psychiatry	684
Levine, Steven R (MD)	Neurology	413
Levine, William (MD)	Sports Medicine	773
Levinson, Arnold (MD)	Allergy & Immunology	96
Levitan, Ruven (MD)	Gastroenterology	233
Levitsky, Lynne Lipton (MD)	Pediatric Endocrinology	572
Levitt, Selwyn (MD)	Urology	833
Levy, Joseph (MD)	Pediatric Gastroenterology	578
Levy, Moise (MD)	Dermatology	192
Levy, Philip (MD)	Endocrinology, Diabetes & Metabolism	210
Levy, Richard Alshuler (MD)	Pediatric Endocrinology	575
Levy, Robert M (MD)	Neurological Surgery	384
Levy, Ronald (MD)	Medical Oncology	314
Lewin, Alan (MD)	Radiation Oncology	721
Lewin, Klaus J (MD)	Pathology	543
Lewis Jr., Frank R. (MD)	Surgery	794
Lewis, Edmund J (MD)	Nephrology	365
Lewis, Hilel (MD)	Ophthalmology	458
Lewis, Ronald W (MD)	Urology	838
Leyden, James (MD)	Dermatology	184
Libby, Daniel (MD)	Pulmonary Disease	694
Libby, Peter (MD)	Cardiology (Cardiovascular Disease)	122
Liberman, Robert Paul (MD)	Psychiatry	687
Libertino, John A. (MD)	Urology	829
Libow, Leslie (MD)	Geriatric Medicine	245
Licata, Angelo A (MD)	Endocrinology, Diabetes & Metabolism	208
Lichtenstein, Michael Joseph (MD)	Geriatric Medicine	250
Lichter, Allen (MD)	Radiation Oncology	723
Lichter, Paul R. (MD)	Ophthalmology	458
Liddle, Rodger Alan (MD)	Gastroenterology	228
Lieberman, James (MD)	Physical Medicine & Rehabilitation	624
Liebman, Jerome (MD)	Pediatric Cardiology	565
Liebmann, Jeffrey (MD)	Ophthalmology	447
Liebowitz, Michael R (MD)	Psychiatry	680
Liem, Pham (MD)	Geriatric Medicine	250
Lieskovsky, Gary (MD)	Urology	849
Light, Richard Wayne (MD)	Pulmonary Disease	699
Light, Terry (MD)	Hand Surgery	273
Lightdale, Charles (MD)	Gastroenterology	224
Lillemoe, Keith Douglas (MD)	Surgery	786
Lindenfeld, JoAnn (MD)	Cardiology (Cardiovascular Disease)	139

ALPHABETICAL LISTING OF DOCTORS

Name	Specialty	Page
Lindor, Keith Douglas (MD)	Gastroenterology	233
Lindsay Jr, Joseph (MD)	Cardiology (Cardiovascular Disease)	127
Lindsey, Stephen M (MD)	Rheumatology	767
Lindstrom, Richard Lyndon (MD)	Ophthalmology	458
Linenberger, Michael (MD)	Hematology	291
Linn, Edward S (MD)	Obstetrics & Gynecology	436
Lipkin, David L (MD)	Physical Medicine & Rehabilitation	626
Lipkowitz, George S. (MD)	Surgery	781
Lippman, Marc E (MD)	Medical Oncology	307
Lipschitz, David Arnold (MD/PhD)	Geriatric Medicine	250
Lipshultz, Larry (MD)	Urology	846
Lipshutz, William H. (MD)	Gastroenterology	224
Lipsitz, Lewis Arnold (MD)	Geriatric Medicine	243
Lipson, Stephen Jay (MD)	Orthopaedic Surgery	476
Lipstate, James Mitchell (MD)	Rheumatology	768
Lisak, Robert Philip (MD)	Neurology	413
Lisman, Richard (MD)	Ophthalmology	448
Lister, George (MD)	Pediatric Critical Care Medicine	569
Litt, Iris F (MD)	Adolescent Medicine	90
Little, Alex G (MD)	Thoracic Surgery	824
Little, John W (MD)	Plastic Surgery	638
Littlejohn, Charles (MD)	Colon & Rectal Surgery	169
Litzow, Mark Robert (MD)	Hematology	289
Livesay, James J (MD)	Thoracic Surgery	822
Livingston, Philip (MD)	Medical Oncology	298
Livingston, Robert B (MD)	Medical Oncology	314
Lloyd Jr, Lewis K (MD)	Urology	838
Lo Gerfo, Frank W (MD)	Vascular Surgery (General)	858
Lobo, Rogerio (MD)	Reproductive Endocrinology	744
Lock, James E (MD)	Pediatric Cardiology	561
Lock, Terrence Ralph (MD)	Orthopaedic Surgery	491
Lockey, Richard (MD)	Allergy & Immunology	99
Lockhart, Jorge L (MD)	Urology	838
Lockshin, Michael Dan (MD)	Rheumatology	759
Lockwood, Charles (MD)	Maternal & Fetal Medicine	343
Lockwood, Ted (MD)	Plastic Surgery	648
Loeffler, Jay Steven (MD)	Radiation Oncology	717
Loeser, John D (MD)	Neurological Surgery	389
Loewenstein, Richard (MD)	Psychiatry	680
Loftus, Christopher M. (MD)	Neurological Surgery	387
Logigian, Eric L (MD)	Neurology	403
Lohr, Jacob (MD)	Pediatrics	618
Long, Donlin M (MD/PhD)	Neurological Surgery	377
Long, Sarah S (MD)	Pediatric Infectious Disease	590
Look, Katherine (MD)	Gynecologic Oncology	260
Lopez, Raul (MD)	Neurology	409
Lorusso, Thomas (MD)	Pulmonary Disease	699
Loscalzo, Joseph (MD)	Cardiology (Cardiovascular Disease)	122
Lott, Ira T (MD)	Child Neurology	156
Loughlin, Gerald M (MD)	Pediatric Pulmonology	604
Louis, Dean (MD)	Hand Surgery	273
Lowe, Franklin (MD)	Urology	833

Name	Specialty	Page
Lowe, Nicholas J (MD)	Dermatology	194
Lowenberg, David W (MD)	Orthopaedic Surgery	497
Lowry, Ann (MD)	Colon & Rectal Surgery	174
Loyd, James Emory (MD)	Pulmonary Disease	700
Lubahn, John D (MD)	Hand Surgery	268
Lublin, Fred (MD)	Neurology	404
Luby, James P (MD)	Infectious Disease	327
Luby, Joan Lida (MD)	Child & Adolescent Psychiatry	668
Luce, Edward (MD)	Plastic Surgery	646
Luchins, Daniel (MD)	Geriatric Psychiatry	674
Luciano, Anthony Adolph (MD)	Reproductive Endocrinology	743
Luck Jr, James Vernon (MD)	Orthopaedic Surgery	497
Ludwig, Stephen (MD)	Pediatrics	617
Lue, Tom F (MD)	Urology	849
Luerssen, Thomas G. (MD)	Neurological Surgery	384
Luggen, Michael (MD)	Rheumatology	765
Luken, Martin (MD)	Neurological Surgery	384
Lumsden, Alan Boyd (MD)	Vascular Surgery (General)	863
Lunsford, L Dade (MD)	Neurological Surgery	377
Lurain, John R (MD)	Gynecologic Oncology	260
Lusk, Rodney (MD)	Pediatric Otolaryngology	602
Lutcher, Charles (MD)	Hematology	287
Luterman, Arnold (MD)	Surgery	791
Luthra, Harvinder Singh (MD)	Rheumatology	765
Lyckholm, Laurel Jean (MD)	Medical Oncology	302
Lyketsos, Constantine G (MD)	Geriatric Psychiatry	672
Lyles, Kenneth W (MD)	Geriatric Medicine	246
Lynch, Joseph P (MD)	Pulmonary Disease	704
Lynch, Thomas (MD)	Medical Oncology	293
Lytle, Bruce Whitney (MD)	Thoracic Surgery	817

M

Name	Specialty	Page
Ma, Dong M (MD)	Physical Medicine & Rehabilitation	625
Mabrey, Jay D (MD)	Orthopaedic Surgery	495
Macchia, Richard (MD)	Urology	833
MacDonald, John (MD)	Medical Oncology	298
MacFadyen, Bruce (MD)	Surgery	798
MacIntyre, Neil Ross (MD)	Pulmonary Disease	700
MacKeigan, John (MD)	Colon & Rectal Surgery	174
MacKenzie, Richard G (MD)	Adolescent Medicine	90
Mackey, William C. (MD)	Vascular Surgery (General)	858
Mackinnon, Susan (MD)	Plastic Surgery	646
Mackool, Richard (MD)	Ophthalmology	448
MacLean, James Andrew (MD)	Allergy & Immunology	95
Macris, Nicholas T (MD)	Allergy & Immunology	96
Maddrey, Willis Crocker (MD)	Gastroenterology	236
Magramm, Irene (MD)	Ophthalmology	448
Maguire, James (MD)	Infectious Disease	317
Maharam, Lewis (MD)	Sports Medicine	773
Mahler, Donald A (MD)	Pulmonary Disease	692
Mahler, Richard J (MD)	Endocrinology, Diabetes & Metabolism	201
Mahon, Kathleen MK (MD)	Ophthalmology	465

ALPHABETICAL LISTING OF DOCTORS

Name	Specialty	Page
Mahoney, Charles Patrick (MD)	Pediatric Endocrinology	577
Mahony, Lynn (MD)	Pediatric Cardiology	566
Mahowald, Mark W (MD)	Neurology	414
Majd, Massoud (MD)	Nuclear Medicine	425
Makaroun, Michel (MD)	Vascular Surgery (General)	861
Make, Barry J (MD)	Pulmonary Disease	707
Maker, Vijay (MD)	Surgery	794
Maki, Dennis G (MD)	Infectious Disease	326
Malik, Ghaus (MD)	Neurological Surgery	384
Malin, Jennifer (MD)	Rheumatology	768
Malkowicz, Bruce (MD)	Urology	834
Mallory, Thomas (MD)	Orthopaedic Surgery	491
Maloney, Mary (MD)	Dermatology	182
Maloney, Robert Keller (MD)	Ophthalmology	466
Manche, Edward Emanuel (MD)	Ophthalmology	466
Mancuso, Anthony (MD)	Diagnostic Radiology	733
Mandel, Susan (MD)	Endocrinology, Diabetes & Metabolism	201
Mandell, Gerald (MD)	Infectious Disease	324
Mandell, Lynda (MD/PhD)	Radiation Oncology	720
Mangat, Devinder Singh (MD)	Otolaryngology	515
Mangiardi, John (MD)	Neurological Surgery	377
Mann, John (MD)	Infectious Disease	320
Manning, Warren (MD)	Cardiology (Cardiovascular Disease)	122
Manoli II, Arthur (MD)	Orthopaedic Surgery	491
Manske, Paul (MD)	Hand Surgery	273
Manson, Paul (MD)	Plastic Surgery	638
March, John (MD)	Child & Adolescent Psychiatry	667
Marchlinski, Francis Edward (MD)	Cardiac Electrophysiology	116
Marcus, Robert A (MD)	Endocrinology, Diabetes & Metabolism	212
Marder, Stephen Robert (MD)	Psychiatry	687
Margolis, James (MD)	Cardiology (Cardiovascular Disease)	131
Marin, Deborah B (MD)	Psychiatry	680
Marini, John Joseph (MD)	Pulmonary Disease	704
Marion, Donald W (MD)	Neurological Surgery	378
Mark, Eugene J. (MD)	Pathology	535
Markman, Maurie (MD)	Medical Oncology	307
Markowitz, Bernard Lloyd (MD)	Plastic Surgery	653
Markowitz, David (MD)	Gastroenterology	224
Marks, Lawrence (MD)	Radiation Oncology	721
Marks, Stanley M (MD)	Medical Oncology	298
Marmor, Michael F (MD)	Ophthalmology	466
Marrs, Richard P (MD)	Reproductive Endocrinology	752
Marsh, Jeffrey L (MD)	Plastic Surgery	646
Marshall, Fray F (MD)	Urology	838
Marshall, John Crook (MD/PhD)	Endocrinology, Diabetes & Metabolism	204
Martell, John Mark (MD)	Orthopaedic Surgery	491
Marten, Timothy James (MD)	Plastic Surgery	653
Martenson Jr, James A (MD)	Radiology	737
Martin, Paul (MD)	Gastroenterology	238
Martin, Richard (MD)	Neonatal-Perinatal Medicine	353
Martin, Richard Jay (MD)	Pulmonary Disease	707

ALPHABETICAL LISTING OF DOCTORS

Name	Specialty	Page
Martin, Rick A (MD)	Clinical Genetics	162
Martinez, Fernando J (MD)	Pulmonary Disease	704
Masket, Samuel (MD)	Ophthalmology	466
Mason, Kristin Denise (MD)	Physical Medicine & Rehabilitation	627
Mason, Wilbert Henry (MD)	Pediatric Infectious Disease	594
Mass, Daniel (MD)	Hand Surgery	273
Massad, L Stewart (MD)	Gynecologic Oncology	260
Massagli, Teresa Luisa (MD)	Physical Medicine & Rehabilitation	631
Massin, Edward Krauss (MD)	Cardiology (Cardiovascular Disease)	140
Massry, Shaul Gourgi (MD)	Nephrology	369
Masters, Gregory (MD)	Medical Oncology	307
Masur, Henry (MD)	Infectious Disease	320
Matar, Fadi (MD)	Interventional Cardiology	145
Matarasso, Alan (MD)	Plastic Surgery	639
Matas, Arthur J (MD)	Surgery	794
Mathes, Stephen (MD)	Plastic Surgery	653
Mathisen, Douglas (MD)	Thoracic Surgery	806
Matthay, Katherine Kurshan (MD)	Pediatric Hematology-Oncology	589
Matthay, Michael Anthony (MD)	Pulmonary Disease	711
Matthay, Richard ()	Pulmonary Disease	692
Matthews, David (MD)	Plastic Surgery	644
Matthews, Dennis Jerome (MD)	Physical Medicine & Rehabilitation	628
Mattox, Douglas (MD)	Otolaryngology	509
Maurer, Janet Rae (MD)	Pulmonary Disease	704
Maurer, William (MD)	Pediatric Endocrinology	576
Max, Mitchell Bruce (MD)	Neurology	404
Maxwell, G Patrick (MD)	Plastic Surgery	644
May Jr, James W (MD)	Plastic Surgery	635
Mayberg, Marc (MD)	Neurological Surgery	384
Mayer, John (MD)	Pediatric Surgery	611
Mayer, Lloyd (MD)	Gastroenterology	224
Mayer, Nathaniel (MD)	Physical Medicine & Rehabilitation	625
Mayes, Maureen Davidica (MD/PhD)	Rheumatology	765
Maytal, Joseph (MD)	Child Neurology	152
Mazow, Jack Bernard (MD)	Pediatric Allergy & Immunology	558
Mazow, Malcolm L. (MD)	Ophthalmology	462
Mazza, David S (MD)	Allergy & Immunology	96
Mazzone, Theodore (MD)	Endocrinology, Diabetes & Metabolism	208
Mc Vary, Kevin (MD)	Urology	842
McAlister, Bill (MD)	Radiology	738
McAninch, Jack (MD)	Urology	849
McAuliffe, John A (MD)	Hand Surgery	270
McCabe, Edward (MD)	Pediatrics	619
McCann, Merle Clements (MD)	Psychiatry	680
McCann, Richard L (MD)	Vascular Surgery (General)	863
McCarley, Dean L (MD)	Medical Oncology	302
McCarthy, Joseph (MD)	Plastic Surgery	639
McCarthy, Patrick McGuane (MD)	Thoracic Surgery	818
McCarthy, Paul L (MD)	Pediatric Rheumatology	608
McCarthy, Shirley (MD/PhD)	Diagnostic Radiology	731
McClamrock, Howard Dean (MD)	Reproductive Endocrinology	744
McComb, J Gordon (MD)	Neurological Surgery	389

ALPHABETICAL LISTING OF DOCTORS

Name	Specialty	Page
McConnell, John Dowling (MD)	Urology	846
McConnell, Robert John (MD)	Endocrinology, Diabetes & Metabolism	201
McCord, Clinton (MD)	Ophthalmology	454
McCormack Jr, Richard R (MD)	Hand Surgery	268
McCormick, Beryl (MD)	Radiation Oncology	720
McCormick, Paul (MD)	Neurological Surgery	378
McCormick, Steven (MD)	Pathology	537
McCormick, Wayne (MD)	Geriatric Medicine	251
McCracken, James Thomas (MD)	Child & Adolescent Psychiatry	670
McCulley, James P (MD)	Ophthalmology	462
McCullough, David L (MD)	Urology	838
McCune, W. Joseph (MD)	Rheumatology	765
McDiarmid, Suzanne V (MD)	Pediatric Gastroenterology	582
McDonald, Charles J (MD)	Dermatology	182
McDonald, Marguerite B. (MD)	Ophthalmology	462
McDonald, Ruth A (MD)	Pediatric Nephrology	599
McDougal, William Scott (MD)	Urology	829
McGlashan, Thomas (MD)	Psychiatry	676
McGovern, Brian Anthony (MD)	Cardiac Electrophysiology	115
McGovern, Francis (MD)	Urology	829
McGowan Jr, John E (MD)	Infectious Disease	324
McGregor, Christopher (MD)	Thoracic Surgery	818
McGuirt, W Fredrick (MD)	Otolaryngology	509
McHugh, Paul (MD)	Psychiatry	680
McKenna Jr, Robert J (MD)	Thoracic Surgery	824
McKeown, Craig A (MD)	Ophthalmology	443
McKinney Jr, Ross E (MD)	Pediatric Infectious Disease	592
McKinney, Peter W. (MD)	Plastic Surgery	646
McLaren, Rodney A (MD)	Maternal & Fetal Medicine	344
McLeod, Allan G W (MD)	Obstetrics & Gynecology	434
McMahon, Marion (MD)	Endocrinology, Diabetes & Metabolism	208
McNeese, Marsha (MD)	Radiation Oncology	725
McNutt, N Scott (MD)	Pathology	538
Meals, Roy Allen (MD)	Hand Surgery	276
Medich, David (MD)	Colon & Rectal Surgery	171
Medina, Jesus (MD)	Otolaryngology	520
Medow, Norman (MD)	Ophthalmology	448
Medsger Jr, Thomas A (MD)	Rheumatology	760
Meek, Rita (MD)	Pediatric Hematology-Oncology	584
Mehlman, David J (MD)	Cardiology (Cardiovascular Disease)	136
Mehta, Atul Chandrakant (MD)	Pulmonary Disease	705
Meier, Diane (MD)	Geriatric Medicine	245
Mellins, Robert (MD)	Pediatric Pulmonology	604
Mellow, Alan M. (MD/PhD)	Geriatric Psychiatry	674
Melman, Arnold (MD)	Urology	834
Melmed, Shlomo (MD)	Endocrinology, Diabetes & Metabolism	212
Melone Jr, Charles P (MD)	Hand Surgery	268
Meltzer, Toby R (MD)	Plastic Surgery	653
Melvin, W Scott (MD)	Surgery	794
Mendell, Jerry R (MD)	Neurology	414
Mendelsohn, Janis (MD)	Pediatrics	619
Mendenhall, Nancy P (MD)	Radiation Oncology	722

Name	Specialty	Page
Mendenhall, William M (MD)	Radiation Oncology	722
Menezes, Arnold (MD)	Neurological Surgery	384
Menkes, John H (MD)	Child Neurology	156
Menninger, W Walter (MD)	Psychiatry	684
Mennuti, Michael (MD)	Maternal & Fetal Medicine	343
Menon, Mani (MD)	Urology	842
Menter, M Alan (MD)	Dermatology	192
Meredith, Travis (MD)	Ophthalmology	458
Merrick III, Hollis W. (MD)	Vascular Surgery (General)	866
Merrick, Frank W (MD)	Obstetrics & Gynecology	436
Merrill, Walter H (MD)	Thoracic Surgery	813
Merritt, Diane (MD)	Obstetrics & Gynecology	436
Mersey, James Harris (MD)	Endocrinology, Diabetes & Metabolism	201
Messer, Joseph V (MD)	Internal Medicine	336
Mesulam, Marek Marsel (MD)	Neurology	414
Metcalfe, Dean D (MD)	Allergy & Immunology	97
Metersky, Mark Lewis (MD)	Pulmonary Disease	692
Mets, Marilyn (MD)	Ophthalmology	458
Metz, David C. (MD)	Gastroenterology	224
Metz, Henry (MD)	Ophthalmology	448
Meyer, Anthony A (MD)	Surgery	791
Meyers, Bryan (MD)	Thoracic Surgery	818
Meyers, Paul (MD)	Pediatric Hematology-Oncology	584
Michalska, Margaret (MD)	Rheumatology	766
Micheli, Lyle J (MD)	Orthopaedic Surgery	476
Michler, Robert (MD)	Thoracic Surgery	818
Middleton, Richard (MD)	Urology	845
Mih, Alexander (MD)	Hand Surgery	273
Mihm Jr., Martin C. (MD)	Dermatology	182
Milad, Magdy P (MD)	Reproductive Endocrinology	749
Milam, Douglas F (MD)	Urology	838
Mildvan, Donna (MD)	Infectious Disease	320
Miles, Brian J (MD)	Urology	846
Milhorat, Thomas H (MD)	Neurological Surgery	378
Miller, Carol A (MD)	Pediatrics	619
Miller, Charles (MD)	Surgery	787
Miller, David Craig (MD)	Thoracic Surgery	824
Miller, Douglas Kent (MD)	Geriatric Medicine	248
Miller, Franklin (MD)	Radiology	738
Miller, Joshua (MD)	Surgery	791
Miller, Kenneth B. (MD)	Hematology	285
Miller, Marilyn T (MD)	Ophthalmology	459
Miller, Neil (MD)	Ophthalmology	448
Miller, Robert (MD)	Pediatric Otolaryngology	602
Miller, Sheldon I (MD)	Addiction Psychiatry	661
Miller, Stanley (MD)	Dermatology	185
Miller, Timothy Alden (MD)	Plastic Surgery	654
Millis, J. Michael (MD)	Surgery	794
Mills, Stacey E (MD)	Pathology	539
Milmoe, Gregory J (MD)	Pediatric Otolaryngology	601
Milsom, Jeffrey (MD)	Colon & Rectal Surgery	171
Mims III, James Luther (MD)	Ophthalmology	462

ALPHABETICAL LISTING OF DOCTORS

Name	Specialty	Page
Minaker, Kenneth (MD)	Geriatric Medicine	243
Minckler, Donald Saier (MD)	Ophthalmology	466
Mindich, Bruce (MD)	Thoracic Surgery	810
Minervini, Donald (MD)	Surgery	791
Minkoff, Howard L (MD)	Obstetrics & Gynecology	432
Minkoff, Jeffrey (MD)	Orthopaedic Surgery	487
Minsky, Bruce (MD)	Radiation Oncology	720
Miro-Quesada, Miguel (MD)	Hematology	291
Miskovitz, Paul (MD)	Gastroenterology	225
Mitchell, Beverly (MD)	Medical Oncology	302
Mitchell, Charles (MD)	Pediatric Infectious Disease	592
Mitchell, James Edward (MD)	Psychiatry	684
Mitchell, Paul Ralph (MD)	Ophthalmology	443
Mitchell, Wendy Gayle (MD)	Child Neurology	156
Mitnick, Hal J (MD)	Rheumatology	760
Mitnick, Julie (MD)	Diagnostic Radiology	732
Miyamoto, Richard (MD)	Otolaryngology	515
Mladick, Richard (MD)	Plastic Surgery	644
Moawad, Atef H (MD)	Obstetrics & Gynecology	436
Mobley, William Charles (MD)	Child Neurology	156
Moder, Kevin Gerard (MD)	Rheumatology	766
Modic, Michael (MD)	Radiology	738
Mohl, Paul C. (MD)	Psychiatry	685
Mohr, Jay Preston (MD)	Neurology	404
Mohsenifar, Z (MD)	Pulmonary Disease	711
Molnar, Joseph (MD)	Plastic Surgery	644
Monaco, Anthony (MD)	Surgery	782
Moncure, Ashby (MD)	Thoracic Surgery	806
Mondino, Bartly John (MD)	Ophthalmology	466
Moneim, Moheb S.A. (MD)	Hand Surgery	274
Mones, Richard (MD)	Pediatric Gastroenterology	578
Money, Samuel (MD)	Vascular Surgery (General)	868
Montague, Drogo K. (MD)	Urology	843
Montie, James (MD)	Urology	843
Montz, Fredrick John (MD)	Gynecologic Oncology	257
Moodie, Douglas (MD)	Pediatric Cardiology	565
Moore, Anne (MD)	Medical Oncology	298
Moore, Constance A. (MD)	Psychiatry	685
Moore, David H (MD)	Gynecologic Oncology	260
Moore, Wesley Sanford (MD)	Vascular Surgery (General)	869
Moores, Russell (MD)	Medical Oncology	302
Morady, Fred (MD)	Cardiac Electrophysiology	117
Moran, John (MD)	Cardiology (Cardiovascular Disease)	136
Morgan, Linda S (MD)	Obstetrics & Gynecology	434
Morgan, Raymond (MD)	Plastic Surgery	644
Morgan, Wayne J. (MD)	Pediatric Pulmonology	606
Morgenlander, Joel Charles (MD)	Neurology	409
Morley, John (MD)	Geriatric Medicine	248
Morrell, Martha J (MD)	Neurology	404
Morris, Colleen A. (MD)	Clinical Genetics	165
Morris, Douglas (MD)	Interventional Cardiology	145
Morris, John (MD)	Neurology	414

Name	Specialty	Page
Morris, Robert Edward (MD)	Adolescent Medicine	91
Morrison, Glenn (MD)	Neurological Surgery	381
Morrow, Charles Paul (MD)	Gynecologic Oncology	264
Morrow, Monica (MD)	Surgery	794
Mortimer, Joanne (MD)	Medical Oncology	307
Morton, Donald Lee (MD)	Thoracic Surgery	825
Moses, Alan Charles (MD)	Endocrinology, Diabetes & Metabolism	198
Moses, Jeffrey W (MD)	Cardiology (Cardiovascular Disease)	127
Moshang Jr., Thomas (MD)	Pediatric Endocrinology	573
Mosher, Deane F (MD)	Hematology	289
Moskowitz, Roland (MD)	Rheumatology	766
Mostwin, Jacek Lech (MD/PhD)	Urology	834
Motzer, Robert J (MD)	Medical Oncology	298
Mulcahy, John J. (MD)	Urology	843
Muldoon, Thomas O (MD)	Ophthalmology	448
Mulliken, John B. (MD)	Plastic Surgery	635
Mullin, Vildan (MD)	Pain Management	530
Mullin, Walter (MD)	Plastic Surgery	644
Mullins, Charles (MD)	Pediatric Cardiology	567
Mundy, Gregory Robert (MD)	Endocrinology, Diabetes & Metabolism	210
Munich, Richard (MD)	Psychiatry	685
Munin, Michael Craig (MD)	Physical Medicine & Rehabilitation	625
Murali, Raj (MD)	Neurological Surgery	378
Muraskas, Erik (MD)	Obstetrics & Gynecology	436
Murphree, A. Linn (MD)	Ophthalmology	466
Murphy, Ana Alvarez (MD)	Reproductive Endocrinology	747
Murphy, Thomas M (MD)	Pediatric Pulmonology	604
Muss, Hyman (MD)	Medical Oncology	293
Mustoe, Thomas (MD)	Plastic Surgery	646
Mutch, David (MD)	Gynecologic Oncology	261
Myerburg, Robert (MD)	Cardiology (Cardiovascular Disease)	131
Myers, Bryan David (MD)	Nephrology	369
Myers, Charles E (MD)	Medical Oncology	302
Myers, Eugene (MD)	Otolaryngology	505
Myerson, Mark (MD)	Orthopaedic Surgery	482
Myerson, Robert J (MD)	Radiation Oncology	724
Myones, Barry Lee (MD)	Pediatric Rheumatology	609

N

Name	Specialty	Page
Naccarelli, Gerald V (MD)	Cardiology (Cardiovascular Disease)	127
Nachman, James (MD)	Pediatric Hematology-Oncology	587
Naclerio, Robert (MD)	Otolaryngology	515
Nadeau, Stephen E (MD)	Neurology	409
Nadler, Lee Marshall (MD)	Medical Oncology	293
Nadol, Joseph (MD)	Otolaryngology	501
Naftolin, Frederick (MD)	Obstetrics & Gynecology	431
Nagey, David Augustus (MD)	Maternal & Fetal Medicine	343
Nagib, Mahmoud (MD)	Neurological Surgery	384
Nagle, Daniel J (MD)	Orthopaedic Surgery	492
Nagler, Harris M (MD)	Urology	834
Nahai, Foad (MD)	Plastic Surgery	645
Nahmias, Jaime Pablo (MD)	Obstetrics & Gynecology	434

ALPHABETICAL LISTING OF DOCTORS

Name	Specialty	Page
Najarian, John S (MD)	Surgery	794
Nakayama, Don Ken (MD)	Pediatric Surgery	613
Nand, Sucha (MD)	Hematology	289
Nardell, Edward (MD)	Pulmonary Disease	692
Nash, Martin (MD)	Pediatric Nephrology	595
Nash, Thomas (MD)	Pulmonary Disease	334
Naslund, Michael (MD)	Urology	834
Natale, Ronald B (MD)	Medical Oncology	314
Nath, Rahul Kamur (MD)	Plastic Surgery	650
Nathwani, Bharat N (MD)	Pathology	543
Nazzaro, Jules M. (MD)	Neurological Surgery	373
Neblett, Wallace W (MD)	Pediatric Surgery	613
Neff, James R (MD)	Orthopaedic Surgery	494
Nelson, Audrey May (MD)	Rheumatology	766
Nelson, Carl (MD)	Orthopaedic Surgery	495
Nelson, Harold (MD)	Allergy & Immunology	102
Nelson, Heidi (MD)	Colon & Rectal Surgery	174
Nelson, J Craig (MD)	Psychiatry	677
Nelson, Joel Byron (MD)	Urology	834
Nelson, Maureen R (MD)	Physical Medicine & Rehabilitation	630
Nemeroff, Charles Barnet (MD)	Geriatric Psychiatry	673
Nemickas, Rimgaudas (MD)	Cardiology (Cardiovascular Disease)	136
Neppe, Vernon Michael (MD)	Psychiatry	687
Nesburn, Anthony B (MD)	Ophthalmology	467
Netterville, James (MD)	Otolaryngology	510
Neu, Josef (MD)	Neonatal-Perinatal Medicine	353
Neuberg, Marcy (MD)	Dermatology	190
Neumann, Ronald D (MD)	Nuclear Medicine	425
Neustrom, Mark Ray (DO)	Allergy & Immunology	102
Nevins, Thomas E (MD)	Pediatric Nephrology	598
New, Maria Iandolo (MD)	Pediatric Endocrinology	573
Newburger, Jane (MD)	Pediatric Cardiology	561
Newell, Kenneth (MD/PhD)	Surgery	795
Newman, Lee (MD)	Pulmonary Disease	707
Newman, Leonard (MD)	Pediatric Gastroenterology	578
Newman, M Haskell (MD)	Plastic Surgery	647
Newman, Nancy Jean (MD)	Neurology	409
Neylan, John Francis (MD)	Nephrology	363
Ngeow, Jeffrey (MD)	Pain Management	528
Nichols, David Gregory (MD)	Pediatric Critical Care Medicine	570
Nickman, Steven L (MD)	Child & Adolescent Psychiatry	664
Niederman, Michael (MD)	Pulmonary Disease	694
Nigra, Thomas P (MD)	Dermatology	185
Nigro, Michael A (DO)	Child Neurology	153
Niloff, Jonathan Mitchell (MD)	Gynecologic Oncology	255
Niparko, John (MD)	Otolaryngology	505
Nisonson, Barton (MD)	Sports Medicine	773
Nissenblatt, Michael (MD)	Medical Oncology	299
Nitti, Victor (MD)	Urology	834
Nivatvongs, Santhat (MD)	Colon & Rectal Surgery	174
Nixon, Daniel (MD)	Medical Oncology	302
Nobunaga , Austin (MD)	Physical Medicine & Rehabilitation	627

ALPHABETICAL LISTING OF DOCTORS

Name	Specialty	Page
Olopade, Olufunmilayo I F (MD)	Medical Oncology	307
Olson, Jack Conrad (MD)	Geriatric Medicine	248
Olsson, Carl (MD)	Urology	835
Omachi, Rodney S (MD)	Nephrology	369
Ontjes, David A (MD)	Endocrinology, Diabetes & Metabolism	204
Opelka, Frank (MD)	Colon & Rectal Surgery	176
Orlow, Seth (MD)	Dermatology	185
Orobello Jr, Peter W (MD)	Otolaryngology	510
Orringer, Mark B (MD)	Thoracic Surgery	818
Ory, Steven (MD)	Reproductive Endocrinology	747
Osborne, Charles Kent (MD)	Medical Oncology	312
Osteen, Robert T (MD)	Surgery	782
Oster, Martin (MD)	Medical Oncology	299
Osterman Jr, Arthur Lee (MD)	Orthopaedic Surgery	482
Ostroff, James Warren (MD)	Gastroenterology	238
Ostrom, Nancy Kay (MD)	Pediatric Allergy & Immunology	559
Othersen, H Biemann (MD)	Pediatric Surgery	614
Ott, David A (MD)	Thoracic Surgery	822
Otto, Pamela (MD)	Diagnostic Radiology	734
Otto, Randal A (MD)	Otolaryngology	520
Ouellette, Elizabeth Anne (MD)	Hand Surgery	270
Ouriel, Kenneth (MD)	Vascular Surgery (General)	866
Ouslander, Joseph (MD)	Geriatric Medicine	246
Ovalle, Fernando (MD)	Endocrinology, Diabetes & Metabolism	204
Owen, William F. (MD)	Nephrology	359
Owsley, John Q (MD)	Plastic Surgery	654
Owyang, Chung (MD)	Gastroenterology	233
Oz, Mehmet Cengiz (MD)	Thoracic Surgery	810
Ozols, Robert Felix (MD/PhD)	Medical Oncology	299

P

Name	Specialty	Page
Pachter, H Leon (MD)	Surgery	787
Pacifico, Albert D (MD)	Thoracic Surgery	814
Pacin, Michael (MD)	Allergy & Immunology	99
Pack, Allan I (MD/PhD)	Pulmonary Disease	694
Packer, Milton (MD)	Cardiology (Cardiovascular Disease)	127
Packer, Roger (MD)	Child Neurology	153
Padma-Nathan, Harin (MD)	Urology	849
Pagani, Francis Domenic (MD)	Thoracic Surgery	818
Paganini, Emil (MD)	Nephrology	365
Page, David L (MD)	Pathology	540
Paget, Stephen (MD)	Rheumatology	760
Pagon, Roberta Anderson (MD)	Clinical Genetics	165
Paidas, Charles Nicholas (MD)	Pediatric Surgery	612
Pairolero, Peter (MD)	Thoracic Surgery	818
Palacios, Igor F (MD)	Cardiology (Cardiovascular Disease)	122
Paletta , George A (MD)	Sports Medicine	774
Paller, Amy Susan (MD)	Dermatology	190
Palmaz, Julio C. (MD)	Radiology	739
Palmberg, Paul (MD/PhD)	Ophthalmology	454
Palmer, Andrew (MD)	Orthopaedic Surgery	482
Palmer, Earl A. (MD)	Ophthalmology	467

ALPHABETICAL LISTING OF DOCTORS

Name	Specialty	Page
Peppard, Terrence Richard (MD)	Physical Medicine & Rehabilitation	626
Peppercorn, Mark (MD)	Gastroenterology	222
Perez Fontan, J Julio (MD)	Pediatric Critical Care Medicine	570
Perez, Carlos A (MD)	Radiation Oncology	724
Perkins, Rodney (MD)	Otolaryngology	522
Perler, Bruce Alan (MD)	Vascular Surgery (General)	861
Perlman, David (MD)	Infectious Disease	320
Perlman, Jeffrey (MD)	Neonatal-Perinatal Medicine	354
Perlmutter, Joel S (MD)	Neurology	414
Perloff, Joseph Kayle (MD)	Cardiology (Cardiovascular Disease)	142
Perret, Phillip Samuel (MD)	Pulmonary Disease	709
Perrone, Ronald (MD)	Nephrology	360
Perry, James (MD)	Orthopaedic Surgery	487
Perry, Michael (MD)	Medical Oncology	307
Perry, Stanton Bruce (MD)	Pediatric Cardiology	561
Perryman, Richard A (MD)	Thoracic Surgery	814
Persky, Mark (MD)	Otolaryngology	505
Peters, Glenn Eidson (MD)	Otolaryngology	510
Peters, Jeffrey Harold (MD)	Surgery	801
Peters, William P (MD/PhD)	Medical Oncology	308
Petersen, Robert Allen (MD)	Ophthalmology	443
Petito, Carol (MD)	Pathology	540
Petito, Frank (MD)	Neurology	404
Petrek, Jeanne (MD)	Surgery	787
Petri, Michelle Ann (MD)	Rheumatology	760
Petrovich, Zbigniew (MD)	Radiology	740
Pettrone, Frank A (MD)	Orthopaedic Surgery	487
Petty, Thomas L (MD)	Pulmonary Disease	707
Philipson, Elliot (MD)	Maternal & Fetal Medicine	346
Phillips III, Harry Rissler (MD)	Cardiology (Cardiovascular Disease)	132
Phillips, Theodore Locke (MD)	Radiation Oncology	727
Pi, Edmond Hsin-Tung (MD)	Psychiatry	687
Piccione, William (MD)	Thoracic Surgery	819
Piccirillo, Jay (MD)	Otolaryngology	516
Pichard, Augusto (MD)	Interventional Cardiology	144
Picken, Catherine A (MD)	Otolaryngology	505
Piel, Ira (MD)	Medical Oncology	308
Pielet, Bruce (MD)	Maternal & Fetal Medicine	346
Piepgras, David (MD)	Neurological Surgery	385
Piepmeier, Joseph (MD)	Neurological Surgery	374
Pierach, Claus (MD)	Internal Medicine	336
Pierce, Lori J (MD)	Radiation Oncology	724
Pierson III, Richard Norris (MD)	Thoracic Surgery	814
Piest, Kenneth L (MD)	Ophthalmology	462
Pile-Spellman, John (MD)	Radiology	736
Pillsbury, Harold Crockett (MD)	Otolaryngology	510
Pimstone, Neville R (MD)	Gastroenterology	238
Pingleton, Susan (MD)	Pulmonary Disease	707
Pinnell, Sheldon (MD)	Dermatology	188
Piraino, Beth Marie (MD)	Nephrology	361
Pisano, Etta Driscoll (MD)	Diagnostic Radiology	733
Pistenmaa, David A (MD)	Radiation Oncology	726

ALPHABETICAL LISTING OF DOCTORS

Name	Specialty	Page
Pisters, Katherine M W (MD)	Medical Oncology	312
Pitlick, Paul T (MD)	Pediatric Cardiology	567
Pitman, Gerald (MD)	Plastic Surgery	639
Pitt, Bertram (MD)	Interventional Cardiology	146
Pitts, Lawrence H (MD)	Neurological Surgery	389
Pizzo, Philip Anthony (MD)	Pediatrics	617
Platt, Lawrence David (MD)	Obstetrics & Gynecology	439
Platzker, Arnold CG (MD)	Pediatric Pulmonology	606
Plehn, Jonathan (MD)	Cardiology (Cardiovascular Disease)	127
Plotnick, Leslie Parker (MD)	Pediatric Endocrinology	573
Plotz, Paul (MD)	Rheumatology	760
Plum, Fred (MD)	Neurology	405
Podoloff, Donald (MD)	Nuclear Medicine	427
Podos, Steven M (MD)	Ophthalmology	449
Podratz, Karl C (MD/PhD)	Gynecologic Oncology	261
Poe, Dennis (MD)	Otolaryngology	501
Poehling, Gary G. (MD)	Orthopaedic Surgery	487
Pohl, Marc (MD)	Nephrology	365
Polan, Mary Lake (MD/PhD)	Reproductive Endocrinology	752
Poliakoff, Steven (MD)	Gynecologic Oncology	258
Polin, Richard (MD)	Neonatal-Perinatal Medicine	352
Polisson, Richard Paul (MD)	Rheumatology	757
Polk Jr, Hiram C (MD)	Surgery	792
Pollack, Ian (MD)	Neurological Surgery	378
Pollack, Jed (MD)	Radiation Oncology	720
Pollard, Zane F (MD)	Ophthalmology	454
Pollock, Stephen (MD)	Ophthalmology	455
Polonsky, Kenneth S (MD)	Endocrinology, Diabetes & Metabolism	208
Polsky, Bruce (MD)	Infectious Disease	321
Pomer, Sydney Lawrence (MD)	Psychiatry	687
Pomerantz, Marvin (MD)	Thoracic Surgery	820
Pongracic, Jacqueline (MD)	Pediatric Allergy & Immunology	557
Ponton, Lynn Elisabeth (MD)	Child & Adolescent Psychiatry	670
Pope Jr, Harrison G (MD)	Psychiatry	677
Pope, Richard M (MD)	Rheumatology	766
Popovich Jr, John (MD)	Pulmonary Disease	705
Portenoy, Russell (MD)	Pain Management	528
Porter, Co-burn Joseph (MD)	Pediatric Cardiology	565
Porter, John M. (MD)	Vascular Surgery (General)	869
Porth, Karen (MD)	Neurology	414
Posner, Jerome (MD)	Neurology	405
Posnick, Jeffrey Craig (MD/DMD)	Plastic Surgery	639
Poss, Robert (MD)	Orthopaedic Surgery	477
Post, Kalmon (MD)	Neurological Surgery	378
Postma, Gregory N (MD)	Otolaryngology	510
Potkul, Ronald (MD)	Gynecologic Oncology	261
Potsic, William Paul (MD)	Pediatric Otolaryngology	601
Powderly, William (MD)	Infectious Disease	326
Powell, Bayard Lowery (MD)	Medical Oncology	303
Powell, Nelson Bert (MD/DDS)	Otolaryngology	522
Powers, Alvin C (MD)	Endocrinology, Diabetes & Metabolism	205
Powers, Eric Randall (MD)	Cardiology (Cardiovascular Disease)	132

ALPHABETICAL LISTING OF DOCTORS

Name	Specialty	Page
Powers, Pauline (MD)	Psychiatry	683
Prager, Joshua Philip (MD)	Pain Management	531
Prakash, Udaya (MD)	Pulmonary Disease	705
Preisler, Harvey D (MD)	Hematology	290
Prensky, Arthur (MD)	Child Neurology	154
Present, Daniel (MD)	Gastroenterology	225
Press, Joel (MD)	Physical Medicine & Rehabilitation	627
Press, Oliver William (MD/PhD)	Medical Oncology	314
Pressman, Peter (MD)	Surgery	787
Pribaz, Julian (MD)	Plastic Surgery	636
Price, Ronald (MD)	Ophthalmology	459
Prinz, Richard (MD)	Surgery	795
Prosnitz, Leonard (MD)	Radiation Oncology	722
Pruitt, David B. (MD)	Child & Adolescent Psychiatry	666
Pryor, Jon L. (MD)	Urology	843
Prystowsky, Eric Neal (MD)	Cardiac Electrophysiology	118
Puccetti, Diane (MD)	Pediatric Hematology-Oncology	587
Puckett, Charles Linwood (MD)	Plastic Surgery	647
Pula, Thaddeus (MD)	Neurology	405
Putnam Jr, Joe B (MD)	Thoracic Surgery	822
Putnam, Matthew Douglas (MD)	Hand Surgery	274
Putterman, Allen M. (MD)	Ophthalmology	459

Q

Quaegebeur, Jan Modest (MD)	Pediatric Surgery	612
Quatela, Vito Charles (MD)	Otolaryngology	506
Quigley, Harry Alan (MD)	Ophthalmology	449
Quinn, Graham Earl (MD)	Ophthalmology	449
Quinn, Suzanne Lorraine (MD)	Endocrinology, Diabetes & Metabolism	205
Quintessenza, James (MD)	Thoracic Surgery	814
Quismorio Jr, Francisco P (MD)	Rheumatology	769
Quittell, Lynne (MD)	Pediatric Pulmonology	604
Quivey, Jeanne Marie (MD)	Radiation Oncology	727

R

Raab, Edward (MD)	Ophthalmology	449
Rabins, Peter (MD)	Geriatric Psychiatry	673
Racz, Gabor (MD)	Pain Management	531
Rader, Janet Sue (MD)	Gynecologic Oncology	261
Raffin, Thomas Alfred (MD)	Pulmonary Disease	712
Raghu, Ganesh (MD)	Pulmonary Disease	712
Ragnarsson, Kristjan (MD)	Physical Medicine & Rehabilitation	625
Rahal, James (MD)	Infectious Disease	321
Rahko, Peter (MD)	Cardiology (Cardiovascular Disease)	137
Rahn, Daniel W (MD)	Rheumatology	762
Raiford, David S (MD)	Gastroenterology	229
Raja, Srinivasa (MD)	Pain Management	528
Rajfer, Jacob (MD)	Urology	849
Rakowski, Thomas A (MD)	Nephrology	361
Ramamurthy, Somayaji (MD)	Pain Management	531
Ramee, Stephen Robert (MD)	Cardiology (Cardiovascular Disease)	140
Ramenofsky, Max (MD)	Pediatric Surgery	612

Name	Specialty	Page
Ramirez, Oscar M (MD)	Plastic Surgery	639
Ramsey, Bonnie W (MD)	Pediatric Pulmonology	606
Ranawat, Chitranjan (MD)	Orthopaedic Surgery	483
Rand, Richard Pierce (MD)	Plastic Surgery	654
Rao, Nalini (MD)	Infectious Disease	321
Rao, Narsing Adupa (MD)	Ophthalmology	467
Rao, Satish S C (MD)	Gastroenterology	233
Rapoport, Judith (MD)	Child & Adolescent Psychiatry	666
Rappaport, Leonard (MD)	Pediatrics	617
Raskin, Philip (MD)	Endocrinology, Diabetes & Metabolism	210
Rasmussen, Steven A (MD)	Psychiatry	677
Rassman, William Richard (MD)	Surgery	801
Ratain, Mark J (MD)	Medical Oncology	308
Ratner, Robert (MD)	Endocrinology, Diabetes & Metabolism	201
Ratts, Valerie Sue (MD)	Reproductive Endocrinology	749
Ratzan, Kenneth (MD)	Infectious Disease	324
Ravich, William Jay (MD)	Gastroenterology	225
Rayan, Ghazi M. (MD)	Hand Surgery	275
Raz, Shlomo (MD)	Urology	849
Ready, L Brian (MD)	Pain Management	531
Reaman, Gregory (MD)	Pediatric Hematology-Oncology	585
Reasner, Charles A (MD)	Endocrinology, Diabetes & Metabolism	210
Recht, Abram (MD)	Radiation Oncology	717
Rechtine, Glenn (MD)	Orthopaedic Surgery	487
Redding , Gregory (MD)	Pediatric Pulmonology	607
Reddy, Daniel (MD)	Vascular Surgery (General)	866
Reder, Anthony T (MD)	Neurology	414
Redlich, Carrie (MD)	Pulmonary Disease	692
Reed, Richard J (MD)	Pathology	541
Reed, Robert L (MD)	Neurology	415
Regan, Joan (MD)	Pediatrics	352
Reichelderfer, Mark (MD)	Gastroenterology	233
Reichman, Lee Brodersohn (MD)	Pulmonary Disease	694
Reilly Jr, John Joseph (MD)	Pulmonary Disease	693
Reilly, Donald T. (MD)	Orthopaedic Surgery	477
Reilly, Raymond J (MD)	Obstetrics & Gynecology	431
Reinisch, John F (MD)	Plastic Surgery	654
Reintgen, Douglas Scott (MD)	Surgery	792
Reisberg, Barry (MD)	Geriatric Psychiatry	673
Reisman, Robert E (MD)	Allergy & Immunology	97
Reiss, Craig (MD)	Cardiology (Cardiovascular Disease)	137
Reitz, Bruce Arnold (MD)	Thoracic Surgery	825
Rennels, Margaret (MD)	Pediatric Infectious Disease	591
Resnick, Lawrence (MD)	Endocrinology, Diabetes & Metabolism	201
Resnick, Martin (MD)	Urology	843
Resnick, Neil M. (MD)	Geriatric Medicine	243
Retik, Alan (MD)	Urology	830
Reuben, David (MD)	Geriatric Medicine	251
Reul, George J (MD)	Thoracic Surgery	822
Reus, Victor Ivar (MD)	Psychiatry	687
Rex, Douglas Kevin (MD)	Gastroenterology	233
Reynolds, James D. (MD)	Ophthalmology	449

ALPHABETICAL LISTING OF DOCTORS

Name	Specialty	Page
Reynolds, Marleta (MD)	Pediatric Surgery	615
Reynolds, R Kevin (MD)	Gynecologic Oncology	261
Rezai, Ali R (MD)	Neurological Surgery	385
Rhoads, Jon Marc (MD)	Pediatric Gastroenterology	579
Rhoton Jr, Albert L (MD)	Neurological Surgery	381
Rice, Dale (MD)	Otolaryngology	523
Rich, Stuart (MD)	Cardiology (Cardiovascular Disease)	137
Rich, Tyvin Andrew (MD)	Radiation Oncology	722
Richard, George (MD)	Pediatric Nephrology	596
Richard, James Marshall (MD)	Ophthalmology	463
Richards, Jon (MD/PhD)	Medical Oncology	308
Richardson, James David (MD)	Surgery	792
Richardson, Mark A. (MD)	Pediatric Otolaryngology	601
Richert, John R (MD)	Neurology	405
Richie, Jerome (MD)	Urology	830
Richman, Douglas (MD)	Infectious Disease	329
Richter, Joel (MD)	Gastroenterology	234
Ricotta, John (MD)	Vascular Surgery (General)	861
Riddle, Mark A (MD)	Child & Adolescent Psychiatry	666
Ries, Andrew (MD)	Pulmonary Disease	712
Riew, K Daniel (MD)	Orthopaedic Surgery	492
Rigel, Darrell (MD)	Dermatology	185
Rikkers, Layton F (MD)	Surgery	795
Riles, Thomas (MD)	Vascular Surgery (General)	861
Rimoin, David L (MD/PhD)	Clinical Genetics	165
Ringel, Steven (MD)	Neurology	416
Rink, Richard C ()	Urology	844
Riordan, John William (MD)	Nephrology	369
Ristow, Brunno (MD)	Plastic Surgery	654
Ritch, Robert (MD)	Ophthalmology	450
Ritchie, James L. (MD)	Cardiology (Cardiovascular Disease)	143
Rivera, Frank James (MD)	Diagnostic Radiology	734
Rizk, Norman Wade (MD)	Pulmonary Disease	712
Rizza, Robert Alan (MD)	Endocrinology, Diabetes & Metabolism	208
Robb, Richard M (MD)	Ophthalmology	443
Robbins, Robert Clayton (MD)	Thoracic Surgery	825
Robbins, Thomas (MD)	Otolaryngology	511
Robert, Nicholas J (MD)	Medical Oncology	303
Roberts, James A (MD)	Gynecologic Oncology	264
Roberts, Patricia L (MD)	Colon & Rectal Surgery	169
Roberts, William (MD)	Pathology	541
Robertson, Gary Lee (MD)	Endocrinology, Diabetes & Metabolism	209
Robertson, Rose Marie (MD)	Cardiology (Cardiovascular Disease)	132
Robins, Perry (MD)	Dermatology	185
Robinson, Dwight R. (MD)	Internal Medicine	333
Robinson, Lawrence (MD)	Physical Medicine & Rehabilitation	631
Rocchini, Albert P (MD)	Pediatric Cardiology	565
Roche, James Kenneth (MD/PhD)	Gastroenterology	229
Rochester, Carolyn (MD)	Pulmonary Disease	693
Rock, John A (MD)	Reproductive Endocrinology	747
Rockswold, Gaylan (MD)	Neurological Surgery	385
Rockwood Jr, Charles A (MD)	Orthopaedic Surgery	495

Name	Specialty	Page
Rodgers, Bradley Moreland (MD)	Pediatric Surgery	614
Rodman, David (MD)	Pulmonary Disease	707
Rogers Jr, James Henry (MD)	Pediatric Cardiology	567
Rogers, Arvey (MD)	Gastroenterology	229
Rogers, Douglas G (MD)	Pediatric Endocrinology	576
Rogers, Gary L (MD)	Ophthalmology	459
Rogers, James N (MD)	Pain Management	531
Rogers, Joseph (MD)	Cardiology (Cardiovascular Disease)	137
Rogers, Lisa R (DO)	Neurology	415
Rogers, Robert M (MD)	Pulmonary Disease	694
Roguska-Kyts, Jadwiga (MD)	Nephrology	366
Rohrich, Rodney James (MD)	Plastic Surgery	650
Roland, Peter S (MD)	Otolaryngology	520
Roman-Lopez, Juan J (MD)	Gynecologic Oncology	263
Romo III, Thomas (MD)	Otolaryngology	506
Roos, Raymond (MD)	Neurology	415
Ropper, Allan (MD)	Neurology	398
Rose, Cecile (MD)	Pulmonary Disease	708
Rose, Christopher Marshall (MD)	Radiation Oncology	727
Rose, Eric A (MD)	Thoracic Surgery	810
Rosen, Charles Burke (MD)	Surgery	795
Rosen, Mark J (MD)	Pulmonary Disease	695
Rosen, Paul Peter (MD)	Pathology	538
Rosen, Peter J (MD)	Medical Oncology	314
Rosen, Richard (MD)	Ophthalmology	450
Rosen, Steven T (MD)	Medical Oncology	308
Rosenbaum, Jerrold Frank (MD)	Psychiatry	677
Rosenbaum, Kenneth (MD)	Clinical Genetics	160
Rosenberg, Michael A (MD)	Ophthalmology	459
Rosenberg, Steven (MD)	Surgery	787
Rosenberg, Thomas D (MD)	Orthopaedic Surgery	494
Rosenblum, Mark (MD)	Neurological Surgery	385
Rosenfeld, Richard M (MD)	Pediatric Otolaryngology	601
Rosenfield, Robert (MD)	Pediatric Endocrinology	576
Rosenman, Julian (MD)	Radiation Oncology	722
Rosenthal, Amnon (MD)	Pediatric Cardiology	565
Rosenthal, David (MD)	Vascular Surgery (General)	864
Rosenwaks, Zev (MD)	Reproductive Endocrinology	745
Rosenwasser, Lanny Jeffrey (MD)	Allergy & Immunology	102
Rosenwasser, Melvin (MD)	Orthopaedic Surgery	483
Roses, Daniel F (MD)	Surgery	787
Rosier, Randy (MD/PhD)	Orthopaedic Surgery	483
Roskes, Saul David (MD)	Pediatric Nephrology	595
Rosner, Howard L (MD)	Pain Management	528
Rosoff, Phillip Martin (MD)	Pediatric Hematology-Oncology	586
Rosomoff, Hubert L (MD)	Neurological Surgery	381
Ross, Lawrence S (MD)	Urology	844
Ross, Merrick I (MD)	Surgery	798
Rosse, Richard B (MD)	Psychiatry	681
Roth, Bennett E (MD)	Internal Medicine	337
Roth, Bruce Joseph (MD)	Medical Oncology	303
Roth, David (MD)	Nephrology	364

ALPHABETICAL LISTING OF DOCTORS

Name	Specialty	Page
Roth, Elliot (MD)	Physical Medicine & Rehabilitation	628
Rothbaum, Robert Jay (MD)	Pediatric Gastroenterology	581
Rothenberg, Mace (MD)	Medical Oncology	303
Rothenberger, David (MD)	Colon & Rectal Surgery	175
Rothman, Richard (MD)	Orthopaedic Surgery	483
Rothman, Steven Alan (MD)	Cardiac Electrophysiology	116
Rothrock, John (MD)	Neurology	409
Rowbotham, Michael Charles (MD)	Pain Management	532
Roy-Byrne, Peter (MD)	Psychiatry	688
Roye, David (MD)	Orthopaedic Surgery	483
Rubin, Lewis (MD)	Pulmonary Disease	712
Rubin, Susan (MD)	Neurology	415
Ruckdeschel, John C (MD)	Medical Oncology	303
Rudnick, Paul Arthur (MD)	Endocrinology, Diabetes & Metabolism	212
Ruge, John (MD)	Neurological Surgery	385
Rusch, Valerie (MD)	Thoracic Surgery	811
Rush Jr, Augustus John (MD)	Psychiatry	685
Russak, Sidney (MD)	Child & Adolescent Psychiatry	670
Russell Jr, Richard (MD)	Cardiology (Cardiovascular Disease)	132
Russell, Andrew Thomas (MD)	Child & Adolescent Psychiatry	670
Ryan, Neal David (MD)	Child & Adolescent Psychiatry	666

S

Name	Specialty	Page
Saag, Michael S (MD)	Infectious Disease	324
Saal, Howard (MD)	Clinical Genetics	162
Sacchi, Terrence J (MD)	Cardiology (Cardiovascular Disease)	127
Sachar, David (MD)	Gastroenterology	225
Sachs, Greg (MD)	Geriatric Medicine	249
Sack, Kenneth Edward (MD)	Rheumatology	769
Saclarides, Theodore John (MD)	Colon & Rectal Surgery	175
Sadock, Benjamin (MD)	Psychiatry	681
Sadock, Virginia (MD)	Psychiatry	681
Sadowsky, Carl Howard (MD)	Neurology	410
Safai , Bijan (MD)	Dermatology	185
Saffle, Jeffrey (MD)	Surgery	796
Safi, Hazim Jawad (MD)	Vascular Surgery (General)	868
Safian, Robert D (MD)	Cardiology (Cardiovascular Disease)	137
Sagalowsky, Arthur I (MD)	Urology	846
Sage, Jacob (MD)	Neurology	405
Sagel, Stuart Steven (MD)	Diagnostic Radiology	733
Saha, Sukamal (MD)	Surgery	795
Sahn, Steven A. (MD)	Pulmonary Disease	700
Sailer, Scott (MD)	Radiation Oncology	722
Saiman, Lisa (MD)	Pediatric Infectious Disease	591
Salant, David (MD)	Nephrology	360
Saleh, Saleh (MD)	Nephrology	369
Salem, Philip Adeeb (MD)	Medical Oncology	312
Salem, Ronald (MD)	Surgery	782
Salky, Barry A (MD)	Surgery	788
Sallent, Jorge (MD)	Pediatric Pulmonology	605
Saltzman, Charles Louis (MD)	Orthopaedic Surgery	492
Salvati, Eduardo Augustin (MD)	Orthopaedic Surgery	483

Name	Specialty	Page
Salvati, Eugene (MD)	Colon & Rectal Surgery	171
Salvatierra, Oscar (MD)	Urology	850
Salz, James Joseph (MD)	Ophthalmology	467
Sampson, Hugh (MD)	Pediatric Allergy & Immunology	555
Samson, Duke (MD)	Neurological Surgery	387
Samuels, Brian Louis (MD)	Medical Oncology	308
Samuels, Louis (MD)	Thoracic Surgery	811
Samuels, Martin Allen (MD)	Neurology	398
Samuelson, Thomas ()	Ophthalmology	460
Sanchez, Miguel (MD)	Pathology	538
Sandborn, William Jeffery (MD)	Gastroenterology	234
Sanders, Georgiana (MD)	Allergy & Immunology	101
Sanders, Stephen Pruett (MD)	Pediatric Cardiology	563
Sanders, William Holt (MD)	Urology	839
Sandler, Martin P (MD)	Nuclear Medicine	427
Sangeorzan, Bruce J. (MD)	Orthopaedic Surgery	498
Sanger, James (MD)	Plastic Surgery	647
Sanz, Luis E (MD)	Obstetrics & Gynecology	433
Sapir, Daniel Gustave (MD)	Nephrology	361
Sargent III, A John (MD)	Child & Adolescent Psychiatry	669
Sarnaik, Ashok P (MD)	Pediatric Critical Care Medicine	570
Sarosi, George (MD)	Internal Medicine	336
Sasaki, Clarence T (MD)	Otolaryngology	501
Sataloff, Robert (MD)	Otolaryngology	506
Sato, Thomas Tad (MD)	Pediatric Surgery	615
Saudek, Christopher D (MD)	Endocrinology, Diabetes & Metabolism	202
Sauer, Mark (MD)	Reproductive Endocrinology	745
Saul, Robert (MD)	Clinical Genetics	161
Savino, Peter (MD)	Ophthalmology	450
Scandling Jr, John David (MD)	Nephrology	369
Scarborough, Mark (MD)	Orthopaedic Surgery	487
Scardino, Peter (MD)	Urology	835
Schaberg, Dennis Ray (MD)	Internal Medicine	335
Schaefer, Steven (MD)	Otolaryngology	506
Schaeffer, Anthony (MD)	Urology	844
Schafer, Michael F (MD)	Orthopaedic Surgery	492
Schaff, Hartzell (MD)	Thoracic Surgery	819
Schanberg, Laura Eve (MD)	Pediatric Rheumatology	609
Schapiro, Randall (MD)	Neurology	415
Schatz, Norman Joseph (MD)	Neurology	410
Schatzberg, Alan F (MD)	Psychiatry	688
Schechter, David Louis (MD)	Sports Medicine	775
Scheel Jr, Paul Joseph (MD)	Nephrology	361
Scheff, Alice M (MD)	Nuclear Medicine	427
Scheinberg, David (MD/PhD)	Medical Oncology	299
Scheinman, Melvin M (MD)	Cardiology (Cardiovascular Disease)	143
Scheithauer, Bernd (MD)	Pathology	540
Schelbert, Heinrich R (MD/PhD)	Nuclear Medicine	428
Scheld, William Michael (MD)	Infectious Disease	324
Scheller, Arnold (MD)	Orthopaedic Surgery	477
Schellhammer, Paul (MD)	Urology	839
Schenck, Robert Roy (MD)	Hand Surgery	274

ALPHABETICAL LISTING OF DOCTORS

Name	Specialty	Page
Schenken, Robert S (MD)	Reproductive Endocrinology	751
Scher, Howard (MD)	Medical Oncology	299
Scher, Richard K (MD)	Dermatology	185
Schiff, Eugene (MD)	Gastroenterology	229
Schiff, Isaac (MD)	Reproductive Endocrinology	744
Schiff, Peter B (MD/PhD)	Radiation Oncology	720
Schiffer, Charles Alan (MD)	Medical Oncology	308
Schiller, Alan (MD)	Pathology	538
Schiller, Joan H ()	Medical Oncology	309
Schindler, Robert Allen (MD)	Otolaryngology	523
Schink, Julian C (MD)	Gynecologic Oncology	261
Schirmer, Bruce David (MD)	Surgery	792
Schlaepfer, William W (MD)	Pathology	538
Schlaff, William D (MD)	Reproductive Endocrinology	751
Schlegel, Peter (MD)	Urology	835
Schluger, Neil (MD)	Pulmonary Disease	695
Schmalzried, Thomas P (MD)	Orthopaedic Surgery	498
Schmidt, Joseph (MD)	Urology	850
Schmidt, Warren Norman (MD)	Gastroenterology	234
Schnabel, Freya (MD)	Surgery	788
Schneider, Lon S (MD)	Geriatric Psychiatry	675
Schnitt, Stuart (MD)	Pathology	536
Schnittger, Ingela (MD)	Cardiology (Cardiovascular Disease)	143
Schnur, Paul (MD)	Plastic Surgery	650
Schoen, Robert Taylor (MD)	Rheumatology	757
Schoetz, David (MD)	Colon & Rectal Surgery	169
Schold Jr., S. Clifford (MD)	Neurology	405
Schooley, Robert Turner (MD)	Internal Medicine	336
Schottenfeld, Richard (MD)	Addiction Psychiatry	661
Schreiber, James (MD)	Reproductive Endocrinology	750
Schrier, Robert William (MD)	Nephrology	367
Schrock, Theodore R (MD)	Colon & Rectal Surgery	177
Schroeder, John S (MD)	Cardiology (Cardiovascular Disease)	143
Schuberth, Kenneth Charles (MD)	Pediatric Allergy & Immunology	555
Schuckit, Marc A (MD)	Addiction Psychiatry	662
Schuger, Claudio David (MD)	Cardiac Electrophysiology	118
Schuller, David (MD)	Otolaryngology	516
Schulman, Steven Paul (MD)	Cardiology (Cardiovascular Disease)	128
Schulze, Konrad S (MD)	Gastroenterology	234
Schurman, David J (MD)	Orthopaedic Surgery	498
Schuster, Michael (MD)	Hematology	286
Schusterman, Mark A (MD)	Plastic Surgery	650
Schwab, Richard (MD)	Surgery	788
Schwab, Steve Joseph (MD)	Nephrology	364
Schwartz, Allan (MD)	Cardiology (Cardiovascular Disease)	128
Schwartz, Burton (MD)	Medical Oncology	309
Schwartz, Cindy Lee (MD)	Pediatric Hematology-Oncology	585
Schwartz, David A (MD)	Pulmonary Disease	700
Schwartz, Gary Lee (MD)	Internal Medicine	336
Schwartz, Peter (MD)	Gynecologic Oncology	255
Schwartz, Robert P (MD)	Pediatric Endocrinology	574
Schwartz, Robert S (MD)	Geriatric Medicine	249

Name	Specialty	Page
Schwartz, Stanley (MD)	Endocrinology, Diabetes & Metabolism	202
Schwarz, Donald F. (MD)	Adolescent Medicine	89
Schwarz, Kathleen (MD)	Pediatric Gastroenterology	578
Schwarz, Marvin Ira (MD)	Pulmonary Disease	708
Schwarz, Steven M (MD)	Pediatric Gastroenterology	579
Schwenk, Thomas L (MD)	Sports Medicine	774
Scialli, Anthony R (MD)	Obstetrics & Gynecology	433
Sciarra, John J (MD)	Obstetrics & Gynecology	437
Scott, Gwendolyn (MD)	Pediatric Infectious Disease	592
Scott, R. Michael (MD)	Neurological Surgery	374
Scott, Richard David (MD)	Orthopaedic Surgery	477
Scott, W Norman (MD)	Orthopaedic Surgery	483
Scott, William (MD)	Ophthalmology	460
Scudera, Peter (MD)	Gastroenterology	229
Sculco, Thomas Peter (MD)	Orthopaedic Surgery	484
Seagren, Stephen L (MD)	Radiation Oncology	727
Seashore, Margretta (MD)	Clinical Genetics	159
Seaver, Laurie Heron (MD)	Clinical Genetics	161
Seeger, James M (MD)	Vascular Surgery (General)	864
Seely, Ellen Wells (MD)	Endocrinology, Diabetes & Metabolism	198
Seftel, Allen D (MD)	Urology	844
Segal, Bernard L (MD)	Cardiology (Cardiovascular Disease)	128
Seibert, Joanna J (MD)	Radiology	739
Seidner, Steven Richard (MD)	Neonatal-Perinatal Medicine	355
Seifter, Julian L (MD)	Nephrology	360
Sekhar, Laligam N (MD)	Neurological Surgery	381
Selby, Richard N (MD)	Neurology	421
Selch, Michael T (MD)	Radiation Oncology	727
Selkoe, Dennis (MD)	Neurology	398
Selman, Warren R (MD)	Neurological Surgery	385
Selwyn, Peter (MD)	Internal Medicine	334
Semenkovich, Clay F (MD)	Endocrinology, Diabetes & Metabolism	209
Senagore, Anthony (MD)	Colon & Rectal Surgery	175
Senzer, Neil Nathan (MD)	Radiation Oncology	726
Sepkowitz, Kent (MD)	Infectious Disease	321
Serafano, Donald Natale (MD)	Ophthalmology	467
Seremetis, Stephanie (MD)	Internal Medicine	334
Sergott, Robert C (MD)	Ophthalmology	450
Session, Donna Ruth (MD)	Reproductive Endocrinology	750
Sessoms, Sandra Lee (MD)	Rheumatology	768
Sethi, Kapil (MD)	Neurology	410
Seward, James Bernard (MD)	Cardiology (Cardiovascular Disease)	137
Sexson, Sandra G B (MD)	Child & Adolescent Psychiatry	667
Sexton, Daniel John (MD)	Infectious Disease	325
Seybold, Marjorie (MD)	Neurology	421
Seyfer, Alan (MD)	Plastic Surgery	654
Shaban, Stephen F (MD)	Urology	839
Shackelford, Penelope Greta (MD)	Pediatric Infectious Disease	593
Shadick, Nancy A (MD)	Rheumatology	757
Shaffrey, Christopher I (MD)	Neurological Surgery	390
Shah, Dhiraj (MD)	Vascular Surgery (General)	861
Shah, Jatin P (MD)	Surgery	788

ALPHABETICAL LISTING OF DOCTORS

Name	Specialty	Page
Shah, Prediman K (MD)	Cardiology (Cardiovascular Disease)	143
Shaha, Ashok (MD)	Surgery	788
Shahian, David (MD)	Thoracic Surgery	806
Shalita, Alan (MD)	Dermatology	186
Shani, Jacob (MD)	Cardiology (Cardiovascular Disease)	128
Shank, Brenda (MD/PhD)	Radiation Oncology	727
Shapiro, Charles L (MD)	Medical Oncology	309
Shapiro, Eugene D (MD)	Pediatric Infectious Disease	590
Shapiro, Gail Greenberg (MD)	Pediatric Allergy & Immunology	559
Shapiro, Lawrence R (MD)	Clinical Genetics	160
Shapiro, Ron (MD)	Surgery	788
Shapiro, William R. (MD)	Neurology	418
Sharlip, Ira Dorian (MD)	Urology	850
Sharma, Om Prakash (MD)	Pulmonary Disease	712
Shaw Jr, Byers Wendell (MD)	Surgery	796
Shaw, Edward Gus (MD)	Radiation Oncology	722
Shaw, William Wei-Lien (MD)	Plastic Surgery	655
Shaywitz, Bennett (MD)	Child Neurology	151
Shaywitz, Sally Epstein (MD)	Pediatrics	617
Shea, Thomas (MD)	Medical Oncology	303
Shear, Mary Katherine (MD)	Psychiatry	681
Shearer, William T (MD)	Pediatric Allergy & Immunology	558
Sheehan, Myles (MD)	Geriatric Medicine	249
Sheen, Jack (MD)	Plastic Surgery	655
Shelbourne, K Donald (MD)	Orthopaedic Surgery	492
Shellito, Judd Ernest (MD)	Pulmonary Disease	709
Shellito, Paul C (MD)	Colon & Rectal Surgery	170
Shenaq, Saleh (MD)	Plastic Surgery	650
Shenk, Ian (MD)	Gastroenterology	229
Shennib, Hani (MD)	Thoracic Surgery	811
Shepard, Alexander D (MD)	Vascular Surgery (General)	866
Shepherd, Gillian M (MD)	Allergy & Immunology	97
Sherertz, Elizabeth F (MD)	Dermatology	188
Sherman, David (MD)	Neurology	418
Sherman, James (MD)	Pediatric Pulmonology	605
Sherman, Orrin (MD)	Orthopaedic Surgery	484
Sherman, Randolph (MD)	Plastic Surgery	655
Sherry, David (MD)	Pediatric Rheumatology	610
Sherwin, Robert (MD)	Endocrinology, Diabetes & Metabolism	198
Shields, Jerry (MD)	Ophthalmology	450
Shields, William Donald (MD)	Child Neurology	156
Shipley, William (MD)	Radiation Oncology	717
Shively, Robert A (MD)	Sports Medicine	774
Shlofmitz, Richard A (MD)	Cardiology (Cardiovascular Disease)	128
Shore, Bernard L (MD)	Internal Medicine	336
Shorr, Norman (MD)	Ophthalmology	467
Shortliffe, Linda (MD)	Urology	850
Shoulson, Ira (MD)	Neurology	405
Shucart, William A (MD)	Neurological Surgery	374
Shuck, Jerry M (MD)	Surgery	795
Shuldiner, Alan Rodney (MD)	Endocrinology, Diabetes & Metabolism	202
Shults, Clifford Walter (MD)	Neurology	422

Name	Specialty	Page
Shumway, Norman Edward (MD)	Thoracic Surgery	825
Shupack, Jerome L (MD)	Dermatology	186
Shure, Deborah (MD)	Pulmonary Disease	700
Shwayder, Tor A (MD)	Dermatology	190
Sicard, Gregorio Arquel (MD)	Vascular Surgery (General)	867
Siddique, Teepu (MD)	Neurology	415
Siegel, Barry (MD)	Nuclear Medicine	427
Siegel, Gordon J (MD)	Otolaryngology	516
Siegel, Jerome (MD)	Gastroenterology	225
Siegel, Stuart E (MD)	Pediatric Hematology-Oncology	589
Sigal, Leonard H (MD)	Rheumatology	760
Sigman, Mark (MD)	Urology	830
Sillers, Michael (MD)	Otolaryngology	511
Sills, Edward M (MD)	Pediatric Rheumatology	608
Silver, Michael (MD)	Pulmonary Disease	705
Silverman, Norman A (MD)	Thoracic Surgery	819
Silverman, William Bruce (MD)	Gastroenterology	234
Silverstein, Herbert (MD)	Otolaryngology	511
Silverstein, Janet H (MD)	Pediatric Endocrinology	575
Silverstein, Melvin J (MD)	Surgery	801
Silverstein, Roy (MD)	Hematology	286
Simon, John W (MD)	Ophthalmology	450
Simon, Michael (MD)	Orthopaedic Surgery	492
Simon, Robert Isaac (MD)	Psychiatry	681
Simpson, George M (MD)	Psychiatry	688
Simpson, Joe Leigh (MD)	Obstetrics & Gynecology	438
Singer, Peter Albert (MD)	Endocrinology, Diabetes & Metabolism	212
Singer, Robert (MD)	Plastic Surgery	655
Singer, Samuel (MD)	Surgery	782
Singh, Nalini (MD)	Pediatric Infectious Disease	591
Singletary, S Eva (MD)	Surgery	798
Sinha, Uttam Kumar (MD)	Otolaryngology	523
Sirdofsky, Michael D (MD)	Neurology	406
Sisung, Charles (MD)	Physical Medicine & Rehabilitation	628
Sivak, Michael (MD)	Gastroenterology	234
Sivina, Manuel (MD)	Vascular Surgery (General)	864
Sivit, Carlos (MD)	Radiology	738
Sizemore, Glenn (MD)	Endocrinology, Diabetes & Metabolism	209
Skinner, Donald George (MD)	Urology	850
Skinner, Eila C (MD)	Urology	850
Skoner, David Peter (MD)	Pediatric Allergy & Immunology	555
Skyler, Jay S (MD)	Endocrinology, Diabetes & Metabolism	205
Slankard, Marjorie (MD)	Allergy & Immunology	97
Slap, Gail (MD)	Adolescent Medicine	89
Slavin, Raymond (MD)	Allergy & Immunology	101
Sleasman, John W (MD)	Pediatric Rheumatology	609
Sledge Jr, George W (MD)	Medical Oncology	309
Sliwa, James (DO)	Physical Medicine & Rehabilitation	628
Slomowitz, Marcia (MD)	Child & Adolescent Psychiatry	668
Slonim, Alfred (MD)	Pediatric Endocrinology	573
Sly, Ridge Michael (MD)	Pediatric Allergy & Immunology	555
Small, Gary William (MD)	Geriatric Psychiatry	675

ALPHABETICAL LISTING OF DOCTORS

Name	Specialty	Page
Smalley, Stephen R (MD)	Radiation Oncology	725
Smalling, Richard Warren (MD/PhD)	Interventional Cardiology	147
Smedira, Nicholas (MD)	Thoracic Surgery	819
Smego, Douglas (MD)	Surgery	782
Smith Jr, Sidney C (MD)	Cardiology (Cardiovascular Disease)	132
Smith, Arthur D (MD)	Urology	835
Smith, Barbara Lynn (MD)	Surgery	782
Smith, Craig R (MD)	Thoracic Surgery	811
Smith, Daniel (MD)	Gynecologic Oncology	257
Smith, Donna Marie (MD)	Gynecologic Oncology	262
Smith, James P (MD)	Pulmonary Disease	695
Smith, Joanne (MD)	Pain Management	530
Smith, Joseph (MD)	Urology	839
Smith, Lee (MD)	Colon & Rectal Surgery	171
Smith, Leon G (MD)	Infectious Disease	321
Smith, Peter Kent (MD)	Thoracic Surgery	814
Smith, Robert B (MD)	Urology	850
Smith, Ronald E (MD)	Ophthalmology	468
Smith, Thomas Joseph (MD)	Medical Oncology	304
Smith, Wade S (MD/PhD)	Neurology	422
Smith, Yolanda (MD)	Reproductive Endocrinology	750
Sninsky, Charles (MD)	Gastroenterology	229
Snustad, Diane Gail (MD)	Geriatric Medicine	246
Snyder III, Howard M (MD)	Urology	835
Snyder III, William Henry (MD)	Surgery	798
Snyder, Peter Joseph (MD)	Endocrinology, Diabetes & Metabolism	202
Sobel, Jack (MD)	Infectious Disease	326
Sobel, Michael (MD)	Vascular Surgery (General)	861
Sobel, Stuart (MD)	Dermatology	188
Socinski, Mark A (MD)	Medical Oncology	304
Socol, Michael (MD)	Obstetrics & Gynecology	437
Sodt, Peter (MD)	Pediatric Cardiology	566
Sokol, Mae Sandra (MD)	Child & Adolescent Psychiatry	669
Sokoloff, Daniel (MD)	Dermatology	188
Sola, Augusto (MD)	Neonatal-Perinatal Medicine	355
Solberg, Lawrence (MD)	Hematology	287
Solin, Lawrence (MD)	Radiation Oncology	721
Sollinger, Hans W (MD)	Surgery	795
Solomon, Gary (MD)	Rheumatology	761
Solomon, Robert A (MD)	Neurological Surgery	379
Soloway, Mark (MD)	Urology	839
Somerville, James (MD)	Nephrology	366
Sondel, Paul M (MD)	Pediatric Hematology-Oncology	587
Sonnenblick, Edmund (MD)	Cardiology (Cardiovascular Disease)	128
Sonntag, Volker (MD)	Neurological Surgery	387
Sontheimer, Richard (MD)	Dermatology	190
Soper, Nathaniel (MD)	Surgery	796
Sorrell, Michael (MD)	Gastroenterology	235
Sorrentino, Robert A. (MD)	Cardiac Electrophysiology	117
Sosa, R Ernest (MD)	Urology	835
Sostman, H Dirk (MD)	Diagnostic Radiology	732
Soules, Michael Roy (MD)	Reproductive Endocrinology	752

Name	Specialty	Page
Sparling, Philip Frederick (MD)	Infectious Disease	325
Spear, Scott L (MD)	Plastic Surgery	639
Speeg, Kermit Vincent (MD/PhD)	Gastroenterology	237
Speer, Kevin (MD)	Sports Medicine	774
Spektor, Zorik (MD)	Otolaryngology	511
Spence, Alexander Morton (MD)	Neurology	422
Spencer, Dennis D (MD)	Neurological Surgery	374
Spencer, Susan S (MD)	Neurology	399
Spencer, Thomas (MD)	Child & Adolescent Psychiatry	664
Spengler, Dan M (MD)	Orthopaedic Surgery	487
Sperling, Mark Alexander (MD)	Pediatric Endocrinology	573
Spetzler, Robert (MD)	Neurological Surgery	387
Speyer, James (MD)	Medical Oncology	299
Spiegel, David (MD)	Psychiatry	688
Spielvogel, Richard Lee (MD)	Dermatology	186
Spiera, Harry (MD)	Rheumatology	761
Spindler, Kurt Paul (MD)	Orthopaedic Surgery	488
Spinelli, Henry M (MD)	Plastic Surgery	640
Spivak, Jerry L. (MD)	Hematology	286
Sponseller, Paul D (MD)	Orthopaedic Surgery	484
Spray, Thomas L (MD)	Pediatric Surgery	612
Springfield, Dempsey (MD)	Orthopaedic Surgery	484
Staas Jr, William E (MD)	Physical Medicine & Rehabilitation	625
Staats, Peter (MD)	Pain Management	528
Stamos, Michael Jerry (MD)	Colon & Rectal Surgery	177
Stankiewicz, James (MD)	Otolaryngology	516
Stanley, James (MD)	Vascular Surgery (General)	867
Stanley, John R (MD)	Dermatology	186
Stansell, John Dee (MD)	Pulmonary Disease	712
Staples, Edward D (MD)	Thoracic Surgery	814
Stapleton, F Bruder (MD)	Pediatric Nephrology	599
Stark, Walter J (MD)	Ophthalmology	450
Starnes, Vaughn Alden (MD)	Thoracic Surgery	825
Steed, David Luther (MD)	Vascular Surgery (General)	862
Steege, John Francis (MD)	Obstetrics & Gynecology	434
Steele, Glenn D (MD/PhD)	Surgery	796
Steers, William D (MD)	Urology	840
Steiger, David (MD)	Pulmonary Disease	695
Stein, Elliott (MD)	Geriatric Psychiatry	673
Stein, Mark R (MD)	Allergy & Immunology	99
Stein, Murray Brent (MD)	Psychiatry	688
Steinberg, Gary K (MD)	Neurological Surgery	390
Steinberg, Harry (MD)	Pulmonary Disease	695
Steiner, Hans (MD)	Child & Adolescent Psychiatry	670
Steinert, Roger F (MD)	Ophthalmology	444
Steinhagen, Randolph (MD)	Colon & Rectal Surgery	171
Steinherz, Peter G (MD)	Pediatric Hematology-Oncology	585
Steinhorn, Robin (MD)	Neonatal-Perinatal Medicine	353
Steinkampf, Michael (MD)	Reproductive Endocrinology	747
Stern, Jeffrey L (MD)	Gynecologic Oncology	264
Stern, Kathleen (MD)	Ophthalmology	451
Stern, Matthew (MD)	Neurology	406

ALPHABETICAL LISTING OF DOCTORS

Name	Specialty	Page
Stern, Peter (MD)	Hand Surgery	274
Stern, Robert C (MD)	Pediatric Pulmonology	605
Sternberg Jr, Paul (MD)	Ophthalmology	455
Stevenson, David K (MD)	Neonatal-Perinatal Medicine	355
Stevenson, Lynne W (MD)	Cardiology (Cardiovascular Disease)	122
Stevenson, Roger E (MD)	Clinical Genetics	161
Stevenson, Thomas Ray (MD)	Plastic Surgery	655
Stevenson, William G. (MD)	Cardiac Electrophysiology	115
Stewart, Ronald Mack (MD)	Surgery	799
Stewart, William (MD)	Cardiology (Cardiovascular Disease)	138
Stieg, Philip E (MD/PhD)	Neurological Surgery	379
Stiehm, E Richard (MD)	Pediatric Allergy & Immunology	559
Stiff, Patrick J (MD)	Hematology	290
Stiles, Alan (MD)	Neonatal-Perinatal Medicine	353
Stimmler, Mary McMillen (MD)	Rheumatology	770
Stinnett, James (MD)	Psychiatry	681
Stock, Richard (MD)	Radiation Oncology	721
Stoller, James (MD)	Pulmonary Disease	705
Stoller, Marshall Leedy (MD)	Urology	851
Stone, Anthony (MD)	Urology	851
Stone, Edwin (MD)	Ophthalmology	460
Stone, Joel (MD)	Medical Oncology	304
Stone, Richard Maury (MD)	Hematology	285
Stout, J Timothy (MD/PhD)	Ophthalmology	468
Stover-Pepe, Diane E (MD)	Pulmonary Disease	695
Strand, William (MD)	Urology	847
Strashun, Arnold M (MD)	Nuclear Medicine	426
Strassner, Howard T (MD)	Maternal & Fetal Medicine	346
Stratta, Robert (MD)	Surgery	792
Strauch, Robert (MD)	Hand Surgery	269
Straus, Stephen (MD)	Infectious Disease	321
Strauss, H William (MD)	Nuclear Medicine	428
Streeter Jr, Oscar E (MD)	Radiation Oncology	727
Stringer, Scott Pearson (MD)	Otolaryngology	511
Strober, Warren (MD)	Allergy & Immunology	97
Strom, Eric Alan (MD)	Radiation Oncology	726
Strome, Marshall (MD)	Otolaryngology	516
Strong III, Michael D (MD)	Thoracic Surgery	811
Strongwater, Allan (MD)	Orthopaedic Surgery	484
Strunk, Robert (MD)	Pediatric Allergy & Immunology	557
Stryker, Steven J (MD)	Colon & Rectal Surgery	175
Stuart, Richard Scott (MD)	Thoracic Surgery	811
Stulberg, Samuel David (MD)	Orthopaedic Surgery	493
Stulting, R. Doyle (MD)	Ophthalmology	455
Stumpf, David A (MD)	Child Neurology	154
Stuzin, James M (MD)	Plastic Surgery	645
Stylianos, Steven (MD)	Pediatric Surgery	613
Suarez, Carlos (MD)	Pediatric Hematology-Oncology	587
Suen, James (MD)	Otolaryngology	520
Sugarbaker, David John (MD)	Thoracic Surgery	806

Sugarbaker, Paul H (MD)	Surgery	788
Suit, Herman (MD)	Radiation Oncology	718
Suki, Wadi (MD)	Nephrology	367
Sullivan, Patrick Kevin (MD)	Plastic Surgery	636
Sultan, Mark (MD)	Plastic Surgery	640
Sunderland, Trey (MD)	Geriatric Psychiatry	673
Sundt III, Thoralf Mauritz (MD)	Thoracic Surgery	820
Sundy, John Sargent (MD/PhD)	Rheumatology	762
Supiano, Mark A. (MD)	Geriatric Medicine	249
Surawicz, Christina (MD)	Gastroenterology	238
Surks, Martin (MD)	Endocrinology, Diabetes & Metabolism	202
Surrey, Eric Shire (MD)	Reproductive Endocrinology	751
Sussman, Norman (MD)	Psychiatry	681
Sutherland, David (MD)	Surgery	796
Swaid, Swaid (MD)	Neurological Surgery	381
Swanson, David A (MD)	Urology	847
Swarm, Robert A (MD)	Pain Management	530
Swartz, Richard D (MD)	Nephrology	366
Sweet, Michael (MD)	Pulmonary Disease	701
Sweet, Richard Lance (MD)	Obstetrics & Gynecology	433
Swerdloff, Ronald Sherwin (MD)	Endocrinology, Diabetes & Metabolism	213
Swerdlow, Charles Dennis (MD)	Cardiac Electrophysiology	119
Swerdlow, Michael (MD)	Neurology	406
Swerdlow, Steven Howard (MD)	Pathology	538
Swiontkowski, Marc F (MD)	Orthopaedic Surgery	493
Szabo, Robert (MD)	Hand Surgery	276
Szachowicz II, Edward H (MD)	Otolaryngology	516

T

Tabak, Brian (MD)	Dermatology	194
Tabbal, Nicolas (MD)	Plastic Surgery	640
Taft, Timothy (MD)	Orthopaedic Surgery	488
Takahashi, Masato (MD)	Pediatric Cardiology	567
Taleisnik, Julio (MD)	Hand Surgery	276
Tamaroff, Marc A (MD)	Allergy & Immunology	103
Tamborlane, William V (MD)	Pediatric Endocrinology	572
Tamer, Dolores (MD)	Pediatric Cardiology	563
Tan, Merita R.C. (MD)	Obstetrics & Gynecology	437
Tanguay, Peter (MD)	Child & Adolescent Psychiatry	667
Tanner, Caroline M (MD/PhD)	Neurology	422
Tapper, David (MD)	Pediatric Surgery	616
Tapson, Victor (MD/PhD)	Pulmonary Disease	701
Targan, Stephan Raoul (MD)	Gastroenterology	238
Tashkin, Donald P (MD)	Pulmonary Disease	713
Taylor Jr., Peyton T. (MD)	Gynecologic Oncology	259
Taylor, Lloyd M (MD)	Vascular Surgery (General)	869
Taylor, Marie E (MD)	Radiation Oncology	724
Taylor, R Stan (MD)	Dermatology	192
Taylor, Robert N (MD)	Reproductive Endocrinology	752
Teal, James S (MD)	Diagnostic Radiology	732

ALPHABETICAL LISTING OF DOCTORS

Torti, Frank M (MD)	Medical Oncology	304
Toskes, Phillip (MD)	Gastroenterology	230
Totonchi, Emil (MD)	Urology	844
Toufanian, Ahmad (MD)	Pediatric Surgery	614
Towne, Jonathan (MD)	Vascular Surgery (General)	867
Traboulsi, Elias Iskan (MD)	Ophthalmology	460
Tranbaugh, Robert (MD)	Thoracic Surgery	811
Trastek, Victor (MD)	Thoracic Surgery	822
Trauner, Doris Ann (MD)	Child Neurology	156
Treadwell, Marjorie Clarke (MD)	Maternal & Fetal Medicine	346
Treadwell, Patricia (MD)	Dermatology	190
Treat, Joseph (MD)	Medical Oncology	300
Treem, William R (MD)	Pediatric Gastroenterology	579
Tremaine, William John (MD)	Gastroenterology	234
Trento, Alfredo (MD)	Thoracic Surgery	825
Trese, Michael T (MD)	Ophthalmology	460
Trick, Lorence Wain (MD)	Orthopaedic Surgery	495
Troner, Michael (MD)	Medical Oncology	304
Troost, Bradley Todd (MD)	Neurology	410
Trulock, Elbert (MD)	Pulmonary Disease	706
Trumble, Thomas (MD)	Hand Surgery	276
Tsai, Tsu-Min (MD)	Hand Surgery	271
Tse, David (MD)	Ophthalmology	455
Tucci, Debara Lyn (MD)	Otolaryngology	511
Tunkel, David Eric (MD)	Pediatric Otolaryngology	601
Turk, William (MD)	Child Neurology	153
Turner, James (MD)	Vascular Surgery (General)	862
Turner, Roderick Randolph (MD)	Pathology	543
Turner, Stephen Gordon (MD)	Ophthalmology	468
Turner, William F (MD)	Thoracic Surgery	822
Turrentine, Mark W (MD)	Thoracic Surgery	820
Turrisi III, Andrew Thomas (MD)	Radiation Oncology	723
Tychsen, Lawrence (MD)	Ophthalmology	460
Tyson, Jon Edward (MD)	Neonatal-Perinatal Medicine	355
Tzakis, Andreas (MD)	Surgery	792

U

Uehling, David T (MD)	Urology	844
Uhde, Thomas W (MD)	Psychiatry	684
Ulshen, Martin H (MD)	Pediatric Gastroenterology	579
Umans, Jason (MD/PhD)	Nephrology	362
Umetsu, Dale T (MD/PhD)	Pediatric Allergy & Immunology	559
Underwood, Louis (MD)	Pediatrics	618
Ungerleider, Ross M (MD)	Thoracic Surgery	815
Unni, K Krishnan (MD)	Pathology	540
Upton, Joseph (MD)	Hand Surgery	267
Urbaniak, James R (MD)	Hand Surgery	271
Uribe, John (MD)	Orthopaedic Surgery	488
Urist, Marshall (MD)	Surgery	792
Urken, Mark (MD)	Otolaryngology	506

ALPHABETICAL LISTING OF DOCTORS

Urschel Jr, Harold C (MD)	Thoracic Surgery	823

V

Vail, Thomas Parker (MD)	Orthopaedic Surgery	488
Valenstein, Edward (MD)	Neurology	410
Valentino, Joseph (MD)	Otolaryngology	511
Valentino, Leonard A (MD)	Pediatric Hematology-Oncology	587
Valero, Vicente (MD)	Medical Oncology	312
Valji, Karim (MD)	Radiology	740
Van Der Horst, Charles (MD)	Infectious Disease	325
van der Kolk, Bessel (MD)	Psychiatry	677
Van Heertum, Ronald Lanny (MD)	Nuclear Medicine	426
Van Nagell Jr., John R. (MD)	Gynecologic Oncology	259
Van Thiel, David (MD)	Gastroenterology	235
Vance, Mary Lee (MD)	Internal Medicine	335
Vander Ark, Condon R (MD)	Cardiology (Cardiovascular Disease)	138
Vander Kolk, Craig Alan (MD)	Plastic Surgery	640
Vander Laan, Ronald Lee (MD)	Cardiology (Cardiovascular Disease)	138
Vander Salm, Thomas (MD)	Thoracic Surgery	806
Vapnek, Jonathan M (MD)	Urology	835
Vas, George A (MD)	Neurology	406
Vasconez, Luis O (MD)	Plastic Surgery	645
Vaughan, Edwin D (MD)	Urology	836
Vaughey, Ellen (MD)	Pulmonary Disease	701
Veith, Frank James (MD)	Vascular Surgery (General)	862
Veith, Richard (MD)	Geriatric Psychiatry	675
Velcek, Francisca (MD)	Pediatric Surgery	613
Veldhuis, Johannes D (MD)	Endocrinology, Diabetes & Metabolism	205
Venkat, K K (MD)	Nephrology	366
Verrier, Edward (MD)	Thoracic Surgery	826
Vetrovec, George (MD)	Cardiology (Cardiovascular Disease)	132
Vicini, Frank A (MD)	Radiation Oncology	724
Vicioso, Belinda Angelica (MD)	Geriatric Medicine	250
Vierling, John Moore (MD)	Gastroenterology	238
Vignola, Paul (MD)	Cardiology (Cardiovascular Disease)	133
Vining, Eugenia (MD)	Otolaryngology	501
Vinuela, Fernando (MD)	Radiology	740
Vitek, Jerrold Lee (MD)	Neurology	410
Voelkel, Norbert F (MD)	Pulmonary Disease	708
Vogel, Stephen Burton (MD)	Surgery	792
Vogelzang, Nicholas (MD)	Medical Oncology	309
Vogt, Peter (MD)	Plastic Surgery	647
Vokes, Everett Emmett (MD)	Medical Oncology	309
Volberding, Paul Arthur (MD)	Medical Oncology	314
Volkmar, Fred R (MD)	Child & Adolescent Psychiatry	664
Vollmer, Timothy Lee (MD)	Neurology	399
Volpe, Joseph J. (MD)	Child Neurology	151
Volpe, Peter Anthony (MD)	Colon & Rectal Surgery	177
Volshteyn, Oksana (MD)	Physical Medicine & Rehabilitation	628
Von Eschenbach, Andrew C (MD)	Urology	847

ALPHABETICAL LISTING OF DOCTORS

|---|---|---|
| Von Sternberg, Thomas (MD) | Geriatric Medicine | 249 |
| Voorhees, John (MD) | Dermatology | 190 |

W

Waagner, David (MD)	Pediatric Infectious Disease	594
Wackym, Phillip (MD)	Otolaryngology	517
Waggoner, Steven (MD)	Gynecologic Oncology	262
Wagner-Weiner, Linda (MD)	Pediatric Rheumatology	609
Wahl, Richard (MD)	Nuclear Medicine	427
Wain, John (MD)	Thoracic Surgery	806
Wait, Susan Braynard (MD)	Psychiatry	682
Wajsman, Zew Lew (MD)	Urology	840
Wald, Arnold (MD)	Gastroenterology	225
Wald, Ellen (MD)	Pediatric Infectious Disease	591
Wald, Jeffrey A (MD)	Allergy & Immunology	102
Waldbaum, Robert (MD)	Urology	836
Waldo, Albert (MD)	Cardiac Electrophysiology	118
Walker lll, R Dixon (MD)	Urology	840
Walker, David H (MD)	Pathology	541
Walker, Marion L. (MD)	Neurological Surgery	386
Walkup, John (MD)	Child & Adolescent Psychiatry	667
Wallace Jr, Richard James (MD)	Infectious Disease	328
Wallace, Jeanne Marie (MD)	Pulmonary Disease	713
Wallach, Edward Eliot (MD)	Reproductive Endocrinology	745
Wallach, Robert C (MD)	Gynecologic Oncology	257
Waller, John F (MD)	Orthopaedic Surgery	484
Walsh, B Timothy (MD)	Psychiatry	682
Walsh, Edward Patrick (MD)	Pediatric Cardiology	561
Walsh, Joseph (MD)	Ophthalmology	451
Walsh, Nicolas Eugene (MD)	Physical Medicine & Rehabilitation	630
Walsh, Patrick (MD)	Urology	836
Walters, Mark (MD)	Obstetrics & Gynecology	437
Walton, David S (MD)	Ophthalmology	444
Walton, Robert Lee (MD)	Plastic Surgery	647
Waner, Milton (MD)	Otolaryngology	520
Wang, Frederick (MD)	Ophthalmology	451
Wanner, Adam (MD)	Pulmonary Disease	701
Wapner, Keith Leslie (MD)	Orthopaedic Surgery	485
Wapner, Ronald (MD)	Maternal & Fetal Medicine	343
Wara, Diane Wickizer (MD)	Pediatric Allergy & Immunology	560
Warady, Bradley (MD)	Pediatric Nephrology	598
Ward, Barbara (MD)	Surgery	783
Ward, John Harris (MD)	Medical Oncology	310
Ward, Robert (MD)	Otolaryngology	506
Waring III, George Oral (MD)	Ophthalmology	455
Warnke, Roger Allen (MD)	Pathology	544
Warren, Robert Hughes (MD)	Pediatric Pulmonology	606
Warren, Robert Wells (MD)	Pediatric Rheumatology	609
Warren, Russell (MD)	Orthopaedic Surgery	485
Warshaw, Andrew L (MD)	Surgery	783

ALPHABETICAL LISTING OF DOCTORS

ALPHABETICAL LISTING OF DOCTORS

Weiss, Lawrence M (MD)	Pathology	544
Weiss, Martin Harvey (MD)	Neurological Surgery	390
Weiss, Robert M (MD)	Urology	830
Weiss, Sharon (MD)	Pathology	540
Weissler, Jonathan C (MD)	Pulmonary Disease	709
Weissler, Mark Christian (MD)	Otolaryngology	512
Weissman, Peter (MD)	Endocrinology, Diabetes & Metabolism	205
Welch, Peter (MD)	Infectious Disease	321
Wells, James H (MD)	Plastic Surgery	655
Wener, Mark (MD)	Rheumatology	770
Wenger, Nanette Kass (MD)	Cardiology (Cardiovascular Disease)	133
Wenzel, Sally E (MD)	Pulmonary Disease	708
Werner, Phillip Ladd (MD)	Endocrinology, Diabetes & Metabolism	209
Wesson, Donald (MD)	Nephrology	368
West, Sterling (MD)	Rheumatology	767
Weston, William Lee (MD)	Dermatology	191
Wexner, Steven (MD)	Colon & Rectal Surgery	173
Weyman, Arthur Edward (MD)	Cardiology (Cardiovascular Disease)	123
Weymuller, Ernest (MD)	Otolaryngology	523
Wheeland, Ronald (MD)	Dermatology	192
Wheeler, Thomas M (MD)	Pathology	542
Whelan, Alison (MD)	Clinical Genetics	163
Whelan, Richard (MD)	Colon & Rectal Surgery	171
Whisler, Walter W (MD)	Neurological Surgery	386
Whitaker, John N (MD)	Neurology	411
Whitaker, Linton A (MD)	Plastic Surgery	640
White, Barbara (MD)	Rheumatology	761
White, Carl W (MD)	Interventional Cardiology	146
White, Charles (MD)	Diagnostic Radiology	732
White, David P (MD)	Pulmonary Disease	693
White, Dorothy (MD)	Pulmonary Disease	696
White, Neil H (MD)	Pediatric Endocrinology	576
White, Peter (MD)	Hematology	290
White, Rodney Allen (MD)	Vascular Surgery (General)	869
Whitington, Peter (MD)	Pediatric Gastroenterology	581
Whittemore, Anthony D (MD)	Vascular Surgery (General)	858
Whyte, Richard (MD)	Thoracic Surgery	826
Wicha, Max S (MD)	Medical Oncology	310
Wickiewicz, Thomas (MD)	Orthopaedic Surgery	485
Wiedel, Jerome D (MD)	Orthopaedic Surgery	494
Wiedemann, Herbert P (MD)	Pulmonary Disease	706
Wiener, Eugene (MD)	Pediatric Surgery	613
Wiener, Jerry M (MD)	Child & Adolescent Psychiatry	667
Wiesel, Sam W (MD)	Orthopaedic Surgery	485
Wiet, Richard James (MD)	Otolaryngology	517
Wigley, Frederick M (MD)	Rheumatology	761
Wilansky, Susan (MD)	Cardiology (Cardiovascular Disease)	140
Wilber, David James (MD)	Cardiac Electrophysiology	118
Wilcox, Benson (MD)	Thoracic Surgery	815
Wilcox, Christopher S (MD)	Nephrology	362

Wolinsky, Jerry (MD)	Neurology	418
Wong, Johnson T (MD)	Allergy & Immunology	95
Wong, Westley Douglas (MD)	Colon & Rectal Surgery	171
Woo, Peak (MD)	Otolaryngology	507
Wood Molo, Mary (MD)	Reproductive Endocrinology	750
Wood, Beverly (MD)	Radiology	740
Wood, Douglas (MD)	Thoracic Surgery	826
Wood, John (MD)	Allergy & Immunology	102
Wood, Lawrence Crane (MD)	Internal Medicine	333
Wood, R Patrick (MD)	Surgery	799
Wood, Robert Alan (MD)	Pediatric Allergy & Immunology	556
Wood-Smith, Donald (MD)	Plastic Surgery	641
Woodruff, James M. (MD)	Pathology	538
Woodson, Gayle Ellen (MD)	Otolaryngology	512
Wooten, George Frederick (MD)	Neurology	411
Wormser, Gary (MD)	Infectious Disease	322
Wright, Cameron (MD)	Thoracic Surgery	806
Wright, Harry (MD)	Child & Adolescent Psychiatry	668
Wright, Kenneth W (MD)	Ophthalmology	468
Wright, Robert B (MD)	Neurology	415
Wunderink, Richard (MD)	Pulmonary Disease	701
Wylen, Michele (MD)	Obstetrics & Gynecology	433
Wyllie, Elaine (MD)	Child Neurology	154
Wyllie, Robert (MD)	Pediatric Gastroenterology	581

Y

Yaffe, Bruce (MD)	Internal Medicine	334
Yager, Joel (MD)	Psychiatry	686
Yancovitz, Stanley (MD)	Infectious Disease	322
Yannuzzi, Lawrence (MD)	Ophthalmology	451
Yao, James (MD)	Vascular Surgery (General)	867
Yates, Alayne (MD)	Child & Adolescent Psychiatry	671
Yee, Billy (MD)	Reproductive Endocrinology	753
Yeh, Timothy S (MD)	Pediatric Critical Care Medicine	571
Yellin, Albert E (MD)	Vascular Surgery (General)	870
Yonkers, Kimberly A (MD)	Psychiatry	677
Yoon, Sydney (MD)	Radiology	736
Yordan, Edgardo (MD)	Gynecologic Oncology	262
Yoshikawa, Thomas T (MD)	Infectious Disease	329
Yoshizumi, Marc Osamu (MD)	Ophthalmology	468
Young, Anne (MD)	Neurology	399
Young, Iven (MD)	Endocrinology, Diabetes & Metabolism	203
Young, James B (MD)	Cardiology (Cardiovascular Disease)	138
Young, Keith Randall (MD)	Pulmonary Disease	701
Young, Ming-Lon (MD)	Pediatric Cardiology	564
Young, Robert Henry (MD)	Pathology	536
Young, Vernon Leroy (MD)	Plastic Surgery	647
Younge, Brian R (MD)	Ophthalmology	460
Younger, J Benjamin (MD)	Reproductive Endocrinology	747
Yousem, Samuel A. (MD)	Pathology	539

ALPHABETICAL LISTING OF DOCTORS

CASTLE CONNOLLY ORDER FORM

I want to order the following Castle Connolly Guides:

Top Doctors:
    New York Metro Area   # ___ of books at $24.95 $_____

How to Find the Best Doctors:
    Chicago Metropolitan Area   # ___ of books at $24.95 $_____
    Florida   # ___ of books at $24.95 $_____

The Buyer's Guide to Choosing
the Best Healthcare   # ___ of books at $12.95 $_____

The ABCs of HMOs: How To
Get The Best From Managed Care   # ___ of books at $11.95 $_____

                                                  Subtotal $_____

              *NY residents, please add 8.25% sales tax $_____
              **NJ residents, please add 3% sales tax $_____

     Add $3 per book for shipping and handling #___ of books x $3 $_____

                                                    TOTAL $_____

Please fill in the following information (please print):

Name: _____

Address: _____

City: _____

State: _____ Zip: _____

Phone (day): _____

Phone (eve): _____

E-mail: _____

___ Check or Money Order enclosed
    (payable to Castle Connolly Medical Ltd.)

___ Credit Card: please circle one   Amex   MC   Visa

Card #: _____

Exp. Date: _____ Today's Date: _____

Signature: _____

Mail or fax to:
Castle Connolly Medical Ltd. 60 East 56th Street, New York, NY 10022
Fax: (212) 980-1716   www.castleconnolly.com   AOL keyword: Castle Connolly

RATE A PHYSICIAN

The purpose of this questionaire is to enable you to rate physicians who have cared for you. Please feel free to duplicate this form in order to rate multiple physicians.

Doctor's First Name:_____   Doctor's Last Name:_____

Specialty:_____   Hospital:_____

Phone:(_____)_____-_____   Doctor's Address:_____

City:_____   State:_____

Please rate your doctor in the following areas (leave blank if not applicable):

	Poor	Fair	Good	Very Good	Excellent
Waiting room time	____	____	____	____	____
Doctor availability	____	____	____	____	____
Returns calls in a timely fashion	____	____	____	____	____
Personal attention during visit	____	____	____	____	____
Shows caring & compassion	____	____	____	____	____
Ability to communicate	____	____	____	____	____
Explanation/coordination of medications	____	____	____	____	____
Willingness to make referrals	____	____	____	____	____
Quality of referrals	____	____	____	____	____
Professionalism of staff	____	____	____	____	____
Accuracy of billing	____	____	____	____	____
Cleanliness of office	____	____	____	____	____
Overall quality of care	____	____	____	____	____

Would you recommend this doctor to a friend or relative?   Yes____   No____

Mail or fax to:
Castle Connolly Medical Ltd. 60 East 56th Street, New York, NY 10022
Fax: (212) 980-1716   www.castleconnolly.com   AOL keyword: Castle Connolly

ACKNOWLEDGMENTS

The publishers would like to thank the entire staff for their many hours and days of intense and precise work on this guide in order to further its goal of assisting consumers in making the best healthcare choices. Our special thanks go to the Vice President for Research, Jean Morgan, M.D.; Senior Advisors Ina Bendis, M.D., Ph.D., M.S.M. and Sebastian Dovi, M.D.; Research Associates, Robert Franz, Maryann Hynd, Monica Joaquin and Jonathan Pincus; Director of Content Development, Arline Lane, J.D., M.P.S.; Director of Internet Operations, Russell Hodgson; Director of Management Information Systems, Michael T. Pitkin; Publications Coordinator, Tina Jacoby; Vice President for Operations and CFO, Patti Quinn; Director of Public Relations, Diane Bender; Vice President of Business Development, William Liss-Levinson, Ph.D.; Supervisor/Information Associate Alethea Brown; Information Associate Lekisha Clardy and Administrative Assistant/Receptionist Tina Williams. We would also like to thank the following individuals: Robert Brown; Deborah Carrera-Bly; Barbara Chisolm; Josh Comers; Sereima Hasty; Donna Love; Danielle Myers; Tajh Pelzer; Gregory Rider; Marc Samuels; Willie Sutton; Valda Walker and Sheldon Watts. Additionally, we are grateful to Kathy Freeman of Health and Fitness Concepts and Mike Schlegel of Ziment Associates for their assistance with this project.

We also would like to extend our gratitude to the American Board of Medical Specialties (ABMS) for allowing us to use excerpts, especially the descriptions of medical specialties and subspecialties, from the text of their publication "Which Medical Specialist for You?"

OTHER PUBLICATIONS FROM CASTLE CONNOLLY MEDICAL LTD.:
Top Doctors: New York Metro Area
How to Find the Best Doctors: Chicago Metropolitan Area
How to Find the Best Doctors: Florida
The Buyer's Guide to Choosing the Best Healthcare
The ABCs of HMOs: How To Get The Best From Managed Care

To order, see form on prior pages

For further information on physicians and hospitals please visit the Castle Connolly Web site at
www.CastleConnolly.com   AOL keyword: Castle Connolly
or at
www.AmericasTopDoctors.com